Medical-Surgical Nursing

CRITICAL THINKING FOR COLLABORATIVE CARE

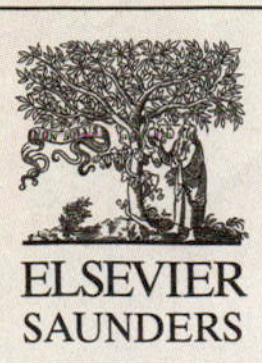

5

FIFTH EDITION

Medical-Surgical Nursing

CRITICAL THINKING FOR COLLABORATIVE CARE

Donna D. Ignatavicius, MS, RN, C
Presenter and Consultant for Nursing Programs
President, DI Associates, Inc.
Placitas, New Mexico

M. Linda Workman, PhD, RN, FAAN
Gertrude Perkins Oliva Professor of Oncology
Frances Payne Bolton School of Nursing
Case Western Reserve University
Cleveland, Ohio

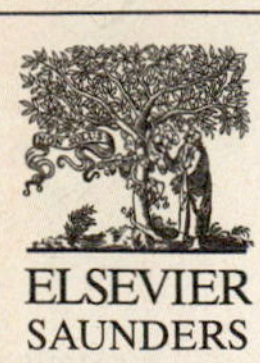

ELSEVIER
SAUNDERS

11830 Westline Industrial Drive
St. Louis, Missouri 63146

MEDICAL-SURGICAL NURSING: CRITICAL THINKING FOR COLLABORATIVE CARE

NOTICE

Nursing is an ever-changing field. Standard safety precautions must be followed, but as new research and clinical experience broaden our knowledge, changes in treatment and drug therapy may become necessary or appropriate. Readers are advised to check the most current product information provided by the manufacturer of each drug to be administered to verify the recommended dose, the method and duration of administration, and contraindications. It is the responsibility of the licensed health care provider, relying on experience and knowledge of the patient, to determine dosages and the best treatment for each individual patient. Neither the publisher nor the editor assumes any liability for any injury and/or damage to persons or property arising from this publication.

ISBN-13: 978-0-7216-0446-6 (Single Vol.)
ISBN-10: 0-7216-0446-3 (Single Vol.)
ISBN-13: 978-0-7216-0671-2 (2-Vol. Set)
ISBN-10: 0-7216-0671-7 (2-Vol. Set)

Executive Publisher: Barbara Nelson Cullen
Editor: Lee Henderson
Developmental Editor: Laura Sieh Chu, Robin Richman
Publishing Services Manager: Deborah L. Vogel
Senior Project Manager: Jodi M. Willard
Book Designer: Teresa McBryan

Printed in United States of America

Last digit is the print number: 9 8 7 6 5 4 3

DEDICATION

To Charles and Stephanie
Thanks for your unending support, love, and understanding during every edition; I could not do this without you!

Donna

To my mother, Eunice Workman, from whom I inherited the creativity and persistence to pursue my dream of being an author.

Linda

About the Authors

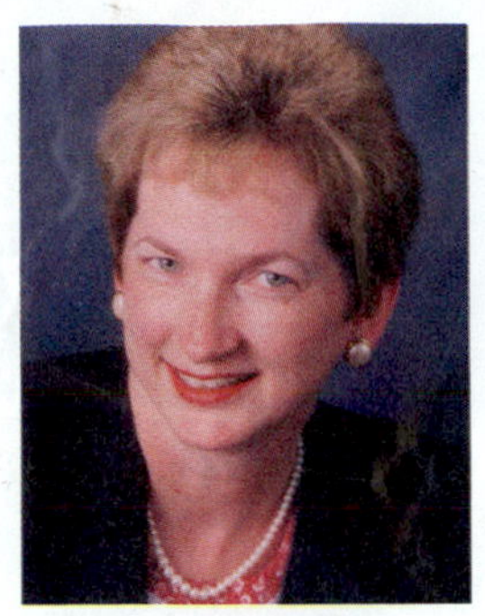

Donna D. Ignatavicius received her diploma in nursing from the Peninsula General School of Nursing in Salisbury, Maryland. After working as a staff and charge nurse in medical-surgical nursing, she became an instructor in Staff Development at the University of Maryland Medical Center. She then received her BSN from the University of Maryland School of Nursing. For 5 years she taught in several schools of nursing while working toward her MS in Nursing, which she received in 1981. Ms. Ignatavicius then taught in the BSN program at the University of Maryland for 6 years, after which she continued to pursue her interest in gerontology and accepted the position of Director of Nursing of a major skilled-nursing facility in her home state of Maryland. She has been a certified gerontologic nurse since 1989 and was certified in nursing case management by the American Nurses Credentialing Center in 1998. Recently she has taught in both diploma and associate degree nursing programs. Through her consulting and seminar business, Ms. Ignatavicius has gained national recognition in nursing education and critical thinking. She is currently the President of DI Associates, Inc. (http://www.diassociates.com/), a company dedicated to improving health care through education and consultation for both faculty and clinicians.

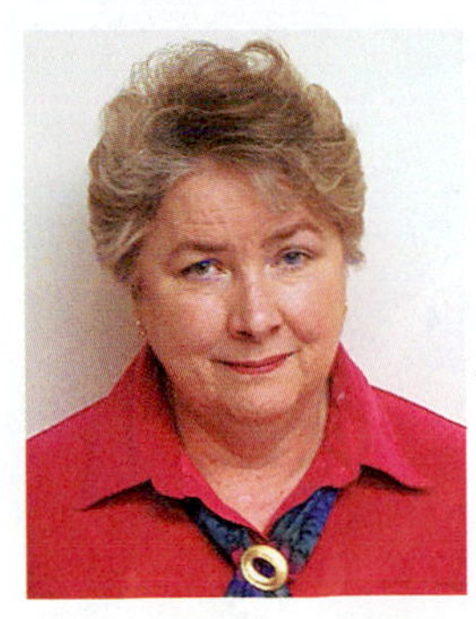

M. Linda Workman received her BSN from the University of Cincinnati College of Nursing and Health. After serving in the U.S. Army Nurse Corps and working as an Assistant Head Nurse and Head Nurse in civilian hospitals, Dr. Workman, a native of Canada, earned her MSN from the University of Cincinnati College of Nursing and Health and a PhD in Developmental Biology from the University of Cincinnati College of Arts and Sciences. Dr. Workman's 25 years of academic experience include teaching at the diploma, associate degree, baccalaureate, and master's levels. Her areas of teaching expertise include medical-surgical nursing, physiology, pathophysiology, genetics, oncology, and immunology. Dr. Workman has been recognized nationally for her teaching expertise and was inducted into the American Academy of Nursing in 1992. She received the Excellence in Teaching award at the University of Cincinnati in 2001 and at Case Western Reserve University in 2004. She is a former American Cancer Society Professor of Oncology Nursing and currently is senior faculty at the Frances Payne Bolton School of Nursing, Case Western Reserve University, where she occupies an endowed chair in oncology.

Consultants

ELAINE BISHOP KENNEDY, EdD, RN
Professor, Department of Nursing
Wor-Wic Community College
Salisbury, Maryland
Concept Maps
Plans of Care

MICHELLE M. BYRNE, PhD, RN, CNOR
Associate Professor
Department of Nursing
North Georgia College and State University
Dahlonega, Georgia
Culture consultant

RICHARD LINTNER, RT(R), (CV), (MR), (CT), ARRT
Program Director
School of Interventional Radiology;
Manager
Interventional Radiology
Kansas University Medical Center
Kansas City, Kansas
Consultant for interventional radiology

Contributors

RICHARD B. ARBOUR, MSN, RN, CCRN, CNRN
Guest Lecturer, Graduate Program
LaSalle University School of Nursing;
Staff Nurse/Clinical Researcher
Albert Einstein Healthcare Network
Philadelphia, Pennsylvania

DEANNE A. BLACH, MSN, RN
Coordinator, CE Programs and Senior Health & Education
University of Arkansas for Medical Sciences
AHEC-NW at Harrison
Harrison, Arkansas

MARCIA M. BOEHMKE, DNS, RN, ANPc
Research Assistant Professor, School of Nursing
University of Buffalo, The State University of New York
Buffalo, New York

MICHELLE M. BYRNE, PhD, RN, CNOR
Associate Professor
Department of Nursing
North Georgia College and State University
Dahlonega, Georgia

LINDA J. CAPUTI, EdD, MSN, RN
Professor, Department of Nursing
College of DuPage
Glen Ellyn, Illinois

JOHN M. CLOCHESY, PhD, RN, FAAN, FCCM
Independence Foundation Professor of Nursing Education
Case Western Reserve University
Cleveland, Ohio

TAMMY L. COFFEE, MSN, ACNP
Acute Care Nurse Practitioner
Metro Health Medical Center
Cleveland, Ohio

JANICE CUZZELL, RN, MA, CWS
Certified Wound Specialist
Savannah, Georgia

KARRIE K. DIETZEN, MSN, RN, CGRN
Assistant Professor, Associate's of Science in Nursing Program
Ivy Tech State College, East Central Region
Muncie, Indiana;
PRN: Staff RN Medical/Surgical Unit & Endoscopy Lab
Community Hospital-Anderson
Anderson, Indiana

MARY R. HERON EVANS, MS, RN, ONC
Assistant Professor, School of Nursing
Gulf Coast Community College;
Staff, Gulf Coast Medical Center
Panama City, Florida

CHRISTINE A. GATES, BS, CRT
Certified Respiratory Therapist
Cincinnati, Ohio

JACQUELYN R. GIBBS, MSN, RN
Assistant Professor, Department of Nursing
Raymond Walters College, University of Cincinnati
Cincinnati, Ohio

GAYLE K. GILMORE, RN, MA, MIS, CIC
Consultant, Infection Control Education and Consultation
Duluth, Minnesota

LYNN C. HADAWAY, MEd, RNC, CRNI
President, Lynn Hadaway Associates, Inc.
Milner, Georgia

WADE HAGAN, MSN, RN, PHN, CCRN
Instructor, Nursing Department
Mt. San Jacinto Community College District
Menifee, California;
Faculty Associate
California State University
Dominguez Hills, California

KATHY A. HAUSMAN, PhD, RN, C
Assistant Professor, School of Nursing
University of Maryland
Baltimore, Maryland

MARY K. KAZANOWSKI, PhD, ARNP, CHPN, BC
Professor, Department of Nursing
Saint Anselm College;
Level III RN
VNA Hospice
Manchester, New Hampshire

ELAINE BISHOP KENNEDY, EdD, RN
Professor, Department of Nursing
Wor-Wic Community College
Salisbury, Maryland

LINDA A. LaCHARITY, PhD, RN
Assistant Professor, College of Nursing
University of Cincinnati
Cincinnati, Ohio

LINDA LASKOWSKI-JONES, RN, MS, APRN, BC, CCRN, CEN
Director, Trauma, Emergency & Aeromedical Services
Christiana Care Health System—Christiana Hospital
Newark, Delaware

RUTH LINDQUIST, PhD, RN, APRN, BC
Professor, School of Nursing;
Senior Associate Dean for Academic Affairs and Administration
University of Minnesota
Minneapolis, Minnesota

DEITRA LEONARD LOWDERMILK, PhD, BSN, RNC, MEd
Clinical Professor, Women's Health, School of Nursing
University of North Carolina at Chapel Hill
Chapel Hill, North Carolina

JUDY MALKIEWICZ, PhD, RN
Professor, School of Nursing
University of Northern Colorado
Greeley, Colorado

JANICE HOOT MARTIN, PhD, RN, GNP
Professor Emeritus, School of Nursing
University of Northern Colorado
Greeley, Colorado

CYNTHIA KINDLER MATZKO, MSN, RN, APRN, BC
Master's Prepared Advanced Practice Nurse;
Rheumatology Clinical Nursing Specialist
Geisinger Medical Center
Danville, Pennsylvania

LORA McGUIRE, RN, MS
Professor, Department of Nursing
Joliet Junior College
Joliet, Illinois

M. ELAINE McLEOD, MSN, APRN, BC-ADM, APRN-BC, CDE
Clinical Nurse Specialist, Diabetes
Tennessee Valley Healthcare System
Nashville, Tennessee

MADELINE B. MURPHY, MSN, NP-C
Coordinator, Adult NP Program
Breen School of Nursing
Ursuline College;
Clinical Faculty, Department of Medicine
University Hospitals of Cleveland
Cleveland, Ohio

CATHY A. MURRAY, MSN, RN, CNS, ONC
Assistant Professor, Department of Nursing
Ivy Tech State College—Community College of Indiana;
PRN Staff Nurse Orthopedics
Ball Memorial Hospital
Muncie, Indiana

FRANK EDWARDS MYERS III, MA, CIC, CPHQ
Manager of Clinical Epidemiology and Safety Systems
Scripps Mercy Hospital/Scripps Health
San Diego, California

KAREN NOVAK, MSN, RN, OCN, ACNP
Nurse Practitioner
Northwestern Medical Faculty Foundation
Chicago, Illinois

REBECCA M. PATTON, MSN, RN, CNOR
Director of Perioperative Services
EMH Regional Healthcare System
Elyria, Ohio

TOMMIE WRIGHT PNIEWSKI, MSN, RN, CNAA
Associate Professor, Department of Nursing
Hopkinsville Community College;
Education Coordinator of Special Projects
Christian Health Center/Christian Church Homes of Kentucky
Hopkinsville, Kentucky

SUZANNE K. POWELL, BSN, RN, MBA, CCM, CPHQ
Editor-in-Chief
Lippincott's Case Management: The Journal for Professional Practice
Lippincott, Williams & Wilkins
Philadelphia, Pennsylvania;
Director, Acute Care Quality Improvement Program
Health Services Advisory Group
Phoenix, Arizona

ANGELA SAMMARCO, PhD, RN
Assistant Professor, Department of Nursing
College of Staten Island, City University of New York
Staten Island, New York

JAMES G. SAMPSON, ND, MSN, ANP-C
Assistant Professor, Adjunct
University of Colorado School of Nursing;
Adult Nurse Practitioner
Denver Health Medical Center
Denver, Colorado

MARIAH SNYDER, PhD, FAAN
Professor Emeritus, School of Nursing
University of Minnesota
Minneapolis, Minnesota

KAREN L. TOULSON, BSN, RN, CEN
Nurse Manager, Emergency Department
Christiana Care Health Systems
Newark, Delaware

SHIRLEY E. VAN ZANDT, MS, MPH, CRNP
Instructor, School of Nursing
Johns Hopkins University
Baltimore, Maryland

CONSTANCE VISOVSKY, PhD, RN, ACNP
Assistant Professor, Frances Payne Bolton School of Nursing
Case Western Reserve University;
Nurse Practitioner, Ireland Cancer Center
University Hospitals of Cleveland
Cleveland, Ohio

CHRIS WINKELMAN, PhD, RN, CNP, CCRN
Assistant Professor, Frances Payne Bolton School of Nursing
Case Western Reserve University;
Staff Nurse, Trauma and Critical Care
MetroHealth Medical Center
Cleveland, Ohio

PAMELA C. ZICKAFOOSE, EdD, MSN, RN, CAN, BC
Instructor, Department of Nursing
Delaware Technical & Community College;
Educator
Bayhealth Medical Center
Dover, Delaware

Reviewers

JOAN P. ANDERSON, MA, RN, MALS
Suffolk County Community College
Selden, New York

MICHELE AUGUST-BRADY, DNSC, RN
Moravian College
Bethlehem, Pennsylvania

GAYLE A. BERO, MSN, RN, FNP, NCC
St. Joseph's Hospital Health Center
St. Joseph's College of Nursing
Syracuse, New York

SANDRA BRANNAN, MSN, RN
Lamar University
Beaumont, Texas

MICHELE BUNNING, MSN, RN
Good Samaritan College of Nursing and Health Science
Cincinnati, Ohio

PAMELA R. CANGELOSI, PhD, RN
George Mason University
College of Nursing and Health Science
Fairfax, Virginia

BARBARA CELIA, EdD, RN
Drexel University
College of Nursing and Health Professions
Philadelphia, Pennsylvania

CATHERINE M. CONCERT, MS, RN, APRN, BC, FNP, CGRN
Wyckoff Heights Medical Center;
Long Island University
Brooklyn, New York

PATSY ELAINE CRIHFIELD, MSN, RN, CCRN, APRN, BC, NP-C
Dyersburg State Community College
Dyersburg, Tennessee

DORIS DENISON, MSN, RN, NP, ACNP
Wayne State University
College of Nursing
Detroit, Michigan

CLAIRE P. DONAGHY, PhD, RN, APN C, CCRN, ACNP
County College of Morris
Randolph, New Jersey;
St. Clare's Health Services;
Morris Anesthesia Group
Denville, New Jersey

SHEILA A. DUNN, MSN, RN, C-ANP
St. Louis VA Medical Center
Belleville, Illinois;
St. Louis University
St. Louis, Missouri

JAYNE EDMAN, MSN, RN
Brookdale Community College
Lincroft, New Jersey

ANN E. FRONCZEK, MSN, RN, NP
Binghamton University
Decker School of Nursing
Binghamton, New York

DAVID GOEDE, MS, RN, APRN, BC
Monroe Community College;
University of Rochester
Strong Memorial Hospital
Rochester, New York

SHARRON E. GUILLETT, PhD, RN
Marymount University
Arlington, VA

ANNETTE GUNDERMAN, EdD, MSN, RN
Bloomsburg University
Bloomsburg, Pennsylvania

SUZY HARRINGTON, MS, RN, CHES
Central Colorado Area Health Education Center
Denver, Colorado

CONNIE S. HEFLIN, MSN, RN
West Kentucky Community and Technical College
Paducah, Kentucky

SARAH M. HOWELL, MSN, RN
Mississippi University for Women
Columbus, Mississippi

SUSAN J. LAMANNA, MA, MSN, RN, ANP
Onondaga Community College
Syracuse, New York

SUSAN B. LEIGHT, EdD, RNCO, CRNP
West Virginia Wesleyan College
Buckhannon, West Virginia

CAROL T. LEMAY, RN
University of Massachusetts, Amherst
Amherst, Massachusetts

JANIE LIPPS, MSN, APRN C, CDE
Vanderbilt University Medical Center
Nashville, Tennessee

JAYNE HANSCHE LOBERT, MS, RN, CS, NP
Oakland Community College
Waterford, Michigan

MARGARET A. LYNCH, MSN, FNP
The Cambridge Hospital
Cambridge, Massachusetts

CYNTHIA GLAWE MAILLOUX, PhD, RN
Pennsylvania State University, Worthington Scranton
Dunmore, Pennsylvania

DOROTHY MATHERS, MSN, RN
Pennsylvania College of Technology
Williamsport, Pennsylvania

ELIZABETH J. MILLER, MSN, MPH, APRN-BC, ABD
John Dingell Detroit VA Medical Center
Detroit, Michigan

IRIS L. MULLINS, PhD, RN
Radford University
School of Nursing
Radford, Virginia

MARIO R. ORTIZ, PhD, RN, FNP
University of Portland
School of Nursing
Portland, Oregon

AMY B. SHARRON, MS, RN, CS, GNP
United Health Care
Evercare
Auburndale, Massachusetts

MARY VIRGINIA SHINDLE, MSN, RNBC, HNC
Shepherd University
Shepherdstown, West Virginia

DARRELL R. SPURLOCK JR., MSN, RN, CCRN, CEN
Mount Carmel College of Nursing
Columbus, Ohio

PATRICIA SWEENEY, MS, APRN, BC
Pennsylvania State University, Worthington Scranton
Dunmore, Pennsylvania;
Emergency Services PC
Scranton, Pennsylvania

SUZANNE E. TATRO, MS, BSN, RN
York Technical College
Rock Hill, South Carolina

JOYCE B. VAZZANO, MSN, RN, CMSRN
John Hopkins University
School of Nursing
Baltimore, Maryland

SHARON HENRY WALICEK, MEd, MSN, RN, CCRN, CCNS, ANP-BC
Elgin Community College;
Elgin Cardiology Associates
Elgin, Illinois

COLEEN WEIL, MSN, RN, C
Wor-Wic Community College
Salisbury, Maryland

JOAN DOMIGAN WENTZ, MSN, RN
Assistant Professor
Jewish Hospital College of Nursing and Allied Health
St. Louis, Missouri

DIANE M. WHEELER, RNCS, ANP
Upper Care Internal Medicine
Falmouth, Massachusetts

CHERYLE I. WHITNEY, MSN, RN, BC
Tomball College
Tomball, Texas

CECILIA ELAINE WILSON, MS, RN, CPN
Texas Woman's University
College of Nursing
Dallas, Texas

RITA E. M. WISE, MSN, RN
Reading Hospital
School of Nursing
West Reading, Pennsylvania

Preface

The first edition of this text, entitled *Medical-Surgical Nursing: A Nursing Process Approach*, received widespread acclaim in the 1990s. The following three editions built on that achievement and further solidified the book's position as a major trendsetter for the practice of adult health nursing. Now in its fifth edition, "Iggy" charts an essential course for the future of adult nursing–a course reflected in its current title: *Medical-Surgical Nursing: Critical Thinking for Collaborative Care.*

This title was carefully chosen to emphasize the importance of developing and enhancing critical thinking skills to help today's nursing students function in interdisciplinary teams in a variety of health care settings, including both acute care and community-based settings.

KEY THEMES FOR THE 5TH EDITION

As in the extraordinarily successful fourth edition, a key theme of this edition–reflected in the book's subtitle–is critical thinking. To help achieve that emphasis on critical thinking, case-based Critical Thinking Challenges are interspersed throughout the text. These exercises provide a safe and effective means of practicing the on-the-spot decision making that students will face in the fast-paced world of medical-surgical nursing. Suggested answer guidelines for these Critical Thinking Challenges are provided on the text's Evolve website.

In addition to this key theme of critical thinking, the fifth edition also emphasizes "readiness"–readiness for the NCLEX® Examination, readiness for major emergencies such as we saw in the aftermath of the events of 9/11, readiness for safe drug administration, and readiness for the new world of genetics that is unfolding before us.

As the nursing shortage becomes more acute, it is more critical than ever that students be ready to pass the licensure exam on the first try. To help both students and faculty in reaching that goal, the fifth edition includes an innovative end-of-chapter feature called "Get Ready for the NCLEX Examination!" These unique learning aids consist of a list of Key Points *organized by NCLEX Client Needs Category* as found in the NCLEX test plan. Also included in these "Get Ready for the NCLEX Examination!" sections are highlighted reminders to go to the Student CD-ROM for "Review Questions for the NCLEX Examination" and to the Evolve website for "Integrated Management of Care Questions for the NCLEX Examination." The Review Questions for the NCLEX Examination (found on the Student CD-ROM) are keyed to the Learning Outcomes at the start of each chapter–one question per Learning Outcome. The "Integrated Management of Care Questions for the NCLEX Examination" (on the Evolve website) focus on delegation and supervision, assignment, and prioritization/decision making. These questions are aimed at stimulating and validating critical thinking to help students understand and apply the material covered in the text and integrate it with material they have learned elsewhere in the curriculum.

To help prepare students for both common medical-surgical emergencies and mass-casualty events such as the terrorist acts and natural disasters that seem to be increasingly in the news, this edition features an entirely new unit–Unit 3 (Concepts of Emergency Nursing)–which consists of two emergency care chapters. Chapter 12 (Emergency and Mass Casualty Nursing) provides an introduction to emergency and mass casualty nursing. At the end of this chapter, the reader is "walked through" a case scenario related to bioterrorism and the response of the emergency health care team. Chapter 13 (Interventions for Clients with Common Environmental Emergencies) describes selected environmental emergencies, such as heatstroke, spider bites, and near-drowning. The first-response/emergency interventions and continuing care are discussed for each emergency.

To promote readiness for safe drug administration, the fifth edition provides Pharmacology Review Questions on the Evolve website. These questions, which are keyed to the text with distinctive "Evolve Pharm Review" icons, give students practice in concepts of safe medication administration–a major theme of the NCLEX Examination.

To promote readiness for the emerging genetic basis of many diseases and disorders, we provide a new chapter, Genetic Concepts for Medical-Surgical Nursing (Chapter 11), as well as Genetic Considerations boxes and "Etiology and Genetic Risk" headings wherever appropriate.

Additional themes carried over from the previous edition are an emphasis on women's health issues, cultural considerations, complementary and alternative therapies, and the special needs of older adults. In addition, concepts of case management and community-based care are interwoven throughout to help the reader understand these growing roles and trends.

CLINICAL CURRENCY AND ACCURACY

To ensure this text's currency and accuracy, we listened to the readers of the previous editions–their impressions of and experiences with the text. Based on this input, we formulated our revision plan. We assembled a team of clinical experts to revise, rewrite and, in some cases, draft entirely new chapters.

We also commissioned in-depth reviews of selected chapters by clinicians and instructors from across the United States and Canada and used their reviews to guide us in revising the chapters into their final form. A nursing expert in cultural issues reviewed the entire fourth edition and made recommendations for how to best present illustrations, research findings, and incidence/prevalence data. For this edition we also enlisted the assistance of an interventional radiologist to ensure the accuracy of selected diagnostic testing procedures and associated client care.

The results are reflected in the fifth edition's strong, consistent focus on critical thinking, collaborative care, pathophysiology, drug therapy, and community-based care; its foundation of relevant research; and its emphasis on the critical "need to know" information that nurses must master in order to provide safe, effective care based on solid scientific evidence. This base of scientific evidence is emphasized throughout the text and is highlighted in our Best Practice charts. In addition, our Evidence-Based Practice for Nursing boxes now designate the *level of evidence* reflected in the reported research as based on a national standard described in Chapter 1.

OUTSTANDING READABILITY

The fifth edition has been carefully revised from cover to cover for improved readability. Today's students need to be able to read information once and understand it; they do not have time to repeatedly re-read the same information. To achieve this level of readability, we took two steps: (1) We revised the text into a direct-address style, wherever appropriate, that speaks directly to the reader; and (2) we kept sentences as short as possible consistent with the complexity of the content.

Reading level is highly influenced by the length of sentences and the length of words. Thus, while we can control the length of the sentences, medical terms are often 4 to 5 syllables long and will tend to skew a chapter's reading level. Nevertheless, the result of our efforts for the fifth edition is a med-surg text of consistently outstanding readability. The average reading level is 10th-11th grade, with a few chapters above and below that threshold.

It is important to note that reducing the reading level of this edition did not reduce the quality or depth of content that students need to know. Instead, the content is clear and focused.

EASE OF ACCESS

To make the text as easy to use as possible, we have maintained the fourth edition's approach of smaller chapters of more uniform length. The fifth edition has 80 chapters.

We also have maintained the fourth edition's unit structure, with vital body systems (cardiovascular, respiratory, and neurologic) appearing earlier in the book. In these three units, we have continued to provide critical care content in separate chapters that discuss managing critically ill clients with coronary artery disease, respiratory problems, and neurologic problems.

To help break up long blocks of text and also to highlight key information, we have included numerous headings, bulleted lists, tables, charts, and in-text highlights. We end each chapter with a Selected Bibliography (with classic sources before 2000 noted with an asterisk [*]). Key Terms are in boldface type and are defined in the text to foster the learning of need-to-know vocabulary.

A COLLABORATIVE APPROACH

As in the previous four editions, we take a collaborative approach to client care. We believe that in the real world of health care, nurses, clients, and other health care providers (including physicians, advanced-practice nurses, and physician's assistants) *share* responsibility for the management of client problems. Thus we present client care in a collaborative management framework. In this framework we make no artificial distinctions between medical treatment and nursing care. Instead, under each Collaborative Management heading we cover the entire range of approaches taken by health care practitioners of all disciplines when dealing with client problems.

New to this edition are 7 additional Concept Maps (for a total of 15) that underscore this collaborative approach. Also known as *clinical correlation maps,* these Concept Maps now begin with a case scenario. They then demonstrate visually how a complex health problem is addressed. Each Concept Map spells out the steps of the nursing process and related concepts to illustrate the relationships among disease processes, medical treatments, nursing interventions, and more. Identifying these relationships not only underscores the collaborative nature of health care but also stimulates critical thinking and fosters learning.

Although our approach is collaborative, the text is first and foremost a *nursing* text. We therefore use a nursing process approach to organize discussions of client health problems and their management. Discussions of key health problems follow a full nursing process format, with the following structure:

- [Health problem]
  - Pathophysiology
    - Etiology and Genetic Risk
    - Incidence/Prevalence
  - Collaborative Management
    - Assessment
    - Analysis
      - Common Nursing Diagnoses and Collaborative Problems
      - Additional Nursing Diagnoses and Collaborative Problems
    - Planning and Implementation
      - Nursing Diagnosis/Collaborative Problem
        - Planning: Expected Outcomes
        - Interventions
    - Community-Based Care
      - Health Teaching
      - Home Care Management
      - Health Care Resources
    - Evaluation: Outcomes

The nursing diagnoses used in this edition are the 2003-2004 NANDA-approved diagnoses–the most recently approved diagnoses at the time of this revision.

Discussions of less common or less complex disorders, although not given this complete subhead structure, nonetheless follow the same basic format: a discussion of the problem itself (including pertinent information on pathophysiology) followed by a section on collaborative care of clients with the disorder. Common nursing diagnoses/collaborative problems are often identified as well.

Integral to this collaborative management approach is a clear delineation of just who is responsible for what. When a responsibility is primarily the nurse's, the text says so. When a decision must be made jointly by the client, nurse, physician, and physical therapist, for example, this is clearly stated. When different health care practitioners in different care settings might be involved in the client's care, this is stated.

To further emphasize the nurse's role, we have integrated pertinent components of the Nursing Interventions Classification (NIC) system and the Nursing Outcomes Classification (NOC) system. These systems were developed by the Center for Nursing Classification to standardize nursing interventions and outcomes and the terminology used to describe them. Where appropriate for health problems that receive full nursing process coverage, NIC interventions are clearly identified with a NIC symbol NIC. Selected activities associated with each identified intervention are listed in NIC Intervention Activities charts.

The expected outcomes for client care in this edition are consistent with the NOC system. However, NOC continues to be developed and refined to ensure that outcomes are evidence-based. We have therefore included NOC outcomes and specified indicators when appropriate, as well as other outcome statements validated empirically by clinical practice. Those statements that are particularly consistent with NOC language are identified with a NOC symbol NOC.

ORGANIZATION

The 80 chapters of *Medical-Surgical Nursing: Critical Thinking for Collaborative Care* are grouped into 17 units. Unit 1, Health Promotion and Illness, lays the foundation for the health care concepts incorporated throughout the text. Unit 2 covers important biopsychosocial concepts related to health care, including pain and rehabilitation. Chapter 11 is a new chapter in this unit and introduces the major concepts of genetics and related nursing implications for client care. A new unit, Unit 3, consists of two emergency care chapters as previously described.

Unit 4 consists of six chapters on the management of clients with fluid, electrolyte, and acid-base imbalances. This unit includes an expanded chapter on infusion therapy (Chapter 17) and is supplemented with an online fluid and electrolyte tutorial on the companion Evolve website.

Unit 5 presents the perioperative nursing content that medical-surgical nurses need to know. This content provides a solid foundation to help the student better understand the specific surgeries covered throughout the remainder of the text.

Unit 6 provides core content on health problems related to immune system function. This content includes normal inflammation and the immune response, altered cell growth and cancer development, and interventions for clients with connective tissue disease, HIV infection, and other immunologic disorders, cancers, and infections.

The remaining 11 units cover medical-surgical content by body system. Each of these units begins with an Assessment chapter and continues with one or more Interventions chapters for clients with specific health problems in that body system.

MULTINATIONAL, MULTICULTURAL, MULTIGENERATIONAL FOCUS

To reflect the increasing diversity of our society, *Medical-Surgical Nursing: Critical Thinking for Collaborative Care* takes a multinational, multicultural, and multigenerational focus. Addressing the needs of both U.S. and Canadian readers, we have included examples of trade names of drugs available in the United States and those available in Canada. Drugs that are available only in Canada are designated with a ✱ symbol.

To help nurses provide quality care for clients whose cultural background may differ from their own, numerous Cultural Considerations boxes highlight important aspects of culturally competent care throughout the text. A revised cultural health chapter (Chapter 6) is also included in this edition. Located inside the back cover is an innovative Communication Quick Reference for Spanish-Speaking Clients. This Quick Reference helps ensure clear communication between native English speakers and the rapidly growing population who speak Spanish as a first language.

Increases in life expectancy and the "graying" of the baby-boom generation add up to a steadily increasing older adult population. To help equip nurses for this challenge, the fifth edition continues to feature expanded coverage of the care of older adults. It includes a greater number of Nursing Focus on the Older Adult charts and highlights laboratory values and drug dosages typical for older clients. Charts specifying normal physiologic changes to expect in the older population are included in each Assessment chapter. In addition, Considerations for Older Adults boxes are included throughout the text to emphasize key points to keep in mind when caring for these clients.

Also appearing throughout the text is an increased number of Women's Health Considerations boxes, which address topics of concern to women and their health care providers. These in-text highlights alert the reader to gender-related differences in assessment parameters and in the incidence, severity, and treatment of common health problems.

ADDITIONAL LEARNING RESOURCES

As in previous editions, the fifth edition continues to include a rich array of "andragogic" learning aids–learning aids geared toward adult learners–to help students quickly identify and understand key information and to serve as study aids. Several of these features are new to this edition.

- Written in "client-friendly" language, Client Education Guide charts provide the types of instructions that nurses must learn to provide to clients and their families to help them cope with life changes caused by illness.
- Laboratory Profile charts summarize important information on laboratory tests commonly ordered to evaluate health problems. Information typically includes normal ranges of laboratory values (including differences for older adults, when appropriate) and the possible significance of abnormal findings.
- Drug Therapy charts summarize important information about commonly used drugs. These charts include both U.S. and Canadian trade names for typically used drugs, usual dosages (including dosages for older clients, as

appropriate), and nursing interventions with rationales. In addition, "Med Error Alerts" have been added for this edition where common mistakes could be made in medication administration. Medication errors are a major health problem in health care today, and our goal with this new feature is to help students administer drugs safely.

- Key Features charts highlight the clinical manifestations of important health problems.
- Evidence-Based Practice for Nursing boxes, provided in nearly every chapter, give synopses of recent nursing research articles and other scientific articles applicable to nursing. Each box provides a summary of the article, a brief critique, the level of evidence (new to this edition), and a summary of implications for nursing practice. The goal of this feature is to help students identify the strengths and weaknesses of the research and see how research can help guide nursing practice.
- Nursing care plans remain significant tools with which the nursing student must be familiar. The fifth edition therefore includes selected examples of these care-planning tools. It has been retitled "Plan of Care" and incorporates NIC and NOC language. Nursing Plans of Care continue to include a distinctive icon (D) to designate interventions that can be delegated to assistive nursing personnel.
- New to this edition, Home Care Assessment charts serve as a convenient summary of essential assessment points for clients who need follow-up home health nursing care.
- Assessment Using Gordon's Functional Health Patterns charts provide a convenient one-stop list of relevant questions to ask clients regarding the impact of health conditions on everyday function.
- Meeting *Healthy People 2010* Objectives boxes suggest specific activities that nurses can undertake to promote achievement of the specific numbered objectives of the *Healthy People 2010* program.
- Resource Management boxes (formerly "Cost of Care" boxes) provide an important financial/resource context for medical-surgical nurses when managing resources for client care. Nurses must increasingly understand cost and other resource factors in order to help clients work toward wellness.
- Legal/Ethical Issues boxes introduce students to some of the dilemmas they will face in the increasingly high-tech world of medical-surgical nursing.

AN INTEGRATED MULTIMEDIA RESOURCE BASED ON PROVEN LEARNING STRATEGIES

Medical-Surgical Nursing: Critical Thinking for Collaborative Care, 5th edition, is the hub of a comprehensive package of electronic and print publications that break new ground in the application of proven learning strategies and evidence-based educational practice. This integrated multimedia resource actively engages the student in problem solving and critical thinking. Every effort has been made to correlate content among the text and its companion publications. Unlike many textbook authors, we have personally been involved in the development of most of the companion publications to ensure consistency and cohesion between the textbook and the companion publications.

RESOURCES FOR INSTRUCTORS

Resources for instructors include a printed Instructor's Resource Manual, an Instructor's Electronic Resource CD-ROM/DVD, and Evolve Learning Resources for faculty.

The printed Instructor's Resource Manual, written by Susan Behmke and Sharon Souter, along with contributions from four expert authors, continues to serve as a touchstone for new and seasoned faculty alike. The IRM for the 5th edition features a simplified new format as well as four new introductory chapters. The introductory chapters cover evaluation of critical thinking, test construction, incorporation of technology into the classroom, and teaching strategies for students with a variety of learning styles. IRM chapters now correspond directly to textbook chapters and feature Concept Map Case Studies that correspond to the 15 Concept Maps in the text.

The Instructor's Electronic Resource CD-ROM/DVD consists of a Test Bank, Image Collection, Lecture Slides, ready-to-use narrated PowerPoint Lectures, and a Faculty Development Video.

- The Test Bank is a robust 2500-item bank that includes both traditional and NCLEX Examination "alternate" item types, and each question is coded for correct answer, rationale, cognitive type, nursing process step, and NCLEX Client Needs Category. The Test Bank is provided in ExamView, Blackboard, and ParTest formats.
- The expanded Image Collection now consists of 700 images from the text and are delivered in a format that makes incorporation into lectures and presentations easier than ever.
- The Lecture Slides (formerly "LectureView") are a collection of 1200 text slides developed to correspond to each chapter in the text.
- The new, ready-to-use PowerPoint Lectures are narrated lectures by co-author Linda Workman on topics that faculty find particularly challenging.
- The new Faculty Development Video, delivered on DVD-ROM as part of the Instructor's Electronic Resource, is a 60-minute video by Donna Ignatavicius that addresses the implications of changes in the NCLEX Examination for faculty. Excerpted from one of Donna Ignatavicius's popular seminars, this DVD is a unique resource for faculty.

For the convenience of faculty, all of these resources except the Faculty Development Video are also available online on a secure instructor area of the Evolve website entitled Evolve Learning Resources.

RESOURCES FOR STUDENTS

Resources for students include a free Student CD-ROM, a thoroughly revised and updated Critical Thinking Study Guide, a Clinical Companion, a Virtual Clinical Excursions workbook/CD-ROM, and Evolve Learning Resources.

The new Student CD-ROM features Review Questions for the NCLEX Examination–one for each Learning Outcome at the beginning of the chapter. Also included on the

Student CD-ROM are animations and video clips (each keyed to the text by a distinctive "clapboard" icon, as well as a new Audio Glossary. The Audio Glossary includes the definitions of all Key Terms from the text, along with audio files for difficult pronunciations. The Student CD-ROM also includes Audio Clips that allow students to hear key sounds in health assessment.

The *Critical Thinking Study Guide* has been carefully revised and updated under the authorship of Julie S. Snyder for an increased emphasis on critical thinking and rigorous accuracy. The Study Guide features a simplified format and a greater variety of question types. Multiple-choice questions are now written in NCLEX format and emphasize the NCLEX priorities of delegation, management of care, and pharmacology. The use of Case Studies is expanded in this edition, and a new chapter on study tips is included.

The pocket-sized *Clinical Companion,* authored by Kathy A. Hausman, retains the alphabetical organization and streamlined format that made it so popular in previous editions. The new edition is printed in color and in a smaller page size for easier portability, and it includes a quick reference to nursing care after incidents of chemical terrorism and bioterrorism. The *Clinical Companion* is a pocket-sized "Iggy" for students going into clinicals and is written by an author who actively supervises clinicals and who knows firsthand what students in clinicals are being asked to know about their clients.

The *Virtual Clinical Excursions* workbook/CD-ROM package, featuring an updated and easy-to-navigate "virtual" clinical setting, will once again be available for the fifth edition. This unique learning tool guides the student through a virtual clinical environment and helps the student apply textbook content in a "safe" context. The clinical simulations and workbook represent the next generation of research-based learning tools to promote critical thinking and meaningful learning.

Also available for students in a dynamic collection of Evolve Learning Resources, available at http://evolve.elsevier.com/Iggy/. Evolve resources include the following:

- Pharmacology Review Questions (keyed to icons in the textbook)
- Integrated Management of Care Questions for the NCLEX Examination
- Answer Guidelines for Critical Thinking Challenges
- Answer Guidelines for Study Guide Case Studies
- "Building" Concept Maps ("building" versions of the 15 Concept Maps from the text)
- Concept Map Creator (a handy tool for creating customized Concept Maps)
- Fluid & Electrolyte Tutorial (a complete self-paced tutorial on this perennially difficult content)
- WebLinks (a dynamic library of Internet links, updated regularly for currency)
- Content Updates
- Health Assessment Image Collection (supplemental images of common assessment findings)
- The Audio Glossary, Audio Clips, Animations, and Video Clips from the Student CD-ROM.

For more information on any of these innovative companion publications, contact your Elsevier sales representative, visit http://www.us.elsevierhealth.com/, or contact Elsevier Faculty Support at 1-800-222-9570 or sales.inquiry@elsevier.com.

• • •

In summary, *Medical-Surgical Nursing: Critical Thinking for Collaborative Care,* 5th edition, together with its fully integrated multimedia ancillary package, provides the tools you will need to meet the challenge of nursing in the first decade of the 21st century and beyond. The only elements that remain to be added to this package are those that you alone can provide–your diligence, your commitment, your innovation, *your nursing care.*

Donna D. Ignatavicius
M. Linda Workman

Acknowledgments

Publishing a textbook and ancillary package of this depth and breadth would not be possible without the combined efforts of many people. Our contributing authors once again provided consistently excellent manuscripts in a timely fashion. Special thanks to Elaine Kennedy, who developed all of our new case-study-based Concept Maps. Our reviewers–expert clinicians and instructors from around the United States and Canada–provided invaluable suggestions and encouragement throughout the book's development.

The staff of W.B. Saunders/Elsevier once again provided us with crucial guidance and support throughout the planning, writing, revision, and production of the fifth edition. In particular, Executive Publisher Barbara Nelson Cullen and Editor Lee Henderson worked closely with us from the early stages of this edition to help us hone and focus our revision plan, and Lee oversaw the project from start to finish. Developmental Editor Laura Sieh Chu and Managing Editor Robin Richman then worked with us step-by-step to bring the fifth edition from vision to publication. Maureen Iannuzzi held the reins of our complex ancillary package and worked with a gifted group of writers and content experts to provide an outstanding library of resources to complement and enhance the text. Special thanks to Senior Editor's Assistant Marie Thomas, who handled the countless administrative details associated with a project of this size. She is without peer among editorial assistants.

Senior Project Manager Jodi Willard was once again a joy to work with. If, as is said, the mark of a good copy editor is that her work is invisible to the reader, then Jodi is the consummate copy editor. Her unwavering attention to detail, flexibility, and conscientiousness not only helped to make this edition the most consistently readable ever, but also made the entire production process incredibly smooth and headache-free.

Special thanks also to Publishing Services Manager Debbie Vogel. For two editions now, Debbie has worked quietly behind the scenes to help bring the book to publication precisely on schedule and with a very high level of quality.

Designer Teresa McBryan is responsible for the beautiful cover and interior design of the fifth edition. The praise of a book designer's work is often unsung, but Teresa's work on this edition has cast important features in exactly the right light, with neither too much nor too little emphasis, making this edition not only practical and easy to read, but beautiful.

Our acknowledgments would not be complete without recognizing Karen McKie, Bob Boehringer, Jo Beth Griffin, our dedicated team of sales representatives, and other key members of the Sales and Marketing staff who helped to put this book into your hands.

Finally, we wish to thank Executive Vice President, Nursing and Health Professions, Sally Schrefer. Sally's personal leadership style continues to create a unique publishing environment in which authors and editors have the freedom to interact creatively to produce the best books in the field.

Donna D. Ignatavicius
M. Linda Workman

Contents

UNIT ONE

HEALTH PROMOTION and ILLNESS

UNIT FOUR

MANAGEMENT of CLIENTS with FLUID, ELECTROLYTE, and ACID-BASE IMBALANCES

CHAPTER 14

CHAPTER 15

CHAPTER 16

CHAPTER 17

CHAPTER 18

UNIT SEVEN

PROBLEMS of OXYGENATION

Management of Clients with Problems of the Respiratory Tract

UNIT EIGHT

PROBLEMS of CARDIAC OUTPUT and TISSUE PERFUSION

Management of Clients with Problems of the Cardiovascular System

CHAPTER 36

CHAPTER 37

CHAPTER 38

CHAPTER 39

CHAPTER 40

CHAPTER 41

UNIT NINE

PROBLEMS of TISSUE PERFUSION

Management of Clients with Problems of the Hematologic System

UNIT TEN

PROBLEMS of MOBILITY, SENSATION, and COGNITION

Management of Clients with Problems of the Nervous System

CHAPTER 51

Assessment of the Ear and Hearing, 1111

JUDY MALKIEWICZ

CHAPTER 52

Interventions for Clients with Ear and Hearing Problems, 1125

JANICE HOOT MARTIN

UNIT TWELVE

PROBLEMS of MOBILITY

Management of Clients with Problems of the Musculoskeletal System

CHAPTER 53

Assessment of the Musculoskeletal System, 1144

CATHY A. MURRAY

CHAPTER 54

Interventions for Clients with Musculoskeletal Problems, 1157

CATHY A. MURRAY

CHAPTER 55

Interventions for Clients with Musculoskeletal Trauma, 1189

MARY R. HERON EVANS

UNIT THIRTEEN

PROBLEMS of DIGESTION, NUTRITION, and ELIMINATION

Management of Clients with Problems of the Gastrointestinal System

UNIT SIXTEEN
PROBLEMS of EXCRETION
Management of Clients with Problems of the Renal/Urinary System

UNIT SEVENTEEN
PROBLEMS of REPRODUCTION
Management of Clients with Problems of the Reproductive System

CHAPTER 77
Interventions for Clients with Breast Disorders, 1791
ANGELA SAMMARCO

CHAPTER 78
Interventions for Clients with Gynecologic Problems, 1823
KAREN NOVAK

CHAPTER 79
Interventions for Male Clients with Reproductive Problems, 1856
LINDA J. CAPUTI

CHAPTER 80
Interventions for Clients with Sexually Transmitted Diseases, 1883
SHIRLEY E. VAN ZANDT

Guide to Special Features

ASSESSMENT USING GORDON'S FUNCTIONAL HEALTH PATTERNS

BEST PRACTICE

BEST PRACTICE for EMERGENCY CARE

CLIENT EDUCATION GUIDE

CONCEPT MAPS

DRUG THERAPY

EVIDENCE-BASED PRACTICE for Nursing

FOCUSED ASSESSMENT

HOME CARE ASSESSMENT

KEY FEATURES

LABORATORY PROFILE

LEGAL/ETHICAL ISSUES

Meeting HEALTHY PEOPLE 2010 Objectives

NIC INTERVENTION ACTIVITIES

NURSING FOCUS on the OLDER ADULT

PLAN of CARE

RESOURCE MANAGEMENT

Reference Guide for Student CD-ROM

The Student CD-ROM provided with this text contains the following features:

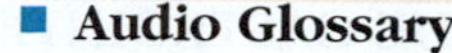

- Review Questions for the NCLEX Examination
- Health Assessment Audio Clips
- Health Assessment Images
- Audio Glossary
- Health Assessment Video Clips
- Animations

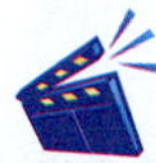

Look for this multimedia icon in the margins of the text. This icon highlights related animations and health assessment video clips on your Student CD-ROM.

HEALTH ASSESSMENT AUDIO CLIPS

UNIT SIX MANAGEMENT OF CLIENTS WITH PROBLEMS OF THE IMMUNE RESPONSE

CHAPTER 26

Stridor

UNIT SEVEN MANAGEMENT OF CLIENTS WITH PROBLEMS OF THE RESPIRATORY TRACT

CHAPTER 30

Bronchial breath sounds
Bronchovesicular breath sounds
Vesicular breath sounds
High-pitched crackles
Low-pitched crackles
High-pitched wheeze
Low-pitched wheeze
Pleural friction rub

UNIT EIGHT MANAGEMENT OF CLIENTS WITH PROBLEMS OF THE CARDIOVASCULAR SYSTEM

CHAPTER 36

Single S1
S1 at various locations
Single S2
S2 at various locations
The fourth heart sound (S4)
The third heart sound (S3)
Murmurs: High, medium, and low
Murmurs: Blowing, harsh or rough, and rumble
Systolic murmur
Diastolic murmur
Pericardial friction rub

HEALTH ASSESSMENT VIDEO CLIPS

UNIT SEVEN MANAGEMENT OF CLIENTS WITH PROBLEMS OF THE RESPIRATORY TRACT

CHAPTER 30

Inspection: Nose (adult female)
Inspection and palpation: Breathing and respiratory excursion, anterior chest (adult male)
Inspection and palpation: Respirations, respiratory excursion, and tactile fremitus, posterior chest (adult male)
Palpation: Tactile fremitus, posterior chest (adult female)
Inspection and percussion: Diaphragmatic excursion (adult male)
Percussion: Anterior thorax (adult male)

UNIT EIGHT MANAGEMENT OF CLIENTS WITH PROBLEMS OF THE CARDIOVASCULAR SYSTEM

CHAPTER 36

Inspection and palpation: Cardiac, anterior chest (adult female)
Inspection and palpation: Cardiac, auscultatory landmarks (adult male)
Auscultation: Cardiac, with diaphragm (adult male)
Auscultation: Cardiac, with bell (adult male)
Auscultation: Cardiac, with diaphragm and bell (adult female)
Auscultation: Carotid artery (adult male)
Inspection and palpation: Pulses, lower extremities (adult female)

UNIT TEN MANAGEMENT OF CLIENTS WITH PROBLEMS OF THE NERVOUS SYSTEM

CHAPTER 44

Evaluation: Smell, cranial nerve I–olfactory nerve (adult male)
Evaluation: Central vision and visual acuity, cranial nerve II–optic nerve (adult male)
Evaluation: Pupil responses, direct and accommodation, cranial nerves III, IV, and VI–oculomotor, trochlear, and abducens nerves (adult male)
Evaluation: Sensory, light touch; face, upper, and lower extremities, cranial nerve V–trigeminal nerve (older adult female)
Inspection: Fine motor coordination, upper extremities (older adult male)
Inspection: Fine motor coordination, lower extremities (older adult female)
Evaluation: Sensory, face, and upper extremities
Evaluation: Deep tendon reflex, patellar tendon (adult male)

UNIT ELEVEN MANAGEMENT OF CLIENTS WITH PROBLEMS OF THE SENSORY SYSTEM

CHAPTER 49

Inspection and palpation: External eye (adult male)
Evaluation: Central vision and visual acuity (adult male)
Evaluation: Pupil responses, direct and consensual (older adult female)

CHAPTER 51

Inspection and palpation: External ear (older adult male)
Inspection: Ear canal (adult male)

UNIT TWELVE MANAGEMENT OF CLIENTS WITH PROBLEMS OF THE MUSCULOSKELETAL SYSTEM

CHAPTER 53

Inspection: Gait (older adult female)
Inspection: General muscle strength (adult male)
Inspection and palpation: Muscular development (adult male)

UNIT THIRTEEN MANAGEMENT OF CLIENTS WITH PROBLEMS OF THE GASTROINTESTINAL SYSTEM

CHAPTER 56

Auscultation: Abdomen, bowel sounds (adult male)
Auscultation: Percussion: Abdomen (adult male)
Percussion: Liver (adult male)
Percussion: Spleen (adult male)
Palpation: Abdomen, superficial and deep (adult male)

UNIT SEVENTEEN MANAGEMENT OF CLIENTS WITH PROBLEMS OF THE REPRODUCTIVE SYSTEM

CHAPTER 76

Inspection: External genitalia (younger adult female)
Inspection: Speculum examination (younger adult female)
Palpation: Bimanual examination (younger adult female)
Inspection and palpation: Standing position (younger adult male)
Inspection and palpation: Standing position, clip 2 (younger adult male)
Palpation: Inguinal hernia evaluation (younger adult male)

CHAPTER 77

Inspection: Female breasts (sitting position, adult female)
Inspection: Female breasts (supine position, adult female)

HEALTH ASSESSMENT IMAGES

UNIT SEVEN MANAGEMENT OF CLIENTS WITH PROBLEMS OF THE RESPIRATORY TRACT

CHAPTER 30

Anterior lobes of the lung
Posterior lobes of the lung
Chest landmarks
Pleural effusion diagram

CHAPTER 33

Bronchitis diagram
Emphysema diagram

CHAPTER 34

Pneumonia diagram
Atelectasis diagram

CHAPTER 35

Client with pneumothorax

UNIT EIGHT MANAGEMENT OF CLIENTS WITH PROBLEMS OF THE CARDIOVASCULAR SYSTEM

CHAPTER 39

Rubor phase of Raynaud's disease
Cyanotic phase of Raynaud's disease

UNIT NINE MANAGEMENT OF CLIENTS WITH PROBLEMS OF THE HEMATOLOGIC SYSTEM

CHAPTER 42

Pale skin with anemia

UNIT TEN MANAGEMENT OF CLIENTS WITH PROBLEMS OF THE NERVOUS SYSTEM

CHAPTER 44

Sensory pathways of CNS
Major motor pathways of CNS
Reflex arc

CHAPTER 47

Facial presentation of Bell's palsy
Residual slight muscle weakness post-Bell's palsy

UNIT ELEVEN MANAGEMENT OF CLIENTS WITH PROBLEMS OF THE SENSORY SYSTEM

CHAPTER 49

Anatomy of the middle ear
Anatomy of the inner ear
Pathways of hearing

CHAPTER 50

Hordeolum
Chalazion
Acute conjunctivitis

CHAPTER 52

Otitis externa
Causes of conductive hearing loss
Causes of sensorineural hearing loss

UNIT THIRTEEN MANAGEMENT OF CLIENTS WITH PROBLEMS OF THE GASTROINTESTINAL SYSTEM

CHAPTER 56

Abdominal auscultation sites
Abdominal structures that may be palpable
Referred abdominal pain–anterior
Referred abdominal pain–posterior

CHAPTER 57

Lymph nodes–head and neck
Lymph nodes–tongue
Lymph nodes–ear

CHAPTER 60

Inguinal hernia pathway
Femoral hernia pathway

UNIT FOURTEEN MANAGEMENT OF CLIENTS WITH PROBLEMS OF THE ENDOCRINE SYSTEM

CHAPTER 66

Addison's disease

CHAPTER 67

Anterior view of thyroid in Asian female with goiter

UNIT FIFTEEN MANAGEMENT OF CLIENTS WITH PROBLEMS OF THE SKIN, HAIR, AND NAILS

CHAPTER 69

Distribution of eccrine and apocrine sweat glands
Ecchymosis caused by injury from falling on a hard object

CHAPTER 70

Contact dermatitis of hands due to prolonged exposure to bleach
Atopic dermatitis on the cheeks of an infant
Urticaria
Anatomical distribution of psoriasis
Cherry angioma

UNIT SEVENTEEN MANAGEMENT OF CLIENTS WITH PROBLEMS OF THE REPRODUCTIVE SYSTEM

CHAPTER 80

Anatomic distribution of secondary syphilis

ANIMATIONS

UNIT SEVEN MANAGEMENT OF CLIENTS WITH PROBLEMS OF THE RESPIRATORY TRACT

CHAPTER 30

Pulmonary circulation
Anatomic location of sinuses
Percussion tones throughout the chest
Patterns of respiration

UNIT EIGHT MANAGEMENT OF CLIENTS WITH PROBLEMS OF THE CARDIOVASCULAR SYSTEM

CHAPTER 36

Cardiac cycle during systole and diastole
Blood flow: Circulatory system
Pulse variations
Auscultation of heart valves

UNIT TEN MANAGEMENT OF CLIENTS WITH PROBLEMS OF THE NERVOUS SYSTEM

CHAPTER 44

Functional areas of the brain
Reflex arc
Sensory pathways and clinical evaluation of the central nervous system
Motor pathways and clinical evaluation of the central nervous system

UNIT ELEVEN MANAGEMENT OF CLIENTS WITH PROBLEMS OF THE SENSORY SYSTEM

CHAPTER 51

Weber test

UNIT TWELVE MANAGEMENT OF CLIENTS WITH PROBLEMS OF THE MUSCULOSKELETAL SYSTEM

CHAPTER 53

Classification of joints: Hinge joint
Classification of joints: Gliding joint–hand
Classification of joints: Condyloid joint

UNIT SEVENTEEN MANAGEMENT OF CLIENTS WITH PROBLEMS OF THE REPRODUCTIVE SYSTEM

CHAPTER 76

Lymphatic drainage of breast
The menstrual cycle

CHAPTER 79

Rectal examination

UNIT ONE

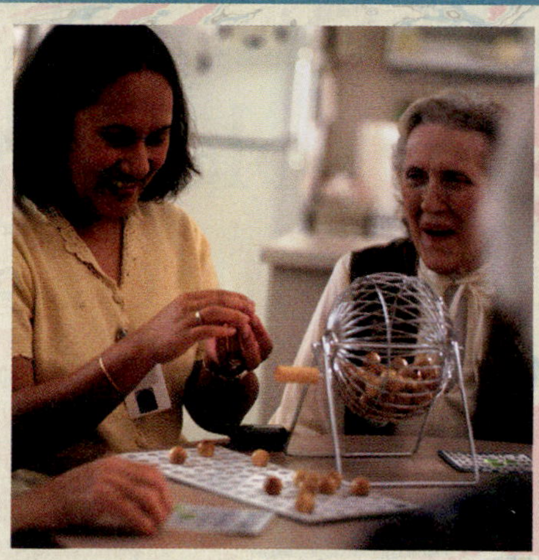

HEALTH PROMOTION and ILLNESS

CHAPTER 1

Critical Thinking in the Role of the Medical-Surgical Nurse

DONNA D. IGNATAVICIUS

LEARNING OUTCOMES

After studying this chapter, you should be able to:

1. Explain why critical thinking is an essential part of medical-surgical nursing.
2. Compare and contrast common definitions of health.
3. Explain why some populations are more likely to experience health problems than others.
4. Explain the purpose of Healthy People 2010.
5. Differentiate the three levels of illness prevention and provide at least one example of each level.
6. Identify the major roles of the medical-surgical nurse.
7. Explain the relationship between critical thinking and evidence-based practice.
8. Assess factors that may affect the teaching-learning process.
9. Describe best practice interventions for promoting adult learning.
10. Review the key components of the nursing process.
11. Describe the difference between a nursing diagnosis and a medical problem.
12. Identify best practice interventions for clinical documentation.

Go to your Student CD-ROM for Review Questions for the NCLEX Examination keyed to these Learning Outcomes.

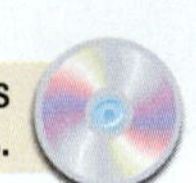

The purpose of medical-surgical nursing, sometimes called adult health nursing, is to promote health and prevent illness in individuals from 18 to older than 100 years of age. Nurses who practice medical-surgical nursing are generalists who must have a broad knowledge base to meet the needs of clients in a variety of health care settings. Rapid advances in technology, massive increases in knowledge, and dramatic changes in the health care delivery system require that medical-surgical nurses use expert critical thinking skills to provide complex, holistic health care.

CRITICAL THINKING

Critical thinking, sometimes referred to as clinical reasoning or judgment, is an essential competency that all nurses need to provide quality, cost-effective client care. Alfaro-LeFevre (2003) describes critical thinking as purposeful, outcome-directed thinking that aims to make judgments based on scientific evidence, rather than on tradition or conjecture (guesswork). The best source of evidence is the result of research. Nursing has increased its research findings on which to base its practice.

Evidence-Based Practice

The term **evidence-based practice** is often used to describe the care that nurses provide based on research and identified standards. Throughout this text, Evidence-Based Practice for Nursing boxes summarize and critique some of the most current research for medical-surgical nursing.

However, available nursing research is limited and often does not represent the highest level of evidence. As seen in Table 1-1, the highest level of evidence, or LOE-1, is based on a meta-analysis of multiple well-designed randomized controlled studies. A significant amount of nursing research consists of small pilot studies at LOE-7 or LOE-8. The findings of these studies cannot be generalized, but they provide a basis for future larger and better controlled research. Each study in this text's Evidence-Based Practice for Nursing boxes is rated by level of evidence using the scale in Table

TABLE 1-1 Level of Evidence (LOE) Rating Scale and Origins of Evidence

LOE	Origin of Evidence
Highest	
LOE-1	Meta-analysis of multiple well-designed randomized controlled trials (RCTs) of adequate quality
LOE-2	At least one properly designed RCT of appropriate size (more than 100 subjects, multiple sites)
LOE-3	Well-designed trial without randomization (e.g., single pretest and post-test, cohort, time series, or meta-analysis of cohort studies)
Moderate	
LOE-4	Well-conducted qualitative systematic review (integrative review on nonexperimental design studies)
LOE-5	Well-conducted case control study
LOE-6	Poorly controlled study (RCT with major flaws) Uncontrolled studies (e.g., correlational descriptive study, case series)
Lowest (Weakest)	
LOE-7	Conflicting evidence with the weight of evidence supporting the recommendation of meta-analysis showing a trend that did not reach statistical significance NIH Consensus Reports Published practice guidelines from professional organizations, health organizations, or federal agencies (e.g., Centers for Disease Control and Prevention)
LOE-8	Qualitative designs with few participants Opinion from expert authorities, agencies, or committees Case studies

Modified from Hadorn, D., et al. (1996). Rating the quality of evidence for clinical practice guidelines. *Journal of Clinical Epidemiology, 49*(7), 749-753; and Rosswurm, M., & Larrabee, J. (1999). A model for change to evidence-based practice. *Image: The Journal of Nursing Scholarship, 31*(4), 317-322.

1-1. Nursing implications are also discussed to help you consider these findings for daily practice.

Critical Thinking Skills and Behaviors

Alfaro-LeFevre (2004) also developed **Critical Thinking Indicators (CTIs)** that identify the behaviors and skills of a critical thinker. The CTIs are divided into the three aspects of critical thinking: knowledge, affective or emotional behaviors, and cognitive behaviors. Examples of each of these aspects of critical thinking are listed in Table 1-2. Medical-surgical nurses should use all of these behaviors and skills to provide high-quality, excellent care.

Critical Thinking Challenges are threaded throughout this book to help you apply critical thinking for a variety of clinical case scenarios. Additional critical thinking activities may be found at http://www.evolve.elsevier.com/Iggy/.

HEALTH

Beliefs about health and illness are a major feature of every known culture. How one views himself or herself as a person and as a part of the environment affects how health is defined.

TABLE 1-2 Examples of Critical Thinking Indicators

Behaviors Demonstrating Critical Thinking Characteristics and Attitudes

Open and fair-minded: Shows tolerance for different viewpoints; questions how own viewpoints are influencing thinking

Creative: Offers alternative solutions and approaches; comes up with useful ideas

Proactive: Anticipates consequences, plans ahead, acts on opportunities

Behaviors Demonstrating Knowledge and Intellectual Skills

Knowledge
- Clarifies reasons behind interventions and diagnostic studies
- Clarifies personal values, beliefs, needs
- Demonstrates focused physical assessment skills (e.g., breath sounds or IV site assessment)

Intellectual Skills/Competencies
- Sets priorities and makes decisions in a timely way; includes key stakeholders in making decisions
- Distinguishes normal from abnormal; identifies risks for abnormal
- Considers multiple explanations and solutions

Data obtained from Alfaro-LeFevre, R. (2003). *Critical thinking in nursing: A practical approach* (3rd ed.). Philadelphia: W.B. Saunders.

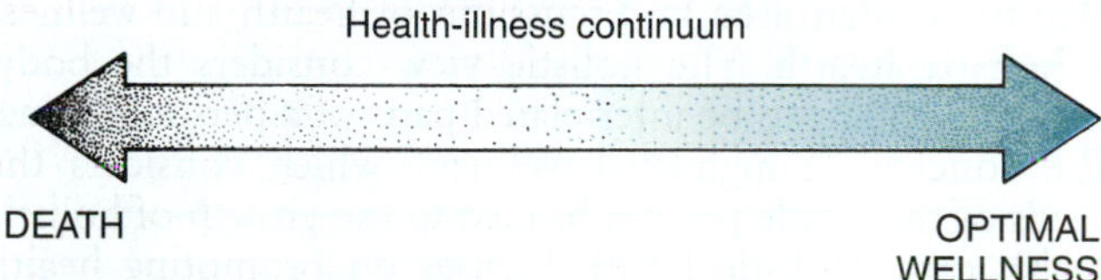

Figure 1-1 ■ Common concept of health as a continuum ranging from optimal wellness at one end to illness culminating in death at the other end.

Health is often viewed as a continuum on which optimal wellness, at one end, is the highest level of function, and illness, at the other end, results in death (Figure 1-1). Every person is somewhere on the continuum. As a person's health state changes, his or her location on the continuum changes.

Although the term *health* is used every day, no universally accepted definition has been established. Over time, the focus and expression of health have varied depending on knowledge, theories, and beliefs. Some individuals view health and disease as a reward or punishment for their actions. Others consider health to be a wholeness of the body; this view is often referred to as holistic health.

Definitions of Health

A typical dictionary may define health in terms of a person's ability to function in society. Some definitions also describe health as a disease-free state or condition. Definitions such as these do not make clear what constitutes health and illness and seem to present an "either/or" situation; that is, a person is either healthy or ill.

WORLD HEALTH ORGANIZATION DEFINITION OF HEALTH

As science has progressed, the definition of **health** has evolved. One of the most commonly quoted definitions is the one presented in 1947 by the World Health Organization (WHO), in which health is defined as "a state of complete physical, mental, and social well-being and not merely the absence of disease or infirmity" (WHO, 1947, p. 1). According to WHO, to be healthy a person must be in a state of physical, mental, and social well-being. Some health care professionals have found this concept problematic because achieving a state of "health" seems to be an unrealistic goal. This definition does not allow for degrees of health or illness, and it fails to reflect the dynamic, ever-changing nature of health.

SOCIOLOGIC DEFINITIONS OF HEALTH

Sociologists view health as a condition that allows for the pursuit and enjoyment of desired cultural values. Researchers who have polled laypersons for their definitions of health concur that health is the absence of symptoms and a feeling of well-being. "Good health" includes the ability to carry out "normal" daily activities, such as going to work and performing household chores.

HOLISTIC HEALTH

One term often used in discussions of health and wellness is **holistic health.** The holistic view considers the body, mind, and spirit to be interrelated parts of a person's being. The concept of high-level wellness, which considers the needs of the whole person, has led to the growth of holistic health care. Holistic health focuses on promoting health and preventing illness, with an emphasis on the person's responsibility to achieve high-level wellness. There is also concern with bringing the person's mind, body, and spirit into harmony with the environment. Various alternative and complementary therapies have been used for many years to promote mind-body-spirit harmony. Chapter 4 describes some commonly used therapies and how they can be incorporated into medical-surgical nursing practice. Additional discussions of these therapies can be found under the text for various disorders throughout the text.

DEFINITION OF HEALTH USED IN THIS TEXT

In this text, health is defined as a person's "level of wellness." This level of wellness is a process in which a person strives to attain his or her full potential. Health reflects a person's biologic, psychological, and sociologic state (Figure 1-2). The *biologic* (physical) state refers to the structure of body tissues and organs as well as to the biochemical interactions and functions within the body. The *psychological* state includes a person's mood, emotions, and personality. The *sociologic* (social) state involves the interaction between a person and the environment.

Spiritual health is sometimes considered to be part of sociologic health but may be described as a separate aspect of the overall health state. Spiritual health often affects both the client's biologic and psychological health state. A study by Narayanasamy & Owens (2001) found that nurses are often confused about the meaning of spirituality and their role related to spiritual health. However, the study sample believed that clients' faith produced a positive effect on clients and families. (See the Evidence-Based Practice for Nursing box above.)

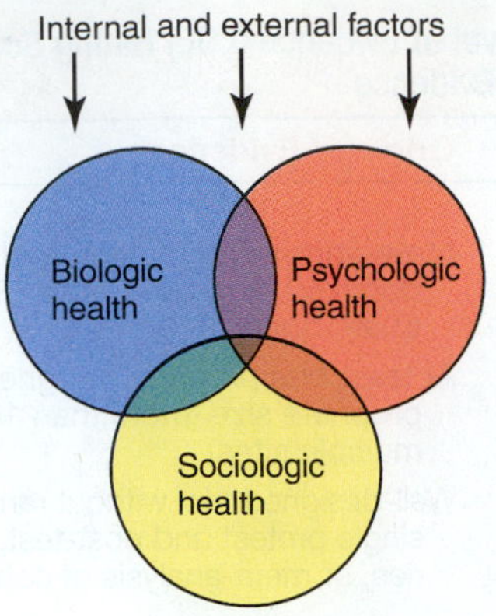

Figure 1-2 ■ Textbook definition of health–a person's biologic, psychological, and sociologic health state. Internal and external factors affect a person's level of wellness.

EVIDENCE-BASED PRACTICE for Nursing

How do nurses intervene to promote spiritual health of clients?

Narayanasamy, A., & Owens, J. (2001). A critical incident study of nurses' responses to the spiritual needs of their patients. *Journal of Advanced Nursing, 33*(4), 446-455.

The purpose of this study was to determine what nurses identify as spiritual needs of clients in an acute care setting and to explore how they responded to those needs. Critical incidents were obtained from 115 volunteer nurses. These data were subjected to content analysis and themes were identified that answered the study questions. The themes were "personal," "procedural," "culturalist," and "evangelical." The findings suggest that nurses are confused about the domain of spiritual health and what it means. They recognized that spirituality plays a positive role in health promotion and the clients' trust in the staff. Nurses did feel that promoting spiritual health was important, but they differed in their approach.

Level of Evidence: 6—Uncontrolled study, but serves as pilot research for nurses' understanding of spiritual health.

Critique. Nurses in acute care often become focused on technical tasks and give less attention and time to meeting other types of needs. This study confirms that nurses believe that spiritual health is an important domain for health promotion, but demonstrates the variety of beliefs and approaches related to spirituality. The data from this convenience sample prevent generalizing these findings, but show the need for further research and education in this area.

Implications for Nursing. Nurses need to recognize the importance of spiritual health in the promotion of overall health. The meaning of spirituality differs from person to person, and nurses need to ask about what it means for each client. Then, a mutual plan for meeting spiritual health needs should be implemented.

A high level of wellness is achieved when these biopsychosocial needs are met. One of the primary functions of nursing is to assist clients in reaching this high level of wellness. It is therefore essential that you understand the concept of health and wellness. As you assess clients, be aware of factors that affect a person's health state, and select nursing interventions that promote and maintain an optimal level of wellness (Figure 1-3).

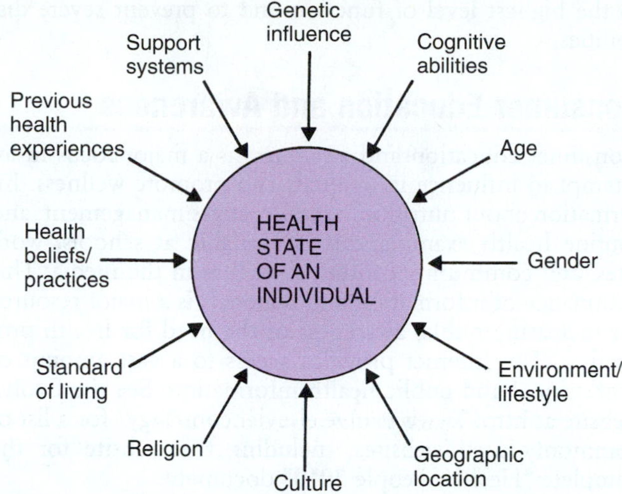

Figure 1-3 ■ Multiple variables influence health and illness.

Quality of Life

Over the past two decades, the concept of **quality of life (QOL)** has emerged as a broad, multidimensional description of a client's health and functional status. Cella (1994) proposed two domains for QOL measurement: subjectivity and multidimensionality. *Subjectivity* refers to clients' perceptions of satisfaction with their functional level, including activities of daily living (e.g., dressing) and independent living skills (e.g., shopping). Older adults typically equate their health status with how well they can function on a daily basis. *Multidimensionality* refers to physical, functional, emotional, and social well-being.

Through her classic nursing research with cancer clients, Ferrell (1996) conceptualized QOL as having four domains: physical, psychological, social, and spiritual well-being. When caring for any client with a major health problem, consider the importance of all domains. Medical-surgical nurses often become focused only on the physical aspects of care, but the other domains are equally important to clients.

A holistic nursing specialty that emphasizes the relationship between spirituality and health is **parish nursing** (Tuck, Wallace, & Pullen, 2001). Parish nurses are generally affiliated with one or more churches, and foster health promotion and education for members of the church, especially those with identified health care needs. Some nurses provide their services on a part-time volunteer basis, whereas others are paid for their services.

Health Promotion and Protection

Health promotion and protection refers to activities that are directed toward developing a person's resources to maintain or enhance well-being as a protection against illness. Reversing the emphasis from curing a disease to promoting health provides a more positive orientation for health care. Illness no longer needs to be the primary focus of health care. In addition, illness care is much more expensive than health promotion.

In 1990, the U.S. Department of Health and Human Services (DHHS) joined the world mission to promote health in its "Healthy People 2000" campaign. The expectation was that individuals would be healthier and would be practicing healthier lifestyles by the year 2000. In particular, the agenda called for health care access for everyone, a longer life expectancy, and equal life expectancy for individuals of all cultures. These goals have not been met. For example, some ethnic groups in the United States–especially Hispanics, black individuals, Asian Americans, and Pacific Islanders–continue to have shorter life expectancies than other groups.

"Healthy People 2010" (DHHS, 2000) has been published to revise these goals and present a more aggressive plan to improve the nation's health by focusing on health promotion practices. This plan has two overall national health goals:

- Increase quality and years of healthy life
- Eliminate health disparities among different demographic groups in the United States

The Healthy People (HP) initiative focuses on 28 areas devoted to an array of diseases, conditions, and public health challenges. Each focus area lists specific health objectives to meet by 2010. These objectives target interventions designed to reduce or eliminate illness, disability, and premature death. This text contains special boxes entitled "Meeting Healthy People 2010 Objectives" that list some of the key objectives from the document and the interventions that nurses can use to help meet those national health objectives.

Several nursing theorists have developed health promotion models for nursing. One of the best known models is that advocated by Pender. In her classic model, Pender (1987) makes a distinction between health promotion and illness prevention: Health promotion is not "health problem specific," but illness prevention (most recently called health protection) is. Pender believes that health promotion is a positive activity, whereas illness prevention is an avoidance activity.

Although this text integrates health promotion and illness prevention (health protection), it recognizes that the two concepts are somewhat different. The goal of both types of activities is to improve or maintain the client's health.

Part of the health promotion movement in nursing is reflected in the use of the term *client* rather than *patient.* The word *patient* is associated with a dependent position in a hospital, whereas the word *client* suggests an active partnership in the process of health care delivery and maintenance in any setting. Therefore *client* is the term used for the health care consumer, or "customer," in this text.

PRACTICES TO PROMOTE HEALTH

Researchers have found that certain health practices have a positive correlation with health promotion in adults. These general health practices include the following:

- Eating well-balanced meals that incorporate foods from the food pyramid, as recommended (see Figure 64-2)
- Eating moderately to maintain ideal weight and prevent obesity
- Exercising moderately on a routine schedule
- Sleeping regularly, about 8 hours each day
- Limiting alcohol consumption to a moderate amount
- Not smoking
- Keeping exposure to the sun to a minimum

These practices have been associated with high-level wellness regardless of gender, age, or economic status. The greater the number of these practices followed in a consistent, routine manner, the better the health state.

PRACTICES TO PREVENT ILLNESS

Illness prevention is related to health protection and maintenance. Prevention is essential for decreasing the occurrence of illness. Preventive health behavior is described as a voluntary action taken by a person or group to decrease the potential or actual threat of illness and its harmful consequences. Ethnic groups vary in the ways that they promote health, especially prevention and early detection. Throughout this text, these cultural considerations are discussed where appropriate.

Individuals must be motivated and educated to make health-related changes. However, each individual must choose whether or not to make these changes. Three levels of illness prevention are summarized in Table 1-3: primary, secondary, and tertiary.

Primary Prevention

Primary prevention is used to avoid or delay the actual occurrence of a specific disease. Strategies for health maintenance raise the general level of health and well-being of a person, family, or community. Attending smoking cessation clinics, receiving immunizations, and using seat belts are examples of primary prevention strategies.

Secondary Prevention

The purpose of **secondary prevention** is early detection of a disease or condition, sometimes before the signs and symptoms are evident. The emphasis is on early diagnosis and treatment as well as on intervention to prevent or limit permanent disability or death. Screening procedures, such as obtaining a Papanicolaou (Pap) smear for detecting cervical cancer, are examples of secondary prevention.

Tertiary Prevention

Tertiary prevention involves rehabilitation and begins when the disease or condition has stabilized and no further healing is expected. An example is cardiac rehabilitation after a myocardial infarction. The goal is to return the person to the highest level of function and to prevent severe disabilities.

TABLE 1-3 Examples of Health Behaviors for the Three Levels of Illness Prevention

Level	Examples of Behaviors
Primary prevention	Wearing seat belts Eating well-balanced meals Not smoking Consuming no or minimal alcohol Being immunized Maintaining ideal body weight
Secondary prevention	Having yearly Papanicolaou (Pap) smear tests Performing a monthly breast or testicular self-examination Having mammograms as recommended Having routine tonometry tests to detect glaucoma
Tertiary prevention	Following a cardiac rehabilitation program Pursuing rehabilitation programs for stroke, head injury, or arthritis

Consumer Education and Awareness

Consumer education and awareness is a major focus in an attempt to influence individuals and promote wellness. Information about nutrition, exercise, stress management, and routine health examinations is available at schools, work sites, and community centers, as well as in the media. This abundance of information and materials is a major resource for increasing public awareness of the need for health promotion. The Internet provides access to a vast amount of professional and public health information. See the Evolve website at http://www.evolve.elsevier.com/Iggy/ for a list of commonly used websites, including the website for the complete "Healthy People 2010" document.

ROLE OF THE MEDICAL-SURGICAL NURSE

Medical-surgical nursing is one of the many specialties in nursing, yet its scope is much broader than other specialties such as cardiovascular or orthopedic nursing. In 1991, the Academy of Medical-Surgical Nurses (AMSN) was formed as the first specialty organization for this group of nurses. AMSN has published standards for medical-surgical nursing and a core curriculum. The official journal of the AMSN is *MEDSURG Nursing: The Journal of Adult Health.*

The focus of **medical-surgical nursing** is on the adult client with acute or chronic illness in any health care setting or on the client who is at risk for illness (Figure 1-4). Nurses who specialize in medical-surgical nursing need to have a broad knowledge of the biologic, psychological, and social sciences because their clients have a range of needs. The overall outcome of care is similar to that for any other specialty—the achievement of an optimal level of wellness and the prevention of illness.

Because the typical client is usually older than 65 years of age, medical-surgical nurses need a strong background in **gerontology,** or the care of older adults. In this text, charts

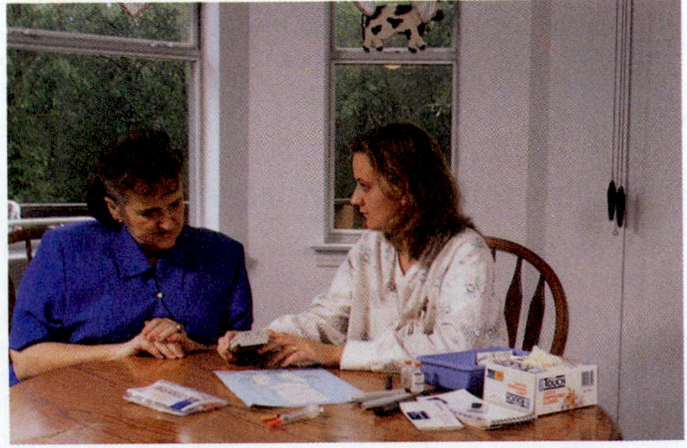

Figure 1-4 ■ Medical-surgical nurses care for adult clients in various settings with such chronic disorders as diabetes mellitus. (From Harkreader, H.C. [2004]. Fundamentals of nursing: Caring and clinical judgment [2nd ed.]. Philadelphia: W.B. Saunders.)

entitled Nursing Focus on the Older Adult highlight the special nursing interventions required for this group of clients. In addition, Considerations for Older Adults are discussed as appropriate throughout this text.

As medical-surgical nursing meets changing health care needs, the expectations for providing client care expand and increase. Medical-surgical nurses assume various roles and functions within a number of health care settings (Figure 1-5). Although each role is associated with specific responsibilities, some aspects are interrelated and are common to all nursing positions and specialties. All roles require the use of critical thinking skills and behaviors.

Coordinator of Care

You cannot provide all of the care that a client needs. As a **care coordinator,** collaborate with the health care team to help the client meet expected outcomes identified as part of the interdisciplinary plan of care. Interdisciplinary clinical rounds and other methods for communication facilitate the process of planning and implementation.

Caregiver

Another role commonly associated with the medical-surgical nurse is that of **caregiver.** In this role, nurses assess clients, analyze collected information to determine clients' needs, develop nursing diagnoses and collaborative problems, plan care and carry out the plan with the health care team, and evaluate the care given. This process, which is referred to as the nursing process (discussion begins on p. 10), is used throughout this text as an organizational and practice framework.

As a caregiver, the nurse provides physical care through skills such as administering medications and performing comprehensive assessments. Some nursing tasks and activities may be delegated to assistive nursing personnel–unlicensed nursing staff members such as patient care technicians (PCTs) or patient care assistants (PCAs). Interventions that you may delegate are indicated throughout this text and in the Client Care Plans. The nurse also implements psychosocial and spiritual interventions, such as encouraging the client to discuss concerns with a clergyperson or offering measures to reduce anxiety.

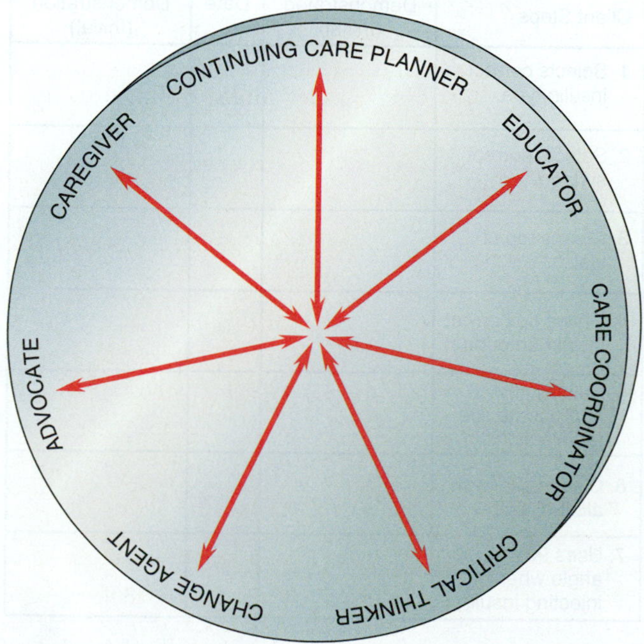

Figure 1-5 ■ Major roles of the medical-surgical nurse.

Activities performed by the nurse caregiver are often categorized as *collaborative* (interdependent) or *independent.* **Collaborative** functions include the following:

- Those that are mutually determined by the nurse and the physician or other health care team member, such as setting activity limitations or providing a special diet
- Those that are directed or prescribed by the health care provider (physician, nurse practitioner, or physician's assistant) but require nursing judgment to perform (e.g., administering medications)

Independent nursing functions are initiated and carried out by the nurse without direction from the health care provider. Examples include the following:

- Weighing a client
- Listening to breath sounds
- Elevating the head of the bed to facilitate breathing

This text discusses both types of functions–collaborative and independent–in an interrelated framework under the heading *Collaborative Management.* Charts entitled Best Practice for Nursing identify the most important nursing care for clients with selected health problems.

Continuing Care Planner

Because health care continues to emphasize early discharge from the hospital, nursing home, and home care, the role of the medical-surgical nurse as a continuing care planner has become increasingly important. This process involves an assessment of the client's health needs across the health care continuum. A large part of this process is health teaching and assessment of the home (or other setting to which the client is discharged) for available resources, support systems, and equipment, if needed.

Continuing care planning may be coordinated by a case manager or by a designated discharge planner employed by the agency in collaboration with the staff nurse. The discharge planner or case manager is usually a nurse or social worker. Chapter 3 describes case management in detail. If the agency does not employ designated discharge planners, you may be responsible for the continuing care planning. Throughout this text, sections entitled Community-Based Care are included to facilitate planning and describe settings in which continuing care may be needed (see also Chapter 2).

Educator

Client education is a major component of medical-surgical nursing care. In collaboration with the interdisciplinary health team, the nurse tries to improve health by facilitating client learning regarding health promotion, disease and illness, and specific treatment. As educators, nurses work with individual clients and family members or other caregivers. The role of education has become increasingly important because clients are discharged "quicker and sicker" from the hospital, subacute unit, or nursing home. Nurses often become frustrated when they feel they do not have the time they need to teach in these fast-paced settings.

THE TEACHING-LEARNING PROCESS

In collaboration with other members of the health care team, assess the client's learning needs and barriers to learning. A client with a disease of 20 years' duration may need as much teaching as one with a newly diagnosed condition. Make no assumptions; instead assess each client individually. Determine the client's goals and willingness to learn. If the client has no interest in learning, wait for another time or setting before beginning client education. Chart 1-1 summarizes the most important teaching-learning principles for adults.

Teaching may occur in a spontaneous, informal manner, or it may follow a more structured, formal approach based on written teaching plans. Most facilities provide written teaching plans and tools for the interdisciplinary team to ensure that every client receives the same accurate information.

The nurse documents on the appropriate record what was taught and what the client learned (Figure 1-6). Some health care agencies use a lay version of the clinical pathway as a learning tool that outlines care in a sequential manner for the client (see Developing the Collaborative Plan of Care, p. 14). In general, a summary of the teaching-learning process for each client becomes a part of the client's medical record. A copy is also given to the client or family member or significant other at discharge. Each Community-Based Care section within this text includes a subsection entitled Health Teaching. Client Education Guides for teaching clients are also included as appropriate throughout the text.

FACTORS AFFECTING THE TEACHING-LEARNING PROCESS

As interdisciplinary team members assess the teaching-learning needs of each client, they evaluate many factors that may enhance or impede learning. Some of the most important factors include the client's educational level, socioeconomic level, support system, age, and culture.

CHART 1-1

BEST PRACTICE for Adult Learning

- Assess the client's goals and willingness to learn.
- Before beginning teaching, assess how the client is feeling (e.g., a client in acute pain is unlikely to learn).
- Include family and significant others in teaching as appropriate.
- Assess factors that may influence the client's ability or motivation to learn, such as educational level, socioeconomic status, and cultural background.
- Provide pictures or other types of visual aids to reinforce learning.
- Break complex information or skills into small parts until the client learns them.
- Provide the client with "hands-on" experience for psychomotor skills, and request a return demonstration by the client (e.g., insulin administration, dressing change, colostomy care).
- Provide the client with a health resource contact for follow-up questions or concerns.

Educational Level

The client's educational level will directly affect your plans for teaching. In the United States it is estimated that more than one third of adults do not have a high school diploma. Consequently, illiteracy in the United States is widespread. Therefore information written for the public should not be above the sixth grade reading level, and it often needs to be lower.

For illiterate clients and for those with limited reading skills, use other types of visual aids (e.g., pictures and videos). When possible, explain and interpret information for clients rather than merely offering them a booklet or instruction sheet.

Socioeconomic Level

Consider the clients' financial resources when teaching them how to care for themselves at home. For example, if a client needs to perform muscle-strengthening exercises using small weights, do not expect the client to purchase expensive commercial weights. Instead, suggest the use of 1- or 2-pound coffee cans or bags, bags of sugar or flour, or similar household items.

Another concern is the cost of required medications, equipment, or supplies. Clients who do not qualify for medical assistance but work for an employer that does not provide group health insurance may not be able to afford the necessary medical items or follow-up care. As part of continuing care planning, attempt to locate resources that can provide the necessary items, such as community health organizations, churches, or lay organizations, such as the Lions Club. Clinics that specialize in providing care for working and uninsured clients are available in some parts of the United States. Some of these clinics are nurse-managed community centers.

Teaching-Learning Record for Insulin Self-Administration			
Client Steps	Taught/ Demonstrated (Initial)	Date	Return Demonstration (Initial)
1. Selects correct insulin type.			
2. Selects correct syringe.			
3. Cleans top of vial.			
4. Draws up correct insulin amount(s).			
5. Selects appropriate site for injection.			
6. Cleans skin with alcohol swipe.			
7. Uses 90-degree angle when injecting insulin.			

Figure 1-6 ■ A sample teaching-learning record for the self-administration of insulin.

Support Systems

Assess the client's support systems, including part or all of these systems in client education. Examples of support systems include families, significant others, churches, and social community clubs and organizations. In general, individuals tend to be more compliant with their health regimen if they have the encouragement of others. Support is particularly important when the client must follow many lifestyle restrictions. For instance, a farmer who is accustomed to eating fried foods and red meat may find it difficult to change to a low-fat, low-sodium diet. If the farmer's wife has always been the cook in the home, the nurse includes her in the teaching process to help ensure compliance with the new dietary restrictions.

Age

Age also affects the teaching-learning process. An older adult may take longer to process information or may have visual or hearing deficits (Chart 1-2). Provide small amounts of information at a time and check with the client before proceeding to make sure that he or she has understood. Too much information is difficult to comprehend and absorb, and this usually results in frustration and noncompliance.

Cultural Considerations

Consider the client's cultural background before teaching. If the client does not clearly understand the primary language, locate resources that can help with the teaching process. For example, many individuals who immigrated to the United States in the 1940s have attempted to retain their language and culture and not become too "Americanized." As a result, when interacting with health care professionals, they may need someone to interpret for them.

Another factor to consider during health teaching is the health practices of various cultures. For example, Mexican Americans, particularly those living near the Mexican border, often use *curandismo* (folk medicine) either because they cannot afford Westernized health care or because they prefer their own medical traditions. These clients may also avoid the health care system because of limitations in speaking, reading, or writing English or Spanish.

The nurse also considers spiritual and religious differences. A client whose spiritual beliefs forbid taking medication is not likely to comply with instructions about drug therapy. This type of information is essential so you can incorporate cultural beliefs and practices into the teaching-learning process.

CHART 1-2

NURSING FOCUS on the OLDER ADULT

Facilitating Learning

- Ensure that the client wears glasses or hearing aids if needed.
- Be sure that the area for teaching has ample lighting and minimal distraction.
- Provide most of the teaching in the morning (after breakfast), before the client becomes too fatigued.
- Speak slowly and provide small amounts of new information at a time.
- Ask the client to repeat the information to make sure that he or she has learned it.
- Provide written information so the client can refer to it later if needed.

Advocate

As a client advocate, the medical-surgical nurse assists the client and family in interpreting information from other health care team members. Offer additional assistance that the client needs in making decisions about health care. Such assistance may include explaining the implications of the client's decisions and ensuring that the client receives appropriate care. For example, a client scheduled for a total knee replacement may not understand that the knee joint will be removed and replaced with a prosthesis. *If the client does not fully understand the operative procedure, notify the surgeon of the need for additional preoperative education.* The information is reinforced even if another health team member has provided it.

Change Agent

The medical-surgical nurse serves as a change agent within the work setting and within the profession. The role of the change agent involves planning and implementing a system to change the client's health-related behaviors. In the work setting, the nurse assesses the health behaviors of the client and family and identifies those that need altering. The most important factor in this process is assessing the client's readiness to change. If the client is not ready, he or she will not comply with the change, and the nurse will be ineffective in this role.

Within the community, medical-surgical nurses serve as role models and assist consumers in bringing about changes to improve the environment, work conditions, or other factors that affect health. Nurses also work together to bring about change through legislation. For example, they provide and support legislative bills that can affect a person's health status, such as those that mandate a client's bill of rights.

THE CONCEPT OF CARING

A critical attribute for medical-surgical nurses is caring. Nurse caring has been broadly described as a process, a set of actions, and an attitude that conveys physical care and emotional concern for others. Nurses have been studying and practicing caring for many years, yet confusion remains about a precise definition of caring. Debate also continues among nursing theorists and researchers regarding the best method for measuring human caring (Beck, 1999).

The results of a classic study by Barr and Bush (1998) found four factors or broad examples of caring in critical care nurses:

- Support from colleagues (nurses they work with)
- Nurses modeling care (and caring)
- Observable client progress and positive client and family interaction
- Economic/bureaucratic factors (negative factors that nurses must overcome)

When providing client care, the nurse subjects in the study stated that listening and caring were key caring techniques. Today's medical-surgical nurses who work in hospitals often feel they do not have time to listen to or show caring toward their clients. The focus of client care is often on technical tasks rather than on outcomes or psychosocial interventions such as caring. However, in keeping with the definition of health and the role of the nurse, clients need to have their biopsychosocial needs met to promote health and prevent illness.

PRACTICE SETTINGS FOR MEDICAL-SURGICAL NURSES

Medical-surgical nurses have opportunities to provide health care in a variety of settings, including hospitals, long-term care facilities, and community-based settings (Figure 1-7). Most acute care hospitals and fewer long-term or community settings are voluntarily accredited by the Joint Commission on Accreditation of Healthcare Organizations (JCAHO). This group sets standards that assure quality health care. The hospital setting is described in this chapter. Chapter 2 discusses community-based settings.

Hospitals, or **acute care facilities**, have historically been the largest employers of nurses, with slightly more than half of all nurses working within hospitals. This percentage is declining as hospitals continue to "rightsize" and as care continues to move into the community. Few hospitals are freestanding today. Most are part of an integrated health care system (IHS) or integrated health care delivery system (IHDS) that typically comprises inpatient and ambulatory facilities, and may include long-term care and home health agencies.

In the United States, most hospital care costs are paid for by third-party payers, either managed care organizations or traditional insurers. Medicare Part A (in-hospital coverage), a federal program, pays for most of the acute care given to individuals who are older than 65 years of age or who have been disabled for at least 2 years. State medical assistance programs, often managed care Medicaid, pay for some of the health care provided to clients of any age who are indigent. Chapter 3 describes managed care and case management.

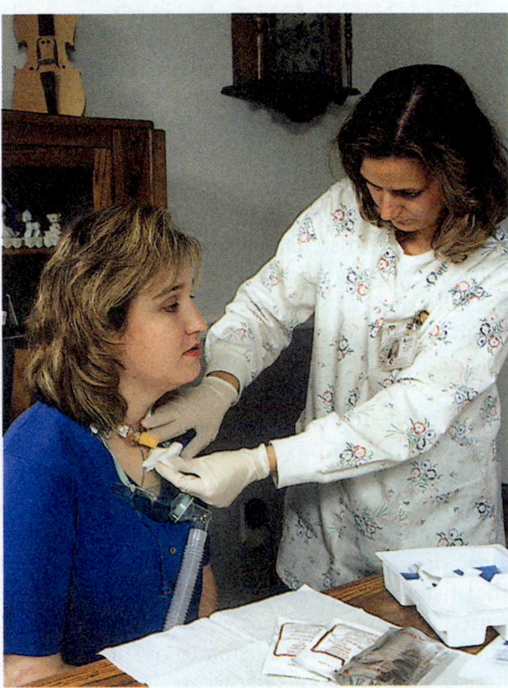

Figure 1-7 ■ Nurses often care for clients in the home. (From Harkreader, H.C. [2004]. Fundamentals of nursing: Caring and clinical judgment [2nd ed.]. Philadelphia: W.B. Saunders.)

In Canada, all individuals are entitled to free comprehensive health care for life. The Canadian government started this system in the 1960s with the belief that health care should be accessible to all Canadian citizens.

There are three general types of inpatient units in most hospital settings:

- Critical care units
- Intermediate or specialty care units
- Long-term care units (including subacute units)

Critical Care Units

Critical care units are areas for the complex, intense care of critically ill clients. Examples are surgical or medical intensive care units, shock trauma and "step-down" units, and neurosurgical intensive care units. Emergency and operating departments are also considered critical care areas because of the acute and intense nature of the care provided in these parts of the hospital. Critical care areas require nurses who thrive in crisis situations and who work effectively under high stress. Nurses in these areas must be highly skilled in making accurate observations of clients' conditions and in interpreting findings quickly and correctly. The nurse-to-client ratio in critical care units is typically 1:2 or 1:3 depending on the acuity of the clients. Critical care nursing is a subspecialty of nursing practice.

Intermediate or Specialty Care Units

Intermediate care units have changed dramatically over the past two decades. The clients in these units are much sicker today than in the past. Examples of specialty intermediate care areas are neuroscience (neurology) units, urology units, and orthopedic units. In hospitals that are too small to separate clients by specialty, intermediate care units provide treatment for a combination of multiple medical and surgical health problems.

Nurses in intermediate care areas must be able to adapt to caring for various types of illness and must be competent in health teaching and discharge planning. As in critical care areas, nurses must also be highly skilled in critical thinking and psychomotor tasks.

Long-Term Care Units

Long-term care (LTC) units may be found within or adjacent to a hospital for clients with chronic illnesses or health problems that require a finite period of medical care or rehabilitation. These units may also be referred to as transitional care units, skilled nursing facilities (SNFs), or subacute units. Most long-term care, though, is provided in freestanding nursing homes. Chapter 2 describes long-term care in more detail.

OVERVIEW OF THE NURSING PROCESS

The nursing process is an organized, systematic approach used by medical-surgical nurses to meet the individualized health care needs of their clients, families, and communities. The term nursing process emerged in the mid-1960s. As nursing became more recognized and respected as a profession, there was a growing need to define more clearly what nurses do.

Comparison of the Nursing Process with the Scientific Method

The **nursing process** is a decision-making approach that requires critical thinking. Many textbooks compare the nursing process with the scientific method of solving problems. The steps in these two approaches are similar–they both proceed from identification of the problem to evaluation of the solution. One difference is that the scientist identifies the problem first and then collects the data, whereas the nurse collects the data first and then determines the problem.

Intuitive Judgment in Nursing Practice

Over the past 20 years, research has shown that nurses sometimes use (and should use) intuitive judgment in clinical practice (Benner & Tanner, 1987). **Intuition** is the ability to understand immediately without using formal analysis; it is based on experience and knowledge, and is therefore used by experts (Alfaro-LeFevre, 2003). Intuition helps the nurse to act quickly if necessary, particularly in critical care settings or emergency situations in which he or she must assess the client and intervene at once.

The authors of this text use the nursing process as the organizing framework for its content. We do not believe that the nursing process is merely a technical skill with rules that apply in all situations but rather that nurses need to use critical thinking based on current evidence and intuition when the situation demands it.

Steps of the Nursing Process

Most literature citations list five steps for the nursing process: assessment, analysis (nursing diagnosis), planning, implementation, and evaluation. The steps are usually followed in sequence, from assessment to evaluation. However, once the nursing process begins, it is continuous or cyclic (Figure 1-8). For example, if the client's outcomes are not met on the basis of the initial evaluation, the nurse may need to reassess the client or implement new actions to help achieve the desired outcomes. To understand the nursing process as a whole, it is first necessary to briefly review each step and its associated activities. A more detailed discussion of the nursing process may be found in basic nursing textbooks.

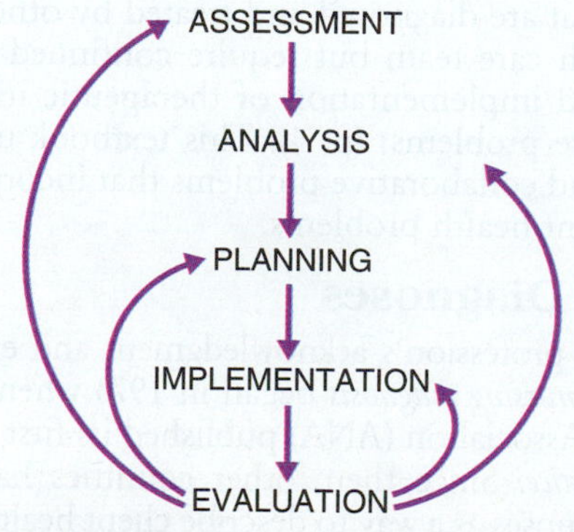

Figure 1-8 ■ The nursing process cycle.

ASSESSMENT

Assessment, the first step of the nursing process, is a systematic method of collecting data about the client, family, or community for the purpose of identifying actual and potential health problems. The **database** is the organization of assessment data and often refers to the tool or chart form used to record the data.

Admission/First Visit Database

The complete database includes a thorough health history, physical assessment, and psychosocial assessment. In the acute care setting, the admission database is usually completed during the first 8 hours after a client's admission to the hospital. Assessments are updated at least every shift throughout the client's stay. In the home or ambulatory care setting, complete the database during the first visit and update it during subsequent visits.

In the skilled nursing unit or nursing home, the admission nursing assessment is documented within the first 24 hours. The federally mandated and standardized interdisciplinary Minimum Data Set (MDS) requires initial completion within 5 days of admission.

The information collected by the nurse is *not* a repetition of the medical history recorded by the health care provider. A *medical* history is obtained by the health care provider to determine the presence of a pathologic condition and to provide a basis for planning medical care. A **nursing history** is obtained by the nurse and focuses on the meaning of the illness and/or hospitalization to the client and family. It is used as a basis for planning nursing care.

Data may be organized in one of a variety of methods. In clinical practice, data are often collected by body system. In a few health care settings, human response patterns or functional health patterns are used as a framework. Some nursing programs also teach students to organize and collect data by one of these methods.

This text incorporates Gordon's (2002) **Functional Health Patterns** in the Assessment chapters (Table 1-4). In addition, the first page of each unit illustrates the relationship of health patterns, common health concepts, and major health problems discussed in this text.

Episodic, or Problem-Centered, Database

An episodic database is collected for a limited or short-term problem. It focuses on one problem, and the data collected are associated with the problem. For example, an older hospitalized woman falls while trying to get out of bed and

TABLE 1-4 Gordon's Functional Health Patterns

- Health Perception—Health Management Pattern
- Nutritional-Metabolic Pattern
- Elimination Pattern
- Activity-Exercise Pattern
- Sleep-Rest Pattern
- Cognitive-Perceptual Pattern
- Self-Perception—Self-Concept Pattern
- Role-Relationship Pattern
- Sexuality-Reproductive Pattern
- Coping—Stress—Tolerance Pattern
- Value—Belief Pattern

Data from Gordon, M. (2002). *Manual of nursing diagnosis* (10th ed.). St. Louis: Mosby.

complains of hip pain. The nurse's history focuses on how the fall occurred, which parts of the client's body made contact with the floor, and what position she assumed after she fell. The physical assessment is centered on the neurologic and musculoskeletal systems, especially the head, hip, and knee. These data are usually recorded on a variance form, or incident report, according to agency policy.

In other situations, the nurse documents assessment findings on a flow sheet at frequent intervals during the day. For example, the client who is receiving epidural analgesia must be monitored continuously to determine whether the intervention is successful and whether adverse effects occur.

Sources of Data

Obtain and document data from several sources in the client's medical record according to the policies of the health care agency.

CLIENT

The client is the primary source of data. This information is direct and firsthand and is collected during an interview. Interviewing is a communication skill by which you can explore the thoughts, feelings, and perceptions of the client. As in the teaching-learning process, the interview process is affected by many variables, including timing, environment, and demographic factors such as age. Chart 1-3 provides tips for interviewing an older adult.

FAMILY AND SIGNIFICANT OTHERS

The client's family members or significant others are secondary sources of data and can often supplement or verify information provided by the client. They may also be able to offer information about the client before the illness, provide a family history related to health and illness, and describe the client's home environment.

CHART 1-3

NURSING FOCUS on the OLDER ADULT

Interviewing

- Review old records and the medical history, if available, before interviewing the client.
- Provide as much privacy as possible.
- Ask the client whether family or significant others should be present during the interview.
- Refer to the client by his or her last name (e.g., Mrs. Brown) unless he or she prefers another name.
- Make sure that eyeglasses, contact lenses, and hearing aids are available and working properly (if the client wears these devices).
- Conduct the interview when the client is not experiencing pain and after basic comfort needs have been met.
- Before conducting the interview, allow the client to adjust to a new environment.
- Sit at the client's eye level during the interview.
- Speak clearly, slowly, and in a low-pitched voice; do not shout.
- Be aware that the client may not be able to distinguish soft consonant blends such as "sh" or "ch."
- Interview in the morning, after breakfast, or in the early afternoon, after the client has rested.
- Whenever possible, use open-ended questions to gather more information; avoid questions that can be answered "yes" or "no."
- Consider the client's education, culture, and age when phrasing questions, especially about sensitive or controversial issues.
- Observe the client's nonverbal behavior as well as what he or she says.

MEDICAL RECORDS

Previous medical histories, laboratory records, vital signs, and diagnostic reports provide pertinent data. These data can validate information identified in the current history and physical examination or can serve as a comparison to indicate changes in the client's health condition. Records from previous hospital admissions supply additional pieces of information. The client's health care provider usually requests the old records from the agency's medical records department or other health care facility where the client has sought health care.

INTERDISCIPLINARY COLLABORATION

A nurse often gathers client information in collaboration with other members of the health care team. The physician or nurse practitioner is a key source of information. A case manager or home care nurse who has worked with the client can also contribute valuable information.

When a client is admitted to the hospital from another health care facility, such as a nursing home, the hospital nurse should contact the nurse who cared for the client in the previous facility for specific client information. Most nursing homes supply a transfer form that accompanies the client to the hospital or other facility. This form describes the client's abilities and limitations, drug therapy, diet therapy, and past and current health state. This information is particularly helpful when the client cannot communicate and when no family is available.

ANALYSIS

The second step of the nursing process is the analysis of data. In this phase, summarize and analyze the data, and draw conclusions to determine what health problems the client may have or is at risk for. Compare client data with "normal" findings and behaviors for the client's age, education, and cultural background. Review abnormal data to determine patterns of altered functioning. Client health problems are identified and categorized as potential problems requiring prevention or as actual problems being managed or requiring interventions.

In their classic book, Aspinall and Tanner (1981) state that nurses make two types of judgments or conclusions about the health state of a client: (1) those health problems that nurses, "by virtue of their education and experience, are licensed and able to treat" (nursing diagnoses), and (2) those problems that are diagnosed and treated by other members of the health care team but require continued nursing assessment and implementation of therapeutic interventions (collaborative problems) (p. 4). This textbook uses nursing diagnoses and collaborative problems that incorporate both types of client health problems.

Nursing Diagnoses

The nursing profession's acknowledgment and endorsement of the term *nursing diagnosis* began in 1973 when the American Nurses Association (ANA) published its first *Standards of Nursing Practice.* Since then, other countries have adopted nursing diagnoses as a way to describe client health problems.

Although many definitions of nursing diagnosis have been proposed by various nursing leaders, the authors of this text recognize the official definition approved by the North American Nursing Diagnosis Association (NANDA) at its Ninth Conference in 1990: "A nursing diagnosis is a clinical judgment about an individual, family, or community response to actual or potential health problems/life processes which provides the basis for definitive therapy toward achievement of outcomes for which the nurse is accountable" (Carpenito, 1995, p. 65).

Unlike medical diagnoses, which identify illness, nursing diagnoses identify the *responses* to health problems and life processes such as aging or death. A medical diagnosis is the basis for medical interventions; a nursing diagnosis is the basis for nursing interventions. Nursing diagnoses are not diagnostic tests, medical treatments, or problems experienced by the nurse while caring for the client (Table 1-5).

Since 1973, the list of nursing diagnoses has expanded. In 2003, there were 167 NANDA-approved nursing diagnoses (NANDA International, 2003). Even though these diagnoses are heavily emphasized in nursing programs, many health care facilities do not use them as they are stated in practice. JCAHO-accredited health care agencies are mandated to use an interdisciplinary, collaborative approach to client care. Therefore both collaborative problems and nursing diagnoses are discussed in this text.

Collaborative Problems

Collaborative problems, as identified in this text, are potential health problems for which the nurse monitors and helps to prevent. They often require interdisciplinary interventions. Through keen assessment skills, detect the health problem as early as possible if it occurs and notify the health care provider. Then, in collaboration with members of the interdisciplinary care team, carry out interventions to resolve the problem. An example of a collaborative problem is Potential for Hypoglycemia for a client with diabetes.

PLANNING

The planning step follows the analysis step of the nursing process. Throughout the planning process, the nurse performs several important functions: setting priorities and expected outcomes, selecting nursing interventions, and determining resources.

Setting Priorities and Outcomes

After analyzing the needs of the client to identify client health problems, decide on the urgency of these problems. This step is vital because some problems are more critical than others. Problems of higher priority require more immediate intervention than problems of lower priority. Setting priorities helps you to organize and plan care to solve the most urgent problems first.

ESTABLISHING PRIORITIES

In determining the priority of the problems, consider their impact on the client. Priorities may fluctuate as the client's level of wellness changes. Consider both actual and potential problems when establishing priorities. Actual problems are usually more important than potential problems; however, potential problems may at times be more important. For example, in a client who has had a stroke (brain attack), the Risk for Aspiration related to impaired swallowing is potentially more life threatening than the actual problem of Constipation related to immobility. Ensuring that any client has an effective airway is always the most important priority when rendering care. To help you learn and practice priority setting, the critical thinking challenges in this text ask you to establish priorities in specific clinical scenarios.

ESTABLISHING OUTCOMES

If possible, the client and the nurse then try to reach a mutual decision regarding expected outcomes on the basis of identified nursing diagnoses and collaborative problems. Outcomes serve as guides for selecting nursing interventions and for determining criteria for evaluating nursing interventions. The purpose of writing **expected outcomes** is to assist in evaluating the client's progress and in determining the resolution of the client's problem if possible.

Expected outcomes have the following characteristics:

- Client-centered
- Realistic in terms of the client's potential for achievement and the nurse's ability to help the client achieve them
- Specific and measurable to the extent possible, using **indicators**

Moorhead, Johnson, and Maas (2004) updated the Nursing Outcomes Classification (NOC) system, which lists evidence-based expected outcomes with indicators that determine whether outcomes were met. Like the NANDA nursing diagnoses, the outcomes are alphabetized using broad labels. For example, Aspiration Prevention is an NOC outcome that is defined as "personal actions to prevent the passage of fluid and solid particles into the lung (Moorhead, Johnson, & Maas, 2004, p. 153). Two of the indicators for Aspiration Prevention are:

- Positions self upright for eating/drinking
- Selects food according to swallowing ability

For a specific client who is at risk for aspiration, the nurse can rate whether or not the client demonstrated the indicators

TABLE 1-5 Differentiation Between Medical and Nursing Diagnoses

Medical Diagnosis	Nursing Diagnosis
Identifies the pathologic basis for an illness	Identifies a response to illness
Focuses on the physical condition of the client	Focuses on the physical, psychosocial, and spiritual needs of the client
Addresses actual, existing problems	Addresses actual and potential problems
Is not validated with the client	Is validated with the client if possible
Uses standardized goals and treatments	Uses individualized outcomes and interventions
May not be resolvable	Is usually resolvable

using a rating scale of 1 to 5 (5 being the best). If the client received a 4 or 5 for the desired indicators, the outcome of Aspiration Prevention was met. Otherwise, the outcome was not met.

This text incorporates NOC outcomes where appropriate and presents selected indicators to help you determine if the outcomes were met. The rating scales are not included due to space constraints, but you can refer to the NOC text reference listed in this chapter's Selected Bibliography (Moorhead, Johnson, & Maas, 2004) for that information.

Selecting Nursing Interventions

After determining the outcomes, develop strategies to accomplish them. Nursing interventions, also known as nursing actions or measures, are designed to assist the client in achieving the desired outcomes. They are based on the client's health problems and define activities required to promote, maintain, or restore health.

McCloskey and Bulechek (2000) define an **intervention** as "any treatment, based upon clinical judgement and knowledge, that a nurse performs to enhance patient/client outcomes" (p. 3). In 1992 these authors published the results of the first phase of the Iowa Intervention Project. This research produced a Nursing Interventions Classification (NIC) system of 336 standardized nursing interventions. The newest update includes 514 evidence-based interventions that have been supported by a number of nursing specialty organizations (Dochterman & Bulechek, 2004).

As with the development of nursing diagnoses and NOC, NIC is intended to help nurses standardize their terminology and practice.

Using NIC, the primary intervention for a Risk for Aspiration related to impaired swallowing is Aspiration Precautions. This intervention is defined as "prevention or minimization of risk factors in the [client] at risk for aspiration" (Dochterman & Bulechek, 2004, p. 175). A number of specific activities are associated with this intervention, such as the following:

- Maintain an airway.
- Monitor pulmonary status.
- Feed in small amounts.
- Cut food into small pieces.

These actions direct the nurse or other health care team member in providing evidence-based client care.

NIC interventions and activities are included throughout the Interventions chapters of this text as appropriate and space allows. Refer to the NIC text reference listed in the Selected Bibliography (Dochterman & Bulechek, 2004) for more information.

Developing the Collaborative Plan of Care

The Joint Commission on Accreditation of Healthcare Organizations (JCAHO) mandates that its accredited agencies establish a collaborative plan of care for its clients. The **collaborative plan of care (POC)** is an interdisciplinary document that outlines the essential aspects of client care, often across a time sequence. One format that may be used is a clinical pathway, which is also called a critical path, care map, or coordinated POC.

The **clinical pathway (CP)** delineates what care must be provided, who will provide the care, and when the care will be provided. It is a guideline for care that can be individualized if needed. Most pathways also list expected outcomes for the client, which may be hourly, daily, or weekly depending on the nature of the health care setting. CPs are typically used in acute care, subacute care, and rehabilitation settings. This text provides several samples of clinical pathways on the Evolve website.

A number of health care agencies do not use pathways, and instead use interdisciplinary care plans, similar in format to traditional nursing care plans. Various members of the health care team develop the plan of care as appropriate for the client, and all members monitor the client's progress in meeting expected outcomes.

This text includes sample Client Care Plans. Although these plans of care are not interdisciplinary, they are helpful for beginning students to learn the steps of the nursing process and to identify the rationale (scientific evidence) for selected nursing interventions. Interventions that the nurse can delegate to assistive nursing personnel are specified. This format is no longer used in most clinical practice settings because JCAHO does not require the use of columnar care plans. Instead JCAHO requires evidence that nurses plan and implement care on the basis of identified client health problems and in collaboration with the interdisciplinary team.

To save time and duplication, a number of computer programs and books have been developed to create standardized plans of care or clinical pathways that can be individualized as needed. As technology advances, these programs should be more widely available to nurses in all health care settings.

This text also provides examples of visual plans of care known as **concept maps,** sometimes referred to as clinical care maps or clinical correlation maps. These concept maps present assessment data, nursing diagnoses/collaborative problems, and collaborative care for clients with complex health problems. NIC and NOC categories are included as needed. The maps show the relationships among these components, thus enabling you to see the "big picture" regarding the client's interdisciplinary care. Concept maps are not used in the clinical practice setting, but they provide a learning tool for summarizing client care and stimulating critical thinking (Ignatavicius, 2004).

Determining Resources

When planning nursing interventions, determine what resources are necessary for implementation of these interventions. The client is a valuable source of information about health care resources that were successful in the past. For example, the client with an irritated stoma may mention that an enterostomal therapist was helpful with previous problems. Including the client and family in planning care often promotes their cooperation during the implementation phase.

Other nurses and health care team members are valuable resources. An interdisciplinary conference or "walking rounds" during which health care team members identify problems and the resources to solve them may be very helpful, especially in planning community-based care.

When the financial feasibility of the plan is explored, consider the availability of other resources for the client, such as equipment, time, personnel, and money. The client's value system is also considered. For instance, if the client requires dialysis in the home, the type of system implemented depends on the home water supply, electrical capability, space, available money, spiritual beliefs, and personal support system.

IMPLEMENTATION

Implementation involves the actual carrying out of a specific, individualized POC. This step of the nursing process is the action phase, in which the nurse assumes responsibility for implementing the POC based on the nursing diagnosis and collaborative problems. Best practice interventions are based on scientific evidence, identified standards of care and, at times, intuitive judgment. Best Practice for Nursing interventions are summarized in charts throughout this text. Because planning and implementation are closely related, this text discusses them under one heading, Planning and Implementation, with expected outcomes and interventions clearly labeled.

EVALUATION

Evaluation, the fifth step of the nursing process, is a cognitive activity that completes the nursing process by indicating the degree to which the client's expected outcomes have been met.

Although evaluation is given as the final step of the nursing process, it is an ongoing and integral part of each step of the process (see Figure 1-8). Review the data to determine whether sufficient information was collected and whether the appropriate behaviors were identified. Nursing diagnoses and collaborative problems are evaluated for their accuracy and completeness. Examine the expected outcomes, indicators, and interventions to determine whether they were realistic, achievable, and effective.

The result of evaluation may be one or a combination of the following:

- The client responded as expected and the problem is resolved. No additional nursing actions are needed.
- Client behaviors indicate that the client's problem has not been resolved. Re-evaluation will continue.
- Client behaviors are similar to those present initially. Little or no evidence is available to show that the problem has been resolved. Reassessment and replanning are needed.
- Client behaviors indicate a new problem. Assessment, planning, and implementation of an additional plan of action are needed to resolve the problem.

In this text, NOC outcomes are listed under the Planning and Implementation and Evaluation: Outcomes sections.

Documentation

Documentation of each phase of the nursing process is essential and is accomplished by various means. Two general, traditional methods of documentation are still used in many health care settings: (1) source-oriented charting, which usually includes narrative notes that organize varied data and are entered into the medical record by health care professionals (e.g., nurses' notes, physicians' progress notes, dietary notes), and (2) the problem-oriented record (POR), in which a master health problem list is developed. Each problem is numbered, and all chart entries refer to one of the problems identified on the list. This system is used less often.

In the POR system, all health care professionals may record their notes in a SOAP, SOAPIER, or PIE format (or one of its many variations) and on the same progress note form in the chart. The initials represent **S**ubjective data, **O**bjective data, **A**nalysis, **P**lan of action, **I**nterventions, **E**valuation, and **R**evision of the plan. This technique of documentation is systematic and limits data to only pertinent information related to the identified problem. Although this system assists the nurse in addressing each step of the nursing process, it is very time consuming and promotes duplication of record keeping. Some physicians, social workers, and dietitians still use the SOAP format, but new systems for nursing documentation have been and are being developed.

DOCUMENTATION SYSTEMS

Focus Charting

A useful format in documentation is focus charting. Focus charting is not limited to specific client health problems but instead encourages nurses to document any significant changes in the client's condition, any client concern, or any significant client event. As seen in Figure 1-9, the record has three columns. The actual notes are divided into **D**ata, **A**ction, and **R**esponse information. An **E** may be added for documenting client **E**ducation. This technique helps locate desired information but still uses the familiar narrative approach to recording pertinent data.

Charting by Exception

Another system is charting by exception (CBE). CBE was started at St. Luke's Hospital in Milwaukee, Wisconsin, in an attempt to save nursing time. It incorporates three basic components (Burke & Murphy, 1988):

- Comprehensive flow sheets that list normal findings and require the nurse to initial them if they are present. If the findings are not present, the nurse writes an entry into the notes.
- References to preestablished nursing standards. The nurse initials the appropriate space when they are completed.

Date/Time	Focus/Problem	Notes
4/11/05 2:15 P.M.	Fever	D: T = 102.2° (R); face flushed; diaphoretic A: Give Tylenol 2 tab as ordered. Recheck temp. in 1 hr. *R. Jones, RN*
4/11/05 3:15 P.M.	Fever	R: T = 100.2° (R); face not flushed; not diaphoretic *D. Ignas, LPN*
4/12/05 3:30 A.M.	Impaired skin	D: 2-cm reddened area over coccyx; blanches A: Positioned on (L) side *N. Smith, RNC*

Figure 1-9 ■ A sample of focus charting.

- Bedside accessibility of forms. All flow sheets are kept at the bedside, which prevents wasting the nurse's time in looking for a client's chart. Bedside charting also prevents transcription of data from one form to another, which can lead to errors and wasted time. The information is available for any health care professional to read.

Many acute care facilities have a modified form of CBE and use a variety of flowsheets. Many agencies do not have bedside charting due to recent federal laws and regulations that protect the client's privacy.

Computerized Nursing Information Systems (NIS)

One major advantage of documentation systems such as CBE is the ability to transfer the concept to computerization. **Electronic charting**, also known as point-of-care charting and online documentation, is common in hospitals, nursing homes, home care agencies, and ambulatory care settings. The literature suggests that the major advantages of point-of-care documentation are accuracy and time savings. Electronic charting at the bedside also increases the time that the nurse spends in the client's room. The goal of any system should be to streamline or diminish paperwork and save valuable time, giving nurses more time for direct client care. Some health care facilities are adding NANDA diagnoses, NOC, and NIC to their documentation systems.

LEGAL ASPECTS OF DOCUMENTATION

Regardless of the type of documentation system used, remember that the client's chart is a legal document. Chart 1-4 lists basic charting guidelines that all nurses should follow. Further discussion of documentation can be found in basic fundamental nursing texts.

CHART 1-4

BEST PRACTICE for Nursing Documentation

- Write clearly and legibly.
- Do not erase or "white-out" any part of the client's record.
- To correct an error, use one line to cross out the incorrect entry, then initial the change.
- Use only standard and facility-approved abbreviations and symbols.
- Document significant information as close as possible to the time it is collected instead of waiting until the end of a shift.
- Transcribe physicians' orders carefully and correctly.
- If using nurses' notes or progress notes, do not leave blank spaces between entries.
- Time and date each entry on the client's record.
- Use only blue or black ink (it visualizes best for copies or microfilm).
- Document like a reporter: State facts objectively and avoid judgment or criticism.
- Do not state that "an incident report has been completed" or refer to any unusual occurrence or special event as an "incident."
- Follow all facility policies for documentation.
- To add one or two words, use a caret (^) and insert the words, then initial the change; if agency policy does not allow this practice, write a late entry.
- To make a late entry, begin by stating that it is a "Late entry for (date and time);" if the entry is more than a day late, state the reason for the late entry (e.g., "on vacation for 3 days").
- If an order is discontinued on the record as indicated by a highlighter, be sure that the original can still be read, especially on copies.

GET READY for the NCLEX Examination!

KEY POINTS

- Critical Thinking is purposeful, outcome-directed thinking involving judgment based on sound, scientific evidence.
- Evidence-based practice is the care that nurses should provide that is grounded in research and other sources of science.
- Health is a continuum from wellness to death; holistic health considers the interrelationship of the mind, body, and spirit.
- Health promotion and protection (illness prevention) refers to activities that the nurse and other health care professionals implement to maintain or enhance wellness.
- Healthy People 2010 is a set of goals for individuals in the United States to improve health for all.
- Three levels of illness prevention—primary, secondary, and tertiary—are available to help clients stay healthy or achieve optimal wellness (see Table 1-3).
- The medical-surgical nurse functions as a coordinator of care, caregiver, continuing care planner, educator, client advocate, and change agent.
- The teaching-learning process is affected by a person's educational level, age, socioeconomic level, support systems, and culture.
- The information in Chart 1-1 and Chart 1-2 summarizes the important points related to the adult learning process, including special needs of older adults.
- The steps of the nursing process are assessment, analysis (nursing diagnoses), planning Nursing Outcomes Classification), implementation (Nursing Interventions Classification), and evaluation. Gordon's Functional Health Patterns help to organize data collection during the client interview (see Table 1-4).
- Chart 1-4 summarizes important information regarding the legal aspects of clinical documentation.

ADDITIONAL STUDY RESOURCES

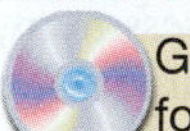

Go to your Student CD-ROM for Review Questions for the NCLEX Examination.

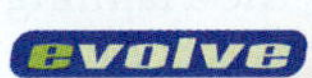

Go to http://evolve.elsevier.com/Iggy/ for Integrated Management of Care Questions for the NCLEX Examination.

SELECTED BIBLIOGRAPHY

Asterisk indicates a classic or definitive work on this subject.

Ackley, B.J., & Ladwig, G.B. (2002). *Nursing diagnosis handbook: A guide to planning care*. St. Louis: Mosby.

Alfaro-LeFevre, R. (2002). *Applying the nursing process: Promoting collaborative care*. Philadelphia: J.B. Lippincott.

Alfaro-LeFevre, R. (2003). *Critical thinking in nursing: A practical approach* (3rd ed.). Philadelphia: W.B. Saunders.

Alfaro-LeFevre, R. (2004). Critical thinking indicators: 2004 evidence-based version. www.alfaroteachsmart.com.

*Allen, K.M., & Phillips, J.M. (1997). *Women's health across the life-span: A comprehensive perspective.* Philadelphia: Lippincott-Raven.

*Aspinall, M.J., & Tanner, C. (1981). *Decision-making for patient care.* Norwalk, CT: Appleton & Lange.

*Barr, W.J., & Bush, H.A. (1998). Four factors of nurse caring in the ICU. *Dimensions of Critical Care Nursing, 17*(4), 214-223.

*Beck, C.T. (1999). Quantitative measurement of caring. *Journal of Advanced Nursing, 30*(1), 24-32.

*Benner, P., & Tanner, C. (1987). How expert nurses use intuition. *American Journal of Nursing, 87*, 23-31.

*Bower, F. (1972). The process of planning nursing care. St. Louis: Mosby.

*Burke, L.J., & Murphy, J. (1988). *Charting by exception: A cost-effective, quality approach.* New York: John Wiley & Sons.

*Carpenito, L.J. (1995). *Nursing care plans and documentation: Nursing diagnoses and collaborative problems.* Philadelphia: J.B. Lippincott.

*Cella, D.F. (1994). Quality of life: The concept and definition. *Journal of Pain and Symptom Management, 6*, 186-192.

Coyle, G.A., & Heinen, M. (2002). Scan your way to a comprehensive electronic record. *Nursing Management, 33*(12), 56-60.

*Davis, C.M., & Curley, C.M. (1999). Disparities of health in African Americans. *Nursing Clinics of North America, 34*(2), 345-355.

Dochterman, J.M., & Bulechek, G.M. (2004). *Nursing Interventions Classification (NIC)* (4th ed.). St. Louis: Mosby.

*Dunn, H.L. (1980). *High level wellness.* Thorofare, NJ: Charles B. Slack.

*Eggland, E.T. (1995). Charting smarter: Using new mechanisms to organize your paperwork. *Nursing95, 25*(9), 34-41.

*Facione, N.C., & Facione, P.A. (1996). Externalizing the critical thinking in knowledge development and clinical judgment. *Nursing Outlook, 44*(3), 129-136.

*Ferrell, B.R. (1996). The quality of lives: 1,525 voices of cancer. *Oncology Nursing Forum, 23*(6), 907-916.

*Flaskerud, J.H., & Kim, S. (1999). Health problems of Asian and Latino immigrants. *Nursing Clinics of North America, 34*(2), 359-380.

Gordon, M. (2002). *Manual of nursing diagnosis* (10th ed.). St. Louis: Mosby.

Ignatavicius, D.D. (2001). Six critical thinking skills for at-the-bedside success. *Nursing Management, 32*(1), 37-39.

Ignatavicius, D.D. (2004). From traditional care plans to innovative concept maps. In *Annual Review of Nursing Education.* New York: Springer.

Jarvis, C. (2004). Physical examination and health assessment (4th ed.). Philadelphia: W.B. Saunders.

Lew, P.S., & Latney. C. (2002). Achieve best practices with an evidence-based approach. *Nursing Management, 33*(12), 24-30.

McCloskey, J.C., & Bulechek, G.M. (2000). *Nursing interventions classification (NIC)* (3rd ed.). Philadelphia: W.B. Saunders.

Mohide, E.A., & King, B. (2003). Building a foundation for evidence-based practice: Experiences in a tertiary hospital. *Evidence-Based Nursing, 6*(4), 100-103.

Moorhead, S., Johnson, M., & Maas, M. (2004). *Nursing outcomes classification (NOC)* (3rd ed.). St. Louis: Mosby.

NANDA International (2003). *NANDA nursing diagnoses: Definitions and classification 2003-2004.* Philadelphia: Author.

Narayanasamy, A., & Owens, J. (2001). A critical incident study of nurses' responses to the spiritual needs of their patients. *Journal of Advanced Nursing, 33*(4), 446-455.

Nay, R. (2003). Evidence-based practice: Does it benefit older people and grerontic nursing? *Geriatric Nursing, 24*(6), 338-342.

*Pender, N.J. (1987). *Health promotion in nursing practice* (2nd ed.). Norwalk, CT: Appleton & Lange.

Thurmond, V.A. (2001). The holism in critical thinking. A concept analysis. *Journal of Holistic Nursing, 19*(4), 375-389.

Tuck, I., Wallace, D., & Pullen, L. (2001). Spirituality and spiritual care provided by parish nurses. *Western Journal of Nursing Research, 23*(5), 441-453.

U.S. Department of Health and Human Services, Public Health Service. (2000). *Healthy People 2010: National health promotion and disease prevention objectives.* Washington, DC: U.S. Government Printing Office.

Wilkinson, J.M. (2000). Nursing diagnosis handbook with NIC interventions and NOC outcomes (7th ed.). Upper Saddle River, NJ: Prentice Hall Health.

*World Health Organization. (1947). *Constitution of the World Health Organization: Chronicle of the World Health Organization.* Geneva: Author.

Young, K.M. (2003). Where's the evidence? *American Journal of Nursing, 103*(10), 11.

CHAPTER

2

Community-Based Care

DONNA D. IGNATAVICIUS

LEARNING OUTCOMES

After studying this chapter, you should be able to:

1. Explain the primary purpose of ambulatory care.
2. Identify the unique features of nursing primary care.
3. Discuss the growth of home care in the United States.
4. Describe the role of the nurse in home care.
5. Identify interventions for which Medicare typically pays in home care.
6. State the purpose of OASIS in home care.
7. Compare and contrast the common types of long-term care settings.
8. Differentiate assisted-living from other types of long-term care.
9. Describe the term *transitional care.*

Go to your Student CD-ROM for Review Questions for the NCLEX Examination keyed to these Learning Outcomes.

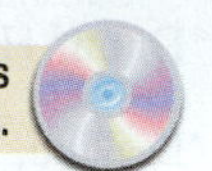

Care for medical-surgical clients can be provided in a number of settings. Community-based care may be needed after a hospital stay or as an alternative to inpatient hospital care. The current trend is toward care in alternative settings, such as ambulatory care, home care, and long-term care in rehabilitation centers, nursing homes, and chronic care facilities. This chapter provides a brief description of each of these settings, which provide varying opportunities for nursing employment.

This text covers care for clients in numerous settings in which medical-surgical nurses practice. The Community-Based Care sections that follow the discussions of major health problems highlight the most important aspects of care in nonhospital environments.

AMBULATORY CARE

Ambulatory health care is a general term for client care provided in a number of community settings, such as physician offices, hospital or freestanding outpatient clinics, freestanding surgicenters, and health maintenance organizations (a type of managed-care organization) (see Chapter 3). The purpose of ambulatory care is health promotion, health protection (illness prevention), short-term treatment (e.g., surgery), and follow-up for existing health problems.

Client visits to ambulatory care settings are episodic and based on need. For example, clients may visit their health care provider for annual physical examinations (health promotion). In some cases, they seek out providers for acute health care problems, chemotherapy, or selected surgeries, such as cataract removal or laparoscopic cholecystectomy (removal of the gallbladder). Still others are monitored periodically for chronic health conditions such as diabetes mellitus and hypertension.

Clients discharged from the hospital are often followed in one or more ambulatory care settings. Many health care providers in these settings are advanced practice nurses (APNs), such as nurse practitioners and clinical nurse specialists. The cost of ambulatory care is typically far less than that of a long-term or home care agency.

Role of the Nurse in Ambulatory Care

One of the major roles of the nurse working in an ambulatory care setting is performing health promotion activities, including client education, health screening, and comprehensive assessment. In a surgicenter, for example, the nurse provides preoperative teaching to prepare clients for the surgical procedure and postoperative expectations. Their vital signs and general condition are assessed to ensure that they are ready for the surgery.

Many physicians employ nurses to assist in their office practice. These nurses often triage clients by telephone; that is, they decide which clients need priority care and intervene accordingly. In some parts of the country, large physician practices employ nurse case managers who monitor high-risk, high-cost, problem-prone clients throughout the continuum of health care in all settings. Some may also participate in **telephonic case management**. In this case, the nurse provides information to help the client receive care in the appropriate setting. Case management is discussed in Chapter 3.

Nursing Primary Care

Nursing primary care takes place in ambulatory care settings, sometimes called community centers. Health care is provided by nurses, often in underserved areas of the country. Although the organizational structure and services provided vary among centers, most of them are affiliated with large university schools of nursing. The primary health care providers are typically nurse practitioners, nurse midwives, clinical nurse specialists, and students preparing to become one of these advanced practice specialists. The funding for nursing primary care varies. Some funding comes from city, state, and federal governments, whereas other funding comes from grants obtained by university faculty.

HOME CARE

Home care in the United States and other countries is a diverse industry. For many clients the home not only is the preferred health care setting but is also the lowest cost setting. **Home care** is part of a continuum of comprehensive health care in which health services are provided to individuals and families in their place of residence. The goal is to promote, maintain, or restore health or to maximize the level of independence while minimizing the effects of disability and illness, including terminal illness (Marrelli & Krulish, 1999).

Historical Perspective and Trends in Home Care Nursing

Modern home care nursing has its roots in public health and community health nursing models. In the mid-1880s, visiting nurse associations (VNAs) evolved in Philadelphia, Boston, and Buffalo, New York. The traditions of Lillian Wald, who is regarded as the founder of public health nursing, began with the Henry Street Settlement in New York City in 1893. During the early twentieth century, most of the home care in the United States was provided by VNAs and the nursing divisions of governmental health agencies. Public health principles and practices, as well as components of family and community care, were integrated into home health nursing services. Nurses provided health promotion services to individuals, families, and communities while continuing to provide nursing care to the sick.

Many factors have contributed to the acceptance of home care, including the following:

- A continued shift from inpatient-based care to community-based care and home care, including palliative care (care of dying clients)
- Increased acceptance by the medical community and the consumer community that home care is often a viable alternative to institutional care
- Baby boomers who, as they get older, are becoming more educated about health care alternatives and are becoming more involved in the decision-making process
- An aging population that has increased the need for health care for older adults
- Technology such as mobile x-ray machines, apnea monitors, and electrocardiographs, which allow clients to remain safely at home while having their health needs monitored; the introduction of telehealthcare services allows even more ways for clients to be monitored from their home (Kinsella, 2003)
- The generally lower cost of home care (compared to institutional care)
- The increase in managed care, which dictates a lower cost care environment

Although there has been significant growth in home care since the 1960s, the number of Medicare-certified agencies has decreased. The National Association for Home Care (NAHC) believes this recent decline to be the direct result of changes in Medicare home care reimbursement, which is now based on a prospective payment system. The amount of reimbursement using this method has declined to the point that some home care agencies have closed.

Types of Home Care

The term *home care* is used to describe a variety of products and services. There are different specialty areas within the home care industry, and nurses may work in any one of these areas. Some companies may provide all or just one of these home care services. There are generally four types of services provided by the home care industry:

1. *Skilled home care service.* This is the largest type of service, with these agencies employing most of the home care nurses and other health care professionals to provide care as needed. Skilled home care services are provided by home care organizations that are usually Medicare certified and provide two or more of the following services:
   - Nursing (RN and LPN)
   - Physical therapy (LPT, LPTA)
   - Occupational therapy (OTR, COTA)
   - Speech/language pathology
   - Social services (MSW, BSW)
   - Home care aides

   The organization may also provide respiratory therapy and other specialty services (e.g., enterostomal therapy, behavioral health nursing), depending on the specialty programs of the organization. In general, Medicare, Medicaid, and other insurance or managed care programs cover these skilled services when the qualifying criteria of the insurance program are met.
2. *Personal care or private duty service.* This type of service may provide "shifts" of nurses or home care aides to clients in their homes. It may also provide additional services such as homemaker services, transportation, respite for caregivers, meal preparation, and sitter services. Some insurance programs may pay for a limited amount of these services related to health care, but most of them are paid privately by the client or family.
3. *Home medical equipment (HME) service.* This service can also include durable medical equipment (DME). HME companies provide hospital beds, wheelchairs, bath benches, oxygen and related equipment and services, walkers, and other equipment. In general, Medicare and other insurance or managed care programs pay for HME when the qualifying criteria of the insurance program are met.
4. *Home infusion or intravenous service.* Companies providing this type of service have pharmacists that mix the infusion therapies. The company then delivers the infusion, sets it up in the home, trains the client/family on proper administration, and sometimes administers the infusion therapies. Therapies can be enteral or parenteral and can include tube feedings, antibiotics, hyperalimentation, blood and blood products, tocolytic therapy, antineoplastics,

opioid analgesics, and catecholamines. Nursing services for activities such as observation and assessment, therapy administration, site care, and line maintenance may be covered by Medicare and other insurance or managed care programs. The therapies may or may not be covered by the insurance or managed care program depending on the coverage criteria of the specific insurance program.

Role of the Nurse in Home Care

Despite all that is changing in the home care environment, one thing has remained the same: nursing is an essential component. A knowledgeable and experienced nurse is able to draw on existing resources and to "create" resources through the use of family and community support systems. This knowledge and experience, coupled with the fact that nursing is an essential component of home care, makes it possible for nurses to direct and manage home care effectively. Nurses can continue to support client advocacy by promoting nursing's unique contribution to the care of the client and caregivers.

Home care has come to mean a variety of specialized and generalized nursing care provided to clients whose primary site for health care is their home. Adult health (medical-surgical) care, child (pediatric) care, perinatal care, older adult (geriatric) care, behavioral health care, and many other specialties are practiced routinely by home care nurses. Effective home care nursing incorporates the aspects of comprehensive assessment skills with current technology and the "high-touch" care of skilled nurses. Home care *case management* uses the client care plan in conjunction with effective care coordination and ongoing communication to ensure that the client is receiving appropriate care. Collaborative communication among team members and active and ongoing client participation ensures that clients are truly equal partners in their health care. Table 2-1 compares nursing in the home care setting to nursing in the inpatient setting.

Home Visits

Home care provided by private duty or personal care companies is often rendered in "hours" or "shifts" of service delivery. In general, intermittent home care is provided in "visits" by Medicare-certified agencies. The actual visit time is the time spent in the client's home for the provision of the ordered care. The length of the visit depends on the complexity of the care being provided, the type of visit (e.g., the admission visit is typically longer because of the increased amount of data being collected and documented), how well the client tolerates the care, and how efficient the nurse is in providing the care. Although the actual visit time is the time spent in the client's home, several components go into effective visit provision:

- Visit preparation, including phone calls to the physician to clarify orders
- Phone calls to other providers involved in the client's care to coordinate care delivery
- Gathering of required documentation and supplies (wound dressings, catheter, venipuncture)
- Phone calls to insurance companies for visit authorization or care delivery updates
- Travel time to the client's home
- Completion of all necessary documentation
- Further care coordination with the physician and/or other members of the health care team

The number of visits nurses are expected to make per day varies from agency to agency. The average is four to six visits per day. The range depends on the geographic location of the clients, the complexity of the care being rendered, the type of visits, and other factors such as weather. Inclement weather poses another challenge to home care staff. Many staff use four-wheel drive vehicles, boats, and other alternate means of transportation. In areas of extremely heavy snowfall, nurses have even been known to use skis, snowmobiles, or snowshoes to ensure that they can reach their clients. Staff assignments are generally based on the geographic location of the client, the client diagnosis, and/or the service to be delivered (e.g., infusion services, cardiac services, rehabilitative services).

Client Plan of Care

As with other care settings, a physician's order is needed for care interventions and care plan changes. Because home care nursing practice is more autonomous than many inpatient settings, it is imperative that orders be obtained from physicians for care and care changes. Sometimes the physician does not see the client for months and therefore relies on the nurse's assessments and reports to assist with devel-

TABLE 2-1 Major Differences Between Nursing Care in the Home and in Inpatient Settings

Home Setting	Inpatient Setting
Nurse is more autonomous and is many times the "eyes and ears" of the physician.	Nurse relies heavily on physician directives.
Environment is controlled by the client/caregiver. Circumstances are often less than optimal for the provision of skilled care.	Environment is controlled by the facility and its staff.
Nurse must be knowledgeable about the care of all types and ages of clients.	Nurse is typically knowledgeable about the care of specific types of clients, often based on diagnosis.
Nurse must know and understand various reimbursement requirements and document accordingly.	Financial officer and accounting department usually handle reimbursement.
For older adults, only selected skilled and nonskilled services are reimbursed by Medicare.	For older adults, hospital care is largely reimbursed by Medicare.
There is limited direct supervision of assistive staff, such as home care aides.	There is continuous direct supervision of assistive staff. Nurse and staff work as a single unit.

opment and revision of the care plan. Verbal and telephone orders are a large part of the home care practice and communication with physicians. For Medicare clients, agencies generally use the Form 485 from the Centers for Medicare and Medicaid Services as the client plan of care (Figure 2-1). This plan of care is developed with input from the client/caregiver, physician, and other members of the health care team. The plan of care must be signed by the physician before the agency bills for the services rendered under the plan of care.

Medicare usually pays for home care services when the beneficiary meets one or more of certain qualifying conditions:

- The client is confined to the home.
- Services are provided under a plan of care established and approved by a physician.
- The client is under the care of a physician.
- The client needs skilled nursing care on an intermittent basis or needs physical therapy or speech-language pathology services.
- The client has a continued need for occupational therapy services.

Once client eligibility has been established, Medicare usually pays for any or all of the following skilled nursing services:

- Observation and assessment of the client's condition when only the specialized skills of a medical professional can determine a client's status
- Management and evaluation of a client care plan
- Teaching and training activities
- Administration of medications and IV fluids
- Nasopharyngeal and tracheostomy suctioning
- Urinary catheters
- Wound care

Department of Health and Human Services
Health Care Financing Administration

Form Approved
OMB No. 0938-0357

HOME HEALTH CERTIFICATION AND PLAN OF CARE

1. Patient's HI Claim No.	2. Start Of Care Date	3. Certification Period From: To:	4. Medical Record No.	5. Provider No.

6. Patient's Name and Address	7. Provider's Name, Address and Telephone Number
8. Date of Birth 9. Sex ☐ M ☐ F	10. Medications: Dose/Frequency/Route (N)ew (C)hanged
11. ICD-9-CM Principal Diagnosis Date	
12. ICD-9-CM Surgical Procedure Date	
13. ICD-9-CM Other Pertinent Diagnoses Date	
14. DME and Supplies	15. Safety Measures:
16. Nutritional Req.	17. Allergies:

18.A. Functional Limitations

1 ☐ Amputation
2 ☐ Bowel/Bladder (Incontinence)
3 ☐ Contracture
4 ☐ Hearing
5 ☐ Paralysis
6 ☐ Endurance
7 ☐ Ambulation
8 ☐ Speech
9 ☐ Legally Blind
A ☐ Dyspnea With Minimal Exertion
B ☐ Other (Specify)

18.B. Activities Permitted

1 ☐ Complete Bedrest
2 ☐ Bedrest BRP
3 ☐ Up As Tolerated
4 ☐ Transfer Bed/Chair
5 ☐ Exercises Prescribed
6 ☐ Partial Weight Bearing
7 ☐ Independent At Home
8 ☐ Crutches
9 ☐ Cane
A ☐ Wheelchair
B ☐ Walker
C ☐ No Restrictions
D ☐ Other (Specify)

19. Mental Status: 1 ☐ Oriented 2 ☐ Comatose 3 ☐ Forgetful 4 ☐ Depressed 5 ☐ Disoriented 6 ☐ Lethargic 7 ☐ Agitated 8 ☐ Other

20. Prognosis: 1 ☐ Poor 2 ☐ Guarded 3 ☐ Fair 4 ☐ Good 5 ☐ Excellent

21. Orders for Discipline and Treatments (Specify Amount/Frequency/Duration)

22. Goals/Rehabilitation Potential/Discharge Plans

23. Nurse's Signature and Date of Verbal SOC Where Applicable:	25. Date HHA Received Signed POT
24. Physician's Name and Address	26. I certify/recertify that this patient is confined to his/her home and needs intermittent skilled nursing care, physical therapy and/or speech therapy or continues to need occupational therapy. The patient is under my care, and I have authorized the services on this plan of care and will periodically review the plan.
27. Attending Physician's Signature and Date Signed	28. Anyone who misrepresents, falsifies, or conceals essential information required for payment of Federal funds may be subject to fine, imprisonment, or civil penalty under applicable Federal laws.

Figure 2-1 ■ Centers for Medicare and Medicaid Services Form 485.

- Ostomy care
- Rehabilitation nursing
- Psychiatric evaluation, therapy, and teaching

Medicare principles governing reasonable and necessary skilled nursing services include the following (Health Care Financing Administration [HCFA], 1996):

- A skilled nursing service is a service that must be provided by a registered nurse (or a licensed practical [vocational] nurse under the supervision of a registered nurse) to be safe and effective.
- A service is not considered a skilled nursing service merely because it is performed by or under the direct supervision of a licensed nurse. A service is not considered a skilled nursing service if it can be performed safely and effectively by the average nonmedical person (or self-administered) without direct nursing supervision.
- If a service requires the skills of a licensed nurse to be provided safely and effectively, it continues to be a skilled service even if it is taught to the client/caregiver.
- The skilled nursing service must be reasonable and necessary to the diagnosis and treatment of the client's illness or injury within the context of the client's unique medical condition.

Documentation and Home Care

Reimbursement for home care relies heavily on the documentation of care. In many home care and other community-based settings, the research-based **Omaha Problem Classification System** may be used instead of the nursing diagnoses from the North American Nursing Diagnosis Association. The Omaha system delineates four general areas that represent community and home care practice and provide organizational groupings for client problems: environmental, psychosocial, physiologic, and health-related behaviors. More than 40 nursing diagnoses with modifiers such as potential deficit, deficit, and health promotion are then listed within their appropriate domains (Barrera, 2003).

Computerization and Home Care

To facilitate the documentation and communication processes, home care agencies have implemented automation. Most agencies have computerized Form 485 (Plan of Care) from the Centers for Medicare and Medicaid Services, and many agencies have implemented an electronic clinical documentation system for their client care staff. Several software products are on the market and use a variety of hardware products, from the handheld to the personal computer. For agencies that have implemented an electronic clinical documentation system, nurses carry a handheld, laptop, or other computer into the clients' homes to document their assessment findings and care delivery. This information is then transmitted to the main agency server.

One advantage of computerization is immediate access to the information by office personnel or other members of the health care team once the nurse has transmitted it to the agency. Another advantage is that the nurse can readily access client medical record information, day or night, without coming into the office. This allows more flexibility in scheduling the day. Many software programs also reduce the amount of times the information must be entered (or written if documentation is done by hand) because it flows to all appropriate locations within the documentation system. Computer literacy is becoming a requirement for nursing practice in many settings, and home care is no exception.

Telehealth and Home Care

A growing trend in home care is the use of telehealth. **Telehealth** can be defined as the "electronic provision of health care and information services for the direct benefit of individual [clients] and their families" (Russo, 2001, p. 3). This technology includes nurse-client and nurse-provider interactions, as well as education and information for nurses and clients. One of the many benefits to telehealth is increased client participation in his or her care.

Examples of technology devices include interactive video systems, monitoring technology using plain old telephones (POTs), and digital subscriber lines and the Internet. The client can contact an on-call nurse any time and set up a video visit to address the problem. Another use of the technology is nursing case management. Nurses can triage clients and prioritize which clients need attention first. The health status of the client can also be monitored. Photos of wounds, for example, allow the nurse an opportunity to track the progress of wound healing (Russo, 2001).

Outcomes and Home Care

In January 1999, new regulations were put into place that require Medicare-certified home care agencies to track and report client outcomes. The research-based tool for outcome tracking is called the **O**utcome and **AS**sessment **I**nformation **S**et (OASIS). These outcome measures are the crux of Outcome Based Quality Improvement (OBQI), a systematic approach that home care agencies can implement and follow for continuous improvement of quality of care.

Before OASIS, there was no uniform data set that agencies could use to track their own outcomes and, perhaps more important, to compare themselves to similar agencies across the United States. In a sense, the OASIS serves as a "report card" for the performance of the home care agency (Wardell, 2003).

LONG-TERM CARE

In clinical practice, long-term care (LTC) has become synonymous with nursing home care, although many clients do not stay for an extended period of time in a nursing home, and not all LTC clients are in nursing homes. Long-term care for adult clients with medical-surgical problems can occur either in the home or in facilities such as nursing homes, transitional care units, chronic care facilities, or rehabilitation centers. In general, **long-term care** implies that clients receive care for a prolonged period of time, usually weeks or months. A small percentage of clients may remain in a facility indefinitely, perhaps a lifetime. The nursing home is the most common type of LTC setting.

Common Types of Long-Term Care Settings

Long-term care settings can be divided into residential (e.g., assisted-living) facilities, nursing homes, and chronic care/extended care facilities. Some are part of retirement communities, and others have specialty units, such as dementia, ventilator, or transitional care/subacute units.

RESIDENTIAL FACILITIES

The most common type of **residential facilities** include assisted-living facilities and group homes. Some of these facilities are small and much like boarding homes before the advent of Medicare (Ignatavicius, 1998). Others are large communities managed by national corporations. Many of the larger complexes are life care or continuing care retirement centers that offer a continuum of services, from independent living to skilled care. The typical resident in a residential facility is fairly independent and is able to perform most or all self-care activities. Employees in these facilities are usually unlicensed staff, although a licensed nurse may be available during the day.

Assisted-living facilities (ALFs) are nonmedical facilities that have grown rapidly over the past 5 years in response to an expanding older adult population. Assisted-living facilities vary somewhat in their requirements for resident function, depending on available services and resources. Some states regulate these facilities as they do nursing homes because sicker and more dependent residents are being accepted.

NURSING HOMES

Nursing home care can be expensive, with annual costs between $30,000 and $45,000 in the United States. Most facilities are profit-making, proprietary organizations. As the proportion of older adults increases from 13% of the population in 2000 to 20% by 2030, the implication for increasing health care expenditures is profound. Older adults use health care services at a far greater rate than do younger adults.

Nursing homes in the United States provide care for clients with physical and cognitive impairments or chronic illness. Clients admitted to a nursing home are called **residents** because the facility is considered their home. The majority of residents are women older than 65 years of age. However, nursing homes are experiencing an increase in the number of younger residents as individuals live longer with debilitating chronic illnesses such as multiple sclerosis and traumatic brain injury (TBI).

Nursing homes have undergone another major change. Most Medicare-certified facilities are increasingly admitting short-term (less than 1 week to 2 weeks) residents for rehabilitation or recovery from an illness or injury and then discharging them to home or another setting. Clients come from hospitals "quicker and sicker," and they often require complex or continuing care. Examples of common health problems that require short-term care in a nursing home include rehabilitation for total joint replacements, serious fractures, and strokes, and continued postoperative care following major surgeries such as a coronary artery bypass graft (CABG).

Nursing homes may provide intermediate or skilled care, or a combination of these levels. Formerly called intermediate care facilities, **nursing facilities (NFs)** provide a custodial, maintenance level of care. Certified, licensed NFs receive Medicaid funding for the care of residents who cannot perform activities of daily living (ADLs) independently. Each state has specific guidelines for reimbursement.

Skilled nursing facilities (SNFs, pronounced "snifs") provide care that requires licensed health care professionals, such as nurses and therapists. Only a small portion of most nursing home residents are categorized as skilled and are therefore eligible for Medicare reimbursement. Examples of skilled care include new tube feedings, daily rehabilitative care for postoperative fractured hips, and care of stage 3 and stage 4 wounds.

Chronic or extended care facilities provide care for long-term, chronically ill clients, such those with severe head injuries or those who need chronic ventilator support. These facilities are often managed by county or state governments.

Role of the Nurse in Long-Term Care

Before 1965, LTC settings were not carefully monitored by external agencies. Poor sanitation, resident abuse, and inadequate care were common in the nursing home industry. Since 1965, nursing homes and other LTC facilities have been carefully scrutinized and highly regulated by both federal and state agencies. Nurses who work in these facilities must be aware of these laws, which are meant to protect both the residents and the staff.

In general, nurses employed in LTC facilities are more autonomous than nurses working in hospitals. Health care providers are usually not present in the LTC facility on a continuous basis, because residents in these facilities are considered to be more medically "stable" than those in acute care. With early discharge from acute care, however, LTC nurses are caring for sicker residents than in the past and therefore need increased skills and knowledge to manage them.

For the past 15 years, geriatric nursing research has helped validate best practice patterns for nurses who care for older adults in a variety of settings. Most notable is the work led by the John A. Hartford Institute for the Advancement of Geriatric Nursing Practice in New York City. Some of the areas studied include pain management, the use of physical restraints, fall prevention, and medication safety (Mezey, Fulmer, & Abraham, 2003) (Table 2-2).

Most nurses in LTC are placed "in charge" of a unit or shift because there are more unlicensed personnel (certified nursing assistants) than professional nurses. Therefore the LTC nurse needs leadership, management, and clinical competencies to function in this interdisciplinary care environment. There may be only one nurse in charge of 30 to 40 residents and a number of certified nursing assistants.

Documentation in Long-Term Care

Documentation in most LTC settings is highly regulated by both federal and state governments. The Minimum Data Set (MDS), for example, is a federally mandated assessment

TABLE 2-2 Examples of Geriatric Nursing Protocols for Best Practice

- Assessment of Function
- Mealtime Difficulties
- Urinary Incontinence
- Assessment of Cognitive Function
- Delirium
- Preventing Falls
- Depression
- Pain Management
- Physical Restraints
- Advance Directives

Data from Mezey, M.D., Fulmer, T., & Abraham, I. (2003). *Geriatric nursing protocols for best practice,* (2nd ed.). New York: Springer.

form that is completed for all nursing home residents regardless of the level of care or reimbursement system. This document is an interdisciplinary tool completed by each member of the health care team.

The team develops an interdisciplinary care plan for all actual or potential resident problems. Depending on the resident's level of care, this plan is updated every 30 to 60 days, or more often as the resident's condition changes.

TRANSITIONAL CARE

Transitional care units (TCU) or **subacute care units (SAC units)** are designed for clients who are too ill to be discharged from the hospital to a traditional nursing home or the client's own home. These units "fill the gap" between the hospital and the traditional long-term care (LTC) facility. Most units are located in hospital settings and provide a skilled level of care.

Little has been published about the role of the nurse in transitional or subacute care. The ratio of licensed to unlicensed staff is usually better than that in traditional homes. Nurses who work in these settings must be knowledgeable about LTC and have medical-surgical, critical care, or rehabilitation skills depending on the type of unit in which they work. Nurses work closely with rehabilitation therapists to help residents meet functional outcomes. Restorative nursing aides may assist the resident in returning to an optimal level of ADL functioning.

REHABILITATIVE CARE

Rehabilitation is designed for clients who have experienced an acute injury or illness or for those who are coping with chronic conditions. Rehabilitation services may be provided in the home setting, nursing home, or rehabilitation unit or center. Chapter 10 discusses in detail the rehabilitation of individuals with chronic or disabling health problems.

GET READY for the NCLEX Examination!

KEY POINTS

- The purpose of ambulatory care is health promotion, health protection (illness prevention), and short-term treatment or follow-up for selected health problems.
- The primary role of the nurse in ambulatory care is client education and assessment.
- Nursing primary care is provided by advanced practice nurses to promote health and prevent illness, especially in underserved areas of the United States.
- Home care has expanded to care for clients who require skilled health care professional services. Examples of skilled nursing services are administering intravenous therapy and medications, assessing and teaching, and providing selected treatments.
- Telehealth is a growing trend in home health care to more easily monitor and assess clients in the home environment.
- The purpose of OASIS is to track clinical outcomes in home health care.
- Long-term care is a general term that includes care in residential facilities, nursing homes, and chronic/extended care settings.
- Assisted-living facilities are nonmedical settings that have grown rapidly in response to an expanding older adult population. Licensed and/or unlicensed staff may be available as needed.
- Transitional care units are designed to "fill the gap" between acute care and traditional long-term care.

ADDITIONAL STUDY RESOURCES

Go to your Student CD-ROM for Review Questions for the NCLEX Examination.

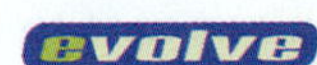

Go to http://evolve.elsevier.com/Iggy/ for Integrated Management of Care Questions for the NCLEX Examination.

SELECTED BIBLIOGRAPHY

Asterisk indicates a classic or definitive work on this subject.

*Abraham, I., et al. (1999). *Geriatric nursing protocols for best practice.* New York: Springer.

*Anderson, A. (1996). Nursing clinics in urban settings. *Home Healthcare Nurse, 14,* 542-546.

Barrera, C., et al. (2003). Nursing care makes a difference: Application of the Omaha System. *Outcomes Management, 7*(4), 181-185.

*Bohny, B.J. (1997). A time for self-care: Role of the home healthcare nurse. *Home Healthcare Nurse, 15*(4), 281-286.

*Boroughs, D.S. (1999). Documentation in the long-term care setting. *Journal of Nursing Administration, 29*(12), 46-49.

*Catanzaro, J., & Serembus, J.F. (1998). High-tech wound and ostomy care in the home setting. *Critical Care Nursing Clinics of North America, 10*(3), 327-338.

Chetney, R. (2003). Home care's challenge: Move the information…not the patient. *Home Healthcare Nurse, 21*(10), 712.

*Congdon, J.G., & Magilvy, J.K. (1998). Rural nursing homes: A housing option for older adults. *Geriatric Nursing, 19*(3), 157-159.

Fermazin, M., et al. (2003). Nursing home compare: Web site offers critical information to consumers, professionals. *Lippincott's Case Management: Managing the Process of Patient Care, 8*(4), 175-183.

*Hammer, R.M. (1999). The lived experience of being at home: A phenomenological investigation. *Journal of Gerontological Nursing, 25*(11), 10-18.

*Health Care Financing Administration. (1996). *Home health agency manual.* Baltimore: Author.

*Health Care Financing Administration. (1998). *OASIS user's manual.* Baltimore: Author.

*Ignatavicius, D.D. (1998). *Introduction to long term care nursing: Principles and practice.* Philadelphia: F.A. Davis.

*Jones, A.M., & Foster, N. (1997). Transitional care: Bridging the gap. *MEDSURG Nursing, 6*(1), 32-38.

*Kinsella, A. (1998). Home telehealthcare services: Their role on home care today. *Home Care Management, 2*(5), 17-22.

Kinsella, A. (2003). Telehealth opportunities for home care patients. *Home Healthcare Nurse, 21*(10), 661-665.

*Marrelli, T., & Krulish, L. (1999). *Home care therapy: Quality, documentation, and reimbursement.* Boca Grande, FL: Marrelli and Associates.

*Martin, K.S., & Scheet, N.J. (1992). *The Omaha system: Applications for community health nursing.* Philadelphia: W.B. Saunders.

*McNeal, G.J. (1998). Care of the critically ill at home. *Critical Care Nursing Clinics of North America, 10*(3), 267-278.

Mezey, M.D., Fulmer, T., & Abraham, I. (2003). *Geriatric nursing protocols for best practice,* (2nd ed.). New York: Springer.

Milone-Nuzzo, P. (2003). Clinical nurse specialists in home care. *Clinical Nurse Specialist, 17*(5), 234-235.

Mitty, E.L. (2003). Policy perspectives: Assisted living and the role of nursing. *American Journal of Nursing, 103*(8), 32-43.

*National Association for Home Care. (1999). *Basic statistics about home care.* Washington, DC: Author.

Russo, H. (2001). Window of opportunity for home care nurses: Telehealth technologies. *Online Journal of Issues in Nursing, 6*(3), 1-10.

Spillman, B.C., & Lubitz, J. (2000). The effect of longevity on spending for acute and long-term care. *New England Journal of Medicine, 342*(19), 1409-1415.

Tappen, R.M., Hall, R.F., & Folden, S.L. (2001). Impact of comprehensive nurse-managed transitional care. *Clinical Nursing Research, 10*(3), 295-313.

*Vaca, K.J., Vaca, B.L., & Daake, C.J. (1998). Review of nursing home regulations. *MEDSURG Nursing, 7*(3), 165-171.

Wallace, M. (2003). Is there a nurse in the house? The role of nurses in assisted living: Past, present, and future. *Geriatric Nursing, 24*(4), 218-221, 235.

Wardell, R.C. (2003). When OASIS becomes our report card. *Home Healthcare Nurse, 21*(6), 415.

CHAPTER 3

Introduction to Managed Care and Case Management

DONNA D. IGNATAVICIUS • SUZANNE K. POWELL

LEARNING OUTCOMES

After studying this chapter, you should be able to:

1. Explain the primary purpose of managed health care, including factors that drive concerns about cost and quality.
2. Contrast the fee-for-service and capitated reimbursement systems for health care.
3. Compare the health maintenance organization (HMO) with the preferred provider organization (PPO).
4. Delineate the overall goals of case management.
5. Explain the role of case management based on national standards.
6. Identify at least three certifications for case managers.
7. Clarify the differences and similarities between case management and disease management.

Go to your Student CD-ROM for Review Questions for the NCLEX Examination keyed to these Learning Outcomes.

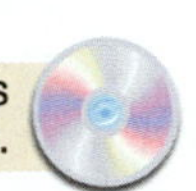

The cost of health care in the United States has dramatically increased over the past 20 years and now accounts for about 15% of the gross national product (GNP). As a result, insurance companies and health care providers have reexamined how health care is paid and how client care is managed. Managed health care has evolved to consider both the quality and the cost of care.

Today managed care has grown to be the largest provider for health care in the United States. **Managed health care** is a system that attempts to control costs by using a select group of providers who have agreed to a set payment *before* delivering care. In this system, client care is outcome driven and is managed by a utilization and/or a case management process. Nurses have many roles in case management and disease management. They work in these roles as they focus on achieving client outcomes while maintaining costs.

There are several factors currently driving concerns about cost and quality in the health care system. These factors include the following (Greenberg, 2003):

- **Aging, chronically ill population:** A large number of Americans are now reaching middle age, bringing chronic illness and higher use of health care services. Availability of new health care technologies and medications, as well as an aging and well-informed population, is driving increased costs in health care.
- **Purchaser pressure to contain costs:** The prices of health care premiums are increasing rapidly. In an effort to manage costs, public and private purchasers are seeking ways to shift the financial burden.
- **Physician and consumer resistance to "tight" management and referral control:** Open access models of health care, such as Preferred Provider Organizations (PPOs), now have the greatest volume of enrollees. Many health care companies no longer rely on utilization management and referral control to manage costs. Financial incentives, personalized care management, and "consumer directed" health care are now used by payers who are attempting to manage care and manage costs.
- **Renewed emphasis on evidence-based practice:** The emergence of disease management reflects a growing trend to align medical practices with evidence-based practice. Health care organizations are seeking to ensure that clients with health care needs are promptly identified and provided with the clinical interventions and resources needed to most effectively manage their illnesses while maintaining health.

MANAGED CARE

The managed care system is very different from the traditional way of paying for health care. Before the managed care movement, hospitals, physicians, and other health care providers were paid by health insurance companies on the basis of what the providers billed for their services. Under this **fee-for-service** arrangement, two physicians could perform identical services but could bill at their own rates. For example, one physician might bill $3000 for a surgical procedure, whereas another might bill $1800 for the same service. Under this fee-for-service system, the financial risk was largely taken by the insurance companies.

Purpose of Managed Care

Managed care organizations (MCOs) standardize and control costs. Under the managed care payment system, health care providers receive a uniform amount of money for each client; this is referred to as a **capitated reimbursement system** (Table 3-1). Unlike the traditional fee-for-service arrangement, the MCO and the providers share the financial risks.

Balancing cost with quality is an important concept for managed care. Health care providers have been concerned that some MCOs may be too focused on saving money rather than on providing high-quality client care (Powell, 2000a). The National Committee for Quality Assurance (NCQA) reviews and accredits MCOs that demonstrate high-quality care.

As discussed in Chapter 1, an important role for the nurse is to advocate for clients to ensure that they receive the necessary and appropriate care. As client advocates, care coordinators, and consumers, nurses need to know about managed care and the need for collaborative management of client care.

Role of Advanced Practice Nurses

Advanced practice nurses, such as nurse practitioners, certified nurse midwives, and clinical nurse specialists, have become more predominant health care providers in the managed care environment because they can deliver more cost-effective health care. In addition, they work from a wellness model, with a focus on empowering clients to stay well and care for themselves. As a result of the increased demand for and success of these advanced practice roles, many schools of nursing are offering new or additional graduate programs.

TABLE 3-1 Glossary of Terms Related to Managed Care and Case Management

authorization The process used by managed health care organizations to grant services for a specified period for reimbursement of specific services

capitation A managed care reimbursement arrangement that prepays the physician or other health care provider a set dollar amount on a per-member, per-month basis for the delivery of services to a specified group of members

deductible The amount of money that an insured person must pay toward health care costs before the insurance company begins reimbursement for health care

disease management A systems-based approach to caring for clients, usually those with high risk or chronic conditions, using standardized treatment strategies that ensure appropriate utilization and high-quality care across the continuum of health care

fee-for-service A reimbursement arrangement in which health care services are paid for as billed by the provider

indemnity An arrangement in which benefits are paid in a predetermined amount in the event of a covered loss

integrated delivery system (IDS) (also know as integrated health care system) A system created to manage or provide health care services ranging from primary to tertiary inpatient care and all other settings for care

risk sharing A mechanism that provides incentives to physicians and other health care providers to deliver cost-effective and efficient services

Types of Managed Care Organizations

Many businesses contract with a variety of MCOs to reduce health benefit costs. Government reimbursement systems have also entered into managed care arrangements to control escalating costs. For example, Medicare, a federal program for older adults and qualified disabled individuals, is expected to become a totally managed care system. Many state Medicaid programs, which pay for health services for the poor, have also entered managed care agreements.

The oldest and most common type of MCO is the **health maintenance organization (HMO)**, which is sometimes referred to as a membership organization. Many models for HMOs are used, but all either employ health care professionals to serve subscribing members (enrollees) in an ambulatory setting, or contract with primary physicians and other providers to treat clients in their private offices. The enrollee usually pays a small copayment, typically $5 or $10, for each visit to the health care provider. A client who wishes to seek services from a specialist typically needs a referral by the primary provider. Hospitalization or other inpatient services are provided by agencies that contract with the HMO.

Another popular type of MCO is the **preferred provider organization (PPO).** PPOs provide contractual arrangements with physicians, hospitals, and other providers who meet their criteria. Clients can seek services from any provider, within or outside of the PPO network, without obtaining a referral from a primary physician. In other words, they can use any of the "preferred" providers who render care to a group of subscribers in the health plan. The co-payment for each office visit to a preferred provider within the PPO network is usually $10 to $20, depending on the PPO.

COLLABORATIVE INTERDISCIPLINARY MANAGEMENT: CASE MANAGEMENT

As the United States moves forward with the managed care system, health care professionals have realized that they must work together as an interdisciplinary team to provide comprehensive, cost-effective care. Although this idea is not new in certain settings (e.g., rehabilitation, home care, and long-term care), health care professionals in hospitals have not always worked in collaborative teams. One of the constraints in acute care is the short-term stay. However, the Joint Commission on Accreditation of Healthcare Organizations (JCAHO) mandates that *all* JCAHO-accredited agencies must provide collaborative, interdisciplinary care for their clients.

This text has advocated collaborative management of care since the publication of its first edition in 1991. This edition continues to discuss client care under Collaborative Management headings. Nurses often take the lead role in the interdisciplinary team because they tend to be with clients for longer periods as they deliver and coordinate comprehensive, holistic care.

Focus on Outcomes

The primary focus of collaborative management is on the outcomes of care. The interdisciplinary team identifies expected outcomes for the client and provides interventions to help the client meet those outcomes. Both clinical and cost outcomes are established. This text identifies common clinical outcomes for clients with a number of diseases and illnesses. When possible, the Nursing Outcome Classification System is used as a guide. However, each client is an individual with unique problems and circumstances that may require modification of the commonly identified expected outcomes.

Resource Management boxes are also found throughout this text to increase awareness of costs and, in some cases, to show how nurses can help manage resources.

Development of Case Management

Although all clients need to have their care managed in a collaborative manner, not all clients need to be case managed. Case management is based on the assumption that certain clients with complex health problems need assistance in using the health care system and its resources effectively.

Case management is not a new concept. Since the turn of the twentieth century, social workers, psychologists, and others have "carried a caseload" of clients in the community for a variety of purposes. For instance, social workers and community health nurses have worked with at-risk older adults to keep them at home rather than admitting them to a nursing home.

In the mid-1980s, Karen Zander and colleagues at the New England Medical Center introduced a nursing case management (NCM) model. In this model, case managers followed up on high-risk, high-cost clients during their hospital stay to coordinate resources and ensure quality outcomes. Physician-nurse collaboration was a primary focus, which increased communication and coordination of care.

The Carondolet integrated health system in Arizona expanded on the NCM model by using case managers across the health care continuum. Sometimes referred to as "beyond the walls" case management, this model incorporated the ethnic values and culture of the community to ensure individualized, holistic care.

Definition and Process of Case Management

Many definitions for case management can be found in the literature. According to the Case Management Society of America (CMSA), "***Case management*** *is a collaborative process of assessment, planning, facilitation and advocacy for options and services to meet an individual's health needs through communication and available resources to promote quality cost-effective outcomes*" (CMSA, 2002). Sometimes case managers meet the health needs of a population rather than a single individual (e.g., all diabetic clients or all asthmatic school-age children in a given community).

The case management process is reserved for clients who have complex health problems (high risk) and incur a high cost to the health care system. An example of a client who could benefit from case management is an older woman with pulmonary emphysema and congestive heart failure who has had repeated admissions to the hospital for pneumonia and lives alone at home. Where appropriate in this text, the role of the case manager is discussed under Community-Based Care sections.

Part of the definition of case management endorsed by CMSA is similar to the steps of the nursing process (Chart 3-1). Similarly, the American Nurses Association (ANA) states that nursing case management includes five components: assessment, planning, implementation, evaluation, and interaction.

Goals of Case Management

The ANA identifies the goals of case management as follows:

- To provide quality health care along a continuum of care
- To decrease fragmentation (and duplication) of care across many health care settings
- To enhance the client's quality of life
- To increase cost containment (through appropriate use of resources)

The goals of case management as outlined by CMSA (2002) are more specific and include the following:

- To enhance an individual's safety, productivity, satisfaction, and quality of life
- To assure that appropriate services are generated in a timely and cost-effective manner

CHART 3-1

BEST PRACTICE for
The Process of Case Management

Needs Assessment
- Assesses/collects data
- Conducts case screening
- Identifies client's support systems and care providers
- Reviews history and determines current health care needs
- Obtains approvals for contracts

Plan Development
- Identifies services and funding options
- Reviews plan for consensus
- Advocates for client as needed
- Develops plan of care as indicated

Implementation and Coordination
- Communicates regularly with clients and support systems
- Coordinates treatment plan
- Promotes coordinated and efficient care
- Identifies needs for additional services

Outcomes Monitoring and Evaluation
- Assesses benefit value to cost and value to quality of life
- Reviews plan for continuity of care
- Evaluates client satisfaction and compliance with treatment plan

Documentation
- Records services and outcomes
- Submits reports and other documentation as needed

- To assist clients to achieve an enhanced level of health, and to maintain wellness and function by facilitating timely and appropriate health services
- To assist clients to appropriately self-direct care, self-advocate, and make informed health care decisions to the highest degree possible
- To maintain cost effectiveness in the provision of health services
- To facilitate appropriate and timely benefit and treatment decisions
- To maintain ongoing documentation and reporting of goal achievement

Types of Case Managers

In some agencies, the case manager is referred to as the care coordinator or care manager. Most case managers are nurses, but some are social workers or mental health/behavioral health workers. Some case managers have little or no clinical health background.

In general, case managers can be considered as having either an internal or an external role. **Internal case managers** are employed by a health care agency and are usually nurses or social workers. Although these individuals manage resources, their primary focus is clinical care. **External case managers** are either employed by a managed care organization (MCO) or traditional insurance company or are self-employed and contract with the MCO or traditional insurance company. The primary focus of external case managers is the utilization of resources for insurance companies.

In the past decades, there has been a growing number of so-called case managers. This "internal versus external" increase of professionals has caused an emerging challenge: how to integrate the care of clients as they move through the health care system. Case management has the same problem as managed care itself–fragmentation. "Through the continuum" case management is one answer to this dilemma. However, "handing off" clients from one setting to another has been a recurring problem (Powell, 2000a).

Complex, integrated health care systems fuel the problem. To resolve this fragmentation problem, some systems insist that *one case manager be assigned the task of being the central point of contact.* If an integrated system includes managed care case managers, acute care case managers, home health case managers, rehabilitation case mangers, and skilled nursing facility case managers, the model still remains fragmented. However, if the primary managed care case manager is ***accountable*** *for the coordination of the big picture;* the other case managers can manage the crises and details while the client resides in his or her respective level of care (Powell, 2000a).

Standards for Case Management Practice

The Case Management Society of America (CMSA) first published its ***Standards of Practice for Case Management*** in 1995. The 2002 revised standards are recognized nationally by health care organizations, certification and accreditation agencies, and individual case managers as voluntary practice guidelines for the case management profession. The standards are intended to identify and address the foundational knowledge and skill sets of a case manager in today's health care environment. Individual case managers, employers, and organizations may use the guidelines across varying case management practice settings and specialty areas (Moreo & Lamb, 2003).

These standards, both in 1995 and 2002, describe responsibilities, delineate expectations, and define accountabilities. The revised standards have also addressed the following issues (American Health Consultants, 2002; Moreo & Lamb, 2003):

- Client confidentiality issues for case managers
- Cultural competency for case management
- Legal issues of consent for case management
- Emerging trends/evolving practice (e.g., population-based practice; evidence-based practice)
- A shift in focus from resource utilization and cost of care to resource management and care management

As the largest professional case management organization, CMSA published standards that specify the recommended preparation for a case manager. As listed in the criteria, the recommended educational preparation is a baccalaureate degree in a health or human service. Although most case managers today are about 40 years of age and are nurses prepared at the associate degree level, it is likely that new case managers will have at least a baccalaureate degree as the twenty-first century unfolds. An increasing number of nursing programs believe that case management is an advanced practice role and offer masters' preparation in a case manager.

According to CMSA, the criteria for preparation as a case manager also includes working toward obtaining a certified case manager (CCM) credential. Since 1997, this certification process has required that the experienced case manager (with at least 2 years' experience) successfully complete a national standardized examination. The CCM designation is a valued credential in the field of case management for any discipline.

A certification is available for nurses who want credentials by their professional organization as a nursing case manager. In October 1997, the first nursing case management examination was given by the American Nurses Credentialing Center (ANCC). This modular test is available to nurses who are already have credentials in another field by the ANCC. Other certifications may also be acquired by case managers, such as the CRRN certification for case managers in rehabilitation nursing (Table 3-2).

Although models for case management vary, all case managers assume a common set of roles and functions. The CMSA *Standards of Practice* outlines the major roles of the case manager, including assessment, planning, facilitation, and advocacy. For nurses, many of the skills needed to fulfill these roles are learned in basic nursing education programs.

As an assessor, the case manager gathers all relevant data from a variety of sources and evaluates this information to identify barriers, clarify or determine realistic outcomes, and seek potential alternatives. The case manager works with the client and family/significant other to develop a plan that ensures that outcomes will be met and costs will be contained. As a facilitator, the case manager uses expert communication skills with all parties involved, including the care providers, client, family, and managed care payer. The client's best interests are represented by the case manager's advocacy for necessary resources, including funding and the coordination of health care services.

TABLE 3-2 The Most Common Types of Case Manager Certifications

Type of Case Manager	Certification Designation
Case manager (generalist)	Certified Case Manager (CCM)
Disability manager	Certified Disability Management Specialist (CDMS), formerly the Certified Insurance Rehabilitation Specialist (CIRS)
Rehabilitation nurse	Certified Rehabilitation Registered Nurse (CRRN)
Occupational health nurse	Certified Occupational Health Nurse (COHN)
Continuity of care manager	Advanced Certification in Continuity of Care (A-CCC)
Vocational evaluator	Certified Vocational Evaluator (CVE)
Drug and alcohol counselor	Masters Addiction Counselor (MAC)
Life care planner	Certified Life Care Planner (CLCP)

Data taken in part from May, V.R., et al. (2000). The life care planning process and certification: Current trends in health care management. *The Journal of Care Management, 6*(1), 38-40, 45-49.

From Case Management to Disease State Management

Case management models vary depending on the country's health care system or specific health care agency. For example, many case managers in the United States practice disease state management, sometimes called disease management. Put simply, disease state management focuses on the care of clients with chronic disease or illness, such as asthma, diabetes, or heart failure. The purpose of this approach is to keep clients with chronic conditions as healthy as possible in the community. Most chronic disease conditions have been "disease managed" in the past 10 years. The following are some of the more common conditions:

- Asthma
- Coronary artery disease (CAD)
- Chronic obstructive pulmonary disease (COPD)
- Heart failure (HF)
- Diabetes
- High-risk pregnancy
- Human immunodeficiency virus (HIV) infection
- Oncology
- Transplants
- Geriatric issues

There has been much debate as to whether disease management is a part of case management or whether case management is a component of disease management. Furthermore, the process is sometimes referred to as "disease-specific case management." One difference is that case management has been traditionally an individual-based approach in *either* acute *or* post-acute care. Disease management is systems based, integrating the clients through multiple levels of care. The essential idea is that disease management is case management at its finest, and case management *can:*

- Be proactive
- Follow a disease-specific population across the continuum of care
- Allow time to fully utilize the critical educational element to promote wellness
- Generate the improved quality of life case that managers seek for their clients

Powell (2000b) suggests that disease management is a system or program, whereas case management is the *process* used in disease management *programs.*

The Role of Clinical Pathways

As mentioned in Chapter 1, the clinical pathway (CP) is one format used as the client's plan of care. It is an interdisciplinary guideline for care that optimally sequences the interventions and expected outcomes for a client. Other names for the pathway include the collaborative plan of care (POC), multidisciplinary action plan (MAP), critical pathway, and care path.

The CP is developed by clinical experts for diagnoses, treatments, procedures, or symptoms that are costly, complex, and variable. The health care team follows the pathway in managing the client's care. If expected outcomes are not met, the case manager, nurse, or other health professional records these variances, or deviations, on a data collection tool. The variances are then analyzed to identify actual or potential problems. An action plan is implemented and followed up to determine whether the problem was resolved or avoided. This sequence of data collection, problem identification, action plan, and follow-up is part of the continuous quality improvement (CQI) process that every health care agency uses to monitor and improve the care that it provides.

CPs were introduced over two decades ago, yet their popularity has waxed and waned. Some hospitals are only *now* beginning to use them, whereas others have seen them come and go. Some facilities have incorporated the best of clinical pathways into their automated case management tools. Still, clinical pathways have an important focus for health care and case management. The forces that initially demanded them remain today (American Health Consultants, 2003):

- Changes in economics in health care
- Initiatives and regulations for quality improvement and best practice from an expanding body of evidence
- The desire for automation of the health care record
- The search for improved methods to involve clients and families

This text provides several examples of CPs with varying formats on the Evolve website. Traditional client care plans are also included in this text to help students identify the difference between a nursing focused care plan and an interdisciplinary plan of care, such as the clinical pathway.

GET READY for the NCLEX Examination!

KEY POINTS

- The primary purpose of managed health care is to provide quality client care while controlling health care costs.
- One major factor that is driving concerns about cost and quality of health care in the United States is its aging, chronically ill population that requires ongoing, high-cost care.

- Under the traditional fee-for-service reimbursement system, the insurance companies paid on the basis of what providers billed for services; under the capitated reimbursement system, each provider agrees to a set amount of payment before rendering services.
- A health maintenance organization (HMO) is a membership program in which enrollees are treated by providers who contract with the HMO. Referral from a primary physician is required if clients seek services from other providers.
- A preferred provider organization (PPO) allows subscribers to acquire health care services from any "preferred" provider that has contracted with the PPO. Clients do not need a referral from a primary physician.
- Case management is a collaborative process used to meet the client's health needs through communication and available resources to promote quality cost-effective outcomes for the client.
- Case management is reserved for clients with complex, high-risk, and/or chronic health problems.
- The primary goals of case management are to ensure that clients receive high-quality health care throughout the continuum, to decrease fragmentation and duplication of services, to enhance the client's quality of life, and to contain costs.
- The primary roles of the case manager include assessment, planning, facilitation, and advocacy, as published by the Case Management Society of America in its 2002 *Standards of Practice for Case Management*.
- Case managers may be certified as a CCM (certified case manager), as a nursing case manager through the American Nurses' Credentialing Center (ANCC), or in a specialty area, such as rehabilitation or disability.
- Disease management is an across-the-continuum, systems-based approach to care for populations of clients with chronic, complex illnesses, such as asthma, HIV infection, and cancer; it uses case management as the process for providing care.

ADDITIONAL STUDY RESOURCES

Go to your Student CD-ROM for Review Questions for the NCLEX Examination.

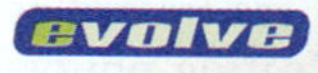

Go to http://evolve.elsevier.com/Iggy/ for Integrated Management of Care Questions for the NCLEX Examination.

SELECTED BIBLIOGRAPHY

Asterisk indicates a classic or definitive work on this subject.

Aliotta, S. (2003). Coordination of care: The Council for Case Management accountability's third state of the science paper. *The Case Manager, 14*(2), 49-52.

American Health Consultants (2002). Revised CMSA standards reflect new CM issues. *Hospital Case Management, 10*(12), 192.

American Health Consultants (2003). Old hat or cutting edge? The state of the art of clinical pathways. *Hospital Case Management, 11*(1), 1-3.

Carr, D.D. (2003). Case management as a triad in long-term care: A collaborative approach. *Lippincott's Case Management: Managing the Process of Patient Care, 8*(5), 224-227.

Case Management Society of America (CMSA). (2002). *Standards of Practice for Case Management–Revised 2002*. Little Rock, AK: Author.

Cesta, T., Tahan, H., & Fink, L. (2003). *The case manager's survival guide* (2nd ed.). St. Louis: Mosby.

Creager, L. (2003). Nine steps to effective and efficient hospital case management. *Care Management, 9*(2), 32-34.

*Engen, C. (1998). Critical thinking in case management. *Inside Case Management, 5*(9), 11-12.

Fick, D.M., et al. (2000). Advance practice nursing care management model for elders in a managed care environment. *Journal of Care Management, 6*(1), 28-30, 33-37, 49.

Finkelman, A.W. (2001). *Managed care: A nursing perspective.* Upper Saddle River, NJ: Prentice Hall.

Greenberg, L. (2003). *Leaping the chasm: A discussion of case management's potential to improve safety and quality.* Retrieved on May 25, 2003, from http://www.cmsa.org/Newsletters/CMSAatWorkForYou.

Huston, C.J. (2002). The role of the case manager in a disease management program. *Lippincott's Case Management: Managing the Role of Patient Care, 7*(6), 221-227.

*Ignatavicius, D.D., & Hausman, K. (1995). *Clinical pathways for collaborative practice.* Philadelphia: W.B. Saunders.

Keim, P. (2003). High-risk population: Evolution of disease management. *Continuing Care, 22*(6), 24-26.

Kelly, T.A. (2003). Critical thinking and case management. *The Case Manager, 14*(3), 70-72.

May, V.R., et al. (2000). The life care planning process and certification: Current trends in health care management. *The Journal of Care Management, 6*(1), 38-40, 45-49.

Moreo, K., & Lamb, G. (2003). Providing relevant guidelines for case management practice: Revised CMSA Standards of Practice for Case Management. *Lippincott's Case Management: Managing the Process of Patient Care, 8*(3), 122-124.

*Mullahy, C.M. (1999). *The case manager's handbook.* (2nd ed.). Gaithersburg, MD: Aspen.

*Nash, D. (1997). Disease management: A bumpy road ahead. *The Journal of Outcomes Management, 4*(1), 2.

Powell, S.K. (2000a). *Nursing case management: A practical guide to success in managed care* (2nd ed.). Philadelphia: Lippincott Williams & Wilkins.

Powell, S.K. (2000b). *Advanced case management: Outcomes and beyond.* Philadelphia: Lippincott Williams & Wilkins.

Powell, S.K., & Ignatavicius, D. (2001). *CMSA core curriculum for case management.* Philadelphia: Lippincott Williams & Wilkins.

Upman, C.M.S. (2003). The evolution of case management. *Care Management, 9*(3), 13-17.

*Zander, K. (1996). *Handbook of nursing case management.* Gaithersburg, MD: Aspen.

CHAPTER

4

Introduction to Complementary and Alternative Therapies in Nursing

RUTH LINDQUIST • MARIAH SNYDER

LEARNING OUTCOMES

After studying this chapter, you should be able to:

1. Describe the purposes of the National Center for Complementary and Alternative Medicine (NCCAM).
2. Identify four examples of mind-body therapies.
3. Discuss the scope of complementary and alternative therapies with particular attention to the cultural aspects of their use.
4. Differentiate manipulative and body-based therapies from biologic-based therapies.
5. Provide examples of herbal therapies, their purpose, and their adverse effects.
6. Identify selected complementary and alternative therapies that nurses can use in providing care to a variety of client populations.
7. Explain the purposes of commonly used therapies in nursing practice.
8. Discuss implications for care of clients using complementary and alternative therapies.

Go to your Student CD-ROM for Review Questions for the NCLEX Examination keyed to these Learning Outcomes.

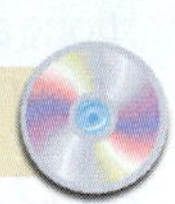

OVERVIEW

Western biomedicine has been the predominant health care system in the United States and other Western countries for the past 100 years. However, during the past 20 years, a growing interest in complementary (additional treatment) and alternative (substitutions for traditional treatment) therapies has evolved. In a national survey in the United States, Eisenberg and colleagues (1998) found that over 40% of Americans used complementary and/or alternative therapies. This number is thought to be a conservative figure in that only English-speaking persons were included and inquiries were only made about the use of 16 therapies. Most persons receiving complementary and alternative therapies pay for them out-of-the pocket, because most third-party payers reimburse for only selected therapies such as chiropractic treatment and acupuncture.

One of the reasons for the increase in nonbiomedical treatments is that individuals wish to be treated in a holistic fashion (Astin, 1998). Biomedicine is based on the Cartesian philosophy in which the body and mind are treated as separate entities. Nurses believe in a holistic, caring philosophy. Therefore complementary and alternative therapies are consistent with nursing and nursing practice.

This chapter describes some of the common therapies used by nurses in a variety of settings. In most cases, no special or advanced training is needed to use these modalities. Some complementary and alternative therapies, such as acupuncture, require specialized education and, in some states, licensure or certification.

NATIONAL CENTER FOR COMPLEMENTARY AND ALTERNATIVE MEDICINE (NCCAM)

Legitimacy was given to complementary and alternative therapies when the National Institutes of Health established the Office of Alternative Medicine in 1992. This office has since been renamed as the National Center for Complementary and Alternative Medicine (NCCAM). The purposes of the center are to:

- Fund studies examining the effectiveness of various complementary therapies
- Advance the knowledge about complementary therapies of health professionals
- Serve as a clearinghouse for information about these therapies.

NCCAM has defined complementary and alternative medicine in the following manner:

Complementary and alternative medicine covers a broad range of healing philosophies, approaches, and therapies that mainstream Western medicine does not commonly use, accept, study, understand, or make available (National Center for Complementary and Alternative Medicine, 2003). NCCAM has also developed a classification system for the more than 1800 therapies (Kreitzer & Jensen, 2000). Table 4-1 presents the five categories in this system and examples of therapies found in each category.

COMMONLY USED THERAPIES IN NURSING

Systems of Care

As indicated in Table 4-1, numerous systems of care exist. Each of these systems is based on a philosophy that guides the practitioner in the assessments to make and the therapies to use. According to Bodeker (2002), the majority of persons in many countries use therapies other than ones in the traditional biomedical system. With the growing immigrant population in the United States, it is imperative that nurses increase their knowledge about other systems of health care.

Numerous therapies that nurses use come from other systems of care such as yoga from Ayurvedic medicine and Qigong from traditional Chinese medicine (TCM). Understanding the philosophic or theoretic base underlying these therapies helps nurses gain a better perspective about the therapy being used. Nyo-Metzger and colleagues (2003) found that knowledge about non-Western health practices assisted health professionals in avoiding misdiagnoses of illnesses in immigrants.

Acupressure, a traditional Chinese medicine therapy, is used in nursing for a number of conditions, particularly in the treatment of pain, nausea, and vomiting. Gach (1990) defines **acupressure** as "an ancient healing art that used the fingers to press certain points on the body to stimulate the body's self-curative abilities" (p. 3). According to the philosophy of TCM, *qi* or energy flows along 12 major meridians. Illness or pain occurs when the flow of *qi* is blocked or diminished (Weiss, 2002). Acupressure is similar to **acupuncture;** pressure instead of needles is used on one of the 365 to 700 **acupoints** that are located on meridians throughout the body. Although most research has been done on acupuncture, studies on the effectiveness of acupressure are increasing.

One acupoint that is often helpful in reducing or eliminating pain is the *hoku* point. This point is on the back of the hand, and is located halfway between the junction of the first and second metacarpal bones. A valley is formed when the thumb is abducted. Pressure (usually with the thumb of the opposite hand) on this point helps alleviate pain. The *hoku* point has also been found to be helpful in stimulating the immune system, in relieving diarrhea, and helping to cure the common cold. There are a number of precautions to observe when using acupressure. Gach (1990) cautions against brisk rubbing or deep pressure in clients with heart disease, cancer, and high blood pressure to prevent sympathetic system stimulation.

Mind-Body Therapies

A huge number of therapies are classified as being mind-body therapies. Because these therapies are based on a holistic philosophy, they fit with the holistic, caring philosophy of nursing. Nurses have traditionally used a number of mind-body therapies such as journaling, imagery, meditation, and animal-assisted therapy.

JOURNALING

Journaling is one of the reflective therapies (Snyder & Lindquist, 2002); it is a tool for recording the process of one's life. Writing provides a vehicle for a person to express feelings, to gain new perspectives, and to pay attention to what is in the unconscious. A number of techniques for journaling can be used: intensive journaling (Progoff, 1975), focused writing (Pennebaker, 1997), and free-flowing (Bolton, 1999).

Free-flowing journaling is the technique most often used. The person writes whatever comes to mind without censoring any thoughts or feelings or correcting grammar or punctuation. The writing done is for oneself and need not be shared. The expectation to share what is written usually places constraints on what is being recorded. Entries are made in a book dedicated to journaling. This may be a loose-leaf notebook or a special journal entry book.

Although journal writing has been done for centuries, little formal research exists to support its use. Spera, Buhrfeind, and Pennebaker (1994) found that persons who had lost their

TABLE 4-1 CCAM Classification for Complementary Therapies and Examples of Therapies in Each Category: Alternative Systems of Care

Category	Examples
Systems of care	Traditional Chinese medicine, Ayurvedic, Native American/American Indian medicine, homeopathy
Mind-body therapies	Imagery, meditation, music, journaling, humor, biofeedback, yoga, prayer
Biologic-based therapies	Herbs, aromatherapy, special diets (Ornish, Pritikin), nutritional and food supplements
Manipulative and body-based therapies	Chiropractic treatment, massage, rolfing, light and color therapies, hydrotherapy
Energy therapies	Healing touch, Reiki, external Qigong, magnets

jobs and used focused-writing about the event were more likely to obtain employment sooner than persons who did not write or who wrote about superficial events. Bolton (1999) reported improved emotional health and less focus on pain connected with a situation or event in persons who recorded their feelings via journaling.

IMAGERY

Imagery has been used for many years in nursing. While changing dressings or doing other procedures that may produce pain, a nurse may ask a client to think about a pleasant event or a beautiful scene. Post-White and Fitzgerald (2002) define **imagery** as "the formation of a mental representation of an object, place, event, or situation that is perceived through the senses" (p. 44). Visualization is sometimes used interchangeably with imagery, but in reality all senses can be used in imagery.

The scientific base for the use of imagery relates to the reduction of stress, which is mediated through psychoneuroimmune interactions (Post-White & Fitzgerald, 2002). Imagery has been used in a wide variety of conditions, including the following:

- Reducing pain (Broome, Rehwaldt, & Fogg, 1998)
- Reducing nausea and vomiting (Troesch et al., 1993)
- Decreasing anxiety (Thompson & Coppens, 1994)
- Promoting comfort during treatment for cancer

Many techniques can be used to help individuals use their senses to create images. Guided imagery in which the client is provided with images or prompts by a nurse, a family member, or a friend, or via a tape is the technique frequently used by nurses. Before suggestions for imagery are presented, provide the client with instructions that will help produce relaxation. These may include tensing and relaxing muscle groups and focusing attention on one's breathing.

When the individual seems relaxed (slower respirations and relaxed muscles), give specific suggestions for imagery. The client may be asked to choose a place he or she enjoys and to think about the sights, smells, tastes, and feelings associated with the place. Time allowed for imagery varies, but it is usually between 15 and 20 minutes. Opportunities are provided for the person to enjoy being in this place; the client is informed that he or she can return to this "place" at anytime. Some clients like to create their own imagery tape to listen to while others prefer listening to commercial tapes or having the nurse or family member guide them through the session. Use of guided imagery has few risks. However, be attentive to any adverse effects such as heightened anxiety or difficulty in breathing.

MEDITATION

Meditation has been a part of many religions and cultures for thousands of years. Although often thought of in terms of religion, meditation, or focusing on the moment, can be used in a nonreligious context. Kreitzer (2002) defined **meditation** as "a self-directed practice for relaxing the body and calming the mind (p. 101). Everly and Rosenfeld (1981) identified four types of meditation:

- Mental repetition such as using a mantra
- Physical repetition such as focusing on breathing or walking
- Problem contemplation such as solving a riddle or *koan*
- Visual concentration that is similar to imagery

Walking meditation, a commonly used type, contains both active and meditative elements. While walking, the person focuses attention on the sound of the foot hitting the ground, the feelings in the muscles and joints, or the movements of the body. This type of meditation may be appealing to persons who are more active and have difficulty concentrating while sitting. The walking meditation should be done for about 20 minutes.

The labyrinth is an ancient form of walking meditation that has attracted renewed attention. Labyrinths are found in many cultures such as Hindu, Hopi Indians, Crete, and medieval European religions. The labyrinth is not a maze. The person walks the circles meditatively. Persons may ask themselves a question and search for answers while walking, they may pray, or they may just focus on feelings they are experiencing.

Meditation has been used to reduce anxiety, reduce pain, relieve symptoms of psoriasis, lower blood pressure, and promote health (Figure 4-1). In early studies, Benson (1975) explored the effectiveness of transcendental meditation (TM) in reducing hypertension. More recently, Kabat-Zinn and colleagues (1998) found that mindfulness meditation was effective in reducing the symptoms of psoriasis. Research on outcomes of meditation continues.

Animal-Assisted Therapy

It is not unusual to see dogs, birds, or other animals when visiting a hospital or nursing home. Since the 1970s, studies have sought to validate the link between animal companionship and positive health outcomes. Jorgenson (2002) differentiates between animal-assisted therapy (AAT) and pet visitation. In AAT, the animal, often a dog, is an integral part of the treatment plan. For example, a dog may be used to assist a client to improve motor skills or increase ability to concentrate. In contrast, the goal of pet visitation is aimed more at increasing socialization or keeping the person in touch with reality.

Animal-assisted therapy has been used with many different client groups including hospice (Chinner & Dalziel, 1991), behavioral health (Barker & Dawson, 1998), and dementia (Batson et al., 1995). Jorgenson (2002) recommends that any facility planning to implement AAT should first develop

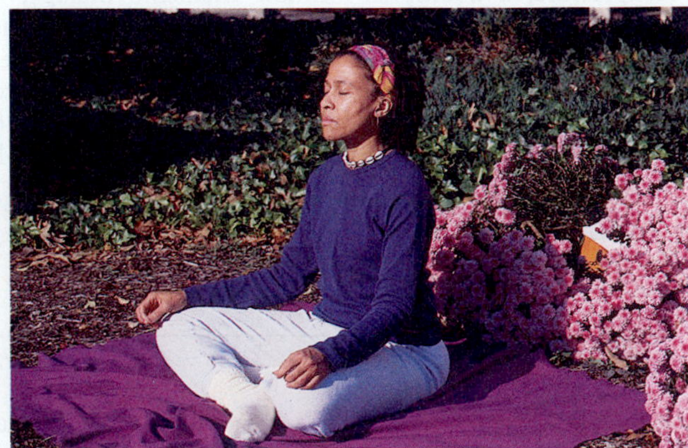

Figure 4-1 ■ Meditation can be used to relax the body and calm the mind. (From Potter, P.A., & Perry, A.G. [2001]. *Fundamentals of nursing* (5th ed.). St. Louis: Mosby.)

guidelines that specify the inclusion and exclusion criteria for clients who might receive AAT, the procedure to be used during the visitation, and the responsibilities of the nursing staff. Some institutions do not allow dogs to be on site for more than 1 hour because the animal becomes exhausted.

Manipulative and Body-Based Therapies

Three large groups of therapies make up the manipulative and body-based NCCAM category: chiropractic, osteopathy, and massage. Movement therapies such as dance and Tai Chi are sometimes also placed in this category. Massage and Tai Chi are common manipulative and body-based therapies that nurses can learn and teach to their clients.

MASSAGE

Massage has a long history within nursing. Until recently, back rubs were a standard nursing procedure administered to all hospitalized clients on a daily basis. **Massage** involves using various strokes and pressure to manipulate soft tissues for therapeutic purposes (Snyder & Lindquist, 2002). Many types of massage exist: Swedish (rather vigorous massage with long, flowing strokes), Esalen (light touch), neuromuscular (deep tissue), Shiatsu (Japanese pressure-point), and reflexology (massage of various points on the foot). Many different strokes are used in massage. Massage can be of the entire body or of selected areas such as foot, hands, shoulder/neck, or back (Figure 4-2).

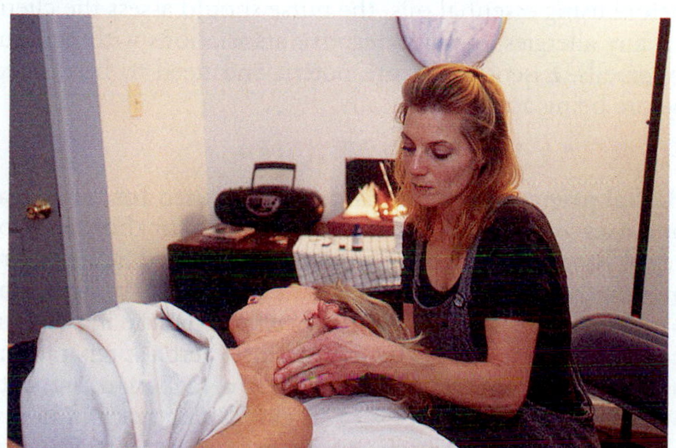

Figure 4-2 ■ Massage therapy can be effectively used to relieve tension. (From Potter, P.A., & Perry, A.G. [2005]. *Fundamentals of nursing* (6th ed.). St. Louis: Mosby.)

Hand massage can be readily used with any client group. Table 4-2 details one technique that can be used. Snyder and colleagues found that hand massage, when used with persons with dementia, produced relaxation and helped to lessen aggressive behaviors (Snyder, Egan, & Burns, 1995).

A growing body of research provides support for massage. As noted in the Evidence-Based Practice for Nursing box on p. 36, back massage produced relaxation in persons undergoing a diagnostic procedure. Massage has been found to reduce pain (Hulme, Waterman, & Hillier, 1999), produce relaxation (Snyder, Egan, & Burns, 1995), and improve sleep (Richards, 1998).

Because of cultural differences related to touch and personal preferences related to touch, the nurse needs to obtain permission of the person before using massage. Massage should not be used over reddened, bruised, or infected areas of skin.

TAI CHI

Tai Chi is a holistic movement therapy that has wide popularity in China, Taiwan, and Japan. **Tai Chi** is a traditional Chinese martial art that has been adapted to be a mind-body exercise. The goal is to integrate body movements, mind concentration, muscle relaxation, and breathing to achieve the desired outcome. Several styles of Tai Chi exist: *chen* (quick and slow large movements), *yang* (slow large movements), *sun* (quick compact), and Tai Chi Chih (simple repetitive movements). The latter is a style that is popular in the United States and originated in the West. Tai Chi is

TABLE 4-2 Directions for Administering Hand Massage

Do not massage the hand if it is injured, reddened, swollen, or infected. Each hand is massaged for about 2½ minutes.

Back of Hand
- Use medium pressure strokes from the wrist to the fingertips.
- Make large half-circle stretching strokes from the center to the side of the hand using moderate pressure.
- Make small circular strokes (like an O) over the entire back of the hand.
- Use light pressure strokes from the wrist to the fingertips.

Palm of Hand
- Make medium pressure strokes from the wrist to the fingertips.
- Use gentle strokes to lift the muscle tissue of the palms.
- Use small circular strokes, applying moderate pressure over the palm.
- Use large stretching strokes from the center of the palm to the sides (like opening up the palm).

Fingers
- Gently squeeze each finger from the base to the tip on both sides using the thumb and index finger.
- Do gentle range of motion.
- Apply gentle pressure on the nail bed.

Completion
- Place the client's hand on yours and cover it with your other hand.
- Gently draw your top hand toward you several times.
- Turn the hand over and gently draw your other hand toward you several times.

Modified from Snyder, M., & Lindquist, R. (Eds.). (2002). *Complementary/alternative therapies in nursing* (4th ed.). New York: Springer.

EVIDENCE-BASED PRACTICE for Nursing

Back massage may reduce stress in clients having cardiac catheterizations

McNamara, M.E., et al. (2003). The effects of back massage before diagnostic cardiac catheterization. *Alternative Therapies in Health and Medicine, 9,* 50-57.

Back massage may be helpful in reducing stress in clients having cardiac catheterizations. The aim of this research was to examine the effects that a 20-minute back massage had on blood pressure, respirations, pain perception, skin temperature, and perceived stress in 46 subjects who were having a diagnostic cardiac catheterization. A repeated measure design was used with a control and an experimental group. Subjects in the control group received the usual care that was provided in the cardiac catheterization laboratory. A 20-minute back massage was administered to the subjects in the experimental group before the test.

Findings showed that subjects receiving the back massage had a 20-mm Hg decline in systolic blood pressure immediately after the massage. The systolic pressure was 7 mm Hg lower than before the catheterization 10 minutes after the completion of the massage. Reductions in pain perception, respirations, and systolic blood pressure and perceived stress occurred in both groups during the waiting period.

Level of Evidence: 5—Well-controlled case study.

Critique. Although this study used a small convenience sample, it was an attempt to examine a nontraditional, yet simple method for minimizing stress in clients having a very stressful procedure. More studies using larger groups of culturally diverse subjects of varying ages need to be done to help generalize findings that can be useful for health care practice.

Implications for Nursing. Back massage could be considered as a possible therapy to use to reduce the stress of clients having cardiac catheterizations and, perhaps, other invasive diagnostic procedures. This intervention requires little time and could be performed by either a nurse or unlicensed nursing personnel before the procedure.

closely tied to the philosophy of traditional Chinese medicine (TCM); the movements promote the flow of *qi* or energy throughout the body.

CONSIDERATIONS FOR OLDER ADULTS

A growing body of research on Tai Chi is evolving. Much of the research on Tai Chi has focused on its use with older adults, particularly in preventing falls (Shih, 1997). Tai Chi has also been shown to promote both physical and mental well-being in older adults (Chen, Snyder, & Kirchbaum, 2001). One notable finding is that many older adults continued to use Tai Chi after the study concluded.

Biologic-Based Therapies

This category of therapies is more similar to the biomedical model. However, the regulations governing herbal preparations and food additives differ from those for pharmaceuticals. This seeming lack of strict regulation has contributed to concerns about these preparations. Use of essential oils in aromatherapy and herbal preparations is becoming more common.

AROMATHERAPY

Aromatherapy is one of the fastest growing areas in complementary therapies. Use of essential oils can be traced back to ancient times. Modern interest in aromatherapy was initiated in France in the 1930s. Clinical **aromatherapy** is defined as "the use of essential oils for their expected outcomes that are measurable" (Buckle, 2002, p. 246). Buckle notes that the term *aromatherapy* conveys that use of the essential oil is via smell. However, essential oils may be applied in compresses, used in baths, or applied topically to the skin. What is common to all of these forms of use is that essential oils, the steam distillate of aromatic plants, are used. Essential oils may be obtained from the flowers, leaves, bark, wood, roots, seeds, or peels of plants.

Numerous essential oils have been identified and used. For example, lavender (*Lavandula officinalis*) and rose (*Rosa damascena)* are two of the oils used to promote relaxation and sleep. Peppermint (*Mentha piperita)* has been used for stimulation and to promote concentration. Sandalwood (*Santalum album)* and lavender (*L. officinalis)* have been used to ease depression. Tea tree has been tested to determine its effectiveness in treating methicillin-resistant *Staphylococcus aureus* (MRSA) infections.

Although only a small body of research on essential oils currently exists, a number of studies are being conducted. Before using essential oils, the nurse should assess the client for any allergies and any negative associations with particular smells. Essential oils are potent and need to be diluted before being applied topically.

HERBAL PREPARATIONS

Herbal preparations are plants that are used for medicinal purposes and have been used by societies for thousands of years. Today they are widely used in the United States where millions of individuals use herbal preparations on a regular basis. In recent years, there has been a dramatic increase in use of herbal remedies by Americans. Herbal preparations have become increasingly popular as a means to promote health, to prevent diseases, or to cure a variety of ailments. For example, herbal preparations are used in an effort to control high blood pressure, relieve abdominal pain, control high serum glucose levels, or manage painful chronic conditions. Several common herbs, their intended purposes, and precautions are listed in Table 4-3.

Herbal preparations are frequently considered an attractive alternative or supplement to conventional health care, and are commonly viewed as "less risky" than conventional drug therapy because they are "natural." However, herbs have pharmacoactive effects that may be serious or deadly as in cases of overuse, inappropriate use, herbal toxicities, and herb-drug and herb-herb interactions. The full range of beneficial and adverse effects of many herbal preparations is not known. Although the effects of some herbs have been studied, others have not. Furthermore, even though herbs have been used for thousands of years, the combination of many of herbs with Western medicine is relatively new (Lu, 2003), and the effects of many herb-drug combinations remain to be determined. Thus with the increased popularity in the use of herbs has come heightened concern about their safety.

There are other drawbacks to herbal therapies. Herbs may be self-administered to treat a serious ailment that could more effectively be treated by conventional medicine, potentially resulting in a delay of diagnosis and treatment by conventional practitioners. In other situations, improper dosages of herbs may be taken when lower dosages or other precautions are indicated due, for example, to a client's

TABLE 4-3 Commonly Used Herbal Preparations

Herb	Intended Effects/Uses	Cautions/Adverse Effects
Gingko biloba	Reduce memory problems, dementia, peripheral vascular disease; has antioxidant and vasodilatory properties.	Use with anticoagulants may cause bleeding; rarely dizziness, headache, GI upset.
Garlic	Lower cholesterol or blood pressure; act as a natural antibiotic; act as an antiplatelet agent.	Bleeding when used with other antiplatelet agents; potentiates antidiabetic drugs; avoid before surgery.
Echinacea	Build immunity; help wound healing.	Not recommended for individuals with immune diseases. May suppress immune function if used for more than 8 weeks.
Ginseng	Promote general well-being; antiaging.	Observe INR with warfarin. Side effects may depend on type of ginseng used.
St. John's wort	Ease mild to moderate depression.	Photosensitivity; avoid use in major depression or with other antidepressants.

INR, International Normalized Ratio; *GI*, gastrointestinal.

poor liver or renal function for detoxification or excretion (Eliopoulos, 1999). In some cases, although herbal intake may contribute to the need for emergency department visits, clients may neglect or choose not to tell their health care providers about their use of herbs.

In the United States, herbal preparations are regulated as food and nutritional supplements by the Food and Drug Administration (FDA). Although regulated by the FDA, regulations are less strict than for drugs. Because herbs are not classified as drugs, they do not receive the same oversight in their preparation and use as drugs. However, even though herbs do not require a prescription, they are the basis of many prescription drugs. It has been observed that of the best selling 150 prescription drugs, 86 contain at least one major active compound from natural sources (Plotnikoff, 2002). Adding to the complexity of herbal therapy, herbal preparations cause a variety of responses depending on the nature of the herb and how it was prepared. There is no guarantee that an herb has been properly prepared, thus there are uncertainties related to product quality. However, herbs that are sold as standardized extracts are viewed as more likely to contain accurate amounts of herbs as reflected on their label and less likely to contain other inactive elements or contamination. Because an herb is natural, it does not mean that it is safe. Because a given herb is considered "safe," it does not mean it is effective. What is on an herbal product's label does not reflect the contents in all cases (Plotnikoff, 2002, p. 263).

Unregulated and unprescribed, herbs may have untoward effects such as liver toxicity; herbs may potentiate other drugs, alter blood pressure, or cause bleeding. Some problems encountered in treating clients who are using herbs with conventional medications and treatments include oversedation, inhibition of coagulation, blood pressure effects (hypertension or hypotension), dysrhythmias, and electrolyte changes.

In any health care setting, it is important to integrate herb usage questions into a client's health history and to interpret findings of physical assessments that are possibly related to the client's herbal use. Ask a client about the intended purpose of herbal use as well as the frequency and dose of the herbs used. If herbal preparations are used, remind the client about the importance of informing future care providers about herbal therapy use. For example, to avoid increased risks of bleeding, one should not use ginkgo, ginseng, and garlic before surgery.

There is increasing need to know the intended effects and side effects of herbal therapies and safety precautions related to their ingestion as the public continues to explore the use of herbs. You can play an important role in the identification of adverse herb effects, herb-herb, and herb-drug interactions, and in the identification and prevention of adverse effects and side effects of herbal therapy. Nurses can inform clients about the use of herbs and discuss dangers of excessive or inappropriate use. You can also explain the importance for clients to monitor their response to herbal preparations over time, so that toxicities and adverse effects may be noted and herbal intake stopped if indicated. Nurses should caution clients about unreliable sources of health information and refer clients to credible resources for herbal remedies. Examples include the National Library of Medicine's PubMed Website: http://www.ncbi.nlm.nih.gov/ PubMed/; the American Botanical Council: http://herbalgram.org; and the Herb Research Foundation: http://www.herbs.org.

Energy Therapies

Energy therapies include both biofield therapies and bioelectromagnetics. Because it is difficult to *see* energy, much skepticism exists about the therapies in this NCCAM category. However, healing touch techniques have a long history of use in nursing. Since the 1970s when Krieger (1976) began her research, nurses have continued to conduct research on the effectiveness of energy therapies in producing positive health outcomes. Umbreit (2002) defined **healing touch** as "a type of complementary therapy that used energy-based techniques to balance and align the human energy field" (p. 165). Healing touch encompasses many techniques. The most well-known energy therapy is therapeutic touch. Therapeutic touch, magnetic unruffling, and magnets are discussed.

THERAPEUTIC TOUCH

According to Quinn (2002), **therapeutic touch** (TT) "is the use of the hands on or near the body with the intention to heal" (p. 183). One of the assumptions upon which TT is based is that illness is an imbalance in the flow of energy or the energy pattern. In TT, the practitioner intervenes in the recipient's energy field to stimulate healing potential.

TT consists of five steps: centering, assessing the energy field, clearing and mobilizing the client's energy field, directing energy for healing, and balancing the energy field. In centering, the practitioner quiets oneself and focuses attention on the client with the intention to heal. The practitioner uses her or his hands to assess the flow of energy in the client; hands are moved from head to foot, noting any blockages in the flow of energy or absences or excesses in energy in a particular spot. In the clearing and mobilizing element, the practitioner holds his or her hands 2 to 4 inches from the client's body and moves the hands with the palms facing the client's, from head to foot in a sweeping motion (Figure 4-3). This process may be repeated. Based on the assessment, the practitioner directs energy so that imbalances are resolved. The practitioner's hands are placed on the client and energy is directed toward the client. Finally, the practitioner seeks to balance the energy in the client by using head-to-toe clearing motions with the intention of smoothing the energy of the client.

TT has been used to achieve numerous health outcomes: reduce anxiety (Quinn & Strelkauskas, 1993), reduce pain (Peck, 1997), improve the immune system (Olson et al., 1997), and improve functional ability (Peck, 1998). Caution should be used in administering TT to the very young and very old.

MAGNETIC UNRUFFLING

Little research has been conducted on **magnetic unruffling.** In this therapy, practitioners move their hands from above the head to past the feet of the client. The practitioner can think of the fingers as magnets collecting excess energy. They may then shake the collected energy from their hands before starting the next sweep. Each sweep takes about 30 seconds. These movements are continued until the body feels like glass (Hover-Kramer, 1999). Magnetic unruffling has been used with clients who have had general anesthesia, have a chemical dependency disorder, are experiencing chronic pain, or have a systemic illness.

MAGNETS

Magnets are another type of energy therapy. One of the prime purposes for using magnets is to relieve chronic pain, particularly back and joint pain. Magnets can be applied via wide belts, orthotics, or in mattresses and pillows. More research is needed about the use of magnets and their effectiveness in managing chronic pain.

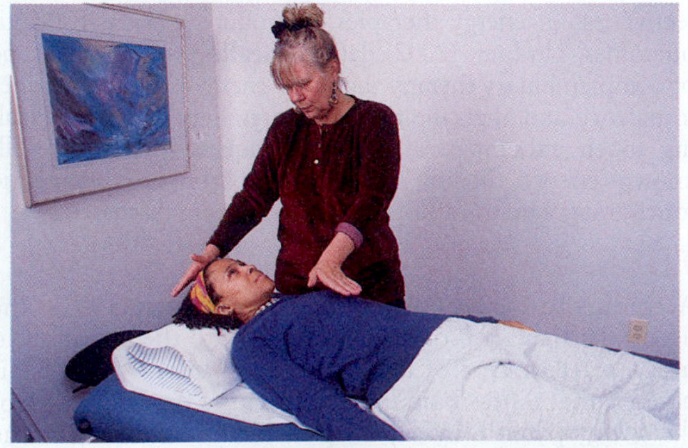

Figure 4-3 ■ In therapeutic touch, the practitioner directs the practitioner's own interpersonal energy to help or heal another. (From Potter, P.A., & Perry, A.G. [2005]. *Fundamentals of nursing.* (6th ed.). St. Louis: Mosby.)

SUMMARY OF IMPLICATIONS FOR NURSING

Complementary and alternative therapies are increasingly being used to promote health, prevent disease, or address illness and symptoms. Increased nursing research is essential to evaluate the usefulness of therapies and their role in medical-surgical nursing practice. Throughout this text, discussions of specific complementary and alternative therapies are included as part of the collaborative management of various diseases and illnesses. These descriptions are labeled with a separate heading to help locate this information.

Nurses have an important role in assessing the clients' use of therapies in order to discuss safety, perceived effectiveness, and satisfaction. Furthermore, the knowledge of clients' use of complementary and alternative therapies is important in the planning of care and in the determination as to how conventional and nonconventional therapies may be safely combined to benefit clients. A better understanding of therapies enhances your ability to educate clients about specific therapies and their effects, to discuss therapies of potential benefit to clients, and to refer clients to appropriate providers for desired therapies.

GET READY for the NCLEX Examination!

KEY POINTS

- Complementary and alternative therapies include a broad range of healing approaches and therapies that are not commonly used as part of Western medicine. Many of these therapies are derived from Eastern medicine, such as traditional Chinese medicine (e.g., acupressure).
- Many individuals living in the United States and other Western countries are using complementary and alternative therapies.
- As part of the National Institutes of Health, the National Center for Complementary and Alternative Medicine is funding research to determine the usefulness of selected therapies.
- Examples of mind-body therapies include journaling, imagery, meditation, and animal-assisted therapy.
- Journaling allows an opportunity for reflection as the individual records thoughts and feelings.
- Imagery is often used for reducing pain, nausea and vomiting, and anxiety.
- Massage is a commonly used manipulative and body-based therapy in nursing, for example, giving a back rub.
- Tai Chi is a popular holistic therapy used in China, Taiwan, and Japan that is gaining interest in the Western sector; it integrates body movements, concentration, and relaxation techniques.
- Aromatherapy and herbal preparations are commonly used biologic therapies; these interventions are used for an assortment of problems (see Table 4-3).
- Therapeutic touch promotes healing by balancing a person's energy field.
- Magnets may be used as an adjunct for chronic pain management, especially for joint and back pain.

ADDITIONAL STUDY RESOURCES

Go to your Student CD-ROM for Review Questions for the NCLEX Examination.

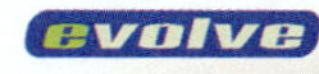

Go to http://evolve.elsevier.com/Iggy/ for Integrated Management of Care Questions for the NCLEX Examination.

SELECTED BIBLIOGRAPHY

Asterisk indicates a classic or definitive work on this subject.

*Astin, J.A. (1998). Why patients use alternative medicine: Results of a national study. *Journal of the American Medical Association, 2799,* 1548-1553.

*Barker, S.B., & Dawson, K.S. (1998). The effects of animal-assisted therapy on anxiety ratings of hospitalizing psychiatric patients. *Psychiatric Service, 49,* 797-801.

*Batson, K., et al. (1995). The effect of a therapy dog on socialization and physiologic indicators of stress in persons diagnosed with Alzheimer's disease. In C.C. Wilson & C.C. Turner (Eds.), *Companion animals in human health* (pp. 203-215). Thousand Oaks, CA: Sage.

*Benson, H. (1975). *The relaxation response.* New York: Avon.

Bodeker, G. (2002). Lessons on integration from the developing world's experience. *British Medical Journal, 322,* 154-167.

*Bolton, G. (1999). *The therapeutic potential of creative writing.* London: Jessica Kingsley Publishers.

*Broome, M.E., Rehwaldt, M., & Fogg, L. (1998). Relationships between cognitive behavioral techniques, temperament, observed distress, and pain reports in children and adolescents during lumbar puncture. *Journal of Pediatric Nursing, 13,* 48-51.

Buckle, J. (2002). Aromatherapy. In M. Snyder & R. Lindquist (Eds.), *Complementary/alternative therapies in nursing* (4th ed., pp. 245-258). New York: Springer.

Chen, K.M., Snyder, M., & Kirchbaum, K. (2001). Clinical use of Tai Chi in elderly populations. *Geriatric Nursing, 22,* 198-200.

*Chinner, T.L., & Dalziel, F.R. (1991). An exploratory study on the viability and efficacy of a pet-facilitated therapy project with a hospice. *Journal of Palliative Care, 7,* 13-20.

*Eisenberg, D.M., et al. (1998). Trends in alternative medicine use in the United States, 1990-1997. *Journal of the American Medical Association, 280,* 1569-1575.

*Eliopoulos, C. (1999). Using complementary and alternative therapies wisely. *Geriatric Nursing, 20,* 139-143.

*Everly, G.S., & Rosenfeld, R. (1981). *The nature and treatment of the stress response.* New York: Plenum.

*Gach, M. (1990). *Acupressure potent points.* New York: Bantam Books.

Hover-Kramer, D. (Ed.). (2001). *Healing touch: A resource for health care professionals.* Albany, NY: Delmar.

*Hulme, J., Waterman, H., & Hillier, V.F. (1999). The effect of foot massage on patients' perception of care following laparoscopic sterilization as day case patients. *Journal of Advanced Nursing, 30,* 460-468.

Jorgenson, J. (2002). Animal-assisted therapy. In M. Snyder & R. Lindquist (Eds.), *Complementary/alternative therapies in nursing* (4th ed., pp. 152-162). New York: Springer.

*Kabat-Zinn, J., et al. (1998). Influence of a mindfulness meditation-based stress reduction intervention on rates of skin clearing in patients with moderate to severe psoriasis undergoing phototherapy (UVB) and photochemotherapy (PUVA). *Psychosomatic Medicine, 60,* 525-632.

Kreitzer, M.J. (2002). Meditation. In M. Snyder & R. Lindquist (Eds.), *Complementary/alternative therapies in nursing* (4th ed., pp. 101-113). New York: Springer.

Kreitzer, M.J., & Jensen, D. (2000). Healing practices: Trends, challenges, and opportunities for nurses in acute and critical care. *AACN Clinical Issues: in Advanced Practice in Acute and Critical Care, 11,* 7-16.

*Krieger, D. (1976). Healing by laying on of hands as facilitators of bioenergetic change: The response of in-vivo hemoglobin. *Psychoenergetic Systems, 1,* 121-129.

Lu, Y. (2003). Herb use in critical care: What to watch for. *Critical Care Nursing Clinics of North America, 15*(3), 313-319.

McNamara, M.E., et al. (2003). The effects of back massage before diagnostic cardiac catheterization. *Alternative Therapies in Health and Medicine, 9,* 50-57.

National Center for Complementary and Alternative Medicine. (2003). Retrieved on June 9, 2003, from www.nccam.gov.

Nyo-Metzger, Q., Massagli, M.P., & Clarridge, B.R. (2003). Linguistic and cultural barriers to care: Perspectives of Chinese and Vietnamese immigrants. *Journal of General Internal Medicine, 18,* 44-52.

*Olson, M., et al. (1997). Stress-induced immunosuppression and therapeutic touch. *Alternative Therapies in Health and Medicine, 3*(2), 68-74.

*Peck, S.D. (1997). The effectiveness of therapeutic touch for decreasing pain in elders with degenerative arthritis. *Journal of Holistic Nursing, 15,* 176-198.

*Peck, S.D. (1998). The efficacy of therapeutic touch for improving functional ability in elders with degenerative arthritis. *Nursing Science Quarterly, 11,* 123-132.

*Pennebaker, J.W. (1997). *Opening up: The healing power of expressing emotions.* New York: Guilford Press.

Plotnikoff, G. (2002). Herbal medicines. In M. Snyder & R. Lindquist (Eds.), *Complementary/alternative therapies in nursing* (4th ed., pp. 259-271). New York: Springer.

Post-White, J., & Fitzgerald, M. (2002). Imagery. In M. Snyder & R. Lindquist (Eds.), *Complementary/alternative therapies in nursing* (4th ed., pp. 43-57). New York: Springer.

*Progoff, I. (1975). *At a journal workshop.* New York: Dialogue House Library.

Quinn, J.F. (2002). Therapeutic touch. In M. Snyder & R. Lindquist (Eds.), *Complementary/alternative therapies in nursing* (4th ed., pp. 183-196). New York: Springer.

*Quinn, J.F., & Strelkauskas, A.J. (1993). Psychoneuroimmunological effects of therapeutic touch on practitioners and recently bereaved recipients: A pilot study. *Advances in Nursing Science, 15*(4), 13-26.

*Richards, K.C. (1998). Effect of a back massage and relaxation intervention on sleep in critically ill patients. *American Journal of Critical Care, 7,* 288-299.

*Shih, J. (1997). Basic Beijing twenty-four forms of Tai Chi exercise and average velocity of sway. *Perceptual and Motor Skills, 84,* 287-290.

Snyder, M., & Lindquist, R. (Eds.). (2002). *Complementary/alternative therapies in nursing* (4th ed.). New York: Springer.

*Snyder, M., Egan, E.C., & Burns, K. (1995). Efficacy of hand massage in decreasing agitation behaviors associated with care activities in persons with dementia. *Geriatric Nursing, 16*(2), 60-63.

Sparber, A. (in press). Complementary therapy in critical care settings. A review of surveys and implication for nurses. *Critical Care Nursing Clinic of North America, 15.*

*Spera, S.P., Buhrfeind, E.D., & Pennebaker, J.W. (1994). Expressive writing and coping with job loss. *Academy of Management Journal, 37,* 722-733.

*Thompson, M.B., & Coppens, N.M. (1994). The effects of guided imagery on anxiety levels and movement of clients undergoing magnetic resonance imaging. *Holistic Nursing Practice, 8*(2), 1179-1185.

*Troesch, L.M., et al. (1993). The influence of guided imagery on chemotherapy-related nausea and vomiting. *Oncology Nursing Forum, 20,* 1179-1185.

Umbreit, A.W. (2002). Healing touch. In M. Snyder & R. Lindquist (Eds.), *Complementary/alternative therapies in nursing* (4th ed., pp. 165-182). New York: Springer.

Weiss, P. (2002). Acupressure. In M. Snyder & R. Lindquist (Eds.), *Complementary/alternative therapies in nursing* (4th ed., pp. 205-220). New York: Springer.

CHAPTER

5 Health Care of Older Adults

DONNA D. IGNATAVICIUS

LEARNING OUTCOMES

After studying this chapter, you should be able to:

1. Identify four subgroups of older adults.
2. Describe nursing interventions for relocation stress syndrome.
3. Discuss common health issues that may concern older adults.
4. Explain why older adults are often at high risk for falls.
5. State common interventions for older clients at high risk for falls.
6. Describe the nursing care required for clients who are restrained.
7. Explain the effects of drugs on the older adult.
8. Compare and contrast delirium and dementia.
9. Interpret the signs and symptoms of elder neglect or abuse.
10. Discuss potential economic issues for older adults.
11. Describe government and community resources that are available for older adults.

Go to your Student CD-ROM for Review Questions for the NCLEX Examination keyed to these Learning Outcomes.

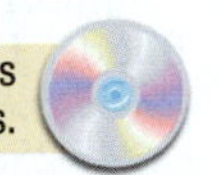

The percentage of individuals older than age 65 years in the United States is about 13%. Women tend to live longer than men. This number is expected to grow as "baby boomers" approach late adulthood in the next 10 to 15 years. As many as 50% to 80% of hospitalized clients on medical-surgical units are over 65 years of age. Health care professionals need to know about the special needs of older adults as they care for them in a variety of settings.

This chapter describes the major health issues associated with late adulthood. The care of older adults (sometimes referred to as elders) with specific health problems, such as pain, acute and chronic illnesses, and surgical procedures, is discussed in appropriate chapters throughout this text. In addition, Nursing Focus on the Older Adult charts and Considerations for Older Adults headings highlight the most important information.

OVERVIEW

Late adulthood can be divided into four subgroups:

- 65 to 74 years of age: the young old
- 75 to 84 years of age: the middle old
- 85 to 99 years of age: the old old
- 100 years of age or more: the elite old

The fastest growing subgroup is the old old, sometimes referred to as the advanced older adult population. The members of this subgroup are sometimes referred to as the "frail elderly," although a number of 85 to 95 year olds are very healthy. In general, the needs and problems of this subgroup are different from those of adults between 65 and 74 years of age. The incidence of chronic disease increases with advanced age. For example, three fourths of all cancer diagnoses occur after age 75 (Loeb, 2003).

About 80% to 85% of all older adults are relatively healthy and live in the community at home, in assisted-living facilities, or in retirement complexes. Men over 65 years of age are less likely to live in a single-person household than women of that age. Five percent of all older adults reside in long-term care facilities (mostly nursing homes), and another 10% to 15% are ill but are cared for at home. Older adults from any setting usually experience one or more hospitalizations in their lifetime. About half of all older adults are admitted for short-term stays in a nursing home.

Many older adults experience one or more relocations during their "senior" years, such as when selling a house to move into a retirement living center. They usually have more difficulty adjusting to major change when compared to younger and middle-aged adults. Being admitted to a hospital or nursing home is a particularly traumatic experience. Older adults often suffer from relocation stress syndrome, also known as relocation trauma. **Relocation stress syndrome** is defined as a nursing diagnosis by the North American Nursing Diagnosis Association (NANDA). It is described as "physiological and/or psychosocial distress following transfer from one environment to another" (NANDA, 2003, p. 147). Examples of physiologic behaviors include sleep disturbance and in-

CHART 5-1

BEST PRACTICE for
Minimizing the Effects of Relocation Stress in Older Adults

- Provide opportunities for the client to assist in decision making.
- Carefully explain all procedures and routines to the client before they occur.
- Ask the family or significant other to provide familiar or special keepsakes to keep at the client's bedside (e.g., family picture, favorite hairbrush).
- Reorient the client frequently to his or her location.
- Ask the client about his or her expectations during hospitalization or nursing home placement.
- Encourage the client's family and friends to visit often.
- Establish a trusting relationship with the client as early as possible.
- Assess the client's usual lifestyle and daily activities, including food likes and dislikes and preferred time for bathing.
- Avoid unnecessary room changes.
- If possible, have a family member, significant other, staff member, or volunteer accompany the client when leaving the unit for special procedures or therapies.

creased physical symptoms, such as gastrointestinal distress. Examples of psychosocial manifestations are withdrawal, anxiety, anger, and depression. The nurse can be very helpful in assisting clients to adjust to their new environment. Chart 5-1 lists nursing interventions that may help to minimize the effects of relocation.

HEALTH ISSUES FOR OLDER ADULTS

Common health issues and problems that can affect older adults in any setting include the following:

- Health promotion
- Self-management
- Nutritional awareness
- Physical fitness and mobility
- Stress management
- Accidents
- Drug use and misuse
- Mental health/behavioral health problems
- Elder neglect and abuse

Health Promotion

Health is a major concern for most older adults. Health status can affect the ability to perform basic activities of daily living and to participate in social roles. A failure to perform these activities may increase dependence on others and may have a negative effect on morale and life satisfaction. When older adults lose the ability to function independently, they often feel empty and worthless. Loss of autonomy is a painful event related to the physical and mental changes of aging, and it can be the result of physical illness (Davidhizar & Shearer, 2000).

Like younger adults, middle and older adults need to practice health promotion and illness prevention to maintain or achieve a high level of wellness. The risk factors that negatively impact "successful" aging are alcohol abuse, smoking, depression, lack of exercise, and obesity. In addition, being nonwhite and uneducated compounds the risk for health problems (Davidhizar, Eshleman, & Moody, 2002).

CHART 5-2

CLIENT EDUCATION GUIDE
Lifestyles and Practices to Promote Wellness

Health-Protecting Behaviors

- Have yearly influenza vaccinations (after October 1).
- Obtain a pneumococcal vaccination. (A routine revaccination may be necessary.)
- Have a tetanus immunization, and get a booster every 10 years.
- Wear seat belts when you are in an automobile.
- Use alcohol in moderation or not at all.
- Avoid smoking.
- If you smoke at home, do not smoke in bed.
- Install and maintain working smoke detectors.
- Create a hazard-free environment to prevent falls; eliminate hazards such as scatter rugs and waxed floors.
- Use medications according to your physician's prescription.
- Avoid over-the-counter medications unless your physician directs you to use them.
- Take one aspirin every day (any dose between 81 and 325 mg) to decrease the risk of myocardial infarction and colon cancer.

Health-Enhancing Behaviors

- Have a yearly physical examination; see your health care provider more often if health problems occur.
- Reduce dietary fat to not more than 30% of calories; saturated fat should provide less than 10% of your calories.
- Increase your dietary intake of complex carbohydrate and fiber-containing food to five or more servings of fruits and vegetables and six or more servings of grain products daily.
- Increase calcium intake to between 1000 and 1500 mg daily.
- Allow at least 10 to 15 minutes of sun exposure two to three times weekly for vitamin D intake; avoid prolonged sun exposure.
- Exercise regularly three to five times a week for 30 minutes per session.
- Manage stress through coping mechanisms that have been successful in the past.
- Get together with individuals in different settings.
- Reminisce about your life.

Chronic illness is a major problem in older adult population (see Chapter 10). The nurse working with these clients in any setting needs to teach them the importance of promoting wellness and strategies for accomplishing this goal (Chart 5-2).

Self-Management

An older person's ability to maintain a positive self-concept and self-control may be hampered by the loss of resources in the late years of life. Older adults may also experience a number of losses that can affect their sense of control over their lives: the death of a spouse and significant others, the loss of social and work roles, and a decrease in physical mobility. The nurse can support older clients' self-esteem and feelings of independence by encouraging them to maintain as much control as possible over their lives, to participate in decision making, and to perform as many tasks as possible.

Regardless of the situation, it is important that older clients direct their lifestyle in a manner that encourages them to feel capable and valued. Most important, they need to find opportunities to be productive and take care of themselves as well as others.

A number of tools are available to the nurse in the community health or home health setting for assessing the self-care or self-management ability of older adults. (See Chapter 10 for discussion of functional assessment.) When older adults are admitted to a hospital or nursing home, the nurse needs to assess self-management capabilities for discharge planning.

Nutritional Awareness

NUTRITIONAL NEEDS IN THE COMMUNITY

A person's need for adequate nutrition remains constant throughout the life span, yet many older individuals are at risk for undernutrition. Inflation, reduced income, and a lack of transportation are factors that may contribute to inadequate nutrition among older adults. Older adults whose diets consist of inappropriate or unbalanced foods (e.g., an excess of carbohydrates) may also be poorly nourished. Some clients reduce their intake of food to near-starvation levels, even with the availability of assistive programs such as food stamps, free food, and Meals on Wheels. The lack of transportation, the necessity of traveling to obtain such services, and the inability to carry large quantities of groceries prohibit some older adults from taking advantage of food programs. Some older adults are too proud to accept free services.

Poor nutrition may also be related to loneliness. Older adults may respond to loneliness, depression, and boredom by not eating, which can lead to undernutrition. Many clients who live alone lose the incentive to prepare or eat balanced diets. Others respond to stress by overeating, which leads to obesity.

NUTRITIONAL REQUIREMENTS

The minimal nutritional requirements of the human body remain consistent from youth through old age, with a few exceptions. Older adults need an increased dietary intake of calcium, vitamin D, vitamin C, and vitamin A because alterations with age disrupt the ability to store, use, and absorb these substances. A sedentary lifestyle and reduced metabolic rate requires a reduction in total caloric intake to maintain an ideal body weight.

PHYSICAL CHANGES AFFECTING NUTRITION

Other physical aging changes influence nutritional status or the ability to consume needed nutrients. Diminished senses of taste and smell often result in a loss of appeal of food. Older adults experience a greater decline in the ability to taste sweet and salt than in the discrimination of bitter and sour. This physiologic change often results in an overuse of table sugar and salt to compensate. Teach the client to substitute herbs and spices to season food or to vary the textures of food substances to achieve satisfaction from food.

Tooth loss and poorly fitting dentures from inadequate dental care can also cause the older adult to avoid important foodstuffs. Older individuals with dentition problems often resort to eating soft, high-calorie foods such as ice cream and mashed potatoes, which lack roughage and fiber. Unless the person carefully chooses more nutritious soft foods, vitamin deficiencies, constipation, and other disorders can result. The extensive use of prescribed and over-the-counter (OTC) drugs, including herbal supplements, may affect appetite, food tolerances, and food absorption and use.

Older adults sometimes respond to problems associated with mobility, prescribed diuretics, and limited bladder capacity by limiting fluid intake, especially in the evening. Teach older adults that fluid restrictions make them susceptible to dehydration and electrolyte imbalances that can cause serious illness or death.

NUTRITIONAL NEEDS IN THE HOSPITAL AND NURSING HOME

In addition to the nutritional needs described for older adults living in the community, those who are in the hospital or nursing home have special needs related to their illness and general health. For example, an older client with a pressure ulcer needs additional protein, vitamin C, and zinc to heal the open skin lesion. The health care provider, nurse, and dietitian collaborate to determine the best sources of these nutrients. The health care provider may prescribe a multivitamin tablet with zinc to be given every day. The dietitian may recommend that a high-calorie, high-protein supplement such as Ensure Plus be given several times a day. The nurse encourages the client to select and eat high-protein foods to promote healing and prevent undernutrition.

Anorexia and weight loss are the most common nutritional problems in both hospitals and long-term care settings. Common causes of undernutrition include drugs, chewing problems, immobility, infections, and Alzheimer's disease. Another issue may be the lack of foods that are culturally specific. For example, a Mexican man may be used to eating enchiladas, rellenos, and tacos, but is served baked chicken and mashed potatoes. Chapter 64 discusses nutrition in detail, including interdisciplinary interventions for the prevention and management of common problems.

Physical Fitness and Mobility

Exercise and activity are important for older adults as a means of promoting and maintaining health (Figure 5-1). Physical activity can help keep the body in shape and main-

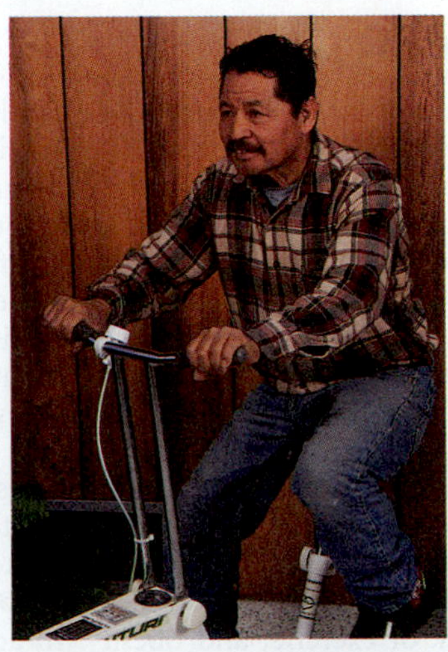

Figure 5-1 ■ Exercise is important to older adults for health promotion and maintenance.

tain an optimal level of functioning. In addition, regular and moderate exercise typically results in feelings of well-being. Numerous studies have shown that exercise has many benefits, including the following (Christmas & Andersen, 2000):

- Decrease falls
- Increase strength
- Reduce arthritis pain
- Reduce depression
- Improve longevity
- Reduce risks for diabetes and coronary artery disease

Nurses and other health care professionals need to teach older adults about the value of physical activity. One of the best exercises for older adults is walking at least 30 minutes, three to five times a week. During the winter, indoor shopping centers and other public places can be used. Swimming is also recommended but does not offer the weight-bearing advantage of walking. Older adults who have been sedentary should start their exercise programs slowly and gradually increase the frequency and duration of activity over time.

A few nursing studies have been conducted to explore exercise habits in the older adult population. One study of Latina older women found that, although the subjects verbalized the benefits of exercise, perceived barriers prevented them from exercising on a regular basis (Juarbe et al., 2002). The common barriers cited were time constraints, spousal and maternal roles, personal health limitations, lack of motivation, and fatigue. External barriers included transportation difficulties and cost. The researchers concluded that health education for this group needed to be culturally relevant, focusing on time and role-constraint barriers.

When any older adult is hospitalized, the opportunity for continuing a program of physical fitness is interrupted, at least temporarily. During severe or prolonged illness, clients are at high risk for complications of decreased physical mobility, such as pneumonia, skin impairment, contractures, muscle atrophy, constipation, and renal calculi. These problems are addressed elsewhere in this text.

Stress Management

FACTORS CONTRIBUTING TO STRESS IN OLDER ADULTS

Stress can speed up the aging process over time, or it can lead to diseases that increase the rate of degeneration. Stress can impair the reserve capacity of older adults and lessen their ability to respond and adapt to changes in their environment.

Although no period of the life cycle is free from stress, the later years can be a time of especially high risk. Frequently observed sources of stress for the older population include rapid environmental changes that require immediate reaction, changes in lifestyle resulting from retirement or physical incapacity, acute or chronic illness, the loss of significant others, financial hardships, and relocation. How individuals react to these stresses depends on their personal coping skills and support networks. The loss of roles experienced by older adults often limits the availability of external support networks. For instance, losses leave many clients without friends to whom they can turn for support and help. As a result, many must rely solely on their personal resources to maintain their mental health/behavioral health. A combination of poor physical health and social problems leaves older adults susceptible to stress overload, which can result in illness and premature death.

COPING WITH STRESS

The ways in which individuals adapt to old age largely depend on the personality traits and coping strategies that have characterized them throughout their lives. Establishing and maintaining relationships with others throughout life is especially important to the older person's happiness. Even more important than having friends is the nature of the friendships. Individuals who have close, intimate, stable relationships with others in whom they confide are more likely to maintain integrity in times of crisis.

A qualitative study by Loeb et al. (2003) found that older adults with at least two chronic illnesses coped by focusing on lifestyle changes to promote health, relying on spirituality and/or religion, and engaging in life. Some older adults sought information about health care, such as asking pharmacists about their medications. A limitation of this study was that all study subjects were white, and coping strategies may be different for various ethnic or racial groups.

ENVIRONMENTAL FACTORS

Most older adults live in and own their own homes. Physical or economic problems may force some to relocate to a retirement center or an assisted-living facility. Family members and facility staff need to be aware that older adults need personal space in their new surroundings. They need to participate in deciding how the space will be arranged and what they can keep in their new home to help offset the feelings of powerlessness. Suggest that the client or family bring in personal items, such as pictures of relatives and friends, favorite clothing, and valued knickknacks to assist in making the new setting seem more familiar and comfortable. This same intervention can be carried out in a hospital setting.

Changes in vision, touch, and motor ability can create difficulties for older adults in any environment. For example, decreased vision in old age, especially the poor perception of distance, may make walking more difficult; the person is less aware of the location of each step. A reduced sense of touch decreases the awareness of body orientation (e.g., whether the foot is squarely on the step). The decreased reaction time that commonly results from age-related changes in the neurologic system may also impair the ability to recognize or move from a dangerous setting.

Accidents

ACCIDENTS IN THE COMMUNITY

Most accidents occur at home. Teach older adults about the need to be aware of safety precautions to prevent accidents, such as falls. Incapacitating accidents are a primary cause of restricted physical fitness and decreased mobility in old age. Some individuals develop **fallophobia** and avoid leaving their homes for fear of falling.

Safeguards such as handrails, slip-proof underpads for rugs, and adequate lighting are essential in the home. Avoiding scatter rugs, slippery floors, and clutter is also important to prevent falls. Remind older adults to avoid going out on days when steps are wet or icy, and to ask for help when ambulating. To minimize sensory overload, advise the older adult to concentrate on one activity at a time. If needed, encourage the use of visual, hearing, or ambulatory assistive devices. High costs and a fear of appearing old sometimes prevent older adults from obtaining or using hearing aids, eyeglasses, walkers, or canes.

ACCIDENTS IN THE HOSPITAL AND NURSING HOME

The most common accident among older clients in a hospital or nursing home setting is falling. A **fall** is an unintentional change in body position that results in the client's body coming to rest on the floor or ground (Resnick, 2003). Some falls result in serious injuries such as fractures and head trauma. Most health care settings require an admission fall risk assessment and a protocol for clients who are at high risk for falls.

Risk Assessment and Interventions for Preventing Falls

Assess the client for risk for falls. Many risk assessment tools have been developed to help the nurse focus on factors that increase an older person's risk of falling (Resnick, 2003). Chart 5-3 lists some of the common risk factors that the nurse should assess and the measures for preventing falls. A history of falling is the single most important predictor for falls.

Once an older client has been identified as being at high risk for falls, choose interventions that help prevent falls and possible serious injury. For clients in the community, Tai Chi exercise is gaining popularity as an important activity to improve balance and functional mobility, as well as to decrease the fear of falling, especially among older women (Taggart, 2002).

Chart 5-3 lists common interventions that should be implemented for all older adults at a high risk for falling. One of the most controversial issues in fall prevention is the use of siderails as a physical restraint, especially in the hospital setting. At this time, hospital staff members are encouraged to evaluate each client as to the need to raise all four rails, two upper rails only, or no rails. In the nursing home, siderails are classified as restraints.

Older clients often have **nocturia** (urination at night) and get out of bed to go to the bathroom. They may forget to ask for assistance and may subsequently fall as a result of disorientation in the darkness in an unfamiliar environment. In some cases, they may crawl over the siderail, which can make the fall more serious. Because of this, siderails are used less often in both hospitals and nursing homes.

Use of Restraints

Similar considerations have been given regarding the use of other physical and chemical restraints. A **restraint** is any device or medication that prevents the client from moving freely. In 1990, the federal government enforced a law that gives nursing home residents the right to be restraint free. Removing physical restraints from nursing home residents has reduced serious injuries, although falls and minor injuries have increased in some cases.

CHART 5-3

BEST PRACTICE for
Assessing Risk Factors and Preventing Falls in Older Adults

Assess for the presence of the following risk factors:
- History of falls
- Advanced age (>80 years)
- Multiple illnesses
- Generalized weakness or decreased mobility
- Disorientation or confusion
- Use of drugs that can cause increased confusion, mobility limitations, or orthostatic hypotension
- Urinary incontinence
- Communication impairments
- Major visual impairments or visual impairment without correction
- Substance abuse
- Location of client's room away from the nurses' station (in the hospital or nursing home)
- Change of shift or mealtime (in the hospital or nursing home)

Implement the following nursing interventions for all clients, regardless of risk:
- Monitor the client's activities and behavior as often as possible, preferably every 30 to 60 minutes.
- Remind the client to call for help before getting out of bed or a chair.
- Help the client to get out of bed or a chair.
- Provide, or remind the client to use, a walker or cane for ambulating.
- Remind the client to wear eyeglasses or a hearing aid if needed.
- Help the incontinent client to toilet every 1 to 2 hours.
- Clean up spills immediately.
- Arrange the furniture in the client's room or hallway to eliminate clutter or obstacles that could contribute to a fall.
- Provide adequate lighting at all times, especially at night.
- Observe for side effects and toxic effects of drug therapy.
- Orient the client to the environment.
- Keep the call light within reach, and ensure that the client can use it.
- Place the bed in the lowest position with the brakes locked.
- Place objects that the client needs within reach.
- Ensure that adequate handrails are present in the client's room, bathroom, and hall.
- Have the physical therapist assess the client for mobility and safety.

For clients at a high risk for falls:
- Implement all interventions listed above.
- Relocate the client for best visibility and supervision.
- Use bed and chair alarms.
- Encourage family members or significant other to stay with the client.

Hospitals have also reduced the use of physical restraints. The Joint Commission on Accreditation of Healthcare Organizations (JCAHO) has specific standards that limit the use of physical restraints in hospitals and nursing homes. Chemical restraints or psychoactive drugs such as haloperidol (Haldol) have sometimes been used in place of physical restraints.

PHYSICAL RESTRAINTS

Experts agree that older adults should not be placed in a physical restraint or sedated just because they are old. Alternatives are used before applying any type of restraint (Chart 5-4). However, if all other interventions (e.g., reminding clients to call for assistance when needed or asking a family member to stay with clients) are ineffective in fall prevention, the nurse may need to use a physical restraint

CHART 5-4

BEST PRACTICE for Restraint Alternatives

- If the client is acutely confused, reorient him or her to reality as often as possible.
- If the client has dementia, use validation to reaffirm his or her feelings and concerns.
- Check the client often, at least every hour.
- If the client pulls tubes and lines, cover them with roller gauze or another protective device.
- Provide activities that keep the client busy, such as an activity pillow or apron, puzzle, or art activity.
- Provide soft, calming music.
- Place the client in an area where he or she can be supervised. (If the client is agitated, do not place him or her in a noisy area.)
- Turn off the television if the client is agitated.
- Ask a family member or friend to stay with the client at night.
- Help the client to toilet every 2 to 3 hours, including during the night.
- Be sure that the client's needs for food, fluids, and comfort are met.
- If agency policy allows, provide the client with a pet visit.
- Provide familiar objects or cherished items that the client can touch.
- Document the use of all alternative interventions.
- If a restraint is applied, use the least restrictive device (e.g., mitts rather than wrist restraints, a roller belt rather than a vest).

for a specified period. Applying a restraint is a serious intervention and should be analyzed for its risk versus its benefit. Check the client in a restraint every 30 to 60 minutes, and release the restraint at least every 2 hours for turning, repositioning, and toileting. Physical restraints such as vests have caused serious injury and even death. If restraint is needed, the least restrictive device should be used.

CHEMICAL RESTRAINTS

Chemical restraints, or psychoactive drugs, are often overused in hospital settings. Clients who are noisy, agitated, abusive, or combative may have an "as needed" order for a psychoactive drug. Such medications include the following:

- Antipsychotic drugs
- Antianxiety drugs
- Antidepressant drugs
- Sedative-hypnotic drugs

These drugs produce serious side effects and toxic effects and therefore should be reserved for clients with a documented mental health or behavioral health problem, such as severe anxiety or psychosis. Clients receiving these medications must be closely monitored for therapeutic and adverse effects.

The most potent group of psychoactive drugs is the antipsychotics. These drugs may be appropriate for the control of certain behavioral symptoms, such as hallucinations, delusions, and violent episodes. However, fewer than half of clients respond to these drugs. If a psychoactive drug is used as a last resort to control behavior, the lowest dose should be given.

Drug Use and Misuse

Drug therapy for the older population in general is another major health issue. Because of the multiple chronic and acute illnesses that occur in this age group, drugs for older adults account for about one third of all prescription drug costs. The term **polypharmacy** has been used to describe the use of multiple drugs by older adults.

Older adults also commonly use nonprescription drugs, such as analgesics, antacids, cold and cough preparations, laxatives, and herbal/vitamin supplements, often without consulting a health care provider. The occurrence of adverse drug reactions is directly related to the number of drugs taken and the frequency with which they are taken. Therefore older adults are at high risk for adverse drug reactions or interactions and are often admitted to the hospital for these problems.

PHYSIOLOGIC CHANGES AFFECTING DRUG USE

Older adults may not tolerate the standard dosage of medications traditionally prescribed for younger adults. The physiologic changes related to aging make drug therapy more complex and challenging. These changes affect the absorption, distribution, metabolism, and excretion of drugs from the body.

Age-related changes that can potentially affect drug absorption from an oral route include an increase in gastric pH, a decrease in gastric blood flow, and a decrease in gastrointestinal motility. Despite these changes, most clients do not have major absorption difficulties because of age-related changes alone.

Age-related changes that affect drug distribution include smaller amounts of total body water, an increased ratio of adipose tissue to lean body mass, a decreased albumin level, and a decreased cardiac output. Increased adipose tissue in proportion to lean body mass can cause increased storage of lipid-soluble drugs. This leads to a decreased concentration of the drug in plasma but an increased concentration in tissue.

Drug metabolism most often occurs in the liver. Age-related changes affecting metabolism include a decrease in liver size, a decrease in liver blood flow, and a decrease in liver enzyme activity. These changes can result in increased plasma concentrations of a drug. Changes in the kidneys can also result in high plasma concentrations of drugs.

The excretion of drugs most often involves the renal system. Age-related changes of the renal system include decreased renal blood flow and reduced glomerular filtration rate. These changes result in a decreased creatinine clearance and thus a slower excretion time for medications. Consequently, serum drug levels can become toxic, and the client can become extremely ill or die.

EFFECTS OF DRUGS ON OLDER ADULTS

Because of age-related physiologic changes, older adults are at a high risk for side effects and toxic effects from drugs. Older adults have less reserve capacity in most organ systems. When chronic disease is added to the physiologic changes of aging, drug reactions have a more dramatic effect and take a longer time to correct. Often a lower dose of medication is necessary to prevent adverse effects. The policy of "start low, go slow" is essential when health care providers prescribe drugs for this group. The physiologic changes of aging are highly individual. Alterations in drug therapy should always be individualized according to the actual physiologic changes present and the occurrence and severity of chronic disease. Common adverse drug reactions are listed in Table 5-1.

Many of these signs and symptoms can be mistakenly attributed to a concurrent illness or assumed to be part of the aging process. Assess all older clients with such symptoms for possible adverse reactions to medications.

SELF-ADMINISTRATION OF MEDICATION

Most individuals older than 65 years of age live at home and are responsible for taking their own medications. Because the risk of drug toxicity is considerably increased in the older population, the nurse should assist clients in assuming this task responsibly. Help prevent problems by educating clients and their caregivers, providing clear and concise directions, and developing ways to assist them in overcoming handicaps or difficulties with self-administration.

Older adults make errors in self-administration for several reasons. First, they may simply forget. In the rush of daily activities, they may not take the drug at all or may take it too often because of an inability to remember when or whether their medications have been taken. It can be helpful for clients to associate pill taking with daily events (e.g., meals) or to keep a simple chart or calendar. Pill boxes have been devised so that a daily, weekly, or monthly supply of medicine can be placed in the appropriate compartments (Figure 5-2). Egg cartons can be very cost-effective pill boxes. Large print on the drug label assists clients who have poor visual acuity. Writing the drug regimen on the top of the bottle with large letters and numbers is also helpful.

A second reason that older adults often commit errors in taking medications is poor communication with health care professionals. These difficulties result from inadequate explanations or explanations that are not understood because of educational limitations or language barriers. Health care professionals often presume that their client has acquired the knowledge if they have told the client about the medications. The nurse or other health care provider needs to help older adults plan their medication schedules.

A third reason for medication errors is attitude and ingrained feelings about taking medicine. Some individuals add to their drug regimen by taking over-the-counter (OTC) drugs, which can interact with prescription drugs and cause serious problems. For example, a client receiving warfarin (Coumadin, Warfilone✱) for anticoagulation may take ibuprofen (Motrin) regularly for arthritis. Because ibuprofen has anticoagulant ability, this combination can cause overt or occult bleeding. When obtaining a medication history, it is important to ask clients about all OTC drugs, including herbal and food supplements.

Other older individuals avoid taking medication whenever they can. The fear of drug dependency or the cost of the drugs may cause many to discontinue their medications too soon. In addition, the actions or side effects of some drugs may not be desirable. For example, diuretics may cause incontinence when clients cannot get to the bathroom quickly enough. Others may think that two pills are twice as effective as one; some older adults take medication that is leftover from a previous illness or take a drug that has been prescribed for someone else.

Health care providers can influence the attitudes of older adults toward their medications and their health problems. One method being tried in some hospitals and nursing homes is supervised drug self-administration, in which clients are allowed to take their own medications under supervision. In this way, the nurse can be sure of a client's understanding and ability to self-administer medications at home or in another health care setting.

TABLE 5-1 Common Adverse Drug Reactions in Older Adults

▪ Edema	▪ Dizziness
▪ Nausea and vomiting	▪ Urinary retention
▪ Anorexia	▪ Diarrhea
▪ Dry mouth	▪ Constipation
▪ Fatigue	▪ Confusion
▪ Weakness	

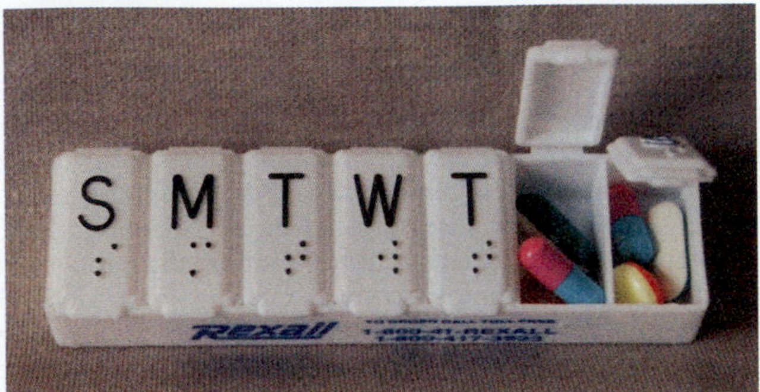

Figure 5-2 ▪ A medication system for safe self-administration.

Mental Health/Behavioral Health

Most older adults are mentally sound and competent. A few changes in cognition have been identified as age related and are linked to specific cognitive functions rather than intellectual capacity. These changes include a decreased reaction time to stimuli and an impairment of memory for recent events. However, gross cognitive impairment, depression, hallucinations, and delusions are not part of the normal aging process.

Two forms of competence exist: legal competence and clinical competence. A person is **legally competent** if he or she is:

- 18 years of age or older
- Pregnant or a married minor
- A legally emancipated (free) minor who is self-supporting
- Not declared incompetent by a court of law

If a court determines that a person is not legally competent, a guardian is appointed to make financial and health care decisions.

A person is **clinically competent** if he or she is legally competent and has decisional capacity. Decisional capacity is determined by an individual's ability to identify problems, recognize options, make decisions, and provide the rationale supporting the decisions.

It is not surprising that mental illness does occur among the older population. Losses in income and physical health, a lack of comprehensive health care and social services, a loss of social roles, and the death of significant others may affect a person's emotional stability. Older adults are often unaware of early symptoms of emotional or mental impairments. Their symptoms may go unnoticed by family and friends and thus progress until crisis results. The three most common cognitive problems among older adults are depression, dementia, and delirium.

DEPRESSION

Depression, the most common mental health/behavioral health disorder among older adults, is a response to multiple life stresses, a single situation (situational depression), a primary disorder, or a problem associated with dementia. It can range from mild, transient feelings of sadness to a severe sense of helplessness and hopelessness. Depression is thought to result from a lack of the neurotransmitters norepinephrine and serotonin in the brain. It is often underdiagnosed by physicians and is therefore undertreated (Kurlowicz, 2003).

Families and nurses are often in a position to suspect depression in an older adult. Several screening tools are available to help determine if the client has clinical depression. The Geriatric Depression Scale–Short Form (GDS-SF) is commonly used and completed by the client. A score of 11 or greater is consistent with a diagnosis of clinical depression (Kurlowicz, 2003).

Without diagnosis and subsequent treatment, depression can result in the following:

- Worsening of medical conditions
- Risk of physical illness
- Alcoholism
- Increased pain and disability
- Delayed recovery from illness
- Suicide (especially among older men)

Older adults have the highest suicide rate of any age-group (Uncapher & Arean, 2000). In their study, Uncapher and Arean (2000) sent two case studies of suicidal, depressed clients to primary care physicians to determine if any bias in treatment would be present. The two cases were the same except for age–one client was age 38 years and the other was age 78 years. The 215 physician responses showed that all providers recognized the depression and suicide risk but were less willing to treat the older client. They believed that suicidal ideation was normal for the older client.

CULTURAL CONSIDERATIONS

White men older than 70 years of age, especially those living alone, are at the highest risk for suicide. Older adults contemplating suicide usually do not talk about their plans and choose a method that will ensure death (e.g., a gunshot).

Elders with depression may experience early morning insomnia, excessive daytime sleeping, poor appetite, a lack of energy, and an unwillingness to participate in social and recreational activities. The primary treatment for depression usually includes drug therapy and psychotherapy. In some parts of the country, electroconvulsive therapy (ECT) may be used either as a last resort or when drugs are not effective.

Selective serotonin reuptake inhibitors (SSRIs) are the first choice for drug therapy, but take 2 to 3 weeks to work. They act by increasing the amount of serotonin and norepinephrine at neuronal synapses in the brain. More information about depression is available in mental health/behavioral health nursing textbooks.

DEMENTIA

Dementia is a broad term used for a syndrome that is characterized by a slowly progressive cognitive decline. Formerly called organic brain syndrome (OBS) and chronic brain syndrome (CBS), dementia represents a global impairment of intellectual function and is generally chronic and progressive. There are many types of dementia, the most common being Alzheimer's disease. Multi-infarct dementia, the second most common dementia, is a vascular disorder and accounts for 20% to 25% of all dementias. Chapter 45 discusses dementias in detail, with a focus on Alzheimer's disease.

DELIRIUM

Whereas dementia is a chronic, progressive disorder, **delirium** is an acute state of confusion. Delirium also differs from dementia in that it is usually short-term and reversible within 3 weeks. It is often seen among older adults in a hospital setting or in a setting with which they are unfamiliar. Behavior typically fits into one of two categories: hyperactivity (most common) or hypoactivity (Ignatavicius, 1999). Hyperactive clients may try to climb out of bed or pull out invasive catheters (e.g., urinary catheters or intravenous cannulas), or they may become quite agitated and combative. Hypoactive clients are quiet, apathetic, and withdrawn. Wakefield (2002) found that most nurses in her study did not realize that acutely confused older adults can be quiet.

Multiple factors can cause delirium, including the following:

- Medication (especially anticholinergic drugs)
- Metabolic disturbances
- Infections
- Surgical operations
- Circulatory, renal, and pulmonary disorders
- Nutritional deficiencies
- Major loss

Acutely confused clients who are discharged from the hospital are at an increased risk for functional decline, falls, and incontinence (Wakefield, 2002). Therefore nurses should assess older clients for acute confusion. A number of assessment tools have been developed, including the Confusion Assessment Method (CAM), Delirium Rating Scale (DRS), and NEECHAM Confusion Scale. Although the CAM is easy to use (Table 5-2), Rapp et al. (2000) found that the most useful tool was the nurse-developed NEECHAM Confusion Scale (see the Evidence-Based Practice for Nursing box on p. 48).

TABLE 5-2 The Confusion Assessment Method (CAM)

1. Acute onset and fluctuating course (e.g., Is there evidence of an acute change in mental status from the client's baseline?)
2. Inattention (e.g., Does the client have difficulty focusing attention or keeping track of what is being said?)
3. Disorganized thinking (e.g., Is the client's thinking and conversation disorganized or incoherent?)
4. Altered level of consciousness (e.g., Is the client lethargic, hyperalert, or difficult to arouse?)

The diagnosis of delirium by the CAM is the presence of features 1 *and* 2 and either 3 *or* 4.

To manage delirium, use a calm voice to reorient the client and to divert the client's attention away from devices or tubes. A number of innovative nursing interventions have been used with some success. For example, playing tapes of soothing music in the client's room may have a calming effect. Giving the client a doll or stuffed animal to "fidget" with may prevent the client from removing important medical instrumentation. Some nurses believe that providing dolls and stuffed animals is treating the adult like a child, but this intervention can sometimes be very effective when used for therapeutic purposes. If the client has a favorite item, such as an afghan blanket or a picture, the nurse asks the family or significant others to provide it for the same purpose.

EVIDENCE-BASED PRACTICE for Nursing

Which tool is best for nurses to use when assessing clients who are acutely confused?

Rapp, C.G., et al. (2000). Acute confusion assessment instruments: Clinical versus research usability. *Applied Nursing Research, 13*(1), 37-45.

Acute confusion (AC), also known as delirium, is a common problem seen by nurses in a variety of health care settings. This study examined five AC assessment tools—Confusion Assessment Method (CAM), Delirium Rating Scale (DRS), Delirium Symptom Inventory (DSI), Mini-Mental State Examination (MMSE), and Neelon/Champagne (NEECHAM) Confusion Scale—to determine the most reliable indicator of acute confusion. The researchers also asked evaluators to identify which tool was the easiest to use. The NEECHAM tool was unanimously selected because it specifically assesses for AC and identifies both at-risk clients and those who actually have AC. They also liked the CAM because it was linked to the criteria for delirium as listed in the *Diagnostic and Statistical Manual,* 4th edition (DSM-IV). A protocol that includes both tools was written, and nurses from the authors' health care system have been trained in its use for screening clients.

Level of Evidence: 6—Poorly controlled study, but helps to validate the use of the CAM.

Critique. The authors evaluated tools that had already been tested for reliability and validity and applied them for use in the practice setting. The NEECHAM tool, the only nurse-designed tool, was selected by the raters. Other authors have reported that this tool can be incorporated into daily practice.

Implications for Nursing. This study validated that nurses need to assess for AC using a standardized screening method, especially for older adults. Early identification of delirium alerts the health care team to the need for modifications in the client's plan of care.

Table 5-3 briefly differentiates delirium and dementia and lists the major nursing considerations for each. The most difficult challenge is caring for a client who is experiencing both problems at the same time.

Elder Neglect and Abuse

Another problem sometimes encountered by older adults is neglect and abuse, both verbal and physical. Some older adults are vulnerable to these problems, especially widowed women who may have difficulty being assertive. Older persons who are neglected or abused are often physically dependent. The abuser is often a family member who becomes frustrated or distraught over the burden of caring for the older adult.

Prolonged caregiving by a family member is a new and unexpected role for adult children, most often women. This new role may result in role fatigue and role conflict. Caregiver Role Strain and Risk for Caregiver Role Strain were added to the list of nursing diagnoses approved by the North American Nursing Diagnosis Association (NANDA). From their research, McCloskey and Bulechek (2000) identified Caregiver Support as a major nursing intervention (Chart 5-5).

Gray-Vickery (2000) described four common types of abuse:

- **Neglect** occurs when a caregiver fails to provide for a client's basic needs, such as food, clothing, or assistance with activities of daily living (ADLs). Whether intentional or unintentional, neglect accounts for almost half of all cases of actual elder abuse.
- **Physical abuse** is the use of physical force that results in bodily injury, especially in the "bathing suit" zone (abdomen, buttocks, genital area, upper thighs). Examples of physical abuse include hitting, burning, pushing, and molesting the client. Approximately one fourth of all cases of actual elder abuse involve physical force.
- **Financial abuse** occurs when the client's property or resources are mismanaged or misused; this is more common than physical abuse.
- **Emotional abuse** is the intentional use of threats, humiliation, intimidation, and isolation toward older adults. It occurs in more than one third of all cases of actual elder abuse.

TABLE 5-3 Differences in the Characteristics of Delirium and Dementia

Variable	Dementia	Delirium
Description	A chronic, progressive cognitive decline	An acute confusional state
Onset	Slow	Fast
Duration	Months to years	Hours to less than 1 month
Cause	Unknown, possibly familial, chemical	Multiple, such as surgery, infection, drugs
Reversibility	None	Usually
Management	Treat signs and symptoms	Remove or treat the cause
Nursing interventions	Reorientation not effective in the late stages; use validation therapy (acknowledge the client's feelings and do not argue); provide a safe environment; observe for associated behaviors, such as delusions and hallucinations	Reorient the client to reality; provide a safe environment

Carefully assess the client for signs of abuse, such as bruises in clusters or regular patterns; burns, commonly to the buttocks or the soles of the feet; unusual hair loss; or multiple injuries, especially fractures. If the older adult is too weak or has no other resources or support systems, he or she may not acknowledge that the abuse is occurring. Neglect may be manifested by pressure ulcers, contractures, dehydration or undernutrition, urine burns, excessive body odor, and listlessness (Gray-Vickery, 1999). Dyer et al. (2000) found that depression and dementia were common in community elders who were abused or neglected.

If physical abuse or neglect is suspected, notify the physician and social worker to investigate the situation. All states in the United States and other Western countries have laws requiring health care professionals to report suspected elder abuse.

ECONOMIC ISSUES FOR OLDER ADULTS

Income

Most adults hope to provide for their own needs throughout their life cycle. One of the greatest fears related to aging is becoming dependent on family, friends, or society. In many cases, older adults have not achieved economic self-sufficiency. One fifth of the total population of the United States is poor, and one fifth of the poor are older than age 65 years.

Most individuals expect their financial resources to decline in their retirement years compared with their working years. They also expect their level of expenses to decline, but this may not occur. In the United States, for example, the inflation that began in the 1970s has reduced the value of financial assets. Older adults have been especially hard hit because most rely on Social Security benefits or pension funds for the bulk of their income. Recent declines in the stock market as a result of terrorism and war have added to the reduction in assets. Many older adults are unable to adjust their income to changing economic circumstances and hence are powerless to combat declining real income.

Health care purchases are paid for in large part by private insurance and federal health and social programs. However, the rising cost of these programs contributes substantially to rising government costs and may result in more out-of-pocket costs for the older health care consumer. Health care costs for older adults is a major issue being debated in the United States by Congress and other political bodies. Many elders take multiple medications that are extremely expensive in the United States, but that can be sometimes obtained in other countries such as Canada and Mexico or ordered on the Internet. The quality of these drugs is not guaranteed, but older adults are looking for ways to comply with their treatment plan, while having enough money to meet their basic needs.

Housing

The popular belief that older adults are frail, dependent, senile individuals living out their last years in an institution has no factual basis. Many older adults live in their own homes and have paid off their mortgages. However, living arrangements are a major problem for some individuals as they age. This issue can increase the client's stress level and have an impact on health care planning.

In many countries, the rising costs of energy and housing have joined the high costs of food and health care as factors that contribute to the economic hardship of older adults. In addition to financial difficulties, housing may be a problem because of a lack of environmental supports that would help older adults to continue residing and participating in the community.

Deterioration of property, escalation of property taxes, and maintenance service costs create many problems for older homeowners wishing to keep their homes. In some areas, older renters are extremely vulnerable to high rents, real estate speculation, and the loss of living quarters because of the removal of substandard, low-rent apartment or hotel buildings. Physical impairments and a lack of available and affordable support services (e.g., household help, transportation, home health care, and meal assistance) prevent some older adults from managing adequately in their own homes.

The need for special housing for older adults has long been recognized. Numbers of government and privately funded experiments in alternative housing have been tested. These projects incorporate variables such as personal care services, special health and safety remedies, and recreation and leisure plans. Although most of these projects provide security, improve life satisfaction, and prove to be cost-effective, many areas of the United States have no overall plan for alternative living arrangements for older adults.

RESOURCES FOR OLDER ADULTS

In the United States, Canada, and other countries, a broad range of government benefits and services is available to assist older adults with problems related to income, health in-

CHART 5-5

NIC INTERVENTION ACTIVITIES for Caregiver Support

Caregiver Support: *Provision of the necessary information, advocacy, and support to facilitate primary client care by someone other than a health care professional.*

- Determine caregiver's level of knowledge.
- Determine caregiver's acceptance of role.
- Teach caregiver stress management techniques.
- Monitor for indicators of stress.
- Identify sources of respite care.
- Teach the caregiver health care maintenance strategies to sustain own physical and mental health.
- Encourage caregiver participation in support groups.
- Educate caregiver about the grieving process.
- Teach caregiver strategies to access and maximize health care and community resources.
- Foster caregiver social networking.

NIC intervention activities selected from Dochterman J.M., & Bulechek, G.M. (Eds.). (2004). *Nursing interventions classification (NIC)* (4th ed.). St. Louis: Mosby.

surance, housing, and social services. Teach older adults and their families about the types of services available to help them achieve a higher quality of life.

Government Resources

INCOME

In the United States, the major portion of federal funds that support programs for older adults is devoted to the Social Security program. The Social Security Act was passed in 1935, when many individuals were economically impoverished after the Depression. Since that time, there has been a gradual shift from a program intended to provide a minimal supplement to retirees' sources of income to one that is the primary source of retirement income for many individuals. Other provisions of this act that are significant for individuals younger than 65 years of age are the disability and survivors' insurance provisions.

HEALTH INSURANCE

Medicare is a federal health insurance program that was enacted as part of the amendments to the Social Security Act of 1965. This program was created to help older adults, individuals receiving dialysis, and disabled individuals of any age to meet the cost of health care. Despite its deficiencies, Medicare has provided a means for older adults to obtain needed health care in times of escalating costs without decimating their total personal savings.

Medicare provides health insurance to individuals 65 years of age and older and to qualified disabled individuals of any age. **Medicare A** primarily pays for most in-hospital care and is paid for by the federal government. It covers only a very small portion of the care required in long-term care and only minimal home care services. Many clients who are enrolled in Medicare are enrolled in managed care organizations (see Chapter 3). **Medicare B** is an optional insurance and requires payment of a monthly premium. Medicare B pays some of the outpatient costs associated with health care provider visits, medication, and home care services. Some older adults also pay for supplemental private insurance to cover what Medicare does not pay.

Medical assistance (Medicaid) is a program designed to provide payment for medical services for the poor, including older adults who are poor. This program supplements the Medicare insurance program for eligible adults 65 years of age and older. Eligibility is related to determination of poverty level, and each state program determines its own criteria for eligibility. A number of states have completed the transition to managed care for their Medicaid recipients.

HOUSING PROGRAMS

The U.S. Congress has passed a number of legislative acts designed to alleviate housing problems for older citizens. Among these programs is rental assistance for low-income families, older adults, and the disabled. Direct low-interest loans are available to individuals to construct special rental housing facilities. For information related to these housing programs, nurses can contact the local public housing authority or the Housing and Urban Development area office in most communities.

CHART 5-6

NURSING FOCUS on the OLDER ADULT

Social Services Provided by the Older Americans Act of 1965

- Senior centers to meet the need for a central place for older adults to congregate, develop new interests, and socialize
- Nutrition programs to provide nutritious meals in a centralized setting as well as to homebound older adults; recreation, education, and health activities incorporated in many sites as a regular part of the program
- Transportation services to accommodate older adults via special fares on existing public transportation systems and the operation of specially equipped vehicles for frail and handicapped older adults
- Information and referral services to direct older adults to the appropriate agency that provides needed services
- In-home services such as household help, telephone reassurance, chore maintenance, and visitation by home care aides to enable impaired older adults to remain living in the community

SOCIAL SERVICES

The Older Americans Act of 1965 provided social services to older adults. Under this legislation, each state created an office to provide leadership in the coordination and development of services for older adults (Office on Aging). Some of the more significant programs and services carried out under this legislation are described in Chart 5-6.

RESEARCH AGENCIES

The National Institute on Aging was established in 1974. Its purpose is to conduct research on the biologic, population-related, and sociologic aspects of aging at its Gerontology Research Center in Baltimore. It also supports research by others at universities and laboratories across the United States.

One division within the National Institute for Mental Health–the Center for Studies of the Mental Health of the Aging–is devoted exclusively to problems of older adults. Its major role is to stimulate, coordinate, and support research training and to offer technical assistance related to aging and mental health/behavioral health. Although it provides no money for programs of service delivery to older adults, it significantly affects the training of those working with older adults in community mental health/behavioral health centers and other service settings.

Community Resources

Over the years it has become evident that government programs cannot provide all of the services needed by older adults. In many areas, private efforts can supply the same services at lower costs and without the red tape involved with some government programs. Transportation is an area in which the private sector and local, state, and federal governments all have roles.

In many urban areas, governments have established Dial-A-Ride or similar services that provide free transportation. The federal government has subsidized the development and operation of transit systems, but the main focus of this aid has been on high-use systems and routes. For occasional travel, particularly in rural areas, the best solution may be for the older adult to rely on a friend or a neighbor. Churches and community groups often help organize this approach by using sign-up sheets and recruiting volunteers to drive each week.

Education, recreation, and cultural activities help maintain a person's physical condition, mental alertness, and social contact. Education helps older adults keep up with a rapidly changing world. Advances in the Internet and in cable and satellite television systems provide a broad range of new educational experiences at home. Nevertheless, the value of person-to-person discussion and the need to focus some educational activities on local issues means that community discussion groups and other informal education will remain important.

Churches and other religious institutions serve older adults in many ways. In addition to their primary role of providing organized worship, they sponsor many activities that bring individuals together with their peers as well as with younger individuals. Clergypersons and other spiritual leaders are often excellent counselors, and other members of the congregation or religious group are sometimes willing to help older members in time of trouble.

Most libraries have community resource books (e.g., those published by the United Way). Area agencies on aging are excellent referral centers. Some of these agencies publish directories of services that are specifically geared toward the older adult. The nurse can help to inform older clients about the community resources they may need depending on their specific life situation.

THE FUTURE OF GERONTOLOGIC NURSING

Nurses in most adult health care settings encounter the challenges of caring for both healthy and ill older adults. In view of the rapidly increasing older population, especially the over-85 age group, nurses in many settings are specializing in gerontologic nursing or geriatric case management. Nurses can practice these specialties in acute care, long-term care, and community-based settings.

Just as nurses can achieve certification in medical-surgical nursing, they can become certified in gerontologic nursing or case management. The American Nurses Credentialing Center (ANCC) provides three gerontology examinations for the certification of those who qualify: gerontologic nurse, gerontologic clinical specialist, and gerontologic nurse practitioner. The ANCC also offers a nursing case management examination that is broad based and not specific for geriatric case management. Other professional organizations also certify case managers, including geriatric case managers.

GET READY for the NCLEX Examination!

KEY POINTS

- The four subgroups of the older adult population are the young old, middle old, old old, and elite old.
- Relocation stress syndrome is the reaction of an older adult when transferred to a different environment; ways to minimize this problem are listed in Chart 5-1.
- Nutrition and physical fitness are two health problems experienced by older adults.
- The biggest concern regarding accidents among older adults in both the community and inpatient setting is falls.
- Risk factors and common nursing interventions to keep older adults from falling are listed in Chart 5-3.
- Physical and chemical restraints should not be used for older adults until all other alternatives have been tried.
- Physiologic changes of aging predispose older adults to toxic effects of medication; drugs are absorbed, metabolized, and distributed more slowly than in younger individuals. Medications are also excreted more slowly by the kidneys.
- Medication use in older adults is often a problem when they commit errors when self-medicating, avoid needed medications, or have problems understanding their medication regimen.
- Depression is the most common, yet most underdiagnosed and undertreated mental health/behavioral health disorder among older adults.
- Delirium is acute confusion that is short-lived; dementia is chronic confusion that progresses slowly and worsens. Table 5-3 compares these two health problems commonly seen in older adults.
- Elder neglect and abuse are serious problems; family caregivers are most commonly the abusers.
- The nurse and other health care professionals need to assess for signs of elder neglect and abuse; if suspected, it should be reported.
- Many older adults are not prepared for retirement in view of increased expenses and income that is not adequate to meet basic needs, health care treatments, and medications.
- The nurse and other health care professionals need to provide information regarding community resources for older adults to help them meet their basic needs.

ADDITIONAL STUDY RESOURCES

Go to your Student CD-ROM for Review Questions for the NCLEX Examination.

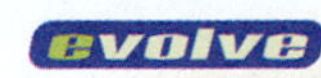

Go to http://evolve.elsevier.com/Iggy/ for Integrated Management of Care Questions for the NCLEX Examination.

SELECTED BIBLIOGRAPHY

Asterisk indicates a classic or definitive work on this subject.

Christmas, C., & Andersen, R.A. (2000). Exercise and older patients: Guidelines for the physician. *Journal of the American Geriatric Society, 48*(3), 318-324.

*Conley, D., Schultz, A.A., & Selvin, R. (1999). The challenge of predicting patients at risk for falling: Development of the Conley Scale. *MEDSURG Nursing: The Journal of Adult Health, 8*(6), 348-354.

Davidhizar, R., & Shearer, R. (2000). Helping elders adjust to losing autonomy. *The Journal of Care Management, 6*(1), 53-54, 69-72.

Davidhizar, R., Eshleman, J., & Moody, M. (2002). Health promotion in aging adults. *Geriatric Nursing, 23*(1), 28-35.

Dochterman, J.M., & Bulechek, G.M. (2004). *Nursing interventions classification (NIC)* (4th ed.). St. Louis: Mosby.

Dyer, C.B., et al. (2000). The high prevalence of depression and dementia in elder abuse or neglect. *Journal of the American Geriatric Society, 48*(2), 205-208.

*Gray-Vickery, P. (1999). Recognizing elder abuse. *Nursing99, 29*(9), 52-63.

Gray-Vickery, P. (2000). Protecting the older adult. *Nursing2000, 30*(7), 34-37.

*Hammond, M., & Levine, J.M. (1999). Bedrails: Choosing the best alternative. *Geriatric Nursing, 20*(6), 297-301.

*Ignatavicius, D.D. (1998). *Introduction to long-term care: Principles and practice.* Philadelphia: F.A. Davis.

*Ignatavicius, D.D. (1999). Resolving the delirium dilemma. *Nursing99, 29*(10), 41-47.

Ignatavicius, D. (2000). Do you help staff rise to the fall-prevention challenge? *Nursing Management, 31*(1), 27-30.

Jacelon, C.S. (2002). Attitudes and behaviors of hospital staff toward elders in an acute care setting, *Applied Nursing Research, 15*(4), 227-234.

Juarbe, T., Turok, X.P., & Perez-Stable, E.J. (2002). Perceived benefits and barriers to physical activity among Latina women. *Western Journal of Nursing Research, 24*(8), 868-886.

Kurlowicz, L.H. (2003). Depression in older adults. In M.D. Mezey, T. Fulmer, & I. Abraham (Eds.), *Geriatric nursing protocols for best practice* (pp. 185-205). New York: Springer.

Loeb, S.J. (2003). The older men's health program and screening inventory: A tool for assessing health practices and beliefs. *Geriatric Nursing, 24*(4), 278-285.

Loeb, S.J., Penrod, J., Falkenstern, S., et al. (2003). Supporting older adults living with multiple chronic conditions. *Western Journal of Nursing Research, 25*(1), 8-29.

McCloskey, J.C., & Bulechek, G.M. (2000). *Nursing interventions classification (NIC)* (3rd ed.). St. Louis: Mosby.

Napierkowski, D. (2002). Using restraints with restraint. *Nursing2002, 32*(1), 58-63.

North American Nursing Diagnosis Association International. (2003). *Nursing diagnoses: Definitions and classification 2003-2004.* Philadelphia: NANDA International.

Rapp, C.G., et al. (2000). Acute confusion assessment instruments: Clinical versus research usability. *Applied Nursing Research, 13*(1), 37-45.

Resnick, B. (2003). Preventing falls in acute care. In M.D. Mezey, T. Fulmer, & I. Abraham (Eds.), *Geriatric nursing protocols for best practice* (pp. 141-164). New York: Springer.

*Schiavento, M. (1997). The Hispanic elderly: Implications for nursing care. *Journal of Gerontological Nursing, 23*(6), 10-15.

Stevens, J.A., & Olson, S. (2000). Reducing falls and resulting hip fractures among older women. *Morbidity and Mortality Weekly Report, 49*(RR02), 1-12.

Taggart, H.M. (2002). Effects of Tai Chi exercise on balance, functional mobility, and fear of falling among older women. *Applied Nursing Research, 15*(4), 235-242.

Theodus, P. (2003). Fall prevention in frail elderly nursing home residents. A challenge to case management: Part I. *Lippincott's Case Management, 8*(6), 246-251.

Uncapher, H., & Arean, P.A. (2000). Physicians are less willing to treat suicidal ideation in older patients. *Journal of the American Geriatric Society, 48*(2), 188-192.

Wakefield, B.J. (2002). Behaviors and outcomes of acute confusion in hospitalized patients. *Applied Nursing Research, 15*(4), 209-216.

Wells, D.L., & Dawson, P. (2000). Description of retained abilities in older persons with dementia. *Research in Nursing and Health Care, 23*(2), 158-166.

UNIT **TWO**

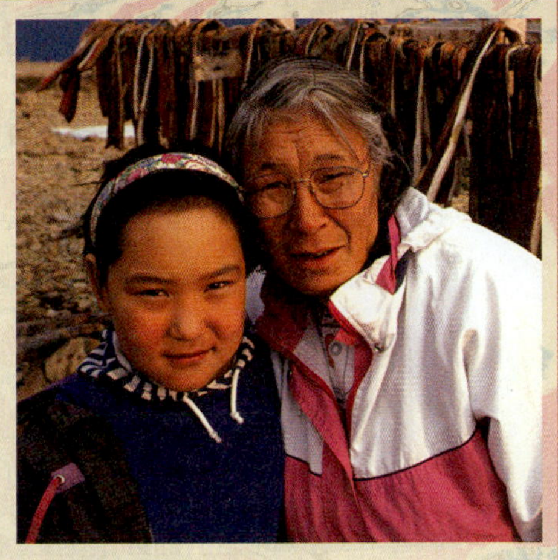

BIOPSYCHOSOCIAL CONCEPTS RELATED to HEALTH CARE

CHAPTER

6 Cultural Aspects of Health

MICHELLE M. BYRNE

LEARNING OUTCOMES

After studying this chapter, you should be able to:

1. Define culture, cultural competence, cultural awareness, and ethnocentrism.
2. Explain the purpose and nursing implications of Healthy People 2010 as related to culture.
3. Identify common factors related to cultural assessment.
4. Describe three methods for cultural assessment.
5. Identify and describe three cultural groups that have often been neglected.
6. Discuss specific cultural practices, such as religion, nutrition, and folk medicine, that the nurse should consider when assessing a client's culture.
7. Describe ways that nurses can communicate sensitively with clients from various cultural groups.

Go to your Student CD-ROM for Review Questions for the NCLEX Examination keyed to these Learning Outcomes.

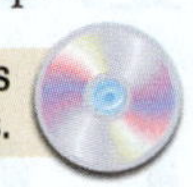

This century, population diversity is rapidly increasing throughout the world. As a result of the Internet, foreign travel, and global industrialization, there is more interaction between different individuals of the world. A myriad of societies and citizens have their own way of doing things and interacting with others, often with unique beliefs and practices. Although there are cultural similarities among many individuals in specific cultures, there are also diverse groups within each culture. As a nurse, cultural diversity is embedded in the relationships with your clients as well as with your coworkers in the workplace setting (Anderson et al., 2003).

THE NEED FOR CULTURAL CONSIDERATIONS OF HEALTH

Many individuals from differing cultures continue to immigrate to North America in large numbers, bringing new and different ideas with them. These individuals have various cultural needs based on their ethnicity, background, and immigration status. According to the U.S. Census Bureau, the estimated figures for the U.S. population in 2000 showed the following percentages for several large cultural groups:

- European Americans: 71.5%
- African Americans: 12.2%
- Hispanics: 12.6%
- Asian Americans/Pacific Islanders: 3.8%

In 2000, the number of minority populations in the United States accounted for 28% of the total population. It is estimated that minority groups are an emerging majority and will make up 43.8% of the population by 2050. This diversity makes culturally sensitive health care imperative.

The U.S. government has an initiative for health care workers and organizations to become culturally competent. There are many definitions for cultural competence. In 2000, the U.S. Department of Health and Human Services (DHHS) developed a widely recognized definition. **Cultural competence** is the ability of health care providers and organizations to understand and respond effectively to the cultural and linguistic needs that clients bring to the health care setting. Among other standards to achieve cultural competence, the DHHS made several suggestions for health care organizations. First, organizations are to ensure that staff members are trained to work respectfully and effectively with clients in culturally diverse health care environments. Second, organizations are to develop procedures to address cross-cultural ethical and legal conflicts in health care delivery, such as culturally insensitive or discriminatory treatment; difficulty in accessing service; or denial of services. For these reasons, the term **cultural sensitivity** is sometimes used to describe the way that one responds to cultural differences.

HEALTHY PEOPLE 2010

Another program created by the U.S. Department of Health and Human Services (2000) is **Healthy People 2010.** The goal by 2010 is to eliminate the differences in six areas of health status experienced by racial and ethnic minorities while trying to continually improve the overall health of all American individuals. The target areas are the following:

- Infant mortality
- Cancer screening and management
- Cardiovascular disease
- Diabetes mellitus
- Human immunodeficiency virus (HIV) infection/acquired immunodeficiency syndrome (AIDS)
- Immunizations

This goal is to be met through research, preventive programs, and inclusion of members of minority groups.

Currently there are significant differences in health and health care access for ethnic or racial groups as compared to the dominant European American group in the United States. The reasons for these differences include the following (Baldwin, 2003; Freire, 2002):

- Poor socioeconomic status
- Health beliefs and behaviors
- Access to health care
- Environmental factors
- Direct and indirect manifestations of discrimination
- Lack of health insurance
- Insufficient transportation
- Geographic location
- Cost of services
- Language barriers

Oftentimes, complex issues such as racism, "classism," ageism, and sexism are embedded in disparities in health care but ignored due to lack of knowledge or awareness by members of the health care team.

CULTURE AND NURSING

Diverse values, beliefs, and practices impact health, illness, professional health care, and folk health care. Nursing has a long history of addressing the physical and emotional needs of individual clients, and currently there is an increased emphasis on taking care of cultural needs. Therefore nurses and nursing students must learn to integrate cultural considerations as part of holistic client care (Figure 6-1).

Definition of Culture

A dictionary definition of **culture** suggests that it is an integrated pattern of human behavior that includes thought, speech, action, and artifacts. Culture is learned and transmitted to succeeding generations. Culture can include things such as language, art, morals, laws, appearance, customs, rituals, technology, economics, and kinship or family systems.

Many individuals in a culture, especially older individuals, spend years teaching about the importance of keeping the traditions of their culture. Beliefs and rituals often vary within a culture, especially when it is made up of distinct subcultures. An example is the Native American population, which consists of many subcultures, or councils, across the United States. For instance, the Lakota Council is made up of several tribes that have specific customs. These customs differ from those of other groups of Native Americans. According to several treaties between the Lakotas and the U.S. government, the Lakotas are American Indians, not Native Americans. For that reason, many Lakotas and other related subcultures refer to themselves as American Indian because that is their legal designated name (Personal communication, Ogala Lakota College, Pine Ridge, SD, August 6, 2003).

Implications for Nursing Practice

Culture also influences health and nursing care. It influences the way individuals think about health, the ways in which they express pain, what they consider to be symptoms, how they seek and accept help and care, and who they consider to be healers. Madeline Leininger, a nurse anthropologist and theorist, has provided a large body of knowledge integrating nursing care and cultural care.

In the 1950s Leininger combined culture and nursing into a new field called **transcultural nursing.** She developed the theory of Culture Care Diversity and Universality. She specified that transcultural nursing is an area of study and practice that focuses on the care, health, and illness patterns of individuals with similarities and differences in their cultural beliefs, values, and practices. The practice of transcultural nurses

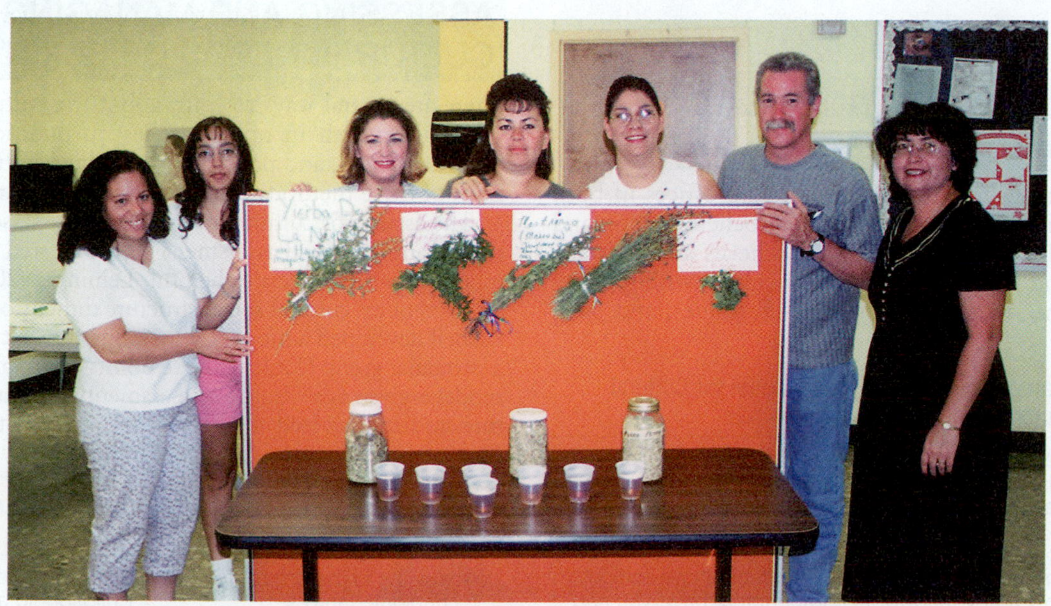

Figure 6-1 ■ Nursing students in an associate degree program learning about the value of herbs for healing in the southwestern part of the United States. (Courtesy Luna Vocational Technical Institute, Las Vegas, NM.)

is to provide care that considers the cultural aspects of the client (Leininger, 2002). Over time, other nurses have become proficient in the field of cultural care, including Andrews, Boyle, Campinha-Bacote, Douglas, Purnell, and Spector.

Cultural considerations should certainly be integrated in the nursing care of all clients. Individuals have diverse needs in health care and may fall into various categories. For example, cultural differences exist between residents of urban and rural areas as well as differing geographic sections of the country. Furthermore, how recently a person has immigrated to the United States can provide insight into cultural variations.

Differences are also found related to age, gender, and sexual orientation. Therefore, it is important that nurses and other health care professionals examine their beliefs and biases about cultural differences (Byrne, 2001, 2002; Byrne et al., 2003). How do you feel about individuals different than yourself? Too often, the term "different" has negative connotations. One of the foundations for becoming culturally competent as a nurse is to examine personal beliefs and biases (Campinha-Bacote, 2001, 2002; Byrne, 2001, 2002; Byrne et al. 2003).

Campinha-Bacote's model of cultural competence includes personal awareness, knowledge, skill, encounters, and desire (Table 6-1). **Cultural awareness** is defined as "the process through which the nurse becomes respectful, appreciative, and sensitive to the values, beliefs, lifeways, practices and problem-solving strategies of a client's culture" (p. 8, 2001). Cultural awareness also includes an examination of one's own prejudice and bias. This awareness is not always easy, in that there is a tendency to be blind to our bias, or ethnocentric in our perspectives. **Ethnocentrism** is the judging of others through the exclusive lens of one's own cultural beliefs. Ethnocentrism has been found to negatively affect client care (Sutherland, 2002). Therefore, explicit examples of bias, stereotypes, and our assumptions may assist health care providers in becoming less ethnocentric in their practice (Byrne, 2001, 2002; Byrne et al., 2003; Sutherland, 2002).

THE CULTURE OF THE HEALTH CARE SYSTEM

Hospitals, nursing homes, and health care offices in both public and private sectors have cultural beliefs, values, and practices, as do nursing programs in schools and universities. Nurses and physicians make up a culture within themselves according to their unique beliefs, values, and practices. If diversity is synonymous with difference, then health care professionals must realize that, if we view a client as different, then a client views us as different as well. Nurses are members of a culture in the health care system. Because each of us has been socialized into the health care team, there are values and belief systems that we hold near and dear to our hearts. We may believe some things so strongly that we do not see our opinions as a value system.

Beliefs can be defined as ideas that a person accepts as true. One belief of health care professionals is a belief of standardization (Spector, 2000). Standardization is implemented through competency statements, policies, procedures, forms, care plans, orders, flow sheets, and critical pathways. Standardization is even embedded in our schooling as we learn via competencies and measurable objectives. However, an emphasis on objectivity and standardization may minimize creativity and individuality.

Another common cultural characteristic found in the health care system is neatness, cleanliness, and timeliness. Disorderliness and disorganization are two attributes that are not highly prized in the health care arena. In addition, perspectives of time among health care workers are future-oriented. Immunizations and prevention measures are directed at minimizing future illnesses. Some cultural groups may blame previous behaviors on present problems or only address health problems that are adversely affecting them at the moment.

Other customs of our health care system is the medicalization of the birthing and dying process. Due to urbanization, reimbursement mandates, and advances in technology, these events usually take place in a hospital setting. Many non-Western cultures do not have the same emphasis on medical intervention during the birth or death of a loved one. It is important to examine the health care culture and determine how our clients may perceive our practices, language, and behaviors as different to bridge cultural differences.

TABLE 6-1 Campinha-Bacote's Asked Model for Cultural Competence

Awareness: Are you aware of your personal biases and prejudices towards cultures different than yours?
Skill: Do you have the skill to conduct a cultural assessment and perform a culturally based physical assessment?
Knowledge: Do you have knowledge of the patient's world view, cultural bound illnesses, and the field of biocultural ecology?
Encounters: How many face-to-face encounters have you had with patients from diverse cultural backgrounds?
Desire: What is your desire to "want to be" culturally competent?

Courtesy of Dr. Josie Campinha-Bacote, expert in cultural nursing.

ASSESSING AND MANAGING THE CULTURAL NEEDS OF CLIENTS

There are several ways to learn about the culture of clients. Cultural research in nursing relies on questioning clients, observing them, and participating in their cultural activities. Each of these methods can also be used in nursing practice.

The aspects of culture that need to be assessed depend on the situation. Several assessment guides created by expert cultural nurses are especially helpful. Leininger (2002) bases her assessment on cultural social structure dimensions (Table 6-2). Purnell developed a model for assessing the cultural aspects of a particular group (Table 6-3). He points out that, although the model is given as a whole for assessment, the situation and culture studied may lead the health care provider to concentrate

TABLE 6-2 Leininger's Factors for Assessing Cultural Groups or Persons

- Worldview of the group
- Technologic factors
- Kinship and social factors
- Economic factors
- Cultural values and lifeways
- Philosophic and religious factors
- Political and legal factors
- Educational factors

on one area before another. In a very religious community, for example, the provider may want to start the assessment with spirituality rather than with another domain.

Many of the same factors are found in various assessment models. Nurses should adapt and integrate assessment models that are most appropriate for their clinical practice arena and types of cultural groups being cared for.

Performing a Cultural Assessment

The three major methods for assessing the culture of a client include observation, interview, and participation. The health care setting often determines the order in which these methods are used.

OBSERVATION

A cultural assessment in the home starts with the observation phase. For example, what are the neighborhood and geographic areas in which the client and family live (Figure 6-2)? Is the street in front of the house a busy one, or is it in a more rural area? Is public transportation available, or do residents have their own cars? Going into the client's house, the nurse observes for Bibles, religious books, and religious symbols on the walls or tables. Evidence of technology, such as air-conditioning, televisions, telephones, kitchen appliances, and computers, is noted. The interactions and communication patterns among family members are also observed.

TABLE 6-3 Purnell's Factors for Assessing Cultural Groups or Persons

■ Nutrition	■ Heritage
■ Communication	■ Pregnancy and childbirth
■ Family roles	■ Death rituals
■ Work issues	■ Spirituality
■ Biocultural ecology	■ Health care practices
■ High-risk behaviors	■ Folk health practices

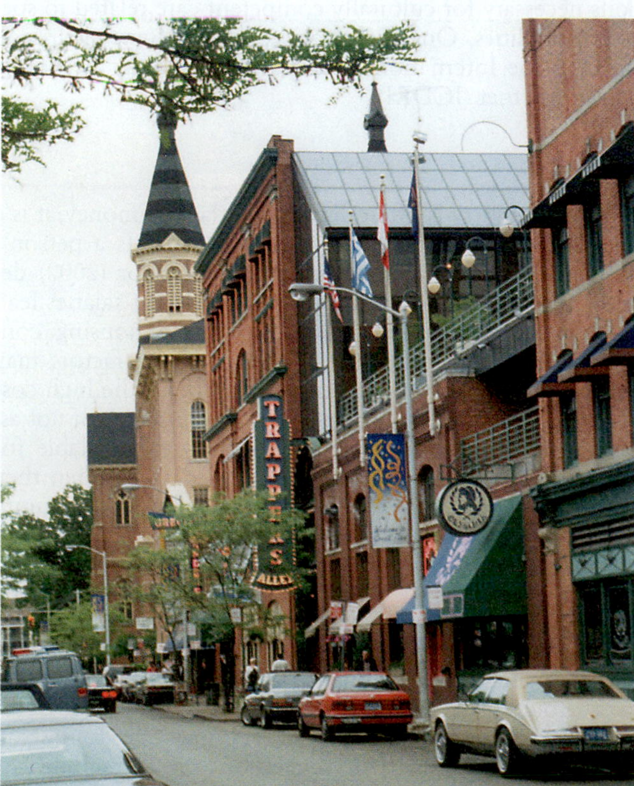

Figure 6-2 ■ Community assessment of Greektown in Detroit, Michigan.

INTERVIEW

Following observation, you should interview the client and possibly the family. Nurses often obtain health histories from their clients, and cultural interviewing is only slightly different. The best questions for cultural interviews are semi-structured and open-ended questions. The nurse usually has an interview guide or an outline for the questions. Spector (2000) has identified nine suggestions for enhancing communication when gathering cultural data:

- Determine the level of fluency in English and arrange for an interpreter if needed.
- Ask how the client prefers to be addressed.
- Allow the client to choose seating for comfortable personal space and eye contact.
- Avoid body language that may be offensive or misunderstood.
- Speak directly to the client, whether an interpreter is present or not.
- Choose a speech rate and style that promotes understanding and demonstrates respect for the client.
- Avoid slang technical jargon and complex sentences.
- Use open-ended questions or questions phrased in several ways to obtain information.
- Determine the client's reading ability before using written materials in the teaching process.

A good interviewer will often deviate from the form if the client shows interest in a particular question. Often more details are learned in such a circumstance. A large amount of information can usually be gleaned from actively listening to a client, whether during an interview or at any other time.

PARTICIPATION

Participation is the third method of collecting data for a cultural assessment. This process is very helpful for understanding a particular cultural population rather than assessing just one client. For example, a nurse may begin working in a community that has had an influx of Hispanic immigrants. To better understand some of the cultural needs of the individual, he or she may begin participating in the community activities.

Trips to local churches can provide insight into the religious life of a culture. Many ethnic communities have festivals with crafts, foods, music, and clothing. Political rallies may also be a good place to interact and learn the beliefs of groups. Similarly, markets held in the community tell a lot about the buying and social habits of a group.

In preparing a cultural assessment, put together the information gathered from the cultural group or from the client about the lifestyles, general beliefs and practices and, specifically, health care beliefs. Cultural data should be integrated in all phases of the nursing process.

Developing the Cultural Care Plan

Use the data gathered about a client or clients from a particular culture to plan, implement, and evaluate culturally competent care. Leininger (2002) has suggested one way of planning cultural care for a client, and this method is used by many nurses. She uses three modes for planning care:

- *Culture care preservation or maintenance* is a way to help "people of a particular culture to retain or preserve relevant care values so they can maintain and/or preserve their well-being, recover from illness, or face handicaps and/or death."
- *Culture care accommodation or negotiation* refers to "professional actions and decisions that help people of a designated culture adapt to or negotiate with others for a beneficial or satisfying health outcome with professional care providers."
- *Culture care repatterning or restructuring* helps clients to "reorder, change or greatly modify their lifeways . . . providing a lifeway more beneficial or healthier than before the changes were co-established with the clients."

Research Applications

It is important for nurses to research the specific health and illness practices for specific cultural groups. One study examined the motivation, health beliefs, and access barriers experienced by older minority women in keeping mammography appointments (Bernstein, Mutschler, & Bernstein, 2000). Minority women have a high mortality rate associated with breast cancer and low rates of routine mammography. The study sample contained mostly African-American women, but also included European American, Hispanic, and Haitian participants. The method used was peer interaction with the participants to educate them about breast health, and offered them a no-cost, next-day appointment for a mammogram. Researchers also assessed their willingness to change behavior. Sixty percent of the study group kept their appointments or had a mammogram within 3 months. According to the authors, the success of the program resulted from the following: (1) the interaction between the women and culturally competent peers who offered education, (2) the use of interpreters for non–English-speaking participants, and (3) the fact that the women in the study group were treated as experts in telling their own experiences and stories related to breast health.

In addition to researching cultural groups, research has explored how nurses respond to the cultural needs of their clients. For example, a sample of 126 United Kingdom registered nurses completed questionnaires that pertained to cultural care (Narayanasamy, 2003). These nurses practiced mostly in adult acute care settings and agreed that their clients presented with cultural needs (80%). However, most nurses focused their cultural assessments and interventions only on religious and dietary practices. The major barriers for culturally focused care identified by this group of nurses was language difficulties, especially the utilization of resources for translation services.

SPECIAL CONSIDERATIONS FOR SELECTED CULTURAL GROUPS

A person's characteristics may be embedded in different cultural groups. For example, there are disabled individuals with Greek-American backgrounds whose cultural care plans would include ethnic and disability characteristics. The same might be true of a lesbian client who is African American. She would need attentive care for her sexual orientation as well as for her ethnicity. Three specific groups in our society–disabled individuals, impoverished persons, and those with diverse sexual orientations–originate from diverse ethnic backgrounds, yet must be assessed from a variety of cultural aspects.

Disability

Disabilities are physical as well as emotional. Some disabilities are visible; others are not. Some disabilities are acquired from various illnesses, conditions, and accidents, whereas others are a result of developmental problems. There are, however, some common themes that describe cultures of individuals with disabilities.

Individuals with disabilities are members of the largest minority group in the United States. Approximately 15% to 20% of U.S. residents have a disabling condition that impacts their life activities (Lipson & Rogers, 2000). Disability activists have argued that health care providers lack knowledge regarding the social nature of disability. Cultural competence must be broadened to include this group (Lipson & Rogers, 2000). Students and nurses should familiarize themselves with the Americans with Disabilities Act, which addresses employment, public services, public accommodations, and telecommunications for these individuals.

It is important for health care professionals to assess their personal attitudes and biases toward clients with disabilities. Nurses can use literature searches to identify specific organizations to assist them in acquiring the knowledge and skills necessary for culturally competent care related to specific disabilities. One such website is http://www.icdri.org, which is the International Center for Disability Resources on the Internet (ICDRI).

Poverty

Although poverty is often defined as a lack of money, it is a much more complex phenomenon that affects a person's health, well-being, and access to care. Spector (2000) describes a cycle of poverty in which insufficient salaries lead to poor nutrition, and densely populated housing contributes to a high incidence of illness. These factors may contribute to a lack of preventive care due to the high cost of health care services. A nurse must be conscious of not assuming that adequate financial resources are available for transportation, prescription, or medical devices when they are not. It is important to be aware of the local community resources for client referral when clients cannot afford nutritious meals, necessary medication, or health care services.

Sexual Orientation

Sexual orientation can influence the delivery of cultural care to a group of individuals. Spinks, Andrews, and Boyle (2000) discuss the provision of cultural care to lesbian clients, but many of their suggestions could include gay men. Unlike a group in which the language, dress, or country of residence give some clue to the culture, the identification of someone in a lesbian or gay community may be more difficult. The nurse may assume incorrectly that a client is heterosexual and thus not provide the unique health care that is needed. A lack of therapeutic communication, along with bias of the health care professional, is often present.

A gay or lesbian client has similar physical health needs in screening and health promotion as most clients but may also have unique issues that need to be addressed. Some examples include whether to have children through adoption, artificial insemination, or intentional heterosexual contact. Substance abuse may be an ineffective coping mechanism because of the inherent stresses in feeling the need to hide one's sexual orientation due societal intolerance. One group in a large city took a proactive role in providing culturally competent care by forming a Feminist Women's Health Center to meet the needs of all women, including lesbian clients (Spinks, Andrews, & Boyle, 2000).

SELECTED CONCEPTS RELATED TO CULTURALLY SENSITIVE NURSING

Specific cultural practices involving spirituality, nutrition, and folk practices should be considered when assessing clients and planning their care.

Religion and Spirituality

The spiritual well-being of clients who practice a religion is an important consideration in nursing in that it has a bearing on many different aspects of health and illness (McEvoy, 2003). Some examples may be the acceptance or nonacceptance of blood products, dietary rules or rituals, the furnishing of religious support for the sick, and beliefs and practices related to birth or death.

In times of crisis, religion often plays a major role in caring for the client. Many individuals are atheists (do not believe in a higher power) or agnostics (question whether there is a God or higher power). It is best to request nonjudgmentally, "Tell me how I can assist you in meeting any religious or spiritual needs you may have." Although Christianity is prevalent in many areas of North America, globalization is bringing together many varied religions that should be considered in planning care. Further discussion of religion and spirituality is found in other fundamental textbooks.

Generic or Folk Medicine

Although many North Americans believe in using the professional medical and nursing system for health care, many more do not seek professional care for many reasons:

- Transportation difficulties
- High cost of care
- Fear and distrust of health care workers
- Poor communication between clients and professionals

Therefore cultural ways of healing might be sought before or while seeking care from the traditional health care system. Although, considered unscientific and strange to many health care workers, it is essential to assess and support clients in their practices when appropriate.

Where do folk health ideas come from? Individuals within certain cultures look at their ideas as ways to preserve both their heritage and their health. Folk health beliefs, practices, and values are learned from experience and observations. They are passed down from generation to generation and have been found to be valuable to cultures and individuals.

Long before there were physicians and nurses, there were systems of caring for and curing individuals. For example, early ancestors found they could prevent or cure disease with plants. Digitalis (which comes from the foxglove plant) and belladonna have been used for many generations to treat heart failure and tuberculosis. Substances other than plants are also used. For example, in the South of the United States (and among Southerners who migrated north), the practice among some black individuals and European Americans from the Appalachian Mountains is to eat clay or dirt to promote maternal wellness. This practice is called **geophagia**. Many southern families have had their own clay banks for years. Some literature suggests that this practice originated in Africa (Spector, 2000). Red clay may be used for anemia, and white clay is preferred for indigestion. White clay consists of kaolin, the same ingredient found in some medications given taken for indigestion today. The cost of these drugs far exceeds that of the natural clay.

There are also numerous hot/cold beliefs related to healing. These beliefs may not necessarily be based on a nurse's definition of temperature. Hot/cold theories of healing are found among Hispanic, Arab, Asian, Southeast Indian, African-American, and Southern Anglo-American cultures. If the nurse provides care to an adult who has some of these beliefs, he or she may find that the client's explanation for the present illness goes back to earlier life. For example, some Hispanic women believe that partaking of "cold" foods and medicines after pregnancy will cause bleeding to stop. They believe this blood is reabsorbed into the body to cause nervousness or insanity later in life. A similar belief is that cold can get into the open vagina after childbirth and stay in the body to cause arthritis in adult life. Health care providers who care for these clients must realize that the client's view of the etiology of the problem may be quite different from the scientific explanation.

The "evil eye" is a prominent belief in some cultures, including Hispanic and Arab cultures. The Spanish term for this belief is *mal de ojo*, and some believe that "the gods" give the evil eye when they become envious or jealous when a person is excessively praised or admired. Another belief is that a person who is angry with another person can "put the evil eye" on him or her. Various amulets are worn to reflect the evil eye back onto the person who caused it (Figure 6-3).

Various methods are used to protect individuals from evil. Garlic or a substance such as asafoetida may be worn around the neck, often in a little red bag. Both of these substances are thought to protect against colds and flu. They both smell so bad that they may indeed work, because other individuals do not want to get close to the wearer.

A very important point to consider with folk medicine is the use of particular phrases to describe health problems. Some African Americans and some Appalachians refer to the blood in various ways that can have several meanings. For example, "high blood" can mean hypertension, or too much blood in the body, or it can mean the movement of

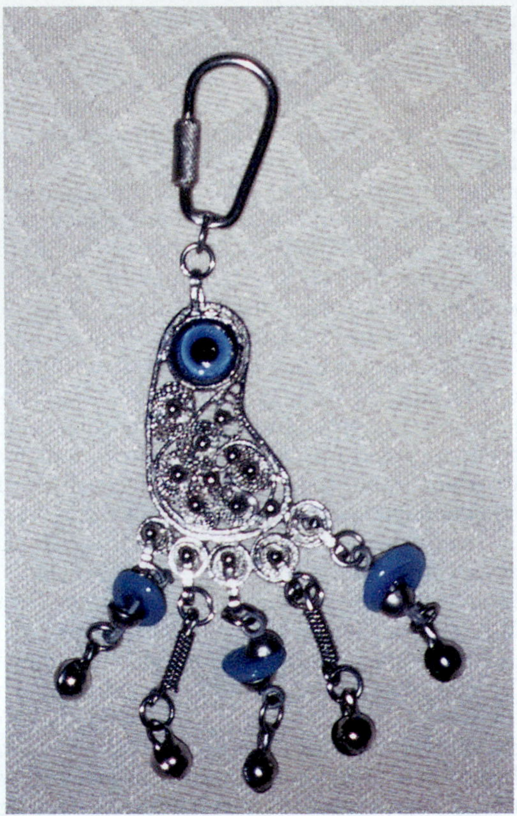

Figure 6-3 ■ "Hand of God" amulet to protect the wearer from the "evil eye."

blood to a higher part of the body such as the brain or head. The movement of blood into the head is commonly believed to cause strokes or nervousness or to make the person "fall out" (faint). A similar situation is "low blood," which can mean low blood pressure or anemia. These different terms can cause communication problems. When taking care of clients, the nurse must sometimes delve deeper into the meaning of certain phrases.

This section has described only a few examples of the generic or folk beliefs that may be found in almost any culture. What must nurses do to help individuals with these beliefs? Most folk practices are not hurtful, but when they are, nurses and physicians must sensitively address them. Belittling of client practices lacks cultural awareness and sensitivity, hence it is imperative for students to learn and appreciate cultural differences.

The subject of folk health is broad; refer to books in the Selected Bibliography for greater detail.

Pain

Pain is universal in all cultures, yet the way in which individuals discuss pain varies greatly among and between cultures. Pain has been labeled the fifth vital sign along with temperature, pulse, respiration, and blood pressure. Nurses routinely assess pain on a Visual Analogue Scale, which is a numerical rating from 0 to 10. Although this technique provides some objectivity among health care providers, it does limit the sensitivity of culturally dependent subjective signs and symptoms of the pain response. Nurses may believe that silent suffering is a valued reaction to pain. Nurses must identify whether they prefer to see self-control in their clients rather than displays of strong feelings related to pain, and how their perceptions impact their nursing interventions addressing pain (Spector, 2000) (see Chapter 7).

The alleviation of pain is also culturally based. Techniques such as acupuncture, long used by the Chinese, have become more widespread in the United States to alleviate pain. Similarly, herbal remedies have been used by many cultures through the ages (see also Chapters 4 and 7). In addition, massage therapy and mind-body techniques of complementary and alternative therapies have also been found to reduce or relieve pain.

Religious practices have a place in pain management and healing. Some Catholics may use their rosaries to guide their prayer. Other denominations in the Christian faith have special healing services either in churches or in the sick room. Jewish clients may ask to speak to a rabbi. Native American/American Indian clients may have shamans who perform religious rituals for healing that involve the client, relatives, and other members of the cultural group. One role of the nurse is to respect and provide privacy for all religious practices.

Nutrition

Culture has a major impact on food and the way in which it is prepared and served. Technology, economics, and religion–all parts of the cultural assessment–influence the food that is eaten by various cultural groups.

Technology affects how food is produced and distributed. High-level technology is involved on large agricultural farms, but very few tools may be necessary to grow a backyard garden. Foods are much less seasonal now than they were before rapid transportation systems could move food from many countries with varying growing seasons.

Economics also affect the production and distribution of food. In some countries, food is produced on small farms. The food that is not needed by the family who produced it is brought to a central market area for sale. Custom also dictates how food is sold. In many European countries, individuals go to specialty stores or markets to buy fresh meat and produce each day. Many economically deprived countries experience famine and starvation.

Religion also dictates what different cultural groups eat and how the food is prepared. Many individuals of the Hindu religion refrain from eating cows; some are lactovegetarians, eating only milk products and vegetables. Some Jewish individuals do not eat pork or shellfish; there are religious rituals for killing the meat to make it kosher. Many Jewish individuals believe that milk and meat should not be eaten at the same meal (Spector, 2000). Religion also influences whether specific things are eaten at different times. Some Christians who are Catholic or Episcopalian "give up" certain foods, commonly meat or desserts, during the Lenten season. Religious holidays may also feature traditional meats, such as the "Christmas turkey" or the "Easter ham."

Beliefs and practices related to the hot/cold theory often involve foods. Illness is often seen as an imbalance between elements, and food or herbs are used to therapeutically restore the body to its natural balance. Therefore curing a "hot" disease such as arthritis may require cold foods or medicines. Beliefs vary about what is hot and what is cold. A similar belief is the Chinese *yin* and *yang* balance of foods for health. When faced with a client who has these beliefs, interview the client and family or refer to books with details about these specific beliefs.

Foods are important in planning care with certain cultural groups. For example, many African and Asian Americans are lactose intolerant and have problems digesting milk and milk products. African Americans also have a tendency to have high blood pressure, which may be diet related. Obesity, overeating, or anorexia nervosa may also have a cultural basis for establishing eating and activity habits.

Communication

One of the stumbling blocks to effective health care is communication. Not only do clients and nurses often speak different languages, there is also miscommunication when nurses use technical language, slang, or jargon. In addition, individuals in every culture have silent ways of expressing themselves through facial expressions, posture, and hand gestures; through the space between individuals; and through touch. Discomfort and a lack of understanding results if efforts are not made to overcome miscommunication or a lack of communication.

When nurses and clients speak an entirely different language, several interventions can be taken to try to effectively communicate with the client and the family. The first step is to assess the population for which care will be provided. If it is primarily a Hispanic group, then learning the language is the ideal answer. Although learning a complete language is often not possible, knowing and using a few words and phrases often goes a long way in making a client comfortable and interested in the care provided.

Interpreters are often used in health care with different cultures. The best situation is to have someone on the health care team act as an interpreter. When this is not possible, arrangements can sometimes be made with individuals in the community. Some health care facilities have found that foreign language professors from nearby schools or colleges can act in this capacity as may the client's friends or family members. An important consideration is the need to maintain confidentiality. With friends and family in the room, the client may be less forthcoming with personal information–information that could be important to diagnosis and treatment.

One helpful resource is the AT&T Language Service ([800] 752-6096). This service offers translation of more than 150 languages. There is a fee for this service, but it can be very helpful.

Another solution is to use pictures identified with both the foreign language word and the English equivalent. For example, Spanish-speaking clients would be shown a picture of a nurse with the words "enfermera" and "nurse" underneath it or a hypodermic syringe and needle with the words "inyección" and "shot" underneath it (Figure 6-4). Many resources are available for nurses to learn Spanish and other languages (Joyce & Villanueva, 2000).

Nonverbal communication can involve space, gestures, posture, and facial expressions, all of which vary with the culture of the person. When someone invades another's personal space, that person can get very uncomfortable and

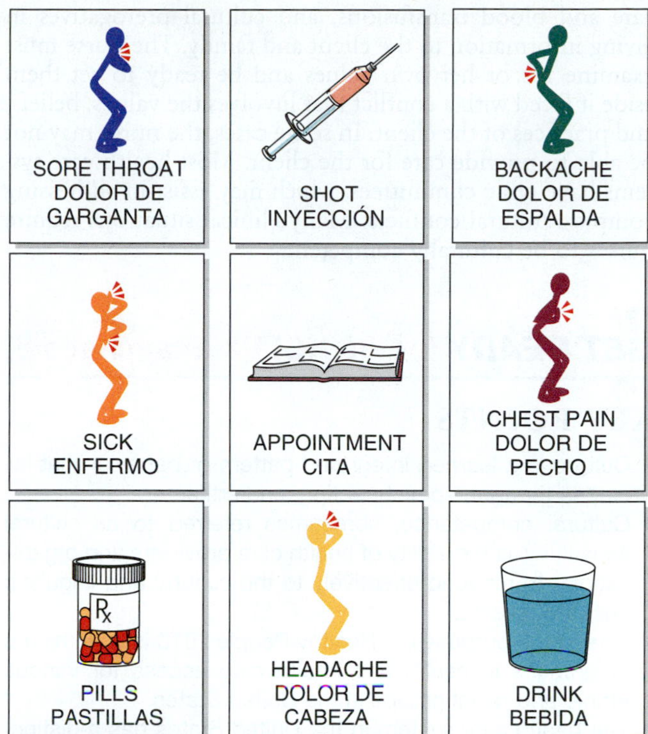

Figure 6-4 ■ English/Spanish pictograph to assist with communication. (Courtesy Anne Grimmer, Xid Design, Tallahassee, FL.)

transmit feelings of discomfort. Understanding that space has culturally embedded relevance can help clients in coping with feelings of being invaded.

Gestures are also culturally embedded ways of communication. They vary between cultures and may be interpreted as unacceptable or threatening depending on the ethnic group. In the European-American culture, the thumb and first finger make a circle and the other fingers are held upright to mean "everything's okay." In some Arab cultures, however, this same hand gesture means a woman's vagina. This example illustrates the concern that the use of certain gestures can cause.

Facial expressions and looking directly at someone can also cause discomfort in certain cultures. Some groups expect their health care providers to be serious and formal, whereas others want a more intimate, personal reaction. European-American nurses value the use of eye-to-eye contact with clients, but some clients may avert their eyes because of cultural differences.

Ethics of Cultural Caring

The ethics of nursing includes, but is not limited to, ensuring client confidentiality, getting informed consent for certain procedures and surgery, and respecting the right of clients to make autonomous decisions about their care. The ethics regarding the cultural care of clients goes further and considers the values of each individual client and his or her cultural beliefs and practices. The nurse must support and advocate for clients to have their unique needs met in the health care system. Some aspects of cultural care involve beliefs related to birth and death, the right to refuse medical care and blood transfusions, and cultural prerogatives in giving information to the client and family. The nurse must examine his or her own values and be ready to set them aside if faced with a conflict that involves the values, beliefs, and practices of the client. In some cases, the nurse may not be able to provide care for the client. Most health care systems have ethic committees, which may assist in addressing complex cultural conflicts. Many clinical situations require nurses to be culturally competent.

GET READY for the NCLEX Examination!

KEY POINTS

- Culture is a learned integrated pattern of behavior that includes thought, speech, action, and artifacts.
- Cultural competence, sometimes referred to as cultural sensitivity, is the ability of health care providers and organizations to respond effectively to the cultural and linguistic needs of clients.
- One of the purposes of Healthy People 2010 is to eliminate differences in health and health care access for various ethnic and racial groups in the United States.
- The health care system in the United States has a distinct culture, including standardization, cleanliness, and medicalization of birthing and dying.
- Factors that are related to cultural assessment are listed in Tables 6-2 and 6-3.
- Three methods of cultural assessment are observation, interview, and participation.
- Special considerations are needed for subcultural groups that may be affiliated with a number of ethnic or racial groups—disabled clients, impoverished persons, and those with diverse sexual orientations.
- Nurses need to be educated in specific cultural practices that affect assessment and planning of client care, including religion, nutrition, and communication.
- Clients may avoid the traditional health care system due to transportation problems, high cost of care, fear and distrust of health care staff, or poor communication between clients and health care providers; generic or folk medicine may be used as an alternative.
- Communication techniques vary among cultural groups and may be misinterpreted; nurses need to learn how groups communicate (verbal and nonverbal) to avoid misperceptions.

ADDITIONAL STUDY RESOURCES

Go to your Student CD-ROM for Review Questions for the NCLEX Examination.

evolve Go to http://evolve.elsevier.com/Iggy/ for Integrated Management of Care Questions for the NCLEX Examination.

SELECTED BIBLIOGRAPHY

Anderson, L., et al., and the Task Force on Community Preventive Services. (2003). Culturally competent healthcare systems: A systematic review. *American Journal of Preventive Medicine, 24*(3S), 68-79.

Baldwin, D. (2003). Disparities in health and health care: Focusing efforts to eliminate unequal burdens. *Online Journal of Issues in Nursing 8*(1), Manuscript 1. Retrieved January 31, 2003, from http://nursingworld.org/ojin/topics20/tpc20_1.htm.

Bernstein, J., Mutschler, P., & Bernstein, E. (2000). Keeping mammography appointments: Motivation, health beliefs, and access barriers experienced by older minority women. *Journal of Midwifery and Women's Health, 45*(4), 308-313.

Byrne, M. (2001) Uncovering racial bias in nursing fundamental textbooks. *Nursing and Health Care Perspectives, 22*(6), 299-303.

Byrne, M. (2002). Instructional bias-awareness and reduction in perioperative education. *AORN Journal, 75*(4), 808-816.

Byrne, M., et al. (2003). The Byrne Guide for Inclusionary Cultural Content. *Journal of Nursing Education, 42*(6), 277-281.

Campinha-Bacote, J. (2001). A model of practice to address cultural competence in rehabilitation nursing. *Rehabilitation Nursing, 26*(1), 8-11.

Campinha-Bacote, J. (2002): *Readings and resources in transcultural health care in mental health* (13th ed.). Cincinnati, OH: Transcultural C.A.R.E. Associates Press.

Freire, G. (2002). Hispanics and the politics of health care. *Journal of Health & Social Policy 14*(4), 21-35.

Joyce, E., & Villanueva, M. (2000): *Say it in Spanish: A guide for health care professionals*. Philadelphia: W.B. Saunders.

Leininger, M. (2002). Culture care theory: A major contribution to advance transcultural nursing knowledge and practices. *Journal of Transcultural Nursing 13*(3), 189-192.

Lipson, J.G., & Rogers, J.G. (2000). Cultural aspects of disability. *Journal of Transcultural Nursing, 11*(3), 212-219.

McEvoy, M. (2003). Culture and spirituality as an integrated concept in pediatric care. *MCN: American Journal of Maternal Child Nursing 28*(1), 39-43.

Narayanasamy, A. (2003). Transcultural nursing: How do nurses respond to cultural needs? *British Journal of Nursing, 12*(3), 185-194.

Purnell, L. (2000). A description of the Purnell model for cultural competence. *Journal of Transcultural Nursing, 11*(1), 40-46.

Spector, R.E. (2000). *Cultural diversity in health and illness* (5th ed.). Upper Saddle River, NJ: Prentice-Hall Health.

Spinks, V.S., Andrews, J., & Boyle, J.S. (2000). Providing health care for lesbian clients. *Journal of Transcultural Nursing, 11*(2), 137-143.

Sutherland, L. (2002). Ethnocentrism in a pluralistic society: A concept analysis. *Journal of Transcultural Nursing, 13*(4), 274-281.

U.S. Department of Health and Human Services, Office of Disease Prevention and Health Promotion. (2000). *Tracking Healthy People 2010* (2nd ed.). Pittsburgh: U.S. Government Printing Office.

CHAPTER 7

Pain: The Fifth Vital Sign

LORA MCGUIRE

LEARNING OUTCOMES

After studying this chapter, you should be able to:

1. Define the concept of pain.
2. Identify three populations at high risk for undertreatment of pain.
3. Discuss the attitudes and knowledge of nurses, physicians, and clients regarding pain assessment and management.
4. Differentiate between addiction, tolerance, and physical dependence.
5. Compare and contrast the characteristics of the major types of pain.
6. Explain the transmission of pain.
7. Describe the components of a comprehensive pain assessment.
8. Describe the use of non-opioid analgesics in pain management.
9. Discuss and compare opioid analgesics, using an equianalgesic chart.
10. Explain the purpose of adjuvant medication in pain management.
11. Differentiate four routes of analgesic administration.
12. Identify special considerations for older adults related to pain assessment and management.
13. Identify physical and cognitive-behavioral therapies for clients experiencing pain.
14. Develop a teaching/learning plan for managing pain as part of community-based care for clients.
15. Describe the role of the nurse as an advocate in pain management.

Go to your Student CD-ROM for Review Questions for the NCLEX Examination keyed to these Learning Outcomes.

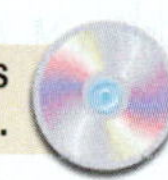

Pain is a universal, complex, subjective experience. It is the most common reason for a client to seek medical care, and the number one reason for a person to take medication. It alters or compromises quality of life more than any other single health-related problem. Despite more than 20 years of work by clinicians and professional and lay organizations, unrelieved and undertreated pain remains a major, yet avoidable public health problem in the United States (Berry & Dahl, 2000).

Your primary role in pain management is to advocate for the client by *believing* reports of pain. Because many practitioners may have difficulty with this concept, it must be emphasized repeatedly that there is no diagnostic test for pain. Even though some nurses with many years of experience think that they can identify clients in pain, it is impossible. To assist in advocating for adequate pain relief, the American Pain Foundation has developed a "Pain Care Bill of Rights" (Table 7-1).

OVERVIEW

Everyone experiences pain at some point in life. Because pain is such a private and personal experience, it may be difficult to describe or explain pain to others. The amount of pain and responses to it vary from person to person; therefore interpreting pain solely on actions or behaviors can be misleading.

Pain is generally related to some type of tissue damage and serves as a warning signal (e.g., pain signals a person to immediately remove a hand from a hot stove). Although pain is familiar to everyone, it is so complex that it cannot be easily described, and there is no single, universal treatment.

Definitions of Pain

Although several attempts have been made to define pain in descriptive or measurable terms, the two most accepted definitions have been put forth by the International Association of Pain (1979) and Margo McCaffery (1979). **Pain** is an unpleasant sensory and emotional experience associated with actual or potential tissue damage.

McCaffery offered a more personal explanation of pain when she stated that pain is whatever the experiencing person says it is and exists whenever he or she says it does. This understanding of pain requires that the client be seen as the authority on the pain and as the only one who can define the experience. In other words, *self-report* is always the most reliable indication of pain. Nurses who approach pain from this perspective can help the client achieve effective pain management by advocating for proper control.

TABLE 7-1 Pain Care Bill of Rights

As a person with pain, you have the right to:

- Have your report of pain taken seriously and to be treated with dignity and respect by doctors, nurses, pharmacists, and other health care professionals.
- Have your pain thoroughly assessed and promptly treated.
- Be informed by your health care provider about what may be causing your pain, possible treatments, and the benefits, risks, and costs of each.
- Participate actively in decisions about how to manage your pain.
- Have your pain reassessed regularly and your treatment adjusted if your pain has not been eased.
- Be referred to a pain specialist if your pain persists.
- Get clear and prompt answers to your questions, take time to make decisions, and refuse a particular type of treatment if you choose.

Although not always required by law, these are the rights you should expect for your pain care.

From American Pain Foundation, Baltimore, MD.

TABLE 7-2 Impact of Unrelieved Pain

Physiologic Impact

- Prolongs stress response
- Increases heart rate, blood pressure, and oxygen demand
- Decreases gastrointestinal motility
- Causes immobility
- Decreases immune response
- Delays healing
- Increases risk for chronic pain

Quality of Life Impact

- Interferes with activities of daily living
- Causes anxiety, depression, fear, anger, and sleeplessness
- Impairs family, work, and social relationships

Financial Impact

- Costs Americans $100 billion per year
- Increases hospital lengths of stay
- Leads to lost income and productivity

Modified from McCaffery, M., & Pasero, C. (1999). *Pain: Clinical manual* (2nd ed.) St. Louis: Mosby.

Scope of the Problem

Pain is a major economic problem and a major cause of disability that hampers the lives of many people. About 9 in 10 Americans regularly suffer pain. Approximately 25 million Americans suffer acute pain related to surgery or injury. Chronic pain is the most common cause of long-term disability, affecting 250 million Americans.

There is overwhelming evidence that pain is undertreated in the United States. In the last decade alone, numerous studies have continued to prove that pain is still not adequately treated in all areas of health care. Populations at the highest risk are older adults, minorities, and addicts. For example, one study of older adults found that 40% to 85% of nursing home residents had undertreated pain. Another study found that Hispanics with pain were half as likely as white clients to receive analgesics (Todd et al., 2000). In clients who are substance abusers, unrelieved pain can contribute to relapses or increased substance use.

Inadequate pain management can lead to many consequences affecting the client and family members. These consequences may affect the client/family physiologically, emotionally, and financially to greatly impair quality of life (Table 7-2).

Types of Pain

There are three main types of pain: acute, chronic cancer pain, and chronic noncancer pain (Tables 7-3 and 7-4). **Acute pain** results from acute injury, disease, or surgery. Chronic pain is divided into two subtypes. **Chronic cancer pain** is pain associated with cancer or another progressive disease such as acquired immunodeficiency syndrome (AIDS). The cause of pain is usually life threatening. **Chronic noncancer pain** is associated with tissue injury that has healed or is not associated with cancer, such as arthritis or chronic back pain. This type of pain is the most common.

TABLE 7-3 Characteristics of Acute and Chronic Pain

Acute	Chronic*
Has short duration	Lasts more than several months (usually greater than 3)
Usually has a well-defined cause	May or may not have well-defined cause
Decreases with healing	Begins gradually and persists
Is reversible	Is exhausting and useless
Ranges from mild to severe intensity	Ranges from mild to severe intensity
May be accompanied by anxiety and restlessness	May be accompanied by depression and fatigue, as well as decreased functional ability

*Includes chronic cancer pain and chronic noncancer pain.

TABLE 7-4 Examples of Acute and Chronic Pain

Acute Pain

- Postoperative
- Trauma
- Burns
- Procedural
- Obstetric

Chronic Cancer Pain

- Tumor invasion
- Nerve compression
- Bone metastasis
- HIV-related pain
- Treatment-related pain (radiation, surgery, chemotherapy)

Chronic Noncancer Pain

- Arthritis
- Low back pain
- Fibromyalgia
- Neuropathic (diabetic neuropathy, phantom limb, post-herpetic neuralgia)
- Complex regional pain syndrome (CRPS)
- Intermittent causes, such as headaches and sickle cell pain

ACUTE PAIN

Almost everyone experiences acute pain at some time. Certain characteristics distinguish this type of pain from the more chronic (long-term) pain often associated with chronic illness. A major distinction between acute and chronic pain is the effect on biologic responses. Acute pain serves a biologic purpose. It acts as a warning signal because it can activate the sympathetic nervous system, causing various physiologic responses. These responses are similar to those found in "fight-or-flight" reactions and include the following:

- Increased heart rate
- Increased blood pressure
- Increased respiratory rate
- Dilated pupils
- Sweating

Behavioral signs of acute pain may include restlessness, an inability to concentrate, apprehension, and overall distress.

Acute pain is usually temporary, of sudden onset, and easily localized. The client can often describe the pain, which may subside with or without treatment. Acute pain often results from sudden, accidental trauma (e.g., fractures, burns, and lacerations) or from surgery, ischemia, or acute inflammation. The pain is usually confined to the affected area. As this area heals, the quality of sensation of the pain changes. Although possibly severe, acute pain is limited over time and generally can be managed successfully. Both the caregiver and the client can see an end to the pain, which makes coping somewhat easier.

Pain that accompanies surgery is one of the most common examples of acute pain, but it is not always well managed. Usually this poorly managed postoperative pain is a result of inadequate drug therapy.

The severity of postoperative pain may be a predictor of long-term pain. The use of **preemptive analgesia** is a technique designed to decrease pain in the postoperative period, decrease the requirements for a postoperative analgesic, improve morbidity, and decrease hospital stay. Preemptive analgesia includes administering local anesthetics, opioids, and nonsteroidal anti-inflammatory drugs (NSAIDs) in the preoperative, intraoperative, and/or postoperative period. This intervention may inhibit changes in the spinal cord—changes that can lead to a central sensitization that results in chronic pain.

In general, intrathoracic and upper intra-abdominal surgical approaches are associated with more severe, steady wound pain and with pain on movement in the postoperative period. Many clients who undergo superficial surgery of the head and neck, chest wall, or limbs report minimal postoperative pain. Muscle-splitting procedures are generally far more painful than muscle-stretching procedures.

CHRONIC PAIN

Chronic pain is defined as pain that persists or recurs for indefinite periods, usually for more than 3 months. The onset is gradual, and the character and quality of the pain change over time. Because chronic pain often involves deep body structures, it is usually poorly localized and often difficult to describe. If the underlying cause cannot be treated medically, controlling the long-term effects of chronic pain may be a difficult clinical challenge.

Because chronic pain persists for extended periods, it can interfere with personal relationships and activities of daily living. It can also result in emotional and financial burdens. Thus the efforts of an interdisciplinary health care team are needed to manage the situation effectively. Inadequately managed pain is an overwhelming, frustrating experience for both the sufferer and the caregiver. Over half of clients with chronic pain become clinically depressed. Although many characteristics of chronic pain are similar in different clients, the nurse should be aware that each situation is unique and requires a highly specialized plan of care.

CHRONIC CANCER PAIN. Approximately two thirds of clients with advanced cancer have moderate to severe pain. What is frustrating is that we have known for over 30 years that 90% of cancer pain can be treated simply by giving adequate amounts of oral opioids around-the-clock. Yet clients with terminal cancer are often inadequately treated for their excruciating pain.

Most cancer pain is caused by the disease itself. The sources of pain include nerve compression, invasion of tissue, and/or bone metastasis. Cancer treatments can also cause pain due to surgery, as well as toxicities from chemotherapy and radiation therapy.

Clients with cancer pain generally have pain in two or more areas, but usually only talk about the primary area of pain. Be sure to perform a complete pain assessment to locate all areas of pain.

CHRONIC NONCANCER PAIN. Chronic noncancer pain is a major health problem. In the United States alone it is estimated that 25% of people, many of them older than 65 years of age, are affected with a chronic illness and chronic pain. Unlike acute pain, chronic pain serves no biologic purpose. After the initial warning signal of pain, the body must learn to adapt to the persistent pain impulses by blocking or adjusting to activation of the sympathetic nervous system (which causes the fight-or-flight reaction in acute pain). Because of this adaptation, the symptoms that may be associated with acute pain are *absent* with chronic pain.

Chronic noncancer pain was formerly called chronic nonmalignant pain. However, most pain experts, and certainly clients who suffer with daily pain, believe that all pain is malignant; thus the newer term.

Chronic noncancer pain may be caused by chronic diseases such as rheumatoid arthritis, lupus erythematosus, sickle cell anemia, fibromyalgia, low back pain, chronic headaches, and osteoporosis (see Table 7-4).

Neuropathic pain is one of the most challenging types of chronic noncancer pains; it results from some type of nerve injury. Examples of causes include diabetic neuropathy, postherpetic neuralgia, radiculopathy (spinal nerve damage), and trigeminal neuralgia. Neuropathic pain is described as burning, shooting, stabbing, and feeling "pins and needles."

Theoretical Bases for Pain

GATE CONTROL THEORY

The **gate control theory** was proposed to explain the observed relationship between pain and emotion. Melzack and Wall (1982) first introduced this theory and concluded that pain is not just a physiologic response. Psychological variables such as behavioral and emotional responses also influence the perception of pain.

According to this theory, a gating mechanism occurs in the spinal cord. Nerve fibers (A delta and C fibers) transmit pain impulses from the periphery of the body. These impulses travel to the dorsal horns of the spinal cord, specifically to the *substantia gelatinosa*. The cells of the substantia gelatinosa can inhibit or facilitate the pain impulses transmitted to the trigger cells (T-cells). When T-cell activity is

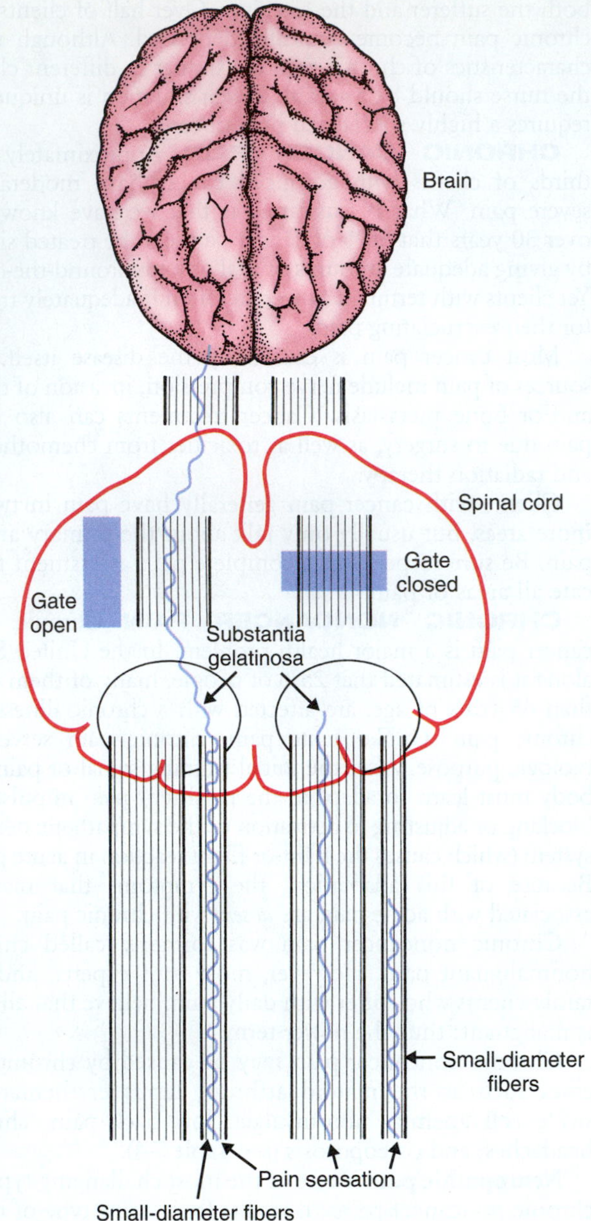

Figure 7-1 ■ The gate control theory of pain.

inhibited, the gate is closed and impulses are less likely to be transmitted to the brain. When the gate is opened, pain impulses ascend to the brain (Figure 7-1).

Similar gating mechanisms exist in the nerve fibers descending from the thalamus and cerebral cortex. These areas of the brain regulate thoughts and emotions, including beliefs and values. When pain occurs, a person's thoughts and emotions can modify perceptual phenomena as they reach the level of conscious awareness.

The gate control theory has helped nurses and other health care professionals to recognize the *holistic* nature of pain. As a result, many cognitive-behavioral therapies (e.g., imagery and distraction (see pp. 84 and 85) are used to help relieve pain.

ANATOMIC AND PHYSIOLOGIC BASES FOR PAIN

PAIN STIMULI. A wide range of sensory input is capable of producing pain. Tissue ischemia and muscle spasm also cause pain. Free nerve endings (receptors capable of responding to painful stimuli) are referred to as nociceptors. Nociceptors are located in various body tissues and are activated by thermal, mechanical, and chemical stimuli. In addition to nociceptors, other receptors in the body respond to almost any type of intense stimulation, which sometimes results in pain.

In most circumstances, painful stimuli cause actual tissue damage, which leads to the release of certain chemical substances called neurotransmitters (e.g., histamine, bradykinin, serotonin, norepinephrine) and certain acids that sensitize nociceptors, including leukotrienes, prostaglandins, and substance P. These chemicals are believed to activate pain receptors.

PAIN FIBERS AND PATHWAYS. Painful stimuli often originate in the periphery (extremities) of the body. To be perceived, the stimuli must be transmitted first to the spinal cord and then to the central areas of the brain, as described by the gate control theory of pain (see Figure 7-1). In the periphery, two specific fibers can transmit stimuli: (1) A delta fibers, which are found primarily in the skin and muscle, and (2) C fibers, which are distributed in muscle, periosteum, and viscera. Both of these nerve fibers are first-order neurons capable of accepting nociceptive stimuli.

A delta fibers are myelinated fibers that carry rapid, sharp, pricking, or piercing sensations. A person feeling these sensations can generally localize them readily to a fairly well-defined area. Because these fibers respond predominately to mechanical rather than chemical or thermal stimuli, they are called mechanical nociceptors.

C fibers are unmyelinated or poorly myelinated fibers that conduct thermal, chemical, and strong mechanical impulses. Pain conduction from C fibers is more diffuse and dull, burning, or achy–quite different from the sensations of A delta fibers. In contrast to the intermittent nature of A delta sensations, C fibers usually produce persistent pain.

Second-order neurons, or pain pathways of the ascending pain tracts, are found in the dorsal horn of the spinal cord and terminate in the thalamus. The spinothalamic tract is divided into two spinal tracts. The lateral, or neospinothalamic, tract is responsible for sensory pain discrimination; it transmits pain stimuli more directly to the sensory cortex, where pain is eventually perceived and interpreted. The paleospinothalamic tract synapses in other parts of the brain, such as the limbic system (emotional center) and the reticular formation (sleep-wake center). The painful stimuli are therefore subjected to emotional and behavioral influences.

CENTRAL NERVOUS SYSTEM PROCESSING. The central processing of pain occurs at three different levels of the brain: the thalamus, midbrain, and cortex. These areas cooperate to raise the awareness of pain, interpret painful stimuli, and produce a response to pain. The thalamus acts as the relay station for sensory input from the spinothalamic tract of the spinal cord. The midbrain signals the cortex to increase awareness of the stimuli. The cortex seems to be involved both in the discrimination of well-localized pain and in the interpretation of the pain experience.

INHIBITORY AND FACILITATORY MECHANISMS. Sensory input to the spinal cord may be influenced by chemical substances known as neuroregulators. Neuroregulators are classified as either neurotransmitters or neuromodulators.

TABLE 7-5 Physiologic Sources of Pain

Physiologic Structure	Characteristics of Pain	Sources of Acute Postoperative Pain	Sources of Chronic Pain Syndromes
Nociceptive Pain			
Somatic Pain			
Cutaneous or superficial: skin and subcutaneous tissues	Sharp, burning	Incisional pain, pain at insertion sites of tubes and drains, wound complications, orthopaedic procedures, skeletal muscle spasms	Bony metastases, osteoarthritis and rheumatoid arthritis, low back pain, peripheral vascular diseases
Deep somatic: bone, muscle blood vessels, connective tissues	Dull, aching, cramping		
Visceral Pain			
Organs and the linings of the body cavities	Poorly localized Diffuse, deep cramping or splitting, sharp, stabbing	Chest tubes, abdominal tubes and drains, bladder distention or spasms, intestinal distention	Pancreatitis, liver metastases, colitis, appendicitis
Neuropathic Pain			
Nerve fibers, spinal cord, and central nervous system	Poorly localized Shooting, burning, fiery, shocklike, sharp, painful numbness	Phantom limb pain, postmastectomy pain, nerve compression	HIV-related pain, diabetic neuropathy, postherpetic neuralgia, chemotherapy-induced neuropathies, cancer-related nerve injury, radiculopathies

Neurotransmitters are the chemicals that exert inhibitory (slowing down) or excitatory (speeding up) activity at postsynaptic nerve cell membranes. Acetylcholine, norepinephrine, epinephrine, dopamine, and serotonin are documented neurotransmitters.

Neuromodulators, also called endogenous opiates, are hormones in the brain. These substances are composed of large amino acid peptides called alpha-**endorphins**, beta-endorphins, and enkephalins. These natural opiate-like substances are responsible for pain relief.

Opioid receptors are binding sites not only for endogenous opiates but also for opioid analgesics taken to relieve pain. There are several types of opioid receptors: mu, kappa, delta, epsilon, and sigma. Mu receptors are found throughout the central nervous system, especially in the brainstem, limbic system, and dorsal horn of the spinal cord. Morphine and morphine agonists bind to mu receptors.

Sources of Pain

There are two major sources of pain–nociceptive and neuropathic. **Somatic pain** (e.g., skin and musculoskeletal structures) and **visceral pain** (body-organ related) are types of **nociceptive pain**. Table 7-5 describes these categories and lists examples of each.

Attitudes and Practices Related to Pain

Negative and mistaken beliefs about pain and its treatment are common in the health care system. Studies have shown that many health care professionals do not have the knowledge and skills to manage pain adequately.

ATTITUDES AND KNOWLEDGE OF NURSES

Nurses' attitudes toward pain influence the way they perceive and interact with clients in pain. Without adequate assessment skills or knowledge of pain and analgesic therapy, nurses may not be able to understand their clients' pain and confidently participate with health care providers and other professionals in its treatment.

Nurses who have little personal experience with pain may not appreciate the magnitude of painful conditions associated with diseases and medical and surgical interventions. They may expect clients with chronic pain to react similarly to those with acute pain. They may assume that reactions to pain fall within a certain norm on the basis of their own cultural values. The more that a client's response varies from these expected norms, the more likely it is that a nurse's attitude toward the client will be positively or negatively biased.

ATTITUDES AND KNOWLEDGE OF HEALTH CARE PROVIDERS

Undertreatment of pain is a serious problem in the United States and elsewhere in the world. Between 50% and 80% of clients with cancer do not receive adequate pain control.

Despite increased education about pain, there are several reasons why many health care providers may underprescribe medication for clients in pain, especially opioids such as morphine. First, cultural and societal attitudes exist regarding opioid use.

Second, fear of regulatory scrutiny may lead to underprescribing of opioids. A physician or other health care provider may be reprimanded by the governing state board for prescribing what the board considers an inappropriate amount or type of pain medication.

Third, there is still a lack of knowledge about the effects of analgesics. Even with knowledge about correct prescribing practices, health care providers may fail to assess and treat the client's pain.

ATTITUDES AND KNOWLEDGE OF CLIENTS

Not only do health care professionals need education about pain management, but the public needs education as well. Nurses can help clients and families maintain successful pain management through education concerning available pain management resources.

Many clients are reluctant to report pain. When they do, they may underestimate its severity (Berry & Dahl, 2000). Clients may not state their pain because they want to be "good" clients or do not want to bother or distract their caregivers from other issues in their care. In clients with a history of cancer, pain can be an unwanted reminder of the disease and its progression.

Clients may also be reluctant to take pain medications, especially opioid analgesics, because they fear becoming addicted to or used to the medication (Berry & Dahl, 2000). These exaggerated fears of addiction must be addressed by the nurse so that the client will comply with the medication regimen.

Pain Perception and Disparities in Care

Many variables affect the perception of and response to pain. Factors such as age, gender, sociocultural background, and even genetics influence the client's ability to process and react to pain. These factors also put clients at risk of undertreatment.

Age can influence how pain is perceived, assessed, and treated. It has been well documented that the incidence of pain in older adults is high, as is risk for undertreatment.

Chart 7-1 addresses key components in assessment and management of pain in older adults.

It is well known that certain painful conditions are more common in either men or women. Seventy-two percent of chronic pain sufferers are women. Women suffer more often from migraine headache, tension headache, rheumatoid arthritis and osteoarthritis, fibromyalgia, and multiple sclerosis. Men suffer more from cluster headache, back pain, gout, peripheral vascular disease, and postherpetic neuralgia.

Women are at a higher risk for undertreatment of pain than men. A classic study by Cleeland et al. (1994) found that female cancer clients were more likely to be undertreated than male clients. It has also been well documented that investigation of chest pain is more extensive in men than women. Researchers are currently exploring gender and cultural differences in response to pain and opioids.

Genetic Considerations

Codeine is a commonly used opioid analgesic used to relieve pain. After ingestion, codeine is converted to morphine in the body's tissues. Thus the morphine is what alters the client's

CHART 7-1

NURSING FOCUS on the OLDER ADULT

Experiencing Pain

Prevalence of Pain

- Recognize that older adults are at great risk for undertreated pain.
- Consider the older adult at risk for the undertreatment of cancer pain because of inappropriate beliefs about pain sensitivity, tolerance, and ability to use opioids.

Beliefs about Pain

- In addition to receiving less analgesia, older adults tend to report pain less often than do younger adults. These findings may be related to beliefs and concerns about pain and the reporting of pain. Many older people hold the following beliefs and concerns about pain:
  - Pain is something that must be lived with.
  - Expressing pain is unacceptable or is a sign of weakness.
  - Complaining of pain will result in being labeled as a "bad" client.
  - Nurses are too busy to listen to complaints of pain.
  - Pain signifies a serious illness or impending death.
- Nurses should be aware of the beliefs of older clients regarding pain management. Nurses and other caregivers often undermedicate these clients and are sometimes reluctant to administer the prescribed analgesics.*

Assessment

- Ask about present pain only.
- Use a standard scale, such as the numerical Faces or Iowa Pain Thermometer rating scales.
- Explain the scale each time it is used.
- Use verbal descriptions other than pain, such as "ache," "sore," and "hurt."
- Use visual representations of pain measures rather than mental images of pain rating scales. Be sure that the client is wearing glasses and hearing aids, if needed and available.
- Alter a written pain scale to include large lettering, adequate space between lines, nonglossy paper, and color for increased visualization.
- Provide adequate lighting and privacy to avoid distracting background noise.

Considerations for Cognitively Impaired Clients

- Assess for nonverbal indicators of pain (facial expressions, grimacing, vocalizations, body movements, behavioral changes).
- Remember to "assume pain is present" (APP) in cognitively impaired clients with diseases and conditions commonly associated with pain.
- Little attention has been given to assessing or managing pain in older adults who are cognitively impaired (confused) and unable to communicate. Feldt (2000) tested a Checklist of Nonverbal Pain Indicators (CNP) to assess cognitively impaired older adults hospitalized for hip fracture. Feldt noted that older adults who were not cognitively impaired received significantly more pain medication in comparison to the impaired group.

Management of Pain

- Use around-the-clock dosing of analgesics.
- Consider an analgesic trial in a cognitively impaired client.
- Beware of adverse effects of acetaminophen (hepatotoxicity and nephrotoxicity) and NSAIDs (GI bleeding nephrotoxicity).
- Start low and go slow with opioid dosing.
- Avoid the use of meperidine, codeine, and propoxyphene (available in combination with acetaminophen, as Darvocet)
- Use methadone and tramadol with caution.
- Older adults and those with renal disease should not take meperidine because of the prolonged half-life of its drug metabolite, normeperidine.
- Use nondrug pain relief measures.

Data is, in part, from The American Geriatrics Society Foundation for Health in Aging. Available at http://www.healthinaging.org; and AGS Panel on Persistent Pain in Older Persons. (2002). The management of persistent pain in older persons. *Journal of the American Geriatrics Society, 50*(6 suppl.), S205-S224.

*Unfounded concerns about overmedication, addiction, and decreases in pain perception may contribute to undermedication (Berry & Dahl, 2000).

pain perception, not the codeine itself. Some clients (as many as 10%) are unable to obtain pain relief from codeine because they have a variation in the gene that codes for the enzyme that converts codeine to morphine (CYP2D6). For these clients, the conversion of codeine is so slow that the drug is excreted before pain is relieved (Burroughs et al., 2002). Therefore when caring for clients who are not obtaining pain relief from codeine, inform the health care provider to determine whether a change to morphine might be appropriate.

CULTURAL CONSIDERATIONS

A person's culture and ethnic background are significant in the meaning of pain and its manifestations. Pain behaviors are learned and influenced by beliefs. Cultural background also influences adherence to treatments.

As mentioned previously, minority clients are at risk for undertreatment of pain. Those at highest risk are clients cared for at centers serving mostly minorities. Different ethnic/racial groups may also experience pain differently. Inadequate and difficult assessment language barriers, attitudes toward pain and opioids, and access to health care may all contribute to undertreatment.

Maintain a nonjudgmental attitude when caring for clients with different cultural backgrounds and avoid stereotyping by ethnic group. Attempt to provide culturally sensitive client-education materials.

It is important to recognize that not all people manifest pain in the same way and that there is no right or wrong way. Accept all clients' expressions of pain, regardless of how different they may be from your own.

Tolerance, Physical Dependence, and Addiction

It is crucial that nurses and other health care professionals not refer to clients as "addict," "clock-watcher," or "drug seeker." These labels have caused biases and impacted the care that these clients have received.

The following descriptions of tolerance, physical dependence, and addiction have come from a consensus document (2001) from the American Academy of Pain Medicine (AAPM), American Pain Society (APS), and American Society of Addiction Medicine (ASAM).

Tolerance is a state of adaptation in which exposure to a drug induces changes that result in a decrease in one or more of the drug's effects over time. **Physical dependence** is the adaptation manifested by a drug-class–specific withdrawal syndrome. It can be produced by abrupt cessation, rapid dose reduction, decreasing blood level of the drug, and/or administration of an antagonist.

Physical dependence occurs in *everyone* who takes opioids over a period of time. It is important to *prevent* physical withdrawal. So-called **withdrawal symptoms** result when a client who is physically dependent on opioids abruptly ceases using them. These symptoms result from autonomic nervous system responses and include nausea and vomiting, abdominal cramping, muscle twitching, profuse perspiration, delirium, and convulsions. When it is necessary to discontinue opioid analgesia for a client who is opioid dependent, a slow tapering (weaning) of the drug dosage lessens or alleviates the physical withdrawal symptoms.

By contrast, **addiction** is a primary, chronic neurobiologic disease with genetic, psychosocial, and environmental factors influencing its development and manifestations. It is characterized by behaviors that include one or more of the following: impaired control over drug use, compulsive use, continued use despite harm, and craving. Addiction occurs over time, not as a result of one hospital stay. The stress of unrelieved pain could cause a relapse in a recovering client or an increase in drug use in the person who is actively using drugs (Nichols, 2003).

Pseudoaddiction is an iatrogenic syndrome created by the undertreatment of pain. It is characterized by client behaviors such as anger and escalating demands for more or different medications, and results in suspicion and avoidance by staff. Pseudoaddiction can be distinguished from true addiction in that the behaviors resolve when pain is effectively treated.

Tolerance, physical dependence, and addiction are separate conditions, but they may coexist. However, it is important to distinguish tolerance and physical dependence from addiction.

The danger of addiction to pain medication is vastly overrated. Although available data on addiction consistently show that it is rarely a result of using opioids for pain relief, health care professionals still have exaggerated fears. Clients and families also have fears related to addiction. Careful explanation of the difference between physical dependence and addiction should be discussed whenever a client starts on opioid therapy.

Clients who are substance abusers often have traumatic injuries and other health problems that cause pain. It is important for the nurse to recognize that substance abusers, typically those abusing opioids, are often tolerant to the pain-relieving effects of opioid analgesics and generally require increased doses. There is always the danger of abrupt physiologic withdrawal when recreational users of opioid agonists are given mixed agonist-antagonists and partial agonists.

Placebos

The clinical use of placebos in non–research-based therapies has not been shown to have a sustained effect on pain relief. McCaffery's definition of a **placebo** is "any medical treatment (medication or procedure, including surgery) or nursing care that produces an effect in a client because of its implicit or explicit or nursing care therapeutic intent and not because of its specific nature (physical or chemical properties)" (1979, p. 160). Placebos are substances or actions that produce an effect regardless of their known intrinsic value. When a client responds favorably to a placebo, it is known as the **placebo effect.** Placebos do not indicate whether or not a client has real pain. Because of the deception involved and the need for informed consent, never administer a placebo to your client.

Health care agencies should develop educational programs to inform professionals about pain management, including the inappropriate use of placebos. Ethics committees should be consulted for assistance in formulating policies and procedures regarding the use of placebos. Because of the Joint Commission's commitment to effective pain control, a policy against the use of placebos is recommended to be in place in all accredited institutions and agencies.

COLLABORATIVE MANAGEMENT

Assessment

HISTORY

Ask the client about the pain experience, including the sequence of events (precipitating and relieving factors); the nature of adjustments, if any, in life or in the family; and beliefs about the cause of the pain and what should be done about it (client's expectations). Personal characteristics (e.g., age and culture) influence attitudes about reporting a pain history. Families and significant others are included in this information-gathering process.

Clients may report pain in the absence of any observable or documented physiologic changes. Respect the client's verbal and nonverbal expressions of pain without making judgments or inferences about the reality of the pain. If clients perceive that health care professionals doubt the existence of their pain, mistrust and other negative feelings can arise and interfere with a therapeutic nurse-client relationship.

Assess the length of time the client has experienced pain. Clients may welcome an opportunity to discuss acute pain with the nurse because it is a relatively short-term experience and is easily described. However, clients with chronic pain can become frustrated when they are unable to adequately describe their vague, diffuse pain experience. Structured interviews using assessment aids (e.g., pain scales and descriptors) often help clients to express their pain.

Information about a client's pain can be helpful in understanding the factors associated with the present pain or previous episodes of pain. If the client is in pain when the nurse is obtaining the history, the session should be kept reasonably short or continued at a later time. Essential data include the following:

- *Precipitating factors.* Does the client associate any activities, food, or other environmental factors with the onset of pain? What does the client think causes the present pain? Was the onset of pain sudden or slow? Has the client done anything or taken anything to relieve the pain? What were the results of the intervention?
- *Aggravating factors.* What factors make the pain worse? What influence has this pain had on the client's activity? What changes of life activity have been affected (e.g., diet, job, sleep)?
- *Localization of pain.* Can the client localize the pain or describe where it travels or radiates?
- *Character and quality of pain.* What words does the client use to describe the pain and its character, quality, or intensity?
- *Duration of pain.* How long has the client experienced this pain?

PHYSICAL ASSESSMENT/CLINICAL MANIFESTATIONS

Although physiologic changes occur in response to acute noxious stimuli, these changes are usually *not* reliable indicators of pain. Acute pain, with its property of warning an individual about harm, *may*, but not always, cause several physiologic manifestations, which are largely a function of sympathetic nervous system stimulation. Clients with acute pain may manifest changes in vital body functions, such as tachycardia and blood pressure changes. Blood pressure is usually increased initially and then decreased. However, not all clients with acute pain have these signs, so *the client's statement of pain is the only reliable indicator.*

Physiologic changes in response to chronic pain are usually adapted to as the body attempts to compensate for and adapt to noxious stimuli. The pain no longer serves as a necessary warning. Chronic pain clients, then, frequently have developed coping skills and may appear to look quite well.

Certain motor or body movements may be associated with either acute or chronic pain. Some may be more exaggerated or obvious than others. Clients in pain may support or shield ("splint"), holding painful body parts while moving, or they may lie listlessly because they are afraid to move. Assess the functional status and degree of impairment in the client with pain.

LOCATION OF PAIN. Assess the pain from two dimensions: the level of pain (deep or superficial) and the position or location of pain. Most clients can usually describe the depth of acute pain or chronic pain. The actual area or location of the pain, however, may not be as easily identified. Ask the client whether the pain is superficial or deep. In general, clients with pain involving superficial or cutaneous (skin) structures describe their pain as superficial and can often localize the pain to a specific area.

Pain may be described as belonging to one of four categories related to its location:

- **Localized pain** is pain confined to the site of origin.
- **Projected pain** is pain along a specific nerve or nerves.
- **Radiating pain** is diffuse pain around the site of origin that is not well localized.
- **Referred pain** is pain perceived in an area distant from the site of painful stimuli.

A client who has difficulty specifying the exact location of pain can be asked to point to the painful areas on his or her own body or on another person. It is sometimes helpful to have the client point to or shade in the painful areas on a diagram on the front and back of the human body (Figure 7-2). Clients who cannot identify the painful areas and state that they just "hurt all over" are encouraged to focus on parts of the body that are *not* painful. Ask the client to concentrate on different body parts, beginning with the hand and fingers of one extremity, and identify the presence or absence of pain. By focusing attention on selected areas of the body, the client is assisted in localizing painful areas. Clients who state that they hurt everywhere often begin to realize that some parts of the body are not painful.

Clients may present with more than one discrete painful site. In fact, about one half of clients with advanced cancer report having pain in more than one location. As painful areas are identified, the nurse helps the client to understand the origin of the pain. This understanding is particularly important for clients with cancer, because every new pain often raises the suspicion of metastasis (spread of disease). The pain may be caused by other reasons, such as immobility or constipation.

OTHER PAIN DATA. After asking the client to locate the pain, ask him or her to describe it. Clients may use one word or a group of words to convey the sensations or feelings of the pain. Avoid suggesting descriptive words for the pain.

Pain is rarely the same at all times. It is perceived differently over time and varies with factors such as physical activity and stress (see the earlier discussion under History).

McGill-Melzack PAIN QUESTIONNAIRE

Patient's name ________________ Age ________

File No. ________________ Date ________

Clinical category (e.g., cardiac, neurologic)

Diagnosis: ____________

____

____

Analgesic (if already administered):

1. Type ________________
2. Dosage ________________
3. Time given in relation to this test ______

Patient's intelligence: circle number that represents best estimate.

1 (low) 2 3 4 5 (high)

****

This questionnaire has been designed to tell us more about your pain. Four major questions we ask are

1. Where is your pain?
2. What does it feel like?
3. How does it change with time?
4. How strong is it?

It is important that you tell us how your pain feels now. Please follow the instructions at the beginning of each part.

Part 1. Where Is Your Pain?

Please mark, on the drawings below, the areas where you feel pain. Put E if external, or I if internal, near the areas you mark. Put EI if both external and internal.

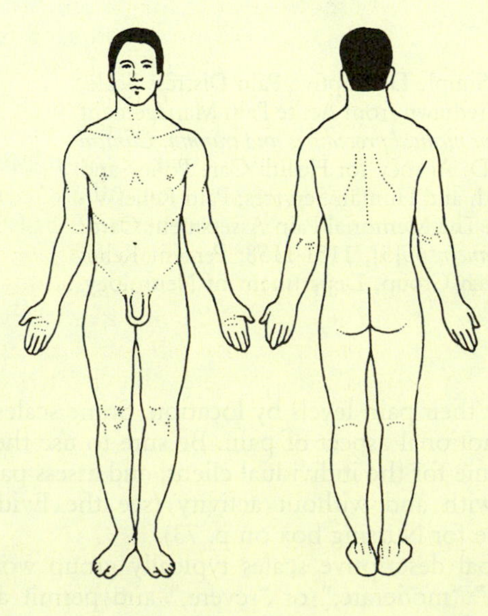

Part 2. What Does Your Pain Feel Like?

Some of the words below describe your *present* pain. Circle *ONLY* those words that best describe it. Leave out any category that is not suitable. Use only a single word in each appropriate category — the one that applies best.

1: Flickering, Quivering, Pulsing, Throbbing, Beating, Pounding

2: Jumping, Flashing, Shooting

3: Pricking, Boring, Drilling, Stabbing, Lancinating

4: Sharp, Cutting, Lacerating

5: Pinching, Pressing, Gnawing, Cramping, Crushing

6: Tugging, Pulling, Wrenching

7: Hot, Burning, Scalding, Searing

8: Tingling, Itchy, Smarting, Stinging

9: Dull, Sore, Hurting, Aching, Heavy

10: Tender, Taut, Rasping, Splitting

11: Tiring, Exhausting

12: Sickening, Suffocating

13: Fearful, Frightful, Terrifying

14: Punishing, Grueling, Cruel, Vicious, Killing

15: Wretched, Blinding

16: Annoying, Troublesome, Miserable, Intense, Unbearable

17: Spreading, Radiating, Penetrating, Piercing

18: Tight, Numb, Drawing, Squeezing, Tearing

19: Cool, Cold, Freezing

20: Nagging, Nauseating, Agonizing, Dreadful, Torturing

Part 3. How Does Your Pain Change With Time?

1. Which word or words would you use to describe the *pattern* of your pain?

1	2	3
Continuous	Rhythmic	Brief
Steady	Periodic	Momentary
Constant	Intermittent	Transient

2. What kind of things *relieve* your pain?
3. What kind of things *increase* your pain?

Part 4. How Strong Is Your Pain?

People agree that the following 5 words represent pain of increasing intensity. They are:

1	2	3	4	5
Mild	Discomforting	Distressing	Horrible	Excruciating

To answer each question below, write the number of the most appropriate word in the space beside the question.

1. Which word describes your pain right now? ____
2. Which word describes it at its worst? ____
3. Which word describes it when it is least? ____
4. Which word describes the worst toothache you ever had? ____
5. Which word describes the worst headache you ever had? ____
6. Which word describes the worst stomachache you ever had? ____

Figure 7-2 ■ The McGill-Melzack Pain Questionnaire. (From Melzack, R. [1975]. The McGill Pain Questionnaire: Major properties and scoring methods. *Pain, 1,* 272-281.)

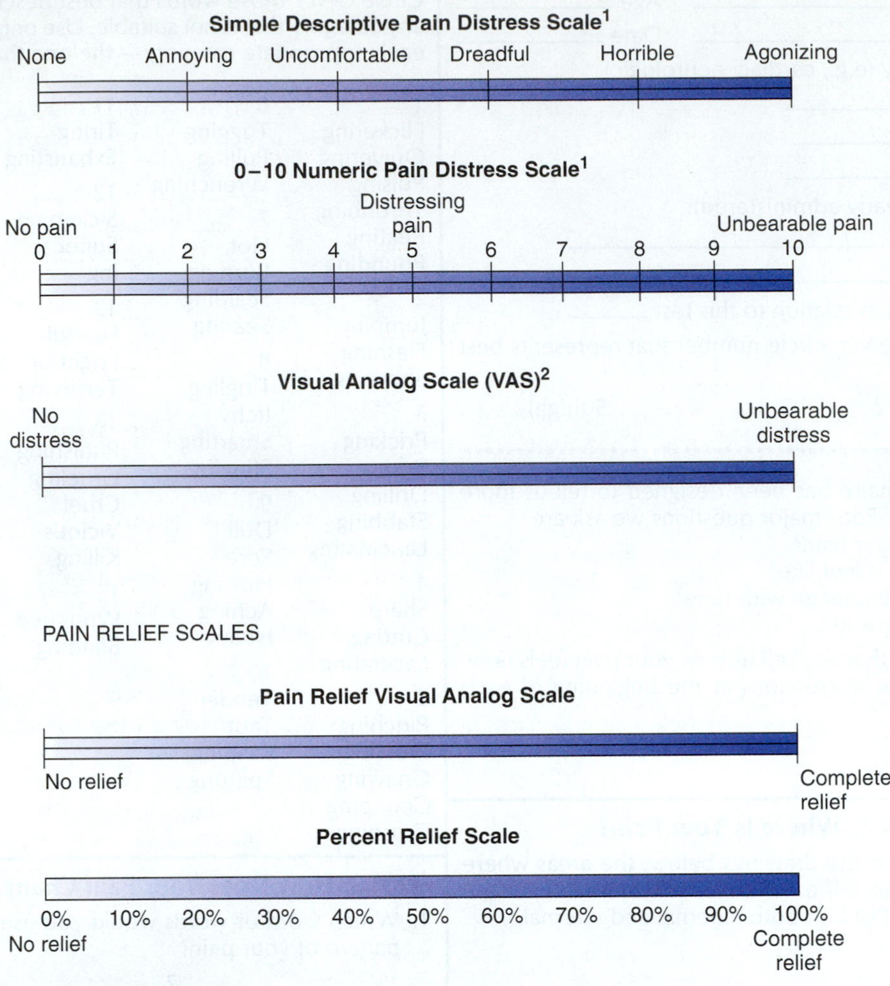

Figure 7-3 ■ Pain rating scales and pain relief scales. (Simple Descriptive Pain Distress Scale, 0-10 Numeric Pain Distress Scale, and Visual Analog Scale redrawn from Acute Pain Management Guideline Panel. [1992]. *Acute pain management: Operative or medical procedures and trauma. Clinical practice guideline.* AHCPR Pub. No. 92-0032. Rockville, MD: Agency for Health Care Policy and Research, Public Health Service, U.S. Department of Health and Human Services; Pain Relief Visual Analog Scale redrawn from Fishman, B., et al. [1987]. The Memorial Pain Assessment Card: A valid instrument for the evaluation of cancer pain. *Cancer, 60*[5], 1151-1158; Percent Relief Scale redrawn from the Brief Pain Inventory. Pain Research Group, Department of Neurology, University of Wisconsin–Madison.)

Subjective measurements of pain intensity by the client are more reliable and accurate than observable qualities of pain. Only the client can determine the amount or severity of pain being experienced. Various visual analog scales (VASs), number rating scales (NRSs), descriptive word scales, and other measures have been designed to help clients communicate the magnitude or severity of pain and to help nurses quantify the pain (Figure 7-3).

Use pain intensity scales to measure pain in the clinical or home setting and to assess and determine the effectiveness of pain relief interventions. The client is presented with a pain scale and asked to rate the amount of painful stimuli. Clients with more than one discrete painful site may wish to specify their pain levels by location. Some scales also assess the emotional aspect of pain. Be sure to use the *same* scale over time for the individual client, and assess pain intensity both with and without activity (see the Evidence-Based Practice for Nursing box on p. 73).

Verbal descriptive scales typically group words such as "none," "moderate," or "severe," and permit an intensity rating of pain. However, the 0 to 10 NRS is most commonly used in clinical practice for adult clients who can communicate in English (see Figure 7-3). For culturally diverse clients with language barriers, the Wong-Baker scale (Faces Pain Rating scale of smile to frown) may be helpful. This scale is also used for children, older adults, and develop-

EVIDENCE-BASED PRACTICE for Nursing

How to assess pain intensity in cognitively impaired African-American older adults

Taylor, L.J. & Jen, K. (2003). Pain intensity assessment: A comparison of selected pain intensity scales for use in cognitively intact and cognitively impaired African American older adults. *Pain Management Nursing, 4*(2), 87-95.

The purpose of this study was to determine the reliability and validity of the Faces Pain Scale, Verbal Description Scale, Numeric Rating Scale, and the Iowa Pain Thermometer for pain assessment in cognitively impaired African-American older adults. Fifty-seven African-American adults participated; 77% had some degree of cognitive impairment, 23% were cognitively intact. All of the participants were able to use all four scales, and both groups preferred the Faces Pain Scale.

Level of Evidence: 6—This study used a small convenience sample. However, it serves as an excellent pilot study to hopefully stimulate further research of larger, randomized groups.

Critique. Very few studies have looked at older African Americans with regard to physical assessment or health care. This study not only used this group as the sample, but also compared cognitively impaired and cognitively intact older adults. In view of growing diversity in the United States, more research of this type is needed to develop best practices for all people of any cultural/ethnic background.

Implications for Nursing. As the population ages, accurate assessment and treatment of pain needs to be a priority. Older and minority clients are each at risk for undertreatment of pain. Use of simple pain scales, such as the Faces Pain Scale, should be a routine part of pain assessment in all clients, both cognitively intact and cognitively impaired.

mentally disabled populations. The book listed in the Selected Bibliography by McCaffery and Pasero (1999) contains 0 to 10 pain rating scales in 25 different languages.

ASSESSING PAIN IN COGNITIVELY IMPAIRED OR CRITICALLY ILL NONVERBAL CLIENTS. Although it seems obvious, nonverbal, intubated, and cognitively impaired clients *do* feel pain! It is important to be proactive and "assume pain is present," or APP (Pasero & McCaffery, 2000).

Clients with painful chronic conditions such as arthritis, osteoporosis, cancer, pressure ulcers, and contractures should receive an analgesic trial of around-the-clock medications. Procedural pain should also be assumed and analgesics given beforehand. Turning, suctioning, drain removal, wound care, and other routine procedures are very painful (Puntillo et al., 2001).

Possible indicators of pain in nonverbal clients include facial expressions, verbalizations, body language, and behavioral changes. There are several behavioral pain indicator checklists or tools available for the nurse to use. In a study of older adults with hip fractures, facial grimaces and restlessness were the two most common pain indicators (Feldt, 2000).

After receiving a 24- to 48-hour analgesic trial, a complete reassessment should be performed. Family members' reports of a client's pain should be incorporated into the plan of care.

PSYCHOSOCIAL ASSESSMENT

ACUTE PAIN. All pain holds significant meaning for the person experiencing it. Clients having acute pain from surgery may interpret their pain as necessary and expected. It may be viewed with relief as a sign that some greater problem has been resolved or alleviated by the surgery. Knowing that the duration of the pain is limited may allow the client to deal with unpleasant sensations without too much difficulty. In contrast, acute chest pain associated with angina may mark the beginning of a life of fear and uncertainty.

CHRONIC PAIN. Various psychosocial factors influence chronic pain. Some factors are similar to those found in the acute pain experience, such as anxiety or fear related to the meaning of the pain. Because chronic pain persists or is perhaps only partially relieved, the client may feel powerless, angry, hostile or desperate. The client is also vulnerable to labels such as "chronic complainer" or "fake."

The status of family and other close relationships, along with the breadth of social resources available to the chronic pain client, must be assessed. The existence of a pain-specific conflict with a spouse or significant other may affect or limit pain coping strategies. Other people may react to chronic pain with depression, social withdrawal, and preoccupation with physical symptoms.

If the chronic pain is associated with a progressive disease such as cancer, rheumatoid arthritis, or peripheral vascular disease, the client may have worries and concerns about the consequences of the illness. Clients with cancer-related pain may fear death or body mutilation. Some may think they are being punished for some wrongdoing in life. Others may attach a religious or spiritual significance to lingering pain.

Ask open-ended questions (e.g., "Tell me how your pain has affected your job or role as a mother") to allow the client to describe personal attitudes about pain and its influence on life. This opportunity can help a client whose life has been changed by pain. However, some clients choose not to share their private information or fears. This decision should be respected. Assess the impact of the pain on their ability to function.

In 2000, the Joint Commission Accreditation of Health Care Organizations (JCAHO) published new pain management standards. The American Pain Society (APS) called pain "the fifth vital sign." Pain documentation as the fifth vital sign is not required by JCAHO or APS, yet most health care agencies use it to ensure all pain is assessed at regular intervals and treated appropriately.

Interventions

Drug Therapy. Medications are the gold-standard form of pain control. However, many nurses and other health professionals have inadequate knowledge regarding the pharmacology of drugs used in pain control. This lack of information, together with the misconceptions and attitudes about pain previously discussed, are the two main reasons why clients have inadequate pain relief.

There are three groups of medications used to manage pain: non-opioids, opioids, and adjuvants. To advocate for your client, a thorough understanding of the medications used to treat pain is necessary (Table 7-6).

Non-Opioid Analgesics. The **non-opioid** (formerly called nonnarcotic) **analgesics** are the first line therapy for mild to moderate pain. The two most common non-opioids are **acetylsalicylic acid (aspirin**, Apo-ASA✱) and **acetaminophen (Tylenol**, Atasol✱). Studies have shown that their analgesic and antipyretic (fever reduction) effects are the same in equal doses. The single optimal dose of aspirin or acetaminophen is between 650 and 1000 mg.

There is a ceiling to the analgesic effect of these non-opioids. In other words, if the dose of the non-opioid analgesic is greater than 1000 mg, there will be no additional analgesic effect, only more side effects. Aspirin can cause bleeding, and acetaminophen can cause hepatotoxicity (liver toxicity).

TABLE 7-6 Examples of Analgesics by Classification

Non-Opioids	Opioids	Adjuvants
Acetaminophen (Tylenol)	Pure agonists:	Tricyclic antidepressants:
NSAIDs (nonselective):	Morphine	Amitriptyline (Elavil)
Aspirin	Fentanyl (Duragesic, Actiq)	Desipramine (Norpramin)
Ibuprofen (Motrin)	Hydrocodone (Vicoden)	Nortriptyline (Pamelor)
Naproxen (Naprosyn)	Oxycodone (OxyContin, Percodan)	Doxepin (Sinequan)
Etodolac (Lodine)	Hydromorphone (Dilaudid)	Anticonvulsants:
Ketoprofen (Toradol)	Meperidine (Demerol) (outdated drug)	Gabapentin (Neurontin)
Piroxicam (Feldene)	Methadone	Valproic acid (Depakene)
Salsalate (Disalcid)	Codeine	Topiramate (Topamax)
NSAIDs (selective):	Agonist/antagonists (not commonly used):	Clonazepam (Klonopin)
Celecoxib (Celebrex)	Pentazocine (Talwin)	Baclofen (Lioresal)
Valdecoxib (Bextra)	Butorphanol (Stadol)	Alpha-2 adrenergics:
	Nalbuphine (Nubain)	Clonidine (Catapres)
	Buprenorphine (Buprenex)	Tizanidine (Zanaflex)
		Local anesthetics:
		Mexiletine (Mexitil)
		Topical lidocaine (Lidoderm)
		NMDA antagonists:
		Ketamine
		Dextromethorphan

Modified from McCaffery, M., & Pasero, C., (1999). *Pain: Clinical manual* (2nd ed.) St. Louis: Mosby.

Many people underestimate the effectiveness of non-opioid analgesics, also referred to as **peripheral-acting analgesics**. For mild pain, the non-opioids aspirin 650 mg and acetaminophen (Tylenol) 650 mg produce pain relief comparable to that of the opioids codeine 32 mg PO and meperidine (Demerol) 50 mg PO. Most non-opioids (other than acetaminophen) are potent anti-inflammatory agents called **nonsteroidal anti-inflammatory drugs (NSAIDs).**

Nonsteroidal Anti-Inflammatory Drugs. Aspirin and other NSAIDs are very effective for inflammatory type pain, such as rheumatoid arthritis, postoperative pain, dental pain, menstrual pain, migraines, low back pain, sunburn, and bone pain. These agents inhibit the synthesis of prostaglandins, which are fatty-acid substances found throughout the body. The release of prostaglandins in tissues causes pain, edema, and inflammation. By inhibiting the synthesis of prostaglandins, anti-inflammatory drugs decrease inflammation and pain. NSAIDs are particularly useful in the management of acute inflammation such as that which causes postoperative pain. **Ketorolac (Toradol)** is one of the most popular NSAIDs prescribed for short-term use in cases of acute pain because it can be given orally, intramuscularly, or by intravenous (IV) push. A newer COX-2 NSAID, **parecoxib (Dynastat),** should soon be available for either IV or intramuscular injection.

Aspirin and other NSAIDs can cause gastrointestinal (GI) disturbances and can prevent platelet aggregation, which results in a tendency toward bleeding. Therefore observe the client for gastric discomfort or vomiting, and bleeding or bruising. Report these problems to the health care provider immediately.

CONSIDERATIONS FOR OLDER ADULTS

Older adults often take over-the-counter (OTC) NSAIDs for common problems, such as osteoarthritis and back pain. However, while they are usually effective in relieving pain, these drugs can increase or decrease the effects of other drugs that the client is taking. The most serious drug-drug interactions are with anticoagulants, oral hypoglycemics, and antihypertensives, including diuretics (Durrance, 2003). To add to these potential problems, normal physiologic changes of aging affect the protein binding, drug distribution, and renal elimination of NSAIDs. King (2000) reported that almost 17,000 deaths occur among clients with arthritis related to long-term NSAID use. In addition, NSAIDs can cause tinnitus and other peripheral and central nervous system symptoms that can contribute to falls in older adults (King, 2000).

NSAIDs also cause renal toxicity; therefore renal function blood tests should be routinely monitored with long-term therapy, especially in the older adult. In addition, NSAIDs can cause sodium and water retention that may lead to congestive heart failure, more often in an older client.

When taking a client history, ask about the use of NSAIDs, keeping in mind that store brand names may not be considered as NSAIDs. For example, Walprofen is Wal-Mart's brand name for ibuprofen; Walproxen is the name for naproxen. Orudis contains ketoprofen, and Aleve contains naproxen. Ask the client or client's family to provide the name of each drug that the client is taking, as well as the daily dosage. Some clients may unknowingly take several types of NSAIDs at the same time, putting them at a high risk for adverse drug effects.

The side effects of individual NSAIDs differ. For example, ibuprofen (Motrin, Actiprofen✱) and naproxen (Naprosyn, Naxen✱) appear to cause fewer GI problems than ketoprofen (Orudis, Rhodis✱). By adding a GI protective drug such as misoprostol (Cytotec), GI side effects may be reduced.

Because of the high incidence of GI bleeding due to NSAID use, particularly in older adults, the American Pain Society Clinical Practice Guidelines (1999) recommend selective cyclooxygenase-2 (COX-2) inhibitors, such as celecoxib (Celebrex) and valdecoxib (Bextra), for long-term use. This newer class of NSAIDs, COX-2 inhibitors, selectively block the COX-2 enzyme responsible for inflammation and the production of substances associated with pain (e.g., prostaglandins). However, all COX-2 inhibitors have recently been associated with increased cardiovascular disease and may have limited use or be unavailable in the future. Most older NSAIDs block both COX-1 and COX-2 enzymes. The COX-1 enzyme is responsible for the gastric and renal side effects associated with older NSAID use. Studies of clients with dental pain, osteoarthritis, and rheumatoid arthritis treated with COX-2 inhibitors demonstrate effective analgesia without GI side effects. There is no difference in the COX-2 analgesic efficacy or in renal side effects, but the decreased risk of GI bleeding makes these drugs more beneficial.

Acetaminophen. Unlike the rest of the non-opioid analgesics, acetaminophen (Tylenol) has few anti-inflammatory properties. Acetaminophen has some advantages over aspirin in that it is available in a liquid form (which is the best way to take oral analgesics) and it can be taken on an empty stomach. Acetaminophen causes no adverse gastrointestinal (GI) effects. Therefore it is preferred for any client who has a history of ulcer disease. Acetaminophen also has no effect on platelet aggregation as most of the other non-opioids do. This drug is also preferred, then, for clients in whom bleeding is likely, such as preoperative or postoperative clients. Acetaminophen is not without its serious side effects, however. The main adverse effects are hepatotoxicity (liver toxicity) and nephro-toxicity (renal toxicity) with long-term use.

Health care providers commonly prescribe acetaminophen for pain. Acetaminophen exerts its analgesic action by blocking peripheral pain receptors, thus increasing the threshold of these receptors to painful stimuli. Reports of liver toxicity have been associated with higher doses of the drug (1000 mg) taken more frequently than every 4 hours for long-term use. Current recommendations restrict the total daily amount of acetaminophen to no more than 4000 mg (4 g). For long-term use, no more than 3600 mg daily should be taken. Less than 2400 mg daily should be used in older adults. Teach clients to be aware of the amount of acetaminophen in combination products such as Vicodin and Darvocet. The acetaminophen in these products limits their use for chronic pain.

Opioid Analgesics. **Opioid analgesics** are the mainstay in the management of all types of pain. Opioids (formerly called **narcotics**) work centrally by blocking the release of neurotransmitters in the spinal cord. Opioids are classified as full agonists (morphine-like), partial agonists, or mixed agonists/antagonists. There are no advantages to the partial or mixed agonists, and they could precipitate a withdrawal if given to a client taking a full agonist.

Full Agonists. The opioid **full agonists** bind to mu receptors and block the release of substance P, preventing the transmission of pain. The full agonists are the most potent of all analgesics.

Most opioid agonists are similar in pharmacologic effects, so a client does not need more than one. Although the oral route is generally the preferred route, most opioids can be administered in many different routes.

There is no ceiling in the dose of a pure opioid agonist. The use of an equianalgesic chart when changing opioids is necessary, though, because these drugs vary in their oral to parenteral dosages (Table 7-7).

Equianalgesic Chart. Nurses should be familiar with a comparison chart of equivalent opioid dosages. This chart is useful when switching opioids or routes of administration of opioids, and it enables the nurse to learn the dosage of the drugs being administered for pain.

The term **equianalgesic** refers to the dose and route of administration of one drug that produces about the same degree of analgesia as the given dose and route of another drug. Most commonly, 10 mg IM of morphine is the standard dose against which other opioids are measured. Equianalgesic opioid drug guides provide only the comparative analgesic potencies among these drugs. Dose modifications may be necessary according to each client's response and as always, with older adults, the guideline is to "start low and go slow" with drug dosing.

Common Opioids. **Codeine** is a short-acting weak opioid. It is considered a pro-drug, meaning an enzyme is necessary to break it down to be effective. It is estimated that 5% to 10% of the population lack this enzyme, which could account for codeine's ineffectiveness in certain clients. Codeine has limited value for severe pain, and should not be used in older adults due to the possible accumulation of a toxic metabolite, as well as constipation.

Hydrocodone is available as a combination product with acetaminophen (Lortab, Vicodin) and ibuprofen (Vicoprofen). Because of this, the dose cannot be escalated due to the toxicities from the non-opioids. Therefore hydrocodone has limited usefulness for chronic, long-term pain.

Oxycodone is available as a single-agent, both in short- and long-acting preparations (OxyContin). It is also available in combination with aspirin (Percodan, Oxycodone✱) or acetaminophen (Percocet, Tylox, Roxicet, Oxycocet✱). Oxycodone is recommended for acute and chronic pain.

Morphine (Duramorph, Roxanol, Avinza, Kadian, Morphitec✱) is the gold standard opioid for both acute and chronic pain (see the Concept Map on p. 77). It is inexpensive, available in many dosage strengths (both short and long acting), and can be given in virtually any route, including rectally. MS Contin, Avinza, and Kadian are examples of long-acting or slow-release forms of the drug. Ten milligrams of morphine intramuscularly equals 30 mg orally.

Hydromorphone (Dilaudid) is eight times more potent than morphine. It is currently only available in the short-acting form. Like morphine, hydromorphone is useful for all types of moderate to severe pain.

Fentanyl (Sublimaze) is a potent opioid available in two special forms, the 72-hour patch known as **Duragesic,** which is useful for chronic pain, and in the oral transmucosal lozenge (Actiq). **Actiq** lozenges are indicated for breakthrough cancer pain and should not be given to opioid-naive clients. **Breakthrough pain** occurs primarily in clients with severe terminal cancer pain. The client experiences pain between scheduled doses of the drug regimen. Other drugs may also be used for this purpose, but lozenges are less invasive for the client. Actiq is also currently being used "off-label" (not FDA approved) for procedural-type pain.

Methadone (Dolophine) is the only full opioid agonist with a dual mechanism of action. It works on both the mu receptors and the NMDA receptors. Because of its long half-life (24 to 36 hours), always assess for sedation (especially days 2 to 3) and use cautiously in older adults. When managing pain in a client in a methadone maintenance program for substance abuse, be sure to increase the methadone dose for pain relief or add a second opioid.

Tramadol (Ultram) is classified as an atypical opioid. It binds weakly to the mu receptors in the central nervous system and inhibits the reuptake of norepinephrine and serotonin. Tramadol can be used for acute pain and chronic neuropathic pain. It should not be given in doses greater than 400 mg daily because it can cause seizures. It should be

TABLE 7-7 Dose Equivalents for Opioid Analgesics in Opioid-Naive Adults[a]

Drug	Approximate Equianalgesic Dose: Oral	Approximate Equianalgesic Dose: Parenteral	Usual Starting Dose for Moderate to Severe Pain: Oral	Usual Starting Dose for Moderate to Severe Pain: Parenteral
Opioid Agonist[b]				
Morphine[c]	30 mg q3-4h (repeat around-the-clock dosing) 60 mg q3-4h (single dose or intermittent dosing)	10 mg q3-4h	30 mg q3-4h	10 mg q3-4h
Morphine, controlled-release[b,d] (MS Contin, Oramorph)	90-120 mg q12h	N/A	90-120 mg q12h	N/A
Hydromorphone[c] (Dilaudid)	7.5 mg q3-4h	1.5 mg q3-4h	6 mg q3-4h	1.5 mg q3-4h
Levorphanol (Levo-Dromoran)	4 mg q6-8h	2 mg q6-8h	4 mg q6-8h	2 mg q6-8h
Meperidine (Demerol)	300 mg q2-3h	100 mg q3h	N/R	100 mg q3h
Methadone (Dolophine, other)	20 mg q6-8h	10 mg q6-8h	20 mg q6-8h	10 mg q6-8h
Oxymorphone[c] (Numorphan)	N/A	1 mg q3-4h	N/A	1 mg q3-4h
Combination Opioid/NSAID Preparations[e]				
Codeine[f] (with aspirin or acetaminophen)	18-200 mg q3-4h	130 mg q3-4h	60 mg q3-4h	60 mg q2h (IM/SC)
Hydrocodone (in Lorcet, Lortab, Vicodin, others)	30 mg q3-4h	N/A	10 mg q3-4h	N/A
Oxycodone (Roxicodone, also in Percocet, Percodan, Tylox, others)	30 mg q3-4h	N/A	10 mg q3-4h	N/A

From Management of Cancer Pain Guideline Panel. (1994) *Management of cancer pain: Clinical practice guidelines.* AHCPR Pub. No. 94-0592. Rockville, MD: Agency for Health Care Policy and Research, Public Health Service, U.S. Department of Health and Human Services.

N/A, Not available; *N/R,* not recommended; *SC,* subcutaneous.

Note: Published tables vary in the suggested doses that are equianalgesic to morphine. Clinical response is the criterion that must be applied for each patient; titration to clinical responses is necessary. Because there is not complete cross tolerance among these drugs, it is usually necessary to use a lower-than-equianalgesic dose when changing drugs and to retitrate to response.

[a]**Caution:** Recommended doses do not apply for adult patients with body weight less than 50 kg.

[b]**Caution:** Recommended doses do not apply to patients with renal or hepatic insufficiency or other conditions affecting drug metabolism and kinetics.

[c]**Caution:** For morphine, hydromorphone, and oxymorphone, rectal administration is an alternate route for patients unable to take oral medications. Equianalgesic doses may differ from oral and parenteral doses because of pharmacokinetic differences.

[d]Transdermal fentanyl (Duragesic) is an alternative option. Transdermal fentanyl dosage is not calculated as equianalgesic to a single morphine dosage. See the package insert for dosing calculations. Doses above 25 mcg/hr should not be used in opioid-naive patients.

[e]**Caution:** Doses of aspirin and acetaminophen in combination opioid-NSAID preparations must also be adjusted to the patient's body weight. Aspirin is contraindicated in children in the presence of fever or other viral disease because of its association with Reye's syndrome.

[f]**Caution:** Codeine doses above 65 mg often are not appropriate because of diminishing incremental analgesia with increasing doses, as well as a higher incidence of nausea, constipation, and other side effects.

used cautiously in clients who are taking antidepressant medications.

Meperidine (Demerol) used to be routinely prescribed in acute care settings. Most health care agencies now have policies in place restricting its use to less than 48 hours, or no more than 600 mg in 24 hours. Many agencies have discontinued its use altogether for older adults due to the resulting toxicities. Because of the accumulation of the toxic metabolite normeperidine, central nervous system toxicities may occur (Waitman & McCaffery, 2001). Repetitive doses of meperidine, particularly in older adults or in people with decreased renal clearance, may cause numbness, twitching, confusion, and seizures. It is never a good idea to give meperidine orally because of its poor bioavailability–75 mg intramuscularly equals 300 mg orally. *Meperidine use is considered to be outdated pain management.*

Agonists-Antagonists. The **agonist-antagonist drugs** are opioid (agonists) that antagonize the pure agonists (counteract opioid effects). These drugs include mixed agonists (pentazocine [Talwin], nalbuphine [Nubain], butorphanol [Stadol]), and partial agonists (buprenorphine [Buprenex]).

Because of their opioid antagonist properties, administering them after a client has been receiving opioids may cause withdrawal symptoms. If agonist-antagonist anal-

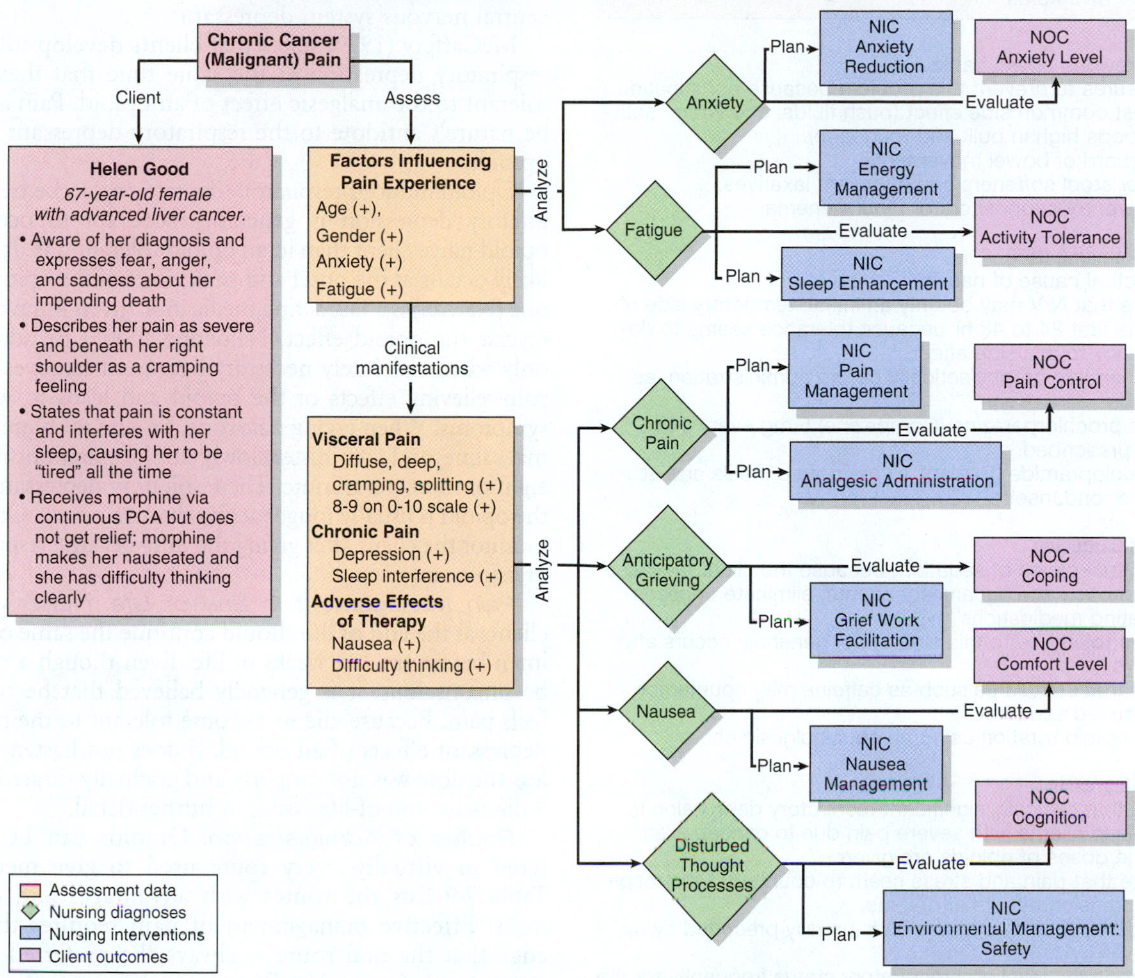

Concept Map by Elaine Bishop Kennedy, EdD, RN

gesics are given together with an opioid, eventually they antagonize opioid analgesia; hence the client has poor pain relief.

The major side effects produced by these drugs are drowsiness, occasional nausea, and psychotomimetic effect such as hallucinations and euphoria. The agonist-antagonist drugs have little place in the management of pain, especially chronic pain. These drugs offer no advantage over morphine-like agonists (American Pain Society, 2003).

Side Effects of Opioids. The most important type of opioid receptor is the mu receptor. **Mu opioids** cause side effects that include constipation, nausea and vomiting, urinary retention, pruritus (itching), sedation, and respiratory depression. These side effects are often mistakenly viewed as allergies, but it is rare to be allergic to morphine-type medications. The side effects (other than constipation) are time limited and easily managed (Table 7-8).

NAUSEA AND VOMITING. Nausea and vomiting often are mistaken for allergic reactions, and clients may be denied opioids. The side effect of nausea or vomiting in clients taking opioids varies from client to client and with opioid to opioid. If a client is nauseated after receiving an opioid, the cause and appropriate treatment must be determined.

Nausea and vomiting may occur initially as a side effect in clients taking opioids for pain relief. Treating the nausea and vomiting with an appropriate antiemetic usually helps. In addition, if client needs to continue the opioid therapy longer than 1 week, the problem usually resolves on its own.

CONSTIPATION. Although constipation may seem like a minor side effect, it is not to the client, especially the older adult. Often the discomfort of constipation is more distressing to the client than the pain itself.

Opioids inhibit peristalsis in the gastrointestinal tract. Clients who take regular doses of opioids almost always become constipated. Also, many clients in pain lack proper exercise and have an inadequate diet, both making the problem of constipation worse.

Whenever a client is started on regular doses of opioids, it is essential that the preventive approach be used. Implement interventions to prevent the problem of constipation (see Table 7-8.)

SEDATION. Because opioids have a depressant effect on the central nervous system, some drowsiness can be anticipated. However, sedation is not always caused by opioids. If the client is still in pain, other causes of sedation should be ruled out before decreasing the opioid dosage or changing medications. For example, other medications, such as hypnotics or tranquilizers (diazepam [Valium], alprazolam [Xanax}, or promethazine [Phenergan], could be causing the

TABLE 7-8 Nursing Interventions to Prevent Side Effects of Opioids

Constipation
- Assess previous bowel habits.
- Use measures to *prevent* this problem because constipation is the most common side effect (push fluids, encourage activity, give foods high in bulk and roughage).
- Keep a record of bowel movements.
- Administer stool softeners and stimulant laxatives.
- If ineffective, try suppository or Fleet's enema.

Nausea and Vomiting (N/V)
- Assess actual cause of nausea.
- Recognize that N/V may be only an initial, temporary side effect for the first 24 to 48 hr because tolerance seems to develop quickly to this side effect.
- Try an antiemetic prophylactically before administration, as prescribed.
- Treat with prochlorperazine (Compazine) 5 mg every 4 hr orally, as prescribed.
- Give metoclopramide (Reglan) 10 mg before meals and at bedtime, or ondansetron (Zofran) 4 mg IV.

Sedation and Confusion
- Assess actual cause of sedation, because the client may also be on hypnotics and antianxiety agents; eliminate unnecessary sedating medications.
- Recall that tolerance to this side effect generally occurs after 2 to 3 days.
- Be aware that stimulants such as caffeine may counteract opioid-induced sedation.
- Consider opioid rotation using an equianalgesic chart.

Respiratory Depression
- Be aware that clinically significant respiratory depression is rarely seen in clients with severe pain due to cancer, even when large doses of opioids are given.
- Recognize that pain and stress seem to counteract the respiratory depression effects of opioids.
- Recall that respiratory depression is usually preceded by sedation.
- Monitor sedation level and respiratory status frequently for the first 24 to 48 hr, especially in opioid-naive clients.
- If increased sedation occurs, decrease opioid dose and attempt to stimulate client.
- Be aware that respiratory rate alone is not indicative of respiratory status.
- If absolutely necessary in an unresponsive client, administer naloxone (Narcan) 0.4 mg diluted in 10 mL of normal saline; push 0.5 mL slowly for 2 min and observe the client.

sedation. Often the elimination of other central nervous system–depressant medications resolves the sedation problem.

Sedation occurs before opioid-induced respiratory depression, so nurse-monitored sedation levels are recommended by use of a sedation scale for opioid-naive clients or clients receiving opioids IV or epidurally. The key to assessing sedation is determining how easily the client is aroused. Assess each client's individual response to the first dose of an opioid. Be sure to assess the client's level of consciousness. Monitor respiratory rate and depth, especially while the client is sleeping.

RESPIRATORY DEPRESSION. A main reason for inadequate pain control is the exaggerated fear of respiratory depression. However, this problem rarely occurs, especially in clients taking opioids for chronic, long-term pain.

The pain, stress, and anxiety experienced by the client are potent respiratory *stimulants* that may override or negate the respiratory depression resulting from the drugs. The nurse also considers that the effect of all opioid analgesics may be greater in a client who is older, has reduced blood volume or renal disease, or has received anesthetic agents or other central nervous system depressants.

McCaffery (1979) states that clients develop tolerance to respiratory depression at the same time that they become tolerant to the analgesic effect of an opioid. Pain appears to be nature's antidote to the respiratory depressant effects of opioids.

Opioid-induced respiratory depression can be treated. Respiratory depression is generally more apt to occur in an opioid-naive client than in an opioid-tolerant one. It also most likely occurs at the onset and peak effect of the opioid. Naloxone (Narcan) is a fast-acting medication given intravenously to reverse the opioid effect. Naloxone should be administered only when absolutely necessary because it removes all of the pain-relieving effects of the opioid and leads to withdrawal symptoms. When giving naloxone, be sure to dilute with normal saline, and administer slowly until respirations increase to eight or more per minute. The respiratory depressant effect of the opioid is usually longer acting than naloxone. Continue to monitor the client after giving the drug because respiratory depression can recur.

Pain Management in End of Life. Nurses caring for clients at the end of life should continue the same opioid regimen before the last weeks of life. Even though a client may be unconscious, it is generally believed that he or she still feels pain. Because clients become tolerant to the respiratory depressant effects of an opioid, it does not hasten death unless the dose was not properly and gradually titrated. Chapter 9 discusses end-of-life issues in further detail.

Routes of Administration. Opioids can be administered in virtually every route used to give medications. Table 7-9 lists the routes with advantages and disadvantages. Effective management of pain requires the knowledge that the oral route is always the preferred route for most types of pain. The IV route is the most efficient route due to its rapid titration. The IM route is no longer acceptable as state-of-the-art pain management, due to its many disadvantages.

PRN Range Orders. Nurses have administered PRN range orders for opioid analgesia for many years. Although this approach is meant to manage the pain of individual clients based on accurate assessments, obvious safety issues are involved.

Patient-Controlled Analgesia. **Patient-controlled analgesia (PCA)** is a common way to combat the problem of inadequate analgesia in the management of acute and chronic pain. This method allows the client to control the dosage of opioid analgesia received. This approach to pain control can improve pain relief and increase client satisfaction. It can also decrease the amount of opioid consumption per day when compared with nurse-administered intermittent dosing methods.

Clients who have ready access to an analgesic are more likely to medicate themselves before the pain becomes severe, and thus they may require a reduced amount. Having such control over drug administration also reduces anxiety, which helps relieve pain.

PCA is achieved through the use of a PCA infusion pump (Figure 7-4). Both stationary pole pumps (for hospital use) and ambulatory pumps (for nursing home or home use) are available. The infusion pump delivers the desired amount of

TABLE 7-9 Routes of Administration

Oral

Advantages
- Preferred route of analgesia
- Allows greater mobility and convenience
- Drug levels peak in 1 to 2 hours
- Greater client satisfaction
- If client is NPO or has a nasogastric or gastrostomy tube, medications can still be given orally
- Cost efficient
- Relatively steady blood levels produced

Disadvantages
- Slow onset
- Long-acting opioids cannot be crushed, broken, or chewed
- Some clients are unable to swallow or are NPO
- Requires functional GI system

Rectal

Advantages
- Good for clients who are NPO, nauseated, or at home
- Easy for clients to self-administer, especially older adults
- Duration of action 4 to 6 hr
- Any opioid can be compounded by a pharmacist for rectal route
- Clinical practice suggests oral and rectal doses of analgesics fairly equal

Disadvantages
- May be more expensive than oral route and difficult to obtain
- Contraindicated in thrombocytopenic clients

Intramuscular

Advantages
- Should be used for acute short-term pain

Disadvantages
- Rapid peak effect but short duration of action and rapid fall-off
- Problems with absorption lead to inconsistent blood levels
- Painful administration
- Not recommended for chronic long-term pain, especially cancer pain
- Client is dependent on others to administer injection
- Not recommended for use with emaciated clients or clients with decreased muscle mass
- Long-term use can cause fibrosis and sterile abscesses

Transdermal

Advantages
- Available as fentanyl (Duragesic)
- Doses of 25, 50, 75, and 100 mcg/hr patches applied every 72 hr
- Noninvasive, easy to use, well accepted by clients

Disadvantages
- Due to gradual increases in plasma concentration, may need to supplement with short-acting analgesics for first 12 to 24 hr after initial application
- Costly
- Difficult to adjust dose
- Febrile clients absorb medication quickly
- Concerns over disposal

OTFC (Oral Transmucosal Fentanyl Citrate)

Advantages
- Good bioavailability, rapid peak effect
- FDA-approved for breakthrough cancer pain
- May be useful off-label for procedural pain

Disadvantages
- Sweetened matrix contains 2 g sugar
- Short-acting, short half-life
- Must be swabbed inside mouth for at least 10 minutes to dissolve completely

Topical

Advantages
- Easy to use
- Little systemic absorption
- Lidoderm patch, EMLA topical cream, capsaicin cream are examples

Disadvantages
- May cause skin reactions
- Capsaicin causes burning initially

Sublingual

Advantages
- Most opioids can be absorbed SL
- Good for clients with no IV access and/or impaired swallowing

Disadvantages
- May not be absorbed or may cause mucosal irritation

Intranasal

Advantages
- Butorphanol (Stadol NS) opioid agonist-antagonist
- Sumatriptan for migraines
- Convenient delivery form
- Good for outpatient use

Disadvantages
- Butorphanol is not to be given to client on pure opioid; can precipitate a withdrawal

Subcutaneous

Advantages
- Available as bolus, continuous infusion, or continuous infusion with PCA
- Avoids need for intravenous access and cheaper than IV
- Readily managed at home
- Recommended for cancer clients who cannot take anything by mouth and in whom IV access is not desirable
- Avoids repetitive injections and is less painful
- Continuous infusion
- Avoids peaks and valleys in bloodstream; maintains steady blood level
- Provides prolonged parenteral administration of opioid
- No delay in drug administration

Disadvantages
- Subcutaneous boluses have slower onset and a lower peak effect than IV boluses
- Requires use of ambulatory infusion pump, which is not always client acceptable

Intravenous
- Available as bolus, continuous infusion, or continuous infusion with PCA IV bolus

Advantages
- Good for acute pain or procedures
- Immediate pain relief
- Provides fastest onset but shortest duration
- Peak in 5 to 15 minutes
- Eliminates anxiety and prevents pain
- Recommended when unable to achieve pain control through oral or rectal routes with high dosages of opioid or unable to use oral/rectal route
- Continuous IV administration provides steady blood level

Disadvantages
- Not recommended for constant pain due to peaks and valleys in bloodstream
- Requires use of infusion pump with an alarm

Continued

TABLE 7-9 Routes of Administration—*cont'd*

Patient-Controlled Analgesia (PCA)

Advantages

- Allows client to receive a predetermined intravenous bolus of an opioid by hitting a syringe pump mechanism
- Gives client sense of control, less anxiety
- Provides quick and consistent pain relief
- Maintains a constant level of pain relief
- Eliminates the need for repeated injections
- Saves time
- Especially recommended for acute pain such as postoperative pain

Disadvantages

- Requires use of a pump
- Requires reinforced client teaching for maximum effectiveness
- Requires two nurses to program to prevent errors (in hospitals)
- Requires designated person to hit button if client cannot

Spinal (Epidural and Intrathecal) Administration

Advantages

- Opioid (usually morphine or fentanyl) administered through catheter into epidural or intrathecal space
- Preservative-free morphine or fentanyl used
- Useful for postoperative pain (abdominal, thoracic, orthopedic) or chronic pain
- May be intermittent bolus or by continuous infusion pump

Disadvantages

- Careful client selection is necessary because procedure is expensive and may be risky
- Side effects include nausea, vomiting, pruritus, sedation, urinary retention, and respiratory depression
- Possible complication of hematoma and infection and/or meningitis

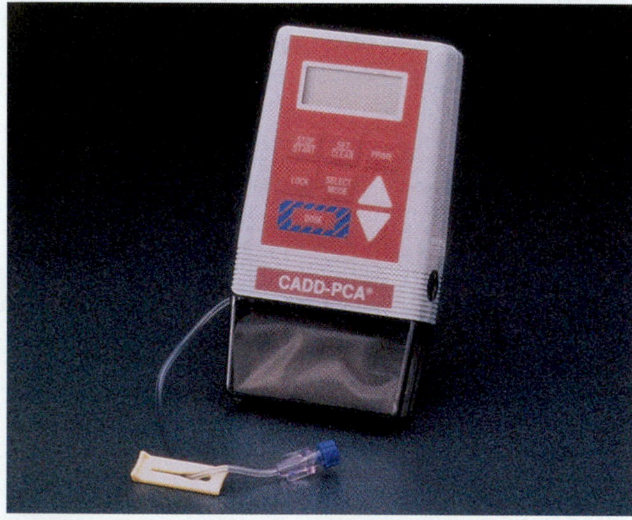

Figure 7-4 ■ An ambulatory patient-controlled analgesia infusion pump. (CADD-PCA is a registered trademark of Pharmacia Deltec, St. Paul, MN.)

medication through a conventional IV route for pain. Morphine is the most commonly used drug for PCA. Meperidine (Demerol) is reserved as a last resort for short-term (usually less than 48 hours) or no more than 600 mg in 24 hours. Its toxic metabolite, normeperidine, may accumulate in the blood and is can induce confusion and seizures. Older adults are particularly at risk. Hydromorphone (Dilaudid) and fentanyl are also used for PCA. Standing or preprinted orders from the health care provider are commonly used for PCA administration.

Drug security to avoid overdosing is achieved through a locked syringe pump system or locked drug reservoir system. The device is programmed to deliver a certain amount of drug (**demand dose**) within a specific interval known as a **lockout interval**. The health care provider specifies the amount of the demand dose. Morphine doses typically range from 1 to 2 mg, hydromorphone from 0.15 to 0.4 mg, and fentanyl from 12.5 to 25 mcg. Doses vary according to the client's degree of pain. The lockout interval is usually 5 to 15 minutes.

To prevent medication errors, it is recommended that two nurses program the dosing parameters into the PCA delivery device. When the client presses the button or pendant (on ambulatory pumps), the appropriate bolus or demand dose is delivered. No drug is administered if the client attempts to access the drug before the designated time interval between doses has elapsed. With this technique, there is little chance that clients will overmedicate themselves.

The PCA regimen may consist of a demand-dosing-only schedule or a continuous infusion or **basal rate** and demand dosing. With demand or self-administered dosing only, the client relies solely on a push of the pendant or bolus feature to seek pain relief. Continuous or basal infusion of the opioid in addition to demand dosing provides more consistent analgesia and allows the client to sleep without fear of missing any pain medication. However, when a continuous infusion is added to the regimen, clients may be at greater risk for opioid-induced side effects (e.g., nausea and vomiting, sedation, respiratory depression), especially if the hourly dose is too much for the client.

Your primary role in caring for clients using PCA is to teach them how to use the device and to report side effects, such as dizziness, nausea and vomiting, and inability to void. As with all opioids, monitor the client's vital signs, particularly respirations, and check sedation level every 2 hours initially.

When a client is cognitively impaired or unable to push the PCA button, another method of administration should be considered. PCA means **patient-controlled**, so having someone else push the button defeats the purpose. More importantly, this practice can cause oversedation and possible serious safety issues. Although controversial, some health care agencies do allow one designee to push the PCA for a client who cannot. If the designee is the nurse, inform the family, visitors, or any health care provider not to push the button. Familiarize yourself with the agency's pain management protocols related to PCA use.

Epidural Analgesia. **Epidural analgesia** (also known as peridural or extradural analgesia) refers to the instillation of a pain-blocking agent, usually an opioid analgesic alone or in combination with a local anesthetic, into the epidural space (the space between the dura mater and the vertebral column). Epidural analgesia is more commonly used for the management acute pain, such as postoperative pain. It has been used since the 1950s but has become more popular as newer and more innovative approaches to acute pain control are explored. Epidural analgesia is used primarily in clients who are predisposed to respiratory complications (including those undergoing thoracic surgery), those with preexisting respiratory disease, and those who are obese.

Intrathecal (subarachnoid) analgesia, in which a pain-blocking agent is introduced into the space between the arachnoid mater and pia mater of the spinal cord (where cerebrospinal fluid is located), may be considered for long-term management of **intractable pain** (chronic pain that cannot be managed using standard therapies). However, it is not used as commonly as epidural analgesia due to increased central nervous system risks.

DESCRIPTION. Morphine (preservative free), hydromorphone (Dilaudid), and fentanyl (Sublimaze) are the most commonly used opioids for epidural administration. Sufentanil (Sufenta), an analogue of fentanyl but more potent, may also be used. A local anesthetic such as bupivacaine (Marcaine), which affects both sensory and motor nerves, may be given alone or in combination with an opioid. *Low* concentrations of local anesthetics are used to prevent significant sensory and motor deficits. The incidence of lower motor weakness is far less common with ropivacaine (Naropin) when compared to bupivacaine because it is more selective for sensory nerves.

Using a combination of opioids, non-opioids, and local anesthetics for postoperative pain (as described above) is sometimes referred to as **multimodal analgesia** or **balanced analgesia**. The advantage of these drug combinations is to provide better pain control at lower doses than any single drug does. Another advantage is that these drugs *decrease* the surgical stress response, which is typically mediated by multiple endocrine and metabolic changes. These changes contribute to increased pain, GI distress, confusion (especially in older adults), and cardiopulmonary complications (Pasero, 2003). Balanced analgesia, then, not only decreases pain, but also helps to decrease other problems that result from the stress of surgery. Balanced analgesia is especially appropriate for clients having complex surgeries, such as those undergoing abdominal or thoracic procedures.

A temporary, externalized epidural catheter is used for acute pain control. This device is not sutured to the skin and is easily dislodged. Be sure to tape the catheter in two places to anchor it properly. Some clinicians do not recommend transparent dressings because the catheter may be dislodged when the dressing is removed. The catheter is generally placed in either the lumbar or the thoracic region. Rarely is the catheter placed above the level of sixth thoracic vertebra, because the diaphragmatic muscle may be affected by the analgesic.

COMPLICATIONS. Complications that occur with epidural analgesia are directly related to catheter placement, catheter maintenance, and the type of analgesic. Infection results from a failure to maintain aseptic technique during catheter placement, direct drug instillation, and infusion solution and tubing changes. Infection also results from a failure to maintain aseptic conditions for indwelling catheters at the site of insertion or at the site of tube junctions. To prevent infections, the nurse ensures that all catheter line connections are secure and that an occlusive sterile dressing is maintained over the catheter site.

Pruritus (itching) and nausea and vomiting are common side effects of epidural opioids. Pruritus is first treated with a small amount of naloxone (Narcan). Because epidural-induced pruritus does not appear to be caused by histamine release, diphenhydramine (Benadryl, Allerdryl✱) may not be effective in relieving itching and may only work via its sedating effects. The health care provider usually prescribes an antiemetic as needed for nausea and vomiting.

Clients who receive epidural opioids are also at risk for respiratory depression resulting from high plasma or cerebrospinal fluid concentrations of the instilled drug. Clients receiving epidural therapy with only a local anesthetic are not at risk for respiratory depression. Because of its potential for greater spread up the spinal cord, morphine is more likely than fentanyl to cause respiratory depression. Morphine is preferred to fentanyl when a larger distribution of analgesia is required (e.g., pain relief from extensive abdominal wounds).

Monitor the client's respirations and sedation level at frequent intervals during and after the administration of epidural opioids and immediately report any concerns to the health care provider. Opioid-induced respiratory depression usually occurs within the first few hours of administering fentanyl, but may not be seen for 12 hours or more when morphine is given. This complication is managed by administering low doses (0.2 mg) of naloxone (Narcan) intravenously.

Urinary retention is another common problem associated with epidural analgesia, but it occurs no more frequently than postoperative urinary retention in clients not receiving epidural analgesia. Although the cause is not clear, this problem usually occurs during the first or second day of analgesia administration and may be treated with bethanechol chloride (Urecholine) or intermittent urinary catheterization. The incidence of this complication is less than 25% and is more likely to occur in men than in woman.

Lower motor weakness is more common when an epidural local anesthetic is used in combination with the opioid. Assist clients who get out of bed for the first time to determine the degree of leg weakness. Do not delegate this activity and assessment to unlicensed assistive personnel.

LONG-TERM USE. Epidural analgesia may also be used for long-term chronic pain relief. Such pain is usually the result of cancer or central sensitization. A permanent epidural catheter may be inserted, and several catheter devices are available for this purpose. The DuPen silastic catheter (Davol) is a commonly used **external catheter**. A portion of the catheter exits the skin. Drugs can be intermittently injected into this portion, or the catheter can be attached to an infusion device for continuous drug administration.

Implantable devices are also used to treat chronic pain. The epidural Port-A-Cath (SIMS Deltec, Inc.) is implanted under the skin, and the catheter portion is inserted into the epidural space. As with the DuPen catheter, this device can be injected with drugs intermittently or can be connected to an infusion device for continuous opioid delivery. Injectable ports have been shown to reduce the incidence of catheter dislodgement and early infection. Systems consisting of either an externalized catheter or a drug delivery device are rarely used for intrathecal drug administration. The SynchroMed pump (Medtronic, Inc.) is a totally implantable system that contains a drug reservoir. The drug reservoir is

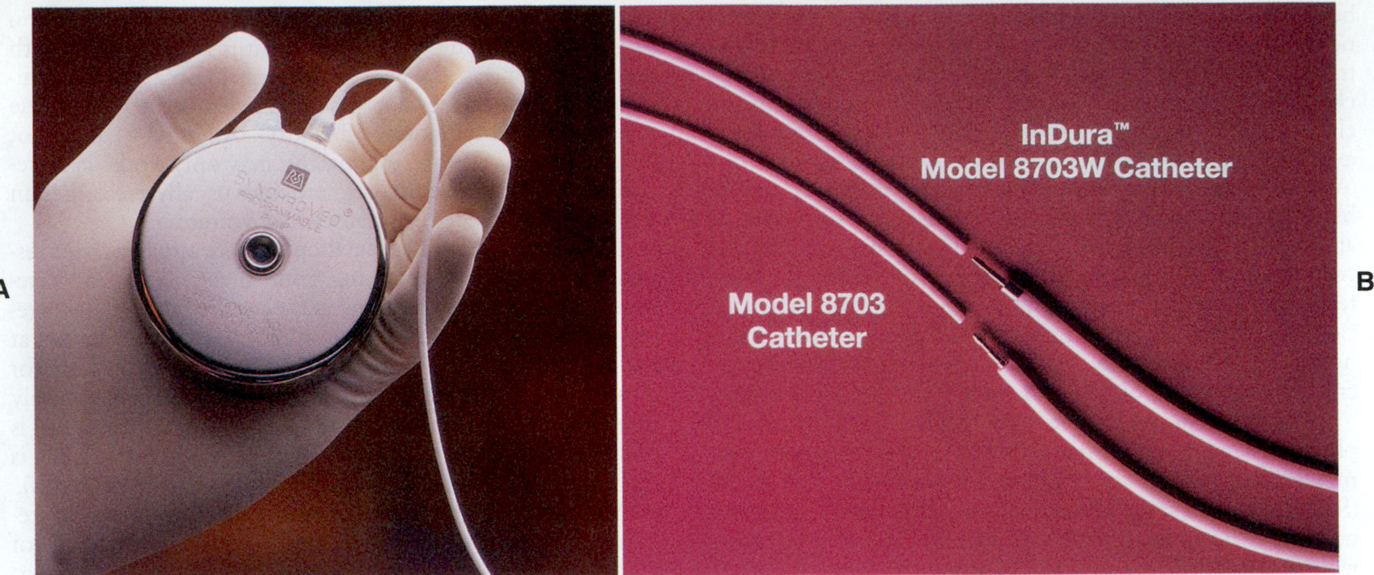

Figure 7-5 ■ A SynchroMed implantable pump **(A)** and spinal catheters **(B)** for delivery of a precise volume of long-term intraspinal analgesia each day. (Courtesy of Medtronic, Inc., Columbia Heights, MN.)

filled on a routine basis and is capable of continuously administering a certain volume of drug each day (Figure 7-5).

The side effects of long-term epidural opioids are common in clients who have had little exposure to opioids. Clients who receive this therapy are usually more tolerant of the effects of opioids and may not require the rigorous monitoring needed for postoperative analgesia. Male clients receiving long-term epidural opioids may complain of sexual dysfunction, decreased libido, and difficulty maintaining an erection; female clients may experience amenorrhea. Testosterone injections seem to help improve sexual function in male clients.

Adjuvant Analgesics. Always consider the use of adjuvant analgesics, especially for clients with chronic pain or complex pain syndromes. Adjuvant analgesics can be helpful for many clients in pain. Although not true analgesics, the **adjuvant medications** relieve pain either alone or in combination with analgesics. These drugs can potentiate or enhance the effectiveness of the analgesic.

Some nurses and other health professionals confuse potentiators with additives. **Additives** are drugs that add an effect, either harmful or beneficial. A common example of this is the drug promethazine (Phenergan). Phenergan is a phenothiazine that has been given for years with opioids such as meperidine (Demerol) to enhance the opioid effects. However, it does just the opposite. Phenergan does not have any analgesic or analgesia-potentiating properties. In fact, it is thought to actually have antianalgesic properties.

The use of adjuvant analgesics not only can provide additional pain relief in some cases but also can help control other discomforts associated with pain (anxiety, depression, nausea, insomnia). Table 7-10 gives examples of adjuvant medications.

Some **antiepileptic drugs** (AEDs or anticonvulsants), such as gabapentin (Neurontin), are effective in treating postherpetic neuralgia and the painful neuropathy associated with diabetes mellitus (Rowbotham et al., 1998; Backonja et al., 1998). They have also been useful in many clients with neuropathic pain from back injuries as well. Doses of gabapentin can be escalated up to 3600 mg daily with few side effects compared to other anticonvulsants. Topiramate (Topamax) is a newer AED with promise for neuropathic pain (Jenson et al., 2002). Because most AEDs can cause hyponatremia, monitor electrolyte values carefully, especially in older adults.

The older **tricyclic antidepressants**, such as amitriptyline (Elavil), nortriptyline (Pamelor), and imipramine (Tofranil), may be beneficial in treating chronic neuropathic pain. Both tricyclic antidepressants and other antidepressants such as trazodone (Desyrel), paroxetine (Paxil), and sertraline (Zoloft) help treat the depression that can accompany chronic pain. They also stimulate the activity of endogenous opiates (endorphins and enkephalins) by increasing levels of the neurotransmitter serotonin. Perhaps the greatest advantage of this group of drugs, particularly the tricyclic antidepressants, is the sedative effect. This effect can be helpful in promoting sleep when administered at bedtime. The tricyclics are contraindicated in clients with a history of seizures or cardiac disease. They should also be used with caution in older adults because they have long-half lives and can cause toxicities.

In some cases, antianxiety agents help relax the client and thus help relieve pain. However, many of these drugs cause confusion, drowsiness, and hypotension; the health care provider selects the drugs with the fewest side effects. Examples of antianxiety agents include alprazolam (Xanax), clorazepate (Tranxene, Novo-Clopate✱), Lorazepam (Ativan), and oxazepam (Serax, Zapex✱). Clonazepam (Klonopin), also used for anxiety, has been shown to be particularly helpful for certain types of nerve injury pain.

Oral local anesthetics, such as mexiletine (Mexitil), act by suppressing the electrical activity of both peripheral nerves and neurons in the central nervous system. They are useful for electric shock–like pain and continuous pain. Mexiletine is contraindicated for clients who have cardiac conduction

TABLE 7-10 Examples of Adjuvant Analgesics

Drug Class	Example	Indications
Tricyclic antidepressants	Amitriptyline (Elavil) Nortriptyline (Pamelor) Desipramine (Norpramin)	Multipurpose; any chronic pain; pain associated with depression
Anticonvulsants	Gabapentin (Neurontin) Carbamazepine (Tegretol) Valproic acid (Depakene) Clonazepam (Klonopin)	First-line recommendation for neuropathic pain Any lancinating, burning, neuropathic pain
Stimulants	Methylphenidate (Ritalin) Dextroamphetamine (Dexedrine) Dronabinol (Marinol)	Lethargy: counteract opioid-induced sedation; used for anorexia with associated weight loss in HIV and cancer clients
Steroids	Dexamethasone (Decadron) Prednisone	Severe bone pain; nerve compression; increased intracranial pressure; soft tissue infiltration
Systemic local anesthetics	Lidocaine (Xylocaine) Mexiletine (Mexitil)	Any lancinating, burning pain
Topical anesthetics	EMLA, Numby Capsaicin Lidoderm patch	Procedural, invasive pain Postherpetic neuralgia; diabetic neuropathy; postmastectomy pain
Miscellaneous	Clonidine Baclofen Calcitonin Tizanidine (Zanaflex)	Nonspecific analgesic; may be helpful for select group of chronic pain clients Trigeminal neuralgia; other neuropathic pains Sympathetically maintained pain; phantom limb pain Alpha$_2$-adrenergics useful for spasticity pain

defects or dysrhythmias or are currently taking cardiac antidisrhythmic medications.

Other agents known to have some effect in relieving mild to moderate chronic pain include dextromethorphan (the active ingredient in many cough syrups) and ketamine. Both of these agents are N-methyl-D-aspartate (NMDA) antagonists. NMDA receptors are involved in the development of tolerance to opioids. The administration of NMDA antagonists is thought to potentiate the action of opioids and prevent the development of opioid tolerance.

Topical Medications. Other topical medications can be useful, particularly for localized neuropathic pain. For example, the Lidoderm patch is approved for postherpetic neuralgia. Up to three patches can be applied at once, or they can be cut to the area of pain. The patch should be put on for 12 hours and removed for 12 hours. There is virtually no systemic absorption of lidocaine.

EMLA and ELA-Max creams are combinations of topical lidocaine and prilocaine. These must be applied to intact skin at least 45 minutes before needle sticks. The topical medications for pain relief have rare side effects of local skin reactions.

Local, short-acting gels and creams may provide **cryotherapy** to decrease pain, especially for muscle aches and pains. Bio-Freeze is an example of a commonly used gel that is often used by physical therapists to "cool down" an area after it has been manipulated. Other products can be bought over-the-counter (OTC) (e.g., Ben Gay). The effects of this type of application last about 1 to 2 hours, depending upon the client.

Other Interventions. There are a number of effective interventions for pain that are nonpharmacologic. These modalities may be used alone, for mild to moderate pain, or in combination with drug therapy for more severe pain. These therapies are classified as either physical measures or cognitive-behavioral measures. Some of these measures may be referred to as part of complementary and alternative medicine (CAM), such as imagery, therapeutic touch, and hypnosis. Chapter 4 discusses CAM in more detail.

Physical Measures. Physical measures may be used instead of or in addition to drug therapy to relieve pain. **Cutaneous (skin) stimulation** strategies to relieve pain have been in use for many years. Various types of stimulation to the skin and subcutaneous tissue produce pain relief. Nurses play an important role in educating clients about these techniques. Methods of cutaneous stimulation include techniques such as the following:

- Transcutaneous electrical nerve stimulation (TENS)
- Application of heat, cold, and pressure
- Therapeutic touch
- Massage
- Vibration

Whichever method is used, several characteristics of cutaneous stimulation must be considered:

- The benefits of these techniques are highly unpredictable and may vary from application to application.
- Pain relief is generally sustained only as long as the stimulation continues.
- Multiple trials may be necessary to establish the desired effects.
- Stimulation itself may aggravate pre-existing pain or may produce new pain.

Despite the drawbacks to cutaneous stimulation, it is effective in the management of both acute pain and chronic pain. These techniques have both physiologic and psychological effects on the client. Cutaneous stimulation techniques also give clients an opportunity to participate actively in the management of their pain.

Physical Therapy. Physical therapy is used for clients experiencing pain to increase function, decrease pain, compensate for decreased function, and prevent further deterioration. Exercises and physical modalities such as heat, cold, massage, or TENS units may be used. Measures of client progress include an increase in the range of motion, strength, and function of the affected area as well as impact of pain on quality of life. Collaborate with the physical therapist to evaluate these treatments.

The physical or occupational therapist may also help to decrease pain by making one or more splints to rest severely inflamed joints. These devices are most commonly used short-term for clients with osteoarthritis or rheumatoid arthritis.

Transcutaneous Electrical Nerve Stimulation. **Transcutaneous electrical nerve stimulation (TENS)** (also referred to as **percutaneous electrical nerve stimulation [PENS]**) involves the use of a battery-operated device capable of delivering small electrical currents to the skin and underlying tissues. This technique is not as widely used as when it first was developed. However, for older adults, it may be safer and just as effective as medications (Resnick, 2003). Electrodes connected to a small box are placed over the painful sites. The voltage or current is regulated by adjusting a dial to the point at which the client perceives a prickly, "pins-and-needles" sensation. The current is adjusted on the basis of the client's degree of pain relief and level of comfort.

The health care provider, nurse, or physical therapist (depending on the health care setting) assists the client in applying the electrodes either on the painful area or above or below it (Figure 7-6). A conducting substance (usually a gel) is placed between the electrode and the client's skin.

The advantages of TENS units are that the client can wear the unit and achieve a level of pain relief while participating in activities of daily living. The unit is easy to use and can be worn for several hours. However, the skin may become irritated at the site of the electrode placement. To prevent this, the nurse teaches the client to rotate electrode sites.

In general, clients can use TENS units for the management of both acute pain and chronic pain. This type of therapy is indicated for localized pain, such as postoperative pain or local chronic pain, particularly low back pain.

Other Cutaneous Techniques. Additional cutaneous stimulation techniques, such as touch, pressure, massage, vibration, and heat and cold application, stimulate the skin and somehow interrupt the pain pathway. These interventions are relatively easy for the client to learn and are fairly economical. Cold applications are especially helpful for inflamed areas. Heat is appropriate when an increased blood flow is desired, such as for clients with arthritis. Paraffin dips for the hands are particularly helpful to those clients to increase movement. Warm showers and compresses that can be done at home are also useful in reducing stiffness and promoting movement in clients with arthritis, especially after awakening.

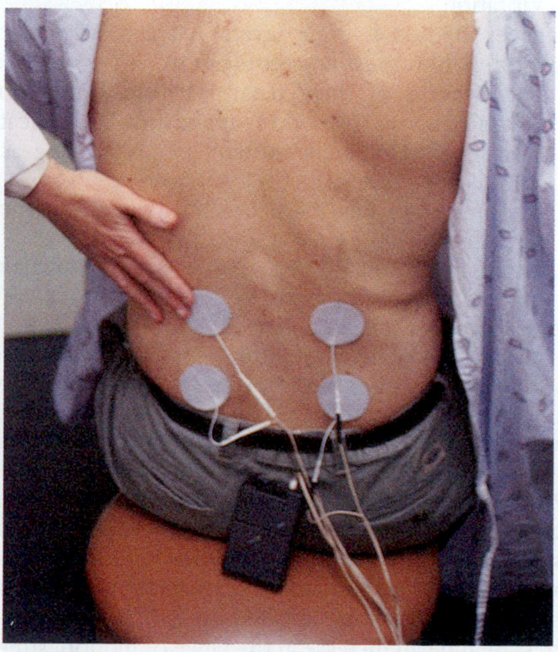

Figure 7-6 ■ Application of a TENS unit.

Cognitive-Behavioral Measures. Cognitive-behavioral strategies to relieve pain (e.g., distraction) have been popular for years, mainly as adjuncts to drug therapy. Theoretic explanations for the effectiveness of these measures reflect the premises of the gate control theory. Examples of cognitive-behavioral measures include distraction, imagery, relaxation, hypnosis, music therapy, aromatherapy, prayer and meditation, and other coping skills (also see Chapter 4).

Distraction. **Distraction** can be an effective method of acute pain relief. Simple measures such as holding a client's hand, taking him or her for a walk, or encouraging deep breathing exercises can divert attention from the pain. Nurses often observe that clients request less pain medication when family members are present and when talking on the phone. After visiting hours are over, many clients request something for pain, because they are no longer distracted.

Instead of viewing distraction as a therapeutic pain relief measure, as they should, some nurses may question the presence or severity of the pain if a client is easily distracted from it. Distraction alters the perception of pain but does not influence the cause or peripheral mechanism of pain. It is a transient method of pain relief and is probably best used with other pain control measures.

You can provide several methods of distraction. For example, visual distractors (e.g., pictures or television) can divert the client's attention to something pleasant or interesting. Auditory distractors, including music or relaxation tapes, can have a calming effect. Changing the environment can remove unpleasant stressors or reminders that may enhance pain. Physical distractions (e.g., deep breathing exercises) help the client concentrate on other physiologic sensations.

Distraction can be particularly useful in the following situations:

- Exacerbations of pain
- Painful procedures (e.g., dressing changes or invasive procedures)
- Interrupting the client's constant perception of pain

Imagery. **Imagery** is a form of distraction in which the client is encouraged to visualize or think about some pleasant or desirable feeling, sensation, or event. Guided imagery occurs when a person, often a nurse, assists the client in sustaining a sequence of thoughts aimed at diverting attention away from the pain. Intense concentration is required to visualize images. Clients who are extremely anxious, agitated, or unable to concentrate may first benefit from mild distraction.

Imagery is particularly useful for chronic pain. Clients who practice this technique can mentally and vividly experience sights, sounds, smells, events, or other sensations. The nurse first assesses the client's level of concentration to determine whether he or she can sustain a particular thought or thoughts for a desired time. The time interval for mental imagery can vary from 5 to 60 minutes. Behaviors that are helpful in assessing a client's capacity for imagery include the following:

- Reading and comprehending the newspaper
- Listening to music or other auditory stimuli
- Having the ability to follow and participate in sustained conversation
- Having an interest in environmental surroundings

When the client has demonstrated some ability to concentrate, assist the client in identifying a pleasant or favorable thought. The client is encouraged to focus on this thought to divert attention away from painful stimuli. Audiotapes may help in forming and maintaining images. The nurse, client, or family may wish to create audiotapes, or commercially available audiotapes may be used. The following is an example of guided imagery instructions: "Imagine yourself on the beach on some deserted island. You can hear the sound of waves rushing onto the shore, the cry of seagulls flying high above, and the rustling of trees as they are brushed gently by the wind. You can feel the warmth of the sun over your body and the cooling breeze."

Imagery works for some clients but not for others. The capacity to become engaged in the reality of the image may be important for the successful use of this therapy.

Relaxation Techniques. Clients may use **relaxation techniques** to reduce anxiety, tension, and emotional stress, all of which may exacerbate pain. Techniques to help clients relax can be both physical and psychological. Physical relaxation techniques include the following:

- Receiving a body massage, back rub, or warm or hot bath
- Modifying the environment to reduce distractions
- Moving into a comfortable position

Psychological relaxation techniques include the following:

- Pleasant conversation
- Music
- Relaxation tapes

Some relaxation tapes assist the client with progressive relaxation of the muscles. Relaxation exercises can be effectively coupled with guided imagery, distraction, and hypnosis.

Hypnosis. **Hypnosis** is defined as an altered state of consciousness in which a person enters a trance and loses an overall sense of reality. Although the person is in a trance, he or she has some sense of awareness and contact with reality and has an understanding of what is actually happening. Hypnosis can be used to treat a variety of pain syndromes, particularly chronic pain. It is used to help clients overcome the emotional consequences of pain and can promote a positive state of mind. Although nurses do not usually teach hypnosis, they are in a key position to help clarify misconceptions, instruct clients about relaxation and distraction, and encourage clients to practice self-hypnosis.

Other Complementary and Alternative Therapies. The data are scarce regarding the usefulness of other pain management techniques, such as magnet therapy, acupuncture, and herbal supplements. Although not supported by research, some clients believe that magnets applied to the skin or worn in shoes can reduce pain. This is a noninvasive therapy, and there is no harm to those who use this modality.

The practice of **acupuncture** originated in China. According to ancient beliefs, the body is divided into sections by lines, or meridians. Specific acupuncture points are located within these meridians. The acupuncturist inserts tiny needles into the skin and subcutaneous tissues at these points, and manual vibration or electrical stimulation is delivered. This technique is used to relieve pain and is thought to cure certain diseases. Several studies have shown that acupuncture can help reduce pain in clients with musculoskeletal problems (Lu, Lu, & Kleinman, 2001; Gilbertson, Wenner, & Russell, 2003).

Acupuncture is still widely acclaimed in China, but is less popular in the West because the physiologic basis for this technique is unclear. Many Western health care professionals are skeptical about its usefulness. Nonetheless, acupuncture is practiced for the treatment of pain and for anesthetic purposes during diagnostic procedures, labor and delivery, and surgery. It is also used to help clients change their behavior (e.g., smoking cessation). Certain parts of the United States (e.g., southwestern states) and other countries are expanding the use of this therapy for various purposes.

Glucosamine is a commonly used supplement for clients who have arthritis. It is believed to restore joint health and thus relieve pain and inflammation. Ask the client about the use of herbal supplements, because some can cause serious interactions with other pharmacologic agents.

Invasive Techniques for Chronic Pain. Invasive techniques are used to interrupt the pain pathways when pain is intractable (not able to be relieved) or severely debilitating. Depending on the technique, some degree of neurologic deficit and nerve destruction is expected. Various invasive techniques are used when chronic or persistent pain can no longer be adequately controlled with drugs or other pain-reducing methods.

Nerve Blocks. **Nerve blocks** can be used for both diagnostic and treatment purposes. These procedures are usually indicated for pain confined to a specific area or nerve distribution. This technique involves localizing a nerve root (or roots) and injecting it with either a local anesthetic for temporary relief or diagnostic evaluations or with a chemical agent (e.g., phenol or alcohol) to achieve permanent **neurolysis** or nerve destruction. Temporary blocks or permanent destruction (neuroablation) might be considered in areas such as the intercostal nerves, celiac plexus, superior hypogastric block, or craniofacial nerves.

The complications associated with nerve block vary. In general, injecting a local anesthetic or chemical agent into a peripheral nerve root leads to decreased sensation in the area; motor function is not affected. Injecting a local anesthetic into the lumbosacral area of the spinal cord area may cause transient motor and bowel and bladder dysfunction. Neurolysis of the lumbosacral nerves can damage motor nerve roots, resulting in lost or impaired bowel, bladder, or sexual function. This procedure is usually reserved for clients with intractable cancer-related pain.

Before permanent neurolysis is considered, a temporary nerve block may be given to determine the degree of relief obtained from disrupting the nerve impulses. Although the intent of neurolysis is to permanently destroy nerve transmission, clients may experience only short-term pain relief because of nerve cell regeneration or the development of alternative pathways capable of transmitting pain. Permanent ablation of nerve roots can be performed with thermal techniques such as **radiofrequency ablation** (uses heat) or **cryoanalgesia** (uses cold).

Because a nerve block is an invasive procedure performed by anesthesiologists, neurosurgeons, surgeons, and neurologists, the health care provider is responsible for informing the client about the procedure and its risks and alternative treatments. The nurse reinforces this information with the client and family.

Spinal Cord Stimulation. Spinal cord stimulator therapy offers a more invasive method of nerve stimulation. This technique involves the use of electrodes implanted under the skin and into the area of the nerve responsible for the pain. At first, a trial of spinal cord stimulation is attempted through the use of temporary externalized electrodes that are implanted and connected to a stimulator device. The amount of electrical current is adjusted to provide pain relief without additional discomfort. If this trial is successful, the client undergoes surgery for placement of a permanent implantable simulator.

Surgical Techniques. The surgical techniques aimed at surgically interrupting the transmission of pain include rhizotomy and cordotomy. These two procedures are not performed as commonly today because of the new, improved pain management measures available (Figure 7-7).

In **rhizotomy,** sensory nerve roots are destroyed where they enter the spinal cord. In a *closed* rhizotomy, a percutaneous catheter is inserted into the area, and the sensory nerve roots are destroyed by chemicals, coagulation, or cryodestruction (extreme cold). A laminectomy is necessary for an *open* rhizotomy. During this surgery, the health care provider isolates and destroys the nerve roots.

In a **cordotomy,** the surgeon cuts the pain pathways at the midline portion of the spinal cord before nerve impulses ascend to the spinothalamic tract. As with the other surgical procedures, clients may experience impaired bowel, bladder, or sexual function. Because of the complexity of the pain experience, the interruption of nerve conduction and pain pathways may not completely interrupt the client's sensation of pain.

After surgical intervention, assess the nature of the neurologic deficits, if any, and teach the client how to adapt to them. If the client has lost sensation in a body area, he or she will need to learn how to protect that area from harm. The nurse also assesses expectations in relation to the surgery and helps the client to express realistic expectations.

Community-Based Care

The pain experience extends beyond hospitalization. Many clients have chronic pain, but are not hospitalized. Others are in nursing homes or assisted-living facilities and have chronic pain, often not well managed. Effective analgesic regimens or pain-relieving strategies should be coordinated before discharge if clients are to leave the hospital still having pain. The nurse ensures that the client, especially one who is on opioids, has enough pain medication to last at least until the first follow-up visit.

HOME CARE MANAGEMENT

Preparation for home care is carried out with the client and family. Together with the client and family, the nurse, discharge planner, or occupational therapist determines whether modifications are necessary for maintaining a reasonably pain-free regimen after discharge. Fatigue heightens the awareness of pain. If physical modifications (e.g., installing a downstairs bathroom) are unrealistic (too expensive or unacceptable to the client or family), suggest schedule changes, role responsibilities, and daily routines to help avoid fatigue.

At home, clients may require a referral for physical therapy, especially to start or continue treatment with cutaneous stimulation, TENS, or heat or cold techniques. Clients may

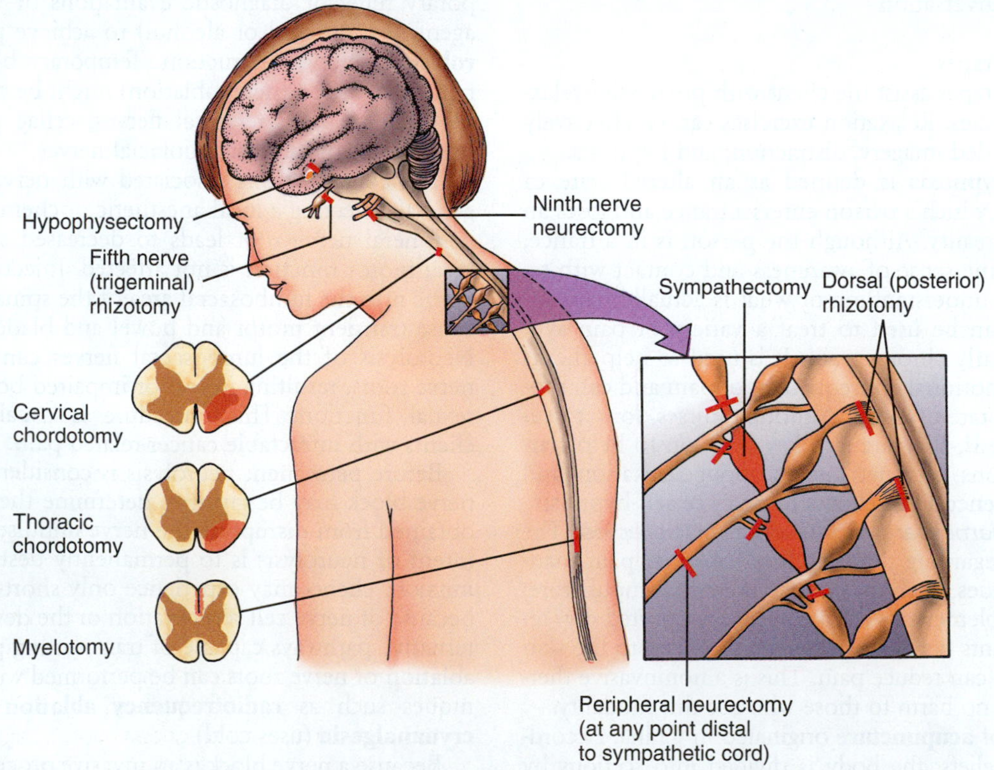

Figure 7-7 ■ Surgical procedures designed to alleviate pain.

need a psychiatric clinical nurse specialist or social worker to assist them in developing coping strategies or maintaining adequate family dynamics. A hospice referral (hospital- or community-based) can help maintain continuity of care in the management of terminally ill clients. Clients with cancer may be at risk for developing uncontrolled pain that results in hospitalization if it cannot be managed at home. It is important that nurses be knowledgeable about palliative care and end-of-life issues so they are better able to manage pain crises (see Chapter 9).

The growing number of home infusion therapy programs provides a wide variety of services to clients who require technology-supported pain care at home. Many of these services depend on approval by the insurance carrier, usually before analgesic options are considered and placement of technology is performed. Well-defined home agency practices and professional support at home are required if clients leave the hospital with infusion therapy for pain management.

HEALTH TEACHING

Direct educational efforts toward involving clients and their families in continuing health care behaviors that relieve pain and improve psychological well-being and overall functional status. Teach the client and family about analgesic regimens, including any technical skills needed to administer or deliver the analgesic, the purpose and action of medications, their side effects or adverse reactions, and the importance of dosage intervals. Also teach the client or family members how to prevent or treat the constipation commonly associated with taking opioid analgesics and other pain medications.

The nurse explains that, ideally, the analgesic regimen should not interfere with the client's sleep, rest, appetite, level of physical mobility, or driving ability. If such interference occurs, encourage the family or significant other to consult with the health care provider or home care nurse.

In clients with pain from advanced cancer, all efforts should be directed toward maximizing pain relief and symptom control at home to eliminate unnecessary readmissions. This may mean that the health care provider prescribes a flexible analgesic schedule that allows the client to adjust analgesics according to the amount of pain. Teach the client and family how to safely increase the medication within the prescribed dosing guidelines.

Evaluate family support systems to assist the client in adhering to and continuing the proposed medical and nursing plans. Family members are informed about and included in activities during and after hospitalization.

To achieve a reasonable level of expectation for the client, suggest ways to continue participation in household, social, sexual, and work-oriented activities after discharge. The nurse can help the client identify important activities and plan them around adequate rest schedules.

The client with chronic pain needs continued support to cope with the anxiety, fear, and powerlessness that often accompany this pain. Help the client and family or significant others to identify coping strategies that have worked in the past. Outside support systems are also identified, such as self-help organizations.

HEALTH CARE RESOURCES

A home care nurse referral is made when it is anticipated that clients will require assistance or supervision with their pain relief regimen at home. This referral should include specific information from the hospital-based staff nurse about the client's overall physical condition, general level of sedation, weakness or fatigue, possible constipation or nutritional problems, sleep patterns, and functional status.

In addition to explaining the client's physical status to the home care nurse, the staff nurse or case manager also describes the client's level of anxiety and general expectations about pain status after discharge. The client's close relationships and available support network are important factors in providing ongoing support for effective pain intervention strategies.

Referral to an advanced practice nurse pain specialist, social worker, or psychologist is an appropriate way to continue providing support to the client and family, reinforce instructions for cognitive-behavioral strategies to deal with pain, and evaluate overall physical and emotional adaptation after discharge. When severe chronic or intractable pain exists, health care professionals should direct the client and family to appropriate resources, such as pain centers or health care providers who specialize in pain management.

Clients with chronic pain often require treatment and support beyond that available in the traditional health care system. For this reason, pain clinics or programs have evolved over the past 25 years. The underlying premise of these resources is to foster independence and self-care behaviors while promoting pain control and maximizing quality of life. These programs use analgesics, adjuvant drug therapy, physical measures, cognitive-behavioral strategies, surgical interventions, and individual and group counseling for clients and family.

GET READY for the NCLEX Examination!

KEY POINTS

- Pain is what the client says it is; self-report is always the most reliable indication of pain.
- Three major types of pain have been identified—acute, chronic cancer, and chronic noncancer.
- Acute pain serves as a warning to the body, causing sympathetic responses, such as increased heart rate, increased blood pressure and pulse, dilated pupils, and sweating.
- Both types of chronic pain do not cause sympathetic reactions; therefore some clients do not appear to be in pain, even when they are (see Table 7-3).
- The gate control theory has helped to explain the mechanism of pain and its management.
- Three populations at risk for undertreatment of pain include older adults, minority clients, and drug addicts.
- Factors that affect pain and its management include age, gender, genetics, and culture.
- Tolerance implies that the client has adapted to a drug and over time its effects decline; physical dependence is manifested by a withdrawal reaction; addiction is a primary, chronic disease that occurs over a long period of time. Behaviors in addiction include craving, compulsive drug use, and continued use despite harm.
- Placebos should never be used on any client; their use in non–research based practice is unethical.
- Assess a client's pain for precipitating factors, aggravating factors, location, character and quality, and duration.

- Standardized pain intensity scales, such as number rating scales and descriptive word scales, are commonly used to quantify the severity of pain.
- Special considerations for older adults experiencing pain are summarized in Chart 7-1.
- Acute and chronic pain can cause anxiety, fear, or depression.
- Non-opioid drugs are the first-line therapy for mild to moderate pain; nonsteroidal anti-inflammatory drugs (NSAIDs) and acetaminophen (Tylenol) are commonly used drugs in this category.
- NSAIDs should be used with caution in older adults due to adverse effects, such as GI disturbances, bleeding, and sodium and water retention.
- Acetaminophen can cause hepatotoxicity with long-term use.
- The opioid full agonists are most effective for both acute and chronic pain management; they bind to mu receptors and block pain transmission.
- Equianalgesic charts are useful when changing from one opioid to another; morphine 10 mg is the standard dose against which other opioids are measured.
- Morphine is the gold standard drug for both acute and chronic pain, and is available in many forms, both short acting and long acting.
- Other commonly used full agonists include codeine, oxycodone, hydromorphone, and fentanyl.
- Meperidine is an outdated drug, but is still sometimes used for acute pain management; its toxic metabolite can cause seizures and confusion.
- Common side effects of opioids include nausea and vomiting, constipation, sedation, and respiratory depression.
- Table 7-9 summarizes the advantages and disadvantages of drug therapy by route of administration.
- Multimodal (balanced) analgesia for epidural pain management is a combination of opioids, non-opioids, and/or local anesthetics to relieve acute pain, usually postoperative pain.
- Sedation is the primary side effect that is assessed for clients receiving PCA or epidural medication.
- Common adjuvant analgesics, as an addition to other drug regimens, are listed in Table 7-10.
- Nonpharmacologic therapies for pain management may be used in place of or in combination with drug therapy; these therapies are classified as physical measures or cognitive-behavioral therapies.
- Examples of physical measures include transcutaneous nerve stimulation (TENS), heat, cold, and massage.
- Distraction, imagery, relaxation techniques, and hypnosis are examples of cognitive-behavioral therapies.
- Acupuncture, magnet therapy, and herbal supplements are examples of other complementary and alternative therapies used for chronic pain management.
- Nerve blocks and surgical techniques are invasive techniques performed by health care specialists to treat chronic pain; rhizotomy and cordotomy are examples of surgeries.
- Pain can be managed in any setting, including the home; some clients require parenteral pain medications at home; therefore health teaching for the client and family is needed.
- Clients whose pain is difficult to manage should be referred to pain specialists and/or pain centers.

ADDITIONAL STUDY RESOURCES

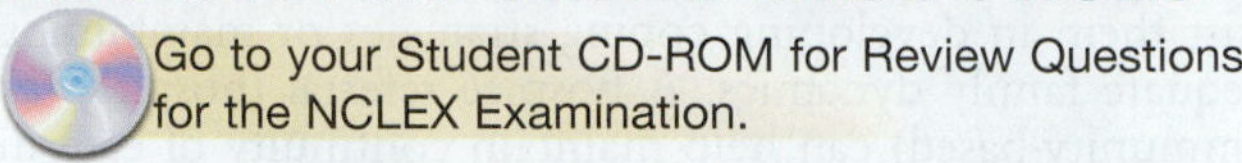
Go to your Student CD-ROM for Review Questions for the NCLEX Examination.

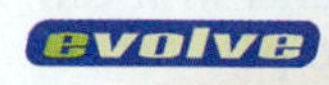

Go to http://evolve.elsevier.com/Iggy/ for Integrated Management of Care Questions for the NCLEX Examination.

SELECTED BIBLIOGRAPHY

Asterisk indicates a classic or definitive work on this subject.

*Acute Pain Management Guideline Panel. (1992). *Acute pain management: Operative or medical procedures and trauma. Clinical Practice Guideline.* AHCPR Pub. No. 92-0032. Rockville, MD: Agency for Health Care Policy and Research, Public Health Service, U.S. Department of Health and Human Services.

AGS, American Geriatric Society. (2002). The management of persistent pain in older persons. *Journal of the American Geriatric Society, 50*(56) 205–224.

*American Pain Society. (1999). *Guideline for the management of pain in osteoarthritis, rheumatoid arthritis, and juvenile chronic arthritis.* Glenview, IL: American Pain Society.

*American Pain Society. (2003). *Principles of analgesic use in the treatment of acute pain and cancer pain* (5th ed.). Glenview, IL: American Pain Society.

American Society of Addiction Medicine. (2001). Definitions related to the use of opioids for the treatment of pain. Consensus document from the American Academy of Pain Medicine, the American Pain Society and the American Society of Addiction Medicine, February 2001. Accessed June 2001 from http://www.asam.org.

Anderson, C. (2000). What's new in pain management. *Home Healthcare Nurse, 18*(10), 649-659.

Ardery, G., et al. Lack of opioid administration in older hip fracture patients. *Geriatric Nursing, 24*(6), 353-359.

*Backonja, M., et al., for the Gabapentin Diabetic Neuropathy Study Group. (1998). Gabapentin for the symptomatic treatment of painful neuropathy in patients with diabetes mellitus. A randomized controlled trial. *Journal of the American Medical Association, 280*(21), 1831-1836.

Berry, P.H., & Dahl, J.L. (2000). The new JCAHO pain standards: Implications for pain management nurses. *Pain Management Nursing, 1*(1), 3-12.

Brookoff, D. (2000). Chronic pain: 1. A new disease. *Hospital Practice, 35,*(7), 306-309.

Burroughs, V.J., et al. (2002). *Cultural and genetic diversity in America: The need for individualized pharmaceutical treatment.* Washington, DC: National Pharmaceutical Council and National Medical Association.

Carter, G., & Galer, B. (2001). Advances in the management of neuropathic pain. *Physical Medicine and Rehabilitation Clinics, 12*(2), 447-459.

Ciccone, D., & Just, N. (2001). Pain expectancy and work disability in patients with acute and chronic pain: A test of the fear avoidance hypothesis. *The Journal of Pain, 2*(3), 181-194.

*Cleeland, C.S., et al. (1994). Pain and its treatment in outpatients with metastatic cancer. *The New England Journal of Medicine, 330*(9), 592-596.

Collins, S., et al. (2000). Antidepressants and anticonvulsants for diabetic neuropathy and postherpetic neuralgia: A quantitative systematic review. *Journal of Pain and Symptom Management, 20*(6), 449-458.

Compton, P., et al. (2000). Pain responses in methadone-maintained opioid abusers. *Journal of Pain and Symptom Management, 20*(4), 237-245.

Coyne, P., & Smith, T. (2002). Nebulized fentanyl citrate improves patients' perception of breathing, respiratory rate, and oxygen saturation in dyspnea. *Journal of Pain and Symptom Management, 23*(2), 157-160.

Dahl, J., & Gordon, D. (2002). Joint commission pain standards: A progress report. *APS Bulletin, 12*(6), 1, 11-12.

Dallocchio, C., et al. (2000). Gabapentin vs. amitriptyline in painful diabetic neuropathy: An open-label pilot study. *Journal of Pain and Symptom Management, 20*(4), 280-285.

Durrance, S.A. (2003). Older adults and NSAIDs: Avoiding adverse reactions. *Geriatric Nursing, 24*(6), 349-352.

Eastman, P. (2003). Better pain control with pharmacogenetics? *Oncology Times, XXV*(1), 26, 27.

Eksterowica, N. (2003). Meperidine-using evidence-based rationale. *ASPMN Pathways, 12*(1), 4-5.

Ellison, N., McPherson, L., & McGuire, L. (2001). Pain report from the Dannemiller Memorial Educational Foundation. San Antonio: Dannemiller.

Fainsinger, R., Gara, C., & Perez, A. (2000). Amputation and prevention of phantom pain. *Journal of Pain and Symptom Management, 20*(4), 308-312.

Feldt, K.S. (2000). The checklist of nonverbal pain indicators (CNPI). *Pain Management Nursing, 1*(1), 13-21.

Ferrell, B., Stein, W., & Beck, J. (2000). The geriatric pain measure: Validity, reliability and factor analysis. *Journal of the American Geriatrics Society, 48*(12), 1669-1673.

Ferrell, B., et al. (2001). Ethical dilemmas in pain management. *The Journal of Pain, 2*(3), 171-180.

Fine, P. (2000). Pain and aging: Overcoming barriers to treatment and the role of transdermal opioid therapy. *Clinical Geriatrics, 8*(12), 1-6.

Frank-Stromborg, M., & Chistensen, A. (2001). A serious look at the undertreatment of pain: Part 1. *Clinical Journal of Oncology Nursing, 5*(5), 235-236.

Freedman, G. (2002). Clinical management of common causes of geriatric pain. *Geriatrics, 57*(5), 36-42.

Furrow, B. (2001). Pain management and provider liability: No more excuses. *Journal of Law, Medicine & Ethics, 29*, 28-51.

Gerstle, D., All, A., & Wallace, D. (2001). Quality of life and chronic nonmalignant pain. *Pain Management Nursing, 2*(3), 98-109.

Gilbertson, B., Wenner, K., & Russell, L.C. (2003). Acupuncture and arthroscopic acromioplasty. *Journal of Orthopaedic Research, 21*(4), 752-758.

Gordon, D., et al. (2001). A nurse-run inpatient pain consultation service. *Pain Management Nursing, 1*(2), 29-33.

Green, C., Wheeler, J., & LaPorte, F. (2003). Clinical decision making in pain management: Contributions of physician and patient characteristics to variations in practice. *The Journal of Pain, 4*(1): 29-39.

Green, C., et al. (2003). Race and chronic pain: A comparison study of young black and white Americans presenting for management. *The Journal of Pain, 4*(4), 176-183.

Guay, D. (2001). Adjunctive agents in the management of chronic pain. *Pharmacotherapy, 21*(9), 1070-1081.

Hazelett, S., Powell, C., & Androulakakis, V. (2002). Patients' behavior at the time of injury: Effect on nurses' perception of pain level and subsequent treatment. *Pain Management Nursing, 3*(1), 28-35.

Heidrich, D. (2001). Controlled-release oxycodone hydrochloride (OxyContin). *Clinical Nurse Specialist, 15*(5), 207-209.

Hutchison, R. (2004). Pain control: COX-2–selective NSAIDs. *American Journal of Nursing, 104*(3), 52-56.

Jacob, E. (2001). The pain experience of patients with sickle cell anemia. *Pain Management Nursing, 2*(3), 74-83.

*Jacox, A.K., et al. (1994). *Management of cancer pain: Adults. Clinical practice guideline No. 9*. AHCPR Pub. No. 94-0593. Rockville, MD: Agency for Health Care Policy and Research, Public Health Service, U.S. Department of Health and Human Services.

Jenson, M.G., et al. (2002). Topiramate for the treatment of neuropathic and chronic pain syndromes: An open label trial. *American Journal of Pain Management, 12*, 16-23.

Katz, N. (2002). The impact of pain management of quality of life. *Journal of Pain and Symptom Management, 24*(1), S38-S47.

Kedziera, P. (2001). Easing elders' pain. *Holistic Nursing Practice, 15*(2), 4-16.

Kessenich, C. (2001). Cyclo-oxygenase 2 inhibitors: An important new drug classification. *Pain Management Nursing, 2*(1), 13-18.

Kettleman, K. (2000). What's so bad about meperidine? *Nursing 2000, 30*(10), 20.

King, S.A. (2000). The use of NSAIDs for geriatric pain. *Geriatric Times, 1*, 1-6.

Knox, K. (2000). PCA patient education: An essential ingredient for success. *Analgesia, 11*(1), 4-6.

LaDike, S. (2002). Ethical issues in pain management. *Critical Care Nursing Clinics of North America, 14*, 165-170.

Laird, M., & Gidal, B. (2000). Use of gabapentin in the treatment of neuropathic pain. *The Annals of Pharmacotherapy, 34*(6), 802-807.

Lee, K., Ray, J., & Dunn, G. (2001). Chronic pain management and the surgeon: Barriers and opportunities. *Journal of the American College of Surgeons, 193*(6), 689-702.

Lu, D.P., Lu, G.P., & Kleinman, L. (2001). Acupuncture and clinical hypnosis for facial and head and neck pain: A single crossover comparison. *American Journal of Clinical Hypnosis, 44*(2), 141-148.

Lynch, M. (2001). Pain as the fifth vital sign. *Journal of Intravenous Nursing, 24*(2), 85-94.

*McCaffery, M. (1979). *Nursing management of the patient with pain* (2nd ed.). Philadelphia: J.B. Lippincott.

*McCaffery, M., & Pasero, C. (1999). Harmful effects of unrelieved pain. *Pain: Clinical Manual* 15-34.

*McCaffery, M., & Pasero, C. (1999). *Pain: Clinical manual* (2nd ed.). St. Louis: Mosby.

McCaffery, M., & Pasero, C. (2001). Stigmatizing patients as addicts. *American Journal of Nursing, 101*(5), 77-79.

McCaffery, M., & Pasero, C. (2003). Breakthrough pain. *American Journal of Nursing, 103*(4), 83-85.

McCaffery, M., & Robinson, E. (2002). Your patient is in pain: Here is how you respond. *Nursing 2002, 32*(10), 36-47.

McNeil, J., et al. (2001). Pain management outcomes for hospitalized Hispanic patients. *Pain Management Nursing, 2*(1), 25-36.

*Melzack, R., Wall, P.D. (1982). *The challenge of pain*. New York: Basic Books.

Merboth, M., & Barnason, S. (2000). Managing pain: The fifth vital sign. *Nursing Clinics of North America, 35*(2), 375-383.

Miller, K., & Miller, M. (2003). Challenges in end-of-life pain management. *Annals of Long-Term Care, 11*(4), 26-32.

Milligan, K. et al. (2001). Evaluation of long-term efficacy and safety of transdermal fentanyl in the treatment of chronic noncancer pain. *The Journal of Pain, 2*(4), 197-204.

Newshan, G. (2000). Pain management in the addicted patient: Practical considerations. *Nursing Outlook, 48*(2), 81-85.

Nichols, R. (2003). Pain management in patients with addictive disease. *American Journal of Nursing, 103*(3), 87, 89.

Pasero, C. (2002). Subcutaneous opioid infusion. *American Journal of Nursing, 102*(7), 61-62.

Pasero, C. (2003). Epidural analgesia for postoperative pain, Part 2. *American Journal of Nursing, 103*(11), 43-45.

Pasero, C., & McCaffery, M. (2000). When patients can't report pain. *American Journal of Nursing, 100*(9), 22-23.

Pasero, C., & McCaffery, M. (2001). Hydromorphone. *American Journal of Nursing, 101*(2), 22-23.

Pasero, C., & McCaffery, M. (2001). Reversing respiratory depression with naloxone. *American Journal of Nursing, 100*(2), 26.

Pasero, C., & McCaffery, M. (2001). The patient's report of pain. *American Journal of Nursing, 101*(12), 73-74.

Pasero, C., & McCaffery, M. (2001). Undertreatment of pain. *American Journal of Nursing, 101*(11), 62, 64, 66.

Pasero, C., & McCaffery, M. (2002). Monitoring sedation. *American Journal of Nursing, 102*(2), 67-69.

Pasero, C., & McCaffery, M. (2002). Pain in the critically ill. *American Journal of Nursing, 102*(1), 56-60.

Pasero, C., & McCaffery, M. (2003). Lidocaine patch 5%. *American Journal of Nursing, 103*(9), 75-78.

Pasero, C., & McCaffery, M. (2003). Tramadol. *American Journal of Nursing, 103*(2), 71, 73.

Pullen, R. (2002). Pain management for chronic nonmalignant neuropathic pain. *Home Healthcare Nurse, 20*(6), 387-392.

Puntillo, K.A., et al. (2001). Patients' perceptions and responses to procedural pain: Results from Thunder Project II. *Am J Critical Care, 10*(4), 238-251.

Resnick, B. (2003). Managing chronic pain in the older patient. *Geriatric Nursing, 24*(6), 373.

Robinson, M., et al. (2001). Gender role expectations of pain: Relationship to sex differences in pain. *The Journal of Pain, 2*(5), 251-257.

*Rowbotham, M., et al. for the Gabapentin Post-Herpetic Neuralgia Study Group. (1998). Gabapentin for the treatment of postherpetic neuralgia: A randomized controlled trial. *Journal of the American Medical Association, 280*(21), 1837-1842.

Sargent, C. (2002). Naloxone: How well do you know this drug? *Clinical Journal of Oncology Nursing, 6*(1), 17-18.

Schaffer, S.D., & Yucha, C.B. (2004). Relaxation and pain management. *American Journal of Nursing, 104*(8), 75-82.

Slaughter, A., Pasero, C., & Manworren, R. (2002). Unacceptable pain levels. *American Journal of Nursing, 102*(5), 75, 77.

Smith, R., Curci, M., & Silverman, A. (2002). Pain management: The global connection, *Nursing Management, 33*(6), 27-30.

Stegman, M. (2001). Control of pain: Every person's right. *Orthopaedic Nursing, 20*(2), 31-36.

Swenson, C. (2002). Ethical issues in pain management. *Seminars in Oncology Nursing, 18*(2), 135-142.

Todd, K.H., et al. (2000). Ethnicity and analgesic practice. *Annals of Emergency Medicine, 35*, 11-16.

Tucker, K. (2001). Deceptive placebo administration. *American Journal of Nursing, 101*(8), 55-56.

Vallerand, A., & Polomano, R. (2000). The relationship of gender to pain. *Pain Management Nursing, 1*(3), S8-15.

Waitman, J., & McCaffery, M. (2001). Meperidine–A liability. *American Journal of Nursing, 101*(1), 57-58.

Watt-Watson, J., et al. (2000). The impact of nurses' empathic responses on patients' management in acute care. *Nursing Research*, 49(4), 191-200.

Wentz, J. (2001). Assessing pain in the cognitively impaired adult. *Nursing 2001, 31*(7), 26.

Wentz, J. (2003). Understanding neuropathic pain. *Nursing 2003, 33*(1), 22.

Young-McCaughan, S., & Miaskowski, C. (2001). Definition of and mechanism for opioid-induced sedation. *Pain Management Nursing , 2*(3), 84-97.

Young-McCaughan, S., & Miaskowski, C. (2001). Measurement of opioid-induced sedation. *Pain Management Nursing, 2*(4), 132-149.

CHAPTER

8

Substance Abuse

TOMMIE WRIGHT PNIEWSKI

LEARNING OUTCOMES

After studying this chapter, you should be able to:

1. Discuss substance abuse as a major health issue in the United States.
2. Explain the effects of substance abuse on the mental and physical health of individuals and society.
3. Describe the relationship between stress and substance abuse.
4. Identify assessment findings associated with use of nicotine, alcohol, stimulants, hallucinogens, depressants, opioids, inhalants, and steroids.
5. Prioritize care for clients who exhibit signs or symptoms of substance abuse.
6. Discuss recent biologic and genetic research in the etiology of substance abuse.
7. Identify symptoms that are indicative of emergency situations associated with the use of the following substances: alcohol, nicotine, stimulants, hallucinogens, depressants, opioids, inhalants, and steroids.
8. Identify the responsibilities of the nurse when a peer or other health care worker is suspected of abusing substances.
9. Identify common medication regimens that are used in the emergency treatment of drug withdrawal and adverse reactions to drugs and alcohol.
10. Prioritize nursing care for clients who are in alcohol withdrawal.

Go to your Student CD-ROM for Review Questions for the NCLEX Examination keyed to these Learning Outcomes.

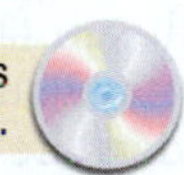

OVERVIEW OF SUBSTANCE ABUSE

Subtance abuse is described as the overindulgence of a chemical substance and the resulting dependence that interferes with life's activities. Each year there are alarming increases in the abuse of mind- and mood-altering substances, such as alcohol, marijuana, cocaine and nontherapeutic use of prescription drugs. The mental and physical health of the individual is affected by substance abuse, which also significantly affects the lives of others. Productivity is drastically reduced, and the costs of abuse to society are enormous. Categories of substances commonly abused include stimulants, hallucinogens, depressants, opioids (narcotics), and other substances that alter the mind. Stimulants are abused by some clients because the need for "faster, better, and longer" exists as a mindset in society. Hallucinogens continue to be popular in various forms but are commonly encountered as mind-altering drugs such as phencyclidine (PCP) and lysergic acid (LSD). Depressants, such as the anxiolytics, are becoming increasingly popular as a maladaptive alternative in responding to the ever-increasing demands of today's busy lifestyles. Opioids and morphine derivatives, although important for therapeutic uses for pain relief, continue to be abused and addictive in the drug community.

Incidence/Prevalence of Substance Abuse

A chronic, long-standing problem, substance abuse continues to be prevalent in the United States. Studies conducted by the National Institute on Drug Abuse (NIDA) (2003) are helpful in assessment of drug abuse. Studies indicate that substance abuse increased from 6.3% of the populations studied in 2000 to 7.1% in 2001. This represents about 15.9 million Americans age 12 years and older being identified as "current users."

Patterns of use among ethnic groups generally remain the same among major racial and ethnic groups. In 2001, the rate among African Americans was 7.4%, white individuals, 7.2%, and Hispanics 6.4%. The highest rates of illicit drug use were among Native Americans/American Indians and Alaskan Natives at 9.9%. The lowest rate of substance use was among Asian Americans at 2.8% (NIDA, 2003).

WOMEN'S HEALTH CONSIDERATIONS

According to the NIDA report, 4 million women in the United States use drugs (Mathias, 2000). Women of all races, ages, educational backgrounds, cultures, and community types are among the drug users in the United States. Drug use

Continued

and abuse data among women are becoming increasingly available as the nursing profession seeks to improve the health of women. Usually women abuse more than one drug. Almost half of all women 15 to 44 years of age have used drugs (including tobacco products and alcohol) at least once in their lifetime. Approximately 2 million women used cocaine and more than 6 million used marijuana in 1999 (Mathias, 2000).

Women are at risk for developing drug dependence as a result of biologic predisposition, stressors in the environment, and availability of quality support services. These factors must be explored during the nursing assessment to be thorough in addressing the specific client's needs.

Cultural Competence Related to Substance Abuse

Culture influences every aspect of the client's life. The nurse needs to demonstrate competence in understanding the cultural influences that are related to drug abuse to plan care that will work for the person with substance abuse problems. In addition, an understanding of the client's culture helps to avoid making assumptions about substance abuse based on the client's body language. Some behaviors (e.g., avoiding eye contact), which are interpreted within the Western culture as negative are considered normal, even reverent, in other cultures (e.g., Asian culture).

Adapt the assessment and subsequent planning of care within the norms of the client's culture. With the stigma associated with substance abuse, be aware of those behaviors and norms that would alienate him or her. Often, substance abuse disorders are a result of interpersonal inadequacies. The user perceives the substance as helpful to reduce stress or assist him or her in coping. Success of drug treatment is often related to the use of external support, forcing the user to rely on other persons rather than the chemical.

Be open to the array of religious preferences to avoid conflicts between treatment modalities and the client's faith. In addition, you need a firm awareness of self to avoid reactive behaviors to the client's beliefs or absence of personal convictions. A posture of judgment is never appropriate and is particularly nontherapeutic when caring for the client with substance abuse. Chapter 6 describes cultural aspects of health in more detail, including how to perform a cultural assessment.

Substance Abuse, Stress, and Addiction

Many clients relate substance abuse to stress relief; however, external situational stress is not the only contributing factor resulting in substance abuse. The role that stress does play in substance abuse occurs more in a biologic response to stress, part of which is a normal response. The introduction of stress in the brain, as perceived by the individual, results in stimulation of the hypothalamus. The hypothalamus, located beneath the thalamus, is the center for emotional responses and houses the limbic system (emotional part of the brain). In addition, the hypothalamus controls the involuntary nervous system and organ functions. Biologic rhythms and internal drives (e.g., sex drive) are directed by the nuclei of the hypothalamus. Perceptions of pleasure, fear, and rage are also found in the hypothalamus. Autonomic nervous system pathways initiate most physical expressions of these emotions, such as a pounding heart, increased blood pressure, pallor, increased perspiration, and a dry mouth.

Responses to external stress (situational or ingested chemicals) or internal stress (disease or withdrawal of drugs) trigger chemical and hormonal responses in the body arising from activity in the hypothalamus. The body reacts to stress by secreting hormones in the blood and neurotransmitters in the brain. Normally, the body secretes stress hormones throughout the day in small amounts. When the body experiences stress, the brain reacts by increasing the level of stress hormones. Corticotropin-releasing factor (CRF) is released into the blood, which carries the CRF to the pituitary gland. This stimulates the release of adrenocorticotropin (ACTH) resulting in stimulation of the release of other hormones, primarily cortisol, from the adrenal glands. Cortisol travels throughout the body, assisting the body to cope with the stress. Cortisol influences the continued response to the stress or reduction depending on the severity of the stressor.

Depending on the source of the stress, the behavioral manifestations frequently have an influence on the quality of the body's response. Stress responses that are frequently triggered can result in a more sensitive response. Continued substance abuse creates a cycle of ever-increasing amounts of the drug to sustain the desired level of response to the drug. As with achieving the desired result, the body also responds with "withdrawal" responses (symptoms of withdrawal) when deprived of the substance. A cyclic ingestion-withdrawal response sets the stage for addiction.

Substance abuse is a documented nursing diagnosis when the following criteria are present:

- The client loses control of use of the drug.
- The client takes the drug even though the drug has caused adverse conditions in the body.
- The client demonstrates cognitive, behavioral, and physiologic disturbances with the abuse of drugs or inhalants.

Dependence is characterized as a condition that causes a habitual, compulsive, and uncontrollable urge to use a substance; and without the substance, the body experiences severe physiologic, psychological, and emotional disturbances. Substance abuse in the presence of medical or surgical problems creates a complicated situation in terms of helping clients to reach their highest level of function.

Genetics of Substance Abuse

Research in the genetic connection between a person's gene makeup and substance abuse has noted associations of genes to cluster and contribute to substance use and/or abuse. A single gene theory has not been substantiated as has the cluster arrangement of groups of genes. A complex interaction between the genetic makeup and the environment has been noted in current research to result in substance abuse and dependence. Even though there have been numerous discoveries by the Human Genome Project, there is still a question as to what mechanisms underlie substance abuse. Drugs that are commonly abused stimulate the reward pathways of the brain.

The exact linkage between genes and their contribution to substance use is not known; however, current projects suggest that there may be activities among genes indicating that one gene influences behavior early in drug use and later another gene may overstimulate the reward center, resulting in "cravings." Current information regarding substance use, abuse, and dependence suggests that common pathways are shared in the reward center of the brain, which perpetuates substance use.

Personality traits are thought to be contributing factors in substance abuse. Genetic factors have been linked to variations in genes among persons with sensation-seeking behavior traits. Persons with the sensation-seeking behaviors have been found to be more susceptible to substance dependence.

Based on clinical research, the strongest risk factor in the assessment of substance use or dependence is the family history. How the individual interprets substance abuse or dependence is important in the planning, intervention, and success of that person. The implication of research linking dependence and drug abuse has profound influence on the perception of the drug user (Hardie, 2002).

Other research findings note that a lack of a specific enzyme (cytochrome P450) may cause more serious reactions to small amounts of "ecstasy" and may be significant in the body's processing of that drug. With further research, there is a potential to predict which persons are at risk for extremely serious reactions to substances such as ecstasy (Tipton, 2003).

Substance abuse, a chronic mental disorder, can be treated effectively, resulting in reduced crime, drug use, and psychological problems associated with drug use. Nursing implications with regard to the genetics of substance use are primarily directed to education in the linkage of substance abuse and genetics.

Substance Abuse and the Hospitalized Client

The client may be hospitalized when he or she can no longer be managed in an ambulatory care setting or when emergencies arise. As part of the comprehensive health assessment, the nurse carefully assesses for any signs, symptoms, or history of substance abuse.

In a comprehensive assessment, alcohol, tobacco, prescription drug, over-the-counter, and illicit drug use must be determined. Obtaining history of herbal treatment is necessary to determine the potential for interactions or symptomatic withdrawal from natural substances. The nurse should be adept in ascertaining substance abuse during the interview process. Failure to include a complete substance use history could have serious adverse effects on the client. The client who habitually uses substances requires closer observation for withdrawal than the occasional user. You need to be knowledgeable of various substances to be alert for signs of complications.

Caring for the client experiencing substance problems includes determining where the client will be going at the time of discharge. If the client has focused on treatment and recovery from the substance, discharge to a residential treatment center may be the environment of choice. If the client's plan includes continuation of the substance use, home may be the choice for discharge. Regardless of the best intentions of health care providers, the client may choose to handle his or her own substance abuse problem. Assist clients in reaching their optimal level of function as determined by both the client and the health care team.

Understanding the influence of abusive substances is an important educational aspect for the hospitalized client. Some chemicals have potentiating effects on therapeutic medications that can lead to serious or life-threatening situations. Room assignment, delegation of personnel, staffing assignments, and other nursing decisions are important with the substance-using client. The course of hospitalization may be altered as a result of substance abuse; treatment, care, and recovery can all be influenced by substance abuse.

Referrals and community-based health resources are important in assisting the client with substance abuse. Emotional support is necessary to help the client cope with the reason for hospitalization, being in the hospital, and dealing with the adverse effects of the substance abuse.

Nurses as Substance Abusers

History has shown a tendency of health care professionals to be susceptible to substance abuse associated with drug availability and job stress. The *ANA Code of Ethics for Nurses* gives a standard of professional behavior that seeks to safeguard and protect the public, as well as preserve integrity within the profession. Nursing practice is governed in each state by a Board of Nursing. In supporting safe and competent nursing, boards of nursing have peer assistance programs to assist in identifying and effectively managing substance abuse in the employment setting. All nurses need to be knowledgeable of their state board of nursing laws and the consequences of unprofessional behavior.

Prescription Drugs and Abuse

Some prescription drugs can easily become addictive because of the nature of their action in the brain. There is a tendency for the client to become comfortable with the effects of the drug long after the therapeutic need is satisfied. Improper use of therapeutic substances can result in addiction; such substances may also be used improperly for pleasure-seeking effects. Examples of therapeutic prescription drugs that can produce addiction or be used for maladaptive purposes are morphine, barbiturates, and benzodiazepines.

Challenges for the health care professional include preparedness to intervene in the risk behaviors created by substance use or abuse. This health problem is not limited to teenagers or to an impoverished population. All age groups and socioeconomic groups are vulnerable to substance abuse. The professional who is knowledgeable about substance abuse will be able to identify and appropriately care for the client experiencing substance use or abuse problems.

CONSIDERATIONS FOR OLDER ADULTS

Substance abuse should not be overlooked in the older adult. The potential for nontherapeutic use or abuse is high because of the number of different types of medications taken. As part the aging process, older adults have more difficulty metabolizing and excreting drugs; therefore toxicity is a common situation. Self-medication is a problem in the older population, increasing the complexity of care. A thorough drug history is necessary for identifying patterns of drug use that are harmful to the client. Misuse of prescription medications can happen quite innocently as memory becomes altered. Regular drug administration times are difficult to remember, resulting in overdosing or underdosing.

Approximately 1 in 4 persons in the United States has a friend or family member with substance abuse problems or a history of drug abuse. Medical-surgical nursing care is affected by substance abuse because of the complications caused by the physical presence or dependence on the substance. Clinical management of client health problems is more complex when the client has an addiction to drugs and/or alcohol.

The following sections describe some of the most common groups of illicit substances and their effects on the body (Table 8-1). Many drugs can cause coma or death. When drug use is suspected, blood and urine testing is done to determine the type of substance ingested. Nursing implications related to assessment and care of clients who abuse drugs and alcohol are also discussed.

STIMULANTS

Stimulants are drugs that excite the cerebral cortex of the brain, producing a variety of behavioral responses (see Table 8-1). Any substance that is introduced into the body that excites or stimulates an increase in body activity is referred to as a stimulant. Examples of stimulants are caffeine, nicotine, amphetamines, and methamphetamines. Although amphetamines and methamphetamines can be used for therapeutic purposes, their use is limited. Agents that are considered to be illicit and abused stimulants are "crack" (a potent form of cocaine), cocaine, and illegally produced methamphetamines. The incidence of stimulant use is varied among age groups and chemicals.

The following are the therapeutic effects of stimulants:

- Increase mental alertness
- Improve one's sense of well-being
- Increase the capacity to work
- Improve the performance of motor skills
- Stimulate general metabolism by increasing respiratory and cardiac function

When a large amount of stimulant is introduced into the body, the effects can cause insomnia, tremor, and restlessness, with resulting loss of motor function. The prolonged and sustained use of a stimulant can result in toxicity; an overdose can cause hallucinations, seizures, and cardiac dysrhythmias.

Amphetamines

OVERVIEW

Amphetamines are stimulants that increase the body's activities. Prescribed therapeutically as psychomotor stimulants, amphetamines and methamphetamines are effective in the treatment of attention deficit hyperactivity disorder (ADHD), obesity, and narcolepsy. When amphetamines are used as for recreation, the desired effect is to achieve a state of euphoria and grandiosity. Names for amphetamines (biphetamine, Dexedrine) in the drug environment include "black beauties," "cross," and "hearts." Knowledge of the "street" names for these drugs assists the nurse in assessment and identification of abusive use of amphetamines. Amphetamines can be ingested by a variety of methods including consumption by mouth, injection, smoking, or sniffing. Amphetamines have a high potential for addiction both physically and psychologically. Use of stimulants results in energy, excitement, relief of fatigue, decreased appetite, insomnia, aggression, and a tendency toward menstrual problems in women.

TABLE 8-1 Commonly Abused Substances

Stimulants
Amphetamines
Methamphetamine
Cocaine
Hallucinogens and Related Compounds
Lysergic Acid (LSD)
Phencyclidine (PCP)
Ketamine
3,4-Methylenedioxymethamphetamine
Marijuana
Depressants
Benzodiazepines
Rohypnol
Gamma hydroxybytyrate (GHB)
Barbiturates
Alcohol
Narcotics: Opioids and Morphine Derivatives
Inhalants
Solvents
Gases
Nitrites
Steroids (Anabolic)

COLLABORATIVE MANAGEMENT

As a result of these effects, assess the client for objective symptoms of stimulant use, overdose, or withdrawal. Table 8-2 lists these clinical manifestations. For both overdose and withdrawal, the priority for care is to maintain a safe environment both physically and psychologically for the client. Close observations are necessary to prevent development of further complications. Supportive communications are necessary to reduce anxiety and fear in the client. A nonjudgmental attitude is essential in establishing a therapeutic rapport. Many times health care providers view substance abuse clients as responsible for their situation and therefore have difficulty maintaining a professional demeanor when providing care.

Methamphetamine

Methamphetamine (Desoxyn) is a powerful substance that is highly addictive. Therapeutically, methamphetamine is available as a Schedule II substance. It is available medically through a prescription for ADHD, narcolepsy, and obesity. Although it is similar to amphetamines, methamphetamine is more powerful and affects the brain more dramatically. High levels of the neurotransmitter dopamine are released as a result of the ingestion of methamphetamine. There is evidence that this drug has neurotoxic effects on the brain, damaging cells that contain other transmitters such as serotonin. Symptoms of parkinsonism can be found in the long-term user. Even small amounts of methamphetamine can result in dramatic results.

Recreational drugs are used to obtain a "rush" or "flash." Commonly known as "chalk," "speed," "crank," "crystal," "glass," and "ice," methamphetamines are manufactured illegally in "meth" labs across the United States. In addition to the results produced by amphetamines, methamphetamine can also produce life-threatening conditions, such as hyperthermia (fever) and convulsions. Irreversible damage to the

TABLE 8-2 Clinical Manifestations and Emergency Care for Clients Who Abuse Stimulants

	Clinical Manifestations	Emergency Care
Stimulant overdose	Respiratory distress Ataxia Fever Convulsions Coma Myocardial infarction Stroke Death	Respiratory support Cooling blanket Anti-epileptic drugs Antipsychotics Ammonium chloride (to acidify urine for excretion of amphetamines [bases])
Stimulant withdrawal	Fatigue Depression Agitation Apathy Anxiety Insomnia Disorientation Craving	Antianxiety medications Antidepressants Dopamine agonists (to reduce tremors)

vessels in the brain can cause strokes. Cardiovascular collapse, resulting in death, can be caused by methamphetamine use.

Assessment findings of methamphetamine use are the same symptoms found in amphetamine use; however, they may be more pronounced or vivid than those for amphetamine use. Nursing care for the client experiencing withdrawal or overdose is the same as that for amphetamine use.

Cocaine

OVERVIEW

Cocaine is a stimulant that is commonly known as "coke," "crack," "flake," "rocks," and "snow." Cocaine, legally used as a Schedule II drug, is valuable as a topical anesthetic or a vasoconstrictor to stop bleeding. The physiologic action of cocaine is interference with the reabsorption process of dopamine. As a chemical messenger related to pleasure and movement, dopamine is released as part of the brain's reward system and is associated with the euphoria achieved with cocaine use. Processing cocaine using ammonia or sodium bicarbonate transforms the cocaine into "crack cocaine," a preparation that can be inhaled. This process is referred to as "freebasing" cocaine. Smoking cocaine is a more direct method of getting the drug to the brain. Physical dependency can occur with psychological dependence being more common. Cocaine use is severely addicting, and withdrawal can be a life-threatening situation. Adverse reactions include all of the reactions listed with stimulant use, including vertigo, nausea, vomiting, abdominal cramps, hypotension or hypertension, chills, fever, tachycardia, and tachypnea, progressing to collapse of the peripheral circulatory system, coma, and death.

COLLABORATIVE MANAGEMENT

Assessment

When caring for the client using cocaine, observe for symptoms that are associated with crack cocaine use. With moderate amounts of this drug, the client may exhibit increased alertness, euphoria, anorexia, high blood pressure, increased heart rate, and dilated pupils. In high doses (overdose), agitation, confusion, hallucinations, panic attacks, paranoia, or convulsions may occur. Withdrawal symptoms include irritability, sluggishness, and prolonged periods of sleep, depression, and nausea. Laboratory results for determining presence in the urine is detectable in the urine 1 to 4 hours after ingestion and may remain in the urine up to 3 days after use. To determine relative time of ingestions, serum levels are necessary.

Interventions

Nursing care of the client with overdose or withdrawal includes astute observation for cardiac symptoms and frequent monitoring of vital signs. Assess for signs of depression and potential suicide gestures during the withdrawal period. Help reduce nausea by ensuring that the environmental temperature is comfortable and that odors are eliminated. Assess nutrition and hydration status due to the tendency of the person to fail to eat or take in fluids during use of the drug.

During the initial and ongoing physical assessment, pay careful attention to the mucous membranes of the nose, because prolonged snorting can deteriorate the membranes and the nasal septum. Nosebleeds are common with snorting the drug and can be a valuable tool in assessment of use. Cardiopulmonary arrest can occur with the first use of cocaine. Generally the medical treatment for cocaine withdrawal or overdose is the same as that for amphetamines.

Nicotine

OVERVIEW

Nicotine is one of the most addictive substances in the United States and is the addictive component of tobacco. Although the U.S. Surgeon General issued a report in 1989 about the health hazards of tobacco and cigarette smoking, tobacco products continue to be used. This report cited nicotine as a major contributing factor to strokes, the third leading cause of death. Today, there is wide use of nicotine products in cigarettes, pipe tobacco, chewing tobacco, and "spit" tobacco (Figure 8-1).

Physiologically, nicotine has both stimulant and sedative properties that affect the central nervous system (CNS). First, nicotine stimulates the discharge of epinephrine from the adrenal cortex, causing a sudden release of glucose. After recovery from the stimulant effects of the nicotine, depressant effects result in feelings of depression and fatigue. Daily

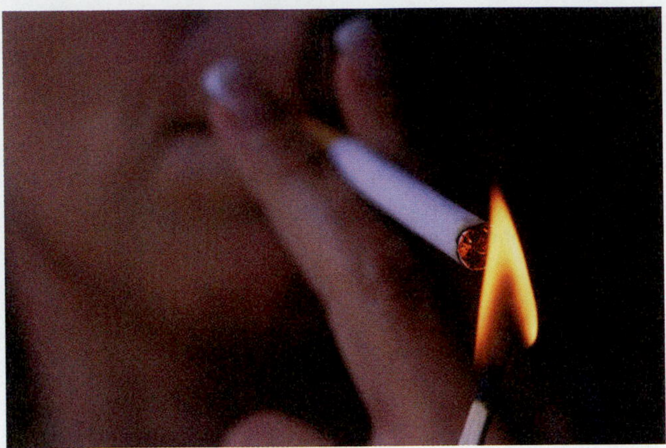

Figure 8-1 ■ The incidence of smoking is increasing among women.

ingestion of nicotine results in accumulation of nicotine in the body, lasting up to 24 hours. Because of the cyclic properties of nicotine, the body begins to require more nicotine usage to maintain the stimulant effects of the drug.

The dependence process begins with the cyclic use of nicotine for continuation of the stimulation experienced by the body. The addictive power of nicotine has been compared to that of cocaine. With the cessation of nicotine use, withdrawal symptoms are observed in the tobacco user. Lack of nicotine use in a 24-hour period can result in aggression, hostility, anger, and inappropriate social interactions. Research into the use of nicotine has resulted in data that show an increased level of dopamine, a neurotransmitter affecting brain pathways that control reward and pleasure. During periods of stress, there is a need for additional nicotine because the stress hormone corticosterone reduces the effects of nicotine. As stress and anxiety increase, the cycle of dependence grows stronger, leading the user to increase consumption of nicotine.

◆COLLABORATIVE MANAGEMENT

As proponents of good health practices, the nurse may help motivate the client to quit using nicotine by describing the negative effects of smoking, including chronic cardiovascular and respiratory diseases. Secondhand smoke affects other people who are exposed to the smoker. The nurse teaches the importance of smoking cessation. A number of community-based support groups and smoking cessation programs, using behavioral methods, hypnosis, acupressure, or other modalities, are available. Smoking cessation is discussed in the cardiovascular unit of this text.

HALLUCINOGENS AND RELATED COMPOUNDS

Chemical substances that possess mind-altering or mental perception–altering properties are known as **hallucinogens** (see Table 8-1). Examples of hallucinogenic substances are lysergic acid (LSD), phencyclidine (PCP), and marijuana. Of these three, the only therapeutic drug is PCP, which is used as a veterinary anesthetic agent. There are no therapeutic uses acceptable for medical treatment today, although marijuana has been used by some to treat cancer pain.

Hallucinogenic compounds are desirable to the drug user because of their thrill-seeking effects, which are caused by an alteration in perception. These drugs produce changes in the neurotransmitters of the brain. Alterations in mood, sensory distortions, delusions, and depersonalization are some of the resulting behaviors. Physical changes experienced by the user are increased pulse, blood pressure, and respirations, as well as pupillary dilation. A psychological dependence may occur, or the client may experience suicidal or psychotic states. Flashbacks are a common phenomenon when psychedelic drugs are used and can occur at any time. The user is returned to the initial drug experience without warning, which can be very disturbing and can create a threat to safety. Observe for objective signs of use, as well as looking for paranoia and suspicious behavior. Addiction to hallucinogens is psychological in nature rather than physical addiction.

Lysergic Acid

OVERVIEW

Lysergic acid (LSD) is the prototype and major hallucinogenic drug, known as "acid" in the drug community. The drug is odorless and colorless with a slightly bitter taste. Usually taken orally, LSD is often distributed on absorbent, decorative paper, making it very attractive to adolescents and children. The health hazards of LSD are unpredictable and are affected by dose, personality and mood of the user, anticipated outcome, and environment at the time of use. Because the exact mechanism of action is not known, further studies in drug research are being conducted by the National Institute on Drug Abuse (Mathias, 2000). LSD is known to influence neurotransmission in the CNS. The effects of the drug can last up to 12 hours and can result in either pleasant or unpleasant experiences, also known as "good trips" or "bad trips."

Introspective thinking may occur with the person experiencing personal revelations about themselves, the truth of the universe, or other bizarre thoughts. Sensory experiences are powerful in LSD use because of the perception of surroundings. Colors seem more vivid and tangible to the person experiencing the effects of LSD. Thoughts and feelings can be so bizarre that a "trip" can result in suicide. LSD use can also result in severe and chronic mental illness, such as schizophrenia. Because LSD does not result in compulsive drug-seeking behaviors, it is not considered addictive, but a strong tolerance can develop. An increased amount of the drug is needed to attain the same level of stimulation as earlier experiences. LSD stimulates the sympathetic nervous system. Some neuromuscular involvement is noted such as tremors and hyperflexia. Effects of LSD can last from 8 to 12 hours.

◆COLLABORATIVE MANAGEMENT

◆Assessment

Observe for intoxication such as:

- Dilated pupils
- Tachycardia
- Palpitations
- Diaphoresis
- Tremors

- Poor coordination
- Elevated temperature
- Increased pulse and respiration

Many psychological symptoms also occur as paranoid ideas, anxiety, depression, and transforming sounds and sights into sensation (hearing colors). Overdose can result in brain damage, psychosis, or death.

Interventions

Treatment options for the person in an LSD crisis include one-to-one observation to keep the client safe and to help the person sort reality as the effects subside. Fears can be comforted and prevent the person from acting on fear or psychotic thoughts. Because there is such a sensory influence on the person, the environment should be calming, at a comfortable temperature with few disturbances. Reducing the stimuli can significantly limit the response to the drug's effects. In an emergency situation, the person is exposed to varied and powerful stimuli that contribute to intense behavioral responses to the powerful stimulus created by LSD. Antianxiety medications (benzodiazepines) or medications to control or eliminate the symptoms of mental illness may be prescribed. Haloperidol (Haldol) has been found to be effective in the treatment of LSD symptoms. Effects created by other hallucinogens such as mescaline and psilocybin (derived from peyote cactus and mushrooms) respond to the same treatment regimen as used with LSD.

Phencyclidine

Phencyclidine, commonly known as PCP, is an animal anesthetic that causes a feeling of detachment in humans. Clients using PCP ("angel dust") are unaware of their surroundings, which causes the detachment. Primarily affecting the CNS, the client exhibits flushing, increased perspiration, aggression, and incoherence. The user may experience feelings of superior strength and physical power. Some users state that their use is related to the numbing effects on the mind. However, the results may progress to a comatose state.

There is no evidence of physical addiction; however, psychological addiction is common. There is evidence to suggest a decrease in the use of PCP, a commonly abused drug in the past. The nurse who suspects PCP abuse assesses for shallow respirations, generalized numbness of the extremities, and psychological effects, including distinct changes in body awareness. High doses of PCP can produce vomiting, loss of balance, visual disturbances, and dizziness. Seizures, coma, and death have resulted from high doses of PCP. Lasting effects of PCP use can include memory loss, speech difficulties, and interference with thinking processes.

Ketamine

Closely associated with PCP, ketamine is a substance classified as a disassociate anesthetic. Because of the short duration, ketamine is sometimes known as "businessman's LSD." Moderate doses produce euphoria, loss of inhibition, confusion, ringing in the ears, a quick burst of energy, and a drunken feeling. Tolerance can occur as well as physical and psychological dependence. Street names for ketamine are "special K," "K", and "kat." Ketamine is also referred to as a "techno" drug because of its attractiveness to the "Rave" culture.

Complications associated with ketamine overdose include the following:

- Tunnel vision
- Shortness of breath
- Loss of balance
- Numbness of the body
- Clinical depression
- No sense of time
- Seizures
- Coma

A calm and stimulus-free environment is important for the client recovering from a ketamine overdose, as well as availability of supportive therapies. Respiratory support is a priority because of the anesthetic effects of the drug.

3,4-Methylenedioxymethamphetamine

OVERVIEW

Amphetamines can be altered to become a hallucinogen, as in the case of **3,4-methylenedioxymethamphetamine (MDMA),** an oral drug that is also called "Adam," "ecstasy," "XTC," "hug," "beans," and the "date rape" drug. Known as the "love drug" in the 1970s and popular in the 1980s in the "Rave" community, MDMA remains an increasingly popular recreational (club drug). MDMA can be ingested orally, smoked, snorted, or injected. The desired effects are development of trust in others, which eases inhibitions between people, and increases in confidence, euphoria, and physical energy. Methylenedioxyamphetamine (MDA) is the parent drug of MDMA, both of which produce psychostimulant and psychedelic effects.

Part of the popularity of the drug includes the relaxation of voluntary muscles and the amnesiac effect for the period in which the drug is most active in the body; hence, the name "date rape" drug. The physiologic effects of MDMA occur at the serotonin receptor sites, which create the inhibition of behaviors. Serotonin plays a vital role in the regulation of aggression, mood, sexual activity, sleep, and pain sensitivity. Action at the serotonin site accounts for the report of heightened sexual experiences and tranquility. Demonstrating a structural relationship to methamphetamine, MDMA also causes a degeneration of neurons containing dopamine, a neurotransmitter, resulting in parkinsonism. MDMA is neurotoxic and can cause brain damage. Interfering with the temperature control mechanism of the body, malignant hyperthermia can also result with the use of MDMA.

COLLABORATIVE MANAGEMENT

Assess the client who has taken MDMA for psychological symptoms, including confusion, depression, sleep disturbances, drug craving, severe anxiety, and paranoia. With moderate doses, other effects are euphoria, nervousness, hyperexcitability, and a rapid heart rate. Physical symptoms of high-dose ingestion are muscle tension, involuntary teeth clenching, nausea, visual disturbances, faintness, and chills or sweating. Abnormal vital signs such as increased heart rate and blood pressure are also observed. Nursing care of the client on MDMA is based on the symptoms that are apparent at the time of assessment.

If acute symptoms are present, the priority for care is safety and symptomatic relief of the psychological manifestations.

Medication regimens are focused on reduction or elimination of the adverse effects of the drug.

Marijuana

OVERVIEW

Marijuana is commonly called "weed," "smoke," "pot," "grass," "Mary Jane," and "herb." Widely used and distributed, this drug is illegal and does not have any accepted legal therapeutic uses. For some clients, it has been used experimentally for chronic pain control. Although there is a considerable and ongoing debate about the uses and need for legalization of marijuana, it remains a contraband substance in the United States. Even though physical dependence for marijuana is seemingly nonexistent, it has a high risk for psychological dependence if it is used over long periods of time. The desired effects of marijuana are sensations of euphoria, sexual arousal, and relaxation. The "high" experience that users feel is a result of the action of tetrahydrocannabinol (THC), the main active substance in marijuana. THC changes the method by which sensory information enters and is processed in the hippocampus. As a component of the brain's limbic system, the hippocampus is necessary for the integration of sensory experiences and emotion, as well as learning and memory. Frequent and long-term use of marijuana can create the same respiratory changes seen in long-term tobacco smokers. Studies of young adults who use marijuana demonstrate that learning and social behavior are affected by heavy marijuana use. Evidence suggests that marijuana use affects critical skills related to attention, memory, and learning. Heavy marijuana users make more mistakes in their work and have more difficulty maintaining attention.

COLLABORATIVE MANAGEMENT

Whether smoked or taken orally, the physical and psychological effects in moderate doses include relaxation, happiness, euphoria, increased heart rate, and impaired short-term memory. High doses produce more pronounced effects such paranoia, restlessness, anxiety attacks, panic attacks, increased appetite, impaired coordination, and altered perceptions. Withdrawal effects include insomnia, decreased appetite, nausea, irritability, and anxiety.

Nursing interventions for the person who is under the influence of marijuana are based on the severity of symptoms presented. A complete physical assessment as well as frequent vital sign assessment is needed to determine stability of the person's physical condition. Communication skills are important to ascertain self-destructive tendencies and the ability to give accurate, relevant data for treatment. Research of marijuana notes that there is no evidence of immediate life-threatening physical complications with use. However, impaired judgment, chromosomal influence on fetuses, and loss of memory are significant long-term effects of marijuana use.

DEPRESSANTS

Drugs that reduce the activity of the central nervous system (CNS) are referred to as **depressants** (see Table 8-1). Benzodiazepines and barbiturates are discussed as depressants because of their activity in the ascending reticular activating system in the CNS. Both classes have valuable therapeutic properties in treating anxiety and emotional disorders. CNS depressants are therapeutically used as adjuncts to sleep and can be used as needed for situational tension. The route of ingestion is either oral or by injection. On the illicit drug market, barbiturates are called "barbs" or "ludes"; depending on the chemical makeup. A commonly abused benzodiazepine, Rohypnol, is referred to as "rophies," "ruffies," "R2s," "Mexican Valium," "rib," "roach," or "Roches." Sometimes Rohypnol (flunitrazepam) is referred to as the "forget me pill" or "forget pill." These are Schedule IV drugs because of their high potential for abuse.

Benzodiazepines

The desired results for the use of prescribed benzodiazepines include relaxation, sleep, seizure control, withdrawal from alcohol, and relief of anxiety. Abuse is present when the client continues to use the drug after the clinical signs have subsided. The street value of benzodiazepines and the drug effects make this drug popular. Physical and psychological dependence on benzodiazepines is prevalent. The user can develop a high tolerance for the drug, causing increasing amounts to be needed to achieve the desired feeling. Benzodiazepines depress the CNS; therefore combination with other CNS substances has a potentiating effect.

ROHYPNOL

Rohypnol (flunitrazepam) is a highly potent benzodiazepine (10 times more potent as diazepam [Valium]) available through a provider prescription. Presently this drug is not available in the United States; however, it is used legally in other countries. Therapeutic use of this drug is for severe sleep disorders and inpatient psychiatric care. Combined with alcohol, this drug is also known to as a date rape drug. It is colorless, tasteless, and is not easily detected in the urine. Rohypnol can be swallowed, inhaled, injected, smoked, or dissolved in a drink. Effects of this drug provide the following:

- Relief from tension
- Anticonvulsant action
- Sedation
- Amnesia
- Muscle relaxation
- Sleep
- Slowing of motor performance, an effect that is greatly increased when combined with alcohol

Young people use this drug to engage in violent or destructive activities without feelings of guilt. Rohypnol has physical and psychological dependence properties. Moderate doses create a loss of inhibition, drunken state, dizziness, tranquility, and slurred speech.

Signs and symptoms associated with withdrawal or overdosing from Rohypnol include the following:

- Headache
- Muscle pain
- Extreme anxiety
- Tension and restlessness
- Confusion and irritability
- Depersonalization
- Hypersensitivity to light, noise, and physical contact
- Delirium

- Convulsions
- Shock
- Respiratory depression
- Cardiovascular collapse

Nursing care should focus on the severity of the symptoms and astute assessment for deterioration in the client's physical condition. Treatment of Rohypnol abuse is aimed at a medical model of detoxification using tapering doses.

GAMMA HYDROXYBUTYRATE

Gamma hydroxybutyrate (GHB) is gaining increased attention as a club drug along with LSD, ecstasy, ketamine, methamphetamine, and Rohypnol. GHB is referred to as "liquid ecstasy." In small amounts, GHB reduces one's social inhibitions and increasing libido. It is produced illegally in the United States and was referred to as the date rape drug of the 1990s. GHB may be inhaled, injected, or swallowed. In small doses, it produces euphoria, anxiety, increased sexual pleasure, impaired judgment, a loss of coordination, and nausea along with the loss of inhibition. Routine urine drug screening does not show GHB, but GHB can be detected if a GHB-specific test is requested.

Results of high doses of GHB range from dizziness to death. Common symptoms of overdose of GHB are respiratory depression, memory loss, bradycardia, muscular fatigue, and coma. The adverse effects of GHB can be devastating. When combined with alcohol, deaths are more prevalent. Anyone presenting at the emergency department in a coma of unknown origin must be evaluated for GHB use.

The nurse needs to be skillful in assessing the client who has taken an overdose of GHB because of the legal ramifications of the drug. Using an open, nonjudgmental approach is necessary to develop a trusting and honest communication. Reactions in the person taking GHB vary with each use and may confuse the client with these different responses.

Barbiturates

Barbiturates are drugs that depress the CNS through action in the cerebral cortex and the reticular formation (helps regulate the sleep-wake cycle). Effects of barbiturates include sedation, drowsiness, and a decrease in motor activity of the body similar to those seen with alcohol use. Therapeutic uses of barbiturates are short-term insomnia, preanesthesia, and anticonvulsant therapy. Because of the aging process, older adults can tolerate only small doses of barbiturates. Dependence on barbiturates can occur in a short time and can lead to withdrawal symptoms if the drug is discontinued abruptly. Initial withdrawal symptoms are anxiety, restlessness, insomnia, irritability, and impaired attention with more severe symptoms if the person has a chronic pattern of use. Physical illness may accompany the withdrawal of barbiturates with nausea, vomiting, abdominal cramping, seizures, and varied behavioral responses. With severe dependence, the effects of withdrawal can be life threatening. Toxic or overdose symptoms include respiratory depression, coma, and pinpoint pupils. Laboratory testing for barbiturates can be done by direct immunoassay from blood, urine, or gastric contents.

Nursing interventions for the client in crisis due to overdose or withdrawal of barbiturates are to ensure safety through frequent vital signs, neurologic checks, and emotional support. Symptomatic treatment such as drug tapering is necessary to avoid the more severe response to drug elimination. Food, fluids, and a calm environment are necessary to achieve the initial outcomes for the client. Because barbiturates are constipating, monitor the client for elimination patterns, being sure to provide high fiber in the diet. Immediate and long-term care of the person with physical addiction requires various members of the health care team to treat and support the planning and implementation of holistic care.

Alcohol

OVERVIEW

Alcohol in various mixed drinks, beer, wine, and liquor provides sedation, relaxation, and release of a person's inhibitions. A substantial number of people in the United States drink alcoholic beverages. For most people, alcohol is used for a pleasure experience. Alcohol acts as a depressant on the CNS and the respiratory system; therefore the signs and symptoms of the effects of alcohol use are primarily neurologic. One of every 13 adults in the United States abuses alcohol (Stewart & Richards, 2003).

Alcoholism (alcohol dependence syndrome) is a disease wherein the person has a strong need or compulsion to consume alcohol, is unable to quit once he or she begins drinking, experiences a physical dependence, and has a need to increase the amount of alcohol to get "high" (high tolerance). Physical dependence occurs when the person experiences withdrawal after alcohol use is stopped after a period of heavy drinking. When drinking alcohol relieves the symptoms of withdrawal, the person has developed a true physical dependence on alcohol, and is considered an alcoholic (Figure 8-2).

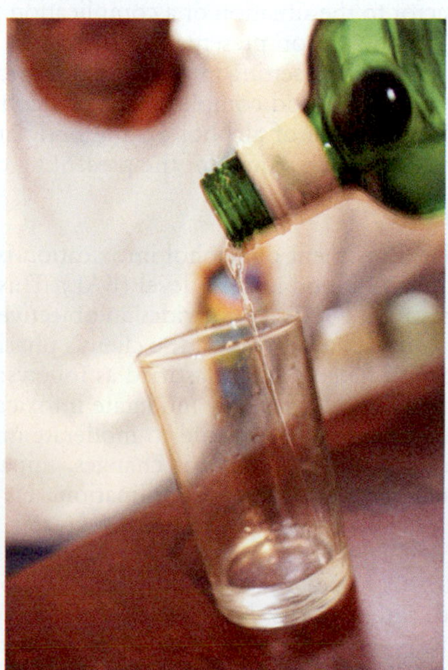

Figure 8-2 ■ Alcohol is commonly used for pleasure and acts as a central nervous system depressant.

Alcohol abuse exists when a person *does not* have a strong craving for alcohol, loss of control, or physical dependence but has problems related to alcohol use. Examples of alcohol abuse are when the person fails to fulfill responsibilities at home, work, or school; when the person drinks in unsafe situations; when the person experiences legal problems that are alcohol related, or when the person continues to drink when problems have been caused or worsened by use of alcohol. When one or more of these events occur within a 12-month period, the person is abusing alcohol.

CONSIDERATIONS FOR OLDER ADULTS

Older adults also face risks for alcohol-related problems. The risk for intoxication and serious drug interactions is increased when alcohol is used in combination with other drugs. Older adults may have experienced a longer history of alcohol use and are at greater risk for severe withdrawal.

Because of the "normal" aging processes, sometimes there is confusion in identification of alcohol withdrawal from expected changes in the aging population. Societal expectations and morés of the older population may make obtaining an accurate substance use history difficult. In treatment of the older person in withdrawal, treatment regimens need to take into consideration the change in function of the aging body. Generally the treatment of the older adult employs adjusted dosages of medications to avoid oversedation and close monitoring for subtle physiologic changes.

COLLABORATIVE MANAGEMENT

Nursing care of the person with alcohol problems or alcoholism is a challenge related to the will of the person and the motivation to reduce or stop alcohol consumption. The person with alcohol problems presents in the emergency department for emergency care when alcohol has been a contributing factor to the situation or a complication to the reason for which the person presents for treatment. The nurse in the medical-surgical setting must be knowledgeable about the signs, symptoms, and complications of alcohol use because of the influence of alcohol on the body and the increase of risk during treatment of the presenting condition.

Assessment

An objective assessment of alcohol intoxication is obtained from obtaining a blood alcohol level (BAL). This measurement is important because it provides an objective reference in which to anticipate severity of the client's physical status.

Toxic levels of alcohol are classified as follows:

- 80 to 200 mg/dL (mild to moderate intoxication). Behaviors consistent with mild to moderate intoxication include mood and behavior changes, impaired judgment, and poor motor coordination. Hypotension may occur in clients with levels greater than 100 mg/dL (Pagana & Pagana, 2002).
- 250 to 400 mg/dL (marked intoxication). Observations noted with this level of intoxication are staggering ataxia and emotional lability. Symptoms may progress to confusion and stupor or coma.
- Greater than 500 mg/dL (severe intoxication). Death is due to respiratory depression.

CHART 8-1

KEY FEATURES of
Disease: Typical Signs and Symptoms of Clients in Alcohol Withdrawal

Objective Symptoms	Subjective Signs
Tremors	No appetite
Jerky movements	Reports "shaking inside"
Vomiting	Nausea
Diaphoresis, tenting skin	Delusional
Undernourished	Hallucinating
Dehydrated	
Increased pulse and blood pressure	
Disoriented to place, time	

The most threatening result of alcohol abuse or alcoholism is withdrawal from the substance. Symptoms of withdrawal range from mild to severe and can progress to death. Alcohol withdrawal can be evaluated by categories according to severity:

- *Minor withdrawal*–restlessness, anxiety, sleeping difficulties, agitation and tremors, tachycardia, low-grade fever, diaphoresis, and elevated blood pressure
- *Major withdrawal*–in addition to the signs and symptoms of mild withdrawal, visual or auditory hallucinations, tremors of the entire body (**delirium tremens,** or **DTs**), heart rate greater than 100 beats/min, diastolic pressure above 100 mm Hg, pronounced diaphoresis, and vomiting
- *Life-threatening withdrawal*–delirium tremens, disorientation times, global confusion, and inability to recognize familiar objects or people

The life-threatening stage of alcohol withdrawal has a 2% to 5% mortality rate, requiring emergency medical interventions. Alcohol seizures may occur 12 to 48 hours after the last drink.

Interventions

When the client is experiencing withdrawal of alcohol–or another depressant–the priority for care is to prevent the client from harming himself or herself or others. Attempt to reorient him or her to reality frequently. The health care provider often prescribes medications to calm or sedate the client according to agency protocol or physician preference. Examples of typical drugs that are used are benzodiazepines, such as chlordiazepoxide (Librium) and diazepam (Valium), to prevent seizures and DTs. Other commonly used drugs include beta-blockers to reduce cravings and decrease pulse and blood pressure, and alpha-adrenergic blockers to decrease withdrawal symptoms. Table 8-2 lists some of the most commonly used medications for alcohol withdrawal. Intravenous fluids and vitamins, such as thiamine, are also prescribed. In collaboration with the dietitian, plan ways to increase protein and calories to address the client's nutritional needs.

Nursing care for the client with alcohol use or abuse includes thorough assessment to identify dependence and frequency of use. Chart 8-1 lists common objective and subjective signs and symptoms of clients in alcohol withdrawal. Chart 8-2 includes nursing activities that you should implement when caring for a client in alcohol withdrawal.

Clients who are alcoholic and their families require extensive rehabilitation and support. Collaborate with the case manager, social worker, or discharge planner to ensure

CHART 8-2

NIC INTERVENTION ACTIVITIES for The Client in Alcohol Withdrawal

Substance Use Treatment: Alcohol Withdrawal: *Care of the client experiencing sudden cessation of alcohol consumption*

- Create a low-stimulation environment.
- Monitor vital signs during withdrawal.
- Monitor for delirium tremens (DTs).
- Administer anticonvulsants or sedatives, as appropriate.
- Medicate to relieve physical discomfort, as needed.
- Address hallucinations in a therapeutic manner.
- Maintain adequate nutrition and fluid intake.
- Administer vitamin therapy as appropriate.
- Provide emotional support to client/family, as appropriate.
- Provide reality orientation, as appropriate.

NIC intervention activities selected from Dochterman, J.M., & Bulechek, G.M. (Eds.) (2004). *Nursing interventions classification (NIC)* (4th ed.). St. Louis: Mosby. No part of this work is to be altered without prior written permission from the Publisher.

that the client and family members are aware of community resources such as Alcoholics Anonymous for clients and Al-Anon for family members and friends. If these programs fail, aversion therapy with disulfiram (Antabuse) may be an option for treatment. Mental health/behavioral health texts discuss psychosocial support and alcohol abuse treatment in more detail.

NARCOTICS: OPIOIDS AND MORPHINE DERIVATIVES

OVERVIEW

Narcotic is a broad term encompassing all drugs that are made from the Asian poppy or produced as a synthetic drug which produces the same effects of the opium plant. A desired (therapeutic) action of narcotics is to reduce the client's perception of pain. Drugs included in this category are codeine, morphine, heroin, methadone, hydromorphone (Dilaudid), meperidine (Demerol), and oxycodone, (OxyContin). These drugs are therapeutically used for relief of severe pain, such as pain experienced in terminal cancer or postoperative pain. Sleep is an added feature of the drug when it is used for pain. Opium and morphine derivatives have become drugs of dependence because of their analgesic and euphoric effects. Common names for heroin and opium in the drug community are "horse" and "smack" for heroin and "Dover's powder" for opium. The sites of action of these drugs are in the brain, binding in the receptor sites of the CNS (causing CNS depression) and in the gastrointestinal system (producing the antidiarrheal effects of opium; Lomotil). Desired effects of substance abuse with these drugs are the escape effect in the mind and analgesia. Aggression and sexual drives are usually minimized with use of the opioids and morphine-like drugs.

A high potential for addiction, tolerance, and dependence occurs with this class of drugs. The withdrawal effects can range from mild withdrawal symptoms to death. According to the National Institute on Drug Abuse, there are four categories of opiate withdrawal (Mathias, 2000):

- Grade 0 is characterized by drug craving, anxiety, and drug-seeking behaviors.
- Grade 1 is characterized by yawning, sweating, lacrimation, and rhinorrhea ("runny nose").
- Grade 2 is characterized by mydriasis (pupillary dilation), gooseflesh, muscle twitching, and anorexia.
- Grade 3, the most dangerous of the grades in opiate withdrawal, is characterized by increased pulse, respiratory rate, and blood pressure; abdominal cramps; diarrhea; vomiting; and weakness.

These drugs may be taken orally, injected, or inhaled. Heroin, a highly addictive drug, is an opiate derivative. Unlike the other opiate drugs noted earlier, heroin has no medical use. The health hazards of heroin are serious and include fatal overdoses and spontaneous abortions. Intravenous use of heroin or other abused substances increases the risk of acquiring infectious diseases such as human immunodeficiency virus infection (HIV) and hepatitis. Short-term effects of heroin are felt immediately and continue for a few hours after a single dose. Heroin users report an immediate feeling of extreme euphoria ("rush"). The person experiences a dry mouth, heavy extremities, and a warm, flushed feeling. Generally, there are alternate sensations of wakefulness and sleep. Common street names for heroin are "horse," "smack," "H," "skag," and "junk." Long-term use of heroin results in many physical problems, such as emaciation, frequent infections, cellulitis, and liver disease. Morphine, heroin, and codeine use can be identified in the urine from 2 hours after ingestion up to 3 days after use.

COLLABORATIVE MANAGEMENT

Care of the client with an opiate or heroin addiction becomes complex because of the physical condition, the addictive behaviors, and the safety concerns both physically and psychologically. The nurse must have an understanding of the withdrawal symptoms to be aware of the severity of the medical condition created by withdrawal from opiates and their derivatives. Implications include the need for current information about addictions and the addictive drug cycle, both physically and mentally.

Assessment

When possible, determine the client's history of drug use, drug of choice, and the last ingestion. A small percentage of clients become addicted to opioids while being treated for severe, chronic pain. For example, clients with sickle cell anemia have episodes of extreme pain during exacerbations of their disease and require large amounts of pain medication.

Three major problems that require emergency intervention may occur when opiates are used: intoxication, overdose, and withdrawal. Assessment findings for each of these conditions are listed in Chart 8-3.

Interventions

Anticonvulsant drugs are commonly prescribed to prevent seizures. Other medications, such as naloxone (Narcan) and naltrexone (ReVia), work as opioid antagonists, competing with opioids at the receptor sites. Midazolam (Versed) may also be given to induce amnesic effects; anxiety-reducing medications (anxiolytics) help to relieve anxiety. In some cases of severe dependence, methadone is prescribed to relieve pain. Other medications may be given to treat symptoms such as diarrhea or nausea.

Provide supportive measures for the client, including nonpharmacologic measures to relieve pain, reduce stimuli, and provide basic comfort measures. Monitor vital signs

CHART 8-3

KEY FEATURES of
Disease: Manifestations of Opiate Use That Require Emergency Interventions

Opiate Intoxication
- Constricted pupils
- Decreased blood pressure
- Decreased respirations
- Drowsiness
- Slurred speech
- Initial euphoria followed by dysphoria (depression)
- Cognitive impairments resulting in judgment and memory losses

Opiate Overdose
- Dilated pupils
- Respiratory depression
- Coma
- Shock
- Convulsions
- Respiratory arrest
- Death

Opiate Withdrawal
- Yawning
- Insomnia
- Irritability
- Rhinorrhea
- Diaphoresis
- Abdominal cramps
- Nausea and vomiting
- Muscle aches
- Chills, cold flashes with goose bumps (referred to as "cold turkey")

frequently and assess for major changes. Pay special attention to alterations in respiratory rate or pattern.

INHALANTS

Breathable chemical vapors that produce psychoactive effects are called **inhalants.** These substances are popular with young people because of their accessibility (in the home) and price. Three categories of inhalants are common household items. **Solvents** produce a "high" when inhaled. Examples of solvents are paint thinners, gasoline, glues, paper correction fluid, felt-tip markers, and electronic contact cleaners. **Gases** are another source of inhalants and include products such as butane lighters, propane tanks, whipping cream aerosols, spray paints, hair or deodorant sprays, chloroform, ether, and nitrous oxide (laughing gas). **Nitrites** are the third source of inhalants and include cyclohexyl nitrite, amyl nitrite, and butyl nitrite. The terms most readily referring to inhalant use are "glue," "kick," "bang," "sniff," "huffing," "poppers," "whippets," and "Texas Shoeshine."

Inhalants produce anesthetic results, consequently slowing body functions. Persons who use inhalants feel intoxicated, less inhibited, and less in control with repeated use. They may inhale to the point of causing unconsciousness. Sniffing highly concentrated chemicals can result in death from cardiac failure. Suffocation can also occur because the inhalant takes the place of oxygen in the lungs and respirations cease. Irreversible effects, including hearing losses, limb spasms, brain damage, and bone marrow suppression, can occur from inhalants. Reversible effects that can occur with inhalants include liver and kidney damage and blood oxygen depletion. Pouring or dispensing the inhalant into a paper bag increases the concentration of the substance, inducing a quicker, more pronounced effect.

Signs of inhalant use follow:
- Slurred speech
- Drunk, dizzy, or dazed appearance
- Chemical smell on the person
- Paint stains on body or face
- Red eyes
- Rhinorrhea

You may come in contact with young adults who have had experience with inhalants. These clients may have been admitted to the hospital for complications of inhalant use or because of medical conditions. Once the client is stabilized, try to determine with the client the reasons for his or her use of inhalants. Management and treatment of chemical ingestions is supportive. There are known antidotes available for inhalant overdose or toxicity.

STEROIDS

Anabolic-androgenic steroids are growing in popularity among young athletes. The term *anabolic* indicates muscle building, and the term *androgenic* refers to increased masculinity. Anabolic steroids are synthetic substances that mimic the actions of testosterone. Steroids are legally available through prescription use for people with hormonal difficulties such as delayed puberty or impotence. Athletes are known to use steroids to increase strength and performance even when it is known to be unhealthy, life threatening, and illegal for use in amateur, professional, and international events. The pressure to become stronger, to achieve, and to succeed many times tempts the person to use steroids to "bulk up" for mastery in selected sports. Misuse of steroids can lead to serious medical problems, some of which are irreversible. Possible effects of steroids include the following:
- For men: shrinking testicles, reduced sperm count, infertility, baldness, development of breasts, and an increased risk for cancer
- For women: growth of facial hair, male pattern baldness, changes or cessation of menses, enlargement of the clitoris, and deepened voice
- For adolescents: premature skeletal maturation and accelerated puberty changes

Aggression is increased by the use of steroids. In addition, there may be a noted increase in mental illness as a result of mood disturbances. Discontinuation of steroids can result in depression.

***GET READY* for the NCLEX Examination!**

KEY POINTS

- Substance abuse interferes with life's activities, which can endanger the client when hospitalized; therefore a complete drug history is essential in identification of substance abuse in the hospitalized client.
- Common drugs of abuse are stimulants, hallucinogens, depressants, opioids, inhalants, and steroids.

- Research findings indicate a link between genetics and substance use. Personality traits are thought to be contributing factors to substance abuse.
- Nursing care of the person using substances must consider the developmental stage, cultural background, and social environment when developing a plan of care for the client.
- Stimulants increase mental alertness, improve a person's sense of well-being, increase the capacity to work, improve performance of motor skills, and increase metabolism through increased respiratory and cardiac function. Examples of stimulants common in the drug culture are amphetamines, methamphetamines, cocaine, and nicotine.
- The following are common slang terms for illicit amphetamine substances:
  Amphetamines: "crosses," "hearts," "black beauties"
  Methamphetamines: "crank," "crystal," "ice," "glass," "speed," "chalk"
  Cocaine: "coke," "snow," "flake," "rocks," "crack"
- Symptoms of stimulant use that require emergency interventions are elevated vital signs (including temperature), dehydration, and neurologic changes, including convulsions or coma.
- Medications common in the treatment of overdose or withdrawal of stimulants include antipsychotics, antiparkinsonism agents, antidepressants, antianxiety medications, and intravenous therapy.
- Hallucinogenic substances, which create an alteration in perception and a subsequent euphoria, include LSD, PCP, ketamine, MDMA (ecstasy), and marijuana. Effects of hallucinogenic substances, such as enhanced sexual arousal, create a safety risk for the person who uses because of the euphoria and false sense of abilities experienced.
- PCP creates a feeling of detachment; referred to as "angel dust," PCP is an animal tranquilizer that creates numbing effects on the mind.
- Depressants, including benzodiazepines, gamma hydroxybutyrate (GHB), barbiturates, alcohol, and narcotics, are among the most popular abused substances.
- Barbiturates are commonly referred to as "barbs" and "ludes"; clients can develop physical withdrawal if they abruptly stop these drugs.
- Alcohol withdrawal is classified as minor, major, and life threatening. Life-threatening symptoms of alcohol withdrawal are delirium tremens (DTs), disorientation, global confusion, and inability to recognize familiar objects or persons.
- Interventions for acute alcohol withdrawal are administration of sedatives, vitamins, magnesium sulfate, anticonvulsants, and folic acid (see Chart 8-2).
- Chart 8-3 summarizes clinical manifestations of alcohol withdrawal that require emergency interventions.
- Minor to moderate symptoms of opiate or narcotic withdrawal are yawning, insomnia, irritability, rhinorrhea, diaphoresis, chills, and "goose bumps."
- The most dangerous grade of opiate withdrawal is characterized by increased pulse and respiratory rates, increased blood pressure, abdominal cramps, diarrhea, vomiting, and weakness. This condition requires emergency intervention to prevent death.
- Interventions for symptoms associated with narcotic withdrawal range from supportive care to use of IV fluids, anticonvulsants, opioid antagonists, methadone substitution, clonidine, and midazolam hydrochloride (Versed).
- Inhalants are used by children and adolescents because of their easy availability; inhalants induce the following effects: slurred speech, drunkenness, dizzy or dazed appearance, red eyes, and rhinorrhea. There may be a chemical odor present or paint smears on the face.
- Inhalants create anesthetic results and slow body functions resulting in feelings of intoxication.
- "Sniffing" can result in unconsciousness and suffocation due to competition for air space in the lungs between the inhalant and oxygen.
- Irreversible effects from inhalant use are limb spasms, brain damage, and hearing loss. Nursing care of the person having used inhalants is symptomatic and supportive.
- Continuous steroid use is found primarily in athletes to build strength and muscle mass. Routine drug screens are helpful in detecting steroids or other drugs that may enhance the athletic ability of a participant.

ADDITIONAL STUDY RESOURCES

Go to your Student CD-ROM for Review Questions for the NCLEX Examination.

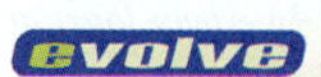

Go to http://evolve.elsevier.com/Iggy/ for Integrated Management of Care Questions for the NCLEX Examination.

SELECTED BIBLIOGRAPHY

Asterisk indicates a classic or definitive work on this subject.

Acello, B. (2000). Controlling pain, facing fears about opioid addiction, *Nursing 2000, 30*(5), 72.

American Nurses Association. (2001). *Code for nurses with interpretative statements.* Washington, DC: American Nurses Association.

Club Drugs: Emergency Room Update, (2001) *SAMHSA News* 9(2), 7-8,

Compton, P. (2002) Caring for an alcohol-dependent patient. *Nursing, 32*(12), 58-63.

Elimination of substance abuse in young people. (2002). International Council of Nurses Position Statement. Available at http://www.icn.ch/psabuse.htm.

Gill, M. (2003). MDMA toxicity: The influence of metabolic genotype at CYP2D6. Available at http://www.tcd.ie/Research/projects/drugs/analsci.html.

*Greenblant, J. (1997). Gamma hydroxy butyrate (GHB) abuse in the United States, SAMHSA, OAS Working Paper. Rockville, MD: SAMHSA's Clearinghouse for Alcohol and Drug Abuse.

Hardie, T. (2002). The genetics of substance abuse. *AACN Clinical Issues, 13*(4), 511-522.

Inhalants: Most popular drug for 12-year-olds. (2001). *SAMHSA News*, 23.

Lehne, R. (2001). *Pharmacology for nursing care* (4th ed.). Philadelphia: W.B. Saunders.

Lesher, A. (2000). A club drug alert. *NIDA, 14*(6), 1-4.

Ludwick, R.E., et al. (2000). Alcohol use in elderly women: Nursing considerations in community settings. *Journal of Gerontological Nursing, 26*(2), 44-49.

Malseed, R. (2004). *Nurse's drug guide.* (5th ed.). Philadelphia: Lippincott Williams & Wilkins.

Marijuana abuse. (2002). *National Institute on Drug Abuse: Research Report Series.* National Institutes of Health Publication No. 03-3859, U.S. Department of Health and Human Services. Available at http://drugabuse.gov/PDF/RRmarijuana.pdf.

Martin, K. (2002). Combining medications may be effective treatment for "speedball" abuse. *NIDA Notes, 17*(3), 11.

Mathias, R. (2000). Cocaine, marijuana, and heroin use up, methamphetamine abuse down. Available at http://drugabuse.gov.

McCloskey, J. (2003). *Unifying nursing languages: The harmonization of NANDA, NIC, and NOC.* Washington, DC: American Nurses Association.

Mioto, K., & Roth, B. (2002). GHB: A club drug to watch. *Substance Abuse Treatment Advisory, 2*(1).

Monitoring the Futures Survey Released, *HHS News (*2001).12.19: Media Advisory, 1-5. Available at www.drugabuse.gov/MedAdv/01/NR12-19.html.

National Institute on Drug Abuse, National Institute of Health, U.S. Department of Health and Human Services. (2003). Available at http://www.nida.nih.gov.

National Priorities II: Healing America's drug users national drug control strategy: 2002. Available at http://www.whitehousedrugpolicy.gov/publicatios/policy/03ndcs/2priorities.html.

Pagana, K., Pagana, T. (2002). *Mosby's manual of diagnostic and laboratory tests.* (2nd ed.). St. Louis: Mosby.

*Perkins, S. (1999). *Drug identification: Designer and club drugs quick reference guide.* Knoxville, TN: Alliance Press.

*Position statement: Abuse of prescription drugs. (1997). Washington, DC: American Nurses Association.

Principles of drug addiction treatment. (2000). Washington, DC: National Institute on Drug Abuse.

Sachse, D. (2000). Emergency: Delirium tremens. *American Journal of Nursing, 100*(5), 41-42.

**Standards of addictions: Nursing practice with selected diagnoses and criteria.* (1988). Washington, DC: American Nurses Association.

Stewart, K.B., & Richards, A.B. (2000). Recognizing and managing your patient's alcohol abuse. *Nursing 2000, 30*(2), 56-59.

*Stocker, S. (1999). Studies link stress and drug addiction. *NIDA Notes, 14*(1), 1-4.

Substance abuse increases in New York City in aftermath of September 11th. (2002). *NIDA.* Available at http://www.drugabuse.gov/Newsroom/02/NR5-28.html.

Substance abuse predicting it, preventing it. (2001). *SAMHSA News 9*(2), 1-27.

Substance abuse treatment advisory, GHB: A club drug to watch. (2002). U.S. Department of Health and Human Services. Available at http://www.samhsa.gov.

Teen smoking dropped dramatically in 2002. (2003). *NIDA Notes, 17*(6).

Tips for teens: The truth about inhalants. (2001). Center for Substance Abuse Prevention, Substance Abuse and Mental Health Services Administration. Available at http://www.health.org.

Tipton, D. (2003). Assessment of the neurotoxicity of "ecstasy." Biochemistry/pharmacology. Available at http://www.tcd.ie/Research/projects/drugs/analsci.html.

Use of marijuana, cocaine, pain relievers and tranquilizers increases according to national household survey on drug abuse. (2002). *NHSDA, 9*(5).

Varcarolis, E. (2002). *Foundations of psychiatric mental health nursing: A clinical approach.* (4th ed.). Philadelphia: W.B. Saunders.

*Viera, A. (1999). Toxic ingestion of gamma-hydroxybutyric acid. *Southern Medical Journal, 92*(4), 404-405.

Williams, J. (2002). Prenatal exposure to ecstasy may impair memory and cognition. *NIDA Notes,* 17(3), 8-9.

Youth marijuana admissions by race and ethnicity. (2002). *The DASIS report*, *9*(2), 1-4. Available at http://www.samhsa.gov/.

Zerwekh, J., & Claborn, J. (2003). *Nursing today: Transitions and trends.* (4th ed.). St. Louis: W.B. Saunders.

Zickler, P. (2002). Brain imaging studies show long-term damage from amphetamine use. *NIDA Notes, 15*(3).

Zickler, P. (2002). Cannabinoid antagonist reduces marijuana's effects in humans. *NIDA Notes, 17*(3), 1, 10.

Zickler, P.(2002) NIDA initiative targets increasing teen use of anabolic steroids. *NIDA Notes, 15*(3), 1, 6.

Zickler, P. (2002). Study demonstrates that marijuana smokers experience significant withdrawal. *NIDA Notes, 17*(3), 7.

CHAPTER 9

End-of-Life Care

MARY K. KAZANOWSKI

LEARNING OUTCOMES

After studying this chapter, you should be able to:

1. Describe the pathophysiology of death.
2. Explain the purpose for advance directives.
3. Discuss the philosophies of palliative and hospice care.
4. Describe the role of the nurse and the interdisciplinary team in end-of-life care.
5. Interpret the common physical and emotional signs of impending death.
6. Identify common symptoms of distress near death.
7. Prioritize interventions for symptoms experienced by the client near death.
8. Describe common psychosocial issues for clients and their families near death.
9. Develop a plan of care to assist clients and families in coping with the dying process.
10. Explain how variations in culture and religious beliefs can impact the experience of dying and death.
11. Describe care of the client after death.
12. Discuss the ethical and legal obligations of the nurse with regard to end-of-life care.

Go to your Student CD-ROM for Review Questions for the NCLEX Examination keyed to these Learning Outcomes.

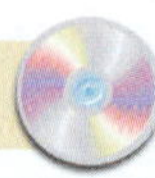

OVERVIEW OF DEATH AND DYING

Death occurs when the lungs and heart cease to function. In general, death is caused by an illness or trauma that overwhelms the compensatory mechanisms of the body. Direct causes of death include respiratory failure and shock, which results in lack of blood flow to meet the demands of vital organs such as the kidneys, brain, and heart.

Multiple Organ Dysfunction Syndrome

Inadequate blood flow to body tissues deprives cells of their source of oxygen, which leads to anaerobic metabolism with acidosis, hyperkalemia, and tissue ischemia. Dramatic changes in vital organs lead to release of toxic metabolites and destructive enzymes. This sequence referred to as **multiple organ dysfunction syndrome (MODS).**

MODS occurs first in the liver, heart, brain, and kidney. MODS also occurs in the lungs in clients with septicemia. A lethal dysrhythmia such as ventricular fibrillation, asystole, or pulseless electrical activity can occur at any point during the process of shock and/or hypoxemia, which ultimately leads to the cessation of cardiac output. Shortly after cardiac arrest, respiratory arrest occurs. When respiratory arrest occurs first, cardiac arrest follows within minutes.

Clinical death refers to the short interval after the cessation of heartbeat and breathing when no evidence of brain function is present. If this termination of function occurs suddenly, as in cardiac arrest or massive hemorrhage, a brief time remains before vital organs lose their viability. Initiation of cardiopulmonary resuscitation (CPR) at this time may be successful in a person with healthy organs. However, CPR is likely to be futile in those with terminal disease.

Incidence of Death

Dying is part of the normal life cycle and more than 2.5 million people die in the United States each year. The most common causes of death in the United States are coronary artery disease and cancer.

Almost 80% of people who die are age 65 years or older (Sheehan & Schirm, 2003). Most of these deaths occur after long, progressively debilitating chronic illnesses, such as cancer, cardiac disease, renal disease, and lung disease. Only 25% of all deaths take place at home, with about 50% occurring in hospitals. The remaining 25% occur in nursing homes, but that number is expected to double by 2020 (Sheehan & Schirm, 2003).

Death as a Natural Process

The U.S. health system is based on the acute care model, which is focused on prevention, early detection, and cure of disease. This focus along with advances in health care makes it difficult for many clients and health care providers to accept death as an outcome of disease. Many view death as a failure of treatment.

These views have led to a major deficiency in the care and quality of life for many Americans at the end of life. In 1995, a landmark study highlighted the poor quality of dying that hospitalized clients experienced at the end of their lives. This SUPPORT study showed that more than 50% of a sample of 9105 individuals with a life-threatening disease had moderate to severe pain during the last days of their lives. In addition, they did not have their wishes met, even when they were made known.

As a result of the SUPPORT study, a major initiative was undertaken to improve care at the end of life. The Institute of Medicine was commissioned to study the problem. Core curricula on end-of-life care were developed and implemented to educate medical and nursing students, physicians, and nurses. These courses focus on death as a natural process and provide information on how to ensure quality end-of-life care. In 1998, the American Association of Colleges of Nursing (AACN) published "Peaceful Death," which outlined 15 undergraduate nursing competencies for providing quality end-of-life care (Table 9-1).

The Institute of Medicine's report on Improving Care at the End of Life addresses the deficiencies in our health care system and its care of dying clients. It concluded that each health care facility should be held accountable for identifying its shortcomings and devising strategies to improve the quality and consistency of care at the end of life. One strategy that has been implemented in select hospitals has been the development of a palliative care team or unit, staffed by nurses and physicians with expertise in end-of-life care.

End-of-life care in long-term care settings has not been addressed in most facilities. In general, the assessment tools (e.g., Minimum Data Set) and regulations for nursing homes do not guide care for residents who are dying. Most staff members are not trained in end-of-life care despite the expected increase in terminally ill residents over the next 10 to 15 years (Sheehan & Schirm, 2003).

TABLE 9-1 Peaceful Death AACN Undergraduate Nursing Competencies

1. Recognize dynamic changes in population demographics, health care economics, and service delivery that necessitate improved professional preparation for end-of-life care.
2. Promote the provision of comfort care to the dying as an active, desirable, and important skill, and an integral component of nursing care.
3. Communicate effectively and compassionately with the client, family, and health care team members about end-of-life issues.
4. Recognize one's own attitudes, feelings, values, and expectations about death and the individual, cultural, and spiritual diversity existing in these beliefs and customs.
5. Demonstrate respect for the client's views and wishes during end-of-life care.
6. Collaborate with interdisciplinary team members while implementing the nursing role in end-of-life care.
7. Use scientifically based standardized tools to assess symptoms experienced by clients at the end of life.
8. Use data from symptom assessment to plan and intervene in symptom management using state-of-the-art traditional approaches.
9. Evaluate the impact of traditional, complementary, and technologic therapies on client-centered outcomes.
10. Assess and treat multiple dimensions, including physical, psychological, social, and spiritual needs, to improve quality of care at the end of life.
11. Assist the client, family, colleagues, and one's self to cope with suffering, grief, loss, and bereavement in end-of-life care.
12. Apply legal and ethical principles in the analysis of complex issues in end-of-life care, recognizing the influence of personal values, professional codes, and client preferences.
13. Identify barriers and facilitators to clients' and caregivers' effective use of resources.
14. Demonstrate skill at implementing a plan for improved end-of-life care within a dynamic and complex health care delivery system.
15. Apply knowledge gained from palliative care research to end-of-life education and care.

Palliative Care

Palliative care is a philosophy that provides a compassionate and supportive approach to clients and families who are living with life-threatening illnesses. This holistic approach neither hastens nor postpones death, but provides relief of symptoms experienced by the dying client (Matzo & Sherman, 2001b). Relieving symptoms, while providing emotional and spiritual support improves the quality of care at the end of life.

THE END-OF-LIFE EXPERIENCE

Advance Directives

An **advance directive** is a written document prepared by a competent individual that specifies what, if any, extraordinary actions a person would want when he or she can no longer make decisions about personal health care. Advance directives such as the durable power of attorney (DPOA) for health care and the living will are usually completed long before a medical crisis. A **DPOA for health care** is a legal document in which a person appoints someone else to make his or her health care decisions in the event he or she becomes incapable of making decisions (Figure 9-1). A **living will** is also a legal document that instructs physicians and family members about what life-sustaining treatment one does or does not want at some future time if a person becomes unable to make decisions.

The Patient Self-Determination Act of 1990 requires that all clients admitted to health care agencies be asked if they have drafted advance directives. Clients who have not drafted advance directives should be given information about the process and the implications of having (or not having) these in place, and should be assisted in drafting them. Nurses should document any discussion regarding a person's decision related to end-of-life care.

Advance directives guide physicians in planning care for seriously ill individuals. If the client has advanced or terminal disease and has indicated that he or she does not want cardiopulmonary resuscitation (CPR) performed, then the physician can initiate a "do not resuscitate" (DNR) order. However, most Americans do not have advance directives in place. Many physicians do not discuss a person's wishes for end-of-life care. Nurses are often in the position of initiating discussions with clients about their wishes regarding CPR, especially when their condition declines quickly. Most agencies require that CPR be initiated on clients whose breathing or heartbeat has ceased unless a physician's order of "do not resuscitate" (DNR) is obtained.

DURABLE POWER OF ATTORNEY FOR HEALTH CARE

Power of Attorney made this __________ day of __________, 20____

1. I, the undersigned hereby appoint (insert name and address of agent)

____

as agent to act for me and in my name to make any and all decisions for me concerning my personal care, medical treatment, hospitalization and health care and to require, withhold or withdraw any type of medical treatment or procedure, even though my death may ensue. My agent shall have the same access to my medical records that I have, including the right to disclose the contents to others. My agent shall also have full power to make a disposition of any part or all of my body for medical purposes, authorize an autopsy and direct the disposition of my remains. (Neither the attending physician nor any other health care provider may act as your agent.)

2. The powers granted above shall be subject to the following rules or limitations (if none, leave blank):

____

____

(The subject of life-sustaining treatment is of particular importance. For your convenience in dealing with that subject some general statements concerning the withholding or removal of life-sustaining treatment are set forth below. If you agree with one of these statements, you may initial that statement; but do not initial more than one.)

(I do not want my life to be prolonged nor do I want life-sustaining treatment
(to be provided or continued if my agent believes the burdens of the treatment
(outweigh the expected benefits. I want my agent to consider the relief of
(suffering the expense involved and the quality as well as the possible extension
______(of my life in making decisions concerning life-sustaining treatment.

(I want my life to be prolonged and I want life-sustaining treatment to be
(provided or continued unless I am in a coma which my attending physician
(believes to be irreversible, in accordance with reasonable medical standards at
(the time of reference. If and when I have suffered irreversible coma, I want
______(life-sustaining treatment to be withheld or discontinued.

(I want my life to be prolonged to the greatest extent possible without regard to
______(my condition, the chances I have for recovery or the cost of the procedures.

3. This power of attorney shall become effective on ______________________

____

4. This power of attorney shall terminate on ______________________

____

5. If any agent named by me shall die, become legally disabled, resign, refuse to act or be unavailable, I name the following (each to act alone and successively, in the order named) as successors to such agent:

____

____

6. If a guardian of my person is to be appointed, I nominate the following to serve as such guardian (if same as agent, leave blank):

____

Figure 9-1 ■ An example of a durable power of attorney for health care.

Continued

7. I am fully informed as to all the contents of this form and understand the full import of this grant of power to my agent.

Signed ______________________
Principal

The principal has had an opportunity to read the above form and has signed the form or acknowledged his or her signature or mark on the form in my presence.

______________________ Residing at ______________________
Witness

(You may, but are not required to, request your agent and successor agents to provide specimen signature below. If you include specimen signature in this Power of Attorney, you must complete the certification opposite the signatures of the agents.)

Specimen signatures of agent (and successors)	I certify that the signature of my agent (and successors) are correct.
______________________ (agent)	______________________ (principal)
______________________ (successor agent)	______________________ (principal)
______________________ (successor agent)	______________________ (principal)

Figure 9-1, *cont'd* ■ An example of a durable power of attorney for health care.

It is now believed that CPR causes pain and that it interferes with a person's ability to have a "good death." A good death is one that is free from avoidable distress and suffering for clients, families, and caregivers; one that is in accord with the client's and family's wishes; and one that is reasonably consistent with clinical, cultural, and ethical standards.

Goals for End-of-Life Care

The goals of care for a client near the end of life are as follows:

- Control symptoms
- Identify client needs
- Promote meaningful interactions between the client and significant others
- Facilitate a peaceful death

Interventions that attend to the physical, psychological, social, and spiritual needs of clients require an interdisciplinary approach to care that is accessible and committed to these goals. The interdisciplinary care of hospice is the most successful approach to end-of-life care to date. Although the perception of hospice is that it provides care for the dying, the emphasis of hospice care is on its provision of quality of life for clients.

Hospice Care

The term **hospice**, which shares the same language root as "hospitality," traces back to medieval times, when it referred to a resting place for weary or ill travelers. In the late 1800s, hospice became synonymous with care of the terminally ill with the founding of Our Lady's Hospice in Dublin by Sister May Aikenhead of the Irish Sisters of Charity, a colleague of Florence Nightingale. In the 1960s, Dame Cicely Saunders, M.D., developed the cornerstone of modern hospice care and opened St. Christopher's Hospice in suburban London. In 1963, Cicely Saunders spoke about hospice at Yale University and, in 1974, Connecticut Hospice began to oversee the care of homebound clients. In 1979, Connecticut Hospice opened the first inpatient hospice in the United States. As of 2002, there were about 3100 hospice programs in the United States.

The concept of hospice came about as a grassroots effort in response to the unmet needs of terminally ill people. As both a philosophy and a system of care, **hospice care** seeks to use an interdisciplinary approach to facilitate both quality of life and a "good" death for clients who are nearing the end of their lives. The hospice system of care is provided in a variety of settings. Hospice programs are often affiliated with home care agencies, providing services to clients at home or in an extended care facility. Some communities also have hospice houses, which admit clients in the terminal phase of their lives and provide a comfortable place where they can die.

In 1983, the Medicare Hospice Benefit passed by Congress defined hospice care in the United States. This benefit pays for hospice services for Medicare recipients who have a prognosis of 6 months or less to live and agree to forgo cu-

TABLE 9-2 General Medical Guidelines for Hospice Appropriateness of Noncancer Clients

- Life expectancy less than 6 months
- No definite terminal diagnosis
- Increasing need for medical care
- Dependence in most ADLs
- Weight loss more than 10% over past 6 months
- Failure to maintain adequate nourishment
- Albumin less than 2.5 g/dL
- Cholesterol less than 156 mg/dL
- Resting tachycardia more than 100 beats/min
- No dialysis or renal transplant

rative treatment for their terminal illness. Historically, clients with terminal cancer have most frequently been the recipients of hospice care. However, clients with other life-limiting conditions with life expectancy of 6 months or less are also appropriate for hospice even if they do not have a definitive terminal diagnosis. Guidelines are available to assist health care providers and families in identifying who is entitled to hospice care under the Medicare hospice benefit (Table 9-2). Clients who are hospice appropriate but do not qualify for Medicare also utilize benefits through private insurance or managed care. In some states, Medical Assistance pays for hospice care.

Not all hospices restrict their services to the terminally ill. Some agencies have bridge programs for clients who have a life-limiting disease, but who are not ready to forgo treatment (and hospitalization) for their disease and/or do not have a prognosis of 6 months or less to live. The advantage of bridge programs is that clients, whose condition may decline, have ready access to expert palliative care. Although treatment of symptoms is the focus of palliative care, no specific therapy is excluded from consideration for clients with a palliative plan of care (Hospice and Palliative Nurses Association, 2002).

SYMPTOMS OF DISTRESS AT END OF LIFE

OVERVIEW

As death nears, clients often have physical symptoms of distress that require treatment to control them until death. Pain, dyspnea, agitation, nausea, and vomiting are common problems at the end of life. Other symptoms include, but are not limited to, fatigue, weakness, constipation, anorexia, and delirium. In general, many symptoms require the use of medications. Once these symptoms occur, medications are usually administered around-the-clock until death to prevent recurrence and attain control. With the appropriate knowledge and resources, the management of symptoms near death can usually be achieved with medication. Most studies show that symptoms of distress (e.g., pain near death) can be effectively controlled in more than 90% of cases when clients have access to palliative care providers.

COLLABORATIVE MANAGEMENT

Assessment

Obtain information about the client's diagnosis, past medical history, and recent state of health to identify the risks for symptoms of distress at end of life. For example, clients with lung cancer, cardiac failure, or chronic respiratory disease are at high risk for respiratory distress and dyspnea near death. Clients with a primary brain tumor or metastasis to the brain are at risk for seizure activity. Those with tumors near major arteries, such as with head and neck cancer, are at risk for hemorrhage. Individuals who have been experiencing pain often continue to have pain, and it may increase, decrease, or remain at the same level of intensity.

PHYSICAL ASSESSMENT/CLINICAL MANIFESTATIONS

Near the end of life, the client often grows weak and lethargic and sleeps for longer periods of time. This lethargy and sleep may progress to the point that the client has a decreased level of consciousness and rouses only to touch. In many cases, the ability of the client to communicate verbally diminishes and level of consciousness decreases, making it difficult to assess the client's perception of symptoms. When caring for clients who are unable to communicate their distress or needs, it is essential that health care providers identify alternative ways to assess symptoms of distress. Professional caregivers should teach family caregivers to watch closely for objective signs of discomfort (e.g., restlessness, grimacing, or moaning). They should also identify when these symptoms occur in relation to positioning, movement, medication, or other external stimuli (Chart 9-1). For example, grimacing when turning from side to side in the bed is indicative of pain or discomfort with movement. When the head of the bed is flat, an increase in respiratory rate and effort indicates shortness of breath and is referred to as orthopnea.

Although the client's point of view is the most valid indicator of comfort or distress, the family's perception of symptoms is also important. The family's perceptions of symptoms should be obtained as part of each client's symptom assessment. Family caregivers, health care providers, and clients may differ in their perceptions of symptoms in terms of intensity, significance, and meaning. Whereas health care providers are often more adept at identifying symptoms of distress, families are often more knowledgeable about client habits and preferences. Health care providers need to incorporate all client-related information into the plan for symptom management and work with clients and families toward a common outcome.

When first recognized, a symptom of distress is assessed in terms of intensity, frequency, duration, quality, exacerbating and relieving factors, and effect on the client's sleep and ability to participate in activities of daily living. A method for rating the intensity of that symptom should be used to facilitate ongoing assessments and evaluate treatment response. A rating scale of 0 to 10 is commonly used, with 0 indicating no distress and 10 indicating the worst possible distress. The intensity of the symptom before and after an intervention (e.g., medication) is documented and is referred to daily to evaluate the client's overall comfort. (See Chapter 7 for a complete discussion of pain assessment.)

Constipation and other problems are typical as a result of immobility and drug effects. These problems are discussed elsewhere in Chapter 10.

As death nears, peripheral circulation decreases and the client's skin often becomes cold, mottled, and cyanotic. Blood pressure decreases, becomes inaudible, and often is

CHART 9-1

CLIENT EDUCATION GUIDE

Common Physical Signs and Symptoms of Approaching Death

Coolness of Extremities

Circulation to the extremities is decreased; the skin may become mottled or discolored.

- Cover the person with a blanket.
- Do not use an electric blanket, hot water bottle, electric heating pad, or hair dryer to warm the person.

Increased Sleeping

Metabolism is decreased.

- Spend time sitting quietly with the person.
- Do not force the person to stay awake.
- Talk to the person as you normally would, even if he or she does not respond.

Fluid and Food Decrease

Metabolic needs have decreased.

- Do not force the person to eat or drink.
- Offer ice chips or small sips of liquids at frequent intervals if the person is alert.
- Use glycerin swabs to keep the mouth moist and comfortable.
- Coat the lips with lip balm or petroleum jelly.

Incontinence

The perineal muscles relax.

- Keep the area clean and dry.
- If the person would be more comfortable, use urine catheters.

Congestion and Gurgling

The person is unable to cough up secretions effectively.

- Suctioning can be used to remove secretions, but this may cause discomfort.
- Medications can decrease the production of secretions.

Breathing Pattern Change

Slowed circulation to the brain may cause the breathing pattern to become irregular, with brief periods of no breathing or shallow breathing.

- Elevate the person's head.
- Position the person on his or her side.

Disorientation

Decreased metabolism and slowed circulation to the brain may occur.

- Identify yourself whenever you communicate with the person.
- Speak softly, clearly, and truthfully.

Restlessness

Decreased metabolism and slowed circulation to the brain may occur.

- Play soothing music.
- Do not restrain the person.
- Massage the person's forehead.
- Reduce the number of people in the room.

Modified from the Hospice of North Central Florida, Inc.

only palpable near death. The dying person's pulse may increase in rate, become irregular in rhythm, gradually decrease, and stop. Meanwhile, respirations become shallow until they, too, stop. Death has taken place when respirations and heartbeat cease.

PSYCHOSOCIAL ASSESSMENT

Individuals facing death may have coping difficulties, fear, and anxiety with regard to their decline and/or impending death. Cultural considerations, values, and religious beliefs of the client and family should be assessed for their influence on the dying experience, control of symptoms, and family bereavement. (See Chapter 7 for cultural considerations in pain management.) Families of individuals near death are also likely to manifest fear, anxiety, and knowledge deficits regarding the process of death and their role in caring for the client.

Assess the client and individual family members for their expectations regarding death and for fear and anxiety. Families may have a preconceived notion about the dying process that may or may not be realistic. Chart 9-2 describes the common emotional signs of approaching death that the nurse should explain to the client, family, or significant others.

CHART 9-2

CLIENT EDUCATION GUIDE

Common Emotional Signs of Approaching Death

Withdrawal

The person is preparing to "let go" from surroundings and relationships.

Vision-like Experiences

The person may talk to people you cannot see or hear and see objects and places not visible to you. These are not hallucinations or drug reactions.

- Do not deny or argue with what the person claims.
- Affirm the experience.

Letting Go

The person may become agitated or continue to perform repetitive tasks. Often this indicates that something is unresolved or is preventing the person from letting go. As difficult as it may be to do or say, the dying person takes on a more peaceful demeanor when loved ones are able to say things such as "It's okay to go. We'll be all right."

Saying Goodbye

When the person is ready to die and you are ready to let go, saying "goodbye" is important for both of you. Touching, hugging, crying, and saying "I love you," "Thank you," "I'm sorry," or "I'll miss you so much" are all natural expressions of sadness and loss. Verbalizing these sentiments can bring comfort both to the dying person and to those left behind.

Modified from the Hospice of North Central Florida, Inc.

Interventions

Common symptoms of distress as death nears are fatigue, pain, dyspnea, nausea and vomiting, restlessness, and agitation. Interventions aim to promote comfort and control the symptoms.

FATIGUE MANAGEMENT. Clients near death frequently have profound fatigue, weakness, and a decreased level of consciousness. Therefore anorexia is common and clients often lose their ability to swallow. If the client is not awake, professional and family caregivers should avoid giving food or liquid orally because of the risk of aspiration. Nurses need to reassure the family that anorexia is often normal and that giving fluid or food can actually lead to discomfort. In general, families have great difficulty accepting that their loved ones are not being fed and may request that intravenous (IV) fluids be initiated. With great sensitivity, reinforce that the cessation of food and liquids is a natural process and that hydration can actually increase discomfort in a person with multisystem slowdown. Discomfort from fluid replacement could lead to respiratory secretions (and distress), increased gastrointestinal secretions, nausea, vomiting, edema, and ascites. Applying emollient to the lips and moistening the mouth and lips with applicators and saturated gauze can help prevent and/or relieve the dry mouth that may occur with a decreased oral intake.

Impaired swallowing near death also presents a problem for medication management because clients lose their ability to swallow their oral medications. Although some pills may be crushed, medications such as sustained-release capsules cannot be taken apart. Scheduled medications can often be discontinued, but medications for pain, dyspnea, agitation, nausea, vomiting, and seizures need to be continued to maintain symptom control until death. In collaboration with a physician and pharmacist experienced in palliative care, identify alternative routes and or alternative medications to maintain control of symptoms. The guiding principle for choice of route in clients near death is to choose the least invasive route with the most effective treatment.

PAIN MANAGEMENT. Pain is the symptom that dying clients fear the most. Although it is not universal, it is common and has many possible causes. Diseases such as cancer often cause tumor pain as a result of the infiltration of malignant cells into organs, nerves, and bones. Other causes of pain in dying clients include "disturbance" pain resulting from headaches, osteoarthritis, muscle spasms, and stiff joints caused by immobility.

Clients who have had their pain controlled with long-acting opioids must continue their scheduled doses of opioids to prevent any recurrence of pain. Depending on the brand of long-acting opioid, oral capsules may be given rectally (same dose and same capsule) when clients are no longer able to swallow. Increases in pain require immediate-relief analgesics (e.g., morphine sulfate immediate-release) and possibly an increase in long-acting opioids. Liquid morphine sulfate can be given sublingually, rectally, or via the buccal mucosa, and it is quick acting, effective, and safe to administer, even to comatose clients. Chapter 7 describes in detail the management of chronic malignant and nonmalignant pain, including complementary and alternative therapies.

DYSPNEA MANAGEMENT. Dyspnea is a subjective experience in which the client experiences an uncomfortable awareness of breathing, breathlessness, or severe shortness of breath. This condition can manifest itself as copious secretions, cough, chest pain, fatigue, or air hunger. It is a common symptom of distress near the end of life, occurring in 50% to 70% of dying clients. Many clients, families, and health care providers consider this to be the worst symptom of distress near death.

Dyspnea can be:

- Directly related to the client's primary diagnosis (e.g., lung cancer, breast cancer, or coronary artery disease)
- Secondary to the primary diagnosis (e.g., pleural effusion, metastasis to the lung or pleura)
- Related to treatment of the primary disease (e.g., heart failure caused by chemotherapy, constrictive pericarditis due to radiation therapy, anemia related to chemotherapy)
- Related to an etiology unrelated to the primary disease (e.g., pneumonia)

Depending on the cause, the pathophysiology of dyspnea can involve the following:

- Obstructive, restrictive, or vascular disturbances in the airways with tumor or nodal involvement
- Pulmonary congestion secondary to fluid overload and/or cardiac dysfunction
- Bronchoconstriction and bronchospasm as seen with respiratory infection, chronic obstructive pulmonary disease (COPD), or airway blockage by a tumor
- A decreased hemoglobin-carrying capacity, as with anemia
- Hyperventilation secondary to neuromuscular disease, with limited movement of the diaphragm

The goal for the client with dyspnea near the end of life is to treat the primary cause and relieve the psychological distress and autonomic response that accompany this symptom. Because diagnostic testing to identify the cause of dyspnea at the end of life is usually inappropriate, the cause is determined by physical assessment and knowledge of the underlying condition. If the cause of dyspnea cannot be treated successfully, interventions are aimed at alleviating the distress.

Opioids. Morphine sulfate is the standard treatment for dyspnea near death. Nurses need to understand that individuals who have not been taking daily opioids should initially receive low doses of morphine (e.g., 5 to 10 mg PO), which can be repeated if necessary. Individuals who have been taking opioids for pain will need to have their breakthrough dose of morphine increased by 50% of their usual dose for effective treatment of dyspnea. If IV access is available, health care providers may prescribe 1 to 2 mg of morphine to be given every 5 to 10 minutes until relief is obtained. However, health care providers should not initiate IV access in dying clients unless it is absolutely necessary.

Morphine via a facial nebulizer is another option for dyspnea near the end of life. Although some research suggests that the nebulized route is no more effective than the oral route, anecdotal reports indicate that nebulized morphine is effective, easy to administer, and has few side effects. The suggested dose for nebulized morphine is 4 mg morphine with 3 mL normal saline (Wrede-Seaman, 2002). If not effective, the concentration should be doubled to 8 mg in 3 mL saline. It should be repeated every 4 hours around-the-clock (ATC) and every 1 hour PRN.

Diuretics and Other Drugs. Individuals with signs of fluid volume excess as manifested by dyspnea, crackles on auscultation, peripheral edema, and other signs of heart failure should be given a diuretic such as furosemide (Lasix) to decrease blood volume, reduce vascular congestion, and reduce the workload of the heart. Furosemide can be administered by mouth, intravenously, subcutaneously, or intramuscularly. IV administration, which is effective in the pulmonary system within minutes, may be preferred for treating congestive heart failure and pulmonary edema.

Bronchodilators such as albuterol or ipratropium bromide via a metered dose inhaler (MDI) or nebulizer may be given for symptoms of bronchospasm (wheezes on auscultation of breath sounds). *Corticosteroids* may also be given for bronchospasm and inflammatory problems within and exterior to the lung. Superior vena cava syndrome and lymphangitis carcinomatosis can cause dyspnea and may respond to corticosteroids.

Antibiotics may be indicated in clients with dyspnea secondary to a respiratory infection. A thorough workup for a respiratory infection is not appropriate in clients in whom death is imminent. However, it is safe to assume an upper respiratory infection is present if dyspnea, an elevated temperature, adventitious breath sounds, and a congested cough have developed. A trial of an appropriate antibiotic should be considered if the client is suffering from the infection.

Secretions in the respiratory tract and oral cavity may contribute to a client's dyspnea near death. Loud, wet respirations (referred to as **death rattle**) are disturbing to family and caregivers even when they do not seem to cause dyspnea or respiratory distress. *Anticholinergics* such as oral or sublingual hyoscyamine (Levsin) or transdermal scopolamine are used to reduce the production of secretions.

Sedatives such as benzodiazepines are commonly used when morphine does not fully control the client's dyspnea. Lorazepam (Ativan) 0.5 mg is commonly administered orally or sublingually every 4 hours PRN or around-the-clock to prevent or control dyspnea and anxiety.

Oxygen. Oxygen for dyspnea near death has not been established as a standard of care for all individuals. However, clients who do not respond promptly to morphine or other medications should be given a trial dose of oxygen (2 to 6 L by nasal cannula) to assess its effect. If it provides relief, it should be continued.

Other Nonpharmacologic Interventions. Pharmacologic interventions should be initiated early in the course of dyspnea near death. Nonpharmacologic interventions can be used in conjunction with, but not in place of, medications. Nonpharmacologic interventions include the following:

- Altering the environment to facilitate the circulation of cool air (e.g., via air-conditioner and fan)
- Applying wet cloths on the client's face
- Positioning the client to facilitate chest expansion
- Encouraging imagery and deep breathing
- Intervening to conserve client energy
- Facilitating the client's rest

Positioning the body with the head of the bed elevated and the upper body supported to facilitate diaphragmatic excursion can be accomplished with a hospital bed or pillows or with the client out of bed and in a chair. Insertion of a Foley catheter to avoid the need for exertion with voiding may be considered if the client will benefit.

NAUSEA AND VOMITING MANAGEMENT. Although not as common a problem as pain or dyspnea, nausea and vomiting are thought to occur in about 40% of terminally ill individuals during the last week of life. It is particularly prevalent in individuals with acquired immunodeficiency syndrome (AIDS) or breast, stomach, or gynecologic cancers.

Common causes of nausea and vomiting at the end of life include the following:

- Initiation of upload therapy (nausea usually lasts a few days)
- Uremia
- Hypercalcemia
- Increased intracranial pressure secondary to brain metastasis
- Vagal stimulation secondary to oral candida
- Stretching of the hepatic capsule
- Constipation or impaction
- Bowel obstruction

If constipation is identified as a problem, a biphosphate enema is administered to release stool quickly. If stool in the rectum cannot be evacuated, a mineral oil enema followed by disimpaction may be required to relieve the client's distress.

Nausea and vomiting related to other causes can generally be controlled by one or more antiemetic agents. Combinations of antiemetics as rectal suppositories, gels, or oral troches can be tried and individualized for maximal relief and control (Chart 9-3).

RESTLESSNESS AND AGITATION MANAGEMENT. Agitation at the end of life requires that you assess for pain or urinary retention, constipation, or other reversible cause. If constipation is ruled out as the cause and if analgesia and catheterization do not relieve the restlessness, sedatives should be administered to provide some relief. Consultation with a spiritual and/or bereavement counselor should be considered to assess for unfinished business or spiritual distress as a possible cause of the agitation.

CONSIDERATIONS FOR OLDER ADULTS

In some cases, agitation and anxiety are part of delirium (acute confusional state), particularly in older adults. Chapter 5 discusses delirium in detail.

Benzodiazepines such as lorazepam (Ativan) or alprazolam (Xanax) are often given for anxiety, restlessness, or myoclonus near death. Lorazepam 1 to 2 mg is often crushed and given sublingually with a few drops of water; this is continued at 0.5 to 2 mg every 6 to 8 hours around-the-clock. If paradoxical agitation occurs, another benzodiazepine is substituted for lorazepam. Until recently, long-acting benzodiazepines such as diazepam (Valium) were not recommended for agitation near death. However, long-acting medications such as diazepam (Valium) and

CHART 9-3

BEST PRACTICE for Symptom Relief

- For unrelieved pain: Morphine solution, 0.25 to 0.5 mL (20 mg/1 mL solution) PO/SL q2-3h PRN
- For unrelieved dyspnea: Morphine solution, 0.25 to 0.5 mL (20 mg/1 mL solution) PO/SL q2h PRN
- For nausea or vomiting: Prochlorperazine, 25-mg suppository PR or 25 mg/0.5 mL transdermal gel to inner wrist q8h PRN
- For unrelieved nausea or vomiting, or for agitation/restlessness: ABH* suppository, 1 PR or 25 mg/0.5 mL transdermal gel to inner wrist q8h PRN
- For severe agitation and restlessness:
  - Determine if client is in pain; treat accordingly
  - Determine if client is constipated or experiencing urinary retention; take appropriate action (Foley catheter)
  - If agitation persists and the safety of the client or caregiver is at risk, administer pentobarbital suppository, 1 PR or 60 mg/0.5 mL gel transdermally q4-6h PRN
- For loud, wet respirations or excessive secretions:
  - Hyoscyamine (Levsin) SL tablets, 1 to 2 PO or SL q4-6h PRN
- For unrelieved respiratory fluid accumulation: Furosemide (Lasix), 40 to 80 mg PO, SC, IM, or IV

Printed with permission from VNA Hospice, Visiting Nurse Services, Manchester, NH.
PR, Per rectum; *SC*, subcutaneous; *SL*, sublingual.
*Many hospice and palliative care organizations use pharmacist-compounded medications which combine the therapeutic effects of several drugs to control symptoms of distress. These medications are compounded as suppositories or gels, which can be administered to clients who cannot swallow. For example, ABH contains Ativan (lorazepam) 1 mg, Benadryl (diphenhydramine) 12.5 mg, and Haldol (haloperidol) 1 mg. Reglan (metoclopramide) is often added to treat nausea and vomiting.

clonazepam (Klonopin) are now considered helpful in controlling anxiety near death.

Barbiturates such as phenobarbital or pentobarbital are given when benzodiazepines fail to control anxiety, delirium, or restlessness near death. The neuroleptic haloperidol (Haldol) may be administered when hallucinations or paranoia occur (see Chart 9-3).

MANAGEMENT OF THE REFRACTORY SYMPTOMS OF DISTRESS. Studies show that most clients with access to palliative care achieve control of symptoms such as pain, dyspnea, and agitation near death. However, a small percentage of clients experience symptoms of distress that are refractory or resistant to treatment. They may require such high doses of analgesia that sedation occurs as a side effect, or they may actually need to be sedated to control symptoms of distress. Although sedation is not ideal, its occurrence as a side effect of treatment for symptoms of distress at the end of life may be acceptable if there is no alternative for comfort. It is important that both health care providers and the public understand that adequate symptom management may at times result in sedation. The sedation that occurs is a side effect of treatment–it is not a treatment goal or an effect meant to hasten death.

The administration of medications for symptoms of distress at the end of life is guided by protocols using doses of medications that are considered safe. These guidelines and protocols are used with the intention of alleviating suffering, not hastening death. The occurrence of an untoward effect of a medication is, however, a risk. According to the Guideline Panel for Management of Cancer Pain (1994), the increased risk of earlier death counts little against the benefit of pain relief and painless death in a client who faces imminent death from progression of a primary disease. The ethical duty of the nurse is to assist in relieving pain or other symptoms of distress in a client near death.

PSYCHOSOCIAL MANAGEMENT. The experience of dying for any person can be extremely difficult for any client and family. But unexpected deaths, particularly in young people, tend to be most traumatic. Dying of a chronic, progressively debilitating illness is also traumatic, but this situation generally presents a different set of issues. Knowledge of the expected outcome of a disease in some ways is helpful, in that it allows health care providers the opportunity to assess client preferences and develop plans of care consistent with these needs. Such a goal requires excellent communication among health care providers, clients, and families.

Whereas death is the termination of life, dying is a process. Individuals facing death may demonstrate emotional signs and symptoms of their response to the dying process through behaviors that equate to saying goodbye or through actual withdrawal. Families need to be educated that such behaviors are normal to the process of dying (see Chart 9-2).

Grief is the emotional feeling related to the perception of the loss. **Mourning** is the outward social expression of the loss. Interventions to assist clients and families in grieving and mourning are based on the cultural beliefs, values, and practices of clients and families. Table 9-3 lists basic beliefs regarding death, dying, and afterlife for some of the major subcultures and religions.

Interventions are aimed at providing appropriate emotional support to allow clients and families to verbalize their fears and concerns. Nurses can also assist by keeping families informed of the client's level of comfort, keeping them involved in health care decisions, and reframing the situation to emphasize the goal of keeping the individual comfortable.

Offering Physical and Emotional Support. Intervene with those grieving an impending death by "being with" as opposed to "being there." "Being with" implies that you are physically and psychologically with the grieving client, empathizing to provide emotional support. Listening and somehow acknowledging the legitimacy of the client and/or family's pain are often more therapeutic than speaking; this concept is sometimes referred to as "presence." Nurses facilitate the expression of grief by giving the person who is mourning permission to express herself or himself. Your manner and words show that these expressions of grief are acceptable and expected. Say something such as, "This must be very difficult for you" or "I'm sorry this is happening."

Being Realistic. The pain of loss cannot be, nor should it be, taken away no matter how committed you may be to the client's comfort. Avoid trite assurances such as, "Things will be fine. Don't cry," or "Don't be upset. She wouldn't want it that way," or "In a year you will have forgotten." Such comments can actually be barriers to demonstrating care and concern. Accept whatever the grieving person says about the situation and remain present, ready to listen attentively and guide gently. In this way, you can help the bereaved prepare for the necessary reminiscence and integration of the loss.

Encouraging Reminiscence. Storytelling through reminiscence and life review can be an important activity for clients who are dying. Life review is a structured process of reflecting on one's life and is often facilitated by an interviewer. Reminiscence is the process of randomly reflecting on memories of events in one's life. The benefits of storytelling through either method include catharsis, the ability to attain perspective, and enhancement of meaning. Suggest that the client and family tape autobiographic stories, record memories in a journal, or develop a scrapbook. If the client does not have enough energy for these activities, familiar objects such as photographs and favorite jewelry pieces can be used to spark ideas for stories that the client may want to tell.

Promoting Spirituality. **Spirituality**, a part of every human being, is the connection to self, others, the environment, and a "higher power" (e.g., God, Allah, spirit). **Religion** can be described as the formal expression of one's spirituality. Studies have shown that religious acts (e.g., prayer, meditation, inspirational reading, recitation of mantras) help clients cope with death and the dying process (Cairns, 1999). Perform a spiritual assessment to identify whether God or religion is important to the client and to facilitate open expression of one's beliefs and needs. Offer and arrange for clergy visits to perform sacred rituals or rites if valued by the client.

Clients who have been alienated from their religious or spiritual community and/or have difficulty in finding meaning in their suffering and approaching death may suffer from spiritual distress. Possible causes include guilt, regrets, lack of meaning, poor relationships, and fear of the unknown. Acknowledge the client's spiritual pain, encourage verbalization, and use a family genogram to elicit relationships, fears, hopes, and unfinished business. Explore issues related to forgiveness for possible resolution.

TABLE 9-3 Basic Beliefs Regarding Death, Dying, and Afterlife for Selected Major Cultures and Religions

African American

One cannot make a definitive statement about the dying and mourning process because of the diversity that exists among different communities.

Funerals tend to be highly involved ceremonies with defined rituals; family, friends, and acquaintances of the deceased make an effort to attend.

Asian—encompasses several countries and religions (e.g., Chinese, Filipino, Japanese, Laotian, Cambodian, Korean, Vietnamese)

There is a traditional strong family and extended family with male dominance.

Herbal medicine plays an important role.

Direct eye contact is considered impolite.

For Southeast Asians, discussing dying brings bad luck, and hospitals and treatments are alien. Some Southeast Asians, especially if uneducated, are likely to avoid visiting terminally ill family members for fear of contracting the disease.

The number or character "4" is avoided because it symbolizes death.

Funeral and burial customs vary greatly depending on culture, religion, and generation involved.

Latino/Hispanic

Many subcultures within this population with diverse cultural variations exist (e.g., Mexico, Central America, the Caribbean, South America).

Catholicism is the predominant religion, but many people depend on folk healers for treatment of ailments.

Death is viewed as a direct result of life; one naturally follows the other.

There is an acceptance of death due to poverty, religion, and culture.

Family and family life are important, especially regarding deaths and funerals.

Expression of grief is open, especially among women.

Native Americans/American Indians

Over 350 distinct tribes in the United States exist with variation in cultural practices.

The focus of identity is on the tribe or council, rather than on ancestry; each tribe has its own belief system.

Most tribes have the belief that spirits are attached to living things.

Indian healers (Shamans) are common.

Family is usually a large extended unit, often including as many as a hundred or more.

Family may not want the client to die at home, but to allow a family member to die alone is also not appropriate.

Material possessions often are dispersed before or after death to friends and family members.

Bereavement follow-up may not be appropriate because some tribes have a taboo against speaking of the dead.

Judaism

This religion encompasses Orthodox, Conservative, and Reformed Jews.

There is a strong belief in the sacredness of life and one, indivisible God.

Funerals have two common themes: honor the dead and comfort the mourners.

The body must not be left unattended until burial which should take place as soon as possible (preferably within 24 hours).

Autopsies and cremation are opposed.

The deceased is often dressed in a white shroud and buried in a plain pine box.

A 7-day mourning period, called Shiva, follows the person's death for the immediate next of kin.

Due to acculturation to American society, there may be variations in funeral and mourning traditions.

Modified from Antelope, T., Eighmy, J., & Nahman, E. (2002). Care of the patient and family. In Hospice and Palliative Nurses Association (Eds.), *Core curriculum for the generalist hospice and palliative care nurse.* (pp. 155-180). Dubuque, IA: Kendall/Hunt.

Fostering Hope. Hope involves picturing a reality that is not yet present and imagining what a situation might be like. This image sets the direction for clients and their families to give them purpose in life and to help them find the strength to go forward, even in the darkest times (Wang, 2000). Foster hope for clients and their families by listening and caring.

Avoiding Explanations of the Loss. Do not try to explain the loss in philosophic or religious terms. Statements such as "Everything happens for the best" or "God sends us only as much as we can bear" are not helpful when the bereaved person has yet to express feelings of anguish or anger. Telling someone too soon that they have other children to rely on or that there are other family members who need them does not diminish the intensity of the grief. In fact, doing so can create feelings of anger and resentment toward the nurse because it reflects an insensitivity to client pain. "Being with" remains important as the weeks or months pass and the funeral crisis supports dissipate. The out-of-town relatives return home, and friends and local relatives resume their own lives. Consider contacting family members after the death to allow them the opportunity to voice their perceptions of the experience. In particular, family caregivers who assumed the role of symptom manager in the home often welcome the opportunity to discuss their experience.

Communicating with the Client. Clients near death are often obtunded and/or withdrawn from the external environment. However, their sense of hearing remains intact until death. Conversation in the room and near the client should be conducted as if the client were alert. Caregivers are encouraged to talk softly to the client and to touch and gently stroke the skin. Although the dying person may not respond, these actions foster a sense of communication between the client and the caregiver.

Providing Referrals to Bereavement Specialists. Bereavement includes grief and mourning–the inner feelings and outward reactions of the survivor. Inform the client and family about bereavement counselors who can assist them to cope both before and after the death. Bereavement counselors are extremely knowledgeable about the grieving process and can be accessed through hospice agencies. Any nurse caring for clients who are dying or have died, should know how to access this resource.

Participation in bereavement support groups by individuals who are grieving a person's pending or past death has been shown to facilitate the grieving process. Being a part of a support group (e.g., Alzheimer caregiver support group) can help people to discover that others have suffered through an experience just as devastating as their own. This discovery makes them more likely to share their feelings with others and work toward some resolution of the experience.

Teaching About the Physical Signs of Death. Although emotionally challenging, witnessing the death of a loved one may actually facilitate the family's acceptance of death. Witnessing how ill a person is makes the event real and enhances an understanding of how disease affects bodily function and decline. If death is anticipated, use nontechnical language to give the client and family or significant others information about the signs of death. The physical signs are described in detail–realistic enough to be unmistakable yet not so graphic as to alarm the listeners. Chart 9-1 describes the common signs and symptoms of approaching death. Such charts are often shared with family and friends who are anticipating the death of a loved one.

Ensuring Palliative Care. Family and friends who are anticipating the death of a loved one often fear that the death will be characterized by pain and suffering. Reassure families that clients will be monitored closely for any sign or symptom of distress. Appropriate medications and other measures will be administered as needed until pain or other symptom of distress is controlled. Families are reassured that significant advances have been made in pain and symptom control.

Most people who choose hospice care prefer the home to other environments during the final episodes of illness. Although there are exceptions, being surrounded by familiar people and things, having ready access to friends and relatives, and having the freedom from institutional restriction make the home setting more comfortable and give the client and family more control. If clients are not able to stay at home until death, they should be offered information about the nearest hospice house. Hospice houses are generally staffed by nurses who provide direct care, and families are allowed to remain with clients. Clients whose cases are being followed by either type of hospice have access to nurses, home health aides, social workers, spiritual and/or bereavement counselors, the medical hospice director, and volunteers, each of whom are members of the interdisciplinary team. Interdisciplinary hospice team meetings are scheduled regularly to review client needs and to review the plan of care initiated by the nurse and client.

To ensure that client and family needs are promptly addressed as they arise, hospices provide 24-hour on-call services. It is not always possible to predict the final phase of the terminal process or the development of symptoms of distress. To address this problem, some hospices have arranged for pharmacies to supply clients with "symptom relief kits by prescription." These kits provide a limited amount of commonly used medications that are effective in treating symptoms near death.

CHART 9-4

HOME CARE ASSESSMENT of
The Client with Physical Manifestations of Death

- No breathing
- No heartbeat
- Release of bowel and bladder contents
- No response to name, environmental sounds, touch, or pain
- Eyelids slightly open
- Pupils enlarged and not constricting in response to light
- Eyes fixed on a certain spot
- No blinking in response to air moving over the eyes or to a light touch on the eye
- Jaw relaxed and mouth slightly open

CHART 9-5

BEST PRACTICE for
Postmortem Care

- Ensure that the nurse or physician has completed and signed the death certificate.
- Ask the family or significant others if they wish to wash or help wash the client.
- Remove or cut all tubes and lines according to health care agency policy.
- Close the client's eyes.
- Replace dentures or other dental appliances, if worn.
- Straighten the client and lower the bed to a flat position.
- Place a pillow under the client's head.
- Wash the client as needed; comb and arrange the client's hair.
- Place pads under the client's hips and around the perineum to absorb feces and urine.
- Clean up the client's room or unit.
- Allow the family or significant others to see the client in private and to perform any religious or cultural customs they wish.
- Notify the hospital chaplain or appropriate community religious leader if requested by the family or significant others.
- Prepare the client for transfer to either a morgue or funeral home; wrap the client in a shroud and attach identification tags per agency policy (if the client is to be transferred to the morgue).

POSTMORTEM CARE

Cessation of breathing is usually noticed by nurses and family at the time of death. Chart 9-4 lists other physical manifestations of death.

Depending on the state or county, the nurse or physician pronounces the client as dead in a health care agency. The nurse or the physician then completes a death certificate, which must accompany the body to the funeral home. Before preparing the body for transfer, ask the physician whether an autopsy will be ordered. When the death is expected, an autopsy will likely be deferred. But when the physician or family members do not know the cause of death, an autopsy may be performed. The nurse or unlicensed assistive personnel prepare the body for immediate postmortem viewing by the family as described in Chart 9-5.

After the family or significant others view the body, follow agency procedure for preparing the client for transfer to either the morgue or a funeral home. In the hospital, a postmortem kit is generally used with a shroud and identification tags.

TABLE 9-4 Definitions of Ethical Concepts Related to Issues at End of Life

Passive euthanasia An act of omission (e.g., withholding or withdrawing treatment) that might prolong the life of a person who cannot be cured by the treatment. In this situation, the withdrawal of the intervention does not directly cause the client's death.

Principle of double effect Involves taking an action (e.g., administering an opioid) intended to have a good effect, which also has a known harmful effect. This is not active euthanasia.

Voluntary active euthanasia An act by which the causative agent in the death of a client is administered directly by another.

Involuntary active euthanasia The action to end the client's life is taken without the client's consent.

Physician-assisted suicide Refers to a practice whereby a physician provides a means (e.g., medication) to a client with the knowledge that the client will use the means to commit suicide.

CULTURAL CONSIDERATIONS

Basic beliefs about death, dying, and afterlife vary among groups. Table 9-3 lists some of these common beliefs and practices in selected cultures and religions.

EUTHANASIA

Nurses spend more time with clients and their families than do any other health care professionals. Therefore they are usually in the best and most immediate position to assist clients with dealing with end-of-life care. This includes assisting in the decision-making process related to end-of-life care, whether it be an immediate need or an issue for the future. To do this, nurses must be knowledgeable about terminology and ethical issues related to death and dying (Table 9-4).

There is a great deal of confusion regarding the concepts of euthanasia. It is essential that everyone understand and articulate the distinction between active and passive euthanasia and assisted suicide versus the appropriate treatment of pain and symptoms of distress. **Passive euthanasia** involves the withdrawal or withholding of a treatment that might prolong the life of a person who cannot be cured by the treatment. In this situation the withdrawal of the intervention does not directly cause the client's death. It is the progression of the client's disease or the poor health status of the client that is the cause of death. Professional organizations such as the American Nurses Association, the American Medical Association, and religious communities such as the Catholic Church support the right of clients and their surrogate decision makers to refuse or stop treatment (e.g., mechanical ventilation, tube feedings, antibiotics, and intravenous fluids), which are medically futile and may actually cause discomfort.

Active euthanasia involves a health care provider taking action that purposefully and directly causes the client's death. Active euthanasia is not supported by most professional organizations, including the American Nurses Association. In the state of Oregon, physician-assisted suicide is legal in certain situations.

Nurses should not be involved in active euthanasia or physician-assisted euthanasia. They do, however, play a major role in clients' end-of- life care by advocating for clients' wishes, and ensuring quality symptom management and support at the end of life.

GET READY for the NCLEX Examination!

KEY POINTS

- Death occurs when the lungs and heart no longer function, causing inadequate blood flow to major organs, acidosis, and tissue ischemia (multiple organ dysfunction syndrome [MODS]).
- Clinical death occurs when there is no brain function present.
- Palliative care is a holistic philosophy that provides compassionate and supportive care to clients and families who are living with life-threatening illnesses.
- An advance directive is a written document prepared by a competent person that specifies what, if any, extraordinary actions that person would want if she or he could no longer make decisions about care; examples are living wills and durable powers of attorney for health care.
- Hospice care is an interdisciplinary approach to help clients have a good quality of life and a "good" death, minimizing symptoms of distress.
- Pain, dyspnea, agitation, nausea, and vomiting are common problems at the end of life.
- Chart 9-2 describes the emotional signs of impending death that the nurse should explain to the client and family.
- Common physical signs of approaching death are listed in Chart 9-1.
- Medications are frequently used for unrelieved dyspnea, pain, agitation, and nausea and vomiting (see Chart 9-3).
- Nursing interventions to manage the psychosocial aspects of death and dying include offering physical and emotional support, being realistic, encouraging reminiscence, promoting spirituality, fostering hope, avoiding explanation of loss, and communicating with the client. Bereavement service referral is also important.
- Postmortem care is described in Chart 9-5.
- Passive euthanasia involves withholding treatment that might prolong a client's life; active euthanasia involves giving a client a treatment or agent that causes death.

ADDITIONAL STUDY RESOURCES

Go to your Student CD-ROM for Review Questions for the NCLEX Examination.

evolve Go to http://evolve.elsevier.com/Iggy/ for Integrated Management of Care Questions for the NCLEX Examination.

SELECTED BIBLIOGRAPHY

Asterisk indicates a classic or definitive work on this subject.

Amella, E. (2003). Geriatrics and palliative care: Collaboration for quality of life until death. *Journal of Hospice and Palliative Nursing, 5*(1), 40-48.

*American Association of Colleges of Nursing. (1998). *Peaceful death: Recommended competencies and curricular guidelines for end-of-life nursing care.* Washington, DC: Author.

*American Nurses Association. (1994a). *Position statement on active euthanasia.* Washington, DC: Author.

*American Nurses Association. (1994b). *Position statement on assisted suicide.* Washington, DC: Author.

*Benzein, E., & Saveman, B. (1998). Nurses' perception of hope in patients with cancer: A palliative care perspective. *Cancer Nursing, 21*(1), 10-16.

*Cairns, A.B. (1999). Spirituality and religiosity in palliative care. *Home Healthcare Nurse, 17*(7), 450-455.

Davis, A.J., & Konishi, E. (2000). End-of-life ethical issues in Japan. *Geriatric Nursing, 21*(2), 89-91.

End-of-Life Nursing Education Consortium (ELNEC). (2000). *ELNEC faculty guide.* Washington, DC: American Association of Colleges of Nursing and City of Hope National Medical Center.

*Escalante, C.P., et al. (1996). Dyspnea in cancer patients: Etiology, resource utilization, and survival implications in a managed care world. *Cancer, 78,* 1314-1319.

*Field, M.J., Cassel, C.K., Committee on Care at the End of Life, Institute of Medicine. (1997). *Approaching Death: Improving Care at the End of Life,* Washington, DC: National Academy Press.

Griffie, J., Nelson-Marten, P., & Muchka, S. (2004). Acknowledging the "elephant": Communication in palliative care. *American Journal of Nursing, 104*(1), 48-58.

*Harwood, K.V. (1999). Dyspnea. In C.H. Yarbro, M.H. Frogge, & M. Goodman (Eds.). *Cancer symptom management* (2nd ed., pp. 45-57). Boston: Jones & Bartlett.

*Hospice and Palliative Nurses Association. (1996). *Clinical practice protocol: Dyspnea.* Pittsburgh: Author.

*Hospice and Palliative Nurses Association. (1997). *Clinical practice protocol: Terminal restlessness.* Pittsburgh, PA: Author.

Hospice and Palliative Nurses Association. (2002). *Core curriculum for the generalist hospice and palliative care nurse.* Dubuque, IA: Kendall/Hunt.

Kessler, T.C., et al. (2003). Assessment of dying. *American Journal of Nursing, 103*(11), 52-57.

*Kubler-Ross, E. (1969). *On death and dying.* New York: Macmillan.

*Management of Cancer Pain Guideline Panel. (1994). *Management of cancer pain. Clinical practice guidelines.* AHCPR Publication No. 94-0592. Rockville, MD: Agency for Health Care Policy and Research, Public Health Service, U.S. Department of Health and Human Services.

*March, P.A. (1998). Terminal restlessness. *The American Journal of Hospice and Palliative Care, 15*(1), 51-53.

Matzo, M.L., & Sherman, D.W. (Eds.). (2001a). *Palliative care nursing: Quality care to the end of life.* New York: Springer.

Matzo, M.L. & Sherman, D.W. (2001b). Palliative care: Ensuring competent care at the end of life. *Geriatric Nursing, 22*(6), 288-293.

*McMillan, S.C. (1996). The quality of life of patients with cancer receiving hospice care. *Oncology Nursing Forum, 23,* 1221-1228.

Norton, S.A., & Talerico, K.A. (2000). Facilitating end-of-life decision-making: Strategies for communicating and assessing. *Journal of Gerontological Nursing, 26*(9), 6-13.

Perrin, K.O. (2001). Ethical issues at the end of life. In *Ethics and conflict.* (pp. 127-151). Thorofare, NJ: Slack.

Pitorak, E.F. (2003). Care at the time of death. *American Journal of Nursing, 103*(7), 42-51.

Robinson, C.B., et al. (2000). Development of a protocol to prevent opioid-induced constipation in patients with cancer: A research utilization project. *Clinical Journal of Oncology Nursing, 4,* 79-84.

Sheehan, D.K., & Schirm, V. (2003). End-of-life care of older adults. *American Journal of Nursing, 103*(11), 48-54.

*Support Study Principal Investigators. (1995). A controlled trial to improve care for seriously ill hospitalized patients. *Journal of the American Medical Association, 274,* 1591-1598.

Travis, S.S., et al. (2001). Terminal restlessness in the nursing facility: Assessment, palliation, and symptom management. *Geriatric Nursing, 22*(6), 308-312.

Virani, R., & Sofer, D. (2003). Improving the quality of end-of-life care. *American Journal of Nursing, 103*(5), 52-55.

Wang, C.H. (2000). Knowing and approaching hope as human experience: Implications for the medical-surgical nurse. *MEDSURG Nursing, 9*(4), 189-192.

Wilkie, D.J. (2001). Toolkit for nursing excellence at end-of-life transition for nurse educators (TNEEL-NE). Seattle, WA: University of Washington.

Wrede-Seaman, L. (2002). *Symptom management algorithms: A handbook for palliative care.* Yakima, WA: Intellicard.

CHAPTER

10 Rehabilitation Concepts for Acute and Chronic Problems

DONNA D. IGNATAVICIUS

LEARNING OUTCOMES

After studying this chapter, you should be able to:

1. Differentiate between impairment, disability, and handicap.
2. Identify the roles of each member of the interdisciplinary rehabilitation team.
3. Interpret physical and psychosocial assessment findings for the client in a rehabilitation program.
4. Describe the major components of a functional assessment.
5. Prioritize nursing diagnoses for the client in a rehabilitation program.
6. Develop a teaching plan for the rehabilitation client who has impaired physical mobility.
7. Explain the role of the interdisciplinary team in managing clients with self-care deficits.
8. Analyze risk factors for skin breakdown in clients who are in rehabilitation settings.
9. Differentiate bladder training techniques for a client with spastic versus flaccid bladder.
10. Assess client outcomes of the interdisciplinary rehabilitation program.
11. Explain the primary concerns for clients being discharged to home after rehabilitation.

Go to your Student CD-ROM for Review Questions for the NCLEX Examination keyed to these Learning Outcomes.

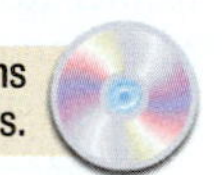

A **chronic illness** or condition is one that has existed for at least 3 months. A **disabling condition** is any physical or mental health/behavioral health problem that can cause disability. This text focuses on physical health problems; mental health/behavioral health problems are discussed in textbooks on mental health/behavioral health nursing.

The rate of chronic and disabling illnesses is expected to increase rapidly as baby boomers approach late adulthood. Medical-surgical nurses care for clients with chronic conditions in a variety of health care settings.

Clients with chronic and disabling conditions often participate in rehabilitation programs to prevent disability, maintain functional ability, and restore as much function as possible. The nurse is a vital member of the rehabilitation team.

OVERVIEW

Chronic and disabling illnesses are a major health problem in the United States, with almost half of the population having one or more chronic conditions. Chronic disease accounts for about 70% of all deaths, and associated medical costs account for over 60% of the nation's health care cost (http://www.ncsl.org/programs/health/phchronic.htm). Some people with chronic and disabling problems are in residential settings, whereas others are managed at home. Disability occurs slightly more often in men than in women and in families with lower incomes (see the Resource Management box on p. 119).

Stroke is the leading cause of disability. Coronary artery disease, cancer, chronic obstructive pulmonary disease (COPD), asthma, and arthritis are other common chronic conditions that may result in varying degrees of disability. Most of these conditions occur in people older than 65 years of age. These health problems are discussed throughout this text.

Chronic and disabling conditions are not always diseases such as heart disease; they may also result from accidents. Accidents are the leading cause of death among young adults and the third leading cause of death in adults 45 to 54 years of age. Increasing numbers of people survive accidents because of advances in medical technology. These survivors are often faced with chronic or disabling conditions, such as traumatic brain injuries (TBIs) and spinal cord injuries (SCIs). Many of them require months to years of follow-up health care after returning to the community. As a result, the need for rehabilitation is on the rise.

RESOURCE MANAGEMENT

CHRONIC AND DISABLING DISEASES IN THE UNITED STATES

Cost of Care

- Direct medical costs for chronic conditions were about $510 billion in 2000.
- Direct costs are expected to increase to almost $2 trillion by 2020 due to the aging baby boomer population.
- The number of Americans with chronic conditions is growing at an explosive rate, with over 125 million having one or more chronic illnesses.
- The most common costly chronic illnesses are diabetes, arthritis, asthma and other chronic lung problems, osteoporosis, mental disorders, Alzheimer's disease, neurologic disorders such as strokes and spinal cord injuries, and hypertension.

Implications for Nursing

Many chronic conditions can be prevented or detected early before they result in life-threatening and costly complications. Health education reduces costs by teaching clients how to care for themselves. Nurses need to be more involved in promoting wellness, even when they are caring for clients who are ill. For example, teach women about ways to minimize risk factors that predispose them to cardiovascular diseases, such as stroke and coronary artery disease. Teach older men about the importance of prostate screening to detect early cancer. Health teaching and promotion interventions are described throughout this textbook.

CONCEPTS RELATED TO REHABILITATION

Rehabilitation is the process of learning to live with chronic and disabling conditions, often those resulting from trauma. The goal of rehabilitation is to return the client to the fullest possible physical, mental, social, vocational, and economic capacity. Rehabilitation is not limited to the return of function in post-traumatic situations. It also includes education and therapy for any chronic illness characterized by a change in a body system function or body structure. Rehabilitation programs related to respiratory, cardiac, and musculoskeletal health problems are common examples that do not involve trauma. Cancer rehabilitation is not as common, but needs to increase as the number of cancer diagnoses and cancer survival rates increase (Beck, 2003).

In any discussion of rehabilitation, it is important to define and distinguish the terms *impairment, disability,* and *handicap*. These terms have been used interchangeably in some settings; for this chapter, the terms are defined according to the classic, but still widely used, *International Classification of Impairments, Disabilities and Handicaps* (World Health Organization, 1980).

Impairment

Impairment is an abnormality of a body structure or structures or an alteration in a body system function resulting from any cause; it represents a disturbance at the organ level. Impairments can be temporary or permanent and may or may not be associated with an active pathologic condition.

Disability

Disability is the consequence of an impairment and is usually described in terms of a client's altered functional ability; it represents a disturbance at the personal level. A variety of diseases or traumas impair mobility and may result in a decreased ability to function.

Handicap

A **handicap** is the disadvantage that a person feels as a result of impairments and disabilities. This disadvantage is based on interactions that the client experiences in society. Although impairments and the disabilities that result from pathologic changes in a body organ are often unpreventable or irreversible, handicaps are both preventable and reversible.

REHABILITATION AS PART OF COMMUNITY-BASED CARE

After the acute condition or injury has been stabilized in a hospital, the client may be discharged to continue the healing process at home, generally under the follow-up care of a nonhospital health care provider (e.g., a family physician). The nurse provides home care preparation, health teaching, psychosocial preparation, and information about various health care resources to help the client resume his or her usual roles in society.

Some health problems require the intermediate step of rehabilitation, which can occur in a number of settings. Rehabilitation starts in the acute care hospital (sometimes called acute rehabilitation) and continues after discharge from the hospital. The nurse's coordination of care from acute care through community-based care is critical to the success of rehabilitation.

Settings for Rehabilitation

For continuing rehabilitation services, the most common settings are freestanding rehabilitation hospitals, rehabilitation units within hospitals, and skilled nursing home units to which the client is typically admitted for 1 to 3 weeks (Figure 10-1). Ambulatory care rehabilitation departments and home rehabilitation programs may be needed for continuing less intensive rehabilitative services.

Some hospitals and nursing homes have converted one or more inpatient units into transitional care units (TCUs). In this way, the client can stay in the same health care system for both acute and continuing rehabilitative care.

After disabled clients become more confident and independent in the inpatient setting, they may choose to live at home or in a group home. Group homes are facilities where clients live independently while together with other disabled adults. Each client or group of clients has a care provider, such as a personal care aide, to assist with the activities of daily living (ADLs) and decisions requiring accurate judgments. The clients may or may not be employed. The goal of these centers is to provide independent living arrangements outside an institution, especially for younger clients with traumatic brain injury (TBI).

The Rehabilitation Team

Successful rehabilitation depends on the coordinated effort of a group of health care professionals, the interdisciplinary rehabilitation team, and the involvement of the client, family, and other support systems in planning and implementing care. The goal of the rehabilitation team is to restore and maintain function.

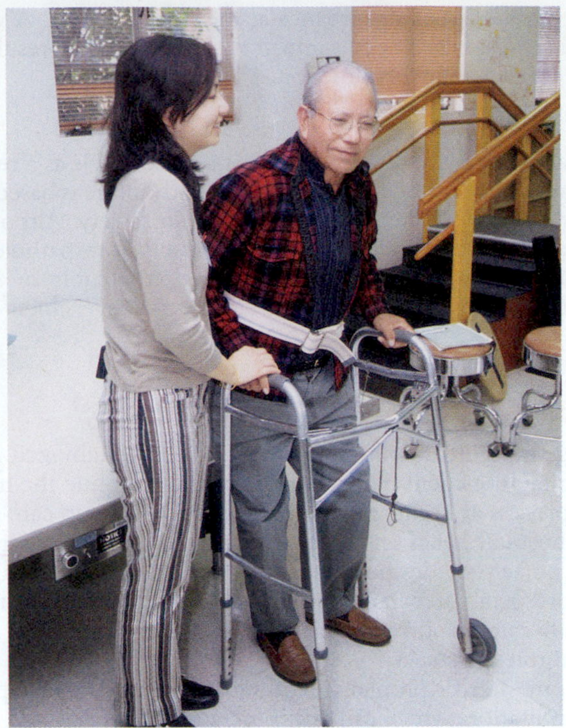

Figure 10-1 ■ A physical therapist helping a client to ambulate.

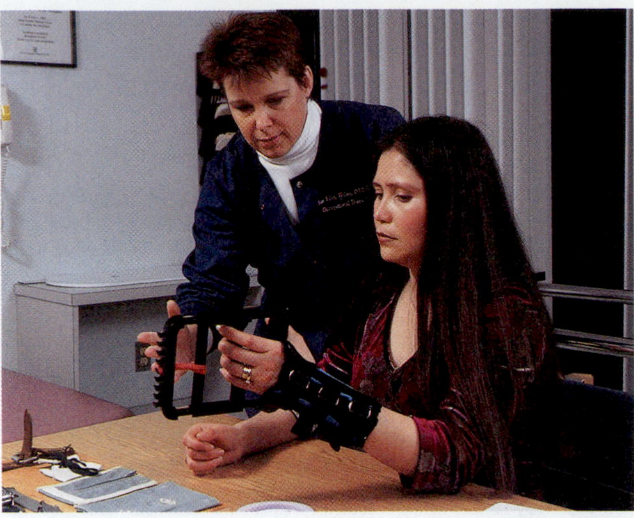

Figure 10-2 ■ An occupational therapist working with a client.

Members of the interdisciplinary health care team in the rehabilitation setting include physicians, nurses, physical therapists, occupational therapists, speech-language pathologists, recreational or activity therapists, cognitive therapists, aides, social workers, psychologists, vocational counselors, clients, and family members or significant others. Not all settings that offer rehabilitation services have all of these members on their team.

A physician who specializes in rehabilitative medicine is called a **physiatrist.** Except for most freestanding skilled nursing facilities, most inpatient rehabilitation settings employ physiatrists.

The **rehabilitation nurse** in the inpatient setting coordinates the efforts of the team members and therefore may be designated as the client's case manager. Nurses and other health care professionals may be designated as **rehabilitation case managers** in the home or in acute care settings. In clients undergoing rehabilitation, health problems are characterized by an altered functional ability and a diminished quality of life. The goal of rehabilitation nursing is to assist in the restoration and maintenance of optimal health. The rehabilitation nurse must be innovative and patient in helping clients regain independence.

Physical therapists (PTs) intervene to help the client achieve mobility (e.g., by facilitating ambulation and teaching the client to use a walker). They may also teach techniques for performing certain ADLs, such as transferring (e.g., moving into and out of bed), ambulating, and toileting.

Occupational therapists (OTs) work to develop the client's fine motor skills used for ADLs, such as those required for eating, maintaining hygiene, dressing, and driving. OTs may also teach skills related to coordination (e.g., hand movements) and cognitive retraining (Figure 10-2).

Speech-language pathologists (SLPs) evaluate and retrain clients with speech, language, or swallowing problems. Speech is roughly defined as the ability to say words, and language is the ability to understand and put words together in a meaningful way. Some clients, especially those who have experienced a head injury or stroke, have difficulty with both speech and language. Clients who have experienced a stroke also typically have dysphagia (difficulty with swallowing). SLPs provide screening and testing for dysphagia. If the client has dysphagia, the SLP recommends appropriate foods and feeding techniques.

Recreational or **activity therapists** work to help clients continue or develop hobbies or interests. These therapists often coordinate their efforts with those of the OT.

Cognitive therapists, usually neuropsychologists, work primarily with clients who have experienced head injuries and have cognitive impairments. These therapists often use computers to assist with cognitive retraining.

Nursing or **therapy assistants** work in the nursing or therapy departments to assist in the care of clients. These members of the rehabilitation team are under the direct supervision of the registered nurse or therapist.

Various counselors are helpful in promoting community reintegration of the client and acceptance of the disability or chronic illness. **Social workers** help clients to identify support services and resources, including financial assistance, and they usually coordinate transfers to or discharges from the rehabilitation setting. Psychologists also counsel clients and families on their psychological problems and on strategies to cope with disability.

Vocational counselors assist with job placement, training, or further education. Work-related skills are taught if the client needs to change careers because of the disability. If the client has not yet completed high school, educational tutors may help with completion of the requirements for graduation.

Interdisciplinary team conferences for the exchange of ideas are held on a regular basis with the client, family members and significant others, and health care providers. Chart documentation is shared and read by all team members.

COLLABORATIVE MANAGEMENT

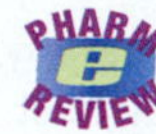

Assessment

HISTORY

Collect the health history, including the history of the client's present condition, any current medications, and any treatment programs in progress. Begin by obtaining general background data about the client and family. These data include financial status, occupations, educational levels, cultural background, and home situation. In collaboration with the occupational therapist, the nurse or case manager addresses the architectural features of the home environment (e.g., the layout of the home). Together they discuss whether the physical layout at home, such as the presence of stairs or the width of doorways, will present a problem to the client. Data are gathered on the client's neighborhood, such as the location of shopping centers and available transportation.

Assess the client's usual daily schedule and habits of everyday living. These include hygiene practices, eating, elimination, sexual activity, and sleep. Ask about the client's preferred method and time of bathing and hygiene activity. In assessing dietary patterns, food likes and dislikes are noted. Information about bowel and bladder function and the normal pattern of elimination is also obtained.

In assessing sexuality patterns, ask about changes in sexual function since the onset of the disability. The client's current and previous sleep habits, patterns, usual number of hours of sleep, and use of hypnotics are also assessed. Question whether the client feels well rested after sleep. Sleep patterns have a significant impact on activity patterns. The assessment of activity patterns focuses on work, exercise, and recreational activities.

PHYSICAL ASSESSMENT/CLINICAL MANIFESTATIONS

Collect the physical assessment data systematically according to major body systems on admission for baseline and every day, according to agency policy and type of setting (Table 10-1). The focus of the assessment related to rehabilitation and chronic disease is on the functional abilities of the client.

CARDIOVASCULAR ASSESSMENT. An alteration in cardiac status may affect the client's cardiac output or cause activity intolerance. Assess the manifestations of decreased cardiac output (e.g., chest pain and fatigue). If present, determine when the client experiences these symptoms and what relieves them. The physician may prescribe a change in medications or may prescribe a prophylactic dose of nitroglycerin to be taken before the client resumes activities. Collaborate with the physician and appropriate therapists to determine whether activities need to be modified.

For the client showing fatigue, the nurse and the client plan methods for using limited energy resources. For instance, frequent rest periods can be taken throughout the day, especially before performing activities. Major tasks could be performed in the morning because most people have the most energy at that time.

A great hindrance to rehabilitation for clients with cardiac disorders is fear. These clients may have survived a life-threatening experience (e.g., myocardial infarction) and are now so afraid of recurrence (and death) that they are unable or unwilling to resume any activity. They usually benefit from participation in a structured cardiac rehabilitation program. (See Chapter 38 for a complete description of cardiac rehabilitation.)

TABLE 10-1 Assessment of Clients in Rehabilitation

Body System	Relevant Data
Cardiovascular system	Chest pain Fatigue Fear of cardiac failure
Respiratory system	Shortness of breath or dyspnea Activity tolerance Fear of inability to breathe
Gastrointestinal system and nutrition	Oral intake, eating pattern Anorexia, nausea, and vomiting Dysphagia Laboratory data (e.g., serum prealbumin level) Weight loss or gain Bowel elimination pattern or habits Change in stool Ability to get to toilet
Renal-urinary system	Urinary pattern Fluid intake Urinary incontinence or retention Urine culture or urinalysis
Neurologic system	Motor function Sensation Cognitive abilities
Musculoskeletal system	Functional ability Range of motion Endurance Muscle strength
Integumentary system	Risk of skin breakdown Presence of skin lesions

RESPIRATORY ASSESSMENT. Ask the client whether he or she is experiencing shortness of breath during or after activity. It is important to determine the level of activity that can be accomplished without experiencing shortness of breath. For example, can the client climb one flight of stairs without shortness of breath, or does shortness of breath occur after climbing only two steps?

The fear associated with any inability to breathe normally can render a person dependent in many aspects of life. Some problems related to disorders of the respiratory system can be resolved or diminished, but some chronic disease, such as emphysema, often continue to worsen.

GASTROINTESTINAL AND NUTRITIONAL ASSESSMENT. Monitor the client's oral intake and pattern of eating. He or she is also assessed for the presence of anorexia, dysphagia (difficulty swallowing), nausea, vomiting, or discomfort that may interfere with oral intake. In collaboration with the physician and the dietitian, review the client's height, weight, hemoglobin and hematocrit levels, and serum prealbumin, and blood glucose concentrations (see Chapter 64 for a complete nutritional assessment). Weight loss or weight gain is particularly significant and may be related to an associated disease or to the illness that caused the disability.

Elimination habits vary from person to person; they are often related to daily job or activity schedules, dietary patterns, and family or cultural background. Elimination habits may be difficult to assess, because many nurses are hesitant to request (and many clients are afraid to volunteer) information pertaining to elimination. When assessing elimination status, the nurse first asks about the client's usual elimination patterns before the injury or the illness.

Note any changes in the client's bowel routine or stool consistency. If the client reports any change in elimination pattern, try to determine whether this alteration is due to a change in diet, activity pattern, or medication use that could cause increased or decreased motility of the gastrointestinal tract. Bowel habits are evaluated on the basis of what is normal for that person.

The nurse also asks whether the client can manage bowel functions independently. Independence in bowel elimination requires cognition, manual dexterity, sensation, muscle control, and mobility. If the client requires help, the nurse determines whether someone is available at home to provide the assistance. The client's (and family's) ability to cope with any dependency in bowel elimination must also be assessed.

RENAL AND URINARY ASSESSMENT. Ask about the client's baseline urinary patterns, including the number of times the client usually voids, and determine whether the client routinely awakens during the night to empty the bladder or has uninterrupted sleep. Fluid intake patterns and volume are recorded, including the type of fluids ingested and the time they were consumed.

The nurse questions whether the client has ever experienced any problems with urinary incontinence or retention. Laboratory reports, especially the results of the urinalysis, are also monitored.

NEUROLOGIC ASSESSMENT. In rehabilitation, the neurologic assessment includes the functional aspects of motor ability, sensation, and cognition. The nurse assesses the client's pre-existing problems, general physical condition, and communication abilities.

The movement of an extremity is compared with the function of the opposite extremity to identify **paresis** (weakness) or **paralysis** (absence of movement). The identification of sensory-perceptual alterations is important in assessing the client's risk for injury. Assess the client's response to light touch, hot or cold temperature, and position change in each extremity and on the trunk. Levels of decreased sensation are identified. For a perceptual assessment, the nurse evaluates the client's ability to receive and understand what is heard and seen and the ability to express appropriate motor and verbal responses. During this portion of the assessment, begin to assess short-term and long-term memory.

The nurse also ascertains the client's cognitive abilities, especially if there is a head injury or stroke. Several tools are available to evaluate cognition. One of the most common is the Mini-Mental State Examination, which is described in detail in Chapter 45.

MUSCULOSKELETAL ASSESSMENT. As with other body systems, the rehabilitation nursing assessment of the musculoskeletal system focuses on function. Assess the client's musculoskeletal status, response to the impairment, and demands of the home, work, or school environment. The client's endurance level is determined, and both active and passive range of motion (ROM) of joints are measured. Review the results of manual muscle testing by physical therapy, which identifies the client's ROM and resistance against gravity. In this procedure, the therapist determines the degree of muscle strength present in each body segment. The grading system usually ranges from 0 (no evidence of muscle contractility) to 5 (normal muscle contractility) (see Chapter 53).

SKIN ASSESSMENT. When assessing a client's skin, the nurse identifies actual or potential interruptions in its integrity.

RISK FOR SKIN BREAKDOWN. To maintain healthy skin, the body must have adequate food, water, and oxygen intake; intact waste removal mechanisms; sensation; and functional mobility. Changes in any of these variables can lead to rapid and extensive skin breakdown. If the client cannot protect or maintain the skin, the nurse must be able to assess and plan for his or her needs. The nurse monitors the client to determine the risk of skin breakdown before it occurs.

Most rehabilitation settings use special skin assessment tools to identify clients at risk for skin breakdown. For example, the classic Braden Scale for Predicting Pressure Sore Risk (see Chapter 70) assesses several areas: sensory perception, skin moisture, activity level, nutritional status, and potential for friction and shear.

Other skin risk assessment tools are available. Some tools also include additional indicators of nutritional status, such as the serum prealbumin. When either of these levels is low, the client is at high risk for pressure ulcers. Some tools include incontinence and altered mental state as risk factors.

ACTUAL SKIN BREAKDOWN. If a pressure ulcer or other change in skin integrity develops, the nurse accurately assesses the problem and its possible causes. If possible, inspect the skin every 2 hours (more often if needed) until the client learns to inspect his or her own skin several times a day. The depth and diameter of the open skin area is measured in centimeters or inches, depending on the policy of the facility. The area around the open lesion must also be assessed to determine the presence of cellulitis or other tissue damage. Chapter 70 includes a widely used classification system for staging skin breakdown. Determine the client's understanding of the cause and treatment of skin breakdown as well as his or her ability to inspect the skin and participate in maintaining skin integrity.

In many health care agencies, a skin assessment and documentation tool ("skin sheet") is used to keep track of each area of skin breakdown. A baseline assessment is conducted on admission to the agency, and the form is updated periodically depending on the agency's policy and the nurse's judgment. In some long-term care, acute care, or rehabilitation settings, and with the client's permission, photographs of the skin are taken on admission and at various intervals to document its condition.

FUNCTIONAL ASSESSMENT

Functional ability refers to the client's ability to perform **activities of daily living (ADLs),** such as bathing, dressing, feeding, and ambulating, as well as independent living skills such as using the telephone, shopping, preparing food, and housekeeping. **Functional assessment** tools are used to assess a client's abilities. Rehabilitation nurses, physiatrists, or therapists complete one or more of these assessment tools on the basis of the client's abilities and the policy of the health care setting. The most commonly used tool is the Functional Independence Measure. Other tools, such as the LORS-II, are referenced in the Selected Bibliography at the end of this chapter.

A uniform data system used for outcome data collection across the United States is the Functional Independence Measure (FIM) developed by Granger and Gresham (1984). As a basic indicator of the severity of a disability, the FIM attempts to quantify what the person actually does, whatever the diagnosis or impairment. It does not measure what a person should do or how the person would perform under a different set of circumstances. To eliminate the bias of a particular discipline, the assessment may be performed by trained clinicians. The entire assessment may be performed by one person, or certain categories may be completed by representatives of various disciplines.

Categories for assessment are self-care, sphincter control, mobility and locomotion, communication, and cognition. Scoring is done with numbers that use predetermined criteria for measurement. The client is evaluated when he or she is admitted to and discharged from a rehabilitation institution and at other specified times to determine client progress. In some settings, it is also being used to help determine staffing levels (Gross, et al., 2001). The FIM assessment system has also been adapted for use in other health care settings, including acute care and home care.

PSYCHOSOCIAL ASSESSMENT

The nurse must understand the theories of body image and self-esteem to assess the client's psychosocial needs adequately. These concepts serve as a basis for understanding psychological responses to chronic illness and the resulting disability. The client's self-esteem and body image are assessed through verbal indicators and descriptions of self-care.

Assess the client's use of defense mechanisms and manifestations of anxiety, such as those noted in facial expressions and communication patterns. To assess the client's response to loss, the nurse asks the client to describe feelings concerning the loss of a body part or function. The presence of any stress-related physical problem is noted. The client may experience symptoms of depression, such as fatigue, a change in appetite, or feelings of powerlessness. See Chapter 9 for a more thorough discussion of loss and grieving.

The nurse assesses the availability of support systems for the client. The major support system is typically the family or significant others. Family interactions and coping patterns are also assessed.

VOCATIONAL ASSESSMENT

The client is assisted in maximizing functional status to allow him or her to resume many usual activities. The nurse should be aware of the appropriate resources for each client in compiling a vocational database. Vocational counselors can help the client find meaningful training, education, or employment after discharge from the rehabilitation setting.

Clients in the United States should be informed about the Americans with Disabilities Act, which was passed by Congress in 1991 to prevent employer discrimination against disabled people. The employer must offer reasonable assistance to a disabled employee to allow him or her to perform the job. For example, if an employee has a severe hearing loss, the employer may need to hire an interpreter for sign language. Workers have a right to ask for special adaptations based on their disabilities.

The rehabilitation team assesses the cognitive and physical demands of the client's job and ascertains whether he or she can return to the former job or whether retraining in another field is necessary. The physical demands of jobs range from light in sedentary occupations (0 to 10 pounds often lifted) to heavy (more than 100 pounds often lifted). The nurse must also consider other aspects of the job, such as strength, mobility, or senses required (e.g., hearing).

Job analysis also involves assessing the work environment of the client's former job. Collaborate with the vocational counselor to determine whether the environment is conducive to the client's return. Union contracts must also be considered, and any job modifications must be noted. If an injured worker requires vocational rehabilitation, refer him or her to vocational rehabilitation personnel to evaluate present skills and learn new skills for employment if needed. In most states, worker's compensation insurance helps to support vocational rehabilitation.

Analysis

COMMON NURSING DIAGNOSES AND COLLABORATIVE PROBLEMS

Regardless of the client's age or specific disability, the following nursing diagnoses are commonly applicable to the client with chronic illness or disability:

1. Impaired Physical Mobility related to neuromuscular impairment, sensory-perceptual impairment, and/or pain
2. Self-Care Deficit (specify deficits) related to neuromuscular impairment and/or perceptual or cognitive impairment
3. Risk for Impaired Skin Integrity related to altered sensation and/or altered nutritional state
4. Impaired Urinary Elimination related to neurologic dysfunction and/or trauma or disease affecting spinal cord nerves
5. Constipation related to neurologic impairment
6. Ineffective Coping related to situational crisis and/or inadequate time to prepare for stressor

ADDITIONAL NURSING DIAGNOSES AND COLLABORATIVE PROBLEMS

Additional nursing diagnoses may apply depending on the client's specific disability. For example, a client with rheumatoid arthritis also experiences Chronic Pain related to chronic physical disability. The client with a spinal cord injury may also have Sexual Dysfunction related to altered body function.

Planning and Implementation

IMPAIRED PHYSICAL MOBILITY

NOC **PLANNING: EXPECTED OUTCOMES.** Most clients with chronic illness or disability are expected to move purposefully in his or her environment with or without assistive device. Not all clients are able to achieve all indicators for this outcome due to physical limitations. Indicators include that the client has noncompromised:

- Balance
- Coordination
- Gait
- Muscle movement
- Body positioning performance
- Transfer performance

INTERVENTIONS. Most problems requiring rehabilitation relate to impaired physical mobility. Clients with neurologic disease or injury, amputations, arthritis, severe burns, and cardiopulmonary disease experience some degree of impaired mobility. Physical and occupational therapists are the key rehabilitation team members in helping clients meet their mobility goals. Depending on the setting, clients often spend several hours every day working in the physical therapy department to regain function and skills.

Transfer Techniques. Clients with decreased mobility may require assistance with transfers, such as from a bed to a chair, commode, or wheelchair. Because the degree of assistance required varies with the client and the specific disability, the nurse carefully assesses mobility status before attempting a transfer. The physical or occupational therapist usually specifies the type of transfer. For example, a quadriplegic client may use a sliding board for transfer, whereas a client with an above-knee amputation may need a wheelchair with removable arms. In any case, the nurse always plans the transfer technique before initiating it. The desired outcome is that the client will eventually be able to transfer independently and safely.

Basic techniques for the nurse to use when assisting in the transfer of the client from a bed to a chair or wheelchair (and vice versa) are identified in Chart 10-1. These techniques are also taught to the family member or other caregiver who will be caring for the client at home. Additional information about transfers can be found in basic nursing textbooks.

CHART 10-1

BEST PRACTICE for
Transfer Techniques

Bed to Wheelchair or Chair

1. Place the chair at an angle to the bed on the client's strong side.
2. Lock the wheelchair brakes or secure the chair position.
3. Assist the client to stand, and move his or her strong hand to the armrest.
4. Keep the client's body weight forward and pivot.
5. When the client's legs touch the chair edge, assist the client in sitting.

Wheelchair or Chair to Bed

1. Place the chair with the client's strong side next to the bed.
2. Lock the wheelchair brakes or secure the chair position.
3. Assist the client to stand, and move his or her strong hand to the armrest.
4. Keep the client's body weight forward and pivot.
5. When the client's legs touch the bed edge, assist the client in sitting and then reclining.

Use of a Sliding Board

1. Place the chair or wheelchair as close to the bed as possible.
2. Remove the armrest from the chair or (if removable) wheelchair.
3. Powder the sliding board.
4. Place the sliding board under the client's buttocks.
5. Instruct the client to reach toward his or her side.
6. Assist the client in sliding gently to the bed.

Alternative Transfer Techniques. Some clients cannot bear weight. For example, a spinal cord injury resulting in quadriplegia involves using either a **sliding board** (which requires balance skills) or, with the nurse or therapist, a "bear hug" technique. The sitting client places his or her arms around the nurse's neck while being lifted from the bed to the chair or vice versa. Another person assists with the transfer by stabilizing the wheelchair and holding onto the client's waist. Most physical therapists recommend that the client wear pants or a **gait belt** so the assistant can hold onto the belt during the transfer.

Potential Problems with Transfers. Before any transfer, the nurse carefully observes for potential problems. Orthostatic, or postural, hypotension is a common problem in rehabilitation and contributes to falls, which are common in any client with impaired mobility. If the client moves from a lying to a sitting or standing position too quickly, his or her blood pressure drops; as a result, he or she becomes dizzy or faints. This problem is worsened by antihypertensive medications, especially in older adults. To prevent this, help the client change positions slowly, with frequent rest periods to allow the blood pressure to stabilize. The nurse may measure blood pressure with the client in the lying, sitting, and standing positions to examine the differences. Orthostatic hypotension is indicated by a drop of more than 20 mm Hg in systolic pressure or 10 mm Hg in diastolic pressure between positions. Notify the physician about this change.

If the client has problems in maintaining blood pressure while out of bed, the physical therapist usually starts the client on a tilt table to gradually increase tolerance. This is a particularly common problem for clients who are quadriplegic.

Weight gain is another potential problem. Because the client undergoing rehabilitation has impaired mobility, he or she tends to gain weight. Excessive weight hinders transfers both for the nurse or the therapist who is assisting and for the client who is learning to transfer independently. Weight is usually checked every week to monitor gains or losses.

Gait Training. The physical therapist works with clients for gait training if they are able to ambulate. While regaining the ability to ambulate, clients may need to use canes or walkers (Figure 10-3). When working with clients who are using such assistive devices, also known as **ambulatory aids,** the physical therapist ensures that there is a level surface on which to walk. The nurse reinforces the physical therapist's instructions and encourages practice, with the goal being to walk independently with or without an assistive device. Older clients typically use a walker for a broader base of support. Younger or minimally impaired clients often progress to the use of a hemi-cane or straight cane. Chart 10-2 outlines how to use assistive devices for ambulation.

Some clients never regain the ability to walk because of their impairment, such as multiple sclerosis or spinal cord injury. They may become wheelchair dependent and need to learn wheelchair mobility skills. With the help of physical and occupational therapy, most clients can learn to move anywhere in the wheelchair.

Prevention of Complications. During the rehabilitation phase, clients are vulnerable to complications of immobility. Table 10-2 lists the common complications and the major strategies the nurse can use to help prevent each complication. Implementing range-of-motion (ROM) routines, adhering to schedules for turning and repositioning, and maintaining skin care are constant components of rehabilitation nursing care to prevent complications of immobility. The key is to increase mobility.

One way to increase mobility, even with clients who are bedridden, is through ROM exercises. ROM techniques are beneficial for any client with decreased mobility (Table 10-3). Although basic ROM techniques are presented in basic nursing textbooks, a few key principles are pertinent to rehabilitation nursing care:

- The human body contains more joints than simply the knees, hips, elbows, and shoulders. For ROM techniques to be effective in preventing musculoskeletal contractures, the client must exercise all joints, including each joint of the fingers, hands, toes, and so forth.
- In performing ROM activities, the nurse or client completes full-range movement of each joint at least five times and completes the entire process at least three times daily.
- The nurse does not move the joints beyond the point at which the client expresses pain or beyond the point at which the nurse perceives stiffness or difficulty.

Clients with decreased mobility who are able to follow directions are taught by the nurse and the physical therapist to perform active or active-assisted ROM exercises.

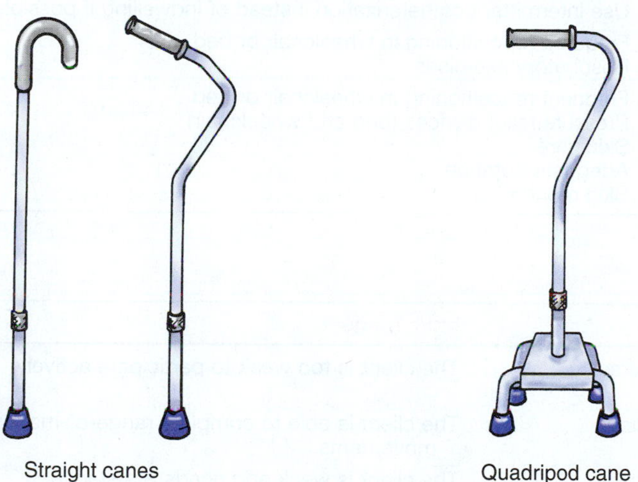

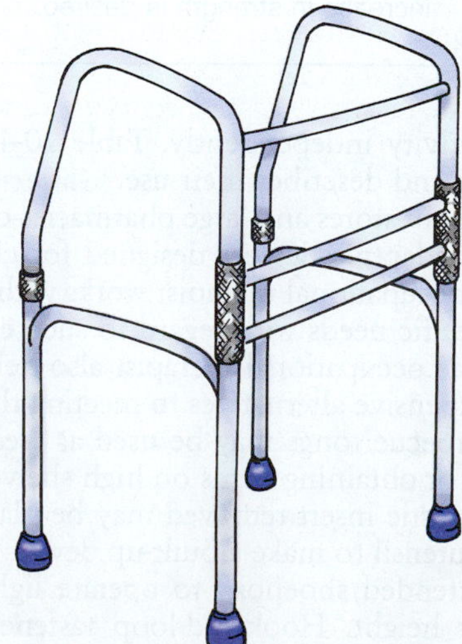

Figure 10-3 ■ Assistive devices for ambulation. Assistive devices vary in the amount of support they provide. A straight cane provides less support than a quadripod cane or walker.

SELF-CARE DEFICIT

NOC **PLANNING: EXPECTED OUTCOMES.** Most clients with chronic illness or disability are expected to perform the most basic physical tasks and personal care activities independently with or without assistive devices. Indicators include that the client demonstrates noncompromised:

- Eating
- Dressing
- Toileting
- Bathing
- Grooming
- Hygiene
- Oral hygiene
- Walking or wheelchair mobility
- Transfer performance
- Positioning of self

INTERVENTIONS. Activities of daily living (ADLs), or self-care activities, include eating, bathing, dressing, grooming, and toileting. Encourage the client to perform as much self-care as possible. The nurse and occupational therapist collaborate to identify ways in which self-care activities can be modified so the client can perform them independently, if possible. For example, the occupational therapist teaches a hemiplegic client to put on a shirt by first placing the affected arm in the sleeve and then putting the unaffected arm in the appropriate sleeve. The nurse reinforces this dressing technique and encourages the client to practice.

CHART 10-2

BEST PRACTICE for
Gait Training

Walker Assisted

1. Apply a gait belt around the client's waist.
2. Assist the client to a standing position.
3. Assist the client in placing both hands on the walker.
4. Ensure that the client is well balanced.
5. Assist the client repeatedly to perform the following sequence:
   a. Lift the walker.
   b. Move the walker 2 feet forward and set it down on all legs.
   c. While resting on the walker, take small steps.
   d. Check balance.

Cane Assisted

1. Apply a gait belt around the client's waist.
2. Assist the client to a standing position.
3. Assist the client in placing his or her strong hand on the cane.
4. Ensure that the client is well balanced.
5. Assist the client to perform the following sequence repeatedly:
   a. Move the cane forward.
   b. Move the weaker leg one step forward.
   c. Move the stronger leg one step forward.
   d. Check balance.

TABLE 10-2 Prevention of the Common Hazards of Immobility

Body System	Complication	Prevention
Musculoskeletal	Contractures	Range-of-motion exercises
	Foot drop	Foot support while in bed, range-of-motion exercises, high-top tennis shoes
	Osteoporosis	Range-of-motion exercises, ambulation if possible (walking)
	Susceptibility to fractures	Weight-bearing exercises
	Muscular atrophy	Passive or active range-of-motion exercises
Gastrointestinal	Constipation	Increased activity level Increased fluid intake, fiber
Cardiovascular	Decreased cardiac output	Range-of-motion exercises
	Increased venous stasis	Exercise, support hose, or antiembolism stockings
	Thrombus formation	Exercise, support hose, or antiembolism stockings
	Embolism	Avoidance of leg massage, low–molecular weight heparin
Neurologic	Disorientation	Sleep-wake schedule in accord with light-dark pattern Reorientation (to person, place, and time) Control of sensory stimulation
	Postural hypotension	Avoidance of sudden position changes, tilt table
Renal/urinary	Calculi	Decreased dietary calcium level Increased fluid intake Maintenance of acidic urine
	Infection	Increase fluids Use intermittent catheterization instead of indwelling if possible
Respiratory	Pneumonia	Frequent repositioning in wheelchair or bed Respiratory exercises
Integumentary	Pressure ulcers	Frequent repositioning in wheelchair or bed Pressure relief devices (bed and wheelchair) Skin care Adequate nutrition Skin monitoring

TABLE 10-3 Types of Range-of-Motion Exercises

Type	Description	Indications
Passive	Exercises are performed by the nurse for the client.	The client is too weak to participate actively.
Active	Exercises are performed by the client.	The client is able to complete range-of-motion movements.
Assisted, or active assisted	Exercises are performed by the client but are guided by the nurse or therapist.	The client is weak and needs assistance.
Resistive	The actions of the client are in opposition to those performed by the nurse or therapist.	The client has full range of motion, and an increase in strength is desired.

In long-term care (LTC) settings (e.g., nursing homes), federal regulations require that residents not lose their functional skills. Therefore most facilities have developed **restorative nursing** programs and have coordinated these programs with rehabilitation therapy and activity therapy. The focus of this coordinated effort includes the following:

- Bed mobility
- Walking
- Transfers
- Dressing
- Grooming
- Active range of motion
- Communication

Nursing assistants in LTC and home health settings are typically involved in restorative programs (Marrelli, 2003).

NIC **Self-Care Assistance.** A variety of **assistive/adaptive devices** are available for clients with chronic illness and disability. An assistive/adaptive device, or self-care support device, is any item that enables the client to perform all or part of an activity independently. Table 10-4 identifies common devices and describes their use.

Many department stores and large pharmacies carry clothing and assistive/adaptive devices designed for clients with disabilities. The occupational therapist works with the client to determine specific needs with regard to such equipment. The nurse and the occupational therapist also help look for creative and inexpensive alternatives to meeting these needs. For example, barbecue tongs may be used as "reachers" for pulling up pants or obtaining items on high shelves. A foam curler with the plastic insert removed may be placed over a pencil or eating utensil to make a built-up device. The client might use an extended shoehorn to operate light switches from wheelchair height. Hook-and-loop fasteners (Velcro) sewn on clothes can prevent the frustrations caused by buttons and zippers. Chart 10-3 lists nursing interventions for clients who need self-care assistance.

Energy Conservation. Fatigue is commonly associated with chronic and disabling conditions. Therefore nurses

TABLE 10-4 Uses of Assistive/Adaptive Devices

Device	Use
Buttonhook	Threaded through the buttonhole to enable clients with weak finger mobility to button shirts Alternative uses include serving as pencil holder or cigarette holder
Extended shoe horn	Assists in the application of shoes for clients with decreased mobility Alternative uses include turning light switches off or on while client is in a wheelchair
Plate guard	Applied to a plate to assist clients with weak hand and arm mobility to feed themselves
Gel pad	Placed under a plate or a glass to prevent dishes from slipping and moving Alternative uses include placement under bathing and grooming items to prevent them from moving
Foam buildups	Applied to eating utensils to assist clients with weak hand grasps to feed themselves Alternative uses include application to pens and pencils to assist with writing or over a button-hook to assist with grasping the device
Hook and loop fastener (Velcro) straps	Applied to utensils, a buttonhook, or a pencil to slip over the hand and provide a method of stabilizing the device when the client's hand grasp is weak
Long-handled reacher	Assists in obtaining items located on high shelves or at ground level for clients who are unable to change positions easily
Elastic shoelaces or Velcro shoe closure	Prevents the need for tying shoes

CHART 10-3

NIC INTERVENTION ACTIVITIES for The Client in Rehabilitation

Self-Care Assistance: *Assisting another to perform activities of daily living*

- Monitor client's ability for independent self-care.
- Monitor client's need for adaptive devices for personal hygiene, dressing, grooming, toileting, and eating.
- Provide assistance until the client is fully able to assume self-care.
- Use consistent repetition of health routines as a means of establishing them.
- Encourage client to perform normal activities of daily living to level of ability.
- Teach family to encourage independence, to intervene only when the client is unable to perform.
- Establish a routine for self-care activities.

NIC intervention activities selected from Dochterman, J.M., & Bulechek, G.M. (Eds.) (2004). *Nursing interventions classification (NIC).* (4th ed.). St. Louis: Mosby.

CHART 10-4

NURSING FOCUS on the OLDER ADULT
Special Considerations in Rehabilitation

- When getting the client out of bed, move him or her (or instruct him or her to move or sit up) slowly to prevent orthostatic hypotension. This problem is most common in older adults who take antihypertensive medications.
- Turn the client more often than every 2 hours, even if it is just a minor position change. Skin becomes thinner and more fragile with age.
- Determine whether the client had any problem with urinary patterns before the illness or rehabilitation. A client with a previous problem may not have a successful bladder training program.
- Be aware that intestinal motility decreases with age, which leads to constipation.
- Assess the client's support system of family and significant others. Many older clients have no spouse or close friends, who would usually serve as a support network.

work with occupational therapists to assess the client's self-care abilities and to determine possible ways of conserving energy. The nurse and the therapist develop strategies for **energy conservation** after evaluating the client's self-care routines. Preparation for ADLs can be helpful in reducing effort and energy expenditure (e.g., gathering all necessary equipment before starting grooming routines). If a client has high energy levels in the morning, he or she can be taught to schedule energy-intensive activities in the morning rather than later in the day or evening. Spacing activities is also helpful for conserving energy. In addition, allowing time to rest before and after eating and toileting decreases the strain on the client's energy level.

RISK FOR IMPAIRED SKIN INTEGRITY

NOC **PLANNING: EXPECTED OUTCOMES.** The client with chronic illness or disability is expected to have structural intactness and physiologic function of the skin as indicated by having none of the following:

- Skin lesions
- Erythema
- Blanching
- Necrosis
- Induration
- Skin flaking

INTERVENTIONS. An enormous variety of topical and mechanical remedies have been used with varying success to prevent and treat pressure ulcers. Pressure reduction is a nursing intervention that may be achieved when the nurse temporarily repositions the client or alters the physical properties of the mattress surface, such as adding a mattress overlay.

Turning and Repositioning. The best intervention to prevent skin impairment is frequent position changes in combination with adequate skin care and sufficient nutritional intake. In general, the nurse turns and repositions the client every 2 hours if the client is unable to perform this activity. This may not be sufficient for people who are frail and have thin skin, especially older adults (Chart 10-4). To determine the best turning schedule, assess the client's skin condition during each turning and repositioning. For example, if the client has been sleeping for 2 hours and the nurse decides to postpone turning for 1 hour, reddened areas over the bony prominences may be present. If such reddened areas do not fade within 30 minutes after pressure relief or do not blanch, they may be classified as preulcer areas, or stage I pressure areas (see Chapter 70).

Clients who sit for prolonged periods in a wheelchair need to be repositioned at least every 1 to 2 hours. Each client is evaluated by the physical or occupational therapist for the best seating pad or cushion that is comfortable yet reduces pressure on bony prominences. Clients who are able are taught to perform "wheelchair push-ups" by using their arms to lift their buttocks off the wheelchair seat for 10 seconds or longer every hour, or more often if needed. The physical therapist helps clients strengthen their arm muscles in preparation for performing wheelchair push-ups.

If the client wears tennis shoes for foot positioning, remove the shoes and assess for pressure areas. Many clients with neurologic problems have decreased or absent sensation and may not be able to feel the discomfort of increased pressure. Also check clients who are sitting in wheelchairs for signs of pressure, especially on the lower legs where the leg of the wheelchair could rub against the skin.

Skin Care. Adequate skin care is an essential component of prevention. The nurse performs or assists clients in completing skin care each time they are turned, repositioned, or bathed. Skin care includes cleaning soiled areas, drying carefully, and applying body lotion. If a client is incontinent, topical barrier creams or ointments can help protect the skin from moisture, which facilitates skin breakdown. Reddened areas are not rubbed because doing so can cause extensive damage to the already fragile capillary system. Instead the nurse carefully observes the areas for further breakdown and relieves pressure on the areas as much as possible. Bed pillows are often good pressure-relieving devices. (See Chapter 70 for a complete discussion of skin care interventions.)

Nutrition. Sufficient nutrition is needed both to repair wounds and to prevent pressure ulcers. The nurse collaborates with the dietitian to assess the client's food selection and ensure that it contains adequate protein and carbohydrates. Both the nurse and the dietitian closely monitor the client's weight and levels of serum prealbumin. If either of these indexes decreases significantly, the client may be given high-protein, high-carbohydrate food supplements (e.g., milkshakes) or commercial preparations (e.g., Ensure Plus) (also see Chapter 64).

Mechanical Devices. Pressure-relieving devices include waterbeds, gel mattresses or pads, air mattresses, low–air loss overlays or beds, and air-fluidized beds. Mattress overlays, such as air and gel types, and replacement mattresses are often effective in reducing pressure. The use of any mechanical device (except air-fluidized beds) does not eliminate the need for turning and repositioning.

Specialty beds are categorized as either "low air loss" or "air fluidized." Air-fluidized therapy (e.g., Clinitron or FluidAir bed) provides the most effective pressure relief; the client is maintained in a nearly pressure-free environment (Figure 10-4). In general, these beds are not used to prevent skin breakdown, because most insurers will not reimburse the agency for the use of the bed. Therefore special beds are usually reserved for severe skin problems that have not healed with the use of a conventional bed or other mechanical device. If optimal nutrition and healing conditions are maintained, skin breakdowns should heal with continued use of air-fluidized therapy. The primary disadvantage of this therapy is its expense, which may exceed several hundred dollars for each day of use. The cost of air-fluidized therapy may be reimbursed by some health insurance providers.

IMPAIRED URINARY ELIMINATION

NOC PLANNING: EXPECTED OUTCOMES. Most clients with chronic illness or disability are expected to have a normal collection and discharge of urine. Not all clients are able to meet the following indicators due to physiologic impairment. Indicators include that the client has noncompromised:

- Elimination pattern
- Adequacy of fluid intake
- Emptying of bladder

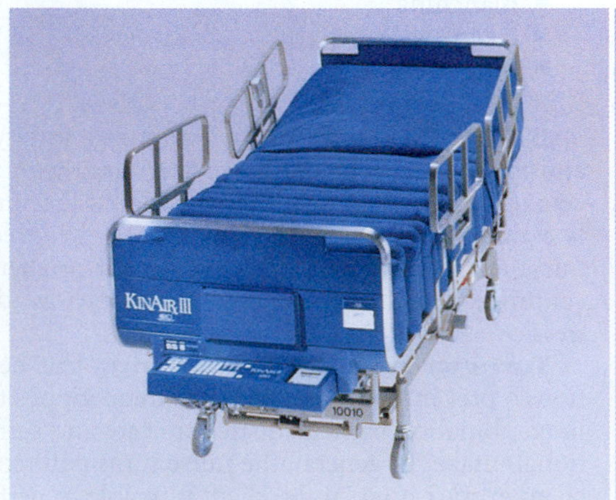

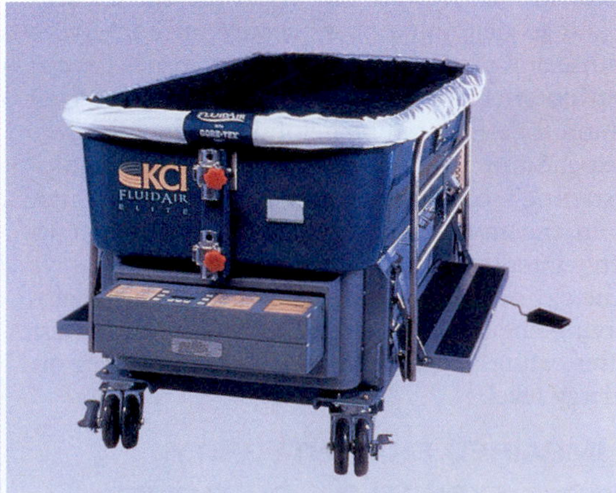

Figure 10-4 ■ Pressure relief devices. *Left,* KinAir III beds provide controlled air suspension to redistribute body weight away from bony prominences. *Right,* FluidAir Elite beds use airflow and bead fluidizations. Both of these beds are covered with Gore-Tex fabric, which resists tearing. This fabric is also waterproof and acts as a barrier against bacteria. (Courtesy Kinetic Concepts, Inc., San Antonio, TX.)

In addition, the client is expected to have none of the following:

- Hesitancy with urination
- Urinary retention
- Urinary incontinence

INTERVENTIONS. Neurologic disabilities may interfere with successful bladder control in a client undergoing rehabilitation. These disabilities result in three basic functional types of neurogenic bladder: reflex (spastic) bladder, flaccid bladder, and uninhibited bladder.

A **reflex** or **spastic** (upper motor neuron) **bladder** causes incontinence that is characterized by sudden, gushing voids. The bladder does not usually empty completely. A reflex bladder is also sometimes referred to as a "spastic" bladder. Neurologic problems affecting the upper motor neuron typically occur with high-level or mid-level spinal cord injuries above the twelfth thoracic vertebra (T12). These injuries result in a failure of impulse transmission from the lower spinal cord areas to the cortex of the brain. When the bladder fills and transmits impulses to the spinal cord, the client is not conscious of the filling sensation. However, because there is no injury to the lower spinal cord and the voiding reflex arc is intact, the efferent (motor) impulse is relayed and the bladder contracts.

A **flaccid** (lower motor neuron) **bladder** results in urinary retention and overflow (dribbling). Injuries that cause damage to the lower motor neuron at the spinal cord level of S2-4 (e.g., multiple sclerosis and spinal cord injury below T12) may directly interfere with the reflex arc or may result in inappropriate interpretation of impulses to the brain. The bladder fills and afferent (sensory) impulses conduct the message via the spinal cord to the cortical region of the brain. Because of the injury, the impulse is not interpreted correctly by the cortical bladder center in the brain, and there is a failure to respond with a message for the bladder to contract.

An **uninhibited bladder** may occur when the client has a neurologic problem that affects the cortical bladder center of the brain (frontal lobe), such as stroke or brain injury. When the bladder needs to empty, the client has little sensorimotor control and cannot wait until he or she is on the commode or bedpan before voiding. The client is incontinent, but the bladder may not completely empty.

Bladder Training. The nurse can teach three techniques to assist the client in "repatterning" voiding (bladder training):

- Facilitating, or triggering, techniques
- Intermittent catheterization
- Consistent scheduling of toileting routines; "timed void"

These techniques may not be as effective in clients with physiologic changes associated with aging.

Facilitating or Triggering Techniques. Facilitating (triggering) techniques are used to stimulate voiding (Table 10-5). If there is an upper motor neuron problem but the reflex arc is intact (reflex bladder pattern), the voiding response can be initiated by any stimulus that sends the message to the spinal cord level S2-4 that the bladder might be full. Such techniques include stroking the medial aspect of the thigh, pinching the area above the groin, pulling pubic hair, massaging the penoscrotal area, pinching the posterior aspect of the glans penis, and providing digital anal stimulation.

When the client has a lower motor neuron problem, the voiding reflex arc is not intact (flaccid bladder pattern), and additional stimulation may be needed to initiate voiding. Two techniques used to facilitate voiding are the Valsalva maneuver and the Credé maneuver. In teaching the Valsalva maneuver, the nurse instructs the client to hold his or her breath and bear down as if trying to defecate. The nurse assists the client in performing the Credé maneuver by placing the client's hand in a cupped position directly over the bladder area and instructing the client to push inward and downward as if massaging the bladder to empty.

Intermittent Catheterization. Intermittent catheterization is often used for disorders that involve a flaccid or spastic bladder. In assisting the client with intermittent catheterization for a flaccid bladder, the nurse initially inserts a urinary catheter every 2 to 3 hours—after the client has attempted voiding and has used the Valsalva and Credé maneuvers. If less than 150 mL of residual urine is obtained, the nurse typically increases the interval between catheterizations. This interval may be up to 3 to 4 hours according to the health care provider's order or health care agency protocol. The interval may be gradually increased to 4 to 6 hours, but the client should not go beyond 8 hours between catheterizations. The exception occurs when the residual urine volume is less than 150 mL each time with an adequate intake of fluids. If the client will be performing intermittent self-catheterization at home after discharge from the rehabilitation facility, the nurse instructs the client about clean (not sterile) technique.

Intermittent catheterizations may also be performed to determine residual urine volumes for the client with a reflex (upper motor neuron) or uninhibited bladder, although this procedure has been largely replaced with the less invasive **bladder ultrasound.** Nurses can perform this test at the bedside to determine postvoiding residuals. The

TABLE 10-5 Management of Impaired Urinary Elimination

Functional Type	Neurologic Disability	Clinical Manifestations	Re-establishing Voiding Patterns
Reflex (spastic)	Upper motor neuron spinal cord injury above T12	Urinary frequency, incontinence	Triggering or facilitating techniques Medications Bedside bladder ultrasound Intermittent catheterization Consistent toileting schedule
Flaccid	Lower motor neuron spinal cord injury below T12 (affects S2-4 reflex arc)	Urinary retention, overflow	Valsalva and Credé maneuvers Medications
Uninhibited	Brain damage from injury or stroke	Frequency, urgency, incontinence, voiding in small amounts	Intermittent catheterization Consistent toileting schedule Regulation of fluid intake

client is catheterized if the bladder volume is greater than 150 mL.

Toileting Schedule. Consistent toileting routines may be the best way to re-establish voiding continence when the client displays an uninhibited bladder pattern (associated with brain damage or head injury). Assess the client's previous voiding pattern and determine his or her daily routine. At a minimum, the nurse assists the client with voiding after awakening in the morning, before and after meals, before and after physical activity, and at bedtime. Most often, the client is toileted every 2 hours during the day and every 4 hours at night.

Consider the client's bladder capacity, which may range from 100 to 500 mL, as well as mobility limitations and restrictive clothing. Bladder capacity is determined by measuring urine output. Ensure that the client is aware of nearby bathrooms at all times or has a call system to contact the nurse or unlicensed assistive personnel for assistance.

Drug Therapy. Medications that may be used for urinary elimination problems include cholinergics (to promote bladder emptying), antispasmodics (to prevent incontinence), and skeletal muscle relaxants (to decrease spasticity, which promotes self-care). Medications are not usually prescribed by the health care provider in the initial management of bladder problems, but may be used to assist with a bladder training program. Report the client's progress in bladder training to the rehabilitation team so that the best decision regarding drug therapy can be made. In general, anticholinergics, antispasmodics, and skeletal muscle relaxants help to promote continence in clients with a reflex (upper motor neuron) bladder. Cholinergics, such as bethanechol chloride (Urecholine), may decrease urinary retention problems resulting from a flaccid bladder. They may also facilitate complete bladder emptying in a client with a large residual volume, which occurs with reflex bladder problems. An uninhibited bladder does not routinely require medications for bladder training programs unless urinary function is affected by additional pathologic changes.

Fluid Intake. Instruct the client to maintain an adequate intake of fluids, at least 2000 to 2500 mL/day. An acidic urine usually minimizes the risk of urinary tract infection and calculus (stone) formation, although this belief is controversial. However, some microorganisms, such as *Escherichia coli,* do grow best in acidic environments. Therefore encourage the client to drink fluids that promote an acidic urine, including large amounts of cranberry juice, prune juice, bouillon, tomato juice, and water. Fluids that promote an alkaline urine are discouraged, including citrus juices, excessive amounts of milk and milk products, and carbonated beverages. Remind the client that drinking water and other liquids helps prevent urinary infection.

In addition, discourage high-calorie fluids for overweight clients. Disabled clients have more difficulty with mobility and self-care if their weight is not controlled.

Prevention of Complications. The client with altered urinary elimination is at risk for skin breakdown from incontinence, urinary tract infection from urinary retention, and urinary calculi from urinary retention and stasis. The nurse keeps the client clean and dry and provides skin care as described under Risk for Impaired Skin Integrity (pp. 127 and 128). (See Chapter 73 for preventive measures for urinary tract infection and calculi.)

CONSTIPATION

NOC **PLANNING: EXPECTED OUTCOMES.** The client with chronic illness or disability is expected to have a normal formation and evacuation of stool. Indicators include that the client has noncompromised:

- Elimination pattern
- Control of bowel movements
- Ease of stool passage
- Comfort of stool passage
- Muscle tone to evacuate stool

INTERVENTIONS. Neurologic problems often affect the client's bowel pattern by causing a reflex (spastic) bowel, a flaccid bowel, or an uninhibited bowel.

Upper motor neuron diseases and injuries, such as a cervical or mid-level spinal cord injury, may result in a reflex (spastic) bowel pattern, with defecation occurring suddenly and without warning. With a reflex pattern, any facilitating or triggering mechanism may lead to defecation if the lower colon contains stool. An example of facilitating or triggering techniques is digital stimulation. For this technique, use a lubricated glove or finger cot and massage the anus in a circular motion for no less than 1 full minute. Digital stimulation should not be used for clients with cardiac disease because of the risk of inducing a vagal response (a rapid decrease in heart rate).

Lower motor neuron diseases and injuries interfere with transmission of the nervous impulse across the reflex arc and may result in a flaccid bowel pattern, with defecation occurring infrequently and in small amounts. The use of facilitating and triggering mechanisms in combination with a toileting schedule, suppository use, and disimpaction yields the best results. Clients may be able to self-administer the suppository or disimpact if necessary.

Neurologic injuries that affect the brain may cause an uninhibited bowel pattern, with frequent defecation, urgency, and complaints of hard stool. Clients may manage uninhibited bowel patterns through a consistent toileting schedule, a high-fiber diet, and the use of stool softeners.

Bowel Training. An overview of management techniques for bowel dysfunction is presented in Table 10-6. In many cases, clients are not able to regain control over their bowel function in the manner previously possible. The rehabilitation team assists in designing a bowel elimination program that accommodates the disability.

The nurse works with clients to schedule bowel elimination as close as possible to their previous routine. For example, a client who had stools at noon every other day before the illness or injury should have the bowel program scheduled in the same way. An exception is the client who prefers another time that best fits into his or her daily routine. If the client is employed during the day, a time-consuming bowel elimination program in the morning may not be reasonable. It may be preferable to change the bowel protocol to the evening, when there is more time.

Drug Therapy. Bowel training programs for clients with neurologic problems are often designed to include a combination of suppository use and a consistent toileting schedule. Although medications should not be a first choice when formulating a bowel training program, consider the need for a suppository if clients do not re-establish defecation habits through a consistent toileting schedule, dietary modification, anal stimulation, and disimpaction.

TABLE 10-6 Management of Bowel Dysfunction

Functional Type	Neurologic Disability	Dysfunction	Re-establishing Defecation Patterns
Reflex (spastic)	Upper motor neuron spinal cord injury above T12	Defecation without warning	Triggering mechanisms Facilitation techniques High-fiber diet Suppository use Consistent toileting schedule
Flaccid	Lower motor neuron spinal cord injury below T12 (affects S2-4 reflex arc)	Infrequent, small stools	Triggering or facilitating techniques High-fiber diet Suppository use Consistent toileting schedule Manual disimpaction
Uninhibited	Brain damage from injury or stroke	Frequency, urgency, and constipation	Consistent toileting schedule High-fiber diet Stool softener use

Bisacodyl (Dulcolax) and glycerin are common agents prescribed by health care providers as suppositories in bowel training programs. Suppositories must be placed against the bowel wall to stimulate the sacral reflex arc and promote rectal emptying. Both agents are equivalent in effect, with results occurring in 15 to 30 minutes. Administer the suppository when the client expects to defecate, for example, after a meal to coincide with the gastrocolic reflex. Administering the suppository every second or third day is usually effective in re-establishing defecation patterns. Depending on each client's need, other medications (e.g., laxatives) may be indicated for bowel training programs.

Nutrition. Bowel elimination is directly related to the type and quality of food and fluid ingested. A high-fiber diet is a mainstay of most bowel training programs and includes whole-grain foods, bran, and fresh and dried fruits. Increasing dietary fiber is effective in facilitating defecation only if the client reduces fat intake. Drinking plenty of fluids also helps with bowel elimination.

Prevention of Complications. Constipation, diarrhea, and flatulence are common complications of any bowel training program. Assess for these complications and modify the bowel training program accordingly in collaboration with the physician and the dietitian.

INEFFECTIVE COPING

NOC **PLANNING: EXPECTED OUTCOMES.** The client with chronic illness or disability is expected to take personal actions to manage stressors that tax the client's resources. Indicators include that the client consistently:

- Identifies ineffective and effective coping patterns
- Verbalizes a sense of control
- Reports decrease in stress
- Seeks information concerning illness and treatment
- Modifies lifestyle as needed
- Adapts to life changes
- Uses available social support

INTERVENTIONS. The client with a disability often has a poor self-concept because of changes in body image from structural or functional changes. The use of an assistive device, such as a wheelchair, also differentiates the client from most other people, and the client may not want to accept the need for the device. Encourage the client to discuss his or her feelings and ask questions to elicit specific information that can help in assessing his or her acceptance of and ability to cope with the disability.

A disability also affects a person's role in society. For instance, a young medical student may fall from a ladder and become a quadriplegic; as a result, plans for a career as a surgeon are altered. A middle-aged farmer may be burned severely when his tractor catches on fire. He can no longer care for his farm, and his wife takes over during his rehabilitation process. An older adult who cares for her grandchildren is crippled with rheumatoid arthritis and can no longer provide child care. Disability requires role changes and always involves losses in the lives of those affected.

In addition to role changes, relationships with people change. Socializing with friends and family may be a strain when a person feels "different." Intimate relationships are affected because sexual dysfunction may result from disability. The nurse should be sensitive to these issues and should not avoid discussing them.

Assess the client's previous coping strategies and support systems so they can be used during rehabilitation if needed. The client is asked what strategies have been used to cope successfully with previous life crises, if any. Spiritual and religious beliefs are important for some people and should not be overlooked when helping to identify sources of support.

Some clients use complementary and alternative medicine (CAM) to cope with chronic disease and disability, especially if chronic pain is a problem. Examples of these therapies include acupuncture, acupressure, imagery, and music. Chapter 4 discusses CAM in detail.

Community-Based Care

Discharge planning begins during the client's admission. If the client is being transferred from a hospital to a rehabilitation unit or facility, orient him or her to the change in routine and emphasize the importance of self-care. When the client is admitted to the rehabilitation unit or facility, the case manager assesses his or her current living situation at home. Together with the client and family members or significant others, the case manager determines the adequacy of the current situation and the potential needs after discharge to home. The client with chronic illness and disability may require home care, assistance with activities of daily living (ADLs), nursing care, or physical or occupational therapy after discharge. The case manager assesses these needs and plans with the client, family or significant other, social worker, physical or vocational therapist, and physician the best ways to meet identified needs.

Other health care professionals may be necessary to meet the unique needs of special populations. For example, clients with brain injury may benefit from life planning, a process that examines and plans to meet lifelong needs. Case managers specializing in life planning may be part of the interdisciplinary rehabilitation team.

HOME CARE MANAGEMENT

Before the client returns home, the nurse assesses his or her readiness for discharge from the rehabilitation facility or hospital. The home may be assessed in multiple ways.

PREDISCHARGE ASSESSMENT. Before discharge, the case manager or occupational therapist may visit the home to assess its layout and accessibility. These professionals may be employed by the health care agency or by a third-party payer, such as a health maintenance organization (see Chapter 3 for a discussion of third-party payers). Because of the stress of hospitalization, a client with a fractured hip who is ambulating well with a walker may neglect to explain to the nurse that the home has three steps at the entrance and that the bathroom is accessible by stairway only. The client may not consider it important to mention that throw rugs, which do not provide a completely level surface on which to use a cane, are scattered throughout the apartment.

During a predischarge visit to the home, the case manager assesses the accessibility of the home in general and of the bathrooms, bedrooms, and kitchen. If the client will be wheelchair dependent after discharge from the facility, ramps are needed to replace steps, and doorways should be checked for adequate width. A doorway width of 36 to 38 inches (slightly less than 1 m) is usually sufficient for a standard-sized wheelchair. Any room that the client needs to use is checked. The bedroom should have sufficient space for the client to maneuver transfers to and from the wheelchair and the bed.

Space requirements depend on the client's need to use a wheelchair, walker, or cane. In the bathroom, grab bars may need to be installed before the client comes home. Bathtub benches can provide support for the client who has difficulty with mobility and, when used in combination with a handheld shower head, can provide easily accessible bathing facilities. Assessment of the kitchen may or may not be critical depending on whether the client has help with cooking and preparing meals. If the client will be responsible for cooking after discharge, the kitchen is assessed for wheelchair or walker accessibility, appliance accessibility, and the need for adaptive equipment.

LEAVE-OF-ABSENCE VISIT. A second method of assessing the client's home is through a brief home visit, also called a leave-of-absence (LOA) visit, by the client before discharge. The nurse explains the need for the trial home visit and assesses the client's comfort level with this idea. The client who has been hospitalized for a lengthy period may feel intense anxiety about returning home. The nurse may allay such anxieties with careful preparation. Before the visit, the rehabilitation nurse meets with the client and family members or significant others to set goals for the visit and to identify specific tasks to be attempted while at home. After the home visit, the client is interviewed to determine the success of the visit and to assess additional education or training needs before final discharge.

Going home may not be an option for everyone. Some clients may not have a support network of family members or significant others. For example, many older adults have no spouse or close friends living nearby. Children may live far away, which can make home care difficult. If no caregiver is available, the family must decide whether care can be provided in the home by an outside resource or whether the client needs to be admitted to a 24-hour supervised health care setting, such as a nursing home. Rehabilitation services are available in most long-term care settings (skilled nursing facilities) at least 5 days a week.

HEALTH TEACHING

Education of the client and the family is the cornerstone of nursing care. Assess every component of care to determine how to teach the client to perform activities of daily living (ADLs) independently. Determine the client's learning potential and cognitive capacity and encourage him or her to perform or direct each skill or technique independently to verify understanding. Written material explaining the steps in the procedure is provided to the client and family members to reinforce learning and to provide support with the technique after discharge. Before distributing written material, the rehabilitation team assesses the reading level of the material and determines whether it is appropriate for the client's reading ability and language skills.

Any chronic illness or disability necessitates changes in lifestyle and body image. The nurse assists in dealing with such changes by encouraging the verbalization of feelings and emotions. A focus on existing capabilities instead of disabilities is emphasized.

The client may fail to relate psychologically to the disability during hospitalization. For example, he or she may display anger or frustration in attempting to perform self-care routines before discharge from the rehabilitation facility. Encourage the client to be open about such feelings and to talk about ways to prevent worries from becoming realities after discharge.

The leave-of-absence home visit assists the client and family members or significant others in psychosocial preparation for discharge. It allows the experience of the home situation while being able to return to the hospital environment after a few hours. Often the client finds that his or her fears were not realized during the home visit but finds new problems in the home that must be addressed before discharge. Review this information with the client in preparation for discharge to the home.

HEALTH CARE RESOURCES

After discharge to the home, various health care resources (e.g., physical therapy, home care nursing, and vocational counseling) are available to the client with chronic illness and disability. Assess the need for additional care and support throughout the hospitalization and collaborate with the case manager and physician in arranging for home services.

Evaluation: Outcomes

The client and rehabilitation team evaluate the effectiveness of interdisciplinary interventions on the basis of the identified nursing diagnoses and collaborative problems. Expected outcomes may include that the client will:

- Move purposefully in his or her environment with or without assistive devices.

- Perform the most basic physical tasks and personal care activities independently with or without assistive devices.
- Have structural intactness and physiologic function of the skin.
- Have normal collection and discharge of urine.
- Have normal formation and evacuation of stool.
- Take personal actions to manage stressors that tax the client's resources.

GET READY for the NCLEX Examination!

KEY POINTS

- Rehabilitation is the process of learning to live with chronic and disabling conditions.
- Clients in a rehabilitation setting are managed by an interdisciplinary team of health care professionals; the client is also a member of the team.
- Assessment of the client in rehabilitation includes the components that are listed in Table 10-1.
- The Functional Independence Measure (FIM) system is used to assess functional ability of the client in rehabilitation.
- The members of the interdisciplinary team teach clients how transfer, bed mobility, and gait training techniques.
- The client is taught how to perform activities of daily living with or without using adaptive devices; the client should be encouraged to be as independent as possible.
- One of the goals of nursing care is to prevent complications of immobility for the client (see Table 10-2).
- Clients in rehabilitation should be assessed for risk factors that make them likely to develop skin breakdown; interventions to prevent skin problems include repositioning and adequate nutrition.
- Clients with bladder and bowel problems are managed by training programs; spastic, flaccid, and uninhibited elimination are managed differently (see Tables 10-5 and 10-6).
- Nurses and other health care team members assist clients to cope with their losses and assess the availability of client support systems.

ADDITIONAL STUDY RESOURCES

Go to your Student CD-ROM for Review Questions for the NCLEX Examination.

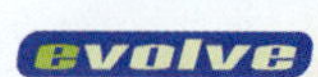
Go to http://evolve.elsevier.com/Iggy/ for Integrated Management of Care Questions for the NCLEX Examination.

SELECTED BIBLIOGRAPHY

Asterisk indicates a classic or definitive work on this subject.

Association of Rehabilitation Nurses. (2000a). *Standards and scope of rehabilitation nursing practice.* Glenview, IL: Author.

Association of Rehabilitation Nurses. (2000b). *The specialty practice of rehabilitation nursing: A core curriculum* (4th ed.). Skokie, IL: Author.

Beck, L.A. (2003). Cancer rehabilitation: Does it make a difference? *Rehabilitation Nursing, 28*(2), 42-47.

*Braden, B.J., & Bergstrom, N. (1992). Pressure reduction. In G.M. Bulechek & J.C. McCloskey (Eds.), *Nursing interventions: Essential nursing treatments* (2nd ed., pp. 94-108). Philadelphia: W.B. Saunders.

Bray, J. (2003). Therapeutic relationships: Building blocks for rehabilitation nursing. *Rehabilitation Nursing, 28*(5), 140.

Dochterman, J.M., & Bulechek, G.M. (2004). *Nursing interventions classification (NIC)* (4th ed.). St. Louis: Mosby.

Gallagner, R.M. (2000). How long-term care is changing. *American Journal of Nursing, 100*(2), 65-67.

Gibson, K.L. (2003). Caring for a patient who lives with a spinal cord injury. *Nursing, 33*(7), 36-41.

Glenn, J. (2003). Restorative Nursing Bladder Training Program: Recommending a strategy. *Rehabilitation Nursing, 28*(1), 15-22.

*Granger, C.V., & Gresham, G.E. (1984). *Functional assessment in rehabilitation medicine.* Baltimore: Williams & Wilkins.

*Granger, C.V., et al. (1993). Performance profiles of the Functional Independence Measure. *Journal of Physical Medicine and Rehabilitation, 72,* 84-89.

Gross, J.C., et al. (2001). Determining stroke rehabilitation inpatients' level of nursing care. *Clinical Nursing Research, 10*(1), 40-51.

*Ignatavicius, D.D. (1998). *Introduction to long term care nursing.* Philadelphia: F.A. Davis.

*Institute of Medicine. (1991). *Disability in America.* Washington, DC: National Academy Press.

*Katz, S., et al. (1963). Studies of illness in the aged. The index of ADL: A standardized measure of biological and psychosocial function. *Journal of the American Medical Association, 185,* 914-919.

Lorig, K.R., Ritter, P.L., & Gonzalez, V.M. (2003). Hispanic chronic disease self-management: A randomized community-based outcome trial. *Nursing Research, 52*(6), 361-369.

Maas, M., Buckwalter, M., Hardy, M., et al. (2001). *Nursing care of older adults: Diagnoses, outcomes, and interventions.* St. Louis: Mosby.

Marrelli, T. (2003). Restorative care and home care: New implications for aide and nurse roles? *Geriatric Nursing, 24*(2), 128-129.

Moorhead, S., Johnson, M., & Maas, M. (2004). *Nursing outcomes classification (NOC)* (3rd ed.). St. Louis: Mosby.

*Nazarko, L. (1999). Rehabilitation. *Nursing Management, 6*(5), 24-27.

Nazarko, L. (2003). Rehabilitation and continence promotion following a stroke. *Nursing Times, 99*(44), 52, 55.

*Neal, L.J. (1995). The rehabilitation nurse in the home care setting: Treating chronic wounds as a disability. *Rehabilitation Nursing, 20*(5), 261-264.

Percentage of deaths due to chronic diseases. (2002). Available at http://ncsl.org/programs/health/phchronic.htm.

*Posavec, E.J., & Carey, R.G. (1982). Using a level of function scale (LORS-II) to evaluate the success of inpatient rehabilitation programs. *Rehabilitation Nursing, 7*(6), 17-19.

Pryor, J. (2000). Creating a rehabilitative milieu. *Rehabilitation Nursing, 25*(4), 141-144.

*Sorensen, B., & Luken, K. (1999). Improving functional outcomes with recreational therapy. *The Case Manager, 10*(5), 48-53.

*Wood, C., & Lui, J. (1999). The evolution of disability care and case management: Identifying core competencies. *The Case Manager, 10*(4), 41-46.

*World Health Organization. (1980). *International classification of impairments, disabilities and handicaps.* Geneva: Author.

CHAPTER

11

Genetic Concepts for Medical-Surgical Nursing

M. LINDA WORKMAN

LEARNING OUTCOMES

After studying this chapter, you should be able to:

1. Describe the structure and forms of DNA.
2. List the events and processes involved in DNA replication.
3. Describe the relationship between genes and proteins.
4. Compare the concept of phenotype with that of genotype.
5. Compare the patterns of inheritance for single gene traits.
6. Explain how genetic variations can induce or affect adult health problems.
7. List 10 adult health problems that have a genetic basis.
8. Identify assessment questions that help obtain information for a genetic assessment.
9. Construct a three-generation pedigree.
10. Identify clients at risk for a genetic predisposition for health problems.
11. Explain how genetic testing is different from other laboratory tests.
12. Describe the role of the medical-surgical nurse in genetic counseling.

Go to your Student CD-ROM for Review Questions for the NCLEX Examination keyed to these Learning Outcomes.

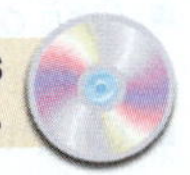

Many scientific advances are leading to better health by preventing illness, disease, or disability and by improving interventions to treat health problems that do occur. For example, 50 years ago only about 15% of clients diagnosed with cancer lived 5 years, and even fewer were cured. Today more than 50% of clients diagnosed with cancer in North America are cured of the disease, and many others will live 5 years or longer. Advances in cancer prevention, diagnosis, and treatment have made these improvements possible.

One of the most important areas of advancement is in the understanding of the influence of genetic factors on adult health and adult illness. These advances, marked by completion of the first phase of the Human Genome Project, led to a whole new era, called **genomic medicine.** Genomic medicine, or "genomics," will lead to drug therapies that take into account each client's genetic differences, allowing a drug regimen to be tailored for a specific client. Genomics also will help to identify clients at risk for specific health problems so that prevention and early detection strategies can be better targeted.

Nursing organizations, such as the American Nurses Association and the American Academy of Nursing, support the need for all nurses to have a basic understanding of genetics to provide the best possible care for clients and families (Grady & Collins, 2003; Lea, 2002a). Many common adult health problems (e.g., hypertension, diabetes, heart disease, cancer, arthritis, and many others) have a genetic basis. Changes in genes (mutations or variations) can have serious results. Gene mutations/variations can increase the risk for a disorder and thus are known as "susceptibility" genes or gene differences. Other gene mutations/variations decrease the risk for a disorder and thus are known as "protective" genes or gene differences. The purpose of this chapter is to help you learn more about basic genetics and how this information relates to adult health care. Table 11-1 defines commonly used genetic terms.

GENETIC BIOLOGY

All living things, including people, animals, plants, and microorganisms, have genes. Genes are the instructions for the making of all the different substances any organism makes. Think of all the hormones, enzymes, and other proteins your body makes. It is the specific genes that tell each cell what protein to make, how to make it, when to make it, and how much to make. Think of each gene as a specific "recipe" for making a certain protein.

So where are these genes? The genes are located in the nucleus of most body cells. As shown in Figure 11-1, the cell nucleus contains the DNA in the form of chromosomes. It is interesting that all cells with a nucleus contain all the

TABLE 11-1 Genetic Terms and Concepts

allele One of possible alternate forms of a gene. Can be due to a variation in a gene sequence or to the existence of many slightly different genes (within a species) coding for the same single trait.

base pairs Nucleotides that pair up loosely together when DNA is double-stranded. They are held together with the relatively weak forces of hydrogen bonds. Normally, adenine and thymine form a pair by sharing two hydrogen bonds; cytosine and guanine form a base pair sharing three hydrogen bonds.

complementary bases The nitrogenous bases that normally pair using hydrogen bonds. Adenine and thymine are complementary to each other. Cytosine and guanine are complementary to each other. Because these pairs are complementary (and faithful), if the sequences of bases for one strand of DNA is known, the complementary strand can be predicted.

chromosome A temporary but consistent state of cellular DNA tightly condensed and coiled into dense bodies that take up stain and are visible under a microscope during metaphase of mitosis.

euploid The normal or expected number of chromosomes for the species.

diploid (2N) This is the complete set of chromosome pairs found in all the individual's somatic cells. The normal diploid chromosome number for humans is 46 (23 pairs). The normal diploid chromosome number for mice is 40 (20 pairs).

haploid (1N) A set of chromosomes consisting of half of each pair. The normal haploid number of human chromosomes is 23. Only the sex cells (ova and sperm) have the haploid number so that fertilization results in the normal diploid number.

centromere The "pinched-in" area of a chromosome where the two chromatids are joined.

chromatid The longitudinal half of a metaphase chromosome (split through the centromere). This structure actually is the original and duplicated DNA that has not yet separated during mitosis.

"p" arm The short "arm" of a chromosome above the centromere.

"q" arm The long "arm" of a chromosome below the centromere.

autosomes The 22 pairs of human chromosomes that do not code for the sexual differentiation of the individual.

sex chromosomes The pair of chromosomes that code for the sexual differentiation of the individual. In males the sex chromosomes are usually an X and a Y. In females the sex chromosomes are usually two Xs.

nucleoside A nitrogenous base of adenine, guanine, cytosine, or thymine attached to a five-sided sugar (ribose sugar).

nucleotide A nucleoside (nitrogenous base attached to a five-sided sugar) connected to a phosphate group. It is this structure that assembles into a single strand of DNA.

concordance The frequency with which a specific trait or condition is found in both members of a natural pair. When such a trait/condition is present in both members of a natural pair (as in the case of "identical" twins), the trait/condition is considered genetic in origin.

monozygotic (MZ) siblings These siblings are the product of one fertilized egg that split into two or more equal parts during embryogenesis. The genetic material is identical for all individuals who develop as a result of this split. This is the origin of "identical" twins or triplets.

dizygotic (DZ) siblings Even though these siblings have shared a womb and are born at the same time, they are the result of different fertilized eggs. Their genetic material is not identical and is no more similar than any other siblings. This is the origin of "fraternal" twins, triplets or other multiple births.

codon Think "code"! Each amino acid that makes up a protein has a specific code in the DNA. This is made up of a three-base sequence. For example, the DNA code (codon) for the amino acid methionine is TAC (for thymine, adenine, and cytosine).

anticodon The "anticodon" is actually the complementary code of an amino acid.

RNA RNA, or ribonucleic acid, is a single strand of nitrogenous bases (adenine, guanine, cytosine, and uracil) constructed during transcription from a segment of DNA containing the gene for a specific protein. The RNA is complementary to the "template" DNA. A major difference in RNA is the use of the base "uracil" in place of thymine.

transcription The process of making a new strand of DNA or RNA that is complementary to the original or "template" DNA. When a cell is dividing, both entire strands of DNA are transcribed so that there is sufficient DNA for each of the two new "daughter" cells. When a protein is going to be made, only the segment of DNA that contains the gene for the protein is transcribed into RNA.

translation The using of a messenger RNA molecule as the directions for proper placement of amino acids during protein synthesis.

ribose A five-sided sugar with a hydroxyl group (OH) on the number 2 carbon. This type of sugar forms an attachment with the bases that compose the RNA nucleotides (adenosine, guanosine, cytidine, and uridine).

deoxyribose A five-sided sugar with a hydrogen molecule (and no oxygen) on the number 2 carbon. This type of sugar forms an attachment with the nitrogenous bases that compose DNA nucleotides (adenosine, guanosine, cytidine, and thymidine).

gene expression The activation of a gene leading to the transcription, translation, and synthesis of a specific protein. The result of gene expression is the observable presence of the specific trait or condition coded for by the gene.

genome The complete set of genes for the species.

gene locus The exact location of a gene on a specific chromosome.

genotype The exact allele pair composition for any given single gene trait. When both alleles are identical *(homozygous),* genotype and phenotype are the same. When a gene's alleles are different from each other *(heterozygous),* the actual genotype may be different from what is observed *(phenotype).*

phenotype The observed expression of any given single trait (e.g., blood type, hair color, presence of male secondary sexual characteristics).

homozygous Having identical alleles (two) at a gene chromosome locus for a specific single gene trait.

heterozygous Having two different alleles at a gene chromosome locus for a specific single gene trait.

mutation An alteration in the base sequence of a gene that has deleterious effects on the function of the gene's product.

polymorphism An alteration in the base sequence of a gene that has minimal effects on the function of the gene's product.

genes. At one time, science tried to explain how different cells have different functions by suggesting that the genes of different cells were unique. For example, you make insulin in the beta cells of your pancreas and nowhere else. Wouldn't it make sense that the reason only the beta cells can make insulin is that they are the only cells that have the gene for insulin? Well, even though that theory makes some sense, it is not the case. In fact *all* human cells with a nucleus have the gene for insulin. The only cell type, however, that allows the insulin gene to be active and make insulin is the beta cell of the pancreas. We have the insulin gene in our skin cells, heart cells, brain cells, and other cells, but only in the beta cells is this gene selectively "turned on" **(expressed)** when you need to make insulin.

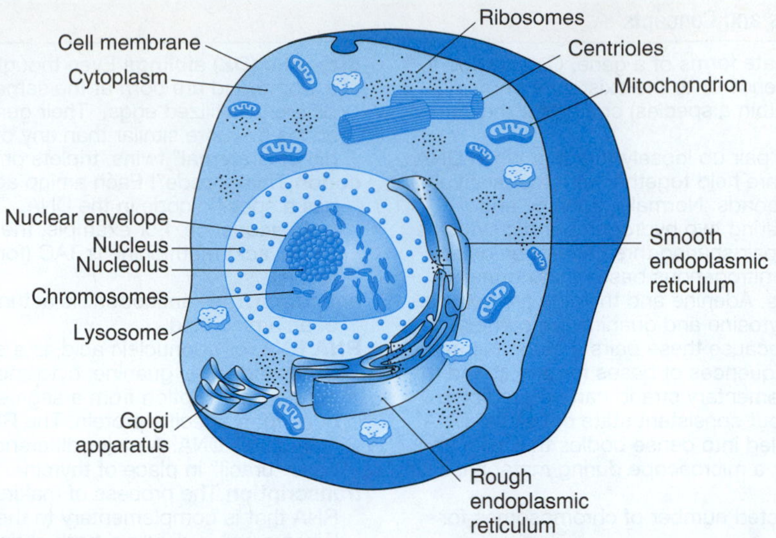

Figure 11-1 ■ Anatomy of a cell.

An important fact to remember is that all human cells with a nucleus each contain the entire set of human genes. This complete set of genes is called the **genome.** The human genome contains about 35,000 individual genes (Collins et al., 2003).

The only exceptions for chromosomes are the mature red blood cells, which have no nucleus, and the sex cells (the eggs and sperm). Sex cells have only one chromosome of each pair (thus 23 chromosomes) so that when an egg is fertilized by a sperm, the chromosomes unite to form a new individual with 46 chromosomes.

One area that is somewhat confusing about genetics is how DNA (deoxyribonucleic acid) is different from the genes and from the chromosomes. DNA, chromosomes, and genes are all the same basic thing; only the structures differ. Figure 11-2 shows that if we pick out any one chromosome in the nucleus, we can "unwind" it and see that the framework of any chromosome is the DNA. Each chromosome has many genes within it. Humans have 23 pairs of chromosomes–46 individual chromosomes. The Y chromosome, a small chromosome, has only 78 genes. Larger chromosomes, such as the number 1 chromosome, contain thousands of genes.

One way to think of it is to consider all the DNA in any cell's nucleus to be a giant "cookbook" containing all the recipes needed to make all the proteins, hormones, enzymes, and other substances your body needs. The chromosome pairs are the different book chapters (so the human genome cookbook has 23 chapters), and the genes are the individual recipes contained within the chapters.

There is a specific chromosome location **(locus)** for every gene. For example, the locus for the gene for blood type is on chromosome 9. The locus for the gene for the beta chain of hemoglobin is on chromosome 11. The first phase of the Human Genome Project determined the exact sequence of DNA and the location of many genes. Figure 11-2 shows that each chromosome is made up of a large chunk of DNA that has been twisted (like a length of rope) until it coils up tightly into a very dense structure. Thus in each cell the DNA is divided into 46 separate chunks.

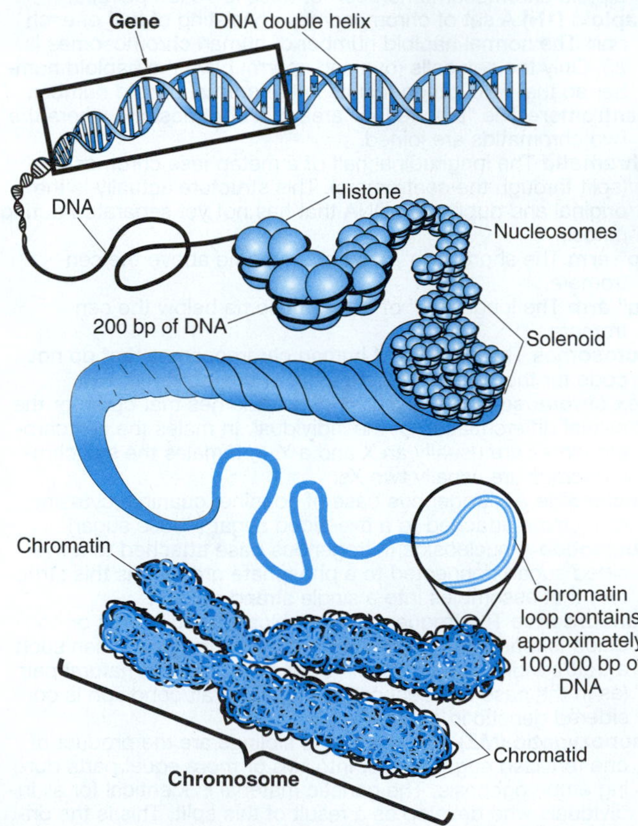

Figure 11-2 ■ Coiling loose DNA tightly into a chromosome.

Deoxyribonucleic Acid

DNA is short for **deoxyribonucleic acid,** which is the basic genetic material in a cell that contains genes. Most DNA (about 99.99%) is in the nucleus. A small amount of DNA is also present in other cell organelles, such as the mitochondria. This chapter focuses on the nuclear DNA.

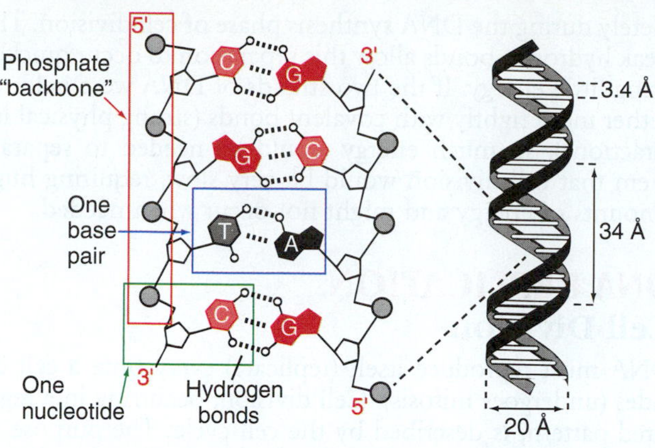

Figure 11-3 ■ The structure of DNA.

DNA STRUCTURE

In humans, DNA is a linear, double-stranded structure composed of multiple units of four different nitrogenous bases, each attached to a sugar molecule. The bases in each strand are connected together by phosphate groups. The two individual strands are held together (loosely) by hydrogen bonds interacting with the base pairs of the two strands.

This double-stranded DNA is arranged like a long set of railroad tracks. The "backbones" of the track are the two long steel rails. For DNA these backbones are the phosphate groups that hold the strand of bases together (like beads on a string with the string being the backbone). The bases are the individual railroad ties (or beads). Think of each tie as having two pieces, one piece attached to the right-handed rail and one piece attached to the left-sided rail.

Figure 11-3 shows a very small piece of double-stranded DNA on the left (containing only four base pairs) taken from the larger piece of DNA on the right. The phosphate groups that hold the nucleotides together as a strand are in the red box. The green box in the lower left-hand section shows a whole nucleotide (a base with the sugar and the phosphate group) in place in the left-hand DNA strand. The blue box in the middle of the two strands shows how the base from the left strand lines up with and pairs to a complementary base in the right strand.

Bases

Many trillions of bases in the double-stranded DNA are found in the nucleus of just one cell. In fact, if you could crack the cell open like an egg, then extract the nucleus (yolk) and open it, the amount of DNA in the nucleus, stretched out, is about 6 feet long. If the DNA in one cell could be made large enough to see and touch (about the width of a tape measure), it would be long enough to stretch out more than 1000 feet! There is much more DNA in each nucleus than is needed for the 35,000 genes. The gene DNA makes up only about 5% of all the DNA in each cell. What is known about all that extra DNA is discussed on p. 139.

The four bases in DNA are adenine (A), guanine (G), cytosine (C), and thymine (T). These four bases are made from vitamins and the nitrogen atoms from amino acids. For example, thymine is made from folic acid and nitrogen. Two of the bases (thymine and cytosine) are called **pyrimidines** because

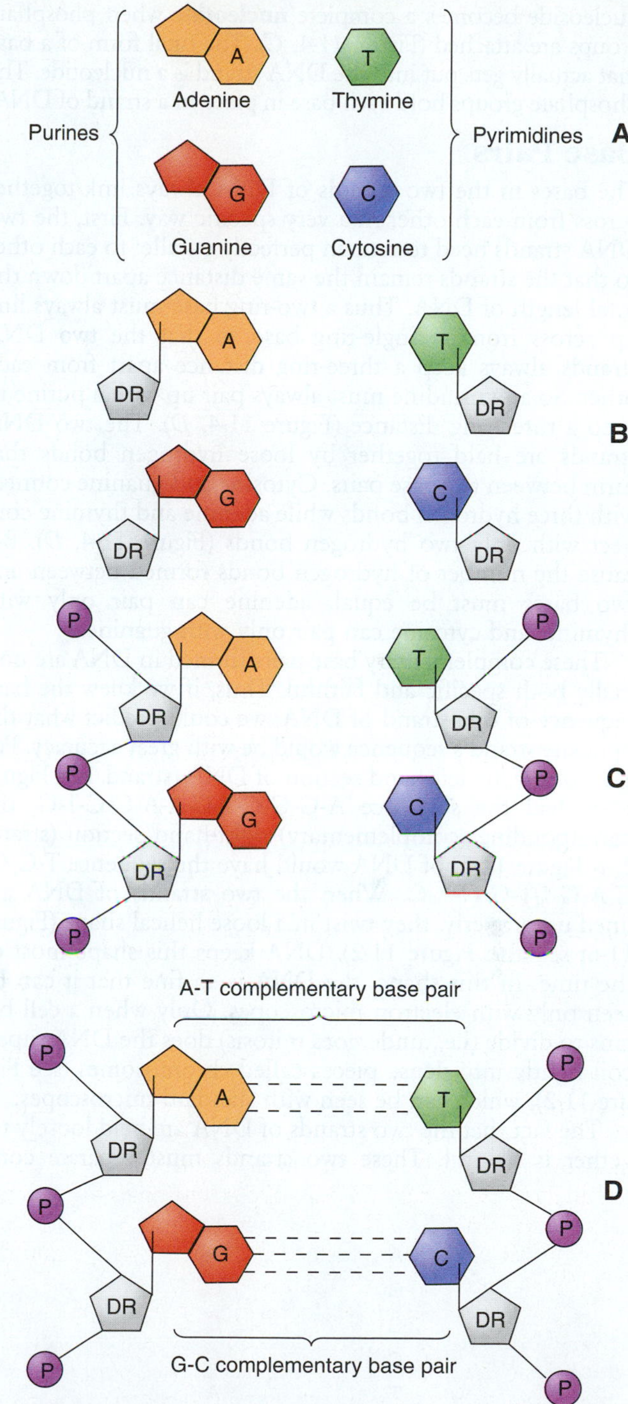

Figure 11-4 ■ Close view of DNA. **A,** The four nitrogenous bases of DNA. **B,** Nitrogenous bases converted into nucleosides by attaching a deoxyribose sugar (DR). **C,** The four nucleosides converted into nucleotides by attaching phosphate groups (P). **D,** Two short strands of DNA held loosely together by hydrogen bonds forming complementary base pairs. ––––, weak hydrogen bonds.

of their single-ringed chemical structures (Figure 11-4, *A*). The other two bases (adenine and guanine) are called **purines** because of their double-ringed chemical structures.

Each base becomes a **nucleoside** when a five-sided sugar (known as a deoxyribose sugar) is attached to it. Figure 11-4, *B* shows how the four bases become four nucleosides. Each nucleoside becomes a complete **nucleotide** when phosphate groups are attached (Figure 11-4, *C*). The final form of a base that actually gets put into the DNA strand is a nucleotide. The phosphate groups hold each base in place in a strand of DNA.

Base Pairs

The bases in the two strands of DNA always link together across from each other in a very specific way. First, the two DNA strands need to remain perfectly parallel to each other so that the strands remain the same distance apart down the total length of DNA. Thus a two-ring base must always line up across from a single-ring base so that the two DNA strands always keep a three-ring distance apart from each other. So a pyrimidine must always pair up with a purine to keep a three-ring distance (Figure 11-4, *D*). The two DNA strands are held together by loose hydrogen bonds that form between the base pairs. Cytosine and guanine connect with three hydrogen bonds while adenine and thymine connect with only two hydrogen bonds (Figure 11-4, *D*). Because the number of hydrogen bonds formed between any two bases must be equal, adenine can pair only with thymine, and cytosine can pair only with guanine.

These complementary base pairs formed in DNA are normally both specific and faithful. Thus, if we knew the base sequence of one strand of DNA, we could predict what the opposite strand's sequence would be with great accuracy. For example, if the left-hand section of DNA (strand 1 in Figure 11-5) had the sequence A-G-G-C-T-C-A-A-C-C-T-G, the corresponding (complementary) right-hand section (strand 2 in Figure 11-5) of DNA would have the sequence T-C-C-G-A-G-T-T-G-G-A-C. When the two strands of DNA are lined up properly, they twist in a loose helical shape (Figure 11-6; see also Figure 11-2). DNA keeps this shape most of the time. In this shape, the DNA is so fine that it can be seen only with electron microscopes. Only when a cell begins to divide (i.e., undergoes mitosis) does the DNA supercoil tightly into dense pieces called chromosomes (see Figure 11-2), which can be seen with standard microscopes.

The fact that the two strands of DNA are held loosely together is helpful. These two strands must separate completely during the DNA synthesis phase of cell division. The weak hydrogen bonds allow this separation to occur quickly, using little energy. If the two strands of DNA were held together more tightly with covalent bonds (strong physical interactions), so much energy would be needed to separate them that cell division would be very slow, requiring huge amounts of energy and might not occur when needed.

DNA REPLICATION

Cell Division

DNA must reproduce itself (replicate) every time a cell divides (undergoes mitosis). Cell division, occurring in a regulated pattern, is described by the cell cycle. The purpose of mitotic cell division is for one cell to reproduce (duplicate) into two new cells. Each of the two new cells is identical to the original cell that started mitosis. In order for each new cell to have exactly the right amount of DNA and genes, the DNA in the dividing cell must exactly replicate. Figure 11-7 shows the phases of the cell cycle.

Living cells that are not actively reproducing are in a reproductive resting state called G_0. During the G_0 period, cells actively carry out their functions but do not divide. Normal cells spend most of their lives in the G_0 state, just as most humans spend the majority of their lives in a nonpregnant state.

Mitotic cell division makes one cell divide into two cells. These two cells are identical to each other and to the origi-

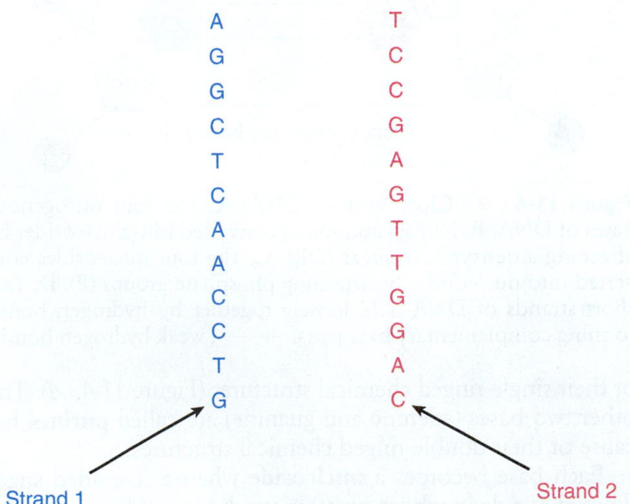

Figure 11-5 ■ Complementary strands of DNA.

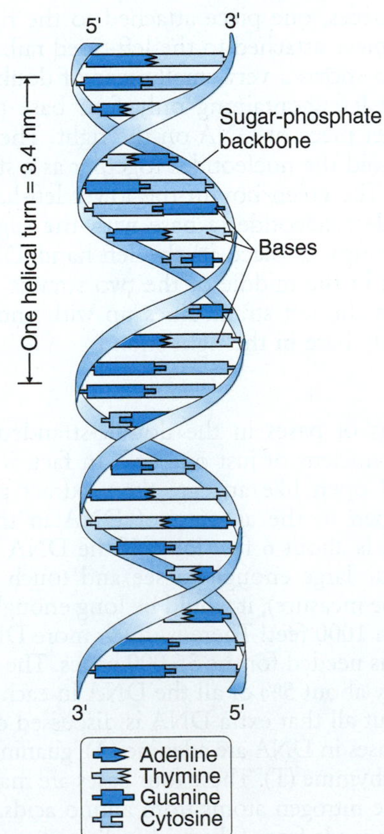

Figure 11-6 ■ Complementary strands of DNA twisted into a loose helical shape.

nal cell that started the mitotic cell division. Cells must go through four phases of the cell cycle to divide:

- ***G_1:*** The cell is getting ready for division by taking on extra nutrients, making more energy, and growing extra membrane. The amount of cell fluid (cytoplasm) also increases.
- ***S:*** Because making one cell into two cells requires twice as much of everything, including DNA, the cell must double its DNA content through DNA synthesis. This process occurs in S phase. First the double strands of DNA must separate. Then enzymes read the sequence of one of the original strands and build a new strand complementary to the original strand. The same thing is happening to the other original strand (Figure 11-8). The process of making a new copy of an entire strand of DNA is called **DNA transcription.**

Numerous enzymes are involved in DNA synthesis. Some of the enzymes "relax" and then "unwind" the double-stranded DNA. Other enzymes separate the two strands and keep them separate. Different enzymes "read" the original DNA strands and determine the order of the bases for the new strands. Special enzymes actually build the new strands by placing and linking nucleotides together. Finally, other enzymes actually "spell check" the new strands of DNA to ensure that each base in the new strand is exactly complementary to its base pair on the original strand.

When DNA synthesis is complete, the result is two sets of double-stranded DNA. Each of the two sets has one old strand and one new strand. Notice in Figure 11-7 that the nucleus during S phase is twice as large as it was during G_1 because it now has twice as much DNA.

During M phase of the cell cycle, one set of DNA will move into one of the two new cells made during mitosis and the second set will move into the other new cell. In this way, every new cell ends up with exactly the right amount of DNA with all the genes.

- ***G_2:*** The cell makes important proteins that will be used in actual cell division and in normal physiologic function after cell division is complete.
- ***M:*** The single cell splits apart into two cells (actual mitosis). It is in this phase, after the DNA has completely replicated itself, that the 46 separate chunks of DNA twist very tightly, bending around small protein balls called histones, to form very dense bodies that can be seen (when stained) using a standard microscope.

These dense bodies are called "chromosomes" because in this form they can take up stain and have color.

Chromosome Formation

It is during M phase that the fact that there is much more DNA in each cell than just the genes is helpful. The delivery of genes to each new cell during mitosis is critical for the new cells to be able to function. Thus, this DNA delivery must be precise and perfect. Having the DNA pack down into chromosomes makes for precise DNA delivery. This works in much the same way that oral drugs do. For example, think about the size of a single aspirin tablet that contains 325 mg of the drug aspirin. This tablet is not very large, only a little over 1 cm in diameter. This tablet also contains some other material that is not aspirin but helps to form the aspirin tablet. Now think about a drug that contains only 1 mg of drug per tablet. If that tablet contained just the 1 mg of drug, the tablet would be too small to handle (about the size of a grain of sand). Thus more material is added with the 1 mg of drug to make the tablet large enough to handle.

If each cell contained only enough DNA to make up the genes, the process of DNA replication and delivery of DNA to the two new cells would be less precise. So there is at least 20 times more DNA than is needed for the 35,000 genes. This extra DNA allows chromosomes to form, which can then be split exactly in half, allowing very precise delivery of DNA to the new cells.

So, as you can see in Figure 11-2, a chromosome is a specific large chunk of double-stranded DNA, with each chunk containing billions of bases and hundreds (and sometimes thousands) of genes. During M phase, each chromosome forms and moves to the center of the cell that is about to divide. Stringlike fibers form from each side of the cell and attach to each chromosome half (chromatid). This action is shown in Figure 11-9 (using just four chromosomes). Just before the cell splits into two cells *(cytokinesis),* each chro-

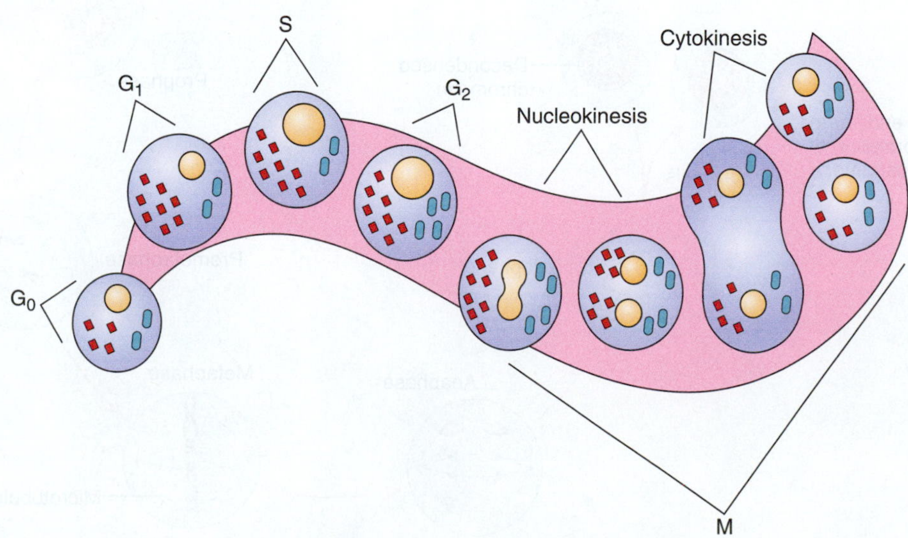

Figure 11-7 ■ The cell cycle.

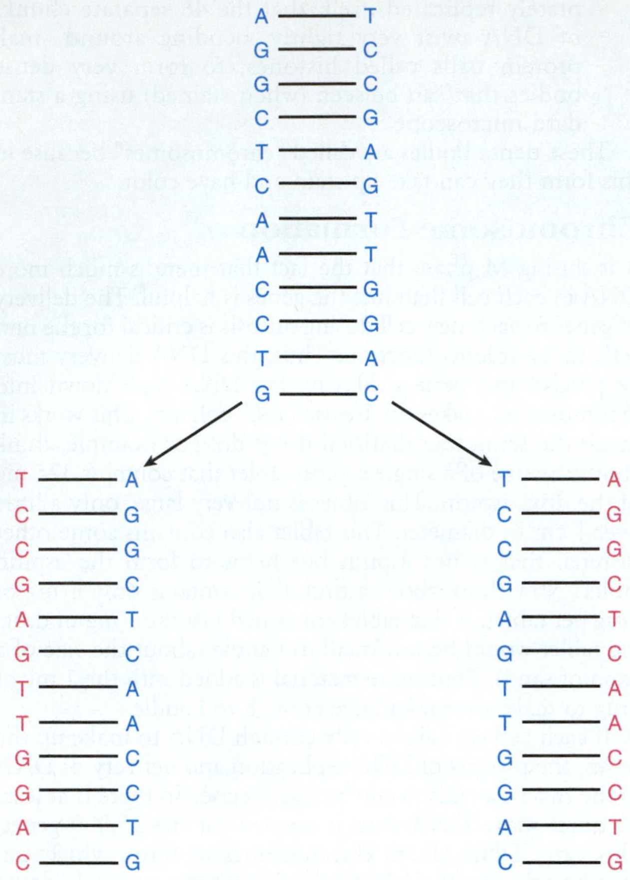

Figure 11-8 ■ DNA replication. *Blue type,* Original DNA; *red type,* newly made (replicated) DNA.

mosome is pulled apart so that half of each chromosome goes into one new cell and the other half goes into the other new cell. The process of pulling the chromosomes apart is called *nucleokinesis.*

Chromosome Function

Chromosomes are temporary structures, but their job is important: precise delivery of DNA to the two new cells. As we have seen, humans have 46 chromosomes divided into 23 pairs. This number is known as the "diploid" number of chromosomes for humans. Remember that each chromosome we view just before cell division actually has twice the DNA in it. This chromosome is going to split down the middle during mitosis, with half of the chromosome going to one new cell and the other half going to the other cell.

Figure 11-10 shows a metaphase chromosome. The "pinched-in" area of the chromosome is the **centromere.** Each longitudinal half of the chromosome is a **chromatid,** shown encircled on the right. The "arms" above the centromere are the short arms, or the "p" arms. The longer arms (not legs) below the centromere are the "q" arms. You may read that a particular gene is located on 9q, meaning that the gene has its location **(locus)** on the long arm of the number 9 chromosome.

The very "tips" of the chromosomes are the **telomeres,** or the telomeric DNA (deep pink area of Figure 11-10 and Figure 11-11). This DNA actually caps each chromosome. Figure 11-11 shows a chromosome lying on its side. The deep pink areas at each end are the telomeres. The inset figure below the chromosome is the enlarged end region and telomere of the chromosome. This region contained many thousands of bases when we were born. With every round of cell

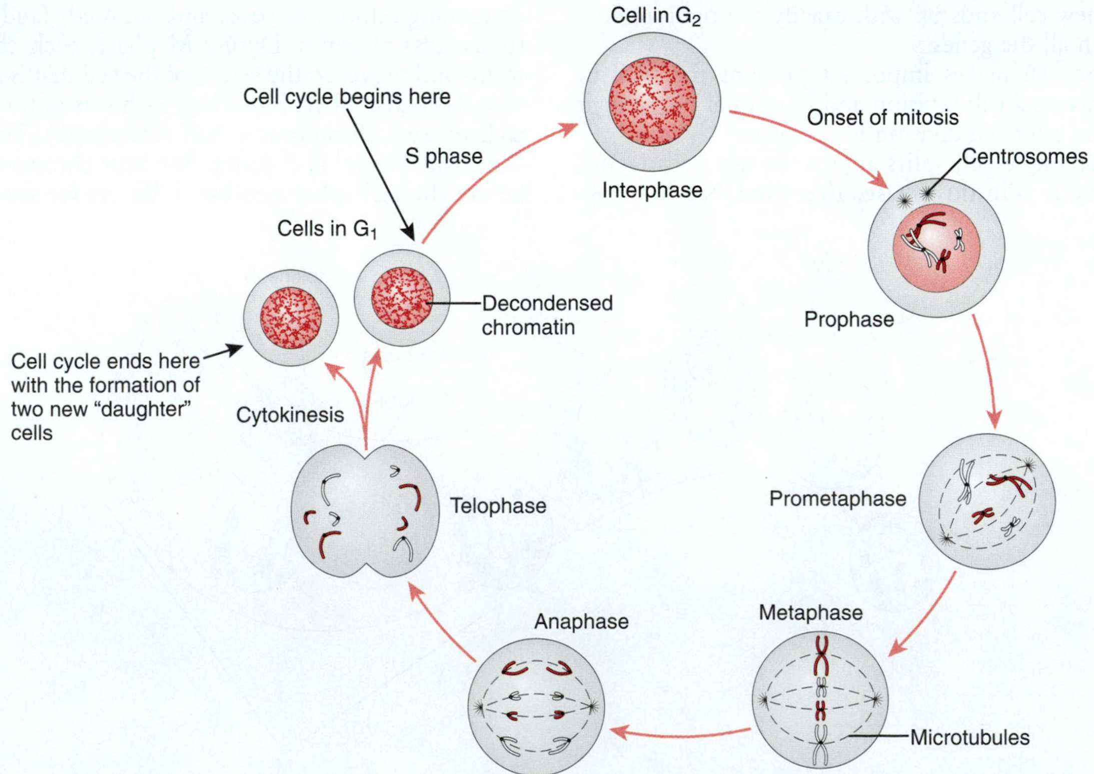

Figure 11-9 ■ DNA changes during the cell cycle. Especially note the four chromosomes lining up during metaphase of mitosis and being pulled apart during anaphase of mitosis.

division, the telomeres of the chromosomes in the cell that just divided are shortened by 50 to 100 bases. Telomeric DNA is not replaced by the cell. As a person ages, the telomeres become shorter. Eventually, the telomere DNA is gone and the chromosomes unravel, which is a signal for the cell to commit "cellular suicide" **(apoptosis)** and die.

Telomeres are related to aging and other important events that happen in the life of the cell. With normal aging, these telomeres shorten until they are gone and the cell then dies. When the cell death rate in any one organ occurs faster than cells can be replaced, the organ cannot function, and death ensues (Novak, 2003). The normal loss of telomeric DNA with each cell division gives all our normal cells a finite life span. The rate at which a person ages is related to the rate of telomere loss. Faster cellular aging occurs with faster rates of telomere loss. Slower cellular aging occurs with slower rates of telomere loss.

Chromosomal Analysis

We can tell some things about a person or their cells by examining chromosomes. It is important to remember that the information that can be obtained by chromosomal analysis is limited because there is a large chunk of DNA in every chromosome. Only very large deletions, additions, or rearrangements of DNA show up at the level of the chromosome. Losses or gains of just a few bases (or even thousands) cannot be detected at the chromosome level. Figure 11-12 shows how the chromosomes of one cell look just before cell division. To analyze chromosomes, they must first be organized into a karyotype.

A **karyotype** is a technique used to make an organized arrangement of all of the chromosomes within one cell during the metaphase section of mitosis (Figure 11-13). A technician first collects the chromosomes into pairs and then lines them up according to size (largest first) and centromere position. This gross organization of DNA can be used to determine missing or extra whole chromosomes and some large structural rearrangements. A missing gene or a mutated gene would not show up at this level of analysis. What we can tell about the person from whom the set of chromosomes in Figure 11-13 was taken is that the person is human, female, and **euploid** (has the correct number of chromosome pairs for the species). We really cannot tell much more than that. This person is chromosomally "normal," although she might have one or more genes that are mutated and "abnormal." If the karyotype is abnormal in any way (had more or less than the normal number or broken chromosomes), the karyotype would be called **aneuploid.**

Autosomes are the 22 pairs of human chromosomes (numbered 1 through 22) that do not code for the sexual differentiation of a person. Autosomal chromosomes contain genes that code for all the structures and regulatory proteins needed for normal function.

Sex chromosomes are the pair of chromosomes that contain the genes for the sexual differentiation of the person. In males the sex chromosomes are an X and a Y. In females the sex chromosomes are two XXs (see Figure 11-13).

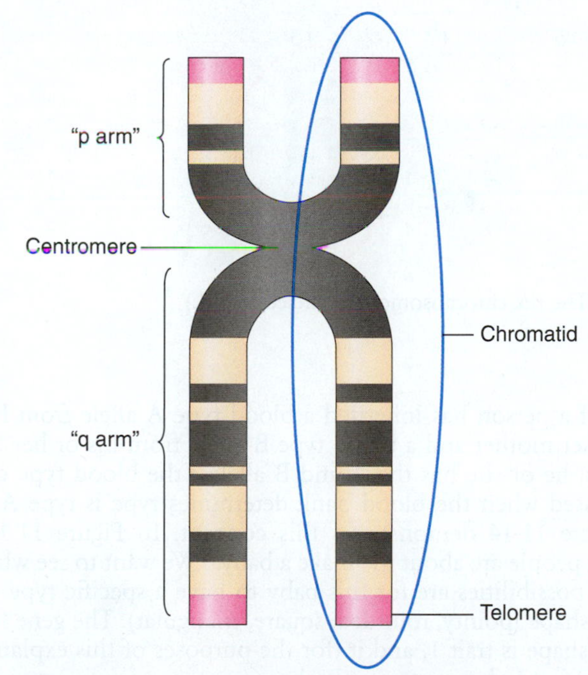

Figure 11-10 ■ A single metaphase chromosome.

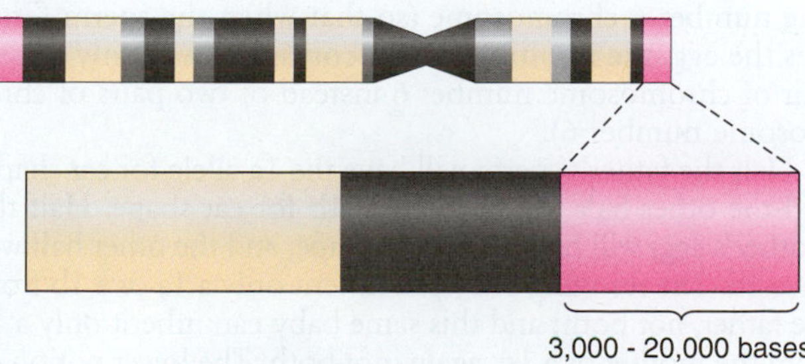

Figure 11-11 ■ Telomeric DNA.

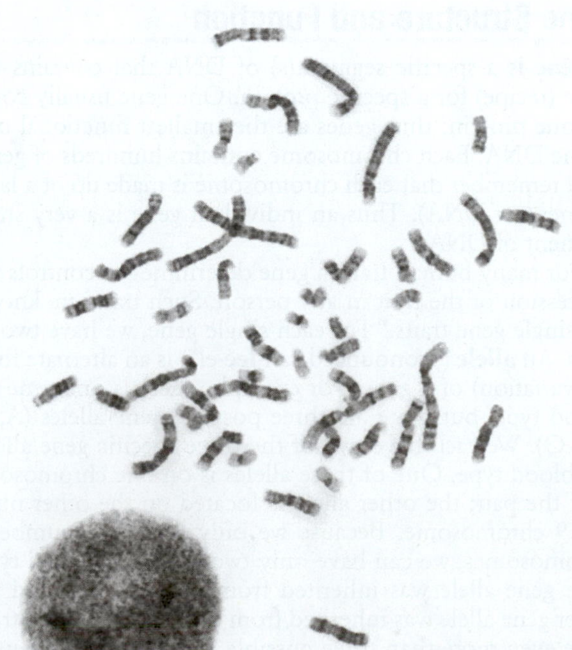

Figure 11-12 ■ A spread of chromosomes from one cell during metaphase of mitosis. (The dark spot in the lower left-hand corner is the nucleus of another cell.)

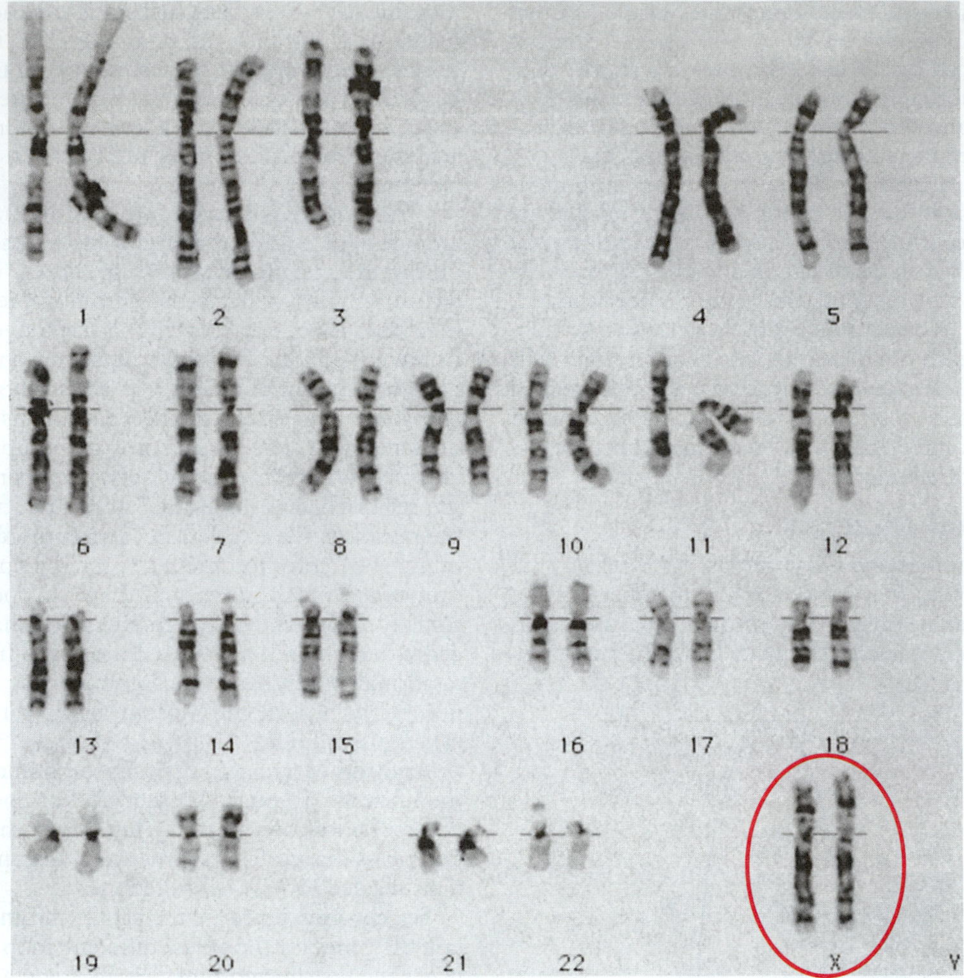

Figure 11-13 ■ A karyotype of a normal female. (The sex chromosomes are circled in red.)

Gene Structure and Function

A **gene** is a specific segment(s) of DNA that contains the code (recipe) for a specific protein. One gene usually codes for one protein; thus genes are the smallest functional unit of the DNA. Each chromosome contains hundreds of genes (and remember that each chromosome is made up of a large segment of DNA). Thus an individual gene is a very small segment of DNA.

For many human traits a gene determines or controls the expression of the trait in any person. Such traits are known as "single gene traits." For each single gene, we have two alleles. An **allele** (pronounced "ah-**lee**-el") is an alternate form (or variation) of a gene. For example, there is one gene for blood type, but there are three possible gene alleles (A, B, and O). We each have two of the three specific gene alleles for blood type. One of these alleles is on one chromosome 9 of the pair; the other allele is located on the other number 9 chromosome. Because we only have two number 9 chromosomes, we can have only two alleles for blood type. One gene allele was inherited from our mothers, and the other gene allele was inherited from our fathers. (Some traits have even more than three possible alleles, but each person only has two.) Which gene alleles we inherit from our parents determines our blood type.

If a person has inherited a blood type A allele from his or her mother and a blood type B allele from his or her father, he or she has the A and B alleles; the blood type expressed when the blood bank determines type is type AB. Figure 11-14 demonstrates this concept. In Figure 11-14, two people are about to "make a baby." We want to see what the possibilities are for this baby to have a specific type of ear shape (pointy, rounded, square, triangular). The gene for ear shape is trait 1, and it (for the purposes of this explanation) is on chromosome number 6.

Each of the father's sperm contains only one number 6 chromosome, and each of the mother's eggs contains only one number 6 chromosome (so that when the sperm fertilizes the egg, the resulting person conceived will only have a pair of chromosome number 6 instead of two pairs of chromosome number 6).

Half the father's sperm will have the 1a allele for ear shape, and the other half will have allele 1b for ear shape. Half the mother's eggs will have 1c for ear shape, and the other half will have 1d. The resulting baby can inherit only a 1a or a 1b from the father, not both; and this same baby can inherit only a 1c from the mother or a 1d, again, not both. The lower potion of Figure 11-14 shows all the combinations possible for each ear shape gene alleles for any child created by these two people.

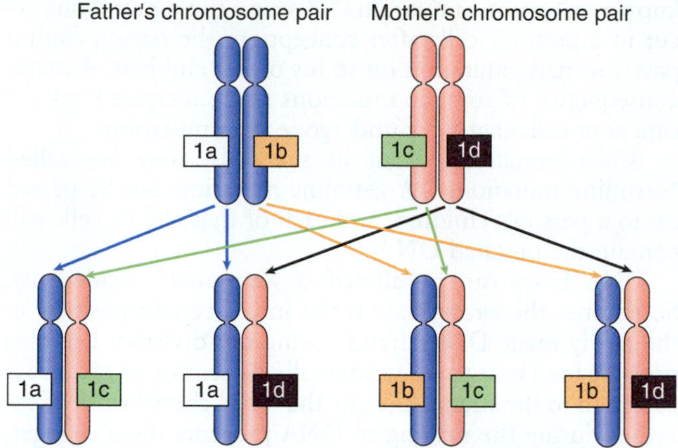

Figure 11-14 ■ Inheritance of four possible alleles for the single gene trait 1. (Any one person can have only two alleles for a single gene trait.)

If a person has two identical alleles for a single gene trait, that person is said to be *homozygous* for that trait. So if a person has an A blood-type gene allele on one number 9 chromosome and an A blood-type gene allele on the other number 9 chromosome, he or she is homozygous for that trait and will express the A blood type.

If a person has two different alleles for a single gene trait, he or she is *heterozygous* for that trait. So if a person has an A blood-type gene allele on one number 9 chromosome and a B blood-type gene allele on the other number 9 chromosome, that person is heterozygous for that trait and will express the AB blood type. Because the A and B alleles are equally dominant *(co-dominant)*, they will both be expressed in the actual blood type.

There are differences in expression of the alleles for a trait depending on whether an allele is dominant or is recessive. If a person has an A blood-type gene allele on one number 9 chromosome and an O blood-type gene allele on the other number 9 chromosome, that person is heterozygous for that trait and expresses only the A blood type. Because the A allele is dominant and the O allele is recessive, they will not both be expressed in the actual blood type. Only the dominant allele is expressed, and the recessive allele is "silent." We will learn more about dominant, recessive, and co-dominant expression later under Patterns of Inheritance on p. 146.

PHENOTYPE

The **phenotype** of any gene for a person is what characteristic can actually be observed or, in some cases, determined by a laboratory test. For example, the person who has the AO gene alleles for blood type has the phenotype of type A blood. A person with curly hair has a curly hair phenotype regardless of whether he or she has two alleles for curly hair or one allele for curly hair and one allele for straight hair.

GENOTYPE

The **genotype** for a person's single gene trait is what the actual alleles are for that trait, not just what can be observed. A person with a phenotype of type A blood could have either an AA genotype or an AO genotype. The person who has type O blood would be known to have an OO genotype. When a person has homozygous alleles for a trait, the genotype and phenotype are the same. When a person has heterozygous alleles for a trait, the phenotype and the genotype are not the same. Recessive traits are expressed only when the person is homozygous for the alleles. Thus for recessive traits phenotype and genotype are the same. Dominant traits are expressed when the person is homozygous for the alleles or heterozygous for the alleles. Thus for dominant traits phenotype and genotype can be the same but do not have to be the same.

Gene Expression

The purpose of a gene is to code for the making of a specific protein used by a cell, tissue, or organ within a person. For example, the hormone insulin is a protein. When a person's blood glucose level starts to rise, the beta cells of the pancreas rapidly make insulin to meet the immediate needs of the person for blood glucose homeostasis.

To continue the cookbook analogy, each gene is the recipe needed to make a specific protein. All the "stuff" that our body makes–every hormone, every enzyme, every growth factor, every biologic chemical needed to keep us functioning–is a protein. These proteins are "gene products" because they are produced when the right gene is "turned on" or "expressed." The following are just a few examples of gene products: insulin, hemoglobin, erythropoietin, angiotensin, and estrogen.

Protein Synthesis

Protein synthesis is the process by which we use genes to make proteins that are needed for proper physiologic function. As you may remember from your science classes, proteins are made up of individual amino acids hooked together like beads on a string. There are 22 different amino acids. Every protein has a specific amount of the amino acids and a specific order in which they are put together. If even one amino acid is out of order or completely deleted from the sequence, the protein will be incorrect and unable to do its job in the body.

For example, the hormone insulin is a protein that contains 51 amino acids in a specific sequence. If some of the amino acids are missing or are in the wrong position, the protein made would be different from real insulin and could not reduce blood glucose levels. Therefore the actual order of the amino acids is critical for the final function of any protein.

Within the DNA there is a code for each amino acid (Table 11-2). Each amino acid code is three bases (nucleotides) long. A gene is the recipe for making a specific protein. It contains all the amino acid codes in exactly the right order for that specific protein. For example, the final active form of the protein insulin has 51 amino acids. Thus the minimum number of bases needed in the gene for insulin would be 153 (three bases per amino acid X 51 amino acids). Figure 11-15 shows an example of short protein made up of only seven amino acids.

Figure 11-16 shows the model of using DNA to make proteins. To think of this process in terms of the cookbook, the entire genome in each cell is the giant cookbook in the library. When a specific protein needs to be made, the chapter for that protein is opened (the chromosome), and the right recipe is found (the gene). The recipe is copied (transcribed) onto a note card (messenger ribonucleic acid, or mRNA) and taken to the kitchen (endoplasmic reticulum). In the kitchen, all the ingredients (amino acids) are put together (translated) in the right order with the help of bowls, ovens, pans, potholders, and other kitchen tools (adapter and transfer molecules). Some foods may need to be altered a little before serving, such as carved, frosted, or peeled (removing extra amino acids to activate the protein).

Many of the steps of protein synthesis use the same enzymes and similar processes as in DNA synthesis, although there are a few differences. During DNA synthesis, the entire DNA strand is transcribed into a new DNA strand. For protein synthesis only the area of the DNA that contains the gene for the specific protein needed is transcribed into RNA.

RNA itself is similar to DNA with a few differences. First the sugar attached to the base is a ribose sugar (hence the name "ribo"nucleic acid). In addition, thymine does not exist in RNA. Instead a similar base called uracil is placed in RNA instead of thymine. This means there is a specific three-base RNA code (called a codon) for each amino acid (see Table 11-2). These RNA codes are complementary to the DNA amino acid codes, with uracil in place of thymine. In addition to the amino acid codes, RNA contains some "stop" codes that tell the process when the protein is finished. Last, RNA is single-stranded instead of double-stranded (Figure 11-17).

Mutations

Mutations are DNA changes that are passed from one generation to another and thus are *inherited.* An inherited mutation does not have to mean that the mutation is passed from one human generation to another. It can mean that the mutation is passed from one *cell* generation to another and thus might affect only certain tissues within a person rather than be a problem within a family. These types of mutations occur in general body cells (somatic cells) and are known as "somatic mutations." Because these mutations occur in a person's cells after conception, the person cannot pass a somatic mutation on to his or her children. A major consequence of somatic mutations is the increased risk for cancer in cells that have undergone such mutations.

When mutations occur in sex cells, they are called "germline mutations." A germline mutation can be passed on to a person's children, and each of that child's cells will contain the mutated DNA.

DNA bases can be altered or "mutated" accidentally. Sometimes the wrong base is put into a certain position in the newly made DNA strand during cell division. It is also possible for a base to be accidentally deleted or an extra base placed in to the strand. Usually the "spell check" work of enzymes during the making of DNA prevents these changes, although some changes probably occur daily in any one person. If these changes occur in a gene area of the DNA, the change can alter the expression of that gene, and an incorrect gene product (protein) might result.

The genes for most proteins are generally the same in all people. Sometimes a base in one person's gene for a specific protein is not the same as that in most people. This difference can be either a variation known as a *single nucleotide polymorphism, or SNP* ("snip"), or it can be a mutation. When a base difference allows the protein to be made but there are differences in how well the protein works, the difference is called a variation or a **polymorphism.** When a base difference causes a loss of protein function, it is called a **mutation.**

TABLE 11-2 Examples of DNA Codes and RNA Codons for Selected Amino Acids

Amino Acid	DNA Code(s)	RNA Codons
Alanine	CGA, CGG, CGT, CGC	GCU, GCC, GCA, GCG
Glycine	CCA, CCG, CCT, CCC	GGU, GGC, GGA, GGG
Isoleucine	TAA, TAG, TAT	AUU, AUC, AUA
Lysine	TTT, TTC	AAA, AAG
Tryptophan	ACC	UGG
Tyrosine	ATA, ATG	UAU, UAC
Start		AUG
Stop		UAA, UAG, UGA

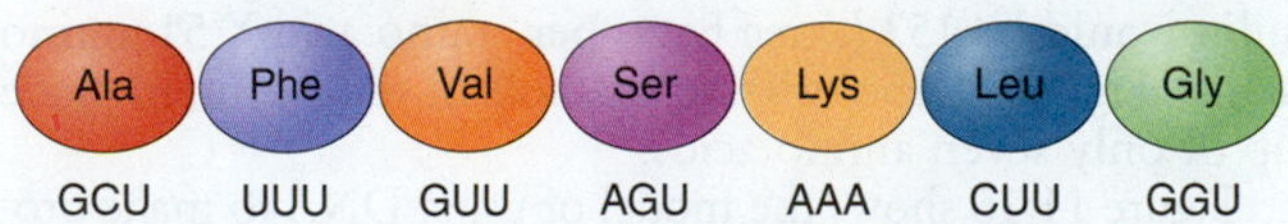

Figure 11-15 ■ A sample protein composed of seven amino acids. The RNA codons for the individual amino acids are listed below each amino acid.

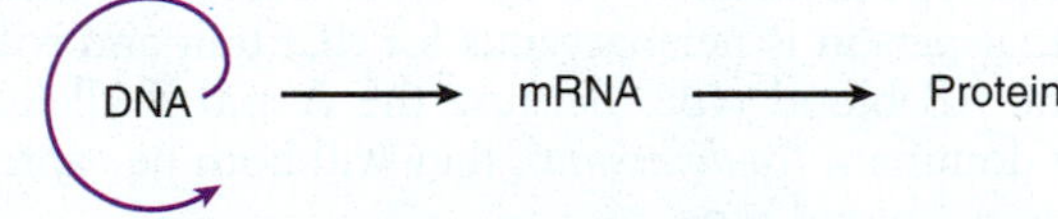

Figure 11-16 ■ The genetic model for protein synthesis.

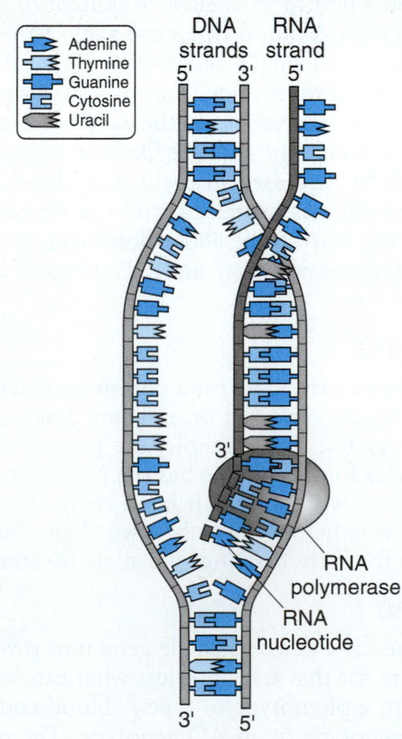

Figure 11-17 ■ RNA transcription for protein synthesis.

POINT MUTATION

The two types of mutations are point mutations and frameshift mutations. **Point mutations** are the substitution of one base for another. A change has been made at a single point of DNA, and the type of change is a base substitution, not a deletion or addition. So the triplets, or three-base codes, remain intact, although one may be incorrect. This change may or may not alter amino acid position or protein synthesis.

Below is an analogy to a point mutation. The top sentence represents the "reading sequence" for a specific gene:

THE BIG DOG ATE THE CAT

THE BIG DOG ATE THE CAP

A point mutation, as seen in the bottom sentence, has changed the *t* in cat to a *p*. The coded message is similar but not exactly the same.

Sometimes a point mutation can change the protein (gene product) a little, but it can still "sort of" work. Sometimes, however, a point mutation changes the protein just enough that it does not work at all. It all depends on how critical the amino acid that changed was to the function of the protein.

For example, the beta chain of hemoglobin in healthy people has the amino acid glutamine in the sixth position (shown in Figure 11-18 in the red box with the DNA code of CTC, the RNA codon of GAG). People who have sickle cell disease have a single base substitution in the gene for the beta chain of hemoglobin, replacing the T with an A (shown in the blue box in Figure 11-18). This results in the DNA code of CAC (instead of CTC), the RNA codon of GUG (instead of GAG), and the placement of valine instead of glutamine in the sixth amino acid position. The altered beta chain will function adequately as part of hemoglobin as long as plenty of oxygen is present. However, when hypoxia occurs in people who have valine rather than glutamine in both of the beta chains of hemoglobin, the chain pulls in on itself and distorts the red blood cell into a sickle shape (see Figure 43-1 in Chapter 43). This shape change causes blood cells to clump and obstruct blood flow to tissues, leading to cell damage and death. So this mutation does not completely disrupt hemoglobin function (which would be incompatible with life) but reduces its efficiency and can have severe consequences.

HbA	1	2	3	4	5	6
DNA	CAC	GTG	GAC	TGA	GGA	CTC
RNA	GUG	CAC	CUG	ACU	CCU	GAG
AAs	val	his	leu	thr	pro	glu

HbS	1	2	3	4	5	6
DNA	CAC	GTG	GAC	TGA	GGA	CAC
RNA	GUG	CAC	CUG	ACU	CCU	GUG
AAs	val	his	leu	thr	pro	val

Figure 11-18 ■ A clinical example of the consequences of a point mutation. *AAs,* Amino acids; *HbA,* adult hemoglobin; *HbS,* sickle cell hemoglobin.

Sometimes an SNP or base substitution does not change the amino acid sequence. For example, Figure 11-19, *A,* shows the original (and correct) DNA codes in a short gene sequence. In Figure 11-19, *B,* there is a point mutation in which the third G in the third DNA code is substituted with a C. Both GGG and GGC code for the amino acid proline, however, and there is no resulting amino acid change in the final protein. This is an example of a "silent" mutation. The mutation did not affect the amino acid sequence of the protein. In Figure 11-19, *C,* a point mutation in the first DNA code substitutes a C in place of a G. This will cause a different amino acid to be placed in the protein. Usually, a different amino acid at least reduces the effect of the protein and may make it nonfunctional altogether. This type of mutation is a "missense" mutation. Some missense mutations cause mild dysfunction or problems and others cause major dysfunction or problems. A nonsense mutation is one in which a single base change, as in Figure 11-19, *D,* results in a "stop" codon; so translation will stop at this point, and a complete protein is not made.

FRAMESHIFT MUTATION

In a **frameshift mutation** a base is added or deleted. This type of mutation always alters amino acid position, disrupts the reading frame, and stops protein synthesis. These changes ruin the reading sequence of the gene from the mutation on down. These changes are very serious because a normal product cannot be made from a gene with such a mutation.

The following is an analogy to a frameshift mutation. The top sentence represents the correct "reading sequence" for a specific gene.

THE BIG DOG ATE THE CAT

THB IGD OGA TET HEC AT

THE PBI GDO GAT ETH ECA T

DNA code	ACG	CTA	GGG	CAC	a. Original DNA codes and amino acids
Amino acid	Cys	Asp	Pro	Val	
DNA code	ACG	CTA	GGC	CAC	b. Silent mutation in which a base substitution does not change the amino acid
Amino acid	Cys	Asp	Pro	Val	
DNA code	ACC	CTA	GGG	CAC	c. Missense mutation in which a base substitution changes the amino acid
Amino acid	Trp	Asp	Pro	Val	
DNA code	ACT	CTA	GGG	CAC	d. Nonsense mutation in which a base substitution causes an early stop signal and an incomplete, nonfunctional protein
Amino acid	Stop	Asp	Pro	Val	

Figure 11-19 ■ Types of point mutations.

A base deletion mutation, as seen in the middle sentence, has removed the *E* in "THE," shifting the rest of the bases to the left (for the three base codes) and disrupting the reading frame. A base addition mutation, as seen in the bottom sentence, has added a *P* to "BIG," shifting the three-base reading codes to the right and disrupting the reading frame. The coded message (recipe) has been lost completely.

Why are we talking about mutations and variations? Changes in genes, even small changes, can have serious results. Some changes would inactivate a protein. Other changes may alter how often or how well a group of cells divides. Gene variations may cause one person to have a greater than normal risk for developing a disease. A different variation in the same gene may cause another person to have a smaller than normal risk for developing the same disease.

PATTERNS OF INHERITANCE

For every single gene trait we each inherit one allele for that gene from our mothers and one allele from our fathers. How these traits are expressed depend on whether one or both alleles are "dominant" or whether one or both alleles are "recessive." Expression also depends on whether the gene for the trait is located on an autosome or on a sex chromosome.

It is possible to determine how the gene for a specific trait is **transmitted** (passed from one human generation to the next). By looking at how that trait is expressed through several generations of a family, patterns emerge that indicate whether that gene is dominant or recessive and whether it is located on an autosomal chromosome or on one of the sex chromosomes. This information can be determined through pedigree analysis. Determining inheritance patterns for a specific trait makes it possible to predict the risk for any one person to have a trait or transmit that trait to his or her children.

Pedigree

A **pedigree** is a graph of a family history for a specific trait or health problem over several generations. Figure 11-20 shows a typical three-generation pedigree. Figure 11-21 shows the accepted symbols used when creating a pedigree. Although the term *pedigree* is the correct genetic term, some clients are offended by this term. You may want to use the term *family tree* in place of pedigree when talking with clients. When analyzing a pedigree, note the answers to the following questions:

- Is any pattern of inheritance present, or does the trait appear sporadic?
- Is the trait expressed equally among males and females or unequally?
- Is the trait present in every generation, or does it skip one or more generations?
- Do only affected individuals have children affected with the trait, or do unaffected individuals also have children who express the trait?

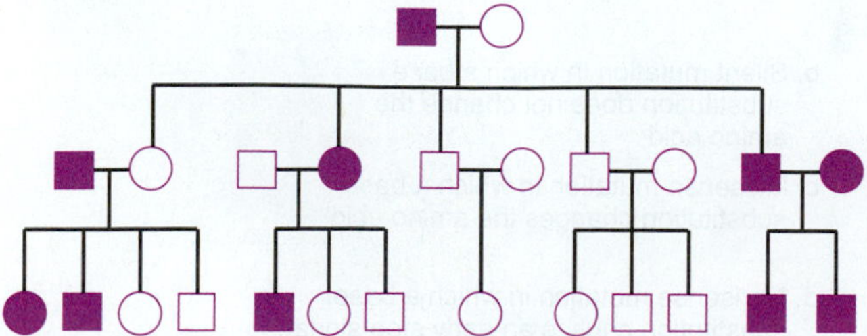

Figure 11-20 ■ A three-generation pedigree showing an autosomal dominant pattern of inheritance.

The four types of inheritance patterns associated with single gene–controlled traits include autosomal dominant, autosomal recessive, sex-linked dominant, and sex-linked recessive. Each inheritance pattern has specific defining criteria. Table 11-3 lists the patterns of inheritance for some disorders that either are identified in adults or may be identified in children who live to adulthood.

Some traits and disorders cluster within a family but do not follow any known pattern of inheritance. Although no specific gene has yet been found for some of these disorders, the clustering suggests a genetic basis. It is thought that for

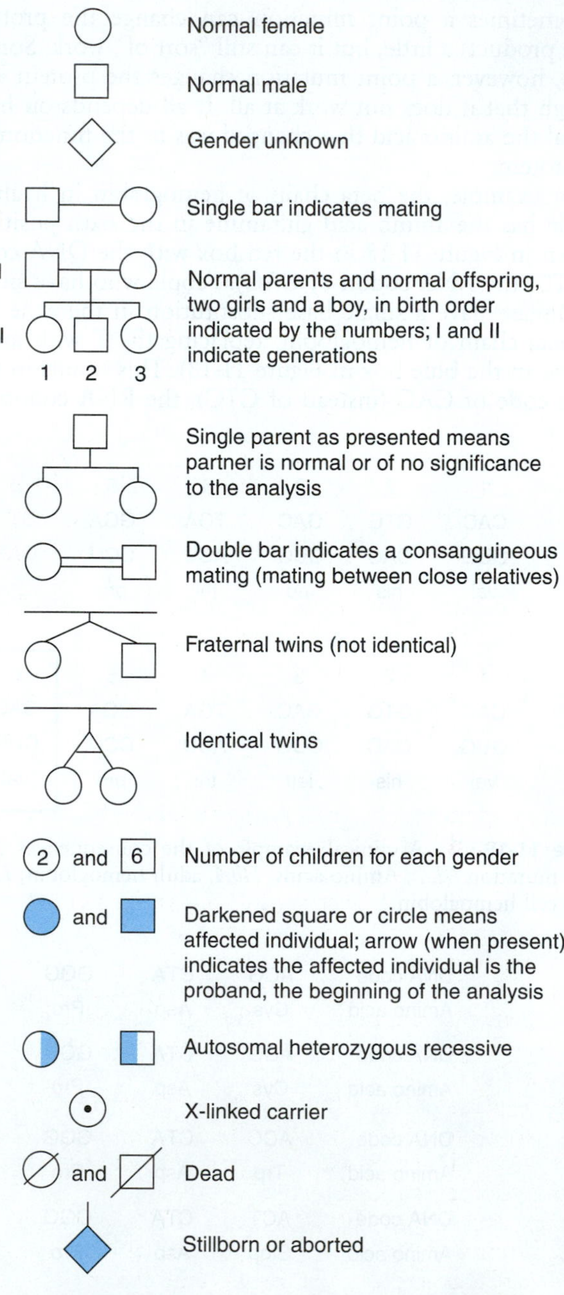

Figure 11-21 ■ Standard pedigree symbols.

some of the disorders that show familial clustering, environmental factors may modify a genetic predisposition. Continued genetic research may solve the familial clustering gene puzzle.

Autosomal Dominant Pattern of Inheritance

Autosomal dominant (AD) single gene traits require that the gene alleles controlling the trait be located on an autosomal chromosome. A dominant gene allele is expressed even when only one allele of the pair is dominant. Other criteria for AD patterns of inheritance include the following:

- The trait appears in every generation with no skipping.
- The risk for an affected person to pass the trait to his or her children is 50% with each pregnancy.
- Unaffected people do not have affected children; therefore their risk is essentially 0%.
- The trait is found equally in males and females.

An example of an AD trait is blood type A. If a person is homozygous for the blood type A allele, he or she will express type A blood (with genotype being identical to the phenotype). If a person is heterozygous for the blood type A allele, with the other allele being type O (which is a recessive trait), he or she will also express type A blood. In this case, however, the phenotype is not identical to the genotype. *When a dominant allele is paired with a recessive allele, only the dominant allele is expressed.* The blood type B allele is also a dominant allele. When a B allele is paired with an O allele, B blood type is expressed. When a person has one blood type A allele and a blood type B allele, however, both alleles are expressed (because they are equally dominant) and the person has type AB blood.

When a person actually has a specific gene allele, he or she is said to "carry" that gene allele. This issue is different from being a "carrier" of a recessive allele. Carrier status is discussed under Autosomal Recessive Patterns of Inheritance on p. 148.

Some health problems are inherited as an autosomal dominant (AD) single gene trait. These problems may not be apparent at birth but develop as the person ages (see Table 11-3). Two factors that affect the expression of some AD single gene traits are penetrance and expressivity.

PENETRANCE

The term **penetrance** describes how often or how well, within a population, a gene is expressed when it is present. Some genes are more penetrant than others. For example, the gene for Huntington disease (HD) is transmitted as an autosomal dominant trait. Therefore, if a person has one HD allele, he or she is at risk for developing HD. This gene is "highly penetrant" (sometimes called "fully penetrant"). This means that if a person has the HD gene allele, his or her risk of expressing the gene and developing the disease is about 99.99%.

Some gene alleles have "reduced" penetrance. This means that even if a person has the gene mutation, his or her risk for this gene being expressed and actually developing the disorder is less than 100%.

Penetrance is calculated by examining a population of people known to have the gene mutation and assessing the percentage that go on to express the gene by developing the disorder. For example, the *BRCA2* gene mutation increases a person's risk for breast cancer. This gene is not fully penetrant, so some women (and men) who have the gene do not develop breast cancer. The penetrance rate for this gene mutation is calculated to be between 60% and 80%, meaning that a person who has the gene mutation has a 60% to 80% risk for developing breast cancer. Although this risk is far higher than among people who do not have this mutant gene, the risk is not 100%. Having the gene mutation does not absolutely predict that the person will develop breast cancer, just that the risk is high.

EXPRESSIVITY

Expressivity is the degree of expression a person has when a specific autosomal dominant gene is present. The gene is always expressed, but some people have more severe results than do other people. For example, the gene mutation for one form of neurofibromatosis (NF1) has an autosomal dominant pattern of inheritance. Some people with this gene have only a few light brown skin tone areas known as café au lait spots. These skin lesions can be so minor that the person may

TABLE 11-3 Patterns of Inheritance for Genetic Disorders Among Adults

Pattern of Inheritance	Disorder
Autosomal dominant	Breast cancer* (mutation of *BRCA1* or *BRCA2* genes) Diabetes mellitus type 2* Familial adenomatous polyposis Familial melanoma Familial hypercholesterolemia Hereditary nonpolyposis colon cancer (HNCC) Huntington disease Long QT syndrome and sudden cardiac death Malignant hyperthermia (MH) Marfan syndrome Myotonic dystrophy Neurofibromatosis (types 1 and 2) Ovarian cancer* (mutation of *BRCA1* genes) Polycystic kidney disease† (types 1 and 2) Retinitis pigmentosa† von Willebrand's disease
Autosomal recessive	Albinism Alpha-1 antitrypsin deficiency Beta thalassemia Bloom syndrome Cystic fibrosis Hereditary hemochromatosis Sickle cell disease Xeroderma pigmentosum
Sex-linked recessive	Glucose-6-phosphate dehydrogenase deficiency Hemophilia Red-green color-blind
Familial clustering	Alzheimer's disease Autoimmune disorders Bipolar disorder Parkinson disease Schizophrenia Hypertension Rheumatoid arthritis

*Some disorders have both a genetic and nongenetic form.
†Some disorders have more than one genetic form and can also be autosomal recessive.

not even be aware that they are present. Other people with the same gene mutation develop hundreds of tumors (neurofibromas) that protrude through the skin. Expressivity accounts for some variation in genetic disease severity.

Autosomal Recessive Pattern of Inheritance

Autosomal recessive (AR) single gene traits require that the gene controlling the trait be located on an autosomal chromosome. The trait can be expressed only when both alleles are present. Table 11-3 lists common adult disorders that have an AR pattern of inheritance. Figure 11-22 shows a typical pedigree for an AR disorder. Criteria for AR patterns of inheritance include the following:

- The trait may not appear in all generations of any one branch of a family.
- The trait or characteristic usually first appears only in siblings rather than in the parents themselves.
- About 25% of a family will be affected and express the trait.
- The children of an affected father and an affected mother will *always* be affected (risk is 100%).
- Unaffected people who are carriers (heterozygous for the trait) and do not express the trait themselves can transmit the trait to their children if their partner is either also a carrier or is affected.
- The trait is found equally in males and females.

An example of an AR trait is type O blood. The blood-type O allele is recessive, and both alleles must be type O (homozygous) for the person to express type O blood. If only one allele is a type O allele and the other allele is either type A or type B, the dominant allele will be expressed and the O allele, although present, is not expressed. For AR single gene traits, phenotype and genotype are always the same.

A person who has one mutated allele for a recessive genetic disorder is a **carrier.** A carrier, even though he or she may have one mutated allele, does not usually have any manifestations of the disorder but can pass this mutated allele on to his or her children. For some autosomal recessive disorders, a carrier may have very mild manifestations. One example is sickle cell trait. A person with two sickle cell alleles has the disease and has many associated health problems. A carrier with one sickle cell allele may be healthy most of the time and have manifestations only under conditions of severe hypoxia.

Sex-Linked Recessive Pattern of Inheritance

Some genes are present only on the sex chromosomes. The Y chromosome has only a few genes that are not also present on the X chromosome. These few genes are important for male sexual development. The X chromosome, however, has many single genes that are not present on the Y or elsewhere in the human genome. Some of these genes are specific for female sexual development, but there are also several hundred other genes on the X chromosome that code for other functions. Thus sex-linked patterns of inheritance issues are really issues of X-linked patterns of inheritance. Few traits or disorders have an X-linked dominant pattern of expression, and they are not discussed in this chapter.

Because the number of X chromosomes in males and females is not the same (1:2), the number of X-linked chromosome genes in the two genders is also unequal. Males have only one X chromosome, a condition called hemizygosity for any gene on the X chromosome. As a result, X-linked recessive genes have a dominant expressive pattern of inheritance in males and a recessive expressive pattern of inheritance females. This difference in expression is because males do not have a second X chromosome to balance the expression of any recessive gene on the first X chromosome.

Sex-linked (X-linked) recessive single gene traits require that the gene allele be present on both of the X chromosomes for the trait to be expressed in females (homozygous) and on only one X chromosome for the trait to be expressed in males (hemizygous). Figure 11-23 shows a typical pedigree for an X-linked recessive disorder. Features of X-linked recessive pattern of inheritance include the following:

- The incidence of the trait is much higher among males in a kinship than among females.
- The trait cannot be transmitted from father to son.
- Transmission of the trait is from father to all daughters (who will be carriers).
- Female carriers have a 50% risk (with each pregnancy) of transmitting the gene to their children.

Familial Clustering

Some disorders appear in families at a rate higher than normal and greater than can be accounted for by chance alone; however, no specific pattern occurs within a family. Although clusters suggest a genetic influence, it is likely that additional factors, such as gender and the environment, also influence disease development or disease severity. Such disorders include Alzheimer's disease, Parkinson disease, type 1 diabetes, and many others. These disorders are often called "multifactorial" because although an increased genetic risk

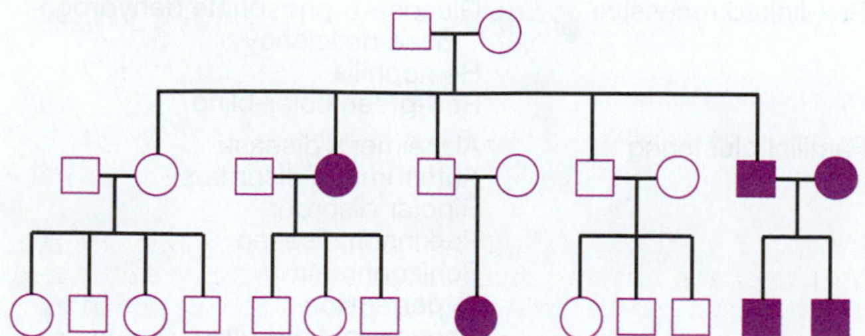

Figure 11-22 ■ A typical pedigree showing an autosomal recessive pattern of inheritance.

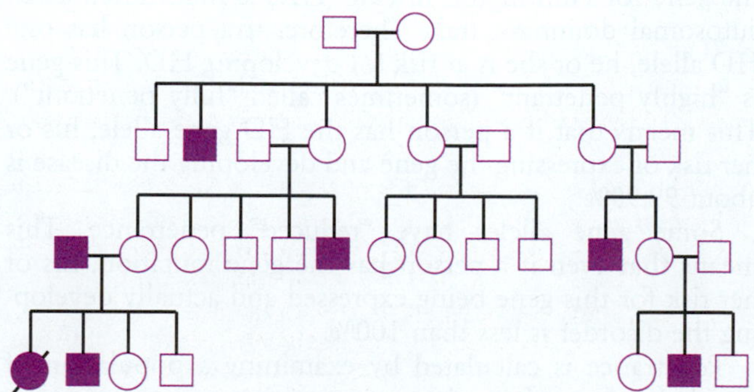

Figure 11-23 ■ A typical pedigree showing a sex-linked (X-linked) recessive pattern of inheritance.

may be present, the risk is changed by diet, lifestyle, exposure to toxins, infectious agents, and other factors.

GENETIC TESTING

PURPOSE OF TESTING

With completion of the first phase of the Human Genome Project, many people are eager to have genetic testing but also are fearful of genetic testing. The lay public often believes that a single genetic test can "tell everything about a person." Although the potential for genetic testing to be all inclusive exists, this is not currently the case. Some people want to identify family members who might have "bad genes." Some people want to identify people with "perfect genes." It is important to remember that no single person is genetically perfect.

Genetic testing can be performed with many different techniques. Some genetic tests are very specific for a disease or disorder. Others may show a gene variation but the significance of the variation may not be known. At times unexpected information is found during genetic testing. Some ordinary tests, such as blood typing and tissue typing, provide genetic information. Laboratory tests that measure the amount of an enzyme or protein a person makes actually provide genetic information.

Actual genetic testing can be performed at many levels. Cellular or biochemical tests provide information about gene products made by a cell, tissue, or organ. Chromosomes can be assessed for missing, extra, or broken chromosomes. Chromosome segments can be analyzed for abnormalities or changes from normal positions. The sequence of an individual gene can be examined to determine variation or mutation. At present not all genes can be analyzed, and the analysis of even one gene is limited by expense and availability. Specific base pairs can be evaluated for mutations. Again, these tests are currently expensive and the results may not be conclusive. Table 11-4 lists purposes of genetic testing for adults.

BENEFITS AND RISKS OF TESTING

Genetic testing is different from any other type of testing for many reasons. *It is important to remember that just because the technology exists does not mean it should be used in all cases.* Informed consent is required before genetic testing is undertaken. At present the person tested is the one who gives consent. Because genetic testing *always* gives information about a family and family members, not just the client, however, there is some debate about who else should give consent.

BENEFITS

Genetic testing can be useful to confirm a diagnosis or to test people who are at risk for a health problem but do not as yet have any symptoms. Presymptomatic testing can help a person, family, and their health care provider develop an appropriate plan of care or screening for early detection. For example, in the case of a strong genetic predisposition of colon cancer, identifying a client before symptoms appear allows interventions to prevent disease development or diagnosis earlier, when cure is more likely.

RISKS

Unlike most tests, genetic testing results do not change. This means that a positive test result cannot be "taken back." Genetic tests pose some unusual risks. The risks of genetic testing may include psychological or social risks as well as a risk for family disruption. Often genetic tests are expensive and may not be covered by insurance. Some genetic tests have limited value for predicting future risk. Testing may identify a client at great risk for the future development of a serious health problem that cannot be prevented. Some disorders, such as Huntington disease (HD), currently have no treatment. Knowing positive test results in these situations can lead to depression, blame, and guilt.

Another risk of genetic testing is that positive results may be used to discriminate against a person or a family. Some protection is in place to prevent health insurance companies from failing to insure a person or dropping the coverage of a person who is at high risk for developing a serious illness (e.g., breast or ovarian cancer). However, there are no protections against rate hikes or exclusions of specific treatments. Clients often fear workplace discrimination and even personal discrimination if positive test results are known.

GENETIC COUNSELING

Genetic testing is not a standard test that any person should have performed without knowing the advantages and disad-

TABLE 11-4 Purposes of Genetic Testing for Adults

Purpose Type	Definition
Carrier testing	Determining whether a client without symptoms has an allele for a recessive disorder that could be transmitted to his or her children. Disorders for which carrier testing is common include sickle cell disease, hemophilia, hereditary hemochromatosis, cystic fibrosis, beta thalassemia, and Tay-Sach's disease.
Diagnostic testing	Determining whether a client has or does not have a mutation that increases the risk for a specific genetic disorder.
Symptomatic	Client has clinical manifestations; test results confirm a diagnosis.
Presymptomatic	Client has no clinical manifestations but is at high risk for inheriting a specific genetic disorder for which there is no known prevention or treatment. A disorder for which presymptomatic testing is commonly performed is Huntington disease.
Predisposition	Family history or genetic testing indicates risk is high for a known genetic disorder. The client does not have any manifestations but wants to know whether he or she has the specific mutation and what the chances are that it will be expressed. Disorders for which predisposition testing is often performed include hereditary breast/ovarian cancer and hereditary colorectal cancers. The advantage of predisposition testing is that the client can then engage in heightened screening activities or medical and surgical interventions that reduce risk.

vantages. Counseling clients before, during, and after testing is critical. Entire families may be a part of the genetic evaluation and follow-up. In fact, it may be difficult to determine just which person is the client. For example, a 45-year-old woman has breast cancer. In her family, her mother, grandmother, brother, and one sister have all had breast cancer. This woman's older daughter wonders whether she has a gene mutation for breast cancer and asks to be tested. This daughter is called the **proband** because she is the person who brought the family's issue to the attention of genetic professionals. When she and her younger sister are tested, the older daughter does not have the mutation but the younger sister does. Thus, although the older sister was considered the client, the younger sister is the one who has a gene mutation.

Genetic counseling is a process, not a single session or a single recommendation. This process should begin when the client or family is first identified as potentially having a genetic problem. The process continues through actual testing, if the decision to test is made, and it continues through interpretation of results and follow-up. Steps in the process are listed in Table 11-5.

Often a client may request genetic testing even when there is no indication of need for the test (evaluation does not indicate an increased risk for a genetic disorder). Genetic counseling and evaluation can help clients understand whether any useful information could be obtained from testing.

Counseling should be performed by a professional or a team that has defined expertise in interpretation of genetic testing results. Such professionals include advanced-practice nurses with specialization in one or more aspects of genetics, certified genetic counselors, clinical geneticists, medical geneticists, and laboratory geneticists. Each of these professionals has a different level of preparation in genetics and thus has different skills and roles in the counseling process (Table 11-6). For example, an advanced-practice nurse may be appropriate to counsel a client about the Huntington disease gene mutation because this test is not ambiguous and the gene is highly penetrant. A person who has a variation or mutation in an unusual gene region or when penetrance is reduced may best be served by counseling from a clinical or medical geneticist.

No matter which professional is involved in genetic counseling, a key feature of this counseling is to be "nondirective." The counselor provides as much information as possible about the risks and benefits but does not in any way influence the client's decision to test or not to test. Once the client has made the decision, the counselor supports the client and the decision. Chart 11-1 lists NIC intervention activities for adult clients considering or having genetic testing.

TABLE 11-5 Steps Involved in the Process of Genetic Testing and Counseling

Pre-testing Assessment and Client Education (may take multiple sessions)
- Determining client understanding and why testing or counseling is being sought
- Determining whether testing is reasonable (considering cost of the test, specificity, probable risk, accuracy of testing)
- Establishing a trusting professional relationship
- Assuring privacy and confidentiality
- Reviewing informed consent procedures
- Assessing the client's ability to communicate accurately (including language issues, cognitive function, and sensory perception)
- Assessing the client's psychosocial status and availability of social support
- Taking a detailed client health history (including drugs, diet, exercise, hormonal history, and lifestyle issues)
- Obtaining physical assessment data relevant to the at-risk disorder
- Taking a detailed family history and constructing a three-generation pedigree (minimum)
- Obtaining and verifying information obtained from the following:
  - Client
  - Family members
  - Medical records
  - Pathology reports
  - Death certificates
- Interpreting the family history
- Discussing the consequences of testing
- Discussing client rights and obligations regarding disclosure of information
- Discussing testing options
- Assessing to determine whether coercion is occurring
- Obtaining material to be tested (usually blood)

Test Result Presentation
- Re-assessing the client's wish to know or not know the test results
- Respecting the client's decision not to know the test results
- Assuring privacy and confidentiality
- Presenting the test results
- Interpreting the test results
- Assessing the client's perception of the test results

Follow-up
- Supporting the client's decision to disclose or not disclose the information to other family members
- Discussing the potential risks for other family members
- Assuring privacy and confidentiality
- Addressing the client's concerns
- Discussing prevention, early detection, and treatment options
- Discussing family concerns
- Addressing psychosocial issues
- Discussing available resources for information, support, further counseling
- Providing summary of results and consultation to the client

ETHICAL ISSUES

THE RIGHT TO KNOW VERSUS THE RIGHT NOT TO KNOW

Many ethical issues must be considered with genetic testing. Individual clients do have a right to know their genetic risk, and they also have a right to choose not to know. Sometimes a client's right to know has an impact on the right of another family member not to know. For example, your maternal grandfather had Huntington disease (HD) and you want to know whether you have that gene, so you are tested. Your mother does not want to know whether she has the gene. If you are tested and found to have the gene, because HD is autosomal dominant, the only way you could have the gene is if your mother also has it. Thus when you find out you are positive and tell your mother your status, your mother will learn that she is also positive, even if she did not want to know.

CONFIDENTIALITY

The results of a genetic test must therefore remain confidential to the client. Currently the results cannot be given to a family member, other health care provider, or insurance

TABLE 11-6 Genetic Professionals

Professional	Educational and Professional Requirements
Certified Genetic Counselor	Master's degree in human genetics or genetic counseling from a program accredited by the American Board of Genetic Counselors. Includes clinical and laboratory training. Successful completion of a certification examination. May specialize in prenatal genetics, cancer genetics, neurogenetic disorders, psychiatric disorders, artificial reproduction, cardiology, or public health.
Clinical Geneticist	Medical doctor (MD) or MD/PhD. Classroom preparation in molecular biology, cytogenetics, biochemical genetics, immunogenetics, and population genetics. Residency in internal medicine, pediatrics, obstetrics, or other area. Completion of an American Board of Medical Genetics fellowship program (usually at least 2 yr). Successful completion of a general certification examination.
Medical Geneticist	PhD; Medical doctor (MD); or MD-PhD. Classroom preparation in molecular biology, cytogenetics, biochemical genetics, immunogenetics, and population genetics. Additional preparation in forensic, pharmaceutical, pathology, and genetic technologies. Completion of an American Board of Medical Genetics genetics fellowship program (usually at least 2 yr). Successful completion of a general certification examination. May also have completed an additional specialty examination.
Advance Practice Nurse with a specialty in genetics	Master's degree in nursing with 16 to 20 semester credits in genetics and counseling. May be eligible to certify through the International Society of Nurses in Genetics (ISONG) after a specified number of clinical practice hours. Current certification is by portfolio.

Data from http://www.kumc.edu/gec/prof/career.html.

CHART 11-1

NIC INTERVENTION ACTIVITIES for The Adult Client with or at Risk for a Genetic Problem

Genetic Counseling: *Use of an interactive helping process focusing on assisting an individual, family, or group, manifesting or at risk for developing or transmitting a birth defect or genetic condition, to cope*

- Provide privacy and ensure confidentiality.
- Establish a therapeutic relationship based on trust and respect.
- Determine the client's purpose, goals, and agenda for the genetic counseling session.
- Determine knowledge base, myths, perceptions, and misperceptions related to a birth defect or genetic condition.
- Determine presence and quality of family support, other support systems, and previous coping skills.
- Provide estimates of client's risk based upon phenotype (client characteristics), family history (pedigree analysis), calculated risk information, or genotype (genetic testing results).
- Provide estimates of occurrence or recurrence risks for client and at-risk family members.
- Provide information on the natural history of the disease or condition, treatment and/or management strategies, and preventions strategies, if known.
- Provide information about the risks, benefits, and limitations of treatment/management options, as well as options for dealing with recurrence risk in a nondirective manner.
- Provide decision-making support as clients consider their options.
- Prioritize areas of risk reduction in collaboration with the individual, family, or group.
- Monitor response when client learns about own genetic risk factors.
- Allow expression of feelings.
- Support client's coping process.
- Institute crisis support measures as needed.
- Provide referral to genetic health care specialists, as necessary.
- Provide referral to community resources, including genetic support groups, as needed.
- Provide client a written summary of genetic counseling session, as indicated.

Coping Enhancement: *Assisting a client to adapt to perceived stressors, changes, or threats that interfere with meeting life demands and roles*

- Appraise the impact of the client's life situation on roles and relationships.
- Appraise the client's understanding of the disease process.
- Appraise and discuss alternative responses to situation.
- Use a calm, reassuring approach.
- Help client to identify the information he/she is most interested in obtaining.
- Provide factual information concerning diagnosis, treatment, and prognosis.
- Evaluate the client's decision-making ability.
- Discourage decision making when the client is under severe stress.
- Acknowledge the client's spiritual/cultural background.
- Confront client's ambivalent (angry or depressed) feelings.
- Arrange situations that encourage client's autonomy.
- Encourage the identification of specific life values.
- Support the use of appropriate defense mechanisms.
- Encourage verbalization of feelings, perceptions, and fears.
- Discuss consequences of not dealing with guilt and shame.
- Appraise the client's needs/desires for social support.
- Determine the risk of the client inflicting self-harm.
- Encourage family involvement, as appropriate.
- Assist the client to clarify misconceptions.

NIC intervention activities selected from Dochterman, J.M., & Bulechek, G.M. (Eds.). (2004). *Nursing interventions classification (NIC)* (4th ed.). St. Louis: Mosby.

carrier without the client's permission. This issue is controversial, as described below under Sharing of Information.

COERCION

The final decision to have genetic testing or to not have rests with the client. Family members or a primary care provider may be urging the client to have the test. However, the client must make the decision without such pressures.

SHARING OF INFORMATION

The client makes the final decision to share the information with family members. Some clients choose not to share this information even when other family members may also be at risk. An area of controversy is one in which the health care provider knows the client has a positive test result for a serious inherited condition, such as hereditary, non-polyposis colon cancer (HNPCC). This condition has an autosomal dominant inheritance pattern, and each child of the client has a 50% risk for having the gene. If the client chooses not to tell his or her grown children, they then do not have the opportunity for increased screening to find the cancer at an early stage when cure is possible. An ethical dilemma arises when the health care provider wants to inform the children of their risk. Different states have different views on whether or not the health care provider has an obligation to inform other family members.

THE ROLE OF THE MEDICAL-SURGICAL NURSE IN GENETIC COUNSELING

Medical-surgical nurses help clients during the assessing, testing, and counseling processes in many areas, although they do not provide in-depth genetic counseling. Clients often feel most comfortable sharing information with nurses and asking nurses to clarify information.

Nurses may be the first health care professionals to identify a client at genetic risk. Some of the following are indicators that a client may have an increased genetic risk for a disease or disorder:

- The disease or disorder occurs at a higher incidence within the family than among the general population.
- The client or close family members have another identified genetic problem.
- The incidence of a specific disease or disorder occurs in the client or in family members at an unusually early age.
- A rare disease is present in two or more family members.
- More than one type of cancer in present in any one person.
- The presence of clinical manifestations is associated with one or more genetic disorders (unusual freckling or skin pigmentation, bicuspid aortic valve, deafness)

A nurse may be the health care professional that verifies information that can bring a genetic problem to light. For example, during an assessment, the client may tell you that her mother died of bone cancer when she was 40 years old. Bone cancer is quite rare among adults; thus you might then ask, "Did your mother ever have any other type of cancer?" Often the client may then tell you that her mother had breast cancer some years before that (and the "bone cancer" was really breast cancer that had spread to the bones). Breast cancer at an early age can indicate a genetic predisposition.

Clients may ask questions that indicate an interest in genetic testing. The following are examples of questions that may be cues that the client has genetic concerns:

- Will my children get this disease?
- Because my sister has this problem, what are the chances I might also develop it?
- Is there a way to test and see whether my chances of getting this disease (or having this problem) are high?

Areas of responsibility for any medical-surgical nurse in working with a client who is considering or having genetic testing include communication, privacy and confidentiality, information accuracy, client advocacy, and support.

COMMUNICATION

As a nurse, you must ensure that communication between the client and whomever is providing the genetic information is clear. First assess the client's ability to receive and process information. Can the client see and hear clearly, or are assistive devices needed? Does the client understand English, or will an interpreter be needed? Is the client's cognition at the time of meeting with the genetic professional adequate, or is it impaired by medication, disease, anxiety, or fear?

If you think the client does not understand terms or jargon during a discussion between the client and a genetic professional, ask the professional to use common terms and examples for the client. Verify with the client that he or she understands.

After any discussion about genetic risk or genetic testing, assess the client's understanding of what was said. Ask the client to explain to you, in his or her own words, what the issue means and what his or her expectations are.

PRIVACY AND CONFIDENTIALITY

All conversations regarding potential diagnoses or genetic testing must occur in a private environment. The client has the right to determine who may be a part of the discussion. The client can decide to exclude his or her primary physician and any family member from the discussion with a genetic professional. It is important that health care professionals who may be present during such discussion do not disclose information, formally or informally, without the client's permission. It is your responsibility to protect this information from improper disclosure to family members, other health care professionals, other clients, insurance providers, or anyone not specifically named by the client.

INFORMATION ACCURACY

As a medical-surgical nurse, you can help correct myths about genetic disorders and teach clients about the nature of genetic testing. In addition, you can help clients to find accurate and helpful resource materials or websites. Medical-surgical nurses are not genetics experts and would not be expected to be the final source of definitive information; however, you can help ensure that the client is referred to the correct level of genetic counseling. If you have been present during the client's discussions with a genetics professional, you can assess whether he or she understands the issues regarding his or her health problem.

CLIENT ADVOCACY

As a client advocate, you must ensure that the client's rights are not neglected or ignored. Ask the client privately what his or her wishes are regarding genetic testing. Ask whether another person or agency is insisting on the testing. Remind the client that he or she does not have to agree to testing. Determine whether the client has signed an informed consent statement for the test.

SUPPORT

Considering or having genetic testing is a stressful experience. The client and family require strong support and may need help to find the best way to cope (see Chart 11-1). Genetic testing should be performed only after genetic counseling has first occurred and should be followed with an opportunity for more counseling.

Clients may feel anger, depression, guilt, or hopelessness. Clients who have positive results from genetic testing may have issues of role changes, risk for early death or disability, and the possibility of having passed the risk for a health problem on to their children. Clients who have an ambiguous test result or one of unknown significance may feel that they have agonized over a decision, spent money, and still have no clear answer or direction. Even clients who have negative genetic test results need counseling and support. Some clients may have an unrealistic view of what a negative result means for their general health. Others may feel guilty that they were "spared" when siblings were not.

Assess the client's response to genetic test results. Ask about how the client may have used coping mechanisms in the past. If the client has disclosed information to family members, assess whether they can help provide client support or need support themselves. Refer the client to appropriate support groups and general counseling services.

GET READY for the NCLEX Examination!

KEY POINTS

- DNA, genes, and chromosomes are different forms of the same substance.
- All human cells with a nucleus contain all the genes.
- Every time a cell divides, it must replicate its DNA.
- The normal human chromosome number is 46.
- The purpose of a gene is to serve as the instructions for making a specific protein.
- Mutations can change the activity of a protein and have adverse effects on health.
- Many common adult diseases or disorders have a genetic basis (hypertension, diabetes, cancer) although some of these diseases also may occur among people with no genetic risk.
- A pedigree with at least three generations is needed when performing a genetic risk assessment.
- Each child of a person who has an autosomal dominant genetic problem has a 50% risk of inheriting the gene for the problem.
- Having a gene for a disorder does not necessarily mean that the disorder will ever develop.
- Genetic testing requires informed consent.
- The results of genetic tests do not change.
- There is no single genetic test that can provide information about all aspects of a client's health risks.
- Genetic testing reveals information about the client and his or her family members.
- Genetic testing is expensive and might not be covered by insurance.
- Genetic testing requires individual genetic risk assessment.
- Just because a genetic test is available does not mean that it is right or necessary that any given client should have the test.
- Clients having genetic testing should have genetic counseling before the testing and follow-up counseling after testing.

ADDITIONAL STUDY RESOURCES

Go to your Student CD-ROM for Review Questions for the NCLEX Examination.

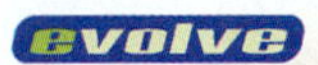

Go to http://evolve.elsevier.com/Iggy/ for Integrated Management of Care Questions for the NCLEX Examination.

SELECTED BIBLIOGRAPHY

American Society of Clinical Oncology. (2003). American Society of Clinical Oncology policy statement update: Genetic testing for cancer susceptibility. *Journal of Clinical Oncology, 21*(12), 2397-2406.

Anionwu, E. (2003). Forum: Genetics is fundamental to quality care. *Nursing Times, 99*(6), 12.

Burke, W. (2002). Genetic testing. *New England Journal of Medicine, 347*(23), 1867-1875.

Burton, H., & Shuttleworth, A. (2003). Genetics education for primary health care nurses. *Primary Health Care, 13*(4), 35-38.

Burton, H., & Stewart, A. (2003). From Mendel to the Human Genome Project: The implications for nurse education. *Nurse Education Today, 23*(5), 380-385.

Calzone, K., Jenkins, J., & Masny, A. (2002). Core competencies in cancer genetics for advanced practice oncology nurses. *Oncology Nursing Forum, 29*(9), 1327-1333.

Cashion, A. (2002). Genetics in transplantation. *MEDSURG Nursing, 11*(2), 91-94.

Cheek, D. (2002). Current issues in genetics. *AACN Clinical Issues: Advanced Practice in Acute and Critical Care, 13*(4), 485.

Cheek, D., & Cesan, A. (2003). Genetic predictors of cardiovascular disease: The use of chip technology. *Journal of Cardiovascular Nursing, 18*(1), 50-56.

Collins, F., et al. (2003). A vision for the future of genomics research. *Nature, 422*(24), 835-847.

Grady, P., & Collins, F. (2003). Genetics and nursing science: Realizing the potential. *Nursing Research, 52*(2), 69.

Greco, K. (2003). Nursing in the genomic era: Nurturing our genetic nature. *MEDSURG Nursing, 12*(5), 307-312.

Guttmacher, A., & Collins, F. (2003). Genomic medicine–A primer. *New England Journal of Medicine, 347*(19), 1512-1520.

Guttmacher, A., Jenkins, J., Uhlmann, W. (2000). Genomic medicine: Who will practice it? A call to open arms. *American Journal of Medical Genetics, 106*(3), 216-222.

Houfek, J., & Atwood, J. (2003). Genetic susceptibility to lung cancer: Implications for smoking cessation. *MEDSURG Nursing, 12*(1), 45-49.

Imperatore, G., et al. (2003). Hereditary hemochromatosis: Perspective of public health, medical genetics, and primary care. *Genetics in Medicine, 5*(1), 1-8.

Jenkins, J. (2002). Genetics competency: New directions for nursing. *AACN Clinical Issues: Advanced Practice in Acute and Critical Care, 13*(4), 486-491.

Jenkins, J. (2000). An historic perspective on genetic care. *Nursing World/Online Journal of Issues in Nursing, 5*(3), 1-17.

Jenkins, J., & Collins, F. (2003). Are you genetically literate? *American Journal of Nursing, 103*(4), 13.

Jenkins, J., & Lea, D. (2005). Nursing care in the genomic era: A case-based approach. Boston: Jones & Bartlett.

Lea, D. (2002a). Position statement: Integrating genetics competencies into baccalaureate and advanced nursing education. *Nursing Outlook, 50*(4), 167-168.

Lea, D. (2002b). What nurses need to know about genetics. *DCCN: Dimensions of Critical Care Nursing, 21*(2), 50-61.

Lea, D., & Williams, J. (2002). Genetic testing and screening: Use them as a part of routine nursing practice. *American Journal of Nursing, 102*(7), 36-43, 49-50.

Lessick, M., et al. (2001). Advances in genetic testing for cancer risk. *MEDSURG Nursing, 10*(3), 123-127.

Loud, J., et al. (2002). Applications of advances in molecular biology and genomics to clinical cancer care. *Cancer Nursing, 25*(2), 110-122.

Middleton, L., et al. (2002). The role of the nurse in cancer genetics. *Cancer Nursing, 25*(3), 196-208.

Nicol, M. (2003). The variation of response to pharmacotherapy: Pharmacogenetics–A new perspective to "the right drug for the right person." *MEDSURG Nursing, 12*(4), 242-249.

Novak, K. (2003). Telomeres and telomerases in cancer. *Medscape General Medicine, 5*(1), 1-5.

Nussbaum, R., McInnes, R., & Willard, H. (2001). *Thompson & Thompson: Genetics in medicine* (6th ed.). Philadelphia: W.B. Saunders.

Olsen, S., et al. (2003). Creating a nursing vision for leadership in genetics. *MEDSURG Nursing, 12*(3), 177-183.

Peska, E. (2003). Genomics offers opportunities for nurses. *Journal of Continuing Education in Nursing, 34*(5), 195-196.

Peters, J., et al. (2001). Cancer genetics fundamentals. *Cancer Nursing, 24*(6), 446-461.

Prows, C., & Prows, D. (2004). Medication selection by genotype. *American Journal of Nursing, 104*(5), 60-70.

Read, C. (2002). Pharmacogenomics: An evolving paradigm for drug therapy. *MEDSURG Nursing, 11*(3), 122-124.

Rieger, P. (2000). The gene genies. *The American Journal of Nursing, 100*(10), 87-90.

Smith, K., (2001). Genetic disease, genetic testing, and the clinician. *Journal of the American Medical Association, 285*(1), 91.

Spahis, J. (2002). Human genetics: Constructing a family pedigree. *The American Journal of Nursing, 102*(7), 44-50.

Varmus H. (2002). Getting ready for gene-based medicine. *New England Journal of Medicine, 347*, 1526-1527.

Williams, J. (2002). Education for genetics and nursing practice. *AACN Clinical Issues: Advanced Practice in Acute and Critical Care, 13*(4), 492-500, 590-595.

Williams, J., & Lessick, M. (2001). Historical evolution of nursing in genetics. *MEDSURG Nursing, 10*(6), 301-307.

Winkelman, C. (2004). What every critical care nurse needs to know about the genetic contribution to critical illness. *Critical Care Nurse, 24*(3), 34-45.

Wung, S. (2002). Genetic advances in coronary disease. *MEDSURG Nursing, 11*(6), 296-300.

UNIT **THREE**

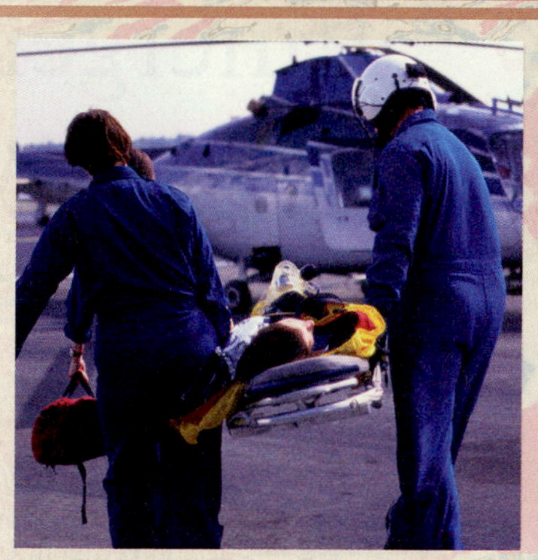

CONCEPTS of EMERGENCY NURSING

CHAPTER 12

Emergency and Mass Casualty Nursing

LINDA LASKOWSKI-JONES • KAREN L. TOULSON

LEARNING OUTCOMES

After studying this chapter, you should be able to:

1. Describe the emergency department (ED) environment, including special populations, cultural considerations, and interdisciplinary team members.
2. Plan and implement best practices to maintain staff and client safety in the ED.
3. Explain the core competencies that nurses need to function in the ED.
4. Identify types of certification that ED nurses can obtain to demonstrate or develop their expertise.
5. Triage clients into emergent, urgent, and nonurgent categories.
6. Prioritize resuscitation interventions based on the primary survey of the ED client.
7. Describe the general process of admission through disposition of a client in the ED.
8. Contrast the triage process under usual conditions with triage in a mass casualty.
9. Identify the components of an Emergency Preparedness and Response Plan.
10. Compare the key personnel roles in an Emergency Preparedness and Response Plan.
11. Differentiate two types of debriefing that occur after a mass casualty incident.
12. Describe the general process that occurs in the ED when a client is suspected of a bioterrorism agent, such as anthrax.

Go to your Student CD-ROM for Review Questions for the NCLEX Examination keyed to these Learning Outcomes.

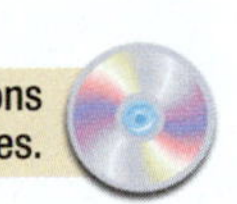

Emergency department (ED) visits in the United States have increased 14% between 1997 and 2000 (McCaig & Ly, 2002). During this same period of time, the number of EDs has decreased from 4005 to 3934. Thus the remaining EDs are encountering more clients with fewer facilities. To add to this problem, about 41 million people in the United States do not have health insurance and use the ED as their primary health care provider.

The ED is fast paced. Clients seek treatment for many physical, psychological, spiritual, and social reasons. At the height of activity, the ED may appear quite chaotic. In general, nurses are drawn to this environment because they dislike routines and thrive in challenging, stimulating work settings.

THE EMERGENCY DEPARTMENT ENVIRONMENT OF CARE

In the emergency care environment, rapid change is the rule. Although most EDs have treatment areas that are designated for certain populations such as clients with trauma, cardiac, psychiatric, or gynecologic problems, care can actually take place anywhere in this environment. In an overcrowded ED, many clients receive initial treatment outside of the usual treatment rooms, including the waiting room and hallways.

Client care areas are typically alive with activity and noise, although the pace can slow at times. Emergency nurses can expect background sounds that include ringing telephones, monitor alarms, vocal clients, crying children, and radio transmissions between ED staff and incoming ambulance or helicopter personnel. Interruptions are the norm.

Demographic Data

Staff members in the ED provide care for clients across the life span with a broad spectrum of issues, illnesses, and injuries—as well as various cultural and religious values. During a given shift, for example, the emergency nurse may function as a cardiac nurse, a pediatric nurse, a psychiatric nurse, a trauma nurse, and even a maternity nurse. Because of the multispecialty nature of the environment, EDs play a unique role within the U.S. health care system. Between 1992 and 2001, the number of ED visits rose from 89.8 million to 107.5 million visits per year (McCaig & Burt, 2003). The most common reasons that clients seek ED care include chest pain, abdominal pain, headache, and fever. The average age of a person who enters the ED is 35.7 years of age;

clients 75 years of age or older generate the highest ED visit rate (McCaig & Burt, 2003).

Special Populations

The ED serves as an important safety net for clients who are ill or injured but lack access to health care. Especially vulnerable populations include those with Medicare and Medicaid, minorities, and those who are underinsured or uninsured. Because the current health care system is complex, expensive, and difficult to navigate, some clients view the ED as an easy access route to basic health care services. Clients may also use the ED as a temporary bridge to establishing a relationship with a primary care provider or a clinic. A small percentage of clients actively attempt to manipulate the system to their advantage. These clients are commonly referred to as "frequent flyers" by frustrated staff. Some are drug seekers. Others are noncompliant with follow-up instructions that they receive upon discharge. They actively elect not to pursue a relationship with another appropriate health care provider and continue to use the ED for virtually all of their health care needs.

CULTURAL CONSIDERATIONS

The emergency nurse needs to be aware of the various cultural and religious values of clients that may impact emergency department care. Many individuals have distinct beliefs that must be respected in the health care setting. For example, Mexican Americans are typically modest and do not like to have their bodies exposed. They are also family oriented and affectionate toward each other. A religious belief system can affect the delivery of trauma care. For example, Jehovah's Witness clients do not accept blood transfusions. Clients with language barriers also present a challenge for the emergency nurse. The Spanish speaking population in the United States, for instance, is rapidly increasing. When a bilingual staff member is not available to competently interpret, the emergency nurse can employ resources such as telephone language lines and dedicated interpreters contracted by the hospital.

Special Nursing Teams

Many EDs have specialized teams that deal with high-risk populations of clients. One example of this concept is the forensic nurse examiner team. **Forensic nurse examiners** are educated to obtain client histories, collect forensic evidence, and offer counseling and follow-up care for victims of rape, child abuse, and domestic violence. They are trained to recognize evidence of abuse and to intervene on the client's behalf. Interventions may include providing information to the client about developing a safety plan or how to escape a violent relationship. The forensic nurse examiner documents injuries and collects physical and photographic evidence. Nurses from this team may also provide testimony in court as to what was observed during the examination and information about the type of care rendered.

The **psychiatric crisis nurse team** is another example of an ED specialty team. These nurses interact with clients and families in crisis. The sudden illness, serious injury, or death of a loved one may have precipitated the crisis. This team also evaluates individuals with psychiatric complaints or disorders and facilitates the client's follow-up or admission to an appropriate psychiatric facility.

Interdisciplinary Team Members

The **emergency nurse** is one member of the large interdisciplinary team who provides care for clients in the emergency department (ED). A team approach to emergency care is considered a standard of practice. In this setting, the emergency nurse must interact in a professional manner with all levels of health team providers, from prehospital emergency medical services (EMS) personnel to physicians, hospital technicians, and professional and ancillary staff.

PREHOSPITAL CARE PROVIDERS

Prehospital care providers are typically the first caregivers encountered by the client if he or she is transported to the ED by an ambulance or helicopter (Figure 12-1). Local protocols define the skill level of the EMS responders dispatched to render assistance to the client. **Emergency medical technicians (EMTs)** offer basic life support (BLS) interventions such as oxygen, basic wound care, splinting, spinal immobilization, and monitoring of vital signs. Some units carry automatic external defibrillators (AEDs) and may be authorized to administer selected medications such as an EpiPen or nitroglycerin based on established medical control protocols. For clients who require care that exceeds BLS resources, paramedics are usually dispatched. **Paramedics** are advanced life support (ALS) providers who can perform advanced techniques, which may include cardiac monitoring, advanced airway management and intubation, establishing intravenous access, and administering drugs en route to the ED (Figure 12-2).

The prehospital provider is a key source for valuable client data. Emergency nurses rely on these providers to be the eyes and ears of the health team in the prehospital set-

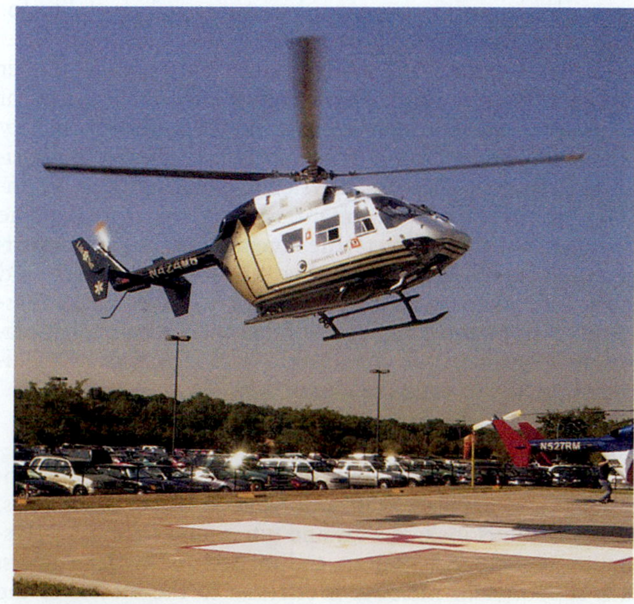

Figure 12-1 ■ Advanced life support helicopter arriving at emergency department landing zone. Helicopters are used to rapidly transport critically ill and injured clients to the hospital for emergent care.

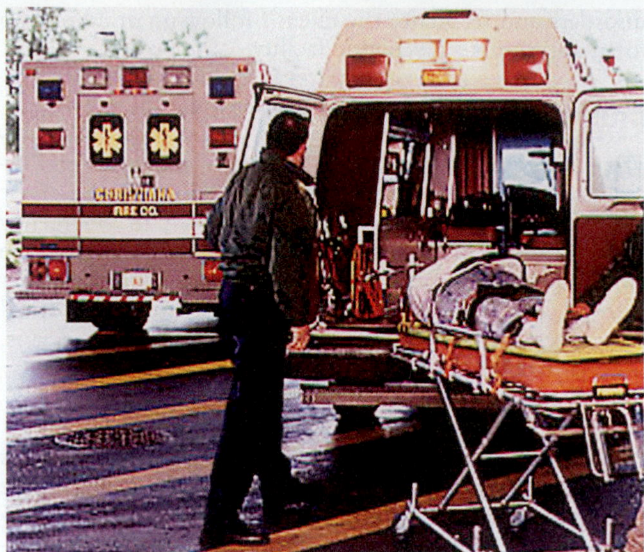

Figure 12-2 ■ Prehospital providers unload a client from the ambulance to be brought into the emergency department.

ting. The emergency nurse must pay close attention to the information that is shared to ensure continuity of care.

PHYSICIANS

Another integral member of the emergency health care team is the **emergency medicine physician**. These doctors receive specialized education and training in emergency client management. In the past, physicians of all types with varying competencies rotated through the ED. As emergency care became increasingly complex and specialized, emergency medicine became a recognized physician specialty practice, complete with board certification requirements. Today, there are emergency medicine residency programs throughout the United States that formally prepare emergency physicians to competently assume responsibility for the emergency client population.

The emergency nurse routinely interacts with a number of staff and community physicians involved in the care of ED clients. On an ongoing basis, however, the emergency nurse works most closely with emergency medicine physicians. Even though other physician specialists may be involved in ED client treatment, the emergency medicine physician typically directs the overall care in the department. Many EDs also employ nurse practitioners and physician's assistants to assume designated roles in client assessment and treatment. These individuals act in collaboration with or under the supervision of the emergency medicine physician to expedite emergency care delivery.

SUPPORT STAFF

The emergency nurse also interacts on a regular basis with professional and ancillary staff who function in support roles. These personnel include x-ray and ultrasound technicians, respiratory therapists, laboratory technicians and social workers. Each support staff member is essential to the success of the emergency health team. It is important for the emergency nurse to gain an understanding of the individual roles and responsibilities of these personnel. The emergency nurse is accountable for communicating pertinent staff considerations, client needs, and restrictions to support staff, such as physical limitations or isolation precautions, to assure that ongoing client and staff safety issues are addressed–and for assuring that clients are properly prepared for diagnostic or therapeutic intervention. Each interaction with a support team member can be viewed as a learning opportunity. These professionals possess unique bodies of knowledge and skill sets that can augment the efforts of the emergency nurse. For example, the respiratory therapist can assist the emergency nurse to trouble shoot mechanical ventilator issues. Laboratory technicians can offer advice regarding specimen collection procedures. During the discharge planning process, social workers can be tremendous client advocates in locating community resources, including temporary housing, durable medical goods, drug and alcohol counseling, health insurance information, prescription services, and health care provider referrals.

INPATIENT UNIT STAFF

The emergency nurse's interactions extend beyond the walls of the ED. Essential to continuity of care is communication with staff nurses from the inpatient units. Providing a concise but comprehensive report of the client's ED experience, including relevant medical history, assessment and diagnostic findings, interventions, and the client's response to those interventions is integral to the transfer process and client safety. Both emergency nurses and nurses on inpatient units should strive to understand the unique aspects of their two practice environments to prevent conflicts. For example, nurses on inpatient units can be critical of the push to move clients out of the ED setting quickly, particularly when the unit activity is high. Similarly, the emergency nurse may be critical of the inpatient unit's lack of understanding or enthusiasm for accepting admissions rapidly. Effective interpersonal communication skills and respectful negotiation can optimize teamwork between the emergency nurse and the inpatient unit nurse. For instance, when ED client volume or acuity is overwhelming, the unit nurse can volunteer to assist the ED nurse by moving a monitored client to the hospital bed. By the same token, the emergency nurse can elect to delay sending admitted clients to inpatient units during change of shift or crisis periods such as a cardiac arrest on the unit whenever possible.

Staff and Client Safety Considerations

In the emergency department (ED) setting, client and staff safety is an ever-present concern for the emergency nurse (Chart 12-1). Some of the most prevalent safety issues involve the following:

- Appropriate client identification
- Fall risk
- Skin breakdown in vulnerable populations
- High risk for medical errors or adverse events due to the emergent nature of care delivery

Staff safety concerns are primarily centered on the potential for transmission of disease and for personal safety when dealing with aggressive, agitated, or violent clients and visitors.

CLIENT IDENTIFICATION

Client identification is a focal point of care in the ED. All clients are issued an identification bracelet at their point of entry of the ED–generally at the triage registration desk or at the bedside if emergent needs exist. For clients with an unknown identity and those with emergent conditions that prevent the proper identification process (e.g., unconscious

CHART 12-1

BEST PRACTICE for
Maintaining Client and Staff Safety in the Emergency Department

Safety Consideration	Interventions to Minimize Risk
Client identification	Provide an ID bracelet for each client. Use two unique identifiers (e.g., name, date of birth). If client identity is unknown, use a special identification system.
Injury prevention for clients	Keep rails up on stretcher. Keep stretcher in lowest position. Remind the client to use call light/bell for assistance. Reorient confused clients frequently. If client is confused, ask a family member or significant other to monitor the client. Implement skin prevention measures for clients at risk for skin breakdown.
Risk for errors and adverse events	Obtain a thorough client and family history. Check the client for a medical alert bracelet or necklace. Search the client's belongings when he or she has altered mental status.
Injury prevention for staff	Use standard precautions at all times. Anticipate hostile, violent client and family behavior. Plan options if violence occurs, including assistance from the security department.

client without identification or emergent trauma client), hospitals commonly use a "Jane/John Doe" or other identification system. Whatever method is used, the emergency nurse is accountable for verifying the client's identity before each intervention and before medication administration. The fast pace of the ED often complicates assuring proper identification. However, the emergency nurse must adhere to client identification standards to optimize client safety and to reduce personal liability risk.

CLIENT SAFETY

The nurse must also ensure that the client is safe in the environment while receiving care. Two primary safety considerations are to protect clients from falls and to prevent skin breakdown.

CONSIDERATIONS FOR OLDER ADULTS

Clients who are on beds or stretchers should have all side rails up and the bed or stretcher in the lowest position. Access to a call light or bell is especially important; the client is instructed to call for the nurse if assistance is needed rather than attempt independent ambulation. Older clients may become confused and need reorientation. In some cases, the nurse should ask a family member, significant other, or sitter to stay with the client to prevent falls.

Some clients spend a lengthy time on stretchers while awaiting inpatient unit bed availability. Protecting skin integrity begins in the ED. Emergency nurses should assess the skin frequently and implement preventive interventions into the ED plan of care, especially when caring for older adults. Interventions that promote clean, dry skin for incontinent clients, mobility techniques that decrease shearing forces when moving the immobile client, and routine turning aid in the prevention of skin breakdown.

RISK FOR ERRORS AND ADVERSE EVENTS

A significant risk for all clients who enter the emergency care environment involves the potential for medical errors or adverse events. Causative factors stem from the episodic and often chaotic nature of emergency management. Clients arrive in the ED with urgent or emergent needs that must be addressed rapidly. They may not know—or even be able to relate—key elements of their medical history such as medical conditions, allergies, or current medications. Gaps in information can lead to prescribing and treatment errors. To reduce the error potential, the emergency nurse makes every attempt to obtain essential medical history information from the client, family, or reliable significant others as necessary. When dealing with clients who arrive with an altered mental status, a quick survey to determine whether the client is wearing a medical alert bracelet or necklace is an important aspect of initial care to gain critical medical information. In addition, a two-person search of client belongings may yield medication containers, the name of a physician, pharmacy, family contact person, or a medication list. In this case, the nurse serves as a detective to find clues, which may not only promote client safety, but which may also help determine the diagnosis and influence the overall emergency treatment plan.

Lastly, emergency nurses need to be aware of their own personal safety while caring for clients. The emergency nurse must use standard precautions at all times when there is a potential for contamination by blood or other body fluids. Clients with tuberculosis can be preferentially placed in a negative pressure room; the nurse can wear a positive air-purifying respirator (PAPR) before engaging in any close interaction.

Hostile behavior also poses a significant injury risk to ED staff members. Recognizing volatile situations or individuals who show evidence of violent tendencies is critical to planning an escape route or attempting de-escalation strategies before harm can occur. Many EDs have at least one security guard in their settings at all times for assistance with these situations.

SCOPE OF EMERGENCY NURSING PRACTICE

The scope of emergency nursing practice encompasses management of clients across the life span—from birth through death—and all health conditions that prompt an individual of any age to seek emergency care. It is the breadth and depth of knowledge as well as the emergency care skills that attract and provide ongoing challenge to nurses who enter into this specialty.

Education

Nurses come to work in the ED in a variety of ways. Traditionally, hospital employers have required nurses to have 6 months to 1 year of experience in an acute care medical-surgical or critical care unit setting before working in the ED.

The rationale for this requirement was that nurses would have developed competencies in basic nursing care and organizational skills before entering ED specialty practice.

The nursing shortage has inspired many emergency nurse leaders to rethink the philosophy of hiring only experienced acute care nurses into the ED when sufficient numbers of them are not available to fulfill staffing needs. Today, many nurses are entering the ED upon graduation from nursing school. Strategies to bridge the knowledge and experience gap include emergency nursing course work and clinical rotations incorporated into senior-level nursing school curricula, extended hospital ED orientation programs, and emergency nursing internship programs (Gurney, 2002).

Core Competencies

Emergency nursing practice requires that nurses be skilled in client assessment, priority setting and critical thinking, multitasking, and communication. A sound knowledge base is essential. Flexibility and adaptability are essential traits of the nurse because situations within the ED, as well as individual clients, can change rapidly.

ASSESSMENT

First and foremost, the foundation of the emergency nurse's skill base is assessment (Twedell, 2000). The emergency nurse not only must rapidly and accurately discern normal from abnormal, but also must categorize assessment findings according to acuity and age. For example, mottling of the extremities may be a normal finding in a newborn, but it may indicate poor peripheral perfusion and a shock state in an older child. The significance of pre-existing disease states, or **comorbidities**, must also be factored into the emergency nurse's assessment in regard to how the condition might adversely affect or complicate a seemingly unrelated health problem. For example, a trauma client who has rib fractures and a past medical history of chronic obstructive pulmonary disease (COPD) may not be able to maintain adequate oxygenation without endotracheal intubation and mechanical ventilatory support in the ED. Another common assessment scenario involves the Type I diabetic client who presents to the ED with an altered mental status after a fall–Is the altered mental status due to hypoglycemia or to intracranial injury? The nurse must quickly act to assess blood glucose in this case, as well as follow trauma protocols for managing a potential head injury.

PRIORITY SETTING/CRITICAL THINKING SKILLS

Another essential skill for the emergency nurse is priority setting, which is inherent in the triage process and is described later in this chapter. Priority setting depends on accurate assessment as well as critical thinking skills. These skills are generally gained through hands-on clinical experience in the ED. However, discussion of case studies and the use of simulation software can help prepare nurses to acquire this skill base in a nonthreatening environment and then apply it in the actual clinical situation.

KNOWLEDGE OF EMERGENCY CARE

The knowledge base for emergency nurses is broad and encompasses not only typical client presentations of common medical and surgical disease entities, but also the less common ones, such as poisonous snake and insect bites, heat stroke, hypothermia, and hazardous materials contamination. These emergency care nursing principles extend to recognition, management, and legal implications of societal problems such as child abuse, domestic violence, elder abuse, and sexual assault.

Although most EDs have physicians available around the clock who are physically located within the ED, the emergency nurse often initiates interdisciplinary protocols to expedite life-saving interventions such as application of cardiac monitoring, oxygen therapy, insertion of intravenous catheters, and infusion of appropriate parenteral solutions. In many EDs, nurses function under medical protocols that allow them to initiate drug therapy for emergent conditions such as anaphylactic shock and cardiac arrest. Emergency care principles extend to knowing what essential laboratory and diagnostic tests may be needed and, when necessary, obtaining them. The Emergency Nurses Association's *Emergency Nursing Core Curriculum* (2000a) is an excellent reference that outlines the fundamental body of knowledge that encompasses the emergency nurse's knowledge and skill base.

TECHNICAL SKILLS

The emergency nurse must also be proficient in performing a variety of technical skills (multitasking), sometimes in a stressful, high-pressure environment such as a cardiac or trauma resuscitation. In addition to basic skills, the emergency nurse may also need to be proficient with equipment most often found in the critical care environment, such as invasive pressure monitoring devices. EDs that are components of a Level I trauma center typically have such critical care equipment in the ED setting.

The emergency nurse assists the physician with a number of procedures. Knowledge and skills related to procedural setup, client preparation, teaching, and post-procedural care are also essential facets of emergency nursing practice. Common ED procedures include the following:

- Simple and complex suturing for wound closure
- Foreign body removal
- Central line insertion
- Endotracheal intubation
- Transvenous pacemaker insertion
- Lumbar puncture
- Pelvic examination
- Chest tube insertion
- Peritoneal lavage
- Fracture management

More than one emergency nurse may be necessary to assist with some procedures. For example, if conscious sedation is used to produce a state of amnesia and relaxation during fracture manipulation, one nurse assists the physician with the actual procedure, while the other nurse is dedicated to monitoring the client before, during, and after the conscious sedation medications are administered.

COMMUNICATION

Finally, an essential aspect of the emergency nurse's skill base is communication. The ED environment is complex–barriers to effective communication exist at virtually all levels of interaction. Overcrowding and insufficient nursing personnel to meet the demand for services create difficulties with communication of pertinent client information and quality of written documentation. The high-stress ED environment also threatens positive, effective interpersonal behaviors, particularly when nurses must deal with hostile, violent, or demanding clientele as well as negative co-workers (Keough, Schlomer & Bollenberg, 2003). Despite the obstacles, the emergency nurse should seek to uphold professional standards of communication to the best of his or her ability when confronted with adversity–and seek administrative support when barriers cannot seem to be overcome. Sometimes practice modifications need to be made based upon overwhelming client volume or acuity, but the nurse should strive to maintain both client safety and dignity and invoke additional resources to manage the burden when possible.

CERTIFICATION

Two general types of certification are referred to in emergency nursing practice: the "certification," which marks successful completion of a particular course of study and emergency nursing specialty certification (Table 12-1). As part of the orientation and employment requirements for staff nurses in most U.S. EDs, successful completion of the Health Care Provider Basic Cardiac Life Support (BCLS) and Advanced Cardiac Life Support (ACLS) provider courses through the American Heart Association (Cummins, 2003) is necessary. These courses provide instruction in fundamental, evidence-based management theory and techniques for cardiopulmonary resuscitation (CPR); course participants include physicians, nurses, and prehospital personnel. BCLS emphasizes hands-on, noninvasive assessment and management skills to restore an effective airway, breathing, and circulation. The participant performs basic airway maneuvers and CPR. The ACLS course builds on the BCLS content to include advanced concepts in cardiac monitoring, invasive airway management skills, pharmacologic and electrical therapies, intravascular access techniques, special resuscitation situations, and postresuscitation management considerations.

Many emergency nurse leaders also require emergency nurses who care for children to successfully complete the Pediatric Advanced Life Support (PALS) course offered jointly by the American Academy of Pediatrics and the American Heart Association (2002). This course teaches the essential concepts of neonatal and pediatric resuscitation to physicians, nurses, and paramedics. Another option for establishing a defined pediatric emergency nursing knowledge base is the Emergency Nurses Association Emergency Nursing Pediatric Course (ENPC) (Eckle, Haley, & Baker, 1998), which offers a broad content area related to nursing management of pediatric conditions, not only resuscitation principles.

For nurses who are employed in EDs that are components of trauma centers, successful completion of the Emergency Nurses Association (2000c) Trauma Nursing Core Course, or a similar program, may be required for employment in addition to BCLS, ACLS, and PALS training. This course includes both lecture and skills stations, and focuses on concepts related to the nursing assessment and management of injuries, particularly during the initial phase of trauma care.

Unlike the "certification" courses, emergency nursing specialty certification through the Emergency Nurses Association's Board Certification for Emergency Nursing (BCEN) program constitutes professional certification in the truest sense of the word. Individuals who both qualify to take the examination and achieve a passing score are authorized to use the initials "CEN"–Certified Emergency Nurse–as part of their professional credentials after their name.

EMERGENCY NURSING PRINCIPLES

Triage

Triage is derived from the French word "trier," which means "to sort" or "to choose" (Gilboy, 2003). The concept of emergency department (ED) **triage** is based upon sorting or classifying clients into priority levels depending on illness or injury severity. The organization of emergency care and even the ED is structured through triage principles. The key concept is that clients who present to the ED with the highest acuity needs receive the quickest evaluation, treatment, and prioritized resource utilization such as x-ray studies, laboratory work, and computed tomography (CT) scans. These clients also have priority for hospital service areas, such as the operating room or cardiac catheterization laboratory. An individual with a lower acuity problem may wait longer in the ED, because the higher acuity client is moved to the "head of the line."

The triage nurse is the gatekeeper in the emergency care system. When clients present to the ED, regulatory standards dictate that a registered nurse (RN), physician, or physician's assistant perform a rapid assessment to determine triage priority (Joint Commission Resources, 2003). The RN is typically the individual assigned to perform the triage function in most hospitals, however. In fact, the Emergency Nurses Association (2001) *Standards of Emergency Nursing Practice* clearly delineate the registered nurse as the health care provider who should triage each ED client. The triage nurse should have appropriate training and experience in both emergency nursing and triage decision-making concepts. Typically, the RN determines the client's triage priority independently. In rare instances, the triage nurse may seek the input of an emergency physician, physician's assistant, or advanced practice nurse to help establish the acuity level if the client's presentation is highly unusual.

TABLE 12-1 Descriptions of Certifications for Emergency Nursing

Certification	Description
Basic Cardiac Life Support (BCLS) (required)	Noninvasive assessment and management skills for airway maintenance and CPR
Advanced Cardiac Life Support (ACLS) (usually required)	Invasive airway management skills, pharmacology, and electrical therapies, special resuscitation
Pediatric Advanced Life Support (PALS) (may be required)	Neonatal and pediatric resuscitation
Certified Emergency Nurse (CEN) (optional)	Validates core emergency nursing knowledge base

Based upon the triage priority, clients may be rushed into a treatment room, directed to a lower acuity area within the ED (e.g., a **"fast track"**), or asked to sit in the waiting room. Variations on this theme include triage nurse–initiated protocols for laboratory work or diagnostic studies that may be performed before the client is actually evaluated by a physician, or even initiation of care on a stretcher in the hallway of an overcrowded ED.

EMERGENT, URGENT, AND NONURGENT CATEGORIES

There are many triage schemes that may be appropriately used by a hospital ED. Whatever scheme is used, it must be applied consistently by all triage nursing staff and endorsed by the emergency medicine physician staff. A basic example of a triage scheme is the commonly used three-tiered model of "emergent, urgent, and nonurgent." In this model, for instance, a client experiencing crushing substernal chest pain, shortness of breath, and diaphoresis would be classified as "emergent" and triaged immediately to a treatment room within the ED. Similarly, a critically injured trauma client or an individual with an active hemorrhage would also be prioritized as "emergent." The **emergent triage** category implies that a condition exists that poses an immediate threat to life or limb.

The **urgent triage** category indicates that the client should be treated quickly, but that an immediate threat to life does not exist at the moment. Reassessment must occur if a physician cannot evaluate the client in a timely manner. In individuals with evidence of clinical deterioration, triage priority may be upgraded from "urgent" to "emergent." Examples of clients who typically fall into the "urgent" category include those with a new onset of pneumonia (as long as respiratory failure does not appear imminent), abdominal pain, renal colic, complex lacerations not associated with major hemorrhage, displaced fractures or dislocations, a history of a seizure before arrival, and temperature greater than 101° F (37° C).

Those categorized as **"nonurgent"** can generally tolerate waiting several hours for health care services without a significant risk of clinical deterioration. Conditions within this classification include clients with sprains and strains, simple fractures, simple lacerations or soft tissue injuries, viral or "cold" symptoms, and skin rashes.

OTHER MULTITIERED MODELS

To further stratify client conditions within an acuity classification or triage priority system, four- and five-tier triage models also exist. Such models are either based on comprehensive lists of conditions that indicate the particular triage priority to which a client should be assigned, or the nature of resources that a client will use in the ED setting. A given client complaint may generate various triage classifications in different hospitals depending upon the triage priority system used at that particular institution. Some schemes may even take into account the presence of pre-existing conditions such as a history of warfarin (Coumadin) use, diabetes, heart disease, and organ transplantation when determining triage priority.

Surprisingly, there is no universally accepted triage system recognized in the United States. Thus there is no standardization of triage acuity data to compare client acuity between hospitals (Travers, 2003). With that said, the Emergency Nurses Association endorses a standardized five-level model known as the **Emergency Severity Index (ESI)** that categorizes both client acuity and resource utilization. "The triage algorithm yields rapid, reproducible, and clinically relevant stratification of clients into five groups, from level 1 (most urgent) to level 5 (least urgent)" (Gilboy et al., 2003). This five-level ESI triage model was found to be safer and provided better discrimination, reliability, sensitivity, and specificity than a three-level triage system in one study involving 15,324 clients at a southeastern tertiary ED (see the Evidence-Based Practice for Nursing box below) (Travers, et al. 2002).

The Primary Survey and Resuscitation Interventions

Perhaps the hallmark public image of emergency nursing is the resuscitation scene as viewed on television where the emergency team acts rapidly and competently to save a human life. This drama is actually played out daily in EDs across the country. Although only a relatively small percentage of clients who seek emergency services actually require this level of care, emergency nurses often define their roles in terms of their resuscitation skills and experience. The opportunity to participate in resuscitation on a regular basis is a primary reason many nurses choose to work in the ED setting. There is much pride in the frequently heard emergency nurse's statement that "we save lives."

Even for the experienced emergency nurse, however, resuscitation can be challenging due to the critical nature of the client's illness or injuries as well as the impact of other issues intrinsic to the emergency environment. There is also

EVIDENCE-BASED PRACTICE for Nursing

Is another triage system better than the traditional three-level triage model?

Travers, D.A., et al. (2002). Five-level triage system more effective than three-level in tertiary emergency department. *Journal of Emergency Nursing, 28,* 395-400.

This retrospective study involved chart reviews at two different times to determine which of two triage systems was the most valid, reliable, and sensitive. At Time I, 305 records were reviewed; at Time II, 303 records were reviewed. Spearman correlations compared the two triage systems. The results showed that the five-level Emergency Severity Index (ESI) was superior to the traditional method—it was more reliable, valid, and stable.

Level of Evidence: 4—Well-conducted qualitative systematic review.

Critique. This study provided evidence that the traditional triage system needs to be revised. The ESI was developed in the United States in the late 1990s. Although this system had strong reliability in other studies, no other study to compare two systems had been published. A retrospective study was the most efficient way to examine large numbers of client records, although all records were from one large medical center. The study should be repeated in other sized hospitals for comparison with this study's results.

Implications for Nursing. Emergency nurses could better depend on the newer system to accurately triage their clients. Emergency departments could start piloting the ESI and collect data on its outcomes, as recommended by the Emergency Nurses Association.

a high risk to the nurse of contamination with blood and body fluids. For this reason, standard precautions attire must be worn in all resuscitation situations and consists an impervious cover gown, gloves, proper eye protection, a face mask, and even a surgical cap and shoe covers if *significant* blood loss is anticipated (e.g., during performance of an ED thoracotomy or when managing a client with gastrointestinal (GI) bleeding).

To remain focused on priorities and keep the situation under control, an organized approach is essential. This approach is applicable for *every* resuscitation situation and promotes rapid identification and intervention techniques to address the most immediate life threats. Although both medical and trauma resuscitation scenes may appear chaotic and complex to the lay person, if performed according to widely accepted protocols and standards, they are actually highly planned events that are based on established priorities of care. These priorities are addressed in order as part of the initial assessment termed the "primary survey." The **primary survey** organizes the approach to the client so that immediate threats to life are rapidly identified and effectively managed. The primary survey is based on a standard "ABC" mnemonic with a "D" and "E" added for trauma clients: airway/cervical spine (**A**), breathing (**B**), circulation (**C**), disability (**D**), and exposure (**E**). Resuscitation efforts occur simultaneously with each element of the primary survey (Cummins, 2003; American College of Surgeons, 1997; Emergency Nurses Association, 2000a). Even though the resuscitation team may encounter multiple clinical problems or injuries, issues identified in the primary survey must be managed before the team engages in interventions of lower priority, such as splinting fractures and dressing wounds.

A: AIRWAY/CERVICAL SPINE

The highest priority intervention in the primary survey is to establish a patent airway. Even minutes without an adequate oxygen supply in humans can lead to cerebral injury that can progress to anoxic brain death. The airway must be cleared of any secretions or debris with either a suction catheter or manually if necessary. The cervical spine must be protected in any trauma client with the potential for spinal injury by manually aligning the neck in a neutral, in-line position and using a jaw thrust maneuver when establishing an airway. Supplemental oxygen is required for all individuals who require resuscitation. In general, a non-rebreather mask is best for the spontaneously breathing client. Bag-valve-mask (BVM) ventilation with the appropriate airway adjunct and a 100% oxygen source is indicated for the individual who needs ventilatory assistance during resuscitation. A client with significantly impaired consciousness, indicated by a Glasgow Coma Score less than or equal to 8, requires a definitive airway such as an endotracheal tube (American College of Surgeons, 1997) (Figure 12-3). After endotracheal intubation, a mechanical ventilator is employed. Initially, oxygen in high concentration (F_{IO_2} 100%) is administered; lower concentrations may be ordered after the client's condition has improved.

B: BREATHING

After the airway is successfully secured, breathing becomes the next priority in the primary survey. This assessment determines whether or not ventilatory efforts are effective–not only whether or not the client is breathing. The focus is on auscultation of breath sounds and evaluation of chest expansion, respiratory effort, and any evidence of chest wall trauma or physical abnormalities. Both apneic clients and those with poor ventilatory effort need bag-valve-mask (BVM) ventilation for support until endotracheal intubation is performed and a mechanical ventilator is used. If cardiopulmonary resuscitation (CPR) becomes necessary, the mechanical ventilator must be disconnected and the client manually ventilated with a BVM device to better sequence ventilations with chest compressions, as well as to assess lung compliance through sensing the degree of difficulty in ventilating the client with the BVM.

Another life-saving intervention that may be performed in this phase is chest decompression, either with a needle or chest tube to vent trapped air. The main indication for chest decompression is clinical evidence of a tension pneumothorax, which can pose a critical threat to both breathing and circulation: decreased to absent breath sounds over the affected side, respiratory distress, hypotension, jugular vein distention, and tracheal deviation. If unrelieved, a tension pneumothorax causes mediastinal shift, cardiovascular collapse, and death. Causes of tension pneumothorax include barotrauma from BVM ventilation or other positive-pressure ventilation, blunt or penetrating chest trauma, and expansion of a simple pneumothorax.

Chest decompression is performed in two ways: needle thoracostomy and tube thoracostomy. **Needle thoracostomy** is a quick, temporary maneuver used in an emergency

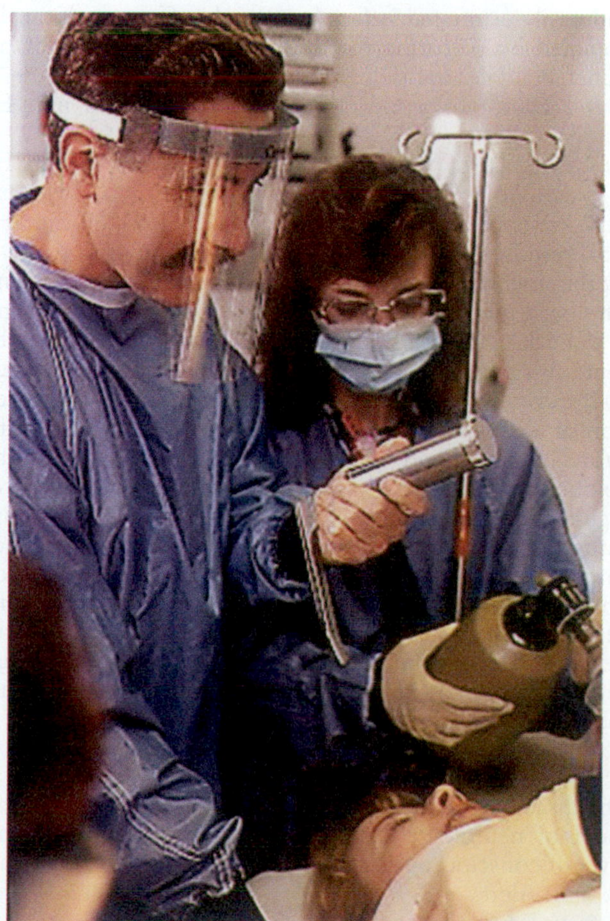

Figure 12-3 ■ Emergency department trauma resuscitation room. Wearing standard precautions attire, trauma team members prepare to intubate the injured client.

to vent trapped air pending chest tube insertion. A large-bore needle (14 or 16 gauge IV catheter, 3 to 6 cm in length) is inserted into the second intercostal space in the midclavicular line; a "rush of air" is expected as the trapped air is expelled from the pleural space under pressure (American College of Surgeons, 1997). Documentation of the air rush out of the catheter confirms the presence of a tension pneumothorax. After needle thoracostomy, a chest tube is inserted **(tube thoracostomy)** in the fifth intercostal space, just anterior to the midaxillary line. Chest tube placement in this anatomic position promotes both air and fluid drainage.

C: CIRCULATION

When effective ventilation is assured, the priority shifts to circulation. The adequacy of heart rate, blood pressure, and overall perfusion become the focus of this element of the primary survey. Common threats to circulation include cardiac arrest, myocardial dysfunction, and hemorrhage leading to a shock state. Interventions are targeted at restoring effective circulation through cardiopulmonary resuscitation, hemorrhage control, intravenous vascular access with fluid and blood administration as necessary, and pharmacologic agents. *External* hemorrhage is best controlled with firm, direct pressure on the bleeding site with thick, dry dressing material. *Internal* hemorrhage is a more covert threat that must be suspected in injured clients or those who present in a shock state.

In a resuscitation situation, blood pressure can be quickly and easily estimated before a manual cuff pressure can be obtained by palpating for the presence or absence of peripheral and central pulses:

- Presence of a radial pulse: BP at least 80 mm Hg systolic
- Presence of a femoral pulse: BP at least 70 mm Hg systolic
- Presence of a carotid pulse: BP at least 60 mm Hg systolic

By the time hypotension occurs, compensatory mechanisms employed by the body in an attempt to maintain vital signs in a shock state have been exhausted. Timely, effective intervention is critical to preserve life and vital organ function.

Intravenous access is best achieved initially with insertion of large-bore peripheral intravenous lines in the antecubital fossae (bend of the elbow). Additional access can be obtained via central veins in the femoral, subclavian, or jugular sites using large-bore (≥8.5 Fr) central venous catheters. Resuscitation solutions of choice are lactated Ringer's and 0.9% normal saline (NS). Fluids and blood products should be warmed before administration to prevent hypothermia. A good rule of thumb is to consider the need for blood product administration in a hemorrhagic shock state when significant hypotension persists after infusion of 2 L of solution.

D: DISABILITY

The disability examination provides a rapid baseline assessment of neurologic status. A simple method to evaluate level of consciousness is the "AVPU" mnemonic:

- A: Alert
- V: Responsive to voice
- P: Responsive to pain
- U: Unresponsive

Another well established means of assessing and documenting level of consciousness that is both objective and widely accepted is the **Glasgow Coma Scale,** which scores eye opening, verbal response, and motor response. The lowest score is 3, which indicates a totally unresponsive client; a normal GCS is 15. Metabolic abnormalities, hypoxia, neurologic injury, and intoxicants can impair level of consciousness. Frequent reassessment is essential to enable rapid intervention in the event of neurologic compromise or deterioration.

E: EXPOSURE

The final component of the primary survey is exposure. All clothing is removed to allow for thorough assessment. In a resuscitation situation, clothing should be cut away to gain rapid access to the body. If evidence preservation is an issue, items should be handled per institutional policy. Evidence may include articles of clothing, impaled objects, weapons, drugs, and bullets. Emergency nurses are often called upon to provide testimony in court regarding their recollections of the presentation and treatment of clients in the ED. Examples of types of cases in which evidence collection is vital include rape, child abuse, domestic violence, homicide, suicide, drug overdose, and assault.

Once clothing is removed, hypothermia (body temperature less than or equal to 36° C) poses a significant risk. In particular, hypothermia complicates management of the injured client by causing vasoconstriction, difficulty with venous access and arterial assessment, impaired oxygenation and ventilation, coagulopathy, increased bleeding, and slowed drug metabolism in the liver (Sedlak, 1995). Interventions to prevent hypothermia are basic: remove wet sheets or clothing, cover the client with blankets, infuse only warm solutions and blood products, set the room temperature at 75° to 80° F, and employ devices such as heat lamps and warming blankets. Table 12-2 highlights the primary survey and associated resuscitation interventions.

The Secondary Survey and Resuscitation Interventions

After the ED resuscitation team addresses the immediate life threats, other activities that the emergency nurse can anticipate include insertion of gastric tubes for decompression of the GI tract to prevent vomiting and aspiration, insertion of a urinary catheter to allow careful measure of urine output, and preparation for diagnostic studies such as bedside ultrasound, 12-lead electrocardiogram (ECG), radiologic studies, and laboratory analysis of blood. The resuscitation team also performs a more comprehensive head-to-toe assessment, known as the **secondary survey,** to identify other injuries or medical issues that need to be managed or that might impact the course of treatment. The client may be transported immediately to the operating room or cardiac catheterization laboratory directly from the ED depending on the nature of the medical problem or injury.

Care of the Emergency Department Client

Most people who come to the ED do not need resuscitation; they come for a variety of reasons. For instance, they are afraid that symptoms they are experiencing may indicate

TABLE 12-2 The Primary Survey and Resuscitation Interventions

Priorities of the Primary Survey	Examples of Specific Interventions
A: Airway/cervical spine	Establish a patent airway by positioning, suctioning, and oxygen, as needed. Protect the cervical spine by maintaining alignment. If the Glasgow Coma Scale (GCS) is ≤8 or the client is at risk for airway compromise, prepare for endotracheal intubation and mechanical ventilation.
B: Breathing	Assess breath sounds and respiratory effort. Observe for chest wall trauma or other physical abnormality. Prepare for chest decompression, if needed.
C: Circulation	Monitor vital signs, especially blood pressure and pulse. Maintain vascular access using a large bore catheter. Use direct pressure for external bleeding.
D: Disability	Evaluate the client's level of consciousness (LOC) using the AVPU system and the GCS. Re-evaluate the client's LOC frequently.
E: Exposure	Remove all clothing for a complete physical assessment. Prevent hypothermia, such as by covering the client with blankets, using heat lamps, and infusing warm solutions.

a very serious condition such as a stroke or heart attack. They have an acute illness, an exacerbation of a chronic illness, or an injury that requires urgent intervention (e.g., asthma, appendicitis, a fracture or laceration). Clients may have nagging problems that they just cannot tolerate until they get an appointment with a primary care physician like a urinary tract infection. Some individuals use the ED as a clinic to meet their episodic health needs in the absence of a primary health care provider.

Because clients have a variety of health care needs in the ED setting, the nursing care needs are highly variable as well. However, certain commonalties for the care of all emergency clients exist. After triage, the emergency nurse assigned to the individual reviews or completes a nursing assessment. Based upon established treatment protocols in some emergency departments (EDs), the nurse may take action when necessary. These interventions may include application of oxygen, cardiac monitoring, intravenous access, and collection of blood or urine specimens, even before the client is seen by a physician.

The client should be undressed to allow for an appropriate examination. Maintaining privacy and dignity, as well as maintaining confidentiality of information, is essential to the ethical provision of nursing care as well as client satisfaction. In a busy ED environment with overcrowding issues, maintaining dignity, privacy, and confidentiality can be challenging, especially when care may sometimes take place on stretchers in the hallway. Keeping voices low when discussing client information, employing alternative areas for clients to undress when no treatment room is available, such as a bathroom or an office with a locking door, and providing two client gowns (one to wear as a robe over the first gown) and a sheet or blanket as a cover are all appropriate strategies. Being creative when confronted with such challenges is a key role expectation of the emergency nurse.

After the physician has evaluated the client, the nurse is responsible for implementing orders. Medication administration, collection of specimens, assistance with bedside procedures such as laceration repair or lumbar puncture, and procuring diagnostic procedures are all in the domain of the emergency nurse. It is the emergency nurse's role to reassess and reprioritize needs whenever necessary, because the client's condition can improve or deteriorate.

Disposition

At the conclusion of the workup, the physician must make a decision regarding client disposition. Should the client be admitted to the hospital or discharged to home with instructions for continued care and follow-up? Usually, the answer is straightforward. A client who has an evolving myocardial infarction, stroke, or acute surgical need will be admitted. Sometimes, though, the ED disposition decision is less clear. Often the emergency nurse and physician discuss this decision collaboratively. The nurse may have a greater sense of how well a client will fare in a home setting depending upon whether or not other family members or friends are available to assist and are reliable. For example, an individual with a minor head injury has suffered a loss of consciousness. Typically, someone is expected to remain with that client for the first 12 to 24 hours after injury to be sure that he does not show any evidence of deterioration. Another common scenario involves the risk to the client in cases of actual or suspected domestic violence or child abuse. If discharge to home is not deemed safe, the client may be admitted to the hospital until resources can be organized to provide for a safe environment. Social workers or case managers are usually consulted to investigate resource needs and to plan accordingly.

Case Management

Some EDs employ registered nurse case managers who can screen ED clients and intervene when necessary to arrange appropriate referral and follow-up. This is a new and evolving role in the ED setting which can be beneficial in the provision of comprehensive care and as a strategy to avoid inappropriate use of resources in an era of profound ED overcrowding.

ED case managers, supported by computer-based information systems, can review the ED census on both a "real-time" as well as on a retrospective basis to determine which clients have visited the ED frequently in a given period of time. The case manager can then determine the reasons why they sought emergency services, such as lack of a primary health care provider, exacerbation of a chronic condition, or lack of health education. Case management interventions include facilitating referrals to primary care providers who are accepting new clients or to subsidized community-based health clinics for individuals or families in need of routine services.

For those with needs related to chronic conditions, the ED case manager can arrange referral into appropriate disease management programs in the community if available (see Chapter 3). Disease management programs are specific to a particular condition such as asthma, COPD, diabetes, hypertension, heart failure, and renal failure. They help clients learn how to properly manage their condition on a day-to-day basis to prevent exacerbations or clinical deterioration. The main goal is to keep the client out of the hospital as long as possible. Health teaching is a key component of these programs. For other health teaching needs, the ED case manager can direct the client to the appropriate educational resources such as a health educator, nutritionist, or organization (e.g., the American Cancer Society, the American Heart Association).

Other functions of the ED case manager might include working with staff to plan disposition for homeless individuals, locating a safe environment for victims of domestic violence or elder abuse, and providing information on community resources for low-cost prescription plans and health insurance.

Client/Family Health Teaching

A key role of the emergency nurse is health teaching. At the most basic level, emergency nurses review discharge instructions with the client and family before signing them out of the department.

> **CULTURAL CONSIDERATIONS**
>
> Most discharge instructions are either preprinted or computer generated, and can be customized to address the individual client's needs. The client's ability to read as well as understand English must be taken into account. Many hospitals have teaching information available in Spanish and other regional languages. However, interpreters may be necessary to assist the health care provider to customize the information appropriately. The emergency nurse may need to demonstrate how to care for a wound, for example, or how to measure the correct dose of a medication. When follow-up is necessary, specific information regarding the timing and type of follow-up must be communicated.

Beyond discharge instructions, the ED environment and community-at-large present many opportunities for health teaching by the nurse. Lassman (2001) asserts that "injury prevention should be an integral part of emergency care" (p. 171) and advocates that emergency nurses are obligated as health care professionals to educate the public about wellness and injury prevention. If the client presented after a motor vehicle crash, for instance, this is an ideal time to reinforce the need to wear seat belts or use child safety seats correctly. ED visits that result from mishaps in the home provide an excellent opportunity to discuss home safety issues, such as the need for smoke detectors and carbon monoxide detectors, and fall prevention tips, such as the need for proper lighting and removal of throw rugs. Safety tips may be based on the developmental stage of children in the home. For example, instructing parents to cover electrical outlets during the toddler years may prevent an electrical injury.

Injury is not the only topic that affords a teaching opportunity. A new onset or an exacerbation of a medical condition also allows for education, such as how to measure blood glucose and ways to control blood pressure or reduce the risk of heart disease.

MASS CASUALTY PRINCIPLES

Mass casualty incidents occur yearly in the United States due to events such as severe weather phenomenon, earthquakes, fire, catastrophic building collapse, and transportation disasters such as plane crashes and train derailments. Emergency preparedness training and drills have been standard functions of EDs and hospitals for many years. The Joint Commission on Accreditation of Health Care Organizations requires that hospitals have an emergency preparedness plan that is tested through drills or actual participation in a real event at least twice yearly, no less than 4 months but no more than 8 months apart. One of these drills or events must involve community-wide resources to assess the efficacy of collaborative efforts and command structures (Joint Commission Resources, 2003).

Even though emergency preparedness is considered a regulatory requirement for hospital accreditation, the degree to which many employees seriously participated in such drills in the past was highly variable. On September 11, 2001, however, the concept of emergency preparedness changed the American way of life and dramatically changed traditional hospital and community disaster planning.

With the catastrophic collapse of the twin towers of the World Trade Center after the terrorist-driven airplanes crashed into them, and the subsequent real and perceived threat of domestic terrorism including anthrax exposure, hospital emergency preparedness concepts became integrated into daily operations of EDs. Suddenly, weapons of mass destruction (WMD) were on the forefront of public health risk to the general population. The term **"NBC"** was coined to refer to nuclear, biologic, and chemical weapons of mass destruction. Hospital ED decontamination facilities and all levels of personal protective gear to protect staff from various types of contaminants are under review and are being upgraded to handle nuclear, chemical, and biologically contaminated clients.

ED physician and nursing staff undergo not only hazardous materials training, but how to recognize patterns of illness in clients who present for treatment that could be indicative of biologic terrorism agents, such as anthrax or smallpox. Protocols for the pharmacologic treatment of infectious disease agents, as well as stockpiles of antibiotics and nerve agent antidotes, are readily available. The most immediate advantage of this intense focus on enhancing emergency preparedness plans is that the ability to competently handle the more typical community mass casualty incident such as a bus crash, tornado, or building collapse has greatly improved in many systems.

Triage

Triage concepts in a mass casualty incident differ from the "civilian triage" covered earlier in this chapter that is practiced during usual ED operations (Table 12-3). In mass casu-

TABLE 12-3 Comparison of Triage Under Usual versus Mass Casualty Operations

Triage Under Usual Conditions	Triage Under Mass Casualty Conditions
Emergent (immediate threat to life)	Emergent or Class I (red tag) (immediate threat to life)
Urgent (major injuries that require immediate treatment)	Urgent or Class II (yellow tag) (major injuries that require immediate treatment)
Nonurgent (minor injuries that do not require immediate treatment)	Nonurgent or Class III (green tag) (minor injuries that do not require immediate treatment)
	Expectant or Class IV (black tag) (expected and allowed to die)

alty or disaster situations, a military form of triage is implemented with the overall goal of doing the greatest good for the greatest number of people (Bracken, 2003). This concept means that clients who are critically ill or injured who might otherwise receive the benefit of an attempted resuscitation during usual operations could be triaged into an "expectant" category and allowed to die. Classic examples of black-tagged clients include those with massive head trauma, extensive full-thickness body burns, and high cervical spinal cord injury requiring mechanical ventilation. The rationale for this seemingly heartless decision is that the limited resources must be dedicated to saving the most lives, rather than expending valuable personnel time, equipment, and supplies to save one life at the possible expense of others.

Triage functions may be performed by emergency medical services (EMS) providers in the field, such as emergency medical technicians (EMTs) and paramedics, nurse and physician field teams who are called from the hospital into a mass casualty scene to assist EMS providers, and nurse and physician hospital teams to assess and reassess incoming clients. Before going to the incident in the field, it is important that nurses and physicians have adequate training to prepare them to recognize risks inherent in an unstable multicasualty environment (e.g., potential for structural collapse; becoming the secondary target of a terrorist attack). They must take measures to protect themselves so that they do not become victims as well.

Mass casualty triage practices can vary in different localities, but some concepts are fairly universal. Most mass casualty teams both in the field and in the hospital setting use a disaster triage tag system that categorizes triage priority by color and number: emergent (class I) clients are identified with a red tag; urgent (class II) clients are marked with a yellow tag; nonurgent (class III) clients are given a green tag; individuals who are expected to die or are dead are issued a black tag (class IV) (Bracken, 2003). In general, red-tagged clients have immediate threats to life such as airway compromise or hemorrhagic shock that require immediate treatment. Yellow-tagged clients have major injuries such as open fractures and large wounds that need treatment within a 30-minute to 2-hour time frame. Green-tagged clients have minor injuries that can be managed in a delayed fashion, generally in more than 2 hours. Examples of minor "green tag" injuries include closed fractures, sprains, strains, contusions, and abrasions.

These green-tagged clients are often referred to as the "walking wounded"; they may actually evacuate themselves from the mass casualty scene and go to the hospital in a private vehicle. Green-tagged clients usually constitute the greatest number in most large-scale multicasualty situations and can overwhelm the system if provisions are not made to handle them as part of the disaster plan. The other issue is that because green-tagged clients may take it upon themselves to come the hospital in their own way, the hospital may not be able to get a sense from the emergency medical providers at the scene just how many actual casualties will arrive at the hospital. A related concern is that green-tagged clients who self-transport may unknowingly carry contaminants from a nuclear, biologic, or chemical incident into the hospital environment with potentially disastrous consequences. ED staff must anticipate these issues and devise emergency response plans accordingly.

A special bracelet with a disaster number is typically applied to each individual in the triage area. Preprinted labels with this specific disaster number can be applied to the client's chart forms and personal belongings; they can even be used as a means to track client movement through the ED (Newberry, 2002). After the client's name has been confirmed, the standard hospital identification bracelet may be used.

Systems Notification/Activation of Emergency Preparedness

A **mass casualty incident** or disaster is commonly defined based on the resource availability of a particular community or hospital facility. When the number of casualties exceeds the resource capabilities, a **disaster** situation is recognized to exist. What may be a routine day in the emergency department (ED) of a large urban trauma center could be defined as a disaster for a small rural community hospital if the same number of clients were to arrive. Each facility, then, must define its own parameters to identify when a disaster situation is present. Flexibility is needed because resources may change by time of day and by day of the week. For instance, hospitals typically have the fewest human resources available after midnight on the weekend. An incident that occurs in this time frame may require activation of the emergency preparedness plan to bring extra resources into the hospital, whereas the same incident during weekday business hours might be handled with on-site personnel alone without activation of the plan.

Notification that a mass casualty situation exists usually occurs by means of radio communication between the ED and EMS providers at the scene. A state or regional emergency management agency may also notify the ED of the event. Each hospital has its own policy that specifies *who* has the authority to activate and *how* to activate the disaster or emergency preparedness plan. Group paging systems, telephone trees, and instant computer-based alert messages constitute the most common means of notifying essential personnel of a mass casualty incident or disaster.

A catastrophic event of great magnitude, such as a devastating earthquake or tornado, or even a terrorist incident involving weapons of mass destruction (WMD) also necessitates volunteer assistance from all levels of health care providers in the region. In this case, the media may be contacted to broadcast messages to the health care community-at-large via television and radio announcements. For such incidents, the National Guard, the American Red Cross, the Public Health Department, various military units, and even a **Disaster Medical Assistance Team (DMAT)** can be activated by state and federal government authorities.

A DMAT is a medical relief team made up of medical, paraprofessional, and support personnel that is deployed to a disaster area with enough medical equipment and supplies to sustain operations for 72 hours (Riley, 2003). DMATs are part of the National Disaster Medical System (NDMS) in the United States and function to provide relief services ranging from primary health care and triage to evacuation and staffing to assist health care facilities that have become overwhelmed with casualties (Riley, 2003). Because licensed health care providers such as nurses act as federal employees when they are deployed, their professional licenses are recognized and valid in all states.

Hospital Emergency Preparedness: Personnel Roles and Responsibilities

The roles and responsibilities of hospital personnel in a mass casualty incident or disaster are defined within the institution's emergency response or preparedness plan (Table 12-4). Each plan can be as individual as the particular hospital's operations. However, virtually all plans identify certain key functions. One of the primary roles to be established at the onset of an incident is the role of a **hospital incident commander** who assumes overall leadership for implementing the institutional plan. This individual is usually either a physician in the ED or a hospital administrator who has the authority to activate resources. The hospital incident commander's role is to take a global view of the entire situation and facilitate client movement through the system as well as bring in both human and supply resources to meet client needs. For example, a hospital incident commander might dictate that all clients due to be discharged from an inpatient unit be moved to a lounge area immediately to free up hospital beds for mass casualty victims. He or she could also direct departments such as physical therapy or a surgical clinic to cancel their usual operations and then convert the space into a minor treatment area to handle numerous "walking wounded" clients. The incident commander assists in the organization of hospital-wide services to rapidly expand hospital capacity, recruit paid or volunteer staff to assume clinical or support assignments, and assure the availability of medical supplies to treat clients.

Another typical role defined in hospital emergency preparedness plans is that of the **medical command physician**. This individual focuses on determining the number, acuity, and medical resource needs of victims arriving from the incident scene to the hospital and organizing the emergency health care team response to the injured or ill clients. Responsibilities include identifying the need for and calling in specialty-trained providers such as the following:

- Trauma surgeons
- Neurosurgeons
- Orthopedic surgeons
- Pulmonologists
- Plastic surgeons
- Burn surgeons
- Infectious disease physicians
- Industrial hygienists
- Radiation safety personnel

In smaller hospitals with limited specialty resources, the medical command physician would also help determine which clients would be transported out of the facility to a higher level of care.

Closely affiliated with the medical command physician is the **triage officer.** Again, this individual is generally a physician in a large hospital who is assisted by triage nurses. When physician resources are limited, a nurse may assume this role. The triage officer rapidly evaluates each individual who presents to the hospital, even those who come in with triage tags in place. Client acuity is re-evaluated for appropriate disposition to the area within the ED or hospital best suited to meet the client's medical needs.

The ED charge nurse, trauma program manager, and other ED nursing leadership personnel act in close collaboration with the medical command physician and triage officer to organize nursing and ancillary services to meet client needs. Telephone trees can be activated to call in off-duty emergency nurses. Nurses from medical-surgical nursing units can be recruited to provide care for stable ED clients, thus freeing up emergency nurses to aid mass casualty victims. Critical care unit nurses can supplement emergency nurses in the resuscitation setting or assist in monitored care and transport to critical care units. Emergency nurse leaders also typically direct the ancillary departments to deliver supplies, instrument trays, medications, food, and personnel to meet service demands.

Many other roles and responsibilities can be defined within the institutional emergency response plan, and may include the supply officer, the communications officer, the infection control officer, and the community relations/public information officer, to name a few. The community

TABLE 12-4 Key Personnel Roles and Functions for Emergency Preparedness and Response Plan

Personnel Role	Personnel Function
Hospital incident commander	Physician or administrator who assumes overall leadership for implementing the emergency plan
Medical command physician	Physician who decides the number, acuity, and resource needs of clients
Triage officer	Physician or nurse who rapidly evaluates each client to determine priorities for treatment
Community relations or public information officer	Person who serves as a liaison between the medical center and media

relations or public information officer is an especially important role to delineate in advance because mass casualty incidents tend to attract a large amount of media attention. This staff member can draw media away from the clinical areas so that essential hospital operations are not hindered. He or she can also serve as the liaison between hospital administration and the media to release only appropriate and accurate information.

Hospital staff of all levels may be required to alter their routine operations to accommodate a high volume of clients. Some plans dictate specific actions by staff members, such as who should be called when the plan is activated, who should report, where to report, what supplies or equipment carts should be brought to a predesignated location, and what type of paperwork or system should be implemented for client identification in a large-scale event. Some staff may even have their roles changed completely, for example, nurses who work in other departments, such as the performance improvement department or case management, may be reassigned to fulfill a clinical responsibility for staffing of a nursing unit. The key concept is that staff members are expected to remain flexible in a mass casualty situation and perform at their highest level to address both the needs of the health care system and those of the clients. The greatest good for the greatest number of people is still the organizing principle when considering roles and responsibilities in mass casualty events, not necessarily individual staff preferences.

Event Resolution

When the last major casualties have been treated and no more are anticipated to arrive in numbers that could overwhelm the health care system, it is time for the incident commander to consider "standing down" or deactivating the emergency response plan. However, although the casualties may have left the ED, other areas in the hospital may still be under great stress and need the support of the supplemental resources brought in by emergency plan activation. Before terminating the response, it is essential to assure that the needs of the other hospital departments have been met and all are in agreement to resume normal operations.

A key consideration in event resolution is staff and supply availability. If nursing staff and other personnel were called in from home during their off hours, or if they worked well beyond their scheduled shifts to meet client and departmental needs, some provision for an adequate rest period should be made. Exhaustion poses a risk not only to client safety but also to the emergency nurse when he or she must drive home. Sleeping quarters at the hospital might be necessary in this case, especially if the disaster event contributed to treacherous travel conditions.

Creativity and flexibility of nursing leaders and emergency nursing staff come together to provide staffing coverage of the ED. A personal emergency preparedness plan for each emergency nurse can help in such situations. It should consist of the preplanned specific arrangements that are to be made for child care, pet care, and elder care if the need arises and the emergency nurse is unable to return home for an extended period of time. Emergency contact names, addresses, and telephone numbers should be included for optimal usefulness in a crisis.

Severe shortages of supplies also pose a threat to normal operations at the conclusion of a mass casualty incident. Taking inventory and restocking the ED are high priority assignments. Close collaboration between the ED and the central supply department are essential to resolving stock availability problems. Instrument trays must be washed, packaged, and resterilized. Critical supplies that have been depleted from hospital stores must be reordered and delivered to the hospital quickly. Contracts with key vendors outlining emergency resupply expectations and arrangements should be a part of the hospital's overall emergency preparedness plan.

Debriefing

CRITICAL INCIDENT STRESS DEBRIEFING

There are two general types of **debriefing** that occur after a mass casualty incident or disaster. The first type of debriefing entails bringing in critical incident stress debriefing (CISD) teams to provide sessions for small groups of staff to promote effective coping strategies. The second type of debriefing involves an administrative review of staff and system performance during the event to determine whether or not opportunities for improvement in the emergency management plan exist.

The concept of CISD began in 1983 as a crisis stress management intervention to decrease the effects of traumatic events and facilitate recovery of high-risk workers such as emergency medical personnel, firefighters, and police officers (Mitchell, Sakraida & Kameg, 2003). CISD is now only one component of a much broader **Critical Incident Stress Management (CISM)** program. CISM programming addresses precrisis through postcrisis interventions for small to large groups, including communities (Everly & Mitchell, 1999). After working through the turmoil and the emotional impact of the incident as well as the aftermath, emergency staff may find it difficult to "get back to normal." Without intervention, staff may develop **post-traumatic stress disorder (PTSD),** which can lead to multiple characteristic psychological and physical effects: flashbacks, avoidance, diminished interest in previously enjoyable events, detachment, and physical manifestations including rapid heart rate, insomnia, and other physiologic effects of anxiety (Mitchell, Kameg & Sakraida, 2003). Individuals suffering from PTSD can have great difficulty relating in their usual way to family and friends. Ultimately, professional "burnout" can stem from the inability to cope with the stress effectively.

A CISD team is comprised of two to three specially trained individuals who come together quickly when called to deal with the emotional needs of health team members after a particularly devastating or disturbing incident. The CISD team leader typically has background in a mental health/behavioral health field; the co-leader is ideally a peer of the group being debriefed (Mitchell, Sakraida & Kameg, 2003). Thus if nurses are to be debriefed, then a nurse member of the CISD team is generally assigned to the session. CISD-trained physicians, police, firefighters, EMTs, and paramedics may also be used depending on the needs of the group. The third member of the team is known as the "doorkeeper" and is responsible for keeping inappropriate individuals out (e.g., media, spectators) and talking with anyone who leaves the session early in an effort to have them return or accept follow-up (Mitchell, Sakraida & Kameg, 2003). Staff involved in the incident need protected time to undergo stress debriefing, which generally lasts from 1 to 3 hours per session.

Typical "ground rules" for stress debriefing include strict confidentiality of information shared during the session and unconditional acceptance of the thoughts and feelings expressed by individuals within the group. The usual arrangement for the most effective group interaction consists of a circular configuration of chairs in a private setting. Food should be available so that hunger is not a distraction. CISD group leaders encourage group discussion through asking a series of questions designed to make everyone involved tell his or her own story about the incident and explain the personal impact. The group leaders enable participants to place the incident into perspective and dispel any feelings of blame or guilt. They also educate participants about self-care concepts and coping strategies to use immediately. Individuals who require more than a CISD session may need referral for mental health/behavioral health counseling. Evidence-based research efforts using meta-analysis techniques have produced mixed results regarding the efficacy of CISD; however, the technique is perceived to be clinically effective (Mitchell, Sakraida & Kameg, 2003).

ADMINISTRATIVE REVIEW

The second type of debriefing is an administrative function directed at analyzing the hospital's response to the event while it is still in the forefront of the minds of everyone who participated in it. The goal of this type of debriefing is to discern what went right and what went wrong during activation and implementation of the emergency preparedness plan so that changes can be made. Typically, representatives from all departments that were involved in the incident come together soon after plan activation has been discontinued. They each are given an opportunity to hear and express both positive and negative comments related to their experiences with the event. Although drills are important, implementing the emergency preparedness plan during an actual mass casualty event is the most effective means of "reality testing" the plan's utility. Information gleaned from participants can be used to modify or revise the plan in preparation for future events. Lessons learned serve as the best catalyst for improvements in the overall system of disaster management.

EMERGENCY DEPARTMENT CASE SCENARIO: POSSIBLE ANTHRAX EXPOSURE

Case Presentation

M.C., a 34-year-old woman, presents to the triage desk of a large suburban emergency department (ED) bearing a box with a dusting of white powder on it. M.C. quickly explains to the triage nurse that she is afraid an employee at her office has contaminated the box with anthrax. She exhibits signs of severe anxiety while she relates that this employee was born in an Arab country and obviously "hates America." Nearly sobbing now, she expresses her fears that she has been deliberately exposed to anthrax by a terrorist and needs treatment.

The triage nurse immediately notifies security and escorts the client outside of the building. The client is confused and angry as to why she cannot be placed in a treatment room. She wants the substance on the box tested to determine if it is indeed anthrax. The emergency nurse instructs M.C. to place the box on the ground in a grassy area outside of the ED. She then asks that the security guard establish a safe perimeter around the box and place calls to both the local law enforcement agency as well as the Department of Public Health. The agency will take possession of the box, investigate the woman's claim, and engage in appropriate testing of the white powder.

In the meantime, the emergency nurse also activates the ED's hazardous materials decontamination plan. Nursing staff don appropriate protective attire which includes an impervious gown, gloves, face mask, and eye protection, and prepare the decontamination facility (Figure 12-4). When ready to begin decontamination, M.C. is directed to enter the decontamination room through the outside door from the parking lot to avoid the potential for contamination of the ED. Staff assist M.C. to remove all of her clothing. She is directed into a shower stall and washed thoroughly with soap and water. When decontamination is complete, she is given a hospital gown, robe, and slippers, and is placed in a wheelchair for transport to an ED treatment room in the "fast track" area for low acuity clients.

Upon arrival to the treatment room, M.C. appears much less anxious. A physician examines her and determines that she has no clinical evidence of infectious disease. For this reason, and because an actual exposure to anthrax has not yet been confirmed by the Public Health Department, the physician elects *not* to prescribe the typical 60-day course of a prophylactic antibiotic for *Bacillus anthracis* such as doxycycline or ciprofloxacin (Cipro). The emergency physician explains that her plan is to discharge the client to home with referral for outpatient follow-up at the Public Health Department. M.C. again becomes tearful and demands that she be given a prescription for an antibiotic because she is afraid she will die. She contends that she will sue the hospital if anything should happen to her.

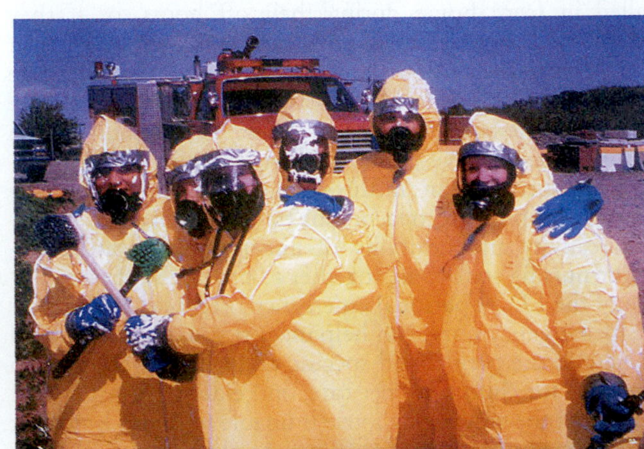

Figure 12-4 ■ Hazardous materials team members wearing protective clothing and respirators prepare to decontaminate individuals exposed to toxic chemicals in an outdoor decontamination area.

The emergency physician and nurse actively engage MC in discharge teaching about anthrax. With compassion and empathy, they explain that taking antibiotics unnecessarily will promote the growth of resistant bacteria and may cause serious drug-related side effects. They tell M.C. that the Department of Public Health will analyze the substance on the box, and if it is found to be *B. anthracis*, she will be notified right away. She will then be re-evaluated by the Public Health Department and started on appropriate postexposure prophylactic antibiotics. M.C. is reassured and offered the services of a community mental health/behavioral health clinic if she desires counseling to address her anxiety about this situation as well as her perceived threat from the Arab employee at her work site. After this teaching episode, M.C. appears to have her anxiety and anger under control. Because M.C.'s own clothing was confiscated and placed in a hazardous materials container for disposal during the decontamination process, the emergency nurse contacts the social worker to request that female apparel be made available from the hospital's supply of donated clothing so that she can get dressed. The client is given written discharge instructions.

Case Discussion

Although it may seem odd that the emergency nurse escorted M.C. outside of the building, this action prevented the potential spread of *B. anthracis* into the ED and potentially the hospital environment. Contamination of innocent bystanders as well as the hospital environment with a hazardous material can force the closure of key areas within the facility and can necessitate evacuation of clients and staff. Because M.C. was a "walk-in" client, she accessed the triage area before undergoing decontamination. Had M.C. been a known potentially contaminated client before arrival (e.g., if she was treated by an ambulance crew), she would have been taken to the decontamination facility upon arrival. Decontamination should precede triage; only the most basic life-sustaining interventions should be performed before or during decontamination (Newberry, 2002). M.C. also brought a potentially contaminated item into the ED. It is important to realize that the ED has no ability to conduct "point of care" testing to determine whether the unknown white powder substance was actually *B. anthracis*, the bacterium responsible for causing anthrax infection. Such testing is the domain of the Public Health Department.

Local, state, and federal law enforcement agencies also must become involved in the overall investigation of an actual or potential bioterrorism event so that the suspected perpetrators can be apprehended, even in the event of a hoax or practical joke. Hoaxes are not taken lightly by law enforcement in this era of heightened terrorist awareness. The practical jokers may find themselves prosecuted as criminals and serving prison time for their actions. More common, however, are the panicked reactions from innocent people like M.C. who come to the ED believing that they have suffered an exposure to a bioterrorism agent.

M.C. was sent into the decontamination room through an outside door. Most ED decontamination facilities have both outside and inside doors. The client enters from the outside, is decontaminated, and is then transported into the ED. Containment tanks to collect wastewater run-off from the decontamination process and separate air handling systems are typical components of new facility designs. Potentially contaminated clothing is removed from the victim and destroyed.

According to Centers for Disease Control and Prevention (2001) guidelines, unless the client exhibits clinical evidence of disease, or the substance under question tests positive for *B. anthracis*, antibiotics are not indicated. Anthrax can manifest disease in three forms: cutaneous, gastrointestinal, and inhalational or pulmonary. Cutaneous anthrax is caused by direct contact with *B. anthracis*. It presents as a pruritic papular lesion that turns into a vesicle, which, in 2 to 6 days, becomes a lesion with depressed black eschar; this form of anthrax is generally nonfatal if treated with antibiotics (CDC, 2001). Gastrointestinal anthrax is caused by ingestion of contaminated food and is characterized by abdominal pain, nausea, vomiting (hematemesis), fever, bloody diarrhea, and sepsis in late stages. There is a high mortality rate, especially after the client exhibits sepsis. Pulmonary or inhalational anthrax stems from inhalation of anthrax spores. This illness begins as a flu-like syndrome with fever and drenching sweats that progresses rapidly to respiratory failure. Classic radiographic evidence consists of a widened mediastinum and pleural effusions on a chest radiograph; these findings may not appear until later in the course of illness (CDC, 2002). Unless treatment is instituted very early in the prodromal stage, mortality rates are exceptionally high.

Once in the fast track setting in this case scenario, attention was directed at reducing the anxiety level of the client and providing effective health teaching. The psychosocial harm that occurs with actual or potential victims of bioterrorism events cannot be underestimated. When large groups of individuals are involved in a potential exposure, there is great potential for hysteria to occur. Effective interventions include calmly providing factual information about the potential threat and offering follow-up with both public health and mental health/behavioral health professionals as needed to address both physical and mental health/behavioral health issues.

GET READY for the NCLEX Examination!

KEY POINTS

- Emergency departments (EDs) are fast-paced and overcrowded environments that process clients across the life span with a variety of health problems.
- The most common reasons that clients seek ED care include chest pain, abdominal pain, headache, and fever.
- The interdisciplinary ED team includes prehospital providers, physicians, nurses, and support (ancillary) staff.
- Use the best practices listed in Chart 12-1 to maintain safety in the ED.
- Core competencies for the ED nurse include assessment, priority setting/critical thinking, knowledge of the ED, technical skills, and communication.
- The most commonly used triage system used under usual conditions is the three-level model: emergent, urgent, and nonurgent.
- Implement the steps of the primary survey and resuscitation interventions outlined in Table 12-2.
- Client education as part of the discharge plan is an important part of ED nursing practice.

- All medical centers must have an emergency preparedness and response team in case of mass casualty.
- The typical triage system for a mass casualty situation includes an additional category for those clients allowed to die (black-tagged).
- Special roles are assigned in a mass casualty incident as identified in Table 12-4.
- In a situation wherein exposure to a biologic agent is suspected, the decontamination team wears special, protective gear and decontaminates the clients who were exposed. Those clients are separated from others in the ED.

ADDITIONAL STUDY RESOURCES

Go to your Student CD-ROM for Review Questions for the NCLEX Examination.

evolve Go to http://evolve.elsevier.com/Iggy/ for Integrated Management of Care Questions for the NCLEX Examination.

SELECTED BIBLIOGRAPHY

Asterisk indicates a classic or definitive work on this subject.

American Academy of Pediatrics & American Heart Association. (2002). *PALS provider manual.* Dallas: American Heart Association.

*American College of Surgeons Committee on Trauma. (1997). *Advanced trauma life support course for physicians student manual* (6th ed.). Chicago: Author.

Bitterman, R. (2000). Overview of hospital and physician responsibilities mandated by EMTALA, In R. Bitterman (Ed.), *Providing emergency care under federal law: EMTALA.* (pp. 15-22). Dallas: American College of Emergency Physicians.

Bracken, J. (2003). Triage. In L. Newberry (Ed.), *Sheehy's emergency nursing principles and practice* (5th ed., pp. 75-83). St. Louis: Mosby.

Case, J., Mowery, M., & Welebob, E. (2002). *The nursing shortage: Can technology help?* Oakland, CA: California Healthcare Foundation.

Centers for Disease Control and Prevention. (2001). Update: Investigation of bioterrorism-related anthrax and interim guidelines for clinical evaluation of persons with possible anthrax. November 02, 2001. *MMWR* 2001, *50*, 941-948. Retrieved September 11, 2003, from http://www.cdc.gov/mmwr/preview/mmwrhtml/mm5043al.htm.

Centers for Disease Control and Prevention. (2002). Clinical issues in the prophylaxis, diagnosis, and treatment of anthrax. *Emerging Infectious Diseases*, *8*(2). Retrieved September 11, 2003, from http://www.cdc.gov/ncidod/EID/vol8no2/01-0521.htm.

*Craig, P.A. (1998). Risk management issues in the emergency department. In B.J. Youngberg (Ed.). *The risk manager's desk reference.* (pp. 1-24). New York: Aspen.

Cummins, R.O. (Ed.). (2003). *ACLS: Principles and practice.* Dallas: American Heart Association.

*Dame, L.A. (1998). The Emergency Medical Treatment and Active Labor Act: The anomalous right to health care. *Health Matrix: Journal of Law Medicine*, *8*, 1.

*Eckle, N., Haley, K., & Baker, P. (Eds.). (1998). *ENPC provider manual* (2nd ed.). Park Ridge, IL: Emergency Nurses Association.

*Emergency Medical Treatment and Active Labor Act, 42 U.S.C.SS 1395dd. (1996).

Emergency Nurses Association. (2000a). *Emergency nursing core curriculum* (5th ed.). Philadelphia: W.B. Saunders.

Emergency Nurses Association. (2000b). *Orientation to emergency nursing: Concepts, competencies & critical thinking* (2nd ed.). Des Plaines, IL: Author.

Emergency Nurses Association. (2000c). *Trauma nursing core course provider manual* (5th ed.). Park Ridge, IL: Author.

Emergency Nurses Association. (2001). *Standards of emergency nursing practice* (4th ed.). Des Plaines, IL: Author.

Emergency Nurses Association. (2002). *Emergency Nurses Association position statements: Stress management strategies.* Retrieved September 23, 2003, from http://www.ena.org/about/position/stressmanagement.asp.

*Everly, G.S., & Mitchell, J.T. (1999). *Critical incident stress management (CISM): A new era and standard of care in crisis intervention.* Ellicott City, MD: Chevron Publishing.

Gilboy, N. (2003). The evolution of triage. In N. Gilboy, et al. (Eds.). *The Emergency Severity Index: Implementation handbook.* (pp. 2-5). Des Plaines, IL: Emergency Nurses Association.

Gilboy, N., et al. (Eds.) (2003). *The Emergency Severity Index: Implementation handbook.* Des Plaines, IL: Emergency Nurses Association.

Gurney, D. (2002). Developing a successful 16-week "Transition ED Nursing" program: One busy community hospital's experience. *Journal of Emergency Nursing, 28*, 505-514.

Heinrich, J. (2001, June 22). EMTALA implementation and enforcement issues. *FDCH Government Account Reports*, Retrieved February 10, 2002, from http://ehostvgw12.epnet.com.

*Hyman, D. (1998). Patient dumping and EMTALA: Past imperfect/future shock. *Health Matrix: Journal of Law Medicine, 8*, 29-57.

Joint Commission Resources. (2003). *Accreditation issues for emergency departments.* Oakbrook Terrace, IL: Joint Commission on Accreditation of Health Care Organizations.

Kamoie, B. (2000). EMTALA: Reading beyond the emergency room to expand hospital liability. *Journal of Health Law, 33*, 25-55.

Kelly, L.Y. & Joel, L. A. (2001). *The nursing experience: Trends, challenges, and transitions* (4th ed.). New York: McGraw-Hill.

Keough, V.A., Schlomer, R.S., & Bollenberg, B.W. (2003). Serendipitous findings from an Illinois ED nursing educational survey reflect a crisis in emergency nursing. *Journal of Emergency Nursing, 29*, 17-22.

Lassman, J. (2001). Teachable moments: A paradigm shift. *Journal of Emergency Nursing, 27*, 171-175.

Litvak, E., et al. (2001). Emergency department diversion: Causes and solutions. *Academic Emergency Medicine, 8*, 1108-1110.

*Mayer, T.A., & Zimmerman, P.G. (1999). ED customer satisfaction survival skills: One hospital's experience. *Journal of Emergency Nursing, 25*, 187-191.

McCaig, L.F., & Burt, C.W. (2003). National hospital ambulatory medical care survey: 2001 emergency department summary. *Advance Data from Vital Health Statistics, 335*, Hyattsville, MD: National Center for Health Statistics.

McCaig, L. F. & Ly, N. (2002). National hospital ambulatory medical care survey: 2000 emergency department summary. *Advance Data from Vital Health Statistics, 326*, Hyattsville, MD: National Center for Health Statistics.

Mitchell, A.M., Kameg, K., & Sakraida, T.J. (2003). Post-traumatic stress: Clinical implications. *Disaster Management & Response, 1*(1), 14-18.

Mitchell, A.M., Sakraida, T.J., & Kameg, K. (2003). Critical incident stress debriefing: Implications for best practice. *Disaster Management & Response, 1*(2), 46-51.

Newberry, L. (2002). Practical suggestions for helping emergency nurses handle mass casualties. *Disaster Management & Response, Premier Issue*, 15-17.

Riley, J.M. (2003). Providing nursing care with federal disaster-relief teams. *Disaster Management & Response, 1*(3), 76-79.

*Sedlak, S.K. (1995). Hypothermia in trauma: The nurse's role in recognition, prevention, and management. *International Journal of Trauma Nursing, 1*(1), 19-26.

Travers, D. (2003). Triage acuity systems. In N. Gilboy, et al. (Eds.). *The emergency severity index: Implementation handbook.* (pp. 6-11). Des Plaines, IL: Emergency Nurses Association.

Travers, D.A., et al. (2002). Five-level triage system more effective than three-level in tertiary emergency department. *Journal of Emergency Nursing, 28*, 395-400.

Twedell, D.M. (2000). Nursing process: Assessment and priority setting. In Emergency Nurses Association. *Emergency nursing core curriculum* (5th ed.). Philadelphia: W.B. Saunders.

CHAPTER

13

Interventions for Clients with Common Environmental Emergencies

LINDA LASKOWSKI-JONES

LEARNING OUTCOMES

After studying this chapter, you should be able to:

1. Assess clients for common types of heat-related injuries.
2. Teach clients how to prevent heat-related injuries.
3. Prioritize first aid interventions for clients who have heat-related injuries.
4. Prioritize first aid interventions for clients experiencing snakebites.
5. Differentiate care for clients who have arthropod bites and stings.
6. Develop a plan of care for a client who is allergic to bees and experiences a bee sting.
7. Teach clients how to prevent arthropod bites and stings.
8. Prioritize care for clients who have been struck by lightning.
9. Teach clients how to avoid cold injuries.
10. Explain the rationale for interventions when warming clients who have cold injuries.
11. Describe best practices for clients who are at risk for or experience altitude-related illnesses.
12. Develop a plan of care for a client with near-drowning.

Go to your Student CD-ROM for Review Questions for the NCLEX Examination keyed to these Learning Outcomes.

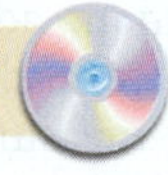

Recreational pursuits as well as home and work responsibilities summon people of all ages to leave the shelter of their homes for the great outdoors. Seemingly harmless outside activities can have associated environmental risks. Some of these hazards, such as insect bites or stings, reptile bites, and environmental conditions, may also pose threats indoors. This chapter gives an overview of selected environmental emergencies and presents management concepts to address immediate emergency care needs as well as acute care interventions for these hazards. Common sense illness and injury prevention strategies for nurses to incorporate into their own lifestyle and health teaching opportunities are also discussed. The information contained in this chapter is pertinent to everyone who has close encounters with the summer and winter elements, whether driving to work or taking part in an adventure sport.

HEAT-RELATED ILLNESSES

There are several notable predisposing environmental and physical factors associated with heat-related illnesses. High environmental temperature (>95° F) and high humidity (>80%) constitute the most common environmental factors. Physical factors range from extremes of age to a client's current health status. For example, dehydration, fatigue, lack of sleep, obesity, heart disease, fever, strenuous exercise, seizures, and all degrees of burns (even sunburn) cause individuals to become more susceptible to heat stress. In addition, the use of drugs such as anticholinergic agents, beta-adrenergic blockers, angiotensin-converting enzyme (ACE) inhibitors, diuretics, cocaine, and amphetamines also increases the risk of heat-related illness (Auerbach, Donner, & Weiss, 2003). Before participating in any hot weather activity, clients at risk should be taught to consider these risk factors and take the necessary steps to eliminate or minimize them whenever possible.

HEALTH PROMOTION/ILLNESS PREVENTION

Chart 13-1 lists heat-related illness prevention strategies. These strategies are important to incorporate into health teaching opportunities with clients who participate in warm weather activities, as well as those with health risk factors that may predispose them to heat-related illness.

Heat Exhaustion

PATHOPHYSIOLOGY

Heat exhaustion is a syndrome primarily caused by dehydration. It stems from heavy perspiration as well as inadequate fluid and electrolyte consumption during heat exposure over hours to days. Clients complain of feeling quite ill, and their clinical presentation resembles having the flu. Although not considered a true emergency condition, if untreated, heat exhaustion can be a precursor to heat stroke.

COLLABORATIVE MANAGEMENT

In heat exhaustion, clients have a normal mental status in the presence of a flu-like syndrome with headache, weakness, fatigue, anorexia, nausea, and vomiting. The client should be assessed for orthostatic hypotension and tachycardia. It is important to note that the client's body temperature is *not* significantly elevated in this condition. He or she may continue to perspire despite the effects of dehydration.

Treatment consists of immediately terminating physical activity and moving the individual to a cool place. Constrictive clothing should be removed. An oral rehydrating solution such as a sports drink should be provided. Salt tablets should never be given without first crushing and dissolving them in adequate quantities of water–salt tablets alone cause stomach irritation, nausea, and vomiting. Effective cooling measures consist of placing cold packs on the neck, chest, abdomen, and groin; soaking the person in cool water; or fanning the individual while spraying water on the skin (Auerbach, Donner, & Weiss, 2003). If the characteristic signs and symptoms persist, an ambulance should be called to transport the client to the hospital.

CHART 13-1

CLIENT EDUCATION GUIDE

Heat-Related Illness Prevention

- Ensure adequate intake of nutritious foods and fluids such as commercially available sports bars and drinks that contain carbohydrates, sodium, and other essential electrolytes before, during, and after exercise.
- Prevent overexposure to the sun; use a sunscreen with an SPF of at least 30.
- Take time to get used to the heat by gradually increasing time spent working or playing in a hot environment.
- Rest frequently when working in a hot environment. Plan to limit activity at the hottest time of day.
- Wear clothing suited to the environment. Lightweight, light-colored, and loose-fitting clothing is best.
- Pay attention to your personal physical limitations; modify activities accordingly.

In the clinical setting, vital sign assessment and temperature monitoring are necessary. The client is typically rehydrated with intravenous (IV) 0.9% saline solution if nausea or vomiting is present. Blood is drawn for serum electrolyte analysis. Hospital admission is typically indicated for clients with significant comorbid conditions that have been worsened by the heat-related illness or for those with unresolved signs and symptoms after a period of treatment and observation.

Heat Stroke

PATHOPHYSIOLOGY

Heat stroke is a true medical emergency with a mortality rate that can approach 80% for individuals not effectively treated in a timely manner (Auerbach, Donner, & Weiss, 2003). The victim's heat regulatory mechanisms fail and are unable to compensate for a critical elevation in body temperature, which may exceed 105° F (40.5° C). If uncorrected, organ dysfunction and death will ensue.

Two types of heat stroke are (1) exertional and (2) classic. **Exertional heat stroke** has a sudden onset and is typically due to strenuous physical activity in hot, humid conditions. Lack of proper acclimatization to the hot weather and wearing clothing too heavy for the environment are common contributing factors. Conversely, **classic heat stroke** occurs over a period of time as a result of chronic exposure to a hot, humid environment, such as a home without air-conditioning in the high heat of the summer. It generally affects ill and older adults. The body's ability to dissipate heat effectively is significantly impaired in this disorder. All of the risk factors for heat-related illness previously described play an important role in the incidence of heat stroke.

COLLABORATIVE MANAGEMENT

Assessment

Victims of heat stroke have a profoundly elevated body temperature (>105° F or 40.5° C). This disorder is also characterized by mental status changes, which occur as a result of thermal injury to the brain. Typical mental status changes are evidenced by the appearance of anxiety, confusion, bizarre behavior, loss of coordination, hallucinations, agitation, seizures, and coma. Vital sign abnormalities may include hypotension, tachycardia, and tachypnea. Although the client's skin is classically described as hot and dry, the presence of sweating does *not* rule out heat stroke–persons may continue to perspire in this state.

Dematte et al. (1998) studied the sequelae of near-fatal classic heat stroke in 58 clients admitted to a Chicago intensive care unit during a sustained heat wave. They found that multiorgan dysfunction with neurologic impairment developed in 100% of these clients. Approximately one-half had moderate to severe renal insufficiency and disseminated intravascular coagulation (DIC), and 10% experienced acute respiratory distress syndrome. The in-hospital mortality rate was 21% for this group. Related complications that have been widely reported include electrolyte and acid-base disturbances, rhabdomyolysis, cerebral edema, and cerebral hemorrhage.

Interventions

Heat stroke must be recognized and treated immediately and aggressively for optimal client outcome (Chart 13-2).

FIRST AID. In the prehospital setting, rapid cooling is the first priority of care after ensuring a patent airway. According to Auerbach, Donner, and Weiss (2003), the faster the cooling, the lower the morbidity and mortality rates of heat stroke. Methods for rapidly cooling the client include the following:

- Stripping away clothing
- Placing ice packs on the neck, axillae, chest, and groin
- Immersing the victim in cold water
- Wetting the client's body with tepid water and then fanning rapidly to aid in cooling by evaporation.

Immersion in ice is contraindicated because shivering generates additional body heat and increases oxygen consumption. No food or liquid should be given by mouth because vomiting and aspiration are risks in the presence of neurologic impairment. Immediate medical care is essential. An ambulance with advanced life support capabilities should be summoned as soon as possible.

HOSPITAL CARE. Once in a clinical setting, monitor and support the client's airway and circulatory status. Initiation of high concentration oxygen therapy and IV lines with 0.9% saline solution are indicated. Ringer's lactate solution should be avoided because the liver may be unable to metabolize lactate effectively while the client is hyperthermic (Morris, 2003). Aggressive interventions to cool the client must continue until rectal temperature is 102° F or less. Methods include using cooling blankets and applying iced gastric and peritoneal lavage (Morris, 2003). Use a continuous temperature monitoring device, such as a rectal probe or temperature-monitoring urinary bladder catheter, to prevent overcorrection of the desired body temperature and hypothermia. If shivering occurs during the cooling process, chlorpromazine (Thorazine) 25 to 50 mg IM or IV may be prescribed.

Seizures pose a serious problem because seizure activity further elevates body temperature. Be sure that a benzodiazepine such as diazepam is immediately available for IV administration. Admission to a critical care unit for continued support and hemodynamic monitoring is usually indicated because complication and mortality rates for heat stroke are high.

CHART 13-2

BEST PRACTICE for
Emergency Care of the Client with Heatstroke

EMERGENCY CARE

At the Scene

- Ensure a patent airway.
- Remove the client from the hot environment (into air-conditioning or into the shade).
- Remove the client's clothing.
- Pour or spray water on the client's body and scalp.
- Fan the client (not only the person providing care, but all surrounding people should fan the client with newspapers or whatever is available).
- If ice is available, place ice in cloth or bags and position the packs on the client's scalp, in the groin area, under the neck, and in the armpits.
- Get the client to the nearest emergency department.

At the Hospital

- Give oxygen by mask or nasal cannula.
- Start at least one IV with a large-bore needle or cannula.
- Administer normal saline (0.9% sodium chloride) as rapidly as possible, using cooled solutions if available.
- Use a cooling blanket.
- **Do not give aspirin or any other antipyretics.**
- Insert a rectal probe to measure core body temperature continuously or use a rectal thermometer and assess temperature every 15 minutes.
- Insert a Foley catheter.
- Monitor vital signs at least every 15 minutes.
- Obtain the following laboratory tests as quickly as possible: serum electrolytes, cardiac enzymes, liver enzymes, and complete blood count (CBC).
- Assess arterial blood gases.
- Administer muscle relaxants (benzodiazepines) if the client begins to shiver.
- Measure urine output and specific gravity to determine fluid needs.
- Slow cooling interventions when core body temperature is reduced to 102° F (38.8° C).

SNAKEBITES

More often than not, people have a fear of snakes. Although most snake species are nonvenomous and harmless, there are one or more species of poisonous snakes found in every U.S. state except Maine, Alaska, and Hawaii. The two families of indigenous poisonous snakes in North America are the Crotalidae and the Elapidae.

The Crotalidae are the "pit vipers," named for the characteristic depression between each eye and nostril that serves as a heat-sensitive organ for locating warm-blooded prey. They include various species of rattlesnakes, copperheads, and water moccasins (also known as "cottonmouths") and account for the vast majority of the poisonous snakebites in the United States (Figures 13-1 and 13-2).

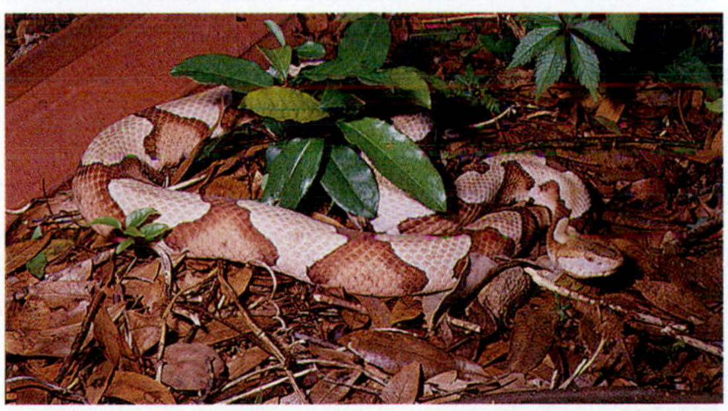

Figure 13-1 ■ Southern copperhead *(Agkistrodon contortrix contortrix)* has markings that make it almost invisible when lying in leaf litter. (From Auerbach, P., Donner, H.J., & Weiss, E.A. [2003]. *Field guide to wilderness medicine* [2nd ed., plate 7]. St. Louis: Mosby.)

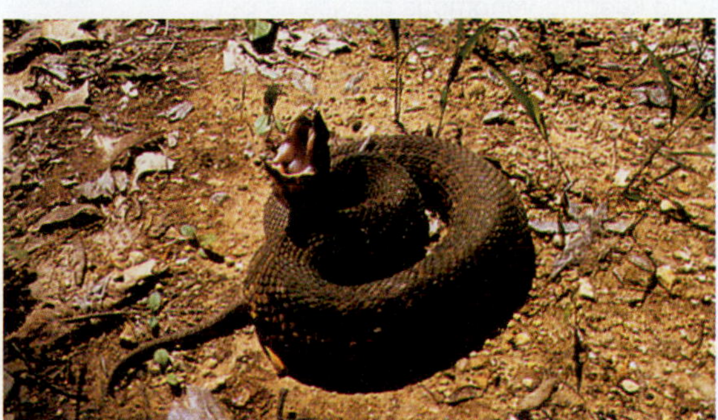

Figure 13-2 ■ Cottonmouth water moccasin *(Agkistrodon piscivoris)*. The open-mouthed threat gesture is characteristic of this semiaquatic pit viper. (From Auerbach, P.S., Donner, H.J., & Weiss, E.A. [2003]. *Field guide to wilderness medicine* [2nd ed., plate 6]. St. Louis: Mosby.)

The Elapidae include the coral snakes, which are found from North Carolina to Florida, and in the Gulf states through Texas and Arizona. Coral snakes are accountable for less than 1% of the snakebites in the United States (Lee, 1997). Coral snakes have broad bands of red and black rings, separated by yellow or cream rings. These nonaggressive snakes have short, fixed fangs and inject neurotoxic venom into prey via a chewing motion.

Of the 5000 snakebites that occur each year in the United States, nearly 25% are inflicted by venomous snakes (Holstege et al., 1997). Fatalities are few, but tend to occur in older adults and in individuals who are inadequately treated. Most bites are reported between April and October, with a peak incidence in July and August. This time frame corresponds to an increase in both human and reptile activity in the outdoor environment during the warm weather months. Most snakes fear humans and attempt to avoid contact with them. Sudden, unexpected confrontations at close range are the usual precursors to defensive strikes. Awareness is the key to snakebite prevention.

HEALTH PROMOTION/ILLNESS PREVENTION

Chart 13-3 provides common sense considerations to avoid being bitten by a poisonous snake.

North American Pit Vipers

North American pit vipers can be differentiated from harmless snakes by noting the following key anatomic features:

- The heat-sensing "pit" described on p. 175
- A triangular head that indicates the presence of venom glands
- Two retractable, curved fangs that have canals for venom flow (fangs retract posteriorly when the snake's mouth is closed)
- Up to three sets of developing "replacement" fangs behind the primary fangs

CHART 13-3

CLIENT EDUCATION GUIDE
Snakebite Prevention

- Avoid keeping venomous snakes as pets.
- Be extremely careful in locations that may harbor snakes such as tall grass, rock piles, ledges and crevices, wood piles, brush, swamps, and caves. Snakes are most active on warm nights.
- Don protective attire such as boots, heavy pants, and leather gloves. When walking or hiking, use a walking stick or trekking poles.
- Inspect suspicious areas before placing hands and feet in them.
- Do not harass any snakes you may encounter. Striking distance is at least the length of the snake. Young snakes still pose a threat; they are capable of envenomation from birth.
- Be aware that newly dead or decapitated snakes can inflict a bite for 20 to 60 minutes after death due to persistence of the bite reflex.
- Use extreme caution if attempting to transport the snake with the victim to the medical facility for identification purposes. Ensure that the snake is placed in a sealed container.

Unlike copperheads and water moccasins, rattlesnakes also have interlocking horny rings in their tails that vibrate and serve as a characteristic warning signal to predators. Pit vipers can regulate the amount of venom flow through their fangs depending, in part, on the size of the prey. The quantity of venom injected in defensive bites on humans is highly variable. Approximately 25% of pit viper bites are actually "dry"; that is, there is no envenomation (venom release), yet there are distinctive fang marks on the client (Table 13-1). In contrast, harmless snakes do *not* have venom glands or fangs.

PATHOPHYSIOLOGY

When providing emergency care to a victim of snakebite, the key question is whether or not envenomation has actually occurred. Understanding venom's purpose and function is essential to recognizing the manifestations of envenomation and planning appropriate interventions. The primary functions of venom are to immobilize, kill, and aid in digestion of prey. Venom causes local and systemic toxic effects. The enzymes in venom break down human tissue proteins, alter membrane integrity, and impair blood clotting mechanisms. Not surprisingly, then, the pathophysiologic effects of pit viper envenomation can lead to local tissue necrosis, massive tissue swelling, intravascular fluid shifts and hypovolemic shock, pulmonary edema, renal failure, and hemorrhagic complications from disseminated intravascular coagulation (DIC).

COLLABORATIVE MANAGEMENT

Assessment

The clinical manifestations of envenomation are based on the type and amount of venom injected, the bite location, as well as the age, size, and health status of the victim. Puncture wounds in the skin are a key *local* sign of pit viper envenomation. One or more puncture wounds may be present, depending upon how many fangs the snake has and how many times the snake struck the client. Severe pain, swelling, and redness or ecchymosis (bruising) in the area around the bite are common. Hours later, vesicles or hemorrhagic bullae may form. *Systemic* responses to venom must be distinguished from the psychophysiologic effects of anxiety and panic related to being bitten by a snake. Commonly reported complaints include a minty, rubbery, or metallic taste in the mouth and tingling or paresthesias of the scalp, face, and lips. Other effects include muscle fasciculations and weakness, nausea, vomiting, hypotension, seizures, and coagulopathy (clotting abnormalities) or disseminated intravascular coagulation (DIC). If the bite site

TABLE 13-1 Grades of Pit Viper Envenomation

Envenomation Characteristics

- None. Fang marks, but no local or systemic reactions
- Minimal. Fang marks, local swelling and pain, but no systemic reactions
- Moderate. Fang marks and swelling progressing beyond the site of the bite; systemic signs and symptoms, such as nausea, vomiting, paresthesias, and hypotension
- Severe. Fang marks present with marked swelling of the extremity, subcutaneous ecchymosis, severe symptoms, including manifestations of coagulopathy

From Auerbach, P.S., Donner, H.J., & Weiss, E.A. (2003). Field guide to wilderness medicine (2nd ed.). St. Louis: Mosby.

does not show evidence of local tissue swelling or redness within 8 hours, systemic effects are unlikely to develop.

Interventions

FIRST AID. First aid interventions for snakebite should begin in the field and can improve the victim's outcome. The first priority is to move the person to a safe area away from the snake and encourage rest to decrease venom circulation. Next, jewelry and constricting clothing are removed before swelling becomes significant. Immobilizing the affected extremity in a position of function with a splint is another intervention to limit the spread of the venom. The extremity should be kept below the level of the heart. Keep the individual warm and provide calm reassurance. Do not offer any alcohol or stimulants such as caffeinated beverages because these may speed the absorption of venom (Gold & Wingert, 1994).

HOSPITAL CARE. Acute care in a hospital is warranted as soon as possible. However, if transportation and definitive treatment will be delayed, a 2- to 4-cm constricting band may be applied proximal to an extremity wound to impede venom circulation via lymphatic flow, but it should not be tight enough to impair venous drainage or arterial flow. This band should *not* be used as a tourniquet. Placement of the band may worsen the local tissue necrosis by retaining venom in the tissues–the risk of increased limb damage must be weighed against the consequences of systemic venom effects (Auerbach, Donner, & Weiss, 2003). Assess distal circulation frequently. The band should be loosened if edema renders it too tight. The wound should *not* be incised and sucked, or have ice applied to it. However, a commercially available device called the Sawyer extractor has been found to remove significant amounts of venom if used within 3 minutes of envenomation and left in place for at least 30 minutes (Auerbach, Donner, & Weiss, 2003).

Initial Interventions. Envenomation is a medical emergency. Acute care management in the hospital involves supportive care, which includes supplemental oxygen, two large-bore IV lines, and infusion of crystalloid fluids such as normal saline solution or lactated Ringer's solution. Continuous cardiac and blood pressure monitoring are necessary to quickly detect clinical deterioration. Because envenomation can cause severe pain at the bite site, opioid pain medication is indicated. Snakebite also poses tetanus and wound infection risks. Therefore tetanus prophylaxis, attention to wound care, and broad-spectrum antibiotics must be incorporated into the management plan.

Severe pit viper envenomation causes coagulopathy (clotting abnormalities) and promotes hemorrhage and tissue destruction. Along with typical baseline laboratory studies, a coagulation profile, complete blood count, creatinine kinase, type and crossmatch, and urinalysis should be anticipated. An electrocardiogram (ECG) is necessary to detect evidence of myocardial ischemia or other cardiac abnormalities. Pertinent client history related to the event includes a full account of the snake's appearance, the time the bite was inflicted, prehospital interventions, and any past incidence of snakebite or antivenom use. To accurately assess the development of tissue edema at the bite site, the circumference of the bitten extremity should be measured and recorded every 15 to 30 minutes.

Drug Therapy. Venom potency varies. Not all snake bite victims need antivenom administration. The decision whether or not to give antivenom is based upon the severity of the envenomation. Table 13-1 provides a classification scheme for grading envenomation severity. Conventional pit viper antivenom is most effective within 4 hours of the bite, less effective after 12 hours, but may reverse coagulopathy beyond 24 hours (Gold & Wingert, 1994). Best practice is to contact the regional poison control center so that toxicologists can provide advice in antivenom dosing and medical management.

Until the newest antivenom known as CroFab was introduced in the year 2001, Antivenin Crotalidae Polyvalent was the most commonly used antivenom to treat bites of all North American and South American crotalids (e.g., rattlesnakes, copperheads, and water moccasins). It is considered to be *conventional* antivenom therapy and continues to play a role on a more limited basis in the management of venomous snakebite. The drug is most effective when administered within the first 4 hours of envenomation, but it may reverse coagulopathy even after 24 hours.

The usual dosing regimen is for the drug to be administered over 2 to 4 hours in the following manner:

- Mild envenomation–5 vials
- Moderate envenomation–10 vials
- Severe envenomation–15 to 20 vials

Each vial of powder comes with a bottle of diluent. Do not shake the solution when reconstituting the drug; this action destroys the antivenom proteins and renders the agent ineffective. The vials should be gently rolled to dissolve the powder into the solution, which may take 10 minutes per vial.

The solution from the reconstituted vials is then injected into 250 mL of normal saline. The infusion is begun slowly at a rate of 1 to 5 mL/hr. In general, the rate can be doubled every minute if there is no evidence of an allergic response. The rate of infusion, then, is 10 to 20 minutes per vial. The total infusion time is typically 1 to 2 hours.

Because Antivenin Crotalidae Polyvalent (conventional antivenom) is made from horse serum, there is a high risk of hypersensitivity reactions of varying severity, including life-threatening anaphylactic shock. Administration of this drug requires care in following all dosing guidelines for dilution and infusion. Intradermal skin testing, which was routinely recommended to detect an allergy to horse serum before antivenom administration, is now considered to be inaccurate and not helpful in medical management decisions (Norris & Bush, 2001). Diphenhydramine, epinephrine, and resuscitation equipment must be immediately available to treat anaphylaxis if it occurs. Serum sickness, a type III hypersensitivity reaction, typically follows 7 to 14 days after drug administration and presents as a flu-like syndrome with a skin rash and joint pain. Serum sickness is generally treated with antihistamines and steroids.

Manifestations of an allergic reaction may include anxiety, chills, weakness, wheezing, stridor, vomiting, dyspnea, diaphoresis, throat constriction, sneezing, or red streaking at the IV site. If an allergic reaction is suspected, stop the infusion. Epinephrine may be prescribed if indicated. Other agents to manage the allergic response include IV diphenhydramine (Benadryl) and cimetidine (Tagamet). Both H1 and H2 antagonists are required to treat the reaction effectively. Other measures include further dilution of the antivenom or restarting at a slower rate.

The initial dosage of conventional antivenom is repeated every 2 hours until the progression of local signs ceases and systemic signs resolve. Pregnancy is *not* a contraindication to treatment (Lee, 1997). CroFab or Crotalidae Polyvalent Immune Fab (Ovine) is the newest IV product indicated for the treatment of minimal to moderate crotalid envenomation (First New Management, 2001). CroFab is made from the blood of healthy sheep immunized with North American snake venom. CroFab consists of specific antibody fragments that bind, neutralize and redistribute toxins in crotalid venom so that they may be removed from the client's body ("First New Management," 2001).

CroFab appears to be safer than conventional antivenom therapy. Mild to moderate allergic reactions such as pruritus and urticaria can occur, but anaphylaxis is rare. Skin testing before administration is not necessary. CroFab should be given to clients as soon as possible. The optimal timing is within 6 hours of envenomation ("First New Management," 2001; Hutchinson & Shahan, 2002). Over the first 10 minutes, the infusion should be slow (25 to 50 mL/hr). Monitor the client closely for evidence of an allergic reaction. If symptoms are not effectively controlled with the first dose, including coagulopathy, an additional four to six vials are recommended. Once the client's symptoms are under control, two vials of CroFab are administered every 6 hours for a total of 18 hours of administration (Hutchinson & Shahan, 2002).

If the client has a known hypersensitivity to ovine (sheep) products, CroFab is contraindicated. CroFab is also contraindicated if the client has an allergy to papain or papaya, which is used during the manufacturing process. Give CroFab cautiously to clients who have the following:

- Had an allergic reaction to conventional antivenom therapy in the past
- A hypersensitivity to bromelain (a pineapple-derived enzyme)
- Renal or hepatic impairment
- Pregnancy
- Sensitivity to mercury-containing products (contains ethyl mercury)

At this time, research is limited regarding the efficacy of CroFab with severe envenomation as well as with copperhead envenomation. Finally, if clinical symptoms and coagulopathy recur after the initial infusion, repeat dosing is required.

Coral Snakes

PATHOPHYSIOLOGY

North American coral snakes are found in the southeastern United States and in Texas and Arizona (Figure 13-3). These snakes burrow into the ground and are characteristically nonaggressive. Their ability to inject venom is less efficient than that of the pit vipers. Their maxillary fangs are small and fixed in an upright position. The coral snake must use a chewing motion to inject venom from venom glands through its maxillary fangs. Most bites occur when people attempt to handle the snake. Coral snake venom lacks the complexity of pit viper venom, but can be extremely potent. It has only two primary components: a postsynaptic neurotoxin and a myotoxin. The amount of venom in an adult coral snake is enough to kill a human.

Coral snakes can be recognized by bands of black, red, and yellow coloration that completely encircle the body of the snake. If a black band lies between the red and yellow bands, the snake is most likely nonvenomous. There are several harmless species that closely mimic the appearance of the coral snake. A helpful memory aid for identifying coral snakes is "red on yellow can kill a fellow" and "red and black, venom lack" (Norris & Bush, 2001).

COLLABORATIVE MANAGEMENT

Assessment

Manifestations of coral snake envenomation (venom release) are most closely related to the neurotoxic properties of coral snake venom. The physiologic effect is to block the binding of acetylcholine at the postsynaptic junction (Norris & Bush, 2001). Unlike pit viper envenomation, pain at the bite site may be only mild and transient. Swelling is unlikely. Fang marks may be difficult to visualize due to the coral snake's small teeth. Coagulopathy does not occur as a result of coral snake envenomation. The toxic effects of coral snake venom also may be delayed up to 12 to 13 hours after a bite, but then produce rapid clinical deterioration. Early signs and symptoms consist of nausea, vomiting, headache, pallor, and abdominal pain. Assess for neurologic manifestations, such as paresthesias, numbness, and mental status changes, as well as cranial nerve and peripheral nerve deficits. Total flaccid paralysis may occur later. The client may have difficulty speaking, swallowing, and breathing.

Respiratory insufficiency and cardiovascular collapse can occur in severe cases. Arterial blood gas analysis reveals evidence of respiratory insufficiency. The myotoxic component of the venom can cause an elevation in creatinine kinase (CK) levels due to muscle breakdown and produce myoglobinuria. Despite the pronounced clinical effects, death is rare if the client receives timely management.

Interventions

FIRST AID. Because several varieties of harmless snakes mimic the appearance of the coral snake, the first priority, if possible, is to definitively identify the snake as a coral snake. Identification can be facilitated if the snake is captured and brought to the health care facility with the victim. However, if the snake cannot be caught or positively identified, the vic-

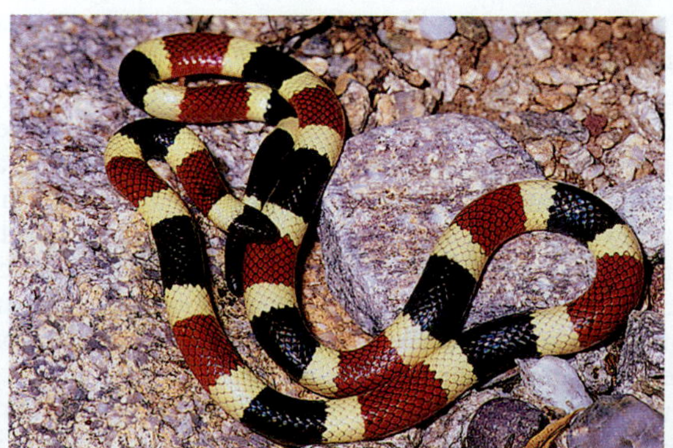

Figure 13-3 ■ Sonoran coral snake *(Micruroides euryxanthus)* is also known as the Arizona coral snake. No documented fatality has followed a bite by this species. (From Auerbach, P.S., Donner, H.J., & Weiss, E.A. [2003]. *Field guide to wilderness medicine* [2nd ed., plate 8]. St. Louis: Mosby.)

tim should be treated as if envenomation has occurred. The field care is the same for that of a pit viper bite without the added concern over tissue necrosis if a constricting band is used, because coral snake venom does not destroy tissue. A field method called the "Australian compression and immobilization technique" in which the extremity is encircled snugly with a roller gauze dressing to impede lymphatic flow and then splinted also may be useful to slow the systemic spread of venom in coral snake bites (Auerbach, Donner, & Weiss, 2003). This compression bandage must not be so tight as to impair arterial flow nor should it be removed until the victim is being managed at an acute care facility.

HOSPITAL CARE. Once in an acute care setting, clients who have had an actual or potential coral snake envenomation should have continuous cardiac, blood pressure, and pulse oximetry monitoring. Prepare to provide aggressive airway management via endotracheal intubation if respiratory insufficiency or severe neurologic impairment occurs. Aspiration of secretions presents a significant risk for this client.

Antivenom administration is recommended even in the absence of clinical evidence of envenomation (Norris & Bush, 2001). The onset of symptoms after coral snake envenomation can be delayed for several hours. However, a delay in antivenom administration can lead to ineffective treatment of neurotoxicity once it develops. The antivenom indicated for the treatment of North American coral snake envenomation is Antivenin *Micrurus fulvius* (Wyeth-Ayerst) made from horse serum. It is effective against the venom of all coral snake species within the United States except the small Sonoran coral snake found in Arizona. No fatalities have been reported as a result of a Sonoran coral snake envenomation; only supportive care is recommended for this type of bite (Norris & Bush, 2001).

The same clinical precautions are applicable when administering coral snake antivenom as with Crotalinae (pit viper) antivenom. The most significant risk to the client is an anaphylactic response to the antivenom. Skin testing is considered inaccurate and not beneficial (Norris & Bush, 2001). Therefore ensure that the client's IV lines are patent and that emergency drugs such as epinephrine as well as resuscitation equipment are immediately available. Premedication with H1- and H2-blocking antihistamines such as diphenhydramine and cimetidine should be anticipated. The adult dose is three to six vials.

Begin the infusion slowly, then increase to enable the entire infusion to be completed within about 2 hours. If an allergic reaction occurs, stop the infusion while the client is treated with epinephrine and/or more antihistamines. The infusion is then restarted at a slower rate. For severe reactions, the physician must determine whether to continue antivenom administration. The initial dose of coral snake antivenom may need to be repeated if neurotoxicity continues to progress. A poison control center should be contacted for assistance with client management and antivenom dosing.

ARTHROPOD BITES AND STINGS

There are several clinically significant insects found in North America that are members of the phylum Arthropoda. These insects include notable species of spiders, scorpions, bees, and wasps. Spiders are carnivorous arthropods that belong to the arachnid class. Unlike snakes, almost all species of spiders are venomous to some degree–most are not harmful to humans either because their mouthparts are too small to pierce human skin, or the quantity of their venom is inadequate to produce significant consequences. However, the venom of some spiders indigenous to the United States does produce significant pathologic effects. Spiders of particular clinical interest are the brown recluse, black widow, and tarantula. Scorpions, bees, and wasps are other venomous arthropods that produce toxic reactions in humans.

Brown Recluse Spider

PATHOPHYSIOLOGY

The brown spiders of the *Loxosceles* genus are known for producing bites that result in ulcerative lesions. In the United States, the brown recluse spider *(L. reclusa)* is the best known culprit of these genera. Brown recluse spiders, also known as "fiddlebacks" or "violin spiders," are medium-sized spiders (body length 8 to 15 mm) that are light brown in color and have a dark brown, fiddle-shaped mark that extends from their eyes down their back (Figure 13-4). Like their name implies, brown recluse spiders are shy and hide in areas that are dark and secluded, such as boxes, closets, basements, sheds, garages, luggage, shoes, clothing, and even bed sheets. Most indoor bites occur when people are sleeping, reaching into boxes or closets, or donning clothing that contains the spider. Few people ever get a look at the spider that bit them. The only evidence may be the characteristic skin lesion and, less often, systemic effects from the injected toxin (commonly referred to as "necrotic arachnidism" or "loxoscelism" in medical literature).

COLLABORATIVE MANAGEMENT

Assessment

Brown recluse spider venom produces cytotoxic effects on tissue. The initial bite has been variously described as painless or stinging to sharp and painful. Some victims are unaware that they were bitten until the telltale lesion with intense local aching and pruritus develops over minutes to hours. The central bite site may appear as a bleb or vesicle surrounded by edema and erythema, which may expand

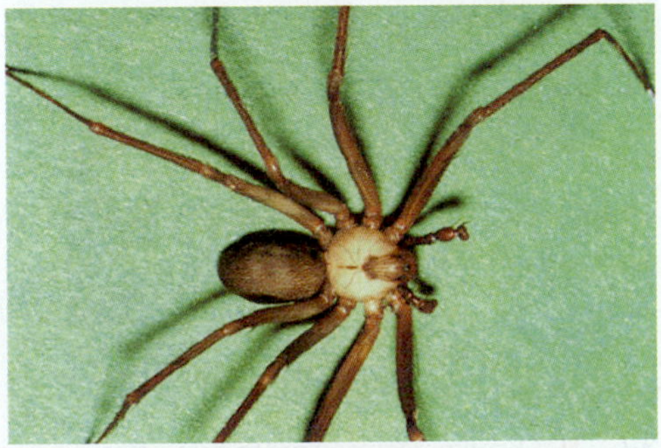

Figure 13-4 ■ Brown recluse spider *(Loxosceles reclusa)*. (From Auerbach, P.S., Donner, H.J., & Weiss, E.A. [2003]. *Field guide to wilderness medicine* [2nd ed., plate 12]. St. Louis: Mosby.)

over the course of hours as the toxin spreads to surrounding tissues. Over the next 1 to 3 days, the central lesion typically becomes dark and necrotic (Figure 13-5). Eschar eventually forms. When the eschar sloughs, an open wound or ulcer can remain for weeks to months. Surgical intervention is often necessary to promote wound healing and reduce scarring. Skin grafting may be required for large wounds. In rare cases, some persons may also exhibit manifestations of systemic toxicity to brown recluse spider bites. These can include fever, chills, nausea, vomiting, malaise, joint pain, and petechiae (Morris, 2003). At the extreme end, hemolytic reactions, renal failure, and death have been reported.

Interventions

FIRST AID. The basic first aid for a brown recluse spider bite is to apply cold compresses intermittently during the first 4 days after the bite (Auerbach, Donner, & Weiss, 2003). The cold compress helps decrease the enzymatic activity of the venom and may limit tissue necrosis. Heat should *never* be used because it increases the enzymatic activity and potentially worsens the wound. Rest and elevation of the affected extremity are also recommended (Morris, 2003).

HOSPITAL CARE. For clients with wounds that appear infected, a topical antiseptic and a sterile dressing are necessary; antibiotics are also indicated (Auerbach, Donner, & Weiss, 2003). For severe wounds, therapy with Dapsone may be considered. Dapsone, administered orally in doses of 50 mg twice daily, is a polymorphonuclear leukocyte inhibitor that is effective in treating crater lesions in adults (Morris, 2003). Because there is a risk of blood dyscrasias in persons with glucose-6-phosphate-dehydrogenase G6PD deficiency, G6PD screening and careful monitoring of blood studies are important to detect abnormalities. Methemoglobinemia is another potential adverse effect of Dapsone. An evaluation by a surgeon is usually necessary for clients whose wounds require interventions beyond conservative management. Debridement and skin grafting may be required in order for severe wounds to heal.

Black Widow Spider

PATHOPHYSIOLOGY

Black widow spiders can be found in every state in the United States except Alaska. They have a notorious reputation for inflicting deadly bites. The black widow belongs to the genus *Latrodectus* and prefers a cool, damp environment like outdoor log piles, vegetation, and under rocks. They also commonly inhabit barns, sheds, and garages. The female spider is about 12 to 16 mm in length and is best identified by her shiny black color and the red hourglass pattern on her ventral abdomen. Male spiders are smaller in size and lighter in color with white and gray markings. The hourglass pattern is faint in males. Black widow spiders carry neurotoxic venom. Their usual prey is another arthropod but may include small lizards and snakes. Bites to humans are defensive in nature when the spider is at risk of being crushed.

The initial bite of a black widow spider is variously described as nearly painless to sharply painful. Typically, the client notices a tiny papule or small red punctate mark. The client may experience intense pain, which seems out of proportion to the lesion. In many cases, the symptoms do not progress beyond a local reaction in the area of the bite site. If systemic signs and symptoms do occur, they generally develop within 1 hour and involve the neuromuscular system.

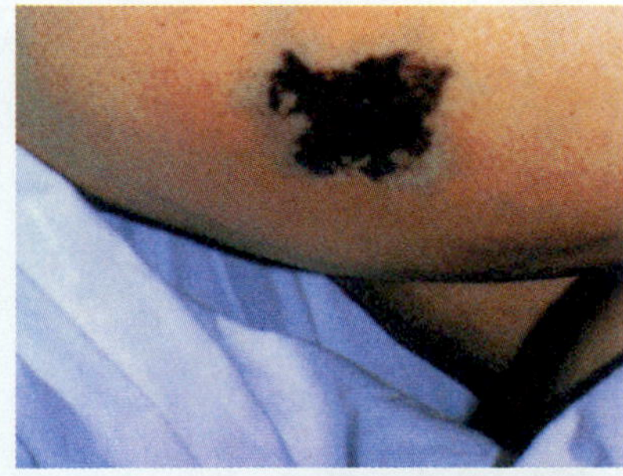

Figure 13-5 ■ Brown recluse spider bite after 24 hours, with central ischemia and rapidly advancing cellulitis. (From Auerbach, P.S., Donner, H.J., & Weiss, E.A. [2003]. *Field guide to wilderness medicine* [2nd ed., plate 13]. St. Louis: Mosby).

COLLABORATIVE MANAGEMENT

Assessment

Envenomation by a black widow spider produces a clinical syndrome known as latrodectism. The neurotoxic venom causes neurotransmitter release from nerve terminals. Severe abdominal pain, muscle rigidity and spasm, hypertension, and nausea and vomiting constitute the classic clinical presentation. In fact, some clinicians erroneously identify the problem as an acute abdomen and consider surgical consultation due to the similar clinical features as peritonitis. The muscle spasms commonly involve the large muscles of the abdomen, back, and limbs. Other noteworthy signs include facial edema (*Latrodectus* facies), ptosis, diaphoresis, weakness, increased salivation, priapism (sustained erection), respiratory difficulty, increased respiratory secretions, fasciculations, and paresthesias. The effects of the bite are self-limited and generally resolve in a few days. However, older adults with significant comorbid conditions such as cardiovascular disease are at much higher risk for a complicated course.

Interventions

FIRST AID. The primary first aid intervention for a black widow spider bite in the prehospital setting is to apply an ice pack. Ice inhibits the action of the neurotoxin. The client should be monitored for evidence of systemic toxicity as described above. If signs or symptoms develop, intervene to support the client's airway, breathing, and circulation. Clients should be transported to a medical facility as soon as possible for advanced life support care.

HOSPITAL CARE. Clients require close monitoring of vital signs, with special attention to blood pressure and respiratory function. Supportive therapy in the hospital includes administration of opioid pain medication and muscle relaxants such as diazepam (Valium). Calcium gluconate (10 mL of a 10% solution) also may be given for muscle spasms, rigidity, and pain. Tetanus prophylaxis is necessary. The client must be observed for the development of seizures related to a rapidly rising blood pressure (Auerbach, Donner,

& Weiss, 2003). Antihypertensive agents may be needed. Although relapses may occur, symptoms usually subside in 48 hours (Morris, 2003). Less often, pulmonary edema, uncontrollable hypertension, and shock ensue. These clients require critical care management. Hospital admission is recommended for all pregnant women and those with a history of hypertension (Boyer, McNally, & Binford, 2001). Antivenom is available for black widow spider bites. However, this agent is rarely used because it carries its own significant risk of anaphylaxis and serum sickness. It is generally administered to treat only severe reactions in which respiratory arrest, seizures, or uncontrolled hypertension occurs. Because pregnant women may have uterine contractions from a black widow spider bite that can cause a premature delivery, antivenom is also indicated for them. The typical dose is one to three ampules. A poison control center can assist in antivenom dosing and client management under these circumstances.

Tarantulas

PATHOPHYSIOLOGY

Tarantulas are members of the Theraphosidae family, the largest sized spiders in the arachnid class. They mainly can be found in the tropical and subtropical areas of the United States and on all continents of the world. However, a number of species are also found in dry, arid states, such as New Mexico and Arizona. Tarantulas can grow to 10 cm in length and live for up to 25 years (Boyer, McNally, & Binford, 2001). These spiders possess venom that paralyzes prey and causes muscle necrosis. However, most bites to humans result in only local effects. A more serious issue is that several genera of tarantulas have *urticating hairs* in their dorsal abdominal area that can be launched into the air as a defensive maneuver and onto a victim. Thousands of these barbed hairs may land on an individual, penetrate skin and eyes, and induce a severe inflammatory reaction.

COLLABORATIVE MANAGEMENT

Assessment

Tarantula bites typically produce pain at the bite site, variously described as mild to moderate to severe. Swelling, redness, numbness, and lymphangitis constitute the usual local effects. Tarantulas found in the United States are not implicated in producing systemic reactions. However, venom from tarantulas in other parts of the world may induce systemic illness. As described earlier, the more troubling aspect of tarantula exposure may be contact with urticating hairs thrown from the spider or rubbed onto a victim's skin during handling. The hairs produce an inflammatory response in skin and mucous membranes consisting of edematous papules that are associated with intense pruritus that can last several weeks. If hairs come into contact with the eyes–sometimes through transfer with hairs on a victim's hands–severe ophthalmic complications can occur (Boyer, McNally, & Binford, 2001).

Interventions

Supportive management is generally all that is required to manage clients who have suffered a venomous bite or exposure to urticating hairs of a tarantula. Pain at the bite site is treated through administration of analgesics appropriate to the level of pain the client is experiencing. The involved extremity can also be immobilized and elevated to decrease pain and swelling. The bite can be expected to heal without sequelae.

Urticating hairs are best removed as soon as possible through repeated use of sticky tape applied to the skin and then removed to pull the hairs from the skin, followed by thorough irrigation (Boyer, McNally, & Binford, 2001). For eye exposure, copious irrigation with saline is required. Oral antihistamines and topical or systemic steroids may be used to treat the intense pruritus associated with urticating hair exposure (Auerbach, Donner, & Weiss, 2003).

Scorpions

PATHOPHYSIOLOGY

Scorpions are found in many states within the United States, although not typically in the Midwest or New England. However, stings are always possible when people keep scorpions as pets or when scorpions are inadvertently transported to nonindigenous areas in baggage and packaging. Unlike spiders that envenom their prey by inflicting a bite, scorpions inject venom through a stinging apparatus on their tail. Most scorpion stings produce a relatively mild reaction characterized by local pain, inflammation, and mild systemic symptoms. These effects are typically self-limiting and best treated by analgesics, supportive management, and basic wound care.

One species of scorpion found in the United States that can inflict a sting associated with a severe, potentially fatal systemic response is the *Centruroides exilicauda,* or the bark scorpion (Figure 13-6). It is often found in trees, wood piles, and around debris. Humans are most often stung when this scorpion gets into clothing, shoes, blankets, and personal items left on the ground. The small bark scorpion is about 5 cm (2 inches) in length and may be solid yellow, brown, or tan in color. There are also some striped varieties, though not as common. While many scorpions have thick claws and thick tails, distinctive features of the bark scorpion

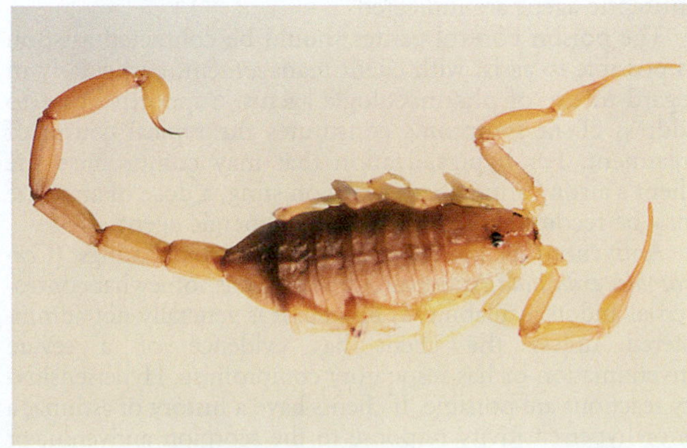

Figure 13-6 ■ *Centruroides exilicauda (C. sculpturatus),* the bark scorpion of Arizona. (From Auerbach, P.S., Donner, H.J., & Weiss, E.A. [2003]. *Field guide to wilderness medicine* [2nd ed., plate 17]. St. Louis: Mosby.)

include thin pincers and a thin tail, as well as the presence of a tubercle, called a subaculeate tooth, at the base of the stinger. This scorpion is found throughout Arizona and in some areas of New Mexico, Texas, Nevada, and California. The venom of the bark scorpion is neurotoxic.

COLLABORATIVE MANAGEMENT

Assessment

Because bark scorpion venom is neurotoxic, manifestations typically involve the cranial nerves and/or the musculoskeletal system. The sting site may or may not show evidence of the envenomation. There may be no redness or other obvious sign of inflammation. Suchard and Connor (2001) advocate the "tap test," that is, a gentle tap at the potential sting site while the client is not looking greatly increases the pain and serves as a confirmatory test for a bark scorpion sting. The severity of the bark scorpion sting is highly variable, from local pain to systemic manifestations, such as respiratory failure, pancreatitis, musculoskeletal dysfunction, and cranial nerve involvement.

Symptoms usually begin immediately after the sting and reach maximum intensity in 5 hours (Suchard & Connor, 2001). Although the symptoms may start to resolve after 9 to 30 hours, the pain and paresthesias can remain for up to 2 weeks.

Interventions

The first priority of client management is vital sign assessment and continuous monitoring for several hours in a hospital emergency department or critical care unit to enable rapid intervention if progression of symptoms occurs. The client may require intubation and mechanical ventilation if signs of respiratory failure occur. Supplemental oxygen and IV fluid replacement should be instituted immediately. Apply an ice pack to the sting site to control pain. Give analgesic and sedative agents with caution in the nonintubated, spontaneously breathing client. Potent opioids, benzodiazepines, and barbiturates can cause loss of airway reflexes and precipitate respiratory failure. Fever is treated with acetaminophen and application of a cooling blanket as needed. Because scorpion stings produce a puncture wound, tetanus prophylaxis and basic wound care with an antiseptic agent are indicated.

The poison control center should be contacted as soon as possible to assist with client management, particularly in regard to use of pharmacologic agents. Supportive care to address client symptoms constitutes the typical course of treatment. For hypersalivation that may compromise the client's airway after a bark scorpion sting, a dose of atropine may be recommended as an anticholinergic agent.

Antivenom is available for bark scorpion stings (*Centruroides exilicauda* Antivenin), but its use is somewhat controversial and its availability is limited. It is generally not administered unless the client has evidence of a severe envenomation or has respiratory compromise. Hypersensitivity reactions are possible. If clients have a history of asthma, a prior hypersensitivity response to the scorpion antivenin, or allergies to goats or goat products, or if the client takes beta blockers or angiotensin-converting (ACE) inhibitors, then antivenom use is contraindicated (Suchard & Connor, 2001). The poison control center should be consulted for preparation and dosing of the antivenom if it is both available and indicated for the client. Be sure that advanced life support equipment is readily available to treat an anaphylactic response to the antivenom if it should occur. Serum sickness may develop after antivenom administration and is generally treated with antihistamines and tapering regimen of corticosteroids.

Bees and Wasps

PATHOPHYSIOLOGY

Bees and wasps are venomous arthropod members of the Hymenoptera order. Stings can produce a wide range of reactions from discomfort at the sting site, to severe pain and life-threatening anaphylaxis in allergic individuals. Bees and wasps are capable of stinging repeatedly when disturbed. Only the honeybee does not have this tendency. "Africanized" or "killer bees" are a very aggressive bee species found in the southwestern states that are known to attack in groups. When an individual sustains multiple stings, reactions are more severe and may be fatal because venom doses have cumulative toxic effects.

HEALTH PROMOTION/ILLNESS PREVENTION

Chart 13-4 lists actions that may help prevent arthropod bites and stings.

COLLABORATIVE MANAGEMENT

Assessment

The client who is stung by a bee or wasp first experiences a local reaction that is characterized by immediate pain and a wheal-and-flare reaction. Swelling can be extensive and involve an entire limb or body area. Systemic effects can then develop based upon the individual's sensitivity to the venom. These effects may include generalized edema, nausea, vomiting, and diarrhea. If the client has an allergy to the

CHART 13-4

CLIENT EDUCATION GUIDE

Arthropod Bite/Sting Prevention

- Wear appropriate protective clothing, including gloves and shoes, when working in areas known to harbor venomous arthropods, such as spiders, scorpions, bees, and wasps.
- Cover garbage cans. Bees and wasps are attracted to uncovered garbage.
- Use screens in windows and doors to prevent flying insects from entering buildings.
- Inspect clothing, shoes, and gear for insects before putting on these items.
- Shake out clothing and gear that has been on the ground to prevent arthropod "stowaways" and inadvertent bites and stings.
- Consult an exterminator to control arthropod populations in and around the home. Eliminating insects that are part of the arthropod's food source may also limit their presence.
- Identify nesting areas such as yard debris and rock piles; remove them whenever possible.
- Do not place unprotected hands where the eyes cannot see.
- Avoid handling insects or keeping them as "pets."
- Carry prescription epinephrine preparations and antihistamines if known to be allergic to bee and wasp stings.

venom, then urticaria, pruritus, and swelling of the lips and tongue may ensue. An allergic response can progress to an anaphylactic reaction rapidly in highly sensitive clients. Anaphylaxis is evidenced by respiratory distress with bronchospasm and laryngeal edema, hypotension, deterioration in mental status, and cardiac dysrhythmias. This type of reaction constitutes a true medical emergency that is imminently life threatening and may lead to cardiac arrest.

Interventions

FIRST AID. Basic emergency care for bee and wasp stings includes quick removal of the stinger and application of an ice pack. Honeybees and yellow jackets are most likely to leave a stinger. Most sources strongly advise against using tweezers to remove a stinger to avoid pinching the venom sac in the stinger and causing additional venom to be injected during removal; the commonly preferred method is to remove the stinger by gently scraping or brushing it off with the edge of a knife blade, credit card, or needle.

HOSPITAL CARE. Advanced emergency care interventions must be prioritized to assure that airway, breathing, and circulation are maintained. First, it is essential to determine whether the client has a history of allergic reactions to bee stings and whether an epinephrine kit has been prescribed. These kits sometimes contain an antihistamine tablet as well. In the presence of a severe allergic reaction characterized by wheezing, facial swelling, and respiratory distress, epinephrine must be administered without delay. Allergic clients typically carry an "EpiPen" (adult). This device enables epinephrine to be administered simply and quickly in an emergency because it delivers the right dose intramuscularly with just a click of a button. Other kits contain a prefilled epinephrine syringe. The standard epinephrine dose for adults is 0.3 to 0.5 mg of a 1:1000 solution given intramuscularly. The IM route is recommended over the subcutaneous route because it has more predictable and rapid absorption (Project Team of the Resuscitation Council [UK], 1999). Usually, directions on the epinephrine delivery device specify that the dose should be repeated in 15 minutes if signs and symptoms persist.

After epinephrine administration, an antihistamine such as diphenhydramine (Benadryl, Allerdryl✱) or chlorpheniramine (Chlor-Trimeton, Novopheniram✱) should also be given immediately. In the field setting, oral liquid diphenhydramine (available over the counter) may be easier for the victim to swallow than the tablet form if there is tongue or pharyngeal edema. For reactions that cause just pruritus and urticaria, only an antihistamine may be indicated initially. It is imperative that the emergency medical system be activated by calling 911 and that the client be transported to a medical facility as soon as possible.

Once in a clinical setting, clients who sustain serious reactions to bee or wasp stings need supplemental oxygen and continuous cardiac and blood pressure monitoring. Establish an IV infusion with normal saline solution to support blood pressure. Advanced life support drugs and equipment should be made immediately available. If epinephrine IM fails to relieve the life-threatening reaction, epinephrine 0.1 mg of a 1:10,000 solution may be ordered as a very slow IV bolus. IV epinephrine administration carries a much greater risk of adverse cardiovascular effects than IM epinephrine. Use the IV form of epinephrine with extreme caution, especially in older adults with cardiovascular disease. Bronchospasm may be treated with albuterol via inhalation or a similar bronchodilating agent.

Parenteral antihistamines and corticosteroids are also commonly prescribed to decrease the immune response. The toxin in the bee and wasp venom may outlast the effects of the initial doses of epinephrine and antihistamines and cause a recurrence of the allergic reaction over time. Corticosteroids prescribed in tapered doses are usually given to manage or prevent delayed allergic effects as well as serum sickness. Anyone who develops an allergic reaction to bee or wasp stings should be strongly encouraged to always carry a prescription epinephrine emergency kit and wear a medical alert tag or bracelet.

LIGHTNING INJURIES

PATHOPHYSIOLOGY

Lightning is a year-round weather problem. It is caused by an electric charge generated within thunderclouds that may propagate downward to become cloud-to-ground lightning, the most dangerous form to people or structures on the ground (Krider & Uman, 1995). Between 1980 and 1995, there were 1318 deaths attributed to lightning in the United States, yielding an average of 82 deaths per year (MMWR, 1998). Males accounted for 85% of the victims of lightning-related death; the majority (68%) were in the 15- to 44-year-old age range (MMWR, 1998). Most lightning-related injuries occur in the summer months due to increased thunderstorm activity and greater numbers of people spending time outdoors. Anyone without adequate shelter, including golfers, hikers, campers, beach goers, and swimmers, are at risk. Lopez and Holle (1995) found that 92% of fatal lightning strikes happened in the months of May through September; of those, 73% occurred in the afternoon and early evening hours.

Lightning has an enormous magnitude of energy and a much shorter duration of contact and a different current flow than a typical high-voltage electric shock. *High-voltage* electricity is considered to exceed 1000 volts. The energy in a single lightning stroke can exceed 1 million volts. The duration of contact, however, is nearly instantaneous, resulting in a flashover phenomenon–an effect that may explain the relatively low overall mortality rate. Because water is a conductor of electricity and current takes the path of least resistance to the ground, any wetness on the body increases the flashover effect of a lightning strike. Lightning flashover can produce an explosive force powerful enough to damage or blow off the victim's clothing and shoes (Cooper, et al., 2001).

Lightning can produce injury by directly striking a victim, by splashing or side flashing off a nearby strike area, and by traveling through the ground–also known as "step voltage" (Cherington, 2003). Although only 30% of victims die, 74% are left with permanent disabilities (MMWR, 1998).

HEALTH PROMOTION/ILLNESS PREVENTION

Perhaps the best remedy for lightning injuries is avoidance. Injuries due to lightning strike are highly preventable. Chart 13-5 lists common sense prevention strategies.

CHART 13-5

CLIENT EDUCATION GUIDE
Lightning Strike Prevention

- Observe weather forecasts when planning to be outside.
- Seek shelter when you hear thunder. Safe areas include the nearest building or an enclosed vehicle. Isolated sheds and the entrances to caves are dangerous, however. Do not stand under an isolated tall tree or structure (e.g., ski lift, flag pole, boat mast, power line) in an open area such as a field, ridge or hilltop; lightning seeks the highest point. A stand of dense trees offers better protection.
- Leave the water immediately (including an indoor shower or bathtub) and move away from any open bodies of water.
- Avoid metal objects: put down tools, fishing rods, garden equipment, golf clubs, and umbrellas; stand clear of fences, exposed pipes, motorcycles, bicycles, tractors, and golf carts.
- If camping in a tent, stay away from the metal tent poles and wet walls.
- Once inside a building, stay away from open doors, windows, fireplaces, metal fixtures, and plumbing.
- Turn off electrical equipment including computers, televisions, and stereos.
- Stay off the telephone. Lightning can enter through the telephone line and produce head and neck trauma, including cataracts and tympanic membrane disruption. Death can result.
- If you are caught out in the open and cannot seek shelter, attempt to move to lower ground such as a ravine or valley; stay away from any tall trees or objects that could result in a lightning strike splashing over to you; place insulating material between you and the ground (e.g., sleeping pad, rain parka, life jacket) and bend down on your knees, bend forward and place your hands on your knees. A lightning strike is imminent if your hair stands on end, you see blue halos around objects, and hear high-pitched or crackling noises. If you cannot move away from the area immediately, crouch on the balls of your feet and tuck your head down to minimize the target size; do not lie down on the ground or have hand contact with the ground.

Data from Auerbach, P.S., Donner, H.J., & Weiss, E.A. [2003]. Field guide to wilderness medicine (2nd ed.). St. Louis: Mosby.

COLLABORATIVE MANAGEMENT

Assessment

Both the cardiopulmonary and the central nervous systems are profoundly affected by lightning injuries. The most lethal initial effect of the massive current discharge on the cardiopulmonary system is either asystole or ventricular fibrillation. It is important to understand that cardiac cells are autorhythmic. An effective cardiac rhythm may return spontaneously. However, prolonged respiratory arrest from impairment of the medullary respiratory center can produce hypoxia and, subsequently, a second cardiac arrest (Cooper, et al., 2001). Therefore the principle of "reverse triage" is the rule when attempting to manage multiple victims of a lightning strike: those who are in cardiopulmonary arrest should be afforded priority resuscitation measures with immediate airway and ventilatory management, chest compressions, and other appropriate life support interventions (Cherington, 2003; Cooper, et al., 2001). Individuals who exhibit signs of life immediately after a lightning strike may be treated in a less emergent fashion because they have the best chance of recovery. Despite survival, victims of lightning strike can suffer serious myocardial injury, which may be manifested by ECG and myocardial perfusion abnormalities. The initial appearance of mottled skin and decreased to absent peripheral pulses usually arises from arterial vasospasm. These findings most often resolve spontaneously in several hours without the need for intervention (Cooper, et al., 2001).

Central nervous system (CNS) injury is a significant result of lightning strike. Typical CNS effects include an immediate but temporary paralysis, known as keraunoparalysis or "muscular stunning," which can persist for minutes to hours, loss of consciousness, amnesia, confusion or disorientation, photophobia, and seizures (Fahmy, et al., 1999). Intracranial hemorrhage, cerebral infarction, encephalopathy, cerebellar dysfunction, and spinal cord injury may also occur (Cherington, 2003). Fatigue and cognitive impairments as well as post-traumatic stress disorder are long-term neuropsychological consequences reported in survivors of lightning injuries (van Zomeren, et al., 1998). Other lightning strike-related effects include ruptured tympanic membranes, blindness, cataracts, and retinal detachment, which may be due to both blast effect and intense heat production (Espaillat, Janigian, & To, 1999).

Lightning strike also causes skin burns. Most burns are superficial and heal without incident. Clients may have punctate full-thickness burns, charring, and contact burns from overlying metal objects. An uncommon but characteristic cutaneous manifestation of lightning is the appearance of branching or ferning marks on the skin called **Lichtenberg figures**, also known as keraunographic markings or erythematous arborization.

Interventions

FIRST AID. Because of lightning's powerful impact to the body, clients are at great risk for the entire spectrum of multisystem trauma. The full extent of injury may not be known until thorough monitoring and diagnostic evaluation can be performed in the hospital. Initial care must include spinal immobilization with attention to stabilization of airway, breathing, and circulation through standard basic and advanced life support measures. As a reminder, reverse triage will potentially do the greatest good for the greatest number of victims in a lightning strike that results in mass casualties. CPR should be performed immediately when a client is in cardiac arrest. In the presence of cardiopulmonary or central nervous system injury, skin burns are an initial priority. However, if time and resources permit, a sterile dressing may be applied to cover the sites. Victims of lightning strike are *not* electrically charged; the rescuer is in no danger from physical contact. Nonetheless, the storm can present a continued threat to everyone in the vicinity who lacks adequate shelter. Contrary to popular belief, lightning can and does strike in the same place more than once.

HOSPITAL CARE. Once in the acute care hospital setting, the client requires advanced life support management, including cardiac monitoring to detect cardiac dysrhythmias. Airway, breathing, and circulatory support are indicated as needed. The client may require a period of mechanical ventilation until spontaneous breathing returns. A thorough physical and diagnostic evaluation to identify both obvious and occult traumatic injuries is important because the client may have suffered a fall or blast effect during the strike. A creatinine kinase (CK) measurement may be ordered to detect skeletal muscle damage resulting from the lightning strike. In severe cases, rhabdomyolysis (muscle destruction) and kidney failure can occur. Burn wounds should be assessed and treated according to standard burn care protocols. Tetanus prophylaxis is necessary. Care of the client is supportive as recovery ensues. Some institutions transfer these clients to a burn center for subsequent management.

COLD INJURIES

Two common cold injuries are hypothermia and frostbite. Both types of injuries can be prevented by implementing protection from the cold. Teach clients at risk ways to prevent these injuries, which can range from mild discomfort to major systemic complications.

HEALTH PROMOTION/ILLNESS PREVENTION

When participating in cold weather activities, clothing choices are critical to the prevention of hypothermia and frostbite. Synthetic clothing is best because it wicks away moisture from the body and dries fast. Cotton clothing, especially as an underlayer, holds moisture, becomes wet, and contributes to the development of hypothermia. Cotton clothing should be strictly avoided in a cold outdoor environment; this rule applies to gloves and socks as well. The mountaineering adage that "cotton kills" is important to remember. Wet socks and gloves promote frostbite in the toes and fingers. Wearing too many pairs of socks can impair circulation and predispose the client to frostbite.

Clothing should be layered so that it can be easily added or removed as the temperature changes. The inner layers should provide warmth (insulation). Polyester fleece is a good choice. The outer layer's purpose is to block the wind and protect the client from moisture. This layer is best made of a windproof, waterproof, breathable fabric such as Gore-Tex. A hat is an essential clothing item that significantly decreases body heat through the head. Face protection with a face mask should be considered on particularly cold days when wind chill poses a risk. Sunscreen (at least SPF 30) and sunglasses are also important to protect skin and eyes from the harmful rays of the sun.

When driving in winter cannot be avoided, water, extra clothing, and food should be kept in the car in case the vehicle becomes stranded. Maintaining personal fitness and conditioning are also important considerations to prevent hypothermia and frostbite. Individuals should not diet or restrict food or fluid intake when participating in winter outdoor activities. Malnutrition and dehydration contribute to cold-related illnesses and injuries. Finally, it is imperative for individuals to know their physical limits and to come in out of the cold when these limits have been met.

Hypothermia

PATHOPHYSIOLOGY

Hypothermia is generally defined as a core body temperature less than 95° F (35° C). An understanding of the etiologies and risk factors involved in the development of hypothermia is key to both recognition and prevention. Predisposing conditions that promote the development of hypothermia include the following:

- Cold water immersion
- Illness
- Injury
- Shock states
- Immobilization
- Weather
- Extremes of age
- Selected medications (e.g., phenothiazines, sedatives, anxiolytics, meperidine, and vasodilating agents)
- Alcohol intoxication
- Malnutrition
- Inadequate clothing or shelter

An important point, however, is that an environmental temperatures less than 82° F can produce hypothermia in any susceptible individual. Therefore clients are actually at risk on a *year-round* basis in most areas of the world. Wind chill is a significant factor: heat loss increases as wind velocity rises. Wet conditions further heat loss through evaporation. Weather is the most notable cause of hypothermia for outdoor sports enthusiasts and for those with inadequate clothing or shelter. The mortality rate for hypothermia exceeds 50% when body temperature falls below 32° C (90° F), and nears 100% in victims who have concurrent illness or injuries (Bowman, et al., 2003).

COLLABORATIVE MANAGEMENT

Assessment

Hypothermia is divided into the categories of *mild* (32° C to 35° C), *moderate* (28° C to 32° C), and *severe* (<28° C). In the injured client, hypothermia exists when the body temperature is 36° C or below (American College of Surgeons, 1997). Treatment decisions are based on the degree of hypothermia present. *Mild* hypothermia is manifested by shivering, dysarthria, muscular incoordination, and impaired cognitive abilities (i.e., mental slowness) and "cold diuresis." Cold diuresis results from peripheral vasoconstriction and shunting of blood to the core of the body. With core hypervolemia, glomerular filtration rate accelerates causing an increase in urine output. Dehydration occurs and exacerbates the hypothermic condition due to impaired circulation. Shivering and an increased metabolic rate are the body's compensatory mechanisms to stimulate heat production. Early cardiopulmonary manifestations include tachycardia and increased respiratory rate.

Clients with *moderate* (28° C to 32° C) to *severe* hypothermia (<28° C) have obvious motor impairment and weakness. They become uncoordinated and may stumble or fall. Their cognitive abilities and mental processes deteriorate. Confusion and apathy progress to irrationality and incoherence, stupor, and unconsciousness. Shivering stops at this point. Victims may even erroneously perceive warmth and engage in "paradoxical undressing" in which they disrobe, an action that aggravates their already perilous hypothermic condition (Auerbach, Donner, & Weiss, 2003). Vital signs become depressed. Bradycardia and hypotension ensue. Respiratory rate and effort, and cardiac output decline. Prolongation of the P-R, QRS, and Q-Tc intervals occur; J waves or Osborn waves may appear on the ECG (Auerbach, Donner, & Weiss, 2003). A cold heart is an irritable heart; atrial and ventricular dysrhythmias are common. The ventricular fibrillation threshold is decreased. Deterioration to ventricular fibrillation and asystole is easily precipitated by rough handling or jolting of the client's body, as well as by performance of some medical procedures and central line insertion. In severe hypothermia (<28° C), neurologic reflexes and responsiveness to pain are absent. Profound hypotension, acid-base abnormalities, ventricular fibrillation, and asystole are characteristic.

In moderate to severe hypothermia, laboratory values may reveal **coagulopathy**, or blood clotting abnormalities, and platelet dysfunction. Clotting factor function is temperature dependent and is reduced in hypothermia (Watts, 1998). Platelet aggregation is impaired; thrombocytopenia develops due to destruction of platelets in the liver and spleen (Watts, 1998). Prolonged bleeding times result. A very important concept is that hypothermia causes coagulopathy over a range of temperatures–the greater the degree of hypothermia, the more likely the client will hemorrhage from injury or invasive procedures. This concept has especially critical implications for the injured client in a shock state who requires resuscitation: hypothermia must be identified and treated effectively to prevent further blood loss.

Interventions

FIRST AID. Treatment of mild hypothermia is straightforward: the individual needs to be sheltered from the cold environment, have all wet clothing removed, and undergo passive or active external rewarming. Passive methods involve applying warm clothing or blankets. Active methods incorporate heating blankets, warm packs, and convective air heaters or warmers to speed rewarming. If a heating blanket is used, Gentilello (1999) advises that the blanket should be placed on top of the client instead of underneath because greater heat loss occurs from above the body by convection and radiation. In addition, the individual may have a reduced risk of burn injury with this arrangement.

In a camping or wilderness setting, a rescuer can share the same sleeping bag with a hypothermic victim to promote transfer of body heat as a primitive but effective means of active external rewarming. Both the rescuer and the victim should be only minimally clothed to facilitate heat transfer. In the case of mild, uncomplicated hypothermia as the only health problem, having the client drink warm high-carbohydrate liquids that do not contain alcohol or caffeine can aid in rewarming. Alcohol is a peripheral vasodilator; both alcohol and caffeine are diuretics. The effects of these agents can potentially worsen dehydration and hypothermia.

HOSPITAL CARE. Treatment of moderate to severe hypothermia differs from that of mild hypothermia in that active, external rewarming methods are contraindicated. Core temperature "afterdrop" can occur. **Afterdrop** is defined as a continued decrease in core body temperature after the victim is removed from the cold environment due to equilibration of core and peripheral blood temperature and countercurrent cooling of blood perfusing cold tissue (Tisherman, 2002). Applying external heat promotes afterdrop by producing peripheral vasodilation, which stimulates the return of cold blood from the periphery to the warmer core.

Several general management principles apply to both moderate and severe hypothermia. The client should be protected from further heat loss and handled gently to prevent ventricular fibrillation. The client is best kept in a horizontal position to prevent orthostatic changes in blood pressure from cardiovascular instability. Only core rewarming methods are indicated to treat moderate to severe hypothermia. For moderate hypothermia, core rewarming methods include administration of warm IV fluids, heated oxygen or inspired gas to prevent further heat loss via the respiratory tract, and heated peritoneal or pleural lavage (Gentilello, 1999). Even though they are commonly employed, gastric, colonic, and bladder lavage are less effective because of the smaller surface area for heat exchange (Gentilello, 1999). Active rewarming with externally applied heating devices is dangerous in this population because it produces vasodilation in the extremities.

In addition to rewarming interventions, standard resuscitation efforts are indicated with special attention to maintenance of airway, breathing, and circulation. Administer drugs with caution because metabolism is unpredictable in hypothermic conditions. Drugs can accumulate without obvious therapeutic effect while the client is cold, but will become active and potentially lead to drug toxicity as effective rewarming is underway. CPR should be initiated for ventricular fibrillation and asystole. Defibrillation attempts may be ineffective until the core temperature is above 30° C (86° F) (Auerbach, Donner, & Weiss, 2003).

The client who is severely hypothermic is at high risk of cardiac arrest. For these clients, the treatment of choice is to employ extracorporeal rewarming methods such as cardiopulmonary bypass, hemodialysis, or continuous arteriovenous rewarming (CAVR). The advantage of CAVR for the trauma client with hemorrhage is that heparin is not required. A limitation is that the client's systolic blood pressure must be greater than 60 mm Hg for blood to flow through the circuit. Cardiopulmonary bypass is the fastest rewarming technique. It supports the circulation and allows for timely correction of fluid, electrolyte, and metabolic abnormalities. However, this device is not available in all hospitals. It requires specialized personnel and resources to operate it properly. Complications can occur after weaning from cardiopulmonary bypass as well. Common complications include acute respiratory distress syndrome (ARDS), acute renal failure and pneumonia.

A long-standing principle in the treatment of clients with hypothermic cardiac arrest is that "no one is dead until they are warm and dead." There is a factual basis to this statement when considering the number of survivors who have suffered a prolonged hypothermic cardiac arrest. Clinical judgment must always take precedence, however. Prolonged resuscitation efforts may not be reasonable in cases in which survival appears highly unlikely, such as in an anoxic event followed by a hypothermic cardiac arrest. If the arrest victim is rewarmed to a core temperature of 30° to 32° C but continues to have no cardiac activity and dilated nonreactive pupils, consideration should be given to terminating resuscitative efforts (Cummins, 2003).

Frostbite

PATHOPHYSIOLOGY

Another significant cold-related injury that may or may not be associated with hypothermia is frostbite. A principal predisposing factor is inadequate insulation against cold weather, that is, either the skin is exposed to the cold or the individual's clothing offers insufficient protection. Wet clothing, in particular, serves as a poor insulator and facilitates the development of frostbite. Fatigue and poor nutrition are other contributing factors. Clients who smoke, consume alcohol, or have impaired peripheral circulation have a higher incidence of frostbite. These factors aggravate cold injuries. Any previous history of frostbite further increases a client's susceptibility.

COLLABORATIVE MANAGEMENT

Assessment

Frostbite is classified as superficial or mild ("frostnip"), or deep. **Frostnip** may produce initial pain, numbness, and pallor of the affected area, but is easily remedied with application of warmth and does not induce tissue injury. Frostnip typically develops on skin areas such as the face, nose, finger, or toes. The American College of Surgeons (1997) characterizes deep frostbite by the degree of tissue freezing. Like burns, frostbite injuries can be partial or full thickness. First-degree frostbite, the least severe type of deep frostbite, involves hyperemia of the involved area and edema formation. In second-degree frostbite, large fluid-filled blisters develop with a partial thickness skin necrosis (Figure 13-7). Third-degree frostbite appears as small blisters that contain dark fluid and an affected body part that is cool, numb, blue, or red and does not blanch. Full thickness and subcutaneous tissue necrosis occurs and require debridement. In fourth-degree frostbite, there are no blisters or edema; the part is numb, cold, and bloodless. The full thickness necrosis extends into the muscle and bone. At this stage, gangrene develops, which may necessitate amputation of the affected part.

Interventions

FIRST AID. Recognition of frostbite is essential to early, effective intervention and prevention of further tissue damage. Asking a partner to frequently observe for early signs of frostbite such as a white, waxy appearance to exposed skin, especially on the nose, cheeks, and ears, is an effective strategy to identify the problem before it worsens. In this case, the best remedy is to have the individual seek shelter from the wind and cold and to attend to the affected body part. Superficial frostbite is easily managed in the prehospital setting using body heat to warm the affected area. Clients can be taught to place their warm hands over the affected areas on their face or to place cold hands under the arms in the axillary region.

HOSPITAL CARE. Clients with deep frostbite need aggressive management. For all degrees of deep frostbite, rapid rewarming in a water bath at a temperature range of 38° C to 41° C is indicated to thaw the frozen part (Tisherman, 2002). Because clients experience severe pain during the rewarming process, this intervention is best accomplished in a medical facility; however, it may be done in another setting if no other options exist for prompt transport or rescue. Analgesic agents, especially IV opiates, are an essential aspect of this client's care plan as soon as possible. Dry heat should never be applied, nor should the frostbitten areas be rubbed as part of the warming process. These actions produce further tissue injury.

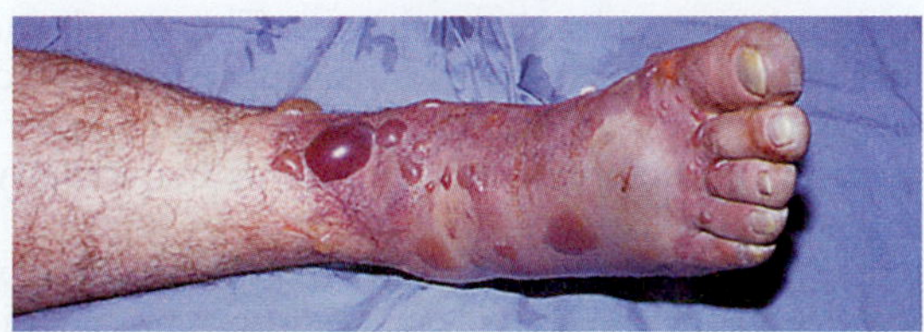

Figure 13-7 ■ Edema and blister formation 24 hours after frostbite injury occurring in an area covered by a tightly fitted boot. (From Auerbach, P.S., Donner, H.J., & Weiss, E.A. [2003]. *Field guide to wilderness medicine* [2nd ed., plate 1]. St. Louis: Mosby.)

When the rewarming process is complete, elevate the extremity above heart level if possible to decrease tissue edema. Frostbite destroys tissue and produces a deep tetanus-prone wound; the client should be immunized for tetanus prophylaxis (Kanzenbach & Dexter, 1999). Once a client's frozen part has been thawed, do not allow it to refreeze, which worsens the injury. Surgical intervention is ultimately indicated to evaluate tissue viability and provide wound management in cases of deep frostbite. Debridement of necrotic tissue will be necessary. Amputation may be indicated for clients with severe injuries or for those who develop gangrene.

ALTITUDE-RELATED ILLNESSES

PATHOPHYSIOLOGY

High altitude, generally defined as elevations above 5000 feet, can produce a range of physiologic consequences in the body. Some of these effects can be quite deleterious to a person's health and, in extreme cases, can be fatal. Because so many people visit mountainous areas for sport and recreation such as skiing and hiking, it is important to have an understanding of altitude physiology and the ability to recognize the most common emergency situations that may be induced by altitude effects on the human body.

As altitude increases, barometric pressure decreases. Oxygen constitutes 21% of the barometric pressure. Therefore as barometric pressure falls, the partial pressure of oxygen decreases, resulting in less available oxygen to humans. The physiologic consequence is hypoxia. Hypoxia becomes more pronounced as elevation increases. High altitude is considered to be about 5000 to 11,500 feet–the same elevation as most Western ski areas in the United States. Very high altitude is defined as altitudes between about 11,500 feet and 18,000 feet. The peaks of some Western ski areas are in the 12,000- to 13,000-foot range. Elevations of greater than 18,000 feet constitute extreme altitude. Supplemental oxygen is necessary at these altitudes to prevent altitude-related illness, including death, from occurring during abrupt ascent.

The process of adapting to high altitude is called **acclimatization**. Acclimatization involves physiologic changes that help the body to compensate for less available oxygen in the atmosphere. As the carotid bodies sense a decline in PaO_2 at about 5000 feet, the respiratory rate increases to improve oxygen delivery. This mechanism is called the hypoxic ventilatory response. Increased respiratory rate causes hypocapnia (decreased carbon dioxide) and respiratory alkalosis, which limits further increases in respiratory rate. At this point, sleep disturbances characterized by periodic respirations are common. REM (rapid eye movement) sleep is impaired. Hypoxia can occur from periods of apnea. Within 24 to 48 hours of being at high altitude, the kidneys excrete the excess bicarbonate and enable the pH to return to normal, and ventilatory rate to again increase as an important compensatory response. Greater sympathetic nervous system activity increases heart rate, blood pressure, and cardiac output. Pulmonary artery pressure rises as an effect of generalized hypoxia-induced pulmonary vasoconstriction. Cerebral blood flow increases to maintain cerebral oxygen delivery. Hypoxia also induces red blood cell production by stimulating the release of erythropoietin. The result is an increase in hemoglobin concentration. Over time, polycythemia can develop in individuals who remain in a high altitude environment.

People who plan to ascend to high altitudes are advised to ascend slowly, over the course of days or even weeks, depending on the degree of elevation. Ascending too rapidly is the primary cause of altitude-related illness, mediated by the effects of hypoxia on the body. Altitude-related illness is more common in individuals who sleep at elevations above 8000 feet.

The three most significant clinical conditions that pose a risk to people at high altitude are acute mountain sickness (AMS), high altitude cerebral edema (HACE), and high altitude pulmonary edema (HAPE). These conditions may overlap in the same individual. The underlying pathophysiology is hypoxia. Although each syndrome has somewhat unique manifestations, the basic assessment and management approach is the same.

COLLABORATIVE MANAGEMENT

Assessment

Acute mountain sickness (AMS) is often the precursor to high altitude cerebral edema (HACE) and/or high altitude pulmonary edema (HAPE). AMS most often occurs in individuals who make a rapid ascent without acclimatization to altitudes above 8000 feet from altitudes below 5000 feet (Hackett & Roach, 2001). Again, the most important altitude effects occur when an individual who is not acclimated sleeps at elevations over 8000 feet. Assessment of the typical client with AMS reveals complaints of throbbing headache, anorexia, nausea, and vomiting. Feeling chilled, irritable, and apathetic are also symptoms associated with AMS. The syndrome produces effects similar to an alcohol-induced hangover. The client may relate a feeling of extreme illness. Vital signs are variable: the client can be tachycardic or bradycardic, have normal blood pressure, or have postural hypotension. The client may experience dyspnea both on exertion and at rest. Exertional dyspnea is expected as an individual adjusts to high altitude. However, dyspnea at rest is abnormal and may signal the onset of high altitude pulmonary edema.

If AMS progresses to **high altitude cerebral edema (HACE),** which is the extreme form of this disorder, the client will be physically unable to perform activities of daily living and will exhibit extreme apathy. A key sign of HACE is the development of ataxia without focal signs (Hackett & Roach, 2001). Clients have a change in mental status with confusion and impaired judgment. Cranial nerve dysfunction and seizures may occur. If untreated, a further decline in the client's level of consciousness ensues. Stupor, coma, and death can result from brain swelling and the subsequent damage caused by increased intracranial pressure over the course of 1 to 3 days.

High altitude pulmonary edema (HAPE) often appears in conjunction with HACE, but may occur during the progression of AMS within the first 2 to 4 days of a rapid ascent to high altitude, commonly on the second night. It is the most frequent cause of death associated with high altitude (Hackett & Roach, 2001). Clients notice poor exercise tolerance and a prolonged recovery time after exertion. Fatigue and weakness, as well as other signs and symptoms of AMS, are present. Important clinical indicators of HAPE include a persistent dry cough and cyanosis of the lips and nail beds. Tachycardia and tachypnea occur at rest. Rales may be auscultated in one or both lungs. Pink, frothy sputum is a late sign of HAPE. A chest x-ray demonstrates pulmonary infiltrates and pulmonary edema. Arterial blood gas analysis shows respiratory alkalosis and hypoxemia (decreased oxygen). Pneumonia also may be a concurrent finding. If a pulmonary artery catheter is inserted for hemodynamic monitoring, pulmonary artery pressure will be significantly elevated. The client may also have an elevated body temperature.

Interventions

FIRST AID. The most important intervention to manage serious altitude-related illnesses is descent to a lower altitude. Clients must be monitored carefully for any evidence of symptom progression. With mild AMS, the client should be allowed to rest and acclimate at the current altitude. The client must be instructed not ascend to a higher altitude, especially for sleep, until symptoms dissipate. If symptoms persist or worsen, the client should be moved to a lower altitude as soon as possible. Even a descent of about 1600 feet to 3300 feet may improve the client's condition and reverse altitude-related pathologic effects. Oxygen should also be administered if available to effectively treat symptoms of AMS.

HOSPITAL CARE. The oral medication acetazolamide (Diamox, Apo-Acetazolamide✱) is used to both prevent and treat AMS. Acetazolamide is a carbonic anhydrase inhibitor. It acts by causing a bicarbonate diuresis, which rids the body of excess fluid, and induces metabolic acidosis. The acidotic state increases respiratory rate and decreases the occurrence of periodic respiration during sleep at night. In this way it helps clients to acclimate faster to a high altitude. For best results, acetazolamide should be taken 24 hours before ascent and be continued for the first 2 days of the trip. Dosing regimens vary. The most common regimens involve taking 125 mg to 250 mg PO twice daily, or one 500 mg sustained-release capsule daily. Acetazolamide is a sulfa drug. It may cause hypersensitivity reactions in allergic individuals.

The other drug that may be helpful in the treatment of moderate to severe AMS is dexamethasone (Decadron, Deronil✱) 4 mg to 8 mg either orally or intramuscularly as an initial dose, then 4 mg every 6 hours while the client is undergoing descent to a lower altitude. This drug's mechanism of action is unclear for AMS treatment. It does not appear to speed acclimatization like acetazolamide, but it does relieve the symptoms of AMS. Symptoms may recur when the drug is stopped.

For the treatment of HACE, early recognition of ataxia or a change in level of consciousness should prompt a rapid descent by rescuers or companions to a lower altitude. While undergoing descent, the client can be given supplemental oxygen and dexamethasone 4 mg to 8 mg initially as an oral, IM, or IV dose, followed by 4 mg every 6 hours if available. If mental status is severely impaired and the client's airway is at risk, all drugs should be given parenterally. Loop diuretics such as furosemide (Lasix) may be prescribed to decrease brain swelling. Ultimately, the client with HACE must be admitted to the hospital. Critical care management may be necessary.

Like HACE, early recognition of HAPE is essential to improve the client's chance for survival. This is a serious condition that requires prompt evacuation to a lower altitude, oxygen administration, and bedrest to save the client's life. If descent must be delayed because of weather conditions or other factors, oxygen administration is essential as soon as possible. Cold stress must be avoided because it can increase pulmonary artery pressure. Keep the client warm at all times. Drugs are not substitutes for descent and oxygen. However, the treatment of HAPE may include administration of diuretics such as furosemide to reduce pulmonary edema, morphine, and vasodilators to decrease pulmonary vascular resistance. Hospital admission is warranted. In uncomplicated cases of HAPE, recovery occurs quickly but effects such as weakness and fatigue may persist for 2 weeks.

Chart 13-6 provides best practice strategies for preventing, recognizing, and treating altitude-related illnesses.

NEAR-DROWNING

PATHOPHYSIOLOGY

Drowning is a leading cause of accidental death in the United States. The victim dies by suffocation from submersion in a liquid medium (usually water). Although suffocation most commonly results from aspiration of fresh or salt water into the lungs, about 10% to 20% of victims experience laryngospasm with subsequent glottic closure followed by asphyxiation. **Near-drowning** is defined as recovery after submersion. Victims are typically children or adolescents. Males—more often engaged in risk-taking behavior—have a significantly greater incidence of drowning/near-drowning episodes than females.

HEALTH PROMOTION/ILLNESS PREVENTION

Prevention is key to avoiding near-drowning events. Common sense health teaching should include the following points:

- Maintain constant surveillance of children in or around water.
- Do not swim alone.
- Test the water depth before diving in head first; never dive into shallow water.
- Avoid alcoholic beverages when swimming, boating or while in proximity to water.
- Assure that water rescue equipment, such as life jackets, floatation devices, and rope, is immediately available when around water.

CHART 13-6

BEST PRACTICE for
Preventing, Recognizing, and Treating Altitude-Related Illnesses

- Plan a slow ascent to allow for acclimatization.
- Learn to recognize clinical manifestations of altitude-related illnesses.
- Avoid overexertion and overexposure to cold; rest at present altitude.
- Ensure adequate hydration and nutrition.
- Avoid alcohol and sleeping pills when at high altitude.
- For progressive or advanced acute mountain sickness (AMS), recognize symptoms and implement an immediate descent; provide oxygen at high concentration.
- To prevent the occurrence of AMS, discuss the use of acetazolamide (Diamox) with your health care provider.
- Protect skin and eyes from the sun's harmful ultraviolet rays at high altitude. Wear sunscreen (at least SPF 30) and high quality wraparound sunglasses or goggles.

COLLABORATIVE MANAGEMENT

Assessment

When water is aspirated into the lungs, the composition of the water is a key factor in the pathophysiology of the near-drowning event. Aspiration of fresh water causes surfactant to wash out of the lungs. Surfactant reduces surface tension within the alveoli, increases lung compliance and alveolar radius, and decreases the work of breathing. Loss of surfactant from fresh water aspiration destabilizes the alveoli and leads to increased airway resistance. Conversely, salt water—a hypertonic fluid—creates an osmotic gradient that draws protein-rich fluid from the vascular space into the alveoli. The consequences of both types of aspiration include impaired alveolar ventilation and resultant intrapulmonary shunting, which further compound the hypoxic state. Another concern is water quality during the near-drowning event. Client outcome may be negatively impacted by contaminants in the water such as chemicals, algae, microbes, sand, and mud. These substances can worsen lung injury and cause a lung infection.

Factors that help predict outcome for victims of near-drowning include the length of time submerged underwater, the degree of damage to the brain caused by hypoxia, the water temperature, client age, and health status. Very cold water seems to have a protective effect—especially for children. Successful resuscitations have been reported even after prolonged arrest intervals. Hypothermia offers some protection to the hypoxic brain by reducing cerebral metabolic rate. The diving reflex is a physiologic response to asphyxia, which produces bradycardia, a reduction in cardiac output, and vasoconstriction of vessels in the intestine, skeletal muscles, and kidney. These physiologic effects reduce myocardial oxygen consumption and enhance blood flow to the heart and cerebral tissues. Survival may be linked to some combination of the effects of hypothermia and the diving reflex.

The cause of the submersion should also be discerned if possible. The client may have suffered a medical condition or injury that precipitated the near-drowning event such as a seizure, myocardial infarction, stroke, or spinal cord injury while in the water. Injuries sustained from diving into shallow water or body surfing such as cervical spine trauma can also increase the difficulty of rescue and resuscitation efforts.

Interventions

FIRST AID. Immediate emergency care should focus on a safe rescue of the victim. Potential rescuers must consider their own swimming abilities and limitations as well as any natural or man-made hazards before attempting to save the victim; failure to do so could place additional lives in jeopardy. Once rescuers gain access to the victim, priorities include safe removal from the water while maintaining spine stabilization with a board or floatation device, and initiating airway clearance and ventilatory support measures. If hypothermia is a concern, gentle handling of the victim is essential to prevent ventricular fibrillation. There is no indication for attempts to get the water out of the victim's lungs. Abdominal thrusts should only be delivered if airway obstruction is suspected.

HOSPITAL CARE. Once the victim is safely removed from the water, airway and cardiopulmonary support interventions should ensue including oxygen administration, endotracheal intubation, and CPR if necessary. In the clinical setting, gastric decompression with a nasogastric or orogastric tube is indicated to prevent aspiration of gastric contents and improve ventilatory function. After a period of artificial ventilation by mask, the client typically has a distended abdomen, which impairs movement of the diaphragm and inhibits lung ventilation if it is not decompressed as described. Clients who experience near-drowning require complex care to support their body systems. The full spectrum of critical care technology may be needed to manage the physiologic derangements and sequelae of near-drowning, including pulmonary infection, acute respiratory distress syndrome (ARDS) and central nervous system impairment. The client's outcome may be difficult to predict in the early stages of care.

GET READY for the NCLEX Examination!

KEY POINTS

- Heat-related injuries can be mild (heat exhaustion) to severe (heat stroke), and can be easily prevented (see Chart 13-1).
- The priority for first aid for heat stroke, after a patent airway is established, is to cool the client as quickly as possible.
- North American pit vipers can be characterized by the triangular-shaped head and retractable fangs; nonpoisonous snakes do not have these features.
- The management of a client who has a snakebite depends on the severity of envenomation (see Table 13-1); both local and systemic manifestations can occur.
- The priority for first aid when a client has a snakebite is to decrease the venom circulation; do *not* use a tourniquet.
- Antivenom drugs are available for most types of poisonous snakebites; monitor for an allergic response when these medications are given.
- The bite of a brown recluse spider can cause tissue necrosis; in rare cases systemic manifestations can occur, including death.
- Cold applications, such as ice, should be used as first aid for poisonous spider bites.
- The venom of a bark scorpion is neurotoxic; monitor the client for signs of respiratory failure that may require mechanical ventilation.
- Single bee and wasp stings cause local reactions unless the person is allergic to them or received multiple stings.
- Arthropod bites and stings may be prevented through client education (see Chart 13-4).
- Epinephrine is the drug of choice for bee and wasp sting allergic reactions, followed by an antihistamine drug.
- The best way to prevent lightning injuries is to avoid places where lightning is likely to strike (see Chart 13-5).
- Lightning causes central nervous system and cardiovascular complications, as well as skin burns.
- Two common cold injuries are hypothermia and frostbite; both can be prevented by selecting appropriate layered clothing; cotton should not be worn.
- In moderate to severe cases of hypothermia, coagulopathy (abnormal clotting) or cardiac failure can occur.
- The priority for care of a client with a cold injury is warming; alcohol should be avoided.
- Frostbite can be mild (frostnip) to serious (fourth degree); severe frostbite can result in amputation due to tissue necrosis and gangrene.
- High altitude can cause a range of physiologic consequences in the body, primarily due to hypoxia.
- The priority for care of the client with illness related to high altitude is descent to a lower altitude.
- Acetazolamide (Diamox, Apo-Acetazolamide✱) is the drug of choice for prevention of mild altitude-related illness.
- Chart 13-6 outlines best practice strategies for preventing, recognizing, and treating altitude-related illnesses.
- Near-drowning victims often require cardiopulmonary support, including CPR.
- The client who has nearly drowned is at risk for pulmonary infection, ARDS, and central nervous system impairment.

ADDITIONAL STUDY RESOURCES

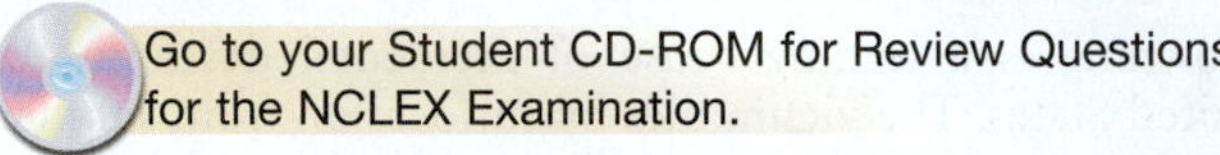

Go to your Student CD-ROM for Review Questions for the NCLEX Examination.

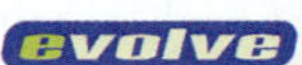

Go to http://evolve.elsevier.com/Iggy/ for Integrated Management of Care Questions for the NCLEX Examination.

SELECTED BIBLIOGRAPHY

Asterisk indicates a classic or definitive work on this subject.

*American College of Surgeons Committee on Trauma. (1997). *Advanced trauma life support.* Chicago: Author.

Auerbach P.S. (2001). *Wilderness medicine: Management of wilderness and environmental emergencies* (4th ed.). St. Louis: Mosby.

Auerbach, P.S., Donner, H.J., & Weiss, E.A. (2003). *Field guide to wilderness medicine.* (2nd ed.). St. Louis: Mosby.

Bowman, W.D., et al. (Eds.). (2003). *Outdoor emergency care: Comprehensive prehospital care for nonurban settings* (4th ed.). Boston: Jones and Bartlett.

Boyer, L.V., McNally, J.T., & Binford, G.J. (2001). Spider bites. In P.S. Auerbach (Ed.), *Wilderness medicine* (4th ed., pp. 807-838). St. Louis: Mosby.

*Cacy, J., & Mold, J.W. (1999). The clinical characteristics of brown recluse spider bites treated by family physicians. *Journal of Family Practice, 48*(7), 536-542.

Cherington, M. (2003). Neurologic manifestations of lightning strike. *Neurology, 60,* 182-185.

Cooper, M.A., et al. (2001). Lightning injuries. In P.S. Auerbach (Ed.), *Wilderness medicine* (4th ed., pp. 73-110). St. Louis: Mosby.

Cummins, R.O. (Ed.). (2003). *ACLS: Principles and practice.* Dallas: American Heart Association.

*Dematte, J.E., et al. (1998). Near-fatal heat stroke during the 1995 heat wave in Chicago. *Annals of Internal Medicine, 129*(3), 173-181.

*Dinakaran, S., Desai, S.P., & Elsom, D.M. (1998). Telephone-mediated lightning injury causing cataract. *Injury, 29*(8), 645-646.

*Espaillat, A., Janigian, R., & To, K. (1999). Cataracts, bilateral macular holes, and rhegmatogenous retinal detachment induced by lightning. *American Journal of Ophthalmology, 127*(2), 216-217.

*Fahmy, S.F., et al. (1999). Lightning: The multisystem group injuries. *Journal of Trauma, 46*(5), 937-940.

First new management for poisonous snakebites in more than 50 years is now available: Biotechnology product provides safe and effective therapy for poisonous snake bites. (2001). *Clinical Nurse Specialist, 15*(3):121-123.

*Gentilello, L.M. (1999). Hypothermia in trauma. In D.D. Trunkey & F.R. Lewis (Eds.), *Current therapy of trauma* (4th ed., pp. 325-328). St. Louis: Mosby.

*Gold, B.S., & Wingert, W.A. (1994). Snake venom poisoning in the United States: A review of therapeutic practice. *Southern Medical Journal, 87*(6), 579-589.

Hackett, P.H., & Roach, R.C. (2001). High-altitude medicine. In P.S. Auerbach (Ed.), *Wilderness medicine* (4th ed., pp. 2-43). St. Louis: Mosby.

*Hoey, J. (1998). Hypothermia. *Canadian Medical Association Journal, 158*(2), 237.

*Holstege, C.P., et al. (1997). Crotalid snake envenomation. *Critical Care Clinics, 13*(4), 889-921.

Hutchinson, T.A., & Shahan, D.R. (Eds.). (2002). Polyvalent crotalid antivenin ovine Fab, *DRUGDEX(R) System.* Greenwood Village, CO: *MICROMEDEX.*

*Kanzenbach, T.L., & Dexter, W.W. (1999). Cold injuries. *Postgraduate Medicine, 105,*(1), 72-78.

*Krider, E.P., & Uman, M.A. (1995). Cloud-to-ground lightning: Mechanisms of damage and methods of protection. *Seminars in Neurology, 15*, 227-232.

*Laskowski-Jones, L. (1999). Responding to winter emergencies. *Dimensions of Critical Care Nursing, 18*(6), 13-21.

Laskowski-Jones L. (2000). Responding to summer emergencies. *Dimensions of Critical Care Nursing, 19*(4):2-12.

*Lazar, H.L. (1997). The treatment of hypothermia. *The New England Journal of Medicine, 337,* 1545-1547.

*Lee, R.C. (1997). Injury by electrical forces: Pathophysiology, manifestations, and therapy. *Current Problems in Surgery, 34*(9), 677-764.

*Lee, S. (1997). Envenomations II: Reptiles. *Toxtalk: A Publication of the Poison Control Center, 8(*1/2), 1-8. Philadelphia: Poison Control Center.

*Lewis, A.M.E. (1997). Understanding the principles of lightning injuries. *Journal of Emergency Nursing, 23*(6), 535-541.

*Lopez, R.E., & Holle, R.L. (1995). Demographics of lightning casualties. *Seminars in Neurology, 15*, 286-295.

**Morbidity & Mortality Weekly Report(MMWR)* (1998, May 22). Lightning-associated deaths–United States. *47*(19), 391-394.

Morris, J. (2003). Environmental emergencies. In L. Newberry (Ed.). *Sheehy's Emergency Nursing Principles and Practice* (5th ed., pp. 612-632). St. Louis: Mosby.

Norris, R.L., & Bush, S.P. (2001). North American venomous reptile bites. In P.S. Auerbach (Ed.), *Wilderness medicine* (4th ed., pp. 896-951). St. Louis: Mosby.

*Project Team of the Resuscitation Council (UK). (1999). Consensus guidelines: Emergency medical treatment of anaphylactic reactions. *Resuscitation, 41*, 93-99.

*Resnik, B.I., & Wetli, C.V. (1996). Lichtenberg figures. *American Journal of Forensic Medicine and Pathology, 17*(2), 99-102.

Suchard, J.R., & Connor, D.A. (2001). Scorpion envenomation. In P.S. Auerbach (Ed.), *Wilderness Medicine* (4th ed., pp. 839-862). St. Louis: Mosby.

Tisherman, S.A. (2002). Hypothermia, cold injury and drowning. In Peitzman, A.B., et al. (Eds.), *The trauma manual* (2nd ed., pp. 404-410). Philadelphia: Lippincott-Raven.

*van Zomeren, A.H., et al. (1998). Lightning stroke and neuropsychological impairment: cases and questions. *Journal of Neurology, Neurosurgery & Psychiatry, 64*(6), 763-769.

*Visscher, P.K., Vetter, R.S., & Camazine, S. (1996). Removing bee stings. *Lancet, 348*(9023), 301-302.

*Walpoth, B., et al. (1997). Outcome of survivors of accidental deep hypothermia and circulatory arrest treated with extracorporeal blood warming. *New England Journal of Medicine, 337*(21), 1500-1505.

*Watts, D.D. (1998). Hypothermic coagulopathy in trauma: Effect of varying levels of hypothermia on enzyme speed, platelet function, and fibrinolytic activity. *Journal of Trauma, 44,* 846-854.

UNIT **FOUR**

MANAGEMENT of CLIENTS with FLUID, ELECTROLYTE, and ACID-BASE IMBALANCES

CHAPTER 14

Fluid and Electrolyte Balance

M. LINDA WORKMAN

LEARNING OUTCOMES

After studying this chapter, you should be able to:

1. Explain why women and older adults have less total body water than do men and younger adults.
2. Interpret whether a client's serum electrolyte values are normal, elevated, or low.
3. Describe the expected blood volume responses when isotonic, hypertonic, or hypotonic intravenous fluids are infused.
4. Describe the expected blood osmolarity responses when isotonic, hypertonic, or hypotonic intravenous fluids are infused.
5. Explain the relationships between antidiuretic hormone, urine output volume, and osmolarity.
6. Analyze a client's hydration status on the basis of physical assessment findings.
7. Evaluate a client's food choices for sodium content.
8. Evaluate a client's food choices for potassium content.
9. Evaluate a client's food choices for calcium content.

Go to your Student CD-ROM for Review Questions for the NCLEX Examination keyed to these Learning Outcomes.

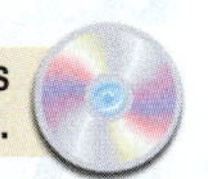

HOMEOSTASIS

The human body works best when some conditions are kept within a narrow range of normal. Examples of such conditions include body temperature, blood electrolyte values (e.g., sodium, potassium, and calcium), blood pH, and blood volume. No body system works well if 2 liters of blood volume are gained or lost. To keep conditions as close to normal as possible (a situation called **homeostasis**), the body has many safeguards or control mechanisms **(homeostatic mechanisms)** to prevent dangerous changes. For example, if a person is in a hot room (e.g., 110° F) and does not have good homeostatic mechanisms, his or her body temperature could go as high as 110° F, resulting in death. The homeostatic mechanisms of sweating to cool by evaporation and dilating blood vessels to expel body heat help to prevent body temperature from rising much more than 1° F above the normal 98.6° F, keeping body temperature in the normal range.

One very important area for homeostasis is maintaining the body's normal fluid volume and composition. Water is the most common substance in the body, making up about 55% to 60% of total adult body weight. This water (fluid) is divided into two spaces or compartments, the **extracellular fluid (ECF)** and the fluid inside the cells, the **intracellular fluid (ICF).** The ECF space contains about one third (15 L) of total body water. This space includes **interstitial fluid** (fluid between cells, sometimes called the "third space"), blood, lymph, bone, and connective tissue water, and the transcellular fluids. **Transcellular fluids** are the fluids in special body spaces and include cerebrospinal fluid, synovial fluid, peritoneal fluid, and pleural fluid. ICF contains the remaining two thirds (25 L) of total body water. Figure 14-1 shows the normal distribution of total body water.

Water is needed to deliver dissolved nutrients, electrolytes, and other substances to all organs, tissues, and cells. Most physiologic processes occur only in a watery environment. In the healthy adult, the volume of water in the fluid compartments remains within the normal range although the water moves constantly between compartments. Changes in either the amount of water or the amount of electrolytes in body fluids can affect the functioning of all cells, tissues, and organs. For proper function, the volume of all body fluids and the types and amount of dissolved substances must be carefully controlled.

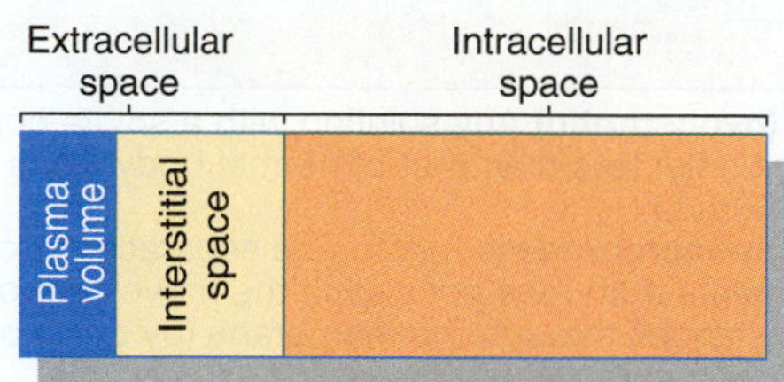

Figure 14-1 ■ Normal distribution of total body water.

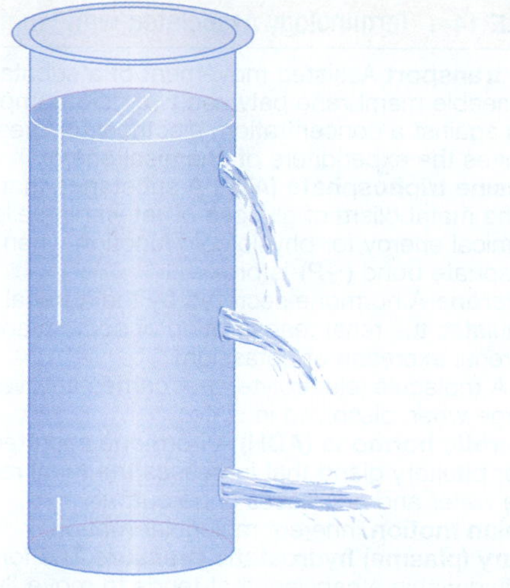

Figure 14-2 ■ Hydrostatic pressure. The pressure that water molecules exert against the sides of the container is highest where the weight of the water is greatest. (From Nave, C., & Nave, B. [1985]. Hydrostatic pressure. In *Physics for health sciences* [3rd ed.]. Philadelphia: W.B. Saunders.)

ANATOMY AND PHYSIOLOGY REVIEW

Physiologic Influences on Fluid and Electrolyte Balance

Many processes control normal fluid and electrolyte balance. These processes work together to maintain balance so the internal environment remains stable even when the external environment changes.

Knowing the terms related to solutions helps to understand the processes involved in fluid and electrolyte balance (Table 14-1). Body fluids are composed of water and particles dissolved or suspended in water. The **solvent** is the water portion of fluids. **Solutes** are the particles dissolved or suspended in the water. Solutes vary in type and amount from one fluid space to another. Proper function is dependent on keeping the correct balance of fluid and electrolytes within each body fluid space.

Important processes involved in fluid and electrolyte balance include filtration, diffusion, osmosis, and active transport. These processes determine how, when, and where fluids and particles move across cell membranes.

FILTRATION

Definition

Filtration is the movement of fluid through a cell or blood vessel membrane because of hydrostatic pressure differences on both sides of the membrane. Basically, filtration depends on differences in water volume pressing against confining walls.

All fluid has weight. Fluid weight in a confined space is related to the amount of fluid present in that area. Water molecules in a confined space constantly press outward against the confining walls. **Hydrostatic pressure** is the force of the weight of water molecules pressing against the confining walls of a space. Hydrostatic pressure is a "water-pushing" pressure, because it is the force that pushes water outward from a confined space through a membrane (Figure 14-2).

Physiologic Activity

Water is the largest part of any body fluid. The amount of water in any body fluid space determines the hydrostatic pressure of that space. The amount of water in a fluid is inversely (negatively) related to the **viscosity** (thickness) of that fluid. Thus more water and less solute decrease viscosity, and less water with more solute increases viscosity. Blood, a viscous fluid ("thicker" than water), is confined within the blood vessels. Blood has hydrostatic pressure because of its weight and volume and because the heart is pumping blood into the arterial circulation.

The hydrostatic pressures of two fluid spaces can be compared whenever a **permeable** (porous) membrane separates the two spaces. If the hydrostatic pressure is the same in both fluid spaces, a state of **equilibrium** (no difference between the two spaces) exists for hydrostatic pressure. If the hydrostatic pressure is not the same in both spaces, **disequilibrium** exists. This means that the two spaces have a **gradient,** or a graded difference, of hydrostatic pressure: one space has a higher hydrostatic pressure than the other. Because the human body constantly seeks equilibrium, a gradient forces movement on both sides of the membrane until an equilibrium exists (Figure 14-3).

In most instances, substances move from the greater amount of pressure or concentration to the lesser amount. Thus when a hydrostatic pressure gradient exists between two fluid spaces, fluid from the space with the higher hydrostatic pressure moves **(filters)** through the membrane into the space with the lower hydrostatic pressure. This filtration continues only as long as the hydrostatic pressure gradient exists. Equilibrium is reached when enough fluid leaves one space and enters the other space to make the hydrostatic pressure in both spaces equal.

When the two spaces are in equilibrium for hydrostatic pressure, a gradient no longer exists between them. Although water molecules may be exchanged evenly between two spaces in equilibrium, no net filtration of fluid occurs. In equilibrium, neither space gains nor loses water molecules, and the hydrostatic pressure in both spaces remains the same.

Clinical Function and Significance

Blood pressure is a hydrostatic filtering force measured in millimeters of mercury (mm Hg). It moves whole blood from the heart to tissue areas where filtration can occur. Filtration is important for the exchange of water, nutrients, and waste products when blood arrives at the tissue capillaries. One factor that determines whether or not fluid leaves the

TABLE 14-1 Terminology Associated with Fluid and Electrolyte Balance

active transport Assisted movement of a substance through a permeable membrane between two fluid compartments; occurs against a concentration, electrical, or pressure gradient; requires the expenditure of chemical energy

adenosine triphosphate (ATP) A substance that is generated by the metabolism of glucose or fat within cells and releases chemical energy for physiologic function when a high-energy phosphate bond (~P) is broken

aldosterone A hormone secreted by the adrenal cortex that stimulates the renal reabsorption of sodium and water and the renal excretion of potassium

anion A molecule (electrolyte) that carries an overall negative charge when dissolved in water

antidiuretic hormone (ADH) A hormone secreted from the posterior pituitary gland that increases the renal reabsorption of pure water and decreases urine output

brownian motion Inherent molecular motion

capillary (plasma) hydrostatic pressure The force generated by fluid within a capillary that tends to move fluid out from the capillary and into the interstitial space

capillary (plasma) osmotic pressure The force generated by the concentration of plasma solutes (osmotic and oncotic pressures) that tends to retain fluid within the capillary or move fluid from the interstitial space into the capillary

cation A molecule (electrolyte) that carries an overall positive charge when dissolved in water

cofactor A substance required to enhance the activity of an enzyme or a physiologic reaction

colloidal oncotic pressure The osmotic pressure exerted by the concentration of colloids (proteins) within a solution

diffusion Unimpeded movement of a substance through a permeable membrane between two fluid compartments; occurs down a concentration gradient; does not require the expenditure of chemical energy

disequilibrium A state in which two fluid compartments are unequal in at least one characteristic

electrolytes Substances that carry an electrical charge when dissolved in water

electroneutrality A state in which a body fluid has an equal number of cations and anions so that the fluid does not express an electrical charge

equilibrium A state in which two fluid compartments are equal in one or more characteristics

extracellular fluid (ECF) Body fluid present outside of cells; includes plasma, interstitial fluid, and transcellular fluid

facilitated diffusion Assisted movement of a substance through a permeable membrane between two fluid compartments; occurs down a concentration gradient; does not require the expenditure of chemical energy

filtration The movement of fluid through a biologic membrane as a result of hydrostatic pressure differences on the two sides of the membrane

gradient A graded difference in some characteristic between two fluid compartments

hydrostatic pressure The force of pressure exerted by static water in a confined space—"water-pushing" pressure

hypertonic (hyperosmotic) Any solution with a solute concentration (osmolarity) greater than that of normal body fluids (>310 mOsm/L)

hypotonic (hyposmotic) Any solution with a solute concentration (osmolarity) less than that of normal body fluids (<270 mOsm/L)

impermeable membrane A membrane separating two fluid compartments that does not permit the movement of one or more substances through the membrane (by diffusion) from one compartment to the other

insensible fluid loss Unregulated fluid losses from the skin, gastrointestinal tract, wounds, and pulmonary epithelium

interstitial fluid Fluid present in tissues between cells

intracellular fluid (ICF) Fluid found inside cells

isotonic (isosmotic) Any solution with a solute concentration equal to the osmolarity of normal body fluids or normal saline (0.9% NaCl), about 300 mOsm/L

natriuretic peptide (NP) A hormone secreted by cardiac atrial cells that increases the renal excretion of sodium and water

obligatory urine output The minimal amount of urine output necessary to ensure the excretion of metabolic wastes (about 400 mL/day)

osmolality The concentration of solute within a solution as measured by the amount of solute osmoles per kilogram of solvent

osmolarity The concentration of solute within a solution as measured by the amount of solute osmoles per liter of solution

osmoreceptor Specialized sensory nerve cells in the thalamus or hypothalamus that are sensitive to changes in the osmolarity of extracellular fluid

osmosis Diffusion of water (no other substance) through a selectively permeable membrane from an area of lower osmotic pressure to an area of greater osmotic pressure

osmotic pressure The pressure exerted by a solution that contains a relatively high concentration of solute; this pressure draws water from areas or compartments with lower concentrations of solute into the areas or compartments with higher concentrations of solute—"water-pulling" pressure

permeable membrane A membrane separating two fluid compartments that permits the movement of one or more substances through the membrane (by diffusion) from one compartment to the other

solubility The degree to which any given solute completely dissolves (dissociates) in water

solute The solid particles dissolved in a solution

solvent The fluid (water) portion of a solution

tissue hydrostatic pressure (THP) The force generated by fluid within the interstitial spaces that tends to move fluid into the capillary from the interstitial space

tissue osmotic pressure (TOP) The force generated by the concentration of interstitial fluid solutes that tends to retain fluid in the interstitial space or move fluid from the capillary into the interstitial space

transcellular fluid Extracellular fluid confined to a specific area or region of the body (cerebrospinal fluid, pericardial fluid, visceral fluid, aqueous humor, peritoneal fluid, and pleural fluid)

viscosity Gumminess or thickness of the molecules in a solution, causing friction within that solution

blood vessels and enters the tissue spaces **(interstitial fluid)** is the difference between the hydrostatic pressure of capillary blood and that of the interstitial fluid.

The lining of the capillaries is only one cell layer thick. Therefore the "wall" that holds blood in the capillaries is thin. Large spaces **(pores)** between the cells in the capillary membrane help water filter freely through capillary membranes in either direction if a hydrostatic pressure gradient is present (Figure 14-4).

Edema (tissue swelling with fluid collection) develops with changes in normal hydrostatic pressure differences, such as in clients with right-sided heart failure. In this con-

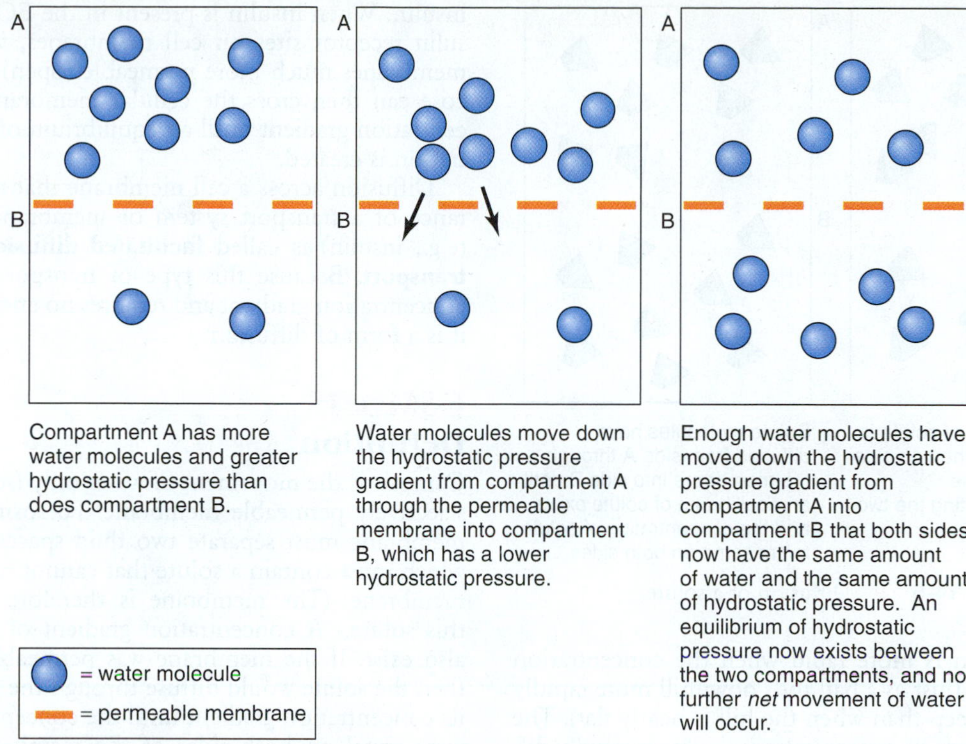

Figure 14-3 ■ The process of filtration. (© 1992. M. Linda Workman. All rights reserved.)

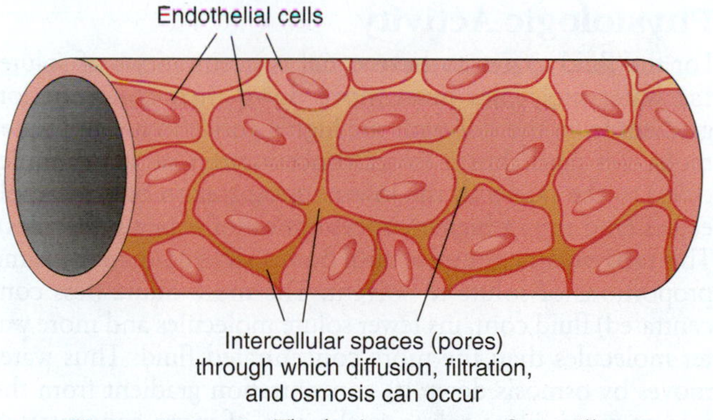

Figure 14-4 ■ The basic structure of a capillary.

dition, the volume of blood in the right side of the heart increases greatly because the right ventricle is too weak to pump blood efficiently into the pulmonary blood vessels. As blood backs up into the venous system, venous hydrostatic pressure rises. The increased venous pressure causes capillary hydrostatic pressure to increase until it is higher than the hydrostatic pressure in the interstitial space. Excess filtration of fluid from the capillaries into the interstitial tissue space occurs, forming visible edema.

DIFFUSION

Definition

Diffusion is the free movement of particles (solute) across a permeable membrane down a **concentration gradient,** that is, from an area of higher concentration to an area of lower concentration. Diffusion controls the movement of solute particles in solution across various body membranes.

Physiologic Activity

The diffusion of particles into and out of cells and body fluid spaces occurs via **brownian motion,** the kinetic energy of molecular motion. Brownian motion is the vibration of single molecules caused by electrons orbiting at the core of each molecule. Such motion causes totally random movement of molecules, which collide or bump into each other within a confined space. Each collision increases the speed of molecular movement.

As a result of the collisions, molecules in a solution spread out evenly through the available space. They move from an area of higher amounts (concentration) of molecules to an area of lower amounts until equal amounts are present in all areas. The number of collisions is related to the concentration of molecules in a confined space. Spaces with many molecules have more collisions and faster molecule movement than spaces with fewer molecules.

A concentration gradient exists when two fluid spaces have different amounts of the same type of molecules. Brownian motion of the molecules causes them to move down the concentration gradient. As a result of brownian motion, any membrane that separates two spaces is struck repeatedly by molecules. When the molecule strikes a pore in the membrane that is large enough for it to pass through, diffusion occurs (Figure 14-5). The chance of any single molecule colliding with the membrane and going through a pore is much greater on the side of the membrane with a higher molecule concentration.

The speed of diffusion is related to the concentration gradient (difference in amount) between the two sides of the membrane. The degree of concentration difference is known as the *steepness* of the gradient: The larger the concentration difference between the two sides, the steeper the

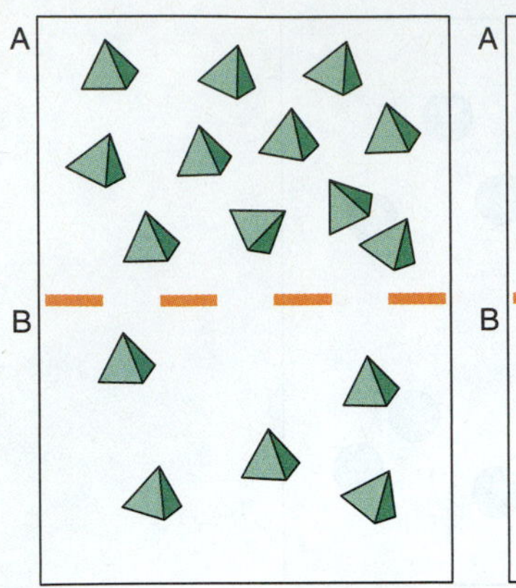

The concentration of solute is greater on side A than on side B, with a permeable membrane separating the two compartments.

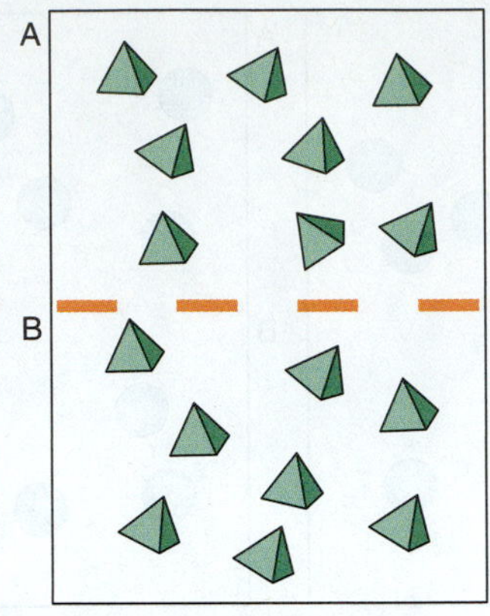

Solute molecules have diffused from side A through the membrane into side B until an equilibrium of solute exists and the concentration of solute is the same on both sides.

Figure 14-5 ■ Diffusion of a solute.

gradient. Diffusion is more rapid when the concentration gradient is steeper (just as a ball rolls downhill more rapidly when the hill is steep than when the hill is nearly flat). The greater the difference in concentration, the more rapidly diffusion occurs from the area of higher concentration to the area of lower concentration.

Diffusion of solute particles continues through the membrane as long as a concentration gradient exists between the two sides of the membrane. *When the concentration of solute is the same on both sides of the membrane, an equilibrium exists and only an equal exchange (not a net movement) of solute continues.*

Clinical Function and Significance

Diffusion is important in the transport of gases and in the movement of most electrolytes, atoms, and molecules through cell membranes. Unlike capillary membranes, which permit the diffusion of most small-sized substances down a concentration gradient, cell membranes are *selective.* They permit the movement of some substances and inhibit the movement of other substances. Some molecules cannot move across a cell membrane, even when a steep "downhill" gradient exists, because the membrane is **impermeable** (not porous) to that molecule. Thus the concentration gradient is maintained across the membrane.

Impermeability and special transport systems cause differences in the concentrations of specific substances from one fluid compartment to another. For example, usually the fluid outside of the cells, the **extracellular fluid (ECF),** contains almost 10 times more sodium ions than the fluid inside the cell, the **intracellular fluid (ICF).** This extreme concentration difference is caused by the impermeability of the cell membrane to sodium and from a special "sodium pump" that moves any extra sodium out of the cell "uphill" against its concentration gradient and back into the ECF.

In some instances diffusion cannot occur without help, even down steep concentration gradients, because of membrane selectivity. A clinical example is the fact that, even though the amount of glucose is much higher in the ECF than in the ICF (creating a steep gradient for glucose), glucose cannot cross most cell membranes without the help of insulin. When insulin is present in the ECF, it binds to insulin receptor sites on cell membranes, which makes the membranes much more permeable (open) to glucose. Glucose can then cross the cellular membrane down its concentration gradient until an equilibrium of glucose concentration is created.

Diffusion across a cell membrane that requires the assistance of a transport system or membrane-altering system (e.g., insulin) is called **facilitated diffusion** or **facilitated transport.** Because this type of transport occurs down a concentration gradient and requires no energy from the cell, it is a form of diffusion.

OSMOSIS

Definition

Osmosis is the movement of water only (solvent) through a selectively permeable membrane. For osmosis to occur, a membrane must separate two fluid spaces, at least one of which must contain a solute that cannot move through the membrane. (The membrane is therefore impermeable to this solute.) A concentration gradient of this solute must also exist. If the membrane was permeable to this solute, then the solute would diffuse through the membrane down its concentration gradient until the concentrations of solute were equal on both sides of the membrane. Because the membrane is impermeable to the solute, these particles cannot cross the membrane, but water molecules can.

Physiologic Activity

For the fluid spaces to have equal concentrations of solute, the water molecules must move down their concentration gradient from the side with the higher concentration of water molecules (and thus a lower concentration of solute molecules) to the side with the lower concentration of water molecules (and thus a higher concentration of solute molecules). This movement continues until both spaces contain the same proportions of solute to solvent. The more dilute (less concentrated) fluid contains fewer solute molecules and more water molecules than the more concentrated fluid. Thus water moves by osmosis down its concentration gradient from the area of more dilute solute to the area of more concentrated solute until a new equilibrium occurs (Figure 14-6).

At this point, the concentrations of solute in the fluid spaces (the proportion of solute to solvent) on both sides of the membrane are equal, even though the total numbers of solute and volume of water may be different. This equilibrium occurs by the movement of water molecules rather than the movement of solute molecules.

Factors that determine whether and how fast osmosis occurs include the overall concentration of particles (solute) in solution, how easily the solute dissolves in water **(solubility),** and the amount of membrane available for osmosis.

CONCENTRATION OF SOLUTE

The concentration of particles in body fluids is expressed in milliequivalents per liter (mEq/L), millimoles per liter (mmol/L), and milliosmoles per liter (mOsm/L). Osmoles and milliosmoles are used to describe the total amount of solute particles (including electrolytes) contained in a solution. The number of milliosmoles present in body fluids is expressed as either osmolarity or osmolality.

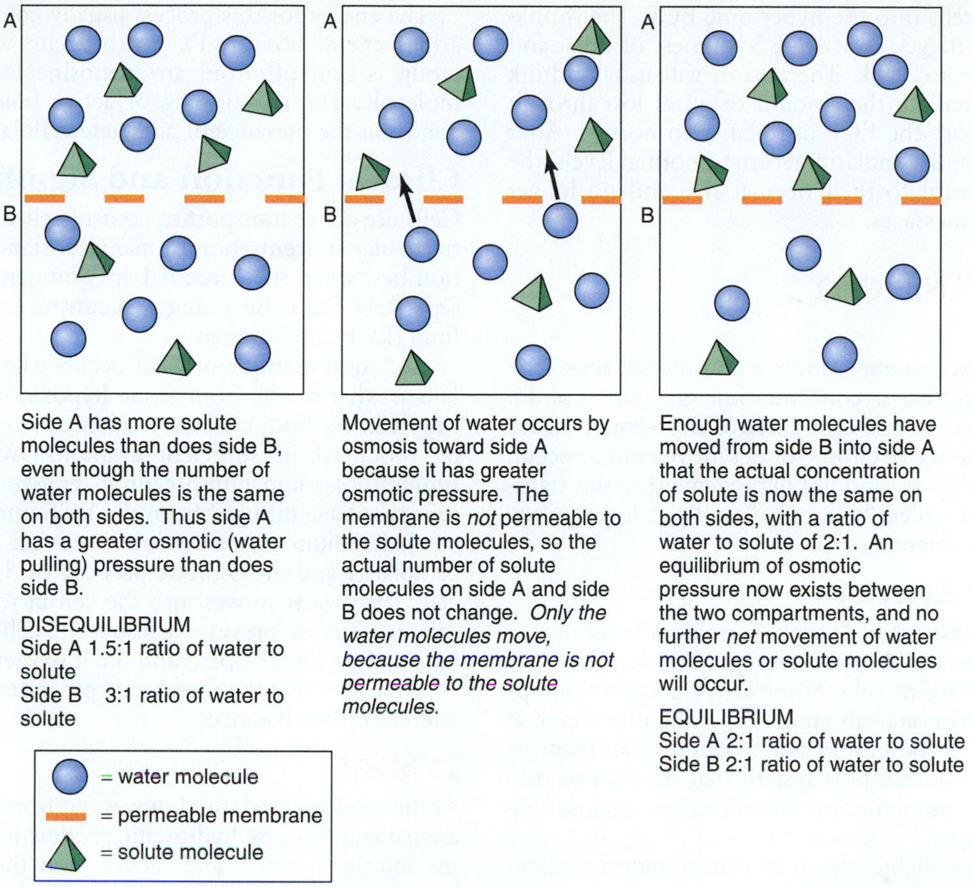

Side A has more solute molecules than does side B, even though the number of water molecules is the same on both sides. Thus side A has a greater osmotic (water pulling) pressure than does side B.

DISEQUILIBRIUM
Side A 1.5:1 ratio of water to solute
Side B 3:1 ratio of water to solute

Movement of water occurs by osmosis toward side A because it has greater osmotic pressure. The membrane is *not* permeable to the solute molecules, so the actual number of solute molecules on side A and side B does not change. *Only the water molecules move, because the membrane is not permeable to the solute molecules.*

Enough water molecules have moved from side B into side A that the actual concentration of solute is now the same on both sides, with a ratio of water to solute of 2:1. An equilibrium of osmotic pressure now exists between the two compartments, and no further *net* movement of water molecules or solute molecules will occur.

EQUILIBRIUM
Side A 2:1 ratio of water to solute
Side B 2:1 ratio of water to solute

= water molecule
= permeable membrane
= solute molecule

Figure 14-6 ■ The process of osmosis.

Osmolarity is the number of milliosmoles in a *liter* of solution; **osmolality** is the number of milliosmoles in a *kilogram* of solution. The normal osmolarity value for plasma and other body fluids ranges from 270 to 300 mOsm/L.

The body functions best when the osmolarity of the fluids in all body fluid spaces is close to 300 mOsm/L. Many mechanisms work to keep the solute concentration at or near optimum levels. When all body fluids have this solute concentration, the osmotic pressures (water-pulling) of the two fluid compartments are equal, and no *net* water movement occurs. In this situation, the body fluids are **isosmotic** to each other. Another term with the same meaning is **isotonic** (sometimes called **normotonic**). Examples of specific intravenous (IV) solutions with overall solute concentrations equaling 270 to 300 mOsm/L include 0.9% sodium chloride in water and Ringer's lactate in water. Because these solutions are isotonic (or isosmotic) to plasma, their addition to plasma does not change the osmolarity or osmotic pressure of the plasma.

Fluids with osmolarities (solute concentrations) greater than 300 mOsm/L are **hyperosmotic,** or **hypertonic,** compared with isosmotic fluids. Hyperosmotic fluids have a greater osmotic pressure than do isosmotic fluids and tend to pull water from the isosmotic fluid space into the hyperosmotic fluid space until an osmotic balance occurs.

Fluids with osmolarities of less than 270 mOsm/L are **hypo-osmotic,** or **hypotonic,** compared with isosmotic fluids. Hypo-osmolar fluids have a lower or smaller osmotic pressure than isosmotic fluids. As a result, water tends to be pulled from the hypo-osmotic fluid space into the isosmotic fluid space until an osmotic balance occurs.

SOLUBILITY OF SOLUTE

Solubility is the degree to which a solute dissolves in water. Solubility is related to osmotic pressure: The greater the solubility of the solutes in a fluid, the higher the osmotic pressure of that fluid.

AMOUNT OF AVAILABLE MEMBRANE

The greater the amount of membrane available for osmosis, the faster the rate of osmosis. More membrane increases the chances that water molecules will hit the membrane at a point where penetration is possible.

Clinical Function and Significance

Osmosis and filtration act together in capillary fluid dynamics to control both extracellular fluid (ECF) and intracellular fluid (ICF) volumes. The thirst mechanism is an example of how osmosis helps maintain homeostasis. The feeling of thirst is caused by the activation of cells in the brain that respond to changes in extracellular fluid (ECF) osmolarity. These cells are so sensitive to changes in ECF osmolarity that they are called *osmoreceptors.* When a person loses body water but most of the solute remains, such as through excessive sweating during exercise, ECF volume is decreased and osmolarity is increased (hypertonic conditions exist). The cells in the thirst center shrink as water moves from the cells into the hypertonic ECF. The shrinking of these cells triggers a person's awareness of thirst and increases the urge to drink. The person will usually drink enough fluid to replace the amount of water lost through sweating and restore the ECF osmolarity to normal. After the ECF volume and osmolarity return to normal levels, the osmoreceptors return to their normal size and no longer send stimulatory messages.

ACTIVE TRANSPORT

Definition

A cell must use extra energy to move a substance across the cell membrane against a concentration gradient (uphill). This type of movement is called **active transport** because the cell must make active efforts for net movement to occur. Because of its energy use and uphill movement, active transport is sometimes called "pumping," and the mechanisms are known as membrane pumps.

Physiologic Activity

Active transport systems or "pumps," are usually located in the cell membrane and act as "gatekeepers" to maintain special environments inside cells. Some active transport pumps can carry more than one substance across the membrane at the same time. The sodium-potassium pump is an example of a common active transport system that moves two substances at the same time in opposite directions against concentration gradients.

Sodium diffuses slightly down its concentration gradient into the intracellular fluid (ICF) because it has such a high extracellular fluid (ECF) concentration compared with its ICF concentration. Similarly, because potassium has such a high concentration inside the cells compared with its concentration in ECF, it diffuses slightly down its concentration gradient into the ECF. The action of the sodium-potassium pump moves the extra sodium out of the cell and returns the lost potassium back into the cell. The sodium-potassium pump requires the use of cellular energy.

The energy for this process usually comes from breaking a high-energy bond (~P), which occurs when a phosphate group is split off from an adenosine triphosphate (ATP) molecule. The functioning of active transport pumps depends on the presence of adequate cellular ATP.

Clinical Function and Significance

Cells use active transport to control cell volume and the intracellular concentration of many substances. All cells function best when their internal environments are maintained separately from the changes occurring in the extracellular fluid (ECF) environment.

A clinical example of what occurs when active transport fails is what results from tissue **hypoxia** (decreased oxygen supply in the body). Without adequate oxygen, ATP cannot be produced in sufficient amounts. Without ATP, the sodium-potassium pump cannot remove the extra sodium ions that have diffused from the ECF into the cell. The increased sodium concentration inside the cell increases the osmolarity and the osmotic pressure of the fluid inside the cell. Then water moves into the cell in response to the increased osmotic pressure, causing the cell to swell and perhaps to **lyse** (break open) and die if oxygen is not provided.

Table 14-2 lists the membrane processes involved in fluid and electrolyte balance.

LYMPH

At the capillary level, fluid moves out from the capillary at its arterial end (because hydrostatic pressure is greater there) into the interstitial space, and moves from the interstitial space back into the capillary at the venous end. In most cases, not all of the fluid that leaves the capillary at the arterial end and enters the interstitial space is returned to the capillary at the venous end. A small amount remains in the tissues. If this situation is not balanced by another mechanism to return the fluid to the systemic circulation, blood volume would become depleted and the interstitial areas would constantly be edematous. Instead, this extra fluid leaking out from the capillaries is returned to the systemic circulation as **lymph.**

TABLE 14-2 Summary of Membrane-Fluid Actions

Action	Definition	Specific Characteristics
Filtration	The movement of fluid through a biologic membrane as a result of hydrostatic pressure differences on both sides of the membrane	Does not require energy Is limited to solvent and low–molecular weight solute Usually occurs from capillaries to the interstitial fluid Depends on hydrostatic pressure differences Occurs more rapidly with steep gradients
Diffusion	The free movement of substances across a permeable membrane and down a concentration gradient	Does not require energy Is not pressure dependent Moves solute and solvent down their individual gradients Occurs more rapidly with steep gradients Is directly related in speed to the amount of membrane available Occurs in both directions across capillary and cell membranes Is responsible for maintaining tissue nutrition
Osmosis	The process by which only the *solvent* diffuses through a selectively permeable membrane	Does not require energy Involves movement of water only Depends on hydrostatic and osmotic pressures Occurs more rapidly with steep gradients
Active transport	The movement of a substance across a selectively permeable membrane and against a concentration, electrical, or pressure gradient	Requires energy Requires a transport system (pump) Helps to maintain a special intracellular environment

Lymph fluid is similar to blood plasma (from which it is formed) but contains far less protein. It is returned to the circulation by lymph vessels, or **lymphatics.** Lymphatics begin as small, thin-walled, veinlike vessels that join to form larger lymphatic vessels. Two large groups of lymphatic vessels connect the entire lymph system with the general circulatory system. The left thoracic lymph duct drains lymph from the abdomen, gastrointestinal tract, pelvis, lower extremities, left side of the thorax, left arm, and left side of the head and neck into the left subclavian vein at the point where it joins the left internal jugular vein (Figure 14-7). Lymph from the right arm, right side of the chest, and right side of the head and neck drains into the right subclavian vein through three lymph ducts. Lymph nodes are situated along the lymphatic paths and filter the lymph fluid.

Lymphatics carry lymph fluid in one direction: toward the heart. Lymph flow is slower than blood flow because lymph has no pump. Lymph flow is enhanced by skeletal muscle contractions, intrathoracic pressure changes during breathing, and a peristalsis-like motion in the lymph vessels.

Hormonal Regulation of Fluid and Electrolyte Balance

The endocrine system helps control fluid and electrolyte balance. Three hormones that help control these critical balances are aldosterone, antidiuretic hormone (ADH), and natriuretic peptide (NP).

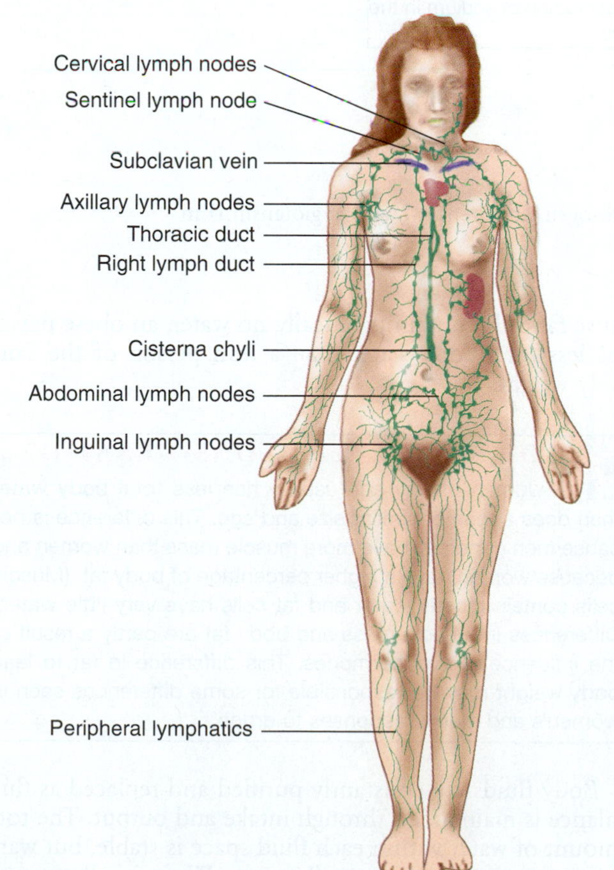

Figure 14-7 ■ Patterns of lymph drainage. (From Guyton, A., & Hall, J. [1996]. *Textbook of medical physiology* [9th ed.]. Philadelphia, W.B. Saunders.)

ALDOSTERONE

Aldosterone is a hormone secreted by the adrenal cortex. Aldosterone secretion is stimulated by either a decreased sodium level in the extracellular fluid (ECF) or an increased sodium level in urine. The secretion and function of aldosterone, angiotensinogen, and angiotensin are outlined in Figure 14-8. Aldosterone protects sodium balance by preventing sodium loss. Because sodium in body fluids exerts osmotic (water-pulling) pressure, water attempts to follow sodium in proportionate amounts. As a result of this sodium-water relationship, aldosterone secretion also helps regulate water balance.

In the kidney, blood is supplied to the nephrons via the afferent arteriole. Specialized cells **(juxtaglomerular cells)** inside the afferent arteriole near the nephron glomerulus are sensitive to changes in blood sodium levels. This area of the afferent arteriole touches a special area of the distal convoluted tubule (the **macula densa**). Together, the juxtaglomerular cells and the macula densa form the **juxtaglomerular complex.** When this complex senses that blood sodium levels are lower than normal or that the total blood volume is low, the macula densa triggers juxtaglomerular cells to secrete **renin.**

Renin acts on a plasma protein called **renin substrate** (formerly called **angiotensinogen),** converting it to angiotensin I. Angiotensin I is then further converted into angiotensin II by an enzyme called angiotensin-converting enzyme (ACE). **Angiotensin II** constricts many blood vessels and stimulates aldosterone secretion from the adrenal cortex.

Aldosterone acts on the distal tubules of the nephrons, triggering these areas to reabsorb sodium from the urine back into the blood. This action increases blood osmolarity. Aldosterone secretion increases when blood osmolarity or sodium levels are low, and its presence is normally needed to prevent excessive renal excretion of sodium. Aldosterone secretion also helps prevent blood potassium levels from becoming too high. Aldosterone secretion is stopped when blood osmolarity or serum sodium levels are greater than normal.

ANTIDIURETIC HORMONE

Antidiuretic hormone (ADH), or **vasopressin,** is produced in the brain and stored in the posterior pituitary gland. ADH release from the posterior pituitary gland is controlled by the hypothalamus in response to changes in blood osmolarity. The hypothalamus contains specialized cells **(osmoreceptors)** that are sensitive to changes in blood osmolarity. Increased blood osmolarity, especially an increase in the level of plasma sodium, results in a slight shrinkage of these cells and triggers ADH release from the posterior pituitary gland.

ADH acts directly on kidney tubules and collecting ducts, making them more permeable to water. As a result, more water is reabsorbed by these tubules and returned to the blood, decreasing blood osmolarity by making it more dilute. When blood osmolarity decreases, especially when the plasma sodium level is below normal, the osmoreceptors swell slightly and inhibit ADH release. Less water is then reabsorbed and more is lost from the body in the

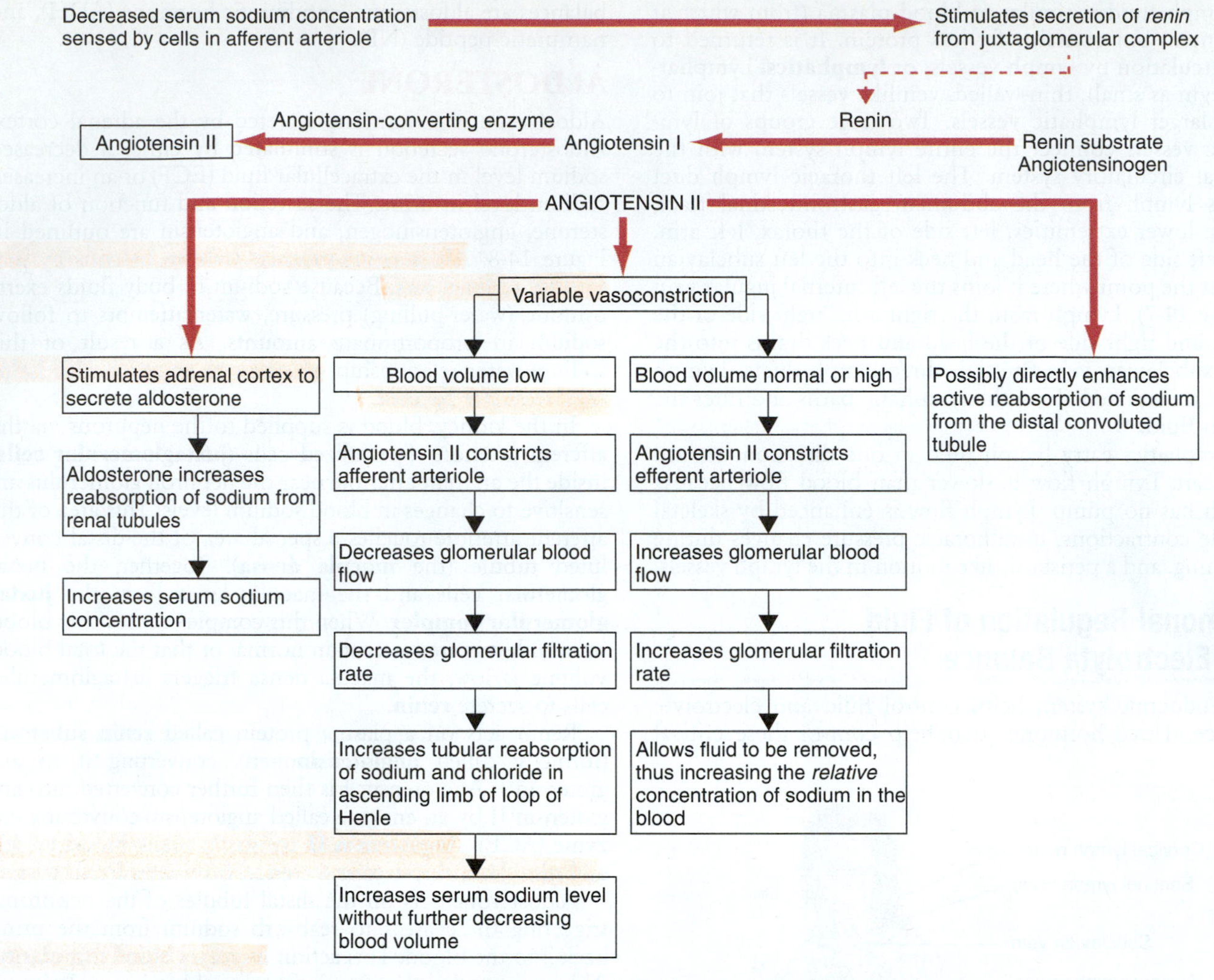

Figure 14-8 ■ The role of aldosterone, angiotensinogen, angiotensin I, and angiotensin II in the renal regulation of water and sodium.

urine. As a result, the amount of water in the extracellular fluid (ECF) decreases, bringing osmolarity to normal.

NATRIURETIC PEPTIDES

Natriuretic peptides (NPs) are hormones secreted by special cells that line the atria of the heart (atrial natriuretic peptide, or ANP) and the ventricles of the heart (brain natriuretic peptide, or BNP). They are secreted in response to increased blood volume and blood pressure, which stretch the heart tissue. NP binds to receptor sites in the nephrons, creating effects that oppose the renin-angiotensin system. When either ANP or BNP is secreted, kidney reabsorption of sodium is inhibited at the same time that glomerular filtration is increased. The outcome is increased output of urine with a high sodium content, which results in decreased circulating blood volume and decreased blood osmolarity.

Body Fluids

A person's age, gender, and ratio of lean mass to body fat affect the amount and distribution of body fluids. An older adult has less total body water than a younger adult. Because fat cells contain practically no water, an obese person has less total body water than a lean person of the same body weight.

WOMEN'S HEALTH CONSIDERATIONS

A woman of any age usually has less total body water than does a man of similar size and age. This difference is because men generally have more muscle mass than women and because women have a higher percentage of body fat. (Muscle cells contain mostly water and fat cells have very little water.) Differences in muscle mass and body fat are partly a result of the influence of sex hormones. This difference in fat to lean body weight may be responsible for some differences seen in women's and men's responses to drugs.

Body fluids are constantly purified and replaced as fluid balance is maintained through intake and output. The total amount of water within each fluid space is stable, but water moves continually among all spaces. Water in all spaces is exchanged continually while maintaining constant fluid volume. Table 14-3 lists the key points regarding fluid and electrolyte balance.

TABLE 14-3 Summary of Key Points Regarding Fluid and Electrolyte Balance

- All plasma electrolyte values must remain within a narrow range for proper physiologic functioning.
- The plasma is the entrance and exit site for all fluids and electrolytes.
- The primary organs or tissues of fluid and electrolyte regulation are the hypothalamus, kidney, adrenal glands, posterior pituitary gland, thyroid gland, and parathyroid glands.
- The total number of positive charges within a solution must be balanced by an equal number of negative charges to maintain electroneutrality.
- Although the specific types and concentrations of substances (solute) dissolved in body fluid vary from one fluid compartment to another, the total concentration of all solutes is the same in all fluid compartments (270 to 300 mOsm/L).
- Whenever possible, the body's regulatory mechanisms attempt to create or maintain an osmolar equilibrium in all body fluid compartments.
- A fluid compartment that is hyposmolar (hypotonic) to normal body fluids expels water from the compartment.
- A fluid compartment that is hyperosmolar (hypertonic) to normal body fluids draws water into it.

SOURCES OF FLUID INTAKE

Fluid intake is regulated through the thirst drive. Fluids enter the body primarily as liquids (Table 14-4). Because solid foods contain up to 85% water, some fluid also enters the body with ingested solid foods. In addition, water is a by-product of metabolism. This metabolic water accounts for about 300 mL of the daily water requirement. A rising blood osmolarity or a decreasing blood volume triggers the sensation of thirst. Sensations such as mouth dryness or the thought that a person has not had a drink recently also trigger the thirst drive. An adult drinks an average of 1500 mL of fluid per day and ingests an additional 800 mL of fluid from food.

ROUTES OF FLUID LOSS

The body has several ways to remove excess water and waste products (see Table 14-4). Of all the water loss pathways, the kidney is the most important and the most sensitive. Water loss by the kidney is closely regulated and is adjustable. The volume of urine excreted daily varies depending on the amount of fluid intake and the body's need to conserve fluids.

The minimum amount of urine per day needed to dissolve and excrete toxic waste products is 400 to 600 mL. This minimal volume is called the **obligatory urine output.** If the 24-hour urine output falls below the obligatory output amount, wastes are retained and can cause lethal electrolyte imbalances, acidosis, and a toxic buildup of nitrogen. This urine is maximally concentrated, with a **specific gravity** (the weight of the liquid compared with the weight of pure water) of 1.032 or higher and an osmolarity of at least 1400 mOsm/L.

Urine can also become very dilute, with a specific gravity of 1.005 and an osmolarity of 200 mOsm/L. Dilution normally results from a large fluid intake and is reflected in a large volume of urine output. The ability of the kidneys to make either concentrated or very dilute urine helps maintain fluid and electrolyte balance. With the influence of aldosterone, antidiuretic hormone (ADH), and natriuretic peptides, the kidney is able to respond when extracellular fluid concentrations, volumes, or pressures change.

TABLE 14-4 Routes of Fluid Ingestion and Excretion

Intake	Output
Measurable	
Oral fluids	Urine
Parenteral fluids	Emesis†
Enemas*	Feces†
Irrigation fluids*	Drainage from body cavities
Not Measurable	
Solid foods	Perspiration
Metabolism	Vaporization through the lungs

*Measured by subtracting the amount returned from the amount instilled.
†Measurement is accurate only when these substances are excreted in liquid form.

Other normal water loss occurs through the skin, the lungs, and the gastrointestinal tract. Additional water losses can occur via salivation, drainage from fistulas and drains, and gastrointestinal suction.

Water loss from the skin, lungs, and stool—called **insensible water loss,** because it cannot be controlled—can be significant. In a healthy adult, insensible water loss is about 15 to 20 mL/kg/day. Insensible water loss increases dramatically in hypermetabolic states such as thyroid crisis, trauma, burns, states of extreme stress, and fever. For every degree increase in body temperature, insensible water loss increases by about 10%. Insensible water loss also increases when the environment is hot and dry. Examples of clients at risk for increased insensible water loss include those being mechanically ventilated and those with rapid respirations (tachypnea). Insensible water loss (not including sweat) is pure water and does not contain electrolytes. Therefore excessive insensible water loss results in a more hypertonic extracellular fluid (ECF) with a smaller volume. If this loss is not balanced by intake, the hypertonic ECF and dehydration can lead to **hypernatremia** (elevated serum sodium level).

Loss by sweating is variable and can reach a maximum rate of about 2 L/hr. Although it contains electrolytes, sweat is slightly hypotonic compared to blood. The amount of sweating is controlled by the autonomic nervous system, body temperature, and blood flow in the skin.

Water loss through stool is normally minimal. However, this loss can increase greatly with severe diarrhea or excessive fistula drainage. Clients with ulcerative colitis can have a diarrheal fluid loss of several liters per day. Diarrheal fluid contains water, potassium, sodium, bicarbonate, and chloride. Thus with diarrhea, fluid and some electrolytes are lost.

Electrolytes

Electrolytes, or **ions,** are substances in body fluids that carry an electrical charge. **Cations** have positive charges; **anions** have negative charges. Body fluids are electrochemically neutral, which means that the number of positive ions is balanced by an equal number of negative ions. However, the distribution of ions differs between the extracellular fluid (ECF) and the intracellular fluid (ICF) (Figure 14-9).

Most electrolytes have different concentrations in the ICF and ECF. This concentration difference helps maintain membrane excitability and allows nerve impulse transmission. The

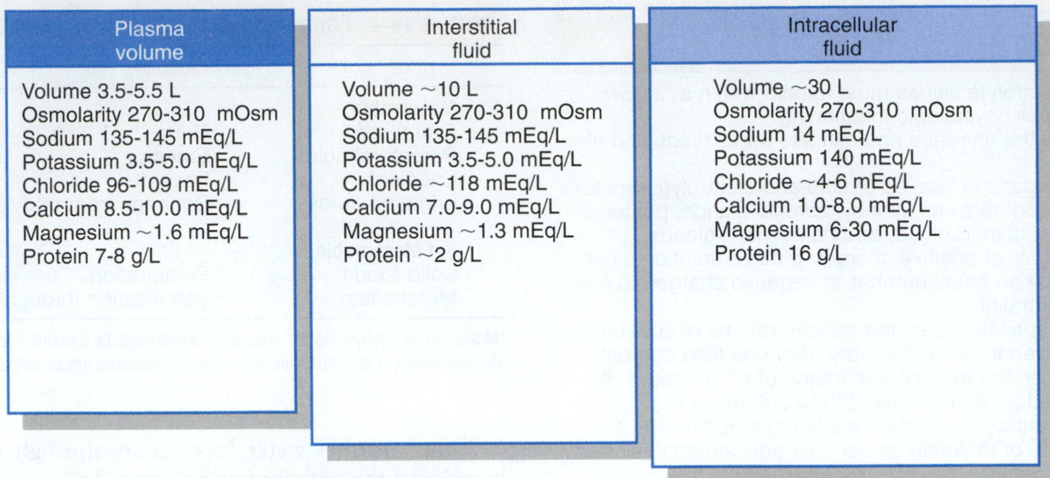

Figure 14-9 ■ The composition of various body fluids.

TABLE 14-5 Major Serum Electrolyte Concentrations and Functions

Electrolyte	Reference Range	International Recommended Units	Functions
Sodium (Na^+)	136-145 mEq/L	136-145 mmol/L	Maintenance of plasma and interstitial osmolarity Generation and transmission of action potentials Maintenance of acid-base balance Maintenance of electroneutrality
Potassium (K^+)	3.5-5.0 mEq/L	3.5-5.0 mmol/L	Regulation of intracellular osmolarity Maintenance of electrical membrane excitability Maintenance of plasma acid-base balance
Calcium (Ca^{2+})	9.0-10.5 mg/dL	2.25-2.75 mmol/L	Cofactor in blood-clotting cascade Excitable membrane stabilizer Adds strength/density to bones and teeth Essential element in cardiac, skeletal, and smooth muscle contraction
Chloride (Cl^-)	98-106 mEq/L	98-106 mmol/L	Maintenance of plasma acid-base balance Maintenance of plasma electroneutrality Formation of hydrochloric acid
Magnesium (Mg^{2+})	1.3-2.1 mEq/L	0.66-1.07 mmol/L	Excitable membrane stabilizer Essential element in cardiac, skeletal, and smooth muscle contraction Cofactor in blood-clotting cascade Cofactor in carbohydrate metabolism Cofactor in DNA and protein synthesis
Phosphorus (P*i*)	3.0-4.5 mg/dL	0.97-1.45 mmol/L	Activation of B-complex vitamins Formation of adenosine triphosphate and other high-energy substances Cofactor in carbohydrate, protein, and lipid metabolism

Data from Pagana, K., & Pagana, T. (2002). *Mosby's manual of diagnostic and laboratory tests* (2nd ed). St. Louis: Mosby.

normal ranges of electrolyte concentration are very narrow. Thus even small changes in these concentrations can cause major problems.

Table 14-5 lists major electrolytes, their normal serum concentrations, and main functions. Most electrolytes enter the body in ingested food.

Electrolyte homeostasis is controlled by balancing the dietary intake of electrolytes with the renal excretion or reabsorption of electrolytes. For example, the plasma level of potassium is maintained between 3.5 and 5.0 mmol/L. In theory, the potassium in common foods could greatly increase the ECF potassium level and lead to major problems. Usually, however, the kidney excretion of potassium keeps pace with potassium intake and prevents major changes in the blood potassium level.

SODIUM

Sodium (Na^+) is the major cation in the extracellular fluid (ECF) and is responsible for maintaining ECF osmolarity. The activity of the sodium-potassium pump keeps the sodium level of the intracellular fluid (ICF) low (about 14 mmol/L) while maintaining high sodium levels in blood and other extracellular fluids. Maintaining this difference in sodium levels is vital for the following functions:

- Skeletal muscle contraction
- Cardiac contractions

TABLE 14-6 Sodium Values of Common Foods*

Food Source	Amount (mg)
Table salt (1 tsp)	2000
Cheddar cheese (1 oz)	176
Cottage cheese (4 oz)	457
American cheese (1 oz)	439
Whole milk (8 oz)	120
Skim milk (8 oz)	126
Butter (1 tsp)	123
White bread (1 slice)	123
Whole-wheat bread (1 slice)	159
Soy sauce (1 tbsp)	1029
Ketchup (1 tbsp)	156
Mustard (1 tbsp)	188
Beef, lean (4 oz)	60
Pork, lean, fresh (4 oz)	60
Pork, cured (4 oz)	850
Chicken, light meat (4 oz)	70
Chicken, dark meat (4 oz)	70

Data from Pennington, J. (2004). *Bowe's and Church's food values of portions commonly used* (18th ed.). Philadelphia: J.B. Lippincott.
*U.S. Department of Agriculture recommended daily allowance for adults: 1100-3300 mg.

- Nerve impulse transmission
- Normal ECF osmolarity
- Normal ECF volume

The ECF sodium level determines whether water is retained, excreted, or moved from one fluid space to another.

To maintain electrical balance, the sodium (a cation) level within a body fluid must be matched by an equal number of anions (negatively charged substances). Each positive charge in the ECF must be balanced by a negative charge so the fluid does not carry either an overall positive or an overall negative charge. When this balance is present, a state of **electroneutrality** exists in that fluid. Changes in the plasma sodium level seriously change fluid volume and the distribution of other electrolytes.

The normal plasma sodium level ranges between 136 and 145 mEq/L or mmol/L (see Table 14-5). Sodium enters the body through the ingestion of many foods and fluids (Table 14-6). The average dietary intake of sodium is about 6 to 14 g/day. Sodium is also stored deep within the kidney tissues and can be released to the ECF as needed. Despite variation in sodium intake from one day to the next, the serum sodium level usually remains within the normal range. Serum sodium balance is regulated by the kidney under the influences of aldosterone, antidiuretic hormone (ADH), and natriuretic peptide (NP).

Low serum sodium levels inhibit the secretion of ADH and NP and trigger aldosterone secretion. Together these actions increase serum sodium levels by increasing kidney reabsorption of sodium and enhancing kidney loss of water.

High serum sodium levels inhibit aldosterone secretion and directly stimulate secretion of ADH and NP. Together these hormones increase kidney excretion of sodium and kidney reabsorption of water.

POTASSIUM

Potassium (K^+) is the major cation of the intracellular fluid (ICF). The normal plasma potassium level ranges from 3.5 to 5.0 mEq/L or mmol/L (see Table 14-5). The normal ICF potassium level is about 140 mEq/L (mmol/L). Because of its high concentration inside cells, potassium has some control over intracellular osmolarity and volume. Keeping this large difference in potassium concentration between the ICF and the extracellular fluid (ECF) is critical for excitable tissues to generate action potentials and transmit impulses. Functions of potassium include the following:

- Regulation of protein synthesis
- Regulation of glucose use and storage
- Maintenance of action potentials in excitable membranes

Because potassium levels in the blood and interstitial fluid are so low, any change seriously affects physiologic activities. For example, a decrease in blood potassium of only 1 mEq/L (from 4 mEq/L to 3 mEq/L) is a 25% difference in total ECF potassium concentration. In contrast, a 1-mEq/L decrease in blood sodium level (from 140 mEq/L to 139 mEq/L) is, overall, a much smaller change (less than 1%) in total ECF sodium concentration.

Potassium drifts out of cells down its concentration gradient into the ECF. Almost all foods contain potassium (Table 14-7). Potassium intake is about 2 to 20 g/day. Despite heavy potassium intake and the drifting of potassium from cellular storage sites into the ECF, the healthy adult keeps plasma potassium levels within the narrow range of normal values needed for physiologic function.

The main controller of ECF potassium level is the sodium-potassium pump within the membranes of all body

TABLE 14-7 Potassium Values of Common Foods*

Food Source	Amount (mg)
Corn flakes (1¼ c)	26
Cooked oatmeal (¾ c)	99
Egg (1 large)	66
Codfish, raw (4 oz)	400
Salmon, pink, raw (3½ oz)	306
Tuna fish (4 oz)	375
Apple, raw with skin (1 medium)	159
Banana (1 medium)	451
Cantaloupe (1 c pieces)	494
Grapefruit (½ medium)	175
Orange (1 medium)	250
Raisins (½ c)	700
Strawberries, raw (1 c)	247
Watermelon (1 c pieces)	186
White bread (1 slice)	27
Whole-wheat bread (1 slice)	44
Beef (4 oz)	480
Beef liver (3½ oz)	281
Pork, fresh (4 oz)	525
Pork, cured (4 oz)	325
Chicken (4 oz)	225
Veal cutlet (3½ oz)	448
Ham (4 oz)	328
Whole milk (8 oz)	370
Skim milk (8 oz)	406
Avocado (1 medium)	1097
Carrot (1 large)	341
Corn (4-inch ear)	196
Cauliflower (1 c pieces)	295
Celery (1 stalk)	170
Green beans (1 c)	189
Mushrooms (10 small)	410
Onion (1 medium)	157
Peas (¾ c)	316
Potato, white (1 medium)	407
Spinach, raw (3½ oz)	470
Tomato (1 medium)	366

Data from Pennington, J. (2004). *Bowe's and Church's food values of portions commonly used* (18th ed.). Philadelphia: J.B. Lippincott.
*U.S. Department of Agriculture recommended daily allowance for adults: 1875-5625 mg.

cells. This pump removes three sodium ions from the fluid inside the cell for every two potassium ions that it returns to the cell. In this way, the levels of both serum sodium and cellular potassium remain high.

Some potassium control also occurs through kidney function. The kidney is the excretory route for ridding the body of ECF potassium (80% of potassium removed from the body occurs via the kidney). Unlike sodium, no hormone has been identified that directly controls kidney reabsorption of potassium; thus the kidney does not conserve potassium directly.

CALCIUM

Calcium (Ca^{2+}) is a mineral with functions closely related to those of phosphorus and magnesium. Calcium is a **divalent cation** (an ion having two positive charges) that exists in the body in two forms: bound and ionized (unbound or free).

Bound calcium is usually attached to serum proteins, especially albumin. Ionized calcium is present in the blood and other extracellular fluid (ECF) as free calcium. Free calcium is the active form and must be kept within a narrow range in the ECF. The body functions best when blood calcium levels are maintained between 9.0 and 10.5 mg/dL, or between 2.25 and 2.75 mmol/L (see Table 14-5). Because the amount of calcium in the intracellular fluid (ICF) is low, calcium has a steep gradient between ECF and ICF. Calcium is important in the following actions:

- Bone strength and density
- Activation of enzymes or reactions
- Skeletal muscle contraction
- Cardiac muscle contraction
- Nerve impulse transmission
- Blood clotting

Calcium enters the body by dietary intake and absorption through the intestinal tract (Table 14-8). Absorption of dietary calcium requires the active form of vitamin D. Calcium is stored in the bones. When both plasma calcium levels and stored calcium levels are adequate, intestinal absorption of dietary calcium is reduced and urine excretion of excess calcium increases. When more calcium is needed, **parathyroid hormone (PTH)** is released from the parathyroid glands (Table 14-9). PTH causes serum calcium levels to increase in the following ways:

- Releasing free calcium from bone storage sites directly into the ECF **(resorption)**
- Stimulating vitamin D activation, thus increasing intestinal absorption of dietary calcium
- Inhibiting kidney excretion of calcium and stimulating kidney reabsorption of calcium

When excess calcium is present in plasma, PTH secretion is inhibited and the secretion of **thyrocalcitonin (TCT)**, a hormone secreted by the thyroid gland, is increased. TCT causes the plasma calcium level to decrease in the following ways:

- Inhibiting bone resorption of calcium
- Inhibiting activation of vitamin D, causing decreased gastrointestinal uptake of calcium
- Increasing kidney excretion of calcium in the urine

PHOSPHORUS

Phosphorus (P) is in the body in both inorganic and organic forms. Normal serum levels of phosphorus range from 3.0 to 4.5 mg/dL, or 0.97 to 1.45 mmol/L (see Table 14-5). Most phosphorus (80%) can be found in the bones. Phosphorus is the major anion in the intracellular fluid (ICF), and its concentration inside cells is much higher than in extracellular fluid (ECF). Phosphorus is needed for the following cellular activities:

- Activating B-complex vitamins
- Forming and activating adenosine triphosphate (ATP)

TABLE 14-8 Calcium Values of Common Foods*

Food Source	Amount (mg)
Cheddar cheese (1 oz)	204
Cottage cheese (4 oz)	68
American cheese (1 oz)	174
Whole milk (8 oz)	288
Skim milk (8 oz)	302
Yogurt, low-fat (1 c)	415
Broccoli, raw (½ c)	75
Carrot (1 large)	37
Collard greens, raw (3 oz)	200
Green beans (1 c)	62
Rhubarb (1 c)	266
Spinach, raw (3½ oz)	93
Tofu (3 oz)	100

Data from Pennington, J. (2004). *Bowe's and Church's food values of portions commonly used* (18th ed.). Philadelphia: J.B. Lippincott.

*U.S. Department of Agriculture recommended daily allowance for adults: 800-1200 mg.

TABLE 14-9 Hormonal Regulation of Calcium

Hormone	Action
Parathyroid Hormone (PTH) Secreted in response to low or low-normal serum calcium levels Secretion results in a rise in serum calcium concentration	Increases bone resorption of calcium (leaching of stored calcium) Increases the absorption of ingested calcium from the gastrointestinal tract into the extracellular fluid Increases the renal reabsorption of calcium at the proximal convoluted tubule
Thyrocalcitonin (TCT) Secreted by the thyroid gland in response to high or high-normal serum calcium levels Secretion results in a reduction of the serum calcium concentration	Increases bone uptake of calcium Inhibits the absorption of calcium from the gastrointestinal tract so that ingested calcium is excreted from the body in the feces Inhibits the renal reabsorption of calcium at the proximal convoluted tubule so that more calcium is excreted in the urine

- Assisting in cell division
- Cooperating in carbohydrate metabolism
- Cooperating in protein metabolism
- Cooperating in lipid (fat) metabolism

Other phosphorus functions include acid-base buffering and calcium homeostasis. The average North American diet is high in phosphorus (1 to 2 g/day). Table 14-10 lists food sources of phosphorus.

Phosphorus balance and calcium balance are intertwined. Normally, plasma levels of calcium and phosphorus exist in a balanced, reciprocal relationship, which means that the product of the plasma concentrations remains constant. Therefore a change in the amount of plasma phosphorus results in an equal and opposite change in the amount of plasma calcium (and vice versa).

The regulation of ECF phosphorus occurs through the activity of parathyroid hormone (PTH). Increased PTH levels cause a net loss of phosphorus. Reduced PTH levels enhance kidney reabsorption of phosphorus, resulting in increased plasma levels of phosphorus.

MAGNESIUM

Magnesium (Mg^{2+}) is a mineral that forms a cation when dissolved in water. Adults have an average total body level of 25 g of magnesium, most of which (60%) is stored in bones and cartilage. Little magnesium is present in the extracellular fluid (ECF). Plasma levels of free magnesium range from 1.3 to 2.1 mg/dL, or 0.65 to 1.05 mmol/L (see Table 14-5). Much more magnesium is present in the intracellular fluid (ICF), and it has more functions inside the cells than in the blood. Magnesium is critical for the following intracellular reactions or activities:

- Skeletal muscle contraction
- Carbohydrate metabolism
- Adenosine triphosphate (ATP) formation
- B-complex vitamin activation
- Deoxyribonucleic acid (DNA) synthesis
- Protein synthesis

Extracellular magnesium regulates blood coagulation and skeletal muscle contractility.

The daily magnesium requirement for adults is about 300 mg. Table 14-11 lists food sources of magnesium.

Magnesium regulation occurs through the kidney and the gastrointestinal tract although the exact mechanisms are not known. When blood magnesium levels are low, ingested magnesium is rapidly absorbed in the small intestine and kidney excretion of magnesium stops. When blood magnesium levels are high, little if any magnesium is absorbed from food and the kidney increases magnesium excretion.

CHLORIDE

Chloride (Cl^-) is the major anion of the extracellular fluid (ECF) and works with sodium to maintain ECF osmotic pressure. Chloride is important in the formation of hydrochloric acid in the stomach. The normal plasma concentration of chloride ranges from 98 to 106 mEq/L or mmol/L (see Table 14-5).

Only a small amount of chloride is present inside the cells because negative charges on the cell membrane repel chloride and prevent it from crossing the membrane. However, extracellular chloride can enter cells when exchanged for another anion that is leaving the cell. This situation, called a **chloride shift,** decreases plasma chloride without a net body loss of chloride. Bicarbonate (HCO_3^-) is the anion most commonly exchanged for chloride.

Chloride enters the body through dietary intake. Because chloride (along with sodium, potassium, and many other minerals) is a part of a salt, most diets contain enough chloride to meet the normal needs of the body.

Fluid and Electrolyte Changes Associated with Aging

Only 45% to 50% of the body weight of older adults is water, compared with 55% to 60% in younger adults. This decrease occurs because of a loss of muscle mass and a reduced ratio of

TABLE 14-10 Phosphorus Values of Common Foods*

Food Source	Amount (mg)
Rolled oats, cooked (¾ c)	133
Egg (1 large)	90
Codfish (3 oz)	175
Tuna fish, white, canned (6½ oz)	405
Raisins (½ c)	75
White bread (1 slice)	26
Whole-wheat bread (1 slice)	23
Cheddar cheese (1 oz)	145
American cheese (1 oz)	211
Whole milk (8 oz)	228
Skim milk (8 oz)	247
Yogurt, low-fat (8 oz)	326
Beef (4 oz)	215
Beef liver (4 oz)	375
Pork, fresh (4 oz)	325
Chicken (4 oz)	200
Almonds (1 oz)	141
Peanuts (1 oz)	110

Data from Pennington, J. (2004). *Bowe's and Church's food values of portions commonly used* (18th ed.). Philadelphia: J.B. Lippincott.

*U.S. Department of Agriculture recommended daily allowance for adults: 800 mg.

TABLE 14-11 Magnesium Values of Common Foods*

Food Source	Amount (mg)
Rolled oats, cooked (¾ c)	42
Tuna fish, white, canned (6½ oz)	59
Raisins (½ c)	25
Beef (4 oz)	24
Pork (4 oz)	30
Chicken (4 oz)	26
Whole milk (8 oz)	33
Skim milk (8 oz)	28
Yogurt, low-fat (8 oz)	40
Peanut butter (1 tbsp)	22
Avocado (1 medium)	70
Broccoli (1 stalk)	24
Cauliflower (1 c pieces)	24
Peas (¾ c)	35
Potato (1 medium)	34
Spinach, raw (3½ oz)	88

Data from Pennington, J. (2004). *Bowe's and Church's food values of portions commonly used* (18th ed.). Philadelphia: J.B. Lippincott.

*U.S. Department of Agriculture recommended daily allowance for adults: 300-350 mg.

CHART 14-1

NURSING FOCUS on the OLDER ADULT

Impact of Age-Related Changes on Fluid and Electrolyte Balance

System	Change	Result
Skin	Loss of elasticity	An unreliable indicator of fluid status
	Decreased turgor	Dry, easily damaged skin
	Decreased oil production	
Renal	Decreased glomerular filtration	Poor excretion of waste products
	Decreased concentrating capacity	Increased water loss
Muscular	Decreased muscle mass	Decreased total body water Greater risk of dehydration
Neurologic	Diminished thirst reflex	Decreased fluid intake, increasing the risk of dehydration
Endocrine	Adrenal atrophy	Poor regulation of sodium and potassium, predisposing the client to hyponatremia and hyperkalemia

CHART 14-2

NURSING FOCUS on the OLDER ADULT

Normal Plasma Electrolyte Values for People Older Than 60 Years of Age

Electrolyte	Reference Range	International Recommended Units
Calcium (Ca^{2+})	9.0-10.5 mg/dL	2.2-2.75 mmol/L
>90 years	8.2-9.6 mg/dL	2.05-2.40 mmol/L
Chloride (Cl^-)	98-106 mEq/L	98-106 mmol/L
>90 years	98-111 mEq/L	98-111 mmol/L
Magnesium (Mg^{2+})	1.2-2.1 mEq/L	0.65-1.5 mmol/L
Phosphorus (P_i)	3-4.5 mg/dL	0.97-1.45 mmol/L
Potassium (K^+)	3.5-5.0 mEq/L	3.5-5.0 mmol/L
Sodium (Na^+)	136-145 mEq/L	136-145 mmol/L
>90 years	132-146 mEq/L	132-146 mmol/L

Data for adults <90 years from Pagana, K., & Pagana, T. (2002). *Mosby's manual of diagnostic and laboratory tests* (2nd ed). St. Louis: Mosby.
Data for adults >90 years from Tietz, N.W. (Ed.). (1995). *Clinical guide to laboratory tests* (3rd ed.). Philadelphia: W.B. Saunders.

lean body weight to total body weight. This decrease in total body water places older adults at greater risk for dehydration.

Skin **turgor** (the normal resiliency of a pinched fold of skin) is not always an accurate assessment of extracellular deficient fluid (ECF) volume (dehydration) in the older adult because the natural aging process decreases turgor (Chart 14-1). Also, the older adult may have a reduced thirst sense and decreased kidney function, both of which increase the risk for dehydration and make assessment more difficult. When working with older clients, it is important to accurately record intake and output and weight, because these measurements reflect hydration status more accurately than does skin turgor.

The normal concentration of blood electrolytes also changes with the aging process. Chart 14-2 lists the normal electrolyte values for people older than 60 years of age.

CHART 14-3

Fluid and Electrolyte Assessment

USING GORDON'S FUNCTIONAL HEALTH PATTERNS

Nutritional-Metabolic Pattern

- What is your typical daily food intake? Describe a day's meals, snacks, and vitamins.
- How much salt do you typically add to your food? Do you use salt substitutes?
- How is your appetite?
- Do you have any difficulty chewing or swallowing?
- What is your typical daily fluid intake? What types of fluids (water, juices, soft drinks, coffee, tea)? How much?
- Have you had any recent change in your weight? Weight gain? Weight loss? How much?
- Have you noticed a change in tightness of your rings or shoes? Tighter? Looser?

Elimination Pattern

- What is your usual bowel elimination pattern? Frequency? Character? Discomfort? Laxatives?
- What is your usual urinary elimination pattern? Frequency? Amount? Color? Odor? Control?
- Have you noticed a change in the amount of urine?
- Do you have any problem with excessive perspiration?
- Do you have any other type of drainage?

Based on Gordon, M. (2002). Manual of nursing diagnosis (10th ed.). St. Louis: Mosby.

Electrolyte balance may be more difficult to maintain in older adults. Small changes in the levels of potassium and calcium may have serious results. Although the ranges of electrolytes in plasma and intracellular fluid (ICF) may remain normal, the balance is fragile and more easily disturbed in an older adult. Part of this fragility is related to decreased regulatory functions that occur with aging. Age-related kidney changes include decreased blood flow, decreased filtration, and decreased numbers of working nephrons. Kidney and capillary changes from hypertension are more likely to be present in the older adult.

ASSESSMENT OF FLUID AND ELECTROLYTE BALANCE

History

One way of organizing history data to assess the client's fluid and electrolyte status is to use Gordon's Functional Health Patterns (Gordon, 2002). The patterns that most affect fluid and electrolyte status are the Nutritional-Metabolic Pattern and the Elimination Pattern (Chart 14-3).

The client's nutritional history can reveal problems that affect fluid and electrolyte balance. Obtain this information directly because the client may not understand the connection between dietary intake and the onset of fluid and electrolyte imbalances.

The guidelines for obtaining a thorough fluid and electrolyte history do not differ from those for assessing any other system; however, the information collected is more specific. For example, exact intake and output volumes are important, as are serial daily weight measurements. You may need to guide the client in reporting accurately the amount of fluid ingested and changes in urine patterns. Also assess the types of fluids and foods ingested to determine amount and osmolarity. Many clients do not know that solid foods contain liquid. Solid foods such as ice cream, gelatin, and ices are liquids at body temperature, and these must be included when calculating fluid intake.

Output includes losses not only as urine but also as sweat, diarrhea, and insensible loss during fevers. Ask specific questions about prescribed and over-the-counter drugs and check the dosage, the length of time taken, and the client's adherence with the drug regimen. A client who is taking diuretics can have an imbalance of fluid, potassium, sodium, or hydrogen ions when other water loss occurs through vomiting or excessive sweating.

Older adults often use laxatives, which can disturb fluid and electrolyte balance. Misuse and overuse of these drugs can lead to serious imbalances.

Other important areas of the client history include body weight changes, thirst or excessive drinking, exposure to hot environments, and the presence of other disorders, such as kidney or endocrine diseases (e.g., Cushing's disease, Addison's disease, diabetes mellitus, and diabetes insipidus). Assess the client's level of consciousness and mental status, because changes in mental status occur with fluid imbalance. In such cases, you may need to check the accuracy of information with family members.

Physical Assessment

Hydration is the state of fluid balance. A normally hydrated adult is alert, has moist eyes and mucous membranes, has a urine output nearly the same as the amount of fluid ingested (with a urine specific gravity of about 1.015), and good skin turgor.

Assess skin turgor by pinching a fold of skin. This pinched fold should return immediately to its original shape after release. Decreased turgor, a sign of dehydration, is present when the fold remains in a pinched shape after being released and rebounds slowly **(tenting)** (Figure 14-10). Skin turgor is best assessed in body areas that have little fat tissue, such as over the sternum, on the forehead, or on the back of the hand. An older person has poor skin turgor on the hands and feet because of the loss of tissue elasticity related to aging; thus state of hydration is more difficult to assess in an older adult than in a younger adult. The best areas for assessing turgor in the older adult are over the sternum and on the forehead.

Skin hydration assessment also includes an examination for dryness. The mucous membranes and the conjunctiva are normally moist. An assessment of fluid balance always includes an examination of the eyes, nose, and oral mucous membranes. A dry, sticky, "cottony" mouth; the absence of tearing; weight loss; and decreased urine output all indicate deficient fluid volume.

Accurate measurement of fluid intake and output is needed to assess fluid and electrolyte status. Use volumetric devices to accurately measure actual fluid intake and output.

Include behavioral and neurologic assessment in fluid assessment because fluid imbalance can change neurologic function. In hypertonic states, neuron shrinkage may induce serious nervous system excitability and hyperactivity, and convulsions may occur. Another variable to assess is the degree of thirst, but this may be difficult to gauge in a confused older client.

Estimate insensible water loss (e.g., sweat) in every client. Consider possible fluid loss from other routes, including the following:

- Fluid losses from wounds
- Gastric or intestinal drainage
- Blood loss from hemorrhage
- Drainage of body secretions, such as bile and pancreatic juices through fistulas

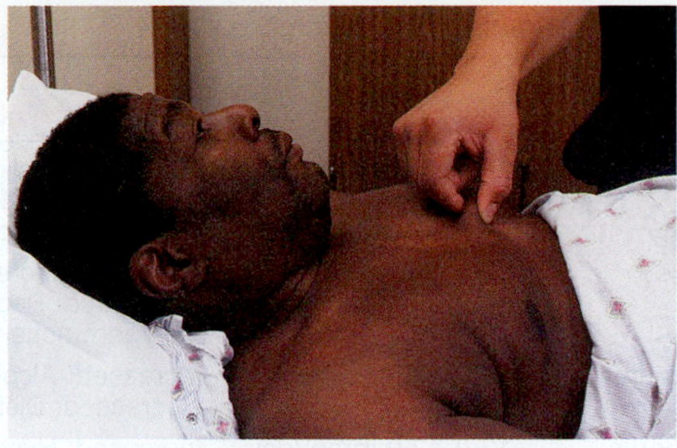

Figure 14-10 ■ Examining the skin turgor of an older client.

Electrolytes control the activity of excitable membranes, and electrolyte imbalances alter excitable membrane function. Electrolyte assessment includes a complete neuromuscular assessment of muscle tone and strength, movement, coordination, and tremors. Assessment of other systems, including the cardiac system (heart rate, the strength of contractions, and the presence of dysrhythmias) and gastrointestinal system (peristalsis), may indicate changes of excitable membrane function.

Your assessment must also focus on changes from previous findings (including mental status, physical examination data, and laboratory data). Fluid and electrolyte imbalances can occur quickly; therefore you must be familiar with the client's baseline assessment data to detect any changes.

Psychosocial Assessment

Psychosocial assessment related to fluid and electrolyte status includes both psychological and cultural factors that might influence balance. Depressed clients may refuse fluids or forget to drink adequate fluids. Clients with bulimia or anorexia nervosa (eating disorders) may abuse laxatives or may induce vomiting, causing fluid and electrolyte imbalances. Also assess social practices. For example, alcohol or drug abuse may cause fluid or electrolyte imbalance.

Diagnostic Assessment

Laboratory results help identify specific fluid and electrolyte imbalances or disorders that alter fluid and electrolyte status. Normal serum electrolyte values are listed in Table 14-5, and normal values for adults older than 60 years of age appear in Chart 14-2. Other laboratory values that are helpful in assessing fluid and electrolyte status include blood urea nitrogen level (BUN), blood glucose level, creatinine level, pH, bicarbonate level, osmolarity, hemoglobin, and hematocrit.

Urine test results may be helpful in assessing fluid status (Table 14-12). If a laboratory report is not available, you can perform some tests using a dipstick to help determine fluid and electrolyte status, including detecting substances normally not present in the urine, such as glucose, acetone, protein, and blood. Urine pH and specific gravity also can be determined in this way.

TABLE 14-12 Normal Urine Electrolyte Values

Electrolyte/ Characteristics	Normal Value*	Significance of Abnormal Value†
Calcium	2.5-7.5 mmol/day	Increased: Malignancy, thyrotoxicosis, hyperparathyroidism, osteoporosis, vitamin D intoxication Decreased: Hypoparathyroidism, rickets, kidney disease, hypothyroidism
Chloride	110-250 mEq/day 110-250 mmol/day	Increased: Increased salt intake, drug-induced diuresis, adrenocortical insufficiency Decreased: Reduced salt intake, water retention, vomiting, cerebral edema, adrenocortical hyperfunction
Magnesium	3.0-5.0 mmol/day	Increased: Alcohol intake, diuretics, corticosteroid therapy, cisplatin therapy Decreased: Dietary insufficiency
Phosphorus	12.9-42.0 mmol/day	Increased: Hyperparathyroidism, renal tubular damage, immobility, nonrenal acidosis Decreased: Hypoparathyroidism
Potassium	25-100 mmol/day (varies with diet)	Increased: Early starvation, hyperaldosteronism, metabolic acidosis Decreased: Addison's disease, renal disease
Sodium	40-220 mEq/day 40-220 mmol/day	Increased: Increased dietary intake, adrenal failure, diuretic therapy Decreased: Low sodium intake, sodium and water retention, adrenocortical hyperfunction, excessive diaphoresis, diarrhea
Osmolarity (osmolality) random	50-1200 mOsm/kg water	Increased: Dehydration, SIADH Decreased: Diabetes insipidus, primary polydipsia
Specific gravity	1.015-1.025	Increased: Dehydration, SIADH, diabetes mellitus, toxemia of pregnancy Decreased: Chronic renal insufficiency, diabetes insipidus, lithium toxicity, early renal disease

Data from Tietz, N. (Ed.). (1995). *Clinical guide to laboratory tests* (3rd ed.). Philadelphia: W.B. Saunders; & Pagana, K., Pagana, T. (2002). *Mosby's manual of diagnostic and laboratory tests* (2nd ed.). St. Louis: Mosby.
SIADH, Syndrome of inappropriate antidiuretic hormone.
*Based on a 24-hr total volume urine sample.
†Common conditions associated with abnormal values.

GET READY for the NCLEX Examination!

KEY POINTS

Safe Effective Care Environment

- Ensure access to adequate fluids for clients who are unable to talk or who have limited mobility.
- Evaluate the accuracy of intake and output measurements taken by unlicensed assistive personnel.

Health Promotion and Maintenance

- Encourage all clients to maintain an adequate fluid intake (minimum of 3 L per day) unless another condition requires fluid restriction.
- Teach all people to increase fluid intake when exercising, in hot or dry environments, or during conditions that increase metabolism (such as fever).
- Teach clients how to determine electrolyte content of processed foods by reading labels.

Psychosocial Integrity

- Check the hydration status of any client who has a sudden change in mental status.
- Identify changes in a client's mental status.

Physiological Integrity

- Use volumetric devices to measure intake and output for any client at risk for fluid volume deficits or excesses.
- Assess skin turgor on the forehead or the sternum of older clients.
- Use daily weights to determine fluid gains or losses.
- Ask clients about the use of drugs such as diuretics, laxatives, salt substitutes, and antihypertensives that may alter fluid and electrolyte status.
- Check the osmolarity, electrolyte composition, and flow rate of any intravenous solution.
- Correctly interpret laboratory electrolyte values.

ADDITIONAL STUDY RESOURCES

Go to your Student CD-ROM for Review Questions for the NCLEX Examination.

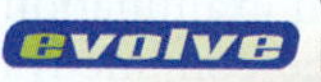

Go to http://evolve.elsevier.com/Iggy/ for Integrated Management of Care Questions for the NCLEX Examination.

SELECTED BIBLIOGRAPHY

Asterisk indicates a classic or definitive work on this subject.

Berne, R., et al. (2004). *Physiology* (5th ed.). St. Louis: Mosby.

Call-Schmidt, T. (2001). Interpreting lab results: A primer. *MEDSURG Nursing, 10*(4), 179-184.

Ebersole, P., Hess, P., & Luggen, A. (2004). *Toward healthy aging: Human needs and nursing response* (6th ed.). St. Louis: Mosby.

Elgart, H. (2004). Assessment of fluids and electrolytes. *AACN Clinical Issues, 15*(4), 607-621.

Gordon, M. (2002). *Manual of nursing diagnosis* (10th ed.). St. Louis: Mosby.

Jarvis, C. (2004). *Physical examination and health assessment* (4th ed). Philadelphia: W. B. Saunders.

McConnell, E. (2002). Measuring fluid intake and output. *Nursing2002, 32*(7), 17.

Mead, M. (2000). Serum calcium. *Practice Nurse, 20*(2), 112.

*O'Donnell, M. (1995). Assessing fluid and electrolyte balance needs in elders. *American Journal of Nursing, 95*(1), 41-46.

Pagana, K., & Pagana, T. (2002). *Mosby's manual of diagnostic and laboratory tests* (2nd ed). St. Louis: Mosby.

Pennington, J. (2004). *Bowe's and Church's food values of portions commonly used* (18th ed.). Philadelphia: J.B. Lippincott.

*Stark, J. (1998). A comprehensive analysis of the fluid and electrolytes system. *Critical Care Nursing Clinics of North America, 10*(4), 471-475.

Trissel, L. (2003). *Handbook on injectable drugs* (12th ed.). Bethesda, MD: American Society of Health-System Pharmacists.

CHAPTER 15

Interventions for Clients with Fluid Imbalances

M. LINDA WORKMAN

LEARNING OUTCOMES

After studying this chapter, you should be able to:

1. Identify clients at risk for fluid imbalances.
2. Use laboratory data and clinical manifestations to assess fluid balance and imbalance.
3. Apply appropriate nursing techniques to promote comfort and safety in the client with dehydration.
4. Prioritize nursing care for the client with dehydration.
5. Explain why different types of intravenous fluids are used to treat different types of dehydration.
6. Develop a community-based teaching plan to prevent dehydration in the older client at continuing risk for fluid loss.
7. Analyze changes in clinical manifestations to determine the effectiveness of therapy for the client with dehydration.
8. Prioritize nursing care for the client with overhydration.
9. Analyze changes in clinical manifestations to determine the effectiveness of therapy for the client with overhydration.

Go to your Student CD-ROM for Review Questions for the NCLEX Examination keyed to these Learning Outcomes.

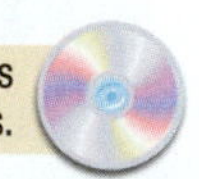

Proper body fluid balance is needed for normal functioning. All clients are at risk for some degree of fluid imbalance because many health problems can disrupt fluid intake or output. Fluid imbalances can occur in any setting. Although imbalances of fluid can involve electrolyte imbalances, this chapter focuses on client problems related to fluid imbalances.

DEHYDRATION

PATHOPHYSIOLOGY

In **dehydration,** fluid intake is less than what is needed to meet the body's fluid needs, resulting in a **fluid volume deficit.** Three basic types of dehydration are possible (Figure 15-1):

- **Isotonic dehydration,** in which water and dissolved electrolytes are lost in equal proportions
- **Hypertonic dehydration,** in which water loss is greater than electrolyte loss
- **Hypotonic dehydration,** in which electrolyte loss is greater than water loss

Dehydration is a condition rather than a disease and can be caused by many factors. Dehydration may be an *actual* decrease in total body water caused by either too little intake of fluid or too great a loss of fluid. Dehydration also can occur without an actual loss of total body water, such as when water shifts from the plasma into the interstitial space. This condition is called *relative* dehydration.

The actual incidence of dehydration is not known; however every ill client is at risk and the cost of treating dehydration is significant. (See the Resource Management box on p. 213.) Older clients are at high risk because they have less total body water than younger adults. Conditions affecting fluid intake in the older adult include decreased thirst sensation and difficulty with walking or other motor skills needed for ingesting fluids. Many older clients also take drugs such as diuretics and antihypertensives that increase fluid excretion.

Isotonic Dehydration

Isotonic dehydration is the most common type of fluid volume deficit. It involves loss of isotonic fluids from the extracellular fluid (ECF) space, including both the plasma and the interstitial spaces. Because isotonic fluid is lost, plasma osmolarity remains normal while volume is reduced. This type of dehydration does not cause a shift of fluids between spaces, so the intracellular fluid (ICF) volume remains normal. Isotonic dehydration decreases circulating blood volume **(hypovolemia)** and leads to inadequate tissue perfusion. Problems caused by isotonic dehydration result from loss of plasma volume. The body's defenses compensate during dehydration to maintain adequate blood flow to vital organs in spite of decreased vascular volume (Figure 15-2).

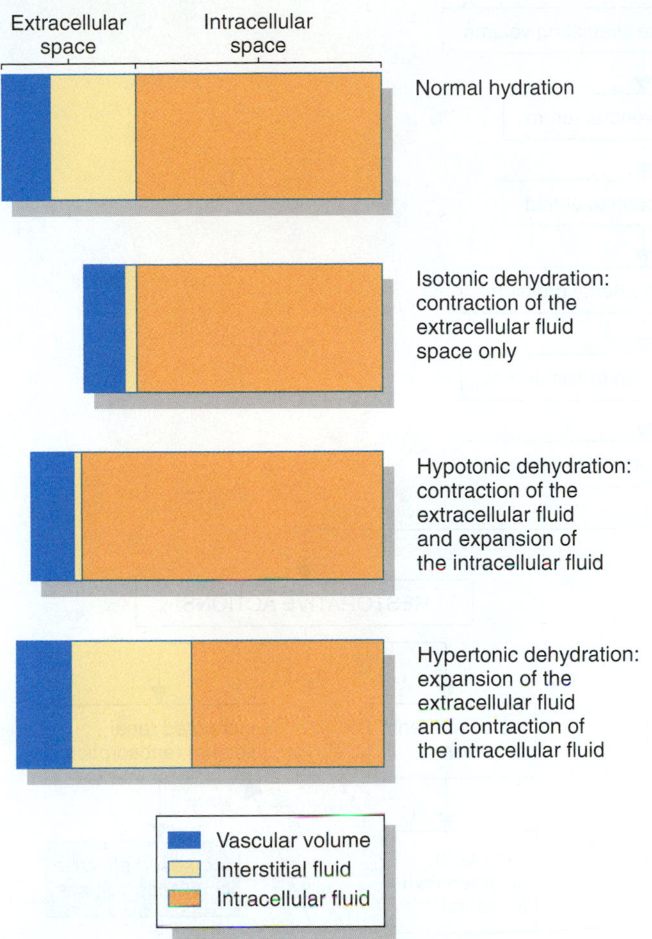

Figure 15-1 ■ Three types of dehydration. (© 1992 M. Linda Workman. All rights reserved.)

RESOURCE MANAGEMENT

PREVENTION OF DEHYDRATION

Cost of Care

- Dehydration is a common occurrence among older adults (in the community and in nursing home environments), clients who are somewhat cognitively impaired, and clients who have mobility problems.
- Dehydration is among the 10 most frequently reported diagnoses for Medicare hospitalizations.
- Treatment of dehydration and dehydration associated complications among clients older than 65 years of age accounts for nearly 2 million hospital days per year in the United States alone, with an estimate cost of $1.2 billion.
- Complications of dehydration can lead to increased morbidity and mortality rates.
- Most cases of dehydration are totally preventable.
- Most strategies to promote hydration require minimal costs.
- Awareness of dehydration as a health risk is under emphasized by health care personnel and family members.
- Time is a critical factor in ensuring adequate oral intake among older or impaired adults.

Implications for Nursing

Due to the high cost of treating problems associated with dehydration, nurses need to develop individualized plans in conjunction with clients to increase the availability and assistance needed to support adequate hydration, especially among older adults. The issue is not so much that nurses don't believe that hydration is important, it is in finding the time to ensure it happens. Educating unlicensed assistive personnel in the importance of taking the time to encourage older clients to drink fluids with and between meals is crucial in this time of nursing shortage. Using the time of medication administration to ensure that clients receiving oral medications drink 100 to 200 mL with oral medications is a simple way to promote hydration.

Data from Bennett, J. (2000). Dehydration: Hazards and benefits. *Geriatric Nursing, 21*(2), 84-88; Culp, K., Mentes, J., & Wakefield, B. (2003). Hydration and acute confusion in long-term care residents. *Western Journal of Nursing Research, 25*(3), 251-266; and Robinson, S., & Rosher, R. (2002). Can a beverage cart help improve hydration? *Geriatric Nursing, 23*(4), 208-211.

Isotonic dehydration has many causes (Table 15-1). These include poor intake of fluids and solutes, fluid shifts between fluid spaces, and heavy losses of isotonic body fluids.

Hypertonic Dehydration

Hypertonic dehydration is the second most common type of fluid volume deficit. It occurs when water loss from the extracellular fluid (ECF) is greater than electrolyte loss. This water loss increases the osmolarity of the remaining plasma, making it *hypertonic* or *hyperosmolar* compared with normal ECF. The hyperosmolar plasma has an increased osmotic pressure that causes water to move from the intracellular fluid (ICF) into the plasma and interstitial fluid spaces. The fluid shift leads to cellular dehydration and shrinkage. The fluid shift also causes the plasma volume to increase to normal or greater than normal levels. *Thus the compensatory mechanisms and symptoms of hypovolemic shock are not present.* The problems caused by hypertonic dehydration result from changes in the levels of specific electrolytes affecting excitable membrane activity. Compensation mechanisms for hypertonic dehydration occur in response to the increased ECF osmolarity (Figure 15-3).

Hypertonic dehydration is caused by the loss of water or any hypotonic body fluid (low osmolarity, or decreased level of solute particles compared with isotonic body fluid). Common causes of hypertonic dehydration include excessive sweating, hyperventilation, ketoacidosis, prolonged fevers, diarrhea, early-stage renal failure, and diabetes insipidus (see Table 15-1).

Hypotonic Dehydration

Hypotonic dehydration is the least common type of fluid volume deficit. The problems caused by hypotonic dehydration result from fluid shifts between spaces, causing a decrease in plasma volume.

Hypotonic dehydration involves excessive loss of sodium and potassium from the ECF. This loss leads to decreased blood and interstitial fluid osmolarity, making them hypotonic compared with normal ECF. The decreased ECF osmolarity lowers the osmotic pressure of plasma and interstitial fluids to below that of the fluid inside the cells, the ICF. As a result of this difference in osmotic pressure, water moves from the plasma and interstitial spaces into the cells, creating a plasma volume deficit and causing the cells to swell.

Cell swelling causes widespread problems and symptoms. Because brain cells are more sensitive to swelling than the cells of other tissues, neurologic problems often occur with

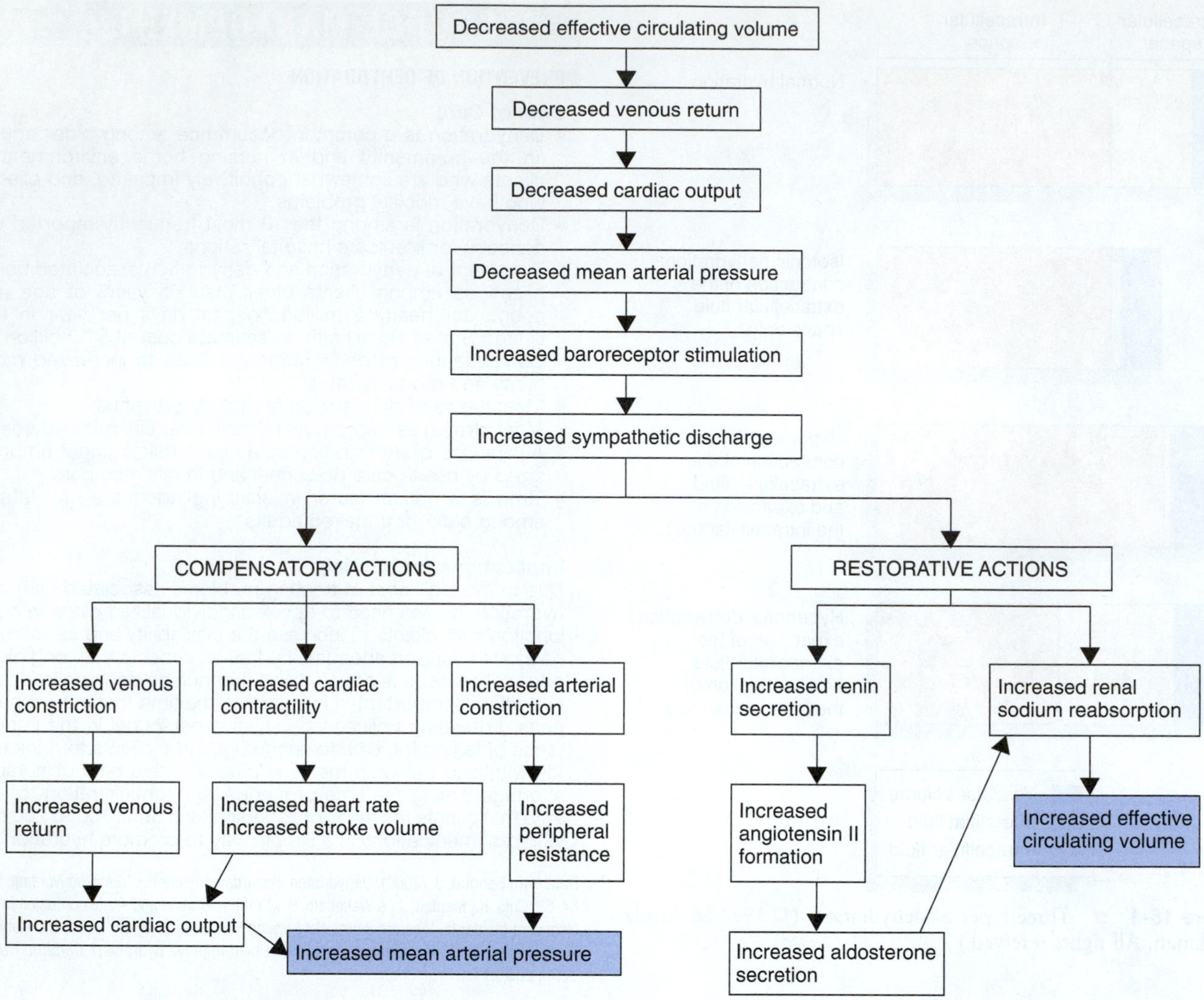

Decreased effective circulating volume
Decreased venous return
Decreased cardiac output
Decreased mean arterial pressure
Increased baroreceptor stimulation
Increased sympathetic discharge
COMPENSATORY ACTIONS
RESTORATIVE ACTIONS
Increased venous constriction
Increased cardiac contractility
Increased arterial constriction
Increased renin secretion
Increased renal sodium reabsorption
Increased venous return
Increased heart rate
Increased stroke volume
Increased peripheral resistance
Increased angiotensin II formation
Increased effective circulating volume
Increased cardiac output
Increased mean arterial pressure
Increased aldosterone secretion

Figure 15-2 ■ Compensatory mechanisms associated with isotonic dehydration.

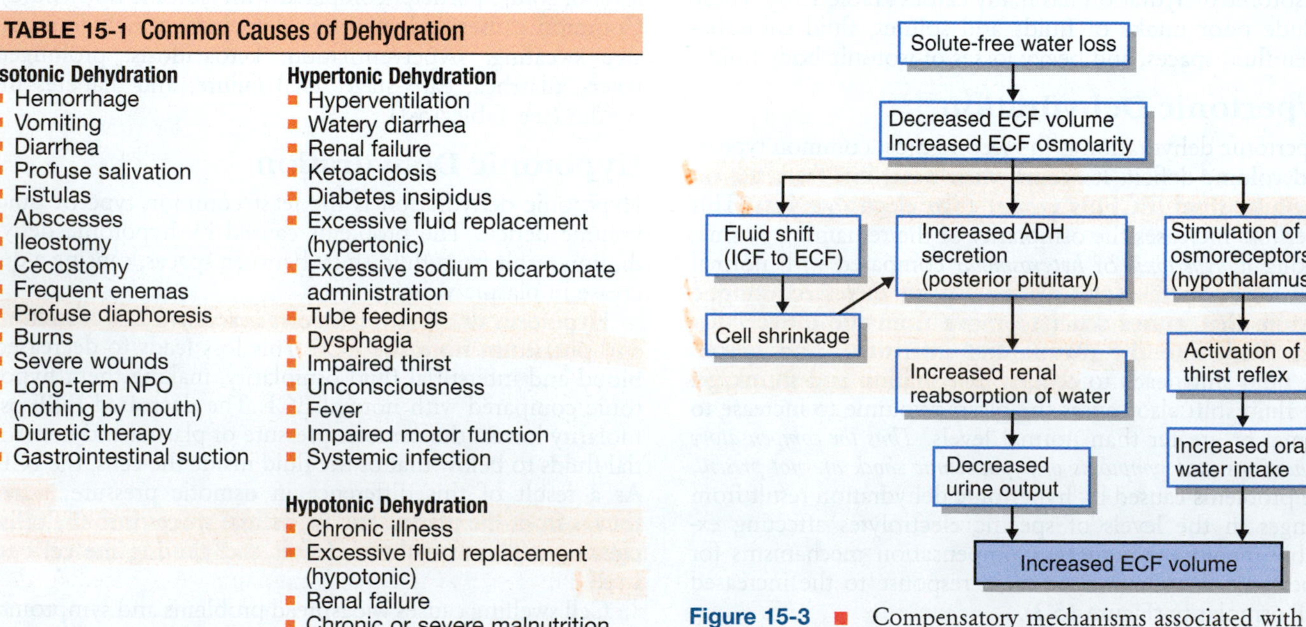

TABLE 15-1 Common Causes of Dehydration

Isotonic Dehydration	Hypertonic Dehydration
■ Hemorrhage ■ Vomiting ■ Diarrhea ■ Profuse salivation ■ Fistulas ■ Abscesses ■ Ileostomy ■ Cecostomy ■ Frequent enemas ■ Profuse diaphoresis ■ Burns ■ Severe wounds ■ Long-term NPO (nothing by mouth) ■ Diuretic therapy ■ Gastrointestinal suction	■ Hyperventilation ■ Watery diarrhea ■ Renal failure ■ Ketoacidosis ■ Diabetes insipidus ■ Excessive fluid replacement (hypertonic) ■ Excessive sodium bicarbonate administration ■ Tube feedings ■ Dysphagia ■ Impaired thirst ■ Unconsciousness ■ Fever ■ Impaired motor function ■ Systemic infection **Hypotonic Dehydration** ■ Chronic illness ■ Excessive fluid replacement (hypotonic) ■ Renal failure ■ Chronic or severe malnutrition

Solute-free water loss
Decreased ECF volume
Increased ECF osmolarity
Fluid shift
(ICF to ECF)
Increased ADH
secretion
(posterior pituitary)
Stimulation of
osmoreceptors
(hypothalamus)
Cell shrinkage
Increased renal
reabsorption of water
Activation of
thirst reflex
Decreased
urine output
Increased oral
water intake
Increased ECF volume

Figure 15-3 ■ Compensatory mechanisms associated with hypertonic dehydration. *ADH,* Antidiuretic hormone; *ECF,* extracellular fluid; *ICF,* intracellular fluid.

hypotonic dehydration. Hypotonic fluid also dilutes the normal electrolyte levels and causes sodium and potassium imbalances.

Hypotonic dehydration occurs more often with chronic illness. Chronic renal failure with sodium wasting leads to hypotonic dehydration. Malnutrition and ingesting excessive amounts of hypotonic fluids also cause hypotonic dehydration.

HEALTH PROMOTION/ILLNESS PREVENTION

Mild dehydration is common among healthy adults and is corrected or prevented easily by matching fluid intake with fluid output. Problems occur when people perform heavy exercise, especially in warm environments, without taking the time to replace excessive fluid losses. Teach all clients to drink more fluids whenever they engage in heavy physical activity.

Moderate to severe dehydration is more likely to occur in people who are unable to obtain fluids without help. Older adults living in long-term care facilities and those adults with cognitive or motor problems are dependent upon others for hydration. Dehydration in this population can be prevented with purposeful hydration programs (see the Evidence-Based Practice for Nursing box at right).

COLLABORATIVE MANAGEMENT

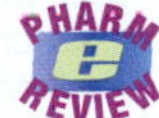

Assessment

HISTORY

Collect data on risk factors and factors causing dehydration (Table 15-2).

AGE. The client's age is important because dehydration in older adults develops quickly in response to small fluid losses. In addition, older people are more likely to have chronic illnesses or to be taking drugs, such as diuretics, that can lead to fluid and electrolyte imbalances.

HEIGHT AND WEIGHT. Measuring height and weight is important for calculating fluid needs. If possible, take these measurements directly. *Because 1 L of water weighs about 2.2 pounds (1 kg), changes in daily weights are the best indicators of fluid losses or gains.* A weight change of 1 pound corresponds to a fluid volume change of about 500 mL.

OTHER CHANGES. Ask the client about changes in ring or shoe tightness. A sudden decrease in tightness may indicate dehydration; an increase may reflect edema. Other related changes include palpitations or light-headedness on moving from a lying or a sitting position to a standing position caused by orthostatic hypotension. **Orthostatic hypotension** (also called **postural hypotension**) is a large drop in blood pressure during the first few seconds to minutes after changing from a sitting or lying position to a standing position.

Ask about any abnormal or excessive fluid losses, such as sweating, diarrhea, bleeding, vomiting, urination, salivation, and wound drainage. Other important information to collect includes history of chronic illnesses, recent acute illnesses, recent surgery, and drug regimens.

Ask specific questions about urine output, including the frequency and amount of voidings. Also ask about the client's usual fluid intake and the intake during the previous 24 hours. It is just as important to assess the *types* of fluids ingested as it is to assess the *amount* of fluids ingested, because fluids vary widely in osmolarity. Ask whether the client has recently engaged in strenuous physical activity and, if so, whether the activity took place in hot or dry environmental conditions.

EVIDENCE-BASED PRACTICE for Nursing

If you come, they will drink it

Robinson, S., & Rosher, R. (2002). Can a beverage cart help improve hydration? *Geriatric Nursing, 23*(4), 208-211.

This study compared the indicators of dehydration in older adults before, during, and after implementation of a dehydration prevention strategy. The dehydration prevention strategy was the use of a beverage cart and a designated "hydration assistant" to increase the fluid intake among 51 nursing home residents. The purpose of the study was to determine the effectiveness of a hydration program to increase fluid intake to a minimum of 1500 mL/day in preventing conditions associated with dehydration (delirium, urinary tract infections, respiratory infections, falls, skin breakdown, and constipation). The study used a quasiexperimental, prospective design. A hydration assistant was educated in the problems associated with dehydration and the techniques for oral fluid administration. A specific hydration needs assessment was performed for each resident to determine special fluid needs (e.g., sugar-free fluids, thickened fluids). A beverage cart was created using colorful pitchers and glasses. The intervention involved offering each resident who participated in the study an 8-oz drink at mid-morning and mid-afternoon. Each resident was offered at least four choices of beverages at each encounter.

Participants served as their own controls. Data regarding indicators of hydration were collected weekly for 9 weeks. These data included bioimpedence analysis of body water, and documentation of the number of bowel movements, laxatives, enemas, falls, episodes of mental status changes, urinary tract infections, respiratory tract infections, and skin breakdown. Additionally, the amount of fluid ingested with the intervention was recorded. Two weeks of data collection occurred before implementing the intervention. The intervention was implemented for the next 5 weeks. Data collection continued for 2 weeks after the intervention was stopped.

Fifty-three percent of the participants consistently achieved the goal of consuming an extra 8 oz of fluid twice each day. During the intervention, the participants had greater total body water volumes and fewer indicators of dehydration than they did before or after the intervention.

Level of Evidence: 3—Well-designed trial without randomization.

Critique. This study demonstrated that an extra 500 mL of fluid intake per day among nursing home residents could provide enough hydration to meet minimal fluid needs and prevent some problems of dehydration. Measuring the utility of a "hydration assistant" was not a stated purpose of this study but may be one of the most important study outcomes. Although it is useful to have participants serve as their own controls, a true control group would have strengthened the study. Additionally, examining daily weights of all participants during the data collection period could have validated the use of this measure as an outcome indicator for adequate hydration.

Implications for Nursing. This study demonstrated the usefulness of purposeful hydration in a nursing home population. Although the study pointed out that having a "hydration assistant" may not be feasible, the costs associated with the prevention of problems associated with dehydration could offset the cost of a hydration assistant. One of the benefits of having a hydration assistant is the amount of time this person could spend with each participant to encourage intake.

TABLE 15-2 Risk Factors for Dehydration

Illnesses
- Vomiting
- Diarrhea
- Burns
- Large, draining wounds
- Liver dysfunction
- Diabetes mellitus
- Diabetes insipidus
- Renal disease
- Hemorrhage
- Major venous obstruction
- Prolonged febrile state

Other Situations
- Extremes of age: older adults, infants
- Unconsciousness
- Motor limitations

Therapies
- Surgery
- Diuretics
- Nothing by mouth
- Excessive hypertonic enemas
- Nasogastric suction

PHYSICAL ASSESSMENT/CLINICAL MANIFESTATIONS

The clinical manifestations of dehydration depend on which body fluid spaces lose fluid, although all body systems are affected to some degree (Chart 15-1). The most obvious and life-threatening problems are seen when dehydration decreases the plasma volume.

CARDIOVASCULAR MANIFESTATIONS. Cardiovascular changes are good indicators of plasma volume changes. Heart rate increases with plasma volume deficits in an attempt to maintain blood pressure with less blood. Peripheral pulses are weak, difficult to find, and easily blocked with light pressure. If interstitial edema occurs with dehydration, the peripheral pulses may not be palpable. The blood pressure also decreases, as does the pulse pressure, with a greater decrease in the systolic blood pressure. Hypotension is more severe with the client in the standing position than with the client in the sitting or lying position (orthostatic or postural hypotension). Because the blood pressure with the client standing may be much lower than in other positions, first measure blood pressure with the client lying down, then sitting, and finally standing. These measures are also called "ortho checks" or "ortho changes."

Another indicator of hydration status is the degree of neck vein and hand vein filling. Normally, hand veins fill and become engorged when the hands are lower than the level of the heart. As the hands are raised above the level of the heart, the veins flatten or collapse (Figure 15-4). Neck veins are normally distended when a client is in the supine position. These veins flatten when the client moves to a sitting position. When dehydration causes a plasma volume deficit, neck and hand veins are flat, even when the neck and hands are not raised above the level of the heart. These cardiovascular changes are not seen in hypertonic dehydration.

RESPIRATORY MANIFESTATIONS. The respiratory rate increases with the degree of fluid loss from plasma volume. The decreased blood volume is perceived by the body as decreased oxygen levels **(hypoxia),** and increased respiratory rate is an attempt to maintain oxygen delivery.

CHART 15-1

KEY FEATURES of Dehydration

Manifestations of Dehydration in General*

Cardiovascular
- Increased pulse rate
- Thready pulse quality
- Decreased blood pressure
- Postural (orthostatic) hypotension
- Flat neck and hand veins in dependent positions
- Diminished peripheral pulses
- Weight loss

Respiratory
- Increased respiratory rate
- Increased depth of respirations

Neuromuscular
- Decreased central nervous system activity (lethargy to coma)
- Fever

Renal
- Decreased urine output
- Increased urine specific gravity

Integumentary
- Skin dry and scaly
- Turgor poor, tenting present
- Mouth dry and fissured, pastelike coating present

Gastrointestinal
- Decreased motility
- Diminished bowel sounds
- Constipation
- Thirst

Manifestations of Hypotonic Dehydration
- Skeletal muscle weakness

Manifestations of Hypertonic Dehydration
- Hyperactive deep tendon reflexes
- Increased sensation of thirst
- Pitting edema

*These manifestations are most severe with hypotonic dehydration.

SKIN MANIFESTATIONS. Changes in skin may indicate a change in hydration. Assess for changes in the skin and mucous membranes that may indicate dehydration, including skin color, moisture, skin turgor, and edema. In older clients this information is less reliable because of poor skin turgor resulting from the loss of elastic tissue and the loss of tissue fluids with aging. Assess skin turgor by checking the following:

- How easily the skin over the back of the hand and arm can be gently pinched between the thumb and the forefinger to form a "tent"
- How soon the pinched skin resumes its normal position after release
- Whether depressions (pits) remain in the skin after a finger is pressed firmly but gently (over the shin, over the sternum, and over the sacrum)
- How deep the depression is (in millimeters)
- How long the depression remains

In generalized dehydration, skin turgor is poor, with the tenting remaining for minutes after pinching the skin, and no skin depressions occur with gentle pressure. The skin is dry and scaly.

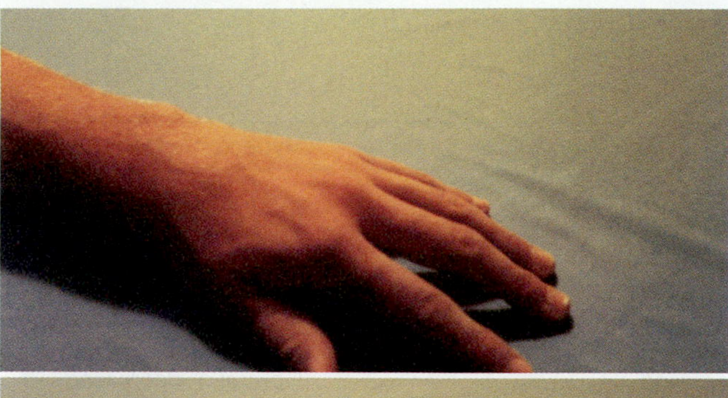

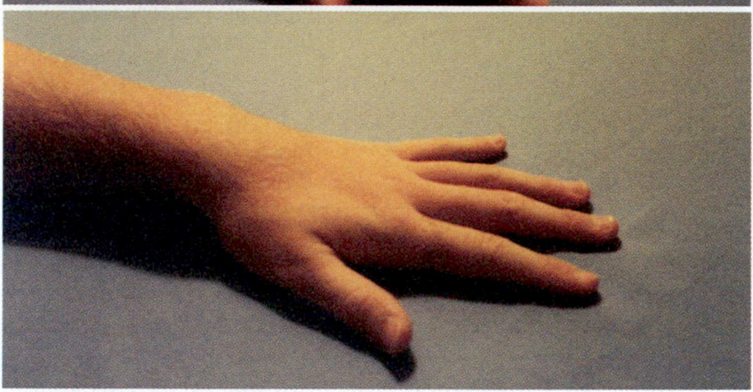

Figure 15-4 ■ Hand veins full and bulging in the dependent position *(top)*. Hand veins collapsed *(bottom)*.

CONSIDERATIONS FOR OLDER ADULTS

Assess skin turgor in an older adult by pinching the skin over the sternum or the forehead, rather than the back of the hand, because these areas more reliably indicate hydration (see Figure 14-10). As a person ages, the skin loses elasticity and tents on hands and arms even when the person is well hydrated.

In dehydration, oral mucous membranes are not moist. They may be covered with a thick, sticky, pastelike coating and may have cracks and fissures. The surface of the tongue may have deep furrows.

NEUROLOGIC MANIFESTATIONS. Dehydration may cause changes in mental status and body temperature status because blood flow in the brain is reduced. Mental status changes, especially confusion, with dehydration are more common among older adults and may be the first indication of a fluid balance problem. Chart 15-2 outlines how to assess mental status quickly. The client with dehydration often has a low-grade fever. One cause of the fever is the blood vessel constriction that occurs as a compensation for hypovolemia. The blood vessel constriction makes heat dissipation more difficult.

Fever can also cause dehydration. A client with a temperature greater than 102° F (39° C) for longer than 6 hours is especially at risk. Older adults, who normally have a body temperature range of 96° to 98° F (35.4° to 36.6° C), are at greater risk for dehydration during episodes of fever.

RENAL MANIFESTATIONS. The volume and the composition of urine output indicate hydration status. Monitor urine output, comparing total output with total fluid intake and daily weights. Accurate intake and output measurement is a major nursing responsibility. Urine output below 500 mL/day for any client without renal disease is cause for concern. Weigh the client each day at the same time and on the same scale. When possible, have the client wear the same amount and type of clothing for each weigh-in. Metabolic weight loss (even in starvation) usually accounts for only about ½ pound of weight loss per day. Any weight loss in excess of this amount is fluid loss.

CHART 15-2

BEST PRACTICE for
Brief Check of Mental Status

- Is the client awake?
- If the client is not awake, what type of stimulation is needed to wake the client?
  - Calling the client's name in a normal voice volume
  - Calling the client's name in a louder voice volume
  - Touching the client's arm or face while calling the client's name
  - Gently tapping or shaking an arm
  - Vigorously shaking a hand or arm
  - Applying a painful stimulus
- If the client is awake, ask questions that require more than a "yes" or "no" response to establish orientation to time and place.
- Avoid the use of nonsense questions (e.g., "Do helicopters eat their young?").
- Ask questions that are reasonable and likely to be known by the client, such as "When is your birthday?" Avoid questions such as "Who was vice president under Truman?"
- Is it necessary to repeat questions to obtain a response?
- Does the response answer the question asked?
- Does the client have difficulty with word choices in forming responses?
- Is the client irritated or upset by the questions?
- Can the client concentrate on a question long enough to provide an appropriate response, or is the attention span short?
- Can the client count by threes?
- Can the client count backward from 100 by threes?
- Does the client know the names of immediate family members?
- Does the client know who the questioner is (not necessarily the questioner's name but that person's role in the client's care, such as nurse, doctor, chaplain, therapist)?
- Does the client know his or her immediate location (e.g., home, hospital, clinic)?
- Does the client know the year?

PSYCHOSOCIAL ASSESSMENT

Observe the client for behavioral changes that occur with dehydration. At first, a dehydrated client may have a flat affect and may seem unconcerned about his or her health and possible treatment regimens. As dehydration worsens, the client may become anxious, restless, lethargic, and confused (especially an older adult client). These changes are more obvious in hypertonic and hypotonic dehydration because of intracellular fluid (ICF) shifts in brain cells, resulting in shrinkage or swelling of the cells. If dehydration continues, blood flow to the brain becomes so impaired that delirium and coma can occur.

LABORATORY ASSESSMENT

No single laboratory test result confirms or rules out dehydration. Instead, dehydration is determined by laboratory findings along with clinical manifestations. Laboratory findings depend on the type of dehydration present (Chart 15-3). Isotonic and hypotonic dehydration with plasma volume deficits show **hemoconcentration** (elevated levels of hemoglobin,

CHART 15-3

LABORATORY PROFILE
Dehydration

Values*	Isotonic Dehydration	Hypotonic Dehydration	Hypertonic Dehydration
Blood Values			
BUN	Normal or increased	Increased	Increased
Creatinine	Normal or increased	Increased	Increased
Sodium	Normal	<120 mEq/L (mmol)	>150 mEq/L (mmol)
Osmolarity	Normal	Decreased	Increased
Hematocrit	Increased	Increased	Normal or decreased
Hemoglobin	Increased	Increased	Normal or decreased
WBCs	Increased	Increased	Normal or decreased
Protein	Increased	Increased	Increased
Urine Values			
Specific gravity	>1.010	<1.010	>1.030
Osmolarity	Increased	Increased	Increased
Volume	Decreased	Decreased	Decreased

BUN, Blood urea nitrogen; *WBC*, white blood cell.
*All values reflect dehydration states alone and not the underlying pathologic changes or disease states contributing to the dehydration.

hematocrit, serum osmolarity, glucose, protein, blood urea nitrogen, and various electrolytes) because only the water is lost and other substances remain. Hemoconcentration is not present when dehydration is caused by hemorrhage, because loss of all blood and plasma products occurs together.

Specific urine laboratory values can help confirm dehydration if the client does not have renal dysfunction. Usually the urine of the client with dehydration is concentrated, with a specific gravity greater than 1.030. Volume is decreased, and osmolarity is greatly increased. The color is dark amber and has a strong odor.

Critical Thinking Challenge

The client is a 45-year-old, obese woman with type 1 diabetes who is brought to the emergency department in a coma. Her daughter tells you that the client has had pain and burning on urination for the past 3 days and that she has stopped drinking fluids so that she would not have to go to the bathroom as often. The daughter also tells you that the client has not taken her insulin for at least 2 days. The client's laboratory results are as follows: Blood glucose level is 540 mg/dL, white blood cell count (WBC) is 22,000/mm^3, hematocrit is 52%, serum potassium is 7 mmol/L, serum sodium is 140 mmol/L, blood osmolarity is 380 mOsm/L, and urine is positive for ketones.

1. What type of dehydration does she have?
2. What is the relationship between this type of dehydration and diabetes? (See Chapter 68.)
3. Would you expect her to have poor skin turgor or pitting edema? Why or why not?
4. Would you expect her to have hypotension? Why or why not?

evolve For suggested answer guidelines, go to http://evolve.elsevier.com/Iggy/.

Analysis

COMMON NURSING DIAGNOSES AND COLLABORATIVE PROBLEMS

The following are priority nursing diagnoses for clients with dehydration:

1. Deficient Fluid Volume related to excessive fluid loss or inadequate fluid intake
2. Decreased Cardiac Output related to decreased plasma volume
3. Impaired Oral Mucous Membrane related to inadequate oral secretions

The primary collaborative problem is Potential for Dysrhythmias.

ADDITIONAL NURSING DIAGNOSES AND COLLABORATIVE PROBLEMS

In addition to the common nursing diagnoses and collaborative problems, clients with dehydration may have one or more of the following:

- Constipation related to decreased body fluids
- Risk for Falls related to orthostatic (postural) hypotension
- Deficient Knowledge (medication regimen and preventive measures) related to lack of exposure or lack of interest in learning
- Risk for Impaired Skin Integrity related to deficiencies of interstitial fluid and inadequate tissue perfusion
- Ineffective Airway Clearance related to thick, sticky secretions
- Potential for Hypovolemic Shock
- Potential for Electrolyte Imbalances

Planning and Implementation

DEFICIENT FLUID VOLUME

NOC **PLANNING: EXPECTED OUTCOMES.** The client with dehydration is expected to have body fluid levels restored to normal as indicated by:

- Maintaining blood pressure and pulse (rate and quality) within normal limits
- Having 24-hour fluid intake balance with 24-hour fluid output
- Having urine specific gravity <1.030
- Having good skin turgor (no tenting when skin is pinched up)

INTERVENTIONS. Management of dehydration aims to prevent further fluid losses and increase fluid compartment volumes to normal ranges.

NIC **Fluid Management.** Diet therapy, oral rehydration therapy, and drug therapy are used to correct fluid volume deficit (Chart 15-4).

CHART 15-4

NIC INTERVENTION ACTIVITIES for The Client with Deficient Fluid Volume

Fluid Monitoring: *Collection and analysis of client data to regulate fluid balance*

- Monitor serum and urine electrolyte values, as appropriate.
- Monitor blood pressure, heart rate, and respiratory status.
- Monitor orthostatic blood pressure and change in cardiac rhythm, as appropriate.
- Monitor weight.
- Monitor intake and output.
- Note presence or absence of vertigo on rising.
- Monitor color, quantity, and specific gravity of urine.

Fluid Management: *Promotion of fluid balance and prevention of complications resulting from abnormal or undesired fluid levels*

- Administer IV therapy, as prescribed.
- Give fluids, as appropriate.
- Promote oral intake (e.g., provide a drinking straw, offer fluids between meals, change ice water routinely), as appropriate.
- Distribute the fluid intake over 24 hours, as appropriate.
- Encourage significant other to assist client with feedings, as appropriate.
- Offer snacks (e.g., frequent drinks and fresh fruits/fruit juice), as appropriate.

Oral Health Restoration: *Promotion of healing for a client who has an oral mucosa or dental lesion*

- Encourage frequent rinsing of mouth with any of the following: sodium bicarbonate solution, warm saline, or hydrogen peroxide solution.
- Monitor lips, tongue, mucous membranes, tonsillar fossae, and gums for moisture, color, texture, presence of debris, and infection, using good lighting and a tongue blade.
- Instruct client to avoid commercial mouthwashes.
- Monitor client every shift for dryness of the oral mucosa.
- Increase mouth care to every 2 hours and twice at night, if stomatitis is not controlled.
- Avoid use of lemon-glycerin swabs.
- Increase liquids on the meal tray.

Diet Therapy. Mild to moderate dehydration is corrected with oral fluid replacement if the client is alert enough to swallow and can tolerate oral fluids. Encourage and measure fluid intake. The specific type of fluid needed for replacement varies with the type of dehydration.

Gain the client's cooperation in drinking oral replacement fluids by using fluids he or she enjoys and by carefully timing the intake schedule. Dividing the total amount of fluids needed by nursing shifts helps to meet fluid needs more evenly over 24 hours with less danger of overhydration. Offer the conscious client small volumes of fluids every hour to increase intake.

Oral Fluid Rehydration Therapy. Oral rehydration therapy (ORT) is the most cost-effective way to replace fluids for the client with dehydration. Specifically formulated solutions containing glucose and electrolytes are absorbed even when the client is vomiting or has diarrhea. Fluid losses from diarrhea are usually 2 to 3 L/day and should be replaced liter for liter, especially in older clients. A typical prescription might be "Resol 1 L every 8 hours." Table 15-3 lists commercially available ORT solutions.

Drug Therapy. Drug therapy for dehydration is directed at restoring fluid balance and controlling the causes of dehydration. Whenever possible, fluids are replaced by the oral route. When dehydration is severe or life threatening, or the client is unconscious, intravenous (IV) fluid replacement is needed. Calculation of how much fluid to replace is based on the client's weight loss and clinical manifestations. The rate of fluid replacement depends on the degree of dehydration and the presence of other cardiac, pulmonary, or renal problems.

The type of fluid prescribed by the health care provider varies with the type of dehydration and the client's cardiovascular status. Usually the client receives IV infusions of water with whatever solutes (especially electrolytes) are needed on the basis of laboratory values. Table 15-4 lists the osmolarity, caloric content, and tonicity of common IV fluids. Generally, isotonic dehydration is treated with isotonic fluid solutions, hypertonic dehydration is treated with hypotonic fluid solutions, and hypotonic dehydration is treated with hypertonic fluid solutions. The two most important areas to monitor during rehydration are pulse rate and quality and urine output.

Drug therapy corrects the causes of the dehydration. Antidiarrheal drugs are prescribed when diarrhea causes dehydration. Antimicrobial therapy may be used in clients with bacterial diarrhea. Antiemetics to control vomiting may be needed when vomiting induces dehydration. Antipyretics to reduce temperature are helpful when fever makes dehydration worse.

DECREASED CARDIAC OUTPUT

NOC **PLANNING: EXPECTED OUTCOMES.** The client with dehydration is expected to have cardiac output restored to normal levels and to maintain adequate oxygenation to vital organs as indicated by:

- Having blood pressure and pulse (rate and quality) within the client's normal range
- Maintaining a urine output of at least 30 mL/hr

INTERVENTIONS. Interventions of drug and oxygen therapy aim to increase circulating fluid volume, support compensatory mechanisms, and prevent complications.

Drug Therapy. Drug therapy to increase body fluid volume and prevent excessive fluid loss is the same as that for the client with fluid volume deficit. Drugs to increase venous return or improve cardiac contractility are used only when a cardiac problem also is present.

TABLE 15-3 Commercial Solutions for Oral Rehydration Therapy

Brand Name	Na^+ (mEq/L)	K^+ (mEq/L)	Cl^- (mEq/L)	Citrate (mEq/L)	Sugar or Starch	Calories (kcal/L)
Ricelyte (Mead-Johnson)	50	25	45	34	Rice syrup (30 g)	126
Resol (Wyeth-Ayerst)	50	20	50	34	Dextrose (20 g)	84
Rehydralyte (Ross Labs)	75	20	65	30	Dextrose (25 g)	100
Pedialyte (Ross Labs)	45	20	35	30	Dextrose (25 g)	100
Gastrolyte (Rorer)	60	20	60	10	Dextrose (17.8 g)	75
Rapolyte (Richmond)	90	20	80	30	Dextrose (20 g)	84
Lytren (Mead-Johnson)	50	25	45	30	Dextrose (20 g)	84
Oralyte (Rugby)	45	20	25	48	Dextrose (25 g)	100
Kao Lectrolyte (Pharmacia & UpJohn)	50	20	—	30	Dextrose (20 g)	84

Data from United States Pharmacopeia Dispensing Information (USP DI): Vol I. (2000). *Drug information for the health care professional* (20th ed.). Englewood, CO: Micromedex.

TABLE 15-4 Characteristics of Common Intravenous Therapy Solutions

Solution	Osmolarity (mOsm/L)	pH	Calories* (kcal)	Tonicity
0.9% saline	308	5	0	Isotonic
0.45% saline	154	5	0	Hypotonic
5% dextrose in water (D_5W)	272	3.5-6.5	170	Isotonic†
10% dextrose in water ($D_{10}W$)	500	3.5-6.5	340	Hypertonic†
5% dextrose in 0.9% saline	560	3.5-6.5	170	Hypertonic†
5% dextrose in 0.45% saline	406	4	170	Hypertonic†
5% dextrose in 0.225% saline	321	4	170	Isotonic†
Ringer's lactate	273	6.5	9	Isotonic
5% dextrose in Ringer's lactate	525	4-6.5	179	Hypertonic†

Data from Trissel, L. (2003). *Handbook on injectable drugs* (12th ed.). Bethesda, MD: American Society of Hospital-System Pharmacists.

*Calories are calculated on the basis of a volume of 1000 mL.

†*Solution tonicity at the time of administration.* Within a short time after administration, the dextrose is metabolized, and the tonicity of the infused solution decreases in proportion to the osmolarity or tonicity of the nondextrose components (electrolytes) within the water.

Oxygen Therapy. Oxygen is delivered by mask or nasal cannula to the client with dehydration. Give the client water-nebulized oxygen at the rate or amount specified by the health care provider's prescription.

NIC **Fluid Monitoring.** Monitoring vital signs and level of consciousness is important when caring for clients with dehydration (see Chart 15-4). Monitor the pulse, blood pressure, pulse pressure, central venous pressure, respiratory rate, and skin and mucous membrane color every 15 minutes. Monitor urine output at least every hour until the fluid imbalance is resolved.

Critical Thinking Challenge

The client with diabetic ketoacidosis and dehydration is prescribed to receive intravenous normal saline (0.9% sodium chloride) at 1000 mL/hr for the first 2 hours. Ten (10) units of regular insulin are given immediately IV push and a continuous insulin infusion of 10 units/hr is prescribed until the ketosis has stopped.

1. What is the osmolarity of the normal saline solution? Is this considered hypotonic, isotonic, or hypertonic?
2. What would be the rationale for giving this client saline when her serum sodium level is in the normal range?
3. Why is the client not prescribed oral replacement fluids?
4. Should the care of this client be assigned to an RN, LPN/LVN, or assistive nursing personnel? (Explain your rationale for the caregiver assignment.)
5. What criteria would you use to determine whether the fluid replacement is adequate?
6. How often should this client be assessed? Why?

evolve For suggested answer guidelines, go to http://evolve.elsevier.com/Iggy/.

IMPAIRED ORAL MUCOUS MEMBRANE

NOC **PLANNING: EXPECTED OUTCOMES.** With appropriate intervention, the client with dehydration is expected to have moist mucous membranes as indicated by:

- Absence of cracks or fissures on lips and tongue
- Absence of coating on tongue

INTERVENTIONS. Interventions for oral health include drug therapy, fluid replacement, and good oral hygiene, as well as the early diagnosis and prevention of complications (see Chart 15-4).

Drug Therapy. Drug therapy to increase fluid volume and prevent fluid loss is the same as that discussed earlier for deficient fluid volume (p. 218). Saliva substitutes, such as

Salivart, can reduce the sensation of mouth dryness. *To prevent aspiration, do not use such agents in an unconscious client.*

Oral Hygiene. Nursing actions to promote oral hygiene can increase the client's comfort. Keep the lips clean and moist. Offer mouth care at least every 8 hours to reduce the thick, sticky coating on the tongue and mouth during dehydration.

Mouth care includes gentle toothbrushing several times a day and rinsing hourly. Teach the client to avoid mouthwashes and swabs that contain alcohol or glycerin because these products dry the oral mucosa further and may sting open areas of the mucosa. Rinsing the mouth with dilute solutions of hydrogen peroxide two times per day is a good form of oral hygiene; however, when used more often, it increases oral dryness. Tap water and normal saline rinses can be used safely as often as the client wishes.

Prevention of Complications. A dry mouth can cause sores and fissures in the mucosa, increasing the risk for infection. The thick, sticky coating also is an excellent breeding ground for organisms. A complication of mouth dryness is a wide variety of oral infections. Chart 15-4 lists NIC interventions for mouth care.

POTENTIAL FOR DYSRHYTHMIAS

NOC **PLANNING: EXPECTED OUTCOMES.** The client with dehydration is expected to maintain his or her normal cardiac rhythm.

INTERVENTIONS. Interventions are aimed at correcting the dehydration and recognizing dysrhythmias so that appropriate drug therapy can be initiated.

Drug Therapy. Drug therapy to increase body fluid volume and prevent excessive fluid loss is the same as that discussed earlier for deficient fluid volume (p. 218).

Elevated potassium or calcium levels can cause life-threatening dysrhythmias. Drug therapy to reduce these electrolytes may be prescribed. If potassium levels are high, a combination of 20 units of regular insulin in 100 mL of 20% dextrose may be prescribed to promote movement of potassium from the blood into the intracellular fluid (ICF). Drugs such as etidronate (Didronel) and plicamycin (Mithracin) may be prescribed to reduce high serum calcium levels.

Monitoring. Monitor the client for signs and symptoms of cardiac dysrhythmias every 15 minutes until he or she is fully rehydrated. Assess the rate, rhythm, and quality of the apical pulse and compare those findings with the client's baseline measurements. Assess for fatigue, chest discomfort or pain, and shortness of breath. Assess hand grasps and deep tendon reflexes, and record changes from baseline.

Clients at risk for dysrhythmias are monitored using electrocardiography (ECG). The pattern may show tall T waves or a shortened ST segment. Immediately report any change from the client's baseline ECG to the health care provider.

Community-Based Care

No extensive home care preparations are necessary for clients with mild dehydration or for those with dehydration of sudden onset. The imbalance is corrected before discharge from the facility and is unlikely to recur. Clients who are most likely to be discharged before the imbalance is completely corrected and who are susceptible to recurrent episodes are those with chronic problems, such as renal disease, diabetes, cancer, adrenal insufficiency, and many endocrine disorders. These clients often need long-term diet and drug therapy.

CHART 15-5

HOME CARE ASSESSMENT of The Client at Risk for Dehydration

Assess cardiovascular status.
- Vital signs, including apical pulse, pulse pressure, presence or absence of orthostatic hypotension, and quality and rhythm of peripheral pulses
- Presence or absence of peripheral edema
- Hand vein filling in the dependent position
- Neck vein filling in the recumbent and sitting positions
- Weight gain or loss

Assess cognition and mental status.
- Level of consciousness
- Orientation to time, place, and person
- Can the client accurately read a seven-word sentence containing no words greater than three syllables?

Assess condition of skin and mucous membranes.
- Presence or absence of skin tenting over the sternum or the forehead
- Moistness of skin, most reliable on chest and back
- Presence or absence of coating on tongue or teeth
- Can the client spit?

Assess neuromuscular status.
- Reactivity of patellar and biceps reflexes
- Oral temperature
- Handgrip strength
- Steadiness of gait

Assess renal system.
- Observe urine specimen for color, odor, cloudiness, and amount

Ask about the following:
- 24-hour fluid intake and output
- 24-hour diet recall
- 24-hour activity recall
- Over-the-counter and prescribed medications the client has taken

Assess client's understanding of illness and compliance with treatment.
- Signs and symptoms to report to health care provider
- Medication plan (correct timing and dose)

Perform a focused assessment (Chart 15-5) and a mental status check at every home visit to a client at risk for dehydration. Review drugs, manifestations of dehydration, and health care resources with the client and family.

Education is important in the prevention and early detection of dehydration. Teach the client at risk for dehydration about diet, drug regimens, and the manifestations of dehydration. Explain the meaning of changes found on assessment.

Stress the importance of recording accurate daily weights in assessing hydration status. Instruct clients to weigh themselves on the same scale daily, close to the same time each day, and with about the same amount of clothing on each time. Keeping a chart comparing the recorded weights from one day to the next can help the client recognize early-stage dehydration.

Instruct clients to take drugs as prescribed and not increase the use of diuretics. Explain that if a diuretic is not taken one day, the next day's dose should not be doubled. Teach clients how and where to assess skin turgor. Teach them how to measure their own peripheral pulse and obtain a return demonstration.

If the client has any mobility impairment, instruct the family to keep fluids in places that the client can access. Teach them to modify containers, such as opening zip-top cans and covering them with foil, to ensure that the client can easily open container lids. "Sipper" containers not only provide easy access but also are unbreakable and reduce spillage.

Critical Thinking Challenge

Your diabetic client has had her dehydration and diabetic ketoacidosis corrected. She is going home and will be managed at the diabetes clinic.

1. What specific areas of teaching will you emphasize to her?
2. What fluids would be most useful in preventing a recurrence of the dehydration?

evolve For suggested answer guidelines, go to http://evolve.elsevier.com/Iggy/.

Evaluation: Outcomes

Evaluate the care of the client with dehydration on the basis of the identified nursing diagnoses and collaborative problems. The expected outcomes include that the client should:

- Ingest at least 1500 mL of hypotonic fluids each day
- Maintain a fluid output approximately equal to fluid intake
- Have urine output volumes and specific gravity within normal limits
- State that oral mucosal discomfort is relieved
- Experience no oral mucosal complication

Specific indicators for these outcomes are listed for each nursing diagnosis and collaborative problem under the Planning and Implementation section (see earlier).

OVERHYDRATION

PATHOPHYSIOLOGY

Overhydration, also called fluid overload, is an excess of body fluid. It is not a disease but rather a clinical sign of a problem in which fluid intake or retention is greater than the body's fluid needs. Overhydration may be either an actual excess of total body fluid or a relative fluid excess in one or more body fluid spaces. The three basic types of fluid volume excess are isotonic overhydration, hypotonic overhydration, and hypertonic overhydration (Figure 15-5).

Most problems caused by overhydration are related to fluid volume excess in the vascular space or to dilution of specific electrolytes and blood components. Clinical manifestations vary with the type and degree of overhydration (Chart 15-6). The conditions leading to overhydration (fluid overload) are related to excessive intake or inadequate excretion of fluid. Table 15-5 lists common causes of overhydration.

Isotonic Overhydration

Isotonic overhydration is also called **hypervolemia** because the problems result from excessive fluid in the extracellular fluid (ECF) space. In isotonic overhydration, isotonic fluids are ingested or retained, so that osmolarity remains normal. Only the ECF compartment expands, and fluid does not shift between the spaces. The problems caused by severe isotonic overhydration are circulatory overload and edema. Figure 15-6 outlines the compensation that occurs in response to mild or moderate isotonic overhydration. When isotonic overhydration is severe, or when it occurs in a person with poor cardiac function, overhydration can lead to heart failure and pulmonary edema.

Hypotonic Overhydration

In hypotonic overhydration (water intoxication), the excess fluid is hypotonic to normal body fluids. Thus the osmolarity of the ECF decreases, and hydrostatic pressure increases. Fluid moves into the intracellular space because of the decreased plasma osmotic pressure, and all fluid spaces expand (see Figure 15-5). Because the excess fluid is hypotonic, electrolyte imbalances caused by dilution occur with hypotonic overhydration.

Hypertonic Overhydration

Hypertonic overhydration is rare and is caused by an excessive sodium intake. The hyperosmolarity of the plasma and interstitial compartments draws fluid from the intracellular fluid (ICF) compartment. Thus the ECF volume expands, and the ICF volume contracts (see Figure 15-5).

COLLABORATIVE MANAGEMENT

Assessment

Manifestations of overhydration vary with the specific type, the body fluid spaces involved, and the degree of overhydration. Clients with isotonic overhydration or hypertonic overhydration have circulatory overload and pitting edema (Figure 15-7). Clients with hypotonic overhydration have problems

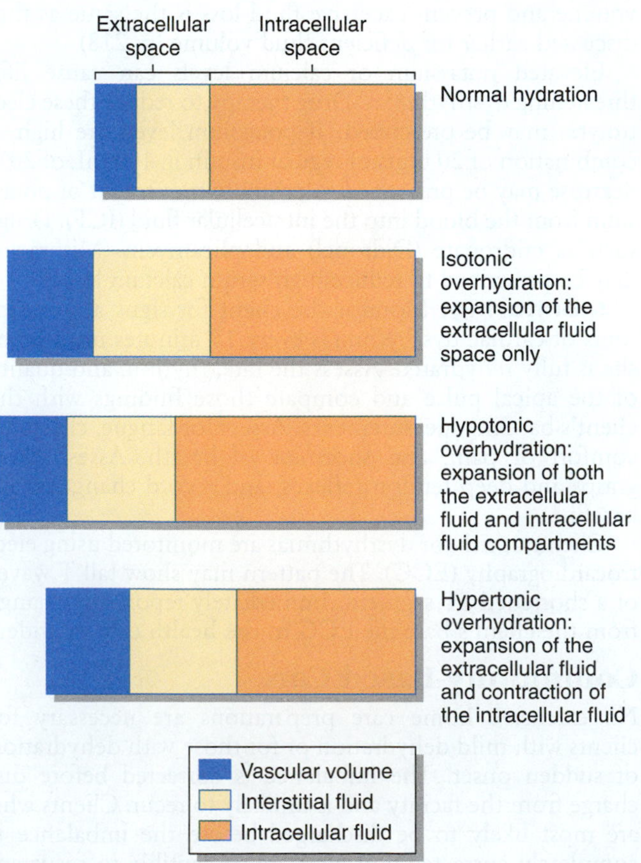

Figure 15-5 ■ Three types of overhydration. (© 1992 M. Linda Workman. All rights reserved.)

CHART 15-6

KEY FEATURES of Overhydration

Manifestations of Overhydration in General

Cardiovascular
- Increased pulse rate
- Bounding pulse quality
- Peripheral pulses full
- Elevated blood pressure
- Decreased pulse pressure
- Elevated central venous pressure
- Distended neck and hand veins
- Engorged venous varicosities
- Weight gain

Respiratory
- Respiratory rate increased
- Shallow respirations
- Dyspnea increases with exertion or in the supine position
- Moist crackles present on auscultation

Integumentary
- Pitting edema in dependent areas
- Skin pale and cool to touch

Neuromuscular
- Altered level of consciousness
- Headache
- Visual disturbances
- Skeletal muscle weakness
- Paresthesias

Gastrointestinal
- Increased motility

Manifestations of Isotonic Overhydration
- Liver enlargement
- Ascites formation

Manifestations of Hypotonic Overhydration
- Polyuria
- Diarrhea
- Nonpitting edema
- Cardiac dysrhythmias associated with electrolyte dilution
- Projectile vomiting

with cellular swelling and electrolyte dilution. Chart 15-6 lists the common manifestations of overhydration.

A diagnosis of overhydration is based on assessment findings and the results of laboratory tests. In isotonic overhydration, serum electrolyte values are normal, but decreased hemoglobin, hematocrit, and serum protein levels may result from **hemodilution** (excessive water in the vascular space). In hypertonic overhydration caused by kidney failure, electrolytes, blood urea nitrogen (BUN), and creatinine levels are elevated. Hypotonic overhydration decreases the complete blood count, serum proteins, and electrolyte levels.

Common Nursing Diagnoses and Collaborative Problems

Nursing diagnoses and collaborative problems that may apply to clients with overhydration include the following:

- Excess Fluid Volume related to compromised regulatory mechanisms (inability of the kidneys to maintain body fluid balance)

TABLE 15-5 Common Causes of Overhydration

Isotonic Overhydration
- Poorly controlled IV therapy
- Renal failure
- Long-term corticosteroid therapy

Hypotonic Overhydration
- Early renal failure
- Congestive heart failure
- Syndrome of inappropriate antidiuretic hormone
- Poorly controlled IV therapy
- Replacement of isotonic fluid loss with hypotonic fluids
- Psychogenic polydipsia
- Irrigation of wounds and body cavities with hypotonic fluids

Hypertonic Overhydration
- Excessive sodium ingestion
- Rapid infusion of hypertonic saline
- Excessive sodium bicarbonate therapy

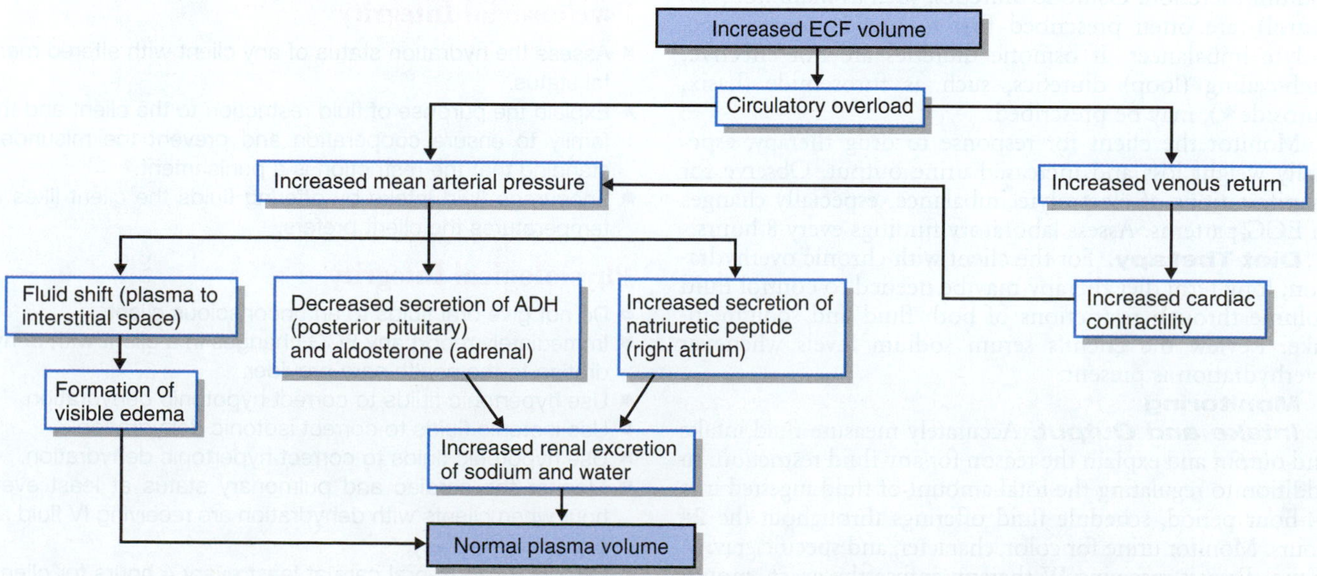

Figure 15-6 ■ Compensatory mechanisms associated with hypervolemia. *ADH,* Antidiuretic hormone; *ECF,* extracellular fluid.

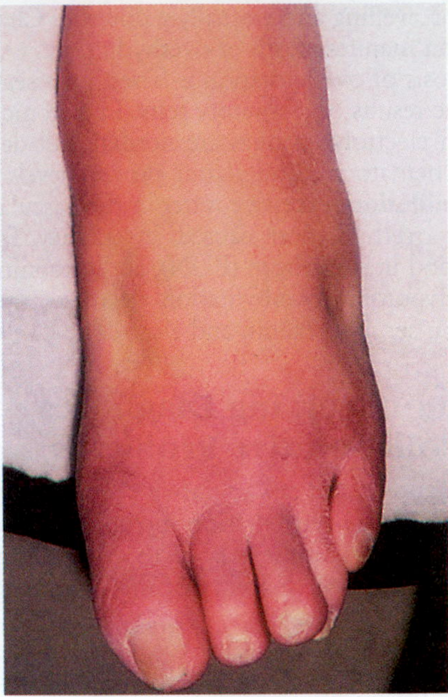

Figure 15-7 ■ Pitting edema.

- Deficient Knowledge (fluid restrictions, drug therapy, and manifestations of fluid excess) related to lack of exposure or lack of interest in learning
- Potential for Electrolyte Imbalances
- Potential for Hypertension
- Potential for Pulmonary Edema

Interventions

Interventions for clients with fluid volume excess aim to restore normal fluid balance, provide supportive care until the imbalance is resolved, and prevent future fluid overload. Drug and diet therapies are the basis of intervention.

Drug Therapy. Diuretics may be prescribed for clients with overhydration if renal failure is not the cause. Diuretics work on the kidneys to increase the water or sodium excretion. Osmotic diuretics, such as mannitol (Osmitrol), are often prescribed first to prevent severe electrolyte imbalances. If osmotic diuretics are not effective, high-ceiling (loop) diuretics, such as furosemide (Lasix, Furoside✱), may be prescribed.

Monitor the client for response to drug therapy, especially weight loss and increased urine output. Observe for manifestations of electrolyte imbalance, especially changes in ECG patterns. Assess laboratory findings every 8 hours.

Diet Therapy. For the client with chronic overhydration, long-term diet therapy may be needed to control fluid volume through restrictions of both fluid and sodium intake. Review the client's serum sodium levels whenever overhydration is present.

Monitoring

Intake and Output. Accurately measure fluid intake and output and explain the reason for any fluid restriction. In addition to regulating the total amount of fluid ingested in a 24-hour period, schedule fluid offerings throughout the 24 hours. Monitor urine for color, character, and specific gravity. If the client is receiving IV therapy, infuse the exact amount prescribed. Monitor for indicators of increased fluid overload (increased pulse quality, increasing neck vein distention, presence of crackles in lungs, increasing peripheral edema).

Weight. Fluid retention may not be visible. A sudden weight gain, however, indicates fluid retention. Metabolism can account for no more than a half pound of weight gain in one day. Each pound of weight gained (after the first half pound) equates to 500 mL of retained water. Weigh the client at the same time every day (before breakfast), using the same scale. Whenever possible, have the client wear the same type of clothing for each weigh-in.

GET READY for the NCLEX Examination!

KEY POINTS

Safe Effective Care Environment

- Monitor all intravenous infusions at least once per hour.
- Use a pump or controller to deliver intravenous fluids to clients with overhydration.
- Assess the oral mucous membranes at least every shift for clients with dehydration.

Health Promotion and Maintenance

- Instruct clients at risk for fluid imbalance to weigh themselves on the same scale daily, close to the same time each day, and with about the same amount of clothing on each time, and to monitor these daily weights for changes or trends.
- Encourage all clients to maintain an adequate fluid intake (minimum of 3 L/day) unless another condition requires fluid restriction.
- Instruct clients who exercise heavily (athletes) to take scheduled fluid replacement breaks.
- Instruct caregivers of older adults who have cognitive impairments or mobility problems to schedule offerings of fluids at regular intervals throughout the day.
- Teach people who are concerned about incontinence that reducing fluid intake does not help incontinence.

Psychosocial Integrity

- Assess the hydration status of any client with altered mental status.
- Explain the purpose of fluid restriction to the client and the family to ensure cooperation and prevent the misunderstanding that the restriction is a punishment.
- Encourage fluid intake by offering fluids the client likes at temperatures the client prefers.

Physiological Integrity

- Do not give oral fluids to an unconscious client.
- Immediately report any ECG changes in a client with dehydration to the health care provider.
- Use hypertonic fluids to correct hypotonic dehydration.
- Use isotonic fluids to correct isotonic dehydration.
- Use hypotonic fluids to correct hypertonic dehydration.
- Monitor the cardiac and pulmonary status at least every hour when clients with dehydration are receiving IV fluid replacement therapy.
- Offer or perform oral care at least every 4 hours for clients with dehydration.

ADDITIONAL STUDY RESOURCES

Go to your Student CD-ROM for Review Questions for the NCLEX Examination.

evolve Go to http://evolve.elsevier.com/Iggy/ for Integrated Management of Care Questions for the NCLEX Examination.

SELECTED BIBLIOGRAPHY

Asterisk indicates a classic or definitive work on this subject.

Ackley, B., & Ladwig, G. (2002). *Nursing diagnosis handbook: A guide to planning care* (5th ed.). St. Louis: Mosby.

Bennett, J. (2000). Dehydration: Hazards and benefits. *Geriatric Nursing, 21*(2), 84-88.

Brown, J., & Marland, G. (2002). Hydration in older people with mental health problems. *Nursing Times, 98*(3), 38-39.

Call-Schmidt, T. (2001). Interpreting lab results: A primer. *MEDSURG Nursing, 10*(4), 179-184.

Cannon, J. (2004). Recognizing chronic renal failure. *Nursing2004, 34*(1), 50-53.

Culp, K., Mentes, J., & Wakefield, B. (2003). Hydration and acute confusion in long-term care residents. *Western Journal of Nursing Research, 25*(3), 251-266.

Dochterman, J.M., & Bulechek, G.M. (Eds.). (2004). *Nursing interventions classification (NIC)* (4th ed.). St. Louis: Mosby.

Ebersole, P., Hess, P., & Luggen, A. (2004). *Toward healthy aging: Human needs and nursing response* (6th ed). St. Louis: Mosby

Hamilton, S. (2001). Detecting dehydration and malnutrition in the elderly. *Nursing2001, 31*(12), 56-57.

Kraft, P. (2000). The osmotic shift. *Journal of Intravenous Nursing, 23*(4), 220-224.

Krantz, M., & Baker, W. (2002). ECG challenge: Test your interpretive skills. *Consultant, 42*(14), 1757-1763.

Maintaining oral hydration in older people. (2001). *Best Practice, 5*(1), 1-6.

McCance, K., & Huether, S. (2002). *Pathophysiology: The biologic basis for disease in adults and children* (4th ed). St. Louis: Mosby.

McConnell, E. (2002). Measuring fluid intake and output. *Nursing2002, 32*(7), 17.

Mentes, J., Lyon, S., & Titler, M. (2000). Hydration management protocol. *Journal of Gerontological Nursing, 26*(10), 6-14.

Moorhead, S., Johnson, M., & Maas, M. (Eds.). (2004). *Nursing outcomes classification (NOC)* (3rd ed.). St. Louis: Mosby.

Pagana, K., & Pagana, T. (2002). *Mosby's manual of diagnostic and laboratory tests* (2nd ed.). St. Louis: Mosby.

Robinson, S., & Rosher, R. (2002). Can a beverage cart help improve hydration? *Geriatric Nursing, 23*(4), 208-211.

Suhayda, R., & Walton, J. (2002). Preventing and managing dehydration. *MEDSURG Nursing, 11*(6), 267-279.

*Stark, J. (1998). A comprehensive analysis of the fluid and electrolytes system. *Critical Care Nursing Clinics of North America, 10*(4), 471-475.

*Tietz, N.W. (Ed.). (1995). *Clinical guide to laboratory tests* (3rd ed.). Philadelphia: W.B. Saunders.

Trissel, L. (2003). *Handbook on injectable drugs* (12th ed.). Bethesda, MD: American Society of Health-System Pharmacists.

Yen, P. (2000). Focus on fluids. *Geriatric Nursing, 21*(4), 222-223.

CHAPTER 16

Interventions for Clients with Electrolyte Imbalances

M. LINDA WORKMAN

LEARNING OUTCOMES

After studying this chapter, you should be able to:

1. Identify clients at risk for imbalances of potassium.
2. Use laboratory data and clinical manifestations to assess potassium balance and imbalance.
3. Prioritize nursing care for the client with potassium imbalance.
4. Develop a community-based teaching plan to prevent deficiencies or excesses of potassium in the older adult client at risk for potassium imbalance.
5. Explain the effects of potassium imbalances on the activity of digoxin.
6. Differentiate diuretics that increase potassium loss from those that reduce potassium loss.
7. Analyze changes in clinical manifestations to determine the effectiveness of therapy for the client with potassium imbalance.
8. Identify clients at risk for imbalances of sodium.
9. Use laboratory data and clinical manifestations to assess sodium balance and imbalance.
10. Identify drugs that contain large amounts of sodium.
11. Prioritize nursing care for the client with sodium imbalance.
12. Develop a community-based teaching plan to prevent deficiencies or excesses of sodium in the older adult client at risk for sodium imbalance.
13. Analyze changes in clinical manifestations to determine the effectiveness of therapy for the client with sodium imbalance.
14. Identify clients at risk for imbalances of calcium.
15. Use laboratory data and clinical manifestations to assess calcium balance and imbalance.
16. Prioritize nursing care for the client with calcium imbalance.
17. Develop a community-based teaching plan to prevent deficiencies or excesses of calcium in the older adult client at risk for calcium imbalance.
18. Analyze changes in clinical manifestations to determine the effectiveness of therapy for the client with calcium imbalance.

Go to your Student CD-ROM for Review Questions for the NCLEX Examination keyed to these Learning Outcomes.

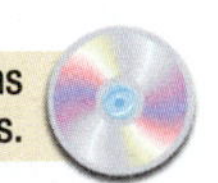

Electrolyte imbalances can occur in healthy people as a result of changes in fluid intake and output. These imbalances are usually mild and are easily corrected. Severe electrolyte imbalances are life threatening and can occur in any setting. People at greatest risk for severe imbalances are older clients, clients with chronic renal or endocrine disorders, clients who are mentally impaired, and clients who are taking drugs that alter fluid and electrolyte levels. Ill people are at some risk for electrolyte imbalances.

POTASSIUM IMBALANCES

Hypokalemia

PATHOPHYSIOLOGY

Because 98% of total body potassium (K^+) is inside cells, minor changes in extracellular potassium levels cause major changes in cell membrane excitability and in other cellular processes. **Hypokalemia** is a serum potassium level below

3.5 mEq/L (mmol/L). A common electrolyte imbalance, hypokalemia can be life threatening because every body system is affected.

Low serum potassium levels increase the difference in the amount of potassium between the fluid inside the cells **(intracellular fluid [ICF])** and the fluid outside the cells **(extracellular fluid (ECF])**. This increased difference reduces the excitability of cells. As a result, the cell membranes of all excitable tissues, such as nerve and muscle, are less responsive to normal stimuli.

The severity of problems caused by hypokalemia is related to how rapidly the serum potassium level drops. When the loss of ECF potassium is gradual, cells adjust and cellular potassium decreases in proportion to the ECF potassium level. In this situation, the potassium difference between the two fluid compartments remains unchanged and symptoms of hypokalemia may not appear until the potassium loss is extreme. Rapid reduction of serum potassium levels can cause dramatic changes in function.

Etiology

Hypokalemia may result either from an *actual* total body potassium loss or from the movement of potassium from the ECF to the ICF, causing a *relative* decrease in extracellular potassium level. Table 16-1 lists the common causes of hypokalemia.

Actual potassium depletion occurs when potassium loss is excessive or when potassium intake is not adequate to match normal potassium loss. Relative hypokalemia occurs when total body potassium levels are normal but the potassium distribution between fluid spaces is abnormal. Conditions that increase cell uptake of potassium, leading to hypokalemia, include metabolic alkalosis and insulin use.

Incidence/Prevalence

The actual incidence of hypokalemia is not known, although it is a common occurrence in acute care and long-term care settings. Mild hypokalemia, caused by dilution when a person drinks a large amount of fluid that does not contain potassium, occurs often but is corrected easily and quickly by diet.

COLLABORATIVE MANAGEMENT

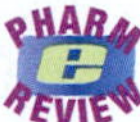

Assessment

HISTORY

Collect data from clients at risk as well as from those with actual hypokalemia.

AGE. Age is important because renal urine concentration decreases with aging, which increases potassium loss. Older adults are more likely to use drugs that lead to potassium loss.

DRUGS. Ask the client about drugs, especially diuretics, corticosteroids, and beta-adrenergic agonists or antagonists. These drugs increase potassium loss through the kidneys. A common cause of hypokalemia is the use and misuse of diuretics. In clients taking digoxin (Lanoxin, Novodigoxin✱), hypokalemia increases the sensitivity of the cardiac muscle to the drug and may result in digoxin toxicity, even when the digoxin level is within the therapeutic range.

Ask whether the client takes a potassium supplement, such as potassium chloride (KCl). The client may not be taking the supplement as prescribed because of its unpleasant taste.

TABLE 16-1 Common Causes of Hypokalemia

Actual Potassium Deficits

Excessive Potassium Loss

- Inappropriate or excessive use of drugs
  - Diuretics
  - Digitalis
  - Corticosteroids
- Increased secretion of aldosterone
  - Cushing's syndrome
- Diarrhea
- Vomiting
- Wound drainage (especially gastrointestinal)
- Prolonged nasogastric suction
- Heat-induced excessive diaphoresis
- Renal disease impairing reabsorption of potassium

Inadequate Potassium Intake

- Nothing by mouth

Relative Potassium Deficits

Movement of Potassium from Extracellular Fluid to Intracellular Fluid

- Alkalosis
- Hyperinsulinism
- Hyperalimentation
- Total parenteral nutrition

Dilution of Serum Potassium

- Water intoxication
- IV therapy with potassium-poor solutions

OTHER FACTORS. Any acute or chronic disease may lead to potassium loss. Ask the client about recent illnesses and medical or surgical interventions. A thorough diet history, including a typical day's food and beverage intake, helps identify clients at risk for hypokalemia.

PHYSICAL ASSESSMENT/CLINICAL MANIFESTATIONS

The clinical manifestations of hypokalemia are seen as altered function of many systems (Chart 16-1).

MUSCULOSKELETAL MANIFESTATIONS. Skeletal muscles become weak in response to hypokalemia, and a stronger stimulus is needed to begin muscle contraction. A client may be so weak that he or she is unable to stand. Hand grasps are weak, and **hyporeflexia** (a decreased response to deep tendon reflex stimulation) may be seen. Severe hypokalemia causes flaccid paralysis. Assess for muscle weakness and determine the client's ability to perform activities of daily living (ADLs).

RESPIRATORY MANIFESTATIONS. The respiratory system can be seriously affected by hypokalemia through weakness of the muscles needed for breathing. Skeletal muscle weakness results in shallow respirations. *Thus respiratory status should be assessed first in any client who might have hypokalemia.* Assess the client's breath sounds, ease of respiratory effort, color of nail beds and mucous membranes, and rate and depth of respiration. Assess respiratory status at least every 2 hours because respiratory insufficiency is a major cause of death.

CARDIOVASCULAR MANIFESTATIONS. Assess the cardiovascular system by first palpating the peripheral pulses. In the client with hypokalemia, the pulse is usually thready and weak. Palpation is difficult, and the pulse is easily blocked with light pressure. The pulse rate can range from very slow to very rapid, depending on whether a **dysrhythmia** (irregular heartbeat) also is present. Measure blood pressure with the client in the lying, sitting, and standing positions because orthostatic (postural) hypotension occurs with hypokalemia.

NEUROLOGIC MANIFESTATIONS. The neurologic manifestations of hypokalemia include changes in mental status. The client may have short-term irritability and anxiety followed by lethargy that progresses to confusion and coma as hypokalemia worsens. Severe hypokalemia decreases sensory awareness. For example, the client may not be able to identify mild pain, touch, heat, and cold.

GASTROINTESTINAL MANIFESTATIONS. Hypokalemia decreases smooth muscle contractions within the gastrointestinal (GI) system, which leads to decreased peristalsis. The client has hypoactive bowel sounds and may have nausea, vomiting, constipation, and abdominal distention. Assess distention by measuring abdominal girth. Auscultate for bowel sounds in all four abdominal quadrants to assess the extent of decreased peristalsis. Severe hypokalemia can cause **paralytic ileus** (the absence of peristalsis).

PSYCHOSOCIAL ASSESSMENT

Behavioral changes caused by hypokalemia can occur quickly. You may need to obtain information about the client's behavior from close family members or friends if the client is confused.

Collect data about the onset and duration of behavioral changes as well as their association with any physical change. The client may be lethargic and unable to perform simple problem-solving tasks such as counting backward from 100 by threes. As hypokalemia progresses, the client may become more confused, especially to time and place. In severe hypokalemia, coma may develop.

LABORATORY ASSESSMENT

Hypokalemia is confirmed by a serum potassium value below 3.5 mEq/L (mmol/L). However, this value alone does not determine whether potassium loss has occurred or whether potassium has moved from the blood into the cells.

OTHER DIAGNOSTIC ASSESSMENTS

A baseline electrocardiogram (ECG) and continuous cardiac monitoring may be prescribed for a client with severe hypokalemia. Hypokalemia causes electrical conduction changes in the heart, including ST-segment depression, flat or inverted T waves, and increased U waves. Dysrhythmias can lead to death, particularly in older adults who are taking digoxin.

CHART 16-1

KEY FEATURES of Hypokalemia

Cardiovascular Manifestations
- Variable pulse rate, more often rapid
- Pulse quality thready and weak
- Peripheral pulses difficult to palpate
- Orthostatic (postural) hypotension
- Electrocardiographic abnormalities
  - ST depression
  - Inverted T wave
  - Prominent U wave
  - Heart block

Respiratory Manifestations
- Shallow, ineffective respirations resulting from profound weakness of the skeletal muscles of respiration
- Diminished breath sounds

Neuromuscular Manifestations
- Anxiety, lethargy, confusion, coma
- Loss of tactile discrimination
- General skeletal muscle weakness
- Deep tendon hyporeflexia
- Eventual flaccid paralysis

Gastrointestinal Manifestations
- Decreased motility
- Hypoactive to absent bowel sounds
- Nausea
- Vomiting
- Abdominal distention
- Paralytic ileus
- Constipation

Renal Manifestations
- Decreased ability to concentrate urine
- Polyuria
- Decreased specific gravity

Critical Thinking Challenge

The client is a 75-year-old woman who fell when she attempted to get up during intermission while attending a concert with a friend. When asked whether she takes any drugs, she tells you that she has been taking Diuril for 20 years to manage her high blood pressure. The only other drugs she takes are an aspirin each day and a multivitamin. She is alert and just a little anxious. Her vital signs are as follows: T 98.4; P 102, thready, slightly irregular; R 30 and shallow; BP 98/50; O_2 saturation 95%.

1. What other assessment data should you obtain?
2. What question should you ask about her drug regimen?
3. Should you apply oxygen? Why or why not?
4. Should she be monitored by electrocardiography? Why or why not?

evolve For suggested answer guidelines, go to http://evolve.elsevier.com/Iggy/.

Analysis

COMMON NURSING DIAGNOSES AND COLLABORATIVE PROBLEMS

The following are priority nursing diagnoses for clients with hypokalemia:

1. Risk for Falls related to skeletal muscle weakness
2. Constipation related to smooth muscle atony

The primary collaborative problem is Potential for Respiratory Insufficiency.

ADDITIONAL NURSING DIAGNOSES AND COLLABORATIVE PROBLEMS

In addition to the common nursing diagnoses and collaborative problems, clients with hypokalemia may have one or more of the following:

- Impaired Physical Mobility related to skeletal muscle weakness
- Total Self-Care Deficit related to skeletal muscle weakness
- Decreased Cardiac Output related to dysrhythmia

Critical Thinking Challenge

The 75-year-old client with hypokalemia tells you that she took two doses of Diuril today because she and her friend were going to a Chinese restaurant after the concert and she was afraid the salty food would make her hypertension worse. She has not eaten in the last 7 hours and has only had one cup of coffee in the past 4 hours. She says she last saw her doctor 6 months ago and that the blood work done at that time was "okay."

1. Is she at risk for any other fluid or electrolyte imbalance?
2. If so, what specific imbalance is she at risk for and why?

evolve For suggested answer guidelines, go to http://evolve.elsevier.com/Iggy/.

Planning and Implementation

RISK FOR FALLS

NOC **PLANNING: EXPECTED OUTCOMES.** The client with hypokalemia is expected to avoid falls and have a return to a normal serum potassium level.

INTERVENTIONS. Interventions for hypokalemia aim to prevent potassium loss, increase serum potassium levels, and provide a safe environment for the client. (See Chart 16-2 for NIC interventions for hypokalemia.) Drug and diet therapies help restore normal serum potassium levels.

Drug Therapy. Drug therapies for the treatment and prevention of hypokalemia include additional potassium and drugs to prevent potassium loss.

Potassium Supplements. Most potassium supplements are potassium chloride, potassium gluconate, potassium citrate, or a combination of these salts. The amount and the route of potassium replacement depend on the degree of potassium loss. A client with a serum potassium level of 3 mEq/L needs 100 to 200 mEq of potassium supplement; a client with a serum potassium level of 2.0 mEq/L needs 500 to 600 mEq.

Potassium is given intravenously for severe hypokalemia. A dilution of no more than 1 mEq/10 mL of solution is recommended. *The maximum recommended infusion rate is 5 to 10 mEq/hr; this rate is never to exceed 20 mEq/hr under any circumstances.* Older clients may not be able to handle this rate. Because rapid infusion of potassium can cause cardiac arrest, potassium is not given by intravenous (IV) push.

Potassium is a severe tissue irritant and is never given by intramuscular or subcutaneous injection. Tissues damaged by potassium can become necrotic and slough, causing loss of function and requiring reconstructive surgery. IV potassium solutions irritate veins and can cause phlebitis. Check the orders carefully to ensure that the client receives the correct amount of potassium. Assess the IV site every 2 hours and ask the client whether he or she feels burning or pain at the site. *Stop the IV solution immediately if infiltration occurs.*

Oral potassium preparations may be taken as liquids or solids. Potassium has a strong, unpleasant taste that is difficult to mask. Because potassium chloride can cause nausea and vomiting, advise clients not to take it on an empty stomach.

Potassium-Sparing Diuretics. Diuretics that increase the renal excretion of potassium can cause hypokalemia. These classes of diuretics include high-ceiling (loop) diuretics (e.g., furosemide [Lasix, Furoside✱], bumetanide [Bumex], and ethacrynic acid [Edecrin]) and the thiazide diuretics (chlorothiazide [Diuril], hydrochlorothiazide [Esidrix, HydroDIURIL, Urozide✱], and quinethazone [Hydromox]). Avoid these drugs in clients with actual hypokalemia and in those who are at risk for hypokalemia. A potassium-sparing diuretic may be prescribed for clients with hypokalemia who need diuretic therapy. Potassium-sparing diuretics increase urine output without increasing potassium loss. Potassium-sparing diuretics include spironolactone (Aldactone, Novospiroton✱), triamterene (Dyrenium), and amiloride (Midamor).

Diet Therapy. Consult with the dietitian in teaching the client how to increase dietary potassium intake. Eating foods that are naturally rich in potassium helps to restore normal potassium levels and prevent further loss. Table 14-7 lists the potassium content of common foods.

CHART 16-2

NIC INTERVENTION ACTIVITIES for The Client with Hypokalemia

Electrolyte Management: Hypokalemia: *Promotion of potassium balance and prevention of complications resulting from serum potassium levels lower than desired*

- Monitor lab values associated with hypokalemia (e.g., elevated glucose, metabolic alkalosis, reduced urine osmolality, urine potassium, hypochloremia, and hypocalcemia).
- Administer prescribed supplemental potassium (PO, NG, or IV), per policy.
- Prevent/reduce irritation from potassium supplement (e.g., administer PO or NG potassium supplements during or after meals to minimize GI irritation, dilute IV potassium adequately, administer IV supplement slowly, and apply topical anesthetic to IV site), as appropriate.
- Administer potassium-sparing diuretics (e.g., spironolactone [Aldactone] or triamterene [Dyrenium]), as appropriate.
- Avoid administration of alkaline substances (e.g., IV sodium bicarbonate and PO or NG antacids), as appropriate.
- Monitor neurologic manifestations of hypokalemia (e.g., muscle weakness, altered level of consciousness, drowsiness, apathy, lethargy, confusion, and depression).
- Monitor cardiac manifestations of hypokalemia (e.g., hypotension, broad T wave, U wave, ectopy, tachycardia, and weak pulse).
- Monitor renal manifestations of hypokalemia (e.g., acidic urine, reduced urine osmolality, nocturia, polyuria, and polydipsia).
- Monitor GI manifestations of hypokalemia (e.g., anorexia, nausea, cramps, constipation, distention, and paralytic ileus).
- Monitor pulmonary manifestations of hypokalemia (e.g., hypoventilation and respiratory muscle weakness).
- Monitor for symptoms of respiratory failure (e.g., low Pa_{O_2} and elevated Pa_{CO_2} levels and respiratory muscle fatigue).
- Monitor for rebound hyperkalemia.

NIC intervention activities selected from Dochterman, J.M., & Bulechek, G.M. (Eds.). (2004). *Nursing interventions classification (NIC)* (4th ed.). St. Louis: Mosby.

GI, Gastrointestinal; Pa_{O_2}, partial pressure of arterial oxygen; Pa_{CO_2}, partial pressure of arterial carbon dioxide.

Safety. For a client with muscle weakness from hypokalemia, use safety measures, eliminate hazards, and assist with ambulation. Remove obstacles or slippery areas from the ambulation path, and make certain the client wears nonslip footgear. Be sure to have the client wear a gait belt when ambulating with assistance.

CONSTIPATION

NOC **PLANNING: EXPECTED OUTCOMES.** The client with hypokalemia is expected to have a normal bowel elimination pattern as indicated by:

- Stool amount appropriate for the diet
- Stools are soft and formed
- No discomfort when stool is passed

INTERVENTIONS. Interventions aim to restore normal serum potassium levels and induce gastric motility. Interventions include drug and diet therapies to restore serum potassium levels to normal values (discussed earlier under Drug Therapy and Diet Therapy [Risk for Falls], p. 229, stimulate intestinal peristalsis, and prevent constipation.

Drug Therapy. Laxatives that add bulk or fiber may be used to stimulate peristalsis. Other drugs that enhance gastric emptying and stimulate gastrointestinal (GI) motility, such as metoclopramide (Reglan, Maxeran✱), are used to treat constipation associated with hypokalemia.

Diet Therapy. Provide high-fiber foods and plenty of liquids for the client who is not on fluid restrictions. To ensure cooperation, prepare a list of foods that contain high concentrations of fiber and ask the client to select favorite items from that list.

Comfort Measures. Provide privacy when the client uses the toilet or bedpan. Close the door, draw the privacy curtains, and ask visitors to step out of the room. Because physical activity promotes gastric motility, encourage the client to walk whenever his or her condition permits. A bedridden client can benefit from frequent position changes and mild bed exercises.

POTENTIAL FOR RESPIRATORY INSUFFICIENCY

NOC **PLANNING: EXPECTED OUTCOMES.** The client with hypokalemia is expected to have a breathing pattern adequate to maintain gas exchange as indicated by:

- Pulse oximetry within the normal range
- Absence of cyanosis or pallor

INTERVENTIONS. Monitor the client's respiratory rate and depth at least once per hour, noting in particular increased rate and decreased depth. Assess respiratory muscle effectiveness by checking the client's ability to cough. Examine the face, oral mucosa, and nail beds for pallor or cyanosis. Evaluate arterial blood gas values for **hypoxemia** (decreased blood oxygen levels) and **hypercapnia** (increased arterial carbon dioxide levels). See Chapter 30 for respiratory assessment techniques.

Critical Thinking Challenge

Your client's serum potassium level is 2.4 mEq/L and her serum sodium is 142 mEq/L. In addition, her hematocrit is 47%. She is prescribed to receive 1 L of normal saline (0.9% sodium chloride) with 40 mEq of potassium added. The rate of administration prescribed is 200 mL/hr.

1. What vein should you choose to start this IV? Why?
2. How many mEq of potassium will she be receiving per hour at this infusion rate?
3. What safety precautions should you take with this prescription and why?
4. Should the care of this client be assigned to an RN, LPN/LVN, or assistive nursing personnel? (Explain your rationale for the caregiver assignment.)
5. What assessment data would you need to determine whether the interventions are effective?

evolve For suggested answer guidelines, go to http://evolve.elsevier.com/Iggy/.

Community-Based Care

No special home care preparations are needed for clients with mild hypokalemia or sudden-onset hypokalemia. The imbalance is corrected before discharge and, with teaching, is unlikely to recur. Clients with chronic diseases are more likely to be discharged before the imbalance is completely corrected and are at risk for recurrence. These clients often need long-term diet and drug therapy. Health teaching for prevention and early detection is a major nursing responsibility.

Instruct the at-risk client (especially one using diuretics or corticosteroids) about the proper use of drugs, the symptoms of hypokalemia, when to seek medical help, and which foods are rich in potassium. Teach the client to assess the rate, rhythm, and quality of the peripheral pulses at least once each day and whenever any symptoms of hypokalemia appear. For clients at chronic risk for hypokalemia, stress how often serum potassium levels should be checked.

A home care aide may be needed to assist with hygiene and ensure a safe environment. Weekly visits by a nurse may also be needed to assess changes and ensure adherence with the drug regimen. Perform a focused assessment at every home visit to a client at risk for hypokalemia (Chart 16-3). Review drugs, the symptoms of hypokalemia, and health care resources with the client and family.

Critical Thinking Challenge

After restoration of fluid volume and serum potassium levels, your client with hypokalemia is discharged to home and advised to make an appointment with her usual health care provider. She tells you that years ago she tried taking potassium supplements but found the taste too unpleasant to continue.

1. What should you teach this client to prevent a recurrence of the imbalance?
2. What should you teach this client to reduce her risk for falling?
3. How could this client increase her intake of potassium without using potassium supplements?

evolve For suggested answer guidelines, go to http://evolve.elsevier.com/Iggy/.

Evaluation: Outcomes

Evaluate the care of the client with hypokalemia on the basis of the identified nursing diagnoses and collaborative problems. The expected outcomes are that the client should:

- Return to and maintain a normal serum potassium level (between 3.5 and 5.0 mEq/L)
- Adhere to prescribed drug and diet therapies
- Identify the early manifestations of hypokalemia
- Avoid falls

CHART 16-3

HOME CARE ASSESSMENT of
The Client at Risk for Hypokalemia

Assess respiratory status.
- Rate, depth, rhythm of respiration
- Color of lips, tongue, nail beds
- Can the client complete a sentence without taking a breath?

Assess cardiovascular status.
- Vital signs, including apical pulse, pulse pressure, presence or absence of orthostatic hypotension, and quality and rhythm of peripheral pulses
- Presence or absence of peripheral edema
- Hand vein filling in the dependent position
- Neck vein filling in the recumbent and sitting positions
- Weight gain or loss

Assess cognition and mental status.
- Level of consciousness
- Orientation to time, place, and person
- Can the client accurately read a seven-word sentence containing no words greater than three syllables?

Assess condition of skin and mucous membranes.
- Presence or absence of skin tenting over the sternum or the forehead
- Moistness of skin (most reliable on chest and back)
- Presence or absence of coating on tongue or teeth
- Can the client spit?

Assess neuromuscular status.
- Reactivity of patellar and biceps reflexes
- Oral temperature
- Handgrip strength
- Steadiness of gait

Assess renal system.
- Observe urine specimen for color, odor, cloudiness, and amount.

Ask about the following:
- 24-hour fluid intake and output
- 24-hour diet recall
- 24-hour activity recall
- What over-the-counter and prescribed medications has the client taken?
- Has the client experienced any dizziness or lightheadedness?
- Does the client have a headache (what time of day, associated with what activities)?
- Muscle twitches, cramps, pain, or spasms

Assess the client's understanding of illness and adherence to treatment.
- Signs and symptoms to report to health care provider
- Medication plan (correct timing and dose)

- Have normal bowel elimination patterns
- Maintain adequate gas exchange
- Maintain regular cardiac rate and rhythm

Specific indicators for these outcomes are listed for each nursing diagnosis and collaborative problem under the Planning and Implementation section (see earlier).

Hyperkalemia

PATHOPHYSIOLOGY

Hyperkalemia is a serum potassium level greater than 5.0 mEq/L (mmol/L). Because the range of normal serum potassium values is narrow, even slight increases above normal values can affect excitable tissues, especially the heart.

A high serum potassium level decreases the potassium difference between the intracellular fluid (ICF) and the extracellular fluid (ECF). This decreased difference increases cell excitability; as a result, excitable tissues respond to less intense stimuli and may even discharge spontaneously.

TABLE 16-2 Common Causes of Hyperkalemia

Actual Potassium Excesses
Excessive Potassium Intake
- Overingestion of potassium-containing foods or medications
  - Salt substitutes
  - Potassium chloride
- Rapid infusion of potassium-containing IV solution
- Bolus IV potassium injections
- Transfusions of whole blood or packed cells

Decreased Potassium Excretion
- Adrenal insufficiency (Addison's disease, adrenalectomy)
- Renal failure
- Potassium-sparing diuretics

Relative Potassium Excesses
Movement of Potassium from Intracellular Fluid to Extracellular Fluid
- Tissue damage
- Acidosis
- Hyperuricemia
- Uncontrolled diabetes mellitus

Hyperkalemia alters the function of all excitable membranes to some degree. The excitable membrane in the heart is very sensitive to serum potassium increases and the most serious complications of hyperkalemia are altered cardiac function.

The problems that occur with hyperkalemia are related to how rapidly ECF potassium levels increase. Sudden rises in serum potassium cause severe problems at potassium levels between 6 and 7 mEq/L. When serum potassium rises slowly, problems may not occur until potassium levels reach 8 mEq/L or higher.

Hyperkalemia may result from an actual increase in total body potassium or from the movement of potassium from the cells into the blood. Table 16-2 lists common causes of hyperkalemia.

Hyperkalemia is rare in people with normal kidney function. Most cases of hyperkalemia occur in hospitalized clients and in those undergoing medical treatment. Those at greatest risk for hyperkalemia are chronically ill clients, debilitated clients, and older adults.

COLLABORATIVE MANAGEMENT

Assessment

HISTORY

Age is important because renal function decreases with aging. Ask about chronic illnesses (particularly renal disease and diabetes mellitus), recent medical or surgical treatment, and urine output, including frequency and amount of voidings. Ask about drug use, particularly potassium-sparing diuretics and angiotensin-converting enzyme (ACE) inhibitors. Obtain a diet history to determine the intake of potassium-rich foods or the use of salt substitutes (which contain potassium).

Collect data regarding symptoms related to hyperkalemia. Ask if the client has had palpitations, skipped heartbeats, other cardiac irregularities, muscle twitching, weakness in the leg muscles, or unusual tingling or numbness in the hands, feet, or face. Ask about recent changes in bowel habits, especially diarrhea.

CHART 16-4

KEY FEATURES of
Hyperkalemia

Cardiovascular Manifestations
- Irregular heart rate, usually slow
- Decreased blood pressure
- Electrocardiographic abnormalities
  - Tall T waves
  - Widened QRS complexes
  - Prolonged PR intervals
  - Flat P waves
- Ectopic beats
- Late; dysrhythmias, ventricular fibrillation, cardiac arrest in diastole

Respiratory Manifestations
- Unaffected until late, when profound weakness of the skeletal muscles causes respiratory failure

Neuromuscular Manifestations
- Early phase, or mild, hyperkalemia
  - Muscle twitches, cramps
  - Paresthesias
- Late phase, or severe, hyperkalemia
  - Profound weakness
  - Ascending flaccid paralysis in distal to proximal direction; involves the arms and legs

Gastrointestinal Manifestations
- Increased motility
- Hyperactive bowel sounds
- Diarrhea

PHYSICAL ASSESSMENT/CLINICAL MANIFESTATIONS

The manifestations of hyperkalemia are listed in Chart 16-4. Cardiovascular changes are the most severe problems from hyperkalemia and are the most common cause of death in clients with hyperkalemia. Cardiac manifestations of hyperkalemia include bradycardia, hypotension, and electrocardiographic (ECG) changes of tall, peaked T waves, prolonged PR intervals, flat or absent P waves, and wide QRS complexes (Figure 16-1). As serum potassium levels rise, **ectopic beats** (beats generated outside the normal conduction system in the ventricles) may appear. Complete heart block, asystole, and ventricular fibrillation are life-threatening complications of severe hyperkalemia.

The neuromuscular response to hyperkalemia has two phases. Skeletal muscles twitch in the early stages of hyperkalemia, and the client may be aware of unusual nerve sensations (e.g., tingling and burning) that are followed by numbness in the hands and feet and around the mouth **(paresthesia).** As hyperkalemia worsens, muscle twitching changes to weakness followed by flaccid paralysis. The weakness moves up from the hands and feet and first affects the muscles of the arms and legs. Trunk, head, and respiratory muscles are not affected until serum potassium levels reach lethal levels.

The smooth muscle of the gastrointestinal (GI) tract has increased motility. As a result, the client may have diarrhea and spastic colonic activity. Listen to bowel sounds and observes stools. Bowel sounds are hyperactive, with audible rushes and gurgles. Bowel movements are frequent and watery.

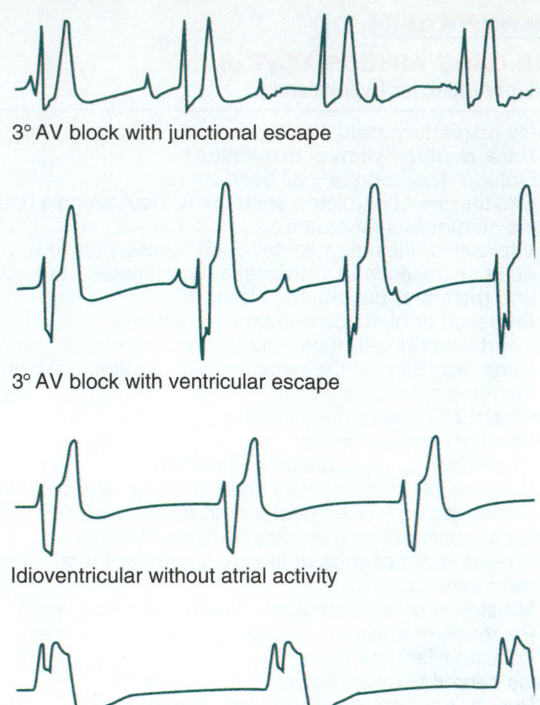

Figure 16-1 ■ Electrocardiographic (ECG) changes associated with hyperkalemia. (Modified with permission from John M. Clochesy.)

LABORATORY ASSESSMENT

A serum potassium level over 5.0 mEq/L confirms hyperkalemia. If hyperkalemia results from dehydration, levels of other electrolytes, hematocrit, and hemoglobin also are elevated. Hyperkalemia caused by renal failure occurs with elevated serum creatinine and blood urea nitrogen, decreased blood pH, and normal or low hematocrit and hemoglobin levels.

Interventions

Interventions for hyperkalemia are aimed at rapidly reducing the serum potassium level. Drug therapy can restore normal potassium balance by enhancing potassium excretion and promoting the movement of potassium from the extracellular fluid (ECF) into the cells. Monitoring the client's response to intervention is another major nursing responsibility. (See Chart 16-5 for NIC interventions for hyperkalemia.)

Eliminate extra potassium by stopping potassium-containing infusions. Keeping the IV catheter open is useful in managing hyperkalemia. Withhold oral potassium supplements and provide a potassium-restricted diet.

Increasing potassium excretion helps reduce hyperkalemia if renal function is normal. Potassium-excreting diuretics, such

CHART 16-5

NIC **INTERVENTION ACTIVITIES for**
The Client with Hyperkalemia

Electrolyte Management: Hyperkalemia: *Promotion of potassium balance and prevention of complications resulting from serum potassium levels higher than desired*

- Administer electrolyte-binding and electrolyte-excreting resins (e.g., Kayexalate) as prescribed, if appropriate.
- Monitor lab values for changes in oxygenation or acid-base balance, as appropriate.
- Administer prescribed medications to shift potassium into the cell (e.g., 50% dextrose and insulin, sodium bicarbonate, calcium chloride, and calcium gluconate), as appropriate.
- Avoid potassium-sparing medications (e.g., spironolactone [Aldactone] and triamterene [Dyrenium]), as appropriate.
- Maintain potassium restrictions.
- Administer prescribed diuretics, as appropriate.
- Monitor fluid status, including intake and output, as appropriate.
- Monitor potassium levels after diuresis.
- Monitor cardiac manifestations of hyperkalemia (e.g., decreased cardiac output, heart blocks, peaked T waves, fibrillation, or asystole).
- Respond to cardiac arrest.

NIC intervention activities selected from Dochterman, J.M., & Bulechek, G.M. (Eds.). (2004). *Nursing interventions classification (NIC)* (4th ed). St. Louis: Mosby. No part of this work is to be altered without prior written permission from the Publisher.

as furosemide, are prescribed. For a client with renal problems, drug therapy to increase potassium excretion includes cation exchange resins that promote intestinal sodium absorption and potassium excretion, such as sodium polystyrene sulfonate (Kayexalate). However, this therapy may take many hours to reduce potassium levels. If potassium levels are dangerously high, additional measures, such as dialysis, are needed.

Movement of potassium from the extracellular fluid (ECF) to the intracellular fluid (ICF) can help reduce serum potassium levels temporarily. Potassium movement into the cells is enhanced by insulin. Insulin increases the activity of the sodium-potassium pumps, which move potassium from the ECF into the cell (see Chapter 14). IV fluids containing glucose and insulin are prescribed to help decrease serum potassium levels (usually 100 mL of 10% to 20% glucose with 10 to 20 units of regular insulin). These IV solutions are hypertonic and are infused through a central line or in a vein with a high blood flow to avoid local vein inflammation. Observe the client for manifestations of hypokalemia and hypoglycemia during this therapy.

Cardiac monitoring allows for the early recognition of dysrhythmias and other manifestations of hyperkalemia on cardiac muscle. Compare recent ECG tracings with the client's baseline tracings or with tracings obtained when the client's serum potassium level was close to normal.

Health teaching is key to the prevention of hyperkalemia and the early detection of complications. The teaching plan for the client at risk for hyperkalemia includes diet, drugs, and recognition of the manifestations of hyperkalemia. Diet education includes knowledge of foods to avoid (those high in potassium) and permissible foods containing little potassium (Chart 16-6). Instruct the client to read the labels on drug and food packages to determine the potassium content. Warn clients to avoid salt substitutes, which contain potassium.

CHART 16-6

CLIENT EDUCATION GUIDE
Dietary Management of Hyperkalemia

You Should Avoid

- Meats, especially organ meat and preserved meat
- Dairy products
- Dried fruit
- Fruits high in potassium
  - Bananas
  - Cantaloupe
  - Kiwi
  - Oranges
- Vegetables high in potassium
  - Avocados
  - Broccoli
  - Dried beans or peas
  - Lima beans
  - Mushrooms
  - Potatoes (white or sweet)
  - Seaweed
  - Soybeans
  - Spinach

You May Eat

- Eggs
- Breads
- Butter
- Cereals
- Sugar
- Fruits low in potassium (fresh, frozen, or canned)
  - Apples
  - Apricots
  - Berries
  - Cherries
  - Grapefruit
  - Peaches
  - Pineapple
  - Cranberries
- Vegetables low in potassium
  - Alfalfa sprouts
  - Cabbage
  - Carrots
  - Cauliflower
  - Celery
  - Eggplant
  - Green beans
  - Lettuce
  - Onions
  - Peas
  - Peppers
  - Squash

Data from Pennington, J. (2004). *Bowe's and Church's food values of portions commonly used* (18th ed.). Philadelphia: Lippincott-Raven.

SODIUM IMBALANCES

Hyponatremia

PATHOPHYSIOLOGY

Hyponatremia is a serum sodium (Na^+) level below 136 mEq/L (mmol/L). Because sodium is the major cation of the blood and interstitial fluid and maintains the osmolarity of these fluids, sodium imbalances often occur with fluid volume imbalances.

The problems caused by hyponatremia involve two mechanisms. The first mechanism is a change in cell excitability. As the sodium level in the blood and other extracellular fluid

TABLE 16-3 Common Causes of Hyponatremia

Actual Sodium Deficits

Increased Sodium Excretion
- Excessive diaphoresis
- Diuretics (high-ceiling diuretics)
- Wound drainage (especially gastrointestinal)
- Decreased secretion of aldosterone
- Hyperlipidemia
- Renal disease (scarred distal convoluted tubule)

Inadequate Sodium Intake
- Nothing by mouth
- Low-salt diet

Relative Sodium Deficits

Dilution of Serum Sodium
- Excessive ingestion of hypotonic fluids
- Psychogenic polydipsia
- Freshwater drowning
- Renal failure (nephrotic syndrome)
- Irrigation with hypotonic fluids
- Syndrome of inappropriate antidiuretic hormone secretion
- Hyperglycemia
- Congestive heart failure

(ECF) decreases, the difference in sodium levels between the ECF and the cellular fluid also decreases. Less sodium is present to move across the excitable membrane, resulting in slower membrane depolarization. The second mechanism is the movement of water from the ECF space into the cells. Cells swell, and their functions are impaired.

Many conditions can lead to hyponatremia (Table 16-3). Hyponatremia can result from the loss of total body sodium, the movement of sodium from the blood to other fluid spaces, or the dilution of serum sodium from excessive water in the plasma.

CHART 16-7

KEY FEATURES of Hyponatremia

Cardiovascular Manifestations*
- Normovolemic
  - Rapid pulse rate
  - Normal blood pressure
- Hypovolemic
  - Rapid pulse rate
  - Pulse quality thready and weak
  - Hypotension
  - Central venous pressure normal or low
  - Flat neck veins in supine position
- Hypervolemic
  - Rapid, bounding pulse
  - Central venous pressure normal or elevated
  - Blood pressure normal or elevated

Respiratory Manifestations
- Late manifestations related to skeletal muscle weakness
  - Shallow, ineffective respiratory movements
- Hypervolemia
- Pulmonary edema
  - Rapid, shallow respiration
  - Moist crackles

Neuromuscular Manifestations
- Generalized skeletal muscle weakness
- Diminished deep tendon reflexes

Cerebral Manifestations
- Personality changes
- Headache

Renal Manifestations
- Increased urine output
- Decreased urine specific gravity

Gastrointestinal Manifestations
- Increased motility
- Nausea
- Hyperactive bowel sounds
- Diarrhea

*Symptoms vary with changes in vascular volume.

COLLABORATIVE MANAGEMENT

Assessment

The manifestations of hyponatremia are caused by its effects on excitable cellular activity. The cells especially affected are those involved in cerebral, neuromuscular, and gastric smooth muscle functions (Chart 16-7).

CEREBRAL MANIFESTATIONS. Changes in cerebral function are the most obvious problems of hyponatremia. Because these changes may be seen as either depressed activity or excessive activity (and sometimes both), establishing the client's usual cognitive and behavioral patterns is essential. Behavioral changes result from cerebral edema and increased intracranial pressure. Closely observe and document the client's behavior and level of consciousness.

NEUROMUSCULAR MANIFESTATIONS. Assess the client's neuromuscular status during each nursing shift for changes from baseline. The neuromuscular response to hyponatremia is general muscle weakness. Muscle tone and deep tendon reflexes diminish.

Muscle weakness occurs bilaterally and is worse in the legs and arms. Assess deep tendon reflexes by lightly tapping the patellar (knee) tendons and Achilles (heel) tendons with a reflex hammer and document the degree of reflex movement. The technique for assessing motor strength and reflexes is described in depth in Chapter 44.

GASTROINTESTINAL MANIFESTATIONS. The smooth muscle of the gastrointestinal (GI) system responds to decreased serum sodium levels with increased motility, causing nausea, diarrhea, and abdominal cramping. Assess the GI system by listening to bowel sounds and observing stools. Bowel sounds are hyperactive, with rushes and gurgles over the splenic flexure and in the lower left quadrant. Bowel movements are frequent and watery. Peristaltic movements may be palpated through the abdominal wall and may even be visible on the abdominal surface.

CARDIOVASCULAR MANIFESTATIONS. Hyponatremia has little direct effect on cardiac muscle contractility; however, cardiac output is changed with hyponatremia. When hyponatremia occurs with changes in blood volume, these fluid changes alter cardiac function. The cardiac responses to hyponatremia and **hypovolemia** (decreased plasma volume, or fluid deficit) are a rapid, weak, thready pulse. Peripheral pulses are difficult to palpate and are easily blocked with light pressure. Neck veins are flat when the client is in the supine position. Blood pressure, especially diastolic pressure, is decreased. The client may have severe hypotension when moving from a

CHART 16-8

NIC INTERVENTION ACTIVITIES for The Client with Sodium Imbalances

Electrolyte Management: Hyponatremia: *Promotion of sodium balance and prevention of complications resulting from serum sodium levels lower than desired*

- Monitor for electrolyte imbalances associated with hyponatremia (e.g., hypokalemia, metabolic acidosis, and hypoglycemia), as appropriate.
- Monitor for renal loss of sodium (oliguria).
- Monitor intake and output.
- Weigh client daily and monitor trends.
- Monitor for indications of fluid overload/retention (e.g., crackles, elevated CVP or PCWP, edema, neck vein distention, and ascites), as appropriate.
- Administer hypertonic (3% to 5%) saline at 3 mL/kg/hr or per policy for rapid correction of hyponatremia, as appropriate.
- Maintain fluid restriction, as appropriate.
- Monitor for neurologic and/or neuromuscular manifestations of hyponatremia (e.g., lethargy, increased ICP, confusion, headache, seizures, coma, fatigue, tremors, apprehension, muscle weakness, and hyperreflexia).
- Monitor for cardiovascular manifestations of hyponatremia (e.g., elevated blood pressure, cold and clammy skin, and hypo- or hypervolemia).

Electrolyte Management: Hypernatremia: *Promotion of sodium balance and prevention of complications resulting from serum sodium levels higher than desired*

- Monitor for indications of dehydration (e.g., decreased sweating, decreased urine, decreased skin turgor, and dry mucous membranes).
- Monitor vital signs, as appropriate.
- Weigh client daily and monitor trends.
- Provide comfort measures to decrease thirst.
- Maintain patent IV access.
- Monitor intake and output.
- Provide frequent oral hygiene.
- Administer isotonic (0.9%) saline, hypotonic (0.45%) saline, hypotonic (5%) dextrose, or diuretics, as appropriate, based on fluid status and urine osmolality.
- Maintain sodium restrictions.

NIC intervention activities selected from Dochterman, J.M., & Bulechek, G.M. (Eds.). (2004). *Nursing interventions classification (NIC)* (4th ed.). St. Louis: Mosby. No part of this work is to be altered without prior written permission from the Publisher.
CVP, Central venous pressure; *ICP,* intracranial pressure.

lying or sitting position to a standing position. The central venous pressure is low.

When hyponatremia occurs with **hypervolemia** (increased plasma volume or fluid excess), cardiac changes include a full pulse with normal or high blood pressure. Central venous pressure is normal or high depending on how well the left ventricle handles the extra fluid. Peripheral pulses are full and difficult to block; however, they may not be palpable if edema is present.

Interventions

Interventions with drug therapy and diet therapy aim to restore serum sodium levels to normal and prevent complications. Chart 16-8 lists NIC interventions for electrolyte management of hyponatremia.

Drug Therapy. Drug therapy can restore serum sodium levels to normal. Drug therapy regimens vary depending on whether or not fluid imbalance occurs with hyponatremia and how fast the imbalance has developed. In chronic hyponatremia, sodium is replaced slowly.

When hyponatremia occurs with a fluid deficit (hypovolemia), IV saline infusions are prescribed to restore both sodium and fluid volume. Severe hyponatremia may be treated with small-volume infusions of hypertonic (2% to 3%) saline. The infusions are delivered through a controller to prevent accidental increases in infusion rate. Monitor the infusion rate and the client's response.

When hyponatremia occurs with fluid excess, drug therapy includes giving osmotic diuretics that promote the excretion of water rather than sodium, such as mannitol (Osmitrol). Assess the client hourly for signs of excessive fluid loss, potassium loss, and increased sodium levels.

Drug therapy for hyponatremia caused by inappropriate secretion of antidiuretic hormone (ADH) includes agents that antagonize ADH, such as lithium and demeclocycline (Declomycin).

Diet Therapy. Diet therapy can help restore normal sodium balance in mild hyponatremia. Table 14-6 lists the sodium content of common foods. Collaborate with the dietitian to teach the client about which foods to increase in the diet. Therapy involves increasing oral sodium intake and restricting oral fluid intake. Fluid restriction may be needed long-term when overhydration is the cause of the hyponatremia or when renal fluid excretion is impaired. Measure fluid intake and output and reinforce the purpose of the fluid restriction.

Hypernatremia

PATHOPHYSIOLOGY

Hypernatremia is a serum sodium level over 145 mEq/L. High serum sodium levels can be caused by or can cause changes in fluid volumes. Table 16-4 lists common causes of hypernatremia.

As serum sodium level rises, a larger difference in sodium levels occurs between the extracellular fluid (ECF) and the intracellular fluid (ICF). More sodium is present

TABLE 16-4 Common Causes of Hypernatremia

Actual Sodium Excesses

Decreased Sodium Excretion
- Hyperaldosteronism
- Renal failure
- Corticosteroids
- Cushing's syndrome or disease

Increased Sodium Intake
- Excessive oral sodium ingestion
- Excessive administration of sodium-containing IV fluids

Relative Sodium Excesses

Decreased Water Intake
- Nothing by mouth

Increased Water Loss
- Increased rate of metabolism
- Fever
- Hyperventilation
- Infection
- Excessive diaphoresis
- Watery diarrhea
- Dehydration

to move rapidly across cell membranes during depolarization. With mild hypernatremia, most excitable tissues are excited more easily. This condition is called **irritability** and excitable tissues overrespond to stimuli. In addition, the osmolarity of the ECF increases as the level of sodium increases. This problem causes water to move from the cells into the ECF to dilute the hyperosmolar ECF. Therefore when hypernatremia persists or worsens, compensatory actions cause severe cellular dehydration. The dehydrated excitable tissues may no longer be able to respond to stimuli.

CHART 16-9

KEY FEATURES of Hypernatremia

Cardiovascular Manifestations
- Decreased myocardial contractility
- Diminished cardiac output
- Heart rate and blood pressure respond to vascular volume

Respiratory Manifestations
- Problems associated with pulmonary edema when hypernatremia is accompanied by hypervolemia

Central Nervous System Manifestations*
- Hypernatremia and normovolemia or hypovolemia
  - Increased neural activity
  - Agitation, confusion, seizures
- Hypernatremia and hypervolemia
  - Decreased neural activity
  - Lethargy, stupor, coma

Neuromuscular Manifestations
- Mild or early hypernatremia
  - Spontaneous muscle twitches
  - Irregular contractions
- Severe or late hypernatremia
  - Skeletal muscle weakness
  - Diminished or absent deep tendon reflexes

Renal Manifestations
- Decreased urine output
- Increased urine specific gravity

Integumentary Manifestations
- Dry, flaky skin
- Presence or absence of edema related to accompanying fluid volume changes

*Upper neural function changes are related to volume changes as well as sodium increases.

COLLABORATIVE MANAGEMENT

Assessment

The manifestations of hypernatremia vary with the severity of imbalance and whether a fluid imbalance is also present. Rapid increases in serum sodium cause more obvious and severe symptoms. Gradual increases in serum sodium may produce no observable physical changes, even when sodium levels increase to ranges that are well above normal. The manifestations of hypernatremia involve changes in excitable membrane activity, especially cerebral, neuromuscular, and cardiac function (Chart 16-9).

CENTRAL NERVOUS SYSTEM MANIFESTATIONS. Altered cerebral function is the most common problem of hypernatremia. Assess the client's mental status for attention span, recall of recent events, and cognitive function. In hypernatremia with normal or decreased fluid volumes, the client may have a short attention span and be agitated or confused about recent events. Manic episodes or seizures may occur if serum sodium continues to rise. When hypernatremia occurs with blood volume overload, the client may be lethargic, drowsy, stuporous, and even comatose.

NEUROMUSCULAR MANIFESTATIONS. Skeletal muscles responses vary with the degree of sodium increases. Mild rises cause muscle twitching and irregular muscle contractions. As hypernatremia worsens, the muscles and nerves are less able to respond to a stimulus. The muscles become progressively weaker with rigid paralysis. Deep tendon reflexes are reduced or absent. Muscle weakness occurs bilaterally and has no specific pattern. Assess neuromuscular status by observing for twitching in muscle groups. Assess muscle strength by having the client perform handgrip and arm flexion against resistance. Assess peripheral nerve responses by lightly tapping the patellar (knee) tendons and Achilles (heel) tendons with a reflex hammer and measuring the movement.

CARDIOVASCULAR MANIFESTATIONS. Increased serum sodium slows the movement of calcium into the heart cells, which decreases contractility. Assess cardiac status by measuring blood pressure and the rate and quality of the apical and peripheral pulses. Pulse rate and blood pressure may be normal, above normal, or below normal, depending on the fluid volume and how rapidly the imbalance occurred.

Pulse rate is increased in clients with hypernatremia and hypovolemia. Peripheral pulses are difficult to palpate and are easily blocked. Hypotension and severe orthostatic (postural) hypotension are present, and pulse pressure is reduced.

Clients with hypernatremia and hypervolemia have slow to normal bounding pulses. Peripheral pulses are full and difficult to block. Neck veins are distended, even with the client in the upright position. Blood pressure, especially diastolic blood pressure, is increased.

Common Nursing Diagnoses and Collaborative Problems

Nursing diagnoses and collaborative problems that may apply to clients with hypernatremia include the following:

- Excess Fluid Volume related to excess sodium intake
- Decreased Cardiac Output related to poor cardiac contractility
- Risk for Falls related to skeletal muscle weakness
- Impaired Memory related to fluid and electrolyte imbalances
- Readiness for Enhanced Nutrition related to the need for dietary sodium restrictions
- Potential for Pulmonary Edema

Interventions

Drug and diet therapies aim to prevent further increases in serum sodium and decrease high serum sodium levels. Chart 16-8 lists NIC interventions for electrolyte management of hypernatremia. Other interventions used when sodium levels become life threatening include hemodialysis and blood ultrafiltration.

Drug Therapy. When hypernatremia is caused by fluid loss, drug therapy is used to restore fluid balance. Hypotonic IV infusions, usually 0.225% or 0.45% sodium chloride, are prescribed. Hypernatremia caused by fluid and sodium losses require fluid replacement with IV infusions of isotonic sodium chloride (NaCl) solutions. Hypernatremia caused by poor renal excretion of sodium requires drug therapy with diuretics that promote sodium loss, such as furosemide (Lasix, Furoside✱), bumetanide (Bumex), and ethacrynic acid (Edecrin). Assess the client hourly for symptoms of excessive fluid, sodium or potassium losses.

Diet Therapy. Mild hypernatremia can be prevented or corrected by ensuring adequate water intake among older adults or those who may not have self-access to water. Dietary sodium restriction may be needed to prevent sodium excess when renal problems are present. In addition, fluids must often be restricted. Collaborate with the dietitian to teach the client how to determine the sodium content of foods, beverages, and drugs. Stress the importance of adhering to the diet.

CALCIUM IMBALANCES

Hypocalcemia

PATHOPHYSIOLOGY

Hypocalcemia is a total serum calcium (Ca^{2+}) level below 9.0 mg/dL or 2.25 mmol/L. Calcium is stored in bone, with only a small amount of total body calcium present in extracellular fluid (ECF). Because the normal blood level of calcium is so low, any change in calcium levels has major effects on function.

Calcium is an excitable membrane stabilizer, regulating depolarization and the generation of action potentials. Calcium decreases sodium movement across excitable membranes, decreasing the rate of depolarization. Low serum calcium levels increase sodium movement across excitable membranes, allowing depolarization to occur more easily and at inappropriate times.

TABLE 16-5 Common Causes of Hypocalcemia

Actual Calcium Deficits

Inhibition of Calcium Absorption from the Gastrointestinal Tract

- Inadequate oral intake of calcium
- Lactose intolerance
- Malabsorption syndromes
  - Celiac sprue
  - Crohn's disease
- Inadequate intake of vitamin D
- End-stage renal disease

Increased Calcium Excretion

- Renal failure—polyuric phase
- Diarrhea
- Steatorrhea
- Wound drainage (especially gastrointestinal)

Relative Calcium Deficits

Conditions That Decrease the Ionized Fraction of Calcium

- Hyperproteinemia
- Alkalosis
- Calcium chelators or binders
  - Citrate
  - Mithramycin
  - Penicillamine
  - Sodium cellulose phosphate (Calcibind)
  - Aredia
- Acute pancreatitis
- Hyperphosphatemia
- Immobility

Endocrine Disturbances

- Removal or destruction of parathyroid glands
  - Thyroidectomy
  - Irradiation of thyroid
  - Strangulation
  - Neck injuries

Hypocalcemia is caused by many chronic and acute conditions as well as medical or surgical treatments. Table 16-5 lists the common causes of hypocalcemia.

Actual calcium loss (a reduction in total body calcium) occurs when the absorption of calcium from the gastrointestinal (GI) tract slows or when calcium is lost from the body. Relative calcium loss causes total body calcium amounts to remain normal while serum calcium levels are low. This type of hypocalcemia occurs when the free or ionized (unbound) calcium in the body is reduced or when parathyroid gland function is decreased.

CULTURAL CONSIDERATIONS

Many black and Asian clients have a lactose intolerance caused by a deficiency of the enzyme lactase. These clients cannot use the nutrients in milk and have cramping, diarrhea, and abdominal pain after ingesting dairy products. Dairy products, especially milk, are common and rich source of both calcium and vitamin D. Clients with lactose intolerance may, therefore, have difficulty obtaining enough calcium and vitamin D from other sources to maintain normal calcium levels in the blood and bones.

WOMEN'S HEALTH CONSIDERATIONS

Postmenopausal women are at risk for calcium loss. This problem is related to reduced weight-bearing activities and a decrease in estrogen levels. In general, women are

Continued

smaller framed than men and the female skeleton does not bear as much weight as the male skeleton. As they age, many women decrease weight-bearing activities such as running and walking. Osteoporosis occurs when weight-bearing activity decreases or is limited. In addition, the estrogen secretion that protects against osteoporosis diminishes. All of these factors increase the risk for calcium loss in postmenopausal women.

CONSIDERATIONS FOR OLDER ADULTS

Older adults are at risk for most electrolyte imbalances as a result of age-related organ changes. For example, older adults have less total body water than younger adults, and therefore are more at risk for fluid imbalances. Older adults are more likely to be taking drugs that affect fluid or electrolyte balance. Some older adults have dietary calcium or vitamin D deficits because of reduced income or problems with obtaining, preparing, or eating food.

COLLABORATIVE MANAGEMENT

Assessment

The diet history is important to assess for the risk of hypocalcemia. Ask the client about his or her intake of calcium-containing foods and whether a calcium supplement is taken regularly (see Table 14-8).

One indicator of hypocalcemia is a report of frequent, painful muscle spasms ("charley horses") in the calf or foot during rest or sleep. Other information that indicates possible hypocalcemia is a history of recent orthopedic surgery or bone healing. Endocrine disturbances and treatments are risk factors for hypocalcemia. A history of thyroid surgery, therapeutic irradiation of the upper middle chest and neck area, or a recent anterior neck injury increase the risk for hypocalcemia. The most common manifestations of hypocalcemia are caused by overstimulation of the nerves and muscles (Chart 16-10).

NEUROMUSCULAR MANIFESTATIONS. The client usually notices symptoms in the limbs, with changes occurring first in the hands and feet. Paresthesias occur at first, with sensations of tingling and numbness. If hypocalcemia continues or worsens, actual muscle twitching or painful cramps and spasms occur. Paresthesias may also affect the lips, nose, and ears. These problems may signal the onset of neuromuscular overstimulation and tetany.

Assess for hypocalcemia by testing for **Trousseau's** and **Chvostek's signs.** To test for Trousseau's sign, place a blood pressure cuff around the upper arm, inflate the cuff to greater than the client's systolic pressure, and keep the cuff inflated for 1 to 4 minutes. Under these hypoxic conditions, a positive Trousseau's sign occurs when the hand and fingers go into spasm in palmar flexion (Figure 16-2). To test for Chvostek's sign, tap the face just below and in front of the ear (over the facial nerve) to trigger facial twitching of one side of the mouth, nose, and cheek (Figure 16-3).

CARDIOVASCULAR MANIFESTATIONS. With hypocalcemia, the heart rate may be slower or slightly faster than normal, with a weak, thready pulse. Severe hypocalcemia causes severe hypotension and electrocardiographic (ECG) changes, including a prolonged ST interval and a prolonged QT interval.

INTESTINAL MANIFESTATIONS. Hypocalcemia increases peristaltic activity. Auscultate the abdomen for hyperactive bowel sounds. The client may report painful abdominal cramping and diarrhea.

Common Nursing Diagnoses and Collaborative Problems

Nursing diagnoses and collaborative problems that may apply to clients with hypocalcemia include the following:

- Acute Pain related to hypocalcemia-induced muscle spasms and hyperactive gastric motility
- Decreased Cardiac Output related to hypocalcemia-induced dysrhythmias or reduced myocardial contractility

CHART 16-10

KEY FEATURES of Hypocalcemia

Cardiovascular Manifestations
- Decreased heart rate
- Decreased myocardial contractility
- Diminished peripheral pulses
- Hypotension
- Electrocardiographic abnormalities
  - Prolonged ST interval
  - Prolonged QT interval

Respiratory Manifestations
- Not directly affected
- Respiratory failure or arrest can result from decreased respiratory movement because of muscle tetany or seizure activity

Neuromuscular Manifestations*
- Anxiety, irritability, psychosis
- Paresthesias followed by numbness
- Irritable skeletal muscles—twitches, cramps, tetany, seizures
- Hyperactive deep tendon reflexes
- Positive Trousseau's sign
- Positive Chvostek's sign

Gastrointestinal Manifestations
- Increased gastric motility
- Hyperactive bowel sounds
- Abdominal cramping
- Diarrhea

*The neuromuscular system is most profoundly affected by hypocalcemia.

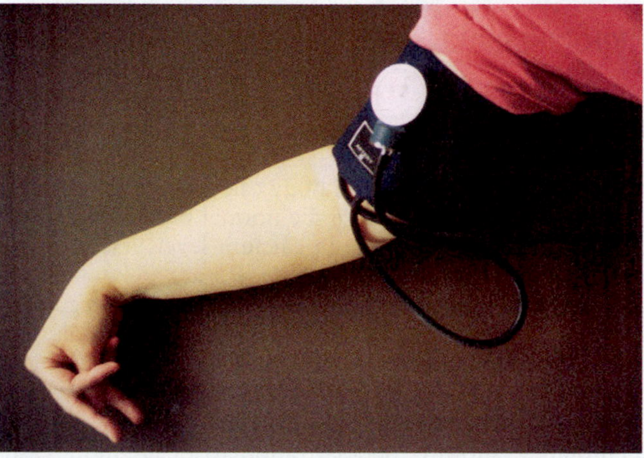

Figure 16-2 ■ Palmar flexion–positive Trousseau's sign in hypocalcemia.

- Deficient knowledge (dietary calcium) related to lack of exposure
- Risk for Injury related to bone density loss
- Readiness for Enhanced Nutrition related to the need to increase oral calcium intake

Interventions

Interventions aim to restore normal calcium levels and prevent complications. Chart 16-11 lists NIC interventions for electrolyte management of hypocalcemia. Interventions include drug therapy, diet therapy, reducing environmental stimuli, and preventing injury.

Drug Therapy. Drug therapy for hypocalcemia includes direct calcium replacement, drugs that enhance the absorption of calcium, and drugs that decrease nerve and muscle responses. Chart 16-12 lists the different drug types used to manage hypocalcemia.

Diet Therapy. A high-calcium diet is needed for clients with mild hypocalcemia and for those with chronic conditions that cause them to be at continuous risk for hypocalcemia. Collaborate with the dietitian to assist the client in selecting calcium-rich foods. The calcium content of common foods is listed in Table 14-8.

Environmental Management. The excitable membranes of the nervous system and the skeletal system are overstimulated in hypocalcemia. Therefore you must reduce the stimulation of these systems.

Use seizure precautions for the client with hypocalcemia. Such precautions include padding the siderails of the bed and keeping emergency equipment (e.g., oxygen and suction) at the bedside. Keep an emergency cart equipped with emergency drugs and an endotracheal tray just outside the client's room.

Injury Prevention. The client with long-standing calcium loss may have brittle, fragile bones that fracture easily and cause little pain. When lifting or moving a client with fragile bones, use a lift sheet rather than pulling the client. Observe for normal range of joint motion and for any unusual surface bumps or depressions over bony areas.

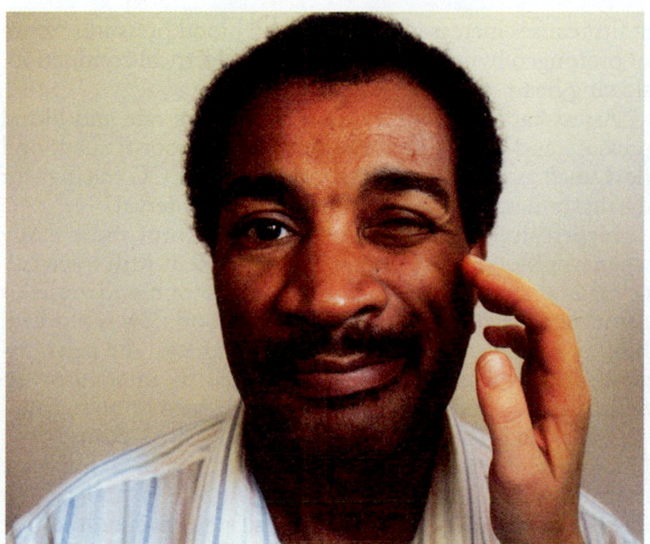

Figure 16-3 ■ Facial muscle response–positive Chvostek's sign in hypocalcemia.

Hypercalcemia

PATHOPHYSIOLOGY

Hypercalcemia is a total serum calcium level above 10.5 mg/dL or 2.75 mmol/L. Because the normal range for serum calcium is so narrow, even small increases have severe effects. Although the effects of hypercalcemia occur first in excitable tissues, all systems are affected to some degree.

Hypercalcemia means either that the amount of serum calcium is so great that the normal calcium-controlling mechanisms cannot keep pace or that at least one mechanism is not functioning properly. Hypercalcemia causes excitable tissues to be less sensitive to normal stimuli thus requiring a stronger stimulus to function. The excitable tissues affected most by hypercalcemia are the heart, muscles, nerves, and intestinal smooth muscles.

CHART 16-11

NIC INTERVENTION ACTIVITIES for The Client with Calcium Imbalances

Electrolyte Management: Hypocalcemia: *Promotion of calcium balance and prevention of complications resulting from serum calcium levels lower than desired*

- Monitor trends in serum levels of calcium (e.g., ionized calcium), as available.
- Monitor fluid status, including intake and output, as appropriate.
- Administer appropriate prescribed calcium salt (e.g., calcium carbonate, calcium chloride, and calcium gluconate), as indicated.
- Monitor for side effects of IV administration of ionized calcium (e.g., calcium chloride), such as thrombophlebitis, soft tissue damage with extravasation, clotting, and thrombus formation, as appropriate.
- Encourage intake of calcium (e.g., dairy products, seafood, nuts, broccoli, spinach, and supplements), as appropriate.
- Provide adequate intake of vitamin D (e.g., vitamin supplement and organ meats) to facilitate GI absorption of calcium, as appropriate.
- Monitor for neuromuscular manifestations of hypocalcemia (e.g., tetany, muscle twitching, cramping, grimacing, seizure, altered deep tendon reflexes, and spasm).
- Monitor for cardiovascular manifestations of hypocalcemia (e.g., decreased contractility, decreased cardiac output, hypotension, lengthened ST segment, and prolonged QT interval).
- Monitor for overcorrection and hypercalcemia.

Electrolyte Management: Hypercalcemia: *Promotion of calcium balance and prevention of complications resulting from serum calcium levels higher than desired*

- Monitor intake and output.
- Monitor trends in serum levels of calcium (e.g., ionized calcium), as available.
- Monitor for fluid overload resulting from hydration therapy (e.g., daily weight, urine output, jugular vein distention, lung sounds, and right atrial pressure), as appropriate.
- Monitor for neuromuscular manifestations of hypercalcemia (e.g., weakness, malaise, paresthesias, myalgia, hypotonia, decreased deep tendon reflexes, and poor coordination).
- Administer indomethacin (Indocin), calcitonin, or plicamycin (Mithracin), as appropriate.
- Encourage mobilization to prevent bone resorption.
- Monitor for recurring hypercalcemia 1 to 3 days after cessation of therapeutic measures.

NIC intervention activities selected from Dochterman, J.M., & Bulechek, G.M. (Eds.). (2004). *Nursing interventions classification (NIC)* (4th ed.). St. Louis: Mosby.
GI, Gastrointestinal.

CHART 16-12

DRUG THERAPY for Hypocalcemia

Drug	Precautions
Oral Calcium Supplements	
Calcium carbonate Calcium citrate Calcium gluconate Calcium lactate	Dose must be increased in older clients because of decreased intestinal absorption. Use with thiazide diuretics can increase the risk for hypercalcemia. Use with phenytoin decreases the bioavailability of both drugs; phenytoin should not be given within 3 hours of calcium administration.
Intravenous Calcium	
Calcium acetate Calcium chloride Calcium gluconate	All must be administered slowly, not to exceed 27 g/min. Clients should be monitored for electrocardiographic changes during administration. Observe the client for infiltration; calcium is a severe tissue irritant/vesicant. There is a potential for hypercalcemia and hypomagnesemia. The injection should be warmed to body temperature before administration.
Agents That Increase Calcium Absorption	
Aluminum hydroxide	This agent reduces serum phosphorus levels, causing the countereffect of increasing calcium levels; there is a potential for hypophosphatemia. Signs and symptoms include bradycardia, decreased deep tendon reflexes, shortness of breath, and confusion.
Vitamin D Alfacalcidol✱ Calcifediol Calcitriol Dihydrotachysterol	This agent increases the intestinal absorption of calcium; there is a potential for hypercalcemia. This is a fat-soluble vitamin and is stored to some degree; there is a risk for vitamin D toxicity resulting in renal failure and/or cardiac failure.
Agents That Reduce Nerve and Skeletal Muscle Excitability	
Magnesium sulfate	This agent is a tissue irritant; the preferred route of administration is intravenous. There is a potential for hypermagnesemia; signs and symptoms of toxicity include bradycardia, flushing, headache, nausea, vomiting, shortness of breath, hypotension.
Methocarbamol Robaxin Carbacot Metaxalone Skelaxin Orphenadrine Banflex Flexoject Myolin Diazepam Valium Vivol✱ E-Pam✱ Carisoprodol Soma Vanadom	These agents act at the level of the central nervous system to decrease skeletal muscle activity. All have some sedative effect. All have some risk for psychological dependency and abuse.

Calcium is needed by many of the enzymes involved in blood-clotting. Hypercalcemia causes faster clotting times. Clots may form when they are not needed to control bleeding. Excessive clotting related to hypercalcemia occurs more easily in vessels with slow or blocked blood flow.

Causes of hypercalcemia include increased absorption of calcium, decreased excretion of calcium, and increased bone resorption of calcium (Table 16-6).

COLLABORATIVE MANAGEMENT

Assessment

The manifestations of hypercalcemia are related to both the severity of the imbalance and how quickly the imbalance occurred. The client with a mild but rapidly occurring calcium excess usually has more severe problems than the client whose hypercalcemia is severe but has developed slowly. Chart 16-13 lists the common manifestations of hypercalcemia.

CARDIOVASCULAR MANIFESTATIONS. The most serious and life-threatening problems of hypercalcemia are changes in cardiac function. Mild hypercalcemia at first causes increased heart rate and blood pressure. Severe or prolonged hypercalcemia depresses electrical conduction, slowing heart rate.

Assess cardiac status by measuring pulse rate and blood pressure and observing for indications of poor tissue blood flow, such as cyanosis and pallor. Examine ECG tracings for dysrhythmias, especially a shortened QT interval.

Hypercalcemia allows blood clots to form more easily whenever blood flow is poor. Thus the client with hypercalcemia is at risk for clot formation in areas of blood vessel or tissue damage and in vessels in which blood flow is blocked. Blood clotting is more likely in the lower legs, the pelvic region, areas where blood flow is blocked by internal or external constrictions, and where venous obstruction occurs.

Assess each client for slowed or impaired blood flow. Measure and record calf circumferences with a soft tape measure. Ask the client to alternately dorsiflex and plantar flex the ankles and state whether calf pain occurs in either position **(Homan's sign).** Assess the feet for temperature, color, and capillary refill to determine the blood flow to and from the area.

TABLE 16-6 Common Causes of Hypercalcemia

Actual Calcium Excesses

Increased Calcium Absorption
- Excessive oral intake of calcium
- Excessive oral intake of vitamin D

Decreased Calcium Excretion
- Renal failure
- Use of thiazide diuretics

Relative Calcium Excesses

Increased Bone Resorption of Calcium
- Hyperparathyroidism
- Malignancy
    - Direct invasion (cancers of breast, lung, prostate, and osteoclastic bone and multiple myeloma)
    - Indirect resorption (liver cancer, small cell lung cancer, and cancer of the adrenal gland)
- Hyperthyroidism
- Immobility
- Use of glucocorticoids

Hemoconcentration
- Dehydration
- Use of lithium
- Adrenal insufficiency

NEUROMUSCULAR MANIFESTATIONS. The neuromuscular manifestations include severe muscle weakness and decreased deep tendon reflexes without paresthesia. Central nervous system manifestations include an altered level of consciousness that can range from confusion and lethargy to coma. Psychiatric problems also can occur.

INTESTINAL MANIFESTATIONS. Decreased peristalsis is an early manifestation of hypercalcemia. The client may have constipation, anorexia, nausea, vomiting, and abdominal pain. Bowel sounds are hypoactive or absent. Assess the intestinal tract by listening for bowel sounds in all four abdominal quadrants. The abdomen increases in size because the intestinal contents remain in the tract instead of being moved forward. Assess abdominal size by measuring abdominal girth with a soft tape measure in a line circling the abdomen at the umbilicus.

RENAL MANIFESTATIONS. Hypercalcemia causes increased urine output and leads to dehydration. Chronic hypercalcemia may cause renal **calculi** (stones) to form in the kidney, because the excess calcium precipitates out of solution. Measure intake and output, assess voided urine for blood or cloudiness, and strain the urine for stones.

Interventions

Interventions for hypercalcemia aim to reduce serum calcium levels through drug therapy and dialysis. Chart 16-11 lists NIC interventions for electrolyte management of hypercalcemia.

Drug Therapy. IV solutions containing calcium are stopped. Discontinue giving oral drugs containing calcium or vitamin D (e.g., calcium-based antacids).

Fluid volume replacement can help restore normal serum calcium levels. IV normal saline (0.9% sodium chloride) is usually prescribed because sodium increases the excretion of calcium in the urine.

Thiazide diuretics are discontinued and are replaced with diuretics that enhance the excretion of calcium, such as furosemide (Lasix, Furoside✱). Calcium chelators (calcium binders) help lower serum calcium levels. Such drugs include plicamycin (Mithracin) and penicillamine (Cuprimine, Pendramine✱).

CHART 16-13

KEY FEATURES of
Hypercalcemia

Cardiovascular Manifestations
- Increased heart rate (early phase)
- Increased blood pressure
- Bounding, full peripheral pulses
- Electrocardiographic abnormalities
    - Shortened ST segment
    - Widened T wave
- Potentiation of digoxin-associated toxicities
- Decreased clotting time
- Late phase
    - Bradycardia
    - Cardiac arrest, sinus arrest

Respiratory Manifestations
- Ineffective respiratory movement related to profound skeletal muscle weakness

Neuromuscular Manifestations
- Disorientation, lethargy, coma
- Profound muscle weakness
- Diminished or absent deep tendon reflexes

Renal Manifestations
- Increased urine output
- Dehydration
- Formation of renal calculi

Gastrointestinal Manifestations
- Decreased motility
- Hypoactive bowel sounds
- Anorexia, nausea
- Abdominal distention
- Constipation

Drugs to prevent hypercalcemia include agents that inhibit calcium resorption from bone, such as phosphorus, calcitonin (Calcimar), bisphosphonates (etidronate), and prostaglandin synthesis inhibitors (aspirin, nonsteroidal anti-inflammatory drugs).

Dialysis. When severe hypercalcemia causes life-threatening cardiac problems, drug therapy may not reduce serum calcium levels fast enough to prevent death. Dialysis (either hemodialysis or peritoneal dialysis) or blood ultrafiltration may be necessary.

Cardiac Monitoring. Continuously monitor clients with hypercalcemia to identify dysrhythmias and decreased cardiac output. Compare recent electrocardiogram (ECG) tracings with the client's baseline tracings. Especially look for changes in the T waves and the QT interval as well as changes in rate and rhythm.

PHOSPHORUS IMBALANCES

Hypophosphatemia

PATHOPHYSIOLOGY

Hypophosphatemia is a serum phosphorus level below 3.0 mEq/L. Even though the serum phosphorus level has a narrow range of normal (3.0 to 4.5 mEq/L), body functions are not usually impaired with rapid, wide changes in serum phosphorus levels. Reduced function occurs more often with chronic hypophosphatemia.

Most of the effects of hypophosphatemia are related to decreased energy metabolism and imbalances of other electrolytes and body fluids. Because of the reciprocal relationship between phosphorus and calcium, decreases in serum phosphorus levels cause increases in serum calcium levels.

Three main processes lead to decreased serum phosphorus levels: decreased absorption of phosphorus, increased excretion of phosphorus, and intracellular phosphorus shift (Table 16-7).

COLLABORATIVE MANAGEMENT

Assessment

The manifestations of hypophosphatemia occur when low serum phosphorus levels are severe or prolonged. Acute manifestations of hypophosphatemia are related to the decreased amounts of high-energy compounds (e.g., adenosine triphosphate [ATP]) needed to perform normal metabolic functions. Manifestations are most apparent in the cardiac, musculoskeletal, hematologic, and central nervous systems (Chart 16-14).

CARDIOVASCULAR MANIFESTATIONS. Cardiac changes include decreased stroke volume and decreased cardiac output. Peripheral pulses are slow, difficult to find, and easy to block. Cardiac depression is caused by low stores of intracellular energy. Without sufficient energy in myocardial cells, contractions are weak and ineffective. Prolonged hypophosphatemia causes progressive but reversible cardiac muscle damage.

MUSCULOSKELETAL MANIFESTATIONS. Hypophosphatemia weakens skeletal muscles and may cause acute muscle breakdown **(rhabdomyolysis).** The weakness is generalized, and paresthesias usually are not present. When skeletal muscle weakness becomes profound, respiratory movements are ineffective, leading to respiratory failure. Assess for muscle strength and observe respiratory effort.

The manifestations of chronic hypophosphatemia are most evident in the skeletal system. Bone density is decreased, which leads to fractures and changes in bone shape. These changes are caused by the bone calcium loss that occurs with hypophosphatemia. Assess the client for unusual lumps or depressions over bony areas that indicate bone fractures.

CENTRAL NERVOUS SYSTEM MANIFESTATIONS. Central nervous system manifestations are not apparent until hypophosphatemia is severe. These first appear as irritability and may progress to seizure activity followed by coma.

Interventions

Discontinue drugs that promote hypophosphatemia (e.g., antacids, osmotic diuretics, and calcium supplements). Oral replacement of phosphorus along with a vitamin D supplement may correct moderate hypophosphatemia or prevent hypophosphatemia in at risk clients. IV phosphorus is given only when serum phosphorus levels fall below 1 mg/dL and the client has serious manifestations. Infuse IV phosphorus slowly because the problems caused by hyperphosphatemia are equally serious.

Diet therapy involves increasing the intake of phosphorus-rich foods while decreasing the intake of calcium-rich foods (Chart 16-15).

TABLE 16-7 Common Causes of Phosphorus Imbalance

Hypophosphatemia

Insufficient Phosphorus Intake
- Malnutrition
- Starvation
- Use of aluminum hydroxide-based antacids
- Use of magnesium-based antacids

Increased Phosphorus Excretion
- Hyperparathyroidism
- Hypercalcemia
- Renal failure
- Malignancy

Intracellular Shift
- Hyperglycemia
- Hyperalimentation
- Respiratory alkalosis
- Uncontrolled diabetes mellitus
- Alcohol abuse

Hyperphosphatemia
- Decreased renal excretion resulting from renal insufficiency
- Tumor lysis syndrome
- Increased intake of phosphorus
- Hypoparathyroidism

CHART 16-14

KEY FEATURES of Hypophosphatemia

Cardiovascular Manifestations
- Decreased contractility
- Cardiomyopathy (reversible)

Respiratory Manifestations
- Shallow respirations

Musculoskeletal Manifestations
- Weakness
- Rhabdomyolysis
- Decreased deep tendon reflexes

Central Nervous System Manifestations
- Irritability
- Confusion
- Seizures

Hematologic Manifestations
- Increased bleeding
- Decreased platelet aggregation
- Immunosuppression

CHART 16-15

CLIENT EDUCATION GUIDE
Dietary Management of Hypophosphatemia

You Should Avoid	You May Eat
Milk	Fish
Cheese	Beef
Yogurt	Chicken
Collard greens	Pork
Rhubarb	Organ meats
	Nuts
	Whole-grain breads and cereals

Hyperphosphatemia

PATHOPHYSIOLOGY

Hyperphosphatemia is a serum phosphorus level above 4.5 mEq/L. Serum phosphorus levels above normal are well tolerated by most body systems.

The problems caused by hyperphosphatemia center on the hypocalcemia that results when serum phosphorus levels increase. These problems include increased membrane excitability to the extent that membranes depolarize spontaneously.

Causes of increased serum phosphorus levels include renal insufficiency, certain cancer treatments, increased phosphorus intake, and hypoparathyroidism. Table 16-7 lists specific common causes of hyperphosphatemia.

COLLABORATIVE MANAGEMENT

Hyperphosphatemia causes few direct problems with body function. However, hypocalcemia is usually present because calcium and phosphorus ions exist in the blood in a balanced reciprocal relationship: when one increases, the other decreases. The hypocalcemia greatly alters many body system functions and can cause life-threatening side effects. Thus the management of hyperphosphatemia entails the management of hypocalcemia.

MAGNESIUM IMBALANCES

Hypomagnesemia

PATHOPHYSIOLOGY

Hypomagnesemia is a serum magnesium (Mg^{2+}) level below 1.2 mEq/L. Most problems leading to hypomagnesemia are caused by decreased magnesium intake or increased magnesium loss. As a result, hypomagnesemia reflects a decrease in the total body magnesium content.

TABLE 16-8 Common Causes of Magnesium Imbalance

Hypomagnesemia

Insufficient Magnesium Intake
- Malnutrition
- Starvation
- Diarrhea
- Steatorrhea
- Celiac disease
- Crohn's disease

Increased Magnesium Excretion
- Drugs (diuretics, aminoglycoside antibiotics, cisplatin, amphotericin B, cyclosporine)
- Citrate (blood products)
- Ethanol ingestion

Intracellular Movement of Magnesium
- Hyperglycemia
- Insulin administration
- Sepsis
- Alkalosis

Hypermagnesemia
- Increased magnesium intake
  - Magnesium-containing antacids and laxatives
  - IV magnesium replacement
- Decreased renal excretion of magnesium resulting from renal insufficiency

The effects of hypomagnesemia are caused by increased membrane excitability and the accompanying serum calcium and potassium imbalances. Excitable membranes, especially nerve cell membranes, may depolarize spontaneously.

Hypomagnesemia is caused by decreased absorption of dietary magnesium or increased renal magnesium excretion. Table 16-8 lists the specific causes of hypomagnesemia.

COLLABORATIVE MANAGEMENT

Assessment

Common clinical manifestations of hypomagnesemia are seen in the neuromuscular, central nervous, and intestinal systems (Chart 16-16).

NEUROMUSCULAR MANIFESTATIONS. The neuromuscular manifestations cause increased nerve impulse transmission. Normally, magnesium inhibits nerve impulse transmission at synapse areas. Decreased magnesium levels increase impulse transmission from nerve to nerve or from nerve to skeletal muscle. The client with hypomagnesemia has hyperactive deep tendon reflexes (+4), painful paresthesia (numbness and tingling), and tetanic muscle contractions. Positive Chvostek's and Trousseau's signs may be present because hypomagnesemia may occur with hypocalcemia (see the earlier discussion of these assessment signs under Neuromuscular Manifestations [Hypocalcemia], p. 238). Skeletal muscle weakness is present if intracellular magnesium levels

CHART 16-16

KEY FEATURES of Hypomagnesemia

Cardiovascular Manifestations
- Electrocardiographic changes
  - Tall T waves
  - Depressed ST segments
- Dysrhythmias
  - Ectopic beats
  - Ventricular tachycardia
  - Ventricular fibrillation
- Hypertension

Gastrointestinal Manifestations
- Decreased motility
- Anorexia
- Nausea
- Abdominal distention
- Decreased bowel sounds

Respiratory Manifestations
- Shallow respirations

Neuromuscular Manifestations
- Fasciculations
- Twitches
- Paresthesias
- Positive Trousseau's sign
- Positive Chvostek's sign
- Hyperreflexia
- Tetany
- Seizures

Central Nervous System Manifestations
- Irritability
- Confusion
- Psychosis

are also decreased. The client may have tetany and seizures as hypomagnesemia worsens.

CENTRAL NERVOUS SYSTEM MANIFESTATIONS. Central nervous system (CNS) manifestations are caused by increased nerve impulse transmission. Increased CNS irritability may present as psychological depression, psychosis, and confusion.

INTESTINAL MANIFESTATIONS. Intestinal manifestations are intestinal smooth muscle contraction. Clients have decreased gastric motility, anorexia, nausea, constipation, and abdominal distention. A paralytic ileus may occur when hypomagnesemia is severe.

Interventions

Interventions for hypomagnesemia aim to correct the magnesium imbalance and manage the specific problem that caused the hypomagnesemia. In addition, because hypocalcemia often occurs with hypomagnesemia, interventions also aim to restore normal serum calcium levels.

Discontinue drugs that promote magnesium loss, such as high-ceiling (loop) diuretics, osmotic diuretics, aminoglycoside antibiotics, and drugs containing phosphorus. Magnesium is replaced intravenously with magnesium sulfate ($MgSO_4$) when hypomagnesemia is severe. The IV route is used because $MgSO_4$ causes pain and tissue damage when injected intramuscularly. Assess deep tendon reflexes at least hourly in the client receiving IV magnesium to monitor effectiveness and prevent hypermagnesemia. Oral magnesium often causes diarrhea and can increase magnesium loss. If hypocalcemia is also present, drug therapy to increase serum calcium levels is prescribed.

Diet therapy consists of increasing the intake of foods that contain high amounts of magnesium (see Table 14-11).

Hypermagnesemia

PATHOPHYSIOLOGY

Hypermagnesemia is a serum magnesium level above 2.1 mEq/L. Magnesium is a membrane stabilizer. When magnesium excess occurs, excitable membranes are less excitable and need a stronger-than-normal stimulus to respond. With severe hypermagnesemia, excitable membranes may not respond to any stimulus.

Hypermagnesemia results from increased intake of magnesium coupled with decreased renal excretion of magnesium. Table 16-8 lists the specific causes of hypermagnesemia.

COLLABORATIVE MANAGEMENT

Assessment

Most manifestations of hypermagnesemia occur as a result of reduced membrane excitability. Manifestations usually are not apparent until serum magnesium levels exceed 4 mEq/L. The most common manifestations are seen in the cardiac, central nervous, and neuromuscular systems.

The cardiac manifestations include bradycardia, peripheral vasodilation, and hypotension. These problems become more severe as serum magnesium levels increase. Electrocardiographic (ECG) changes show a prolonged PR interval with a widened QRS complex. Bradycardia can be severe and cardiac arrest is possible. Hypotension with a wide pulse pressure is also severe, with a diastolic pressure lower than normal. *Clients with severe hypermagnesemia are in grave danger of cardiac arrest.*

Central nervous system manifestations result from depressed nerve impulse transmission. Clients may be drowsy or lethargic. Coma may occur if the hypermagnesemia is prolonged or severe.

Neuromuscular manifestations result from decreased nerve impulse transmission to the skeletal muscles. Deep tendon reflexes are reduced or even absent. Voluntary skeletal muscle contractions become progressively weaker and finally stop.

Hypermagnesemia has no direct effect on the lungs; however, when the respiratory muscles are weak, respiratory insufficiency can lead to respiratory failure and death.

Interventions

Interventions for hypermagnesemia aim to reduce the serum magnesium level and correct the underlying problem that caused the hypermagnesemia.

All oral and parenteral magnesium are discontinued. When renal failure is not present, giving magnesium-free IV fluids can reduce serum magnesium levels. High-ceiling (loop) diuretics such as furosemide (Lasix, Furoside✱) can further reduce serum magnesium levels. When cardiac problems are severe, giving calcium may reverse the cardiac effects of hypermagnesemia.

Diet therapy can prevent hypermagnesemia when other chronic conditions increase the risk for excess serum magnesium. Dietary restrictions involve limiting meat, nuts, legumes, fish, vegetables, and whole-grain cereal products. To prevent the recurrence of hypermagnesemia, teach the client to avoid drugs that increase magnesium, such as magnesium-containing antacids, laxatives, or enemas.

GET READY for the NCLEX Examination!

KEY POINTS

Safe Effective Care Environment

- Do not give intravenous potassium at a rate greater than 20 mEq/hr.
- Never give potassium supplements by the intramuscular or subcutaneous routes.
- Use a pump or controller when giving intravenous potassium-containing solutions.
- Use a gait belt when assisting a client with muscle weakness to walk.
- Collaborate with the dietitian to teach clients about diets that are restricted in potassium, sodium, or calcium.
- Use a lift sheet to move or reposition a client with hypocalcemia.

Health Promotion and Maintenance

- Teach all clients to take drugs as prescribed, especially diuretics, antihypertensives, and cardiac drugs.
- Teach clients who are taking digoxin to measure their pulse for rate, rhythm, and quality.
- Teach clients who are taking diuretics to measure their pulse for rate, rhythm, and quality.

- Include the person who prepares the client's meals when teaching about dietary electrolyte restrictions.

Psychosocial Integrity

- Assess clients who have a sudden change in cognition for electrolyte imbalances.
- Determine the client's food preferences and dislikes when planning an electrolyte restricted diet.

Physiological Integrity

- Clearly mark the IV bag that contains potassium.
- Assess the IV site of a person receiving IV solutions containing potassium at least every 2 hours.
- Document the condition of the IV site of a person receiving intravenous potassium infusions at least every 2 hours.
- Immediately stop the infusion of potassium-containing solutions if infiltration or extravasation is suspected.
- Avoid administering magnesium sulfate by the intramuscular route.
- Assess all clients with hyperkalemia for cardiac dysrhythmias and ECG abnormalities, especially tall T waves, conduction delays, and heart block.
- Assess the respiratory status of all clients with hypokalemia.
- Monitor the hydration status of clients who have hypernatremia, hyperkalemia, or hypercalcemia.
- Assess the bowel sounds; deep tendon reflexes; heart rate, rhythm and quality; and hand grasps to evaluate the client's responses to therapy for an electrolyte imbalance.

ADDITIONAL STUDY RESOURCES

Go to your Student CD-ROM for Review Questions for the NCLEX Examination.

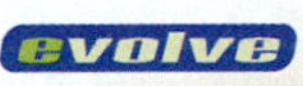

Go to http://evolve.elsevier.com/Iggy/ for Integrated Management of Care Questions for the NCLEX Examination.

SELECTED BIBLIOGRAPHY

Asterisk indicates a classic or definitive work on this subject.

Adams, M., & Pelter, M. (2004). Electrolyte imbalances. *American Journal of Critical Care, 13*(1), 85-86.

Adrogue, H., & Madias, N. (2000). Primary care: Hypernatremia. *The New England Journal of Medicine, 342*(20), 1492-1499.

*Ahern-Gould, K., & Stark, J. (1998). Quick resource for electrolyte imbalance. *Critical Care Nursing Clinics of North America, 10*(4), 477-490.

Burger, C. (2004). Emergency: Hypokalemia. *American Journal of Nursing, 104*(11), 61-65.

Call-Schmidt, T. (2001). Interpreting lab results: A primer. *MEDSURG Nursing, 10*(4), 179-184.

Call-Schmidt, T., & Williams-Evans, S. (2000). How to recognize hypokalemia. *Nursing2000, 30*(2), 22.

Castiglione, K. (2000). Hyperkalemia. *American Journal of Nursing, 100*(1), 55.

*Chmielewski, C. (1998). Hyperkalemic emergencies: Mechanisms, manifestations, and management. *Critical Care Clinics of North America, 10*(4), 449-457.

Collins, N. (2002). Take the guesswork out of sodium restrictions. *Nursing2002, 32*(8), 32hn7-32hn8.

Criner, J., et al. (2002). Rhabdomyolysis: The hidden killer. *MEDSURG Nursing, 11*(3), 138-143.

Dochterman, J.M., & Bulechek, G.M. (Eds.). (2004). *Nursing interventions classification (NIC)* (4th ed). St. Louis: Mosby.

Ebersole, P., Hess, P., & Luggen, A. (2004). *Toward healthy aging: Human needs and nursing response* (6th ed). St. Louis: Mosby.

Francis, J. (2001). ECG challenge–hypocalcemia. *Emergency Medicine, 33*(8), 41-42.

*Gosling, P. (1999). Fluid balance in the critically ill: The sodium and water audit. *Care of the Critically Ill, 15*(1), 11-16.

Guyton, A., & Hall, J. (2000). *Textbook of medical physiology* (10th ed.). Philadelphia: W.B. Saunders.

Hadaway, L. (2001). How to safeguard delivery of high-alert drugs. *Nursing2001, 31*(2), 36-41.

Held-Warmkessel, J. (2000). Test your knowledge: Altered calcium metabolism. *Clinical Journal of Oncology Nursing, 4*(3), 139-140.

Incredibly easy! Understanding hypokalemia. (2002). *Nursing2002, 32*(3), 65.

Innerity, S. (2000). Hypomagnesemia in acute and chronic illness. *Critical Care Nursing Quarterly, 23*(2), 1-19.

Jordan, K. (2000). Fluid resuscitation in acutely injured patients. *Journal of Intravenous Nursing, 23*(2), 81-87.

Kraft, P. (2000). The osmotic shift. *Journal of Intravenous Nursing, 23*(4), 220-224.

Krantz, M., & Baker, W. (2002). ECG challenge: Test your interpretive skills. *Consultant, 42*(14), 1757-1763.

Kugler, J., & Hustead, T. (2000). Hyponatremia and hypernatremia in the elderly. *American Family Physician, 61*(12), 3623-3630.

McCance, K., & Huether, S. (2002). *Pathophysiology: The biologic basis for disease in adults and children* (4th ed). St. Louis: Mosby.

Moorhead, S., Johnson, M., & Maas, M. (Eds.). (2004). *Nursing outcomes classification (NOC)* (3rd ed). St. Louis: Mosby.

*O'Donnell, M. (1995). Assessing fluid and electrolyte balance needs in elders. *American Journal of Nursing, 95*(1), 41-46.

Pagana, K., & Pagana, T. (2002). *Mosby's manual of diagnostic and laboratory tests* (2nd ed). St. Louis: Mosby.

Ruholl, L. (2002). Managing medications for older patients. *Nursing2002, 32*(3), 32hn6-32hn8.

*Stark, J. (1998). A comprehensive analysis of the fluid and electrolytes system. *Critical Care Nursing Clinics of North America, 10*(4), 471-475.

Trissel, L. (2003). *Handbook on injectable drugs* (12th ed.). Bethesda, MD: American Society of Health-System Pharmacists.

Webster, A., Brady, W., & Morris, F. (2002). Recognizing signs of danger: ECG changes resulting from an abnormal serum potassium concentration. *Emergency Medicine Journal, 19*(1), 74-77.

CHAPTER 17

Infusion Therapy

LYNN C. HADAWAY

LEARNING OUTCOMES

After studying this chapter, you should be able to:

1. Categorize the purpose and types of intravenous (IV) infusion therapy.
2. Identify the types and characteristics of vascular access devices (VADs).
3. Evaluate clients for vascular access needs.
4. Distinguish the components of an infusion system.
5. Differentiate the types of rate control devices and nursing considerations for their use.
6. Prioritize nursing interventions for maintaining an infusion system.
7. Assess, prevent, and manage complications related to infusion therapy and VADs.
8. Determine special needs of older adults receiving IV therapy.
9. Identify nursing considerations for intra-arterial, intraperitoneal, subcutaneous, intraosseous, epidural, and intrathecal infusion therapy.

Go to your Student CD-ROM for Review Questions for the NCLEX Examination keyed to these Learning Outcomes.

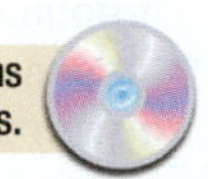

Infusion therapy is the delivery of parenteral medications and fluids through a wide variety of catheter types and locations using multiple techniques and procedures. Intravenous (IV) and intra-arterial therapy delivers the solution into the vascular system. The peritoneal cavity can be used for infusion of certain types of oncology medications. Subcutaneous therapy and hypodermoclysis slowly infuse certain fluids and medications into the subcutaneous tissue; other medications can be delivered to the central nervous system through the epidural or intrathecal space. The intraosseous space can be used for emergency access in infants, children, and adults. This chapter focuses on access for and administration of all types of infusion therapy.

INTRODUCTION TO INFUSION THERAPY

Virtually all clients will require some type of infusion therapy during their hospital stay. Although less common, infusion therapy is also seen in community-based settings, including the client's home. The number of vascular access devices (VADs) inserted annually in the United States now exceeds seven million. Infusion therapy is also delivered in all health care settings, including home care, ambulatory clinics, physician's offices, and long-term care facilities. Infusion therapy is the center of the treatment plan for many clients, and it spans all age groups from birth to death.

The services of a specialized team of infusion nurses has the highest recommendation from the Centers for Disease Control as a strategy to reduce complications and improve client outcomes (O'Grady et al., 2002). This specialty practice encompasses the management of infusion therapy services for a facility or agency, including the following:

- Policy and procedure development
- Insertion of several types of peripheral and central venous catheters
- Monitoring clinical outcomes
- Serving as an educational resource for staff nurses
- Consulting on a variety of clinical and management issues, such as product selection and purchasing decisions

The rapid advances in technology for infusion therapy have driven the need for nurses specializing in vascular access and infusion therapy; however, not all health care agencies have an infusion therapy team. All nurses who provide direct client care are expected to perform basic infusion therapy procedures, although there are wide variations in responsibilities among facilities.

Several professional organizations strive to improve clinical outcomes with infusion therapy and vascular access through educational opportunities and publications. The Infusion Nurses Society (INS), formerly the Intravenous Nurses Society, publishes standards of practice intended to serve as the framework for policy and procedure development in all health care settings. These standards establish the performance criteria for all nurses delivering infusion therapy (Intravenous

Nurses Society, 2000). The Infusion Nurses Certification Corporation (INCC) offers a written certifying examination. Nurses who successfully complete this examination have mastered an advanced body of knowledge in this specialty and may use the initials *CRNI,* which stand for "certified registered nurse infusion." The Association for Vascular Access (AVA) is a multidisciplinary organization focusing on advanced practices with vascular access. The Oncology Nursing Society (ONS) writes guidelines about chemotherapy and biotherapy administration, and the American Society of Parenteral and Enteral Nutrition (ASPEN) writes standards and guidelines for all types of nutrition.

TYPES OF INFUSION THERAPY FLUIDS

Infusion therapy encompasses many types of parenteral fluids for multiple purposes. These fluids may be administered through several routes, but the most common route is via a vein (IV route). The primary goals of infusion therapy include the following:

- Achieving normal fluid and electrolyte balance
- Achieving optimal nutrition status
- Maintaining hemostasis through blood and blood component administration
- Treating numerous conditions with medications

Intravenous Fluids

Currently more than 200 IV fluids are available from commercial manufacturers that meet the requirements established by the United States Pharmacopeia (USP). Each solution is classified by its tonicity and pH. Tonicity is categorized by comparison to normal blood plasma. Normal plasma osmolarity is about 290 mOsm/L. Parenteral fluids close to this value are considered **isotonic;** those above 350 mOsm/L are considered **hypertonic;** and those below 250 mOsm/L are considered **hypotonic.** The pH of the IV fluids measures the acidity or alkalinity and usually ranges from 3.5 to 6.2. Extremes of both osmolarity and pH can cause vein damage leading to phlebitis and thrombosis. Therefore fluids and medications with a pH value less than 5 and greater than 9 and osmolarity greater than 500 mOsm/L should not be infused through a peripheral vein (Intravenous Nurses Society, 2000).

Parenteral Nutrition

Parenteral nutrition formulas include dextrose, protein, fat, vitamins, and numerous trace elements tailored to the specific metabolic needs of their client. Parenteral nutrition should be used *only* when the gastrointestinal (GI) tract cannot be used. The GI tract produces a better physiologic response and is less expensive and easier to manage. The osmolarity of all parenteral nutrition fluids is greater than 500 mOsm/L, requiring a central venous catheter for infusion of all formulas. Infusion of low-dextrose formulas through a peripheral vein leads to high rates of vein damage and subsequent phlebitis, thrombosis, and extravasation injury. Repeated peripheral venipunctures are usually needed when short peripheral catheters are used, thus increasing the rate of complications and the cost of therapy. (See Chapter 64 for a complete discussion of parenteral nutrition.)

Blood Transfusion and Other Components

Blood transfusion is accomplished using packed red blood cells, created by removing a large portion of the plasma from whole blood leaving the oxygen carrying red blood cells. Other blood components include platelets, fresh frozen plasma, albumin, and several specific clotting factors. Each component has detailed requirements for blood-type compatibility and infusion techniques. Facilities that are accredited by the Joint Commission on Accreditation of Healthcare Organizations (JCAHO) are required to ensure that blood components are properly ordered, handled and dispensed, and administered along with appropriate client monitoring. Positive client identification is essential before any blood component is administered. An acute hemolytic transfusion reaction due to an incompatible blood transfusion is a sentinel event requiring an intense analysis of the cause and corrective action. Established policies and procedures must be rigidly followed to ensure a safe transfusion and reduce the risk of complications. (See Chapter 43 for a complete discussion of blood transfusions.)

Medications

IV medications provide a rapid therapeutic effect but can also lead to immediate serious reactions. Hundreds of medications are available for infusion by a variety of techniques, mandating easy access to a reliable nursing reference written specifically for IV administration of medications. As with all drug administration, you must be knowledgeable about drug indications, proper dosage, contraindications, and precautions. However, IV administration also requires knowledge of appropriate dilution, rate of infusion, pH and osmolarity, compatibility with other IV medications, and specific aspects of client monitoring because of the immediate effect. Regardless of familiarity with the drug, never assume that IV administration is the same as giving that drug by other routes. New information is continuously being published, and new drugs are rapidly being introduced.

Medication safety is of paramount importance in all health care settings today. JCAHO now produces client safety goals annually. One major goal is improving the safety of high-alert medications. An example is concentrated electrolyte solutions (e.g., potassium chloride), which require restricted access, prominent warnings about the concentration, and storage in a secured location. Other strategies to reduce medication errors include limiting available concentrations of drugs and dispensing all drugs, including catheter flush solutions, in single-dose containers.

PRESCRIBING INFUSION THERAPY

An order for infusion therapy written by a physician or authorized prescriber is necessary before you begin IV therapy. To be complete, the order for infusion fluids must include the following:

- Specific type of fluid
- Rate of administration written in milliliters per hour, or the total amount of fluid and the total number of hours for infusion (e.g., 125 mL/hr or 1000 mL/8 hr)

- Medications and the specific dose to be added to the fluid such as electrolytes or vitamins

A medication order must include the following:

- Medication name, preferably by generic name
- Specific dose and route
- Frequency of administration

Some continuously infused medications, such as those for pain management, are prescribed as milligrams per hour. The type and volume of dilution for infusion medications may be included in the order; however, the infusion pharmacist may determine these factors for medication admixture.

You are responsible for determining that the order is appropriate for the client and clarifying any questions before administration. An example is an order for 5% dextrose in water to keep vein open (KVO). This order does not specify the rate of infusion and is not considered complete (Intravenous Nurses Society, 2000).

VASCULAR ACCESS DEVICES

A catheter, also known as a **vascular access device (VAD),** is a plastic tube placed in a blood vessel to deliver fluids and medications. Therapy characteristics determine whether the infusion can be given safely through peripheral veins or if the large central veins of the chest are needed. Advances in catheter materials and insertion techniques have radically expanded the types of VADs currently used. This discussion includes the description and uses for seven types: short peripheral catheters, midline catheters, peripherally inserted central catheters (PICC), nontunneled percutaneous central catheters, tunneled catheters, implanted ports, and hemodialysis catheters.

Technologic improvements have caused a change in how we approach vascular access. Repeated venipunctures with short peripheral catheters should not be done. Instead the goal is to assess the client's needs for vascular access and choose the device that has the best chance of infusing the prescribed therapy for the required length of time while using the minimal number of catheters.

Short Peripheral Catheters

Short peripheral catheters are composed of a plastic cannula built around a sharp stylet extending slightly beyond the cannula (Figure 17-1). The stylet allows for the venipuncture, and the cannula is advanced into the vein. These catheters are designed with a safety mechanism to house or cover the sharp end of the stylet after it is removed from the client. These stylets are hollow-bore, blood-filled needles that carry the highest risk of exposure to bloodborne pathogens if needle stick injury occurs. A federal law enacted in 2000 amended the Bloodborne Pathogen Standards from the Occupational Safety and Health Administration (OSHA) requiring the use of catheters with an engineered safety mechanism.

INSERTION

Short peripheral catheters are inserted into superficial veins of the hand and forearm. In emergent situations, these catheters can also be used in the external jugular vein of the neck. In infants the feet can be used, although the use of veins in the feet of adults should be avoided because of an increased risk of deep vein thrombosis.

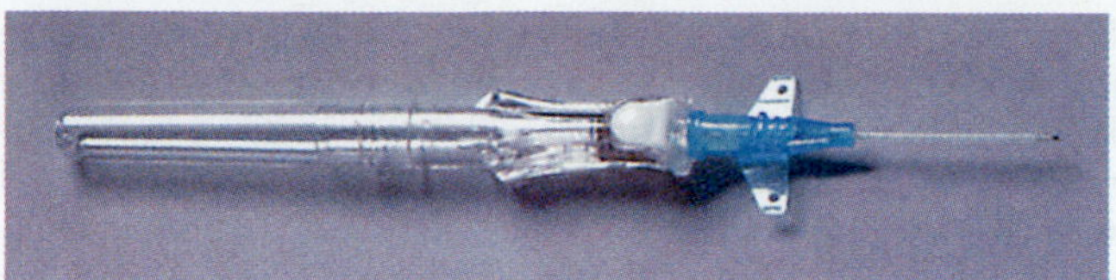

Figure 17-1 ■ Insyte AutoGuard IV catheters. With the push of a button, the needle instantly retracts, reducing the risk of accidental needle stick injuries. (Courtesy Becton Dickinson Infusion Therapy Systems, Sandy, UT.)

These catheters range in length from ¾ inch to 1¼ inch with gauge sizes from 26 gauge (the smallest) to 14 gauge (the largest). The smallest gauge catheter capable of delivering the prescribed therapy should be chosen. Current design allows for a thin-wall construction, providing a larger lumen without increasing the outer diameter. This design improves the capacity for fluid flow through the catheter while using a smaller gauge and thereby decreasing the possibility of vein irritation from a large catheter. For example, a thin-walled 24-gauge Insyte (BD Medical, Sandy, UT) catheter has about the same flow-rate capabilities as a 22-gauge non–thin-walled Angiocath (BD Medical, Inc.) Larger gauge sizes will always allow for faster flow rates but also cause phlebitis more often. Table 17-1 lists each gauge size and its common uses.

Short peripheral catheters are allowed to dwell for 72 to 96 hours and then require removal and insertion at another venous site. If the length of the client's therapy is expected to be longer than six days, a midline catheter or PICC should be chosen (O'Grady et al., 2002). When selecting the site for insertion of a peripheral catheter, consider the client's age, history, and diagnosis; the type and duration of the prescribed therapy; and, whenever possible, the client's preference. Chart 17-1 lists the major criteria for the placement of peripheral VADs.

PLACEMENT

The most appropriate veins for peripheral catheter placement include the dorsal venous network, basilic, cephalic, and median veins, as well as their branches (Figure 17-2). Veins on the hand may not be appropriate in older clients with a loss of skin turgor and poor vein condition or for active clients receiving infusion therapy in an ambulatory clinic or home care. Mastectomy, axillary lymph node dissection, lymphedema, paralysis of the upper extremity, and the presence of dialysis grafts or fistulas alter the normal pattern of blood flow through the arm. Cannulation of veins in the extremity affected by these conditions requires a physician's order. Short peripheral catheters are not recommended for obtaining routine blood samples (Intravenous Nurses Society, 2000).

Veins on the palm side of the wrist should be avoided because the median nerve is located close to veins in this area, making the venipuncture more painful and difficult to stabilize. The cephalic vein begins above the thumb and extends up the entire length of the arm. This vein is usually large and prominent, appearing as a prime site for catheter insertion. Research has shown, however, that the sensory branch of the median nerve can intersect with the cephalic vein up to three times from its origin to about 4 to 5 inches up the lateral aspect of the arm (Vialle et al., 2001). Transection of the nerve can result in permanent loss of function, and local nerve

TABLE 17-1 Choosing the Gauge Size for Peripheral Catheters

24- and 26-gauge	Use for neonates, pediatric, and older clients Recommended when extremely small-diameter veins are the only choice Blood return in the flash chamber may be slower Suitable for most infusions, but flow rates are slower May be used for blood transfusion ***without an infusion pump;*** a unit of packed red blood cells should be divided into two bags to accommodate the extended infusion time
22-gauge	Used for all infusions including blood and blood products Infusion rates will be slightly slower Recommended for most adults, especially those with small or fragile veins Not appropriate when rapid flow rates are required such as trauma or surgery
20-gauge	Used for all infusions including blood and blood products suitable for minor surgical procedures Most commonly used size
18-gauge	Trauma and surgery Rapid flow rates Requires a large vein to allow room for blood to flow in the vein around the catheter Irritation to the vein wall and phlebitis results when the catheter is too large for the chosen vein
16- and 14-gauge	High-risk surgical procedures and trauma Large volumes and rapid flow Requires a large vein Mechanical irritation and phlebitis are likely

CHART 17-1

BEST PRACTICE for
Placement of Short Peripheral Venous Catheters

- Verify that the order for infusion therapy is complete and appropriate for infusion through a short peripheral catheter.
- For adults, choose a site for placement in the upper extremity.
- Choose the client's nondominant arm when possible.
- Choose a distal site and make all subsequent venipunctures proximal to previous sites.
- Do not use the arm on the side of a mastectomy, lymph node dissection, arteriovenous shunt or fistula, or paralysis.
- Avoid choosing a site in an area of joint flexion.
- Avoid choosing a site in a vein that feels hard or cordlike.
- Avoid choosing a site close to areas of cellulitis, dermatitis, or areas of complications from previous catheter sites.

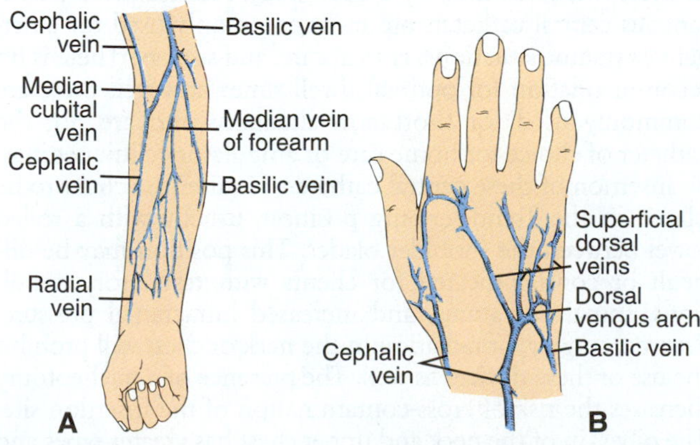

Figure 17-2 ■ Common IV sites. **A,** Inner arm. **B,** Dorsal surface of hand.

damage can become a chronic systemic pain syndrome. Complaints of tingling, feeling "pins and needles" in the extremity, or numbness during the venipuncture procedure can indicate nerve puncture. The procedure should be stopped immediately, the catheter removed, and a new site chosen.

Winged needles may be placed in the veins of the hand and forearm. Although these devices are easy to insert, they are associated with a high frequency of infiltration. They are most commonly used for injection of single-dose medications or for drawing blood samples. Like a short peripheral catheter, winged needles should also have an engineered safety mechanism to house the needle when removed.

Midline Catheters

INDICATIONS

Midline catheters are 6 to 8 inches long and are inserted through the veins of the antecubital fossa. The basilic vein is preferred over the cephalic vein because of its larger diameter, and it will allow greater hemodilution of the fluids and medications being infused. The catheter tip is located in the upper-arm level with the axilla. These catheters are used for therapies lasting from 1 to 4 weeks; however, there are no recommendations for the optimal dwell time (O'Grady et al., 2002). Because of the extended dwell time, sterile technique is used for insertion of a midline catheter. Additional education and skill assessment are required for the nurse to be considered qualified to insert midline catheters.

A midline catheter can be used when skin integrity or limited peripheral veins make it difficult to maintain a short peripheral catheter. Other indications include the following:

- Fluids for hydration
- Five to 10 days of antibiotics to treat urosepsis or pneumonia
- Heparin infusions for deep vein thrombosis
- Bronchodilators, such as aminophylline
- Steroids

Limiting venipunctures in clients who have received anticoagulation agents is desirable to avoid excessive bruising and hematoma formation. Metabolic changes in steroid-dependent clients results in changes in the skin and vein conditions, making repeated venipuncture difficult.

The fluids and medications infused through a midline catheter should have a pH between 5 and 9 and a final osmolarity of less than 500 mOsm/L (Intravenous Nurses Society, 2000). The pH and osmolarity outside these parameters increase the risk of complications like phlebitis and thrombosis.

Midline catheters should not be used for infusion of **vesicant medications,** which are drugs that will cause tissue damage if they escape into the subcutaneous tissue **(extravasation).** At this tip location, larger amounts of the drug can extravasate before the problem is detected. All parenteral nutrition formulas, including those with low concentrations of dextrose, have an osmolarity greater than 500 mOsm/L and should not be infused through a midline catheter. Blood sampling from a midline catheter should not be routinely performed (Intravenous Nurses Society, 2000). Midline catheters should not be placed in extremities affected by mastectomy with lymphedema, paralysis, or dialysis grafts and fistulas.

Midline catheters may be designed with pressure-sensitive valves located near the internal catheter tip (e.g., Groshong, made by Bard Access Systems, Salt Lake City, UT) or in the external catheter hub (e.g., PASV, made by Boston Scientific, Natick, MA). These valves open when pressure is applied, allowing for infusion and aspiration; however, when no pressure is applied, they are closed to prevent blood refluxing into the lumen or air entering the bloodstream. The manufacturers of both catheters state that saline only can be used to flush these lines, eliminating the need for heparin to maintain lumen patency.

Peripherally Inserted Central Catheters

PLACEMENT

A peripherally inserted central catheter (PICC) is a long catheter inserted through the veins of the antecubital fossa or the middle of the upper arm. In adults the catheter length ranges from 40 to 65 cm, with the tip residing in the superior vena cava (SVC). Placement of the catheter tip in veins distal to the SVC should be avoided. This inappropriate tip location, often called mid-clavicular catheters, are associated with much higher rates of thrombosis than when the tip is located in the SVC (Kearns, Coleman, & Wehner, 1996). Mid-clavicular tip locations should be used only when anatomic or pathophysiologic changes prohibit advancement of the catheter into the SVC (National Association of Vascular Access Networks, 1998).

PICCs should be inserted early in the course of therapy, before veins of the extremity have been damaged from multiple venipunctures and infusions. Insertion methods using guidewires and ultrasound greatly improve insertion success. The basilic vein is the preferred site for insertion; however, the cephalic vein can be used if necessary. Sterile technique is used for insertion to reduce the risk of bloodstream infections. A chest radiograph indicating that the tip resides in the lower SVC is required before the catheter can be used for infusion. PICCs are available in single-, dual-, or triple-lumen configurations and are available with both Groshong and PASV valves.

PICCs have lower complication rates because of the insertion site in the upper extremity. The dry skin of the arm has fewer types and numbers of microorganisms, leading to lower rates of infection. Inadvertent arterial puncture or excessive bleeding can be controlled by direct pressure. Insertion complications such as pneumothorax associated with other central venous catheters do not occur with PICCs. In addition, PICC lines are less expensive than central catheters (Smelling et al., 2001).

INDICATIONS

PICCs can accommodate the infusion of all types of therapy because the tip resides in the SVC where the rapid blood flow will quickly dilute the fluids being infused. Therefore, there are no limitations on the pH or osmolarity of fluids that can be infused through a PICC. Clients requiring lengthy courses of antibiotics, antineoplastic agents, parenteral nutrition formulas, vasopressor agents, and numerous other fluids can benefit from a PICC. PICCs have been reported to dwell successfully for months or even years; however, the optimal dwell time is not known (O'Grady et al., 2002).

PICCs can be used for blood sampling; however, lumen sizes of 4F or larger are recommended. Using lumens with small diameters may not yield a sample capable of producing the needed test results. Transfusion of blood through a PICC usually requires the use of an infusion pump. Packed red blood cells are cold and viscous. The length of the PICC adds resistance and may prevent the blood from infusing within the 4-hour limitation.

Teach clients with a PICC to perform normal activities of daily living; however, they should avoid excessive physical activity. Muscle contractions in the arm from physical activity like heavy lifting can lead to catheter dislodgment and possible lumen occlusion.

PICC insertion is commonly performed in the client's hospital room, an outpatient treatment facility, or the radiology department. Nurses placing these catheters require a high level of skill with venipuncture and central venous catheter management. Additional education, along with documented competency assessment, is required.

Nontunneled Percutaneous Central Catheters

Nontunneled percutaneous central catheters are inserted through the subclavian vein in the upper chest or the jugular veins in the neck using sterile technique. They are usually 15 to 20 cm long and have dual or triple lumens. The tip resides in the SVC, confirmed by a chest x-ray. Nontunneled percutaneous central catheters are most commonly used for emergent or trauma situations, critical care, and surgery. There is no recommendation for optimal dwell time; however, these are commonly used for short-term situations and are not the catheter of choice for home care or ambulatory clinic settings.

Insertion of these central catheters requires the client to be placed in the Trendelenburg position, usually with a rolled towel between the shoulder blades. This position may be difficult or contraindicated for clients with respiratory conditions, spinal curvatures, and increased intracranial pressure. Trauma, surgery, or radiation in the neck or chest will prohibit the use of these devices as well. The presence of a tracheotomy increases the risk of cross-contamination of the insertion site. The oily skin of the neck and upper chest has greater types and numbers of microorganisms, resulting in greater numbers of bloodstream infections with this type of catheter.

Tunneled Central Catheters

Tunneled central venous catheters have a portion of the catheter lying in a subcutaneous tunnel, separating the points where the catheter enters the vein from where it exits the skin. This separation is intended to prevent the organisms on the skin from reaching the bloodstream (Figure 17-3). The catheter has a cuff made of a rough material that is positioned inside the subcutaneous tunnel. The tissue granulates into this cuff, providing a mechanical barrier to microorganisms and anchoring the catheter in place. This design requires surgical techniques for insertion. Single, dual, and triple lumens are available. These catheters were originally named for the physicians who designed them, including Broviac, Hickman, and Leonard catheters. These names are now trade names and should be used when referring to those particular brands.

Tunneled catheters are used primarily when the need for infusion therapy is frequent and long-term. Clients needing parenteral nutrition for months, years, or the remainder of their life commonly choose a tunneled catheter. Tunneled catheters are also chosen when several weeks or months of infusion therapy are needed and a PICC is not a good choice. For example, paraplegic clients needing 6 to 8 weeks of antibiotics are not good candidates for a PICC because of the excessive use of the upper extremities for mobility. Some oncology clients may prefer a tunneled catheter instead of an implanted port because they cannot tolerate the needle sticks required for accessing those devices.

Implanted Ports

Implanted ports consist of a portal body, a dense septum over a reservoir, and a catheter (Figure 17-4). A subcutaneous pocket is surgically created to house the port body. The catheter is inserted into the vein and attached to the portal body. The septum is made of self-sealing silicone and is located in the center of the port body over the reservoir. The catheter extends from the side of the port body. The incision is closed, and no part of the catheter is visible externally; therefore this device has the least impact on body image.

PLACEMENT

Venous ports may be placed on the upper chest or the upper extremity. The venous catheter may enter either the subclavian or internal jugular vein and is available as a single- or double-lumen device. Although an implanted port is most commonly used in the venous system, the catheter may be placed in arteries, the epidural space, or the peritoneal cavity, with the port pocket located over a bony prominence.

MAINTENANCE

Implanted ports are accessed by using a noncoring needle specially designed with a deflected tip. This design slices through the dense septum without coring out a small piece of it, thus preserving the integrity of the septum. Port bodies placed in the chest have a larger septum and will usually tolerate about 2000 punctures. Port bodies placed in the upper extremity are smaller and are rated to tolerated about 750 punctures. Before puncture, the port is palpated to locate the septum. Carefully palpate to feel the shape and depth of the port body to ensure puncture of the septum, not the attached catheter. Noncoring port access needles, also called **Huber needles,** may have a straight shaft or may be bent at a right angle. Some have attached extension sets and wings to stabilize the needle. One important feature is an engineered safety mechanism to contain the needle when it is removed from the septum. Because the dense septum holds tightly to the needle, there can be a rebound when it is pulled from the septum, often resulting in needle stick injury to the nurse (Figure 17-5).

An implanted port needs to be flushed after each use and at least once a month between courses of therapy. When not accessed, there is no external catheter requiring a dressing. Puncture of the skin over the port is required to gain access to the port body, causing pain for some clients. Topical anesthetic creams can be used to make the access procedure more tolerable for the client.

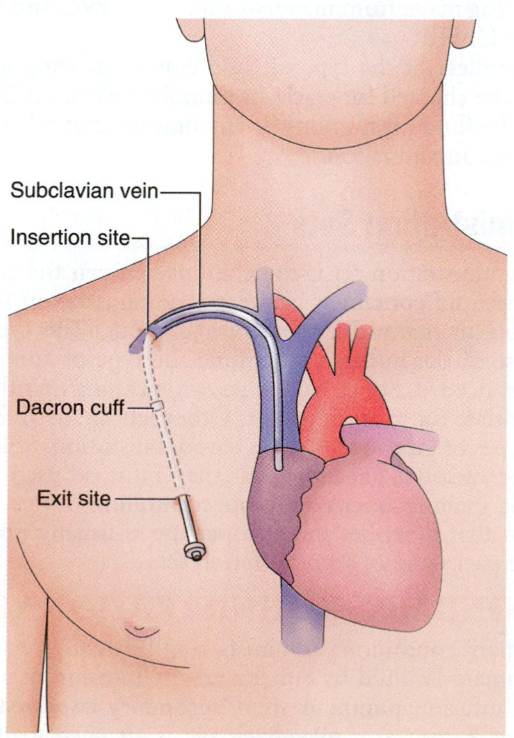

Figure 17-3 ■ Tunneled catheter. A portion of this catheter lies in a subcutaneous tunnel, separating the points where the catheter enters the vein from where it exits the skin.

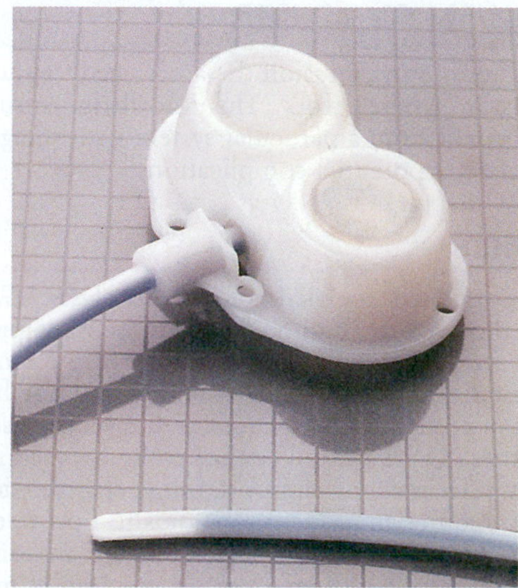

Figure 17-4 ■ A dual-lumen implanted port for venous access. (Courtesy of HMP-Horizon Medical Products Inc., Manchester, GA.)

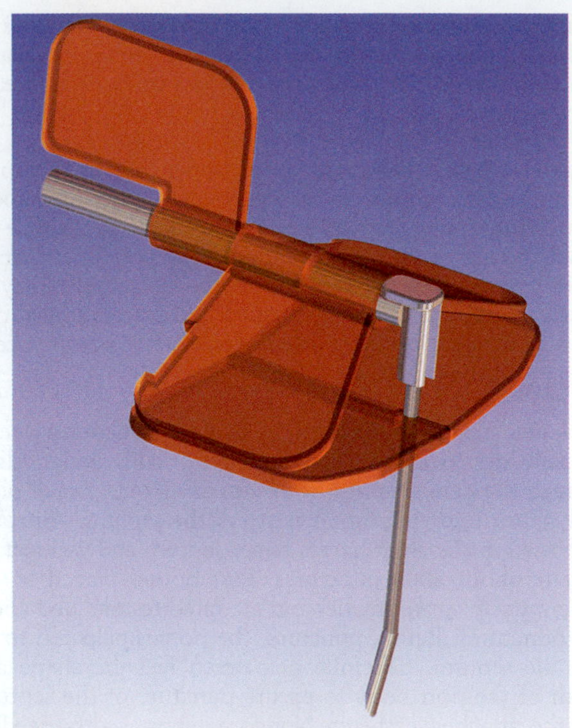

Figure 17-5 ■ Huber Plus Noncoring Needle. The safety mechanism traps the needle to prevent needle stick injury. (Courtesy of NowMedical, Chadds Ford, PA.)

Dialysis Catheters

Dialysis catheters have very large lumens to accommodate the hemodialysis procedure or a pheresis procedure that harvests specific blood cells. They may be tunneled for long-term needs or nontunneled for short-term needs. A dialysis catheter is critical to the client's management of renal failure and must function well. Bloodstream infection and vein thrombosis are common problems; therefore this catheter should not be used for administration of other fluids or medications, except in an emergency.

INFUSION SYSTEMS

Nurses administering infusion therapies need to understand how infusion systems work. This knowledge ensures that you can benefit from a particular system's advantages while minimizing any potential complications.

Containers

Infusion containers are made of glass or plastic. *Glass* bottles were the original fluid container to be mass produced. They are easily sterilized; it is easy to read the amount of fluid remaining in the bottle; and they do not have the problems of compatibility with some drugs like plastic does. Glass bottles are heavy and cannot easily be used in many situations, such as client transport during emergencies. Glass bottles do require an air vent for fluids to flow freely from them. The most common method is to use an administration set with a special filtered vent. Some bottles may have a straw tube open to the room air through the rubber stopper in the bottle and extending to above the level of the fluid. Bottles with a venting straw do not have a barrier to prevent contaminants in the air from entering the fluid.

Plastic containers are considered **closed systems** because they do not rely on outside air to allow the fluid to infuse. Instead, atmospheric pressure pushes against the flexible sides of the container, allowing the fluid to flow by gravity. For this reason, plastic containers do not require vented administration sets. These containers are lightweight, unbreakable, and easy to use in emergency conditions.

Plastic containers are commonly made of polyvinyl chloride (PVC). To increase flexibility and strength, PVC requires the addition of plasticizers. The most common chemical used as a plasticizer is di-2-ethylhexyl-phthalate or DEHP. There has been growing concern in the past few years over the exposure of clients to this chemical. DEHP does not chemically bind to the PVC and can leach from the plastic fluid container or tubing and can be infused to the client with the IV fluid or medication.

Plastic containers present incompatibility issues with insulin, nitroglycerin, lorazepam (Ativan), fat emulsions, and lipid-based drugs. Nitroglycerin and insulin adhere to the walls of the PVC container, making it impossible to know exactly how much medication the client is receiving.

Another concern with plastic bags is the accuracy of reading the amount of fluid remaining in the container. The middle graduations have been shown to be 10% above or below the actual amount of fluid, but the first and last markings could be inaccurate by as much as 40% (Perucca, 2001).

Semirigid containers are made of plastic but offer some of the benefits of glass, such as the absence of plasticizers and drug compatibility problems. These containers are lightweight and unbreakable but are more bulky and less flexible. They also require an air vent to allow the fluid to flow freely. Recent changes have led to a traditional flexible plastic bag made from materials other than PVC and do not require DEHP.

Regardless of the type of fluid container being used, it should be checked for cracks or pinholes before use. Always check the fluid for turbidity or any unusual color that could indicate contamination.

Administration Sets

The administration set is the conduit between the catheter and the fluid container. Numerous administration sets are available in many different configurations. The type and purpose of the infusion determine the type of administration set needed. Some sets are *generic,* meaning that they are appropriate for most infusions. Other sets are used for specific types of infusions, such as blood transfusion. Still other sets are *dedicated,* meaning that they must be used with a specific manufacturer's infusion controlling device. Information that describes their proper use is usually provided on the packaging of administration sets.

SECONDARY ADMINISTRATION SETS

A primary continuous administration set is used to infuse the primary IV fluid by either a gravity infusion or an electronic infusion pump. A short **secondary administration set,** also known as a **piggyback set,** is attached to the primary set at a Y-injection site and is used to deliver intermittent medications. Chart 17-2 shows the procedure for pig-

CHART 17-2

BEST PRACTICE for
Piggybacking an Intermittent Medication

1. Verify the order from the health care provider.
2. Check the compatibility between the medication and the large-volume parenteral (LVP) infusion and its additives.
3. Spike the medication minibag with the secondary set.
4. Prime the secondary set, close the roller clamp, and hang the mini-bag on the other arm of the IV pole.
5. Place the hanger that comes with the secondary set on the IV pole with the LVP.
6. Cleanse the Y-site injection port on the LVP administration set.
7. Attach the secondary set to the Y-site.
8. Lower the level of the LVP by hanging it from the hanger. Do not adjust the LVP roller clamp. (The rate will decrease and then stop when the secondary set is opened.)
9. Open the roller clamp on the secondary set and regulate the flow to the desired rate.
10. When the intermittent infusion completes, the LVP will automatically begin again. Hang the LVP from the IV pole, and adjust the roller clamp to deliver the prescribed rate.

CHART 17-3

BEST PRACTICE for
Backpriming Method for Infusing an Intermittent Medication

- The backpriming method allows multiple medications to be infused through the same secondary set.
- Assess the primary fluid container for admixed medications. If present, these medications *must* be compatible with the secondary medication.
- Lower the empty secondary container and allow fluid to flow into it from the primary container.
- Close the clamp and disconnect the secondary container.
- Attach the new secondary container with the next dose of medication.
- Hang and adjust the rate or set the infusion pump as indicated. If using an infusion pump, follow the specific manufacturer's guidelines to backprime the secondary set.

gybacking an intermittent medication. Once attached, these sets should remain connected together as an infusion system. If multiple intermittent medications are required, it may be possible to use only one secondary set rather than a secondary set for each medication. This depends on the compatibility of the medications. Chart 17-3 explains the sets to use one secondary set to infuse multiple medications using the backpriming method. This process eliminates the costs of using multiple secondary sets and allows you to adhere to the Infusion Nurses Society (INS) standards of practice. These sets are changed every 72 to 96 hours (Intravenous Nurses Society, 2000; O'Grady et al., 2002).

INTERMITTENT ADMINISTRATION SETS

An intermittent administration set is used to infuse multiple doses of medications when no primary continuous fluid is being infused through a catheter that has been capped with a needleless connection device. The medication container from the previous dose is removed and the new one attached. The sterile cap covering the distal end of the set is removed, and the set is attached to the catheter. Because both ends of the set are being manipulated with each dose, the INS standards of practice state that this set should be changed every 24 hours. If a secondary administration set is detached from the primary set, it should be considered an intermittent set and changed every 24 hours (Intravenous Nurses Society, 2000).

Administration sets are sterile in the fluid pathway and under the sterile caps on each end of the set. The set is not packaged as a completely sterile product and cannot be added to a sterile field. Careful attention is required to maintain the sterility of the spike and the connection end of the tubing to prevent introduction of microorganisms into the catheter and bloodstream.

ADD-ON DEVICES

Several other types of add-on devices include short extension sets, injection caps, and filters. Extension sets may be packaged as a sterile product for adding to a sterile field; however, you should always check the product label to ascertain this information.

Administration sets have two ways to connect to the catheter hub: a slip lock or a Luer-Lok. The *slip lock* is a male end that slips into the female catheter hub. A *Luer-Lok* connection has the same male end with a threaded collar that requires twisting onto the corresponding threads of the catheter hub. All set connections should have a Luer-Lok design to ensure that the set remains firmly connected. Loose connections lead to fluid leakage and increase the risk of contamination and subsequent bloodstream infection. When using a central venous catheter, a Luer-Lok connection is critical to reduce the risk of air embolism. Tape is not considered an adequate mechanism for securing set connections.

Filters may be integral to the administration set or may be separate add-on pieces. Their purpose is to remove particulate matter, microorganisms, and air from the infusion system. Filter sizes depend on the pore size, with common sizes being 5 microns intended to remove gross particles, 1.2 microns used to filter lipid-containing parenteral nutrition, and 0.22 microns intended to remove all particles and microorganisms. Filters should be placed as close to the catheter hub as possible.

Particulate matter in the IV fluid, a primary reason to use filters, comprises undissolved, unintended substances and may include rubber pieces, glass particles, cotton fibers, drug particles, paper, and metal fibers. These particles become trapped in the small circulation of the lungs. A red blood cell is about 5 microns in diameter and is the largest size that can pass through the pulmonary capillary bed, and yet IV fluids may contain particles larger than this. For clients receiving infusion therapy for long periods, there could be a significant amount of particles that block the blood flow through the pulmonary circulation (Weinstein, 2001). Microcirculation in the spleen, kidneys, and liver could also be affected. Particulate matter has also been implicated in the development of phlebitis in peripheral veins (O'Grady et al., 2002).

Other concerns with using filters include the possibility for filter rupture, their use with certain drugs that bind to the filter surface, using the correct size of filter for drugs with large molecules, and choosing a filter that will tolerate the pressure exerted by infusion pumps. Rupture of the filter is most commonly associated with the exertion of high pressure exceeding the limit tolerated by the specific filter. Some drugs cannot be filtered because they are retained inside the filter because of their chemical nature or molecule size. For these reasons, medication filtration during the process of admixing is now used as an alternative to final filtration at the bedside. Drugs of a very small quantity should be administered below the filter.

Filters used on blood administration sets have much larger pore size and are not interchangeable with filters used for fluids and medications. A standard blood filter ranges from 170 to 220 microns and removes microclots and other debris caused by blood collection and storage. Microaggregate filters have a pore size of 20, 40, or 80 microns and are used to remove degenerating platelets, white blood cells, and fibrin strands present in blood within 5 days of storage. Leukocyte removal filters are used to remove white blood cells that cause febrile and allergic blood transfusion reactions, cytomegalovirus, and some herpes viruses. They are measured by efficiency rather than pore size (Weir, 2001).

NEEDLELESS CONNECTION DEVICES

In July 1992 the Occupational Safety and Health Administration (OSHA) published guidelines entitled *Occupational Exposure to Bloodborne Pathogens, Final Rule.* This document requires health care organizations to initiate engineering controls "that isolate or remove the bloodborne pathogen hazard from the workplace." This standard was amended in 2000 with the passage of the Needlestick Safety and Prevention Act, which requires the use of devices engineered with safety mechanisms and mandates the involvement of staff performing these tasks directly with selecting products. It also requires each employer to maintain a sharps injury log with details of each incident. Many products are designed to minimize health care workers' exposure to contaminated needles. Blunt cannulas injected through a pre-slit septum and luer-activated valves are the prevailing designs of these products.

Although these devices have reduced the incidence of accidental needle sticks for health care professionals, concern remains about a possible increase in the risk of infection to the client. Several early studies compared these needleless devices with the conventional use of needles to connect tubing together. Also, studies have been done that compare the infection risk of various designs of needleless devices. According to the Centers for Disease Control, when these systems are used according to the manufacturer's instructions, they do not increase the risk of bloodstream infection to your client. All injection sites must be adequately cleaned with an alcohol pad before connecting an IV set or syringe (O'Grady et al., 2002).

The original needleless injection devices have become a source of concern because of their tendency to promote blood reflux into the catheter lumen when the administration set or syringe is disconnected. Over time this small amount of blood can lead to lumen occlusion from a thrombus (Hadaway, 1998). To overcome this blood reflux or negative fluid displacement, positive pressure flushing techniques must be used. This can be accomplished by one of two methods:

- As you flush the last 0.5 mL of fluid into the catheter, withdraw the blunt cannula from the injection port or
- After flushing all fluid into the catheter, continue to hold your thumb on the syringe plunger while closing a clamp on the catheter or extension set and then disconnect the syringe.

New designs of needleless systems overcome this problem by causing a positive fluid displacement within the catheter lumen (Figure 17-6). The device holds a small amount of fluid in a reservoir. When the syringe or administration set is disconnected, this fluid is automatically pushed out to the catheter tip to prevent blood moving into the catheter lumen. When a positive fluid displacement needleless connector is used, positive pressure flushing techniques cannot be used because these techniques defeat the internal mechanism. Some of these devices allow for the elimination of heparinized saline as the final catheter flush; therefore the catheter can be flushed with normal saline only.

Rate-Controlling Devices

The ability to regulate the rate and volume of infusions is critical to the safe and accurate administration of medications and fluids to clients. Nurses have a choice of numerous devices designed to regulate infusions. Infusion devices can be mechanically or electronically regulated.

Mechanically regulated systems include elastomeric balloons, spring-coiled syringes and containers, and a multichambered fluid container placed in a mechanical roller. These devices are commonly used to deliver intermittent medications such as antibiotics in alternative care settings. They are powered by positive pressure from the collapsing balloon or roller returning to its coiled position. Fluid volume is determined by the size of the fluid container; however, most hold 50 to 100 mL. They deliver a preset infusion rate determined by the size of the opening in the tubing connected to the fluid container; therefore additional tubing is not required. These small, portable devices do not require power sources such as batteries or electricity.

Electronic infusion devices fall into two categories: controllers and pumps, based on the mechanism of operation.

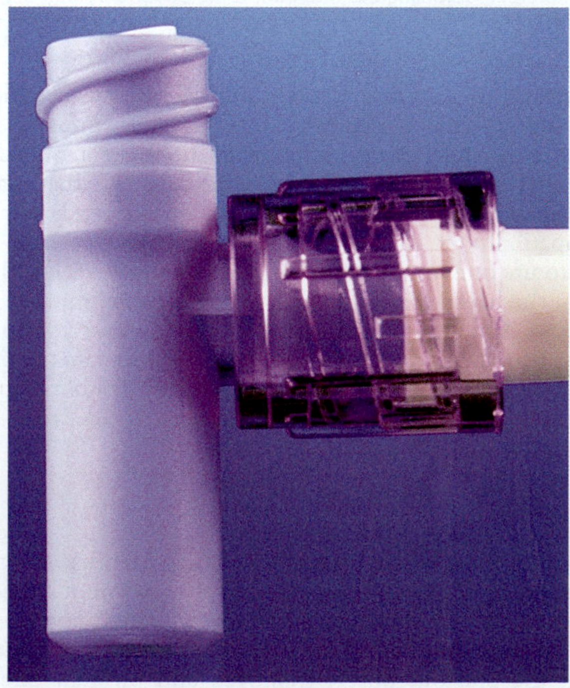

Figure 17-6 ■ The new design of the CLC2000 causes a positive fluid displacement within the catheter lumen. (Courtesy of ICU Medical, San Clemente, CA.)

Nurses and clients who use these electronic infusion devices reap the benefits of some of the latest computer technology. Electronic infusion devices can save nursing time, prevent clients from receiving too much infusion solution, and keep infusion access devices patent; however, the nurse must remember that the use of these devices does not decrease the practitioner's responsibility to monitor carefully the client's infusion site and the infusion rate.

A **controller** is a stationary, pole-mounted electronic device that uses a sensor to monitor fluid flow and to detect when flow has been interrupted. Controllers rely completely on gravity to create fluid flow and do not create pressure. Because controllers rely on counting drops, which vary in size and therefore volume, controllers are not as accurate as pumps.

Pumps may be either large and pole-mounted or ambulatory and portable. As their name indicates, these devices actually pump medications or fluids under pressure. They accurately measure the volume of fluid being infused by using one of three mechanisms:

- A syringe-type mechanism that fills and empties
- A wavelike, peristaltic action that pushes fluid along the tubing
- A series of microchambers that fill and empty

Regardless of the pumping mechanism, these devices require dedicated cassette tubing designed to match the pump.

Syringe pumps use a battery-powered piston to push the plunger continuously at a selected milliliter-per-hour rate. The use of syringe pumps is limited to small-volume continuous or intermittent infusions and is dependent on the syringe size. Antibiotics and patient-controlled analgesia are frequently delivered with syringe pumps. Pediatric clients and those requiring fluid restrictions can also benefit from using a syringe pump because smaller yet accurate volumes can be used to dilute medications. Syringe pumps are generally not appropriate for continuous administration of larger volumes because they require frequent syringe changes.

Ambulatory pumps are generally used for home care clients and allow them to return to their usual activities while receiving infusion therapy. They have a wide range of sizes, with some requiring a backpack, but they usually weigh less than 6 pounds. They are used to deliver accurately continuous infusions such as parenteral nutrition or many programmable medication schedules. Frequent battery recharging or replacement is usually necessary.

Electronic infusion devices can be programmed in many different ways and require a thorough knowledge of the specific brand being used. Infusion rate and the volume to be infused are usually entered in single milliliter increments, but some can be programmed as fractions of a milliliter for use in infants. Some pumps allow the rate to be programmed to taper or ramp up and down at the beginning and ending of the infusion. Secondary syringe infusion, secondary infusion rate, remote site programming, adjustable infusion pressure, and integration into the nurse call system are also possible.

Electronic infusion devices have a variety of alarms, such as air-in-line, upstream and downstream occlusion, infusion complete, and low-battery or power warnings. All devices must have some mechanism to prevent free flow of the infusing fluid or medication. When the cassette or tubing is removed from the pump, this mechanism will automatically stop fluid flow until it is properly replaced in the pump. This prevents accidental rapid infusion of large amounts of fluid or medication leading to serious clinical problems.

CATHETER CARE AND MAINTENANCE

Educating the Client

Before catheter insertion, educate the client about the following:

- The type of catheter to be used
- The therapy required
- Alternatives to the catheter and therapy
- Client activity limitations
- Any signs or symptoms of complications that should be reported to a health care professional

Whereas written information should be provided before placement of a long-term catheter, you should continue to assess the client's understanding of the information and provide more information or answers as needed. Most manufacturers of PICCs, tunneled catheters, and implanted ports provide information booklets written for clients; however, specific information about the chosen procedures and supplies may be required. The booklets may be useless to clients who cannot read or have a low reading level.

Confirming Tip Location

All central venous catheters require a postinsertion chest radiograph to document the tip location. The initial verbal and subsequent written report should contain specific information about the catheter tip location in relation to anatomic structures. Your knowledge of accurate tip location is required before beginning infusion through the catheter. Repeating the chest radiograph during catheter use may be necessary if the client complains of unusual pain or sensation.

Performing the Nursing Assessment

Nursing assessment of all infusion systems should be systematic. Begin with the insertion site and work upward. Know the type of catheter your client has in place. Complications are frequently seen at or near the catheter; however, you will need to know the length of catheter, the insertion site, and tip location to do a complete assessment. Assess the insertion site by looking for redness, swelling, hardness, or drainage. Lightly palpate the area over the dressing. When a midline catheter or PICC is used, assess the entire extremity and upper chest of signs of phlebitis and thrombosis. When a tunneled catheter is used, assess the exit site, the entire length of the tunnel, and the point where the catheter enters the vein. For a well-healed catheter, it may not be possible to detect the vein entrance site; however, on newly inserted catheters there could be a small puncture site with a suture. For implanted ports, assess the incision and surgically created subcutaneous pocket.

Assess the integrity of the dressing, making sure it is clean, dry, and adherent to the skin on all sides. Check all connections on the administration set and ensure that they are secure. Check the rate of infusion for all fluids by either counting drops or checking the electronic infusion pump.

Assess the amount of fluid that has infused from the container. Is it accurate, or is it infusing too fast or too slow? Adjust the rate to the prescribed flow rate. Check all labels on fluid containers for the client's name and fluid or medication.

Avoid taking blood pressures in an extremity with any type of catheter in place. If a short peripheral catheter is being used for continuous infusion, the compression while taking the blood pressure can increase venous pressure, causing fluid to overflow from the puncture site, resulting in an infiltration. When a midline catheter or PICC is being used, compression from the blood pressure cuff could increase vein irritation and lead to phlebitis.

Venipuncture for blood sampling should be performed in the extremity opposite from all catheters. Blood samples should not be drawn from a venipuncture site proximal to an infusing peripheral catheter because the infusing fluid could alter the results of the test to be performed. Venipuncture at or near the insertion site of a midline catheter or PICC could inadvertently damage the catheter and add to areas of venous inflammation.

A

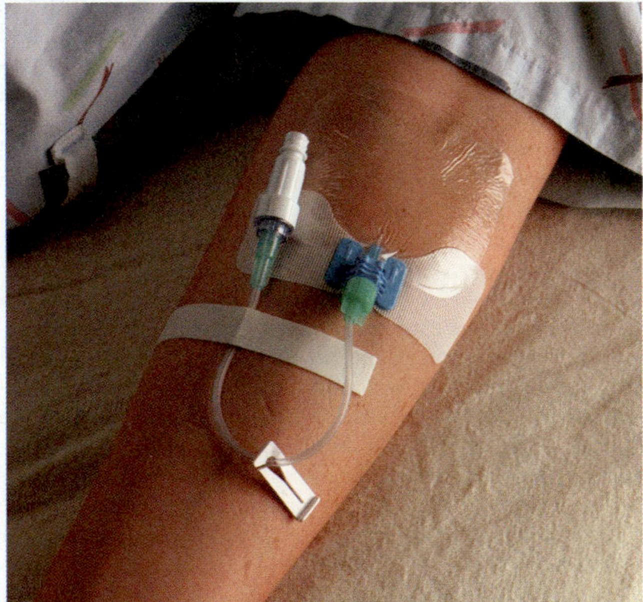

B

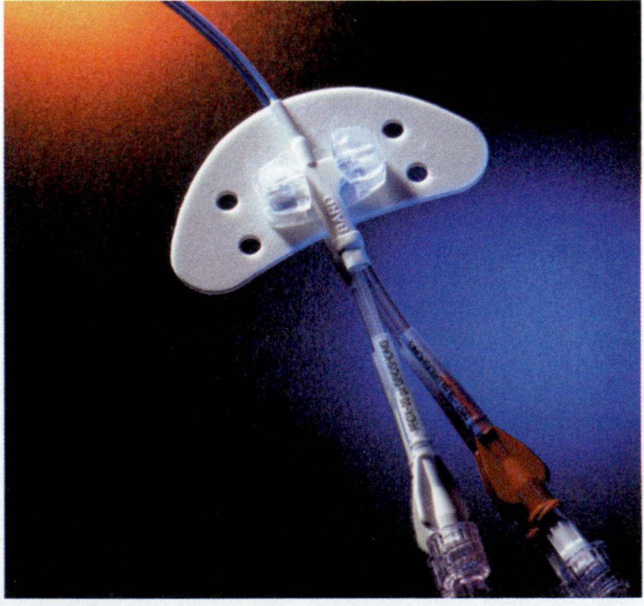

Figure 17-7 ■ The Statlock provides a standardized method to prevent catheter movement. (Courtesy of Venetec International, San Diego, CA.)

Securing and Dressing the Catheter

Adequate catheter securement is vital to prevent many complications. Tape, sutures, and specially designed securement devices can be used for this purpose. For a short peripheral catheter, tape strips are most common; however, the tape should be *clean*. Tape strips from a peripheral IV start kit are preferred. Strips of tape should not be taken from rolls of tape moved between client's rooms, from other procedures, or from uniform pockets. Precutting tape and placing it on the client's bedrails or other object should also be avoided.

Securement devices are designed for all catheter types and provide a standardized method to prevent catheter movement (Figure 17-7). PICCs and nontunneled percutaneous central catheters may be sutured in place; however, this creates additional breaks in the skin that could become infected. If these sutures are loose or broken, the physician must be notified to replace them or some additional securement method must be used. Tunneled catheters usually have sutures placed near the skin exit site that are removed after the tunnel has healed. The incision over a port pocket will have sutures until it has healed also.

Dressings used over the insertion site protect the skin and puncture site. For a short peripheral catheter, the transparent membrane dressings do not require routine changes but rather may remain until the catheter is removed. Tape and gauze or a transparent membrane dressing can be used for midline catheters and all types of central venous dressings. Tape and gauze dressings should be changed every 48 hours. Transparent membrane dressings are changed once or twice weekly. The initial dressing on a midline catheter or PICC is usually tape and gauze changed within 24 hours after insertion because some bleeding is likely. Transparent membrane dressings can be used for subsequent dressing.

Site protection may be needed for short peripheral catheters or for port access needles. Plastic shields can be placed over the site to prevent accidental bumping or pressure from clothing (Figure 17-8).

Remove the dressing by pulling laterally from side to side. It can also be removed by holding the external catheter

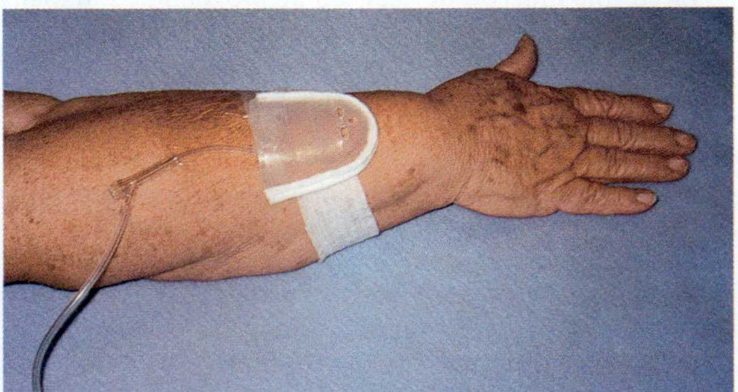

Figure 17-8 ■ I.V. House, a commercially available safety device used for IV site protection, guards the integrity of the older adult's skin while helping to secure the site. (Courtesy I.V. House, Hazelwood, MO.)

and pulling it off toward the insertion site. Never pull it off by pulling away from the insertion site because this could dislodge the catheter.

After removing the dressing from a midline catheter or any central venous catheter, take note of the external catheter length. Compare this length with the original length at insertion. If this length has changed, the catheter tip location has also changed and may no longer be in a vein appropriate for infusion. This situation may require a repeat chest radiograph and careful assessment of the type of therapy and remaining length of therapy required.

The external catheter, dressing, and all attached tubing must be protected from water because water is a source of contamination. While bathing, the extremity should be covered. Plastic trash bags can be taped over the extremity; however, devices specially designed for this purpose are usually more convenient for your client to use.

Changing Administration Sets and Needleless Connectors

Primary and secondary administration sets are usually changed every 72 or 96 hours; however, certain types of fluids require more frequent change. These include lipid emulsion, blood products, and drugs such as propofol.

All connections must be secured by using a luer-locking device. Do not rely on tape to secure connections. Tape residue attracts organisms and increases the risk of infection.

Plan the change of administration sets and fluid containers to occur at the same time, if possible, to minimize the number of times the system is opened. For short peripheral catheters, the administration set and catheter should also be changed at the same time to avoid excessive manipulation of the catheter.

Needleless connector devices can be changed when the administration set is changed. If it is being used for intermittent infusions, the device should be changed at least once per week. Fluid leakage from the device indicates the integrity has been compromised, and it should be changed immediately.

Precautions to prevent air emboli are required when changing the set or connectors attached to any catheter; however, central venous catheters require special attention. The client should be lying flat to ensure that the catheter exit site is at or below the level of the heart. Some catheters may have a pinch clamp that can be closed during this procedure. Ask the client to perform a Valsalva maneuver by holding his or her breath and bearing down while you disconnect the old set and reconnect the new. This will prevent air from entering the lumen, the heart, and pulmonary circulation.

Controlling Infusion Pressure

Fluid flow through the infusion system requires that the pressure on the external side be greater than the pressure at the catheter tip. Fluid flow can be slowed or obstructed by many causes. At or above the catheter hub, kinked tubing, tubing or syringe diameter, and fluid temperature or viscosity could create resistance to flow. Inside the catheter lumen, resistance is created by the catheter length and diameter or by deposits of fibrin, thrombus, or drug precipitate. Near the catheter tip, resistance to flow comes from the catheter tip impinging on the vein wall, thrombus, or venous spasm.

All catheter manufacturers have warnings about the use of excessive pressure. Gravity and infusion pumps do not exert pressure too high for the catheter to handle; however, excessive pressure from syringes can lead to catheter damage. For this reason, use of 10-mL syringes is often recommended for use with central venous catheters. Although these larger syringes will generate less pressure, it is still possible to reach excessive pressure levels if great force is applied against a syringe attached to a catheter that is partially occluded. Catheter patency must be carefully assessed before each use. Attach a 10-mL syringe filled with saline and attempt to flush the catheter without excessive force. If resistance is felt, *always stop the flush! Never forcefully flush any catheter with any size of syringe.* Catheter rupture or forcing a blood clot into circulation could result.

Flushing the Catheter

Catheter flushing prevents contact between incompatible drugs and maintains patency of the lumens. Normal saline alone or normal saline followed by heparinized saline may be used. When using valved catheters and certain positive fluid-displacement needleless devices, normal saline alone is acceptable because these devices have mechanisms that prevent the backflow of blood into the catheter lumen. When one of these products is not being used, the final flush should be normal saline followed by heparinized saline.

Before using any catheter, you should flush with normal saline to remove the heparinized saline left from the previous use and to determine lumen patency. Apply slow, gentle pressure to the syringe plunger. *If you feel any resistance, stop the procedure immediately.* During the flushing procedure, always aspirate for a brisk blood return from the catheter lumen. If the catheter will not yield a blood return, further diagnostic studies may be needed to determine the cause of the problems. Heparin is incompatible with many other medications, and the normal saline prevents contact between drugs and prevents drug precipitate from forming.

For short peripheral catheters, usually 3 mL normal saline is adequate to flush the catheter. For all other catheters, 5 to 10 mL of preservative-free normal saline is needed. Bacteriostatic normal saline is limited to no more than 30 mL in a 24-hour period in adults. By using 10 mL before and after each dose of medication, it is easy to exceed this limitation.

The concentration of heparinized saline ranges from 10 to 100 units/mL. The chosen concentration should not affect the client's clotting factors. Lower concentrations are used when the catheter is needed for frequent intermittent infusions; however, for infrequent use, 100 units/mL is preferred. Be sure that you know the policy and procedure established by your facility. Hemodialysis catheters may have larger concentrations of heparin used, such as 5000 units/mL; however, the heparin is aspirated before catheter use.

The volume of heparinized saline for catheter flushing should be a quantity that is twice the volume of the catheter lumen and the extension set or connectors added on, usually 3 to 5 mL.

Heparin use for catheter flushing is the cause of growing concern. It is often difficult for clients to remember the sequence of multiple flush solutions, adding to the need for repeated education of clients in home care. As mentioned previously, heparin is incompatible with many other drugs. Heparin may also interfere with obtaining blood samples taken from the catheter lumen, especially when coagulation studies are needed. Heparin-induced thrombocytopenia can also result from small doses used to flush catheters, resulting in loss of an extremity from blood clots and even death.

Catheters should be flushed immediately following each use. Delay in disconnecting the intermittent administration set and flushing the catheter could cause lumen occlusion from blood that backflows into the lumen when the infusion pressure is lower than venous pressure.

All fluids used to flush catheters should be obtained from single-dose containers or prefilled syringes. Vials used for multiple doses contribute to medication errors and increase the risk of contamination.

Obtaining Blood Samples from the Catheter

Short peripheral and midline catheters should not be routinely used for obtaining blood samples. This additional manipulation could lead to vein irritation that requires removal of the catheter. Central venous catheters can be used for obtaining blood samples after a careful assessment of the risk versus the benefits. If your client has no peripheral venipuncture sites or is fearful of needles, using the central venous catheter may be appropriate. The risks associated with obtaining blood samples from a central venous catheter are numerous. This procedure calls for additional hub manipulation, which is a major cause of bloodstream infection. Consider the laboratory tests needed and the types of fluids that have recently been infused. Heparin interferes with coagulation studies; electrolytes in the fluid may alter the results of serum electrolytes; and antibiotics such as vancomycin may interfere with measuring the peak serum levels of the drug.

If blood sampling from a central venous catheter is the best alternative, use methods that do not require the use of needles. Vacuum tubes attached directly to the catheter hub eliminate the need to transfer the blood from a syringe into the tubes. For small-diameter catheters, the vacuum in the tube may cause the catheter to temporarily collapse, preventing the backflow of blood into the tube. In this situation, small syringes should be used because they create less pressure on aspiration, the opposite of what small syringes do on injection. Transfer of the blood from the syringe to the vacuum tube requires the use of a special transfer device to avoid the use of needles.

Removing the Catheter

Short peripheral catheters are usually removed 72 or 96 hours after insertion. If a complication develops, they should be removed immediately. Lift opposite sides of the transparent dressing and pull laterally to remove the dressing from the site while stabilizing the catheter. Slowly withdraw the catheter from the skin, and immediately cover the puncture site with dry gauze. Do not use an alcohol pad because this will interfere with coagulation. Hold pressure on the site until hemostasis is achieved.

Removal of midline catheters and PICCs must be performed with the same slow, gentle techniques used to insert the catheter. Veins can develop venospasms when rapid or forceful techniques are used. After explaining to the client that this procedure will not be painful, remove the dressing and withdraw the catheter in short segments by pulling from the insertion site. If you feel resistance, always stop and never apply force to the catheter. Extreme traction or force could cause the catheter to break and embolize to the heart or pulmonary circulation.

Simple distraction techniques and deep breathing may be sufficient to relax the client and remove the catheter. If these fail, replace the dressing and apply heat; allow time for the vein wall to relax. Keeping the extremity warm and dry and asking the client to drink warm liquids could facilitate removal. Use of medications to relax the vein wall may be required if the catheter cannot be removed after several hours. Radiographic studies may also be needed to determine whether the cause is a thrombosis instead of venospasm.

Nontunneled percutaneous central catheters are removed by clipping any sutures and withdrawing the catheter in short segments. Venospasm does not commonly occur when removing these catheters because the vein diameter is large.

For all catheters, immediately after the catheter comes out of the skin, apply digital pressure with a dry gauze dressing to stop any bleeding. Apply a sterile occlusive gauze dressing with an antiseptic ointment. When a central venous catheter is removed, a tract between the skin and vein creates a conduit for air to be pulled into the vein. The ointment seals off the tract. After removal, measure the catheter length and compare it with the length documented on insertion. If the entire catheter length was not removed, contact the physician immediately.

Removal of tunneled catheters and implanted ports requires surgical techniques and is usually performed by nurse practitioners or physicians.

COMPLICATIONS OF INFUSION THERAPY

Complications from infusion therapy can be minor and limited or life threatening. Serious life-altering or life-threatening complications are dramatically increasing in frequency and severity and present a tremendous financial burden to the U.S. health care system. Catheter-related bloodstream infections (CRBSIs) are an excellent example. In critical care units in U.S. hospitals, about 80,000 CRBSIs occur annually. When the entire hospital is included, that number escalates to 250,000, and if the entire health care system is considered, the number soars to 500,000. Using the 250,000 that occur in hospitals, studies have estimated that 12% to 25% of clients die from these infections. Estimates of the cost for treating one episode of CRBSI range from $34,000 to $56,000. The annual costs for treating all CRBSIs range from $296 million to $2.3 billion (O'Grady et al., 2002).

Local complications of IV therapy occur at or near the catheter. A priority for care of clients with intravenous therapy is to prevent, assess, and detect these complications. In some cases, nurses also manage these problems. Definitions, causes, signs and symptoms, treatment, and prevention of local complications are summarized in Table 17-2. **Systemic complications** of IV therapy involve the entire vascular system or multiple systems. Information on common systemic complications can be found in Table 17-3. For central venous catheters, complications can occur during the insertion procedure or during the dwell time; these problems are described in Tables 17-4 and 17-5.

Text continued on p. 266

TABLE 17-2 Local Complications of Intravenous Therapy

Complication	Definition	Cause	Signs and Symptoms	Treatment	Prevention
Infiltration	Leakage of a nonvesicant IV solution or medication into the extravascular tissue	Peripheral catheter has punctured the vein in a second location Obstruction of blood flow causing increased pressure and fluid overflow from peripheral puncture site Inflammatory process causing fluid leakage at the capillary level Fibrin sheath fully encasing a central venous catheter leading to retrograde flow and leakage from venipuncture site Damaged septum of implanted port Dislodged port access needle	IV rate slows down; increasing edema at or above the insertion site; client may complain of skin tightness; blanching or coolness of skin; burning, tenderness or general discomfort at the insertion site; fluid leaking from puncture site; presence or absence of a blood return is not reliable diagnostic tool on a short peripheral catheter	Stop infusion and remove short peripheral catheter immediately after identification of problem. Apply sterile dressing if weeping from tissue occurs. Apply cold compresses. Elevate extremity if it increases client comfort. Insert a new catheter in the opposite extremity. For all central venous catheters, obtain a dye study to determine the cause of the problem. For implanted port, remove and insert a new port access needle.	Stabilize short peripheral catheter well; use smallest catheter that will accomplish the infusion; avoid placement over area of flexion; use handboard if sites in an area of flexion must be used; avoid placing restraints in the area of an IV site; make successive venipunctures proximal to the previous site; monitor site frequently; educate client about activities and signs and symptoms. For all central venous catheters, always obtain a brisk blood return before using the catheter for infusion. Frequently assess proper positioning of port access needle. Stabilize it well and protect from clothing.
Extravasation	Leakage of a vesicant IV solution or medication into the extravascular tissue	Same as infiltration	Same as infiltration Tissue sloughing appears in 1 to 4 wk	Stop infusion and disconnect administration set. Aspirate drug from short peripheral catheter or port access needle. Leave short peripheral catheter or port access needle in place to deliver antidote, if indicated by established policy. If possible, aspirate residual drug from the exit site of a central venous catheter. Administer antidote according to established policy. Apply cold compresses for all drugs EXCEPT vinca alkaloids and epipodophyllotoxins. Photograph site. Monitor at 24 hr, 1 wk, 2 wk, and as needed. Surgical interventions may be required. Provide written instructions to client and family.	Same as infiltration. Know the vesicant potential before giving any IV medication.

Continued

TABLE 17-2 Local Complications of Intravenous Therapy—*cont'd*

Complication	Definition	Cause	Signs and Symptoms	Treatment	Prevention
Phlebitis and post-infusion phlebitis	Inflammation of the vein Post-infusion phlebitis presents within 48 to 96 hr after the catheter has been removed	Mechanical cause from insertion technique, catheter size, and lack of catheter securement Chemical cause from extremes of pH and/or osmolarity of the fluid or medication Bacterial cause from a break in aseptic technique, poor securement, and extended dwell time	Client may complain of pain at the IV site; nurse may observe that vein appears red and inflamed along the length; vein may become hard and cordlike (see Table 17-6)	Remove short peripheral catheter at the first sign of phlebitis; use warm compresses to relieve pain. Monitor frequently. Document using Phlebitis Scale. Restart a new catheter using the opposite extremity. Mechanical phlebitis occurring in the first week after PICC insertion may be treated without catheter removal. Apply continuous heat; rest and elevate the extremity. Significant improvement is seen in 24 hr and complete resolution is seen within 72 hr. Remove catheter if treatment is unsuccessful.	Choose the smallest gauge catheter for the required therapy. Avoid sites of joint flexion or stabilize with a handboard. Avoid infusing fluids or medications with a pH below 5 or above 9 through a peripheral vein. Avoid infusing fluids or medications with a final osmolarity above 500 mOsm/L through a peripheral vein. Rotate sites every 72 to 96 hr according to established policy. Adequately secure the catheter. Use aseptic technique. For PICCs, teach client to avoid excessive physical activity with the extremity.
Thrombosis	Blood clot inside the vein	Traumatic venipuncture Multiple venipuncture attempts Use of catheters too large for the chosen vein Contact between the catheter and the vein wall, especially at or near the central venous catheter tip Fluid volume deficits in clients with a central venous catheter	Slowed or stopped infusion rate Swollen extremity Tenderness and redness Engorged peripheral veins of the ipsilateral chest and extremity Difficulty moving the neck or jaw	Stop infusion and remove short peripheral catheter immediately. Apply cold compresses to decrease blood flow and stabilize the clot. Elevate extremity. Surgical intervention may be required. For central venous catheters, notify the physician and obtain orders for a diagnostic study. Low-dose thrombolytic agents can be used to lyse the clot.	Use good venipuncture technique. Make only 2 attempts to perform venipuncture. Choose the smallest-gauge catheter in the largest vein possible. Secure catheter adequately. Use handboards if short peripheral catheters are placed in areas of joint flexion. Ensure adequate hydration to avoid changes in blood composition and flow. Prophylactic low-dose warfarin (Coumadin, Warfilone✱) may be prescribed for clients with a central venous catheter.
Thrombophlebitis	The presence of a blood clot and vein inflammation	Same as phlebitis and thrombosis	Same as phlebitis and thrombosis	Same as phlebitis and thrombosis. Apply cold compresses initially followed by warm.	Same as phlebitis and thrombosis.
Ecchymosis and hematoma	Ecchymosis is the infiltration of blood into the surrounding tissue Hematoma is the uncontrolled bleeding from a venipuncture site creating a painful lump	Venipuncture by unskilled person Venipuncture attempts into veins that cannot be seen or palpated Anticoagulated and steroid-dependent clients are at the greatest risk Using fragile veins or areas of poor skin turgor Excessive pressure or failure to apply direct pressure for the required time when removing a catheter	Swelling usually seen first Bruising at the insertion site Pain or tenderness	Remove IV device and apply light pressure; excessive pressure could cause other fragile veins in the area to rupture. For hematoma, apply direct pressure until bleeding has stopped. See treatment for infiltration.	Avoid veins that cannot be easily seen or palpated. Know your client's history. Use good venipuncture technique. Apply direct pressure long enough to control bleeding.

Site infection	Localized redness and hardness at the IV site caused by invasion of microorganisms in the absence of simultaneous bloodstream infection	Break in aseptic technique during insertion or the handling of sterile equipment Lack of proper hand hygiene and skin antisepsis	Site appears red, swollen, and warm; client may complain of tenderness at the site; may observe purulent or malodorous exudate	Clean exit site with alcohol, expressing drainage if present. For short peripheral, midline catheter or PICC, remove using sterile technique and avoid contact between skin and catheter. Amputate catheter tip into a sterile container. Send catheter tip for culture, if ordered. Clean site with alcohol and cover with dry sterile dressing; physician to evaluate for septic phlebitis and need for antimicrobial therapy or surgical intervention.	Use strict aseptic technique when inserting, maintaining, or removing catheters. Practice good hand hygiene. Ensure dressing remains clean, dry and adherent to skin at all times.
Venous spasm	A sudden contraction of the vein or artery	Catheter advancement immediately after tourniquet removal Infusion of cold fluids such as blood Sudden changes in the infusion pressure Removal of a midline catheter or PICC	Cramping or pain at or above the insertion site Numbness in the area Slowing of the infusion rate Inability to withdraw midline catheter or PICC	Temporarily slow infusion rate. Apply warm compress. Does not require immediate removal of short peripheral catheter. If occurring during midline catheter or PICC removal, do not apply tension or attempt forceful removal. Reapply a dressing, apply heat, encourage client to drink warm liquids, and keep extremity covered and dry. 12 to 24 hr may be required before catheter can be removed.	Allow time for vein diameter to return to normal after tourniquet removal and before advancing catheter. Infuse fluids at room temperature, if possible. For a midline catheter or PICC, gently withdraw the catheter in short segments.
Nerve damage	Inadvertent piercing or complete transection of a nerve	Venipuncture near known nerve locations Unanticipated nerve locations	Complaints of tingling or feeling pins and needles at or below the insertion site Numbness at or near the insertion site	Immediately stop the insertion procedure if the client complains of extreme pain. Remove the catheter if complaints of discomfort do not improve when the catheter is secured.	Avoid using the cephalic vein near the wrist. Avoid using veins on the palm side of the wrist. Adequately secure the catheter but avoid tape that is too tight. Support areas of joint flexion with an armboard.

PICC, Peripherally inserted central catheter.

TABLE 17-3 Systemic Complications of Intravenous Therapy

Complication	Definition	Cause	Signs and Symptoms	Treatment	Prevention
Circulatory overload	Disruption of fluid homeostasis with excess fluid in the circulatory system	Infusion of fluids at a rate greater than the client's system can accommodate	Client may complain of shortness of breath and cough; client's blood pressure is elevated, and there is puffiness around the eyes and edema in dependent areas; client's neck veins may be engorged, and nurse may hear moist breath sounds.	Slow the IV rate and notify physician; raise client to an upright position; monitor vital signs and administer oxygen as ordered; administer diuretics as ordered.	Monitor intake and output carefully and notify physician as soon as an imbalance is noticed between the client's intake and output.
Speed shock	Systemic reaction to the rapid infusion of a substance unfamiliar to the client's circulatory system	Rapid infusion of drugs or bolus infusion, which causes the drug to reach toxic levels quickly	Client may complain of lightheadedness or dizziness and chest tightness; nurse may note that client has a flushed face and an irregular pulse; without intervention, client may lose consciousness and go into shock and cardiac arrest.	Immediately discontinue the drug infusion and hang D_5W to keep the vein open; monitor vital signs carefully and notify physician for further treatment orders.	Be aware of the appropriate infusion rate of medications and adhere to them; use of infusion control devices assists in prevention of speed shock.
Allergic reaction	Local or general response to an allergen	May be a response to tape, cleansing agent, drug, solution, or IV device	A client having a local reaction may exhibit a wheal, redness, or itching at the IV site; in the case of a general reaction, client may complain of itching, running nose, and tearing; nurse may note bronchospasm, wheezing, and a truncal rash; without treatment, client may experience anaphylaxis.		
Catheter embolism	A shaving or piece of catheter breaks off and floats freely in the vessel	May occur if the needle of an over-the-needle catheter is reinserted into the catheter or if the needle of a through-the-needle catheter is inadvertently pulled back through the catheter	Client will experience a decrease in blood pressure and complain of pain along the vein; pulse becomes weak, rapid, and thready, and nurse may note cyanosis of the nail beds and circumorally; client may lapse into unconsciousness.	Discontinue catheter and apply a tourniquet high on the limb of the catheter site; inspect catheter for any rough edges; an x-ray is taken to determine the presence of any catheter piece; surgical intervention may be necessary.	When inserting over-the-needle catheters, never reinsert the needle into the catheter; avoid pulling a through-the-needle catheter back through the needle during insertion.

TABLE 17-4 Insertion-Related Complications of Central Venous Catheter

Problem	Definition	Possible Causes	Signs and Symptoms	Treatment	Prevention
Pneumothorax	Collection of air in the pleural space (space between the lung and chest wall)	Puncture of the pleural covering of the lung by the introducer on insertion of a direct subclavian approach	Chest pain Dyspnea Apprehension Cyanosis Decreased breath sounds on the affected side Abnormal chest x-ray findings	Remove catheter or assist with removal. Assess client by monitoring vital signs, and assess breath sounds. Notify physician immediately if suspected after insertion. Administer oxygen as ordered. Assist with insertion of a chest tube.	Use jugular or upper extremity insertion sites instead of subclavian sites. Use ultrasound to locate veins.
Hemothorax	Collection of blood in the pleural cavity	Result of puncture or transection of the subclavian vein or artery	Similar to pneumothorax; usually see dyspnea first and then tachycardia Decreased hemoglobin because of blood pooling	Same as for pneumothorax. Apply pressure on insertion site after introducer needle and catheter are removed.	Use jugular or upper extremity insertion sites instead of subclavian sites. Use ultrasound to locate veins.
Chylothorax	Lymph (chyle) enters the pleural cavity	Transection of the thoracic duct on the left side	Same as in hemothorax Usually noted on insertion with withdrawal of a milklike substance	Same as for pneumothorax.	Use right side for subclavian insertion. Use jugular or upper extremity insertion sites. Use ultrasound to locate veins.
Hydrothorax	Infusion of IV fluids directly into the thoracic cavity	Transection of the subclavian vein and placement of the catheter into the thoracic cavity	Same as in pneumothorax with absence of vesicular breath sounds and a murmur with a flat sound over the location	Same as for pneumothorax with removal of the catheter and aspiration of fluid.	Use jugular or upper extremity insertion sites instead of subclavian sites. Use ultrasound to locate veins.
Air embolism	Air enters the central venous system	Air is introduced into the central venous system during catheter insertion, tubing changes, catheter rupture, and catheter removal	Chest pain, dyspnea, hypoxia Anxiety, tachycardia, hypotension Nausea Light-headed, dizzy Loud churning heard over the pericardium on auscultation is possible but not always heard	Clamp catheter immediately. Place client in lateral Trendelenburg position on left side. Notify physician immediately. Oxygen therapy. Arterial blood gases. Electrocardiogram.	Lie client flat when changing administration sets or needleless connectors. Close slide clamp on catheter extension, if present. Ask client to perform a Valsalva maneuver, if possible. Use Luer-Lok connections on all catheters. Apply occlusive dressing with antiseptic ointment when removing a central venous catheter. Allow to remain in place for at least 24 hr.
Arterial puncture	Cannulation of an artery	Accessed the artery instead of the vein	Pulsating of bright red blood from the introducer needle	Remove needle immediately and apply pressure to the site. Secure a pressure dressing for 5-10 min.	Use ultrasound to locate veins during insertion procedure.
Nerve injury	Damage to one of the ulnar, median, or radial cords	Ineffective cannulation of the vein	Tingling to sensory motor deficit to complete paralysis	Immediate removal of catheter.	Use ultrasound during cannulation.
Malpositioned catheters	Catheter has passed into the jugular vein, the right atrium, the azygos vein or several other tributary veins	Improper client positioning during insertion Insertion of catheter length that is too short or too long for client	No signs or symptoms may be experienced before detection on initial chest radiograph to confirm tip location Ear, neck, or back pain Palpitations or dysrhythmias Inability to irrigate	Place client in semi-Fowler's position and flush with 20 to 50 mL of saline. Notify physician to reposition catheter by guidewire exchange. Refer to radiology for repositioning under fluoroscopy.	Insertion under fluoroscopy. Proper client measurement for catheter length. Proper client positioning.

PICC, Peripherally inserted central catheter; *SVC*, superior vena cava.

TABLE 17-5 Complications During the Dwell of Central Venous Catheters

Complication	Definition	Possible Causes	Signs and Symptoms	Treatment	Prevention
Catheter migration	Movement of a properly placed catheter tip to another vein No change in the external catheter length	Changes in intrathoracic pressure caused by coughing, vomiting, sneezing, heavy lifting, and congestive heart failure	For migration to the jugular vein complaints of hearing a running stream or gurgling sound on the side of catheter insertion For migration to the azygos vein, back pain between the shoulder blades Neurologic complications if medications are infused	Stop all infusions and flush catheter. Notify physician. Obtain a chest radiograph to assess tip location. Spontaneous repositioning back to the SVC is possible. Repositioning by radiology may be required.	Catheter tip properly placed in the lower third of the SVC near the junction with the right atrium. Instruct client to perform normal activities of daily living but to avoid excessive physical activity.
Catheter dislodgment	Movement of catheter into or out of the insertion site	Inadequate catheter securement Excessive physical activity with a PICC	External catheter length has changed, also changing the internal tip location No other signs or symptoms may be immediately noticed	Stop all infusions and flush catheter. NEVER readvance the catheter into the insertion site. Determine the amount of external catheter length and compare with the length documented on insertion. Notify the physician or nurse inserting the catheter for further assessment.	Proper catheter securement. Instruct client to perform normal activities of daily living but to avoid excessive physical activity.
Catheter rupture	Catheter is broken, damaged, or separated from hub or port body	Forcefully flushing a catheter with any size syringe against resistance Using scissors to remove a dressing Catheter compression of a subclavian inserted catheter between the clavicle and first rib. Also known as pinch-off syndrome	Fluid leaking from insertion site Pain or swelling during infusion Reflux of blood into the catheter extension Inability to aspirate blood from catheter	Repair of the damaged segment; depends on the availability of a repair kit designed for the specific brand of catheter being used; repair may be considered a temporary measure instead of a permanent treatment. Catheter exchange using several special techniques. Remove catheter.	NEVER use excessive force when flushing a catheter, regardless of syringe size. On injection, small syringes generate more pressure than larger syringes. Use of a 10-mL syringe is generally recommended for flushing procedures. Catheter insertion through jugular or upper extremity sites instead of subclavian site.
Lumen occlusion	Catheter lumen is partially or totally blocked	Drug or mineral precipitate (calcium, diazepam, and phenytoin are common) Lipid sludge from long-term infusion of fat emulsion Blood clots and fibrin sheath caused by blood reflux into lumen Allowing administration sets to remain connected for extended periods after medication has infused	Infusion stops or pump alarm sounds Inability or difficulty administering fluids Inability or difficulty drawing blood Increased resistance to flushing of the catheter	Assess history of catheter use. A suddenly developing problem may indicate contact between incompatible medications. A problem that develops over an extended period may indicate a gradual clot formation. For drug precipitate, determine the pH of the precipitated drug. Use hydrochloric acid for acidic drug. Use sodium bicarbonate for alkaline drugs. For blood clot, use thrombolytic enzymes such as alteplase.	Always flush with normal saline between, before, and after each medication given through the catheter. Use positive-pressure flushing techniques when a negative fluid displacement needleless connector is being used. Use a positive fluid displacement needleless connector. Flush catheters immediately when medication infusion is complete.

Phlebitis	Inflammation of the vein wall	Mechanical phlebitis is common with PICC lines and will appear within 7 days after insertion Chemical phlebitis may be seen with catheter rupture	Pain, redness, slight swelling May progress to cellulitis and palpable cord or collateral circulation	Mechanical phlebitis: conservative measures, warm compresses applied for 20 min four times daily for about 48-72 hr. Mild exercise. Chemical: change catheter or medication.	
Thrombosis	Formation of a blood clot in a vessel within the neck, chest, or arms that occurs in the presence of a central venous catheter	Stasis, vessel wall injury, or hypercoagulability	Chest pain, earache, or jaw pain Edema of neck, supraclavicular area, or extremities Edema at puncture site Jugular distention Collateral circulation on the affected side	Anticoagulant therapy. Possible catheter removal.	
Exit, port pocket, or tunnel infection	Infection may be localized at the insertion site or in the catheter or may progress to systemic infection	Failure to maintain sterile technique during catheter insertion or care Wet or soiled dressing remaining on site Immunosuppression Contaminated catheter or solution	Redness, warmth, tenderness, swelling at the insertion site Cellulitis Possible exudate of purulent material Local rash or pustules Fever, chills, malaise Leukocytosis Nausea and vomiting Elevated urine glucose level	Monitor vital signs closely. Monitor culture site. Redress with sterile technique. Treat systemically with antibiotics or antifungals, depending on culture results. Blood cultures. Remove catheter.	
Bloodstream infection	Invasion of pathogenic organisms enter the client's circulation	Inadequate skin antiseptic agents and application techniques Manipulation of the catheter hub leading to intraluminal contamination Inadequate hand hygiene	Early symptoms include fever, chills, headache, and general malaise; if left, client may experience severe infection, which may lead to vascular collapse and death	Change the entire infusion system from solution to IV device; notify physician, obtain cultures, and administer antibiotics as prescribed; if the infusate is the suspected cause, send a specimen to the laboratory for evaluation.	Same as for local infection above.

PICC, Peripherally inserted central catheter; *SVC*, superior vena cava.

TABLE 17-6 Phlebitis Scale from INS Standards of Practice

Grade	Criteria
0	No symptoms
1	Erythema with or without pain
2	Pain at access site with erythema and/or edema
3	Pain at access site with erythema and/or edema Streak formation Palpable cord
4	Pain at access site with erythema and/or edema Streak formation Palpable venous cord >1 inch long Purulent drainage

Data from Intravenous Nurses Society: Infusion Nursing Standards of Practice (2000). *Journal of Intravenous Nursing, 23*(65), 556.

OLDER ADULT CARE

The aging process causes numerous changes in all body functions, and yet aging occurs differently in each person. Nutrition, environment, genetics, social factors, and education are just a few of the factors that influence the older adult's needs. Because all body functions are affected, infusion therapy can be affected by these changes.

Skin Care

Aging skin becomes thinner and loses subcutaneous fat, decreasing the skin's ability for thermal regulation. Fewer nerve endings mean the decreased ability to feel pain. Your client *may* not perceive pain from traumatic venipuncture requiring excessive probing or multiple attempts; however, this action increases the risk of fluid leakage and subsequent infiltration or extravasation injury. Inserting and removing a catheter and dressing could tear the skin layers.

Skin antisepsis is extremely important because of the possible compromised immune status of the older client. Lipids are normally found in skin as a protective agent, and alcohol easily dissolves lipids. Whereas greater numbers of organisms may be killed, the skin can also become excessively dry and cracked. Current recommendations call for using friction when cleaning the skin to penetrate the layers of the epidermis. Excessive friction may damage fragile skin. Chlorhexidine gluconate is now the preferred agent, and the product currently available contains alcohol. Check for allergies to iodine before using iodine or iodophors. Iodophors such as povidone-iodine require contact with the skin for a minimum of 2 minutes to be effective. All antiseptic solutions must be thoroughly dry before applying the dressing or tape.

Skin should never be shaved before venipuncture, but excessive amounts of hair can be clipped away. Shaving causes microabrasions that can lead to infection. Skin of an older client may be more delicate and therefore more easily nicked while shaving.

Skin integrity can easily be compromised by the application of tape or dressings. Use of skin protectant solutions puts a protective barrier between the skin and dressing and improves the adherence of the dressing to the skin. Removal of tape and dressings may require adhesive remover solutions or an alcohol pad may accomplish the same purpose.

Vein and Catheter Selection

Vein and catheter selection are of highest importance in older adults. Insertion sites must be chosen carefully after consideration of skin integrity, vein condition, and activities of daily living. The general principle of starting with the most distal sites usually indicates use of hand veins. Fragile skin and small tortuous veins on the back of the hand (dorsum) should be avoided, and the initial IV site should be higher on the arm.

Venous distention must be accomplished with a flat tourniquet; however, the veins may require longer to distend. Allowing a tourniquet to remain in place for extended periods causes an overfilling of the vein and can result in a hematoma when the vein is punctured. On extremely fragile skin, the tourniquet application can lead to ecchymotic areas. A tourniquet may not be required in veins that are already distended; however, these veins must be carefully palpated to determine their condition. Hard, cordlike veins should be avoided. Blood pressure cuffs can also be used for venous distention. Inflate the cuff and release until the pressure is slightly less than diastolic pressure. Other methods to distend veins include the following:

- Light tapping, but avoid forceful slapping
- Asking the client to open and close the fist so the muscles can force blood into the veins. Make sure the hand is relaxed when the venipuncture is attempted.
- Placing the extremity lower than the heart
- Heat applied to the entire extremity for 10 to 20 minutes and removed just before making the venipuncture

As with all clients, venipuncture technique requires adequate skin and vein stabilization during the puncture and complete catheter advancement. Veins of an older adult are more likely to roll away from the needle. Low angles of 10 to 15 degrees between the skin and catheter will improve your success with venipuncture.

As soon as the catheter enters the vein, it may be necessary to release the tourniquet. Release of venous pressure from the puncture can lead to ecchymosis. Allowing the tourniquet to remain in place during the complete catheter advancement could increase this problem.

Catheter securement may mean that the administration sets are placed out of easy reach of a confused client. Using flexible netting over the extremity may prevent the client from pulling at the dressing or tubing while allowing you easy assess to the site. Rolled bandages should not be used to cover the extremity because they will prevent easy visualization of the site, allowing complications to progress to an advanced state before recognition.

Choosing a midline catheter or PICC may be best in older clients with poor skin turgor, limited venous sites, or veins that are fragile, tortuous, or hard. These catheters are placed in the upper extremity, where venous distention techniques can be used. Inserting nontunneled percutaneous central catheters in older adults may be a great challenge. Venous distention for insertion requires the Trendelenburg position and a well-hydrated client. Fluid volume deficit prevents adequate distention of the subclavian or jugular veins. Respiratory conditions like chronic obstructive pulmonary disease, spinal curvatures, and increased intracranial pressure may contraindicate this position. Tunneled catheters and implanted ports may be appropriate after consideration of the surgical techniques required to insert these catheters.

Cardiac and Renal Changes

Because of changes in cardiac and renal status, the accuracy of infusion volume and flow rate measurements is very important in the older adult. The health care provider's order for infusion therapy should be assessed for appropriateness for the client's condition. Electronic controlling devices may be required to ensure the necessary accuracy. When fluid restrictions are required, medications could be diluted in small quantities and delivered using a syringe pump or a manual IV push. For instance, 1 g of an antibiotic could be diluted in 10 mL normal saline instead of the more common 50 mL. This would allow the client to have more fluid to drink. Serum sodium levels should be considered when normal saline is routinely used for dilution in clients with hypertension or cardiac problems. For a poorly controlled diabetic client, dextrose solutions for dilution may not be preferred, although well-controlled diabetic clients may not have a problem with the small amount of dextrose in the solution. Consultation with the pharmacist and prescriber may be needed to answer these questions.

ALTERNATIVE SITES FOR INFUSION

Many reasons drive the need for infusion through sites other than the venous circulation. Through numerous technologic advances, we are now capable of infusion into arteries, peritoneum, bone marrow, epidural and intrathecal space, and subcutaneous tissue.

Arterial Therapy

DESCRIPTION

Catheters are placed into arteries to obtain repeated arterial blood samples, to monitor various hemodynamic pressures continuously, and to infuse antineoplastic agents. Catheters placed in the radial, brachial, or femoral arteries are used for obtaining blood samples or arterial pressure monitoring. Pulmonary artery pressure measures the function of the left heart and is accomplished by advancing a catheter through the central venous system, through the right heart chambers, and into the pulmonary artery.

Arterial waveforms and pressures are converted to digital values displayed on attached monitors. Between the catheter and the monitor is a special administration set capable of handling high infusion pressure, a pressurized fluid container with heparinized solution, a continuous flush attachment, a three-way stopcock, and a transducer. The transducer is positioned at the level of the client's atrium and secured to an IV pole to enable correct arterial pressure measurements.

Catheters used for pressure monitoring are inserted percutaneously through veins of the upper extremity or the subclavian or jugular sites. Insertion procedures are similar to the procedures used for venous cannulation. Removal requires the deflation of arterial balloons, if used, and applying digital pressure for longer than when removing a venous catheter.

Antineoplastic agents administered arterially allow infusion of a high concentration of drug directly to the tumor site before it is diluted in the circulatory system or metabolized by the liver or kidneys. Drug infusion through the same blood supply feeding the tumor optimizes cell kill at the tumor site while minimizing systemic side effects. The most common arterial sites include the hepatic and celiac arteries for liver tumors, although the carotid artery for tumors of the head, neck, or brain and pelvic arteries for cervical tumors have been used. Necrotizing pancreatitis has also been treated with infusion of protease inhibitors and antibiotics (West, 1998).

Arterial catheter insertion can be either a surgical procedure or an interventional radiologic procedure. Implanted ports are commonly used for extended therapies. For short-term therapy, an external catheter may be used for 3 to 7 days, although longer periods result in high complication rates.

One other device used for arterial infusion of antineoplastic agents is an implanted pump with an attached catheter. These small devices hold 50 mL of fluid in an upper chamber. The lower chamber exerts pressure when the upper chamber is filled, causing the drug to flow at 1 to 2 mL/day. Changes in blood pressure, body temperature, and altitudes alter the flow rate. The client must return for refilling the fluid chamber every 14 days.

NURSING CONSIDERATIONS

All arterial catheters require close attention to securing all junctions on the administer sets with luer-locked devices. When an infusion pump is used, it should have a pumping pressure high enough to overcome arterial pressure. Observe the insertion site and involved extremity closely. Assess for warmth, sensation, capillary refill, and pulse. When the carotid artery is involved, perform neurologic assessments. When a femoral catheter is used, anti-embolic stockings or other measures are indicated.

Complications from arterial catheters are similar to those from venous catheters, including infection, bleeding from the insertion site, catheter migration, infiltration, and catheter lumen or arterial occlusion.

Intraperitoneal Infusion

DESCRIPTION

Intraperitoneal (IP) therapy is the administration of antineoplastic agents into the peritoneal cavity. IP therapy is used to treat intra-abdominal malignant tumors such as ovarian or colorectal tumors that have moved to the peritoneum after surgery.

Catheters used for IP therapy may be an implanted port for long-term treatment or an external catheter for temporary use. These catheters, including those attached to an implanted port, have large internal lumens with multiple side-holes along the catheter length to allow for delivery of large quantities of fluid. Administration of IP therapy includes three phases: the instillation phase; the dwell phase, usually 1 to 4 hours; and the drain phase. Because this treatment involves the delivery of biohazardous agents, additional competency is required to handle the infusion properly.

NURSING CONSIDERATIONS

The client is in the semi-Fowler's position for the infusion. Your client may experience nausea and vomiting caused by increasing pressure on the internal organs from the infusing fluid. Pressure on the diaphragm may cause respiratory distress. Reducing the flow rate and treatment with antiemetic drugs is indicated. Severe pain may indicate that the catheter has migrated and an abdominal radiograph is needed to determine its location.

During the dwell and drainage phases, your client may need assistance in frequently moving from side to side to distribute the fluid evenly around the abdominal cavity. After the fluid has drained, the catheter is flushed with normal saline, although heparinized saline may be used in implanted ports. Catheter lumen occlusion is caused by the formation of fibrous sheaths or fibrin clots or plugs inside the catheter or around the tip.

Exit site infection, indicated by redness, tenderness, and warmth of the tissue around the catheter and microbial peritonitis and inflammation of the peritoneal membranes from the invasion of microorganisms, can occur. The client may experience a fever and complain of abdominal pain. Abdominal rigidity and rebound tenderness may be present. This condition is preventable by using strict aseptic technique in the handling of all equipment and infusion supplies. Management includes antimicrobial therapy administered either intravenously or intraperitoneally.

Subcutaneous Infusion

DESCRIPTION

Subcutaneous (SC or Sub Q) therapy has rapidly expanded in the past few years, with many drugs being infused to treat numerous conditions (Table 17-7). SC therapy is often used in palliative care clients who cannot tolerate oral medications, when intramuscular injections are too painful, or when vascular access is not available or is too difficult to obtain. Other studies reveal that SC infusion therapy produces better outcomes compared with IV infusion. A survey of SC infusion practices in hospices in the United States found that 73% used continuous SC infusion, primarily for pain management (Herndon & Fike, 2001).

Hypodermoclysis involves the slow infusion of isotonic fluids into the client's subcutaneous tissue. In the early to mid-twentieth century, this was the acceptable method for infusing parenteral fluids; however, severe reactions related to misuse occurred in the 1950s, causing this method to lose favor with physicians. In the 1980s, hypodermoclysis gained acceptance again because of the growth of the specialties of geriatrics and palliative health care (Slesak et al., 2003).

Hypodermoclysis can be used for short-term fluid volume replacement. The client must have sufficient sites of intact skin without infection, inflammation, bruising, scarring, or edema. The most common sites are the front and sides of the thighs and hips, the upper abdomen, and the area under the clavicle. Unlike IV therapy, the upper extremity should not be used because fluid is absorbed more readily from sites on the torso with larger stores of adipose tissue. Hypodermoclysis should not be used if the fluid replacement needs exceed 3000 mL/day, in emergency situations, or if there are bleeding or coagulation problems (Brown & Worobec, 2000).

TABLE 17-7 Examples of Subcutaneous Infusion Therapy

Disease or Condition	Drug or Therapy
Chronic iron overload	Deferoxamine mesylate (Desferal)
Chronic pain management	Morphine (Morphitec✱) Hydromorphone (Dilaudid) Fentanyl Haloperidol (Haldol, Peridol✱) Midazolam (Versed)
Diabetes, type 1	Insulin
Rheumatoid arthritis	Etanercept (Enbrel)
Head and neck malignant tumors	Amifostine (Ethyol)
Pulmonary arterial hypertension	Treprostinil (Remodulin)
Chronic asthma	Terbutaline (Brethine)
Recurrent preterm labor	Terbutaline (Brethine)

Hyaluronidase 150 units may be mixed with each liter of infusion fluid. This is an enzyme that improves the absorption of the infusing fluids from the SC tissue. An intradermal test dose is required because of the possibility of an allergic reaction. If the enzyme is not used, the infusion may not be well absorbed and redness at the insertion site is more likely (Brown & Worobec, 2000).

A small-gauge winged infusion or "butterfly" needle, a small-gauge short peripheral catheter, or an infusion set specially designed for subcutaneous infusion can be chosen. The SC infusion sets have a small needle extending at a right angle from a flat disk that helps to stabilize the needle.

NURSING CONSIDERATIONS

When choosing the infusion site, consider the client's level of activity. The area under the clavicle or the abdomen may have the least interference with ambulation. Clip excess hair in the area, and clean the chosen site with the antiseptic solution, preferably chlorhexidine gluconate. Prime the infusion tubing and the attached SC infusion set or winged needle. Gently pinch an area of about 2 inches (1 cm) and insert the needle. After securing the needle, cover the site with a transparent dressing. Hydrocortisone cream can be applied to the skin to prevent irritation.

Flow rates for hydration fluids begin at 30 mL/hr. After 1 hour, the rate can be increased if the client has experienced no discomfort. The maximum rate is 75 to 80 mL/hr (Brown & Worobec, 2000). For pain medication infusion, the flow rate is usually 2 or 3 mL/hr. If required for adequate pain control, two subcutaneous sites may be needed (Pasero, 2002).

Assess the site at least twice daily. Redness, heat, leakage, bruising, swelling, and complaints of pain indicate tissue irritation and the infusion needle should be removed. Rotate the SC site at least once per week.

Other complications include pooling of the fluid at the insertion site and an uneven fluid drip rate. Both of these problems may be resolved by restarting the infusion in another location. An infusion pump may also be used. Small ambulatory infusion pumps can be used to allow for greater mobility.

Intraspinal Infusion

The spinal column is covered by three layers: the dura mater, or outermost covering; the arachnoid, or middle layer; and the pia mater, which is closest to the spinal cord. Two spaces used for infusion are the **epidural** space between the dura mater and vertebrae and the **subarachnoid** space. The epidural space consists of fat, connective tissue, and blood vessels that protect the spinal cord. Medications infused into the epidural space must diffuse through the dura mater, and there is the possibility that some drug will be absorbed systemically. **Intrathecal** medications are infused into the subarachnoid space closer to the spinal cord, allowing reduced doses.

DESCRIPTION

Postoperative and chronic pain management are the primary indications for epidural infusion. Opioids administered epidurally slowly diffuse across the dura mater to the dorsal horn of the spinal cord. They lock onto receptors and block pain impulses from ascending to the brain. The client receives pain relief from the level of the injection caudally (toward the toes). Local anesthetics administered epidurally work on the sensory nerve roots in the epidural space to block pain impulses. The physician administers the first dose of medication; then, depending on state law, the type of medication, and facility policies, nurses trained in epidural therapy may administer subsequent doses.

Intrathecal infusion is used for treating cancers that cross the blood-brain barrier and involve the central nervous system (CNS). Some medications used to treat CNS neoplasms, such as methotrexate and cytarabine, are not effective intravenously because they cannot cross the blood-brain barrier. Others must be administered in large doses to cross this natural protective mechanism. It may not be possible to administer large doses of chemotherapeutic agents intravenously because of the severe systemic side effects associated with them. Administration of medications via the intrathecal route eliminates this problem because the medication is administered directly into the cerebrospinal (CSF). Intrathecal infusion is also used to treat spasticity of neurologic diseases such as cerebral palsy, multiple sclerosis, reflex sympathetic dystrophy, or traumatic and anoxic acquired brain injuries.

Temporary catheters used for epidural therapy can be a percutaneous catheter that is secured at the site and extends up the back toward the shoulder. These catheters are used for postoperative pain management and usually dwell for only several hours or a few days. Infection and subsequent meningitis and catheter migration are the possible complications.

Epidural catheters used for longer periods include a tunneled catheter and implanted port. Tunneled catheters are tunneled toward the abdomen and have a subcutaneous cuff to act as a barrier to infection. The external catheter exists the skin on the abdomen, so it can be easily reached for use by the client or caregiver. An epidural implanted port is the same design as an IV implanted port and is accessed with the same noncoring needle. The catheter extends from the lumbar puncture site to the port pocket and is located over a bony prominence on the abdomen through a subcutaneous tunnel. Surgically implanted pumps, described earlier for intra-arterial infusion, can also be used to deliver epidural and intrathecal infusion.

NURSING CONSIDERATIONS

Intraspinal catheters are usually inserted in the lumbar region. The external portion of a temporary epidural catheter is laid along the back toward the head and usually extends over the shoulder. The entire catheter length is taped for added security. Dressings are usually not routinely changed because they are only used for short periods. If bleeding or fluid leakage requires dressing removal, extreme care is required to prevent dislodging the catheter.

For a tunneled catheter or implanted port, the entire subcutaneous tunnel and port pocket should be frequently assessed. Measurement of an external catheter segment could help identify catheter migration.

An in-line filter is used on all intraspinal infusions to block the infusion of particulate matter. Medications commonly contain preservatives such as alcohol, phenols, or sulfites; however, these are toxic to the CNS. All medications used for intraspinal infusion must be free of preservatives. Alcohol and products containing alcohol should not be applied to the insertion site because the solution could track along the catheter and cause nerve damage. Povidone iodine solutions are preferred for skin antisepsis before insertion and during catheter dwell, including tunneled catheter exit sites and implanted port pockets.

Complications from epidural and intrathecal infusion can be caused by the type of medication being infused or be related to the catheter. It is important to know the specific location of the intraspinal catheter because the doses of medications are quite different. When used for pain management, doses are usually 10 times greater for epidural than for intrathecal infusion. Your client should be assessed for response to the drugs being given, their level of alertness, respiratory status, and itching.

Catheter-related complications include infection, bleeding or leakage of CSF, occlusion of the catheter lumen, and catheter migration. Infection in the client receiving either epidural or intrathecal therapy could be the result of a lack of asepsis when handling the medication or during the administration. There may be local evidence of infection, such as redness or swelling at the catheter exit site. The client may also exhibit neurologic and systemic signs of infection, such as headache, stiff neck, or temperature higher than 101° F (38.3° C).

Intraosseous Therapy

DESCRIPTION

Intraosseous (IO) therapy allows access to the rich vascular network located in the long bones. This vascular network is more prominent in children younger than 6 years of age. Thus IO is typically regarded as a pediatric procedure, but it can be used in adults also. Victims of trauma, burns, cardiac arrest, and other life-threatening conditions benefit from this therapy because often clinicians are unable to access these clients' vascular systems for traditional IV therapy. Research indicates that absorption rates of large-volume parenteral (LVP) infusions and medications administered via the IO route are similar to those achieved with peripheral or central venous administration. IO should be used only during the immediate period of resuscitation and should not be used longer than 24 hours. After establishing IO access, efforts should continue to obtain IV access as well.

Theoretically, any needle can be used to provide therapy and access the medullary space. In children, an 18-gauge needle is chosen, whereas adults require a 15- or 16-gauge needle. Needles specifically designed for IO are preferred because they have the following:

- A needle with a removable stylet that screws into the cannula to keep the needle from retracting during insertion
- A short shaft to eliminate accidental dislodgment after placement
- An adjustable guard to stabilize the needle at skin level
- Graduations along the needle to guide the practitioner during insertion

Sites chosen include the distal or proximal tibia and the distal femur. The sternum is not recommended because it is too thin to accommodate a needle; it could lead to pneumothorax and may interfere with other resuscitation efforts.

NURSING CONSIDERATIONS

If IV access cannot be obtained within the first few minutes of resuscitation procedures, IO may be attempted. The leg is restrained, and the site is cleaned with an antiseptic agent. After successful insertion, the needle must be secured to prevent movement out of the bone. The same doses of fluids and medications can be infused IO as IV. An infusion pump may be used for rapid flow rates.

Improper needle placement is the most common complication of IO therapy. An accumulation of fluid under the skin at either the insertion site or on the other side of the limb indicates that the needle is either not far enough in to penetrate the bone marrow or is too far into the limb and has protruded through the other side of the shaft. Needle obstruction occurs when the puncture has been accomplished but there has been a delay in flushing. This delay may cause the needle to become clotted with bone marrow.

Osteomyelitis is a serious complication of IO therapy that occurs in fewer than 1% of clients. This bone infection is unusual but is generally caused by allowing the IO needle to remain in place for a lengthy period or by the use of hypertonic solutions (West, 1998).

Compartment syndrome is a condition in which increased tissue pressure in a confined anatomic space causes decreased blood flow to the area. The decreased circulation to the area leads to hypoxia and pain in the area. This is rare in IO therapy, but the nurse should monitor the site carefully and alert the physician promptly if the client exhibits any signs of decreased circulation to the limb, such as coolness, swelling, mottling, or discoloration. Without improvement in perfusion to the limb, the client may require amputation of the limb.

GET READY for the NCLEX Examination!

KEY POINTS

- Infusion therapy is the delivery of parenteral medications and fluids through a wide variety of catheters and locations.
- Infusion therapy is used for establishing fluid and electrolyte balance, achieving optimum nutrition, maintaining hemostasis, and treating or preventing illnesses with medications.
- Vascular access devices (VADs) are catheters that are used to deliver fluids and medications.
- Common types of VADs include short peripheral catheters, midline catheters, peripherally inserted central catheters (PICCs), nontunneled percutaneous and tunneled central catheters, implanted ports, and hemodialysis catheters.
- The type of VAD that is used depends on the reason for infusion therapy, the client's condition, and the length of therapy.
- PICCs, tunneled central catheters, and implanted ports are commonly used for long-term infusion therapy.
- Devices engineered with safety mechanisms are required by the Occupational Safety and Health Administration (OSHA) to prevent injuries from needles, thus preventing bloodborne pathogen hazards.
- Infusion controllers and pumps are electronic devices used to regulate the flow of infusion fluids and medications.
- Nursing care for clients receiving IV therapy includes using sterile technique when starting the therapy and when changing part of the infusion system, changing and securing the site dressing, and assessing the site for local complications (see Table 17-2).
- Most catheters are flushed with either normal saline or heparinized saline on a periodic basis per agency policy.
- Older adults present special challenges when infusion therapy is used; physiologic changes of the skin and cardiac/renal systems must be taken into consideration.
- Small catheters should be used for older adults and should be inserted using a 10- to 15-degree angle to prevent rolling of the vein.
- Nurses are also responsible for detecting and managing systemic complications of infusion therapy as outlined in Tables 17-3, 17-4, and 17-5.
- Arterial therapy is used primarily for the administration of antineoplastic agents directly into a tumor site; the liver is the most common arterial site for this purpose.
- Intraperitoneal therapy is used for antineoplastic agent administration into the peritoneal cavity, especially for ovarian and colorectal tumors that have metastasized into the peritoneum.
- Subcutaneous therapy of fluids (hypodermoclysis) involves a slow infusion for a short time; the thighs, hips, and abdomen are commonly used sites.
- Epidural and intrathecal administration of medications is the common use for intraspinal infusion. Epidural infusions are most commonly for pain management; intrathecal infusions are usually antineoplastic agents used for cancers that cross the blood-brain barrier into the central nervous system.
- Intraosseous therapy allows fluids and medications to be absorbed by the rich vascular network of the long bones; it is used most often in children, but it can be used for adults as well.

ADDITIONAL STUDY RESOURCES

Go to your Student CD-ROM for Review Questions for the NCLEX Examination.

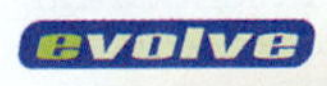

Go to http://evolve.elsevier.com/lggy/ for Integrated Management of Care Questions for the NCLEX Examination.

SELECTED BIBLIOGRAPHY

Asterisk indicates a classic or definitive work on this subject.

Brown, M., & Worobec, F. (2000). Hypodermoclysis: Another was to replace fluids. *Nursing 2000, 30*(5), 58-59.

Brunelle, D. (2003). Impact of a dedicated infusion therapy team on the reduction of catheter-related nosocomial infections. *Journal of Infusion Nursing, 26*(6), 362-366.

CDRH. (2001). *Safety assessment of Di(2ethylhexyl)phthalate (DEHP) released from PVC medical devices.* Rockville, MD: Center for Devices and Radiological Health, Food and Drug Administration.

Chernecky, C., et al. (2003). Preferences in choosing venous access devices by intravenous and oncology nurses. *Journal of Vascular Access Devices, 8*(1), 35-40.

Crosby, C., & Mares, A. (2001). Skin antisepsis: Past, present and future. *Journal of Vascular Access Devices, 6*(1), 26-31.

Fong, N., et al. (2001). Peripherally inserted central catheters: Outcome as a function of the operator. *Journal of Vascular and Interventional Radiology, 12*, 723-729.

Galloway, M. (2002). Using benchmarking data to determine vascular access device selection. *Journal of Infusion Nursing, 25*(5), 320-325.

Gorski, L.A. (2003). Central venous access device occlusions. Part 2: Nonthrombotic causes and treatment. *Home Healthcare Nurse, 21*(3), 168-171.

*Hadaway, L.C. (1998). Thrombotic and nonthrombotic complications: Loss of patency. *Journal of Intravenous Nursing, 21*(5S), S143-S160.

*Hadaway, L.C. (1999a). I.V. Rounds: Choosing the right vascular access device, Part 1. *Nursing 99, 29*(2), 18.

*Hadaway, L.C. (1999b). IV Rounds: Choosing the right vascular access device, Part 2. *Nursing, 99, 29*(7), 28.

*Hadaway, L.C. (1999c). Vascular access devices: Meeting patient's needs. *MedSurg Nursing, The Journal of Adult Health, 8*(5), 296-303.

Hadaway, L.C. (2001). IV Rounds: Managing a vasovagal reaction. *Nursing 2001, 31*(4), 73.

Hadaway, L.C. (2003). Skin flora and infection. *Journal of Infusion Nursing, 26*(1), 44-48.

Herndon, C., & Fike, D. (2001). Continuous subcutaneous infusion practices of United States hospices. *Journal of Pain Symptom Management, 22*(6), 1027-1034.

Hunter, M.R. (2003). Development of a vascular access team in an acute care setting. *Journal of Infusion Nursing, 26*(92), 86-91.

Intravenous Nurses Society (INS). (2000). Infusion nursing standards of practice. *Journal of Intravenous Nursing, 23*(6S).

*Kearns, P.J., Coleman, S., & Wehner, J.H. (1996). Complications of long arm catheters: A randomized trial of central vs peripheral tip location. *Journal of Parenteral and Enteral Nutrition, 20*(1), 20-24.

Monarch, K. (2002). Legal aspects of infusion practice: Trends and issues. *Journal of Infusion Nursing, 25*(6 Suppl): S21-30.

*National Association of Vascular Access Networks (NAVAN). (1998). Position paper: Tip location of peripherally inserted central catheters. *Journal of Vascular Access Devices, 3*(2), 8-10.

O'Grady, N., et al. (2002). Guideline for the prevention of intravascular catheter-related infections. *Morbidity and Mortality Weekly Report, 51*(RR10), 1-26.

Pasero, C. (2002). Subcutaneous opioid infusion. *American Journal of Nursing, 102*(7), 61-62.

Perucca, R. (2001). Infusion therapy equipment: Types of infusion therapy equipment. In J. Hankins et al. (Eds.), *Infusion therapy in clinical practice* (2nd ed.). Philadelphia: W.B. Saunders.

Rosenthal, K. (2004). Where did this patient's I.V. therapy go awry? *Nursing 2004, 34*(5), 56-57.

Ryder, M. (2001). *The role of biofilm in vascular catheter-related infections.* Physicians & Scientists Publishing Co. Retrieved February 5, 2002, from http://www.medpub.com/cme.htm.

Santolucito, J.B. (2001). A retrospective evaluation of the timeliness of physician-initiated PICC referrals. *Journal of Vascular Access Devices, 6*(3), 20-26.

Slesak, G., et al. (2003). Comparison of subcutaneous and intravenous rehydration in geriatric patients: A randomized trial. *Journal of the American Geriatric Society, 51*(2), 155-160.

Smelling, R., et al. (2001). Central venous catheters for infusion therapy in gastrointestinal cancer. A comparative study of tunneled centrally placed catheters and peripherally inserted central catheters. *Journal of Intravenous Nursing, 24*(1), 38-47.

Trimble, T. (2003a). IV Rounds. Peripheral I.V. starts: Insertion techniques. *Nursing 2003, 33*(8), 17.

Trimble, T. (2003b). IV Rounds. Peripheral I.V. starts: Vein preparation tips. *Nursing 2003, 33*(7), 17.

Viale, P.H. (2003). Complications associated with implantable vascular access devices in the patient with cancer. *Journal of Infusion Nursing, 26*(2), 97-102.

Vialle, R., et al. (2001). Anatomic relations between the cephalic vein and the sensory branches of the radial nerve: How can nerve lesions during vein puncture be prevented? *Anesthesia and Analgesia, 93*, 1058-1061.

Weinstein, S. (2001). *Plumer's principles and practice of intravenous therapy* (7th ed.). Philadelphia: J.B. Lippincott.

Weir, J. (2001). Blood component therapy. In J. Hankins et al. (Eds.), *Infusion therapy in clinical practice* (2nd ed., pp. 156-175). Philadelphia: W.B. Saunders.

*West, V. (1998). Alternative routes of administration. *Journal of Intravenous Nursing, 21*(4), 221-231.

Zwicker, C.D. (2003). The elderly patient at risk. *Journal of Infusion Nursing, 26*(3), 137-143.

CHAPTER

18 Acid-Base Balance

M. LINDA WORKMAN

LEARNING OUTCOMES

After studying this chapter, you should be able to:

1. Describe the relationship between free hydrogen ion level and pH.
2. Explain the role of bicarbonate in the blood.
3. Explain the concept of compensation.
4. Compare the role of a buffer in conditions of acidosis and alkalosis.
5. Compare the roles of the respiratory system and the renal system in maintaining acid-base balance.
6. Describe the role of oxygen in maintaining acid-base balance.
7. Interpret whether the client's arterial blood gas values are normal, elevated, or low.

Go to your Student CD-ROM for Review Questions for the NCLEX Examination keyed to these Learning Outcomes.

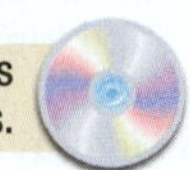

Acid-base balance occurs through control of hydrogen ion (H^+) production and elimination. Body fluid **pH** is a measure of the body fluid's free hydrogen ion level. The free hydrogen ion level, or pH, has the narrowest range of normal and the tightest control mechanisms of all electrolytes. The level of free hydrogen ions, formed from acids, must be rigidly controlled for proper function. Even small changes in the free hydrogen ion level, or pH, of body fluids can cause major problems in function. Keeping the pH within the normal range involves balancing acids and bases in body fluids.

The normal free hydrogen ion level of blood and other body fluids is quite low (less than 0.0001 mEq/L) compared with the body fluid levels of other electrolytes (see Chapters 14 and 16). Because it is so low, free hydrogen ion level is measured in pH units, calculated as the negative logarithm of the concentration in milliequivalents per liter (Figure 18-1). Normal pH ranges from 7.35 to 7.45 for arterial blood and from 7.31 to 7.41 for venous blood.

Because pH is calculated in negative logarithm units, the value of pH is inversely related (negatively related) to the level of free hydrogen ions. In other words, the lower the pH value of a fluid, the higher the level of free hydrogen ions in that fluid. The pH of a solution may range from 1 (as acidic as possible) to 14 (as alkaline as possible), with 7 being neutral. *A change of 1 pH unit actually represents a 10-fold change in free hydrogen ion level.* Therefore even a pH unit change of one tenth (e.g., a change from 7.4 to 7.3) represents a large increase in the free hydrogen ion level. Table 18-1 lists terms used to describe acid-base balance.

Changes from normal blood pH (7.35 to 7.45) interfere with many normal physiologic functions by:

- Changing the shape of hormones and enzymes so that they may no longer perform their normal functions
- Changing the distribution of other electrolytes, causing fluid and electrolyte imbalances
- Altering the responses of excitable membranes so that the heart, nerves, skeletal muscles, and gastrointestinal tract are either less or more active than normal
- Decreasing the uptake, activity, and effectiveness of many hormones and drugs

Fortunately, the body has many mechanisms to ensure minimal changes in free hydrogen ion level.

INTRODUCTION TO ACID-BASE BALANCE

As discussed in Chapters 14 and 16, body fluids are electrically neutral even though they contain ions with overall positive charges (**cations** or **protons**) and ions with overall negative charges **(anions).** When fluids contain an equal number of positive and negative charges, the electrical charge of the fluid remains neutral. The body keeps blood pH between 7.35 and 7.45 in a similar manner; however, this value is not strictly neutral (7.0 is neutral) but rather is slightly alkaline. Normal body fluid pH remains at a near-neutral value when the acids and bases are nearly balanced, limiting the total number of free or unbalanced hydrogen ions. Acid-base balance occurs by matching the rate of hy-

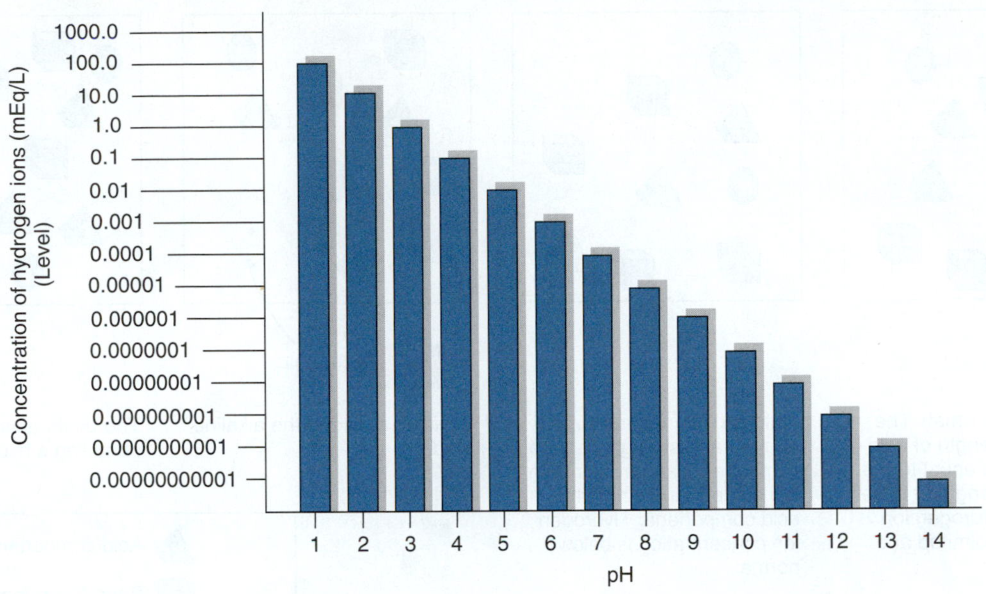

Figure 18-1 ■ Relationship between pH and concentration of hydrogen ions.

TABLE 18-1 Pertinent Acid-Base Balance Terminology

acid Any substance releasing a hydrogen ion when dissolved in water
anaerobic metabolism Cellular metabolism occurring without the presence of oxygen
base Any substance binding a hydrogen ion when dissolved in water
buffer A substance capable of binding a hydrogen ion from body fluids (acting as a base) or releasing a hydrogen ion into body fluids (acting as an acid)
chemoreceptors Special cells in the respiratory center of the brain sensitive to changes in the carbon dioxide concentration of extracellular fluid
pH The concentration of hydrogen ions in a solution, calculated as the negative logarithm of the milliequivalent concentration per liter

drogen ion production with activities for hydrogen ion removal or uptake.

Acid-Base Chemistry

ACIDS

Acids are substances that release hydrogen ions when dissolved in water (H_2O). An acid in solution *increases* the amount of free hydrogen ions in that solution. The strength of an acid is measured by how easily it releases a hydrogen ion in solution. A strong acid, such as hydrochloric acid (HCl), **dissociates** (separates) completely in water and readily releases all of its hydrogen ions:

HCl	+	H_2O	→	H^+	+	Cl^-	+	H_2O
Hydrochloric acid		Water		Hydrogen ion		Chloride ion		Water

A weak acid does not completely separate in water; it releases only some of its hydrogen ions. In the following example, each molecule of acetic acid (CH_3COOH), a weak acid, contains a total of four hydrogen molecules. When acetic acid combines with water, it releases only one of its four hydrogen molecules. The other three hydrogen molecules remain bound to the acetic acid molecule:

$$CH_3COOH + H_2O \rightarrow H^+ + CH_3COO + H_2O$$

BASES

A **base** binds free hydrogen ions in solution. Thus bases are hydrogen acceptors that reduce the amount of free hydrogen ions in solution. Strong bases bind hydrogen ions easily. Examples of strong bases include sodium hydroxide (NaOH) and ammonia (NH_3).

Weak bases bind hydrogen ions less readily. Examples of weak bases include aluminum hydroxide ($AlOH_3$) and bicarbonate (HCO_3^-). Although bicarbonate is a weak base, bicarbonate ions in the body prevent major changes in body fluid pH.

BUFFERS

Buffers can either release a hydrogen ion into a fluid or bind a hydrogen ion from a fluid. Most substances, when dissolved in water, react by either releasing a hydrogen ion (an acid) or binding a free hydrogen ion (a base). Buffers dissolved in water can react in two ways: either as an acid (releasing a hydrogen ion) or as a base (binding a hydrogen ion).

How a buffer reacts when dissolved in water depends on the existing acid-base balance of that fluid. Buffers always try to bring the fluid as close as possible to the normal body fluid pH of 7.35 to 7.45. If the fluid is basic (with few free hydrogen ions), the buffer releases hydrogen ions into the fluid (Figure 18-2). If the fluid is acidic (with many free hydrogen ions), the buffer acts as a base, binding some hydrogen ions. Buffers act like hydrogen ion "sponges," soaking up hydrogen ions when too many are present and squeezing out hydrogen ions when too few are present. Because of this flexibility, buffers are important regulators of body fluid pH, or hydrogen ion level (acid-base balance).

Liquids with a pH of 7.0 are neutral; they have a free hydrogen ion level in which the number and strength of acids and bases are equal. Figure 18-3 represents the concept of

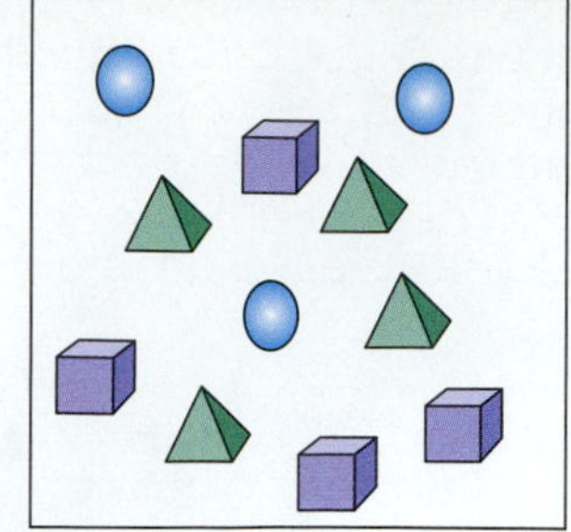

Fluid pH 7.38 (normal). The number and strength of acid components are equal to the number and strength of base components. Hydrogen ion concentration is limited and constant.

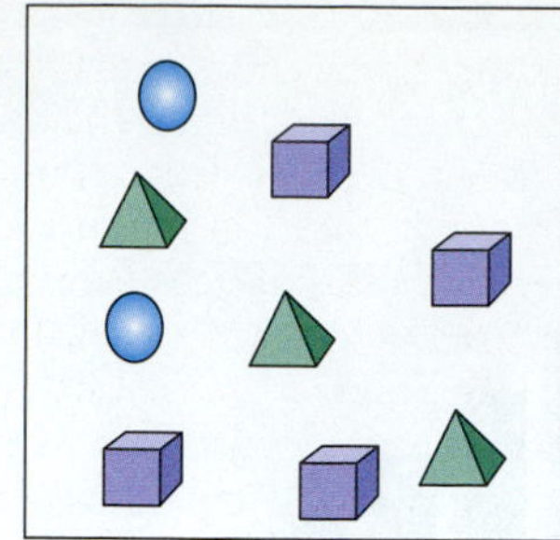

Fluid pH 7.51 (alkaline). The number and strength of base components are greater than the number and strength of acid components. Hydrogen ion concentration is below normal.

Buffer is added to the alkaline fluid.

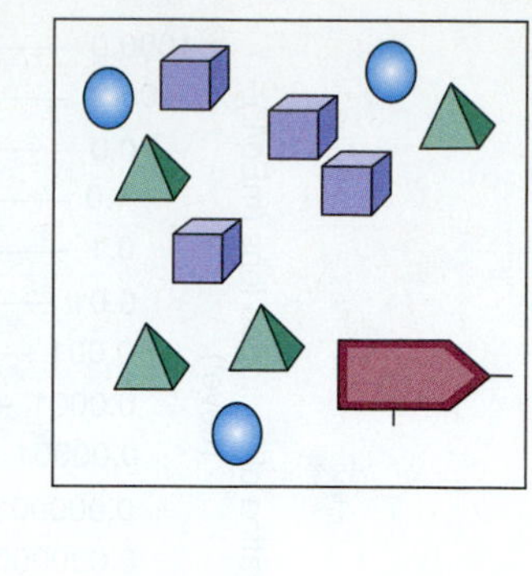

The buffer acts as an acid, releasing a hydrogen ion.

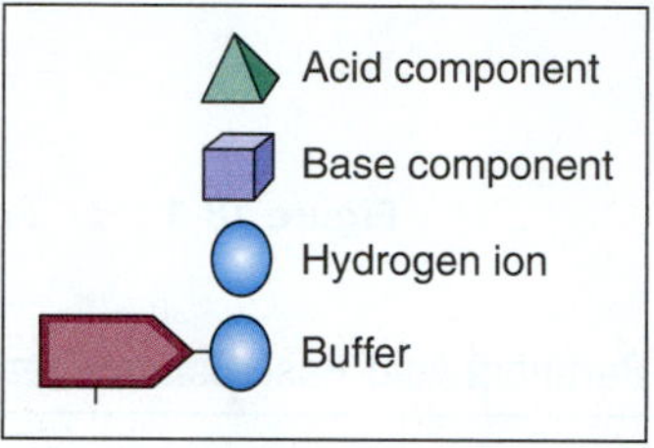

Figure 18-2 ■ Action of buffer in solution. (© 1992 by M. Linda Workman. All rights reserved.)

Neutral	Acidic (acid excess)	Acidic (base deficit)
AAABBB	AAAABBB	AAABB
AAABBB	AAAABBB	AAABB
AAABBB	AAAABBB	AAABB

Figure 18-3 ■ Concept of acidic versus normal pH. **A** = Acid; **B** = base.

Neutral	Alkaline (base excess)	Alkaline (acid deficit)
AAABBB	AAABBBB	AABBB
AAABBB	AAABBBB	AABBB
AAABBB	AAABBBB	AABBB

Figure 18-4 ■ Concept of alkaline versus normal pH. **A** = Acid; **B** = base.

neutral pH. This figure shows that the combined *strength* and *amount* of all acids are equal to the combined *strength* and *amount* of all bases in a given solution. This is not the actual case in human physiology. However, in acid-base homeostasis, the relative amounts and strengths of acids and bases are nearly equal, so the overall free hydrogen ion levels remain constant.

Liquids with a pH ranging from 1.0 to 6.99 have more or stronger (or both) acids compared with the amount or strength (or both) of bases. Such liquids are *acidic* (see Figure 18-3), which means that more free hydrogen ions are being released than bound, increasing the number of free hydrogen ions.

Liquids with a pH ranging from 7.01 to 14.0 have more or stronger (or both) bases compared with the amount or strength (or both) of acids. These liquids are *basic*, which means that more hydrogen ions are being bound than released, decreasing the number of free hydrogen ions (Figure 18-4).

Body Fluid Chemistry

BICARBONATE IONS

Body fluids contain many different types of acids and a few types of bases. The most common base in human body fluid is bicarbonate (HCO_3^-); the most common acid is carbonic acid (H_2CO_3). In health, the body keeps these substances within extracellular fluid (ECF) at a constant ratio of one molecule of carbonic acid to 20 free bicarbonate ions (1:20) (Figure 18-5). To maintain this ratio, both carbonic acid and bicarbonate must be carefully controlled. Both of these substances and their constant ratio are related to the production and elimination of carbon dioxide (CO_2) and hydrogen ions (H^+).

A key concept in understanding acid-base balance is the *carbonic anhydrase equation.* This equation, driven by the enzyme carbonic anhydrase, shows how hydrogen ion levels and carbon dioxide levels are directly related to one another, so that an increase in one causes an equal increase in the other:

$$CO_2 + H_2O \Leftrightarrow H_2CO_3 \Leftrightarrow H^+ + HCO_3^-$$

Carbon dioxide + Water ⇔ Carbonic acid ⇔ Hydrogen ion + Bicarbonate ion

Carbon dioxide is a gas that forms carbonic acid when combined with water. Carbon dioxide is a changeable part

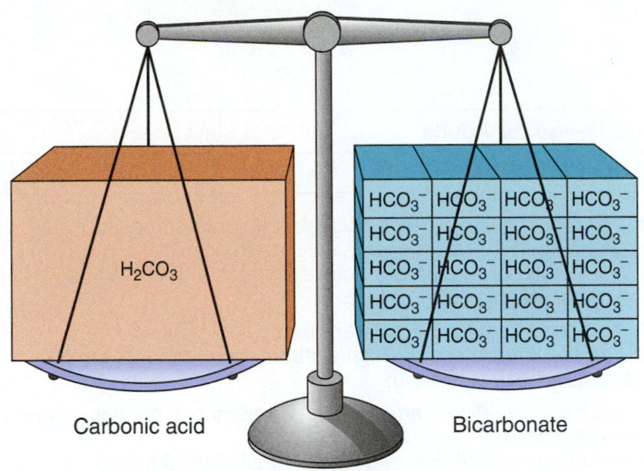

Figure 18-5 ■ Normal ratio of carbonic acid to bicarbonate is 1:20.

of carbonic acid. Carbonic acid is not stable, and the body needs to keep a 1:20 ratio of carbonic acid to bicarbonate. As soon as carbonic acid is formed from water and carbon dioxide, it immediately separates into free hydrogen ions and bicarbonate ions. *Therefore the carbon dioxide content of a fluid is directly related to the amount of hydrogen ions in that fluid. Whenever conditions cause carbon dioxide to increase, more free hydrogen ions are created. Likewise, whenever free hydrogen ion production increases, more carbon dioxide is produced.*

RELATIONSHIP BETWEEN CARBON DIOXIDE AND HYDROGEN IONS

When excess carbon dioxide is produced, the amount of carbon dioxide increases and the carbonic anhydrase equation shifts to the right, causing an increase in hydrogen ions (and a decrease in pH):

$$\mathbf{CO_2} + H_2O \Rightarrow H_2CO_3 \Rightarrow H^+ + HCO_3^-$$

When very little carbon dioxide is produced, no free hydrogen ions are created by the carbonic anhydrase equation.

When excess hydrogen ions are produced or brought into the body, the carbonic anhydrase equation shifts to the left, causing the creation of more carbon dioxide:

$$CO_2 + H_2O \Leftarrow H_2CO_3 \Leftarrow \mathbf{H^+} + HCO_3^-$$

When the amount of free hydrogen ions in body fluids is low, no extra carbon dioxide is produced.

CALCULATION OF FREE HYDROGEN ION LEVEL

The pH is a calculation of the free hydrogen ion level in body fluids. A formula is used because the actual number of free hydrogen ions is not easily measured. The pH calculations come from a mathematical formula (the Henderson-Hasselbalch equation) that shows how three factors are related: the level of free hydrogen ions, the amount of bases, and the strength of acids in a solution. In the body, if two of these three factors are known, the third factor can then be calculated.

Because the normal ratio of carbonic acid and bicarbonate level in ECF is 1:20, the only factor that changes is the carbon dioxide level. Whenever the carbon dioxide level changes, the pH changes to the same degree, in the opposite direction. Thus when the carbon dioxide level of a liquid increases, the pH drops, indicating more free hydrogen ions (more acidic). On the other hand, when the carbon dioxide level of a liquid decreases, the pH rises, indicating fewer free hydrogen ions (more alkaline).

An increase in bicarbonate causes the amount of hydrogen ions to decrease and the pH to increase, or become more alkaline (basic). Conversely, an increase in the carbon dioxide level causes the free hydrogen ion level to increase and the pH to decrease, or become more acidic.

Because the kidneys control bicarbonate levels and the lungs control carbon dioxide levels in the healthy person, pH is also described as the function of the kidneys divided by the function of the lungs:

$$\text{pH} = \frac{\text{Kidneys (bicarbonate)}}{\text{Lungs (carbon dioxide)}}$$

SOURCES OF ACIDS

Acids are formed as normal waste products of carbohydrate, protein, and fat metabolism. Carbohydrate metabolism forms carbon dioxide, which can then be converted to free hydrogen ions. Fat and protein metabolism directly create acids.

GLUCOSE METABOLISM (PRODUCTION OF CARBON DIOXIDE). Carbon dioxide is a waste product of glucose breakdown and other metabolic reactions. (The complete breakdown of one molecule of glucose forms 36 molecules of adenosine triphosphate [ATP], six molecules of water, and six molecules of carbon dioxide.) Because of the relationship between carbon dioxide and free hydrogen ions, any increase in carbon dioxide levels always leads to increased amounts of hydrogen ions. The result is a decrease in pH.

Carbon dioxide is exhaled by the lungs during breathing. One factor that determines blood pH is how much carbon dioxide is produced by body cells during metabolism versus how rapidly that carbon dioxide is removed by breathing.

FAT AND PROTEIN METABOLISM. The breakdown of food for energy results in the formation of *fixed acids*. Protein breakdown forms sulfuric acid. Fat breakdown forms fatty acids and ketoacids.

INCOMPLETE METABOLISM OF GLUCOSE AND FATS. Incomplete breakdown of glucose, which occurs whenever cells metabolize under **anaerobic** (no oxygen) conditions, forms lactic acid. Anaerobic conditions occur with hypoxia, sepsis, and shock. Incomplete breakdown of fatty acids, occurring when large amounts of fatty acids are being metabolized, forms ketoacids (Guyton & Hall, 2000).

DESTRUCTION OF CELLS. Whenever cells are damaged or destroyed, cell membranes are broken and cell contents are released. Some cell structures contain acids that are released into the extracellular fluid (ECF) when this occurs.

SOURCES OF BICARBONATE IONS

Bicarbonate is the primary buffer of the ECF. Bicarbonate comes from the breakdown of carbonic acid, intestinal absorption of ingested bicarbonate, pancreatic production of bicarbonate, movement of cellular bicarbonate into the ECF, and kidney reabsorption of filtered bicarbonate. Once bicarbonate is in the ECF, it is kept at a level 20 times greater than that of carbonic acid.

CHART 18-1

LABORATORY PROFILE
Acid-Base Assessment

	Normal Range for Adults		
Test	**Arterial**	**Venous**	**Significance of Abnormal Findings**
pH >90 yr	7.35-7.45 7.25-7.45	7.31-7.41	Increased: metabolic alkalosis, loss of gastric fluids, decreased potassium intake, diuretic therapy, fever, salicylate toxicity Decreased: metabolic or respiratory acidosis, ketosis, renal failure, starvation, diarrhea, hyperthyroidism
Pao_2 (mm Hg) >90 yr	80-100 >50		Increased: increased ventilation, oxygen therapy, exercise Decreased: respiratory depression, high altitude, carbon monoxide poisoning, decreased cardiac output
$Paco_2$ (mm Hg)	35-45	40-50	Increased: respiratory acidosis, emphysema, pneumonia, cardiac failure, respiratory depression Decreased: respiratory alkalosis, excessive ventilation, diarrhea
Bicarbonate (mEq/L or mmol/L)	22-26	24-29	Increased: bicarbonate therapy, metabolic alkalosis Decreased: metabolic acidosis, diarrhea, pancreatitis
Lactate	3-7 mg/dL 0.3-0.8 mmol/L	5-20 mg/dL 0.6-2.2 mmol/L	Increased: hypoxia, exercise, insulin infusion, alcoholism, pregnancy Decreased: fluid overload

Pao_2, Partial pressure of arterial oxygen; *$Paco_2$*, partial pressure of arterial carbon dioxide.

ACID-BASE HOMEOSTASIS

As long as body cells are healthy, they continually produce acids, carbon dioxide, and hydrogen ions. Despite this production, hydrogen ions, bicarbonate, oxygen, and carbon dioxide levels are kept within normal limits when physiologic function is normal. Chart 18-1 lists normal values for these substances in arterial and venous blood. This homeostasis depends on three factors:

- Hydrogen ion production is consistent and not excessive.
- Carbon dioxide loss from the body through breathing must keep pace with hydrogen ion production.
- The ratio between carbonic acid and bicarbonate must be kept at 1:20.

Acid-Base Regulatory Mechanisms

To keep the free hydrogen ion level (pH) of the ECF within the narrow range of normal, the body has chemical, respiratory, and renal mechanisms for acid-base balance (Table 18-2).

CHEMICAL ACID-BASE CONTROL MECHANISMS

Buffers are the first line of defense against changes in the amount of free hydrogen ions. Because they are always present in body fluids, buffers act fast to reduce or raise the amount of free hydrogen ions to normal. By acting as hydrogen ion "sponges," buffers can bind hydrogen ions when too many are present or release hydrogen ions when not enough are present. Buffers are composed of chemicals or proteins.

CHEMICAL BUFFERS. Chemical buffers are paired mixtures, usually a weak base and an acid salt. The two most common chemical buffer systems are bicarbonate buffers (which are active in both the extracellular fluid [ECF] and intracellular fluid [ICF]) and phosphate buffers (which are active in the ICF).

PROTEIN BUFFERS. Proteins are the largest source of buffers. Proteins in body fluids can either bind or release free hydrogen ions as needed. Both ICF and ECF proteins serve as buffers.

A major cell protein buffer is hemoglobin. Hemoglobin buffers hydrogen ions directly and also buffers acids formed during the production of carbon dioxide. When the amount of free hydrogen ions in the blood increases, some of the excess hydrogen ions cross the membranes of red blood cells and bind to the large numbers of hemoglobin molecules in each red blood cell.

Extracellular protein buffers are albumin and globulins. These proteins buffer carbonic acid and other acids present in the ECF as a result of catabolism.

RESPIRATORY ACID-BASE CONTROL MECHANISMS

When chemical buffers alone cannot prevent changes in blood pH, the respiratory system is the second line of defense against changes. Breathing controls the amount of free hydrogen ions by controlling the amount of carbon dioxide in arterial blood. Carbon dioxide is converted into hydrogen ions through the carbonic anhydrase reaction. Therefore the carbon dioxide level is directly related to the hydrogen ion level. Breathing rids the body of the excess carbon dioxide created through metabolism.

The amount of carbon dioxide in venous blood increases during normal metabolism. This carbon dioxide is moved in the blood to the lung capillaries. Because the amount (pressure) of carbon dioxide is far higher in capillary blood than in the air in the alveoli, carbon dioxide diffuses freely from the blood into the alveolar air. Once in the alveoli, carbon dioxide is exhaled during breathing and is lost from the body. Because the amount (pressure) of carbon dioxide in normal atmospheric air is nearly zero, carbon dioxide usually continues to be exhaled even when breathing is impaired to some degree.

HYPERVENTILATION. Respiratory regulation of acid-base balance is under the control of the central nervous system (Figure 18-6). Special receptors in the respiratory areas of the brain are sensitive to changes in the amount of carbon dioxide in brain tissues. As the amount of carbon dioxide begins to rise above normal in brain blood and tissues, these central receptors trigger the neu-

TABLE 18-2 Acid-Base Regulatory Mechanisms

Mechanism Type	Key Characteristics
Chemical	
Protein buffers	Very rapid response
Extracellular	Provide immediate response to changing conditions
Albumin	Can handle relatively small fluctuations in hydrogen ion production and elimination encountered under normal metabolic and health conditions
Globulins	
Intracellular	
Hemoglobin	
Chemical buffers	
Extracellular	
Bicarbonate	
Intracellular	
Phosphate	
Bicarbonate	
Respiratory	
Increased hydrogen ions	Primarily assist buffering systems when the fluctuation of hydrogen ion concentration is acute
Increased carbon dioxide	
Stimulates central respiratory neurons, leading to increased rate and depth of breathing, causing more carbon dioxide to be lost and decreasing the hydrogen ion concentration	
Decreased hydrogen ions	
Decreased carbon dioxide	
Inhibition of central respiratory neurons, leading to decreased rate and depth of breathing, causing normally produced carbon dioxide to be retained, increasing the hydrogen ion concentration	
Renal	
Mechanisms to decrease pH	The most powerful regulator of acid-base balance
Increased renal excretion of bicarbonate	Respond to large or chronic fluctuations in hydrogen ion production or elimination
Increased renal reabsorption of hydrogen ions	Slowest response (hours to days)
Mechanisms to increase pH	Longest duration
Decreased renal excretion of bicarbonate	
Decreased renal reabsorption of hydrogen ions	

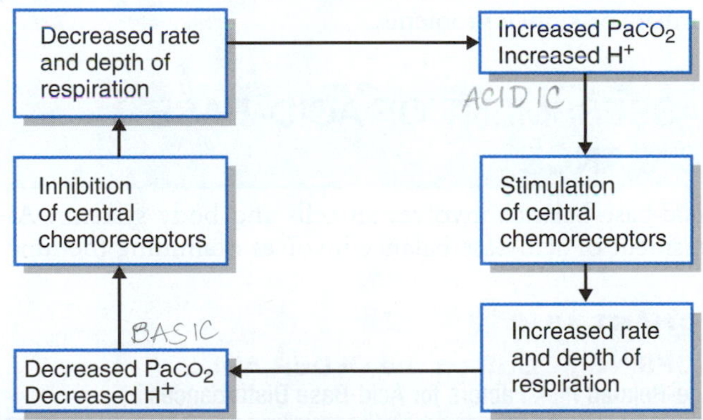

Figure 18-6 ■ Neural regulation of respiration and hydrogen ion concentration. *$PaCO_2$*, Partial pressure of arterial carbon dioxide; *H^+*, hydrogen ion.

rons to increase the rate and depth of breathing. As a result, more carbon dioxide is exhaled ("blown off") from the lungs and the amount carbon dioxide in the ECF decreases. When the amount of arterial carbon dioxide returns to normal, the rate and depth of breathing return to levels that are normal for the person.

HYPOVENTILATION. If the amount of ECF free hydrogen ions is too low, then the amount of carbon dioxide also is too low. Central receptors sense these low carbon dioxide levels and stop or slow the neuron activity in the respiratory centers, decreasing the rate and depth of breathing. As a result, less carbon dioxide is lost through the lungs and more carbon dioxide is retained in arterial blood. This retention of already-formed carbon dioxide, together with the normal production of carbon dioxide from metabolism, results in a rapid return of the arterial carbon dioxide levels (and hydrogen ion levels) to normal. When these levels are normal, the rate and depth of breathing also return to normal levels.

The respiratory system's response in regulating acid-base balance is rapid. Changes in the rate and depth of breathing occur within minutes after changes in the hydrogen ion level or carbon dioxide level of the ECF occur.

RENAL ACID-BASE CONTROL MECHANISMS

The kidneys are the third line of defense against wide changes in body fluid pH. Renal mechanisms are stronger for regulating acid-base balance but take longer than chemical and respiratory mechanisms to completely respond. (They take 24 to 48 hours to respond.) When blood pH changes are persistent, renal mechanisms that increase excretion and reabsorption rates of acids or bases (depending on the direction of the pH changes) begin to operate. These mechanisms are kidney movement of bicarbonate, formation of acids, and formation of ammonium.

KIDNEY MOVEMENT OF BICARBONATE. This first renal mechanism occurs in the kidney tubules in two ways: (1) kidney movement of bicarbonate produced elsewhere in the body and (2) kidney movement of bicarbonate produced in the kidneys. Much of the bicarbonate made in other body areas is excreted in the urine. When blood hydrogen ion levels are high, this bicarbonate is reabsorbed from the kidneys back into circulation, where it can help buffer excess hydrogen ions. When blood hydrogen ion levels are low, the bicarbonate remains in the urine and is excreted. When hydrogen ion excess occurs, the kidney tubules also can make additional bicarbonate that will be reabsorbed.

FORMATION OF ACIDS. The second renal mechanism occurs through the phosphate-buffering system inside the cells of the kidney tubules. When the newly created bicarbonate made in the kidney cells is reabsorbed into the blood along with sodium, the urine has an excess of anions, including phosphate (HPO_4^{2-}). This negatively charged fluid draws hydrogen ions (which carry a positive charge) into the urine. Once the hydrogen ion is in the urine, it binds to phosphate ions, forming an acid, H_2PO_4, which is then excreted in the urine.

FORMATION OF AMMONIUM. In the third renal mechanism, ammonia (NH_3), which is formed during normal protein breakdown, is converted into ammonium (NH_4^+). The ammonia is secreted into the urine, where it can combine with hydrogen ions to form ammonium, stays in the urine, and then is excreted from the body. This "trapping" of hydrogen ions in ammonium prevents the free hydrogen ion level in the urine from becoming so high that it inhibits movement of hydrogen ions from the blood into the urine. The overall result is a loss of hydrogen ions and an increase in blood pH.

COMPENSATION

In the process of *compensation,* the body attempts to correct changes in blood pH. A pH below 6.9 or above 7.8 is usually fatal. The normal pH range for human extracellular fluid (ECF) is 7.35 to 7.45. Both the kidneys and the lungs can compensate for acid-base imbalances, but they are not equal in their compensatory responses. The respiratory system is much more sensitive to acid-base changes and can begin compensation efforts within seconds to minutes after a change in pH. However, these efforts are limited and can be overwhelmed easily. The renal compensatory mechanisms are much more powerful and result in rapid changes in ECF composition. However, these more powerful mechanisms are not fully triggered unless the acid-base imbalance continues for several hours to several days.

RESPIRATORY COMPENSATION. The lungs can usually compensate for acid-base imbalances of a metabolic origin. For example, when prolonged running causes buildup of lactic acid, hydrogen ion levels in the ECF increase and the pH drops. To bring the pH back to normal, breathing is triggered in response to increased carbon dioxide levels. Both the rate and depth of respiration increase. These respiratory efforts cause the blood to lose carbon dioxide with each exhalation, so ECF levels of carbon dioxide and free hydrogen ions gradually decrease. When the lungs can fully compensate, the pH returns to normal.

RENAL COMPENSATION. A healthy kidney can correct or compensate for changes in blood pH when the respiratory system is either overwhelmed or is not healthy. For example, in a person with chronic obstructive pulmonary disease (COPD), the respiratory system cannot exchange gases adequately. Carbon dioxide is retained and the blood pH falls (becomes more acidic). To oppose this process, the kidney excretes more hydrogen ions and increases the reabsorption of bicarbonate back into the blood. As a result, the blood pH remains either within or closer to the normal range. When these backup mechanisms are completely effective, acid-base problems are fully compensated and the pH of the blood returns to normal, even though the levels of oxygen and bicarbonate may be abnormal.

Sometimes, however, the respiratory problem causing the acid-base imbalance is so severe that kidney actions can only partially compensate, and the pH is not quite normal. Even partial compensation is helpful because it prevents the acid-base imbalance from becoming severe or life threatening.

Age-Related Changes in Acid-Base Balance

Older adults are at greater risk for pH problems than are younger people because their lungs and kidneys are less able to respond to minor changes in hydrogen ion production or elimination. In addition, older adults often take drugs that alter normal pH-compensating mechanisms (Chart 18-2).

Gas exchange during breathing is reduced as a person ages. There is less alveolar membrane for gas exchange in older persons, and many also have some degree of blood vessel thickening, which further impairs gas movement through capillaries. These conditions can cause carbon dioxide retention, increasing the free hydrogen ion level.

Because kidney function decreases with age, older adults are less able to excrete hydrogen ions or produce bicarbonate ions. The kidneys may be able to handle ordinary changes resulting from normal metabolism but cannot compensate when health problems such as pneumonia, fever, or infection, interfere with acid-base balance.

Two drugs often prescribed for older clients are diuretics and digoxin. Both agents increase kidney excretion of hydrogen ions, which can result in an increased blood pH.

All older clients are at risk for acid-base disturbances. This risk is even greater for clients with pulmonary, vascular, cardiac, or kidney problems.

ASSESSMENT OF ACID-BASE BALANCE

Acid-base balance involves all cells and body systems. Assessment of acid-base balance involves examining the func-

CHART 18-2

NURSING FOCUS on the OLDER ADULT

Age-Related Risk Factors for Acid-Base Disturbances

Disturbance	Risk Factors
Increased hydrogen ion concentration	Pulmonary diseases Chronic obstructive pulmonary disease (COPD) Pneumonia Dehydration Infection Renal disease Vascular disease Atherosclerosis Arteriosclerosis Angiitis
Decreased hydrogen ion concentration	Overhydration Congestive heart failure Drugs Diuretics (loop and thiazide) Digoxin Insulin Antibiotics Chemotherapeutic agents

tioning of systems responsible for acid-base balance, especially the lungs and kidneys. Assessment also involves examining body responses to changes in the levels of acids or bases. Behavioral and neurologic assessments also are included in assessment of acid-base balance because changes in pH can alter neurologic function.

History

One way of organizing history data to assess the client's acid-base status is the use of Gordon's Functional Health Patterns (Gordon, 2002). The patterns that affect acid-base balance most are Activity-Exercise, Elimination, and Cognitive-Perceptual patterns (Chart 18-3), showing the effectiveness of lung and kidney function.

Physical Assessment

Hydration status can indicate fluid balance. A normally hydrated adult is alert, has moist eyes and mucous membranes, has a urine output nearly the same as the amount of fluid ingested (with a urine specific gravity between 1.010 and 1.030), and has good skin turgor (see Chapter 14). A dry, sticky, "cottony" mouth; the absence of tearing; weight loss; and decreased urine output all indicate either a problem with oral intake or excess fluid loss. Accurate assessment of fluid intake and output can help determine kidney function and acid-base balance.

Hydrogen ions affect the activity of excitable membranes, and acid-base imbalances alter the function of these membranes. Acid-base assessment includes assessment of muscle tone and strength, movement, coordination, and tremors. Assessment of other systems, including the cardiac (heart rate, rhythm, and strength of contractions) and gastrointestinal (motility) systems, may indicate changes in excitable membrane function.

Part of your assessment focuses on changes from previous findings, including mental status, physical examination data, and laboratory data. Acid-base imbalances can occur quickly and you must be familiar with the client's baseline assessment data to detect any changes.

CHART 18-3

Acid-Base Assessment
USING GORDON'S FUNCTIONAL HEALTH PATTERNS

Activity-Exercise Pattern
- Have you had any shortness of breath or difficulty breathing at rest or during activity?
- Have you noticed any changes in your breathing rate or depth?
- Do you have a hard time "catching" your breath?
- Do you have any difficulty clearing excretions?
- Do you feel the need for additional energy to accomplish routine tasks?
- Do you have any difficulty concentrating?
- Have you noticed any changes in your interest in normal daily activities?
- Have you noticed any changes in your leisure activities?

Elimination Pattern
- What is your usual urinary elimination pattern? Frequency? Amount? Color? Odor? Control?
- Have you noticed any changes in the amount of urine?
- Has your urine changed color or odor?
- What is your usual bowel elimination pattern? Frequency? Amount? Control?
- Have you noticed any changes in the number or consistency of your stools?

Cognitive-Perceptual Pattern
- Have you noticed any changes in memory lately?
- Have you noticed an increase in anxiety or feelings of apprehension?
- Are you sleeping more or sleeping less than usual for you?
- Have you noticed any changes in your attention span?
- Have your muscles seemed weak or "twitchy" lately?

Based on Gordon, M. (2002). *Manual of nursing diagnosis* (10th ed.). St. Louis: Mosby.

Diagnostic Assessment

Arterial blood gases (ABGs) are important in identifying specific acid-base imbalances and are discussed fully in Chapter 19 (see also Chart 18-1). Other laboratory values helpful in assessing acid-base balance include serum electrolyte levels, blood urea nitrogen (BUN) level, glucose level, creatinine level, and osmolarity.

Urine test results may be helpful in determining whether a kidney or metabolic problem is affecting acid-base balance. Such tests include glomerular filtration rate and detection of substances that should not be present in the urine, such as glucose, acetone, protein, or blood.

GET READY for the NCLEX Examination!

KEY POINTS

- The normal pH of the body's extracellular fluids (including blood) is 7.35 to 7.45.
- The normal pH of arterial blood is slightly higher (less acidic) than venous blood.
- The more hydrogen ions present, the more acidic the fluid.
- The less hydrogen ions present, the more alkaline the fluid.
- Lower pH values (below 7.35) mean acidosis is present.
- Higher pH values (above 7.45) mean alkalosis is present.
- The pH in the body can be described as the relationship of bicarbonate to carbonic acid, or a 20:1 ratio.
- Carbon dioxide is the most changeable component of carbonic acid.
- The concentration of carbon dioxide is directly related to the concentration of hydrogen ions. Anything that increases the carbon dioxide level in the blood, increases the hydrogen ion content and lowers the pH.
- An acid gives up hydrogen ions in solution; a base binds hydrogen ions in solution.
- Acids are normally formed in the body as a result of metabolism and incomplete oxidation of glucose and fats.
- Acid-base balance is regulated by chemical, respiratory, and renal mechanisms.
- Chemical buffers are the immediate way that acid-base imbalances are corrected.
- The lungs control the amount of carbon dioxide that is retained or exhaled.
- The kidneys regulate the amount of hydrogen and bicarbonate ions that are retained or excreted by the body.
- Compensation is the process in which the body uses its three regulatory mechanisms to correct for changes in the pH of body fluids.

- If a lung problem causes retention of carbon dioxide, the healthy kidney compensates by increasing the amount of bicarbonate that is produced and retained.
- The best way to determine acid-base balance is by analyzing arterial blood gases (ABGs).

ADDITIONAL STUDY RESOURCES

Go to your Student CD-ROM for Review Questions for the NCLEX Examination.

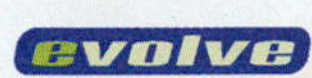

Go to http://evolve.elsevier.com/Iggy/ for Integrated Management of Care Questions for the NCLEX Examination.

SELECTED BIBLIOGRAPHY

Adrogue, H.E., & Adrogue, H.J. (2001). Acid-base physiology. *Respiratory Care, 46*(4), 328-341.

Berry, B., & Pinard, A. (2002). Assessing tissue oxygenation. *Critical Care Nurse, 22*(3), 22-24, 26-30, 32-36.

Call-Schmidt, T. (2001). Interpreting lab results: A primer. *MEDSURG Nursing, 10*(4), 179-184.

Capovilla, J. (2000). Noninvasive blood gas monitoring. *Critical Care Nursing Quarterly, 23*(2), 79-86.

Ebersole, P., Hess, P., & Luggen, A. (2004). *Toward healthy aging: Human needs and nursing response* (6th ed.). St. Louis: Mosby.

Gordon, M. (2002). *Manual of nursing diagnosis* (10th ed.). St. Louis: Mosby.

Guyton, A., & Hall, J. (2000). *Textbook of medical physiology* (10th ed.). Philadelphia: W.B. Saunders.

Jarvis, C. (2004). *Physical examination and health assessment* (4th ed.). Philadelphia: W.B. Saunders.

McCance, K., & Huether, S. (2002). *Pathophysiology: The biologic basis for disease in adults and children* (4th ed.). St. Louis: Mosby.

McConnell, E. (2002). Measuring fluid intake and output. *Nursing2002, 32*(7), 17.

Pagana, K., & Pagana, T. (2002). *Mosby's manual of diagnostic and laboratory tests* (2nd ed.). St. Louis: Mosby.

Simmons, J., & Assell, C. (2001). Acid-base basics. *Support Line, 23*(1), 6-11, 24, 28.

Trissel, L. (2003). *Handbook on injectable drugs* (12th ed.). Bethesda, MD: American Society of Health-System Pharmacists.

Wallace, L. (2000). Using color to simplify ABG interpretation. *MEDSURG Nursing, 9*(4), 205-207.

CHAPTER 19

Interventions for Clients with Acid-Base Imbalances

M. LINDA WORKMAN

LEARNING OUTCOMES

After studying this chapter, you should be able to:

1. Identify clients at risk for acidosis.
2. Use laboratory data and clinical manifestations to determine the presence of acidosis.
3. Analyze arterial blood gases to determine whether acidosis is respiratory or metabolic in origin.
4. Analyze arterial blood gases to determine whether respiratory acidosis is acute or chronic.
5. Prioritize nursing care for the client with acute acidosis.
6. Develop a community-based teaching plan to prevent acidosis in the client at continuing risk for acid-base imbalances.
7. Identify clients at risk for alkalosis.
8. Use laboratory data and clinical manifestations to determine the presence of alkalosis.
9. Analyze arterial blood gases to determine whether alkalosis is respiratory or metabolic in origin.
10. Prioritize nursing care for the client with alkalosis.
11. Develop a community-based teaching plan to prevent alkalosis in the client at continuing risk for acid-base imbalances.

Go to your Student CD-ROM for Review Questions for the NCLEX Examination keyed to these Learning Outcomes.

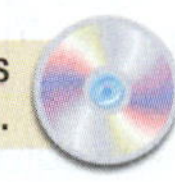

Acid-base imbalances are changes in the blood hydrogen ion level or pH. These changes are caused by problems with the acid-base regulatory mechanisms of the body or by exposure to dangerous conditions. Imbalances in which blood pH is below normal reflect **acidosis,** and imbalances in which blood pH is above normal reflect **alkalosis.** Acid-base imbalances impair the function of many organs and can be life threatening. Table 19-1 lists key points about acid-base imbalances.

ACIDOSIS

PATHOPHYSIOLOGY

In acidosis, the acid-base balance of the blood and other extracellular fluid (ECF) is disturbed by an excess of hydrogen ions (H^+). This problem is reflected as an arterial blood pH below 7.35. The amount or strength (or both) of acids is greater than normal compared with the amount or strength of bases.

Acidosis is not a disease; it is a condition caused by a disorder or pathologic process. Acidosis can be caused by metabolic problems, respiratory problems, or both. Clients at greatest risk for acute acidosis are those with problems that impair breathing. Older adults with chronic health problems are at greater risk for developing acidosis (Chart 19-1).

Acidosis can result from an actual or relative increase in the amount or strength of acids. An actual acid excess results in acidosis by either overproducing acids (and release of hydrogen ions) or undereliminating normally produced acids (retention of hydrogen ions). Examples of problems that increase acid production include diabetic ketoacidosis and seizures. Examples of problems that decrease acid elimination include respiratory or renal impairment.

In *relative* acidosis, the amount or strength of acids does not increase. Instead, the amount or strength (or both) of the bases decreases (to create a *base deficit*), which makes the fluid relatively more acidic than basic. A relative acidosis *(base deficit)* is caused by either overeliminating bases (bicarbonate ions [HCO_3^-]) or underproducing bases (Figure 19-1). Examples of problems that underproduce bases include pancreatitis and dehydration. A condition that overeliminates bases is diarrhea.

Regardless of its origin, acidosis causes major changes in body function. The main problems are related to the fact that hydrogen ions are **cations** (positively charged ions). An

TABLE 19-1 Key Points Related to Acid-Base Imbalances

- Acidosis is an increase in the hydrogen ion concentration (pH) of the blood and is reflected by an arterial blood pH below 7.35.
- Acidosis can result from an actual acid excess or a relative base deficit.
- Metabolic acidosis usually results from a lack of bicarbonate or from excess acid production in the body.
- Respiratory acidosis results from the retention of carbon dioxide in the body, causing increased carbonic acid production.
- Manifestations of acidosis are related to fluid and electrolyte imbalances that accompany acid-base imbalance, such as hyperkalemia.
- Chronic respiratory acidosis is common in the medical-surgical setting as a result of chronic obstructive pulmonary disease, such as emphysema.
- Alkalosis is a decrease in the hydrogen ion concentration of the blood, which is reflected by an arterial blood pH above 7.45.
- Alkalosis can result from an actual base excess or an acid deficit.
- Metabolic alkalosis most often occurs when body acids are lost, such as in prolonged vomiting or nasogastric suctioning.
- Respiratory alkalosis most often occurs when hyperventilation causes excessive loss of carbon dioxide.
- Dehydration and hypokalemia are associated with metabolic alkalosis and account for most of the clinical manifestations seen in this type of acid-base imbalance.
- The goal of management for any type of acid-base imbalance is to restore fluid, electrolyte, and acid-base balance to normal or near-normal.

increase in hydrogen ions creates imbalances of other electrolytes, especially potassium. These electrolyte imbalances then disrupt the functions of nerves, cardiac muscle, and skeletal muscle. The early manifestations of acidosis first appear in the musculoskeletal, cardiac, respiratory, and central nervous systems. Even slight increases in blood hydrogen ion levels reduce the activity of many hormones and enzymes, leading to death. Many drugs are less effective during acidosis.

Acidosis can be caused by metabolic problems, respiratory problems, or combined metabolic and respiratory problems. Specific causes of acidosis are listed in Table 19-2.

Metabolic Acidosis

Four processes can result in metabolic acidosis: overproduction of hydrogen ions, underelimination of hydrogen ions, underproduction of bicarbonate ions, and overelimination of bicarbonate ions.

OVERPRODUCTION OF HYDROGEN IONS

Metabolic processes that increase blood hydrogen ion levels are excessive breakdown of fatty acids, anaerobic glucose breakdown (lactic acidosis), and excessive intake of acids.

Excessive breakdown of fatty acids occurs with diabetic ketoacidosis or starvation. When glucose is not available for fuel, the body breaks down fats (lipids). The products of excessive fatty acid breakdown are strong acids *(ketoacids),* which release large amounts of hydrogen ions.

Anaerobic lactic acidosis occurs when cells are forced to use glucose without adequate oxygen (anaerobic metabolism); as a result, glucose is incompletely broken down and forms lactic acid. Lactic acid molecules leave the cell, enter the blood, and release hydrogen ions, causing acidosis. Lactic acidosis occurs whenever the body has too little oxygen.

CHART 19-1

NURSING FOCUS on the OLDER ADULT

The Older Client Experiencing Acid-Base Imbalance

When Obtaining a Client's History

- Assess risk factors for acid-base imbalance, including medications, chronic health problems (especially renal disease, pulmonary disease), and acute health problems.
- Obtain the history when the client is awake and more familiar with his or her surroundings.
- Ask the client to list all prescribed and over-the-counter medications (especially diuretics and antacids). If the client cannot recall this information or seems confused, ask the significant other to bring medications from home to show the nurse.
- Ask the client to recall what liquids he or she has taken in the past 24 hours and whether he or she has urinated as much as usual.

When Assessing the Client

- Compare the client's mental status with what the family, significant other, or health record states is the client's baseline.
- Observe the rate and depth of respiration.
  - Can the client complete a sentence without stopping to take a breath?
  - Examine the color of the client's nail beds and mucous membranes.
- Obtain a urine specimen and observe for color and character. Test for specific gravity and pH.
- Examine skin turgor for dehydration. Attempt to pinch the skin to form a tent over the sternum and on the forehead. If a tent forms, record how long it remains.
- Measure the rate and quality of the pulse.
- Observe the client's clinical responses and laboratory values carefully while the acid-base imbalance is being corrected.
- Administer IV therapy by pump or controller.

AAABBB AAABBB AAABBB	AAAABBB AAAABBB AAAABBB	AAABB AAABB AAABB
Acid-base balance	Actual acidosis (acid excess)	Relative acidosis (base deficit)

Figure 19-1 ■ Concepts of actual and relative acidosis. **A** = Acid; **B** = base.

Conditions that cause lactic acidosis include heavy exercise, seizure activity, fever, and tissue hypoxia.

Excessive intake of acidic substances floods the body directly with hydrogen ions. Common drugs or agents that cause acidosis when ingested in excess include alcoholic beverages, methyl alcohol (a poison), and acetylsalicylic acid (aspirin).

UNDERELIMINATION OF HYDROGEN IONS

Acidosis can occur when hydrogen ions are produced at the normal rate but are not removed at the same rate they are produced. Most hydrogen ion loss occurs through the lungs and the kidneys. Kidney failure causes acidosis when the kidney tubules cannot secrete hydrogen ions into the urine. As a result, too many hydrogen ions are retained.

UNDERPRODUCTION OF BICARBONATE IONS

As discussed in Chapter 18, bicarbonate is the most common base in the blood and buffers carbonic acid (H_2CO_3). A base-deficit state exists when blood levels of bicarbonate

TABLE 19-2 Common Causes of Acidosis

Pathology	Condition
Metabolic Acidosis	
Overproduction of hydrogen ions	Excessive oxidation of fatty acids ▪ Diabetic ketoacidosis ▪ Starvation Hypermetabolism ▪ Heavy exercise ▪ Seizure activity ▪ Fever ▪ Hypoxia, ischemia Excessive ingestion of acids ▪ Ethanol intoxication ▪ Methanol ingestion ▪ Salicylate intoxication
Underelimination of hydrogen ions	Renal failure
Underproduction of bicarbonate	Renal failure Pancreatitis Liver failure Dehydration
Overelimination of bicarbonate	Diarrhea Buffering of organic acids
Respiratory Acidosis	
Underelimination of hydrogen ions	Respiratory depression ▪ Anesthetics ▪ Drugs (especially opioids) ▪ Poisons ▪ Electrolyte imbalance ▪ Trauma Cerebral edema Spinal cord injuries ▪ Neurologic diseases Guillain-Barré Polio Myasthenia gravis Inadequate chest expansion ▪ Skeletal deformities ▪ Muscle weakness ▪ Nonpulmonary restriction Obesity Fluid Tumor Body casts Chest eschar Airway obstruction ▪ Asthma ▪ Cancer ▪ Bronchiolitis Alveolar-capillary block ▪ Thrombus or embolus ▪ Vascular occlusive disease ▪ Pneumonia ▪ Pulmonary edema ▪ Tuberculosis ▪ Cystic fibrosis ▪ Atelectasis ▪ Acute respiratory distress syndrome (ARDS) ▪ Emphysema ▪ Cancer

are too low. Base-deficit acidosis occurs when hydrogen ion production and removal are normal but too few bicarbonate ions are present to balance the hydrogen ions. Such base deficits occur when bicarbonate ions are not produced at the normal rate. Because bicarbonate is made in the kidneys and in the pancreas, renal failure and reduced hepatic or pancreatic function can cause a base-deficit acidosis (McCance & Huether, 2002).

OVERELIMINATION OF BICARBONATE IONS

Base-deficit acidosis occurs when hydrogen ion production and removal are normal but too many bicarbonate ions have been lost. A common cause of base-deficit acidosis is diarrhea.

Respiratory Acidosis

Respiratory acidosis results when any area of respiratory function is impaired, reducing the exchange of oxygen (O_2) and carbon dioxide (CO_2). This impairment causes carbon dioxide retention. Because any increase in carbon dioxide levels causes a corresponding increase in hydrogen ion levels, carbon dioxide retention leads to acidosis. This relationship is shown by the following carbonic anhydrase equation:

$$CO_2 + H_2O \Longrightarrow H_2CO_3 \Longrightarrow H^+ + HCO_3^-$$

An excess of carbon dioxide forces the equation to the right, first increasing the amount of carbonic acid. The carbonic acid then rapidly separates into hydrogen ions and bicarbonate ions. The increase in free hydrogen ions in the blood is acidosis.

Unlike metabolic acidosis, respiratory acidosis results from only one mechanism: retention of carbon dioxide, causing increased production of free hydrogen ions. All causes of respiratory acidosis lead to an acid-excess acidosis. Four types of problems can cause respiratory acidosis: respiratory depression, inadequate chest expansion, airway obstruction, and reduced alveolar-capillary diffusion.

RESPIRATORY DEPRESSION

Respiratory depression is reduced function of the brainstem neurons that trigger breathing movements. The result is a reduced rate and depth of breathing, which causes poor gas exchange and a retention of carbon dioxide. Respiratory depression may be chemical or physical in origin.

Chemical depression of respiration can occur with anesthetic agents, drugs (especially opioids), and poisons such as methyl alcohol, pesticides, and botulinus toxin that cross the blood-brain barrier. Specific electrolyte imbalances also slow or inhibit these neurons (see Chapter 16 for a discussion of electrolyte imbalances).

Physical depression of respiration occurs in response to many problems. Neurons can be damaged or destroyed by trauma or when problems in other areas of the brain increase the intracranial pressure. Such an increase causes edema, which leads to pressure on the respiratory centers located in the brainstem. Problems causing cerebral edema and respiratory depression include brain tumors, cerebral aneurysm, stroke, overhydration, and hyponatremia.

INADEQUATE CHEST EXPANSION

Any problem that restricts chest movement can reduce gas exchange. Chest expansion can be restricted by skeletal trauma or deformities, respiratory muscle weakness, or external constriction.

Skeletal problems restrict chest wall movement when broken or malformed bones distort the shape of the chest. Broken ribs restrict chest movement because they do not provide the rigid structure needed for chest pressure changes (as in flail chest). Pain from broken ribs may also cause the client to breathe more shallowly.

Respiratory muscle weakness reduces chest movement. This weakness can be caused by electrolyte imbalances, fatigue, muscular dystrophy, muscle damage or breakdown, and inflammatory myositis.

External conditions also can restrict the chest movement needed for full lung expansion. Causes of restricted chest movement include body cast enclosure of the chest, tight scar tissue around the chest, severe obesity, abdominal masses, ascites, and **hemothorax** (blood in the thoracic cavity).

AIRWAY OBSTRUCTION

Prevention of air movement into and out from the lungs through airway obstruction leads to poor gas exchange, carbon dioxide retention, and acidosis. The upper airway can be obstructed externally by clothing, neck edema, and local lymph node enlargement. Internal obstruction of the upper airway can be caused by aspiration of foreign objects, constriction of bronchial smooth muscles, and edema. Internal obstruction of the lower airways is caused by smooth muscle constriction, edema, and excessive mucus, all of which occur in asthma, bronchiolitis, and emphysema.

REDUCED ALVEOLAR-CAPILLARY DIFFUSION

Gas exchange in the lungs occurs by diffusion at the point where the alveolar membranes and capillary membranes meet. Any problem that prevents or slows diffusion causes carbon dioxide retention and acidosis. Some disorders that reduce diffusion include pneumonia, fluid aspiration, pneumonitis, tuberculosis, emphysema, acute respiratory distress syndrome, chest trauma, pulmonary emboli, and pulmonary edema.

Combined Metabolic and Respiratory Acidosis

Metabolic and respiratory acidosis can occur at the same time. Uncorrected acute respiratory acidosis always leads to **anaerobic** (lacking adequate oxygen) metabolism and lactic acidosis (McCance & Huether, 2002). Combined acidosis is more severe than either metabolic acidosis or respiratory acidosis alone. Cardiac arrest is an example of a problem leading to combined metabolic and respiratory acidosis.

COLLABORATIVE MANAGEMENT

The Concept Map below addresses assessment and nursing care issues related to respiratory acidosis.

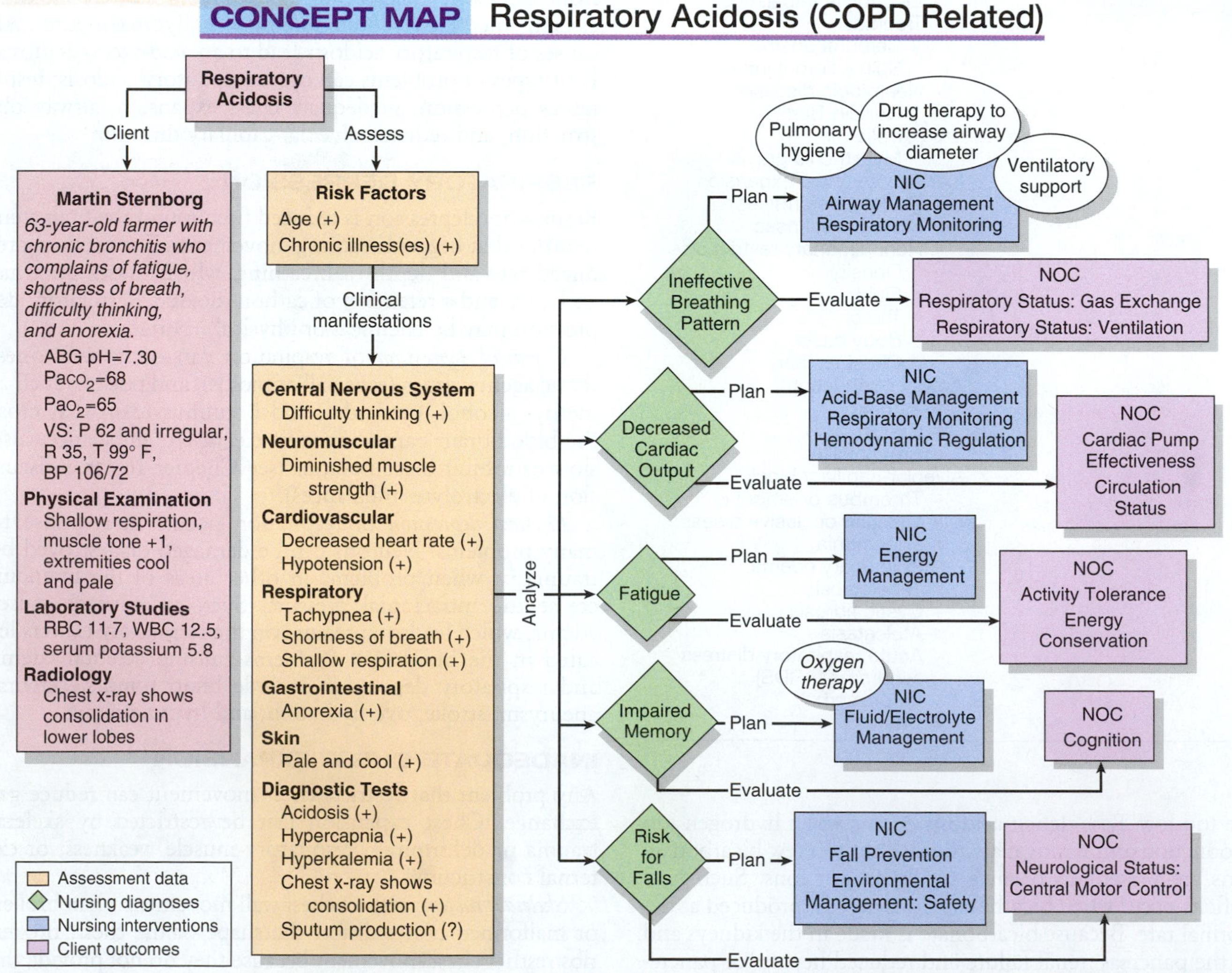

Concept Map by Elaine Bishop Kennedy, EdD, RN

Assessment

HISTORY

When taking the history from any client, collect data about risk factors related to the development of acidosis, specifically age, nutrition, and presenting symptoms.

Older adults are more at risk for problems leading to acid-base imbalance, including cardiac, renal, or pulmonary impairment. In addition, older adults are more likely to be taking drugs that disrupt acid-base, fluid, and electrolyte balance, especially diuretics and aspirin. Ask about specific risk factors, such as any type of breathing problem, kidney failure, diabetes mellitus, diarrhea, pancreatitis, and fever.

Obtain a detailed diet history to determine total caloric intake and the proportions of carbohydrates, fats, and proteins ingested. Ask the client specifically whether he or she has fasted or followed a strict diet within the past week.

Ask the client if he or she has had headaches, behavior changes, increased drowsiness, reduced alertness, reduced attention span, lethargy, anorexia, abdominal distention, nausea or vomiting, muscle weakness, or increased fatigue. Having the client relate activities of the previous 24 hours may help identify activity intolerance, behavior changes, and unexplained fatigue. Because the central nervous system is often depressed in acidosis, you may need to obtain this information from the client's family.

PHYSICAL ASSESSMENT/CLINICAL MANIFESTATIONS

The key clinical manifestations of acidosis are similar whether the cause is metabolic or respiratory (Chart 19-2). Clinical manifestations appear as changes in excitable membrane activity in neurons, skeletal muscle, and gastric smooth muscle.

CHART 19-2

KEY FEATURES of
Acidosis

Central Nervous System Manifestations
- Depressed activity (lethargy, confusion, stupor, and coma)

Neuromuscular Manifestations
- Hyporeflexia
- Skeletal muscle weakness
- Flaccid paralysis

Cardiovascular Manifestations
- Delayed electrical conduction
  - Ranges from bradycardia to heart block
  - Tall T waves
  - Widened QRS complex
  - Prolonged PR interval
- Hypotension
- Thready peripheral pulses

Respiratory Manifestations
- Kussmaul respirations (in metabolic acidosis with respiratory compensation)
- Variable respirations (generally ineffective in respiratory acidosis)

Integumentary Manifestations
- Warm, flushed, dry skin in metabolic acidosis
- Pale to cyanotic and dry skin in respiratory acidosis

CENTRAL NERVOUS SYSTEM MANIFESTATIONS. Depression of central nervous system function is common and may range from lethargy to confusion, especially in older clients. As acidosis worsens, the client may become stuporous and unresponsive. Assess the client's mental status (see Chapter 44).

NEUROMUSCULAR MANIFESTATIONS. An increase in blood hydrogen ion levels, along with hyperkalemia, reduces muscle tone and deep tendon reflexes. Assess muscle strength by having the client do the following:

- Squeeze your hand
- Keep his or her arms flexed while you pull down on the lower arms
- Push both feet against a flat surface while you apply resistance

Muscle weakness from acidosis is bilateral and can progress to flaccid paralysis. Breathing is less effective when skeletal muscles become weak.

CARDIOVASCULAR MANIFESTATIONS. The early cardiac manifestations are increased heart rate and cardiac output. With worsening acidosis or with acidosis and hyperkalemia, electrical conduction through the heart is reduced and heart rate decreases. Peripheral pulses may be hard to find and are easily blocked. The client may have hypotension as a result of vasodilation.

RESPIRATORY MANIFESTATIONS. Assess the client's rate, depth, and ease of breathing. Use pulse oximetry to determine how well oxygen is delivered to the peripheral tissues.

If acidosis is metabolic in origin, the rate and depth of breathing increase in proportion to the rising hydrogen ion level. Breaths are deep, rapid, and not under voluntary control. This pattern is called **Kussmaul respiration.**

If acidosis is respiratory in origin, respiratory efforts are reduced. Respirations are usually shallow and rapid.

SKIN MANIFESTATIONS. With metabolic acidosis, breathing is unimpaired and the rate is increased. This increased gas exchange causes vasodilation and makes the client's skin and mucous membranes appear warm, dry, and pink. With respiratory acidosis, breathing is ineffective and skin and mucous membranes are pale to cyanotic.

PSYCHOSOCIAL ASSESSMENT

It is vital to complete a psychosocial assessment, because behavioral changes may be the first clinical manifestations of acidosis. Observe and document the client's behavior by description (objectively) rather than by interpretation (subjectively). For example, you should state that "the client does not recognize close family members" rather than "the client is confused" or state that "the client spit out the oral drugs" rather than "the client is uncooperative." Ask family members if the client's behavior is typical and establish a baseline for comparison with later assessment findings.

LABORATORY ASSESSMENT

Arterial blood pH is the laboratory value used to confirm acidosis. Acidosis is present when arterial blood pH is less than 7.35. However, this test alone does not indicate what is causing the acidosis or its origin. Manifestations of metabolic acidosis and respiratory acidosis are similar, but their treatments are different. Therefore it is critical to obtain and interpret other laboratory data, such as arterial blood gas (ABG) values and blood levels of electrolytes (Chart 19-3).

METABOLIC ACIDOSIS. The following laboratory data indicate metabolic acidosis:

ABGs

Low pH (<7.35)
Low bicarbonate level (<21 mEq/L)
Normal partial pressure of arterial carbon dioxide ($Paco_2$)

Electrolytes

Elevated serum potassium level
Normal chloride levels (acid excess or high anion gap acidosis)
Elevated chloride levels (base deficit or normal anion gap acidosis)

The pH is low because buffering and respiratory compensation are not adequate to keep the amount of free hydrogen ions at a normal level. The bicarbonate level is below normal for any or all of the following reasons.

- Bicarbonate has been lost, causing a base-deficit acidosis.
- Bicarbonate production is inadequate, causing a base-deficit acidosis
- Bicarbonate may be bound to other substances.

The carbon dioxide level is normal or even slightly decreased because gas exchange is adequate and carbon dioxide retention is not a factor. The oxygen level is normal because gas exchange is adequate.

The serum potassium level is often high in acidosis as the body attempts to maintain electroneutrality during buffering. Figure 19-2 shows the movement of potassium ions as serum pH changes. As the blood hydrogen ion level rises, some of the excess hydrogen ions enter red blood cells for intracellular buffering. The movement of hydrogen ions into the cells creates an excess of positive ions inside the cells. To balance these extra positive charges, an equal number of potassium ions move from the cells into the blood. This increases the blood potassium level, causing hyperkalemia.

RESPIRATORY ACIDOSIS. The following laboratory data indicate respiratory acidosis:

ABGs

Low pH (<7.35)
Elevated $Paco_2$
Low partial pressure of arterial oxygen (Pao_2)

Electrolytes

Elevated serum potassium levels
Variable serum bicarbonate levels

CHART 19-3

LABORATORY PROFILE
Acid-Base Imbalances

Imbalance	Laboratory Value Changes						
	pH	HCO_3^-	Pao_2	$Paco_2$	K^+	Ca^{2+}	Cl^-
Metabolic acidosis	↓	↓	Ø	Ø and ↓	↑	Ø	Ø and ↑
Respiratory acidosis	↓	↑	↓	↑	↑	Ø	↑↓
Combined acidosis	↓	↓↑	↓	↑	↑	Ø	↑
Metabolic alkalosis	↑	↑	Ø	Ø and ↑	↓	↓	↓
Respiratory alkalosis	↑	↓	Ø	↓↓	↓	↓	↑
Combined alkalosis	↑	↑	Ø	↓	↓	↓	↓

↑, Above normal; ↓, below normal; ↑↓, value can increase or decrease depending on other factors; Ø, normal; HCO_3^-, bicarbonate ions; Pao_2, partial pressure of arterial oxygen; $Paco_2$, partial pressure of arterial carbon dioxide; K^+, potassium ions; Ca^{2+}, calcium ions; Cl^-, chloride ions.

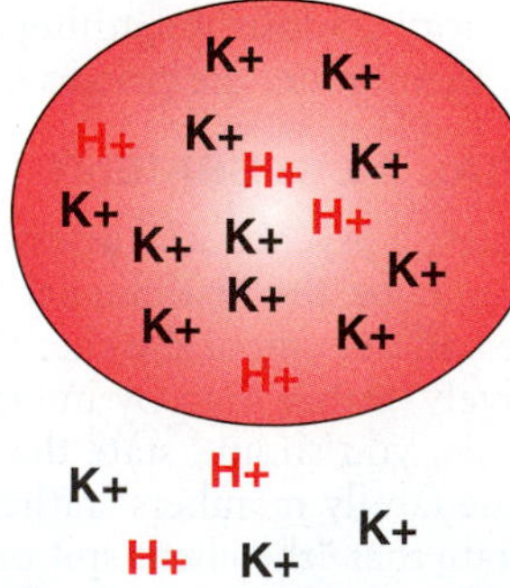

Under normal conditions, the intracellular potassium content is much greater than that of the extracellular fluid. The concentration of hydrogen ions is low in both compartments.

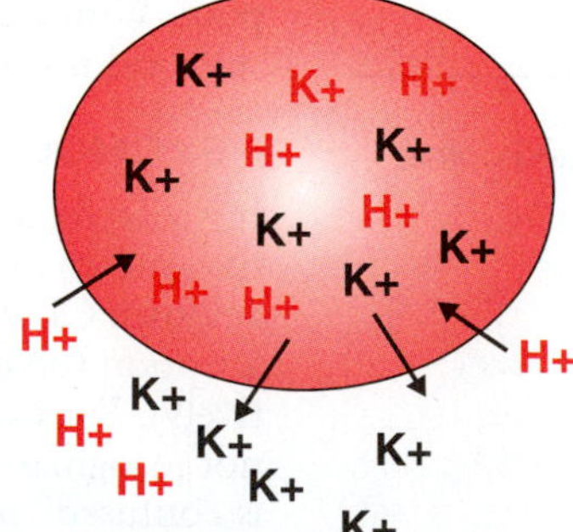

In acidosis, the extracellular hydrogen ion content increases, and the hydrogen ions move into the intracellular fluid. To keep the intracellular fluid electrically neutral, an equal number of potassium ions leave the cell, creating a relative hyperkalemia.

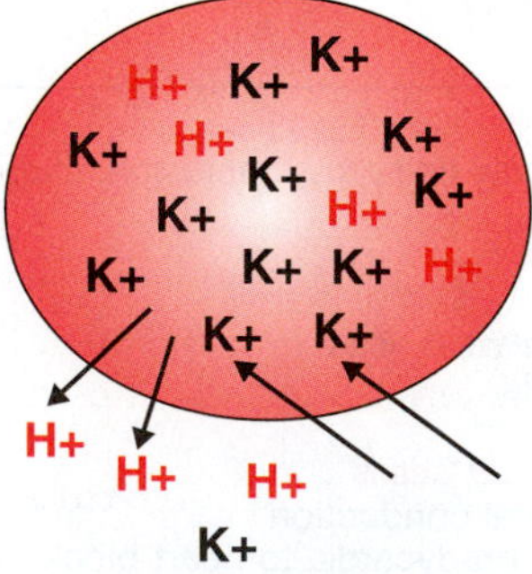

In alkalosis, more hydrogen ions are present in the intracellular fluid than in the extracellular fluid. Hydrogen ions move from the intracellular fluid into the extracellular fluid. To keep the intracellular fluid electrically neutral, potassium ions move from the extracellular fluid into the intracellular fluid, creating a relative hypokalemia.

Figure 19-2 ■ Movement of potassium in response to changes in the extracellular fluid hydrogen ion concentration.

The pH is lowered by the increased amount of free hydrogen ions in the blood. If the kidneys partially compensate for this acidosis, pH is low but not as abnormal as could be expected with the degree of carbon dioxide retention. A client with rapid onset of respiratory acidosis usually has a normal bicarbonate level because kidney compensation has not started. When respiratory acidosis persists for 24 hours or longer, kidney compensation increases the production and retention of bicarbonate. Chronic respiratory acidosis is indicated by an elevated bicarbonate level and increased $Paco_2$.

$Paco_2$ is high and Pao_2 is low because the pulmonary problem impairs gas exchange, causing carbon dioxide retention and poor oxygenation. Carbon dioxide is 20 times more diffusible than is oxygen across the alveolar membrane. Therefore a decreased Pao_2 usually occurs before an increased $Paco_2$.

Serum potassium levels are elevated in acute respiratory acidosis. They are normal or low in chronic respiratory acidosis when renal compensation is present.

> ### Critical Thinking Challenge
>
> The client is a 65-year-old woman with type 1 diabetes mellitus and pneumonia. Her vital signs on admission are as follows: T 103.4; P 122, thready; R 34, shallow.
>
> Her urine is positive for ketones. Her arterial blood gases (ABGs) are as follows: pH 7.21; HCO_3^- 22 mEq/L; $Paco_2$ 50 mm Hg; Pao_2 78 mm Hg.
>
> 1. What type of acid-base imbalance is present?
> 2. Is the origin of the imbalance metabolic or respiratory? Explain your answer.
> 3. Is compensation present or not present? Explain your answer.

evolve For suggested answer guidelines, go to http://evolve.elsevier.com/Iggy/.

Common Nursing Diagnoses and Collaborative Problems

Nursing diagnoses and collaborative problems that may apply to clients with acidosis include the following:

- Deficient Fluid Volume related to dehydration
- Decreased Cardiac Output related to poor cardiac contractility and decreased vascular volume
- Risk for Falls related to skeletal muscle weakness
- Impaired Memory related to fluid and electrolyte imbalances
- Ineffective Breathing Pattern related to reduced gas exchange
- Fatigue related to inadequate tissue oxygenation

Interventions

Interventions for acidosis focus on correcting the underlying problem, increasing aerobic metabolism, and monitoring for changes (Chart 19-4). To ensure appropriate interventions, the specific type of acidosis must first be identified.

METABOLIC ACIDOSIS. Interventions for metabolic acidosis include hydration and drugs or treatments to control the problem causing the acidosis. For example, if the acidosis is a result of diabetic ketoacidosis, insulin is given to correct the hyperglycemia and halt the production of ketone bodies. Rehydration and antidiarrheal drugs are given if the acidosis is a result of prolonged diarrhea. *Bicarbonate is administered only if serum bicarbonate levels are low.*

RESPIRATORY ACIDOSIS. Interventions aim to maintain a patent airway and enhance gas exchange. Such interventions can include drug therapy, oxygen therapy, pulmonary hygiene (positioning and breathing techniques), ventilatory support, and prevention of complications. (See Chapter 33 for a complete discussion of common disorders causing respiratory acidosis.)

Drug Therapy. Drug therapy includes agents to increase the diameter of upper and lower airways and to thin pulmonary secretions. Drug therapy is not aimed directly at altering arterial pH.

Drugs to Increase Airway Diameter. Drugs that relax bronchial smooth muscle increase airway diameter. Many of these agents are adrenergic agonists and methylxanthines. Examples of these drugs include albuterol (Novo-Salmol✱, Proventil, Ventolin), ephedrine, fenoterol (Berotec✱), isoproterenol (Isuprel), metaproterenol (Alupent), pirbuterol (Maxair), terbutaline (Brethine, Bricanyl),

CHART 19-4

NIC INTERVENTION ACTIVITIES for The Client with Acidosis

Acid-Base Management: Metabolic Acidosis: *Promotion of acid-base balance and prevention of complications resulting from serum bicarbonate levels lower than desired*

- Monitor ABG levels for decreasing pH level, as appropriate.
- Maintain patent IV access.
- Monitor intake and output.
- Monitor determinants of tissue oxygen delivery (e.g., Pao_2, Sao_2, and hemoglobin levels and cardiac output), if available.
- Monitor loss of bicarbonate through the GI tract (e.g., diarrhea, pancreatic fistula, small bowel fistula, and ileal conduit), as appropriate.
- Administer fluids as prescribed.
- Administer insulin and fluid hydration (isotonic and hypotonic) for diabetic ketoacidosis, causing metabolic acidosis, as appropriate.
- Prepare client for dialysis (e.g., assist with catheter placement for dialysis), as appropriate.
- Institute seizure precautions.

Acid-Base Management: Respiratory Acidosis: *Promotion of acid-base balance and prevention of complications resulting from serum pCO_2 levels higher than desired*

- Monitor ABG levels for decreasing pH level, as appropriate.
- Monitor determinants of tissue oxygen delivery (e.g., Pao_2, Sao_2, and hemoglobin levels and cardiac output), if available.
- Monitor for symptoms of respiratory failure (e.g., low Pao_2 and elevated $Paco_2$ levels and respiratory muscle fatigue).
- Monitor work of breathing (e.g., respiratory rate, heart rate, use of accessory muscles, and diaphoresis).
- Provide low-carbohydrate, high-fat diet (e.g., Pulmocare feedings) to reduce CO_2 production, if indicated.
- Monitor neurologic status (e.g., level of consciousness and confusion).

NIC intervention activities selected from Dochterman, J.M., & Bulechek, G.M. (Eds.). (2004). *Nursing interventions classification (NIC)* (4th ed.). St. Louis: Mosby.

ABG, Arterial blood gas; *GI*, gastrointestinal; *Pao_2*, partial pressure of arterial oxygen; *Sao_2*, arterial oxygen saturation; *$Paco_2$*, partial pressure of arterial carbon dioxide.

aminophylline (Phyllocontin, Truphylline), and theophylline (Bronkodyl, Theo-Dur).

Some drugs increase bronchodilation by reducing the inflammation of bronchial luminal tissues. These agents are cortisol (steroid) based, such as beclomethasone (Vanceril, Beclovent), dexamethasone (Dexasone), flunisolide (AeroBid, Bronalide✱), and triamcinolone (Azmacort).

Drugs to Thin Bronchial Secretions. Some drugs can break up mucus when thick, sticky lung secretions obstruct airways. These agents are mucolytics; one example is acetylcysteine (Mucomyst, Mucosil). (See Chapter 33 for a discussion of drugs used for chronic airflow limitation [CAL].)

Oxygen Therapy. Oxygen therapy helps promote gas exchange for clients with respiratory acidosis. However, you must use caution when giving oxygen to clients with chronic obstructive pulmonary disease (COPD) and carbon dioxide retention as evidenced by a high $PaCO_2$ level. The only breathing trigger for these clients is a decreased arterial oxygen level. Giving too much oxygen to these clients decreases their respiratory drive and may lead to respiratory arrest.

Pulmonary Hygiene. To promote effective gas exchange, use positioning techniques to enhance the removal of lung secretions, and specific breathing techniques to change airway resistance, keeping alveoli inflated. Help the client assume a Fowler's or semi-Fowler's position to increase lung expansion. Increasing fluid intake may reduce the thickness of lung secretions and assist in their removal.

Ventilation Support. Mechanical ventilation may be needed for clients who are unable to keep their oxygen saturation at 90% or who have respiratory muscle fatigue. Chapters 31 and 35 discuss the criteria for mechanical ventilation and the nursing care needs of clients who are being mechanically ventilated.

Prevention of Complications. Monitoring clients' breathing status is critical in preventing complications. For clients experiencing chronic respiratory acidosis, assess breathing status at least every 2 hours. Auscultate breath sounds and assess the ease with which air moves into and out of the lungs. Examine the client for any muscle retractions, the use of accessory muscles, and whether breathing produces a sound that can be heard without a stethoscope. Assess the color of the nail beds and mucous membranes for cyanosis (a late finding).

Critical Thinking Challenge

The diabetic client with ketoacidosis and respiratory acidosis caused by pneumonia is started on insulin therapy and antibiotic therapy.

1. Should this client receive oxygen therapy? Why or why not?
2. Should this client receive intravenous bicarbonate? Why or why not?
3. What electrolyte imbalance should you be alert for with this client?

evolve For suggested answer guidelines, go to http://evolve.elsevier.com/Iggy/.

ALKALOSIS

PATHOPHYSIOLOGY

In clients with alkalosis, the acid-base balance of the blood is disturbed and has an excess of bases, especially bicarbonate (HCO_3^-). The amount or strength (or both) of the bases is greater than normal compared with the amount or strength of the acids. Alkalosis is a decrease in the free hydrogen ion level of the blood and is reflected by an arterial blood pH above 7.45. Like acidosis, alkalosis is not a disease but rather a manifestation of a problem. Alkalosis can be caused by metabolic problems, respiratory problems, or both (Table 19-3).

TABLE 19-3 Common Causes of Alkalosis

Pathology	Condition
Metabolic Alkalosis	
Increase of base components	Oral ingestion of bases ▪ Antacids ▪ Milk-alkali syndrome Parenteral base administration ▪ Blood transfusion ▪ Sodium bicarbonate ▪ Total parenteral nutrition
Decrease of acid components	Prolonged vomiting Nasogastric suctioning Cushing's syndrome or disease (hypercortisolism) Hyperaldosteronism Thiazide diuretics
Respiratory Alkalosis	
Excessive loss of carbon dioxide	Hyperventilation ▪ Fear ▪ Anxiety ▪ Mechanical ventilation ▪ Central nervous system stimulation Salicylates Catecholamines Progesterone Hypoxemia ▪ Asphyxiation ▪ High altitudes ▪ Shock ▪ Early-stage pulmonary problems Pneumonia Asthma Pulmonary emboli

Alkalosis can result from an actual or relative increase in the amount or strength (or both) of bases. In an actual base excess, alkalosis occurs when base (usually bicarbonate) is either overproduced or undereliminated.

In *relative* alkalosis, the actual amount or strength of bases does not increase. Instead, the amount or strength (or both) of the acids decreases, creating an *acid deficit* and making the blood more basic than acidic. A relative base-excess alkalosis (acid deficit) results from an overelimination or underproduction of acids (Figure 19-3).

The problems of alkalosis are serious and potentially life threatening. Treatment is aimed at correcting the cause of alkalosis after identifying whether it is respiratory or metabolic in origin.

Whether metabolic, respiratory, or both, alkalosis greatly affects specific functions. The pathologic effects are caused by the electrolyte imbalances that occur in response to decreased blood cation levels. The most common problems of alkalosis are related to increased stimulation of the central nervous, neuromuscular, and cardiovascular systems.

Metabolic Alkalosis

Most conditions that result in metabolic alkalosis create the acid-base imbalance through either an increase of bases (base excess) or a decrease of acids (acid deficit).

AAABBB	AAABBBB	AABBB
AAABBB	AAABBBB	AABBB
AAABBB	AAABBBB	AABBB
Acid-base balance	Actual alkalosis (base excess)	Relative alkalosis (acid deficit)

Figure 19-3 ■ Concepts of actual and relative alkalosis. **A** = Acid; **B** = base.

BASE EXCESS

Increases in bases are caused by excessive intake of bicarbonates, carbonates, acetates, citrates, and lactates. Excessive use of oral antacids containing sodium bicarbonate or calcium carbonate can also cause a metabolic alkalosis. Other base excesses can occur during medical treatments, such as citrate excesses during massive blood transfusions, acetate and lactate excesses during hyperalimentation, and IV sodium bicarbonate given to correct acidosis.

ACID DEFICIT

Decreases in acids can be caused by disease processes or medical treatment. Other causes include prolonged vomiting, excess cortisol, and hyperaldosteronism. Medical treatments that promote acid loss causing metabolic alkalosis include thiazide diuretics and prolonged nasogastric suctioning.

Respiratory Alkalosis

The main problem that causes respiratory alkalosis is excessive loss of carbon dioxide through hyperventilation (rapid respirations). Clients may hyperventilate in response to anxiety, fear, or improper settings on mechanical ventilators. Hyperventilation can also result from direct stimulation of central respiratory centers because of fever, metabolic acidosis, central nervous system lesions, and drugs (e.g., salicylates, catecholamines, and progesterone).

COLLABORATIVE MANAGEMENT

Assessment

PHYSICAL ASSESSMENT/CLINICAL MANIFESTATIONS

Clinical manifestations are the same for metabolic or respiratory alkalosis. Many symptoms are the result of the hypocalcemia (low calcium levels) and hypokalemia (low potassium levels) that usually occur with alkalosis (see Figure 19-2). These problems change the function of the central nervous, neuromuscular, cardiovascular, and respiratory systems (Chart 19-5).

CENTRAL NERVOUS SYSTEM MANIFESTATIONS. Overexcitement of the central and peripheral nervous systems is the major cause of the symptoms associated with alkalosis. Clients have dizziness, agitation, confusion, and hyperreflexia, which may progress to seizure activity. Tingling or numbness around the mouth and in the toes may be present. Other indicators of alkalosis with hypocalcemia are positive Chvostek's and Trousseau's signs (see Chapter 16).

NEUROMUSCULAR MANIFESTATIONS. Alkalosis occurs with hypocalcemia and hypokalemia, both of which alter neuromuscular function. Hypocalcemia increases nervous system activity, causing muscle cramps, twitches, and charley horses. Deep tendon reflexes are hyperactive. **Tetany** (continuous contractions) of muscle groups also may be present. Tetany is painful and indicates a rapidly worsening condition.

CHART 19-5

KEY FEATURES of
Alkalosis

Central Nervous System Manifestations
- Increased activity
- Anxiety, irritability, tetany, seizures
- Positive Chvostek's sign
- Positive Trousseau's sign
- Paresthesias

Neuromuscular Manifestations
- Hyperreflexia
- Muscle cramping and twitching
- Skeletal muscle weakness

Cardiovascular Manifestations
- Increased heart rate
- Normal or low blood pressure
- Increased digitalis toxicity

Respiratory Manifestations
- Increased rate and depth of ventilation in respiratory alkalosis
- Decreased respiratory effort associated with skeletal muscle weakness in metabolic alkalosis

Skeletal muscles may contract as a result of nerve overstimulation, but they become weaker because of the hypokalemia. Handgrip strength decreases, and the client may be unable to stand or walk. Respiratory efforts become less effective as the skeletal muscles of respiration weaken.

CARDIOVASCULAR MANIFESTATIONS. Alkalosis increases myocardial irritability, especially when accompanied by hypokalemia. Heart rate increases and the pulse is thready. When hypovolemia (decreased blood volume) is also present, the client may have severe hypotension. The hypokalemia occurring with alkalosis increases myocardial sensitivity to digoxin, which increases the risk for digoxin toxicity.

RESPIRATORY MANIFESTATIONS. Increases in the rate and depth of breathing are the main causes of respiratory alkalosis. Tidal volume (the volume of air inhaled and exhaled with each breath) is nearly normal, but minute volume (the total volume of air inhaled and exhaled in 1 minute) rises with the increased respiratory rate. The increased minute volume may be caused by anxiety or physiologic changes.

LABORATORY ASSESSMENT

Arterial blood pH greater than 7.45 confirms alkalosis, but this test alone does not identify its cause. Because the manifestations of metabolic alkalosis and respiratory alkalosis are similar, it is critical to obtain additional laboratory data, especially arterial blood gas (ABG) values and specific serum electrolytes levels (see Chart 19-3).

METABOLIC ALKALOSIS. The following laboratory data indicate metabolic alkalosis:

ABGs

High pH (>7.45)
Elevated bicarbonate level (>28 mEq/L)
Rising partial pressure of arterial carbon dioxide ($Pa{CO_2}$)
Normal partial pressure of arterial oxygen ($Pa{O_2}$)

Electrolytes

Decreased serum potassium levels
Decreased serum calcium levels

The pH is high because buffering and respiratory compensation are not adequate to maintain the free hydrogen ion level within the normal range. *The hallmark of metabolic alkalosis is an increased bicarbonate level with a rising $PaCO_2$.* The rising $PaCO_2$ compensates for the decreased hydrogen ion level. The serum potassium level decreases as hydrogen ions move out from cells and potassium from the blood moves into cells (see Figure 19-2). As the pH increases, calcium binding increases and the serum calcium level decreases, causing hypocalcemia. Most of the serious problems of alkalosis are caused by the resulting hypocalcemia.

RESPIRATORY ALKALOSIS. The following laboratory data indicate respiratory alkalosis:

ABGs

High pH
Low bicarbonate level
Low $PaCO_2$

Electrolytes

Low serum potassium level
Low serum calcium level

The pH is high because buffering and renal compensation cannot maintain the hydrogen ions at a normal level.

The classic respiratory alkalosis profile is a reduced bicarbonate level (not usually less than 15 mEq/L) along with a very low $PaCO_2$. The carbon dioxide level is low because it is being exhaled more rapidly than it is being produced. The bicarbonate level is low in response to the pH increase. Many blood and cellular buffers release hydrogen ions that combine with the blood bicarbonate ions and form carbonic acid, thus reducing the blood level of bicarbonate.

As in metabolic alkalosis, the blood potassium level is reduced as the body attempts to maintain electroneutrality. Again, as the pH increases, calcium binding increases and the blood level of calcium decreases, causing hypocalcemia.

Common Nursing Diagnoses and Collaborative Problems

Nursing diagnoses and collaborative problems that may apply to clients with alkalosis include the following:

- Acute Pain related to muscle spasms
- Acute Confusion related to excess central nervous system excitation
- Risk for Falls related to skeletal muscle weakness and hypotension

Interventions

Interventions are planned to prevent further losses of hydrogen, potassium, calcium, and chloride ions; to restore fluid balance; and to monitor changes (Chart 19-6).

Drug therapy is used for alkalosis. Drugs are prescribed to resolve the causes of alkalosis and to restore normal fluid, electrolyte, and acid-base balance. For example, the client with metabolic alkalosis caused by diuretic therapy receives fluid and electrolyte replacement. Antiemetic drugs are prescribed if the client is vomiting. Fluids and electrolytes are replaced orally or parenterally. Carefully monitor the client's progress and adjust fluid and electrolyte therapy. Serum electrolyte values are monitored daily until they return to normal or near normal.

CHART 19-6

NIC INTERVENTION ACTIVITIES for The Client with Alkalosis

Acid-Base Management: Metabolic Alkalosis: *Promotion of acid-base balance and prevention of complications resulting from serum HCO_3 levels higher than desired*

- Monitor ABG levels for increased pH level.
- Maintain patent IV access.
- Monitor intake and output.
- Monitor determinants of tissue oxygen delivery (e.g., Pao_2, Sao_2, and hemoglobin levels and cardiac output), if available.
- Avoid administration of alkaline substances (e.g., IV sodium bicarbonate and PO or NG antacids) as appropriate.
- Monitor for electrolyte imbalances associated with metabolic alkalosis (e.g., hypokalemia, hypocalcemia, and hypochloremia), as appropriate.
- Monitor for renal loss of acid (e.g., diuretic therapy), as appropriate.
- Replace extracellular fluid deficit with IV saline, as appropriate.
- Administer antiemetics to reduce loss of HCl in emesis, as appropriate.

Acid-Base Management: Respiratory Alkalosis: *Promotion of acid-base balance and prevention of complications resulting from serum pCO_2 levels lower than desired*

- Monitor ABG levels for increased pH level.
- Monitor for indications of impending respiratory failure (e.g., low Pao_2 level, respiratory muscle fatigue, low Sao_2/Svo_2 level).
- Monitor for hyperventilation resulting in respiratory alkalosis (e.g., hypoxemia, CNS injury, hypermetabolic states, GI distention, pain, and stress).
- Monitor for cardiopulmonary manifestations of respiratory alkalosis (e.g., arrhythmias, decreased cardiac output, and hyperventilation).
- Provide oxygen therapy, if necessary.
- Reduce oxygen consumption to minimize hyperventilation (e.g., promote comfort, control fever, and reduce anxiety), as appropriate.
- Provide mechanical ventilatory support, if necessary.

NIC intervention activities selected from Dochterman J.M., & Bulechek, G.M. (Eds.). (*2004*). *Nursing interventions classification (NIC)* (4th ed.). St. Louis: Mosby. No part of this work is to be altered without prior written permission from the Publisher.

ABG, Arterial blood gas; *HCO_3*, bicarbonate; *Pao_2*, partial pressure of arterial oxygen; *Sao_2*, arterial oxygen saturation; *Svo_2*, venous oxygen saturation; *$Paco_2$*, partial pressure of arterial carbon dioxide; *GI*, gastrointestinal.

GET READY for the NCLEX Examination!

KEY POINTS

Safe Effective Care Environment

- Use caution in giving oxygen to people who have COPD.
- Assess and document the condition of the site from which an arterial blood gas sample was obtained at least every 2 hours for the first 24 hours.

Health Promotion and Maintenance

- Teach all clients to take drugs as prescribed, especially diuretics, antihypertensives, and cardiac drugs.
- Instruct all clients at continuing risk for respiratory acidosis to stop smoking.
- Assist clients interested in smoking cessation to find an appropriate smoking cessation program.

Psychosocial Integrity

- Assess the oxygenation status of any client with acute confusion.
- Monitor the neurologic status at least every 2 hours in clients being treated for an acid-base imbalance.
- Assist clients who have anxiety-induced respiratory alkalosis to identify causes of anxiety.
- Teach clients who have anxiety-induced respiratory alkalosis to use stress management techniques.

Physiological Integrity

- Check the serum potassium level for any client who has acidosis.
- Assess heart rate and rhythm at least every 2 hours for any client with an acid-base imbalance.
- Assess the airway of any client who has acute respiratory acidosis.
- Monitor arterial blood gas values to evaluate the effectiveness of therapy for acid-base imbalances.
- Assess the oxygenation status of any client with acidosis.
- Provide a low carbohydrate, high-fat diet to the client with chronic respiratory acidosis.

ADDITIONAL STUDY RESOURCES

Go to your Student CD-ROM for Review Questions for the NCLEX Examination.

evolve Go to http://evolve.elsevier.com/Iggy/ for Integrated Management of Care Questions for the NCLEX Examination.

SELECTED BIBLIOGRAPHY

Banker, D., Whittier, F., & Rutecki, G. (2003). Acid-base disturbances: 5 rules that can simplify diagnosis. *Consultant, 43*(3), 381, 386-388.

Berry, B., & Pinard, A. (2002). Assessing tissue oxygenation. *Critical Care Nurse, 22*(3), 22-24, 26-30, 32-36.

Call-Schmidt, T. (2001). Interpreting lab results: A primer. *MEDSURG Nursing, 10*(4), 179-184.

Dochterman, J.M., & Bulechek, G.M. (Eds.). (2004). *Nursing interventions classification (NIC)* (4th ed.). St. Louis: Mosby.

Epstein, S., & Singh, N. (2001). Respiratory acidosis. *Respiratory Care, 46*(4), 366-383.

Foster, G., Vaziri, N., & Sassoon, C. (2001). Respiratory alkalosis. *Respiratory Care, 46*(4), 384-391.

Isenhour, J., Slovis, C. (2001). Arterial blood gas analysis: A simple, 3 step approach: Co-oximetry is required for patients with CO poisoning. *Journal of Respiratory Diseases, 22*(5), 289-292, 295-296.

Khanna, A., & Kurtzman, N. (2001). Metabolic alkalosis. *Respiratory Care, 46*(4), 354-365.

Kischner, M. (2002). Additional step in ABG analysis (letter to the editor in response to the Berry & Pinard article). *Critical Care Nurse, 22*(5), 16-17.

Kraut, J., & Madias, N. (2001). Approach to patients with acid-base disorders. *Respiratory Care, 46*(4), 392-403.

McCance, K., & Huether, S. (2002). *Pathophysiology: The biologic basis for disease in adults and children* (4th ed.). St. Louis: Mosby.

McConnell, E. (2002). Measuring fluid intake and output. *Nursing2002, 32*(7), 17.

O'Neill, D. (2001). Making sense of arterial blood gases. *Nursing Times, 97*(27), 36-37, 39.

Pagana, K., & Pagana, T. (2002). *Mosby's manual of diagnostic and laboratory tests* (2nd ed.). St. Louis: Mosby.

Paulson, W. (2000). Problem solving in acid-base diagnosis. Case study: From acid-base disorders to clinical diagnosis. *Journal of Critical Illness, 15*(2), 113-117.

Shoulders-Odom, B. (2000). Using an algorithm to interpret arterial blood gases. *DCCM - Dimensions of Critical Care Nursing, 19*(1), 36-41.

Swenson, E. (2001). Metabolic acidosis. *Respiratory Care, 46*(4), 342-353.

Trissel, L. (2003). *Handbook on injectable drugs* (12th ed.). Bethesda, MD: American Society of Health-System Pharmacists.

UNIT **FIVE**

MANAGEMENT of PERIOPERATIVE CLIENTS

CHAPTER

20

Interventions for Preoperative Clients

REBECCA M. PATTON

LEARNING OUTCOMES

After studying this chapter, you should be able to:

1. Differentiate among the various types and purposes of surgery.
2. Identify personal factors that increase the client's risk for complications during and immediately following surgery.
3. Use effective communication when teaching clients and family members about what to expect during the surgical experience.
4. Assume the role of client advocate.
5. Perform an accurate preoperative assessment of the client's physical and psychosocial status.
6. Identify laboratory value changes that may affect the client's response to drugs, anesthesia, and surgery.
7. Describe the legal implications and proper procedures for obtaining informed consent.
8. Explain the purposes and techniques commonly used for client preoperative preparation.
9. Prioritize teaching needs for the client preparing for surgery.
10. Recognize client conditions or issues that need to be communicated to the surgical and postoperative teams.

Go to your Student CD-ROM for Review Questions for the NCLEX Examination keyed to these Learning Outcomes.

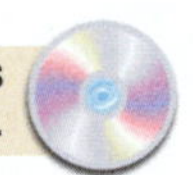

Any client undergoing surgery today receives the benefits of advances in surgical techniques, anesthesia, pharmacology, medical devices, and many supportive interventions. Research defining best practices has resulted in improved outcomes in all areas of the perioperative experience. The technology explosion is responsible for the development of new diagnostic and interventional devices for the use and refinement of new surgical techniques. Examples of such technical advances include the GAMMA knife for brain tumor resections, robotics, and other types of minimally invasive surgeries. Advances in anesthetic agents and techniques also have developed. These changes improve the ways that a surgical client is treated and has made anesthesia safer than ever before.

Cost reduction initiatives by third-party payers are also a driving force as to how the health care community manages the surgical client. Shortened stays and outpatient treatment have become the expected. Ambulatory surgical services are common, with more clients being admitted as inpatients *after* a procedure, rather than before. Some clients may only be observed after surgery and may not be admitted as an inpatient. In response to the ongoing health care delivery changes and the use of multiple settings, nurses have modified their interventions, remaining focused on client care before **(preoperative)**, during **(intraoperative)**, and after **(postoperative)** surgery.

OVERVIEW

The preoperative period begins when the client is scheduled for surgery and ends at the time of transfer to the surgical suite. As a nurse, you must act as an educator, an advocate, and a promoter of health. The surgical environment demands the use of knowledge, judgment, and skills based on the principles of nursing science. Perioperative nursing places special emphasis on safety and client education.

The client's readiness for surgery is critical to the outcome. Care before surgery focuses on client readiness. This care includes education and any intervention needed before surgery to reduce anxiety and complications and to promote cooperation in procedures after surgery. Use adult teaching and learning principles in teaching clients and families before surgery. It is important to validate and clarify information the client has received from the surgeon or other members of the surgical team. In addition, during assessment before surgery it is not uncommon to identify problems that warrant further client assessment and/or intervention before the procedure. Communication and collaboration with the surgical team is essential so that correct actions are taken to achieve the desired outcome.

Categories and Purposes of Surgery

Surgical procedures are categorized according to the following:

- The reason for the surgery
- The urgency of the procedure
- The degree of risk
- The anatomic location
- The extent of surgery required

The primary purposes, or reasons, for surgery can be divided into five general subcategories: diagnostic, curative, restorative, palliative, and cosmetic. **Palliative surgery** makes the client more comfortable, and **cosmetic surgery** reconstructs the skin and underlying structures. The urgency of the procedure can be elective, urgent, and emergent. The degree of risk is classified as minor or major.

Category by location is based on the area of the body on which the surgery occurs (e.g., abdominal surgery, intracranial surgery, or heart surgery). The extent can be simple, modified, or radical. Table 20-1 explains the categories and gives examples of surgical procedures.

Surgical Settings

The term **inpatient** refers to a client who is admitted to a hospital. The client may be admitted the day before or, more often, the day of surgery (often termed same-day admission [SDA]), or the client may already be an inpatient when surgery is needed. The terms **outpatient** and **ambulatory** refer to a client who goes to the surgical area the day of the surgery and returns home on the same day (i.e., same-day surgery [SDS]). Hospital-based ambulatory surgical centers,

TABLE 20-1 Selected Categories of Surgical Procedures

Category	Description	Condition or Surgical Procedure
Reasons for Surgery		
Diagnostic	Performed to determine the origin and cause of a disorder or the cell type for cancer	Breast biopsy Exploratory laparotomy Arthroscopy
Curative	Performed to resolve a health problem by repairing or removing the cause	Laparoscopic cholecystectomy Mastectomy Hysterectomy
Restorative	Performed to improve a client's functional ability	Total knee replacement Finger reimplantation
Palliative	Performed to relieve symptoms of a disease process, but does not cure	Colostomy Nerve root resection Tumor debulking Ileostomy
Cosmetic	Performed primarily to alter or enhance personal appearance	Liposuction Revision of scars Rhinoplasty Blepharoplasty
Urgency of Surgery		
Elective	Planned for correction of a nonacute problem	Cataract removal Hernia repair Hemorrhoidectomy Total joint replacement
Urgent	Requires prompt intervention; may be life threatening if treatment is delayed more than 24-48 hr	Intestinal obstruction Bladder obstruction Kidney or ureteral stones Bone fracture Eye injury Acute cholecystitis
Emergent	Requires immediate intervention because of life-threatening consequences	Gunshot or stab wound Severe bleeding Abdominal aortic aneurysm Compound fracture Appendectomy
Degree of Risk of Surgery		
Minor	Procedure without significant risk; often done with local anesthesia	Incision and drainage (I&D) Implantation of a venous access device (VAD) Muscle biopsy
Major	Procedure of greater risk, usually longer and more extensive than a minor procedure	Mitral valve replacement Pancreas transplant Lymph node dissection
Extent of Surgery		
Simple	Only the most overtly affected areas involved in the surgery	Simple/partial mastectomy
Radical	Extensive surgery beyond the area obviously involved; is directed at finding a root cause	Radical prostatectomy Radical hysterectomy

freestanding surgical centers, physicians' offices, and ambulatory care centers are common. About 70% to 90% of all surgical procedures in North America are performed in ambulatory centers (Bryant, 2002).

One advantage of outpatient surgery is that clients are not separated from the comfort and security of their home and family. With improvements in surgical techniques and anesthesia, more procedures are performed safely on an outpatient basis. Same-day surgery, however, presents new challenges for the client who does not have an adequate or available support system. An older spouse may be unable to assist in care before or after surgery. Clients who are responsible for others may be unable to perform their usual tasks within the family. They may try to continue their family role but jeopardize their own health by doing so. As a result, their stress, fears, and anxieties about the surgical experience and about returning home immediately after surgery may be increased.

COLLABORATIVE MANAGEMENT

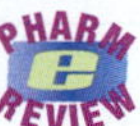

Assessment

HISTORY

Data collection about the client before surgery begins in various settings (e.g., the surgeon's office, the preadmission or admission office, the inpatient unit, and over the telephone). Use privacy to increase the client's comfort with the interview process. Anesthesia and surgery are both physical and emotional stressors. Collect the following data:

- Age
- Use of tobacco, alcohol, or illicit substances, including marijuana
- Current medications
- Use of complementary or alternative medicines, such as herbal therapies, folk remedies, or acupuncture
- Medical history
- Prior surgical procedures and experiences
- Prior experience with anesthesia
- Autologous or directed blood donations
- Allergies, including sensitivity to latex products
- General health
- Family history
- Type of surgery planned
- Knowledge about and understanding of events during the perioperative period
- Adequacy of the client's support system

When taking a history, screen the client for problems that increase the risk for complications during and after surgery. Some problems that increase the surgical risk or increase the risk for complications after surgery are listed in Table 20-2.

AGE. Older clients are at increased risk for complications. The normal aging process decreases immune system functioning and delays wound healing. The frequency of chronic illness increases in older clients. See Chart 20-1 for other changes in older adults that may alter the operative response or risk.

DRUGS AND SUBSTANCE USE. The use of tobacco increases the risk for pulmonary complications because of changes it causes to the lungs and chest cavity. Excessive alcohol and illicit substance use can alter the client's responses to anesthesia and pain medication. Withdrawal of alcohol before surgery may lead to delirium tremens. Prescription and over-the-counter drugs may also affect how the client reacts to the operative experience.

TABLE 20-2 Selected Factors That Increase Surgical Risk or Increase the Risk of Postoperative Complications

Age
- Older than 65 years

Medications
- Antihypertensives
- Tricyclic antidepressants
- Anticoagulants
- Nonsteroidal anti-inflammatory drugs (NSAIDs)

Medical History
- Decreased immunity
- Diabetes
- Pulmonary disease
- Cardiac disease
- Hemodynamic instability
- Multisystem disease
- Coagulation defect or disorder
- Anemia
- Dehydration
- Infection
- Hypertension
- Hypotension
- Any chronic disease

Prior Surgical Experiences
- Less-than-optimal emotional reaction
- Anesthesia reactions or complications
- Postoperative complications

Health History
- Malnutrition or obesity
- Medication, tobacco, alcohol, or illicit substance use or abuse
- Altered coping ability

Family History
- Malignant hyperthermia
- Cancer
- Bleeding disorder

Type of Surgical Procedure Planned
- Neck, oral, or facial procedures (airway complications)
- Chest or high abdominal procedures (pulmonary complications)
- Abdominal surgery (paralytic ileus, deep vein thrombosis)

The potential effects of specific drugs are listed in Table 20-3. Another area of concern is the potential for reaction or serious adverse effects with some herbs, such as those listed in Table 20-4.

MEDICAL HISTORY. Ask the client about his or her medical history. Many chronic illnesses increase surgical risks and need to be considered when planning care. For example, a client with systemic lupus erythematosus may need additional drugs to offset the stress of the surgery. A diabetic client may need a more extensive bowel preparation because of decreased intestinal motility. An infection may need to be treated before surgery.

CARDIAC HISTORY. Ask the client specifically about cardiac disease because complications from anesthesia occur more often in clients with cardiac problems. Cardiac problems that increase surgical risks include coronary artery disease, angina, myocardial infarction (MI) within 6 months before surgery, heart failure, hypertension, and dysrhythmias. These problems impair the client's ability to withstand hemodynamic changes and alter the response to anesthesia. The risk for an MI during surgery is higher in clients with pre-existing heart problems.

CHART 20-1

NURSING FOCUS on the OLDER ADULT

Changes of Aging as Surgical Risk Factors

Physiologic Change	Nursing Interventions	Rationales
Cardiovascular System		
Decreased cardiac output Increased blood pressure	Determine normal activity levels and note when the client tires.	Knowing limits helps prevent fatigue.
Decreased peripheral circulation	Monitor vital signs, peripheral pulses, and capillary refill.	Having baseline data helps detect deviations.
Respiratory System		
Reduced vital capacity Loss of lung elasticity	Teach coughing and deep breathing exercises.	Pulmonary exercises help prevent pulmonary complications.
Decreased oxygenation of blood	Monitor respirations and breathing effort.	Having baseline data helps detect deviations.
Renal/Urinary System		
Decreased blood flow to kidneys Reduced ability to excrete waste products	Monitor intake and output. Assess overall hydration.	Ongoing assessment helps detect fluid and electrolyte imbalances and decreased renal function.
Decline in glomerular filtration rate	Monitor electrolyte status.	
Nocturia common	Assist frequently with toileting needs, especially at night.	Frequent toileting helps prevent incontinence and falls.
Neurologic System		
Sensory deficits Slower reaction time	Orient the client to the surroundings. Allow extra time for teaching the client.	An individualized preoperative teaching plan is developed on the basis of the client's orientation and any neurologic deficits.
Decreased ability to adjust to changes in the surroundings	Provide for the client's safety.	Safety measures help prevent falls and injury.
Musculoskeletal System		
Increased incidence of deformities related to osteoporosis or arthritis	Assess the client's mobility. Teach turning and positioning. Encourage ambulation.	Interventions help prevent complications of immobility.
	Place on fall precautions, if indicated.	Safety measures help prevent injury.

TABLE 20-3 Effects of Routine Medications Taken Preoperatively

Drug	Implications for the Perioperative Experience	Nursing Interventions	Rationales
Antidysrhythmics			
Quinidine gluconate (Quinate✱, Quinaglute Dura-Tabs) Procainamide hydrochloride (Pronestyl, Procan SR)	Antidysrhythmic medications affect the client's tolerance of anesthesia and potentiate anesthetics that are neuromuscular blockers. Antidysrhythmics depress cardiac function by decreasing cardiac output and slowing pulse rate. Antidysrhythmics may cause peripheral vasodilation.	Communicate the use and type of antidysrhythmics to the anesthesia personnel. Monitor vital signs. Obtain a baseline electrocardiogram, as ordered. Assess the client's peripheral circulation.	Cardiac complications during surgery can be life threatening. Ongoing monitoring helps to detect deviations and potential complications.
Antihypertensives			
Methyldopa (Aldomet, Novomedopa✱) Captopril (Capoten) Clonidine hydrochloride (Catapres)	Antihypertensive agents alter the client's response to muscle relaxants and opioid analgesics by inhibiting synthesis and storage of norepinephrine. Antihypertensives may cause a hypotensive crisis intraoperatively and postoperatively.	Monitor blood pressure and pulse frequently. Assess for hypotension during transfer and turning.	Ongoing monitoring helps to detect deviations and potential complications. Hypotensive crisis can occur and may be prevented through timely assessments.
Corticosteroids			
Dexamethasone (Decadron, Dexasone) Hydrocortisone sodium (Solu-Cortef) Prednisone (Deltasone✱, Winpred)	Surgery increases the demand for corticosteroids in the client with no adrenal function. Steroids delay wound healing because of blockage of collagen formation. Steroids increase the serum glucose level and block fibroblast formation. Steroids increase the risk of hemorrhage. Steroids mask the signs and symptoms of infection.	Continue steroid therapy during surgery. Monitor vital signs. Assess for signs of hyperglycemia. Assess for subtle signs of infection and bleeding. Monitor wound healing, support the incision area with binders, and splint the wound when the client is turning, coughing, and deep breathing.	Continuation of steroid therapy avoids problems associated with abrupt withdrawal. Ongoing monitoring helps to detect deviations and potential complications. It is important to detect early signs and symptoms of infection. Specific wound and incision care helps to prevent complications.

aPTT, Partial thromboplastin time, activated; *INR,* International Normalized Ratio; *NPO,* nothing by mouth; *PT,* prothrombin time.

Continued

TABLE 20-3 Effects of Routine Medications Taken Preoperatively—*cont'd*

Drug	Implications for the Perioperative Experience	Nursing Interventions	Rationales
Anticoagulants			
Warfarin sodium (Coumadin, Warfilone sodium✱) Heparin sodium (Leo-Heparin, Hepalean✱) Aspirin (acetylsalicylic acid, Ancasal✱, Astrin✱, Coryphen✱)	Anticoagulant therapy increases the risk of hemorrhage intraoperatively and postoperatively.	Monitor coagulation studies (aPTT, PT, INR). Monitor for signs of bleeding. Gradually discontinue anticoagulants 24-48 hr before surgery, as ordered. Have an antidote (protamine sulfate for heparin and vitamin K [Mephyton] for warfarin sodium) available to reverse the effects of the anticoagulant.	Coagulation studies help detect bleeding disorders. Anticoagulant administration is discontinued to avoid hemorrhage. An antidote needs to be available to prevent complications of bleeding in an emergency situation.
Antiseizure Medications			
Phenobarbital (Luminal, Gardenal✱)	Seizure activity can cause injury to the surgical wound. Antiseizure medications alter the metabolism of anesthetic agents.	Maintain use of the drug. Inform the anesthesia provider to allow for adjustment of the dosage of the anesthetic. Assess for seizure activity. Pad the siderails of the bed. Place suction equipment at the bedside.	Antiseizure medications prevent seizures. Safety measures prevent injury.
Glaucoma Medications			
Demecarium bromide (Humorsol) Echothiophate (Phospholine iodide) Pilocarpine hydrochloride (Isopto Carpine, Pilocar, Miocarpine✱) Timolol maleate (Timoptic)	Glaucoma medications have cumulative systemic effects and can cause respiratory and cardiovascular collapse, especially during surgery.	Consult the physician about stopping Humorsol at least 2 wk before surgery. Monitor respiratory status and cardiac output. Assess for increased intraocular pressure.	Collaboration with the physician helps prevent complications. Ongoing monitoring helps to detect complications.
Antidiabetic Agent			
Insulin	Insulin needs decrease preoperatively when the client is on NPO status. Postoperative insulin demands increase because of IV administration of dextrose. Insulin levels may fluctuate during healing because of dietary and activity restrictions and the physical stress of surgery.	Monitor serum glucose levels. Administer antibiotics and other intermittent medications in normal saline instead of dextrose when possible, as prescribed, or as per facility policy.	Monitoring detects an increased or a decreased need for insulin. The use of normal saline prevents complications.

aPTT, Partial thromboplastin time, activated; *INR,* International Normalized Ratio; *NPO,* nothing by mouth; *PT,* prothrombin time.

PULMONARY HISTORY. Older clients, those with chronic respiratory problems, and smokers are at risk for pulmonary complications because of smoking- or age-related lung changes. Increased chest rigidity and loss of lung elasticity reduce anesthesia excretion. Smoking increases the blood level of **carboxyhemoglobin** (carbon monoxide on oxygen-binding sites of the hemoglobin molecule), which decreases oxygen delivery to organs. Action of cilia in pulmonary mucous membranes decreases, which leads to retained secretions and predisposes the client to infection (pneumonia) and **atelectasis** (collapse of alveoli). Atelectasis reduces gas exchange and causes intolerance of anesthesia.

Chronic lung problems such as asthma, emphysema, and chronic bronchitis also reduce the elasticity of the lungs, which reduces gas exchange. As a result, clients with these problems have reduced tissue oxygenation.

PREVIOUS SURGERY AND ANESTHESIA. The number and type of previous surgical procedures affect the client's readiness for surgery. Previous surgery, especially with complications, may increase fears and concerns about the scheduled surgery. Ask about the client's previous experience with anesthesia and all allergies. These data provide information about tolerance of and possible fears about the use of anesthesia. The family medical history and problems with anesthetics may indicate possible reactions to anesthesia, such as malignant hyperthermia (see Chapter 21).

A sensitivity or allergy to certain substances alerts you to a possible reaction to anesthetic agents or to substances that are used before or during surgery. For example, povidone-iodine used for skin cleansing contains the same allergens found in shellfish. Clients who are allergic to shellfish may have an adverse reaction to povidone-iodine. The client with an allergy to bananas often also has a latex allergy.

TABLE 20-4 Potential Effects of Herbs

Herb	Potential Effect
Black cohosh	Bradycardia, hypotension, joint pains
Bloodroot	Bradycardia, dysrhythmia, dizziness, impaired vision, intense thirst
Boneset	Liver toxicity, mental changes, respiratory problems
Coltsfoot	Fever, liver toxicity
Dandelion	Interactions with diuretics, increased concentration of lithium or potassium
Ephedra	Headache, dizziness, insomnia, tachycardia, hypertension, anxiety, irritability, dry mouth
Feverfew	Interference with blood-clotting mechanisms
Garlic	Hypotension, blood-clotting inhibition, potentiation of diabetes drugs
Ginseng	Headache, anxiety, insomnia, hypertension, tachycardia, asthma attacks, postmenopausal bleeding
Goldenseal	Vasoconstriction
Hawthorn	Hypotension
Kava	Damage to the eyes, skin, liver, and spinal cord from long-term use
Licorice	Hyperkalemia, hypernatremia
Lobelia	Hearing and vision problems
Motherwort	Increased anticoagulation
Nettle	Hypokalemia
Senna	Potentiation of digoxin
St. John's Wort	Antidepressant, photosensitivity
Valerian root	Mild sedative or tranquilizer effect, hepatotoxicity

BLOOD DONATIONS. Clients may donate their own blood **(autologous donations)** for a few weeks just before the scheduled surgery date. If they need blood during or after surgery, an autologous blood transfusion can be given. This practice eliminates transfusion reactions and reduces the risk of acquiring bloodborne disease.

Clients can donate their own blood up to 5 weeks before surgery if they are infection free, have a hemoglobin level greater than 11 g/dL (110 g/L), and have a physician's recommendation. Clients with cardiac disease may need additional clearance from their cardiologist before making an autologous donation. The physician may prescribe supplemental iron before the first donation. Autologous donations can be made as often as every 3 days if other criteria are met. Usually a total of 2 to 4 units is donated. The last donation cannot be made within 72 hours before surgery.

A special tag is placed on the blood bag when an autologous blood donation has been made. The blood donor center gives the client a matching tag that he or she wears or brings to the surgical area before surgery. This procedure helps to ensure that clients receive only their own blood. If the blood is not used, it goes to the blood bank to be used as would any other unit of donated blood.

Clients may wish to have family and friends donate blood exclusively for their use, if needed. This practice (called **directed blood donation**) is possible only if the blood types are compatible and the donor's blood is acceptable. Clients may fear disease transmission from unknown blood and feel more comfortable knowing who gave the blood. Many centers do not accept directed blood, stating that it gives a false sense of security. As with autologous blood donations, a special tag is attached to the blood bag. This tag notes the names of the client and the donor and bears the client's signature.

Ask whether autologous or directed blood donations have been made and document this information in the chart. It is important to know the specific blood collection center where the donation was made and whether the blood has arrived before the client goes into surgery. The hospital receives and stores the blood units until they are used or are no longer needed. Unused blood is returned to the collection center.

PLANNING FOR BLOODLESS SURGERY. Increased use of "bloodless surgery," or minimally invasive surgery, provides alternatives for clients with religious or medical restrictions to blood transfusions. These programs reduce or eliminate the need for transfusion during and after surgery. Some techniques used include limiting blood samples (the number of samples, as well as the volume of blood drawn per sample) before surgery and stimulating the client's own red blood cell production with epoetin alpha (Epogen, Procrit) before, during, and after surgery. Supplemental iron, folic acid, vitamin B_{12}, and vitamin C may be prescribed before surgery to help red blood cell formation. Newer equipment and surgical techniques cause less blood loss than older techniques. Such advances include recycling blood suctioned during surgery and immediately transfusing it back into the client. Assess, monitor, teach, and support the client during the bloodless surgery process.

DISCHARGE PLANNING. Assess the client's home environment, self-care capabilities, and support systems and anticipate postoperative needs before surgery. *All clients, regardless of how minor the procedure or how often they have had surgery, should have discharge planning.* Older clients and dependent adults may need transportation referrals to and from the physician's office or the surgical setting. A home care nurse may be needed to monitor recovery and to provide instructions. All clients with few support systems may need follow-up care at home. Some clients need a planned direct admission to a rehabilitation hospital or center for physical therapy following surgery, such as after a total hip replacement. Shortened hospital stays require adequate discharge planning to achieve the desired outcomes after surgery.

PHYSICAL ASSESSMENT/CLINICAL MANIFESTATIONS

The preoperative client may be any age, with a health status that varies from well to debilitated. Perform a complete assessment before surgery to obtain baseline data. During assessment, identify current health problems, potential complications related to anesthesia, and possible complications that may occur after surgery.

When beginning the assessment, obtain a complete set of vital signs. You may need to obtain vital signs several times for accurate baseline values. Previous vital signs from another admission (if available in the medical record) are helpful to compare against current vital signs. Abnormal vital signs may require postponement of surgery until the problem is treated and the client's condition is stable. Also assess for anxiety, which could increase blood pressure, pulse, and respiratory rate. Document these findings as part of the overall assessment.

Throughout the physical assessment, focus on problem areas identified from the client's history and on all body systems affected by the surgical procedure. The older adult (Chart 20-2; see also Chapter 5) or chronically ill client is at

CHART 20-2

NURSING FOCUS on the OLDER ADULT

Specific Considerations When Planning Care for the Older Preoperative Client

- Greater incidence of chronic illness
- Greater incidence of malnutrition
- More allergies
- Increased incidence of impaired self-care abilities
- Inadequate support systems
- Decreased ability to withstand the stress of surgery and anesthesia
- Increased risk for cardiopulmonary complications after surgery
- Risk of a change in mental status when admitted (related to unfamiliar surroundings, change in routine, drugs given, and so forth)
- Increased risk of a fall and resultant injury

increased risk for complications during and after surgery. Morbidity and mortality during or after surgery are higher in older and chronically ill clients.

Report any abnormal assessment findings to the surgeon and to anesthesiology personnel. In this way, you are a proactive client advocate exercising professional legal responsibility. Often, established protocols or care maps identify what interventions are to be performed before surgery.

CARDIOVASCULAR SYSTEM. Cardiac problems may cause as many as 30% of surgery-related deaths. Check the client for hypertension, which is common, is often undiagnosed, and can affect the response to surgery. Cardiac assessment includes listening to heart sounds for rate, regularity, and abnormalities. Examine the client's hands and feet for temperature, color, peripheral pulses, capillary refill, and edema. Report any problems, such as absent peripheral pulses, pitting edema, or cardiac symptoms, such as chest pain, shortness of breath, and dyspnea, to the physician for further assessment and evaluation. (Cardiac assessment is discussed further in Chapter 36.)

RESPIRATORY SYSTEM. In assessing the client's respiratory status, consider the client's age, smoking history (including exposure to secondhand smoke), and any chronic illness. Observe the client's posture; respiratory rate, rhythm, and depth; overall respiratory effort; and lung expansion. Document any clubbing of the fingertips (swelling at the base of the nail beds caused by a chronic lack of oxygen) or cyanosis. Auscultate the lungs to assess for any abnormal breath sounds (crackles, wheezes, rubs). (More information on respiratory assessment is found in Chapter 30.)

RENAL/URINARY SYSTEM. Kidney function affects the excretion of drugs and waste products, including anesthetic and analgesic agents. If renal function is reduced, fluid and electrolyte balance can be altered, especially in older clients. Ask about problems such as urinary frequency, **dysuria** (painful urination), **nocturia** (awakening during nighttime sleep because of a need to void), difficulty starting urine flow, and **oliguria** (scant amount of urine). Ask the client about the appearance and odor of the urine. Equally important is an assessment of usual fluid intake and degree of continence. If the client has renal or urinary problems, consult with the physician about further workup. (Renal/urinary assessment is discussed further in Chapter 72.)

Kidney impairment decreases the excretion of drugs and anesthetic agents. As a result, drug effectiveness may be altered. Scopolamine (Buscopan✱), morphine, meperidine (Demerol), and barbiturates often cause confusion, disorientation, apprehension, and restlessness when given to clients with decreased kidney function.

NEUROLOGIC SYSTEM. Assess the client's overall mental status, including level of consciousness, orientation, and ability to follow commands, before planning preoperative teaching and care after surgery. A problem in any of these areas affects the type of care needed during the surgical experience. Determine the client's baseline neurologic status to be able to identify changes that may occur later. Also assess for any motor or sensory deficits. (See Chapter 44 for complete nervous system assessment.)

The usual neurologic status of a mentally impaired or older client may be difficult to assess. The client who has been independent and oriented at home may become disoriented in an unfamiliar hospital setting. Family members can often provide information about what the client was like at home.

Assess the client's risk for falling, especially in older clients. Evaluate factors such as mental status, muscle strength, steadiness of gait, and sense of independence to determine the client's risk. Document the client's ability to ambulate and the steadiness of gait as baseline data.

MUSCULOSKELETAL SYSTEM. Musculoskeletal problems may interfere with positioning during and after surgery. For example, clients with arthritis may be able to assume surgical positions but have discomfort after surgery from prolonged joint immobilization. Other anatomic features, such as the shape and length of the neck and the shape of the chest cavity, may interfere with respiratory and cardiac function or require special positioning during surgery.

Ask about a history of joint replacements and document the exact location of any prostheses. During surgery, ensure that electrocautery pads, which could cause an electrical burn, are not placed on or near the area of the prosthesis.

NUTRITIONAL STATUS. Malnutrition and obesity increase surgical risk. Surgery increases metabolic rate and depletes potassium, vitamin C, and B vitamins, all of which are needed for wound healing and blood clotting. In malnourished clients, decreased serum protein levels slow recovery. Negative nitrogen balance may result from depleted protein stores. This problem increases the risk for delayed wound healing, possible dehiscence or evisceration (see Chapter 22), dehydration, and sepsis.

Some older clients may have nutritional imbalances because of chronic illness, diuretic or laxative use, poor dietary planning or habits, anorexia, lack of motivation, or financial limitations. Indications of poor fluid or nutritional status include brittle nails, muscle wasting, dry or flaky skin, hair changes (e.g., dull, sparse, dry), decreased skin turgor, orthostatic (postural) hypotension, decreased serum protein levels, and abnormal serum electrolyte values.

The obese client is often malnourished because of an imbalanced diet. Obesity increases the risk for poor wound healing because of excessive **adipose** (fatty) tissue. Fatty tissue has few blood vessels, little collagen, and decreased nutrients, all of which are needed for wound healing. Obesity stresses the heart and reduces the lung volumes, which can affect the surgery and recovery. In addition, obese clients may need larger doses of drugs and may retain them longer after surgery.

PSYCHOSOCIAL ASSESSMENT

Perform a psychosocial assessment to determine the client's level of anxiety, coping ability, and support systems. Provide information and offer support as needed.

Most clients have some degree of anxiety and fear before surgery. The extent of these reactions varies according to the type of surgery, the perceived effects of the surgery and its potential outcome, and the client's personality. Surgery may be seen as a threat to life, body image, self-esteem, self-concept, or lifestyle. Clients may fear death, pain, helplessness, decreased socioeconomic status, a diagnosis of life-threatening conditions, possible disabling or crippling effects, or the unknown.

Anxiety and fear affect the client's ability to learn, cope, and cooperate with teaching and operative procedures. Anxiety and fear may also influence the amount and type of anesthesia needed and may slow recovery. Be aware of potential fears and anxieties when interviewing the client and planning teaching.

Assess coping mechanisms used by the client under similar situations or in the past when confronted with a stressful situation. Ask open-ended questions about the client's feelings about the entire surgical experience. Factors that influence coping include age; previous surgical or sick-role experiences; and emotional and physical signs of fear, anxiety, or discomfort. Signs of fear and anxiety include anger, crying, restlessness, profuse sweating, increased pulse rate, palpitations, sleeplessness, diarrhea, and urinary frequency.

LABORATORY ASSESSMENT

Laboratory tests before surgery provide baseline data about the client's health and help predict potential complications. The client scheduled for surgery in an ambulatory surgical center or admitted to the hospital on the morning of or day before surgery may have preadmission testing (PAT) performed from 24 hours to 28 days before the scheduled surgery. These test results are usually valid unless there has been a change in the client's condition that warrants repeated testing or the client is taking drugs that can alter laboratory values (such as warfarin [Coumadin], aspirin, or diuretics). Some facilities have time limits for tests, especially pregnancy testing or any other test results that would require altering the surgical plan.

The choice of laboratory testing before surgery varies among facilities and depends on the client's age, medical history, and the type of anesthesia planned. The most common tests are urinalysis, blood type and crossmatch, complete blood count or hemoglobin level and hematocrit, clotting studies (prothrombin time [PT], International Normalized Ratio [INR], activated partial thromboplastin time [aPTT], and platelet count), electrolyte levels, and serum creatinine level. Depending on a female client's age and the nature of the planned procedure, a pregnancy test may also be needed.

Urinalysis is performed to assess abnormal substances in the urine such as protein, glucose, blood, and bacteria. If renal disease is suspected or if the client is older, the physician may request other tests to determine the type and degree of disease present.

Report electrolyte imbalances or other abnormal results to the anesthesia team and the surgeon before surgery. **Hypokalemia** (decreased serum potassium level) increases the risk for toxicity if the client is taking digoxin, slows recovery from anesthesia, and increases cardiac irritability. **Hyperkalemia** (increased serum potassium level) increases the risk for dysrhythmias, especially with the use of anesthesia. *Hypokalemia and hyperkalemia must be corrected before the surgery.*

Other studies may be needed, depending on the client's medical history. For example, baseline arterial blood gas (ABG) values are assessed before surgery for clients with chronic pulmonary problems. Chart 20-3 lists abnormal laboratory findings and their possible causes.

RADIOGRAPHIC ASSESSMENT

A chest x-ray may be requested before surgery. Often, young healthy adults are not required to have a chest x-ray. A chest x-ray determines the size and shape of the heart, lungs, and major vessels and determines the presence of pneumonia or tuberculosis. A chest x-ray also provides baseline data in case of complications. Abnormal x-ray findings alert the surgeon to potential cardiac or pulmonary complications. Heart failure, cardiomyopathy, pneumonia, or infiltrates may cause the cancellation or delay of elective surgery. For emergency surgery, x-ray results assist the anesthesia provider in selecting anesthesia.

Other radiographic studies are based on client need, medical history, and the nature of the surgical procedure. For example, a client with back pain may have computed tomography (CT) or magnetic resonance imaging (MRI) examinations before a **laminectomy** (spinal surgery) to identify the exact location of the problem.

OTHER DIAGNOSTIC ASSESSMENTS

An electrocardiogram (ECG) may be required for all clients older than a specific age who are to have general anesthesia. The age varies among facilities but is often 40 to 45 years. An ECG may also be ordered for clients with a history of cardiac disease or those at risk for cardiac complications. An ECG provides baseline information on new or existing cardiac problems, such as an old myocardial infarction (MI). A client with a known cardiac problem may need a cardiology consultation before surgery. Prophylactic drugs, such as nitroglycerin and antibiotics, may be needed throughout the surgical period to reduce or prevent stress on the heart. Abnormal or potentially life-threatening ECG results may cause the cancellation of surgery until the client's cardiac status is stable.

A focused assessment of the preoperative client is shown in Chart 20-4.

◆Analysis

COMMON NURSING DIAGNOSES AND COLLABORATIVE PROBLEMS

The following are priority nursing diagnoses for preoperative clients:

1. Deficient Knowledge (specific experiences before, during, and after surgery) related to a lack of exposure.
2. Anxiety related to the threat of a change in health status or fear of the unknown

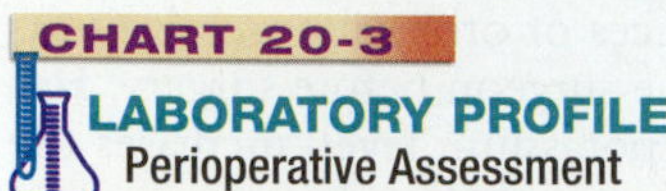

CHART 20-3

LABORATORY PROFILE

Perioperative Assessment

Test	Normal Range for Adults	Significance of Abnormal Findings: Increased in	Decreased in
Potassium (K^+) level	3.5-5.0 mEq/L, or 3.5-5.0 mmol/L	Dehydration Renal failure Acidosis Cellular/tissue damage Hemolysis of the specimen	NPO status when potassium replacement is inadequate Excessive use of non–potassium-sparing diuretics Vomiting Malnutrition Diarrhea Alkalosis
Sodium (Na^+)	≤90 yr: 136-145 mEq/L, or 136-145 mmol/L >90 yr: 132-146 mEq/L, or 132-146 mmol/L	Cardiac or renal failure Hypertension Excessive amounts of IV fluids containing normal saline Edema Dehydration (hemoconcentration)	Nasogastric drainage Vomiting or diarrhea Excessive use of laxatives or diuretics Excessive amounts of IV fluids containing water Syndrome of inappropriate antidiuretic hormone (SIADH)
Chloride (Cl^-)	≤90 yr: 90-110 mEq/L, or 98-106 mmol/L >90 yr: 98-111 mEq/L, or 98-111 mmol/L	Respiratory alkalosis Dehydration Renal failure Excessive amounts of IV fluids containing sodium chloride (NaCl)	Excessive nasogastric drainage Vomiting Excessive use of diuretics Diarrhea
Carbon dioxide (CO_2)	≤60 yr: 23-30 mEq/L, or 23-30 mmol/L 60-90 yr: 23-31 mEq/L, or 23-31 mmol/L >90 yr: 20-29 mEq/L, or 20-29 mmol/L	Chronic pulmonary disease Intestinal obstruction Vomiting or nasogastric suctioning Metabolic alkalosis	Hyperventilation Diabetic ketoacidosis Diarrhea Lactic acidosis Renal failure Salicylate toxicity
Glucose (fasting)	≤60 yr: 70-105 mg/dL, or 4.1-5.9 mmol/L 60-90 yr: 82-115 mg/dL, or 4.6-6.4 mmol/L >90 yr: 75-121 mg/dL, or 4.2-6.7 mmol/L	Hyperglycemia Excessive amounts of IV fluids containing glucose Stress Steroid use Pancreatic or hepatic disease	Hypoglycemia Excess insulin
Creatinine	*Females:* ≤60 yr: 0.5-1.1 mg/dL, or 44-97 μmol/L 60-90 yr: 0.6-1.2 mg/dL, or 53-106 μmol/L >90 yr: 0.6-1.3 mg/dL, or 53-115 μmol/L *Males:* <60 yr: 0.6-1.2 mg/dL, or 53-106 μmol/L 60-90 yr: 0.8-1.3 mg/dL, or 71-115 μmol/L >90 yr: 1.0-1.7 mg/dL, or 88-150 μmol/L	Renal damage with destruction of large number of nephrons Renal insufficiency Acute renal failure Chronic renal failure End-stage renal disease (ESRD)	Atrophy of muscle tissue
Blood urea nitrogen (BUN)	<60 yr: 10-20 mg/dL, or 2.1-7.1 mmol/L 60-90 yr: 8-23 mg/dL, or 2.9-8.2 mmol/L >90 yr: 10-31 mg/dL, or 3.6-11.1 mmol/L	Dehydration Renal failure Excessive protein in diet Liver failure	Overhydration Malnutrition
Prothrombin time (pro time, PT)	11-12.5 sec, 85%-100%, or 1:1.1 client-control ratio	Coagulation defect (bleeding disorder)	Coagulation (clotting) disorder, such as thrombophlebitis or pulmonary embolus
International Normalized Ratio (INR)	0.7-1.8	Anticoagulant therapy (aspirin, warfarin)	Extensive cancer
Partial thromboplastin time, activated (aPTT)	30-40 sec	Coagulation defect (bleeding disorder) Anticoagulant therapy (heparin) Liver disease	Coagulation (clotting) disorder, such as thrombophlebitis or pulmonary embolus Extensive cancer

IRU, International recommended unit; *NPO*, nothing by mouth.

CHART 20-3

LABORATORY PROFILE

Perioperative Assessment—*cont'd*

Test	Normal Range for Adults	Significance of Abnormal Findings: Increased in	Significance of Abnormal Findings: Decreased in
White blood cell (WBC) count (leukocyte count)	Total: 5000-10,000/mm^3, or 7.4 IRU	Infection Inflammation Stress Tissue necrosis	Immune disorder Immunosuppressant therapy
Hemoglobin, total	*Females:* 18-44 yr: 12-16 g/dL, or 117-155 g/L 45-64 yr: 11.7-16.0 g/dL, or 117-160 g/L 65-74 yr: 11.7-16.1 g/dL, or 117-161 g/L *Males:* 18-44 yr: 14-18 g/dL, or 132-173 g/L 45-64 yr: 13.1-17.2 g/dL, or 131-172 g/L 65-74 yr: 12.6-17.4 g/dL, or 126-174 g/L	Dehydration Polycythemia Chronic pulmonary disease Congestive heart failure	Blood loss Anemia Renal failure
Hematocrit	*Females:* 18-44 yr: 35%-45% 45-74 yr: 37%-47% *Males:* 18-44 yr: 42%-52% 45-64 yr: 39%-50% 65-74 yr: 37%-51%	Dehydration Polycythemia High altitude	Blood loss Anemia Renal failure

IRU, International recommended unit; *NPO,* nothing by mouth.

CHART 20-4

FOCUSED ASSESSMENT of The Preoperative Client

As part of the cardiopulmonary assessment, take and record vital signs; report the following:
- Hypotension or hypertension
- Heart rate of less than 60 or more than 120 beats/min
- Irregular heart rate
- Chest pain
- Shortness of breath or dyspnea
- Tachypnea
- Pulse oximetry reading of less than 94%

Assess for and report any signs or symptoms of infection, including the following:
- Fever
- Purulent sputum
- Dysuria or cloudy, foul-smelling urine
- Any red, swollen, draining IV or wound site
- Increased white blood cell count

Assess for and report signs or symptoms that could contraindicate surgery, including the following:
- Increased prothrombin time (PT), International Normalized Ratio (INR), or activated partial thromboplastin time (aPTT)
- Hypokalemia or hyperkalemia
- Client report of possible pregnancy or positive pregnancy test

Assess for and report other clinical conditions that may need to be evaluated by a physician or advanced nurse practitioner before proceeding with the surgical plans, including the following:
- Change in mental status
- Vomiting
- Rash
- Recent administration of an anticoagulant medication

ADDITIONAL NURSING DIAGNOSES AND COLLABORATIVE PROBLEMS

In addition to the common nursing diagnoses, preoperative clients may have one or more of the following:
- Disturbed Sleep Pattern related to internal sensory alterations (e.g., illness and anxiety)
- Ineffective Coping related to the impending surgery
- Anticipatory Grieving related to the effects of surgery
- Disturbed Body Image related to anticipated changes in the body's appearance or function
- Disabled Family Coping related to temporary family disorganization and role changes
- Powerlessness related to the health care environment, loss of independence, and loss of control of one's body

Planning and Implementation

DEFICIENT KNOWLEDGE

NOC **PLANNING: EXPECTED OUTCOMES.** The client is expected to know what to expect during and after surgery and participate in his or her recovery as indicated by:
- Explaining the purpose and expected results of the planned surgery
- Asking questions when a term or procedure is not known
- Adhering to the NPO (nothing by mouth) requirements
- Stating an understanding of preoperative preparations (e.g., skin preparation, bowel preparation)
- Demonstrating correct use of exercises and techniques to be used after surgery for the prevention of compli-

CHART 20-5

NIC INTERVENTION ACTIVITIES for The Preoperative Client

Preoperative Coordination: *Facilitating preadmission diagnostic testing and preparation of the surgical client*
- Review planned surgery.
- Obtain client history, as appropriate.
- Complete a physical assessment, as appropriate.
- Describe and explain preadmission treatments and diagnostic tests.
- Interpret diagnostic test results, as appropriate.
- Determine the client's expectations about the surgery.
- Provide time for the client and significant other to ask questions and voice concerns.
- Discuss postoperative discharge plans.
- Determine ability of caretakers.

NIC intervention activities selected from Dochterman, J.M., & Bulechek, G.M. (Eds.). (2004). *Nursing interventions classification (NIC)* (4th ed.). St. Louis: Mosby. No part of this work is to be altered without prior written permission from the Publisher.

cations (e.g., splinting the incision, coughing/deep breathing, performing leg exercises, ambulating as early as permitted).

INTERVENTIONS. Interventions to increase the client's knowledge level are listed in Chart 20-5. Because the surgical experience is foreign to many people, focus on teaching the client and family members. Preoperative teaching may begin in the surgeon's office for planned or elective surgery. Pamphlets, written instructions, and videotapes may be given or sent to the client. More teaching may occur when the client has preadmission testing. Some facilities hold classes before surgery for groups of clients or show videos for those who are having the same or similar surgical procedures. A tour of the operating suite and the postanesthesia care unit (PACU) may be included.

Explore the client's level of knowledge and understanding. Increased access to information via the Internet may be helpful but is also a concern. Some Internet information may not be accurate or may not apply to a specific client's plan of care.

Information about informed consent, dietary restrictions, specific preparation for surgery (bowel and skin preparations), exercises after surgery, and plans for pain management promote clients' participation and help achieve the desired outcome. A sample educational checklist is shown in Table 20-5. Because education occurs in a variety of settings, coordination of client teaching efforts is challenging. When you care for the client just before surgery (same-day, ambulatory surgery [outpatient] unit or inpatient hospital unit), assess the client's and family members' knowledge and provide additional information as needed.

Ensuring Informed Consent. Surgery of any type involves invasion of the body and requires informed consent from the client or legal guardian (Figure 20-1). Clients deserve, and rightly demand, to be informed and involved in decisions affecting their health care. Consent implies that the client has been given sufficient information to understand the following:
- The nature of and reason for surgery
- Who will be performing the surgery and whether others will be present during the procedure (e.g., students)
- All available options and the risks associated with each option

TABLE 20-5 Preoperative Teaching Checklist

Consider the following items when planning individualized preoperative teaching for clients and families:
- Fears and anxieties
- Surgical procedure
- Preoperative routines (e.g., NPO, enemas, blood samples, showering)
- Invasive procedures (e.g., lines, catheters)
- Coughing, turning, deep breathing
- Incentive spirometer
  - How to use
  - How to tell when used correctly
- Lower extremity exercises
- Stockings and pneumatic compression devices
- Early ambulation
- Splinting
- Pain management

NPO, Nothing by mouth.

- The risks associated with the surgical procedure and its potential outcomes
- The risks associated with the use of anesthesia

Informed consent helps protect the client from any unwanted procedures and protects the surgeon and the facility from lawsuit claims related to unauthorized surgery or uninformed clients. Written record of informed consent is documented on a "consent form," but can also be documented in the physician's notes. The consent form documents the client's consent and signature for the procedure listed.

As a competent adult, it is the client's right to refuse treatment for any reason, even when refusal might lead to death. For example, in the case of Jehovah's Witnesses, some clients will not accept blood transfusions because of their religious convictions.

The surgeon is responsible for having the consent form signed before sedation is given and before surgery is performed. *You, as a nurse, are not responsible for providing detailed information about the surgical procedure. Rather, your role is to clarify facts that have been presented by the physician and dispel myths that the client or family may have about the surgical experience.* You ensure that the consent form is signed and you serve as a witness to the signature, not to the fact that the client is informed. If you believe that the client has not been adequately informed, contact the surgeon and request that he or she see the client for clarification. Document this action in the chart.

Clients who cannot write may sign with an X, which must be witnessed by two persons. In an emergency, telephone or telegram authorization is acceptable and should be followed up with written consent as soon as possible. The number of witnesses (usually two) and the type of documentation vary according to the facility's policy. In a life-threatening situation in which every effort has been made to contact the person with medical power of attorney, consent is desired but not essential. In place of written or oral consent, written consultation by at least two physicians who are not associated with the case may be requested by the physician. This formal consultation legally supports the decision for surgery until the appropriate person can sign a consent form. If the client is not capable of giving consent and has no family, the court can appoint a legal guardian to represent the client's best interests.

Northwest Hospital Center

The hospital centered around its patients.

REQUEST AND AUTHORIZATION FOR MEDICAL AND/OR SURGICAL TREATMENT, BLOOD PRODUCTS ADMINISTRATION

1. I hereby request and authorize Dr.______________________________ and/or his/her associates and whomever they may designate as their assistants, to administer such treatment as is necessary and to perform the following operation____ and such additional operations or procedures as are considered necessary on the basis of conditions that may be revealed during the course of said operation or treatment.
2. The reasons why the above named surgery and/or treatment is considered necessary, its advantages, probability of success, possible complications, and risks, as well as possible alternative modes of treatment were explained to me by Dr.______________________________.
3. I request and authorize the administration of such anesthetics and/or other medications as are necessary.
4. Final disposition of any tissues or parts surgically removed is to be handled in accordance with the customary practices of the hospital.
5. I am aware that the practice of medicine and surgery is not an exact science and I acknowledge that no guarantees have been made to me concerning the results of the operation or procedure.
6. I hereby acknowledge that I have read and fully understand the above request and authorization for medical and/or surgical treatment.
7. I consent to the admittance of permitted observers, the use of closed-circuit television, taking of photographs (including motion pictures), and the preparation of drawings and similar illustrative material, and I also consent to the use of such photographs and other material for scientific purposes, provided my identity is not revealed by the pictures or by the descriptive text accompanying them.
8. I consent to release of my social security number in accordance with the Safe Medical Device Act.

_______________ Date   __________ Time   ____________________ Signature of Patient or Patient Surrogate

_______________ Witness   ____________________ Signature of Physician

CONSENT TO BLOOD/BLOOD PRODUCTS TRANSFUSION

After discussing the risks, benefits and alternatives to transfusion of blood (donor/autologous) (circle one or both) or blood products with my physician or his designee, I consent to the administration of these products.

_______________ Date   __________ Time   ____________________ Signature of Patient or Patient Surrogate

_______________ Witness   ____________________ Signature of Physician

703/1019-3-R-8/97 (40-1331)

Figure 20-1 ■ A surgical consent form. (Courtesy of Northwest Hospital Center, Randallstown, MD.)

A blind client may sign his or her own consent form, which usually needs to be witnessed by two persons. Clients who speak a language other than the general language of the facility require a translator and a second witness. Some facilities have consent forms written in more than one language.

Some surgical procedures, such as intraocular lens implants, sterilization, and experimental procedures, may require a special permit in addition to the standard consent. National and local governing bodies and the individual facility determine which procedures require a separate permit. Separate consents for anesthesia and blood products also may be required.

Surgical procedures that are site specific, such as left, right, or bilateral, require client identification before surgery. The client is asked to mark the site with a marker to ensure the correct site is used and the wrong site is avoided.

Client Self-Determination. Clients receiving medical care have the right to have or to initiate advance directives, such as a living will or durable power of attorney, as mandated by the Patient Self-Determination Act. Advance directives provide legal instructions to the health care providers about the client's wishes and are to be followed. *Surgery does not provide an exception to a client's advance directives or living will.*

Implementing Dietary Restrictions. Regardless of the type of surgery and anesthesia planned, the client is restricted to **nothing by mouth (NPO)** for 6 to 8 hours before surgery. NPO means no eating, drinking (including water), or smoking (nicotine stimulates gastric secretions). It is common practice to begin NPO status at midnight on the night before surgery. This precaution ensures that the stomach contains a limited volume of gastric secretions, which decreases the risk for aspiration. Outpatients and clients who are scheduled for admission to the hospital on the same day that surgery is performed, must receive written and oral instructions about remaining NPO after midnight. *Emphasize the importance of adherence. Failure to adhere can result in cancellation of surgery or increase the risk for aspiration during or after surgery.*

The exact amount of time a client must be NPO before surgery is controversial. Clients, especially older adults, who fast for 8 or more hours may have imbalances of fluids, electrolytes, and blood glucose levels.

Administering Regularly Scheduled Medications. On the day of surgery, the client's usual drug schedule may need to be altered. Consult the medical physician and the anesthesia provider for instructions about drugs, such as those taken for diabetes, cardiac disease, or glaucoma, as well as regularly scheduled anticonvulsants, antihypertensives, anticoagulants, antidepressants, or corticosteroids. The physician may prescribe some drugs, including over-the-counter drugs, such as aspirin, to be stopped until after surgery. The physician may prescribe other drugs to be given by the intravenous (IV) route to maintain the drug level in the blood. *Drugs for cardiac disease, respiratory disease, seizures, and hypertension are commonly allowed with a sip of water before surgery.* Some antihypertensive or antidepressant drugs may be withheld on the day of surgery because of possible adverse effects on blood pressure during surgery.

The diabetic client who takes insulin may be given a reduced dose of intermediate- or long-acting insulin based on the blood glucose level, or may be given regular (fast-acting) insulin in divided doses on the day of surgery. Alternatively, an IV infusion of 5% dextrose in water may be given with the insulin to prevent low blood sugar during surgery. Because of the many treatment approaches to diabetes, clarify drug and IV prescriptions with the physician. (See Chapter 68 for more information about diabetes.)

Intestinal Preparation. Bowel or intestinal preparations are performed to prevent injury to the colon and to reduce the number of intestinal bacteria. Evacuation of the bowel is needed when a client is having major abdominal, pelvic, perineal, or perianal surgery. The surgeon's preference and the type of surgical procedure determine the type of bowel preparation. Table 20-6 shows common bowel preparation regimens and their complications. An enema ordered to be given until return flow is clear is a stressful procedure, especially for the older client. Repeated enemas can cause electrolyte imbalance, fluid volume imbalances, vagal stimulation, and postural (orthostatic) hypotension. Enemas also cause severe anorectal discomfort in clients with hemorrhoids. Some

TABLE 20-6 Complications of Common Bowel Preparations for the Surgical Client

Surgical Site	Preparation	Complications
Stomach, duodenum, and proximal jejunum	Oral laxative (e.g., castor oil preparation or bisacodyl [Dulcolax, Laxit✱]) Clear liquid diet the evening before surgery NPO after midnight	Abdominal cramping Dehydration Electrolyte imbalance Fatigue
Small intestine	Oral laxative (e.g., magnesium citrate) Clear liquid diet the evening before surgery Multiple-position enema the evening before surgery NPO after midnight	Abdominal cramping Dehydration Electrolyte imbalance Fatigue
Large intestine to rectum	Multiple or combination of oral laxatives 12-24 hr before surgery Multiple-position tap water or antibiotic (neomycin) enemas (three times or until the return flow is clear) the evening and morning before surgery Oral antibiotics to sterilize the bowel (e.g., neomycin and erythromycin) 24 hr before surgery Clear liquid diet the day before surgery NPO after midnight	Abdominal cramping Fatigue and weakness Fluid excess or deficit Potassium or sodium deficit Decreased cardiac output from vagal stimulation Irritation of bowel and rectal mucosa from enemas

NPO, Nothing by mouth.

physicians prescribe potent laxatives (e.g., polyethylene glycol electrolyte solution [GoLYTELY]) instead of enemas, especially for older clients. Bowel preparations can be exhausting, and you must take safety precautions to prevent falls.

Skin Preparation. The skin preparation may be embarrassing or uncomfortable for the client, especially if the surgical site is in a sensitive or private body area. Provide a warm, comfortable, and private environment during the procedure. The skin is the body's first line of defense against infection. A break in this barrier increases the risk for infection, especially for older clients. Skin preparation before surgery is the first step in the prevention of surgical wound infection.

EVIDENCE-BASED PRACTICE for Nursing

Gently remove hair at the surgical site

Kjonniken, I., et al. (2002). Preoperative hair removal: A systematic literature review. *AORN Journal, 75*(5), 928-936, 938, 940.

This study was performed in response to the 1999 guidelines of the Centers for Disease Control and Prevention (CDC), which strongly recommends that "hair should not be removed preoperatively unless the hair at or around the incision site will interfere with the surgical procedure. If hair is removed, however, it should be done immediately before surgery, preferably with clippers." This research is an analysis of the evidence regarding preoperative hair removal by shaving, clipping, and the use of depilatories. The authors performed an exhaustive review of the medical and nursing literature from 1966 to 1999 that examined whether or not hair was removed from the surgical site before surgery, the timing of the removal, the method of the removal, and the association of surgical site infections (SSIs). The studies cited as the basis for the CDC guidelines were included in the review, as were many additional randomized and observational studies performed during the designated timeframe.

Ten team members performed the analysis. More than 130 published studies were examined by the team. All members of the team assessed each article independently based on the scale provided by the U.S. Agency for Healthcare Research and Quality. In plenary sessions, all members of the team established the relevance and quality of each published study.

The analysis resulted in conclusions somewhat different from the guidelines recommended by the CDC. No strong evidence supported the decision not to remove hair. Wet or dry shaving the evening before the procedure has a higher rate of SSIs than did the use of either clipper or depilatories. Hair removed with clippers should be performed as close as possible to the surgical procedure.

Level of Evidence: 1—Quantitative systematic review.

Critique. The team used strong research procedures in the assessment and categorization of the existing data. The method used to determine the levels of evidence for categorizing the data was appropriate and applied equally. The review exposes the lack of well-controlled, randomized clinical trials to answer the questions surrounding preoperative hair removal from surgical sites.

Implications for Nursing. There is a lack of clarity regarding the "one best practice" for surgical site preparation with regard to hair removal. Clearly, cleanliness is important and so is the avoidance of skin injury. Shaving, especially dry shaving is known to nick or abrade skin. The degree of skin injury is also, in part, related to the skill of the person doing the shaving. Depilatories, while not nicking skin surfaces, can also cause chemical injury to sensitive skin, resulting in a nonintact skin surface. Whatever hair removal system is used, nurses must use careful handling to reduce or prevent skin injury. In addition, if nurses observe a skin injury at the intended surgical site, documentation is essential.

One or two days before the scheduled surgery, the surgeon may ask the client to shower using an antiseptic solution such as povidone-iodine (Betadine) or hexachlorophene. Instruct the client to be especially careful to clean around the proposed surgical site. If the client is hospitalized before surgery, showering and cleaning are repeated the night before surgery or in the morning before transfer to the surgical suite. This cleaning reduces contamination of the surgical field and reduces the number of organisms at the site. After the final cleaning procedure, especially for an orthopedic surgical procedure, the area may be covered with sterile towels or drapes to prevent contamination.

A controversial step in skin preparation after the cleaning is the shave. Many health care professionals believe that shaving contaminates the surgical area and traumatizes the skin around the area where the incision will be made. Thus whether or not to shave, the timing of the shave, and the equipment used remain controversial (see the Evidence-Based Practice for Nursing box at left).

Factors that predispose to wound contamination include bacteria found in hair follicles, disruption of the normal protective mechanisms of the skin, and nicks in the skin. Shaving of hair creates the potential for infection. Hair clipping with electrical clippers is often used to decrease the problems caused by traditional razors. The Centers for Disease Control and Prevention (CDC) recommend that if shaving is necessary, the hair should be removed using disposable sterile supplies and aseptic principles *immediately* before the start of the surgical procedure. Shaving is performed in the treatment room, the holding area of the operating suite, or the operating room (OR). Figure 20-2 shows areas shaved for various surgical procedures. Shaving, especially of the head or genital area, can be emotionally upsetting to the client, and regrowth of this hair can be uncomfortable.

Preparing the Client for Tubes, Drains, and Vascular Access. Prepare the client for possible placement of tubes, drains, and vascular access devices. Preparation reduces the client's anxiety and fear, and the family's negative reaction. Be careful not to scare the client while providing information about the purpose of each tube.

Tubes. The client may need an indwelling urinary (Foley) catheter before, during, or after surgery to keep the bladder empty and to monitor renal function. The client having abdominal or genitourinary surgery usually has a Foley catheter.

A nasogastric (NG) tube may be inserted before abdominal surgery to decompress or empty the stomach and the upper bowel. More often, however, the tube is placed after the induction of anesthesia, when insertion is less disturbing to the client and is easier to perform.

Drains. Drains are often placed during surgery to help remove fluid from the surgical site. Some drains are under the dressing; others are visible and require emptying. Drains come in various shapes and sizes (see Chapter 22). Inform the client that drains are often used routinely and that generally they are not painful but may cause some discomfort. Discuss the reasons drains should not be kinked or pulled.

Vascular Access. A vascular access (line) is placed for clients receiving a general anesthetic and most clients receiving other types of anesthetics. An access is needed to give drugs and fluids before, during, and after surgery. Clients who

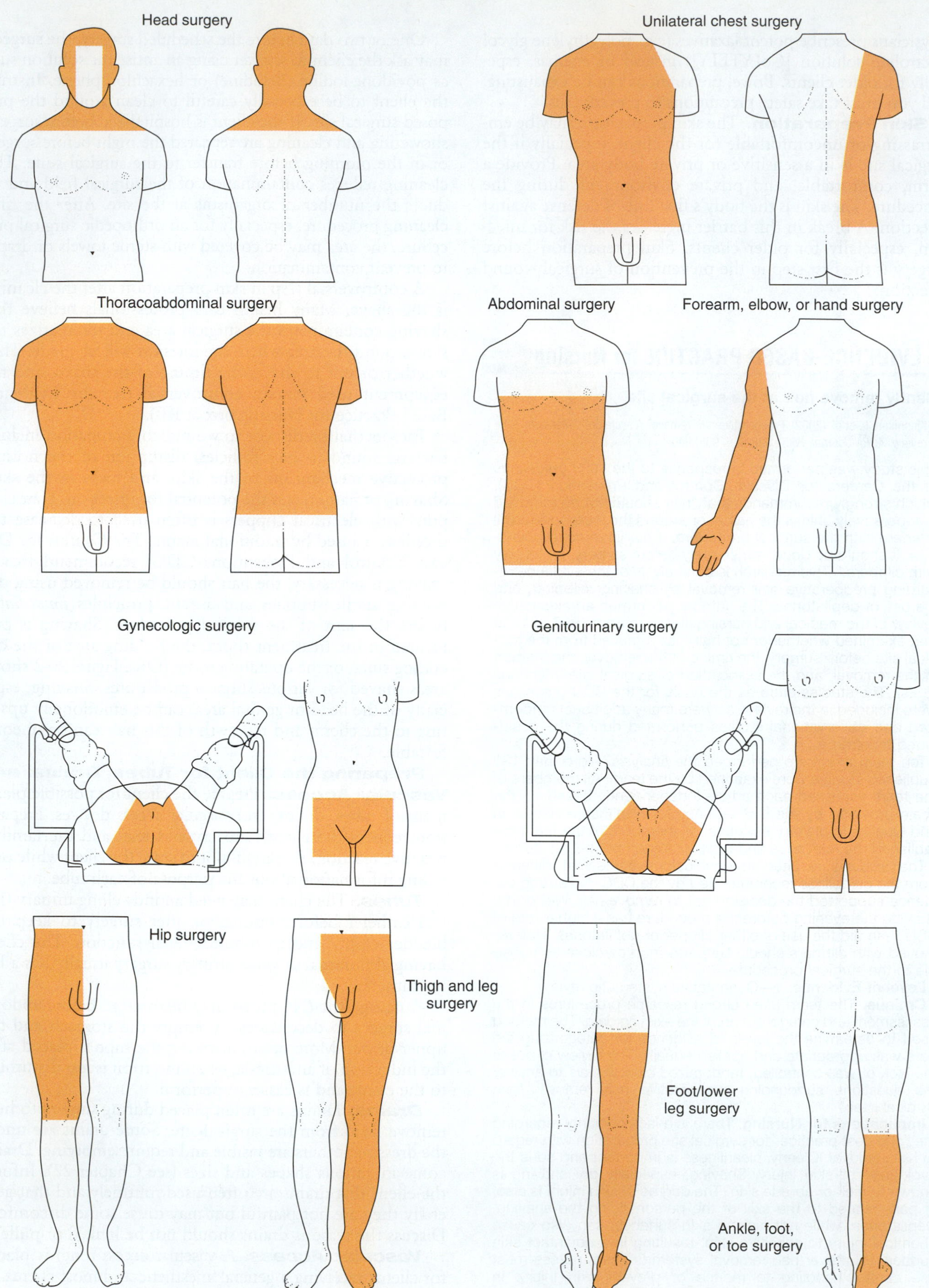

Figure 20-2 ■ Skin preparation of common surgical sites. Shaded areas indicate areas of hair removal.

are dehydrated or at risk for dehydration may receive fluids before surgery.

CONSIDERATIONS FOR OLDER ADULTS

Older adult clients are at greater risk for dehydration because their fluid reserves are lower than those of young or middle-aged adults. Carefully monitor the older adult client and clients with cardiac disease receiving IV fluids. (See Chapter 17 for more information on IV therapy.)

The IV access is usually placed in the arm or the back of the hand using a large, short catheter (e.g., 18-gauge, 1-inch catheter). This type of access provides the least resistance to fluid or blood infusion, especially in an emergency when rapid infusions may be needed. Depending on the client's needs and the facility's policies, the IV access can be placed before surgery when the client is in the hospital room, in the holding or admission area of the surgical suite, or in the OR.

Teaching About Postoperative Procedures and Exercises. Teach the client and family members about exercises and procedures (e.g., checking dressings and obtaining vital signs frequently) to be performed after surgery. Family members can be helpful in reminding clients to perform these exercises. Preoperative teaching reduces apprehension and fear, increases cooperation and participation in care after surgery, and decreases complications.

CHART 20-6

CLIENT EDUCATION GUIDE

Perioperative Respiratory Care

Deep (Diaphragmatic) Breathing

1. Sit upright on the edge of the bed or in a chair, being sure that your feet are placed firmly on the floor or a stool. (After surgery, deep breathing is done with the client in Fowler's position or in semi-Fowler's position.)
2. Take a gentle breath through your mouth.
3. Breathe out gently and completely.
4. Then take a deep breath through your nose and mouth, and hold this breath to the count of five.
5. Exhale through your nose and mouth.

Expansion Breathing

1. Find a comfortable upright position, with your knees slightly bent. (Bending the knees decreases tension on the abdominal muscles and decreases respiratory resistance and discomfort.)
2. Place your hands on each side of your lower rib cage, just above your waist.
3. Take a deep breath through your nose, using your shoulder muscles to expand your lower rib cage outward during inhalation.
4. Exhale, concentrating first on moving your chest, then on moving your lower ribs inward, while gently squeezing the rib cage and forcing air out of the base of your lungs.

Splinting of the Surgical Incision

1. Unless coughing is contraindicated, place a pillow, towel, or folded blanket over your surgical incision and hold the item firmly in place.
2. Take three slow, deep breaths to stimulate your cough reflex.
3. Inhale through your nose, then exhale through your mouth.
4. On your third deep breath, cough to clear secretions from your lungs while firmly holding the pillow, towel or folded blanket against your incision.

When the fear or anxiety level is high, explore the client's feelings before discussing procedures.

Discussion, demonstration with return demonstration, and practice by the client aid in the ability to perform various breathing (Chart 20-6) and leg (Chart 20-7) exercises after surgery. Emphasize the need to begin exercises early in the recovery phase and to continue them, with 5 to 10 repetitions each, every 1 to 2 hours after surgery for at least the first 48 hours. Explain that the client may need to be awakened for these activities.

Breathing Exercises. In deep, or diaphragmatic, breathing, the diaphragm flattens during inspiration, enlarging the chest cavity and expanding the lungs. After you demonstrate and explain the technique, urge the client to practice the five steps of deep breathing.

For clients with chronic lung disease or limited chest expansion, as seen in older clients because of the aging process, expansion breathing exercises are useful. For the client having chest surgery, expansion breathing exercises strengthen accessory muscles and are started before surgery. Expansion breathing may be used after surgery during chest physiotherapy (percussion, vibration, and postural drainage) to help loosen secretions and maintain an adequate air exchange.

Incentive Spirometry. Incentive spirometry is another way to encourage the client to take deep breaths. Its purpose is to promote complete lung expansion and to prevent pulmonary problems. Various types of incentive spirometers are available; some examples are shown in Figure 20-3. With all types, the client must be able to seal the lips tightly around the mouthpiece, inhale spontaneously, and hold his or her breath for 3 to 5 seconds for effective lung expansion. Goals (e.g., attaining specific volumes) can be set according to the client's ability and the type of incentive spirometer. Seeing a light move up a column or a bellows expanding reinforces and motivates the client to continue performance.

Coughing and Splinting. Coughing may be performed along with deep breathing every 1 to 2 hours after surgery. The purposes of coughing are to expel secretions, keep the lungs clear, allow full aeration, and prevent pneumonia and atelectasis. Coughing may be uncomfortable for the client, but when performed correctly, it should not harm the incision. Splinting (e.g., holding) the incision area provides support, promotes a feeling of security, and reduces pain during coughing. The proper technique for splinting the incision site and coughing is described in Chart 20-6. A folded bath blanket or pillow is helpful to use as a splint.

The use of routine coughing exercises after surgery is controversial. Some surgeons believe coughing may harm the surgical wound and that it would be better to use other, safer measures for pulmonary hygiene, such as deep breathing and incentive spirometer exercises. When routine coughing exercises should be avoided for a specific client, such as after a hernia repair, the surgeon usually writes a "do not cough" prescription.

Leg Procedures and Exercises. Antiembolism stockings (TED or Jobst stockings), elastic (Ace) wraps, or pneumatic compression devices (e.g., "sequentials" or "boots") may be used during and after surgery along with leg exercises and early ambulation to promote venous return. Venous stasis can lead to deep vein thrombosis (DVT) or a pulmonary embolus (PE) if the blood clot breaks off and travels to the lungs.

CHART 20-7

CLIENT EDUCATION GUIDE

Postoperative Leg Exercises

Exercise No. 1

1. Lie in bed with the head of your bed elevated to about 45 degrees.
2. Beginning with your right leg, bend your knee, raise your foot off the bed, and hold this position for a few seconds.
3. Extend your leg by unbending your knee, and lower the leg to the bed.
4. Repeat this sequence four more times with your right leg, then perform this same exercise five times with your left leg.

Exercise No. 2

1. Beginning with your right leg, point your toes toward the bottom of the bed.
2. With the same leg, point your toes up toward your face.
3. Repeat this exercise several times with your right leg, then perform this same exercise with your left leg.

Exercise No. 3

1. Beginning with your right leg, make circles with your ankles, first to the left, then to the right.
2. Repeat this exercise several times with your right leg, then perform this same exercise with your left leg.

Exercise No. 4

1. Beginning with your right leg, bend your knee and *push* the ball of your foot into the bed or floor until you feel your calf and thigh muscles contracting.
2. Repeat this exercise several times with your right leg; then perform this same exercise with your left leg.

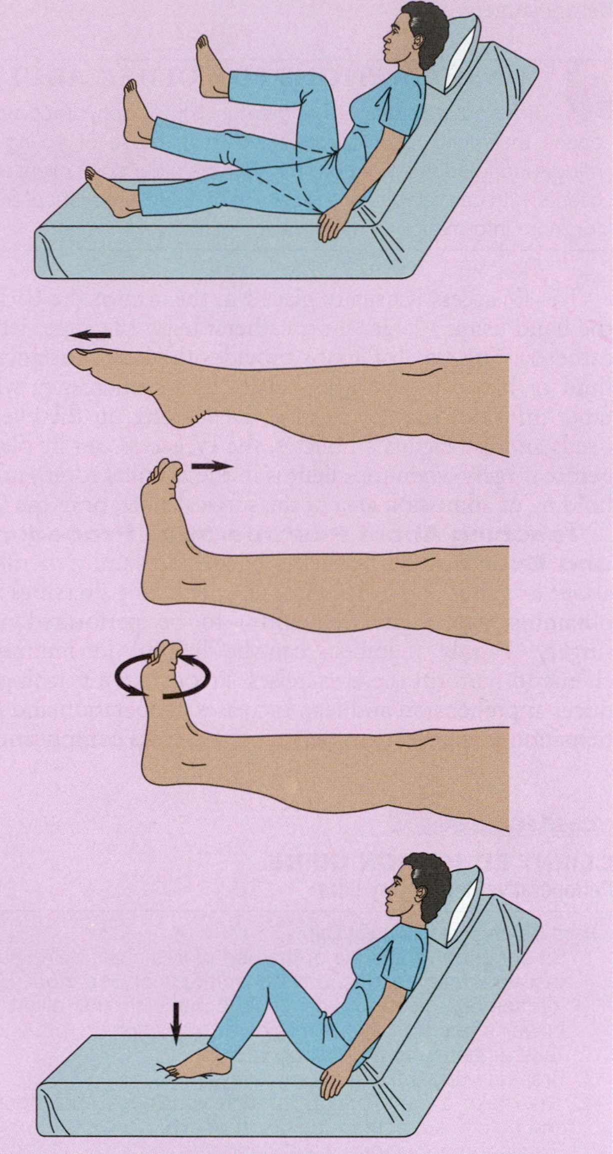

A 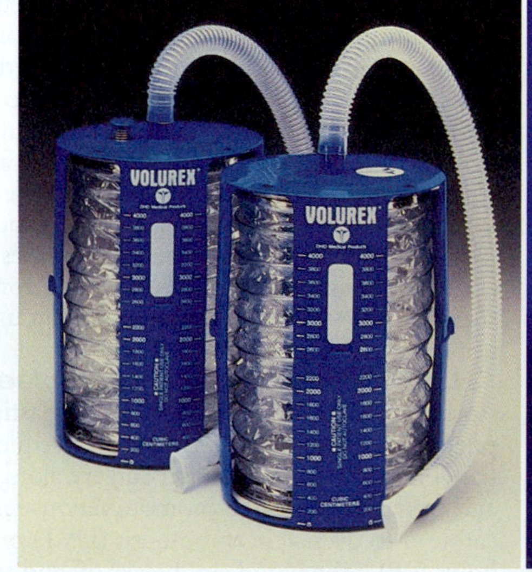

B 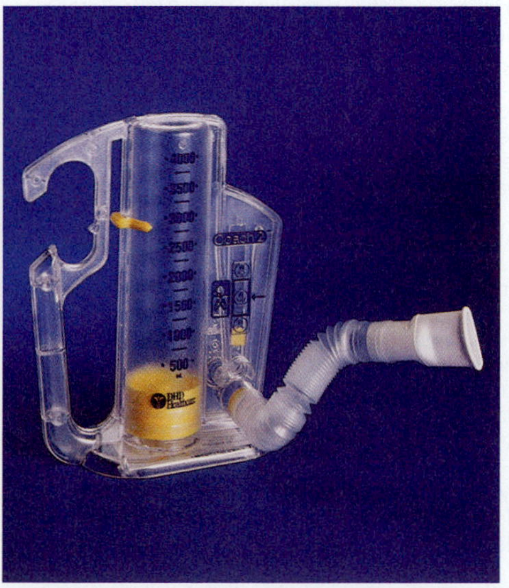

Figure 20-3 ■ Examples of volume incentive spirometers for lung expansion. **A,** A volume displacement incentive spirometer. **B,** A volumetric incentive spirometer. (Courtesy of DHD Healthcare, Canastota, NY.)

Specific interventions depend on the client's risk factors. Clients at greater risk for DVT:

- Are obese
- Are older than 40 years of age
- Have cancer
- Have decreased mobility or are immobile
- Have a leg fracture or leg trauma
- Have a history of DVT, PE, varicose veins, or edema
- Are taking oral contraceptives
- Smoke
- Have decreased cardiac output
- Are undergoing pelvic surgery

Antiembolism Stockings and Elastic Wraps. These stockings and elastic wraps provide graduated compression of the legs, starting at the end of the foot and ankle. Measure the client's leg length and circumference before ordering the stocking size. Elastic wraps are used when the legs are too large or too small for the stockings. Assist the client in applying the devices and ensure that they are neither too loose (are ineffective) nor too tight (inhibit blood flow). The devices need to be worn properly and should be removed one to three times per day for 30 minutes for skin care and inspection.

Pneumatic Compression Devices. Pneumatic compression devices enhance venous blood flow by providing intermittent periods of compression on the legs. Measure the client's legs and order the correct size. Place the boots on the client's legs, then set and check the compression pressures (usually 35 to 55 mm Hg). Figure 20-4 shows various types of sequential devices. Antiembolism stockings may be worn in addition to the boots and may reduce some of the uncomfortable sensations of the boots (e.g., itching, sweating, heat).

Leg Exercises. Leg exercises also promote venous return. Teach the leg exercises outlined in Chart 20-7 and then urge the client to practice these exercises before surgery. The exercises are important, even when other devices are used.

Early Ambulation. Mobility soon after surgery (early ambulation) stimulates intestinal motility, enhances lung expansion, mobilizes secretions, promotes venous return,

A

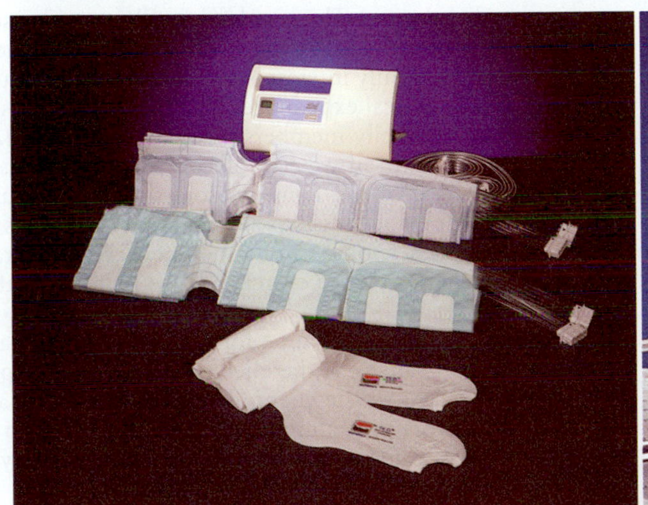

B

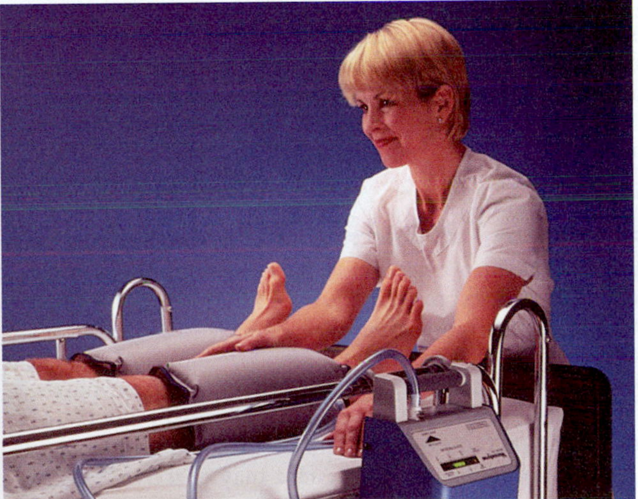

C

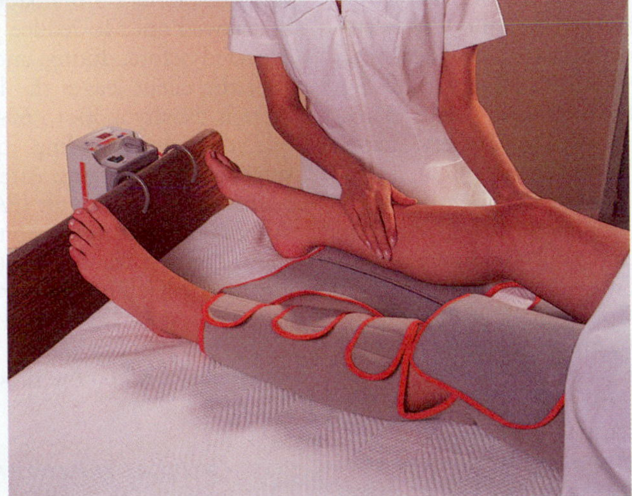

Figure 20-4 ■ Examples of external pneumatic compression devices used to promote venous return and prevent deep vein thrombosis (DVT). **A,** Kendall SCD machine, sleeves, and TED stockings. **B,** Venodyne pneumatic compression system. **C,** Flowtron DVT calf garments. (**A** courtesy of The Kendall Healthcare Company, Mansfield, MA; **B** courtesy of Venodyne, Inc., Norwood, MA; **C** courtesy of Huntleigh Healthcare, Eatontown, NJ.)

prevents joint rigidity, and relieves pressure. For most types of surgery, teach the client to turn at least every 2 hours after surgery while confined to bed. Teach clients how to use the bed siderails safely for turning and how to protect the surgical wound (splinting) when turning. Assure clients that assistance and pain medication will be given as needed to reduce any anxiety and pain they may have with this activity.

For certain surgical procedures, such as some brain, spinal, and orthopedic procedures, the surgeon may prescribe turning restrictions. Ask the surgeon about other interventions to prevent complications of immobility in clients with turning restrictions. Inform the client of anticipated turning restrictions during preoperative teaching.

Many clients are allowed and encouraged to get out of bed the day of or the day after surgery. Assist the client into a chair or with ambulation after the surgery, the next day, or when the surgeon specifies. If a client must remain in bed, help the client turn, deep breathe, and perform leg exercises at least every 2 hours to prevent complications from immobility.

Range-of-Motion Exercises. Passive or active range-of-motion (ROM) exercises help prevent joint rigidity and muscle contracture. The client should perform these exercises three to five times each, three to four times per day while bedridden. Teach the client these procedures and inform the client that he or she will receive help as needed after surgery. (Guidelines for ROM exercises are found in Chapter 22.)

ANXIETY

NOC **PLANNING: EXPECTED OUTCOMES.** Before surgery, the client is expected to have manageable preoperative anxiety as indicated by:

- Expressing a reduced level of anxiety
- Showing an absence of body language indicators of anxiety (e.g., hand wringing, facial tension, dilated pupils, sweating, elevated blood pressure, elevated pulse rate)

INTERVENTIONS. Anxiety often causes restlessness and sleeplessness. The surgical client may perceive the surgical experience as a threat to life and function. Assess the client's level of anxiety, as discussed earlier under Psychosocial Assessment on p. 301. Interventions such as teaching and communicating with the client before surgery, enabling the client to use previously successful coping mechanisms, and giving antianxiety drugs help reduce the anxiety. Incorporate available support systems into the plan of care.

Preoperative Teaching. Assess the client's knowledge about the surgical experience that has been acquired from prior surgical experiences and procedures and from other sources (see earlier discussion under Deficient Knowledge, p. 303). Provide factual information about the surgery and the perioperative experience to promote the client's understanding. Allow ample time for questions. Respond to the questions accurately and refer unanswered questions to the proper person. During the discussion, continually assess the client's responses and anxiety level. Be careful not to provide information that might increase anxiety. Clients have ranked psychosocial support as the most important part of preoperative teaching. The informed, educated client is better able to anticipate events and maintain self-control and is thus less anxious.

Encouraging Communication. Having the client state feelings, fears, and concerns is a technique to reduce anxiety. Develop a trusting relationship with the client so that he or she can express feelings freely without fear of ridicule or judgment. Keep the client informed by clarifying information, answering questions, and allaying fears about the surgery.

Promoting Rest. The stress and anxiety of impending surgery often interfere with the client's ability to sleep and rest the night before surgery. The period before surgery is physically and emotionally stressful. To help the client relax, determine what the client usually does to relax and fall asleep. If the client is able, urge him or her to continue these methods of relaxation. A back rub is relaxing and can be performed by a nurse or family member. The surgeon may prescribe a sedative or hypnotic drug to help the client be well rested for surgery.

Using Distraction. Distraction may be used as an intervention for anxiety, especially in the 24 hours immediately before surgery. Listening to music or audiotapes may decrease anxiety, as may watching television, reading, or visiting with family members.

Teaching Family and Significant Others. Assess the readiness and desire of the family to take an active part in the client's care. The involved family provides support, can assist with the care plan, and helps reduce anxiety. A positive sign of family interest is members' asking of questions about the surgical experience. After family readiness is determined, keep family members informed and encourage their involvement in all aspects of education. Emphasize the important role of the family before surgery but guide discussions and practice sessions so that family members do not dominate the sessions. Family members can encourage and help the client practice exercises to be performed after surgery.

Inform the family of the time for surgery, if known, and of any schedule changes. If the client is an outpatient, provide clear directions to the client and family regarding any specific night-before procedures, what time and where to report, and what to bring with them. Encourage the family to stay with the client before surgery for support.

Most families are anxious about the surgery planned for their loved one. To reduce their anxiety, explain the routines expected before, during, and after surgery. Tell the family that after the client leaves the hospital room or admission area, there is usually a 30- to 60-minute preparation period in the operating area (holding room, treatment area) before the surgery actually begins. After surgery, the client is taken to the postanesthesia care unit (PACU) for 1 to 2 hours before returning to the hospital room or discharge area. Tell the family about the best place to wait for the client or surgeon according to the facility's policy and the physician's preference. Many hospitals and surgical centers have surgical waiting areas so that families can wait in comfortable surroundings and be easily located when the procedure is completed.

Critical Thinking Challenge

The client, a 52-year-old single account executive, has been waiting for 45 minutes to go into surgery for an emergency open reduction with internal fixation of his left ankle. He is about 100 pounds overweight and fractured his ankle in multiple places when he slipped on a wet floor while at work. The client is anxious about having surgery and his ability to get back home to his dog. His constant focus is who will take care of his dog until he gets there. The medical record review documented that he minimized his preoperative teaching since "I only broke my ankle" and appeared disinterested in the cough and deep breathing exercises. During assessment, he told you that he is allergic to strawberries, bananas, tape, and roses. Although he told you he is a nonsmoker, you find him smoking a cigarette when you come back into the room.

1. As the preoperative nurse, how do you decrease this client's anxiety and assess his readiness for surgery?
2. Are any of his allergies important to document or communicate with the rest of the surgical team? Why or Why not?
3. What should you do about the disparity between his statement that he is not a smoker and the fact that you found him smoking?
4. What nursing diagnoses should be anticipated in this client's care?

evolve For suggested answer guidelines, go to http://evolve.elsevier.com/Iggy/.

PREOPERATIVE CHART REVIEW

Review the client's chart to ensure that all documentation, preoperative procedures, and orders are completed. Check the surgical informed consent form and, if indicated, any other special consent forms to see that they are signed and dated, and that they contain the witnesses' signatures. Confirm that the scheduled procedure, including the identification of left versus right when necessary, is what is listed on the consent form. Even though it might be obvious, have the client mark the correct area for surgery. Document allergies according to facility policy. Accurate documentation of height and weight is important for proper dosage calculation of the anesthetic agents. Ensure that the results of all laboratory, radiographic, and diagnostic tests are on the chart. Document any abnormal results and report them to the surgeon and the anesthesia provider. If the client is an autologous blood donor or has had directed blood donations made, those special slips must be included in the chart. Record a current set of vital signs (within 1 to 2 hours of the scheduled surgery time) and document any significant physical or psychosocial observations.

Report special needs, concerns, and instructions (advance directives) to the surgical team. For example, advise the surgical team whether the client is a member of Jehovah's Witnesses and does not accept blood products or whether the client is hard of hearing and does not have his or her hearing aid. This information assists the surgical team in providing continuity of care while the client is in the surgical area.

Critical Thinking Challenge

You are about to send the client, described earlier in the critical thinking exercise, to the surgical suite.

1. How should you communicate this client's allergies?
2. What risk factors does this client have for specific postoperative complications? Why?

evolve For suggested answer guidelines, go to http://evolve.elsevier.com/Iggy/.

PREOPERATIVE CLIENT PREPARATION

Facilities usually require the client to remove most clothing and wear a hospital gown into the operating room (OR); however, underwear may be worn in above-the-waist surgery, and socks may be worn, except in foot or leg surgery. If prescribed by the surgeon, apply antiembolism stockings before surgery. In some ambulatory settings, such as for cataract surgery, minimal clothes are removed.

Clients are advised to leave all valuables at home. If the client has valuables, including jewelry, money, or clothes, they are given to a family member or locked in a safe place, according to the facility's policy. If rings cannot be removed, tape them in place. Remove all pierced jewelry. Religious emblems may be pinned or fastened securely to the client's gown. Some facilities have paper emblems from a religious leader.

The client wears an identification band that clearly gives the first and last name, hospital number, physician, and birth date. An optional bracelet, usually red, identifies any allergies. A bracelet indicating that a blood sample for type and crossmatch has been drawn may be worn, depending on the facility's policy.

Dentures, including partial dental plates, are removed and placed in a labeled denture cup. Denture removal is a safety measure to prevent aspiration and obstruction of the airway. If a client has any capped teeth, document this finding on the checklist.

All prosthetic devices, such as artificial eyes and limbs, are removed and given to a family member or safely stored, as are contact lenses, wigs, and toupees. Check for hairpins and clips, which, if not removed, can conduct electrical current used during surgery and cause scalp burns.

Some facilities allow hearing aids in the surgical suite to help communication before and after surgery. If the client is sent to surgery with a hearing aid, communicate this to the surgical nurse to prevent accidental loss of or damage to the device. Some facilities allow dentures, wigs, and glasses to be worn into the operating suite to prevent embarrassment to the client. These items are removed when absolutely necessary.

The removal of fingernail polish or artificial nails is controversial. Polish is flammable, and artificial nails may affect the accuracy of pulse oximetry readings. In some facilities at least one artificial nail must be removed in order to monitor oxygen saturation by pulse oxymetry.

After the client is prepared for surgery and the operating suite is ready to receive him or her, ask the client to empty the bladder. This action prevents incontinence or overdistention and is a starting point for intake and output measurement. An overly full bladder may hinder access to the surgical site. Answer any questions, offer reassurance as needed, and give any prescribed drugs.

PREOPERATIVE MEDICATIONS

Preoperative drugs may be prescribed regardless of the type of planned anesthesia. Various drugs reduce anxiety, promote relaxation, reduce pharyngeal secretions, prevent laryngospasm, inhibit gastric secretions, and decrease the amount of anesthetic needed for the induction and maintenance of anesthesia. Drug selection is based on the client's age, physical and psychological condition, medical history, and height and weight; other drugs the client takes routinely; test results; and the type and extent of the planned surgical procedure. If more than one response is required, combination therapy may be prescribed. A typical combination consists of a sedative or tranquilizer, an opioid analgesic, and an anticholinergic agent.

Preoperative drugs are often given when the client is "on call" to the surgical suite. After positively identifying the

NORTHWEST HOSPITAL CENTER
PRE-OPERATIVE CHECKLIST

Date of Surgery________________

Addressograph Plate

ALLERGIES

CLINICAL DATA:	YES	NO	COMMENTS
Authorization for Surgical Treatment Completed			
Height & Weight Charted			
History and Physical			
Chest X-Ray			
EKG Report			
Urine Report			
Blood Sugar Within Range of (75-250mg%)			
Hematocrit Within Range of (27-55%)			
Potassium Within Range of (3.2-5.5mEq/L)			
Results Out of Range Reported to Dept. of Anesthesia			

Anesthesiologist Time: By:

PATIENT PREPARATION:	YES	NO	COMMENTS
Jewelry Removed			
Hair Piece, Wig, Hairpin, Barrettes, Beads, Rubberbands Removed			
Loose Teeth or Caps Noted			
Dentures Removed			
Artificial Eye, Contact Lenses, Glasses Removed			
Any Prosthetic Appliance Removed			
Voided or Catheterized - I&O Sheet on Chart			
Identification Bracelet in Place			
Parenteral Fluids Patent & Infusing at cc/hr			
B/P, T.P.R. Charted			
Premedication Given As Ordered			
Side Rails Up-Pt. Care Data & Care Plan on Chart			
Is Patient on Isolation - If Yes, What Type			

COMMUNICATION ASSESSMENT:	Normal	Abnormal	COMMENTS
Vision			
Hearing			
Mental			
Speech			
Other			

Patient's Preferred Name:

Limb For Burial ☐ Yes ☐ No Funeral Home:

R.N. Completing Checklist

702/1091-3-R-4/95 (40-1471) pl/3133N

Figure 20-5 ■ A preoperative checklist. (Courtesy of Northwest Hospital Center, Randallstown, MD.)

client (using the arm band and asking the client to state his or her name) and making sure the operative permit is signed, give the correct drugs. Then raise the siderails, place the call system within easy reach of the client while reminding him or her not to try to get out of bed. Place the bed in a low position. Tell the client that he or she may become drowsy and have a dry mouth as a result of the drugs.

A more common practice is for the preoperative drugs to be given *after* the client is transferred to the operating area. This practice permits the surgical team and anesthesia personnel to make more accurate assessments and have last-minute discussions with a client not yet affected by drugs. In addition, after the client is in the operating area, drugs can be given by the IV route. The oral or intramuscular (IM) route is used less often because of variable absorption rates.

CLIENT TRANSFER TO THE SURGICAL SUITE

In the immediate preoperative period, review and update the client's chart, reinforce teaching, ensure that the client is correctly dressed for surgery, and give prescribed preoperative drugs. Use a preoperative checklist for a smooth, efficient transfer to the surgical suite (Figure 20-5). The client, along with the signed consent form, the completed preoperative checklist, the chart, and the Addressograph plate, is transported to the surgical suite.

Most clients in the hospital setting are transferred to the surgical suite on a stretcher with the siderails up. In special circumstances (e.g., clients requiring traction, those having orthopedic surgery, and those who should be moved as little as possible), the client is transferred in the hospital bed. Other factors that influence the decision to transfer in a bed are the client's age, size, and physical condition. In ambulatory settings, clients either walk or are transferred to the surgical suite on a stretcher or in a wheelchair.

Evaluation: Outcomes

Evaluate the care of the preoperative client on the basis of the identified nursing diagnoses. The expected outcomes include that the client:

- States understanding of the informed consent and preoperative procedures
- Demonstrates postoperative exercises and techniques for prevention of complications
- Has reduced anxiety

Specific indicators for these outcomes are listed for each nursing diagnosis under the Planning and Implementation section (see earlier).

GET READY for the NCLEX Examination!

KEY POINTS

Safe Effective Care Environment

- Ask the client if an advance directive has been completed.
- Ask the client to explain in his or her own words what surgical procedure is being done and why.
- If the client's explanation of the scheduled surgery is not consistent with the documentation, notify the surgeon and request that the surgeon speak to the client.
- Ensure that the client is wearing proper identification.
- Ensure that the client is not asked to sign an operative permit or any other legal document after the preoperative drugs have been given.
- After the client has received preoperative drugs, keep the siderails up and the bed in the "low" position.

Health Promotion and Maintenance

- Teach clients about dietary restrictions and preoperative preparations.
- Teach the client specific interventions to perform after surgery to prevent complications (incision splinting, deep breathing exercises, range of motion exercises, as described in Charts 20-6 and 20-7).

Psychosocial Integrity

- Pace your interview to match the learning needs and style of the individual client.
- Allow the client the opportunity to express fear or anxiety regarding the surgical procedure or its possible outcome.
- Explain all diagnostic procedures, restrictions, and follow-up care to the client scheduled for a surgical procedure.
- Communicate any concerns or fears the client has to the surgeon and anesthesia personnel.

Physiological Integrity

- Communicate to the surgeon and anesthesia personnel any physical or laboratory change that may alter the client's response to drugs, anesthesia, or surgery.
- Check that documentation for any procedure to be performed on one of a paired organ or extremity clearly indicates which organ or extremity is involved.
- Ensure that dentures and any other personal items are removed from the client before the client is transferred to the surgical suite.

ADDITIONAL STUDY RESOURCES

Go to your Student CD-ROM for Review Questions for the NCLEX Examination.

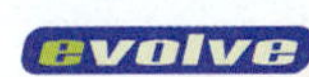

Go to http://evolve.elsevier.com/Iggy/ for Integrated Management of Care Questions for the NCLEX Examination.

SELECTED BIBLIOGRAPHY

Asterisk indicates a classic or definitive work on this subject.

*American Society of Anesthesiologists Task Force. (1999). Practice guidelines for preoperative fasting and the use of pharmacologic agents to reduce the risk of pulmonary aspiration: Application to healthy patients undergoing elective procedures. *Anesthesiology, 90*(3), 896-905.

American Society of PeriAnesthesia Nurses (2004). *Standards, recommended practices, and guidelines.* Denver: Author.

Association of Perioperative Registered Nurses. (2002). Recommended practices for skin preparation of patients. *AORN Journal, 75*(1), 184-187.

Association of Perioperative Registered Nurses. (2003a). ANA code for nurses with interpretive statements: Explications perioperative nursing. In *Standards, recommended practices and guidelines* (pp. 53-83). Denver: Author.

Association of Perioperative Registered Nurses. (2003b). AORN clinical path template. In *Standards, recommended practices and guidelines* (pp. 117-125). Denver: Author.

Beyea, S. (2002). Accident prevention in surgical settings: Keeping patients safe. *AORN Journal, 75*(2), 361-363.

Beyea, S. (2004). Evidence-based practice in perioperative nursing. *American Journal of Infection Control, 32*(2), 97-100.

Bryant, K. (2002). Ambulatory surgery industry takes steps forward. *OR Today, 2*(10), 34-35.

Cogliano, J., & Kisner, D. (2002). Bloodless medicine and surgery in the OR and beyond. *AORN Journal, 76*(5), 830, 832-837, 839.

Dochterman, J., & Bulechek, G. (eds). (2004). *Nursing interventions classification (NIC)* (4th ed.). St. Louis: Mosby.

*Dunn, D. (1998). Preoperative assessment criteria and patient teaching for ambulatory surgery patients. *Journal of PeriAnesthesia Nursing, 13*(5), 274-291.

Dunn, D. (2004). Preventing perioperative complications in an older adult. *Nursing 2004, 34*(11), 36-41.

Ebersole, P., Hess, P., & Luggen, A. (2004). *Toward healthy aging: Human needs and nursing response* (6th ed.). St. Louis: Mosby.

Fort, C. (2002). Get pumped to prevent DVT. *Nursing2002, 32*(9), 50-52.

George-Gay, B., & Parker, K. (2003). Understanding the complete blood count with differential. *Journal of PeriAnesthesia Nursing, 18*(2), 96-117.

Golembiewski, J. (2002). Allergic reactions to drugs: Implications for perioperative care. *Journal of PeriAnesthesia Nursing, 17*(6), 393-398.

Kjonniken, I., et al. (2002). Preoperative hair removal: A systematic literature review. *AORN Journal, 75*(5), 928-936, 938, 940.

McEwen, D. (2002). Ambulatory surgery. In M.H. Meeker & J.C. Rothrock (Eds.). *Alexander's care of the patient in surgery* (12th ed.). St. Louis: Mosby.

Meeker, M.H., & Rothrock, J.C. (2003). *Alexander's care of the patient in surgery* (12th ed.). St. Louis: Mosby.

Moorhead, S., Johnson, M., & Maas, M. (Eds.). (2004). *Nursing outcomes classification (NOC)* (3rd ed.). St. Louis: Mosby.

*Murphy, J. (1999). Preoperative consideration with herbal medicines. *AORN Journal, 69*(1), 173-183.

Pagana, K., & Pagana, T. (2002). *Mosby's manual of diagnostic and laboratory tests* (2nd ed.). St. Louis: Mosby.

Seal, L., & Paul-Cheadle, D. (2004). A systems approach to preoperative surgical patient skin preparation. *American Journal of Infection Control, 32*(2), 57-62.

Tappen, R., Muzic, J., & Kennedy, P. (2001). Preoperative assessment and discharge planning for older adults undergoing ambulatory surgery. *AORN Journal, 73*(2), 464-474.

Walton, J. (2001). Helping high-risk surgical patients beat the odds. *Nursing2001, 31*(5), 54-59.

Wood, B. (2002). Caring for a limited-English proficient patient. *AORN Journal, 75*(2), 305-308.

CHAPTER 21

Interventions for Intraoperative Clients

REBECCA M. PATTON

LEARNING OUTCOMES

After studying this chapter, you should be able to:

1. Discuss nursing interventions to reduce client and family anxiety.
2. Explain procedures to ensure the identity of the client and the accuracy of the planned surgical procedure.
3. Describe the roles and responsibilities of various intraoperative personnel.
4. Identify interventions to ensure the client's safety and dignity during an operative procedure.
5. Identify nursing responsibilities for management of clients receiving anesthesia.
6. Select nursing interventions to prevent skin breakdown for older adults clients during surgery.
7. Recognize the clinical manifestations of malignant hyperthermia.
8. List interventions for the client with malignant hyperthermia.
9. Discuss the potential adverse reactions and complications of specific anesthetic agents.
10. Assess clients for specific problems related to positioning during surgical procedures.

Go to your Student CD-ROM for Review Questions for the NCLEX Examination keyed to these Learning Outcomes.

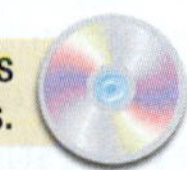

Safety and advocacy for the client during surgery are the main concerns of perioperative nurses. Many hazards can be managed, prevented, reduced, and controlled by nursing actions and observations. The client entering the surgical suite (operating room, or OR) is at risk for infection, impaired skin integrity, increased anxiety, altered body temperature, and injury related to positioning and other hazards. The surgical phase is filled with unfamiliar experiences and uncertain outcomes. Nursing care during this period is critical, because the client's physical needs, spiritual needs, comfort, safety, dignity, and psychological status are dependent on the perioperative nurse. Specific procedures and policies may differ among agencies, but similarities reflect the standards and recommended practices for perioperative nursing, as published by AORN, the Association of periOperative Registered Nurses.

OVERVIEW

Members of the Surgical Team

The surgical team consists of the surgeon, one or more surgical assistants, the anesthesia provider, and the OR staff.

Perioperative, or operating room (OR), nurses include the holding area nurse, circulating nurse, scrub nurse, and specialty nurses. The number of assistants, circulating nurses, and scrub nurses depends on the complexity and projected length of the surgical procedure. For some minor procedures, only a circulating nurse may be needed in addition to the surgeon. More complex procedures may require additional nursing staff to either circulate or scrub.

SURGEON AND SURGICAL ASSISTANT

The **surgeon** is a physician who assumes responsibility for the surgical procedure and any surgical judgments about the client. The **surgical assistant** might be another surgeon (or physician, such as a resident or intern) or a physician's assistant, nurse, or surgical technologist. Under the direction of the surgeon and within the legal scope of practice for each state, the assistant may hold retractors, suction the wound (to improve viewing of the operative site), cut tissue, suture, and dress wounds.

ANESTHESIA PROVIDERS

The **anesthesiologist** is a physician who specializes in giving anesthetic agents. A **certified registered nurse anesthetist (CRNA)** is a registered nurse with additional credentials who delivers anesthetic agents under the supervision of an anesthesiologist, surgeon, dentist, or podiatrist. The anesthesia provider gives anesthetic drugs to induce and maintain anesthesia and delivers other drugs as needed to support the client during surgery.

The anesthesia provider monitors the client during surgery by assessing and monitoring the following:

- The level of anesthesia (i.e., by using a peripheral nerve stimulator or bispectral analysis)
- Cardiopulmonary function (using electrocardiographic [ECG] monitoring, pulse oximetry, end-tidal carbon dioxide monitoring, arterial blood gases [ABGs], and hemodynamic monitoring via arterial lines and/or pulmonary artery catheters)
- Vital signs
- Intake and output

Depending on the client's needs, anesthesia personnel give intravenous (IV) fluids, including blood and blood products.

PERIOPERATIVE STAFF

Perioperative, or OR, staff have several roles during surgery, depending on their education, experience, skill, and job responsibilities. Regardless of their role, the OR nurse uses the nursing process, develops a plan of nursing care, and coordinates care delivery to clients and their family members.

HOLDING AREA NURSE. Some operating suites have a presurgical holding area next to the main ORs. The client waits in this area until the OR is ready. The holding room nurse manages the care while the client is in this area. This nurse greets the client on arrival, reviews the medical record and preoperative checklist, and ensures that the operative consent forms are signed. The nurse assesses the client's physical and emotional status, gives emotional support, answers questions, and provides additional education as needed. The nurse begins documentation on a perioperative nursing record (Figure 21-1).

The holding area is busy, with many staff members performing different procedures before surgery (e.g., starting IV lines or inserting epidural catheters). The holding area nurse maintains an atmosphere to promote comfort, privacy, and confidentiality. Depending on the facility's policy, family members may be able to wait with the client.

CIRCULATING NURSE. The **circulating nurse,** or **circulator** is a registered nurse. This nurse coordinates, oversees, and is involved in the client's nursing care in the OR. The circulating nurse's actions are vital to the smooth flow of events before, during, and after surgery. This nurse is responsible for the activities within that particular OR. The circulator sets up the OR and ensures that supplies, including blood products and diagnostic support, are available as needed. All anticipated equipment is gathered and inspected by the circulator to make certain that it is safe and functional before the surgery. Depending on the procedure and position required, the circulator makes up the operating bed (OR table) with gel pads (to prevent pressure sores) and heating pads (to prevent hypothermia) under the sheets, as indicated.

If there is no holding area nurse, the circulator assumes the responsibilities of that nursing role as well. Even when there is a holding area nurse, the circulator also greets the client and reviews findings with the holding area nurse. The circulator is responsible for continuity of care.

Once the client is ready to be moved into the OR, the circulating nurse assists the OR team in the transfer to the operating bed. The nurse positions the client, protecting bony areas with extra padding while providing comfort and reassurance. While observing the client, the circulating nurse also assists the anesthesia provider with the induction of anesthesia. The circulator then may "prep" (scrub) the surgical site before the client is draped with sterile drapes.

Throughout the surgery, the circulating nurse:

- Monitors traffic in the room
- Assesses the amount of urine and blood loss
- Reports findings to the surgeon and anesthesia provider
- Ensures that the surgical team maintains sterile technique and a sterile field
- Anticipates the client's and surgical team's needs, providing supplies and equipment as needed
- Communicates information regarding the client's status with family members during long or unique procedures
- Documents care, events, interventions, and findings

Depending on facility policy, the circulating nurse may record drugs given, blood, and blood components. (This also may be a function of the anesthesia provider.)

Before the procedure is over, the circulating nurse completes documentation (Figure 21-2; see also Figure 21-1). The presence of drains or catheters, the length of the surgery, and a count of all sponges, "sharps" (needles, blades), and instruments are recorded in the nursing record. The nurse notifies the postanesthesia care unit (PACU) of the client's estimated time of arrival and any special needs.

SCRUB NURSE/SURGICAL TECHNOLOGIST. The **scrub nurse** and/or the surgical technologist sets up the sterile field (Figure 21-3), drapes the client, and hands sterile supplies, sterile equipment, and instruments to the surgeon and the assistant. Knowledge of the surgical procedure allows the scrub nurse to anticipate which instruments and types of sutures the surgeon will need. Anticipating these needs reduces the duration of anesthesia for the client. In addition, the surgeon's anxiety and tension are reduced when the scrub nurse is familiar with the procedure and can anticipate and respond accordingly. Throughout the surgical procedure, the scrub nurse (with the circulating nurse) maintains an accurate count of sponges, sharps, instruments, and amounts of irrigation fluid and drugs used.

A specially trained person who is not a nurse may perform the scrub role. Such people are called **operating room technicians (ORTs)** or **surgical technologists.** Often certified surgical technologists (CSTs) are used in the OR.

SPECIALTY NURSE. The **specialty nurse** is educated in a particular type of surgery (e.g., orthopedic, cardiac, ophthalmologic) and is responsible for nursing care specific to clients needing that type of surgery. The specialty nurse assesses, maintains, and recommends equipment, instruments, and supplies used in that specialty. During surgery the specialty nurse may act as the scrub or circulating nurse.

If the facility uses laser technology, nurses specially trained in the use, care, and maintenance of the laser are needed. This nurse may be called a laser specialty nurse or a laser nurse coordinator. (**Laser** is an acronym for *l*ight *a*mplification by the *s*timulated *e*mission of *r*adiation.) A laser gives off a high-powered beam of light that cuts tissue more cleanly than do scalpel blades. This process creates intense

Our Lady of Lourdes Medical Center
1600 Haddon Avenue Camden, N.J. 08103

PRE-OPERATIVE RECORD

PRE-OPERATIVE

Patient Name ______ Surgeon ______ Date ______

Procedure ______

Arrival ______ **ID** ☐ Verbal ☐ Nameband **Pt Verbalizes** ☐ Procedure Site ☐ Surgeon **NPO** Since ______

Allergies: ☐ NDA ☐ Latex ☐ Other ______ ☐ Drugs ______

Lab Data: ☐ CBC ☐ Urinalysis ☐ Chemistry ☐ Coag Studies ______ ☐ Pregnancy Test

Reports: ☐ EKG ☐ Chest ☐ H & P ☐ Other

Consents: ☐ Surgical ☐ Blood ☐ Anesthesia

Blood Products - # of units In OR ______

Blood Bank ______ ☐ Type and Screen ______ ☐ Type and Cross ______

☐ Autologus ______ ☐ Directed ______ ☐ Homologus ______

Equipment: ☐ IV's ☐ Foley ☐ Ventilator ☐ Cardiac Monitor ☐ IABP ☐ Other ______

Prosthesis: ☐ None ☐ Opthalmic ☐ Otic ☐ Dental ☐ Jewelry Disposition of Prosthesis ______

Orientation: ☐ Awake ☐ Oriented ☐ Sedated ☐ Confused ☐ Agitated ☐ Crying

Implants / Other Comments: ______

______ RN SIGNATURE ______

INTRA-OPERATIVE

Identification: ☐ Verbal ☐ Nameband Scrub Nurse: ☐ Sees Permits ☐ Aware of Allergies

Skin Condition: ☐ Intact ☐ Presence of Lesions - Type / Location ______

Skin Prep: ☐ Betadine ☐ Hibiclens ☐ Other ______

Position: ☐ Supine ☐ Prone ☐ Lithotomy ☐ Lateral ☐ Jackknife ☐ Fracture Table

☐ Other ______ Positioned by ______

Equipment Codes:		**Supports:**
= - Safety Strap	applied by ______	☐ Kidney Rest ______
X - Grounding Pad	applied by ______	☐ Stirrups ______
T - Tourniquet	applied by ______	☐ Arms @ Side ______
Δ - Pressure Pads	applied by ______	☐ Arms on Armboard ______
S - Sandbag	applied by ______	☐ Action Pads ______
R - Roll	applied by ______	☐ Black Leg Positioner ______
A - Action Donut	applied by ______	☐ Bean Bag ______
Z - Zoll Defib Pad	applied by ______	

Tourniquet Unit # ______ mm/Hg ______ Inflated ______ Deflated ______

Warming Blanket Unit # ______ Temp ______ On ______ Off ______

Electrocautery Unit # ______ Coag @ ______ Cut @ ______

Pad # ______ Exp. Date ______ ESU Pad Skin Site ______

Defibrillator # ______ Time / Joules ______

BiPolar Unit # ______ Setting ______ Other Equipment ______

Comments ______

______ RN SIGNATURE ______

FORM #PO1 (REV. 4/96)

Figure 21-1 ■ A perioperative nursing record with areas for charting preoperatively upon the client's arrival in the operating room (OR) suite and upon initial preparation intraoperatively. (Courtesy of Our Lady of Lourdes Medical Center, Camden, NJ.)

Our Lady of Lourdes Medical Center
1600 Haddon Avenue Camden, N.J. 08103

INTRA-OPERATIVE RECORD

Patient Name ______________________ Date ____________ Suite ________

☐ Scheduled ☐ Emergency ☐ Add On In Room ________ Began ________ End ________ Out ________

Surgeon ______________________ Assistant ______________________

Anesthesia ______________________ Perfusion/Other ______________________

Type of Anesthesia: ☐ General ☐ Spinal ☐ Epidural ☐ Regional Block ☐ Local ASB ☐ Local

Scrub ______________________ Circulator ______________________

Relief ______________________ Relief ______________________

Preoperative Diagnosis ______________________

Postoperative Diagnosis ______________________

Procedure ______________________

Clamp/Bypass on ____________ off ____________ EBL ____________

Specimens: Cultures ☐ **Aerobic** ☐ **Anaerobic** ________

Implant Log# ______________________

Irrigation: ______________________

Wound Classification:

Pre-Op	I	II	III	IV
Post-Op	I	II	III	IV
ASA Classification	I	II	III	IV

Medication Dispensed to OR Table **(Include time, drug, amt used, site/route should be prepared by and given by)**

Counts: ☐ Correct ________ ☐ Incorrect ________ Comments: ______________________

Intra-operative X-ray ☐ Yes ☐ No Type ______________________

Drains / Packing: ☐ None ☐ Foley Inserted by ______________________ ☐ Immediate urine output

☐ Jackson Pratt / Davol ________ ☐ Hemovac ________ ☐ Penrose ________ ☐ Packing ________ Other ________

☐ Chest Tubes # and size ______________________ ☐ Pleuravac ☐ Auto transfusion pleuravac

Post Op Skin Condition: ______________________

ESU Pad Skin Site ______________________ Dressing Site ______________________

Receiving Unit ☐ PACU ☐ CVU ☐ ICU / CCU ☐ SDS ☐ Nursing Unit ________ Report given to ________

RN Signature ______________________ Surgeon Signature ______________________

FORM #PO2 (REV. 7/96) White - Original Copy Yellow - O.R. Copy Pink - Surgeon Copy Goldenrod - Pharmacy Copy

Figure 21-2 ■ An interdisciplinary intraoperative record. Names of all personnel involved are listed, and both the circulating nurse's and the surgeon's signatures are required for completion. (Courtesy of Our Lady of Lourdes Medical Center, Camden, NJ.)

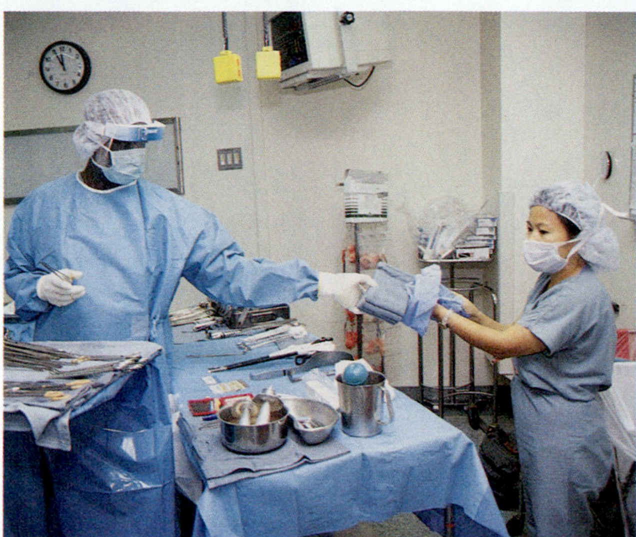

Figure 21-3 ■ Setting up the sterile table.

heat, rapidly clots blood vessels or tissue, and turns target tissue (such as a tumor) into vapor. All personnel must observe safety measures (e.g., wear eye shields, read door signs) during laser procedures to prevent injury to the client and staff.

Preparation of the Surgical Suite and Team Safety

During surgery, the client is unable to protect himself or herself, and all members of the surgical team must provide protection. The operating room (OR) layout prevents infection by reducing contaminants through air exchanges in the room and limiting the traffic and activities in the OR. Safety straps are used for the client, and the operating bed is locked in place. Heating pads are used to prevent hypothermia, and interventions are used to prevent skin breakdown.

The nurse ensures electrical safety through proper placement of grounding pads and use of electrical equipment that meets safety standards. All equipment used during surgery must be functional and in proper working condition as determined by the safety procedure of that facility. Equipment is cleaned and, when required, sterilized so that it can be used as a part of the procedure. The scrub and circulating nurses together ensure a correct count of surgical instruments, sharps, and sponges. Counts are performed before the beginning of the procedure, during the procedure as items are added or at the time personnel are relieved from that assignment, and immediately before complete skin closure.

Fire prevention and prevention of complications from the use of hazardous or toxic substances are concerns of all OR personnel. Ignition sources, oxidizers, and fuels are present in the OR and increase the risk for fires. Such events are rare but can occur during any kind of procedure. A cool room temperature (between 68° and 73° F [21° to 30° C]), with low humidity (30% to 60%) is optimal. The nurse is aware of emergency measures to take in the event of a fire or spill.

LAYOUT

The surgical suite is located out of the mainstream of the hospital and near the PACU and support services (e.g., blood bank, pathology and laboratory departments). Traffic flow is patterned to reduce contamination from outside the suite. Within the suite, clean and contaminated areas are separate. The surgical area is divided into three zones–unrestricted, semirestricted, and restricted–to ensure proper movement of clients and personnel.

The size of a surgical suite depends on the size and surgical capabilities of the facility. Most suites contain staff areas as well as areas related to client care, surgery, and surgical support. Staff areas include locker rooms and staff lounges. Client care areas include an admission or preoperative holding area and operating rooms. Surgical support areas include a number of ORs, cabinets for sterile supplies, separate utility rooms for clean and soiled equipment, and a clean linen room.

Figure 21-4 shows a typical OR. The exact number of tables and equipment used in a room is based on the needs of each client. A communication system links the OR and the main desk of the surgical suite. The system includes an intercom with separate systems for routine and emergency calls.

New OR designs use computers with the surgical equipment, lights, OR bed, and communications. These "hi-tech" rooms are similar to traditional ORs with the addition of computer equipment and panels. These rooms are more efficient for the surgical team with voice-activated commands operating some equipment that used to require manual operation.

HEALTH AND HYGIENE OF THE SURGICAL TEAM

People are a source of bacteria in the surgical setting. Everyone has bacteria on the skin, the hair, and in the airways. Because these organisms can be transmitted to the client, special health standards and dress are needed. Every surgical setting has policies and procedures regarding personnel and attire. Health standards require that all members of the surgical team and other support personnel in the surgical suite be free of communicable diseases. Anyone who has an open wound, cold, or any infection should not participate in surgery.

Good personal hygiene helps prevent and control infection, as does frequent handwashing. Shedding of organisms and skin debris is greatest immediately after showering, so surgical staff should bathe a few hours before changing into OR attire. Jewelry carries many organisms and should be minimal. All personnel must wash their hands between occasions of seeing clients and performing procedures, and more often when indicated. Hands of surgical personnel may be cultured on a regular basis to determine the potential for **nosocomial** (hospital-acquired) infections and to identify sources of pathogens. Further interventions or cultures are needed if quality reports (e.g., through the facility's quality improvement program) indicate a problem. Routine cultures are usually obtained every 3 to 6 months. Surgical attire and the surgical scrub help to prevent contaminations.

SURGICAL ATTIRE

All members of the surgical team and all OR personnel must wear scrub attire for use within the surgical suite. Scrub attire is clean, not sterile. It is worn to reduce contamination from home and areas outside of the surgical setting. Basic surgical attire is a shirt and pants, a cap or hood (Figure 21-5), and shoe

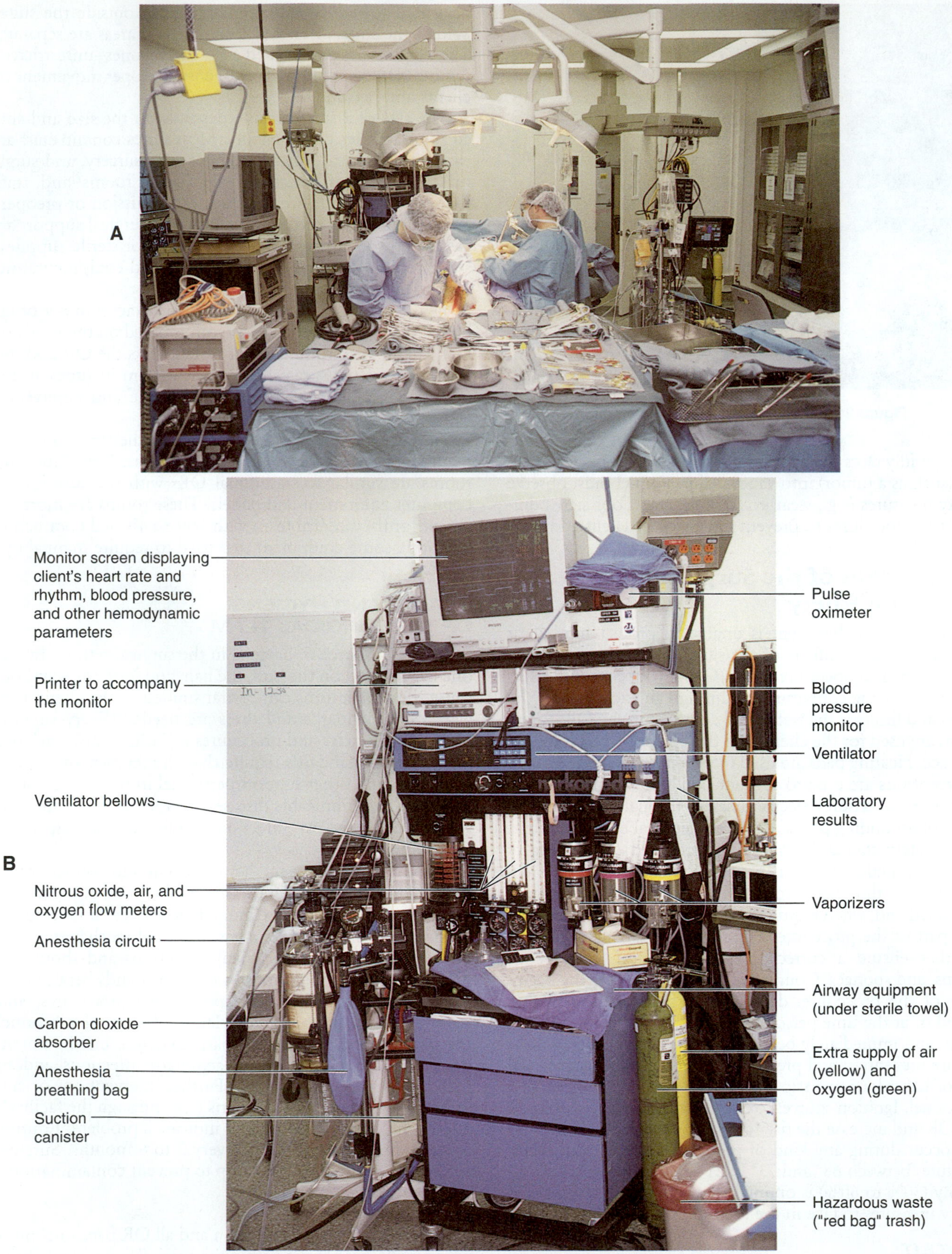

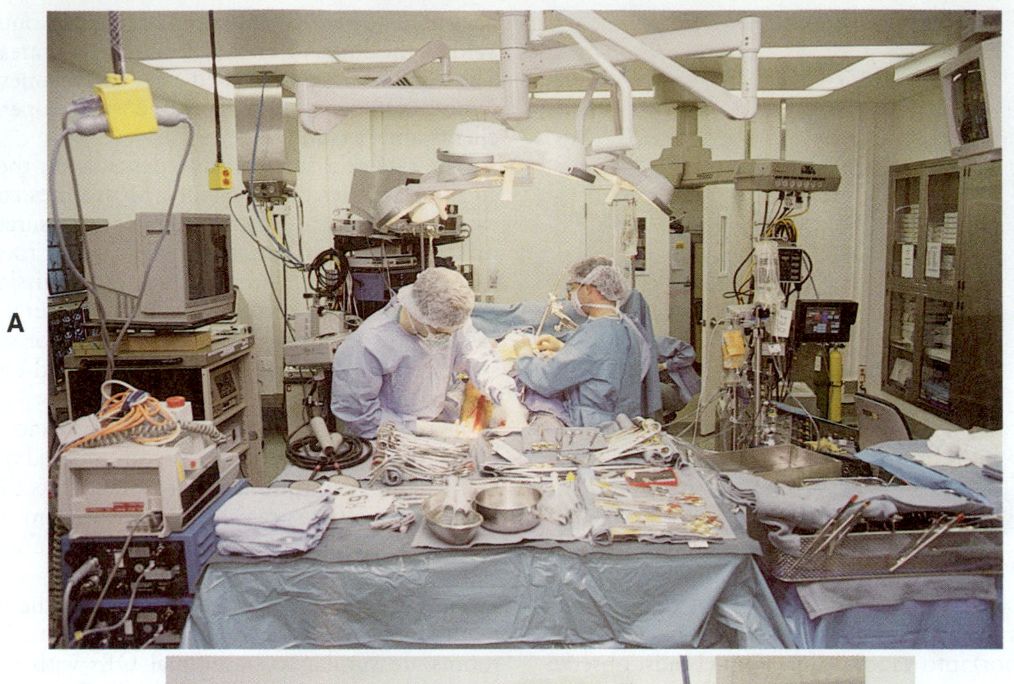

Figure 21-4 ■ **A,** A typical operating room. **B,** A typical anesthesia station with an anesthesia machine.

coverings. *Staff change into clean surgical attire in the OR suite locker rooms, not at home.* All members of the surgical team must cover their hair, including any facial hair.

In addition to basic attire, everyone must wear protective attire. This includes a mask, eyewear, gloves, gown, and shoe covers. Everyone who enters an OR where a sterile field is present must wear a mask. Surgical team members who are scrubbed and at the client's bedside during the surgery must also wear a sterile fluid-resistant gown, sterile gloves, and eye protectors (Figure 21-6). Team members who are *not* scrubbed (e.g., anesthesia provider and circulating nurse) may wear cover scrub jackets (to prevent shedding of organisms from bare arms) and eyewear, as warranted.

SURGICAL SCRUB

The surgeon, all assistants, and the scrub nurse perform a surgical scrub after putting on a mask and before putting on the sterile gown and gloves (Figure 21-7). *The scrub does not make the hands and forearms sterile.* When the scrub is performed correctly, it reduces the number of organisms from the hands, arms, and nails. Rings, watches, and bracelets are removed before scrubbing because they may harbor organisms. Fingernails are kept short, clean, and healthy. Artificial nails are not worn because they, too, can harbor organisms.

A surgical antimicrobial solution is used for the surgical scrub. Vigorous rubbing that creates friction is used from the fingertips to the elbow. The scrub continues for 3 to 5 minutes, followed by a rinse. During the rinse, hands and arms are positioned so that water runs off, rather than up or down, the arms. After scrubbing, personnel enter the OR with their hands held higher than the elbows and thoroughly dry their hands and forearms with a sterile towel. This person is then assisted into a sterile gown **("gowning")** and puts on sterile gloves **("gloving")**.

Gowns, gloves, and materials used at the operative field must be sterile. These items are changed between surgical procedures and as they become contaminated. The areas of the surgical gown considered sterile are the front of the gown from 2 inches below the neck to the waist area, and the elbow to the wrist area. Only when they are properly scrubbed and attired do members of the surgical team handle sterile drapes and equipment.

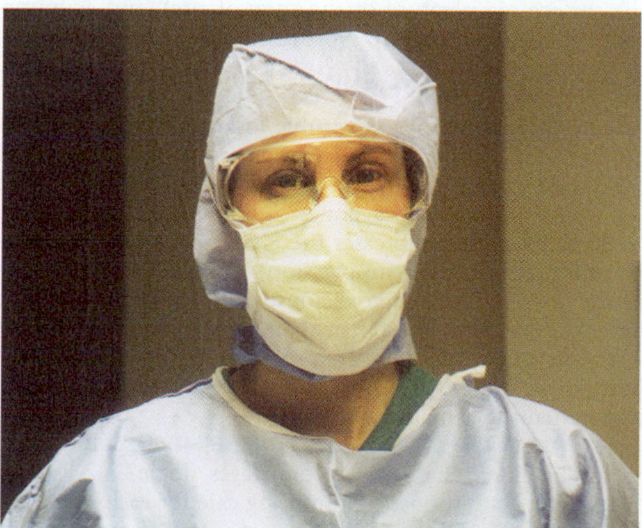

Figure 21-5 ■ An example of a hood-type hair covering that adequately covers facial and scalp hair.

Anesthesia

The word *anesthesia* means "negative sensation." Anesthesia delivery is a precise science. It requires the skill of an anesthesiologist, a certified registered nurse anesthetist (CRNA) working under the direction of an anesthesiologist or another physician, or an anesthesiologist's assistant (AA, similar to a physician's assistant) working under the direction of an anesthesiologist.

Anesthesia is an induced state of partial or total loss of sensation, occurring with or without loss of consciousness. The purpose of anesthesia is to block nerve impulse transmission, suppress reflexes, promote muscle relaxation, and, in some cases, achieve a controlled level of unconsciousness. Anesthesia providers use a separate anesthesia record for documentation (Figure 21-8).

Usually the anesthesia provider selects the anesthesia after consulting with the client and surgeon, and after considering specific client-related factors. The nurse and client communicate client preferences and fears about anesthesia to the anesthesia provider. Client health problems are major factors in the selection and dosage of anesthesia. Selection is also influenced by the following:

- Type and duration of the procedure
- Area of the body having surgery

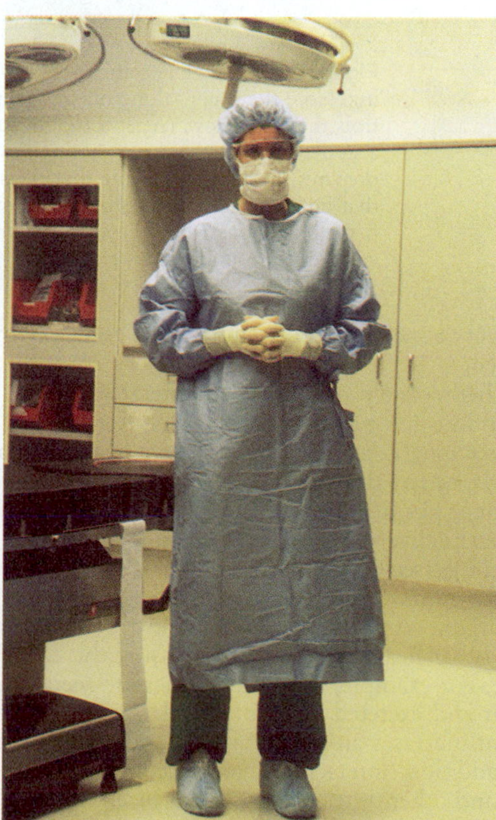

Figure 21-6 ■ Typical attire for all scrubbed personnel. Note complete hair covering, eye shields, mask, sterile gloves over the sleeves of the sterile gown, and shoe coverings. Note that when not in use, the hands are typically folded in front of the body, never below the waist.

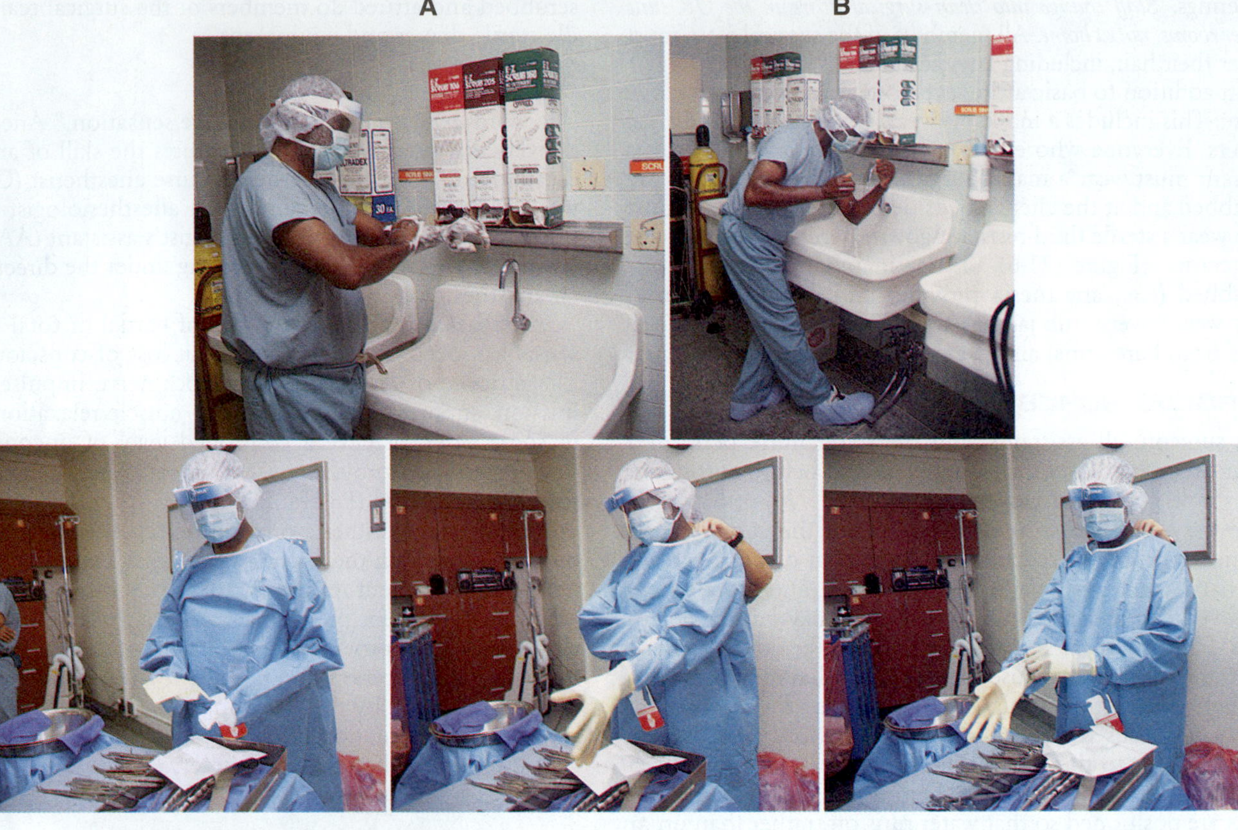

Figure 21-7 ■ The scrubbing, gowning, and gloving process. **A,** The surgical scrub. **B,** Rinsing. Note the water falling off the hands and arms. Also note the foot-operated handle that controls the water flow. (After scrubbing and rinsing, the scrub nurse dries his hands and arms with a sterile towel inside the operating room, then is assisted into a sterile gown.) **C,** The scrub nurse prepares sterile gloves. Note that the scrub nurse's hands are inside the sleeves of the gown and that he is touching the sterile gloves only with the sterile sleeves. **D,** The scrub nurse puts on his first sterile glove while the sterile gown is being tied in the back. Note again that his hand never emerges from under the sterile sleeve. **E,** The scrub nurse puts on his second sterile glove.

- Safety issues to reduce injury, such as airway management
- Whether the procedure is an emergency
- Options for management of pain after surgery
- How long it has been since the client ate, had any liquids, or any drugs
- Client position needed for the surgical procedure

Anesthesia delivery begins with selecting and giving preoperative drugs (see Chapter 20). The nurse must know the actions of commonly used drugs and their effects during and after surgery. Anesthesia affects many systems and can worsen other health problems, increasing the client's need for care. For example, most anesthetics are metabolized by the liver and excreted by the kidneys. Liver or kidney impairment increases anesthetic effects and the risk for toxicity. In addition, interactions may occur between the anesthetics and other drugs the client has received.

Anesthesia can be induced in many ways (Table 21-1):

- General or balanced anesthesia
- Local or regional anesthesia
- Hypnosis or hypnoanesthesia
- Cryothermia
- Acupuncture

Hypnosis or **hypnoanesthesia** (which induces a passive, trancelike state), **cryothermia** (use of cold [e.g., ice] reduces the surface temperature of the surgical site), and acupuncture are not often used in North America.

GENERAL ANESTHESIA

General anesthesia is a reversible loss of consciousness induced by inhibiting neuronal impulses in several areas of the central nervous system (CNS). This state can be achieved with a single agent or a combination of agents. General anesthesia depresses the CNS, resulting in **analgesia** (pain relief or pain suppression), **amnesia** (memory loss of the surgery), and unconsciousness, with loss of muscle tone and reflexes. The client is unconscious and unaware. This type of anesthesia is used most often in surgery of the head, neck, upper torso, and abdomen. It may also be used when clients are unable to cooperate.

STAGES OF GENERAL ANESTHESIA. Induction of general anesthesia involves four stages. Table 21-2 lists the expected client responses and nursing care for each stage.

The speed of **emergence** (recovery from the anesthesia) depends on the type of anesthetic agent, the length of time the client is anesthetized, and whether a reversal agent is

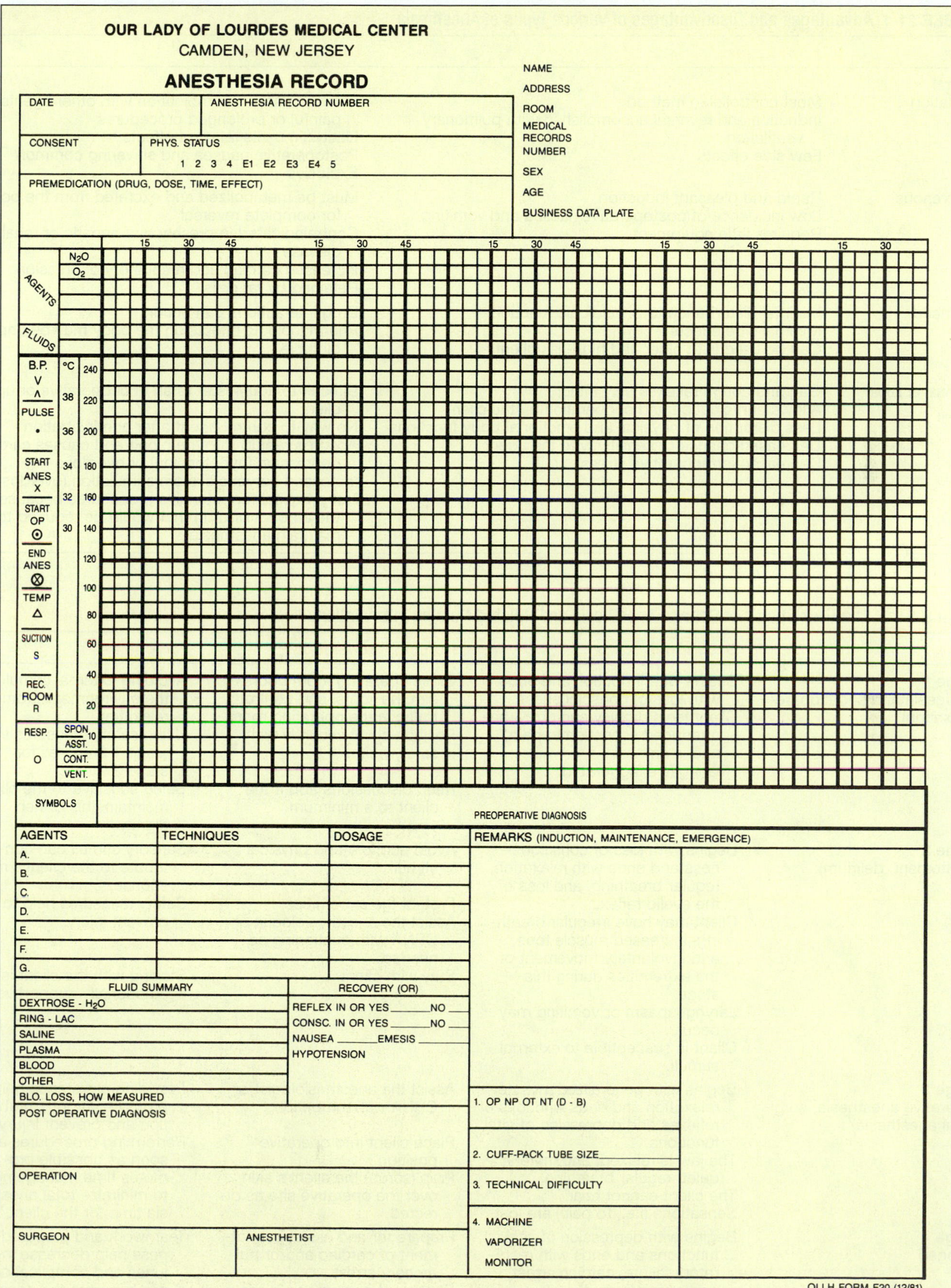
OUR LADY OF LOURDES MEDICAL CENTER
CAMDEN, NEW JERSEY

ANESTHESIA RECORD

DATE | ANESTHESIA RECORD NUMBER

CONSENT | PHYS. STATUS 1 2 3 4 E1 E2 E3 E4 5

PREMEDICATION (DRUG, DOSE, TIME, EFFECT)

NAME
ADDRESS
ROOM
MEDICAL RECORDS NUMBER
SEX
AGE
BUSINESS DATA PLATE

15 30 45 15 30 45 15 30 45 15 30 45 15 30

AGENTS: N_2O, O_2

FLUIDS

B.P. V Λ
PULSE •
START ANES X
START OP ⊙
END ANES ⊗
TEMP △
SUCTION S
REC. ROOM R
RESP. O — SPON, ASST., CONT., VENT.

°C: 38, 36, 34, 32, 30
240, 220, 200, 180, 160, 140, 120, 100, 80, 60, 40, 20, 10

SYMBOLS

PREOPERATIVE DIAGNOSIS

AGENTS	TECHNIQUES	DOSAGE
A.		
B.		
C.		
D.		
E.		
F.		
G.		

REMARKS (INDUCTION, MAINTENANCE, EMERGENCE)

FLUID SUMMARY	RECOVERY (OR)
DEXTROSE - H_2O	REFLEX IN OR YES ____ NO ____
RING - LAC	CONSC. IN OR YES ____ NO ____
SALINE	NAUSEA ____ EMESIS ____
PLASMA	HYPOTENSION
BLOOD	
OTHER	
BLO. LOSS, HOW MEASURED	

POST OPERATIVE DIAGNOSIS

1. OP NP OT NT (D - B)
2. CUFF-PACK TUBE SIZE
3. TECHNICAL DIFFICULTY
4. MACHINE
VAPORIZER
MONITOR

OPERATION

SURGEON | ANESTHETIST

OLLH FORM F20 (12/81)

Figure 21-8 ■ An anesthesia record. (Courtesy of Our Lady of Lourdes Medical Center, Camden, NJ.)

TABLE 21-1 Advantages and Disadvantages of Various Types of Anesthesia

Type	Advantages	Disadvantages
General		
Inhalation	Most controllable method Induction and reversal accomplished with pulmonary ventilation Few side effects	Must be used in combination with other agents for painful or prolonged procedures Limited muscle relaxant effects Postoperative nausea and shivering common Explosive
Intravenous	Rapid and pleasant induction Low incidence of postoperative nausea and vomiting Requires little equipment	Must be metabolized and excreted from the body for complete reversal Contraindicated in presence of hepatic or renal disease Increased cardiac and respiratory depression Retained by fat cells
Balanced	Minimal disturbance to physiologic function Minimal side effects Can be used with older and high-risk clients	Drug interactions can occur Pharmacologic effects on the body may be unpredictable
Regional or Local	Gag and cough reflexes stay intact Allows participation and cooperation by the client Less disruption of physical and emotional body functions Decreased chance of sensitivity to the agent Decreased intraoperative stress	Difficult to administer to an uncooperative or upset client No way to control agent after administration Absorbs rapidly into the blood and causes cardiac depression (hypotension) or overdose Increased nervous system stimulation (overdose) Not practical for extensive procedures because of the amount of drug that would be required to maintain anesthesia

TABLE 21-2 The Four Stages of General Anesthesia and Related Nursing Interventions

Stage	Description	Nursing Interventions	Rationales
Stage 1 (Analgesia and sedation, relaxation)	Begins with induction and ends with loss of consciousness. Client feels drowsy and dizzy, has a reduced sensation to pain, and is amnesic. Hearing is exaggerated.	Close operating room doors, dim the lights, and control traffic in the operating room. Position client securely with safety belts. Keep discussions about the client to a minimum.	Avoiding external stimuli in the environment promotes relaxation. Using safety measures in stage 1 prepares for stage 2. Being sensitive to the client maintains his or her dignity.
Stage 2 (Excitement, delirium)	Begins with loss of consciousness and ends with relaxation, regular breathing, and loss of the eyelid reflex. Client may have irregular breathing, increased muscle tone, and involuntary movement of the extremities during this stage. Laryngospasm or vomiting may occur. Client is susceptible to external stimuli.	Avoid auditory and physical stimuli. Protect the extremities. Assist the anesthesiologist or CRNA with suctioning as needed. Stay with client.	Sensory stimuli can contribute to the client's response. Safety measures help to prevent injury. Staying with the client is emotionally supportive.
Stage 3 (Operative anesthesia, surgical anesthesia)	Begins with generalized muscle relaxation and ends with loss of reflexes and depression of vital functions. The jaw is relaxed, and there is quiet, regular breathing. The client cannot hear. Sensations (i.e., to pain) are lost.	Assist the anesthesiologist or CRNA with intubation. Place client into operative position. Prep (scrub) the client's skin over the operative site as directed.	Providing assistance helps promote smooth intubation and prevent injury. Performing procedures as soon as possible promotes time management to minimize total anesthesia time for the client.
Stage 4 (Danger)	Begins with depression of vital functions and ends with respiratory failure, cardiac arrest, and possible death. Respiratory muscles are paralyzed; apnea occurs. Pupils are fixed and dilated.	Prepare for and assist in treatment of cardiac and/or pulmonary arrest. Document occurrence in the client's chart.	Teamwork and preparedness help decrease injuries and complications, and promote the possibility of a desired outcome for the client.

CRNA, Certified registered nurse anesthetist.

used. Retching, vomiting, and restlessness may occur during emergence although not all clients have these responses. Suction equipment must be available to prevent aspiration. During recovery, shivering, rigidity, and slight cyanosis may occur. These responses are caused by a temporary change in the body's temperature control. The nurse provides warm blankets, radiant light, and oxygen to decrease the effects of emergence.

ADMINISTRATION OF GENERAL ANESTHESIA. General anesthesia is administered by inhalation and IV injection.

INHALATION. Inhalation is an easily controlled method of giving general anesthesia because intake and excretion of the agent occur mainly by the lungs. The client inhales the anesthetic gas or vapor through a mask. The agent then crosses the alveolar membrane to the general circulation. The agent enters the bloodstream and is delivered to many tissues, where it is metabolized.

To improve gas exchange and control the anesthesia, respiration may be assisted or controlled. With **assisted respiration,** an endotracheal (ET) tube is inserted. The ET tube is then connected to the anesthesia machine (see Figure 21-4, *B*). The anesthesia provider overrides, or "assists," the client's own breathing effort and can manually start the breathing cycle.

Controlled respiration uses a mechanical ventilator to automatically inflate the lungs. Controlled ventilation is started after **apnea** (absence of spontaneous respiratory effort) is induced.

The anesthesia provider inserts the ET tube with the help of the circulating nurse. A laryngoscope is used to see the vocal cords, and the tube is placed in the trachea (Figure 21-9). With the ET tube in place, the client has an open airway (through the tube) for the inhaled anesthetic and oxygen.

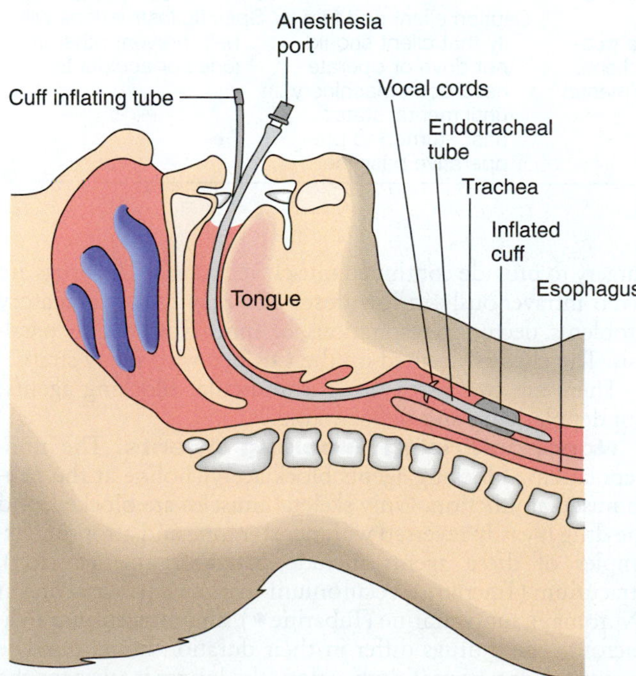

Figure 21-9 ■ An oral endotracheal tube in position. The cuff of the tube was placed just below the vocal cords, then inflated to seal off the airway.

Inhalation anesthetic agents are either gases or volatile agents. Table 21-3 lists the advantages, disadvantages, and nursing implications of inhalation agents.

Gaseous Agents. Nitrous oxide (N_2O) is the most commonly used agent and is usually given with oxygen. It is a colorless, odorless gas that provides analgesia.

Volatile Agents. Liquid agents vaporized for inhalation are "volatile" agents. Oxygen is the carrier, flowing over or bubbling through the liquid in the vaporizer system on the anesthesia machine. All volatile agents cause shivering after surgery because of their effect on the hypothalamus. Awakening is rapid, within 15 to 21 minutes. Table 21-3 lists features and interventions for volatile agents.

INTRAVENOUS INJECTION. IV anesthetic agents are injected, through an IV line, into the blood. The agent rapidly and smoothly spreads through the client's body. The drug is diluted by the blood, but is present at high enough levels in the brain, liver, and kidneys to induce anesthesia. Awakening is related to the client's metabolism. Table 21-4 lists advantages, disadvantages, and nursing implications of IV anesthetic agents.

Barbiturates. Barbiturates are often used for IV induction of anesthesia. These drugs act on the CNS, inducing reactions ranging from mild sedation to deep loss of consciousness. The barbiturate used most often is thiopental sodium (Pentothal). It acts rapidly, causing unconsciousness within 30 seconds. Because this agent depresses breathing and cardiac function, the client's vital signs are monitored continuously until the drug is eliminated.

Ketamine (Ketalar). Ketamine is a **dissociative anesthetic agent** (one that promotes a feeling of separation or dissociation from the environment). Rapid onset of a trancelike, analgesic state occurs. Ketamine is often used for diagnostic and short surgical procedures.

Emergence reactions are common during recovery from ketamine. The OR nurse reports the use of the drug to the PACU nurse so that precautions can be implemented. If the client is combative or restless, the siderails of the bed are padded to prevent injury. External stimuli are reduced until the client awakens. For severe reactions during recovery, small doses of diazepam (Valium, Vivol✱, Novo-Dipam✱) may be needed.

Propofol (Diprivan). Propofol is a short-acting anesthetic agent. Hypnosis occurs in less than 1 minute from the time of injection. The drug is eliminated rapidly and the client becomes responsive within 8 minutes after the infusion ends.

ADJUNCTS TO GENERAL ANESTHETIC AGENTS. Other drugs, such as hypnotics, opioid analgesics, and neuromuscular blocking agents, may be used as part of the anesthesia regimen.

HYPNOTICS. The benzodiazepines may be used for many effects. Common drugs in this class include midazolam (Versed), lorazepam (Ativan, Novolorazem✱), and diazepam (Valium, Vivol✱, Novo-Dipam✱). All have hypnotic, sedative, muscle relaxant, and amnesic effects. Lower doses may be used for sedation before surgery. These drugs also may be used as part of IV conscious sedation for short diagnostic procedures. Higher doses of midazolam can induce general anesthesia. These drugs may be used during surgery along with regional or local anesthesia. Adverse effects include respiratory depression, apnea, and oversedation.

TABLE 21-3 Advantages, Disadvantages, and Related Nursing Implications of Various General Inhalation Anesthetic Agents

Agent	Advantages	Disadvantages	Nursing Interventions	Rationales
Nitrous oxide (N_2O)	Rapid induction and recovery Useful for short procedures When used with other agents, reduces the required concentration of the other agents Minimal cardiovascular and respiratory depression	Relatively weak anesthetic agent May produce hypoxia if the concentration is high Needs addition of other agents for longer procedures	Assess oxygenation via pulse oximetry, physical assessment.	Ongoing assessment leads to early detection and treatment of potential complications.
Halothane (Fluothane)	Rapid and smooth induction Low incidence of postoperative nausea and vomiting Less irritating to the respiratory tract than other inhalation agents	Shivering common postoperatively Malignant hyperthermia possible in susceptible clients Metabolized by the liver Hypotension and bradycardia may occur Can sensitize the myocardium to dysrhythmias	Monitor heart rate for bradycardia. Monitor blood pressure for hypotension. Provide warm blankets, radiant heat.	Ongoing assessment leads to early detection and treatment of potential complications. Warmth helps promote client comfort and decrease shivering.
Enflurane (Ethrane)	Rapid induction and recovery Does not alter heart rate or rhythm	Respiratory depression and hypotension may occur Malignant hyperthermia possible in susceptible clients Lowers seizure threshold	Monitor respiratory rate and depth for hypoventilation. Assess oxygenation via pulse oximetry, physical assessment. Monitor blood pressure for hypotension.	Ongoing assessment leads to early detection and treatment of potential complications.
Isoflurane (Forane)	Rapid induction and recovery Has some muscle relaxant properties Stimulates the heart, which helps keep a stable heart rate Is not significantly metabolized; no renal or hepatic damage	Respiratory depression possible Malignant hyperthermia possible in susceptible clients	Monitor respiratory rate and depth for hypoventilation.	Ongoing assessment leads to early detection and treatment of potential complications.
Desflurane (Suprane)	Rapid induction, recovery, and awakening	May cause coughing and excitement during induction May increase heart rate and blood pressure with deep levels of anesthesia. Malignant hyperthermia possible in susceptible clients May cause changes in mental function	Monitor heart rate and blood pressure. Caution client and family that client should not drive or operate hazardous machinery until mental status has returned to preoperative baseline.	Ongoing assessment leads to early detection and treatment of potential complications. Specific instructions will help prevent other injuries or accidents.

CRNA, Certified registered nurse anesthetist.

OPIOID ANALGESICS. Common opioid analgesics used to enhance anesthesia include morphine sulfate (Statex✱), meperidine (Demerol), fentanyl (Sublimaze), and sufentanil (Sufenta). The use of opioids during surgery helps provide pain relief after surgery. *All opioid analgesics depress respiration.* Breathing is monitored and an open airway is maintained. Reduced dosages are used for older clients, clients with a circulatory problem (e.g., heart failure), and debilitated clients.

Fentanyl and sufentanil induce analgesia in lower doses, but at higher doses they are used to induce anesthesia. Fentanyl is 75 to 125 times more potent than morphine and sufentanil is five times more potent than fentanyl. It is often used in open heart surgery when the sternum must be opened. The client is monitored for bradycardia and decreased cardiac output.

NEUROMUSCULAR BLOCKING AGENTS. The neuromuscular blocking agents are used to relax the jaw and vocal cords immediately after induction so that the endotracheal tube can be placed. These drugs may be used during surgery to provide continued muscle relaxation. The drugs are given intravenously in low doses and may cause circulatory problems, decreased respirations, or apnea from muscle paralysis. The client is secured on the OR bed with safety straps.

There are two types of neuromuscular blocking agents: nondepolarizing and depolarizing.

Nondepolarizing Blocking Agents. The nondepolarizing blocking agents block acetylcholine at the neuromuscular junction. Only skeletal muscles are blocked, and the drug is easily reversed with neostigmine and atropine. Examples of these agents include pancuronium (Pavulon), atracurium (Tracrium), vecuronium (Norcuron), doxacurium (Nuromax), tubocurarine (Tubarine✱), and mivacurium (Mivacron). These drugs differ in their duration of action. The longer the duration of drug action, the longer it takes for the client to recover.

Depolarizing Blocking Agents. The depolarizing blocking agents overstimulate the motor end plate at the neuromuscular junction. In the process, potassium is forced out

TABLE 21-4 Advantages, Disadvantages, and Related Nursing Implications of Various General Intravenous Anesthetic Agents

Agent	Advantages	Disadvantages	Nursing Interventions	Rationales
Barbiturates				
Thiopental sodium (Pentothal) Methohexital sodium (Brevital)	Rapid, pleasant induction and recovery Acts directly on the central nervous system Short acting Low incidence of postoperative nausea and vomiting	Strong respiratory and cardiovascular depressant effect No antagonist medication available Mild to severe local tissue reaction with extravasation Poor analgesic, muscle relaxant effects	Monitor respiratory rate and depth for hypoventilation. Monitor heart rate for bradycardia. Monitor blood pressure for hypotension. Assess IV site.	Ongoing assessment leads to early detection and treatment of potential complications.
Nonbarbiturates				
Ketamine hydrochloride (Ketalar)	Rapid induction Short acting Can be given IM or IV No respiratory depression or loss of muscle tone (protects the airway) Protective reflexes remain intact Stimulates the cardiovascular system Can use for clients with respiratory or cardiac disorders Good amnesic effect Postoperative emergence reactions generally last only 24 hr	Emergence reactions—hallucinations, irrational behaviors, distorted images, unpleasant dreams, restlessness—are common Increased heart rate Increased blood pressure Increased cardiac output Poor muscle relaxant effect Nausea, vomiting, and aspiration possible	Minimize external stimuli: noise, light, touch, movement. Speak in a calm, soothing voice. Reassure client and family that emergence reactions are common and temporary. Have suction equipment near. Monitor blood pressure for hypertension. Monitor heart rate for tachycardia.	Stimuli increase the severity of the emergence reaction. Quiet promotes comfort, decreases anxiety. Reassurance decreases anxiety. Suction may be needed in the event of vomiting to prevent aspiration. Ongoing assessment leads to early detection and treatment of potential complications.
Propofol (Diprivan)	Short acting Rapidly metabolized Client becomes responsive quickly postoperatively Minimal postoperative nausea, vomiting, or sedation	Allergic skin reactions have occurred Client becomes aware of postoperative pain and discomfort sooner than with other anesthetics	Be prepared to administer analgesic medications as prescribed early in the postoperative period. Plan for nonpharmacologic pain interventions (see Chapter 7).	Awareness of pain very early in the postoperative period can be frightening. Pain can increase blood pressure and increase anxiety.
Opioids (As Adjunct)				
Fentanyl (Sublimaze)	Excellent postoperative analgesia Long-acting analgesia	Significant respiratory depression can occur several hours after administration Cardiovascular depression can occur	Monitor respiratory rate and depth for hypoventilation. Monitor blood pressure for hypotension. Have atropine, naloxone (Narcan), vasopressors, and resuscitative equipment nearby.	Ongoing assessment leads to early detection and treatment of potential complications. Having necessary supplies and equipment available provides for prompt response to an emergency.

CRNA, Certified registered nurse anesthetist.

of the muscle cells and into the blood, which can cause hyperkalemia. Clients often have brief muscle twitching, which causes muscle aches after awakening. Other side effects include increased salivation (increasing the risk for aspiration) and increased intraocular pressure (thus the agents may be not be used for clients with glaucoma). An example of a commonly used depolarizing blocking agent is succinylcholine (Anectine). There is no specific antidote for these agents.

BALANCED ANESTHESIA. Balanced anesthesia is a combination of IV drugs and inhalation agents used to obtain specific effects. A combination is used to provide hypnosis, amnesia, analgesia, muscle relaxation, and reduced reflexes with minimal disturbance of physiologic function. This method provides safe and controlled anesthetic delivery, especially for older and high-risk clients. An example of balanced anesthesia is the use of thiopental for induction, nitrous oxide for amnesia, morphine for analgesia, and pancuronium for muscle relaxation. Many combinations are possible, and selection is based on the individual client and the specific surgical procedure.

COMPLICATIONS FROM GENERAL ANESTHESIA. Complications can range from minor and annoying (sore throat) to death. Improvement in anesthesia delivery and surgical techniques has resulted in a decline in anesthesia-related deaths, even among higher-risk clients.

MALIGNANT HYPERTHERMIA. Malignant hyperthermia (MH) is an acute, life-threatening complication of certain drugs used for general anesthesia. The reaction begins in skeletal muscle exposed to specific agents, causing increased calcium levels in muscle cells and increased muscle metabolism. Serum calcium and potassium levels are increased, as is the metabolic rate, leading to acidosis, cardiac dysrhythmias, and a high body temperature.

Onset of MH may occur immediately after induction of anesthesia, several hours into the procedure, or, rarely, even after the anesthetic has been terminated. Clinical features reflect the increased muscle calcium level and the greatly increased body metabolism. Manifestations include tachycardia, dysrhythmias, muscle rigidity (especially of the jaw and upper chest), hypotension, tachypnea, skin mottling, cyanosis, and myoglobinuria (presence of muscle proteins in the urine). The most sensitive indication is an unexpected rise in the end-tidal carbon dioxide level with a decrease in oxygen saturation. Another early indication is sinus tachycardia. *Extremely elevated temperature, as high as 111.2° F (44° C), is a late sign of MH.* Survival depends on early diagnosis and the actions of the entire surgical team. Time is crucial when MH is diagnosed. Dantrolene sodium, a skeletal muscle relaxant, is the drug of choice along with other interventions.

For a known history or risk, the client can be treated before, during, and after surgery with dantrolene to prevent this problem. Chart 21-1 lists best practices for care of the client with MH.

Genetic Considerations

MH is a genetic disorder transmitted as an autosomal dominant trait. The client with a genetic predisposition for MH is at risk for this complication from halothane, enflurane, isoflurane, desflurane, sevoflurane, and succinylcholine. This rare syndrome is most common in young adults. Males are affected more often than females (despite the autosomal dominant pattern of inheritance) because of gender differences in muscle mass. Once a client or family history of MH is known, family members can have a muscle biopsy to determine whether they are at risk.

OVERDOSE. An anesthesia overdose can occur if the client's metabolism and drug elimination are slower than expected. Other drugs (e.g., antihypertensives) also alter metabolism, and interactions can occur between the anesthetic and the client's regular drugs. Accurate information about the client's height, weight, and history, is vital in determining the anesthetic type and dosage. Death during surgery is more often related to pre-existing health problems than to anesthesia overdose.

UNRECOGNIZED HYPOVENTILATION. The respiratory system is most often involved when the client has an anesthesia-induced complication. Failure to exchange gases adequately can lead to cardiac arrest, permanent brain damage, and death. Monitoring standards include the use of an end-tidal carbon dioxide monitor to confirm carbon dioxide in the client's expired gas and a breathing system disconnect monitor to detect any break in the breathing circuit equipment.

COMPLICATIONS OF SPECIFIC ANESTHETIC AGENTS. Specific complications are discussed earlier in the chapter. Older or debilitated clients are at greater risk for complications because of decreased metabolism or poor general physical condition. (For surgical risk factors, see Chapter 20.)

COMPLICATIONS OF INTUBATION. Many complications can occur from intubation (e.g., broken or injured teeth and caps, swollen lip, or vocal cord trauma). Intubation may be difficult because of anatomic variance or disease presence (e.g., small oral cavity, tight jaw joint, or presence of tumor). Improper neck extension during intubation also may cause injury. The surgeon should be in the operating room (OR) during the intubation process in case a tracheostomy is needed when the endotracheal (ET) tube is placed. ET placement causes tracheal irritation and edema. The client may have a sore throat after surgery.

CHART 21-1

BEST PRACTICE for
Care of the Client with Malignant Hyperthermia

- Stop all inhalation anesthetic agents and succinylcholine.
- If an endotracheal (ET) tube is not already in place, intubate immediately.
- Ventilate the client with 100% oxygen, using the highest possible flow rate.
- Administer dantrolene sodium (Dantrium) intravenously at a dose of 2 to 3 mg/kg.
- If possible, terminate surgery. If termination is not possible, continue surgery using anesthetic agents that do not trigger malignant hyperthermia (MH).
- Assess arterial blood gases (ABGs) and serum chemistries for metabolic acidosis and hyperkalemia.
  - If metabolic acidosis is evident by ABG analysis, administer sodium bicarbonate intravenously.
  - If hyperkalemia is present, administer 10 units of insulin in 50 mL of 20% dextrose intravenously.
- Use active cooling techniques.
  - Administer iced saline (0.9% NaCl) intravenously at a rate of 15 mL/kg every 15 minutes for three doses.
  - Apply a cooling blanket over the torso.
  - Wrap or rub extremities with cold, wet towels or ice wrapped in towels.
  - Lavage the stomach, bladder, rectum, and open body cavities (if appropriate) with sterile iced normal saline.
- Monitor core body temperature to assess effectiveness of interventions and avoid hypothermia.
- Monitor cardiac rhythm by electrocardiography (ECG) to assess for dysrhythmias.
- Insert a Foley catheter to monitor urine output.
- Treat any dysrhythmias that do not resolve on correction of hyperthermia and hyperkalemia with antidysrhythmic agents *other than calcium channel blockers*.
- Administer IV fluids at a rate and volume sufficient to maintain urine output above 2 mL/kg/hr.
- Monitor urine for presence of blood or myoglobin.
- If urine output falls below 2 mL/kg/hr, consider using osmotic or loop diuretics, depending on the client's cardiac and renal status.
- Contact the Malignant Hyperthermia Association of the United States (MHAUS) hotline for more information regarding treatment: (800) 644-9373.
- Transfer the client to the intensive care unit (ICU) when stable.
- Continue to monitor the client's temperature, ECG, ABGs, electrolytes, creatine kinase, coagulation studies, and serum and urine myoglobin levels until they have remained normal for 24 hours.
- Instruct the client and family about testing for MH risk.
- Refer the client and family to the Malignant Hyperthermia Association of the United States at (800) 986-4287 or http://www.mhaus.org.
- Report the incident to the North American Malignant Hyperthermia Registry at the University of Pittsburgh: (412) 692-5464.

Data from Malignant Hyperthermia Association of the United States; and Dunn, D. (1997). Malignant hyperthermia. *AORN Journal, 65*(4), 728-762.

LOCAL OR REGIONAL ANESTHESIA

Local or regional anesthesia briefly disrupts sensory nerve impulse transmission from a specific body area or region.

TABLE 21-5 Advantages, Disadvantages, and Related Nursing Implications of Local or Regional Anesthetic Agents

Agent	Advantages	Disadvantages	Nursing Interventions	Rationales
Procaine (Novocain) Tetracaine (Pontocaine) Lidocaine (Xylocaine) Mepivacaine (Carbocaine, Polocaine) Bupivacaine (Marcaine, Sensorcaine)	Easily administered Rapid onset (4-17 min) Can be administered topically or by injection Excellent muscle relaxant effects Protective reflexes (cough, gag) remain intact Client does not lose consciousness Many are available with epinephrine added	Absorbs into the bloodstream Can cause cardiac depression and dysrhythmias with absorption Difficult to control dosage Drug interactions with monoamine oxidase (MAO) inhibitors can cause hypertension Tremors, twitching, shivering, respiratory arrest can occur with absorption	Assess for return of movement and sensation in the area anesthetized. Monitor blood pressure and pulse. Assess administration site for pallor, drainage. Protect area anesthetized until full sensation has returned.	Movement returns first, then sense of touch, pain, warmth, and cold, in that order. Ongoing assessment leads to early detection and treatment of potential complications. Protection prevents injury to the area. Duration of anesthetic is 3-6 hr.

Motor function may or may not be affected. The client remains conscious and able to follow instructions. Because the gag and cough reflexes remain intact, the risk for aspiration is low. Local or regional anesthesia is often supplemented with sedatives, opioid analgesics, or hypnotics to reduce anxiety and increase comfort.

The OR nurse provides the client with information, directions, and emotional support before, during, and after the procedure. Table 21-5 describes local and regional anesthetic agents and related nursing implications.

LOCAL ANESTHESIA. Local anesthesia is delivered topically and by local infiltration. Sometimes when the term *local* is used, it means *any* form of anesthesia that is not general anesthesia.

TOPICAL ANESTHESIA. Topical agents are applied *directly* to the area of skin or mucous membrane surface to be anesthetized. Often the anesthetic is an ointment or spray. This method is often used for respiratory intubation and for diagnostic procedures, such as bronchoscopy or cystoscopy. The onset of action is 1 minute, and the duration is 20 to 30 minutes. Cardiac depression is a potential complication of topical agents applied to the pulmonary tract.

LOCAL INFILTRATION. Local infiltration is the injection of an anesthetic agent directly *into* the tissue around an incision, wound, or lesion. Peripheral nerve function is blocked at its origin. This method is often used during superficial suturing.

REGIONAL ANESTHESIA. Regional anesthesia, a type of local anesthesia, may be used when:

- General anesthesia cannot be used because of medical problems (e.g., dysrhythmias and pulmonary disease)
- The client has had adverse reactions to general anesthesia
- The client has a preference and a choice is possible
- Pain management after surgery is enhanced by regional anesthesia

If the client has eaten and the surgery is an emergency, it may be possible to perform surgery with the client under regional anesthesia (depending on the procedure) to decrease the risk for aspiration. Types of regional anesthesia include field block, nerve block, spinal, and epidural.

FIELD BLOCK. A field block occurs with a series of injections *around* the operative field. Injecting around a specific nerve or group of nerves depresses sensation at a local area. This type of block is used for chest procedures, hernia repair, dental surgery, and some plastic surgeries.

NERVE BLOCK. A nerve block occurs with injection of the local anesthetic agent *into or around* a nerve or group of nerves in the involved area. Nerve blocks disrupt sensory and motor impulse transmission. They prevent pain during a procedure, are used diagnostically to identify the cause of pain, and can be used to relieve chronic pain.

Figure 21-10 shows common nerve block sites. Lidocaine (Xylocaine) or bupivacaine (Marcaine) is often the agent used. A nerve block takes effect within minutes after the injection, and lasts longer than with local infiltration. Epinephrine added to the agent prolongs the effect. Seizures, cardiac depression, dysrhythmias, and respiratory depression may occur if the nerve-blocking agent is injected (by accident) into the bloodstream. The nurse observes for signs of systemic absorption, sensitivity, or overdose.

SPINAL ANESTHESIA. Spinal anesthesia, also called intrathecal block, occurs by injecting an anesthetic agent into the cerebrospinal fluid in the subarachnoid space (Figure 21-11). The drug acts on the nerves as they emerge from the spinal cord and before they leave the spinal canal. This type of block inhibits the autonomic, sensory, and motor nervous systems. The drug is absorbed rapidly into the nerve fibers, producing analgesia with relaxation. This method is often used for lower abdominal and pelvic surgery.

EPIDURAL ANESTHESIA. The anesthetic agent is injected into the epidural space and the spinal cord areas are never entered. Because the agent can diffuse or "float up" the spinal canal, the client can have anesthetic effects as high as the T4 level. Breathing problems may make injection at this high a level less desirable.

Epidural anesthesia is used for anorectal, vaginal, perineal, hip, and lower extremity surgeries. Two advantages of this type of anesthesia are:

- Decreased cardiac and pulmonary complications (especially important for the older client)
- Use of the epidural catheter for pain control after surgery (see Chapter 7)

COMPLICATIONS OF LOCAL OR REGIONAL ANESTHESIA. Complications of local or regional anesthesia are related to client sensitivity to the anesthetic agent (anaphylaxis), incorrect delivery technique, systemic absorption, and overdosage. The nurse observes for central nervous system (CNS) stimulation followed by CNS and cardiac depression, which are signs of a systemic toxic reaction. The nurse also assesses for restlessness, excitement, incoherent

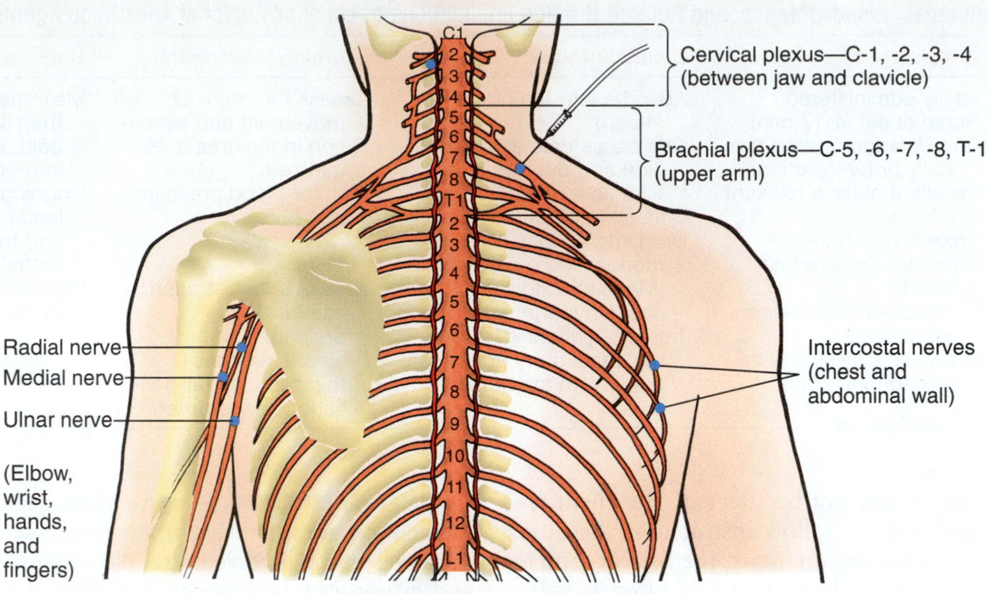

Figure 21-10 ■ Nerve block sites.

speech, headache, blurred vision, metallic taste, nausea, vomiting, tremors, seizures, and increased pulse, respirations, and blood pressure. Interventions include establishing an open airway, giving oxygen, and notifying the surgeon. Usually a fast-acting barbiturate is needed for treatment. If the toxic reaction is untreated, unconsciousness, hypotension, apnea, cardiac arrest, and death may result.

Cardiac arrest may occur as a rare complication of spinal anesthesia. Epinephrine is given to prevent cardiac arrest in clients in whom sudden, unexplained bradycardia develops.

Local complications include edema and inflammation as early problems. Abscess formation, tissue necrosis, and/or gangrene may occur later. Abscesses result from contamination during injection of the agent. Necrosis and gangrene are rare but may occur as a result of prolonged blood vessel constriction in the injected area.

The nurse's role in the delivery of regional anesthesia consists of the following:

- Assisting the anesthesia provider
- Observing for breaks in sterile technique
- Providing emotional support for the client
- Staying with the client
- Offering information and reassurance
- Positioning the client comfortably and safely

CONSCIOUS SEDATION

Conscious sedation is the IV delivery of sedative, hypnotic, and opioid drugs to reduce the level of consciousness but allow the client to maintain a patent airway and to respond to verbal commands. The amnesia action is short and the client usually has a rapid return to activities of daily living. Diazepam (Valium, Vivol✱, Novo-Dipam✱), midazolam (Versed), meperidine (Demerol), fentanyl (Sublimaze), alfentanil (Alfenta), and morphine sulfate are the most commonly used drugs. Conscious sedation is used for endoscopy, cardiac catheterization, closed fracture reduction, cardioversion, and other special but short procedures.

Selection of clients for conscious sedation is based on specific criteria. The physician determines whether the client is a candidate. In most states, a credentialed registered nurse may deliver conscious sedation under physician supervision and within the state-defined scope of nursing practice. Credentialing includes advanced training in IV drug delivery, airway management, and advanced cardiac life support (ACLS).

The nurse monitors the client during and after the procedure for response to the procedure and the drugs. The airway, level of consciousness, oxygen saturation, electrocardiographic (ECG) status, and vital signs are monitored every 15 to 30 minutes until the client is fully awake, oriented, and vital signs have returned to baseline levels.

The client receiving IV conscious sedation can be discharged to go home with a responsible adult. If the client returns to the general medical-surgical nursing unit, the unit staff nurses continue monitoring. The client is expected to be sleepy but arousable for several hours after the procedure. Oral intake is not permitted until 30 minutes after the client has received the sedation or according to the physician's prescription. When fluids are permitted, the nurse makes sure that the client is awake and positioned to avoid aspiration.

COLLABORATIVE MANAGEMENT

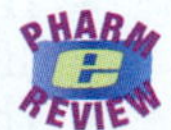

Assessment

HISTORY

On arrival in the surgical suite, the client is taken to the holding area or directly into the operating suite. The holding area nurse or the circulating nurse greets the client on arrival. *Correct identification of the client is the responsibility of every member of the health care team.* The nurse verifies the client's identity with two types of identifiers (name, birth date, medical record number, or social security number). For example, the nurse checks the client's identification bracelet and asks, "What is your name and when were you born?" This prac-

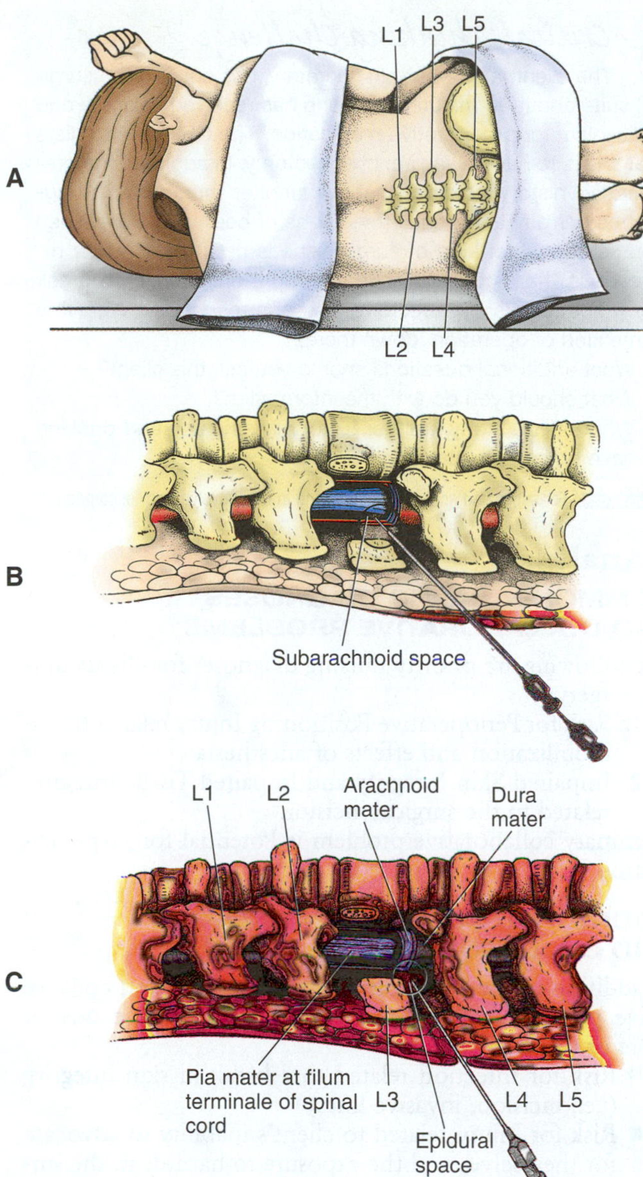

Figure 21-11 ■ Administration of spinal and epidural anesthesia. **A,** Spinal or epidural anesthesia is administered by inserting a spinal needle between the second and third or the third and fourth lumbar vertebrae (L2-3 or L3-4). The client is placed in the flexed lateral (fetal) position (shown here) or seated on the edge of the operating bed with the back arched and the chin tucked to the chest. **B,** Spinal anesthesia (viewed from the side). A large needle is inserted to the surface of the dura mater, and a second, smaller needle is passed through the first to penetrate the dura mater and arachnoid mater. An anesthetic is injected, sometimes through an indwelling catheter, directly into the cerebrospinal fluid in the subarachnoid space. **C,** Epidural anesthesia (viewed from the side). The needle is inserted to the surface of the dura mater, and the anesthetic is injected, usually through an indwelling catheter, into the epidural space.

tice prevents errors by drowsy or confused clients. For example, if a client is asked, "Are you Mr. Gates?" he may respond inappropriately if he is anxious or sedated. The nurse always validates identification using the medical record and identification bracelet, and by asking the client or family.

After completing the identification process, the nurse validates that the surgical consent form has been signed and witnessed. The nurse asks, "What kind of operation are you having today?" to ascertain that the client's perception of the procedure, the operative permit, and the operative schedule are the same. When the procedure involves a specific site, validating the side on which a procedure is to be performed (e.g., for amputation, cataract removal, or hernia repair) is the responsibility of each health care professional before and at the time of surgery. Facilities usually have the client and/or nurse initial the correct surgical site. Before proceeding, each health care professional thoroughly investigates *any* discrepancy and notifies the surgeon and anesthesia provider.

The nurse asks the client about any allergies and determines whether autologous blood was donated. A red allergy bracelet on the client's wrist and the medical record must be verified with what has been communicated.

The nurse checks the client's attire to ensure adherence with facility policy. Dentures and dental prostheses (e.g., bridges and retainers), jewelry (including body piercing), eyeglasses, contact lenses, hearing aids, wigs, and other prostheses are removed. The nurse pays special attention to the removal of dentures, because the denture plate could become loose and obstruct the airway during surgery. At times, the anesthesia provider may request that dentures be left in place to ensure a snug fit of the anesthesia mask. In some facilities, clients may wear eyeglasses and hearing aids until after anesthesia induction.

MEDICAL RECORD REVIEW

The circulating nurse and anesthesia provider review the client's medical record in the holding area or the operating room (OR). The medical record provides information needed to identify client needs during surgery and allows the circulating nurse to assess and plan specific care during and after surgery. The medical record is the main source of information on the type and location of the planned surgery. The nurse checks the medical record to ensure required data are present before surgery is started.

ADVANCE DIRECTIVES AND DO-NOT-RESUSCITATE ORDERS. Ethical dilemmas may occur during or after surgery. As a client advocate, the nurse may have to intervene on behalf of the client's rights and wishes. The nurse must be familiar with the advance directives and do-not-resuscitate (DNR) orders for each client. *These directives are to be honored in the surgical environment regardless of the situation.* It is difficult for some health care providers not to treat the client in the OR for an emergency situation, and they may ignore an advance directive or living will. Some surgical teams suspend DNR orders while a client is undergoing a surgical procedure. The position statement of Association of periOperative Registered Nurses, regarding the care of clients with DNR orders states that suspending a DNR order during surgery undermines a client's right to self-determination (AORN, 2003b).

ALLERGIES AND PREVIOUS REACTIONS TO ANESTHESIA OR TRANSFUSIONS. The nurse asks about allergies and previous reactions to anesthesia or blood transfusions. Allergies to iodine products or shellfish indicate a risk for a reaction to the agents used to clean the surgical area. Latex allergies must be assessed with all clients. Latex-induced anaphylaxis accounts for about 10% of the anaphylactic reactions that occur during surgery (see Chapters 23 and 26). Latex-free equipment and supplies must be used when the client has a latex allergy. The nurse documents the allergy in the medical record and notifies the OR team.

The client's previous experience with anesthesia helps the nurse and anesthesia provider anticipate needs and plan interventions. For example, if a client is restless or agitated as a reaction to anesthesia, the nurse can have padding for the siderails and protective restraints available. The use of blood and blood products during surgery may be influenced by the client's history, religious beliefs, preferences, and past transfusion reactions.

AUTOLOGOUS BLOOD TRANSFUSION. **Autologous blood transfusion** (reinfusing the client's own blood) may be used for surgery. Chapters 20 and 43 discuss autologous transfusion in more detail. Chart 21-2 outlines best practices for autologous blood transfusion during surgery.

LABORATORY AND DIAGNOSTIC TEST RESULTS. The OR nurse reviews the most recent laboratory findings and test results to inform the surgical team about the client's medical condition and to alert them for potential problems. The most recent results are usually obtained within 24 to 28 hours before surgery for hospitalized clients and within 4 weeks for ambulatory surgery clients. The nurse reports all abnormal findings or results to the surgeon and anesthesia provider. Laboratory values greater than or less than the normal range are potentially life threatening for clients having surgery (see Chapter 20). For example, if the hemoglobin level is less than 10 g/dL, oxygen transport capacity is reduced, affecting the amount and type of anesthesia used as well as the impact of blood loss during surgery.

MEDICAL HISTORY AND PHYSICAL EXAMINATION FINDINGS. The OR nurse checks that the medical history and examination findings, including usual pulse and blood pressure, are recorded. This information provides the circulating nurse, surgeon, anesthesia provider, and postanesthesia care unit (PACU) nurse with baseline data to assess the client's reaction to the surgery and anesthesia. Drugs taken before surgery may affect the client's reaction to surgery and wound healing. For example, aspirin reduces platelet action, increasing clotting time and the risk for hemorrhage.

Knowing the client's medical history and age (Chart 21-3) allows the nurse to plan interventions for the care and safety of high-risk clients. The nurse carefully monitors older clients and those with cardiac disease for potential fluid overload.

After completing the medical record review, the nurse may insert an IV catheter and perform a surgical shave. The circulating nurse provides emotional support and explains procedures to the client. *The client is never left unattended.* If the client is in the holding area, he or she is moved to the OR after the preoperative routine is completed.

CHART 21-2

BEST PRACTICE for
Intraoperative Autologous Blood Salvage and Transfusion

- Be aware of the cell-processing method to be used.
- Make sure that collection containers are labeled for the client.
- Assist with sterile setup as necessary.
- Assist with processing and reinfusing procedures as needed.
- Document the transfusion process.
- Monitor the client's vital signs during the transfusion procedure.

Critical Thinking Challenge

The client, a 62-year-old secretary, has entered the surgical suite about 30 minutes after she has received atropine and midazolam for preoperative medication. The OR schedule lists that she is to have a vaginal hysterectomy. In addition, the preoperative history indicates that she smokes three packs of cigarettes per day and drinks three cans of beer each day. When you ask her what kind of surgery she is having today, her response is "I am going to have a hemorrhoidectomy." You ask her if she means hysterectomy and she responds, "Well, it is some kind of operation 'down there.'"

1. What additional questions should you ask this client?
2. What should you do with the information?
3. What effect, if any, will her history of smoking and drinking have on her surgical experience?

evolve For suggested answer guidelines, go to http://evolve.elsevier.com/Iggy/.

Analysis

COMMON NURSING DIAGNOSES AND COLLABORATIVE PROBLEMS

The following are priority nursing diagnoses for clients during surgery:

1. Risk for Perioperative Positioning Injury related to immobilization and effects of anesthesia
2. Impaired Skin Integrity and Impaired Tissue Integrity related to the surgical incision

A primary collaborative problem is Potential for Hypoventilation.

ADDITIONAL NURSING DIAGNOSES AND COLLABORATIVE PROBLEMS

In addition to the common nursing diagnoses and collaborative problems, clients during surgery may have one or more of the following:

- Risk for Infection related to a break in skin integrity (i.e., incision, invasive lines)
- Risk for Injury related to client's inability to advocate for themselves and the exposure to hazards in the surgical environment
- Risk for Disuse Syndrome related to a decreased level of consciousness or to immobilization

CHART 21-3

NURSING FOCUS on the OLDER ADULT
Intraoperative Nursing Interventions

- Allow clients to retain eyeglasses and hearing aids until anesthesia has been administered.
- Use a small pillow under the client's head if his or her head and neck are normally bent slightly forward.
- Lift clients into position to prevent shearing forces on fragile skin.
- Position arthritic and artificial joints carefully to prevent postoperative pain and discomfort from strain on those joints.
- Pad bony prominences to prevent pressure sores.
- Provide extra padding for those clients with decreased peripheral circulation.
- Use head caps to prevent heat loss through the scalp.
- Place stockinette on extremities to conserve body heat.
- Warm prepping solutions and IV and irrigation fluids as indicated.
- Follow strict aseptic technique.
- Carefully monitor intake and output, including blood loss.

- Hypothermia related to evaporation from skin and exposed tissue in a cool environment, body heat loss, changes in the hypothalamus from anesthetic agents, or inadequate body covering
- Fear related to the threat of death, actual or perceived, or anticipation of events posing a threat to self-esteem
- Anxiety related to loss of control or the threat of death
- Deficient Fluid Volume related to decreased intake, evaporative fluid loss through the skin and exposed tissue, or blood loss
- Potential for Peripheral Neurovascular Dysfunction related to intraoperative positioning

Planning and Implementation

RISK FOR PERIOPERATIVE POSITIONING INJURY

NOC **PLANNING: EXPECTED OUTCOMES.** The client is expected to be free of injury as indicated by:

- Capillary refill and peripheral pulses are adequate in all extremities
- Sensory perception and motor function after surgery is at the same level as before surgery
- Absence of skin redness or open skin areas
- Absence of bruising

INTERVENTIONS. Interventions are used to prevent injury from positioning during surgery. Because of anesthesia and the narrow OR bed, the client's normal defense mechanisms cannot guard against nerve or joint damage and muscle stretch or strain. Thus proper positioning is important. The risk for pressure ulcer formation also is greater among clients having surgery than for those hospitalized clients who do not undergo surgery. (See the Evidence-Based Practice for Nursing box at right.) The circulating nurse pads the operating bed with foam and/or silicone gel pads, and properly places the grounding pads. This nurse coordinates the transfer to the operating bed and helps the client to a comfortable position. The nurse assesses the skin, especially of older clients, for bruising or injury, placing extra padding as indicated.

The client is usually in a supine position after transfer to the operating bed. Anesthesia may be given with the client supine, and he or she may then be repositioned for surgery (Figure 21-12).

The circulating nurse coordinates positioning of the client for surgery and modifies the position according to the client's safety and special needs. Factors influencing the *timing* of repositioning include the following:

- The surgical site
- The age and size of the client
- The anesthetic delivery technique
- Pain on movement (conscious client)

Factors influencing the actual *position* include the following:

- The specific procedure being performed
- The surgeon's request
- The client's age, size, and weight
- Any pulmonary, skeletal, or muscular limitations, such as arthritis, joint replacements, or emphysema

Table 21-6 lists complications related to prolonged immobility during surgery and some preventive nursing actions.

The dorsal recumbent, prone, lithotomy, and lateral positions are most often used for surgery. Figure 21-12 shows many surgical positions and the use of protective padding. When general anesthesia is used, the nurse positions the client slowly to prevent hypotension from blood vessel dilation. Proper positioning is ensured by assessing for the following:

- Anatomic alignment
- Interference with circulation and breathing
- Protection of skeletal and neuromuscular structures
- Optimal exposure of the operative site and IV line
- Adequate access to the client for the anesthesia provider
- The client's comfort and safety
- Preservation of the client's dignity

The nurse is aware of potential complications related to specific positions and modifies care as needed. For example, clients in the lithotomy position may develop leg swelling, pain in the legs or back, and reduced sensation or foot pulses. The nurse ensures proper padding and position changes at regular intervals. Throughout the surgery, the nurse prevents obstruction of circulation, respiration, or nerve conduction

EVIDENCE-BASED PRACTICE for Nursing

Pressure ulcers do occur in surgery

Schoonhoven, L., Defloor, T., Grypdonck, M. (2002). Incidence of pressure ulcers due to surgery. *Journal of Clinical Nursing, 11*(4), 479-487.

This descriptive, prospective study sought to determine the incidence of pressure ulcers caused by positioning during surgery. Two hundred and eight subjects from nine different surgical specialties were enrolled in the study as a convenience sample. The sample included 73 women and 136 men, with a mean age of 59 years. Study criteria included that the surgery was planned and expected to have a minimum duration of 4 hours. The population did not contain clients undergoing gynecologic procedures or surgery for trauma. The presence of a pressure ulcer before surgery did not exclude the subject; however, the preexisting ulcers were not included in the analysis. Mean length of the surgical procedures was 6 hours and 38 minutes.

The skin of the subjects was assessed before surgery and the findings documented. Skin was assessed immediately after surgery and daily for 14 days or until discharge. Skin lesions were described, categorized by a standard scale, and photographed. Subjects discharged before 14 days were contacted and asked to describe any skin lesions.

A total of 44 (21.2%) subjects developed one or more pressure ulcers (n = 70) within 48 hours after surgery. An additional 12 subjects developed pressure ulcers on day 3 or later after surgery. The majority of lesions were on the heels with about 15% of lesions forming on the sacral area. Some subjects developed ulcers on the chin and ears as a result of a specific surgical procedure for vertebral surgery that involved a face mask and traction. About 12% of subjects were impaired in some way as a result of their pressure ulcers.

Level of Evidence: 3—Well-designed trial without randomization.

Critique. The prospective nature of the study is a major strength as is the preoperative assessment. The data were collected by four persons trained in the assessment of pressure ulcers, with high inter-rater reliability. Randomization would have added strength to the study. No mention is made of racial or ethnic differences among the subjects. The study was conducted in The Netherlands, where there is a relatively homogeneous ethnic population. While homogeneity limits generalization to other populations, it strengthens the validity of findings within an ethnic population.

Implications for Nursing. Most health care professionals are under the false impression that pressure ulcer formation is a slow process seen in clients who are chronically immobile. This study reinforces the findings of other studies that complete immobility—even for short periods—is a major risk factor for pressure ulcer development. Nurses should take proactive, preventive measures for all clients who are immobilized for 2 hours or longer, no matter what their age or health status.

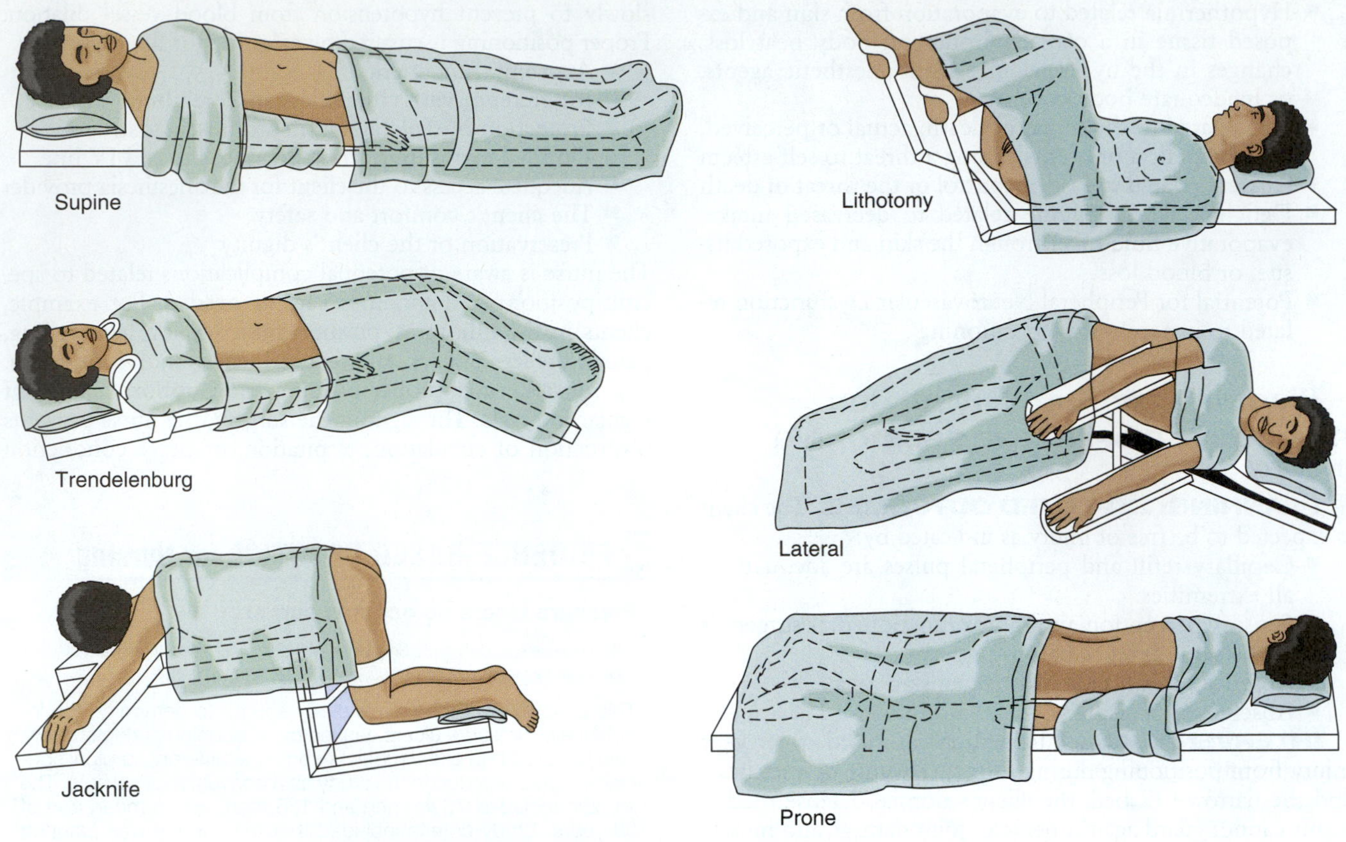

Figure 21-12 ■ Common surgical positions.

TABLE 21-6 Interventions to Prevent Neuromuscular Complications Related to Intraoperative Positioning

Anatomic Area	Complications	Interventions
Brachial plexus	Paralysis Loss of sensation in the arm and shoulder	Pad the elbow. Avoid excessive abduction. Secure the arm firmly on an arm board, positioned at shoulder level.
Radial nerve	Wrist drop	Support the wrist with padding. Do not overtighten wrist straps.
Medial or ulnar nerves	Hand deformities	Place a safety strap above or below the area.
Peroneal nerve	Foot drop	Place a pillow or padding under the knees. Support the lower extremities. Do not overtighten leg straps.
Tibial nerve	Loss of sensation on the plantar surface of the foot	Place a safety strap above the ankle. Do not place equipment on the lower extremities.
Joints	Stiffness Pain Inflammation	Place a pillow or foam padding under bony prominences. Maintain good body alignment. Slightly flex joints and support with pillows, trochanter rolls, or pads.

caused by tight straps, poorly placed pads and pillows, or the position of the bed.

Critical Thinking Challenge

The 62-year-old client about to have a vaginal hysterectomy is brought into the OR. She weighs 96 pounds.

1. In what position should you place this client for a vaginal hysterectomy?
2. What areas on this client are most likely to be injured as a result of poor positioning or inadequate padding?

evolve For suggested answer guidelines, go to http://evolve.elsevier.com/Iggy/.

IMPAIRED SKIN INTEGRITY AND IMPAIRED TISSUE INTEGRITY

NOC **PLANNING: EXPECTED OUTCOMES.** The client is expected to have minimal skin and tissue impairment or infection as a result of surgery as indicated by:

- Absence of inflammation, purulent drainage, or dehiscence of the incision
- Maintenance of a white blood cell count within normal limits

INTERVENTIONS. Surgery places the client at risk for wound complications (such as incisional tears and lacerations), infection, and loss of body fluids. Sterile surgical

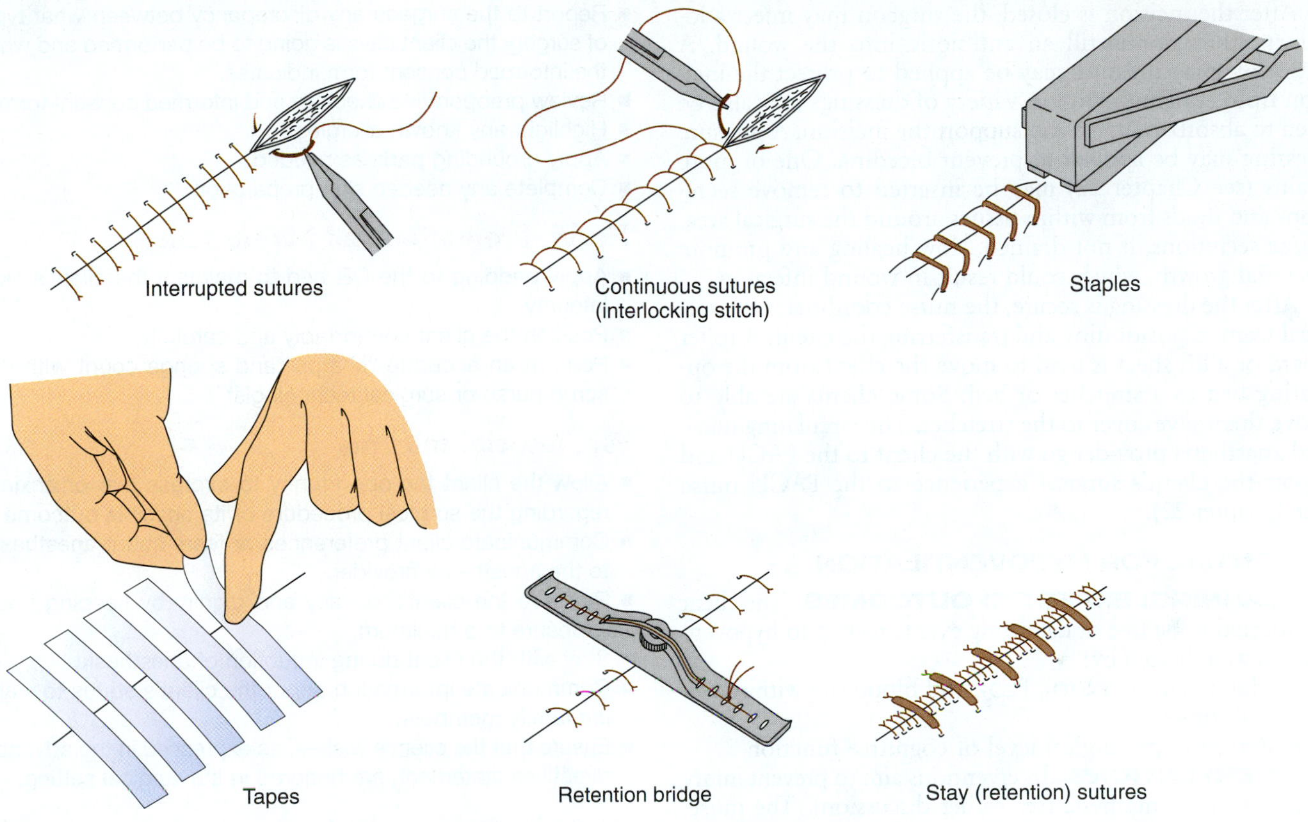

Figure 21-13 ■ Common skin closures.

technique and the use of protective drapes, skin closures, and dressings reduce complications and promote wound healing.

Plastic Adhesive Drape. If a sterile plastic adhesive drape is used, the scrub nurse helps the surgical assistant apply the drape after the surgical site has been cleaned and dried. The plastic drape is applied directly to the client's skin to prevent shifting and exposure of skin edges. *The surgeon makes the incision through the plastic drape.* The cut edge sticks to the skin and creates a seal to reduce bacterial movement into the wound. The scrub nurse and surgical assistant *gently* remove the drape after closure of the incision. Special attention is paid to older clients and those with fragile skin to prevent skin tearing when the adhesive drape is removed.

Skin Closures. Skin and tissue closures, such as sutures and staples, are used to:

- Hold wound edges in place until wound healing is complete
- Occlude blood vessels, preventing hemorrhage and fluid loss
- Prevent wound contamination

The quality of the wound edges and the type of closure material used determine the strength and integrity of the closure. The wound is usually closed in layers to keep tissues together and promote healing with minimal scarring. The surgeon selects the method and type of closures based on the surgical site, the tissue involved, the size and depth of the wound, and the age and medical history of the client. A combination of sutures and clips is commonly used for closure of internal layers of the wound. Staples, retention (stay) sutures, and skin closure tapes (Steri-Strips) are used for closure of superficial skin wounds. Figure 21-13 shows commonly used wound closures.

A suture is one or more strands of material and varies by size, or gauge. The size sequence, from largest diameter to smallest, is 5, 4, 3, 2, 1, 0, 00 (2-0), 000 (3-0), 0000 (4-0), and so forth, to 11-0. Size 0 is thick and often used to close the deep layers of an abdominal wound. The smaller diameter sutures (e.g., 11-0) are used in plastic surgery and eye surgery. Other suture material features, such as type (e.g., nylon, silk, Vicryl), color (e.g., green, blue, black, white, violet), and structure (e.g., twisted, braided), are listed on the package.

Sutures are absorbable or nonabsorbable. **Absorbable sutures** are digested over time by body enzymes. These sutures first lose strength and then gradually disappear from the tissue. Catgut suture, such as "plain gut" and "chromic gut," is a type of natural absorbable suture. Other absorbable sutures are made of synthetic materials. The client's health, the presence of inflammation, and the type of suture used all influence absorption time, which is usually about 2 weeks.

Nonabsorbable sutures become encapsulated in the tissue during the healing process and remain in the tissue unless they are removed. These sutures are made of silk, cotton, steel, nylon, polyester, or other synthetic material. *Body enzymes do not affect nonabsorbable sutures.* Nonabsorbable sutures are used for connecting blood vessels, "wiring" the sternum together after open heart surgery, and closing external wounds. The surgeon may use a double or interlocking stitch to increase closure integrity. Retention (stay) sutures (see Figure 21-13) may be used in addition to standard sutures for clients at high risk for impaired wound healing (those having major abdominal surgery, obese clients, clients with diabetes, and those taking steroids).

After the incision is closed, the surgeon may inject a local anesthetic or instill an antibiotic into the wound. A gauze or spray dressing may be applied to protect the incision from contamination. A variety of dressings may also be used to absorb drainage and support the incision. A pressure dressing may be applied to prevent bleeding. One or more drains (see Chapter 22) may be inserted to remove secretions and fluids from within tissues around the surgical area. These secretions, if not drained, slow healing and promote bacterial growth, which could result in wound infection.

After the dressing is secure, the nurse coordinates the surgical team in positioning and transferring the client. A roller board or a lift sheet is used to move the client from the operating bed to a stretcher or bed. Some clients are able to move themselves over to the stretcher. The circulating nurse and anesthesia provider go with the client to the PACU and report the client's surgical experience to the PACU nurse (see Chapter 22).

POTENTIAL FOR HYPOVENTILATION

NOC **PLANNING: EXPECTED OUTCOMES.** The client is expected to be free of damaging events related to hypoventilation as indicated by:

- Maintenance of SaO_2, PaO_2, and blood pH within normal limits
- Return to presurgical level of cognitive function

INTERVENTIONS. Interventions aim to prevent injury resulting from anesthesia (see earlier discussion). The nurse, surgeon, and anesthesia provider monitor the client according to official standards. These standards, adopted by both the American Society of Anesthesiologists and the American Association of Nurse Anesthetists, include continuous monitoring of breathing, circulation, and cardiac rhythms; blood pressure and heart rate recordings every 5 minutes; and the continuous presence of an anesthesia provider during the case.

Evaluation: Outcomes

The nurse evaluates the care of the client during surgery on the basis of the identified nursing diagnoses and collaborative problems. The expected outcomes are that the client:

- Is safely anesthetized without complications
- Does not experience any injury related to surgical positioning or equipment
- Is free of skin or tissue contamination during surgery
- Is free of skin tears, bruises, redness, abrasion, or maceration over pressure points and elsewhere

Specific indicators for these outcomes are listed for each nursing diagnosis and collaborative problem under the Planning and Implementation section (see earlier).

GET READY for the NCLEX Examination!

KEY POINTS

Safe Effective Care Environment

- Ensure that all personnel entering the OR are wearing proper OR attire for their role.
- Observe for and inform OR personnel of any break in sterile field or sterile technique.
- Check the identity of the client.
- Report to the surgeon any discrepancy between what type of surgery the client says is going to be performed and what the informed consent form indicates.
- Review preoperative checklist and informed consent forms.
- Highlight any known allergies.
- Apply grounding pads as needed.
- Complete any needed skin preparation.

Health Promotion and Maintenance

- Apply padding to the OR bed to maintain the client's skin integrity.
- Position the client comfortably and carefully.
- Perform an accurate "sharps" and sponge count with the scrub nurse or surgical technologist.

Psychosocial Integrity

- Allow the client the opportunity to express fear or anxiety regarding the surgical procedure or its possible outcome.
- Communicate client preferences or fears about anesthesia to the anesthesia provider.
- Preserve the client's privacy and dignity by keeping body exposure to a minimum.
- Stay with the client during induction of anesthesia.
- Communicate information about the client's status to waiting family members.
- Ensure that the client's wishes, as expressed in the advance directives statement, are honored in the surgical setting.

Physiological Integrity

- Ask the client when was the last time he or she had anything to eat or drink.
- Know the expected client responses and side effects to anesthesia induction and awakening produced by the various anesthetic agents.
- Assess the client for tachycardia, increased end-tidal carbon dioxide level, and increased body temperature as indicators of malignant hyperthermia.
- Keep dantrolene sodium available during and after surgery as drug therapy for malignant hyperthermia.
- Monitor the client's airway, level of consciousness, oxygen saturation, ECG, and vital signs during and immediately following conscious sedation.
- Assess all skin areas and document findings before transferring the client to the postanesthesia care unit.

ADDITIONAL STUDY RESOURCES

Go to your Student CD-ROM for Review Questions for the NCLEX Examination.

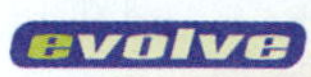

Go to http://evolve.elsevier.com/Iggy/ for Integrated Management of Care Questions for the NCLEX Examination.

SELECTED BIBLIOGRAPHY

Asterisk indicates a classic or definitive work on this subject.

Agarwal, M., Hamilton-Stewart, P., & Dixon, R. (2002). Contaminated operating room boots: The potential for infection. *American Journal of Infection Control, 30*(3), 179-183.

Allen, G. (2002). Supplemental perioperative oxygen to reduce the incidence of surgical-wound infection. *AORN Journal, 76*(2), 330-331.

American Society of PeriAnesthesia Nurses. (2000). *Standards of perianesthesia nursing practice.* New Jersey: Author.

Association of PeriOperative Registered Nurses. (2002). Recommended practices for skin preparation of patients. *AORN Journal, 75*(1), 184-187.

Association of periOperative Registered Nurses. (2003a). Position statement: AORN official statement on RN first assistant. In *Standards, recommended practices and guidelines* (pp. 159-160). Denver: Author.

Association of periOperative Registered Nurses. (2003b). Position statement: Perioperative care of patients with do not resuscitate (DNR) orders. In *Standards, recommended practices and guidelines* (pp. 155-156). Denver: Author.

Association of periOperative Registered Nurses. (2003c). Recommended practices for the care and cleaning of surgical instruments and powered equipment. In *Standards, recommended practices and guidelines* (pp. 291-299). Denver: Author.

Association of periOperative Registered Nurses. (2003d). Recommended practices for disinfection. In *Standards, recommended practices and guidelines* (pp. 227-231). Denver: Author.

Association of periOperative Registered Nurses. (2003e). Recommended practices for documentation of perioperative nursing care. In *Standards, recommended practices and guidelines* (pp. 233-235). Denver: Author.

Association of periOperative Registered Nurses. (2003f). Recommended practices for environmental cleaning for the surgical practice setting. In *Standards, recommended practices and guidelines* (pp. 257-263). Denver: Author.

Association of periOperative Registered Nurses. (2003g). Recommended practices for hazards in the surgical environment. In *Standards, recommended practices and guidelines* (pp. 283-289). Denver: Author.

Association of periOperative Registered Nurses. (2003h). Recommended practices for laser safety in the practice setting. In *Standards, recommended practices and guidelines* (pp. 301-305). Denver: Author.

Association of periOperative Registered Nurses. (2003i). Recommended practices for managing the patient receiving conscious sedation/analgesia. In *Standards, recommended practices and guidelines* (pp. 213-220). Denver: Author.

Association of periOperative Registered Nurses. (2003j). Recommended practices for positioning the patient in the perioperative practice setting. In *Standards, recommended practices and guidelines* (pp. 323-331). Denver: Author.

Association of periOperative Registered Nurses. (2003k). Recommended practices for skin preparation. In *Standards, recommended practices and guidelines* (pp. 339-343). Denver: Author.

Association of periOperative Registered Nurses. (2003l). Recommended practices for sponge, sharp, and instrument counts. In *Standards, recommended practices and guidelines* (pp. 221-226). Denver: Author.

Association of periOperative Registered Nurses. (2003m). Recommended practices for sterile field-maintaining. In *Standards, recommended practices and guidelines* (pp. 351-355). Denver: Author.

Association of periOperative Registered Nurses. (2003n). Recommended practices for sterilization in the practice setting. In *Standards, recommended practices and guidelines* (pp. 357-366). Denver: Author.

Association of periOperative Registered Nurses. (2003o). Recommended practices for surgical attire. In *Standards, recommended practices and guidelines* (pp. 215-219). Denver: Author.

Association of periOperative Registered Nurses. (2003p). Recommended practices for surgical hand scrubs. In *Standards, recommended practices and guidelines* (pp. 277-281). Denver: Author.

Association of periOperative Registered Nurses. (2003q). Recommended practices for traffic patterns in the perioperative practice setting. In *Standards, recommended practices and guidelines* (pp. 373-375). Denver: Author.

Association of periOperative Registered Nurses. (2003r). Recommended practices for use and selection of barrier materials for surgical gowns and drapes. In *Standards, recommended practices and guidelines* (pp. 271-275). Denver: Author.

Bauer, J. (2002). Surgical tape. *RN, 65*(6), 63-65.

Beyea, S. (2002). Accident prevention in surgical settings: Keeping patients safe. *AORN Journal, 75*(2), 361-363.

*Curry, M. (1994). Perioperative nursing care of the elderly patient: A case study. *ACORN Journal, 7*(2), 23-26.

Denault, D. (2002). What counts most in the operating room. *Nursing2102, 32*(4), 32hn8.

Dochterman, J., & Bulechek, G. (Eds.). (2004). *Nursing interventions classification (NIC)* (4th ed.). St. Louis: Mosby.

Documenting postoperative transfer. (2002). *Nursing2102, 32*(3), 82.

Domanovic, M., et al. (2003). Using intraoperative radiation therapy: A case study. *AORN Journal, 77*(2), 412-417.

Dunn, D. (2004). Preventing perioperative complications in an older adult. *Nursing 2004, 34*(11), 36-41.

Ebersole, P., Hess, P., & Luggen, A. (2004). *Toward healthy aging: Human needs and nursing response* (6th ed.). St. Louis: Mosby.

ECRI. (2003). Health devices: Focus on surgical fire safety. 32(1), Plymouth Meeting, PA: Author.

*Entrup, M.H. (1991). Perioperative complications of anesthesia. *Surgical Clinics of North America, 71*(6), 1151-1173.

Flower, J. (2000). Beyond surgery: Predictions for surgery in the next century. *Surgical Services Management, 6*(1), 29-32.

Folin, A., Nyberg, B., & Nordstrom, G. (2000). Reducing blood exposures during orthopedic surgical procedures. *AORN Journal, 71*(3), 573-582.

Garvin, M. (2003). Perioperative hand hygiene: the challenge of integrating rinseless products in the OR. *Infection Control Today, 7*(4), 36-40.

Haslego, S. (2002). Malignant hyperthermia: How to spot it early. *RN, 65*(7), 31-36.

Homa, D., & Palfreyman, M. (2000). Infectious diseases in the O.R. *CRNA: The Clinical Forum for Nurse Anesthetists, 11*(1), 8-14.

Keating, E.M., & Meding, J. (2002). Perioperative blood management practices in elective orthopaedic surgery. *Journal of the American Academy of Orthopaedic Surgeons, 10*(6), 393-399.

Kjonniken, I., et al. (2002). Preoperative hair removal: A systematic literature review. *AORN Journal, 75*(5), 928-936, 938, 940.

Martyn, V., et al. (2002). The theory and practice of bloodless surgery. *Transfusion and Apheresis Science, 27*(1), 29-43.

McEwen, D. (2003). Ambulatory surgery. In M.H. Meeker & J.C. Rothrock (Eds.), *Alexander's care of the patient in surgery* (12th ed., pp. 1189-1210). St. Louis: Mosby.

Meckes, P.F. (2003). Geriatric surgery. In M.H. Meeker & J.C. Rothrock (Eds.), *Alexander's care of the patient in surgery* (12th ed., pp. 1295-1315). St. Louis: Mosby.

Meeker, M.H., & Rothrock, J.C. (2003). *Alexander's care of the patient in surgery* (12th ed.). St. Louis: Mosby.

Meltzer, B. (2003). Seven keys to fast-track anesthesia. *Outpatient Surgery, IV*(3), 52-62.

Mok, E., & Wong, K-Y. (2003). Effects of music on patient anxiety. *AORN Journal, 77*(2), 396-410.

Moorhead, S., Johnson, M., & Maas, M. (Eds.). (2004). *Nursing outcomes classification (NOC)* (3rd ed.). St. Louis: Mosby.

Nussbaum, R., McInnes, R., & Willard, H. (2001). *Thompson & Thompson: Genetics in medicine* (6th ed.). Philadelphia: W.B. Saunders.

Quinn, A. (2002). Cyberknife: A robotic radiosurgery system. *Clinical Journal of Oncology Nursing, 6*(3), 149, 156.

Schoonhoven, L., Defloor, T., Grypdonck, M. (2002). Incidence of pressure ulcers due to surgery. *Journal of Clinical Nursing, 11*(4), 479-487.

Schroeter, K. (2003). Ethics in perioperative practice: Principles and applications. *AORN Journal, 75*(4), 818-824.

Squires, A. (2003). Documenting surgical incision site care. *Nursing2003, 33*(1), 74.

Warnock, K. (2003). Preventing surgical errors: The role of the surgical technologist. *The Surgical Technologist, 35*(6), 15-29.

CHAPTER 22

Interventions for Postoperative Clients

REBECCA M. PATTON

LEARNING OUTCOMES

After studying this chapter, you should be able to:

1. Describe the ongoing head-to-toe assessment of the postoperative client.
2. Prioritize nursing interventions for the client recovering from surgery and anesthesia during the first 24 hours.
3. Prioritize nursing care for the client who has respiratory depression after surgery.
4. Discuss the criteria for determining readiness of the client to be discharged from the postanesthesia care unit.
5. Use proper technique for wound assessment and dressing changes.
6. Recognize wound complications after surgery.
7. Describe steps to take when a client has a surgical wound dehiscence or evisceration.
8. Compare the actions, side effects, and nursing implications for different types of drug therapy for pain management after surgery.
9. Develop a community-based teaching plan for clients after surgery.

Go to your Student CD-ROM for Review Questions for the NCLEX Examination keyed to these Learning Outcomes.

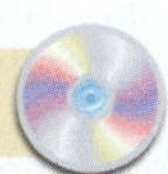

The postoperative period starts at the completion of surgery and transfer of the client to the postanesthesia care unit (PACU), same day surgery unit (ambulatory care unit), or the intensive care unit. Discharge from these areas is based on the stability of the client and the meeting of specific discharge criteria. Many clients are able to be discharged to home shortly after the surgery is completed. They are observed and monitored until discharge criteria are met and are then discharged. Some clients move from the specialized nursing care in the PACU to a hospital inpatient floor or critical care unit for additional nursing care.

The postoperative period continues after the client's condition is stabilized, as well as after the client is discharged from the ambulatory surgery facility or hospital. The actual time spent away from home after surgery varies according to age, physical health, self-care ability, support systems, type and length of surgical procedure, anesthesia, any complications, and community resources.

OVERVIEW

The purpose of a PACU or recovery room is the ongoing evaluation and stabilization of clients, to anticipate, prevent, and treat complications after surgery. The PACU is usually located close to the surgical suite for ease of access and client transfer. The unit is usually a large and open room to provide best observation of clients and easy access to supplies and emergency equipment. Usually, adults are separated from children. The client area may be divided into individual cubicles. Privacy curtains or screens are closed only during bedside procedures. Each cubicle has equipment to monitor and care for the client, such as oxygen, suction equipment, cardiac monitors, airway equipment, and emergency drugs.

After the surgery is completed, the circulating nurse and the anesthesia provider accompany the client to the PACU. When the client is in critical condition, transfer may be directly from the operating room (OR) to the intensive (critical) care unit. On arrival, the anesthesia provider and the circulating nurse give the PACU nurse a verbal report (Table 22-1).

The PACU nurse is skilled in the care of clients with multiple medical and surgical problems immediately after a surgical procedure. This area requires in-depth knowledge of anesthetic agents, pharmacology, pain management, and surgical procedures. The PACU nurse is skilled in assessment and can make quick decisions if emergencies or complications occur. The client is monitored closely. The anesthesia provider and surgeon are consulted as needed.

TABLE 22-1 Report Guidelines on Arrival in the Postanesthesia Care Unit

The anesthesia providers explain the following:
- Type and extent of the surgical procedure
- Type of anesthesia
- Client's tolerance of anesthesia and the surgical procedure
- Client's allergies
- Pathologic condition
- Status of vital signs
- Type and amount of IV fluids and medications administered
- Estimated blood loss (EBL)
- Any intraoperative complications, such as a traumatic intubation

The circulating nurse adds information related to the following:
- Client's primary language and any sensory impairments
- Client's anxiety level before receiving anesthesia
- Special requests that were verbalized by the client preoperatively
- Client's preoperative and intraoperative respiratory function and dysfunction
- Pertinent medical history
- Location and type of incisions, dressings, catheters, tubes, drains, or packing
- Intake and output, including current IV fluid administration and estimated blood loss
- Joint or limb immobility while in the operating room, especially in the older client
- Other intraoperative positioning that may be relevant in the postoperative phase
- Any other important intraoperative occurrences

COLLABORATIVE MANAGEMENT

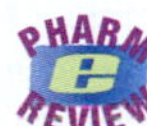

The Concept Map on p. 356 uses a client who is recovering from abdominal surgery as an example for addressing the common assessment and nursing care issues for clients in the postoperative period.

Assessment

HISTORY

Use the surgical team's report to plan the care for an individual client. After receiving the report and assessing the client, review the medical record for information about the client's history, presurgical physical condition, and emotional status. If possible, review this information *before* the client arrives in the PACU. If the client remains as an inpatient, the surgical and postanesthesia information is incorporated into the postoperative plan of care. Chapter 20 identifies situations that increase a client's risk for the following complications:

- Allergic reactions
- Hypothermia
- Hyperthermia
- Hypertension
- Hypotension
- Hypovolemic shock
- Renal failure
- Electrolyte imbalances
- Dysrhythmias
- Chronic heart failure
- Paralytic ileus
- Acute urinary retention
- Deep vein thrombosis (DVT)
- Pulmonary embolism (PE)
- Atelectasis or pneumonia
- Laryngeal edema
- Ventilator dependence
- Gastrointestinal (GI) bleeding
- Disseminated intravascular coagulation (DIC)
- Anemia
- Wound evisceration

PHYSICAL ASSESSMENT/CLINICAL MANIFESTATIONS

Assess the client and record data on a PACU record form (Figure 22-1). Assessment data include level of consciousness, temperature, pulse, respiration, and blood pressure. *The most important area to assess is respiration.* Examine the surgical area for bleeding. Monitor vital signs as often as your facility's policy states, the client's condition warrants, and the surgeon prescribes. Once the client is discharged from the PACU, vital signs are often measured every 15 minutes for four times, every 30 minutes for four times, every 2 hours for four times, and then every 4 hours for 24 to 48 hours if the client's condition is stable. Thereafter, vital signs are assessed according to the facility's policy, the client's condition, and the nurse's judgment.

The health care team determines the client's readiness for discharge from the PACU by the presence of a recovery score rating of at least 10 on the recovery scale (see Figure 22-1). Other criteria for discharge (e.g., stable vital signs; normal body temperature; no overt bleeding; return of gag, cough, and swallow reflexes; and the ability to take liquids) may be specific to the facility. After you determine that all criteria have been met, the client is discharged by the anesthesia provider to the hospital unit or to home. If an anesthesia provider has not been involved, which may be the case with local anesthesia or conscious sedation, the surgeon or nurse discharges the client once the discharge criteria have been met.

Assessment continues from the PACU to the intensive care or medical-surgical nursing unit. If the client is to be discharged from the PACU to home, assessment is continued by home care nurses or by the client or family members after instruction.

RESPIRATORY SYSTEM

AIRWAY ASSESSMENT. *When the client is admitted to the PACU, immediately assess for a patent airway and adequate gas exchange.* An artificial airway, such as an endotracheal (ET) tube, a nasal trumpet, or an oral airway, may be in place. If the client is receiving oxygen, document the type of delivery device and the concentration or liter flow of the oxygen. Continuously monitor pulse oximetry for oxygen saturation while the client is in the PACU.

Assess the rate, pattern, and depth of breathing to determine adequacy of air exchange. A respiratory rate of less than 10 breaths/min indicates anesthetic- or opioid analgesic–induced depression. Rapid, shallow respirations signal cardiac problems, increased metabolic rate, or pain.

BREATH SOUNDS. Listen to the lungs over all lung fields to assess breath sounds. Also check symmetry of breath sounds. If, for example, the client has an ET tube, it could move down into the right mainstem bronchus and prevent left lung expansion. In this case, lung sounds on the left are absent or decreased and only the right chest wall rises and falls with breathing.

OTHER RESPIRATORY ASSESSMENTS. Respiratory assessment includes ongoing inspection of the chest wall for accessory muscle use, sternal retraction, and diaphragmatic breathing. These signs could indicate an excessive anesthetic effect, airway obstruction, or paralysis,

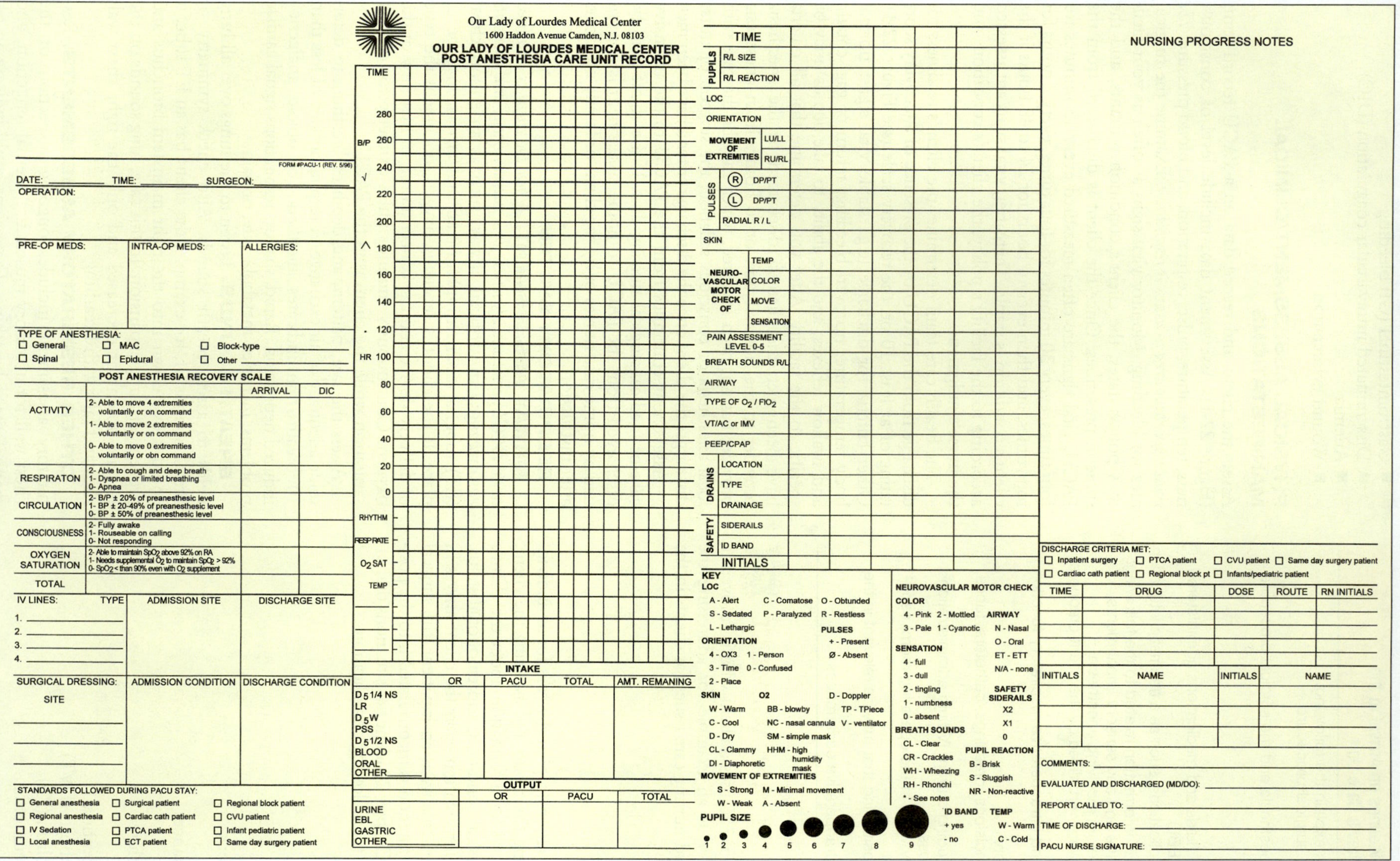

Our Lady of Lourdes Medical Center
1600 Haddon Avenue Camden, N.J. 08103
OUR LADY OF LOURDES MEDICAL CENTER
POST ANESTHESIA CARE UNIT RECORD

FORM #PACU-1 (REV. 5/96)

DATE: ______ TIME: ______ SURGEON: ______
OPERATION:

PRE-OP MEDS: | INTRA-OP MEDS: | ALLERGIES:

TYPE OF ANESTHESIA:
☐ General ☐ MAC ☐ Block-type ______
☐ Spinal ☐ Epidural ☐ Other ______

POST ANESTHESIA RECOVERY SCALE		ARRIVAL	DIC
ACTIVITY	2- Able to move 4 extremities voluntarily or on command 1- Able to move 2 extremities voluntarily or on command 0- Able to move 0 extremities voluntarily or obn command		
RESPIRATON	2- Able to cough and deep breath 1- Dyspnea or limited breathing 0- Apnea		
CIRCULATION	2- B/P ± 20% of preanesthesic level 1- BP ± 20-49% of preanesthesic level 0- BP ± 50% of preanesthesic level		
CONSCIOUSNESS	2- Fully awake 1- Rouseable on calling 0- Not responding		
OXYGEN SATURATION	2- Able to maintain SpO_2 above 92% on RA 1- Needs supplemental O_2 to maintain SpO_2 > 92% 0- SpO_2 < than 90% even with O_2 supplement		
TOTAL			

IV LINES:	TYPE	ADMISSION SITE	DISCHARGE SITE
1.			
2.			
3.			
4.			

SURGICAL DRESSING: SITE	ADMISSION CONDITION	DISCHARGE CONDITION

STANDARDS FOLLOWED DURING PACU STAY:
☐ General anesthesia ☐ Surgical patient ☐ Regional block patient
☐ Regional anesthesia ☐ Cardiac cath patient ☐ CVU patient
☐ IV Sedation ☐ PTCA patient ☐ Infant pediatric patient
☐ Local anesthesia ☐ ECT patient ☐ Same day surgery patient

TIME
B/P 280 260 240 220 200 180 160 140 120
HR 100 80 60 40 20 0
RHYTHM
RESP RATE
O_2 SAT
TEMP

INTAKE	OR	PACU	TOTAL	AMT. REMANING
D 5 1/4 NS				
LR				
D_5W				
PSS				
D 5 1/2 NS				
BLOOD				
ORAL				
OTHER______				

OUTPUT	OR	PACU	TOTAL
URINE			
EBL			
GASTRIC			
OTHER______			

TIME						
PUPILS R/L SIZE						
PUPILS R/L REACTION						
LOC						
ORIENTATION						
MOVEMENT OF EXTREMITIES LU/LL						
MOVEMENT OF EXTREMITIES RU/RL						
PULSES Ⓡ DP/PT						
PULSES Ⓛ DP/PT						
PULSES RADIAL R / L						
SKIN						
NEURO-VASCULAR MOTOR CHECK OF TEMP						
COLOR						
MOVE						
SENSATION						
PAIN ASSESSMENT LEVEL 0-5						
BREATH SOUNDS R/L						
AIRWAY						
TYPE OF O_2 / FIO_2						
VT/AC or IMV						
PEEP/CPAP						
DRAINS LOCATION						
DRAINS TYPE						
DRAINS DRAINAGE						
SAFETY SIDERAILS						
SAFETY ID BAND						
INITIALS						

KEY
LOC
A - Alert C - Comatose O - Obtunded
S - Sedated P - Paralyzed R - Restless
L - Lethargic
PULSES
+ - Present
Ø - Absent
ORIENTATION
4 - OX3 1 - Person
3 - Time 0 - Confused
2 - Place
SKIN
W - Warm
C - Cool
D - Dry
CL - Clammy
DI - Diaphoretic
O2
BB - blowby
NC - nasal cannula
SM - simple mask
HHM - high humidity mask
D - Doppler
TP - TPiece
V - ventilator
MOVEMENT OF EXTREMITIES
S - Strong M - Minimal movement
W - Weak A - Absent
PUPIL SIZE
1 2 3 4 5 6 7 8 9

NEUROVASCULAR MOTOR CHECK
COLOR
4 - Pink 2 - Mottled
3 - Pale 1 - Cyanotic
AIRWAY
N - Nasal
O - Oral
ET - ETT
N/A - none
SENSATION
4 - full
3 - dull
2 - tingling
1 - numbness
0 - absent
SAFETY SIDERAILS
X2
X1
0
BREATH SOUNDS
CL - Clear
CR - Crackles
WH - Wheezing
RH - Rhonchi
* - See notes
PUPIL REACTION
B - Brisk
S - Sluggish
NR - Non-reactive
ID BAND
+ yes
- no
TEMP
W - Warm
C - Cold

NURSING PROGRESS NOTES

DISCHARGE CRITERIA MET:
☐ Inpatient surgery ☐ PTCA patient ☐ CVU patient ☐ Same day surgery patient
☐ Cardiac cath patient ☐ Regional block pt ☐ Infants/pediatric patient

TIME	DRUG	DOSE	ROUTE	RN INITIALS

INITIALS	NAME	INITIALS	NAME

COMMENTS: ______
EVALUATED AND DISCHARGED (MD/DO): ______
REPORT CALLED TO: ______
TIME OF DISCHARGE: ______
PACU NURSE SIGNATURE: ______

Figure 22-1 ■ Example of a postanesthesia care unit record. (Courtesy of Our Lady of Lourdes Medical Center, Camden, NJ.)

which could result in hypoxia. Listen for snoring and **stridor** (a high-pitched crowing sound). Snoring and stridor are signs of airway obstruction resulting from tracheal or laryngeal spasm or edema, mucus in the airway, or blockage of the airway from edema or tongue relaxation. When neuromuscular blocking agents are retained, the client has muscle weakness, which could affect gas exchange. Indicators of muscle weakness include the inability to maintain a head lift, weak hand grasps, and an abdominal breathing pattern.

When the client returns to an inpatient unit, complete an initial assessment on arrival (Chart 22-1) and then continue to assess for indications of respiratory depression or hypoxemia. Auscultate the lungs to check for effective expansion and for abnormal breath sounds. Listen to the lungs at least every 4 hours during the first 24 hours after surgery and then during every nursing shift, or more often, as indicated. Older clients, smokers, and clients with a history of pulmonary disease are at greater risk for respiratory complications after surgery and need more frequent assessment.

CARDIOVASCULAR SYSTEM

VITAL SIGNS. Assess blood pressure, pulse, and heart sounds on admission to the PACU and then at least every 15 minutes until the client's condition is stabile. Automated blood pressure cuffs and cardiac monitoring assist in continuous assessment.

Review vital signs after surgery for upward or downward trends and compare them to those taken before surgery. Report blood pressure changes of more or less than 25% of values obtained before surgery (15- to 20-point difference, systolic or diastolic) to the anesthesia provider or the surgeon. Decreased blood pressure, pulse pressure, and heart sounds indicate possible cardiac depression, fluid volume deficit, shock, hemorrhage, or the effects of drugs (see Chapters 7, 15, and 40). Bradycardia could indicate an anesthesia effect or hypothermia. Older clients are at risk for hypothermia because of age-related changes in the hypothalamus (the temperature regulation center), loss of subcutaneous tissue, and coolness of the operating room (OR) suite. An increased pulse rate could indicate hemorrhage, shock, or pain.

CARDIAC MONITORING. Cardiac monitoring is maintained until the client is discharged from the PACU. For clients at risk for dysrhythmias, monitoring may continue either on telemetry units or on general medical-surgical units. In assessing the vital signs of a client who is not being monitored continuously, compare the rate, rhythm, and quality of the apical pulse with the rate, rhythm, and quality of a peripheral pulse, such as the radial pulse. A **pulse deficit** (a difference between the apical and peripheral pulses) could indicate a dysrhythmia.

PERIPHERAL VASCULAR ASSESSMENT. Anesthesia and positioning during surgery (e.g., the lithotomy position for genitourinary procedures) may impair the peripheral circulation. Compare distal pulses on both feet for the quality of pulsation, observe the color and temperature of extremities, evaluate sensation, and determine the speed of capillary refill. Palpable dorsalis pedis pulses indicate adequate circulation and perfusion of the legs.

Assess the feet and legs for redness, pain, warmth, swelling, and **Homans' sign** (calf pain on dorsiflexion of the foot), which may occur with deep vein thrombosis (DVT). Foot and leg assessment may be performed once during a nursing shift, once daily, or once per visit, depending on the client's risk for complications and the facility's or agency's policy. (See Chapters 20 and 39 for more information on DVT.)

NEUROLOGIC SYSTEM

CEREBRAL FUNCTIONING. Assess cerebral function and the level of consciousness or awareness for *all* clients who have received general anesthesia (Table 22-2) or any type of sedation. Observe for lethargy, restlessness, or ir-

CHART 22-1

FOCUSED ASSESSMENT of
The Client on Arrival at the Medical-Surgical Unit After Discharge from the Postanesthesia Care Unit

Airway
- Is it patent?
- Is the neck in proper alignment?

Breathing
- What is the quality and pattern of the breathing?
- What is the respiratory rate and depth?
- Is the client receiving oxygen? At what setting? What is the pulse oximetry result?

Mental Status
- Is the client awake, able to be aroused, oriented, and aware?
- Does the client respond to verbal stimuli?

Surgical Incision Site
- How is it dressed?
- Mark the amount of drainage on the dressing immediately.
- Is there any bleeding or drainage under the client?
- Are there any drains present?
- Are the drains set properly (e.g., compressed if they should be compressed, not kinked, client not lying on them)?
- How much drainage is present in the drainage container?

Temperature, Pulse, and Blood Pressure
- Are these values within the client's baseline range?
- Are these values significantly different from when the client was in the postanesthesia care unit (PACU)?

Intravenous Fluids
- What type of solution is infusing and with what additives?
- How much solution was remaining on arrival?
- How much solution infused in the transport time from PACU?
- What is the infusion rate supposed to be set at? Is it?

Other Tubes
- Is there a nasogastric or other intestinal tube?
- What is the color, consistency, and amount of drainage?
- Is it set on suction if it is supposed to be? Is it on the right amount of suction?
- Is there a Foley catheter?
- Is the Foley draining properly?
- What is the color, clarity, and volume of urine output?

TABLE 22-2 Immediate Postoperative Neurologic Assessment: Return to Preoperative Level

Order of Return to Consciousness After General Anesthesia
1. Muscular irritability
2. Restlessness and delirium
3. Recognition of pain
4. Ability to reason and control behavior

Order of Return of Motor and Sensory Functioning After Local or Regional Anesthesia
1. Sense of touch
2. Sense of pain
3. Sense of warmth
4. Sense of cold
5. Ability to move

ritability, and test coherence and orientation. Determine awareness by observing responses to calling the client's name, touching the client, and giving simple commands such as "Open your eyes" and "Take a deep breath." Eye opening in response to a command indicates wakefulness or arousability but not necessarily awareness. Determine the degree of orientation to person, place, and time by asking the conscious client to answer questions such as "What is your name?" (person), "Where are you?" (place), and "What day is it?" (time).

CONSIDERATIONS FOR OLDER ADULTS

For an older adult, a rapid return to his or her level of orientation before surgery may not be realistic. Drugs and anesthetics often delay the older client's return of orientation (see Chapters 20 and 21).

Compare the client's baseline neurologic status (obtained before surgery) with the findings after surgery. Clients who had altered cerebral functioning before surgery as a result of another condition continue to have that alteration after surgery. After the client has a satisfactory level of consciousness (and all other criteria have been met), he or she is discharged from the PACU. On the medical-surgical nursing unit, assess the level of consciousness every 4 to 8 hours or as indicated by the client's condition and the facility's policy.

MOTOR AND SENSORY ASSESSMENT. Assess motor and sensory function for all clients who received general or regional anesthesia. General anesthesia depresses all voluntary motor function. Regional anesthesia alters the motor and sensory function of only part of the body. (See Chapter 21 for more information on anesthesia.) *Motor and sensory assessment is very important after epidural or spinal anesthesia.* Evaluate motor function by asking the client to move each extremity. The client who had epidural or spinal anesthesia remains in the PACU until sensory function (feeling) and voluntary motor movement of the legs have returned (see Table 22-2). Also assess the strength of each limb and compare the results on both sides.

Test for the return of sympathetic nervous system tone by gradually elevating the client's head and monitoring for hypotension. Begin this evaluation after the client's sensation has returned to at least the spinal dermatome level of T10. (See Chapter 44 for further neurologic assessment.) After the client is transferred to the nursing unit, continue neurologic assessment as indicated.

FLUID, ELECTROLYTE, AND ACID-BASE BALANCE. Fasting before and during surgery, the loss of fluid during the procedure, and the type and amount of blood or fluid given affect the client's fluid and electrolyte balance after surgery. Fluid volume deficit or fluid volume overload may occur after surgery. Sodium, potassium, chloride, and calcium imbalances also may result, as may changes in other electrolyte levels. Fluid and electrolyte imbalances occur more often in older or debilitated clients and in clients with health problems such as diabetes mellitus, Crohn's disease, or heart failure.

INTAKE AND OUTPUT. Intake and output measurement is part of the operative record and part of the circulating nurse's report to the PACU nurse. Record any intake or output, including intravenous (IV) fluid intake, vomitus, urine, and nasogastric (NG) tube drainage. You must know the total intake and output from both the OR and the PACU to assess fluid balance accurately and to complete the 24-hour intake and output record.

HYDRATION ASSESSMENT. The client's hydration status is assessed in the PACU and the medical-surgical unit. To determine hydration status, inspect the color and moisture of mucous membranes; the turgor, texture, and "tenting" of the skin (test over the sternum or forehead of an older client); the amount of drainage on dressings; and the presence of axillary sweat. Measure and compare total output (e.g., NG tube drainage, urine output, and wound drainage) with total intake to identify a possible fluid imbalance. Consider insensible fluid loss, such as sweat, when reviewing total output. Continue to assess intake and output as long as the client is at risk for fluid imbalances. Some facilities require intake and output to be measured if the client receives IV fluids or has a catheter, drains, or an NG tube.

INTRAVENOUS FLUIDS. Closely monitor IV fluids to promote fluid and electrolyte balance. Isotonic solutions such as lactated Ringer's (LR) and 5% dextrose with lactated Ringer's (D_5/LR) are used for IV fluid replacement in the PACU. After the client returns to the medical-surgical unit, the type and rate of IV infusions are based on need. A typical IV solution for the client being admitted to the nursing unit is 5% dextrose with 0.45% normal saline (D_5 0.45% NS). (See Chapters 15 and 17 for further discussion of IV fluids, electrolyte balance, and hydration assessment.)

ACID-BASE BALANCE. Acid-base balance is affected by the client's respiratory status before and during surgery; metabolic changes during surgery; and losses of acids or bases in drainage. For example, NG tube drainage or vomitus causes a loss of hydrochloric acid and leads to alkalosis. Examine arterial blood gas values and other laboratory values. (See Chapter 19 for more detailed information on acid-base imbalances.)

RENAL/URINARY SYSTEM. Control of urination may return immediately after surgery or may not return for hours after general or regional anesthesia. The effects of drugs, anesthetic agents, or manipulation during surgery can cause urine retention. Assess for urine retention by inspection, palpation, and percussion of the lower abdomen for bladder distention. Assessment may be difficult to perform after lower abdominal surgery. Urine retention is common early after surgery and requires intervention, such as intermittent (straight) catheterization, to empty the bladder.

When the client has an indwelling urinary (Foley) catheter, assess the urine for color, clarity, and amount. If the client is voiding, assess the frequency, amount per void, and any symptoms. Urine output should be close to the total intake for a 24-hour period. Consider other sources of output, such as sweat, vomitus, or diarrhea stools. Report a urine output of less than 30 mL/hr (240 mL per 8-hour nursing shift) to the physician. Decreased urine output may indicate hypovolemia or renal complications. (See Chapter 72 for renal/urinary assessment.)

GASTROINTESTINAL SYSTEM

NAUSEA AND VOMITING. One of the most common reactions after surgery is nausea and vomiting. About 30% of clients who receive general anesthesia have some form of gastrointestinal (GI) upset within the first 24 hours after surgery. Preventive therapy is effective in reducing the incidence. A drug often used is droperidol (Inapsine). Clients with a history of motion sickness are more likely to develop nausea and vomiting after surgery. Obese clients may be at risk because many anesthetics are retained by fat cells and remain in the body longer. Abdominal surgery and the use of opioid analgesics reduce intestinal peristalsis after surgery. These problems increase the risk for prolonged nausea and vomiting after surgery.

Nausea and vomiting can stress and irritate abdominal and GI wounds, increase intracranial pressure in clients who had head and neck surgery, elevate intraocular pressure in clients who had eye surgery, and increase the risk for aspiration. Assess the client continuously for nausea and vomiting. Often clients have nausea as the head of the bed is raised early after surgery. This symptom may occur with or without dizziness. You can help reduce this distressing symptom by having the client in a side-lying position before raising the head slowly.

GASTROINTESTINAL PERISTALSIS. In the PACU and later on the medical-surgical unit, assess for the return of peristalsis. Peristalsis may be delayed because of long anesthesia time, the amount of bowel handling during surgery, and opioid analgesic use. Clients who have abdominal surgery often have decreased peristalsis for at least 24 hours. This problem may persist for several days for those who have GI surgery.

Assessment. Auscultate for bowel sounds in all four abdominal quadrants and at the umbilicus. If NG suction is being used, turn off the suction before listening to prevent mistaking the sound of the suction for bowel sounds. In addition, ask the client whether flatus has been passed. Bowel sounds and flatus passage indicate active peristalsis. Abdominal cramping denotes trapped, nonmoving gas, not peristalsis.

Complications. Decreased peristalsis occurs in clients who have a paralytic ileus. The intestine wall is distended, and there is no movement of the intestinal wall. Assess for the manifestations of paralytic ileus (few or absent bowel sounds, a distended abdomen, abdominal discomfort, vomiting, and no passage of flatus or stool).

The client may also have constipation after surgery as a result of anesthesia, analgesia (especially opioid analgesics), decreased activity, and decreased oral intake. Assess the abdomen by inspection, auscultation, palpation, and percussion and record the elimination pattern to determine whether interventions are needed. Increased dietary fiber intake, the use of mild laxatives or bulk-forming agents, or the use of enemas may be needed.

NASOGASTRIC TUBE DRAINAGE. A nasogastric (NG) tube may be inserted during surgery to decompress and drain the stomach, to promote GI rest, to allow the lower GI tract to heal, and to provide an enteral feeding route. It may also be used to monitor any gastric bleeding and to prevent intestinal obstruction. The Levin tube and the Salem sump tube are two common tubes used. The Salem tube is a double-lumen tube with an air vent to keep the tube from sucking the gastric mucosa. This feature allows easy drainage of the stomach and prevents mucosal damage. The Levin tube is a single-lumen tube with no air vent. To promote drainage, suction (high, medium, or low) is applied to the NG tube. Suction is either continuous (recommended for the Salem tube) or intermittent.

TABLE 22-3 Calculating Nasogastric Tube Drainage

Formula

Drainage in collection device − Amount of irrigant = True (actual) amount of drainage

Example

A client's drainage container was marked at 150 mL at 7 AM. At 3 PM, there was 525 mL in the container. During the nursing shift, the nurse instilled 30 mL of saline as an irrigant into the tube four times, as prescribed by the physician.

525 mL − 150 mL = 375 mL of drainage

30 mL × 4 = 120 mL of irrigant

375 mL − 120 mL = 255 mL of actual drainage

Assessment. Record the color, consistency, and amount of the drained material every 8 hours (Table 22-3). In some instances, an occult blood test (Gastroccult) may be performed. Normal NG drainage fluid is greenish yellow. Red drainage fluid indicates active bleeding, and brown liquid or drainage with a "coffee-ground" appearance indicates old bleeding.

Complications. Assess the client for complications related to NG tube use, such as fluid and electrolyte imbalances, aspiration, and nares discomfort. To prevent aspiration, check the tube placement every 4 to 8 hours and before instilling any liquid into the tube. (See Chapter 59 for information on tube placement and care.) *After gastric surgery, do not move or irrigate the tube without an order from the surgeon.* Fluid and electrolyte imbalances can result from NG drainage and tube irrigation with water instead of saline. Imbalances include fluid volume deficit (see Chapter 15), hypokalemia and hyponatremia (see Chapter 16), hypochloremia, and metabolic alkalosis (see Chapter 19).

SKIN ASSESSMENT. The clean surgical wound heals at skin level in about 2 weeks in the absence of trauma, connective tissue disease, malnutrition, or the use of some drugs, such as steroids. Smokers, older clients, obese clients, diabetic clients, and those with reduced immunity have delayed wound healing. Complete healing of all tissue to presurgical integrity may take 6 months to 2 years. The physical health and age of the client, size and location of the wound, and stress on the wound all affect healing time. Because of the rich blood supply, head and facial wounds heal more quickly than abdominal and leg wounds.

NORMAL WOUND HEALING. During the first few days of normal wound healing, the incised tissue regains blood supply and begins to bind together. Fibrin and a thin layer of epithelial cells seal the incision. After 1 to 4 days, epithelial cells continue growing in the fibrin and strands of collagen begin to fill in the wound gaps. This process continues for 2 to 3 weeks. *At that time, the wound appears to be healed; however, healing is not complete for up to 2 years, until the scar is strengthened.* (See Chapter 70 for discussion of wound healing and wound infection.)

When the client is an inpatient, the surgeon usually removes the original dressing on the first or second day after surgery. Assess the incision on a regular basis, at least every 8 hours, for redness, increased warmth, swelling, tenderness or pain, and the type and amount of drainage. Some drainage, changing from **sanguineous** (bloody) to serosanguineous to

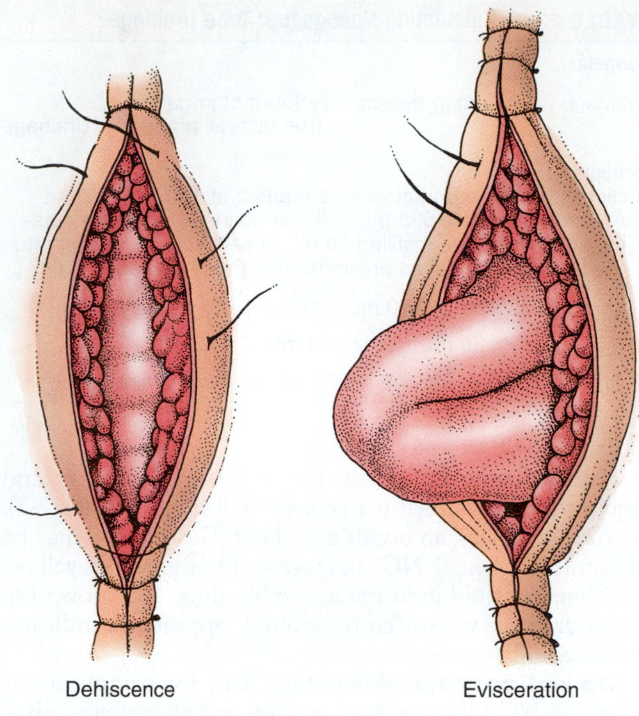

Figure 22-2 ■ Complications of wound healing.

serous (serum-like, or yellow), is normal during the first few days. Serosanguineous drainage continuing beyond the fifth day after surgery alerts you to the possibility of dehiscence, and the surgeon should be notified. Slight crusting on the incision line is normal, as is a pink color to the line itself, which is caused by inflammation from the surgical procedure. Slight swelling under the sutures or staples is also normal. Redness or swelling of or around the incision line, excessive tenderness or pain on palpation, and purulent or odorous drainage indicate wound infection and must be reported to the surgeon.

INEFFECTIVE WOUND HEALING. Ineffective wound healing may be caused by infection, distention from edema or paralytic ileus, stress at the surgical site, and health problems that cause delayed wound healing (such as diabetes). Wound **dehiscence** is a partial or complete separation of the outer wound layers, sometimes described as a "splitting open of the wound." **Evisceration** is the total separation of all wound layers and protrusion of internal organs through the open wound (Figure 22-2). Both of these problems occur most often between the fifth and tenth days after surgery. Wound separation occurs more often in obese clients and those with diabetes or who are using steroids. Dehiscence or evisceration may follow forceful coughing, vomiting or straining, and when not splinting the surgical site during movement. The client may state "Something gave way" or "I feel as if I just split open."

DRESSINGS AND DRAINS. Assess all dressings, including casts and elastic (Ace) bandages, for bleeding or other drainage on admission to the PACU and then hourly thereafter. When the client is on the nursing unit, assess the dressing each time vital signs are taken (at least every shift). During dressing inspection, check for drainage and record its amount, color, consistency, and odor. If drainage is present on a dressing or cast, monitor its progression by outlining it with a pen and indicating the date and time. Check the area underneath the client also, because drainage or blood may leak from the side of the dressing and not appear on the dressing itself. Ensure that the dressing does not restrict circulation or sensation.

The surgeon inserts a drain into or close to the wound if more than a minimal amount of drainage is expected. A Penrose drain (a single-lumen, soft, open, latex tube) is a gravity-type drain under the dressing. Drainage on the dressing is expected with open tube drains but is not expected with closed drainage systems. Assess closed-suction drains, such as Hemovac, VacuDrain, and Jackson-Pratt drains, for maintenance of suction. A T-tube may be placed after abdominal cholecystectomy to drain bile. Figure 22-3 shows commonly used drains.

Assess all drains for patency when the client is admitted to the PACU and every time vital signs are taken. Monitor the amount, color, and type of drainage while the client is in the PACU and at least every 8 hours after the client is transferred to the medical-surgical nursing unit. Large amounts of sanguineous drainage may indicate internal bleeding.

DISCOMFORT/PAIN ASSESSMENT. The client almost always has pain or discomfort after surgery. Pain is a subjective experience and may be more intense than the health care professional can appreciate. Pain after surgery is related to the surgical wound, tissue manipulation, drains, positioning during surgery, presence of an endotracheal (ET) tube, and the client's experience with pain. In assessing the client's discomfort and need for medication, consider the type, extent, and length of the surgical procedure. Assess for physical and emotional signs of acute pain, such as increased pulse and blood pressure, increased respiratory rate, profuse sweating, restlessness, increased confusion (in the older adult), wincing, moaning, and crying. When possible, ask the client to rate the pain before and after drugs are given (e.g., on a scale of 1 to 10, with 1 being no pain and 10 being extreme pain). Plan the client's activities around the timing of analgesia to improve mobility. Observe for a return of normal (baseline) physical behaviors. (See Chapter 7 for further discussion of pain assessment.)

Pain assessment is started by the PACU nurse. After transfer from the PACU, the medical-surgical nurse continues to assess the client's comfort level. Pain usually reaches its peak on the second day after surgery, when the client is more awake, is more active, and the anesthetic agents and drugs given during surgery have been excreted.

PSYCHOSOCIAL ASSESSMENT

Consider the psychological, social, and cultural issues of the client after surgery as you provide physical care. This assessment may be delayed or difficult to perform in the postanesthesia care unit (PACU) when the client is drowsy or incoherent. Consider the client's age and medical history, the surgical procedure, and the impact of surgery on recovery, body image, roles, and lifestyle.

Physical signs of anxiety include restlessness; increased pulse, blood pressure, and respiratory rate; and crying. The client may be anxious and ask questions about the results or findings of the surgical procedure. Reassure the client that the surgeon will speak with him or her after the client is

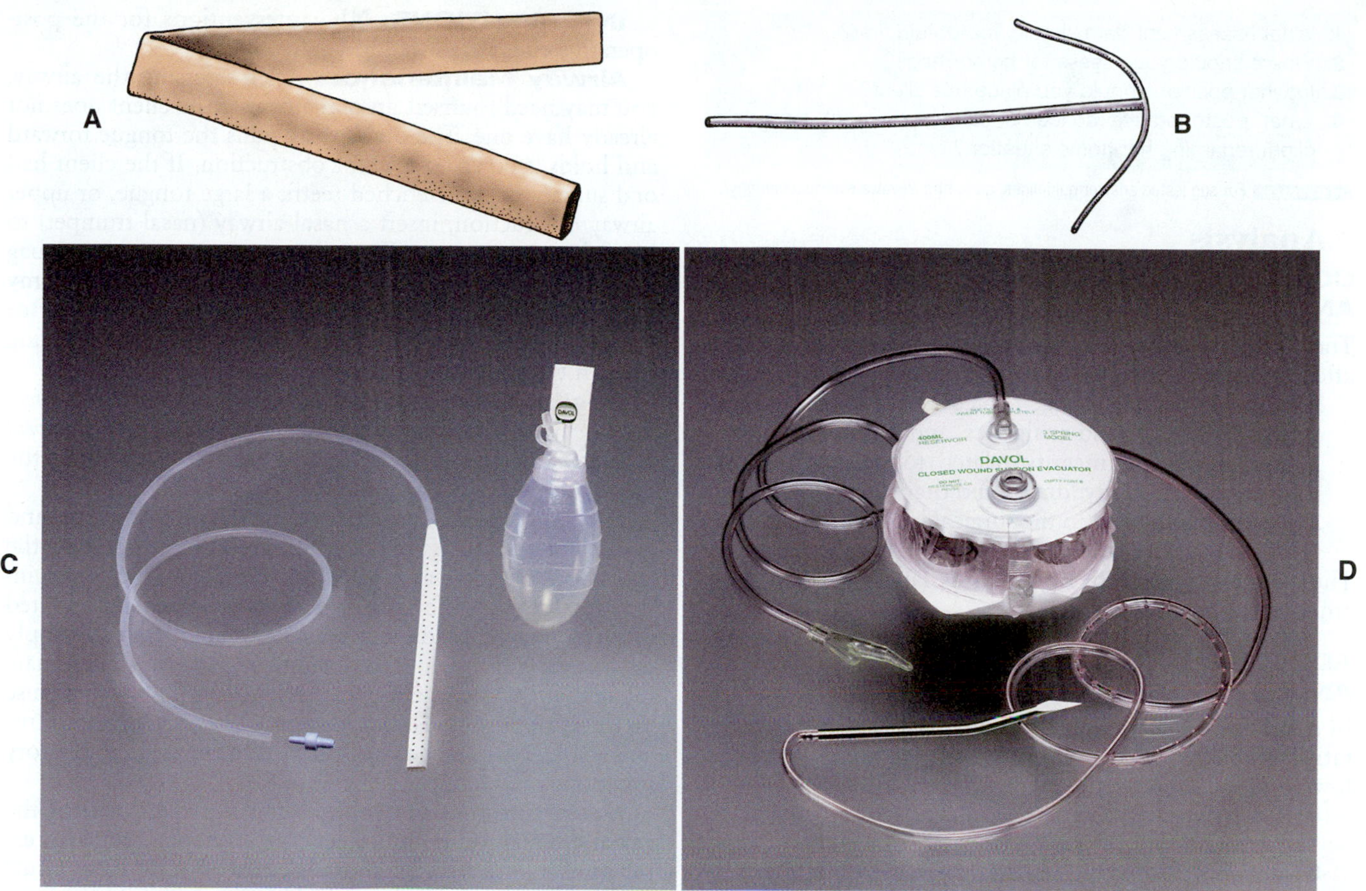

Figure 22-3 ■ Types of surgical drains. Gravity drains, such as the Penrose **(A)** and the T-tube **(B),** drain directly through a tube from the surgical area. In closed wound drainage systems, such as the Jackson-Pratt **(C)** and Hemovac **(D),** drainage collects in a collecting vessel by means of compression and reexpansion of the system. (**C** and **D** courtesy of C.R. Bard, Inc., Covington, GA.)

fully awake. If the surgeon has already spoken with the client, reinforce what was said.

After the client returns to the medical-surgical unit, continue the psychosocial assessment and also assess significant others for psychological discomfort.

LABORATORY ASSESSMENT

Laboratory tests are performed after surgery to monitor for complications. Tests are based on the surgical procedure, the client's medical history, and clinical manifestations after surgery. Common tests include analysis of electrolytes and a complete blood count (see Chart 20-3). A change in laboratory test results (e.g., electrolyte levels, hematocrit, and hemoglobin levels) often occurs during the first 24 to 48 hours after surgery because of blood and fluid loss and the body's reaction to the surgical process. Fluid loss with minimal blood loss may cause hemoconcentration of laboratory values. Such test results are reported as increased, but actually represent a concentrated normal value.

An early indication of infection is an increase in the band cells (immature neutrophils) in the white blood cell differential count. This increase is termed a **left-shift** (sometimes called "bandemia"). The source of infection may be the respiratory system, urinary tract, wound, or IV site. Obtain specimens for culture and sensitivity testing and monitor the culture reports at 24, 48, and 72 hours. Notify the surgeon of positive culture results. (See Chapters 23 and 29 for information on infection and assessment of immune function.)

Arterial blood gas (ABG) tests may be needed for clients who have respiratory or cardiac disease, those undergoing mechanical ventilation after surgery, and those who had chest surgery. Review ABG results and notify the surgeon of any acid-base imbalance or hypoxemia. (For more discussion on arterial blood gases and acidosis, see Chapters 18 and 19.)

Urine and renal laboratory tests also may be obtained (e.g., urinalysis, urine electrolyte levels, and serum creatinine levels). Other laboratory tests depend on the diagnosis, type of surgical procedure, and other health problems. Examples are a serum amylase level for a client who had pancreatic surgery and a blood glucose level for a client with diabetes.

Critical Thinking Challenge

The client is a 62-year-old woman with chronic gallbladder disease who developed biliary obstruction and required an emergency abdominal cholecystectomy. The client is single and lives next door to her 85-year-old mother, for whom she prepares meals and assists with activities of daily living. Her last vital signs before leaving the OR were BP 150/110, P 100, R 12.

She has a Foley catheter, an NG tube to continuous low suction, and a Penrose drain in her wound.

Continued

1. What assessment data should you obtain first?
2. Where should you assess for hemorrhage?
3. In what position should you place this client?
4. What postoperative concerns can you expect from this client regarding her home situation?

evolve For suggested answer guidelines, go to http://evolve.elsevier.com/Iggy/.

Analysis

COMMON NURSING DIAGNOSES AND COLLABORATIVE PROBLEMS

The following are priority nursing diagnoses for the client after surgery:

1. Impaired Gas Exchange related to the effects of anesthesia, pain, opioid analgesics, and immobility
2. Impaired Skin Integrity related to surgical wounds, decreased mobility, drains and drainage, and tubes
3. Acute Pain related to the surgical incision, positioning during surgery, and endotracheal (ET) tube irritation

The primary collaborative problem is Potential for Hypoxemia.

ADDITIONAL NURSING DIAGNOSES AND COLLABORATIVE PROBLEMS

In addition to the common nursing diagnoses and collaborative problems, clients may have one or more of the following problems after surgery:

- Risk for Aspiration related to decreased mobility, anesthesia, and opioid analgesic use
- Ineffective Airway Clearance related to ineffective or absent cough
- Constipation related to decreased mobility, anesthesia, and opioid analgesic use
- Risk for Infection related to surgery and invasive lines, catheters, and tubes
- Urinary Retention related to anesthesia, surgical procedures, and decreased mobility
- Delayed Surgical Recovery related to presence of other health problems (diabetes, obesity), or complications of surgery
- Bathing/Hygiene Self-Care Deficit related to surgical procedures, pain, and decreased mobility
- Disturbed Body Image related to surgical procedures, loss of a body part or function, and pain
- Interrupted Family Processes related to the impact of surgery and illness on the family system
- Potential for Hypovolemic Shock
- Potential for Deep Vein Thrombosis and Pulmonary Embolism

Planning and Implementation

IMPAIRED GAS EXCHANGE

NOC **PLANNING: EXPECTED OUTCOMES.** The client is expected to attain or maintain optimal lung expansion and breathing patterns after surgery as indicated by:

- Partial pressure of arterial oxygen (PaO_2) within normal range
- Partial pressure of arterial carbon dioxide ($PaCO_2$) within normal range
- Oxygen saturation values within normal range

INTERVENTIONS. NIC interventions for the postoperative client are listed in Chart 22-2.

Airway Maintenance. After assessing the airway, you may need to insert an oral airway if the client does not already have one. The oral airway pulls the tongue forward and holds it down to prevent obstruction. If the client had oral surgery or has clenched teeth, a large tongue, or upper airway obstruction, insert a nasal airway (nasal trumpet) to keep the airway open. Keep the manual resuscitation bag and emergency equipment for intubation or tracheostomy nearby. For clients whose only airway is a tracheostomy or laryngectomy stoma, alert other staff members by posting signs in the room and notes on the chart.

Positioning. *In the PACU, immediately position the client in a side-lying position or turn his or her head to the side to prevent aspiration.* Suction the mouth, nose, and throat to keep the airway clear of mucus or vomitus as needed.

Keep the client's head flat to prevent hypotension and possible shock, unless this position is contraindicated by the condition or surgical procedure. (For example, after intracranial surgery, the head of the bed or stretcher is elevated to promote ventilation and prevent cerebral edema.) Apply oxygen via a face tent, nasal cannula, or mask to eliminate inhaled anesthetic agents, increase oxygen levels, and raise the level of consciousness. After the client is fully reactive and stable, raise the head of the bed to promote respiratory function.

Breathing Exercises. After the client regains the gag and cough reflex and meets the agency's criteria for extubation (if intubated), remove the airway or ET tube. Usual extubation criteria are the ability to raise and hold the head up and evidence of thoracic breathing. Help the client to cough (with the incision splinted) and deep breathe to expand the lungs, promote gas exchange, and eliminate inhalation anesthetic agents. Chart 20-6 reviews breathing exercises and splinting of the surgical area. As soon as the

CHART 22-2

NIC INTERVENTION ACTIVITIES for The Postoperative Client

Postanesthesia Care: *Monitoring and management of the client who has recently undergone general or regional anesthesia*

- Administer oxygen, as appropriate.
- Monitor oxygenation.
- Ventilate, as appropriate.
- Monitor quality and number of respirations.
- Encourage client to deep breathe and cough.
- Monitor and record vital signs and perform pain assessment every 15 minutes or more often, as appropriate.
- Monitor urinary output.
- Monitor return of sensorium and motor function.
- Monitor neurologic status.
- Monitor level of consciousness.
- Monitor surgical site, as appropriate.
- Administer narcotic antagonists, as appropriate, per agency protocol.
- Determine client's status for discharge
- Provide client report to the postoperative nursing unit.
- Discharge client to next level of care.

NIC intervention activities selected from Dochterman, J.M., & Bulechek, G.M. (Eds.). (2004). *Nursing interventions classification (NIC)* (4th ed.). St. Louis: Mosby.

client is awake enough to follow commands, urge him or her to cough, use the incentive spirometer, and take deep breaths. Remind the client to continue these activities through out the postoperative period. The client who is unable to remove mucus or sputum requires oral or nasal suctioning. Perform mouth care after removing secretions.

Mobilization. Assist the client out of bed and to ambulate as soon as possible to help remove secretions and promote lung expansion. Even when the client has had extensive surgery, the goal may be to get out of bed the same day of or the first day after surgery. If this is not possible, assist the client to turn at least every 2 hours (side to side) and ensure that breathing exercises and leg exercises are performed (see Charts 20-6 and 20-7). Early ambulation reduces the risk for pulmonary complications, especially after abdominal, pelvic, or spinal surgery. The client may report pain and resist getting up, but you need to stress the importance of activity to prevent complications. When indicated, offer pain medication 30 to 45 minutes before the client gets out of bed.

IMPAIRED SKIN INTEGRITY

NOC **PLANNING: EXPECTED OUTCOMES.** The client is expected to have incision healing without wound complications as indicated by:

- Wound edges remaining together
- Absence of purulent drainage, induration or redness in, from or around the incision

INTERVENTIONS. Nursing assessment of the surgical area is critical (see the discussion of skin assessment on p. 345). Although most wound complications do not require additional surgical intervention, emergency surgical procedures may be needed.

NONSURGICAL MANAGEMENT. Wound care includes changing the dressing, assessing the wound for signs of infection, and caring for drains, including emptying, measuring, and documenting drainage features. Emphasize the importance of early deep breathing exercises to prevent forceful coughing. Encourage hip flexion when the client is in the supine position to reduce tension on a chest or abdominal wound. Remind the client to always splint the incision when coughing. Promote wound healing and protection of the skin in general, especially for the older client. Chart 22-3 lists best practices for skin care of the older client after surgery.

Dressings. The surgeon usually performs the first dressing change to assess the wound, remove any packing, and advance (pull partially out) or remove drains. Before the first dressing change, reinforce the dressing (add more dressing material to the existing dressing) if it becomes wet from drainage. Document the added material, as well as the color, type, amount, and odor of drainage fluid and time of observation. Assess the surgical site every shift and report any unexpected findings to the surgeon.

After removal of the dressing, the surgeon may leave the suture or staple line open to the air, which allows easy assessment of the wound and early detection of poor wound edge adherence, drainage, swelling, or redness. Some surgeons believe that air-drying promotes healing. A draining wound, however, is always covered with a dressing.

Dressing changes are prescribed by the surgeon; however, the facility or unit may have standards or policies that dictate specific protocols for dressing changes and incision care. An unchanged wet or damp dressing is a source of infection. Perform dressing changes using aseptic technique until the sutures or staples are removed.

Dressings vary with the surgical procedure and the surgeon's preference. Common dressings for large incisions consist of gauze or nonadherent pads covered with a larger absorbent pad held in place by tape or by Montgomery straps (Figure 22-4). Some incisions may be covered with a transparent plastic surgical dressing (such as Op-Site) or a spray in the operating room. This type of dressing stays intact for 3 to 6 days and allows direct observation of the wound. It also prevents contamination and eliminates the need for dressing changes.

Wound or suture line care consists of changing gauze dressings at least once during a nursing shift or daily and may include cleaning the area with sterile saline or some other solution. Some suture lines are left open to air without any dressing to cover the incision. The hospital's policy, the unit's standards, and the surgeon's preference determine what solution, if any, is used to clean the wound and how often dressings are changed. For large dressing changes or drain removal, offer the client a prescribed analgesic before the procedure.

Skin sutures or staples are usually removed 6 to 8 days after surgery, and the incision is secured with Steri-Strips. The surgeon or the nurse removes the sutures or staples, depending on the agency's policy. Before removing sutures, examine the condition and healing stage of the wound. If

CHART 22-3

NURSING FOCUS on the OLDER ADULT

Best Practices in Postoperative Skin Care

Improve perfusion to the wound to promote wound healing:
- Keep the client adequately hydrated to maintain cardiac output
- Keep the airway patent and provide adequate oxygenation.
- Keep the client's oxygen saturation on pulse oximetry at greater than 93%.

Conserve the client's energy:
- Allow the client to sleep in a darkened, quiet room.
- Administer medication to combat pain and sleeplessness, as prescribed.
- Provide rest periods throughout the day.
- Control the client's room temperature.
- Assist in activities of daily living.

Place the client on a safety program to prevent falls, if indicated.

Maintain strict aseptic technique in caring for breaks in the integument (IV or other catheters, indwelling urethral catheter, wound).

Maintain the client's psychosocial health:
- Prevent unnecessary stressors.
- Allow the client liberal visitation of supportive others.
- Enable the client to use individual successful coping mechanisms.
- Keep the client well groomed and bathed.

Protect fragile skin:
- Minimize the use of tape on the skin.
- Use hypoallergenic tape or Montgomery straps.
- Change dressings as soon as they become wet.
- Lift the client during transfer or repositioning.

Data from Jones, P.L., & Millman, A. (1990). Wound healing and the aged patient. *Nursing Clinics of North America, 25*(1), 263-277.

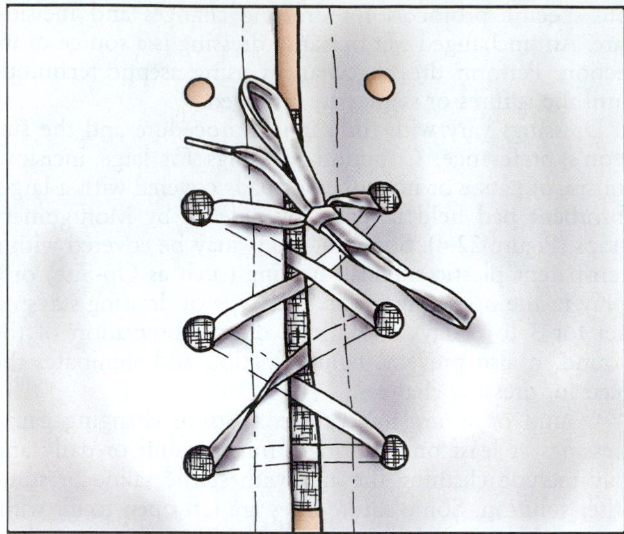

Figure 22-4 ■ Montgomery straps may be used when frequent dressing changes are anticipated. They help prevent skin irritation from frequent tape removal.

the wound does not appear to be healing well, notify the surgeon before removing sutures.

Drains. Drains (see Figure 22-3) may be placed in the wound or through a separate small incision (known as a "stab" wound) close to the incision during surgery. Drains provide an exit route for air, blood, and bile. Drains also help prevent deep infections and abscess formation during healing.

The Penrose drain is placed into the external aspect of the incision and drains directly onto the dressing and skin around the incision. Change a damp or soiled dressing and carefully clean under and around the Penrose drain. Then place absorbent pads distal to the drain to prevent skin irritation and wound contamination. Whether sutured in place or not, the drain can be dislodged or pulled out accidentally during a dressing change. As the wound heals, the surgeon shortens (advances) the drain by pulling it out and cutting the excess external portion until drainage stops.

Jackson-Pratt and Hemovac drains are two self-contained drainage systems that drain wounds directly through a tube via gravity and vacuum. These drains are sutured in place with a suture that seals the area when the drain is removed. Empty the reservoir and record the amount and color of drainage during every nursing shift or more often if prescribed. After emptying and compressing the reservoir, secure the drain to the client's gown (never to the sheet or mattress) to prevent pulling and stress on the surgical wound.

Drug Therapy. Wound infection is a major complication after surgery. It usually results from contamination during surgery, preoperative infection, debilitation, or immunosuppression. A client at risk for wound infection may receive antibiotic therapy with drugs that are effective against organisms common to the specific surgical site. These antibiotics are usually continued for 24 to 72 hours after surgery. The first dose may be given intravenously before or during surgery.

Wounds that become infected and open are treated with dressing changes and systemic antibiotic therapy. Depending on the surgeon's prescription, irrigate the wound (e.g., with sterile saline, hydrogen peroxide, povidone-iodine, or acetic acid), loosely pack it with solution-soaked gauze (e.g., neomycin, gentamicin, iodoform, povidone-iodine, saline, or acetic acid), and cover the wound with dry, sterile dressings. This procedure (wet-to-dry dressings) may be done one to three times daily. The packing promotes healing from within the wound and **debridement** (removal) of the infected tissue as the wound heals.

CHART 22-4

BEST PRACTICE for

Emergency Care of the Client with Surgical Wound Evisceration

EMERGENCY CARE

1. Call for help! Instruct the person who responds to notify the surgeon immediately and to bring any needed supplies into the client's room.
2. Stay with the client.
3. Cover the wound with a nonadherent dressing premoistened with warmed sterile normal saline. **Note:** The supplies needed for this emergency should be in the client's room, especially if the client is at high risk.
4. If premoistened dressings are not available, moisten sterile gauze or sterile towels in a sterile irrigation tray with sterile saline, then cover the wound.
5. If saline is not immediately available, cover the wound with gauze and then moisten with sterile saline using a sterile irrigation tray as soon as someone brings saline.
6. Do not attempt to reinsert the protruding organ or viscera.
7. While covering the wound, note the client's response and assess for manifestations of shock.
8. Place the client in a supine position with the hips and knees bent.
9. Take vital signs and document them. **Note:** If the person who answered the call for help is back in the room before this, instruct that individual to take vital signs while you focus on covering the wound and repositioning the client.
10. Provide support and reassurance to the client.
11. Continue assessing the client, including vital signs assessment, every 5 to 10 minutes until the surgeon arrives.
12. Keep dressings continuously moist by adding warmed sterile saline to the dressing as often as necessary. Do not let the dressing become dry.
13. When the surgeon arrives, report your finding and your interventions. Then follow the surgeon's directions.
14. Document the incident, the activity the client was engaged in at the time of the incident, your actions, and your assessments.

SURGICAL MANAGEMENT

Management of Dehiscence. *If dehiscence (wound opening) occurs, apply a sterile nonadherent (such as Telfa) or saline dressing to the wound and notify the surgeon.* A wound that becomes infected dehisces by itself, or it may be opened by the surgeon through an **incision and drainage (I&D)** procedure. In either case, the wound is left open rather than re-sutured and is treated as described previously.

Management of Evisceration. *An evisceration (a wound opening with protrusion of internal organs or viscera) is a surgical emergency. One nurse tends to the client while another nurse immediately notifies the surgeon.* Chart 22-4 lists best practices for emergency care of the client with surgical wound evisceration. Provide emotional support by explaining what happened and reassuring the client that the emergency will be handled competently.

The surgeon may prescribe a nasogastric (NG) tube to decompress the stomach and relieve internal pressure or to remove the stomach's contents if the client has been eating and general anesthesia is needed. Prepare the client for surgery (see Chapter 20) to close the wound. Regional or local anesthesia may be used, depending on the location and type of the wound. Nausea and vomiting, which stress the already fragile incision, are reduced when regional or local anesthesia is used. To increase the incision's integrity, stay or retention sutures of wire or nylon are used instead of standard sutures or staples (see Figure 21-13).

Prevention. Clients also are at risk for developing pressure ulcers from positioning during surgery, prolonged contact with damp surgical linens, and contact with unpadded surfaces. Pressure ulcers acquired during the surgical period increase lengths of stay and the risk for complications. Addressing early-stage pressure ulcers can prevent progression and limit complications.

Examine the client's skin for areas of redness or lost integrity. Document and report any abnormalities. Use padding and positioning to relieve pressure. Treat any open areas according to facility guidelines and the surgeon's prescription. Ensure that information about the client's skin condition in the PACU is communicated to the medical-surgical nurse.

ACUTE PAIN

NOC **PLANNING: EXPECTED OUTCOMES.** The postoperative client is expected to attain or maintain optimal comfort levels after surgery as indicated by:

- Reporting that pain is controlled
- Absence of physiologic indicators of acute pain (increased heart rate and blood pressure)
- Absence of facial grimacing, teeth clenching
- Willingness to move and participate in self care

INTERVENTIONS. Pain management after surgery includes drug therapy and other methods of management, such as positioning, massage, relaxation techniques, and diversion. Often the client has better pain relief from a combination of approaches. Assess the client's comfort level and the effectiveness of the therapies. See Chapter 7 for discussion of pain assessment and management. The client who has optimal pain control is better able to cooperate with the therapies and exercises to prevent complications and promote rehabilitation. Pain can be a factor in the risk for pulmonary complications after abdominal surgery. (See the Evidence-Based Practice for Nursing Box above.)

Drug Therapy. *The use of opioids or other analgesics for pain management may mask or increase the severity of symptoms of an anesthesia reaction. Therefore give these drugs with caution, especially in the PACU when the client's condition is not stable.* Pain medication in the PACU is usually given intravenously in small doses. After receiving medication for pain, the client remains in the PACU for a defined period (often 30 to 45 minutes). Assess for hypotension, respiratory depression, and other side effects. Within 5 to 10 minutes after an IV injection, assess the effectiveness of the drug (i.e., on a rating scale) in relieving pain.

Opioid analgesics are given during the first 24 to 48 hours after surgery to control acute pain. Around-the-clock scheduling is more effective than "on demand" scheduling because more constant blood levels are achieved. Drugs commonly used include meperidine (Demerol), morphine (Statex✱), hydromorphone (Dilaudid), ketorolac (Toradol), codeine, butorphanol (Stadol), and oxycodone with aspirin (Percodan) or oxycodone with acetaminophen (Tylox, Percocet).

EVIDENCE-BASED PRACTICE for Nursing

Reduce pulmonary complications among older clients after abdominal surgery by managing pain

Shea, R., et al. (2002). Pain intensity and postoperative pulmonary complications among the elderly after abdominal surgery. *Heart & Lung, 31*(6), 440-449.

The purpose of this study was to examine whether pain after abdominal surgery in older adult clients influenced the development of postoperative pulmonary complications (PPCs). This exploratory study is a secondary analysis of data collected as part of a larger prospective study examining factors contributing to PPCs after abdominal or cardiothoracic surgery. The subgroup of subjects for which initial data were reanalyzed consisted of a convenience sample of clients over 60 years of age having open abdominal surgery with general anesthesia and a minimum postoperative stay of 48 hours. Clients with a preexisting pulmonary problem and those requiring more than 10 hours of mechanical ventilation after surgery were excluded from the analysis. PPCs were defined as the presence of any two of the following: new sputum/cough production, new onset of abnormal breath sounds, fever, chest x-ray showing infiltrate or atelectasis, or physician documentation of atelectasis/pneumonia. Pain was defined by self-report and the use of a numeric rating scale.

Data were analyzed for 86 subjects (49 men, 37 women; mean age of 70 years). Two groups were examined: those with a PPC (70 subjects) and those with no PPC (16 subjects). Statistically significant differences between the groups (as determined by analysis of variance) were found for mean pain scores at rest and pain with deep breathing, with the PPC group experiencing greater pain. Pain scores with coughing, movement, and walking were all greater in the PPC group, although these differences did not meet statistical significance. An additional finding was that subjects with a PPC had significantly longer lengths of stay than did subjects in the no PPC group.

Level of Evidence: 3—Well-designed trial without randomization.

Critique. Overall, the methods and analyses were appropriate for the purpose of the study. The criteria for PPC is a strength of the study. The study would be strengthened by randomization and a prospective approach.

Implications for Nursing. Postoperative pulmonary complications after abdominal surgery are costly in terms of morbidity, length of stay, and delayed recovery. Pain may inhibit the client from adequately performing interventions for prevention of pulmonary problems. Additionally, pain triggers the stress response, which reduces immune function, increasing the risk for PPC. Many nurses are hesitant to give opioid analgesics to older clients for fear of increasing confusion or depressing cardiopulmonary function. Ensuring that older clients have adequate pain management in the early postoperative period after abdominal surgery can enhance their participation in preventive interventions and may reduce the incidence of PPC in this population.

Assess the type, location, and intensity of the pain before and after giving medication (see also Discomfort/Pain Assessment on p. 346). Monitor the client's vital signs for hypotension and hypoventilation, after giving opioid drugs. Chart 22-5 lists more information about analgesics used after surgery.

Patient-controlled analgesia (PCA) via IV infusion or internal pump (the catheter is sutured into or near the surgical area) and epidural analgesia are often used for better pain control. In PCA, the client adjusts the dosage of the analgesic on the basis of the pain level and response to the drug. This method allows more consistent pain relief and more control by the client. The maximum dose per hour is "locked

CHART 22-5

DRUG THERAPY for Management of Postoperative Pain

Drug	Usual Dosage	Nursing Interventions	Rationales
Meperidine hydrochloride (Demerol)	50-150 mg PO or IM q3-4h 12.5-25 mg IV Maximum 6-8 doses	Monitor blood pressure. Move and ambulate the client slowly. Monitor pulse rate. Assess for decreased GI motility or GI upset.	Common side effects include decreased blood pressure, orthostatic (postural) hypotension, and bradycardia. Constipation, nausea, and vomiting can occur.
[1]Morphine sulfate (Epimorph✱, Statex✱)	2-15 mg IM or IV incrementally 10-30 mg PO q4h Maximum 6 doses	Monitor respiratory status. Monitor blood pressure. Assess for GI motility and urine output.	Respiratory depression can be severe and require medical intervention. Hypotension, constipation, and urinary retention can occur.
Hydromorphone hydrochloride (Dilaudid)	1-4 mg IV or IM q3-4h 2-4 mg PO q3-4h	Monitor respirations. Monitor blood pressure. Monitor for food intolerance. Monitor fluid and electrolyte balance. Assess GI motility.	Respiratory depression, hypotension, anorexia, nausea, vomiting, and constipation can occur.
Codeine sulfate, codeine phosphate (Paveral✱)	15-60 mg IM or PO q4h Maximum 6 doses	Monitor respiratory status. Monitor for food intolerance. Monitor fluid and electrolyte balance. Assess GI motility.	Respiratory depression, nausea, and vomiting can occur. Constipation is common; prophylactic interventions may be indicated.
Butorphanol tartrate (Stadol)	1-4 mg IM q3-4h 0.5-2 mg IV Maximum 6-8 doses	Monitor neurologic status and changes in level of consciousness. Monitor respiratory status.	Butorphanol can cause increased intracranial pressure and respiratory depression.
Oxycodone hydrochloride and aspirin (Percodan, Endodan✱, Oxycodan✱)	1-2 tablets (5-10 mg) PO q3-4h Maximum 80 mg	Assess GI tolerance of medication. Assess for GI bleeding. Monitor GI motility. Monitor coagulation studies (PT, aPTT). Monitor respiratory status.	The aspirin component can irritate the stomach and could cause GI bleeding. Bleeding times and other coagulation study results may be increased because of the aspirin component. Respiratory depression and constipation can be caused by the oxycodone component.
Oxycodone hydrochloride and acetaminophen (Tylox, Percocet, Endocet✱, Oxycocet✱)	1-2 tablets PO q3-4h Maximum 12 tablets	Monitor blood pressure and respiratory status. Assess for GI motility.	Respiratory depression, hypotension, and constipation can occur.
Ketorolac tromethamine [2](Toradol)	15-60 mg IM or IV q6h Maximum 120 mg 5-day administration maximum	Monitor for GI bleeding. Monitor for renal effects, especially in older adults.	GI bleeding, ulceration, and perforation can occur. Decreased urine output, increased serum creatinine, hematuria, and proteinuria can occur. Ketorolac is cleared more slowly in older adults. Older persons are more sensitive to the renal effects of NSAIDs.
Ibuprofen (Motrin, Amersol✱, Novoprofen✱)	300-800 mg PO q4-6h Maximum 2400 mg daily	Monitor upper GI tolerance of medication. Give with food or milk. Monitor coagulation studies (PT, aPTT). Assess for signs of bleeding or delayed clotting.	Food or milk helps decrease irritation of the stomach. Bleeding times and other coagulation study results may be increased. Monitoring leads to early detection of complications.

PT, Prothrombin time; aPTT, activated partial thromboplastin time; NSAID, nonsteroidal anti-inflammatory drug; GI, gastrointestinal.

[1]**Med Error Alert!** Watch dosage; the dosage of morphine is only one-tenth that of meperidine.

[2]**Med Error Alert!** Do not confuse with Tramadol, a drug used for central analgesia.

CHART 22-6

DRUG THERAPY for
Management of Opioid Overdose

Drug	Usual Dosage	Nursing Interventions	Rationales
Naloxone hydrochloride (Narcan)	0.1-2 mg IV, SC, and IM; repeat every 2-3 min PRN on the basis of the client's response up to 10 mg	Maintain an open airway.	A patent airway maximizes respiratory effort.
		Administer oxygen as prescribed.	Oxygen helps prevent hypoxemia.
		Have suction available.	Vomiting can occur with administration of naloxone; suction prevents aspiration.
		Closely monitor vital signs and pulse oximetry readings until the client responds.	The threat of hypoxemia and respiratory depression or arrest is a concern until the naloxone becomes effective.
		Do not leave the client unattended until he or she is fully responsive.	Staying with the client promotes safety.
		Observe for significant reversal of analgesia.	With reversal of the narcotic's respiratory-depressive effects, analgesic effects will also be reversed.
		Continue to monitor the client for effects of the naloxone for at least 1 hr.	Continued monitoring leads to early detection of hypertension, hypotension, tachycardia, and dysrhythmias, which can be effects of naloxone.

SC, Subcutaneous.

in" to the pump so that the client cannot accidentally overdose. Drugs given by the PCA method include morphine, meperidine, and hydromorphone.

Epidural analgesia can be given intermittently by the anesthesia provider or by continuous drip through an epidural catheter left in place after epidural anesthesia. Drugs given by epidural catheter include the opioids fentanyl (Sublimaze), preservative-free morphine (Duramorph), and bupivacaine (Marcaine).

Take care not to overmedicate or undermedicate, especially with older clients. In assessing for overmedication, monitor vital signs, especially blood pressure and respiratory rate, and level of consciousness. Complications from the use of opioid analgesics include respiratory depression, hypotension, nausea, vomiting, and constipation. An opioid antagonist, such as naloxone (Narcan), may be needed to reverse the acute effects of opioid depression. Because of the short effect of the opioid antagonist, monitor the client's blood pressure and respirations every 15 to 30 minutes until the full effect of the opioid analgesic has passed. You may need to give more doses of the opioid antagonist during this time. (See Chart 22-6 for more information on opioid antagonists.) In addition, the client has breakthrough pain after the opioid antagonist is given, so other interventions to promote comfort are needed.

Assess for undermedication by asking the client about the effects of the drug and observing for nonverbal cues of pain or discomfort (e.g., restlessness, increased confusion, "picking" at bedcovers, and aggressive behaviors). Offer pain medication after checking for hypotension and respiratory depression.

As recovery progresses, reduce the doses and frequency of pain medications. Drugs are changed from injectable or PCA to oral as soon as the client can tolerate oral agents. Nonopioid analgesics, such as acetaminophen (Tylenol, Atasol✱), and nonsteroidal anti-inflammatory drugs (NSAIDs), such as ibuprofen (Motrin, Novo-Profen✱, Amersol✱) and ketorolac (Toradol), are used alone or with an opioid analgesic. Antianxiety drugs, such as hydroxyzine (Vistaril, Novo-Hydroxyzin✱), may be given with an opioid analgesic. This combination decreases pain-related anxiety, reduces muscle tension, and controls nausea.

Complementary and Alternative Therapies. Provide other comfort measures that may lower the amount of pain medication needed. These measures reduce anxiety and allow the client to relax and rest.

Positioning. In positioning the client, consider the position during surgery, the location of the surgical incision and drains, and problems such as arthritis and chronic lung disease. Assist the client to a position of comfort. Support the extremities with pillows. *Place no pillows under the knees, and do not raise the knee gatch, because this position could restrict circulation and increase the risk for thrombophlebitis.* Turn or help the client turn at least every 2 hours while he or she is bedridden to prevent complications caused by immobility.

On the basis of the surgeon's prescription and your assessment of the client's tolerance, encourage the client to increase activity progressively. Activity decreases stiffness, promotes lung expansion, and promotes venous blood return. When the client is first allowed out of bed, assist him or her to the side of the bed and into a chair. Teach the client to splint the surgical wound for support and comfort during the transfer.

Massage. Use gentle massage on stiff joints or a sore back to decrease discomfort. Assist the client to a side-lying position, and apply lotion with smooth, gentle strokes to increase blood flow to the area and promote relaxation. *Do not*

CHART 22-7

BEST PRACTICE for
Nonpharmacologic Interventions to Reduce Postoperative Pain and Promote Comfort

- Control or remove noxious stimuli.
- Cushion and elevate painful areas; avoid tension or pressure on those areas.
- Provide adequate rest to increase pain tolerance.
- Encourage the client's participation in diversional activities.
- Instruct the client in relaxation techniques; use audiotapes and breathing exercises.
- Provide opportunities for meditation.
- Help the client to stimulate sensory nerve endings near the painful areas to inhibit ascending pain impulses.
- Use ice to reduce and prevent swelling, as indicated.
- Find a general position of comfort for the client.
- Help the client stimulate the area contralateral (opposite) to the painful area.

massage the calves, because of the risk of loosening a clot and causing a life-threatening pulmonary embolus.

Relaxation and Diversion. Relaxation and diversion are also used to control acute episodes of pain that may occur during dressing changes and injections. Chapters 4 and 7 discuss how to instruct and guide the client through these pain control methods. Music and noise reduction have also been shown to decrease awareness of discomfort. Chart 22-7 lists other interventions that may help reduce pain and promote comfort.

Critical Thinking Challenge

The client described earlier (a 62-year-old woman who has undergone an abdominal cholecystectomy) has just arrived on the medical-surgical nursing unit. As soon as she is moved to the bed, she vomits a large amount of greenish-yellow liquid. You note that her dressing is completely soaked with serosanguineous drainage. Her vital signs are as follows: BP 102/78, P 132, R 24; pulse oximetry is 95% on room air. She is restless, diaphoretic, and has pulled on her NG tube twice. She received 2 mg of morphine IV about 45 minutes before she was discharged from the PACU.

1. What additional assessment data should you obtain?
2. Should you change her dressing? Why or why not?
3. How should you intervene for her vomiting?
4. Does this client require more frequent or less frequent monitoring than the every 2 hours specified by the facility's policy? Why or why not?

evolve For suggested answer guidelines, go to http://evolve.elsevier.com/Iggy/.

POTENTIAL FOR HYPOXEMIA

NOC **PLANNING: EXPECTED OUTCOMES.** The client is expected to attain or maintain preoperative baseline partial pressure of arterial oxygen (PaO_2) values.

INTERVENTIONS. The key to preventing hypoxemia is to follow the interventions for the nursing diagnoses of Impaired Gas Exchange (p. 348), Ineffective Airway Clearance, and Ineffective Breathing Pattern. After surgery, monitor the client's arterial blood gas (ABG) and pulse oximetry values. A client who received conscious sedation with midazolam (Versed) or lorazepam (Ativan, Nu-Loraz✱) may be overly sedated or have pulmonary depression sufficient to need reversal with flumazenil (Romazicon) (Chart 22-8). Hypothermia after surgery causes shivering that increases oxygen demand and can induce hypoxemia. Many rewarming methods can be used, although prevention is more important. The highest incidence of hypoxemia after surgery occurs on the second postoperative day. Clients who normally have a low PaO_2, such as those with lung disease or older adults, are at higher risk for hypoxemia.

Hypoxemia is treated with oxygen therapy. Depending on the surgeon's preference and established guidelines, oxygen therapy may continue through the second day after surgery. When hypoxemia occurs despite preventive care, interventions to manage the cause of the hypoxemia are prescribed. These may include respiratory treatments and mechanical ventilation (if needed).

Community-Based Care

Many clients are discharged after a brief hospital stay or directly from the PACU to home. Because of the shortened length of hospital stays, discharge planning, teaching, and referral begin before surgery and continue after surgery.

HOME CARE MANAGEMENT

If the client is discharged directly to home, assess information about the home environment for safety, cleanliness, and availability of caregivers. Use the database obtained on admission before surgery to determine the client's needs. For example, if the client is unable or not allowed to climb stairs and lives in a two-story house with only one bathroom, advise the client to rent a bedside commode. Collaborate with the social worker or discharge planner to identify needs related to care after surgery, including meal preparation, dressing changes, and personal hygiene. A referral to a home care nursing agency may be indicated.

The client is usually concerned about complications, pain, changes in the usual activity level, or payment of the hospital bill. The more extensive the surgical procedure is, the more fearful the client is of assuming self-care. Support the client and family members as they make discharge plans. The client with visible scars after surgery may need more emotional support from and acceptance of his or her family. He or she may be angry about the surgical outcome or about role changes. He or she may be concerned about financial matters and work. The surgical outcome may not have met the client's expectations, and further interventions may be necessary to assist in resolving his or her feelings. Ensure that referrals are made for additional counseling as indicated.

HEALTH TEACHING

The teaching plan for the client and family after surgery includes the following:

- Prevention of infection
- Care and assessment of the surgical wound
- Diet therapy
- Pain management
- Drug therapy
- Progressive increase in activity

If dressing changes are needed, instruct the client and family members on the importance of proper handwashing to prevent infection. Explain and demonstrate wound care to

CHART 22-8

DRUG THERAPY for
Management of Benzodiazepine Overdose

Drug	Usual Dosage	Nursing Interventions	Rationales
Flumazenil (Romazicon)	0.2-1 mg IV at rate of 0.2 mg/min; repeat every 2-3 min PRN up to 3 mg in any 1 hr	Maintain an open airway.	A patent airway maximizes respiratory effort.
		Administer oxygen as prescribed.	Oxygen helps prevent hypoxemia.
		Have suction available.	Vomiting can occur with administration of flumazenil; suction prevents aspiration.
		Closely monitor the client's level of sedation, vital signs, and pulse oximetry readings until the client responds.	Hypoventilation may not be fully reversed with flumazenil; sedation, amnesia, and psychomotor effects of the benzodiazepines should be reversed.
		Do not leave the client unattended until fully responsive.	Seizures have occurred with reversal.
		Observe for significant reversal of sedation.	With reversal of the benzodiazepine's sedative and amnesia effect, the client will become more aware of pain/discomfort.
		Observe for up to 2 hr for re-sedation and respiratory depression.	The duration of action of the benzodiazepines is longer than that of flumazenil.

the client and family, who then perform a return demonstration. During teaching sessions, evaluate learning and promote adherence after discharge. At the same time, teach about the manifestations of complications such as wound infection. Also instruct the client and family about what to do if complications occur.

A diet high in protein, calories, and vitamin C promotes wound healing. Supplemental vitamin C, iron, and other vitamins are often prescribed after surgery to aid in wound healing and red blood cell formation. Instruct the client who needs dietary restrictions about the importance of following the prescribed diet while recovering from surgery. Encourage the older adult or debilitated client to continue using dietary supplements, if prescribed, between meals until the wound is completely healed and the energy levels are restored.

Teach the client about drugs for pain, especially about the proper dosage and frequency. Instruct the client to notify the surgeon if pain is not controlled or if the pain suddenly increases. If antibiotics or other drugs are prescribed, stress the importance of completing the entire prescription.

Surgery stresses the body, and time and rest are needed for healing. Teach the client to increase activity level slowly, rest often, and avoid straining the wound or the surrounding area. The surgeon decides when the client may climb stairs, return to work, drive, and resume other usual activities, such as sexual intercourse. The amount of weight that the client can lift safely after surgery is specifically defined by the surgeon (i.e., in pounds or kilograms). Remind clients of the weights of grocery bags, laundry baskets, children, and books.

Instruct the client in the use of proper body mechanics. A client whose work involves a moderate amount of physical labor may return to work about 6 weeks after abdominal surgery. However, he or she may be eager to return to normal activities and may not follow restrictions. Stress the importance of adherence to prevent complications or disability. *The client must receive written discharge instructions to follow at home.* A referral for a visiting nurse may be needed for follow-up.

HEALTH CARE RESOURCES

After returning home, the client may need equipment and assistance with dressing changes, activities of daily living (ADLs), and meal preparation. Referral to a home care agency is made, if needed. Home care may be paid for by third-party insurance payers, including Medicare, if the client is homebound and requires skilled care such as dressing changes or physical therapy. The home care nurse provides skilled nursing assessments, dressing supplies, education in self-care, and referrals for services as needed. Such referrals include Meals on Wheels, support groups, and homemaker services (e.g., for housekeeping and food shopping).

Critical Thinking Challenge

The 62-year-old client who had an abdominal cholecystectomy is getting ready for discharge. After her staples are removed, a 2-cm area of the incision opened and is draining small amounts of serous fluid. She is very upset about this development and is afraid to go home.

1. Is this a major complication? Why or why not?
2. How could you allay her fears?
3. What care for this wound would you recommend?

evolve For suggested answer guidelines, go to http://evolve.elsevier.com/Iggy/.

Evaluation: Outcomes

Evaluate the care of the client after surgery on the basis of the identified nursing diagnoses and collaborative problems. The expected outcomes include that the client:

- Attains and maintains adequate lung expansion and respiratory function.
- Has complete wound healing without complications.
- Has an acceptable comfort level after surgery.

Specific indicators for these outcomes are listed for each nursing diagnosis and collaborative problem under the Planning and Implementation section (see earlier).

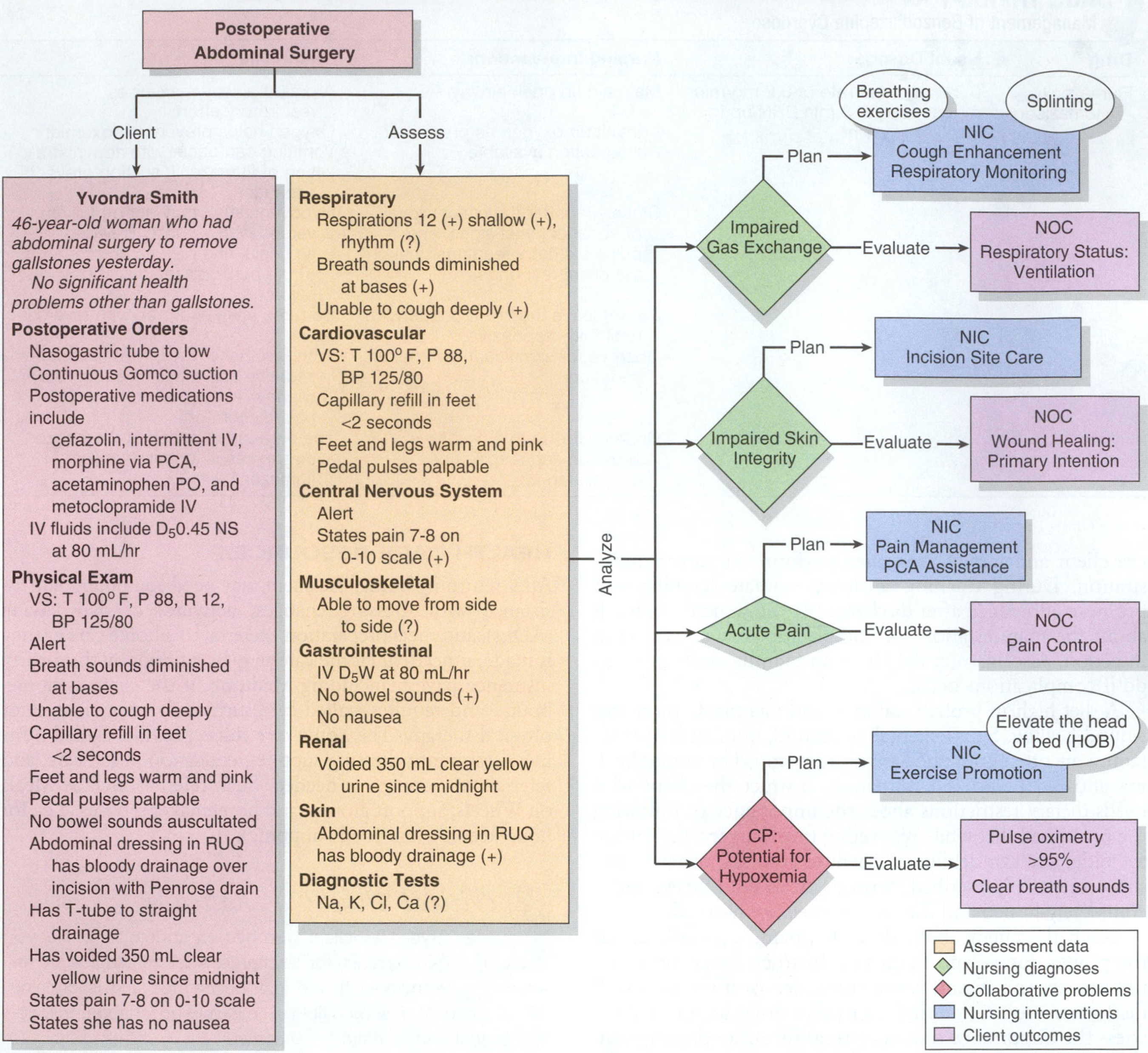

Concept Map by Elaine Bishop Kennedy, EdD, RN

GET READY for the NCLEX Examination!

KEY POINTS

Safe Effective Care Environment

- Use aseptic technique during all dressing changes.
- Use established criteria to determine when a client is ready to leave the postanesthesia care unit (PACU) for discharge to home or a medical-surgical nursing unit.
- Keep suction equipment, oxygen, and artificial breathing equipment near the client in the PACU.

Health Promotion and Maintenance

- Reinforce to the client after surgery the specific interventions to use to prevent complications (incision splinting, deep breathing exercises, range of motion exercises, as described in Chart 20-6).
- Encourage early ambulation.
- Stress the need for following the activity restrictions prescribed by the surgeon.

Psychosocial Integrity

- Explain all procedures, restrictions, drugs, and follow-up care to the client and family.

- Allow the client to verbalizes feelings about any change in physical appearance or lifestyle as a result of surgery.
- Reassure clients that taking pain medication when needed, even opioids, does not make them drug abusers.
- Remain with the client if wound dehiscence or evisceration occurs.
- Offer alternative therapies for relaxation, pain reduction, and distraction, such as massage, music therapy, and guided imagery.

Physiological Integrity

- Begin every assessment of the client after surgery by checking the airway and breathing effectiveness.
- Assess the incision site each shift (on the medical-surgical nursing unit).
- In the event of wound dehiscence or evisceration, have the client lie flat (supine); apply sterile, nonadherent dressing materials to the wound; and follow the steps outlined in Chart 22-4.
- Teach the client about any drugs to be continued after discharge from the facility setting.
- Instruct the client and family about the clinical manifestations of complications and when to seek assistance.

ADDITIONAL STUDY RESOURCES

Go to your Student CD-ROM for Review Questions for the NCLEX Examination.

evolve Go to http://evolve.elsevier.com/Iggy/ for Integrated Management of Care Questions for the NCLEX Examination.

SELECTED BIBLIOGRAPHY

Asterisk indicates a classic or definitive work on this subject.

*Acute Pain Management Guideline Panel. (1992). *Acute pain management in adults: Operative procedures.* AHCPR Publication No. 92-0022. Rockville, MD: Agency for Health Care Policy and Research, Public Health Service, U.S. Department of Health and Human Services.

Allen, G. (2002). Supplemental perioperative oxygen to reduce the incidence of surgical-wound infection. *AORN Journal, 76*(2), 330-331.

American Society of PeriAnesthesia Nurses. (2000). *Standards of perianesthesia nursing practice.* Cherry Hill, NJ: Author.

Aragon, D., Ring, C.A., & Covelli, M. (2003). The influence of diabetes mellitus on postoperative infections. *Critical Care Nursing Clinics of North America, 15*(1), 125-135.

Arnstein, P. (2002). Optimizing perioperative pain management. *AORN Journal, 76*(5), 812-817.

Bryan, S. (2002). Hemolytic transfusion reaction: Safeguards for practice. *Journal of PeriAnesthesia Nursing 17*(6), 399-402.

Bush, N., & Griffin-Sobel, J. (2003). Acute postoperative pain management and malfunctioning epidural catheter. *Oncology Nursing Forum, 30*(2), 227-228.

Candido, L. (2002). Treatment of surgical wound dehiscence. *Dermatology Nursing, 14*(3), 177-178, 181.

Collins, M., & McDonald, V. (2000). Managing postoperative pain at home. *Canadian Nurse, 96*(7), 26-29.

Dang, D., et al. (2002). Postoperative complications: Does intensive care unit staff nursing make a difference? *Heart & Lung, 31*(3), 219-228.

Dixon, L. (2002). Postoperative complications and the older adult. *Geriatric Nursing, 23*(11), 203.

Dochterman, J., & Bulechek, G. (Eds.). (2004). *Nursing interventions classification (NIC)* (4th ed.). St. Louis: Mosby.

Dunn, D. (2004). Preventing perioperative complications in an older adult. *Nursing 2004, 34*(11), 36-41.

Ebersole, P., Hess, P., & Luggen, A. (2004). Toward healthy aging: Human needs and nursing response (6th ed.). St. Louis: Mosby.

Facts and Comparisons. (2001). *Drug facts and comparisons* (55th ed.). St. Louis: Author.

Fort, C. (2002). Get pumped to prevent DVT. *Nursing2002, 32*(9), 50-52.

Golembiewski, J. (2003). Morphine and hydromorphone for postoperative analgesia: Focus on safety. *Journal of PeriAnesthesia Nursing, 18*(2), 120-122.

Golembiewski, J., & O'Brien, D. (2002). A systematic approach to the management of postoperative nausea and vomiting. *Journal of PeriAnesthesia Nursing, 17*(6), 364-376.

Griffis, C., & Gierat, S. (2003). Acute postoperative pain management and malfunctioning epidural catheter. *Oncology Nursing Forum, 30*(2), 227-228.

Hayes, J., Lehman, C., & Castonguay, P. (2002). Graduated compression stockings: Updating practice, improving compliance. *MEDSURG Nursing, 11*(4), 163-167, 191.

Hess, D. (2000). Detection and monitoring of hypoxemia and oxygen therapy. *Respiratory Care, 45*(1), 65-83.

Hrouda, B. (2000). How to remove surgical sutures and staples. *Nursing2000, 30*(2), 54-55.

Jacobs, V. (2000). Informational needs of surgical patients following discharge. *Applied Nursing Research, 13*(1), 12-18.

Kowalczyk, T. (2002). A low-tech approach to venous congestion. *RN, 65*(10), 26-30.

Letizia, M., O'Leary, J., & Vodvarka, J. (2003). Laryngeal edema: Perioperative nursing considerations. *MEDSURG Nursing, 12*(2), 111-115.

*Lusis, S.A. (1996). The challenges of nursing elderly surgical patients. *AORN Journal, 64*(6), 954-955, 957-962.

Mamaril, M. (2003). Standards of perianesthesia nursing practice: Advocating patient safety. *Journal of PeriAnesthesia Nursing, 18*(3), 168-172.

McGaffigan, P. (2002). Advancing sedation assessment to promote patient comfort. *Critical Care Nurse, 22*(1), Supplement 29-36.

Moorhead, S., Johnson, M., & Maas, M. (Eds.). (2004). *Nursing outcomes classification (NOC)* (3rd ed.). St. Louis: Mosby.

Morris, B., Morrison, R., & Yetsko, C. (2002). Venous thromboembolism: Prevention and treatment. *RN, 65*(10), 24hf3-24hf8.

Moz, T. (2004). Wound dehiscence and evisceration. *Nursing 2004, 34*(5), 88.

Pullen, R. (2003). Removing sutures and staples. *Nursing 2003, 33*(10), 18.

Shea, R., Brooks, J., Dayhoff, N., & Keck, J. (2002). Pain intensity and postoperative pulmonary complications among the elderly after abdominal surgery. *Heart & Lung, 31*(6), 440-449.

Sherwood, G., et al. (2003). Changing acute pain management outcomes in surgical patients. *AORN Journal, 77*(2), 374-393.

Squires, A. (2003). Documenting surgical incision site care. *Nursing2003,* 33(1), 74.

Tappen, R., Muzic, J., & Kennedy, P. (2001). Preoperative assessment and discharge planning for older adults undergoing ambulatory surgery. *AORN Journal, 73*(2), 464-474.

Tittle, M., McMillan, S., & Hagan, S. (2003). Validating the Brief Pain Inventory for use with surgical patients with cancer. *Oncology Nursing Forum, 30*(2), 325-330.

Walton, J. (2001). Helping high-risk surgical patients beat the odds. *Nursing2001, 31*(3), 54-59.

Wilson, M. (2000). Giving postanesthesia care in the critical care unit. *Dimensions of Critical Care Nursing, 21*(2), 38-43.

Wood, B. (2002). Caring for a limited-English proficient patient. *AORN Journal, 75*(2), 305-308.

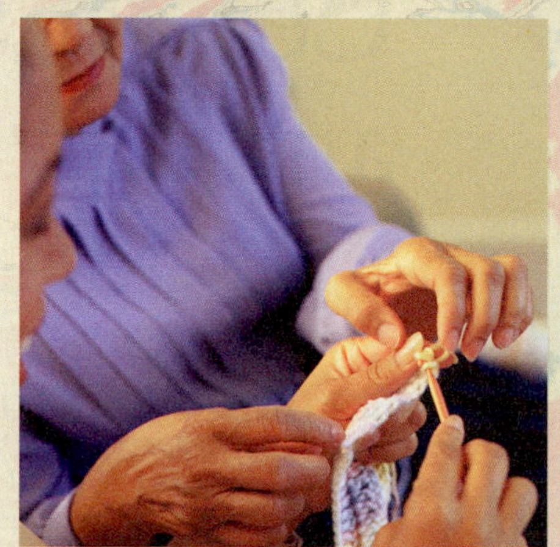

PROBLEMS of PROTECTION

Management of Clients with Problems of the Immune Response

CHAPTER

23

Concepts of Inflammation and the Immune Response

M. LINDA WORKMAN

LEARNING OUTCOMES

After studying this chapter, you should be able to:

1. Describe the concept of self-tolerance.
2. Explain the differences between inflammation and infection.
3. Compare and contrast the cells, purposes, and features of inflammation and immunity.
4. Describe the basis for the five cardinal manifestations of inflammation.
5. Interpret a white blood cell count with differential to indicate no immune problems, an acute bacterial infection, a chronic bacterial infection, or an allergic reaction.
6. Explain how complement activation and fixation assists in protection from infection.
7. Compare the cells, function, and protective actions of antibody-mediated immunity and cell-mediated immunity.
8. Compare the different types of antibody-mediated immunity for their protection effectiveness and duration of immunity.
9. Describe how the immune system responds to the presence of transplanted tissues or organs.
10. Explain the actions and short- and long-term side effects of immunosuppressive drugs.

Go to your Student CD-ROM for Review Questions for the NCLEX Examination keyed to these Learning Outcomes.

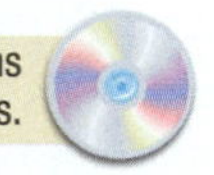

Injury and infectious diseases are common. Most people, however, are healthy more often than they are ill. Inflammation and immunity are the two major defenses that protect a person against diseases and other problems when the body is invaded by organisms. These same defenses also help the body recover after injury or tissue damage. Thus inflammation and immunity are critical to maintaining health and preventing disease. When these defenses are working well, the person is **immunocompetent.**

Immune function is reduced by many diseases, injuries, and medical therapies. Reduction of immune function may be temporary or permanent, but always endangers the client's health.

OVERVIEW

Immunity is composed of many cell functions that protect people against the effects of injury or microscopic invasion. People interact with many other living organisms in the environment. The size of these organisms varies from large (other humans and animals) to microscopic (bacteria, viruses, molds, spores, pollens, protozoa, and cells from other people or animals). As long as organisms do not enter the body's internal environment, they pose no threat to health. The body has some defenses to prevent organisms from gaining access to the internal environment. These defenses are not perfect, and invasion of the body's internal environment by organisms occurs often. Invasion occurs much more often than does an actual disease or illness because of proper immune functioning.

Purpose of Inflammation and Immunity

The purpose of inflammation and immunity is to neutralize, eliminate, or destroy organisms that invade the internal environment. To accomplish this purpose without harming the body, immune system cells use defensive actions only against non-self proteins and cells. Immune system cells can distinguish between the body's own healthy self cells and other, non-self proteins and cells.

Self versus Non-Self

Non-self proteins and cells include infected body cells, cancer cells, and all invading cells and organisms. This ability to recognize self versus non-self, which is necessary to prevent healthy body cells from being destroyed along with the invaders, is called **self-tolerance.** The immune system cells are the only body cells capable of determining self from non-self. Self-tolerance is possible because of the different kinds of proteins present on cell membranes.

All organisms are made up of cells. Each cell is surrounded by a plasma membrane (Figure 23-1). Many different proteins protrude through the cell's membrane. For example, in liver cells, many different proteins are present on the cell membrane surface. The amino acid sequence of each protein type differs from that of all other protein types. Some of these proteins are found on the liver cells of all animals (including humans) that have livers, because these protein types are specific to the liver and serve as a marker for liver tissues. Other protein types are found only on the liver cells of humans, because these protein types are specific markers for humans. Still other protein types are found only on the liver cells of humans with a specific blood type. In addition, each person's liver cells have surface protein types that are specific to that person. These proteins are unique to the person and would be identical only to the proteins of an identical twin. These unique proteins, found on the surface of all body cells of that individual, serve as a "universal product code" or a "cellular fingerprint" for that person. The proteins that make up the universal product code for one person are recognized as "foreign," or non-self, by the immune system of another person. Because the cell-surface proteins are non-self to another person's immune system, they are **antigens,** proteins capable of stimulating an immune response.

Human leukocyte antigens (HLAs) make up this unique universal product code for each person. "Leukocyte antigen" is not a correct term, because these antigens are also present on the surfaces of nearly all body cells, not just on leukocytes. HLAs are a normal part of the person and act as antigens only if they enter another person's body. These antigens specify the **tissue type** of a person. Other names for these personal cellular fingerprints are *human transplantation antigens, human histocompatibility antigens, major histocompatibility antigens,* and *class I antigens.*

Humans have about 40 major HLAs that are determined by a set of genes called the major histocompatibility complex (MHC). The exact number of *minor* HLAs that any person has is not known. The specific antigens that any person has (of a large number of possible antigens) are genetically determined by which MHC genes were inherited from his or her parents.

This universal product code (HLA) is key for recognition and self-tolerance. The immune system cells constantly come into contact with other body cells and with any invader that happens to enter the body. At each encounter, the immune system cells compare the surface protein universal product codes (HLAs) to determine whether or not the encountered cell belongs in the body (Figure 23-2). If the encountered cell's universal product code (HLA) perfectly matches the HLA of the immune system cell, the encountered cell is "self" and is not attacked by the immune system cell. If the encountered cell's universal product code (HLA) does not perfectly match the HLA of the immune system cell, the encountered cell is non-self, or foreign. The immune system cell takes action to neutralize, destroy, or eliminate the foreign invader.

Immune function changes during a person's life, according to nutritional status, environmental conditions, drugs, the presence of disease, and age. Immune function is most efficient when people are in their 20s and 30s and slowly declines with increasing age. Older adults have decreased immune function, increasing their risk for many health problems (Chart 23-1).

Organization of the Immune System

The immune system is not confined to any one organ or area of the body. Most immune system cells come from the bone marrow. Some of these cells mature in the bone mar-

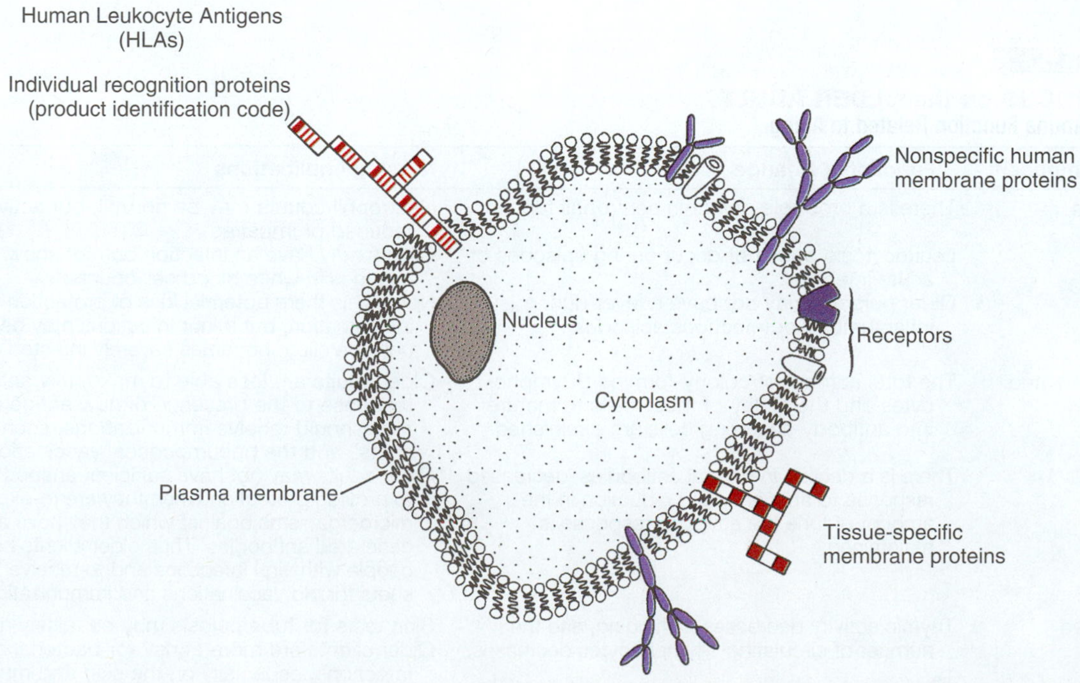

Figure 23-1 ■ Properties of human cell membranes.

row; others leave the bone marrow and mature in different body sites. When mature, most immune system cells are released into the blood, where they circulate to most body areas and have specific effects.

The bone marrow is the source of all blood cells, including immune system cells. The bone marrow produces an immature, undifferentiated cell called a **stem cell** (Abbas & Lichtman, 2003). This immature stem cell is also described as *pluripotent, multipotent,* and *totipotent.* These terms describe the potential future of the stem cell. When the stem cell is first created in the bone marrow, it is undifferentiated. The cell is not yet committed to maturing into a specific blood cell type. At this stage, the stem cell is flexible and could become any one of many mature blood cells. Figure 23-3 shows the possible outcomes for maturation of the pluripotent stem cell. The type of mature cell that the stem cell becomes depends on which pathway it follows.

The maturational pathway of any stem cell depends on body needs at the time, as well as on the presence of specific hormones (cytokines, factors) that direct maturation. For example, **erythropoietin** is made in the kidney. When immature stem cells are exposed to erythropoietin, they commit to the erythrocyte pathway and become mature red blood cells.

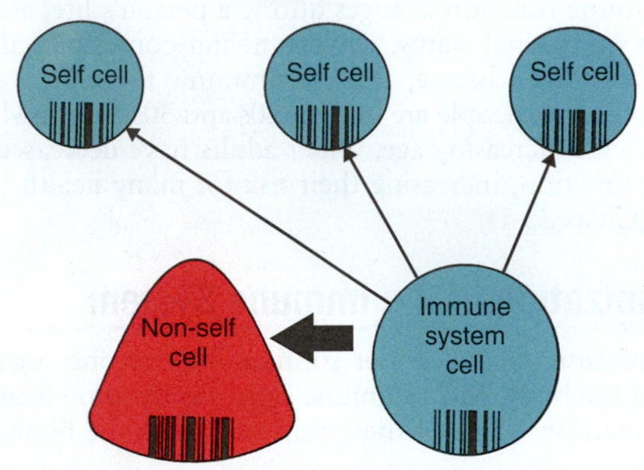

Figure 23-2 ■ Determination of self versus non-self cells.

White blood cells **(leukocytes)** protect the body from the effects of invasion by organisms. These cells are the immune system cells. Table 23-1 lists the functions of different immune system cells. The leukocytes provide protection through many defensive actions (Abbas & Lichtman, 2003). These actions include the following:

- Recognition of self versus non-self
- Phagocytic destruction of foreign invaders, cellular debris, and unhealthy or abnormal self cells
- Lytic destruction of foreign invaders and unhealthy self cells
- Production of antibodies directed against invaders
- Complement activation
- Production of cytokines that stimulate increased formation of leukocytes in bone marrow
- Production of cytokines that increase specific leukocyte growth and activity

The three processes needed for immunity are (1) inflammation, (2) antibody-mediated immunity (AMI), also known as humoral immunity, and (3) cell-mediated immunity (CMI). These processes use different defensive actions, and each process influences or requires assistance from the other two processes (Figure 23-4). *Therefore full immunity* ***(immunocompetence)*** *requires the function and interaction of all three processes.*

INFLAMMATION

Inflammation, sometimes called "natural" immunity, provides immediate protection against the effects of tissue injury and invading foreign proteins. The ability to produce an inflammatory response is critical to health and well-being. Inflammation differs from AMI and CMI in two important ways:

1. Inflammatory protection is immediate but short term against the effects of injury or invading organisms. It

CHART 23-1

NURSING FOCUS on the OLDER ADULT

Changes in Immune Function Related to Aging

Immune Component	Functional Change	Nursing Implications
Inflammation	There is a probable defect in neutrophil function.	Neutrophil counts may be normal, but activity is reduced or impaired.
	Leukocytosis does not occur during episodes of acute infection.	Clients may have an infection but not show expected changes in white blood cell counts.
	Older persons may not have a fever during inflammatory or infectious episodes.	Not only is there potential loss of protection through inflammation, but minor infections may be overlooked until the client becomes severely infected or septic.
Antibody-mediated immunity	The total number of colony-forming B-lymphocytes and the ability of these cells to mature into antibody-secreting cells are diminished.	Older adults are less able to make new antibodies in response to the presence of new antigens. Thus they should receive immunizations, such as "flu shots" and the pneumococcal vaccination.
	There is a decline in natural antibodies, decreased response to antigens, and reduction in the amount of time the antibody response is maintained.	Older adults may not have sufficient antibodies present to provide protection when they are re-exposed to microorganisms against which they have already generated antibodies. Thus older clients need to avoid people with viral infections and to receive "booster" shots for old vaccinations and immunizations.
Cell-mediated immunity	Thymic activity decreases with aging, and the number of circulating T-lymphocytes decreases.	Skin tests for tuberculosis may be falsely negative. Older clients are more at risk for bacterial and fungal infections, especially on the skin and mucous membranes, in the respiratory tract, and in the genitourinary tract.

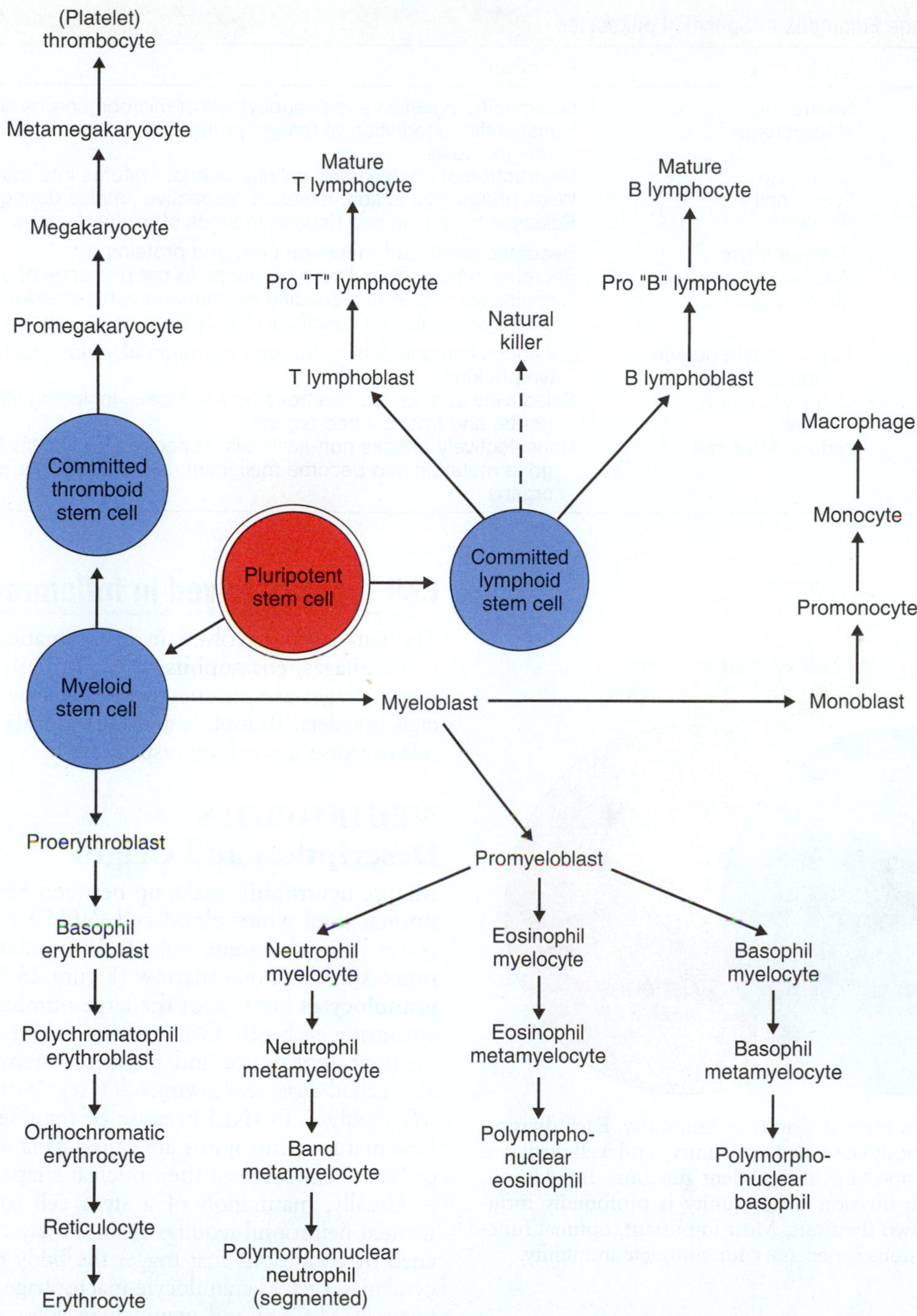

Figure 23-3 ■ Stem cell differentiation and maturation.

does not provide sustained, long-term immunity on repeated exposure to the same organisms.

2. Inflammation is a nonspecific body defense to invasion or injury and can be started quickly by almost any event.

Inflammation is nonspecific; the same tissue responses occur with any type of injury or invasion, regardless of the location on the body or the specific initiating agent. Thus inflammation triggered by a scald burn to the hand is the same as inflammation triggered by excess stomach acid or bacteria in the middle ear. How widespread the symptoms of inflammation are in the body depends on the intensity, severity, duration, and extent of exposure to the initiating injury or invasion. For example, a splinter in the finger triggers inflammation only at the splinter site, whereas a burn injuring 60% of the skin surface results in an inflammatory response involving the entire body.

Purpose

Inflammatory responses start tissue actions that cause visible and uncomfortable symptoms. Despite the discomfort, these actions are important in ridding the body of harmful organisms. However, if the inflammatory response is excessive, tissue damage may result. Inflammatory responses also help start both antibody-mediated and cell-mediated actions to activate a full immune response.

TABLE 23-1 Immune Functions of Specific Leukocytes

Variable	Leukocyte	Function
Inflammation	Neutrophil	Nonspecific ingestion and phagocytosis of microorganisms and foreign protein
	Macrophage	Nonspecific recognition of foreign proteins and microorganisms; ingestion and phagocytosis
	Monocyte	Destruction of bacteria and cellular debris; matures into macrophage
	Eosinophil	Weak phagocytic action; releases vasoactive amines during allergic reactions
	Basophil	Releases histamine and heparin in areas of tissue damage
Antibody-mediated immunity	B-lymphocyte	Becomes sensitized to foreign cells and proteins
	Plasma cell	Secretes immunoglobulins in response to the presence of a specific antigen
	Memory cell	Remains sensitized to a specific antigen and can secrete increased amounts of immunoglobulins specific to the antigen on re-exposure
Cell-mediated immunity	T-lymphocyte helper/inducer T-cell	Enhances immune activity through secretion of various factors, cytokines, and lymphokines
	Cytotoxic/cytolytic T-cell	Selectively attacks and destroys non-self cells, including virally infected cells, grafts, and transplanted organs
	Natural killer cell	Nonselectively attacks non-self cells, especially body cells that have undergone mutation and become malignant; also attacks grafts and transplanted organs

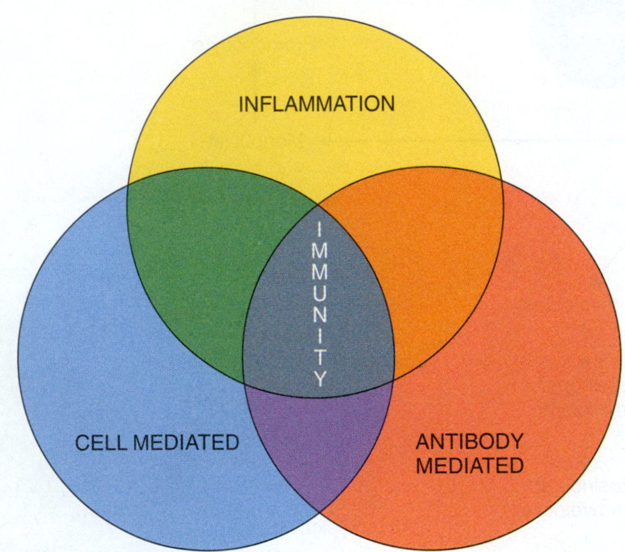

Figure 23-4 ■ The three divisions of immunity. Each division (inflammation, antibody-mediated immunity, and cell-mediated immunity) has an important independent function. In addition, the function of each division of immunity is profoundly influenced by the other two divisions. Most important, optimal function of all three divisions is necessary for complete immunity.

Infection

A confusing issue about inflammation is that this process occurs in response to tissue injury, as well as to invasion by organisms. *Infection is usually accompanied by inflammation; however, inflammation can occur without invasion by organisms.* Examples of inflammation without infection include sprain injuries to joints, myocardial infarction, sterile surgical incisions, thrombophlebitis, and blister formation. Examples of inflammation caused by noninfectious invasion by foreign proteins include allergic rhinitis, contact dermatitis, and other allergic reactions. Inflammations caused by infection include otitis media, appendicitis, bacterial peritonitis, viral hepatitis, and bacterial myocarditis, among many others. *Thus inflammation does not always mean that an infection is present.*

Cell Types Involved in Inflammation

The leukocytes involved in inflammation are neutrophils, macrophages, eosinophils, and basophils. Neutrophils and macrophages use phagocytosis to destroy and eliminate foreign invaders. Basophils and eosinophils act on blood vessels to cause tissue-level responses.

NEUTROPHILS

Description and Origin

Mature neutrophils make up between 55% and 70% of the normal total white blood cell (WBC) count. **Neutrophils** come from the stem cells and complete the maturation process in the bone marrow (Figure 23-5). They are called **granulocytes** because of the large number of granules present inside each cell. Other names for neutrophils are based on their appearance and maturity. Mature neutrophils are also called *segmented neutrophils* ("segs") or *polymorphonuclear cells* ("polys," PMNs,) because of their segmented nucleus. Less mature neutrophils are called *band neutrophils* ("bands" or "stabs") because of their nuclear shape.

Usually, maturation of a stem cell to a functional segmented neutrophil requires 12 to 14 days. This time is shortened by conditions that trigger the body to produce specific cytokines, such as granulocyte-macrophage colony-stimulating factor (GM-CSF) and granulocyte colony-stimulating factor (G-CSF). The purpose and action of cytokines are described later in this chapter under Cytokines, p. 374.

In the immunocompetent healthy person, more than 100 billion fresh, mature neutrophils are released from the bone marrow into the circulation daily (Abbas & Lichtman, 2003). This huge production is needed because the life span of a circulating neutrophil is short, about 12 to 18 hours.

Function

Although the neutrophils are the largest group of circulating leukocytes, each cell is small. This powerful army of small cells is the first internal line of defense against invaders (especially bacteria) in blood and extracellular fluid. It is the granules inside the neutrophils that destroy invaders by phagocytosis.

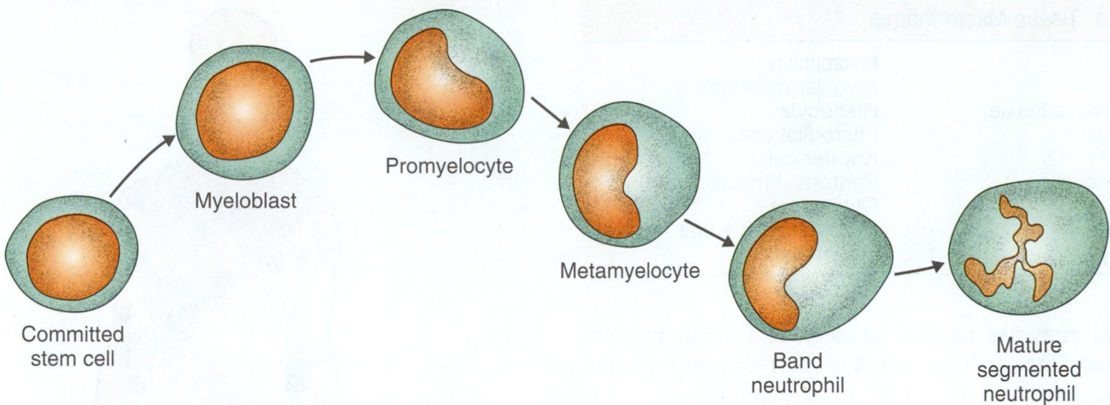

Figure 23-5 ■ Neutrophil maturation.

The mature neutrophil has many granules containing different enzymes that can degrade invaders.

Neutrophils have a small energy supply and no way of replenishing it; neither do they have a way of replenishing the enzymes used in phagocytosis. As a result, each neutrophil can take part in only one episode of phagocytosis before supplies are exhausted.

Mature neutrophils are the only neutrophil stage capable of phagocytosis. Because this cell type is responsible for continuous, instant, nonspecific protection against organisms, the percentage and actual number of mature circulating neutrophils is used to measure a client's risk for infection: the higher the numbers, the greater the resistance to infection. This measurement is the **absolute neutrophil count** (also called the absolute granulocyte count or total granulocyte count).

The differential of a normal white blood cell count shows the number and percent of all the different types of circulating leukocytes (Figure 23-6). This test indicates that most of the neutrophils released into the blood from the bone marrow are segmented neutrophils; only a small percentage are band neutrophils. The less mature neutrophil forms should not be in the blood. Some problems cause the neutrophils in the blood to change from being mostly segmented neutrophils to being less mature forms. This situation is termed a **left shift** or "bandemia" because the segmented neutrophil, which is seen at the far right of the neutrophil pathway (see Figure 23-5), is no longer the greatest number of circulating neutrophils. Instead, more of the circulating cells are "bands," the less mature cell type found farther left on the neutrophil pathway.

A left shift indicates that the client's bone marrow cannot produce enough mature neutrophils to keep pace with the continuing infection and is releasing immature neutrophils into the blood. Unfortunately, most of these immature cells are of no benefit, because they are not capable of phagocytosis.

Differential	%	/mm^3
Total WBC	100	10,000
segs	62	6200
bands	5	500
monos	3	300
lymphs	28	2800
eosin	1.5	150
baso	0.5	50

Figure 23-6 ■ Example of a laboratory slip showing the differential of a normal white blood cell (WBC) count.

MACROPHAGES

Description and Origin

Macrophages come from the committed myeloid stem cells in the bone marrow and form the mononuclear-phagocyte system. The stem cells first form monocytes and are released into the blood at this stage. Until they mature, monocytes have limited activity. Most monocytes move from the blood into body tissues, where they mature into macrophages. Some macrophages become "fixed" in position within the tissues, whereas others can move within and between tissues. Macrophages in various tissues have slightly different appearances and different names. Table 23-2 lists the tissue macrophages. Figure 23-7 shows the distribution of tissue macrophages throughout the body. The liver and spleen contain the greatest numbers of these cells.

Macrophages have long life spans, lasting from months to years. They are large and contain many lytic enzymes.

Function

Macrophages play more than one role in protecting against invasion and tissue injury. These cells are important in immediate inflammatory responses and also stimulate the longer-lasting immune responses of antibody-mediated immunity (AMI) and cell-mediated immunity (CMI). Specific macrophage functions include phagocytosis, repair of injured tissues, antigen presenting/processing, and secretion of cytokines that help control the immune system.

The inflammatory function of macrophages is phagocytosis. Macrophages can easily distinguish between self and non-self and are very effective at trapping invading cells. Unlike neutrophils, macrophages are able to renew their energy

TABLE 23-2 Tissue Macrophages

Tissue	Macrophage
Lung	Alveolar macrophage
Connective tissue	Histiocyte
Brain	Microglial cell
Liver	Kupffer cell
Peritoneum	Peritoneal macrophage
Bone	Osteoclast
Joints	Synovial type A cell
Kidney	Mesangial cell

supplies and enzymes needed to degrade foreign protein. Therefore each macrophage can take part in many phagocytic events.

BASOPHILS

Description and Origin

Basophils come from myeloid stem cells and make up only about 1% of the total circulating WBC count. They are released from the marrow after a short maturation period. These cells cause the manifestations of inflammation.

Function

Basophils have granules containing many chemicals (vasoactive amines) that act on blood vessels. These chemicals include heparin, histamine, serotonin, kinins, and leukotrienes. When released into the blood, most of these chemicals act on smooth muscle and blood vessel walls. Heparin inhibits blood and protein clotting. Histamine constricts small veins and respiratory smooth muscles. Constriction of respiratory smooth muscle narrows airways and restricts breathing. Constriction of veins inhibits blood flow and decreases venous return. This effect causes blood to collect in capillaries and small arterioles. Kinins dilate arterioles and increase capillary permeability. These actions cause blood plasma to leak into the interstitial space **(vascular leak syndrome).**

EOSINOPHILS

Description and Origin

Eosinophils come from the myeloid line and contain many vasoactive chemicals. Usually, only 1% to 2% of the total white blood cell (WBC) count is composed of eosinophils.

Function

Eosinophils act against infestations of parasitic larvae. Eosinophil granules contain many different substances. Some substances induce inflammation when released. In addition, enzymes from eosinophils degrade the vasoactive chemicals released by other leukocytes and can limit inflammatory reactions. This is why the number of circulating eosinophils increases during an allergic response.

Phagocytosis

A key process of inflammation is phagocytosis. **Phagocytosis** is the engulfing and destruction of invaders. This action also rids the body of debris after tissue injury. Neutrophils and macrophages are most efficient at phagocytosis. Phagocytosis involves the seven steps shown in Figure 23-8.

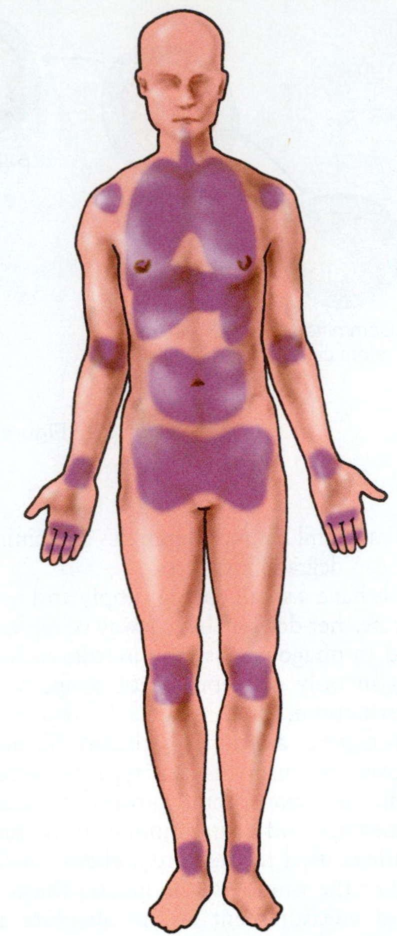

Figure 23-7 ■ Areas of highest concentration of tissue macrophages.

EXPOSURE AND INVASION

Leukocytes that engage in phagocytosis and stimulate inflammation are present in the blood and other extracellular fluids. For phagocytosis to start, leukocytes must first be exposed to organisms, foreign proteins, or debris from damaged tissues. Phagocytosis is triggered by injury or invasion.

ATTRACTION

Phagocytosis can only occur when the WBC comes into direct contact with the target (antigen, invader, or foreign protein). Some substances act as chemical magnets that attract neutrophils and macrophages. These substances are called **chemotaxins** or **leukotaxins.** Damaged tissues and blood vessels secrete chemotaxins. In addition, substances that combine with the surface of invading foreign proteins serve as chemotaxins. This combining (and attracting) mechanism is described next.

ADHERENCE

Because phagocytosis requires direct contact of the leukocyte with its intended target, the phagocytic cell must first bind to the surface of the target. A process called opsonization increases contact of the cell with its target.

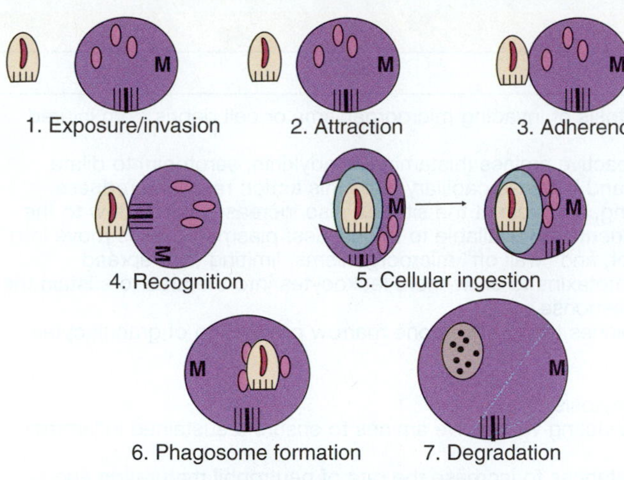

Figure 23-8 ■ Steps of phagocytosis.

Opsonization

The word *opsonin* means "to cover food with a sauce before eating." In inflammation, opsonins coat a target cell (antigen or organism). Coating the target makes it easier for phagocytic cells to stick to it. Many substances can act as opsonins. Some are particles from dead neutrophils, antibodies, and activated (fixated) complement components.

Complement Activation and Fixation

One type of opsonization is complement activation and fixation. Twenty different types of inactive complement proteins are present in the blood. These proteins are made by the liver. With proper stimulation, each complement protein is activated, joins other activated complement proteins, surrounds an antigen, and "fixes" or sticks to the antigen. Complement fixation occurs quickly as a cascade or chain reaction.

RECOGNITION

When the phagocytic cell sticks to the surface of the target cell, it "recognizes" the non-self. The phagocytic cells examine the universal product codes (human leukocyte antigens [HLAs]) of whatever they encounter. Recognition of non-self is made easier by opsonins on the target cell surface. Phagocytic cells start phagocytosis only if the target cell is recognized either as non-self or as debris from damaged self cells.

CELLULAR INGESTION

Because phagocytic destruction occurs inside the cell, the target cell is brought inside the phagocytic cell. The phagocytic cell bends its membrane around to enclose (engulf) the target cell. Once the target is enclosed in the phagocytic cells, a vacuole is formed.

PHAGOSOME FORMATION

When the phagocyte's granules are inside the vacuole, the structure is called a **phagosome (phagolysosome).** These granules break and release enzymes to destroy the ingested target.

DEGRADATION

The enzymes in the phagosome digest the engulfed target. The target is broken into smaller pieces until only small particles of debris remain.

Sequence of Inflammatory Responses

Inflammatory responses occur in a predictable sequence. The sequence is the same regardless of the triggering event. Responses at the tissue level cause the **five cardinal manifestations of inflammation:** warmth, redness, swelling, pain, and decreased function. Inflammatory responses occur in three stages and the timing of the stages may overlap (Table 23-3).

STAGE I (VASCULAR)

In stage I of the inflammatory response, the early effects involve changes in blood vessels. When inflammation results from tissue injury, this stage has two phases.

Phase I

The first phase is rapid but short-term blood vessel constriction caused by trauma to blood vessel smooth muscle. This phase lasts only seconds and may be so short that the person is unaware of it.

Phase II

In the second phase, blood flow to the area increases **(hyperemia)** and swelling **(edema)** forms at the site of injury or invasion. Injured tissues and the leukocytes in this area secrete histamine, serotonin, and kinins that constrict the small veins and dilate the arterioles in the area of injury. These blood vessel changes cause redness and warmth of the tissues. This increased blood flow increases delivery of nutrients to injured tissues.

Capillary leak also occurs, allowing blood plasma to leak into the tissues. This response causes swelling and pain. Edema at the site of injury or invasion protects the area from further injury by creating a cushion of fluid. The extra fluid also can dilute any toxins or organisms that have entered the area. The duration of these responses depends on the severity of the initiating event.

The macrophage is the major cell involved in stage I of inflammation. The action is rapid because macrophages are already in place at the site of injury or invasion. This action is limited because the number of macrophages is so small. To enhance the inflammatory response, the tissue macrophages secrete several cytokines. One cytokine is colony-stimulating factor (CSF), which triggers the bone marrow to increase the rate of white blood cell (WBC) production from 14 days to a matter of hours. Some of the cytokines also increase the release of neutrophils from the bone marrow and attract them to the site of injury or invasion, which leads to the next stage of inflammation.

STAGE II (CELLULAR EXUDATE)

In stage II, **neutrophilia** (increased number of circulating neutrophils) occurs, along with the formation of exudate, commonly called **pus.**

The most active cell in this stage is the neutrophil. Under the influence of cytokines, the neutrophil count can increase up to five times within 12 hours after the onset of inflammation. At the site of inflammation, neutrophils attack and destroy organisms and remove dead tissue through phagocytosis.

In acute inflammation, the healthy person produces enough mature neutrophils to keep pace with invasion and

TABLE 23-3 Stages of Inflammation

Onset	Cells Involved	Actions
Stage I: Vascular		
Minutes after injury or invasion	Tissue macrophages	Limited phagocytosis of invading microorganisms or cell debris from injured tissues Secretion of vasoactive amines (histamine, bradykinin, serotonin) to dilate blood vessels and increase capillary leak; this action results in redness, warmth, swelling, and pain at the site but also increases blood flow to the area; more nutrients are available to the tissues; plasma proteins move into the tissues, clot, and "wall off" microorganisms, limiting their spread Secretion of chemotaxins to draw more leukocytes into the area to sustain the inflammatory response Secretion of cytokines to increase bone marrow production of granulocytes
Stage II: Cellular Exudate		
Hours after injury or invasion	Granular myeloid cells ▪ Neutrophils ▪ Basophils ▪ Eosinophils	Increased phagocytosis Secretion of slow-acting vasoactive amines to ensure a sustained inflammatory response Secretion of substances to increase the rate of neutrophil maturation and macrophage maturation
Stage III: Tissue Repair and Replacement		
Begins at initial injury and continues until new tissues are formed and mature or are functional	Neutrophils Macrophages	Stimulation of mitotically active cells to divide; stimulation of fibroblasts in blood vessels to grow and release collagen to form scaffold on which to build scar tissue

prevent the organisms from growing. At the same time, the WBCs and inflamed tissues secrete cytokines, which allow tissue macrophages to increase and trigger bone marrow production of monocytes. This reaction begins slowly but its effects are long lasting.

During this phase, the arachidonic acid cascade starts to increase the inflammatory response. This action begins by the conversion of fatty acids in plasma membranes into arachidonic acid (AA). Then, enzymes (including cyclooxygenase) convert AA into many chemicals that are further processed into the substances that continue the inflammatory response in the tissues. These substances include histamine, leukotrienes, prostaglandins, serotonin, and kinins. Many anti-inflammatory drugs stop this cascade by preventing cyclooxygenase from converting AA into inflammatory substances.

When an infection stimulating inflammation lasts longer than just a few days, the bone marrow cannot produce and release enough mature neutrophils into the blood to keep pace with the growth of organisms. In this situation, the bone marrow begins to release immature neutrophils, reducing the number of circulating mature neutrophils. This reduction of functional neutrophils limits the helpful effects of inflammation and increases the risk for sepsis.

STAGE III (TISSUE REPAIR AND REPLACEMENT)

Although stage III is completed last, it begins at the time of injury and is critical to the final function of the inflamed area.

Some of the WBCs involved in inflammation start the replacement of lost tissues or repair of damaged tissues by inducing the remaining healthy cells to divide. In tissues that are unable to divide, WBCs trigger new blood vessel growth and scar tissue formation. Because scar tissue does not behave like normal tissue, loss of function occurs wherever damaged tissues are replaced with scar tissue. The degree of function lost is determined by how much tissue is replaced by scar tissue.

Inflammation alone cannot provide immunity. Inflammatory cells must interact with lymphocytes to provide long-lasting immunity. Long-lasting immune actions develop through antibody-mediated immunity (AMI) and cell-mediated immunity (CMI).

ANTIBODY-MEDIATED IMMUNITY

Antibody-mediated immunity (AMI), also known as humoral immunity, involves antigen-antibody interactions to neutralize, eliminate, or destroy foreign proteins. Antibodies are produced by B-lymphocytes (also known as B-cells).

Purpose

The main functions of B-cells are to become sensitized to a specific foreign protein **(antigen)** and to produce antibodies directed specifically against that protein. The antibody (rather than the actual B-cell) causes one of several actions to neutralize, eliminate, or destroy that antigen.

Cell Types Involved in Antibody-Mediated Immunity

The cells with the most direct role in AMI are the B-cells. Macrophages and T-lymphocytes (discussed later under Cell-Mediated Immunity, p. 373) work with B-cells to start and complete antigen-antibody interactions. Therefore, for optimal AMI, the entire immune system must function adequately.

B-cells start as stem cells in the bone marrow, the primary lymphoid tissue. Those stem cells destined to become B-cells commit early to the lymphocyte pathway (see Figure 23-3). At the point of commitment, these stem cells are restricted to lymphocyte development. The lymphocyte stem cells are

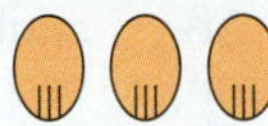
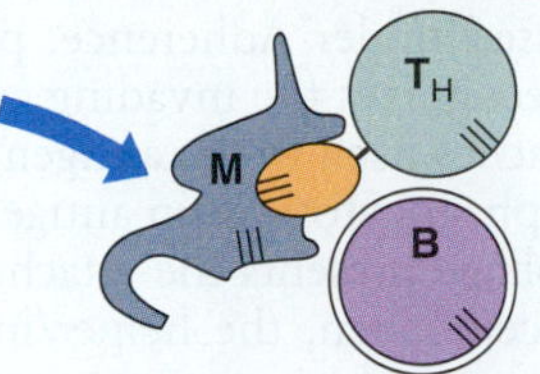

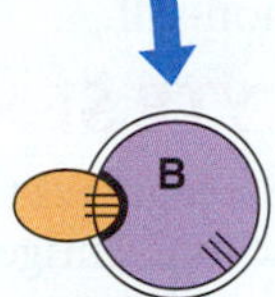

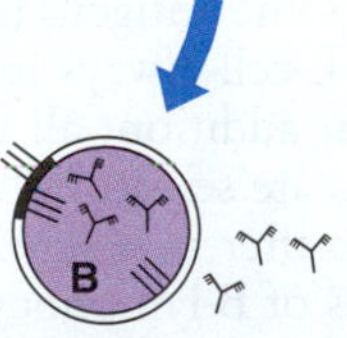

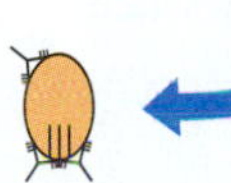
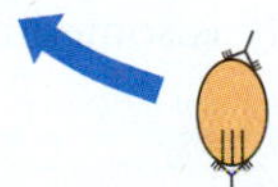

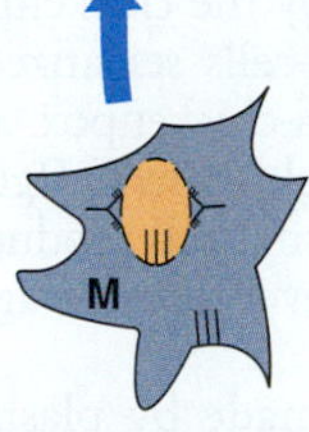

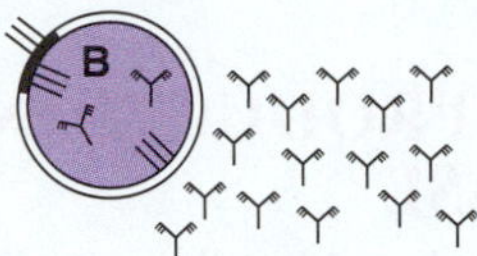

Figure 23-9 ■ Sequence of events stimulating antibody-mediated immunity.

released from the bone marrow into the blood. They then migrate into many secondary lymphoid tissues, where maturation is completed.

The secondary lymphoid tissues for B-cell maturation are the spleen, parts of lymph nodes, tonsils, and Peyer's patches of the intestinal tract.

Antigen-Antibody Interactions

The body learns to make enough of any specific antibody to provide long-lasting immunity against specific organisms or toxins. Seven steps are needed to produce a specific antibody directed against a specific antigen whenever the person is exposed to that antigen. These steps are exposure (invasion), antigen recognition, lymphocyte sensitization, antibody production and release, antigen-antibody binding, antibody-binding reactions, and sustained immunity, or memory (Figure 23-9).

EXPOSURE (INVASION)

Antibody actions occur inside the body or on a few body surfaces. For a person to make an antibody that can exert its effects on a specific antigen, the antigen must first enter the person. Not all exposures or invasions result in antibody production. Invasion by the antigen must occur in such large numbers that some of the antigen evades detection by the body's natural nonspecific defenses or overwhelms the ability of the inflammatory response to get rid of the invader.

Take, for example, a person who has never been exposed to the childhood viral disease chickenpox. This person babysits for three children who develop chickenpox lesions within the next 10 hours. These children, in the pre-eruption stage, shed many millions of live chickenpox virus particles via droplets from the upper respiratory tract. Because small children are often unconcerned about the finer points of infection control, they drink out of the baby-sitter's cup, kiss the baby-sitter directly (and wetly) on the lips, and sneeze and cough directly into the baby-sitter's face. During the 5 hours spent with the children at close range, the baby-sitter is heavily invaded by the chickenpox virus (varicella-zoster) and will become sick with this disease within 14 to 21 days. While the virus is growing and the disease is developing, the baby-sitter's white blood cells are taking part in antibody-antigen actions to prevent the baby-sitter from having chickenpox more than once.

ANTIGEN RECOGNITION

To begin making antibodies against an antigen, the "naive," or "virgin," unsensitized B-cell must first recognize the antigen as non-self. B-cells need the help of macrophages and helper/inducer T-cells to recognize an antigen.

This recognition effort is started by the macrophages. After the antigen surface has been altered by opsonization (previously discussed under Adherence, pp. 366 and 367), the macrophage recognizes the invading antigen as non-self and physically attaches itself to the antigen. This attachment does not result in phagocytosis or in antigen destruction. Instead, the macrophage presents the attached antigen to the helper/inducer T-cell. Then, the helper/inducer T-cell and the macrophage process the antigen to expose the antigen's recognition sites (universal product code). After processing the antigen, the helper/inducer T-cell brings the antigen into contact with the B-cell so that the B-cell can recognize the antigen as non-self.

LYMPHOCYTE SENSITIZATION

Once the B-cell recognizes the antigen as non-self, the B-cell is "sensitized" to this antigen. A single naive B-cell can become sensitized only once. *Therefore each B-cell can be sensitized to only one type of antigen.*

Sensitizing allows this B-cell to respond to any substance that carries the same antigens (codes) as the original antigen. The sensitized B-cell always remains sensitized to that specific antigen. In addition, all cells produced by that sensitized B-cell also are sensitized to that same specific antigen.

Immediately after it is sensitized, the B-cell divides and forms two types of B-lymphocytes, each one remaining sensitized to that specific antigen (Figure 23-10). One new cell becomes a **plasma cell** and immediately starts to produce antibodies against the sensitizing antigen. The other new cell becomes a memory cell. The plasma cell functions immediately and has a short life span. The **memory cell** remains sensitized but does not start to function until the next exposure to the same antigen (discussed later under Sustained Immunity: Memory, p. 372).

ANTIBODY PRODUCTION AND RELEASE

Antibodies are produced by plasma cells. When fully stimulated, each plasma cell can make as much as 300 molecules of antibody per second. Each plasma cell produces antibody specific only to the antigen that originally sensitized the parent B-cell. For example, in the case of the baby-sitter who was exposed to and invaded by the chickenpox virus, the plasma cells derived from the B-cells sensitized to the chickenpox virus can make only anti-chickenpox antibodies. The antibody class (e.g., immunoglobulin G [IgG] or immunoglobulin M [IgM]) that the plasma cell produces may vary, but the antibody can only be forever directed against the chickenpox virus.

Antibody molecules made by plasma cells are released into the blood and other body fluids as free antibody. Each free antibody molecule remains in the blood for 3 to 30 days. Because the antibody is in body fluids (or body "humors") and is separate from the B-cells, this type of immunity is sometimes called **humoral immunity.** *Circulating an-*

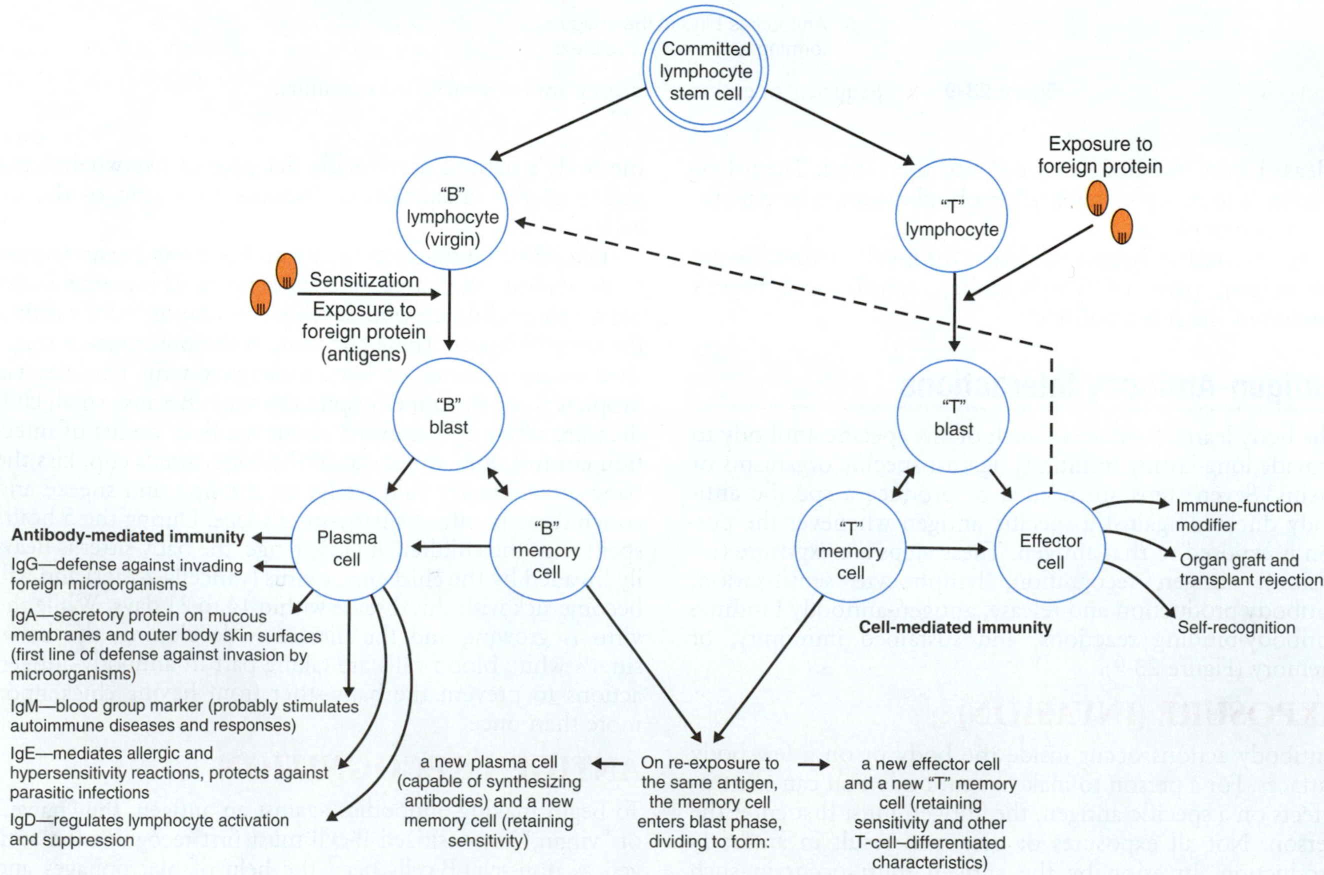

Figure 23-10 ■ Differentiated functions of lymphocytes.

tibodies can be transferred from one person to another to provide the receiving person with immediate immunity of short duration.

ANTIBODY-ANTIGEN BINDING

Antibodies are Y-shaped molecules (Figure 23-11). The tips of the short arms of the Y recognize the specific antigen and bind to it. Because each antibody molecule has two tips (Fab fragments, or arms), each antibody can bind either to two separate antigens or to two areas of the same antigen.

The stem of the Y forms the "Fc fragment." This area can bind to Fc receptor sites on white blood cells (WBCs). The WBC then has not only its own means of attacking antigens, but also has the added power of having surface antibodies that stick to antigens (Figure 23-12).

The actual binding of antibody to antigen is usually not lethal to the antigen. Instead, antibody-antigen binding starts other actions that neutralize, eliminate, or destroy the antigen.

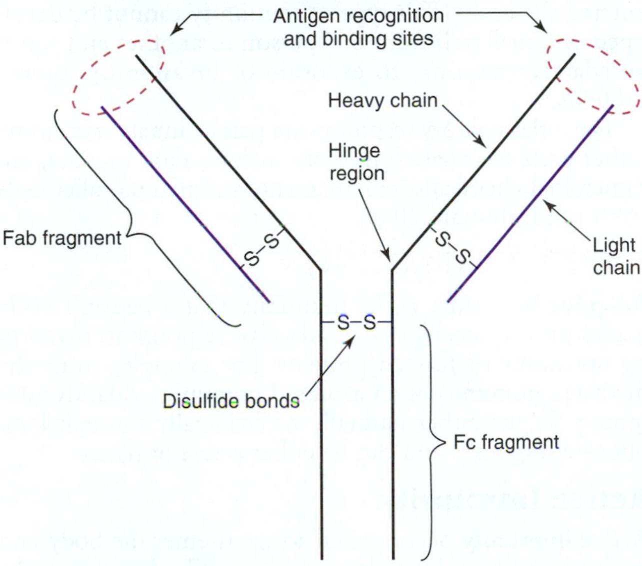

Figure 23-11 ■ Basic antibody structure.

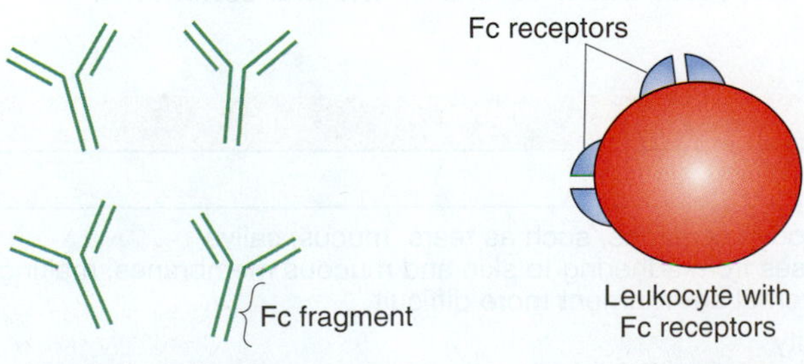

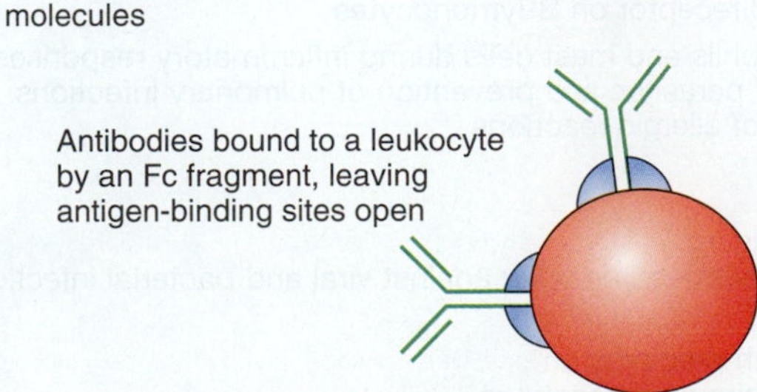

Figure 23-12 ■ Antibody Fc receptors on leukocytes.

ANTIBODY-BINDING ACTIONS

The binding of antibody to antigen triggers reactions that neutralize, eliminate, or destroy the bound antigen. These actions include agglutination, lysis, complement fixation, precipitation, and inactivation or neutralization.

Agglutination

Agglutination is a clumping action that results from the antibody linking antigens together, forming large and small immune complexes (Figure 23-13). Agglutination alone does not directly destroy the antigen. This action starts other defensive effects. First, it slows the movement of the antigen through body fluids. Second, the irregular shape of the antigen-antibody complex (see Figure 23-13) increases the chances of the complex being attacked by other WBCs (e.g., macrophages, neutrophils).

Lysis

Lysis, cell membrane destruction, occurs because of antibody binding to membrane-bound antigens of some invaders. The actual binding makes holes in the invader's membrane, weakening the invader. This response usually requires that complement be activated and "fixed" to the immune complex. Bacteria and viruses are the non-self cells that are damaged most through lysis caused by the binding of antibody to antigens.

Complement Fixation

Some classes of antibodies can remove or destroy antigen through complement activation and complement fixation. (The mechanism by which complement assists in immunity is discussed earlier under Adherence, pp. 366 and 367.) The two classes of antibody that can activate the complement system are IgG and IgM. Binding of antibody from either of these classes to antigen provides a binding site for the first component of complement (C1q). Once C1q is activated, other proteins of the complement system are activated in a cascade.

Precipitation

Precipitation is similar to agglutination. With precipitation, however, antibody molecules bind so much antigen that large, insoluble, antigen-antibody complexes are formed. These complexes cannot stay in suspension in the blood.

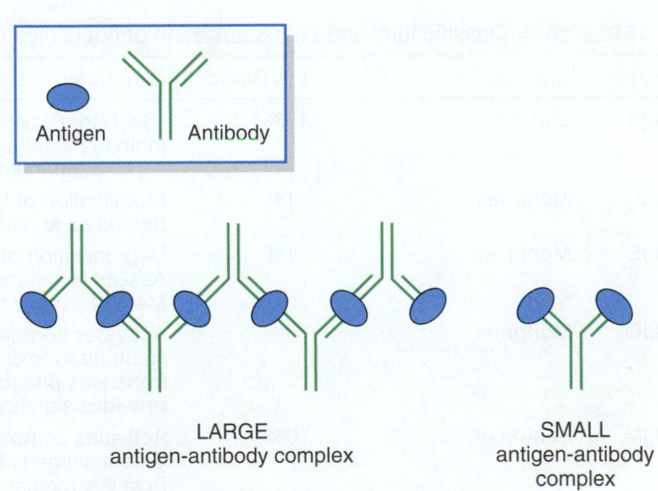

Figure 23-13 ■ Antigen-antibody complexes.

Instead, they form a large precipitate, which can be acted on and removed by neutrophils and macrophages.

Inactivation-Neutralization

Inactivation (neutralization) does not result in the immediate destruction of the antigen. Usually only a small area of the antigen, the **active site,** causes the harmful effects. The rest of the antigen may not be harmful to the host. When an antibody binds to an antigen and covers up the antigen's active site, the antigen is made harmless without destroying it.

SUSTAINED IMMUNITY: MEMORY

The sustained immunity, or memory, function of antibody-mediated immunity (AMI) provides us with long-lasting immunity to a specific antigen. Sustained immunity results from memory B-cells made during the lymphocyte sensitization stage. These memory cells remain sensitized to the specific antigen to which they were originally exposed. On re-exposure to the same antigen, the memory cells rapidly respond. First, the memory cells divide and form new sensitized blast cells and new sensitized plasma cells. The blast cells continue to divide, producing many more sensitized plasma cells. The sensitized plasma cells rapidly make large amounts of the antibody specific for the sensitizing antigen.

This ability of the memory cells to respond on re-exposure to the same antigen that originally sensitized the B-cell allows a rapid and large immune (anamnestic) response to the antigen. So much antibody is made that usually the invading organisms are removed completely, so that the person does not become ill. Because of this process, most people do not become ill with chickenpox or other infectious diseases more than once, even though they are exposed many times to the causative organism. Without the action of memory, people would remain susceptible to specific diseases on subsequent exposure to the organisms, and no sustained immunity would be generated.

General Antibody Classification

All antibodies are **immunoglobulins,** also called **gamma globulins.** These names are based on the structure and function of antibodies. A globulin is a protein that is globular rather than straight. Because antibodies are globular proteins, they are "globulins." The term *immunoglobulin* is used for antibodies because they are globular proteins that provide immunity. Antibodies also are called "gamma globulins" because all free antibodies in the plasma separate out in the gamma fraction of plasma proteins during electrophoresis. The five antibody types are classified by differences in size, timing, and association (Table 23-4).

Acquiring Antibody-Mediated Immunity

Two broad categories of immunity are innate-native immunity and adaptive (acquired) immunity.

INNATE-NATIVE IMMUNITY

Innate-native immunity (sometimes called "natural immunity") is a natural feature of a person. It can be a barrier to prevent organisms from entering the body or can be an attacking force that eliminates organisms that have already entered the body. This type of immunity cannot be developed or transferred from one person to another and is not an adaptive response to exposure or invasion by foreign proteins.

The inflammatory responses are part of innate immunity. Other parts of innate immunity include skin, mucosa, antimicrobial chemicals, complement, and natural killer cells (Abbas & Lichtman, 2003).

ADAPTIVE IMMUNITY

Adaptive immunity is the immunity that a person's body makes (or can receive) as an adaptive response to invasion by organisms or foreign proteins. For example, antibody-mediated immunity is an acquired immunity. Adaptive immunity occurs either naturally or artificially through lymphocyte responses and can be either active or passive.

Active Immunity

Active immunity occurs when antigens enter the body and the body responds by making specific antibodies against the antigen. This type of immunity is active because the body takes an active part in making the antibodies. Active immunity can occur under natural or artificial conditions.

TABLE 23-4 Classification and Characterization of Antibodies

Type	Configuration	Content in Blood	Function
IgA	Dimer	<15%	"Secretory"; present in body secretions, such as tears, mucus, saliva Inhibits bacteria and viruses from adhering to skin and mucous membranes, making penetration into the internal environment more difficult
IgD	Monomer	<1%	Modification of IgM activity Serves as an activated receptor on B-lymphocytes
IgE	Monomer	<1%	Degranulation of basophils and mast cells during inflammatory responses Assists in clearance of parasites and prevention of pulmonary infections Mediates many types of allergic reactions
IgG	Monomer	75%	Activates complement Neutralizes toxins Enhances phagocytosis Provides significant sustained immunity against viral and bacterial infections
IgM	Pentomer	10%	Activates complement Clears antigens through precipitation Possibly mediates autoimmune reactions Mediates ABO incompatibility reactions in blood transfusions

Ig, Immunoglobulin.

NATURAL ACTIVE IMMUNITY

Natural active immunity occurs when an antigen enters the body without human assistance and the body responds by actively making antibodies against that antigen (e.g., chickenpox virus). Most of the time, the invasion that triggers antibody production usually also causes the disease. However, processes occurring in the body at the same time as infection create immunity to that antigen. Thus the person will not become ill after a second exposure to the same antigen. *This type of immunity is the most effective and the longest lasting.*

ARTIFICIAL ACTIVE IMMUNITY

Artificial active immunity is the protection developed by vaccination or immunization. This type of immunity is used to prevent infections or illnesses (e.g., tetanus, diphtheria, polio) that have such serious consequences that avoiding the disease altogether is most desirable. Small amounts of specific antigens are placed as a vaccination into a person. The person's immune system responds by actively making antibodies against the antigen. Because antigens used for this procedure have been specially processed **(attenuated)** to make them less likely to grow in the body, this exposure does not cause the disease. Artificial active immunity lasts many years, although repeated but smaller doses of the original antigen are required as a "booster" to retain the protection.

Passive Immunity

Passive immunity occurs when antibodies against an antigen are in a person's body but were not created there. Rather, these antibodies are transferred to the person's body after being made in the body of another person or animal. Because these antibodies are foreign to the receiving person, the antibodies are recognized as non-self and eliminated quickly. For this reason, passive immunity only provides immediate, short-term protection against a specific antigen.

Natural passive immunity occurs when antibodies are passed from the mother to the fetus via the placenta or to the infant through colostrum and breast milk.

Artificial passive immunity involves injecting a person with antibodies that were produced in another person or animal. This type of immunity is used when a person is exposed to a serious disease for which he or she has little or no actively acquired immunity. Instead, the injected antibodies are expected to inactivate the antigen. This type of immune protection is temporary, lasting only days to a few weeks. Some of the problems in which artificial passive immunity may be used include exposure to rabies, tetanus, and poisonous snake bites.

AMI works with inflammation to protect against infection. However, AMI can provide the most effective, long-lasting immunity only when its actions are combined with those of cell-mediated immunity (CMI).

CELL-MEDIATED IMMUNITY

Cell-mediated immunity (CMI), or cellular immunity, involves many white blood cell (WBC) actions and interactions. This type of immunity is provided by lymphocyte stem cells that mature in the secondary lymphoid tissues of the thymus and pericortical areas of lymph nodes. Certain CMI responses influence and regulate the activities of antibody-mediated immunity (AMI) and inflammation by producing and releasing cytokines. For total immunocompetence, then, CMI must function optimally.

Cell Types Involved in Cell-Mediated Immunity

The WBCs with the most important roles in CMI include several specific T-lymphocytes (T-cells) along with a special population of cells known as natural killer (NK) cells. T-cells have a variety of subsets, each of which has a specific function.

One way of identifying different T-cell subsets is to examine certain "marker proteins" (antigens) on the cell membrane's surface. More than 200 different T-cell proteins have been identified on the cell membrane, and 11 of these (named T1 through T11) are commonly used clinically to identify specific cells. Antibodies have been made against each of these 11 proteins. Thus each T-cell subset can be identified by its reaction to the commercial antibodies. Most T-cells have more than one antigen on their cell membrane. For example, all mature T-cells contain T1, T3, T10, and T11 proteins. Certain T-cells also contain other specific T-cell membrane antigens.

The names used to identify specific T-cell subsets include the specific membrane antigen and the overall actions of the cells in a subset. The three T-lymphocyte subsets that are critically important for the development and continuation of CMI are helper/inducer T-cells, suppressor T-cells, and cytotoxic/cytolytic T-cells.

HELPER/INDUCER T-CELLS

The cell membranes of helper/inducer T-cells contain the T4 protein. These cells are usually called T4+ cells or T_H cells. The most correct name for helper/inducer T-cells is CD4+ (cluster of differentiation 4). The T4 cells may also be referred to as cells that are OKT4 positive or Leu-3 positive because of the specific antigens on the membrane surface.

Helper/inducer T-cells easily recognize self cells versus non-self cells. In response to the recognition of non-self (antigen), helper/inducer T-cells secrete lymphokines that can enhance the activity of other WBCs.

Most lymphokines secreted by the helper/inducer T-cells increase immune function. These lymphokines increase bone marrow production of stem cells and speed up their maturation. Thus helper/inducer T-cells act as organizers in "calling to arms" various squads of WBCs involved in inflammatory, antibody, and cellular defensive actions to destroy or neutralize antigens.

SUPPRESSOR T-CELLS

The membranes of suppressor T-cells contain the T8-lymphocyte antigen; these cells are commonly called T8+ cells or T_S-cells. Suppressor T-cells help regulate CMI.

Suppressor T-cells prevent continuous overreactions **(hypersensitivity)** when a person is exposed to non-self cells or proteins. This function is important in preventing the formation of autoantibodies directed against normal, healthy self cells, which is the basis for many autoimmune diseases.

The suppressor T-cells secrete lymphokines that have an overall *inhibitory* action on most cells of the immune system. These lymphokines inhibit both the growth and activation of immune system cells.

Suppressor T-cells have the opposite action of helper/inducer T-cells. For optimal function of CMI, then, a balance between helper/inducer T-cell activity and suppressor T-cell activity must be maintained. This balance occurs when the helper/inducer T-cells outnumber the suppressor T-cells by a ratio of 2:1. When this ratio increases, overreactions can occur, some of which are tissue damaging as well as unpleasant. When the helper-suppressor ratio decreases, immune function is suppressed, and the person's risk for infections increases.

CYTOTOXIC/CYTOLYTIC T-CELLS

Cytotoxic/cytolytic T-cells are also called T_C-cells. Because they have the T8 protein present on their surfaces, they are a subset of suppressor cells. Cytotoxic/cytolytic T-cells destroy cells that contain a processed antigen's major histocompatibility complex (MHC). This activity is most effective against self cells infected by parasites, such as viruses or protozoa.

Parasite-infected self cells have both self MHC proteins (universal product code) and the parasite's antigens on the cell surface. This allows the person's immune system cells to recognize the infected self cell as abnormal, and the cytotoxic/cytolytic T-cell can bind to it.

When the cytotoxic/cytolytic T-cell binds to the infected cell's MHC complex, the cytotoxic/cytolytic T-cell makes holes in the membrane of the infected cell and delivers a "lethal hit" of enzymes to the infected cell, causing it to lyse and die. Once the lethal hit has been delivered to the infected cell, the cytotoxic/cytolytic T-cell releases the dying infected cell and can then attack and destroy other infected cells that carry the same antigen MHC complex.

NATURAL KILLER CELLS

Natural killer (NK) cells are also known as CD16+ cells and are very important in providing CMI. The actual site of NK cell differentiation and maturation is unknown. Although this cell type has some T-cell features, it is not a true T-cell subset (Abbas & Lichtman, 2003).

NK cells have direct cytotoxic effects on some non-self cells. Unlike cytotoxic/cytolytic T-cells, NK cells can exert these cell killing effects without first being sensitized. Nor do they need to share any of the MHC proteins in common with the non-self cell. The cell killing actions of NK cells are independent of the interactions of other white blood cells. NK cells conduct "seek and destroy" missions in the body to eliminate non-self cells.

NK cells are most effective in destroying unhealthy or abnormal self cells. The non-self cells most often harmed by NK cells are cancer cells and virally infected body cells.

Cytokines

CMI regulates the immune system by the production and activity of cytokines. **Cytokines** are small protein hormones produced by the many WBCs (and some other tissues). Cytokines made by the macrophages, neutrophils, eosinophils, and monocytes are **monokines;** cytokines produced by T-cells are **lymphokines.**

Cytokines work like other types of hormone: one cell produces a cytokine, which in turn exerts its effects on other cells of the immune system. The cells responding to the cytokine may be located close to or remote from the cytokine-secreting cell. The cells that change their activity when a cytokine is present are "responder" cells. For a responder cell to respond to the presence of a cytokine, the responder cell must have a specific receptor to which the cytokine can bind. Once the cytokine binds to its receptor, the responder cell changes its activity (Figure 23-14).

Cytokines control many inflammatory and immune responses (Corwin, 2000a; Corwin, 2000b). Some cytokines are **pleiotropic,** in that the effects are widespread within the immune system, setting into motion many different immune actions. Other cytokines have specific actions limited to only one type of cell. Cytokines include the interleukins, interferons, colony stimulating factors, and tumor necrosis factor. The interleukins are the largest group of cytokines, with interleukin-25 (IL-25) being the most recently defined. Although there are many cytokines, not all are clinically useful at this time. Table 23-5 lists the cytokines that have current clinical importance.

Protection Provided by Cell-Mediated Immunity

Cell-mediated immunity (CMI) helps protect the body through the ability to differentiate self from non-self. The non-self cells most easily recognized by CMI are cancer cells and those self cells infected by organisms that live within host cells. CMI watches for and rids the body of self cells that might potentially harm the body. *CMI is important*

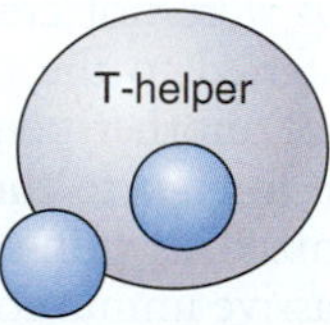

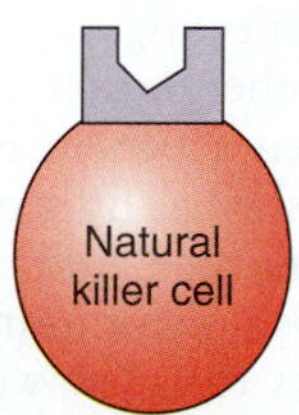

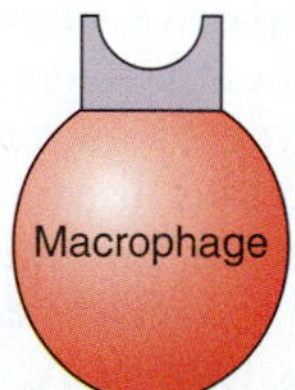

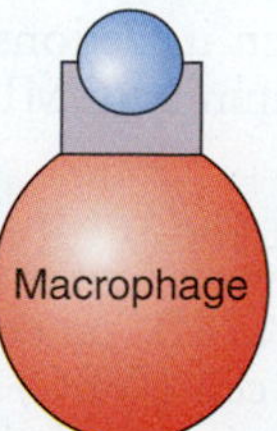

Figure 23-14 ■ Cytokine receptors on leukocytes.

TABLE 23-5 Activity of Selected Cytokines

Cytokine	Cellular Origin	Inducing Event	Cytokine Action
IL-1 (Proinflammatory)	Macrophages Monocytes Natural killer cells	Contact with gram-negative bacterial products Contact with CD4+ cell Presence of TNF	Stimulates increased production of prostaglandins Induces fever Increases proliferation of CD4+ cells Stimulates growth and differentiation of B-lymphocytes Induces further secretion of IL-1 and IL-6
IL-2 (Proinflammatory)	T-helper cells (CD4+ T-cells) CD8+ T-cells	T-cell activation by antigens	Increases growth and differentiation of T-lymphocytes Stimulates increased production of IL-2 from activated lymphocytes Enhances NK activity and activity of tumor-infiltrating lymphocytes
IL-3 (Multilineage CSF)	T-helper cells (CD4+ T-cells)	Infection or antigen invasion	Pluripotent (pleiotropic) stimulation of bone marrow stem cells
IL-4 (B-cell stimulatory factor)	T-helper cells (CD4+ T-cells) Activated mast cells	Presence of anti-Ig antibody	Stimulates growth and differentiation of B-lymphocytes Stimulates increased production of IgG and IgE Induces further secretion of IL-4, IL-5, and IL-6 Suppresses inflammation
IL-5 (B-cell growth factor)	T-helper cells (CD4+ T-cells) Activated mast cells	Helminth infection Pulmonary infection	Stimulates growth and differentiation of eosinophils Stimulates increased production of IgA and IgE
IL-6 (Proinflammatory)	Activated T-cells Fibroblasts Vascular endothelial cells Macrophages Monocytes	Infection or inflammation Presence of IL-1 TNF	Stimulates liver to produce fibrinogen, macroglobulin, C-protein Stimulates growth of activated B-lymphocytes Increases production of bone marrow stem cells
IL-8 (Monocyte chemotactic factor)	Activated T-cells Macrophages Platelets Fibroblasts Endothelial cells	Infection or inflammation	Chemotactic factor for neutrophils, basophils and eosinophils Stimulates neutrophil activation
IL-9	T-helper cells (CD4+ T-cells)	Infection or inflammation	Stimulates mast cell growth Induces IL-4 production Stimulates lymphocyte activation
IL-10	Mature lymphocytes Macrophages Monocytes	Infection or inflammation	Enhances activity of cytotoxic/cytolytic T-cells Suppresses inflammatory response
Interferon-alpha (INF-α)	Macrophages	Viral infection	Decreases viral proliferation
Interferon-beta (INF-β)	Fibroblasts	Viral infection	Decreases viral proliferation
Interferon-gamma (INF-γ)	T-helper cells (CD4+ T-cells) T-suppressor cells (CD8+ T-cells) NK cells	Viral infection	Decreases viral proliferation Activates macrophages Induces differentiation of committed lymphoid stem cells Activates neutrophils Activates NK cells
TNF (Proinflammatory)	Activated macrophages Activated mast cells Activated NK cells Activated T-cells	Infection or inflammation (especially infection with gram-negative microorganisms)	Increases leukocyte adhesion Induces fever Stimulates production of CSF Induces cytolysis of virally infected cells Induces secretion of IL-1 and IL-6
GM-CSF	Activated T-cells Macrophages Fibroblasts Vascular endothelial cells	Infection or inflammation	Increases growth and differentiation of committed myeloid stem cells Slightly activates macrophages
Monocyte-macrophage CSF (M-CSF)	Fibroblasts Vascular endothelial cells	Infection or inflammation	Increases growth and differentiation of committed monocyte-macrophage progenitor cells
G-CSF	Macrophages Vascular endothelial cells Fibroblasts	Infection or inflammation	Increases proliferation and maturation of neutrophils
Erythropoietin	Renal parenchymal cells	Hypoxia	Increases growth and differentiation of erythrocytes

CSF, Colony-stimulating factor; *G,* granulocyte; *GM,* granulocyte-macrophage; *Ig,* immunoglobulin; *IL,* interleukin; *INF,* interferon; *M,* macrophage; *NK,* natural killer; *TNF,* tumor necrosis factor.

in preventing the development of cancer and metastasis after exposure to carcinogens.

Transplant Rejection

Natural killer (NK) cells and cytotoxic/cytolytic T-cells also destroy cells from other people or animals. Although this action is usually helpful, it is also responsible for rejection of grafts and transplanted organs. Because the solid organ transplanted into the host is seldom a perfectly identical match of universal product codes (human leukocyte antigens [HLAs]) between the donated organ and the recipient host, the client's immune system cells recognize a newly transplanted organ as non-self. Without intervention, the host's immune system starts inflammatory and immunologic actions to destroy or eliminate these non-self cells. This activity causes rejection of the transplanted organ. Graft rejection is a result of a complex series of responses that change over time and involve different components of the immune system. Graft rejection can be hyperacute, acute, or chronic.

HYPERACUTE REJECTION

Hyperacute graft rejection begins immediately on transplantation and is an antibody-mediated response. Antigen-antibody complexes form in the blood vessels of the transplanted organ. The host's blood has pre-existing antibodies to one or more of the antigens (including blood group antigens) present in the donated organ. The antigen-antibody complexes adhere to the lining of blood vessels and activate complement. The activated complement in the blood vessel linings triggers the blood clotting cascade, causing small clots to form throughout the new organ. Widespread clotting occludes blood vessels and leads to ischemic necrosis, inflammation with phagocytosis of the necrotic blood vessels, and release of lytic enzymes into the new organ. These enzymes cause massive cellular destruction and graft loss.

Hyperacute rejection occurs mostly in transplanted kidneys. The following clients are at greatest risk for hyperacute rejection:

1. Those who have received donated organs of an ABO blood type different from their own
2. Those who have received multiple blood transfusions at any time in life before transplantation
3. Those who have a history of multiple pregnancies
4. Those who have received a previous transplant

The manifestations of hyperacute rejection are apparent within minutes of attachment of the donated organ to the host's blood supply. The process cannot be stopped once it has started, and the rejected organ is removed as soon as hyperacute rejection is diagnosed.

ACUTE REJECTION

Acute graft rejection occurs within 1 week to 3 months after transplantation. Two mechanisms are responsible. The first mechanism is antibody mediated and results in vasculitis within the transplanted organ. This reaction differs from that of hyperacute rejection in that blood vessel necrosis (rather than thrombotic occlusion) leads to the organ's destruction.

The second mechanism is cellular. Host cytotoxic/cytolytic T-cells and NK cells enter the transplanted organ through the blood, penetrate the organ cells, start an inflammatory response, and cause lysis of the organ cells (Abbas & Lichtman, 2003).

Diagnosis of acute rejection is made by laboratory tests that show impaired function of the donated organ, along with biopsy of the donated organ. Symptoms of acute rejection vary with each client and with the specific organ transplanted. For example, when acute rejection occurs in a transplanted kidney, the client usually has some tenderness in the kidney area and may have other general symptoms of inflammation.

An episode of acute rejection after solid organ transplantation does not automatically mean that the client will lose the new organ. Drug management of host immune responses at this time may limit the damage to the organ and allow the graft to be maintained.

CHRONIC REJECTION

The origin of **chronic rejection** is not clear, but it is similar to chronic inflammation and scarring. The smooth muscles of blood vessels overgrow and occlude the vessels. Functional tissue of the donated organ is replaced with fibrotic, scarlike tissue. Because this fibrotic tissue is not organ tissue, the transplanted organ's function is reduced in proportion to the amount of normal tissue that is replaced by fibrotic tissue. This type of reaction is long-standing and occurs continuously as a response to chronic ischemia caused by blood vessel injury. The results of chronic rejection are unique to different transplanted organs. For example, in transplanted lungs, chronic rejection thickens small airways. In transplanted livers, chronic rejection destroys bile ducts. In transplanted hearts, this process is called **accelerated graft atherosclerosis (AGA)** and is the major cause of death in clients who have survived 1 or more years after heart transplantation (Augustine, 2000).

Although good control over host immune function can delay this type of rejection, the process probably occurs to some degree with all transplanted solid organs. Because the fibrotic changes are permanent, there is no cure for chronic graft rejection. When the fibrosis increases to the extent that the transplanted organ can no longer function, the only recourse is retransplantation.

TREATMENT OF TRANSPLANT REJECTION

Rejection of transplanted solid organs involves all three components of immunity, although cell-mediated immune (CMI) responses are most significant in the rejection process.

Maintenance

The drugs used for routine immunosuppressive therapy after solid organ transplantation are combinations of specific immunosuppressants (cyclosporine [Sandimmune, Neoral, Gengraf]), less specific immunosuppressants (azathioprine [Imuran] or mycophenolate [CellCept, Myfortic]), and one of the corticosteroids, such as prednisone (Apo-Prednisone✱, Deltasone✱) or prednisolone (Delta-Cortef) (Table 23-6). Cyclosporine induces the specific and effective suppression of rejection. This drug, however, induces major long-term adverse actions and is expensive (see the Resource Management box on p. 378.) The dosage of all immunosuppressive agents is ad-

TABLE 23-6 Drugs Used to Prevent or Treat Transplant Rejection

Drug	Action	Problems/Precautions
Immunosuppressants		
Cyclosporine (Sandimmune, Neoral, Gengraf)	Reduces T-lymphocyte production of cytokines important in stimulating T-lymphocyte proliferation and activation (especially interleukin-2)	Has nephrotoxic, neurotoxic, and hepatotoxic properties. Stimulates hyperglycemia—may cause diabetes mellitus. Increases body and facial hair. Causes gingival hyperplasia. Blood levels are sensitive to the presence of other drugs. Must be mixed following strict manufacturer guidelines. Do not administer to clients receiving tacrolimus.
Azathioprine (Imuran)	Converts to an antimetabolite that inhibits DNA synthesis and cell division in T- and B-lymphocytes and myeloid cells	Has hepatotoxic properties. Has high incidence of nausea and vomiting. Suppresses hematologic functions. Use is less frequent compared to mycophenolate mofetil.
Mycophenolate mofetil (CellCept)	Selectively inhibits T- and B-lymphocyte proliferation by interfering with purine synthesis and cell division	Has fewer side effects than azathioprine. Has been demonstrated more effective as part of triple therapy in clients after kidney transplantation. Is less selective than cyclosporine.
Mycophenolate sodium (Myfortic)	Similar to mycophenolate mofetil	Is a different formulation of mycophenolate mofetil. Has fewer gastrointestinal effects than mycophenolate mofetil.
Tacrolimus FK506 (Prograf)	Suppresses T-cell growth and production of interleukin-2	Do not administer with cyclosporine. Has nephrotoxic and neurotoxic properties. Induces hyperglycemia. Has a frequent incidence of nausea, vomiting, and weight loss. May be used as rescue agent in kidney rejection.
Sirolimus (Rapamune)	Suppresses lymphocyte production and B-cell synthesis of antibodies	Induces liver changes, toxicity occurs at lower doses in people with liver impairment. Do not give with grapefruit juice. Increases the risk for infection.
Corticosteroids (prednisone, prednisolone, Decadron, among others)	Directly cytotoxic to circulating lymphocytes Suppresses bone marrow stem cell proliferation	Induces general immunosuppression. Immunosuppression more profound than with other agents. Suppresses adrenal cortical activity. Numerous metabolic and endocrine side effects.
Antibodies		
Interleukin-2 receptor antagonists: Basiliximab (Simulect) Daclizumab (Zenapax)	Binds to interleukin-2 receptors on activated lymphocytes, especially helper/inducer T-cells, preventing proliferation and limiting activation	Used as initial induction therapy, not as continuing therapy. IV administration only. Approved as prophylaxis for kidney transplant only. Synthesized through recombinant DNA technology and contains both human (90%) and mouse (10%) DNA sequences. May induce anaphylaxis. High incidence of flu-like symptoms.
Antithymocyte globulin (Atgam)	Depletes existing T-lymphocytes through antigen-antibody binding actions	Is a polyclonal antibody raised in horses. May induce anaphylaxis or other immune side effects. Side effects increase on re-exposure. Has limited duration of action.
Muromonab-CD3 (Orthoclone OKT3)	Binds to the OKT3 receptor on lymphocytes, down-regulating the receptor action Depletes circulating T-lymphocytes through antigen-antibody binding actions May induce programmed cell death (apoptosis) of bound T-lymphocytes	Is a monoclonal antibody raised in a mouse model. May induce anaphylaxis or other immune side effects. Has limited duration of action. May be inactivated by human antimouse antibodies. Induction of capillary leak syndrome is common. May require premedication with corticosteroids.

justed to the immune response of each client. Treatment with these agents increases the risk for bacterial and fungal infections and for cancer development.

Tacrolimus (Prograf) is used in maintenance therapy and rescue therapy. It is similar to erythromycin and specifically suppresses T-cell actions, including production of interleukin-2 (IL-2). These effects occur through several mechanisms. Without continuous stimulation by IL-2, helper/inducer T-cells and cytotoxic/cytolytic T-cells are slow to reproduce and do not perform their usual functions. Suppression of these two cell populations allows the donated organ to remain free from immunologic destruction. The general immunosuppression is not as profound and the host's risk for infection is not greatly increased. Tacrolimus also prevents activation of unsensitized cytotoxic/cytolytic T-cells.

A newer approach to prevent transplant rejection for clients undergoing kidney transplantation is the use of monoclonal antibodies directed against the IL-2 receptor site on activated T-cells (especially helper/inducer T-cells). These antibodies, basiliximab (Simulect) or daclizumab (Zenapax), are given intravenously within 2 hours before the transplant surgery and within the first few days after the surgery. By binding the antibodies to the IL-2 receptor site, T-cell growth and activation are reduced for several months.

RESOURCE MANAGEMENT

TRANSPLANT REJECTION PROPHYLAXIS

Cost of Care

- The most useful agent in preventing rejection of transplanted solid organs is cyclosporin.
- Cost of maintaining therapeutic levels of this drug for an average-sized adult ranges between $1100 and $1500 per month.
- Clients must take this drug daily for the life of the transplanted organ.
- The effectiveness of this drug is highly dependent on following manufacturer's directions for mixing and administering.
- An antifungal agent, ketoconazole, when taken orally has been demonstrated to slow metabolism of cyclosporin and maintain therapeutic blood levels at lower doses (about 40% to 50% of cyclosporin dose needed when taken without ketoconazole).
- The cost of ketoconazole daily maintenance therapy is about $100 per month.

Implications for Nursing

Because of the high cost of medications to prevent transplant rejection, nurses need to incorporate proper medication administration into their client teaching plans and reinforce this information frequently. Nurses can assist in cost reductions by observing for sustained therapeutic blood levels of cyclosporin in clients and exploring what factors may be contributing to this effect.

Data from Augustine, S. (2000). Heart transplantation: Long-term management related to immunosuppression, complications, and psychosocial adjustments. *Critical Care Clinics of North America, 12*(1), 69-77; Drug Facts and Comparisons. (2004). *Drug facts and comparisons* (58th ed.). St. Louis: Wolters Kluwer; and Personal communication, with CVS Pharmacies, January 2004.

Rescue Therapy

Certain agents are used only to reduce the host's immunologic responses during rejection episodes, especially acute rejection. These agents may be used in addition to or in place of the maintenance drugs in the host's normal treatment regimen.

ANTILYMPHOCYTE GLOBULIN

Antilymphocyte globulin (ALG) is an antibody (or group of antibodies) produced in an animal after the animal has been exposed to human lymphocytes. The globulin can be made more specific by exposing the animal to human T-cells instead of mixed lymphocytes. When these antihuman lymphocyte antibodies are given to humans, the antibodies selectively attack and clear lymphocytes from body fluids, blood, and the transplanted organ. These agents are given only for a short time to combat the acute rejection episode.

Most clients receiving ALG have some immunologic side effects, ranging from low-grade fever and malaise to serum sickness and anaphylaxis. The side effects usually increase in intensity on repeated exposure to ALG.

MUROMONAB-CD3 (ORTHOCLONE OKT3)

Muromonab-CD3 is an antibody directed specifically against the human T-cell cell-surface antigen CD3. This antibody is generated in mice rather than in horses. Because the agent is generated in mice, the clients receiving it rapidly develop antimouse antibodies. These antimouse antibodies attack the CD3 and prevent its anti–T-cell activities. This antibody is most effective against rejection during the first episode in which it is used. Its effect in combating graft rejection decreases with each use.

Antibodies made in other animals, especially mice, cause side effects in humans because the animal proteins in the antibodies are recognized as "foreign" by the human immune system. The incidence of side effects is decreasing because newer antibodies have been "humanized." This process removes most of the mouse-specific proteins from the antibody and replaces them with human specific proteins. The "humanized" antibodies made by mice now contain up to 95% human proteins rather than mouse proteins.

GET READY for the NCLEX Examination!

KEY POINTS

- Inflammation and immunity are provided through the actions and products of white blood cells (WBCs).
- Different types of WBCs provide different types of immune or inflammatory protection.
- The differential of the WBC count can be used to determine the client's risk for infection, the presence or absence of infection, the presence or absence of an allergic reaction, and whether an infection is bacterial or viral.
- WBCs are the only body cells able to recognize non-self cells and try to attack or destroy them.
- Self-tolerance is the special ability of WBCs to recognize healthy self cells and not attempt to attack or destroy them.
- Human leukocyte antigens (HLAs) are an individual's tissue type and are inherited from parents.
- Immunocompetence requires that all three parts of inflammation and immunity have optimal functioning.
- Inflammation is a general, nonspecific protective response.
- The five cardinal manifestations of inflammation are redness, warmth, swelling, pain, and loss of function.
- Inflammation and infection are not the same thing. Infection almost always is accompanied by inflammation but inflammation often occurs without infection.
- The tissue responses to inflammation are helpful if confined to the area of invasion or infection and do not extend beyond the acute phase.
- Chronic inflammation can damage tissues and reduce function.
- The cells and actions of cell-mediated immunity control and coordinate the entire inflammatory and immune responses.
- Inflammation cannot be transferred from one person to another.
- Immune function declines with age, making the older adult at increased risk for infection and cancer development.
- Antibody-mediated immunity (also known as "humoral" immunity) can be transferred from one person (or animal) to another.
- Antibodies transferred from one person into another person have a short-term effect.
- Natural, active immunity is the most beneficial and long-lasting type of immunity.
- Vaccinations cause artificial active immunity and require "boosting" for best long-term effects.
- An individual's normal membrane proteins would be antigens in another person.

- Transplant rejection is a normal response of the immune system that can damage or destroy the transplanted organ.
- Clients who receive transplanted organs (unless from an identical sibling) must take immunosuppressive drugs daily to prevent transplant rejection.
- Clients who take immunosuppressive drugs have an increased risk for infection and for cancer development.

ADDITIONAL STUDY RESOURCES

Go to your Student CD-ROM for Review Questions for the NCLEX Examination.

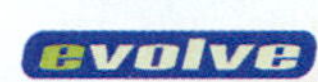

Go to http://evolve.elsevier.com/Iggy/ for Integrated Management of Care Questions for the NCLEX Examination.

SELECTED BIBLIOGRAPHY

Abbas, A., & Lichtman, A. (2003). *Cellular and molecular immunology* (5th ed.). Philadelphia: W.B. Saunders.

Augustine, S. (2000). Heart transplantation: Long-term management related to immunosuppression, complications, and psychosocial adjustments. *Critical Care Clinics of North America, 12*(1), 69-77.

Bauer, S. (2002). Psychoneuroimmunology Part I: Physiology. *Clinical Journal of Oncology Nursing, 6*(3), 167-170.

Branchereau, J. (2002). The long arm of the immune system. *Scientific American, 287*(5), 52-59.

Corwin, E. (2000a). Understanding cytokines part II: Implications for nursing research and practice. *Biological Research for Nursing, 2*(1), 41-48.

Corwin, E. (2000b). Understanding cytokines part I: Physiology and mechanism of action. *Biological Research for Nursing, 2*(1), 30-40.

Facts and Comparisons. (2004). *Drug facts and comparisons* (58th ed.). St. Louis: Author.

Incredibly easy! (2003). Reviewing the immune system. *Nursing2003, 33*(3), 70-71.

McCance, K., & Huether, S. (2002). *Pathophysiology: The biologic basis for disease in adults and children* (4th ed.). St. Louis: Mosby.

Nussbaum, R., McInnes, R., & Willard, H. (2001). *Thompson & Thompson: Genetics in medicine* (6th ed.). Philadelphia: W.B. Saunders.

Otto, S. (2003). Understanding the immune system. *Journal of Infusion Nursing, 26*(2), 79-85.

Parkin, J., & Cohen, B. (2001). An overview of the immune system. *The Lancet, 357*(9270), 1777-1789.

Pierce, J., Cackler, A., & Arnett, M. (2004). Why should you care about free radicals? *RN, 67*(1), 38-42.

Workman, M.L. (2003). The cellular basis of bacterial infection. *Critical Care Clinics of North America, 15*(1), 1-11.

CHAPTER

24 Interventions for Clients with Connective Tissue Disease and Other Types of Arthritis

DONNA D. IGNATAVICIUS • CYNTHIA KINDLER MATZKO

LEARNING OUTCOMES

After studying this chapter, you should be able to:

1. Compare and contrast the pathophysiology and clinical manifestations of osteoarthritis (OA) and rheumatoid disease (RA).
2. Prioritize collaborative interventions for clients with OA and RA.
3. Determine common nursing diagnoses for postoperative clients having total joint replacement surgery.
4. Evaluate the expected outcomes for clients having total joint replacement surgery.
5. Interpret laboratory findings for clients with rheumatoid disease.
6. Identify the nursing implications associated with drug therapy for clients with rheumatoid arthritis.
7. Identify educational needs for clients with arthritis.
8. Differentiate between discoid lupus erythematosus and systemic lupus erythematosus.
9. Describe the priority nursing interventions for clients who have progressive systemic sclerosis.
10. Discuss the treatment of gout based on knowledge of pathophysiology.
11. Explain the differences between polymyositis, systemic necrotizing vasculitis, polymyalgia rheumatica, ankylosing spondylitis, Reiter's syndrome, and Sjögren's syndrome.
12. Describe interventions that clients can use to prevent Lyme disease.
13. Identify the primary concern in care for clients with Marfan syndrome.
14. Describe current treatment strategies for clients with fibromyalgia.

Go to your Student CD-ROM for Review Questions for the NCLEX Examination keyed to these Learning Outcomes.

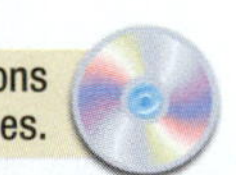

Connective tissue disease (CTD) is the major focus of *rheumatology,* the study of rheumatic disease. A **rheumatic disease** is any disease or condition involving the musculoskeletal system. In this text, CTDs are discussed separately from other musculoskeletal conditions because most CTDs are classified as autoimmune disorders.

Most common CTDs are characterized by chronic pain and progressive joint deterioration, which results in decreased function. Some of these disorders have additional localized clinical manifestations, whereas others are systemic. The economic and social costs of these diseases are staggering and will increase steadily as "baby boomers" continue to age. Client management requires an interdisciplinary approach, including medicine, surgery, nursing, and physical and occupational therapy.

More than 40 million people in the United States (1 in 6) have at least one of more than 100 types of arthritis. **Arthritis** means inflammation of one or more joints. In clinical practice, however, arthritis often refers to either **noninflammatory arthritis** or **inflammatory arthritis.** Noninflammatory arthritis such as OA is not systemic. Systemic autoimmune diseases, such as RA and systemic lupus erythematosus, are connective tissue diseases that are inflammatory.

OSTEOARTHRITIS

PATHOPHYSIOLOGY

Osteoarthritis is the most common arthritis and the second most common cause of disability among adults in the United States. It is also a common cause of disability worldwide (Kee, 2000). **Osteoarthritis (OA)** may be called degenerative joint disease (DJD); however, this term is no longer current. Joint pain and loss of function are common problems with OA.

Osteoarthritis is characterized by the progressive deterioration and loss of cartilage in one or more joints. Weight-bearing joints (hips and knees), the vertebral column, and the hands are primarily affected because they are used most often and, except for the hands, bear the mechanical stress of body weight. Most clients have the *primary (idiopathic)* form of the disease; *secondary* OA can result from other musculoskeletal conditions or from trauma. OA can also be classified as *nodal* (with hand involvement) or *non-nodal* (without hand involvement) (Kee, 2000).

In affected joints, the normal bluish-white, translucent cartilage becomes soft, opaque, and yellow. Fissures, pitting, and ulcerations develop, and the cartilage thins. As cartilage and the bone beneath the cartilage begin to erode, the joint space narrows and **osteophytes** (bone spurs) form (Figure 24-1). Inflammatory enzymes enhance tissue deterioration as a result of altered cartilage metabolism. The repair process is then unable to overcome the rapid process of degeneration. Bone cysts and secondary **synovitis** (synovial inflammation) are common in advanced disease. **Subluxation** (partial joint dislocation) and joint deformities eventually cause marked immobility, pain, muscle spasm and, possibly, inflammation.

Etiology and Genetic Risk

Although the causative mechanisms of *primary* OA at the cellular level have not been well identified, the disease may be initiated by developmental, genetic, metabolic, and traumatic factors. Age is the strongest risk factor, but research does not support that aging is the only cause of the disease. OA is thought to derive from defective chondrocyte metabolism, which explains the lack of a systemic response. Some clients report a family history of OA, which supports a possible genetic cause, especially for women who have the nodal type. Obesity also contributes to the likelihood of degeneration, particularly in the knees.

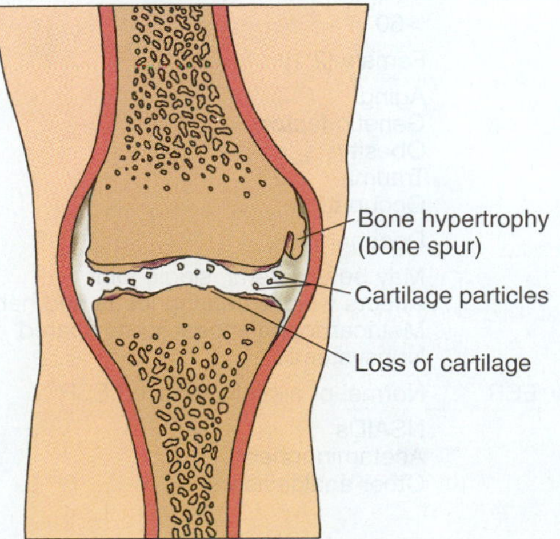

Figure 24-1 ■ Joint changes in degenerative joint disease.

Trauma to the joints from excessive use or abuse predisposes a person to OA. Certain heavy manual occupations (e.g., carpet installation, construction, farming) cause high-intensity or repetitive stress to the joints. The risk of hip and knee OA is also increased in professional athletes, especially football and soccer players, runners, and gymnasts. Lack of exercise can contribute to muscle loss, or **sarcopenia.** Muscle tissue helps to support joints, particularly those that bear weight (e.g., hips and knees).

In a small percentage of people, congenital anomalies, trauma, and joint sepsis can result in *secondary* OA. For example, injuries from motor vehicle accidents can cause OA in later years. Certain metabolic diseases (e.g., diabetes mellitus, Paget's disease of the bone) and blood disorders (e.g., hemophilia, sickle cell disease) can also cause joint degeneration. Inflammatory joint diseases, such as rheumatoid arthritis, can lead to secondary OA.

Incidence/Prevalence

The prevalence of OA varies among different populations but is a universal problem. About three-fourths of people older than 55 years of age have joint changes that can be seen on x-ray examination, although not all of those individuals actually develop OA.

> **WOMEN'S HEALTH CONSIDERATIONS**
>
> Before 50 years of age, more men than women have OA. The disease is much more common in women, especially black women, after 50 years of age; the reason for this difference is not known. Women are more prone to hand involvement, especially in the distal and proximal interphalangeal joints of the fingers, which often produces painful, bony nodes. Women also have a greater number of affected joints compared with men, but men have more hip involvement.

HEALTH PROMOTION/ILLNESS PREVENTION

Several lifestyle considerations can help prevent or slow joint degeneration and subsequent OA. These practices include the following:

- Keep weight within normal limits; obesity causes excess wear on joints, especially hips and knees.
- Avoid or limit activities that promote stress on joints, such as jogging.
- Limit participation in recreational sports that can damage joints, such as football.
- Avoid risk-seeking activities to prevent trauma that can result in OA later in life.

◆COLLABORATIVE MANAGEMENT

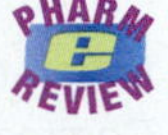

◆Assessment

HISTORY

Ask questions about the course of the disease. Collect information specifically related to osteoarthritis OA, such as the nature and location of joint pain and how much pain is the client experiencing. Use a 0-to-10 scale to assess pain intensity on the day of the interview. Chapter 7 discusses pain assessment in detail.

Other questions to ask include the following:

- If joint stiffness has occurred, where and for how long?
- When and where has any joint swelling occurred?
- What relieves the pain or stiffness?
- Is there any loss of function or difficulty in accomplishing activities of daily living?

Because this disease is observed more often in older women, age, gender, and ethnicity are important factors for the nursing history. Ask clients about their occupation, nature of work, history of trauma, weight history, exercise, and current or previous involvement in sports. A history of obesity is significant, even for clients currently within the ideal range for body weight. A family history of arthritis is also noted. Determine whether the client has a current or previous medical condition that may cause joint manifestations.

PHYSICAL ASSESSMENT/CLINICAL MANIFESTATIONS

In the early stage of the disease, the clinical manifestations of OA may appear similar to those of rheumatoid arthritis (RA). The distinction between OA and RA becomes more evident as the disease progresses. Table 24-1 differentiates the major characteristics of both diseases and their treatments.

JOINT INVOLVEMENT. The typical client with OA is a middle-aged or older woman who complains of chronic joint pain and stiffness. Early in the course of the disease, the pain diminishes after rest and intensifies after activity. Later the pain occurs with slight motion or even when the client is at rest. Because cartilage has no nerve supply, the pain is probably due to joint and soft-tissue involvement and to spasms of the surrounding muscles. During examination of the joints, the nurse can often elicit pain or tenderness by palpation or by putting the joint through range of motion. **Crepitus,** a continuous grating sensation caused by irregular cartilage, may be felt or heard as the joint is put through passive range of motion. One or more joints are affected. The client may also complain of joint stiffness that usually lasts less than 30 minutes after a period of inactivity.

On inspection, the joint is often enlarged because of bony hypertrophy; rarely does a joint appear to be hot and inflamed. The presence of inflammation in clients with OA usually indicates a secondary synovitis. Approximately 50% of clients with hand involvement display the characteristic **Heberden's nodes** (at the distal interphalangeal joints) and **Bouchard's nodes** (at the proximal interphalangeal joints). Although OA is not a bilateral, symmetric disease, these large bony nodes appear on both hands, especially in women. The nodes may be painful and red. Some clients experience pain in developing nodes, which stops once the nodes are fully developed. Others, however, report no nodal pain unless bumped. These nodes tend to be familial and are often a cosmetic concern to clients. The nodes feel hard and cause tenderness when palpated.

OTHER CLINICAL MANIFESTATIONS. Joint effusions are common when the knees are involved. When trying to differentiate the presence of fluid from subcutaneous tissue, you may be able to move fluid from the **infrapatellar notch** (the area directly below the knee) into the **suprapatellar area** (directly above the knee). Other ways to detect fluid in the knee involve grasping the medial and lateral aspect of the knee between the thumb and third finger and pushing down on the top surface of the patella with the forefinger **(ballottement).** If fluid is present, the patella will be able to be pressed down a distance and then rise back up when the forefinger is removed. Subcutaneous tissue cannot be relocated.

Observe any atrophy of skeletal muscle from disuse. The vicious pain cycle of the disease discourages the movement of painful joints, which may result in contractures, muscle atrophy, and further pain. Loss of function may result, depending on which joints are involved. Hip or knee pain may cause the client to limp and restrict walking distance.

TABLE 24-1 Differential Features of Rheumatoid Arthritis and Degenerative Joint Disease

Characteristic	Rheumatoid Arthritis	Osteoarthritis
Typical onset (age)	35-45 yr	>60 yr
Gender affected	Female (3:1)	Female (2:1)
Risk factors or cause	Autoimmune (genetic) Emotional stress (triggers exacerbation)	Aging Genetic factor Obesity Trauma Occupation
Disease process	Inflammatory	Degenerative
Disease pattern	Bilateral, symmetric, multiple joints Usually affects upper extremities first Distal interphalangeal joints of hands spared Systemic	May be unilateral, single joint Affects weight-bearing joints and hands, spine Metacarpophalangeal joints spared Nonsystemic
Laboratory findings	Elevated rheumatoid factor, antinuclear antibody, ESR	Normal or slightly elevated ESR
Common drug therapy	NSAIDs Methotrexate Leflunomide (Arava) Corticosteroids Biological response modifiers Other immunosuppressive agents	NSAIDs Acetaminophen Other analgesics

ESR, Erythrocyte sedimentation rate; *NSAIDs*, nonsteroidal anti-inflammatory drugs.

Osteoarthritis (OA) can often affect the spine, especially the lumbar region at the L3-4 level or the cervical region at C4-6. Compression of spinal nerve roots may occur as a result of vertebral facet bone spurs. The client typically complains of radiating pain, stiffness, and muscle spasms in one or both extremities. Spinal and vertebral arteries may also become compressed.

Severe pain and deformity interfere with ambulation and self-care. In addition to performing a musculoskeletal assessment, conduct a functional assessment of the client with OA to determine mobility and the ability to perform activities of daily living (ADLs). Chapter 10 describes ADLs and functional assessment in depth.

PSYCHOSOCIAL ASSESSMENT

Osteoarthritis (OA) is a chronic condition that may cause permanent changes in lifestyle. An inability to care for oneself in advanced disease prevents socialization and results in role changes and other losses. Therefore the client may exhibit a variety of behaviors indicative of the grieving process, such as anger and depression.

The client may experience a role change in the family, workplace, or both. To identify changes that have been or need to be made, ask the client about his or her roles before the disease developed. Coping strategies to help in living with the disease should also be identified. Kee (1998) found four themes that help people cope with OA. In addition to role changes, joint deformities and bony nodules often cause an alteration in body image and self-esteem. Observe the client's response to body changes. Does the client ignore them or seem overly occupied with them? How does he or she refer to the changes–with anger, degradation, or humor? These clues help to assess the client's acceptance of body alterations.

LABORATORY ASSESSMENT

The health care provider uses the history and physical examination to make the diagnosis of OA The results of routine laboratory tests are usually normal but can be helpful in screening for associated conditions. The erythrocyte sedimentation rate (ESR) and high-sensitivity C-reactive protein (hsCRP) may be slightly elevated when secondary synovitis (synovial inflammation) occurs. ESR also tends to rise with age and infection.

RADIOGRAPHIC ASSESSMENT

Routine x-rays are useful in determining structural joint changes. Specialized views are obtained when the disease cannot be visualized on standard x-ray film but is suspected. A computed tomography (CT) scan may be used to determine vertebral involvement.

OTHER DIAGNOSTIC ASSESSMENTS

The health care provider may order magnetic resonance imaging (MRI) or computed tomography (CT) studies to detect degenerative bony changes, especially in the spine.

Critical Thinking Challenge

You are assigned to care for an older adult in an assisted-living facility. She has long-standing OA of both the hips and knees and a history of diabetes mellitus, heart failure, and hypertension. She is able to care for herself but uses a walker for ambulation because of chronic joint pain and deterioration.

1. How would you perform a physical assessment of this client?
2. What might you expect to find during the physical assessment?
3. How might her other medical diagnoses affect the findings of the physical assessment?

evolve For suggested answer guidelines, go to http://evolve.elsevier.com/Iggy/.

Analysis

COMMON NURSING DIAGNOSES AND COLLABORATIVE PROBLEMS

The following are priority nursing diagnoses for clients with osteoarthritis (OA):

1. Chronic Pain related to muscle spasm, cartilage deterioration, or joint inflammation
2. Impaired Physical Mobility related to pain and muscle atrophy

ADDITIONAL NURSING DIAGNOSES AND COLLABORATIVE PROBLEMS

In addition to the common nursing diagnoses, clients may have secondary problems caused by the pain and immobility common in OA, including one or more of the following:

- Activity Intolerance related to pain and fatigue
- Self-Care Deficit (Partial) related to pain, fatigue, and immobility
- Disturbed Body Image related to the effects of loss of body function
- Impaired Walking related to joint pain
- Ineffective Coping related to chronic pain and decreased function
- Imbalanced Nutrition: More Than Body Requirements related to decreased activity and mobility

Planning and Implementation

CHRONIC PAIN

NOC **PLANNING: EXPECTED OUTCOMES.** The major concern of the client with OA is pain control. Therefore the client is expected to take personal actions to control pain. Indicators include that the client will consistently demonstrate the ability to:

- Recognize pain onset
- Use previous measures that were effective
- Use analgesics appropriately
- Use non-analgesic relief measures
- Report changes in pain symptoms or sites to health care professional
- Report that pain is controlled

INTERVENTIONS. Pain control may be accomplished at home with drug and nonpharmacologic measures. If these measures become ineffective, surgery may be performed to reduce pain. A comprehensive pain assessment should be performed before and after implementing interventions (Chart 24-1).

NONSURGICAL MANAGEMENT. Management of chronic joint pain is difficult for both the client and the health care professional. A combination of modalities is often used, including analgesics, rest, positioning, thermal modalities,

CHART 24-1

NIC INTERVENTION ACTIVITIES for The Client with Osteoarthritis

Analgesic Administration: *Use of pharmacologic agents to reduce or eliminate pain*

- Determine pain location, characteristics, quality, and severity before medicating client.
- Check medical order for drug, dose, and frequency of analgesic prescribed.
- Attend to comfort needs and other activities that assist in relaxation to facilitate response to analgesia.
- Administer analgesics around-the-clock to prevent peaks and troughs of analgesia, especially with severe pain.
- Set positive expectations regarding the effectiveness of analgesics to optimize client response.
- Document response to analgesic and any untoward effects.

Pain Management: *Alleviation of pain or a reduction in pain to a level of comfort that is acceptable to the client*

- Observe for nonverbal cues of discomfort, especially in those unable to communicate effectively.
- Consider cultural influences on pain response.
- Determine the impact of the pain experience on quality of life (e.g., sleep, appetite, activity, cognition, mood, relationships, performance of job, and role responsibilities).
- Evaluate, with the client and the health care team, the effectiveness of past pain control measures that have been used.
- Consider the client's willingness to participate, ability to participate, preference, support of significant others for method, and contraindications when selecting a pain relief strategy.
- Teach the use of nonpharmacologic techniques (e.g., biofeedback, TENS, hypnosis, relaxation, guided imagery, music therapy, distraction, activity therapy, acupressure, hot/cold application, and massage) before, after and, if possible, during painful activities; before pain occurs or increases; and along with other pain relief measures.
- Promote adequate rest/sleep to facilitate pain relief.
- Utilize a multidisciplinary approach to pain management, when appropriate.
- Consider referrals for client, family, and significant others to support groups, and other resources, as appropriate.
- Monitor client satisfaction with pain management at specified intervals.

NIC intervention activities selected from Dochterman, J.M., & Bulechek, G.M. (Eds.). (2004). *Nursing interventions classification (NIC)* (4th ed.). St. Louis: Mosby. No part of this work is to be altered without prior written permission from the Publisher.

weight control, and integrative therapies. Chapter 7 elaborates on methods of pain control for chronic pain.

NIC **Analgesic Administration.** The purpose of drug therapy is to reduce pain and secondary joint inflammation if present. Acetaminophen (Tylenol, Atasol✱) is the primary drug of choice for pain relief; it is not an anti-inflammatory medication. Clients are at risk for liver damage if they take more than 4000 mg daily, have concurrent alcoholism, or have pre-existing liver disease.

Topical salicylates, such as over-the-counter (OTC) Aspercreme, are useful for some clients as a temporary pain reliever. Topical capsaicin products may also be used. This expensive OTC drug works by blocking substance P, a neurotransmitter for pain (Kee, 2000). Tell the client to expect a burning sensation for a short time after applying capsaicin. Recommend the use of plastic gloves for application. To prevent burning of eyes or other body areas, wash hands immediately after applying capsaicin.

If acetaminophen or topical agents are not successful in relieving pain, the analgesic drug class of choice is usually **nonsteroidal anti-inflammatory drugs (NSAIDs)** (see Chart 24-9 later in this chapter). Most NSAIDs work by inhibiting both forms of the enzyme cyclooxygenase, COX-1 and COX-2. COX-1 produces prostaglandins that help regulate normal cell activity, including protecting the lining of the gastrointestinal (GI) tract. COX-2 produces prostaglandins mainly at the sites of inflammation. A subgroup of NSAIDs has been developed to inhibit only the COX-2 enzyme. COX-2–inhibiting medications, such as celecoxib (Celebrex), meloxicam (Mobic), and valdecoxib (Bextra), appear to manage pain and inflammation with fewer adverse side effects of GI distress or bleeding. Clients allergic to sulfa drugs may also be allergic to celecoxib and therefore should not take it. All of the COX-2 inhibiting drugs are thought to cause cardiovascular disease, such as myocardial infarction, and may soon be unavailable on the market.

For temporary relief of pain in a single joint, the health care provider may inject an individual joint with cortisone. Frequently injected joints include the knee, base of the thumb, shoulder, and the trochanteric bursa, which people often identify as the hip.

Other local agents, such as hyaluronate (Hyalgan) and hylan GF 20 (Synvisc), are used as joint injections for OA of the knee. These synthetic joint fluid implants replace or supplement the body's natural hyaluronic acid, which is broken down by inflammation. Muscle relaxants, such as cyclobenzaprine hydrochloride (Flexeril), are sometimes given for painful muscle spasms, especially those occurring in the back. Remind the client not to drive or operate dangerous machinery when taking muscle relaxants. Potent analgesics are not usually appropriate for the client with OA because of the chronic nature of the pain.

NIC **Pain Management.** In addition to analgesics, many nonpharmacologic measures can be used for clients with OA.

Rest. Several types of rest are used to treat clients with OA:

- *Local* rest involves immobilizing a joint with a splint or brace. If a joint becomes acutely inflamed, the joint is rested until inflammation subsides. Rest the joint when painful, but exercise it to maintain mobility and tone. Balance rest and activity. Consult the occupational therapist (OT), who fits the client for the appropriate device and explains its use.
- *Systemic* rest refers to immobilizing the entire body, such as during a nap. Teach the client about the importance of sleeping about 8 to 10 hours and, if possible, resting an additional 1 to 2 hours each day.
- *Psychological* rest is equally important because it allows relief from the daily stresses that can enhance pain.

Positioning. Joints should be placed in their functional position. When the client is in a supine position (recumbent), he or she should use a small pillow under the head or neck but avoid the use of other pillows. The use of large pillows under the knees or head may result in flexion contractures. If needed, the legs may be elevated 8 to 12 inches (20.3 to 30.5 cm) to reduce back discomfort. Remind the client to use proper posture when standing and sitting to reduce undue strain on the vertebral column.

Thermal Modalities. In general, the client with OA uses heat instead of cold to reduce pain. Heat often helps to decrease the muscle tension around the tender joint and thereby decreases pain. Heat is a temporary relief measure that may be used by the client as often as desired. The application of cold is usually reserved for acutely inflamed joints.

Suggest hot showers and baths, hot packs or compresses, and moist heating pads. Regardless of treatment, teach the client to check that the heat source is not too heavy or so hot that it causes burns. A temperature just above body temperature is adequate to promote comfort.

A physical therapist may provide special heat treatments, such as paraffin dips, diathermy (electrical current), and ultrasonography (sound waves). A 15- to 20-minute heat application usually is sufficient to temporarily reduce pain, spasm, and stiffness. Collaborate with the physical therapist to provide comprehensive care.

Weight Control. Contrary to what has been proposed by the media and uninformed authors, there is no "arthritis diet." According to the National Arthritis Foundation, there is no one food that causes or cures arthritis. A well-balanced diet is recommended. Gradual weight loss for obese clients may lessen the stress on weight-bearing joints, decrease pain, and perhaps slow joint degeneration. If needed, collaborate with the dietitian to provide more in-depth teaching about nutrition and meal planning.

Transcutaneous Electrical Nerve Stimulation. Transcutaneous electrical nerve stimulation (TENS) may be particularly helpful for vertebral involvement. The physician or health care provider collaborates with the nurse and physical therapist to determine whether this pain management modality would be beneficial. The client must be able to control the TENS unit for pain relief.

Complementary and Alternative Therapies. Clients may also use acupuncture, acupressure, tai chi, therapeutic touch, hypnosis, magnets, music therapy, and imagery for pain relief (see Chapters 4 and 7). A study by McCaffrey and Freeman (2003) found that music was an effective intervention for controlling pain in community-dwelling older adults (see the Evidence-Based Practice for Nursing box at right).

Cayenne pepper (the source of capsaicin products) and other dietary supplements, gamma-linolenic acid (GLA, Efamol), glucosamine, and chondroitin complement traditional therapies. GLA can be found in evening primrose oil, borage seed oil, and black currant seed oil. GLA is an omega-6 fatty acid, one of the body's essential fatty acids, and is used for both OA and rheumatoid arthritis (RA). Omega-3 fatty acids are found in certain types of fish (e.g., salmon) or may be taken in fish oil capsules. Glucosamine and chondroitin are natural products (also known as nutraceuticals) found in bone cartilage that may help reduce pain and possibly slow the progression of OA. Many clients have reported positive results, especially decreased pain and inflammation, from these dietary supplements and topical analgesics.

Topical creams have gained increased popularity for short-term pain relief. A study by Cohen (2003) found that topical applications of glucosamine and chondroitin sulfate were effective in relieving knee pain due to OA. Other studies have examined herbal ointments and formulas and found improvement in hand and knee pain (Gemmell, Jacobson, & Hayes, 2003).

Stem Cell Therapy. In certain degenerative disorders, such as OA, stem cells are depleted and have decreased the ability to multiply and differentiation. Ongoing research is exploring methods for delivering mesenchymal stem cell preparations from bone marrow to affected knee joints. This treatment has the potential to stimulate regeneration of cartilage and inhibit joint destruction (Barry, 2003).

EVIDENCE-BASED PRACTICE for Nursing

How does music therapy impact pain perception in clients with osteoarthritis?

McCaffrey, R., & Freeman, E. (2003). Effect of music on chronic osteoarthritis in older people. *Journal of Advanced Nursing, 44*(5), 517-524.

The purpose of this clinical trial was to examine the effect of music as a nursing intervention on osteoarthritis (OA) pain in community-dwelling older adults. The control group sat quietly for 20 minutes each day, and the experimental group listened to music for 20 minutes each day. All 66 subjects completed the Short Form McGill Pain Questionnaire on day 1, 7, and 14. The subjects in the experimental group experienced significantly less OA pain that the control group, demonstrating the value of music as an intervention to control pain.

Level of Evidence: 3—This study was a well-designed trial without randomization of the overall sample, but the sample was randomly assigned.

Critique. This study used random assignment of a selected sample for an experimental design. Although the sample was small, it illustrated the importance of the intervention to nursing practice. The study needs to be repeated with larger samples of various cultures and in various settings where older adults reside.

Implications for Nursing. Interventions for pain control other than medication are needed for clients with chronic pain, such as that experienced by clients with OA. Nurses can use this measure in the community when working with older adults or in long-term care, rehabilitation, and assisted living settings. In some cases, clients who are hospitalized may be candidates for music as an intervention.

SURGICAL MANAGEMENT. Surgery may be indicated when all other measures are inadequate to provide pain control for clients with OA. The most common surgical procedure performed for these clients is **total joint arthroplasty (TJA)** (surgical creation of a joint), also know as total joint replacement (TJR). Almost any synovial joint of the body can be replaced with a prosthetic system that consists of at least two parts, one for each joint surface.

A less invasive procedure using arthroscopy may be used to remove damaged cartilage (see Chapter 54). An **osteotomy** (bone resection) may be performed to correct joint deformity, but this procedure is less common because of the success rate of TJR.

Indications. Total joint arthroplasty is a procedure of last resort for pain management; it is used when all other methods of pain relief have been unsuccessful. The hips and knees are the joints most commonly replaced, but replacements of finger and wrist joints, elbows, shoulders, toe joints, and ankles have become more popular in the past 20 years.

Although TJAs are performed most often for clients with OA, other conditions causing joint damage may also require surgery. These disorders include RA, congenital anomalies, trauma, and osteonecrosis. **Osteonecrosis** is bony necrosis secondary to lack of blood flow, usually from trauma or chronic steroid therapy.

Contraindications. The primary contraindications for TJA are infection anywhere in the body, advanced osteoporosis, and severe inflammation. An infection elsewhere in the body or from the joint being replaced can result in an infected TJA and subsequent prosthetic failure. Therefore if a client has a urinary tract infection, for example, the physician treats the infection before surgery. Advanced osteoporosis can cause bone shattering during insertion of the prosthetic device. Acute joint inflammation is treated before surgery because the mechanical stress of the procedure may promote further inflammation and prosthetic failure.

As a group, TJAs are very successful. Many clients who have lived with chronic, unbearable pain for years and could not function independently at home or in the workplace no longer experience pain in the diseased joint. The pain relief and psychological benefit often outweigh the perioperative risks and costs, but the surgeon and client must make that decision with the case manager. When the client is of advanced age, this decision may become an ethical issue in addition to a physical risk and cost-versus-benefit decision (see the Legal/Ethical Issues box below).

Total Hip Arthroplasty. The most commonly replaced joint is the hip. More than 80% of hip replacements last 20 years as a result of improvements in prosthetic design and surgical technology (Branson & Goldstein, 2003). Although clients of any age can undergo total hip replacement (THA), the procedure is performed most often in clients older than 60 years of age. The special needs and normal physiologic changes of older clients often complicate the perioperative period and may result in additional postoperative complications. (See Chapters 20 to 22 for routine perioperative care and the special considerations needed for care of the older client.)

Preoperative Care. As with any procedure, preoperative care begins with assessing the client's level of understanding about the impending surgery. The surgeon explains the procedure and realistic postoperative care expectations during the office visit, but this education may have occurred weeks or months before the scheduled surgery. Older clients in particular may forget some of the information or may not know what questions to ask. Many orthopedic surgeons employ nurses who follow up and address client concerns. An interdisciplinary clinical pathway that outlines expectations during pre-admission, hospitalization, and post-hospitalization phases of care should be reviewed with the client and family or significant other.

In addition, nurse educators or orthopedic nurses may lead formal classes in the hospital or clinic several weeks before surgery to answer questions and clarify information. Pre-admission sessions are an excellent way for nurses to provide education and support and to improve customer satisfaction. During the class, the client sees the prosthesis or a picture of the device and receives written instructions or a teaching booklet to reinforce the information.

In some hospitals or orthopedic office practices, the physical therapist may meet the client before surgery to explain transfers, precautions, ambulation, and postoperative exercises. An occupational therapist may be available to demonstrate assistive/adaptive devices that facilitate independent activities of daily living (ADLs).

Because venous thromboembolism is a serious postoperative complication, especially for hip surgery, the client's risk factors for clotting problems are determined, including history of previous clotting, obesity, and advanced age. Medications that increase the risk of clotting, such as NSAIDs and hormone replacement therapy (HRT), are discontinued before surgery.

Because TJAs are elective procedures, **autologous blood transfusions** are appropriate. The client may donate blood before surgery to be used as needed during and after surgery. This pre-deposit autologous blood donation is a cost-effective blood replacement alternative for clients who are undergoing elective surgeries. It also avoids the risk of blood transfusion reaction.

Operative Procedures. For both total hip and knee arthroplasty, the client is given a dose of intravenous (IV) antibiotics, usually a cephalosporin such as cefazolin (Ancef), at least 1 hour before the initial surgical incision is made or during surgery. Vancomycin (Vancocin) or clindamycin (Cleocin) may be used for clients who are allergic to cephalosporins.

The anesthesiologist or nurse anesthetist places the client having hip or knee replacement under general or **neuroaxial** (epidural/spinal) anesthesia. Neuroaxial induction reduces blood loss and the incidence of deep vein thrombosis. Intraoperative blood loss with hypotensive neuroaxial anesthesia is usually less than that for general anesthesia, thereby decreasing the need for postoperative blood transfusions.

Two types of incisions for hip replacement may be used. The more traditional 8- to 10-inch (20.3 to 24.5 cm) incision is usually longitudinal on the anterolateral thigh. A posterior incision may be used instead to preserve muscle, depending on the surgeon's preference. Some clients are candidates for a minimally invasive two-incision technique, which is gaining popularity. One small incision is used for the acetabular component, and the other is used for the femoral component. Berger (2003) reported that this newer procedure decreased postoperative complications, including hip dislocation. Wenz, Gurkan, and Jibodh (2002) found that their postoperative clients had earlier ambulation and needed less transfer assistance compared with clients who underwent traditional hip surgery. Therefore, hospital stay is shorter.

If the prosthesis is cemented, polymethyl methacrylate (an acrylic fixating substance) is used. During the surgical

LEGAL/ETHICAL ISSUES

QUALITY OF LIFE FOR CLIENTS HAVING TOTAL JOINT REPLACEMENT

Quality of life (QOL) or quality of well-being (QWB) is a difficult concept to define. In general, it is determined by the client's opinion about the importance of certain elements of his or her life and satisfaction with those elements. Few studies have compared the high cost of surgery with QOL following total joint replacement. This *utilitarian* ethical approach is based on the belief that a person deserves resources based on the real or potential productivity that he or she offers to society.

Health economists consider a resource or intervention a bargain for society if it costs less than $30,000 per quality of well year. Lavernia, Guzman, and Gachupin-Garcia (1999) calculated the cost per quality of well year for 100 clients undergoing a total knee replacement. The clients completed the QWB Index before surgery and at 3 months, 6 months, 1 year, and 2 years after surgery. The differences in the scores before and after surgery were multiplied by the client's life expectancy to obtain the cost per quality of well year. The calculated costs were about $30,700 at 3 months but steadily decreased to about $6,600 by 2 years postsurgery. Based on this study, total knee replacement meets the utilitarian approach to ethical decision making and should be considered an appropriate investment by society.

From Lavernia, C.J., Guzman, J.F., & Gachupin-Garcia, A. (1999). Cost effectiveness and quality of life in knee arthroplasty. *Clinical Orthopaedics, 345,* 134-139.

procedure, the operative area is irrigated with a cool solution. To help prevent infection, the surgeon may mix an antibiotic with the cement or plant antibiotic-impregnated beads deep into the wound. The surgeon also inserts one or two wound drains to remove exudate from the tissues, which might serve as a medium for pathogenic growth and cause wound infection.

Although polymethyl methacrylate is an excellent initial fixative, it has a finite life span and deteriorates over time, which loosens the implant and causes pain. When a prosthesis eventually loosens and causes pain, it is replaced in a procedure called a **revision arthroplasty.** Bone grafts **(allografts)** can be placed to fill in the bony defects that result from removing the old prosthesis. During the healing process, the essentially dead bone revascularizes and grafts with the client's own bone. To prevent prosthetic loosening, a number of noncemented devices that do not require a fixating substance are commonly used instead.

Postoperative Care. In addition to providing the routine postoperative care discussed in Chapter 22, assess for and assist in the prevention of possible postoperative complications following a joint replacement. Table 24-2 summarizes common postoperative complications of total hip replacement surgery, including nursing measures for prevention, assessment, and intervention. Chart 24-2 highlights special concerns for the care of older adults in the postoperative period.

Prevention of Dislocation. A common complication of total hip replacement is **subluxation** (partial dislocation) or total dislocation. Therefore correct positioning is maintained at all times. When the client returns from the postanesthesia care unit (PACU), place him or her in a supine position with the head slightly elevated. Place a trapezoid-shaped abduction pillow, wedge, sling, or splint (with or without straps) between the client's legs to prevent adduction beyond the midline of the body. In some hospitals this device is no longer used because it is uncomfortable and unnecessary in most cases. Abduction devices are usually reserved for clients who are restless or are unable to follow instructions, especially older adults. One or two regular bed pillows are used in most cases. For devices with straps, be sure to loosen the straps every 2 hours and check the client's skin for irritation or breakdown.

Place and support the affected leg in neutral rotation. Keep the client's heels off the bed to prevent skin breakdown, particularly likely to occur in older adults. Turning the client is controversial and is dictated by agency policy or surgeon preference. In most cases you are safe to turn the client toward either side as long as the abduction device or other pillow is in place. Some surgeons allow only turning directly onto one side or the other.

Observe for possible signs of hip dislocation, which include increased hip pain, shortening of the affected leg, and leg rotation. If any of these clinical manifestations occur, keep the client in bed and notify the surgeon immediately. The surgeon manipulates and relocates the affected hip after the client receives an analgesic or is anesthetized. The hip is then immobilized by an abduction splint or other device until healing occurs, usually in about 6 weeks.

Prevention of Thromboembolic Complications. The most potentially *life-threatening* complication following THA is venous thromboembolism (VTE), which includes deep venous thrombosis (DVT) and pulmonary embolism (PE). Older clients are especially at increased risk for VTE because of age and compromised circulation before surgery. Obese clients and those with a history of DVT are also at high risk for thrombi. In clients with TJA, thrombi usually develop in the thigh; these thrombi become life-threatening emboli more readily than thrombi in the calf and other areas. For this reason, thigh-high stockings and sequential

TABLE 24-2 Nursing Interventions to Prevent Complications of Total Joint Replacement Surgery

Complication	Prevention/Intervention
Dislocation	Position correctly. For hip, keep legs slightly abducted. For hip, prevent hip flexion beyond 90 degrees. Assess for pain, rotation, and extremity shortening. Report immediately to physician.
Infection	Use aseptic technique for wound care and emptying of drains. Wash hands thoroughly when caring for client. Culture drainage fluid, if change. Monitor temperature. Report excessive inflammation or drainage to physician.
Venous thromboembolism	Have client wear elastic stockings and/or sequential compression device. Teach leg exercises to client. Encourage fluid intake. Observe for signs of thrombosis (redness, swelling, or pain). Observe client for changes in mental status. Administer anticoagulant as prescribed. Do not massage legs. Do not use knee gatch on bed.
Hypotension, bleeding, or infection	Take vital signs at least every 4 hours. Observe client for bleeding. Report excessively low blood pressure or bleeding to physician.

CHART 24-2

NURSING FOCUS on the OLDER ADULT

Total Hip Replacement

- Use an abduction pillow or splint to prevent adduction after surgery if the client is very restless or has an altered mental state.
- Keep the client's heels off the bed to prevent pressure ulcers.
- Do not rely on fever as a sign of infection; older clients often have infection without fever. Decreasing mental status typically occurs when the client has an infection.
- When assisting the client out of bed, move him or her slowly to prevent orthostatic (postural) hypotension.
- Encourage the client to deep breathe and cough, and use the incentive spirometer every 2 hours to prevent atelectasis and pneumonia.
- As soon as permitted, get the client out of bed to prevent complications of immobility.
- Anticipate the client's need for pain medication, especially if he or she is unable to verbalize the need for pain control.
- Expect a temporary change in mental state immediately after surgery as a result of the anesthetic and unfamiliar sensory stimuli. Reorient the client frequently.

compression devices (SCDs) are typically used during the hospital stay (see Chapter 22). Foot-sole pumps (A-V Impulse System) may also be used.

Anticoagulants, such as aspirin (Ecotrin, buffered aspirin), warfarin (Coumadin, Warfilone✱), subcutaneous low-molecular-weight (LMW) heparin, and fondaparinux (Arixtra), are prescribed to prevent VTE. Aspirin may be given to clients with a low risk for VTE. Warfarin may be used for clients who are predisposed to VTE or for those already on the drug for another condition.

During the past decade, the use of LMW heparins has markedly increased for clients with total hip and knee replacements. Examples include enoxaparin (Lovenox), dalteparin (Fragmin), and tinzaparin (Innohep), approved for use in the United States. Other LMW heparins, such as bemiparin (Zibor), are approved for use in other countries. These drugs work to maximize anti-factor Xa and antithrombin to decrease clotting. Given in a low prophylactic dose, they do not affect prothrombin time or activated partial thromboplastin time. However, monitor complete blood count and platelet count because LMW heparins can cause **thrombocytopenia** (decreased platelets). Assess for bleeding, including occult blood in stool and bruising. Protamine can be given as an antidote for all heparins. Be especially alert for signs and symptoms of neurologic dysfunction because spinal and epidural hematomas can occur in clients who received neuroaxial anesthesia.

Fondaparinux (Arixtra) is the first antithrombotic agent that may be prescribed for clients undergoing hip and knee arthroplasty. Its action is similar to that of LMW heparins, and it also has no effect on coagulation tests. Like other drugs, however, the client is at risk for bleeding. No antidote exists at this time for fondaparinux. A complete discussion of nursing care associated with clients taking anticoagulants and VTE can be found in Chapter 39.

The physical therapist (PT) teaches leg exercises, which are begun in the immediate postoperative period and continue until the client is fully ambulatory. These exercises include plantar flexion and dorsiflexion (heel pumping), circumduction (circles) of the feet, gluteal and quadriceps muscle setting, and straight-leg raises (SLRs). The client performs gluteal exercises by pushing the heels into the bed and achieves **quadriceps-setting exercises** ("quad sets") by straightening the legs and pushing the back of the knees into the bed. In addition to preventing clots, these exercises improve muscle tone, which aids restoring the function of the extremity.

Prevention of Infection. Another common potential complication of hip replacement is infection. Infection can occur during hospitalization or for months or years later. Most infections are caused by contamination during surgery.

Monitor the surgical incision and vital signs carefully—every 4 hours for the first 24 hours and every 8 hours thereafter. Observe for signs of infection, such as an elevated temperature and excessive or foul-smelling drainage from the incision. An older client may not have a fever with infection but instead may experience an altered mental state. Obtain a sample of the drainage for culture and sensitivity to determine the offending organisms and the antibiotics that may be needed for treatment.

Assessment of Bleeding and Management of Anemia. Observe the surgical hip dressing for bleeding or other type of drainage at least every 4 hours or when vital signs are taken. Empty and measure the bloody fluid in the drain every shift. The total amount of drainage is usually less than 50 mL/8 hr (possibly more if the client has received a plasma expander such as dextran). The surgeon usually removes the drains and operative dressing 48 to 72 hours after surgery. Clients who have the "mini-incision" surgery may not have a drain. Care must be taken to prevent tape burns when the surgical dressing is removed, especially in older adults.

The surgeon also orders periodic hemoglobin and hematocrit assessments to determine whether the client is anemic and requires blood transfusions. Although some clients receive several units of blood during surgery, the hematocrit and hemoglobin levels may fall below the normal level, in which case additional blood is needed 1 to 2 days after surgery. Blood pressure may be lower than usual because of blood loss during surgery or because cement was used during surgery. (Cement tends to dilate blood vessels and cause hypotension.)

If the client did not donate his or her own blood, another method for blood replacement is intraoperative or postoperative **blood salvage.** The shed blood is collected intraoperatively via aspiration from the surgical site. Using a cell saver, about 50% of the red blood cells are saved for reinfusion. This procedure is used most commonly for bilateral joint replacements or revision surgeries. Blood can be replaced postoperatively by collecting shed blood via suction into a reservoir, filtering the blood, and re-infusing it within a few hours.

Postoperative blood replacement has been standard practice until recently. A preventive alternative is the use of epoetin alfa (Epogen, Procrit, Eprex✱), an approved treatment for anemia that may prevent the necessity of postoperative blood transfusion when given to clients undergoing TJA.

Assessment for Neurovascular Compromise. As with other bone surgery, frequent neurovascular assessments are necessary to monitor for a possible compromise in circulation to the distal extremity. Check and document color, temperature, distal pulses, capillary refill, movement, and sensation. Remember to compare the operative leg with the nonoperative one. Such assessments are performed at the same time the vital signs are checked.

Management of Pain. Although hip arthroplasty is performed to relieve joint pain, the client does experience pain related to the surgical procedure. Many clients state that they have pain after surgery but that it is of a different type and is less excruciating than the pain before surgery. Pain control may be achieved by epidural analgesia, patient-controlled analgesia (PCA), intramuscular opioid analgesia, or a combination of techniques. Chapter 7 contains a chart of commonly used opioid analgesics used for acute pain and related nursing interventions. Keep in mind that the client may also receive other analgesics or anti-inflammatory drugs for chronic arthritic pain in other joints.

Another device for pain control after TJA is a small pump called the Pain Buster. This pump continuously infuses a local anesthetic, such as bupivacaine, directly into the surgical site. The local infusion decreases the amount of opioids that the client needs (e.g., morphine), thus reducing the risk of adverse drug reactions. The device is also ideal for ambulatory surgical clients, who may go home with the device (Kettelman, 2000). After the catheter is removed in 24 to 48 hours, the entire device is discarded and the site is covered with a sterile dressing.

CONSIDERATIONS FOR OLDER ADULTS

Anticipate the older client's need for pain medication if he or she cannot verbalize the need. Many older adults experience several days of increased disorientation or delirium as a result of surgery and anesthesia.

Regardless of the pain management method used, most clients do not require parenteral analgesia after the first 2 days. Oral opioids, such as oxycodone (Supeudol✱) or oxycodone plus acetaminophen (Percocet, Tylox), are then commonly prescribed until the pain can be controlled by NSAIDs such as ketorolac (Toradol, Acular) or ibuprofen (Motrin, Apo-Ibuprofen✱); however, these NSAIDs can impair bone healing (Hutchinson, 2004). Current recommendations are that clients who have orthopedic surgery take NSAIDs on a short-term basis, up to 14 days. More information on pain medication can be found in Chapter 7.

Progression of Activity. The client with a THA is usually allowed to get out of bed the day after surgery, and physical therapy is initiated. Permitted activities differ among surgeons and hospitals, but prolonged bedrest can cause numerous complications (e.g., atelectasis and pneumonia), especially in the older adults. When getting the client out of bed, stand on the same side of the bed as the client's affected leg. After achieving a sitting position, the client stands on the unaffected leg and pivots to the chair with assistance. To prevent hip dislocation, ensure that the client does not flex the hips beyond 90 degrees (Figure 24-2). Raised toilet seats, straight-back chairs, and reclining wheelchairs help prevent hyperflexion.

The surgeon, the type of prosthesis, and the surgical approach determine the resumption of weight bearing on the affected leg. A client with a cemented implant is usually allowed immediate partial weight bearing (PWB) or full weight bearing (FWB) to tolerance. A client with an uncemented prosthesis

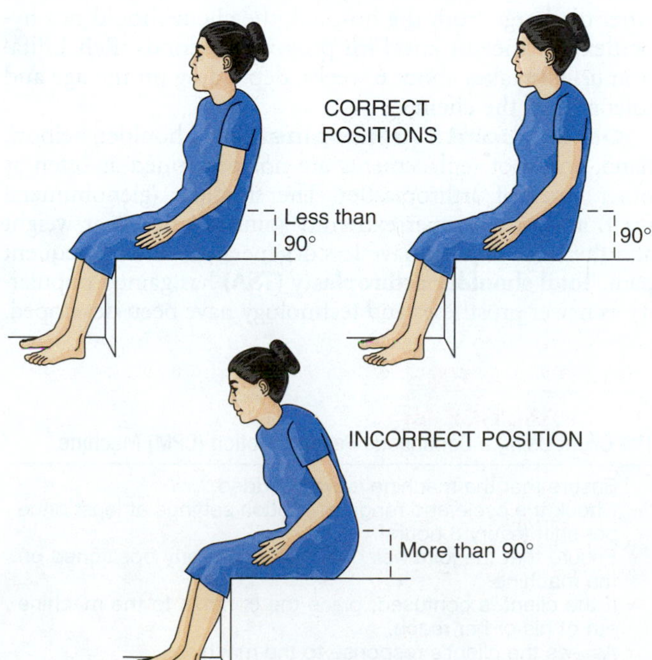

Figure 24-2 ■ Correct and incorrect hip flexion after a total hip replacement.

cannot tolerate FWB until bony ingrowth occurs. Typically, only PWB is permitted for the first few weeks or until there is x-ray evidence of bony ingrowth.

The physical therapist (PT) teaches the client how to follow these weight-bearing restrictions and helps the client progress to FWB status, if possible. Most clients use a walker, but younger clients may use crutches. Clients are usually advanced to a single cane or crutch if they can walk without a severe limp by 1 month after surgery. When the limp disappears, they no longer need an ambulatory/assistive device and are permitted to sit in chairs of normal height, use regular toilets, and drive a car.

Promotion of Self-Care. The hospital's occupational therapy department often supplies assistive/adaptive devices to help with activities of daily living (ADLs). Particularly important for clients are devices designed for reaching to prevent them from bending or stooping and flexing the hips more than 90 degrees. Extended handles on shoehorns and dressing sticks are particularly useful for helping clients achieve independence in ADLs.

For clients who have traditional surgery, the length of stay in the acute care hospital is typically 3 days, but older clients or those experiencing postoperative complications may stay longer. Discharge may be to the home, a rehabilitation unit, transitional care unit, or long-term care facility for rehabilitation or custodial care. For clients who have the "mini-incision" approach, discharge on the surgical day or the next day is typical. The interdisciplinary team provides written instructions for post-hospital care and reviews them with clients and their family members

CHART 24-3

CLIENT EDUCATION GUIDE
Total Hip Replacement

Hip Precautions
- Do not sit or stand for prolonged periods.
- Do not cross your legs beyond the midline of your body.
- Do not bend your hips more than 90 degrees.
- Use an ambulatory aid, such as a walker, when walking.
- Use assistive/adaptive devices for dressing, such as for putting on shoes and socks.
- Resume sexual intercourse as usual upon the advice of your surgeon.

Pain Management
- Report increased hip pain to the physician immediately.
- Take oral analgesics as prescribed and only as needed.
- Do not overexert yourself; take frequent rests.

Incisional Care
- Inspect your hip incision every day for redness, heat, or drainage; if any of these are present, call your physician immediately.
- Cleanse your hip incision with a mild soap and water every day; be sure to dry it thoroughly.

Other Care
- Continue walking and performing the leg exercises as you learned in the hospital.
- Report pain, redness, or swelling in your legs to your physician immediately.
- Report chest pain or shortness of breath to your physician immediately.
- If you are taking an anticoagulant for 4 to 6 weeks, follow the precautions learned in the hospital to prevent bleeding; avoid using a straight razor, avoid injuries, and report bleeding or excessive bruising to your surgeon immediately.

(Chart 24-3). A copy of the post-hospital instructions is sent with clients who are transferred to a facility. Rehabilitation usually takes about 6 weeks, although this time frame depends on the client's age and tolerance as well as the type of prosthesis used.

Total Knee Arthroplasty. After total hip arthroplasty, the second most common total joint arthroplasty procedure involves the knee (total knee arthroplasty, or TKA). The knee is not a simple hinged joint; it is a condylar joint that rotates slightly when flexed and extended. The expected use of a TKA is about 10 to 15 years, but the time is variable depending on the age of the client, type of prosthesis, and activity of the client postoperatively.

Preoperative Care. Only severe symptoms and disability justify TKA in clients with osteoarthritis (OA). Like hip arthroplasty, TKAs are typically avoided in people younger than 60 years of age. The preoperative care for clients undergoing a TKA is similar to that for total hip replacement. The major difference is the teaching, which depends on the postoperative protocol used by the orthopedic surgeon.

Operative Procedures. As with the hip, the knee can be replaced with the client under general or neuroaxial (epidural or spinal) anesthesia. The surgeon typically makes a central longitudinal incision about 8 inches (20.3 cm) long. Osteotomies of the femoral and tibial condyles and of the posterior patella are performed, and the surfaces are prepared for the prosthesis. Noncemented implants are used less for the knee than they are for the hip. The surgeon inserts one or two surgical drains and applies a pressure dressing to prevent bleeding. Some clients have bilateral knee replacements as part of one surgery.

Postoperative Care. Postoperative nursing care of the client with a TKA is similar to that for the client with a total hip arthroplasty; however, maintaining abduction is not necessary. The surgeon usually prescribes a continuous passive motion (CPM) machine, which can be applied in the postanesthesia care unit (PACU) or not used until 1 to 2 days after surgery (Figure 24-3). The CPM keeps the prosthetic knee in motion and prevents the formation of scar tissue, which could impede mobility of the knee and exacerbate postoperative pain. In the immediate postoperative period, the surgeon may also order ice packs or a Hot/Ice Machine to decrease swelling at the surgical site. Swelling and bruising are common with this type of surgery.

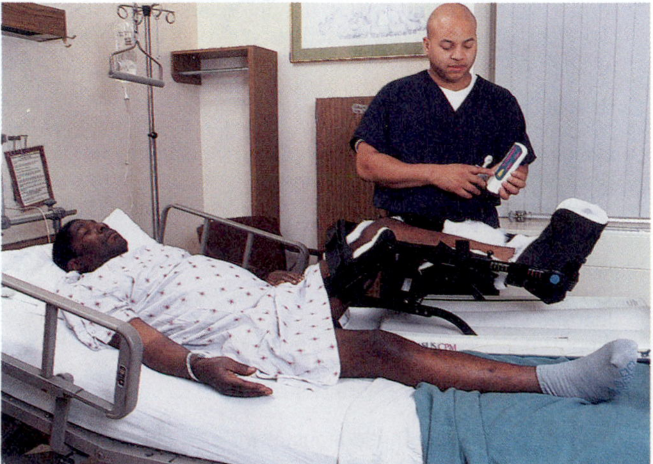

Figure 24-3 ■ A continuous passive motion machine in use.

The surgeon, PT, or technician presets the CPM machine for the appropriate range of motion and cycles per minute. A typical initial setting is 20 to 30 degrees of flexion and full extension (0 degrees) at two cycles per minute, but this setting varies according to surgeon preference. The CPM machine is generally used for 8 to 12 hours per day, with the range of motion increased gradually. The current trend is intermittent use for several hours at a time. Note the client's response to the device and follow the surgeon's protocol for settings.

Some machines do not allow the leg to achieve full extension, thus promoting flexion contractures. One solution is for the client to use the CPM machine during the day and sleep in a knee immobilizer at night to achieve the desired extension. Chart 24-4 outlines the nurse's responsibility when caring for a client using the CPM machine.

In general, pain-control measures for clients with TKA are similar to clients with total hip arthroplasty. Intra-articular morphine for the first 24 hours after surgery is a safe and effective alternative for pain management.

Because dislocation is a rare problem for a client with total knee replacement (TKR), special positioning is usually not required. The knee should be maintained in a neutral position and not rotated internally or externally. Other complications that affect clients with THA may also affect clients with TKA, such as venous thromboembolism, infection, and bleeding. Monitor neurovascular status frequently to check for compromise to the distal operative leg. The preventive and treatment measures described earlier for total hip arthroplasty are also used for TKA (see earlier discussion of postoperative care for total hip arthroplasty, p. 387).

The goal for discharge from the acute hospital unit is that the client should walk independently with a cane or walker and have close to 90 degrees of flexion in the operative knee. The use of a stationary bicycle can help gain flexion. After discharge from the hospital, the client should not hyperflex the knee or kneel for prolonged periods. Rehabilitation usually takes about 6 weeks, depending on the age and tolerance of the client.

Other Joint Arthroplasties. Shoulder, elbow, hand, and foot replacements are not performed as often as other types of arthroplasties. The shoulder (glenohumeral joint) and other upper extremity joints do not bear weight and therefore tend to have less degeneration and subsequent pain. **Total shoulder arthroplasty (TSA)** has gained popularity as newer prostheses and technology have been developed.

CHART 24-4

BEST PRACTICE for

The Client Using a Continuous Passive Motion (CPM) Machine

- Ensure that the machine is well padded.
- Check the cycle and range-of-motion settings at least once per shift (every 8 hours).
- Ensure that the joint being moved is properly positioned on the machine.
- If the client is confused, place the controls to the machine out of his or her reach.
- Assess the client's response to the machine.
- Turn off the machine while the client is having a meal in bed.
- When the machine is not in use, do not store it on the floor.

These procedures usually decrease arthritic pain and increase the client's ability to perform activities of daily living (ADLs). Because the glenohumeral joint is complex and has many **articulations** (joint surfaces), subluxation (or dislocation) can be a complication. A Neer-type prosthesis is commonly used, with or without cement. A **hemiarthroplasty** (replacement of part of the joint), typically the humeral component, may be performed as an alternative to TSA.

The client's operative arm may be placed in a CPM machine shortly after surgery (see Chart 24-4). As an alternative, passive exercises are done to begin shoulder mobilization. As for other total joint arthroplasties, frequent neurovascular assessments are important. Major complications are rare, although a few cases of pulmonary embolism (PE) have occurred. Monitor the client's respiratory rate and rhythm carefully to detect early indications of a PE. The hospital stay is shorter than for a total hip replacement or total knee replacement, usually 1 to 2 days until pain is controlled. Rehabilitation with physical therapy generally takes 2 to 3 months.

Total elbow arthroplasty (TEA) is performed most commonly for clients with rheumatoid arthritis (RA). It is usually successful in increasing range of motion, but infection and loosening may occur because of extensive tissue cutting during surgery. A CPM device may be used postoperatively, or passive exercises are prescribed. In general, elbow motion is allowed as tolerated. Physical therapy may not be necessary, but the need depends on the individual client. Generalized swelling usually resolves in 3 to 6 months.

Any joint of the hand or foot can be replaced **(finger or metatarsal arthroplasties)**, often for clients with RA. Flexible, silicone prostheses are implanted without the use of polymethyl methacrylate because the devices are not ceramic or metal.

For the hand, a bulky dressing is used temporarily after surgery and is then replaced with a dynamic splint, brace, cast, or very small CPM machine. Edema formation is controlled if the client elevates the arm as much as possible. The rehabilitation program for finger arthroplasties may last for weeks, until normal function and strength return. These procedures are typically performed in specialized hand centers. Toe replacements typically require less rehabilitation.

Any bone of the wrist can also be replaced, including the heads of the radius and ulna. The postoperative pressure dressing is removed in 2 to 3 days, and a splint is applied. The client usually regains full function within 6 to 12 weeks, but lifting may be restricted for a longer period. Occupational therapists are usually involved with upper-extremity rehabilitation.

Because the ankles support about 25% of the body's weight and are complex joints, developing an implant that is both small enough and strong enough has been difficult. When a **total ankle arthroplasty (TAA)** is performed, an **arthrodesis** (bone fusion) is usually performed for added stability. Although TAAs have been problematic for more than three decades, newer noncemented prosthetic systems have renewed interest in ankle replacements. Ankle replacements have better client outcomes for clients with RA and OA than has arthrodesis alone.

Postoperative complications include infection, delayed wound healing, nerve injuries, and loosening. Therefore, TAA is not as successful as total hip or knee replacements. Noncemented prostheses seem to be preferred over cemented ones to prevent loosening. The client is allowed to begin weight bearing at about 6 weeks, and rehabilitation continues for about 3 months.

IMPAIRED PHYSICAL MOBILITY

NOC **PLANNING: EXPECTED OUTCOMES.** The client with osteoarthritis (OA) is expected to move purposefully in his or her own environment independently, with or without an assistive device. Indicators include that the client will have noncompromised:

- Balance and coordination
- Gait
- Joint movement
- Transfer performance
- Walking

INTERVENTIONS. Management of the client with OA is an interdisciplinary effort. Collaborate with physical (PT) and occupational therapists (OT) to meet the goal of independent function. Major interventions include therapeutic exercise and the promotion of ADLs and ambulation by teaching about health and the use of assistive devices.

Exercise. Two types of exercise are recommended for the client with OA: recreational and therapeutic. **Recreational exercise** includes hobbies and sports, with no planned purpose other than relaxation. **Therapeutic exercise** includes carefully planned activities that are designed to improve muscle strength, muscle tone, and joint range of motion. Therapeutic exercise can also reduce pain and improve the client's psychological health.

Certain recreational activities may also be therapeutic, such as doing the breaststroke during swimming to enhance chest and arm muscles. Aerobic exercises (e.g., walking, biking, swimming, aerobic dance) are recommended. Usually the PT prescribes exercises for the client with OA, but the nurse reinforces their techniques and principles. The ideal time for exercise is immediately after the application of heat. To prevent further joint damage, clients should rigorously follow the instructions for exercise outlined in Chart 24-5.

Use of Assistive Devices. The PT evaluates the client's need for ambulatory aids such as canes, walkers, or platform crutches. Although many clients do not like to use

CHART 24-5

CLIENT EDUCATION GUIDE

Exercises for Clients with Osteoarthritis or Rheumatoid Arthritis

- Follow the exercise instructions that have been prescribed specifically prescribed for you. There are no universal exercises; your exercises have been specifically tailored to your needs.
- Do your exercises on both "good" and "bad" days. Consistency is important.
- Respect pain. If pain increases as you exercise, stop and report this to your health care provider.
- Use active rather than active-assist or passive exercise whenever possible.
- Reduce the number of repetitions when the inflammation is severe and you have more pain.
- Do not substitute your normal activities or household tasks for the prescribed exercises.
- Avoid resistive exercises when your joints are severely inflamed.

these aids or may forget how to use them, they do help prevent further joint deterioration and pain. An OT evaluates the client's ability to perform ADLs and can provide ideas and devices for assistance.

Community-Based Care

The client with OA is not usually hospitalized for the disease itself but for surgical management. The cost of medical and surgical care for clients with OA has been evaluated (see the Resource Management box below).

HOME CARE MANAGEMENT

If weight-bearing joints are markedly involved, the client may have difficulty going up or down stairs. Making arrangements to live on one floor with accessibility to all rooms is often the best solution. A home care nurse, PT, or OT assesses the need for structural alterations to the home to accommodate ambulatory aids and enable the client to perform activities. For example, a kitchen counter may need to be lowered, or a seat and handrails may need to be installed in the shower. If the client has undergone a total hip replacement, an elevated toilet seat is necessary for several weeks postoperatively to prevent excessive hip flexion.

HEALTH TEACHING

Learning how to protect the joint is the most important feature of client education. Preventing further damage to joints slows the progression of OA and minimizes pain. Explain the general rules of joint protection and cite examples (Chart 24-6).

As with other diseases in which drugs and diet therapy are used, teach the medication protocol, desired and potential side effects, and toxic effects to the client and family. Emphasize the importance of reducing weight and eating a well-balanced diet to promote tissue healing.

Many clients with "arthritis" look for a cure after becoming frustrated and desperate about the course of the disease and treatment. Better control of arthritis is possible, but cure is not yet available. Unfortunately tabloids, books, and the media often cite "curative" remedies. People spend billions of dollars each year on quackery, including liniments, special diets, and copper bracelets. More hazardous substances, such as snake venom and industrial cleaners, are also advertised as remedies. Refer the client to the Arthritis Foundation for up-to-date information about new "cures." The practice of wearing a copper bracelet will not cure arthritis, but it will not hurt the client. If the client is doing something that can be potentially harmful, however, instruct the client to avoid that modality and provide the rationale.

With most types of arthritis and connective tissue disease (CTD), clients must live with a chronic, unpredictable, and painful disorder. Their roles, self-esteem, and body image may be affected by these diseases. Body image is often not as devastating in OA as in the inflammatory arthritic diseases, such as RA. The psychosocial component is discussed in more detail under Psychosocial Assessment (Rheumatoid Arthritis) on p. 395.

HEALTH CARE RESOURCES

The client who has undergone surgery is most likely to need help from community resources. After an arthroplasty, he or she needs extensive assistance with mobility. The client may be discharged to home, a long-term care facility, a transitional care unit, or a rehabilitation unit. Collaborate with the case manager and physician to find the best placement. If the client is discharged to home, home care nurses may be approved for several visits, depending on the concurrent systemic diseases. A nursing assistant may visit the home to help with hygiene-related needs, and a physical therapist may work with ambulatory and mobility skills. A client who has undergone a total hip or knee replacement should not be discharged to home alone. A family member, significant other, or other caregiver

RESOURCE MANAGEMENT

OSTEOARTHRITIS

Cost of Care

- The cost of medical care for older clients with osteoarthritis (OA) is about twice that of older clients with no symptomatic OA.
- The average individual cost of arthritis-related care for clients with rheumatoid arthritis (RA) is about $2200 per year. Medications account for almost two thirds of the cost, and hospital care accounts for 16%. By contrast, the average individual cost for clients with OA is about $550 per year. Medications account for about one third of the cost, and hospital care accounts for close to one half of the cost (most due to total joint arthroplasty).
- Although the individual cost of care for clients with OA is about one fourth of that for clients with RA, the total cost for OA is about seven times greater because the higher prevalence of OA.
- One half of the costs for OA is due to sick days from work: $15.5 billion in the United States.
- Clinical pathways for total hip replacement reduce the length of stay and hospital costs.

Implications for Nursing

Because of the high cost of medications for OA and RA, nurses need to become more familiar with the use of integrative therapies for pain management. Research has shown that some modalities are as effective as analgesics and others serve as excellent adjuncts for pain control. For clients undergoing total joint replacement, extensive staff and client education is needed to follow clinical pathways and ensure positive clinical and cost outcomes.

CHART 24-6

CLIENT EDUCATION GUIDE

Evidence-Based Instructions for Joint Protection

- Use large joints instead of small ones; for example, place your purse strap over your shoulder instead of grasping the purse with your hand.
- Do not turn a doorknob clockwise. Turn it counterclockwise to avoid twisting your arm and promoting ulnar deviation.
- Use two hands instead of one to hold objects.
- Sit in a chair that has a high, straight back.
- When getting out of bed, do not push off with your fingers; use the entire palm of both hands.
- Do not bend at your waist; instead, bend your knees while keeping your back straight.
- Use long-handled devices, such as a hairbrush with an extended handle.
- Use assistive/adaptive devices, such as Velcro closures and built-up utensil handles, to protect your joints.
- Do not use pillows in bed, except a small one under your head.
- Avoid twisting or wringing your hands.

must be in the home at all times for at least the first 4 to 6 weeks—when the client needs the most assistance.

Provide written instructions about the required care, regardless of whether the client goes home or to another inpatient facility. Communication with the new care provider is essential for seamless continuity of care. Arrangements are made for the client to return to the same acute care hospital if needed.

The Arthritis Foundation is an important community resource for all clients with arthritis and CTD. This organization provides information to lay people and health care professionals and refers clients and their families to other resources as needed. Local support groups can help clients and their families cope with these diseases.

Critical Thinking Challenge

Your older client is unable to obtain pain control for OA of the hip and knee and therefore undergoes a left cemented total hip replacement. She returns to the assisted living facility for rehabilitation following a 3-day hospital stay. She is able to ambulate with a walker in her room and wears thigh-high elastic stockings. Her discharge medication orders include Coumadin and Tylox for pain.

1. What teaching should you reinforce with her related to Coumadin?
2. What weight-bearing allowance will she most likely have?
3. What surgical complications is she still at risk for, and how can you help prevent them?

evolve For suggested answer guidelines, go to http://evolve.elsevier.com/Iggy/.

Evaluation: Outcomes

Evaluate the care of the client with OA on the basis of the identified nursing diagnoses. The expected outcomes are that the client:

- Takes personal actions to control pain
- Moves purposefully in his or her own environment independently with or without an assistive device

Specific indicators for these outcomes are listed for each nursing diagnosis under the Planning and Implementation section (see earlier).

RHEUMATOID ARTHRITIS

PATHOPHYSIOLOGY

Rheumatoid arthritis (RA) is one of the most common connective tissue diseases and is the most destructive to the joints. It is a chronic, progressive, systemic inflammatory autoimmune disease process that primarily affects the synovial joints. **Systemic** means this disease affects the body system, affecting many joints and other tissues.

In RA, autoantibodies (rheumatoid factors [RFs]) are formed that attack healthy tissue, especially synovium, causing inflammation. RFs consist mainly of immunoglobulin M and G, and they bind with antigens forming immune complexes. Phagocytes attempt to engulf these complexes and, as a result, release powerful enzymes, such as cytokines. The B- and T-lymphocytes of the immune system are also stimulated and increase the inflammatory response.

Inflammation occurs first in the synovial membrane, which lines the joint cavity. It then begins to involve the articular cartilage, joint capsule, and surrounding ligaments and tendons. Three processes cause cartilage damage in clients with RA (McCance & Huether, 2002):

1. Neutrophils and other cells in synovial fluid are activated and break down the joint cartilage
2. Cytokines, especially interleukin-1 (IL-1) and tumor necrosis factor–alpha (TNFA), cause chondrocytes to attack cartilage. TNF has effects on lipid metabolism, coagulation, insulin resistance, and endothelial function.
3. Synovium digests cartilage, releasing inflammatory substances, such as IL-1 and TNFA. (See Chapter 23 for a complete discussion of the inflammatory response.)

The synovium then thickens and becomes hyperemic, fluid accumulates in the joint space, and a pannus forms. The **pannus** is vascular granulation tissue composed of inflammatory cells; it erodes articular cartilage and eventually destroys bone. As a result, fibrous adhesions, bony ankylosis, and calcifications occur; bone loses density and secondary osteoporosis occurs.

Permanent joint changes can be avoided if RA is diagnosed early. Early, aggressive treatment to suppress synovitis may cause a remission. RA is a disease characterized by natural remissions and exacerbations. Medical treatment helps control the disease to decrease the intensity and number of exacerbations. Preventing RA flares helps prevent joint erosion and permanent joint damage. Advancement of knowledge regarding the disease process and immune system provides many newer treatment options that better control this disease.

Rheumatoid arthritis is a systemic disease; that is, areas of the body besides the synovial joints can be affected. Inflammatory responses similar to those occurring in synovial tissue may be seen in any organ or body system in which connective tissue is prevalent. If blood vessel involvement **(vasculitis)** occurs, the organ supplied by that vessel can be affected. The result is malfunction and eventual failure of the organ or system. These pathologic changes may occur late in the disease process and cause life-threatening problems.

The etiology of RA remains unclear, but research suggests a combination of environmental and genetic factors.

Genetic Considerations

Rheumatoid arthritis shows some familial clustering, suggesting either a genetic predisposition or gene-environment interaction. Gene mutations are associated with RA, especially if they are present in a person with varieties of the tissue type human leukocyte antigen (HLA)-DRB, HLA-DR4, or HLA-DP (McCance & Huether, 2002). For example, the risk for developing the disease in a person with HLA-DRB tissue type who is homozygous for mutations in any one of three susceptibility genes is 30% to 40% for men and 45% to 55% for women (Online Mendelian Inheritance in Man, 2004).

Some researchers suspect that female reproductive hormones influence the development of RA because it affects women more often than men—usually young- to middle-aged women. Others suspect that infectious organisms may play a role, particularly the Epstein-Barr virus (McCance & Huether, 2002). Physical and emotional stresses have been linked to exacerbations of the disorder and may be contributing factors in its development.

CULTURAL CONSIDERATIONS

Despite the common lay belief that warm, dry climates can be beneficial to people with RA, there are no significant differences in its prevalence among geographic locations. The incidence of RA in China is somewhat lower than elsewhere in the world (about 0.3%) and substantially higher among the Pima Indians in North America (about 5%) (Harris, 2001). The cause for these differences is not known.

COLLABORATIVE MANAGEMENT

Assessment

The onset of rheumatoid arthritis (RA) may be acute and severe or slow and insidious; clients may have vague complaints that last for several months before diagnosis. The onset of the disease is more common in the winter months than in the warmer months. The manifestations of RA can be categorized as early or late disease and as articular (joint) or extra-articular (Chart 24-7).

PHYSICAL ASSESSMENT/CLINICAL MANIFESTATIONS

EARLY DISEASE MANIFESTATIONS. The client with RA typically complains of joint stiffness, swelling, pain, fatigue, and may complain of generalized weakness and morning stiffness. Anorexia and a weight loss of about 2 or 3 pounds (1 kg) may occur early in the disease process. Persistent low-grade fever may accompany these complaints. In clients with early disease, the upper-extremity joints are often involved initially, typically the proximal interphalangeal (PIP) and metacarpophalangeal (MCP) joints of the hands. These joints may be slightly reddened, warm, stiff, swollen, and tender or painful, particularly on palpation **(synovitis).** The typical pattern of joint involvement in RA is bilateral and symmetric (e.g., both wrists), and the number of joints involved usually increases as the disease progresses. In early disease, the client may complain of migrating symptoms known as **migratory arthritis.** The presence of only *one* hot, swollen, painful joint (out of proportion to the other joints) may mean the joint is infected. Refer the client to the health care provider (generally the rheumatologist) immediately. Single hot, swollen joints are considered infected until proven otherwise and require immediate long-term antibiotic treatment.

LATE DISEASE MANIFESTATIONS. As the disease worsens, the joints become progressively inflamed and quite painful. The client complains of morning stiffness (also called the **gel phenomenon**), which lasts between 45 minutes and several hours after awakening. On palpation, the joints feel soft and look puffy because of synovitis and **effusions** (joint swelling with fluid, especially the knees). The fingers often appear spindle-like. Note any muscle atrophy (which can result from disuse secondary to joint pain) and a decreased range of motion in the affected joints.

Most or all synovial joints are eventually affected. The temporomandibular joint (TMJ) may be involved in severe disease, but such involvement is uncommon. When the TMJ is affected, the client typically complains of pain when chewing or opening the mouth.

When the spinal column is involved, the cervical joints are most likely to be affected. During clinical examination, gently palpate the posterior cervical spine and identify it as cervical pain, tenderness, or loss of motion. Cervical disease may result in subluxation, especially with the first and second vertebrae. This complication may be life threatening because branches of the phrenic nerve that supply the diaphragm can be compressed, and respiratory function may be subsequently compromised. The client is also in danger of becoming quadriparetic or quadriplegic. If you identify cervical pain or loss of range of motion in the cervical spine of a person with RA, report this information to the client's physician, generally the rheumatologist. Collaboration of such information will assist the physician or other provider to obtain the necessary cervical spine x-ray and may save that client's life. Surgical stabilization is sometimes necessary.

JOINT INVOLVEMENT. Joint deformity occurs as a late, articular manifestation, and secondary osteoporosis can cause bone fractures. Observe common deformities, especially in the hands and feet (Figure 24-4). Extensive wrist involvement can result in carpal tunnel syndrome (see Chapter 54 for assessment and management of carpal tunnel syndrome).

Palpate the tissues around the joints to elicit pain or tenderness associated with other rheumatoid complications. For example, **Baker's cysts** (enlarged popliteal bursae) may occur and cause tissue compression and pain. Tendon rupture is also possible, particularly rupture of the Achilles tendon.

SYSTEMIC COMPLICATIONS. Numerous extra-articular clinical manifestations are associated with advanced disease. Assess other body systems to ascertain systemic involvement. In addition to increased joint swelling and tenderness, moderate to severe weight loss, fever, and extreme fatigue are common in late disease **exacerbations,** often called "flares." Approximately 25% of clients have the

CHART 24-7

KEY FEATURES of
The Client with Rheumatoid Arthritis

Early Manifestations

Joint
- Inflammation

Systemic
- Low-grade fever
- Fatigue
- Weakness
- Anorexia
- Paresthesias

Late Manifestations

Joint
- Deformities (e.g., swan neck or ulnar deviation)
- Moderate to severe pain and morning stiffness

Systemic
- Osteoporosis
- Severe fatigue
- Anemia
- Weight loss
- Subcutaneous nodules
- Peripheral neuropathy
- Vasculitis
- Pericarditis
- Fibrotic lung disease
- Sjögren's syndrome
- Renal disease

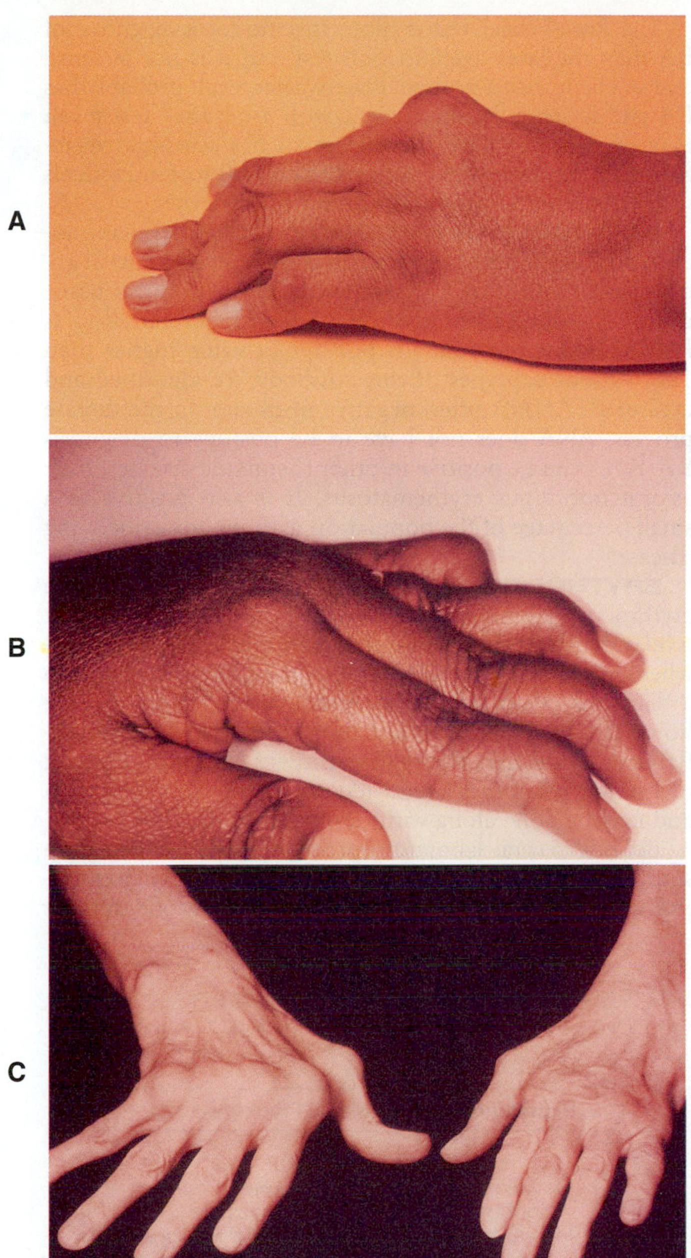

Figure 24-4 ■ Common joint deformities seen in rheumatoid arthritis. **A,** Boutonniere, or buttonhole. **B,** Swan neck. **C,** Ulnar deviation *(on left).* (From the Arthritis Teaching Slide Collection, copyright 1980. Used by permission of the Arthritis Foundation.)

characteristic round, movable, nontender **subcutaneous nodules,** which most often appear on the ulnar surface of the arm, on the fingers, or along the Achilles tendon. These nodules can disappear and reappear at any time and are associated with severe, destructive disease. Rheumatoid nodules are not generally a problem themselves; however, they occasionally open and become infected, and they may interfere with activities of daily living (ADLs). Bumping nodules may cause discomfort or pain. Occasionally nodules are identified within the lungs.

Inflammation of the blood vessels results in vasculitis, particularly of small- to medium-sized vessels. When arterial involvement occurs, major organs and body systems become ischemic and malfunction. Ischemic skin lesions appear in groups as small, brownish spots, most commonly around the nail bed **(periungual lesions).** Monitor the number of lesions, note their location each day, and report vascular changes to the health care provider. An increased number of lesions indicates increased vasculitis, and a decreased number indicates decreased vasculitis. Also carefully assess any larger lesions that appear on the lower extremities; such lesions often lead to ulceration, which heal slowly as a result of decreased circulation. Peripheral neuropathy associated with decreased circulation can cause foot drop and paresthesias (burning and tingling sensations), most often in older adults.

Respiratory complications manifest as pleurisy, pneumonitis, diffuse interstitial fibrosis, and pulmonary hypertension. Cardiac complications include pericarditis and myocarditis. Assess for ocular involvement, which typically manifests as iritis and scleritis. If either of these complications is present, the sclera of one or both eyes is reddened and the pupils have an irregular shape.

ASSOCIATED SYNDROMES. Several syndromes are seen in clients with advanced RA. The most common is **Sjögren's syndrome,** which includes a triad of the following:

- Dry eyes (keratoconjunctivitis sicca [KCS], or the sicca syndrome)
- Dry mouth **(xerostomia)**
- Dry vagina (in some cases)

In Sjögren's syndrome, immune complexes and inflammatory cells are thought to obstruct secretory glands and ducts. The syndrome is usually associated with connective tissue diseases such as RA but may occur alone. Note the client's complaint of dry mouth or dry eyes. Some clients state that their eyes feel "gritty," as if sand is in their eyes. Inspect the mouth for dry, sticky membranes and the eyes for redness and lack of tearing.

Less commonly observed is **Felty's syndrome,** which is characterized by RA, hepatosplenomegaly (enlarged liver and spleen), and leukopenia. **Caplan's syndrome** is characterized by the presence of rheumatoid nodules in the lungs and pneumoconiosis, which is noted primarily in coal miners and asbestos workers. The health care provider diagnoses these syndromes by physical examination and diagnostic testing.

PSYCHOSOCIAL ASSESSMENT

Rheumatoid arthritis (RA) and other inflammatory types of arthritis are chronic diseases that can be crippling if not well controlled. Fear of becoming disabled and dependent, uncertainty about the disease process, altered body image, devaluation of self, frustration, and depression are common psychosocial problems (Smedstad & Liang, 2001). Physical limitations caused by disease may limit activities of daily living (ADLs). These physical limitations result in role changes in the family and society. For example, the person may not be able to cook for the family or be an active sexual partner. In addition, extreme fatigue often causes clients to desire an early bedtime and may result in a reluctance to socialize.

Body changes may also cause poor self-esteem and body image. Because many societies value people with physically fit, attractive bodies, the client with RA may be embarrassed to be seen in public places. The client may grieve or experience degrees of depression. The potential exists for the client to experience a feeling of helplessness accompanied by a loss of control over a disease that can "consume" the body. Fortunately, newer medications have significantly improved the treatment of RA and provide the client with hope and better control of the disease.

Living with a chronic disease and the pain that results may be difficult for the client, family, and significant others. The client may experience a loss of control and independence, especially if he or she is over 65 years of age (Ignatavicius, 2001). Chronic suffering affects quality of life. Assess the client's emotional and mental status in relation to the disease and its problems and evaluate the client's support systems and resources. Help each client gain control of his or her disease. Clients who are knowledgeable about their disease and treatment options will feel emotionally stronger to cope with their disease and better able to discuss treatment options with their physician.

LABORATORY ASSESSMENT

Laboratory tests help to support a diagnosis of RA, but no single test or group of tests can confirm it. Chart 24-8 summarizes the common laboratory tests that the health care provider uses for diagnosing connective tissue diseases.

RHEUMATOID FACTOR. The test for **rheumatoid factor (RF)** measures the presence of unusual antibodies of the immunoglobulin G (IgG) and IgM type that develop in a number of connective tissue diseases. Two methods may be used to ascertain the degree to which these antibodies are present in the body: Rose-Waaler and latex agglutination. In both procedures, values are reported as titers.

The Rose-Waaler test is more specific for a diagnosis of RA than the latex agglutination test, but it is not as sensitive. A client with a positive Rose-Waaler result probably has RA and is seropositive; a client with a negative test result may or may not have the disease or has seronegative inflammatory polyarthritis. Approximately 60% of individuals with RA are seropositive and have a positive titer.

ANTINUCLEAR ANTIBODY TITER. The antinuclear antibody (ANA) test measures the titer of unusual antibodies that destroy the nuclei of cells and cause tissue death. The fluorescent method is sometimes referred to as FANA. If this test result is positive (a value higher than 1:8), various subtypes of this antibody are identified and measured. ANA is often negative until later in the disease process. ANA does not have to be positive to diagnosis RA. ANA can be positive in other rheumatic diseases, such as systemic lupus erythematosus. It is also positive in a small percentage of the population without any underlying disease.

ERYTHROCYTE SEDIMENTATION RATE. The erythrocyte sedimentation rate (ESR) or "sed rate," when it is elevated, can confirm inflammation or infection anywhere in the body. An elevation in the ESR helps point to a diagnosis of an inflammatory connective tissue disease; however, a high ESR does not always relate to severity of inflammatory disease. The high-sensitivity C-reactive protein, or hsCRP, is another useful test to measure inflammation and may be done along with or instead of the ESR.

Because several laboratory procedures are used to measure ESR, normal values will vary; women have higher normal values than men. In general, a value of 20 to 40 mm/hr

CHART 24-8

LABORATORY PROFILE
Connective Tissue Disease

Test	Normal Range for Adults	Significance of Abnormal Findings
Rheumatoid factor		
Rose-Waaler	Negative	Elevations of either titer (increase in number at right of colon) indicative of possible CTD Increased Rose's titer indicative of RA (seropositive); not a sensitive test
Latex agglutination	<1:16	Latex titer not as specific to one disease, but quite a sensitive test
ANA (total)	Negative (if positive, types of ANA identified [e.g., anti-DNA, anti-DNP, anti-RNA] to indicate what part of cells are involved)	Elevations common in SLE, PSS, RA, and other inflammatory CTDs (5% of healthy adults have positive ANA results)
Serum complement (C′ or CH_{50})	Varies greatly among laboratories	Decreased value indicative of active autoimmune disease such as SLE
LE preparation	Negative	A type of ANA (anti-DNP); not reliable because negative result does not rule out SLE; can be used as screening test
SPEP		
Albumin	3.5-5.0 g/dL	Increased levels of gamma globulins indicative of CTD (inflammatory type)
Globulin		
$Alpha_1$ globulin	0.1-0.3 g/dL	Increased level of alpha globulins possible in RA
$Alpha_2$ globulin	0.6-1.0 g/dL	
Beta globulin	0.7-1.1 g/dL	
Gamma globulin	0.8-1.6 g/dL	
HLA testing (HLA-B27)	None	Presence of HLA-B27 indicative of Reiter's syndrome or ankylosing spondylitis

ANA, Antinuclear antibody; *CTD,* connective tissue disease; *DNP,* dinitrophenol; *ESR,* erythrocyte sedimentation rate; *HLA,* human leukocyte antigen; *LE,* lupus erythematosus; *PSS,* progressive systemic sclerosis; *RA,* rheumatoid arthritis; *SLE,* systemic lupus erythematosus; *SPEP,* serum protein electrophoresis.

indicates mild inflammation; 40 to 70 mm/hr, moderate inflammation; and 70 to 150 mm/hr, severe inflammation.

The ESR is not always a reliable indicator but may sometimes be used to monitor a client's response to anti-inflammatory drug therapy. This value should decrease if the drug dosage is effective. The ESR may also be elevated with infection and in older adults.

OTHER LABORATORY TESTS. **Serum complement** attaches to immune complexes in an attempt to destroy them. If a large amount of complement is used in this lytic process, the concentration of free-floating complement in the blood diminishes. Normal values vary considerably, depending on the laboratory technique used. An abnormal finding is indicated by a decrease in serum complement and is seen primarily in clients with vasculitis.

In **serum protein electrophoresis,** the protein fractions of the plasma are measured, and an electrical current is used to separate them. The level of alpha globulin is raised in acute inflammation; in chronic inflammatory conditions such as RA, the level of gamma globulin is increased because of the increase in immunoglobulins.

The **serum immunoglobulins** can be separated into subtypes. In chronic inflammation, IgG is needed to combine with RF. Thus in RA the IgG value is typically elevated.

The presence of most chronic diseases usually causes mild to moderate anemia, which contributes to the client's fatigue. Therefore the client's complete blood count (CBC) is monitored for a low hemoglobin, hematocrit, and red blood cell (RBC) count. An increase in white blood cell (WBC) count is consistent with an inflammatory response. A decrease in the WBC count may indicate Felty's syndrome. Thrombocytosis (increased platelets) is common in clients with RA. Additional laboratory tests may be performed depending on the body systems and organs that may be affected by the disease. For example, if heart involvement is suspected, the health care provider may order cardiac enzymes.

OTHER DIAGNOSTIC ASSESSMENTS

A standard x-ray is used to visualize the joint changes and deformities typical of RA. A computed tomography (CT) scan may help to determine the presence and degree of cervical spine involvement.

An **arthrocentesis** is a diagnostic procedure that may be used for clients with joint involvement. It may be performed at the bedside or in a physician's office or clinic. After administering a local anesthetic, the physician inserts a large-gauge needle into the joint (usually the knee) to aspirate a sample of synovial fluid; this procedure may also relieve pressure. The fluid is analyzed for inflammatory cells and immune complexes, including RF. Fluid from clients with RA shows increased WBCs, turbidity, and volume. After the procedure, monitor the insertion site for bleeding or leakage of synovial fluid. Notify the physician if either of these problems occurs. Teach the client to use ice and rest the affected joint for 24 hours. Often the health care provider will recommend acetaminophen as needed for pain. If increased pain or swelling occurs, have the client notify the health care provider.

A bone scan or joint scan can also assess the extent of joint involvement. Magnetic resonance imaging (MRI) may be performed to assess spinal column disease.

Because RA can affect multiple body systems, tests to diagnose specific systemic manifestations are performed as necessary. For example, electromyography helps to confirm peripheral neuropathy. Pulmonary function tests help to determine the presence of lung involvement.

◆Interventions

As in other types of arthritis, the health care team manages pain by using a combination of pharmacologic and nonpharmacologic measures. Total joint arthroplasty may be indicated when these measures are no longer effective (see earlier discussion of this surgery in the section on Osteoarthritis, p. 385). The Plan of Care on pp. 398 to 402 highlights the most important interdisciplinary interventions for the client with rheumatoid arthritis (RA).

Drug Therapy. Some medications prescribed for RA have analgesic, antipyretic, and anti-inflammatory actions. Other drugs are immunosuppressive and disease modifying, which may cause remission of the illness and prevent erosive joint changes. Biological response modifiers are the newest class of disease-modifying drugs that help reduce signals for the immune system to cause inflammation and thereby reduce the amount of inflammation that the joint receives (see Chart 24-9 on pp. 403-404). These medications have demonstrated superior performance, giving clients additional benefits never before imagined. Clients with inflammatory diseases other than RA are also using various biological response modifying medications successfully. Future genetic research will further advance these medications to give even better control of autoimmune diseases. Although RA is a chronic disease and no cure is yet available, medications now used are better able to control the disease and prevent further deterioration.

Management of Mild Disease. The health care provider, usually a rheumatologist, makes decisions about appropriate drug therapy for clients with rheumatoid disease based on the severity of the disease. Mild disease is usually managed with nonsteroidal anti-inflammatory drugs (NSAIDs) or disease-modifying agents.

Nonsteroidal Anti-Inflammatory Drugs. The NSAIDs are often an initial drug category of choice for inflammatory arthritis to relieve pain and inflammation (see Chart 24-9). The choice of which one to administer depends on the client's needs and the physician's preference. To minimize gastrointestinal (GI) problems, the NSAID may be given with an H2-blocking agent, such as ranitidine (Zantac) or misoprostol (Cytotec). If there is no clinical change after 6 to 8 weeks, the health care provider may discontinue the current NSAID and try another one. This process may be repeated until an effective drug is found for that client. Celecoxib (Celebrex), and valdecoxib (Bextra) are COX-2 inhibiting NSAIDs that are usually preferred over older NSAIDs. COX-2 inhibitors have a decreased incidence of GI side effects associated with older NSAIDs (for further information, see Analgesic Administration [Osteoarthritis], p. 384). However, all COX-2 inhibiting drugs have recently been associated with cardiovascular disease, such as myocardial infarction, and may soon be unavailable on the market.

Salicylates are an older type of NSAID and were previously the drug of choice for pain and inflammation. Within the United States, they are no longer the drug of choice to treat RA because of toxicities, mainly GI bleeding. Salicylates are excellent anti-inflammatory drugs and relatively inexpensive, and therefore they are still used

Text continued on p. 404.

PLAN of CARE MEDICAL DIAGNOSIS: RHEUMATOID ARTHRITIS

NURSING DIAGNOSIS NO. 1 ■ Impaired Physical Mobility

	Expected Outcomes	Nursing Interventions	Rationales
RELATED FACTORS Discomfort Pain Musculoskeletal impairment Intolerance to activity **DEFINING CHARACTERISTICS** Limited ability to perform gross motor skills Limited ability to perform fine motor skills Limited range of motion Difficulty turning	Has full or improved range of motion in all joints Able to turn without assistance Has stable posture during performance of activities of daily living Able to perform fine motor skills Able to perform gross motor skills	NIC **Exercise Therapy: Joint Mobility**	
		Collaborate with physical therapy in developing and executing an exercise program.	Physical therapists are the primary health care professionals responsible for developing and executing an exercise program.
		Initiate pain control measures before beginning joint exercise.	Initiating pain control measures before joint exercise increases the likelihood of client comfort and willingness to engage in the exercise.
		D Dress the client in nonrestrictive clothing.	Nonrestrictive clothing permits full range of joint motion.
		D Protect the client from trauma during exercise.	Stretching exercises may cause the client to be off balance.
		D Assist the client to an optimal body position for passive/active joint movement.	Neutral alignment is optimal positioning for joint movement.
		D Encourage active range-of-motion exercises, according to regular, planned schedule.	Regular active range-of-motion exercise periods maximize the exercise benefit to joints.
		Assist the client to develop a schedule for active range-of-motion exercises.	Regular exercise maximizes the benefit of the exercise.
		D Encourage ambulation, if appropriate.	Ambulation is a form of active joint exercise and also improves cardiovascular tone.
		NIC **Positioning**	
		Provide a firm mattress.	A firm mattress offers support.
		D Encourage the client to get involved in positioning changes, as appropriate.	Involving the client in positioning changes actively exercises the muscles and joints and permits him or her a measure of control in the positioning process.
		Premedicate the client before turning, as appropriate.	Premedicating the client before turning will increase comfort and decrease resistance to repositioning from fear of pain.
		D Position in proper body alignment.	Proper body alignment preserves the functionality of the muscles and bony skeleton.
		Immobilize or support the affected body part, as appropriate.	Immobilization or support of the affected body part will permit healing and decrease further injury.
		D Elevate the affected body part, as appropriate.	Elevation of the affected body part may decrease edema by using gravity to assist with fluid drainage.
		D Avoid placing the client in a position that increases pain.	Repositioning should provide the client with a measure of comfort. Pain may indicate improper body positioning.

D Indicates tasks that can be delegated to unlicensed assistive personnel at the discretion of the nurse.

PLAN of CARE MEDICAL DIAGNOSIS: RHEUMATOID ARTHRITIS—*cont'd*

NURSING DIAGNOSIS NO. 1 ■ Impaired Physical Mobility—*cont'd*

	Expected Outcomes	Nursing Interventions	Rationales
		D Minimize friction and shearing forces when positioning and turning the client.	Friction and shearing forces will cause damage to the skin and underlying tissues.
		Develop a written schedule for repositioning, as appropriate.	A written schedule for repositioning permits all health care workers to participate in repositioning.
		D Use a hand roll or a trochanter roll, as appropriate.	Hand rolls and trochanter rolls are devices to support limbs.
		D Place frequently used objects within reach.	Placing frequently used objects within reach permits the client safe, convenient access.
		D Place the bed-positioning switch within easy reach.	Placing the bed-positioning switch within easy reach permits the client to change position safely and conveniently.
		Other Interventions Instruct in the use of assistive devices.	The client will need instruction in the proper use of canes, crutches, walkers, splints, or other assistive devices.
		Continuing Care Considerations Refer the client to rehabilitative services, as appropriate.	Ongoing support from physical therapists, occupational therapists, and others may be needed to help the client resume activities of daily living.
		Refer the client to a vocational counselor, as appropriate.	Long-term physical impairment may require the client to change employment.
		Collaborate with community organizations to inform the public about injury prevention.	Injury prevention saves the individual and society as a whole an enormous economic burden.

NURSING DIAGNOSIS NO. 2 ■ Chronic Pain

	Expected Outcomes	Nursing Interventions	Rationales
RELATED FACTORS Chronic physical/psychological disability **DEFINING CHARACTERISTICS** Atrophy of involved muscle group Sleep patterns: Change in Fatigue Reduced interaction with people Altered ability to continue previous activities Protective gestures Irritability Self-focus Depression	Denies fatigue Weight remains within ±5 pounds of desired weight No verbal report or observation of alteration in sleep patterns No verbal report or observation of alteration in activity level No verbal report or observation of guarding or protective gestures No verbal report or observation of restlessness No verbal report or observation of irritability	**NIC Pain Management** Perform a comprehensive assessment of pain to include location, characteristics, onset/duration, frequency, quality, intensity or severity of pain, and precipitating factors.	A plan for pain management must be based on the client's unique responses to pain.
		Reduce or eliminate factors that precipitate or increase the pain experience.	Preventing a pain experience is preferred to trying to control or eliminate pain.
		Select and implement a variety of measures to facilitate pain relief, as appropriate.	Pharmacologic, nonpharmacologic, and interpersonal strategies may provide pain relief depending on the client's unique responses to the therapeutic interventions.

Continued

PLAN of CARE MEDICAL DIAGNOSIS: RHEUMATOID ARTHRITIS—*cont'd*

NURSING DIAGNOSIS NO. 2 ■ Chronic Pain—*cont'd*

Expected Outcomes	Nursing Interventions	Rationales
No verbal report or observation of self-focusing behavior	Encourage the client to monitor his or her own pain and to intervene appropriately.	The client is the best person to manage his or her own pain.
No verbal report or observation of depression No verbal report or observation of impaired socialization	Use pain control measures before pain becomes severe.	Medicating the client in a timely manner prevents pain from reaching acutely unpleasant levels.
Denies experiencing pain greater than a 5 on a 0 to 10 pain scale	Teach the use of nonpharmacologic techniques before, after and, if possible, during painful activities; before pain occurs or increases; and along with other pain relief measures.	Nonpharmacologic techniques help the client establish a sense of control over his or her pain experience.
	NIC **Analgesic Administration**	
	Administer analgesics around-the-clock.	Administration around-the-clock prevents peaks and troughs of analgesia, especially with severe pain.
	Evaluate the effectiveness of analgesics at regular frequent intervals after each administration, but especially after the initial dose; also observe for any signs and symptoms of untoward effects.	Frequent evaluation of analgesic effectiveness permits the nurse to adjust the dose and timing interval to the client's need and provides an early warning of adverse responses.
	Implement actions to decrease the untoward effects of analgesics.	Actions taken to prevent predictable but unwanted effects of narcotic analgesics (e.g., constipation) increase client comfort.
	NIC **Progressive Muscle Relaxation**	
	Have the patient tense, for 5 to 10 seconds, each of 8 to 16 major muscle groups.	Tensing the foot muscles for no longer than 5 seconds helps avoid cramping.
	Terminate the session gradually.	Gradual termination maintains the sense of well-being and relaxation.
	Instruct the client to wear comfortable, nonrestrictive clothing.	The client's personal comfort will facilitate relaxation.
	Instruct the client to breathe deeply and to slowly release the breath and tension.	Proper breathing will help the client focus on relaxation rather than external stimuli.
	Instruct the client to focus on the sensations in the muscles both while they are relaxed and while they are tense.	Focusing on the muscle sensations will help build memory that can be called on at later times for relaxation.
	Other Interventions	
	Consider the use of hypnosis, biofeedback, magnetic field therapy, and/or acupuncture to aid in the control of chronic pain.	Cognitive and behavioral strategies may serve as adjuncts to or replacements for pharmacologic or surgical interventions for chronic pain. Each therapy has differing modes of action that may or may not benefit the patient.

D Indicates tasks that can be delegated to unlicensed assistive personnel at the discretion of the nurse.

PLAN of CARE MEDICAL DIAGNOSIS: RHEUMATOID ARTHRITIS—*cont'd*

NURSING DIAGNOSIS NO. 2 ■ Chronic Pain—*cont'd*

	Expected Outcomes	Nursing Interventions	Rationales
		Consider the use of herbals (e.g., ginseng, St. John's wort) after consultation with the client's physician and pharmacist.	Herbals may provide relief from symptoms that often accompany pain, such as fatigue and depression.
		Refer the client to the Pain Advisory Committee.	The Pain Advisory Committee is a multidisciplinary committee with wide expertise in pain relief interventions.
		Continuing Care Considerations	
		Refer the client to an advanced practice nurse pain specialist, social worker, home care nurse, and/or psychologist, as appropriate.	Health team members are able to provide continuing support for the client facing chronic pain.
		Collaborate with health team members to secure a referral to a pain management clinic.	Pain management clinics combine many health care disciplines to focus on the management of chronic pain. The client's individual needs and responses to pain are evaluated, and a unique pain management program is initialed and adjusted.

NURSING DIAGNOSIS NO. 3 ■ Fatigue

	Expected Outcomes	Nursing Interventions	Rationales
RELATED FACTORS Stress Anxiety Depression Disease states: Rheumatoid arthritis **DEFINING CHARACTERISTICS** Energy: Lack of Inability to maintain usual level of physical activity Rest requirements: Increased Inability to maintain usual routines Concentration: Compromised Perceived need for additional energy to accomplish routine tasks Decreased performance Feelings of guilt for not keeping up with responsibilities	No verbal report or observation of being lethargic or listless Denies feeling tired No verbal report or observation of lack of energy Able to maintain usual routines	NIC **Energy Management** Monitor the client for evidence of excess physical and emotional fatigue.	Extended periods of inactivity may place the client at risk for excessive fatigue when carrying out desired activities.
		Monitor nutritional intake.	Ensure that the client has adequate energy resources.
		Arrange physical activities (e.g., avoid activity immediately after meals).	Such an arrangement reduces competition for oxygen supply to vital body functions.
		Encourage alternate rest and activity periods.	This avoids extended periods of either activity or exercise.
		Assist the client to schedule rest periods and avoid care activities during scheduled rest periods.	Rest periods should help restore the client's energy levels.
		D Use passive and/or active range-of-motion exercises.	Exercise relieves muscle tension, and stretching helps diminish muscle spasm.
		Encourage physical activity (e.g., ambulation or performance of activities of daily living, consistent with client's energy resources).	Physical exercise helps build muscle mass and endurance.

Continued

PLAN of CARE MEDICAL DIAGNOSIS: RHEUMATOID ARTHRITIS—*cont'd*

NURSING DIAGNOSIS NO. 3 ■ Fatigue—*cont'd*

	Expected Outcomes	Nursing Interventions	Rationales
		Teach activity organization and time management techniques (e.g., assigning priority to activities to accommodate energy levels, establishing realistic activity goals).	Activity organization and time management techniques are used to prevent fatigue.
		Continuing Care Considerations	
		Avoid overexertion, stress, extremes of temperature, and people with upper respiratory tract infection.	Stressors exacerbate fatigue.

NURSING DIAGNOSIS NO. 4 ■ Disturbed Body Image

	Expected Outcomes	Nursing Interventions	Rationales
RELATED FACTORS Biophysical Psychosocial Illness Illness treatment **DEFINING CHARACTERISTICS** Verbal report of feelings that reflect an altered view of one's body in appearance, structure, or function Nonverbal response to actual or perceived change in body structure and/or function Actual change in structure and/or function Change in social involvement Not looking at body part Preoccupation with change or loss Verbal report: Negative feelings about body (e.g., feelings of helplessness, hopelessness, or powerlessness)	Views, monitors, and acknowledges body Acknowledges loss of significant objects Does not verbalize self-negating statements Denies alteration in relationship with significant other	NIC **Body Image Enhancement** Assist the client to discuss changes caused by illness or surgery, as appropriate.	The client who experiences changes caused by illness or surgery may be reluctant to verbalize his or her feelings.
		Assist the client to separate physical appearance from feelings of personal worth, as appropriate.	The client's feeling of personal worth may be strongly tied to physical appearance so that negative changes in appearance trigger feelings of low self-worth.
		Determine the client's and family's perceptions of the alteration in body image versus reality.	The client's and family's perceptions of the alteration in body image may vary significantly from the reality of the change.
		Determine if a change in body image has contributed to increased social isolation.	A client who experiences a negative change in body image may withdraw from social contact.
		Identify means of reducing the impact of any disfigurement.	The use of clothing, wigs, or cosmetics may reduce the impact of any disfigurement.
		Assist the client to identify actions that will enhance appearance.	Assisting the client to enhance his or her appearance will improve his or her self-concept.
		Other Interventions Provide an atmosphere of caring and acceptance.	A client with traumatic changes in body parts or functioning may be especially sensitive to cues that indicate an aversive reaction.
		Continuing Care Considerations Refer the client to restorative specialists, as appropriate.	Restorative specialists have expertise in body enhancement and techniques to maximize appearance to improve self-concept.
		Refer the client to a support group of others who have experienced the same loss.	The client may receive useful information and support from others who are experiencing the same circumstances.

CHART 24-9

DRUG THERAPY for Arthritis and Connective Tissue Disease*

Drug	Usual Dosage	Nursing Interventions	Rationales
NSAIDs	Dosage varies depending on which drug is being used.	Observe for fluid retention, increased blood pressure, and changes in renal function.	Most NSAIDs cause sodium retention, which can lead to edema, hypertension, renal damage, and congestive heart failure. Drugs should be used with caution in older adults.
		Monitor electrolyte and complete blood count values.	Most NSAIDs cause increased sodium levels and can cause bone marrow suppression.
		Observe for CNS changes (e.g., dizziness or confusion).	Most NSAIDs can cause CNS effects, especially in older adults.
Hydroxychloroquine sulfate (Plaquenil)	Dosage is 200 mg PO daily.	Instruct client to have frequent (every 6-12 mo) ophthalmologic examination.	Drug can cause retinal damage.
Immunosuppressive agents, e.g., azathioprine (Imuran), cyclophosphamide (Cytoxan, Procytox✱), methotrexate (Rheumatrex) (most commonly used)	Dosage varies depending on disease activity and route of drug administration.	Monitor for side effects and toxic effects, including but not limited to nausea/vomiting, bone marrow suppression, alopecia, and increased liver enzymes.	The side effects and toxic effects of these drugs can be devastating.
		Instruct client to avoid crowds and people with infections such as influenza. If ill, seek medical attention.	Bone marrow suppression or immune suppression increases the risk of infection.
Prednisone (Deltasone, Apo-Prednisone✱)	Dosage is 10-150 mg PO daily. For maintenance, attempt to give dose every other day (to allow client's adrenal glands to function).	Observe for cushiongoid changes, such as moon-face, buffalo hump, striae, acne, thin skin, bruising, fluid retention, and increased blood pressure.	These changes are expected and tend to be dose related. Changes diminish as dose decreases.
		Monitor electrolyte and glucose levels. Monitor weight.	Chronic steroid therapy can cause sodium or fluid retention, potassium depletion, and elevated glucose level.
		Observe for long-term effects of chronic steroid therapy, such as osteoporosis, cataracts, hypertension, diabetes, and impaired healing.	These complications may need to be treated with other drugs or modalities.
		Teach client to increase dietary calcium and vitamin D and to take a supplement.	
		Instruct client to avoid crowds and individuals with infections such as influenza.	Drug suppresses immune system (lymphocytes) and increases risk of infection or decreased healing.
Sulfasalazine (Azulfidine)	500 to 3000 mg daily in 2 to 4 doses.	Check for sulfa allergy, or kidney or liver disease.	Drug is a sulfa medication that has potential renal/liver toxicities.
		Teach client to drink adequate fluids.	Failure to drink fluids may cause formation of urine crystals.
		Teach men that the drug can lower sperm count.	Low sperm count may interfere with ability to conceive.
Leflunomide (Arava)	10 to 20 mg daily.	Teach client to get prescribed laboratory tests, usually every 6 to 8 weeks.	Increased liver enzymes and decreased blood count have been reported.
		Remind client to use strict birth control.	Drug can cause birth defects.

CBC, Complete blood count; *CNS*, central nervous system; *COX-2*, cyclooxygenase-2; *CTDs*, connective tissue diseases; *MS*, multiple sclerosis; *NSAIDs*, nonsteroidal anti-inflammatory drugs; *SC*, subcutaneously; *TB*, tuberculosis.

*This is not a comprehensive list; this chart lists only the common drugs used for arthritis and connective tissue disease.

Continued

CHART 24-9

DRUG THERAPY for
Arthritis and Connective Tissue Disease*—*cont'd*

Drug	Usual Dosage	Nursing Interventions	Rationales
Biological response modifiers (BRMs)	Dose typically depends on body weight or response to medication.	Do not give BRMs if client has a serious infection, TB, or MS.	Drugs may exacerbate infections, MS, or lupus.
Etanercept (Enbrel)	Usually 25 mg SC twice weekly	Teach client to report site reaction.	Site reactions can be painful.
Infliximab (Remicade)	Varies from 200 to 400 mg IV each treatment	Refrigerate all BRMs except Remicade.	Refrigeration prevents drug decomposition.
Adalimumab (Humira)	Typically 40 mg SC every 2 wk		
Anakinra (Kineret)	Typically 100 mg SC daily		

CBC, Complete blood count; *CNS,* central nervous system; *COX-2,* cyclooxygenase-2; *CTDs,* connective tissue diseases; *MS,* multiple sclerosis; *NSAIDs,* nonsteroidal anti-inflammatory drugs; *SC,* subcutaneously; *TB,* tuberculosis.
*This is not a comprehensive list; this chart lists only the common drugs used for arthritis and connective tissue disease.

within some countries or when a client has specific needs or restrictions. Salicylates must be taken with food and are sometimes given with GI-acid lowering agents providing GI protection such as proton pump inhibitors. Monitor the client for heartburn, indigestion, stomach discomfort, or black, tarry bowel movements (signs and symptoms of ulceration or GI bleeding). Report such symptoms to the health care provider.

Disease-Modifying Anti-Rheumatic Drugs. **Disease-modifying antirheumatic drugs (DMARDs)**, such as hydroxychloroquine (Plaquenil), sulfasalazine, or minocycline, may be prescribed to slow the progression of mild rheumatoid disease before it worsens (see Chart 24-9).

Hydroxychloroquine (Plaquenil) is an antimalarial drug that helps decrease joint and muscle pain and often helps clients with early RA or other inflammatory autoimmune diseases such as systemic lupus erythematosus (SLE), described later in this chapter. Some health care providers may use Plaquenil as one of the initial treatments for mild disease. The client usually takes 400 mg each evening with a light snack. Occasionally the dose is divided into 200 mg twice daily with food.

Clients generally tolerate Plaquenil quite well. In a few cases, mild stomach discomfort, light-headedness or headache have been reported. The most serious adverse effect of the drug is retinal damage. Teach clients to report blurred vision or headache. Remind clients to have an eye examination every 6 to 12 months to detect changes in the cornea, lens, or retina. If this complication occurs, the health care provider discontinues the drug. Eye complications are rare, but prevention safety is the reason for the recommendation.

Sulfasalazine (Azulfidine) is a medication that may be prescribed for mild to moderate inflammatory arthritis conditions such as RA or psoriatic arthritis (an inflammatory arthritis variant described later). The usual dosage is 1000 mg twice daily taken with breakfast and supper. Starting doses may be less, such as 500 mg once or twice daily, gradually building up to the standard adult dose. Minimization of such GI side effects as sulfa taste, bloating, stomach discomfort, and gas occurs by gradually increasing drug dosing. Monitor the complete blood count (CBC), paying special attention for a decrease in white blood cells (WBCs) or platelet count. Changes in blood counts are rare but severe potential side effects for which the medication must be discontinued. Clients with an allergy to sulfa drugs or aspirin should not take sulfasalazine.

Minocycline (Minocin, a form of the antibiotic tetracycline) is sometimes used to treat mild RA symptoms. Although its mechanism of action is not known, it has both antimicrobial and anti-inflammatory effects. It is also an immune modifier, inhibiting certain chemicals that cause bone and cartilage damage.

Minocycline differs from other agents used for RA in that it has a low incidence of adverse effects. In addition, the client does not develop a resistance to the drug after prolonged use (Sears & Ganger, 2000).

Management of Moderate to Severe Disease. The health care provider selects medications that can slow progression of moderate to severe rheumatoid arthritis (RA). The client may take several of these drugs together, but not in the same drug class. For example, the provider may prescribe methotrexate and infliximab at the same time, along with a NSAID to help relieve pain and inflammation (see Chart 24-9).

Methotrexate (Rheumatrex). Methotrexate, an immunosuppressive medication, in a low, once-a-week dosage (generally 25 mg or less per week), has become the mainstay of therapy for advancing and sustaining RA because it is effective and relatively inexpensive. It is a slow-acting drug, taking 4 to 6 weeks to begin to control inflammatory joint symptoms. Observe for desired drug effects, such as a decrease in joint pain and swelling.

Monitor the client for potential side effects of decreasing WBCs and platelets (as a result of bone marrow suppression) or elevations in liver enzymes or serum creatinine. Remind clients to avoid alcoholic beverages while taking methotrexate to prevent liver toxicity. Teach the client to observe and report other side and toxic effects, which include mouth sores and acute dyspnea from pneumonitis. Rarely, lymph node tumor (lymphoma) has been associated in people who have RA and are taking methotrexate. Folic acid, one of the B vitamins, is often given to clients who are taking methotrexate to help decrease some of the drug's side effects.

Pregnancy is not recommended while taking methotrexate because birth defects are possible. Strict birth control is recommended for childbearing women who are in need of methotrexate to control their RA. If pregnancy is ever desired, the client is informed to consult the rheumatologist as well as their OB/GYN health care provider. Generally, the physician will discontinue the drug at least 3 months before planned pregnancy. Methotrexate may be restarted after birth if the client does not breast feed.

Leflunomide (Arava). Leflunomide is a slow-acting immune-modulating medication that helps diminish inflammatory arthritis symptoms of joint swelling, stiffness, and improves mobility. It is generally prescribed as follows: a loading dose of 100 mg daily for 3 days followed by 20 mg daily thereafter. Inform the client that the drug generally takes 4 to 6 weeks and sometimes up to 3 months before maximum benefit is realized.

Arava is a potent medication that is generally tolerated, but side effects of hair loss, diarrhea, decreased WBCs and platelets, or increased liver enzymes have been reported. Teach clients to report these changes and monitor laboratory results carefully. Remind them to avoid alcohol. Inform them that Arava can cause birth defects, and therefore recommend strict birth control to women of childbearing age. Tell clients to contact the health care provider immediately if pregnancy occurs while taking the drug. Cholestyramine (Questran) is available to help block the drug's action.

Critical Thinking Challenge

A 57-year-old woman has had RA for nearly 10 years. Although she is independent in her activities of daily living (ADLs), she complains of constant pain. She is taking Rheumatrex, Celebrex, Arava, and prednisone, but her disease continues to progress slowly. Because of diabetes mellitus, she can only take a low dose of prednisone. Her husband died 3 years ago, but she has no family who live nearby. When her daughter calls her, the client seems negative, hopeless, and depressed.

1. What are this client's priority nursing diagnoses?
2. What factors are contributing to her emotional state?
3. What outcomes are desired for this client?

evolve For suggested answer guidelines, go to http://evolve.elsevier.com/Iggy/.

Biological Response Modifiers. As a group, biological response modifiers (BRMs) are classified as the newest antiarthritic drugs that neutralize the biologic activity of tumor necrosis factor (TNF) by inhibiting its binding with TNF receptors. Any one of the BRMs may be tried. If one drug is not effective, the health care provider prescribes another drug in the same class. All these medications are extremely expensive at this time, and insurance companies may not completely pay for their use.

Clients with multiple sclerosis or tuberculosis are not given TNF inhibitors. Determine whether the client has had a recent negative purified protein derivative (PPD) test. If not, a PPD skin test is typically administered, and the selected BRM is not started until the results are known to be negative. Collaborate with the client's health care provider to ensure that this process is complete.

Etanercept (Enbrel) is given subcutaneously by injection either as 50 mg once weekly or as 25 mg twice weekly. Immunosuppression with medications such as methotrexate is generally tried before using Enbrel or other biological response modifiers. Methotrexate may also be continued in combination with biologic therapies because the combination may be more effective than either drug alone. Most clients tolerate Enbrel or Enbrel and methotrexate together; however, laboratory monitoring is important. Combination therapy requires complete blood count (CBC), serum creatinine, and a liver panel to be drawn regularly, generally every 4 to 8 weeks. In general, clinical outcomes with Enbrel have been excellent.

Teach the client or family member how to self-administer Enbrel injections. Injection site reactions and infections (especially respiratory) are possible adverse effects. Ice and hydrocortisone 1% cream can be used if the client develops a red itchy rash at the site of an injection. The drug manufacturer cannot yet predict long-term potential side effects regarding severity of infection or cancer risk. To date what has been seen is mild increase in upper respiratory infections with occasional serious infections. The health care provider should be notified if infection or a delay in wound healing occurs.

Infliximab (Remicade), first approved to treat Crohn's disease, is given in a single IV infusion over several hours. The initial dose generally used for RA is 3 mg/kg of body weight. Following the first few weeks of therapy, the drug is repeated at intervals between 2 and 8 weeks, depending on the response of the client. Clients typically take methotrexate before starting Remicade and continue on combination therapy.

Teach the client to report symptoms of infusion reaction: chest discomfort, tachycardia, shortness of breath, or lightheadedness. If any of these symptoms are reported, decrease the IV rate or discontinue it. These symptoms generally subside, but the physician must be notified in case medical assistance is needed. Dose, rate, and interval changes may be needed. Acetaminophen and Benadryl are medications often given to each client before the start of Remicade, and are often used at the time of reported infusion reaction. Clients who experience serious adverse effects, such as hypertension or anaphylaxis, may require permanent discontinuation of the drug.

Adalimumab (Humira) is the first fully human TNF inhibitor and was approved by the federal Food and Drug Association (FDA) in January 2003. Humira is a 40-mg once every 2 weeks subcutaneous injection. Symptoms of inflammatory arthritis tend to decrease with the use of Humira, including less joint swelling, less stiffness, and better movement.

Injection site reactions and adverse effects similar to the other TNF inhibitors have been reported. Careful monitoring, especially with combination therapy of Humira and methotrexate or other immunosuppressive medication, is important and similar to combination therapy with other BRMs.

Anakinra (Kineret) is another biological response modifier. Instead of affecting tumor necrosis factor (TNF), however, it works to inhibit a different protein signal of the immune system called interleukin-1 (IL-1). IL-1 is also a pro-inflammatory protein that signals the immune system to increase inflammation. It is thought that IL-1 is a weaker protein than TNF, but having an alternative medication that targets a different receptor site is helpful when a client is unable to take other biologics. Clients who have multiple sclerosis or tuberculosis can not take TNF inhibitors, but Kineret can be used with this population.

Injection site reactions occur more often with Kineret compared with other BRMs. Ice and hydrocortisone 1% cream are recommended. Remind clients to rotate injection sites. Kineret is administered with a simple jet that the client can use for self-administration. The client has the option to eliminate the simple jet or administer the subcutaneous injection traditionally.

Adjunctive Treatment. Some drugs are given as adjuncts to the previously described medications. It is not unusual for a client to be taking several disease-modifying drugs, such as methotrexate, a BRM, and an adjunct medication. Each drug works differently to relieve symptoms and slow the progression of the disease.

Glucocorticoids (steroids)–usually Prednisone (Deltasone, Medrol)–are given for their fast-acting anti-inflammatory and immunosuppressive effects. Prednisone may be given in high dose for short duration **(pulse therapy)** or as a low chronic dose. Moderate-dose, short-term tapering bridge therapy is commonly used when inflammation is symptomatic and other RA medications are insufficient or have not yet had an effect.

Chronic steroid therapy can result in numerous complications, such as diabetes mellitus, infection, fluid and electrolyte imbalances, hypertension, osteoporosis, and glaucoma. Some drug effects are dose related, whereas others are not. Observe the client for complications associated with chronic steroid therapy and report them to the health care provider. For example, if blood pressure becomes elevated or significant laboratory values change, notify the physician.

Instruct clients taking chronic steroids to take calcium 1200 to 1500 mg daily plus vitamin D 800 mg daily to help prevent osteoporosis. Bisphosphonate medications such as Fosamax or Actonel are often prescribed as well. Bone density measurements are recommended.

Clients with RA may experience one or a few joints that have more pain and inflammation than the others. Cortisone injections in single joints may be used to relieve local pain and inflammation. Have the client ice and rest the joint for 24 hours following the procedure. Oral analgesia is sometimes also needed during that time.

Other Drugs. Other immunosuppressive agents that may be used are azathioprine (Imuran) and cyclophosphamide (Cytoxan). Cyclophosphamide is sometimes given specifically to control RA vasculitis. Such immunosuppressive medications may cause bone marrow suppression and occasionally leukemia or lymphoma. White blood cells are expected to decrease 7 to 14 days following the administration of IV cyclophosphamide; therefore laboratory results are closely monitored to ensure safe limits. Hemorrhagic cystitis is a concern more with oral cyclophosphamide. Instruct the client to drink water and void frequently (about every 2 hours while awake), which dilutes the urine and empties the bladder, thus decreasing opportunity for bladder irritation from residual drug. Hair thinning or loss can be seen with immunosuppressive medications. Cyclophosphamide may also cause sterility; strict birth control is recommended.

Clients should be well informed of each medication's desired and specific potential side effects, the method for taking the medication correctly, and recommended monitoring methods. When taken correctly and monitored, these immunosuppressive medications help control severe autoimmune inflammatory diseases.

Gold therapy is less frequently used to treat RA now that methotrexate and the newer biologic medications are available; however, gold may still sometimes be used to modify RA disease and reduce pain and inflammation. Some clients take gold if they are unable to use other immunosuppressive or biologic medications. The most commonly used parenteral preparation is gold sodium thiomalate (Myochrysine). For intramuscularly administered gold, a test dose of 10 mg is given to detect an allergy to the drug, and weekly gold injections are given thereafter. The dosage increases from 25 to 50 mg weekly. Blood tests must be monitored before each injection. The client's urine is tested for protein level and a CBC is taken. Report any laboratory results outside the normal range to the physician, and hold the gold injection.

If the client responds to gold without having toxic effects (e.g., rash, blood dyscrasias, renal involvement), the injections are slowly tapered to every 2 weeks, then every 3 weeks, and then once a month. If remission does not occur after a total of 1000 mg has been given, the drug is usually discontinued.

Auranofin (Ridaura) is different from IM gold in that it is a form of oral gold that is occasionally used to treat mild RA. Three milligrams twice-daily dosing is generally prescribed. Its major side effects are GI symptoms, especially diarrhea, nausea, and vomiting. Teach the client to report any GI problems to the health care provider.

Analgesic drugs may be prescribed to supplement the pain relief property in anti-inflammatory drugs specific for RA. Some analgesics include acetaminophen (Tylenol), propoxyphene (Darvon), and propoxyphene napsylate (Darvocet-N). Propoxyphene and its associated products can cause headache, dizziness, and drowsiness. In clients with decreased metabolic rates, this slowly excreted drug may accumulate in the body over a long period and can cause death, especially in older adults. Teach the client about the side effects and toxic effects of these drugs and advise the client to report any unusual symptoms or complaints to the physician.

Nonpharmacologic Modalities. Adequate rest, proper positioning, and ice and heat applications are important in pain management (see Pain Management [Osteoarthritis], p. 384). If acute inflammation is present, the physical therapist (PT) or assistive nursing personnel applies ice to the "hot" joints for pain relief until the inflammation lessens. The ice pack should not be too heavy. Heated paraffin (wax) dips may help decrease pain and increase comfort of arthritic hands. Finger and hand exercises are often done more easily following paraffin treatment.

To relieve morning stiffness or the pain of late-stage disease, recommend a hot shower rather than a sponge bath or a tub bath. It is often difficult for the client with RA to get into and out of a bathtub, although special hydraulic lifts and tub chairs may be available. Grab bars and nonskid tread in the tub floor are important safety features to discuss with all clients.

Hot packs applied directly to involved joints may be beneficial. Most physical therapy departments have machines that keep hot packs ready anytime they are needed (Figure 24-5). At home, the client may use the microwave or stovetop heating instructions to warm the heat pack. Teach the client to follow the instructions given with each heating device used.

Plasmapheresis. Plasmapheresis (sometimes called plasma exchange) is an in-hospital procedure prescribed by a health care provider in which the client's plasma is treated to remove the antibodies causing the disease. This procedure may be combined with pulse therapy for clients with severe, life-threatening disease.

Complementary and Alternative Therapies. Some clients may have pain relief from hypnosis, acupuncture, magnet therapy, imagery, or music therapy. Stress management is also popular as a pain relief intervention. Chapters 4 and 7 discuss these therapies in detail.

Good nutrition is an important part of the management of RA. The inflammatory state may place a greater burden on the metabolism of some essential nutrients. This catabolic state may be related to increased cytokine production, specifically tumor necrosis factor (Kremer, 2001). Further research will contribute to future nutritional recommendations. Some attention has been given to specific foods:

- Omega-3 fatty acids (found in coldwater fish such as salmon, sea bass, and tuna) may help decrease inflammation; however, the amount needed may be impractical for human consumption.
- Fish oil capsules containing omega-3 fatty acids at 2.5 to 5 g daily (should not be taken if the client is taking anticoagulant therapy) may be recommended in areas in which coldwater fish are not available.

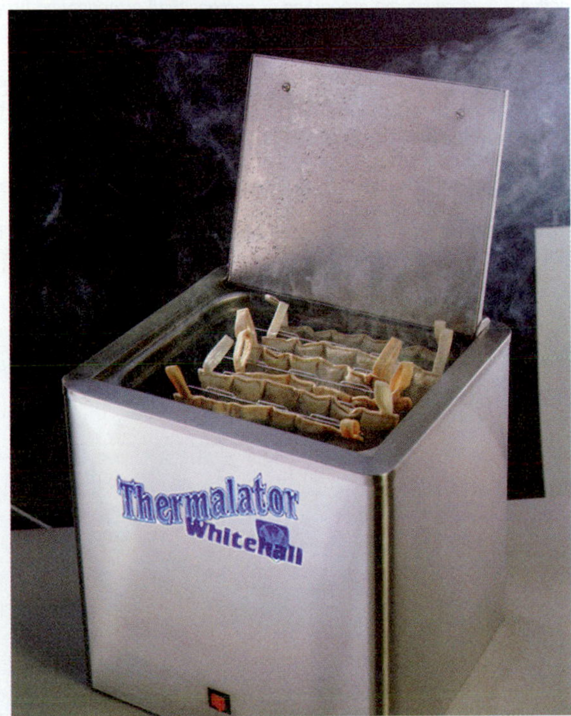

Figure 24-5 ■ Heating units used to keep hot packs warm. (Courtesy Whitehall Manufacturing, City of Industry, CA.)

- Antioxidant vitamins (A,C, E) may help maintain the normal function of the immune system.
- Trace elements such as zinc, selenium, copper, and iron may be needed in sufficient amounts for joint health.

According to the Arthritis Foundation, there is no one food that causes or cures RA; however, healthy nutrition in general is supported. Refer the client to the Arthritis Foundation's pamphlet regarding diet and arthritis. Refer the client to the health care provider or dietitian for vitamin- and nutrition-specific questions or recommendations.

Promotion of Self-Care. Although the physical appearance of a client with severe RA may create the image that independence in activities of daily living (ADLs) is not possible, a number of alternative methods can be used to perform these activities. Do not automatically perform these activities for the client; clients with RA do not want to be dependent. For example, hand deformities often prevent a client from opening packages of food, such as a box of crackers; however, he or she may prefer to use his or her teeth to open the crackers rather than depend on someone else.

In the hospital or long-term care facility, a client may not eat because of the barriers of heavy plate covers, milk cartons, small packages of condiments, and heavy containers. Styrofoam or paper cups may bend and collapse as the client attempts to hold them. A china or heavy plastic cup with handles may be easier to manipulate. Collaborate with the dietitian to allow access to food and total independence in eating.

When fine motor activities (e.g., squeezing a tube of toothpaste) become impossible, larger joints or body surfaces can substitute for smaller ones. For example, teach the client to use the palm of the hand to press the paste onto the brush. Devices such as long-handled brushes can allow clients to brush their hair; dressing sticks can facilitate putting on pants. These examples illustrate the need to assess the problem area, suggest alternative methods, and refer the client to an occupational or physical therapist for special assistive and adaptive devices if necessary.

Management of Fatigue. Nursing interventions depend in part on identifying the factors contributing to fatigue. For example, increases in pain, sleep disturbances, and weakness are positively associated with increased fatigue. Anemia may also be a contributing factor and may be treated with iron (if an iron deficiency anemia is present), folic acid, or vitamin supplements prescribed by the health care provider. Chronic normochromic or chronic hypochromic anemia often occurs in most chronic, systemic diseases. Assess for drug-related blood loss, such as that caused by salicylate therapy or other NSAIDs, by checking the stool for gross or occult blood. Older white women are the most likely clients to experience GI bleeding as a result of taking these medications.

When fatigue results from muscle atrophy, the physician prescribes an aggressive physical therapy program to strengthen muscles and prevent further atrophy. Clients experience increased fatigue when pain prevents them from getting adequate rest and sleep. Measures to facilitate sleep include promoting a quiet environment, giving warm beverages, and administering hypnotics or relaxants as prescribed, if necessary.

In addition to identifying and managing specific reasons for fatigue, determine the client's usual daily activities and teach principles of **energy conservation,** including the following:

- Pacing activities
- Allowing rest periods
- Setting priorities
- Obtaining assistance when needed

Chart 24-10 lists specific suggestions for conserving energy and thus increasing activity tolerance.

Enhancement of Body Image. Body image may be affected by both the disease process and drug therapy. Steroids can cause a moon-faced appearance, acne, striae, "buffalo humps," and weight gain. Determine the client's perception of these changes and the impact of the reactions of family and significant others. The most important intervention is communicating acceptance of the client. When a trusting relationship is established, encourage the client to express his or her feelings.

Another way to improve body image while in the hospital or nursing home is to use personal items. A hospital gown reinforces the sick role. Encourage clients to wear their own clothes, to brush their hair, and to use makeup if desired. Assist the client as needed. The use of colored hair accessories, nail polish, and perfume may improve a female client's image and self-concept.

As a reaction to body image disturbance and the presence of a chronic, painful disease, clients may display behaviors indicative of loss. They may use coping strategies that range from denial or fear to anger or depression. In an attempt to regain control over the effects of the disease process, they may appear to be manipulative and demanding and sometimes may be referred to as having an "arthritis personality." This personality, which has negative connotations, is a myth. Clients are trying to cope with the effects of their illness and should be treated with patience and understanding. Continually assess and accept these behaviors, but remain realistic in discussing goals to improve self-esteem. Emphasize clients' strengths and help them identify previously successful coping strategies.

Community-Based Care

Clients with rheumatoid arthritis (RA) are usually managed at home but may be institutionalized in a long-term care setting if they become restricted to bed or a wheelchair. Some clients may be discharged to a rehabilitation facility for several weeks to aid in developing strategies, techniques, and skills for independent living at home.

HOME CARE MANAGEMENT

The amount of home care preparation depends on the severity of the disease. Structural changes may be necessary if there are deficits in activities of daily living (ADLs) or mobility. Doors must be wide enough to accommodate a wheelchair or walker if one is used. Ramps are needed to prevent the client in a wheelchair from becoming homebound. If the client cannot negotiate stairs, he or she must have access to facilities for all ADLs on one floor. Handrails should be available in the bathroom and halls.

To promote continued homemaking functions, countertops and appliances may require structural changes. The client may also require handrails and elevated chairs and toilet seats, which facilitate transfers (Figure 24-6).

CHART 24-10

CLIENT EDUCATION GUIDE

Energy Conservation for the Client with Arthritis

- Balance activity with rest. Take one or two naps each day.
- Pace yourself; do not plan too much for one day.
- Set priorities. Determine which activities are most important, and do them first.
- Delegate responsibility and tasks to your family and friends.
- Plan ahead to prevent last-minute rushing and stress.
- Learn your own activity tolerance and do not exceed it.

HEALTH TEACHING

Health teaching is a vital role for nurses in the diagnosis and management of arthritis. Many people have signs and symptoms of joint inflammation but do not seek medical attention. Teach clients to seek professional health care to reduce pain and disability (see the Meeting Healthy People 2010 Objectives box below).

Meeting HEALTHY PEOPLE 2010 Objectives

ARTHRITIS AND OTHER RHEUMATIC CONDITIONS

Objective 2.7: Increase the proportion of adults who have seen a health care provider for their chronic joint symptoms.

- Teach clients with suspected arthritis the importance of seeing a health care provider for initial evaluation and follow-up care.
- Educate clients that maintaining functional ability and managing pain can reduce arthritis pain and disability.
- Remind older adults that arthritis is not a normal part of the aging process.
- Assist the client in locating local health care providers who specialize in arthritis management (e.g., rheumatologists, internists).
- Teach clients about the availability of community support groups for people with arthritis.

Objective 2.8: Increase the proportion of persons with arthritis who have had effective evidence-based arthritis education as an integral part of the management of their condition.

- Teach clients about community education programs at local hospitals or through the Arthritis Foundation, such as the Arthritis Self-Help course.
- Educate clients about the value of evidence-based education programs (reduces pain and visits to the health care provider).
- Provide client and family education about arthritis and its management, as needed.

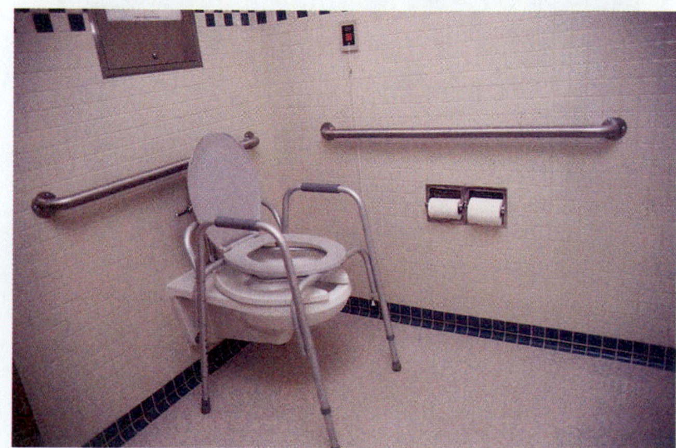

Figure 24-6 ■ Handrails and an elevated toilet seat make transfers easier for the client.

Health teaching is also important for promoting compliance with a treatment plan. A client who understands the disease process and the treatment rationale can better follow and ask questions about the treatment plan.

Teach clients to discuss any questions with their health care provider before trying any over-the-counter or home remedies. Some remedies may be harmful. Check with the Arthritis Foundation for the latest information on arthritis myths and quackery.

Information about drug therapy, joint protection, energy conservation, rest, and exercise should be taught to client, family, and significant others. This information is summarized in Charts 24-5, 24-6, 24-9, and 24-10.

The client with RA often complains of being on an "emotional roller coaster" from coping with a chronic illness every day. Control over one's life is an important human need. The client with an unpredictable chronic disease may lose this control, and this lowers self-esteem. Health care providers must allow the client to make decisions about care. Families and significant others must also include the client in decision-making. Although the client's behavior may be perceived as demanding or manipulative, his or her self-esteem cannot be improved without this important aspect of interpersonal relationships.

Increased dependency also affects a sense of control and self-esteem. Some clients ignore their health needs and portray a tough image for others by insisting that they need no assistance. Emphasize to the client and family that asking for help may be the best decision at times to prevent further joint damage and disease progression.

Rheumatoid arthritis (RA) may also affect work and social roles. The client may have physical difficulty doing tasks that require lifting, climbing, grasp, gross or fine motor activities. The severity of RA disease may cause difficulty with total number of hours worked. Some people with RA are able to do their jobs well without problem; others may have varying degrees of difficulty. Clients who are no longer able to do their job at work may need to discuss having a lighter workload with their employer, but some may need to file for disability with their company and social security.

Arthritis support groups and self-help courses provide the education and the support that clients, families, and friends need; however, refer the client to a psychological counselor or religious or spiritual leader for emotional support and guidance during times of crisis or as needed. Identify and recommend other support systems within the family and community when necessary.

HEALTH CARE RESOURCES

The need for health care resources for the client with RA is similar to that for the client with osteoarthritis. A home care nurse or aide, physical therapist, or occupational therapist may be needed. In collaboration with the discharge planner, the nurse in the hospital or nursing home identifies these resources and makes sure they are available before discharge.

Critical Thinking Challenge

The 57-year-old woman with RA decides to see a new rheumatologist. After a thorough examination and consultation, he wants her to try Enbrel. She is concerned that she will not be able to self-administer the injections and is worried that Medicare and her supplemental insurance will not pay for it. She lives on monthly disability checks for her and her deceased husband.

1. What health teaching will this client require?
2. As her home care nurse, what outcomes would you observe for to determine the effectiveness of the new medication?
3. Why do you think the physician prescribed the new medication?

evolve For suggested answer guidelines, go to http://evolve.elsevier.com/Iggy/.

LUPUS ERYTHEMATOSUS

PATHOPHYSIOLOGY

The word *lupus* is the Latin term for "wolf." In the mid-nineteenth century, the facial rash accompanying this disease was thought to look like bites caused by a wolf. The rash was usually red, and thus the term *erythematosus,* a Latin word meaning "reddened," was added to describe the disease.

There are two main classifications of lupus: **discoid lupus erythematosus (DLE)** and **systemic lupus erythematosus (SLE).** A small percentage of clients with lupus have the DLE type, which affects only the skin.

SLE is a chronic, progressive, inflammatory connective tissue disorder that can cause major body organs and systems to fail. It is characterized by spontaneous remissions and **exacerbations** ("flare-ups"), and the onset may be acute or insidious. The condition is potentially fatal, but the survival rate has improved dramatically most recently in countries where SLE is diagnosed early and treated adequately. Today more than 90% of clients with SLE are living 10 years after diagnosis (Edworthy, 2001). Improvements in determining the cause, diagnosis, and treatment of lupus account for the prolonged survival of these clients.

Lupus is thought to be an autoimmune process; that is, abnormal antibodies are produced and react with the client's tissues. Antinuclear antibodies (ANAs) primarily affect the deoxyribonucleic acid (DNA) within the cell nuclei. As a result, immune complexes form in the serum and organ tissues, which causes inflammation and damage. These complexes invade organs directly or cause **vasculitis** (vessel inflammation), which deprives the organs of arterial blood and oxygen.

Many clients with SLE have some degree of kidney involvement–the leading cause of death. Other causes of death from SLE are cardiac and central nervous system involvement.

In kidney disease, renal biopsies show the following progressive changes within the glomeruli:

- In minimal lupus nephritis, the glomeruli are slightly irregular; immunoglobulins and complement are seen by electron microscopy.
- Focal, or mild, lupus nephritis is characterized by further glomerular changes, and immune complex deposits are common. In this type of lupus, the client begins to show clinical signs of renal impairment.
- In diffuse, severe proliferative nephritis, more than 50% of the glomeruli are affected, and the client is in renal failure.

Lupus affects women between the ages of 15 and 40 years at a rate 8 to 10 times more often than men. Black women have the disease more than white women, but the reason is unknown. The onset of the disease occurs most often during the childbearing years, but it has been reported in young children and older adults. A genetic predisposition is likely based on the trend to develop the disease in twins and the occurrence of autoimmune disease in families of clients who have lupus.

A genetic link between lupus, rheumatoid arthritis, and psoriatic arthritis involves a protein called Runx-1, which helps the thymus gland train cells of the immune system. Research indicates that clients with these diseases have an altered Runx-1 binding site on one of three chromosomes. The interpretation of this finding is not clear, but it demonstrates, in part, the genetic etiology of these autoimmune diseases (Wade, 2003).

A transient lupus-like syndrome can occur in some clients taking selected medications, especially procainamide (Pronestyl) and hydralazine (McCance & Huether, 2003). When these drugs are discontinued, the syndrome usually resolves.

COLLABORATIVE MANAGEMENT

Assessment

It is impossible to describe a typical textbook picture of a client with lupus because of the extreme variability of symptoms. When the disease is in remission, the client may appear healthy and have no activity limitations. When the disease flares, the client may be so ill that admission to a critical care unit is required. Chart 24-11 highlights the clinical manifestations that occur with systemic lupus.

CHART 24-11

KEY FEATURES of Systemic Lupus Erythematosus and Progressive Systemic Sclerosis

Systemic Lupus Erythematosus	Progressive Systemic Sclerosis
Skin Manifestations	
▪ Inflamed, red rash ▪ Discoid lesions	▪ Inflamed ▪ Fibrotic ▪ Sclerotic ▪ Edematous
Renal Manifestations	
▪ Nephritis	▪ Renal failure
Cardiovascular Manifestations	
▪ Pericarditis ▪ Raynaud's phenomenon	▪ Myocardial fibrosis ▪ Raynaud's phenomenon
Pulmonary Manifestations	
▪ Pleural effusions	▪ Interstitial fibrosis ▪ Pulmonary hypertension
Neurologic Manifestations	
▪ CNS lupus	▪ Not common
Gastrointestinal Manifestations	
▪ Abdominal pain	▪ Esophagitis ▪ Ulcers
Musculoskeletal Manifestations	
▪ Joint inflammation ▪ Myositis	▪ Joint inflammation ▪ Myositis
Other Manifestations	
▪ Fever ▪ Fatigue ▪ Anorexia ▪ Vasculitis	▪ Fever ▪ Fatigue ▪ Anorexia ▪ Vasculitis

CNS, Central nervous system.

PHYSICAL ASSESSMENT/CLINICAL MANIFESTATIONS

SKIN INVOLVEMENT. The major skin manifestation of SLE is a dry, scaly, raised rash on the face **("butterfly" rash)** (Figure 24-7). This rash may also appear on the sun exposed upper body. The rash of systemic lupus is generally nonscarring, but it may increase in a lupus flare and disappear when the disease is in remission.

Individual round **discoid** (coinlike) **lesions** are the scarring lesions of discoid lupus. The lesions are especially evident when the client is exposed to sunlight or ultraviolet light.

Alopecia is common in lupus. Observe all skin changes and monitor them daily while the client is in an acute care setting.

MUSCULOSKELETAL CHANGES. In addition to skin changes, **polyarthritis** occurs in 90% of clients with SLE. The initial joint changes are similar to those seen in rheumatoid arthritis (RA), but severe deformities are not common. Small joints and the knees are most commonly involved. **Osteonecrosis** (bone necrosis from lack of oxygen) is often seen in clients with SLE who have been treated for at least 5 years, usually with steroids. Chronic steroid therapy may cause the constriction of small blood vessels supplying the joint, which causes the tissue to die. The hip is most commonly affected, and complaints of pain and decreased mobility result.

Observe for muscle atrophy, which can result from disuse or from skeletal muscle invasion by the immune complexes **(myositis).** Myalgia (muscle pain) may also occur. Inspect and palpate the major muscles, especially those in the extremities.

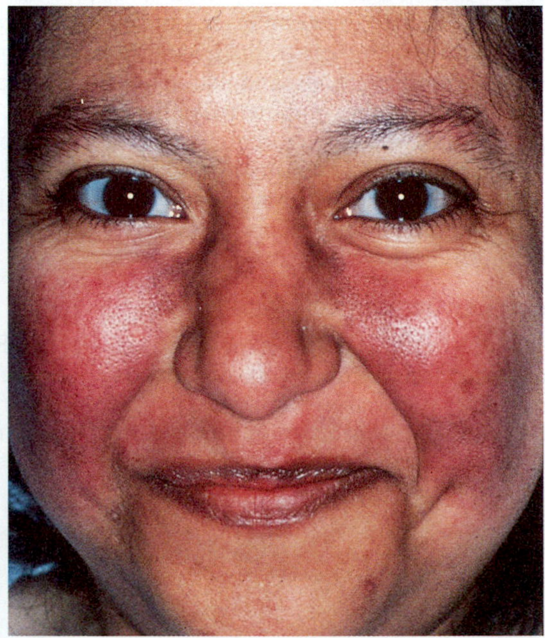

Figure 24-7 ▪ The characteristic "butterfly" rash of systemic lupus erythematosus.

SYSTEMIC MANIFESTATIONS. Because SLE is an inflammatory condition, fever and fatigue are common findings. Fever is the classic sign of a flare, or exacerbation. Various degrees of generalized weakness, fatigue, anorexia, and weight loss occur. These signs may be the only evidence of impending disease, which makes diagnosis by the health care provider difficult. Consequently, some clients have a diagnosis of "probable SLE."

Any or all body systems may be affected by SLE. Because lupus nephritis is the leading cause of death, carefully assess for signs of renal involvement (e.g., changes in urine output, proteinuria, hematuria, and fluid retention). Approximately 50% of clients with SLE have some type of nephritis.

Pleural effusions or pneumonia are found in almost half of all cases of SLE, but **this** complication is usually not life threatening. Pulmonary restrictive or obstructive changes may not result in overt clinical signs; however, progressive involvement can lead to dyspnea and arterial blood gas abnormalities. Perform a complete respiratory assessment to determine any abnormalities in respiratory pattern or breath sounds.

Pericarditis is the most common cardiovascular manifestation and causes tachycardia, chest pain, and myocardial ischemia. Monitor the vital signs at least every 4 hours while the client is in the hospital, and report chest pain immediately to the physician.

Raynaud's phenomenon is noted in 15% of cases of lupus. On exposure to cold or extreme stress, the client with Raynaud's phenomenon complains of the characteristic red, white, and blue color changes and severe pain in the digits; these changes are caused by arteriolar vasospasm. Ask clients whether color changes occur when their hands or feet are exposed to cold or when they are extremely stressed.

Neurologic manifestations are varied. Central nervous system effects include psychoses, paresis, seizures, migraine headaches, and cranial nerve palsies. Peripheral neuropathies are also common. Perform a neurologic assessment as described in Chapter 44.

Monitor abdominal pain, which most often result from serositis (peritoneal involvement). Mesenteric arteritis, pancreatitis from arteritis of the pancreatic artery, and colonic ulcers also can cause abdominal pain with lupus. Note liver enlargement on assessment of the abdomen. Jaundice is rare. More than 50% of clients have lymph enlargement, and 10% have splenomegaly. Palpate the lymph nodes and document findings. Vasculitis affecting any major or small vessels can lead to organ failure.

PSYCHOSOCIAL ASSESSMENT

The psychosocial results of lupus can be devastating. With either DLE or SLE, the rash can be disfiguring and embarrassing. Young adult women who never had a blemish are confronted with a rash that cannot be completely covered with makeup. If chronic steroid therapy is used, side effects such as acne, striae, fat pads, and weight gain intensify the problem of an already altered body image.

Chronic fatigue and generalized weakness may prevent the client from being as active as in the past. He or she may avoid social gatherings and may withdraw from family activities. The unpredictability and chronicity of SLE can cause fear and anxiety. Fear may increase if the client knows another person with the disease, particularly if the other person has more advanced, severe disease. Unfortunately, the myth that lupus is fatal is still common. Inform the client that control of lupus is generally possible with regular medical monitoring, medications, and healthy practices, such as limiting sun exposure to prevent exacerbation of the disease.

Assess the client's feelings about the illness to identify areas requiring intervention. Determine the client's usual coping mechanisms and support systems before developing a plan of care. See Psychosocial Assessment (Rheumatoid Arthritis), p. 395, for additional information about the psychosocial assessment of clients with chronic illness.

LABORATORY ASSESSMENT

Because discoid lupus erythematosus (DLE) is not a systemic condition, the only significant test is a skin biopsy. The physician gently scrapes skin cells from the rash for microscopic evaluation. The characteristic lupus cell and a number of inflammatory cells confirm the diagnosis.

Some of the immunologic-based laboratory tests used to diagnose SLE are the same as those performed for rheumatoid arthritis (RA): rheumatoid factor, antinuclear antibody, erythrocyte sedimentation rate, serum protein electrophoresis, serum complement (especially C_3 and C_4), and immunoglobulins (see Chart 24-8). A false-positive Venereal Disease Research Laboratory (VDRL) syphilis test is common with lupus.

Newer and more specific immunologic tests, such as anti-Ro (SSA), anti-La (SSB), anti-RNP, anti-Smith (anti-Sm), anti-DNA, and anti-phospholipid antibodies (AP) are also performed. High titers of some of these antibodies are associated with lupus (Kuper & Failla, 2000). The rheumatologist generally orders and interprets immunologic tests for clients suspected of having lupus.

In addition to immunologic testing, several tests are performed to evaluate the possible involvement of major organs and body systems. A complete blood count (CBC) commonly shows **pancytopenia** (a decrease of all cell types), probably caused by direct attack of the blood cells or bone marrow by immune complexes. Serum electrolyte levels, renal function, cardiac and liver enzymes, and clotting factors are also routinely assessed to determine other body system functioning.

Interventions

The health care provider often prescribes potent drugs that are used topically and systemically. In addition, precautions are taken to prevent further skin impairment and exacerbations. Many of the skin lesions do not disappear, even with treatment, but they usually fade when the disease is in remission.

Drug Therapy. With DLE, the client's major concern is the rash or discoid lesions. Clients with systemic lupus erythematosus (SLE) may also be concerned about skin changes. Topical cortisone preparations help to reduce inflammation and promote fading of the skin lesions. In addition, the health care provider may prescribe the antimalarial agent hydroxychloroquine (Plaquenil) for some clients to decrease the inflammatory response; other systemic medications are usually not used (see Chart 24-9).

The aim of management of SLE is to treat the disease aggressively until remission. In addition to medications for skin lesions, the health care provider often prescribes chronic steroid therapy to treat the systemic disease process. For renal or central nervous system lupus, the health care provider may also prescribe immunosuppressive agents (e.g., azathioprine [Imuran]), which are sometimes used for clients with RA (see Chart 24-9). Although clinical manifestations improve during remission, maintenance doses of these drugs are usually continued to prevent further exacerbations of the disease. Observe for side effects and toxic effects of these medications and report their occurrence to the physician.

For severe renal involvement, azathioprine or cyclophosphamide (Cytoxan) may be given in combination with steroids. For clients who do not respond to this regimen, IV pulse (high-dose) glucocorticoids, cyclophosphamide, and plasmapheresis may be tried (see discussion under Rheumatoid Arthritis on p. 407). Renal transplantation has been successful for some clients. Recent advances in allogenic stem cell transplantation have improved symptoms in clients who respond poorly to steroids or immunosuppressive drugs (Kuper & Failla, 2000).

Skin Protection. Clients with lupus should avoid prolonged exposure to sunlight and other forms of ultraviolet lighting, including certain types of fluorescent light. Instruct clients that they may need to wear long sleeves and a large-brimmed hat when outdoors. They should use sun-blocking agents with an SPF (sun protection factor) of 30 or higher on exposed skin surfaces.

In addition, teach the client to clean the skin with mild soap (e.g., Ivory) and to avoid harsh, perfumed substances. The skin is rinsed and dried well, and lotion is applied. Excess powder and other drying substances should be avoided. Cosmetics must be carefully selected and should include moisturizers and sun protectors. Consider referring a client to a medical cosmetologist who specializes in applying makeup for skin lesions of all types.

The client's hair should receive special attention because alopecia (hair loss) is common. Recommend the use of mild protein shampoos and the avoidance of harsh treatments (e.g., permanents or highlights) until the hair regrows during remission.

Critical Thinking Challenge

A 32-year-old African-American female visits her physician's office (where you are a nurse) with complaints of a facial rash. On further questioning, you find that she has been more fatigued than usual and has an achy left ankle. Her infant son is 2 months old, and she has just stopped bleeding from her traumatic vaginal delivery (the infant weighed 10 pounds, and she was in labor for 18 hours, causing extended postpartum bleeding).

1. When obtaining a complete history, what other questions should you ask the client?
2. What risk factors does she have for SLE?
3. What laboratory tests will the health care provider most likely order?
4. If the client is diagnosed with SLE, what type of health teaching will she need?

evolve For suggested answer guidelines, go to http://evolve.elsevier.com/Iggy/.

Community-Based Care

Community-based care for the client with lupus is similar to that for RA. In general, the client is home but may need repeated hospitalizations during exacerbations of disease. The client usually does not need rehabilitation or a long-term care facility because severe joint deformity and prolonged immobility are not common.

CHART 24-12

CLIENT EDUCATION GUIDE

Evidence-Based Practice for Skin Protection in Clients with Lupus Erythematosus

- Cleanse your skin with a mild soap, such as Ivory.
- Dry your skin thoroughly by patting rather than rubbing.
- Apply lotion liberally to dry skin areas.
- Avoid powder and other drying agents, such as rubbing alcohol.
- Use cosmetics that contain moisturizers.
- Avoid direct sunlight and any other type of ultraviolet lighting, including tanning beds.
- Wear a large-brimmed hat, long sleeves, and long pants when in the sun.
- Use a sun-blocking agent with a sun protection factor (SPF) of at least 30.
- Inspect your skin daily for open areas and rashes.

Two major differences exist between SLE and RA in terms of education of the client and family or significant others. First, teach the client with SLE how to protect the skin (Chart 24-12). Second, body temperature is monitored carefully with SLE. Fever is the major sign of an exacerbation, during which the client can become seriously ill. Teach the client to report any other unusual or new clinical manifestations to the health care provider immediately.

Many clients become frustrated that family members, significant others, and lay people do not have a good understanding of lupus. When lupus is in complete remission, the client appears to be healthy; however, an exacerbation can necessitate rapid admission to a critical care unit. This unpredictability disrupts the client's life and can cause fear and anxiety. Help the client identify coping strategies and support systems that can help with functioning in the community.

Teach the possible effects of the disease on lifestyle, including fatigue. Women of childbearing age need to know that pregnancy can be a stressor and can cause an exacerbation of the disease, either during pregnancy or after delivery. The pregnant client also has an increased risk of miscarriage, stillbirth, or premature birth. Pregnancy is not recommended for those with cardiac, renal, or central nervous system involvement. Sexual counseling regarding contraception options may be necessary.

Although the Arthritis Foundation is a general resource for all clients with connective tissue disease, the Lupus Foundation is a national organization and has chapters in every state to provide information and assistance for clients with lupus. Local support groups and services are offered free of charge.

PROGRESSIVE SYSTEMIC SCLEROSIS

PATHOPHYSIOLOGY

Progressive systemic sclerosis (PSS), one of a family of diseases, is often referred to as **systemic scleroderma.** *Scleroderma* means hardening of the skin, which is only one clinical manifestation of PSS. Some clients have only skin involvement, or localized scleroderma. As the name implies, PSS is a generalized, systemic disease. It is less common than systemic lupus erythematosus (SLE) but is associated with a higher mortality rate. Chart 24-11 shows a comparison of the clinical manifestations of these two diseases.

Progressive systemic sclerosis is a chronic connective tissue disease characterized by inflammation, fibrosis, and sclerosis of the skin and vital organs. The inflammatory process is so similar to that of lupus that clients are often diagnosed as having probable SLE until the disease progresses or until antibody testing supports the diagnosis. The inflamed tissue undergoes fibrotic and then sclerotic changes. The tissue most obviously affected is the skin, but renal involvement is the leading cause of death. Respiratory involvement and hypertension are also common. Clients with PSS do not respond well to the steroids and immunosuppressants used for lupus, and therefore the mortality rate is higher.

The classification for systemic sclerosis is as follows:

- **Diffuse cutaneous scleroderma**–skin thickening on the trunk, face, proximal and distal extremities.
- **Limited cutaneous scleroderma–**thick skin limited to sites distal to the elbow and knee but also involve the face and neck. Clients have the **CREST syndrome:**

*C*alcinosis (calcium deposits)
*R*aynaud's phenomenon
*E*sophageal dysmotility
*S*clerodactyly (scleroderma of the digits)
*T*elangiectasia (spiderlike hemangiomas)

- **Sine scleroderma**–internal organ manifestations, vascular, and serologic abnormalities, but without clinically detectable skin changes
- **Overlap scleroderma**–any of the preceding three types of scleroderma occurring with lupus, inflammatory muscle disease, or RA
- **Undifferentiated connective tissue disease**–without skin thickening or internal organ abnormalities seen in PSS but with serologic abnormality, Raynaud's phenomenon, or other clinical features of systemic sclerosis (Siebold, 2001)

Little is known about the cause of PSS, but autoimmunity is suspected. The occurrence of more than one case per family is uncommon, but other connective tissue diseases may be noted in the family history.

Progressive systemic sclerosis has been described in people of all races and in all geographic areas. Women are affected three to four times more often than men. The onset of the disease is usually between 30 and 50 years of age. The incidence is higher in coal miners, who have a high incidence of silicosis, a possible predisposing or contributing factor to PSS. Prolonged exposure to other toxins, such as vinyl chloride and epoxy resins, may also predispose an individual to PSS.

◆COLLABORATIVE MANAGEMENT

◆Assessment

PHYSICAL ASSESSMENT/CLINICAL MANIFESTATIONS

Arthralgia (joint pain) and stiffness are common manifestations that you can elicit during the musculoskeletal examination. The acute inflammation that occurs with rheumatoid arthritis (RA) is not common, and deformities are rare.

Findings on inspection of the skin depend on the stage of the scleroderma. Typically there is a painless, symmetric, pitting edema of the hands and fingers; this edema may progress to include the entire upper and lower extremities and face. In this edematous phase, the fingers are described as sausage-like. The skin is taut, shiny, and free of wrinkles. If diffuse scleroderma occurs, swelling is replaced by tightening, hardening, and thickening of skin tissue; this phase is sometimes called the *indurative phase* (Figure 24-8). The skin loses its elasticity, and range of motion is markedly decreased; ulcerations may occur. Joint contractures may develop, and the client may be unable to perform activities of daily living (ADLs) independently.

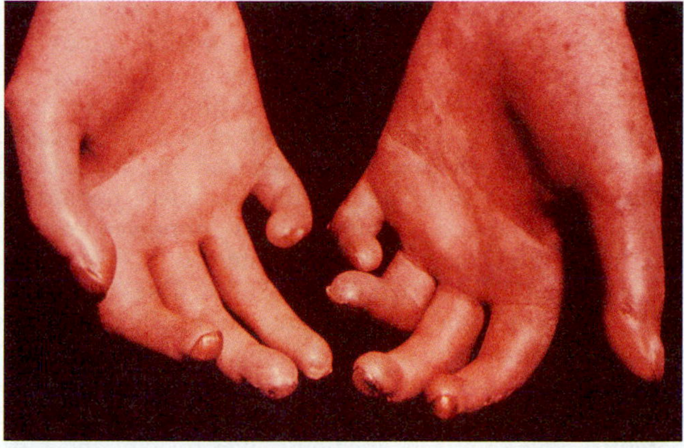

Figure 24-8 ■ Late-stage skin changes seen in clients with progressive systemic sclerosis. (From the Arthritis Teaching Slide Collection, copyright 1980. Used by permission of the Arthritis Foundation.)

Major organ damage is likely to develop with diffuse scleroderma, specifically affecting the following areas:

- Gastrointestinal tract
- Cardiovascular system
- Pulmonary system
- Renal system

Involvement of the gastrointestinal (GI) tract, particularly the esophagus, is common. The esophagus loses its motility, resulting in dysphagia and esophageal reflux. A small, sliding hiatal hernia may be present, and swallowing may be difficult. Reflux of the gastric contents can cause esophagitis and subsequent ulceration, particularly in the lower two thirds of the esophagus. Intestinal changes are similar to those of the esophagus. Peristalsis is diminished, which causes clinical manifestations similar to a partial bowel obstruction. Malabsorption is a common complication, causing malodorous diarrheal stools.

In addition to assessing problems of the digestive tract, observe for cardiovascular manifestations. Raynaud's phenomenon occurs in various degrees in most clients with PSS. On exposure to cold or emotional stress, the small arterioles in the digits of both hands and feet rapidly constrict, which causes decreased blood flow. In severe cases, the client experiences digit necrosis, excruciating pain, and autoamputation of the distal digits (the tips of the digits fall off spontaneously). (See Chapter 39 for a complete discussion of this disorder.) In many clients, vasculitic lesions, often around the nail beds **(periungual lesions),** are evident. Myocardial fibrosis, another common problem, is evidenced by electrocardiographic (ECG) changes, cardiac dysrhythmias, and chest pain.

Lung involvement in the client with PSS may go undetected until late in the disease or sometimes until autopsy.

Fibrosis of the alveoli and interstitial tissues is present in almost all cases of the disease, but clinical manifestations may not be present. Clients with scleroderma and pulmonary arterial hypertension have a more serious prognosis. Recently, bosentan (Tracleer), the first of a new class of drugs called *endothelin receptor antagonists,* demonstrated (in clinical trials) improved walk tests for clients with class III-IV pulmonary arterial hypertension. Various doses improved clients' breathing during exercise, but the potential for liver injury at the highest dose caused recommended doses to be lowered. The client usually takes 62.5 mg twice daily for 4 weeks and then increases the dose to 125 mg twice daily. In clinical practice, clients seem to tolerate bosentan and demonstrate improved breathing. Teach the client the desired and potential adverse effects, including liver toxicity and birth defects.

Renal involvement is an important aspect of the overall disease process and often causes malignant hypertension and death. Assess for signs of impending organ failure, such as changes in urine output and increased blood pressure.

LABORATORY ASSESSMENT

The laboratory findings for PSS are similar to those for SLE. Clinical findings and the client's response to drug therapy help the health care provider differentiate between the two diseases. Additional tests depend on which organs seem to be affected. Upper and lower gastrointestinal series are commonly performed because of the frequency of GI clinical manifestations.

Interventions

The medical management of progressive systemic sclerosis (PSS) aims to force the disease into remission and thus slow disease progression. The health care provider uses drug therapy primarily for this purpose, but it is often unsuccessful. Systemic steroids and immunosuppressants are used in large doses and often in combination (see Chart 24-9).

Local skin protective measures can help to maintain skin integrity. Teach the client to use mild soap and lotions and gentle cleaning techniques. The skin should be inspected daily for further changes or open lesions. Skin ulcers are treated according to their type and location.

In addition to drug therapy to control the overall disease process, specific measures can provide comfort. The client with PSS not only experiences chronic joint pain but also has severe, acute pain during episodes of Raynaud's phenomenon. A bed cradle and footboard keep bed covers away from the skin in severe cases. Adjust the room temperature to prevent chilling, which can precipitate digit vasospasm. The client who can tolerate touching of the affected areas can wear gloves and socks to increase warmth. Because cigarette smoking and extreme emotional stress can also cause symptoms to recur, the client should try to avoid or minimize these factors as much as possible. Chapter 39 describes the management of clients with Raynaud's phenomenon in more detail.

The client with esophageal involvement may need small, frequent meals rather than the traditional three meals daily. He or she should minimize the intake of foods and liquids that stimulate gastric secretion (e.g., spicy foods, caffeine, alcohol). Instruct the client to keep his or her head elevated for 1 to 2 hours after meals. The client may need to be in this position continuously. Histamine antagonists and antacids help to reduce and neutralize gastric acid. To help prevent choking, collaborate with the dietitian for dietary changes (Chart 24-13).

CHART 24-13

BEST PRACTICE for
The Client with Progressive Systemic Sclerosis and Esophagitis

- Keep the client's head elevated at least 60 degrees during meals and for at least 1 hour after each meal.
- Provide small, frequent meals rather than three large meals each day.
- Give the client small amounts of food for each bite, and explain the importance of chewing each bite carefully before swallowing.
- Provide semisoft foods, such as mashed potatoes and pudding or custard; liquids are most likely to cause choking.
- Collaborate with the dietitian about the client's diet.
- Teach the client to avoid foods that increase gastric secretion, such as caffeine, pepper, and other spices.
- Give antacids if the health care provider prescribes them.

Nursing care for the client with joint pain and decreased mobility is very similar to that for the client with rheumatoid arthritis (see Interventions [Rheumatoid Arthritis], p. 397). Nonsteroidal anti-inflammatory drugs are given for inflammation and pain. Joint protection and energy conservation are also important for these clients.

Community-Based Care

Community-based care for the client with PSS is similar to that for the client with lupus. The client is treated at home but may need frequent hospitalizations if major organ involvement occurs during exacerbations. The Arthritis Foundation and Scleroderma Foundation are excellent resources for more information about the disease and how to manage it.

GOUT

PATHOPHYSIOLOGY

Gout, or gouty arthritis, is a systemic disease in which urate crystals deposit in the joints and other body tissues, causing inflammation. The cause and treatment of gout have been firmly established. The classic case of well-advanced disease is seldom seen today unless the client does not comply with the therapeutic regimen. There are two major types of gout: primary and secondary.

Primary gout is the most common type and results from one of several inborn errors of purine metabolism. An end product of purine metabolism is uric acid, which is usually excreted by the kidneys. In primary gout, the production of uric acid exceeds the excretion capability of the kidneys; sodium urate is deposited in synovium and other tissues, resulting in inflammation. Primary gout is inherited as an X-linked trait; males are affected through female carriers. Approximately 25% of clients have a family history of gout. Primary gout affects middle-aged and older men (85% to 90% of clients with gout) and postmenopausal women. The peak time of onset is during a person's 30s and 40s.

Secondary gout involves hyperuricemia (excessive uric acid in the blood) caused by another disease. Secondary gout affects people of all ages. Renal insufficiency, diuretic therapy, and certain chemotherapeutic agents decrease the normal excretion of uric acid and other waste products. Disorders such as multiple myeloma and certain carcinomas result in increased production of uric acid because of a greater turnover of cellular nucleic acids. Treatment involves management of the underlying disorder.

There are four phases of the primary disease process: asymptomatic hyperuricemic, acute, intercritical (intercurrent), and chronic. The client is usually unaware of the **asymptomatic hyperuricemic phase** unless he or she has had a serum uric acid level determination. The serum level is elevated, but no overt signs of the disease are present.

The first "attack" of gouty arthritis begins the **acute phase.** The client experiences excruciating pain and inflammation in one or more small joints, usually the metatarsophalangeal joint of the great toe. Of all clients with gout, 75% experience inflammation of this joint **(podagra)** as the initial manifestation. The erythrocyte sedimentation rate (ESR) and white blood cell count are increased as a result of the inflammatory process.

Months or perhaps years can pass before additional attacks occur; this is the **intercritical,** or intercurrent, **phase** of the disease. The client is asymptomatic, and no abnormalities are found during examination of the joints.

After repeated episodes of acute gout, deposits of urate crystals develop under the skin and within the major organs, particularly in the renal system. The client is then classified as having **chronic tophaceous gout.** In chronic gout, urate kidney stone formation is more common than renal insufficiency.

COLLABORATIVE MANAGEMENT

Assessment

Collect historical data, including age, gender, and a family history of gout. Gout affects more men than women, particularly men who have relatives with gout. A complete medical history is needed to determine whether gout has been caused by another problem. There is a tendency to overuse diuretics, especially among women, which can lead to secondary gout.

ACUTE GOUT

Overt manifestations are present in the acute and chronic phases of gout. You most likely will encounter a client with acute gout; chronic gout is not common in the United States today. Joint inflammation is the most common finding and is usually so painful that the client seeks medical care. Inspect the inflamed area. It is usually too painful and swollen to be touched or moved.

CHRONIC GOUT

With chronic gout, inspect the skin for **tophi,** or deposits of sodium urate crystals (Figure 24-9). Although tophi may occur anywhere, they commonly appear on the outer ear. Other common sites for tophi are the arms and fingers near the joints. The tophi are hard on palpation and are irregular in shape. When the skin over the tophi is irritated, it may break open, and a yellow, gritty substance is discharged. Infection may result.

Other manifestations of chronic gout include signs of renal calculi (stones) or renal dysfunction. Stones develop in about 20% of clients with gout. In some cases, urate kidney stones occur before the arthritis is present.

The health care provider orders determinations of serum uric acid levels to validate hyperuricemia. Because the serum uric acid level can be altered by food intake, serial measurements are usually obtained. A consistent level of more than 8 mg/100 mL is generally considered abnormal. Urinary uric acid levels are also measured; an overproduction of uric acid is confirmed by an excretion of more than 600 mg/24 hr after a 5-day restriction of purine intake.

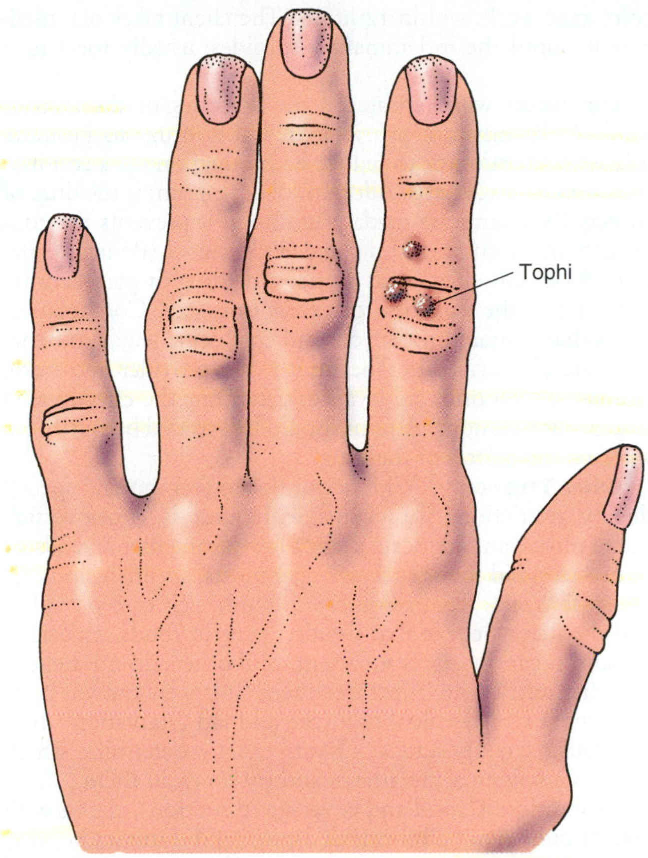

Figure 24-9 ■ Typical appearance of tophi, which may occur in chronic gout, on an index finger.

The health care provider may order renal function tests, such as blood urea nitrogen (BUN) and serum creatinine levels, to monitor possible kidney involvement. A definitive diagnostic test for the disease is synovial fluid aspiration (arthrocentesis) to detect the needle-like crystals that are characteristic of the disorder.

Interventions

Gout is one of the easiest diseases for the health care provider to diagnose and treat in its early phases. If the client receives treatment and complies with drug therapy, he or she should experience no further symptoms and no change in body image or lifestyle. The client with gout is usually treated on an ambulatory basis.

Drug Therapy. Drug therapy is the primary component of management for clients with gout. In acute gouty "attacks," the inflammation subsides spontaneously within 3 to 5 days; however, most clients cannot tolerate the pain for that long. The drugs used for acute gout are different from those used for chronic gout. The health care provider typically prescribes a combination of colchicine (Colsalide, Novocolchicine✱) and a nonsteroidal anti-inflammatory drug (NSAID), such as indomethacin (Indocin, Novomethacin✱) or ibuprofen (Motrin, Amersol✱), for acute gout. IV colchicine works within 12 hours. The client takes oral medications until the inflammation subsides, usually for 4 to 7 days.

For clients with repeated acute episodes or for chronic gout, the health care provider prescribes drugs to promote uric acid excretion or to reduce its production on a continuous, maintenance basis. Allopurinol (Zyloprim) is the drug of choice. As a xanthine oxidase inhibitor, it prevents the conversion of xanthine to uric acid. Probenecid (Benemid, Benuryl✱) is also effective as a uricosuric drug in gout because it promotes the excretion of excess uric acid. Combination drugs that contain probenecid and colchicine (e.g., ColBenemid) are also available. The health care provider and nurse monitor serum uric acid levels to determine the effectiveness of these medications. Aspirin should be avoided because it inactivates the effects of the drug.

Diet Therapy. Whether or not to recommend special dietary restrictions for clients with gout is controversial. Some physicians advocate a strict low-purine diet and advise clients to avoid foods such as organ meats, shellfish, and oily fish with bones (e.g., sardines). Some health care providers and dietitians believe that limiting protein foods, especially red and organ meats, is sufficient. Still others do not believe that diet restrictions affect treatment. It is well known, however, that excessive alcohol intake and fad "starvation" diets can cause a gouty attack. Clients usually determine which foods precipitate acute attacks and try to avoid them.

In addition to food and beverage restrictions, clients with gout should avoid all forms of aspirin and diuretics because they may precipitate an attack. Likewise, excessive physical or emotional stress can exacerbate the disease. Stress-management techniques may be helpful for the client with gout.

Having the client drink more fluids is one of the best measures to prevent the formation of urinary stones. Increasing fluid intake helps to dilute urine and prevent sediment formation. Uric acid is more soluble in urine with a high pH and therefore is less likely to form urinary stones in that environment. The client's urinary pH can be increased with an intake of alkaline ash foods, such as citrus fruits and juices, milk, and certain dairy products. The value of adhering to a strict diet rich in these foods is questionable, however.

The client with a diagnosis of gout is seldom hospitalized unless renal complications develop. If the client follows the prescribed interventions, chronic tophaceous gout should not develop.

OTHER CONNECTIVE TISSUE DISEASES

The care of clients with connective tissue diseases (CTDs) is often similar regardless of the specific diagnosis. This section describes other fairly common diseases that are classified as CTDs.

Polymyositis/Dermatomyositis

Polymyositis is a diffuse inflammatory disease of skeletal (striated) muscle that causes symmetric weakness and atrophy. When a rash accompanies polymyositis, the disease is called **dermatomyositis.** Both diseases vary in their mode of onset and progression and are characterized by spontaneous remissions and exacerbations. Women are affected twice as often as men, and men and women between 30 and 60 years of age are most susceptible to either disease.

In addition to proximal muscle and possible skin involvement, clients typically have polyarthritis, **polyarthralgia** (aching around multiple joints), and Raynaud's phenomenon (see Chapter 39). Clients with dermatomyositis have the characteristic heliotrope (lilac) rash and periorbital (around the eyes) edema. Malignant neoplasms are more common in these clients than in the rest of the population; as many as 30% of clients older than 55 years of age have malignancies. Many clients have difficulty swallowing or talking because of severe muscle weakness.

These conditions are treated with high-dose steroids, immunosuppressive agents, and supportive care. Particular attention is given to nutrition.

Systemic Necrotizing Vasculitis

Necrotizing vasculitis is a term for a group of diseases whose primary manifestation is **arteritis** (inflammation of arterial walls), which causes ischemia in the tissues usually supplied by the involved vessels. The drug of choice for most types of vasculitis is chronic steroid therapy (prednisone), although immunosuppressive drugs may also be used.

Polyarteritis nodosa affects middle-aged men most often and involves every body system. Treatment is similar to that for systemic lupus, but the prognosis is not as promising. Renal disorders and cardiac involvement are the most common causes of death. **Hypersensitivity vasculitis** is the most common form of vasculitis and primarily causes skin lesions as an allergic response to drugs, infections, or tumors. **Takayasu's arteritis,** or the **aortic arch syndrome,** is also called the "pulseless" disease. Women in their 20s, particularly those of Japanese descent, are affected most often. Cerebral ischemia is manifested by visual changes, syncope, and vertigo.

Polymyalgia Rheumatica and Temporal Arteritis

Polymyalgia rheumatica (PMR) is a clinical syndrome characterized by stiffness, weakness, and aching of the proximal musculature (i.e., the shoulder and pelvic girdles). Systemic manifestations such as low-grade fever, arthralgias (aching around joints) and stiffness, fatigue, and weight loss occur in the majority of cases. The most common joints affected are the neck, shoulder, and hip joints. Stiffness is worse in the morning.

Most clients have an increased erythrocyte sedimentation rate (ESR) and a normochromic, normocytic anemia (see Chart 24-8). The disease commonly occurs in women over 50 years of age and typically responds to low-dose steroid therapy in 1 to 3 days (Mikanowicz & Leslie, 2000).

Giant cell arteritis (GCA), or **temporal arteritis (TA),** occurs in as many as 20% of people with PMR. GCA is a systemic vasculitis that affects large and midsized arteries. Clinical manifestations may be classified as systemic, myalgic, and arteritic (Chart 24-14).

The cause of both PMR and GCA is unknown, but a genetic predisposition related to HLA-DRB1 is likely. The dis-

CHART 24-14

KEY FEATURES of
Giant Cell (Temporal) Arteritis

Systemic Manifestations
- Fatigue, malaise
- Fever
- Weight loss
- Night sweats

Myalgic Manifestations (if client has polymyalgia rheumatica [PMR])
- Proximal, symmetric muscle pain
- Stiffness

Arteritic Manifestations
- Erythema
- Pain (especially localized temporal headache)
- Swelling
- Tenderness (especially scalp)
- Amaurosis fugax (temporary vision loss in one eye)
- Diplopia or any vision change (requires urgent management)

order is easy to miss because most clients are older women who complain of declining vision (also an age-related change). GCA is treated *urgently* with high doses of corticosteroids, often as high as 40 to 80 mg daily (Mikanowicz & Leslie, 2000). Taking calcium and vitamin D is important for preventing osteoporosis that can result from steroid therapy, especially in middle-aged women.

Ankylosing Spondylitis

Ankylosing spondylitis (AS) is also known as *Marie-Strümpell disease* or *rheumatoid spondylitis.* The disease affects the vertebral column and causes spinal deformities. Although this disorder is present in both men and women at any age in adulthood, young white men under 40 years of age are most commonly affected. Other features include **iritis** (inflammation of the iris), arthritis or arthralgia (joint aching), and nonspecific systemic manifestations such as malaise and weight loss.

Although the exact cause is unknown, ankylosing spondylitis is associated with the HLA-B27 antigen. Compromised respiratory function caused by a rigid chest wall is the major threat to health. Most clients function normally but live with chronic discomfort. As in other times of inflammatory arthritis, anti-inflammatory drugs, heat applications, and physical therapy are the key components of management (see earlier discussion of pain management for rheumatoid arthritis, p. 397).

Disease-modifying antirheumatic drugs (DMARDs), such as methotrexate (Rheumatrex), have been successful in slowing disease progress. Biological response modifiers (TNF inhibitors), such as infliximab (Remicade), have also been approved for managing ankylosing spondylitis.

Reiter's Syndrome

As with ankylosing spondylitis, **Reiter's syndrome** is associated with the HLA-B27 antigen. This disease most often affects young white men. The complete syndrome is a triad of arthritis, conjunctivitis, and **urethritis** (inflammation of the urethra) resulting from exposure to sexually transmitted disease or dysentery (infectious diarrhea). Urethritis is often the first clinical manifestation.

Although the disease is characterized by this triad of manifestations, other conditions such as **balanitis circinata** (ringlike inflammation of the glans penis) and skin lesions are equally significant for confirmation of the diagnosis.

Management is symptomatic and may be complex if there is organ involvement. NSAIDs and physical therapy are generally prescribed.

Sjögren's Syndrome

With **Sjögren's syndrome,** inflammatory cells and immune complexes obstruct secretory ducts and glands. As a result, the client has dry eyes *(sicca syndrome),* a dry mouth *(xerostomia),* and a dry vagina. Severe cases involve swelling of the parotid and lacrimal areas and systemic manifestations (e.g., fever, fatigue). Of clients with the syndrome, 50% have an associated disease, such as rheumatoid arthritis (RA) or progressive systemic sclerosis (PSS).

Local management includes meticulous care of the mouth, eyes, and perineal areas and the use of artificial tears and saliva. Systemic steroids (prednisone) may also be administered. Pilocarpine is sometimes useful for the eyes. Without treatment, the client can lose vision, and oral ulcerations, dental caries, and difficulty in swallowing or talking may ensue.

Marfan Syndrome

Marfan syndrome is inherited as an autosomal, dominant trait with equal prevalence in males and females. Clients with this syndrome have abnormalities of the skeletal, ocular, cardiopulmonary, and central nervous systems as a result of a basic defect in extracellular microfibrils. Microfibrils are very small fibers within cells.

Clients with the classic form of Marfan syndrome tend to be excessively tall and have elongated hands and feet. The diagnosis of milder forms of Marfan syndrome is often missed in young men, especially athletes involved in sports such as basketball.

Other skeletal abnormalities include scoliosis, a funnel-shaped chest, loss of the normal cervical curve, and hyperextensibility of the joints. Subluxation of the lens is usually bilateral and occurs by the age of 5 years, causing decreased visual acuity or glaucoma.

Cardiovascular problems are responsible for most deaths resulting from Marfan syndrome. The average life span is 32 years. Mitral valve prolapse with regurgitation as well as aortic aneurysm with regurgitation and aortic rupture are common. The client is closely monitored by echocardiography (Holcomb, 2000).

Management is both palliative and preventive and includes careful monitoring, cardiovascular medications, and orthopedic surgery if needed. Genetic counseling should also be part of the treatment plan, especially for women of childbearing age.

Infectious Arthritis

Any infectious agent can invade the joint space and cause inflammation and tissue destruction. Certain pathogens, such as *Staphylococcus aureus,* destroy tissue rapidly; others, especially viruses, do not cause irreversible damage. The cornerstone of management is local or systemic antibiotic therapy for 6 to 8 weeks.

Lyme Disease

Lyme arthritis is a reportable systemic infectious disease caused by the spirochete ***Borrelia burgdorferi*** and results from the bite of an infected deer tick. Signs and symptoms of Lyme disease generally begin with identification of a large "bull's-eye" circular rash along with malaise, fever, headache, and muscle or joint aches. More than 85% of the disease in the United States is seen in New England; the mid-Atlantic states, including Maryland and Virginia; the upper mid-West, including Wisconsin and Minnesota; and northern California, especially during the summer months (Sigal, 2001).

In the early and localized stage I, the client appears with flu-like symptoms, rash (erythema migrans, the "bull's-eye" rash), and pain and stiffness in the muscles and joints. Symptoms begin within 3 to 32 days of the tick bite. Doxycycline, amoxicillin, or cefuroxime is prescribed for 10 to 21 days.

Stage II (early disseminated stage) occurs 2 to 12 weeks after the tick bite. The client experiences carditis with dysrhythmias, dyspnea, dizziness, or palpitations as well as central nervous system disorders such as meningitis, facial paralysis (often misdiagnosed as Bell's palsy), and peripheral neuritis. For severe disease, IV antibiotics (e.g., ceftriaxone or cefotaxime) are given.

If Lyme disease is not diagnosed and treated in the earlier stages, later chronic complications (e.g., arthralgias, fatigue, and memory/thinking problems) can result. This late stage III (chronic persistent stage) occurs weeks to years after the tick bite. For some clients, the first and only sign of Lyme disease is arthritis. In other cases the disease may not respond to antibiotics, and the client develops permanent damage to joints and the nervous system (Sigal, 2001). Prevention is the best strategy for Lyme disease (Chart 24-15).

CHART 24-15

CLIENT EDUCATION GUIDE

Prevention and Early Detection of Lyme Disease

- Avoid heavily wooded areas or areas with thick underbrush.
- Walk in the center of the trail.
- Avoid dark clothing. Lighter-colored clothing makes spotting ticks easier.
- Use an insect repellent on your skin and clothes when in an area where ticks are likely to be found.
- Wear long-sleeved tops and long pants.
- Wear closed shoes and a hat or cap.
- Bathe immediately after being in an infested area, and inspect your body for ticks (about the size of a pinhead); pay special attention to your arms, legs, and hairline.
- Gently remove with tweezers or fingers any tick that you find. Dispose of the tick by flushing it down the toilet (burning a tick could spread infection).
- Wait 4 to 6 weeks after being bitten by a tick before being tested for Lyme disease (testing before this time is not reliable).
- Report symptoms, such as a rash or influenza-like illness, to your physician.
- Obtain a vaccine to prevent disease if you live in a high-risk area.

Pseudogout

Pseudogout is a disease that mimics the clinical manifestations of gout. In this disease, however, the crystals deposited in the joints are calcium pyrophosphate, not sodium urate. These crystals usually migrate to cartilage, but they can also deposit in tendons, ligaments, and synovium.

The client most susceptible to pseudogout is an older hospitalized male. Although the cause is not certain, the incidence is highest in men with metastatic cancer or endocrine imbalances such as hypothyroidism. Nonsteroidal anti-inflammatory drugs (NSAIDs) usually control manifestations of the disease.

Psoriatic Arthritis

Psoriatic arthritis (PsA) affects about 5% to 10% of people who have psoriasis, a skin condition characterized by a scaly, itchy rash, usually on the elbows, knees, and scalp. Fingernail and toenail lifting and pitting may also occur (see Chapter 70 for discussion of this disease). The joint pain associated with psoriasis is often associated with stiffness, especially in the morning. Neck and back pain are particularly common, but various forms of the disease can cause small joint arthritis or involvement of the sacroiliac joints of the spine.

TABLE 24-3 Common Disorders Associated with Arthritis

Crohn's disease	Hyperparathyroidism
Ulcerative colitis	Hyperthyroidism
Tuberculosis	Diabetes mellitus
Hemophilia	Sickle-cell anemia crisis
Whipple's disease	Psoriasis
Intestinal bypass surgery	Infection

Psoriatic arthritis (PsA) occurs most often in people between 20 and 50 in men and women of all races. Nail symptoms are common in clients who have the associated arthritis. Causes may include genetic and environmental factors, infectious agents, and immune system dysfunction.

Although most clients do not experience destructive and deforming arthritis, those who do suffer a major impact on their quality of life. Treatment is focused on managing joint pain and inflammation, controlling skin lesions, and slowing the progression of the disease. Health teaching for skin care is similar to that for lupus. Management of joint inflammation is similar to that for rheumatoid arthritis. Methotrexate (Rheumatrex), sulfasalazine (Azulfidine), and biological response modifiers have been used with success. Further discussion regarding management of psoriasis can be found in Chapter 70.

Other Disease-Associated Arthritis

A number of other diseases can cause secondary arthritis. Tuberculosis, Crohn's disease, ulcerative colitis, hemophilia, and sickle-cell anemia are typical examples. To manage joint involvement, the primary disease is treated. For example, when a client with Crohn's disease is in remission, joint manifestations also subside. Conditions in which joint involvement can occur are presented in Table 24-3.

Fibromyalgia Syndrome

Fibromyalgia syndrome (FMS), also referred to as simply fibromyalgia, was previously known as fibrositis. The name was changed because FMS is now understood to be a

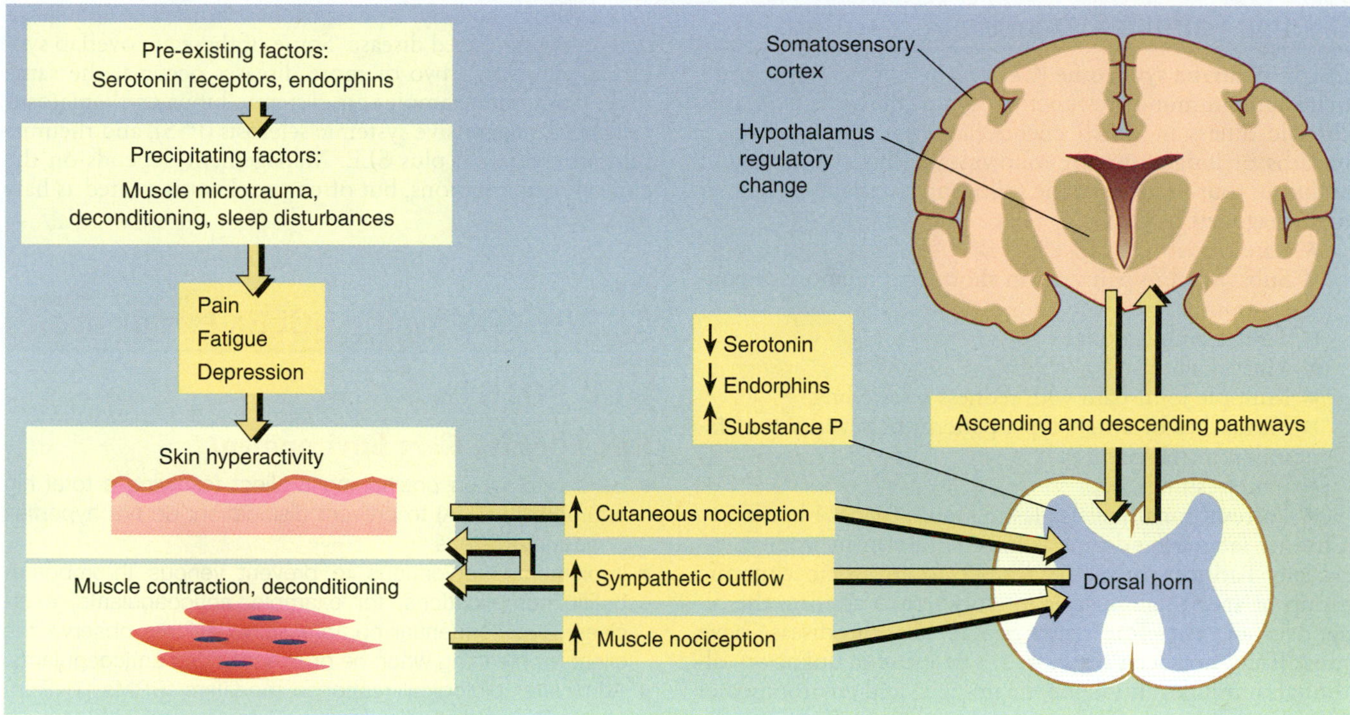

Figure 24-10 ■ Theoretic pathophysiologic model of fibromyalgia.

chronic pain syndrome, not an inflammatory disease. Pain and tenderness are located at specific sites in the back of the neck, upper chest, trunk, low back, and extremities. These tender points are also known as **trigger points** and can typically be palpated to elicit pain in a predictable, reproducible pattern. The pain is typically described as burning and gnawing. As seen in the theoretic pathophysiologic model in Figure 24-10, increased muscle tenderness may be due to the inability to tolerate pain, possibly related to dysfunction in the brain, especially the thalamus and hypothalamus (McCance & Huether, 2002).

The pain and tenderness tend to come and go but typically worsen in response to stress, increased activity, and weather conditions. The client complains of mild to severe fatigue, and sleep disturbances are common. Some clients note numbness or tingling in their extremities, and others are sensitive to noxious odors, loud noises, and bright lights. Headaches and jaw pain are also common.

Other symptoms include the following:

- Gastrointestinal (GI), including abdominal pain, diarrhea and constipation, and heartburn
- Genitourinary, including dysuria, urinary frequency, urgency, and pelvic pain
- Cardiovascular, including dyspnea, chest pain, and dysrhythmias
- Visual, including blurred vision and dry eyes

Many clients with these symptoms become frustrated because they are not properly diagnosed and are in constant pain and discomfort. Some clients are diagnosed as having chronic fatigue syndrome (CFS). CFS, migraine headache, irritable bowel syndrome (IBS), and myofascial pain are often present in clients with FMS. As a result, clients can become depressed and anxious.

Most clients are women between 30 and 50 years of age. It is unlikely that the disease is caused by one factor. Possible precipitating factors include CFS, Lyme disease, trauma, medications, and flu-like illness (McCance & Huether, 2002). FMS may also be aggravated by deep-sleep deprivation. Instruct clients to limit caffeine, alcohol, or other unnecessary substances that could interfere with deep sleep. Establish a regular sleep pattern.

Secondary FMS can accompany any connective tissue disease (CTD), particularly lupus and rheumatoid disease, and may not necessarily be related to sleep patterns. Antidepressive agents such as amitriptyline (Elavil, Apo-Amitriptyline✱) or nortriptyline (Pamelor) may promote sleep and reduce pain or muscle spasm. These drugs should be used with caution in older adults because they can cause confusion and orthostatic hypotension. Trazodone (Desyrel) may be preferred for this population because of its minimal side effects. Selective serotonin reuptake inhibitors (SSRIs), such as sertraline (Zoloft) and escitalopram oxalate (Lexapro), may be prescribed to manage depression. Observe for side effects. Monitor for postural blood pressure changes. Instruct clients to observe for drowsiness and not to operate dangerous machinery or drive if drowsy.

Physical therapy, along with nonsteroidal anti-inflammatory drugs (NSAIDs) and muscle relaxants may be prescribed to help decrease fibromyalgia pain. Instruct the client to exercise at home regularly. Home exercise should include stretching, strengthening, and low-impact aerobic exercise. Walking, swimming, rowing, biking, and water exercise are good examples of low-impact exercise. Complementary and alternative therapies, such as tai chi, acupuncture, hypnosis, and stress management, may help some clients with symptom relief (Taggart, et al., 2003). Refer the client to the land, water, and walking exercise pamphlets produced by the Arthritis Foundation. Inform clients about the National Chronic Fatigue Syndrome and Fibromyalgia Association for additional information.

Chronic Fatigue Syndrome

Chronic fatigue syndrome (CFS), also known as chronic fatigue and immune dysfunction syndrome (CFIDS), is a chronic illness in which clients have severe fatigue for 6 months or longer, usually following flu-like symptoms. In addition, four or more of the following criteria must be met for a diagnosis of CFS:

- Sore throat
- Substantial impairment in short-term memory or concentration
- Tender lymph nodes
- Muscle pain
- Multiple joint pain with redness or swelling
- Headaches of a new type, pattern, or severity (not familiar to the client)
- Unrefreshing sleep
- Postexertional malaise lasting more than 24 hours

Chronic fatigue syndrome is most common in women, especially Latinos, and is not limited to any socioeconomic group or age. There is no laboratory test to confirm the diagnosis, and therefore many people with the disease have most likely not been diagnosed. The cause is unknown, although immune, endocrine, neurologic, and environmental factors are being studied.

Management of the client is challenging in that there is no cure for FMS. Treatment is supportive and focuses on alleviation or reduction of symptoms. For example, NSAIDs may help with body aches and pain. Low-dose antidepressants may also be effective in promoting sleep and preventing or treating depression. Teach the client to follow good health practices, such as adequate sleep, proper nutrition, regular exercise (but not excessive to increase fatigue), stress management, and energy conservation. Complementary and alternative therapies, such as acupuncture, tai chi, massage, and herbal supplements may be helpful for some clients.

Refer the client to the National Chronic Fatigue Syndrome and Fibromylagia Association, American Association for Chronic Fatigue Syndrome, and the Chronic Fatigue and Immune Dysfunction Syndrome Association of America.

Local Inflammatory Disorders

Two of the most common inflammatory conditions, bursitis and tendinitis, are localized to specific connective tissues. Both problems are caused by repetitive motion and overuse related to aging, sports, or work injuries. **Bursitis** is an irritation of subcutaneous tissues and inflammation of the underlying bursae. **Tendinitis** is inflammation of one or more tendon sheaths.

Tight shoes often irritate the heel and cause bursitis. Higher impact aerobic exercise and diseases such as rheumatoid arthritis (RA) and gout can lead to bursitis and tendinitis.

The conservative management for both inflammatory conditions includes rest, ice, and NSAIDs to relieve pain. More aggressive treatment may include corticosteroid injections or surgery to remove the inflamed tissue.

Mixed Connective Tissue Disease

A diagnosis of mixed CTD is made when a client presents with clinical manifestations that are not typical of any one CTD. Approximately 10% of clients with CTDs are classified as having mixed disease. Some of these are overlap syndromes, in which two or more diseases occur at the same time. Common examples are systemic lupus erythematosus (SLE) plus progressive systemic sclerosis (PSS), and rheumatoid arthritis (RA) plus SLE. Management depends on the clinical manifestations, but often the client is treated as having SLE.

GET READY for the NCLEX Examination!

KEY POINTS

Safe Effective Care Environment

- Be careful when positioning a client following a total hip arthroplasty (THA) to prevent dislocation; do not hyperflex or adduct the legs.
- Implement interventions to prevent venous thromboembolitic complications, for example, anticoagulants, exercises, and sequential compression devices; observe the client for bleeding when he or she is taking anticoagulants.
- Administer biological response modifiers (BRMs [TNF inhibitors]) and other disease-modifying agents with caution; do not give TNF inhibitors to clients with tuberculosis or multiple sclerosis.
- Prioritize care for clients with systemic lupus erythematosus (SLE) by monitoring for life-threatening complications, such as renal failure.

Health Promotion and Maintenance

- Teach clients who have osteoarthritis (OA) or are prone to the disease to lose weight (if obese), avoid trauma, and limit strenuous weight-bearing activities.
- Instruct clients with arthritic pain to use multiple modalities for pain relief, including ice/heat, rest, positioning, complementary and alternative therapies, and medications as prescribed.
- Remind clients with arthritis and connective tissue diseases to contact local chapters of the Arthritis Foundation and other disease-specific national groups for information and support groups.
- Teach clients to monitor and report side and adverse effects of drugs used to treat OA and connective tissue diseases.
- Teach clients who are taking hydroxychloroquine (Plaquenil) to have frequent (every 6 months) eye examinations to monitor for retinal changes.
- Reinforce the importance of good health practices, such as adequate sleep, proper nutrition, regular exercise, and stress-management techniques.
- Teach clients with arthritis what exercises to do (Chart 24-5), joint protection techniques (Chart 24-6), and energy conservation guidelines (Chart 24-10).

Psychosocial Integrity

- Recognize that clients with rheumatoid arthritis (RA) may have body image disturbance as a result of potentially deforming joint involvement and nodules.
- Encourage clients with arthritis and connective tissue diseases to "ventilate" about their chronic illness and identify coping strategies that have previously been successful.

- Be aware that chronic, painful diseases affect the client's quality of life and role performance.
- Accept behaviors of clients that may seem manipulative or demanding and emphasize the clients' strengths.
- Teach clients with SLE to avoid sunlight; exacerbations of the disease may be triggered.
- Remind clients with gout to avoid factors that trigger an attack, such as aspirin, organ meats, and alcohol.
- Teach people ways to avoid Lyme disease as listed in Chart 24-15.
- Recognize that clients with fibromyalgia syndrome (FMS) and chronic fatigue syndrome (CFS) are often frustrated because they have not been diagnosed or have been misdiagnosed.
- Teach clients with FMS and CFS that antidepressant drugs can promote sleep and decrease pain as well as prevent or treat the depression that is common with these illnesses.

Physiological Integrity

- Be aware that most of the connective tissue diseases and arthritic disorders have a genetic basis as part of their etiology; most are also classified as autoimmune diseases and have remissions and exacerbations.
- Differentiate that OA is primarily a degenerative joint problem, whereas rheumatoid arthritis RA is a systemic disease.
- Realize that older clients have OA more than younger clients; younger clients have RA more than older adults; other differences between the two diseases are summarized in Table 24-1.
- Monitor laboratory test results for clients with autoimmune connective tissue diseases as highlighted in Chart 24-8.
- Assess for side and adverse effects of medications used for arthritis and connective tissue diseases as specified in Chart 24-9.
- Be aware that disease-modifying antirheumatic drugs (DMARDs) and BRMs slow the progression of connective tissue diseases, especially RA and SLE.
- Assess clients with rheumatoid arthritis for early or late clinical manifestations as listed in Chart 24-7.
- Differentiate clinical manifestations and prognosis for clients with SLE versus progressive systemic sclerosis (PSS), as listed in Chart 24-11.
- Plan interdisciplinary care for clients with arthritis and other diseases in which arthritis is a major manifestation.
- Assess for swallowing ability in clients who have PSS; collaborate with the dietitian for food modifications if needed.
- Monitor for acute joint inflammation for clients with a history of gout; the great toe and other small joints are most typically affected.
- Assess for visual complaints (indicating possible giant cell arteritis) in clients with polymyalgia rheumatica; report changes immediately to the health care provider.
- Be aware that arthritis often accompanies other diseases, such as psoriasis, Crohn's disease, and hemophilia.

ADDITIONAL STUDY RESOURCES

Go to your Student CD-ROM for Review Questions for the NCLEX Examination.

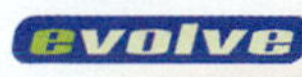

Go to http://evolve.elsevier.com/Iggy/ for Integrated Management of Care Questions for the NCLEX Examination.

SELECTED BIBLIOGRAPHY

Asterisk indicates a classic or definitive work on this subject.

Abelson, A.G., et al. (2002). A common sense guide to rheumatologic tests. *Patient Care for the Nurse Practitioner, 6(Apr).*

Amado, J.A., & Thomas, D.J. (2002). Early Recognition of Marfan's syndrome. *Journal of the American Academy of Nurse Practitioners, 14*(5), 201-204.

American College of Rheumatology Subcommittee on Rheumatoid Arthritis Guidelines. (2002). Guidelines for the management of rheumatoid arthritis. *Arthritis & Rheumatism, 46*(2), 328-342.

Arthritis Foundation. (2003). 2003 Drug guide. *Supplement to Arthritis Today, 1-26.*

Barry, F.P. (2003). Mesenchymal stem cell therapy in joint disease. *Novartis Foundation Symposium, 249*, 86-96.

Berger, R.A. (2003). Total hip arthroplasty using the minimally invasive two-incision approach. *Clinical Orthopedics, 417*, 232-241.

Branson, J.J., & Goldstein, W.M. (2003). Primary total hip arthroplasty. *AORN Journal, 78*(6), 956-969.

Cohen, M., Wolfe, R., Mai, T., & Lewis, D. (2003). A randomized, double blind, placebo controlled trial of a topical cream containing glucosamine sulfate, chondroitin sulfate, and camphor for osteoarthritis of the knee. *Journal of Rheumatology, 30*(3), 523-528.

D'Arcy, Y. (2002). How to treat arthritis pain. *Nursing 2002, 32*(7), 30-31.

*Eaton, L., & Meiner, S.E. (1999). Marfan syndrome: Identification and management. *MEDSURG Nursing, 8*(2), 113-117.

Edworthy, S.M. (2001). Clinical manifestations of systemic lupus erythematosus. In W.N. Kelley et al. (Eds.), *Textbook of rheumatology* (6th ed., pp. 1105-1123). Philadelphia: W.B. Saunders.

*Geier, K. (1998). Perioperative blood management. *Orthopaedic Nursing, 17*(Suppl 1), 6-36.

Gemmell, H.A., Jacobson, B.H., & Hayes, B.M. (2003). Effect of a topical herbal cream on osteoarthritis of the hand and knee: A pilot study. *Journal of Manipulative Physiologic Therapy, 26*(5), 15.

Gever, M.P. (2002). Infliximab: Test your drug IQ. *Critical Care, 33*(1), 32cc6-32cc7.

Goolsby, M.J. (2002). Guidelines for the management of rheumatoid arthritis: 2002 Update. *Journal of the American Academy of Nurse Practitioners, 14*(10), 432-437.

Hahn, B.H. (2001). Management of systemic lupus erythematosus. In W.N. Kelley et al. (Eds.), *Textbook of rheumatology* (6th ed., pp. 1125-1143). Philadelphia: W.B. Saunders.

Harris, E.D. (2001). Treatment of rheumatoid arthritis. In W.N. Kelley et al. (Eds.), *Textbook of rheumatology* (6th ed., pp. 1001-1022). Philadelphia: W.B. Saunders.

Hawke, M. (2002). Scleroderma–conquering the unknown. *Nursing Spectrum,* 12(19DC):10-11.

Holcomb, S.S. (2000). Reviewing Marfan syndrome. *Nursing 2000, 30*(5), 32cc10-32cc12.

Hussar, D. (2002). New drugs 2002–Part III. *Nursing 2002, 32*(7), 60.

Hutchinson, R. (2004). Pain control: COX-2-selective NSAIDs. *American Journal of Nursing, 104*(3), 52-56.

Ignatavicius, D.D. (2001). Rheumatoid arthritis and the older adult. *Geriatric Nursing, 22*(3), 139-142.

Kajs-Wyllie, M. (2002). Lupus cerebritis: A case study. *Journal of Neuroscience Nursing, 34*(4), 176-182.

Karch, A.M., & Karch, F.E.(2003). A Weekly Dosage Taken Daily: Drugs available in new once-weekly formulations require extra vigilance. *American Journal of Nursing, 103*(4), 64.

Kastanek, L. (2002). Using Anakinra for adult rheumatoid arthritis. *The Nurse Practitioner. 27*(4), 62-65.

*Kee, C.C. (1998). Living with osteoarthritis: Insiders' views. *Applied Nursing Research, 11*(1), 19-26.

Kee, C.C. (2000). Osteoarthritis: Manageable scourge of aging. *Nursing Clinics of North America, 35*(1), 199-208.

Kerr, K.L., & Johnson, D.A. (2000). Advanced practice nurses in rheumatology. *Practice View–American College of Rheumatology, 1*(7), 1-8.

Kettelman, K. (2000). Soothing the ache of joint surgery. *Nursing 2000, 30*(7), 14.

Klippel, J.H. (2001). *Primer on the rheumatic diseases* (12th ed.). Atlanta: The Arthritis Foundation.

Kremer, J.M. (2001). Nutrition and rheumatic diseases. In W.N. Kelley, et al. (Eds.), *Textbook of rheumatology* (6th ed., pp. 713-727). Philadelphia: W.B. Saunders.

Kuper, B.C., & Failla, S. (2000). Systemic lupus erythematosus: A multisystem autoimmune disorder. *Nursing Clinics of North America, 35*(1), 253-266.

*Lash, A.A. (1998). Quality of life in systemic lupus erythematosus. *Applied Nursing Research, 11*(3), 130-137.

*Lavernia C.J., Guzman, J.F., & Gachupin-Garcia, A. (1999). Cost effectiveness and quality of life in knee arthroplasty. *Clinical Orthopaedics, 345,* 134-139.

Litton, K.A. (2003). Defenses gone awry. *RN, 66* (3), *53-59.*

Loeser, R.F. (2003). A stepwise approach to the management of osteoarthritis. *Bulletin on the Rheumatic Diseases, 52*(5), 1-4.

Mankin, H.J., & Brandt, K.D. (2001). Pathogenesis of osteoarthritis. In W.N. Kelley, et al. (Eds.), *Textbook of rheumatology* (6th ed., pp. 1391-1407). Philadelphia: W.B. Saunders.

*Matula, P.A., & Shollenberger, D. (1999). Total joint project: Acute care to home care. *MEDSURG Nursing, 8*(2), 92-98.

McCaffrey, R., & Freeman, E. (2003). Effect of music on chronic osteoarthritis pain in older people. *Journal of Advanced Nursing, 44*(5), 517-524.

McCance, K.L., & Huether, S.E. (2002). *Pathophysiology* (4th ed.). St. Louis: Mosby.

*McGrath, A. (1997). Clinical snapshot: Raynaud's syndrome. *American Journal of Nursing, 97*(1), 34-35.

Medication Update Department. (2003). Rheumatoid arthritis treatment approved. *The Nurse Practitioner, 28*(4), 51.

Mikanowicz, C.K., & Leslie, M. (2000). Polymyalgia rheumatica and temporal arteritis: A case presentation. *Nursing Clinics of North America, 35*(1), 245-252.

*Morris, B.A., Colwell, C.W., & Hardwick, M.E. (1998). The use of low molecular weight heparins in the prevention of venous thromboembolic disease. *Orthopaedic Nursing, 17*(6), 23-29.

Pepper, G.A. (2000). Nonsteroidal anti-inflammatory drugs: New perspectives on a familiar class. *Nursing Clinics of North America, 35*(1), 223-244.

Petruzzi, L.M. & Vivino, F.B. (2003). Sjögren's syndrome–implications for perioperative practice. *AORN Journal 77*(3), 611-612, 614, 616-621, 624-628.

*Ritter, M.A., et al. (1999). Intra-articular morphine and/or bupivacaine after total knee replacement. *Journal of Bone and Joint Surgery, 81*(2), 301-303.

Sears, J.R., & Ganger, P.M. (2000). Antibiotics to treat RA. *RN, 63*(1), 41-42.

Sharkey, N.A., Williams, N.I., & Guerin, J.B. (2000). The role of exercise in the prevention and treatment of osteoporosis and osteoarthritis. *Nursing Clinics of North America, 35*(1), 209-222.

Siebold, J.R. (2001). Scleroderma and mixed connective tissue diseases In W.N. Kelley, et al. (Eds.), *Textbook of rheumatology* (6th ed., pp. 1211-1239). Philadelphia: W.B. Saunders.

Sigal, L.H. (2001). Lyme disease. In W.N. Kelley, et al. (Eds.), *Textbook of rheumatology* (6th ed., pp. 1485-1492). Philadelphia: W.B. Saunders.

Sledge, C.B., et al. (2001). The hip. In W.N. Kelley, et al. (Eds.), *Textbook of rheumatology* (6th ed., pp. 1743-1759). Philadelphia: W.B. Saunders.

Smedstad, L.M., & Liang, M.H. (2001). Psychosocial management of rheumatic diseases. In W.N. Kelley et al. (Eds.), *Textbook of rheumatology* (6th ed., pp. 729-734). Philadelphia: W.B. Saunders.

Solomon, L. (2001). Clinical features of osteoarthritis. In W.N. Kelley et al. (Eds.), *Textbook of rheumatology* (6th ed., pp. 1409-1418). Philadelphia: W.B. Saunders.

Strand, C.V., & Keystone, E. (2001). Biologic agents for the treatment of rheumatoid arthritis. In W.N. Kelley et al. (Eds.), *Textbook of rheumatology* (6th ed., pp. 899-911). Philadelphia: W.B. Saunders.

Taggert, H.M., et al. (2003). Effects of t'ai chi exercise on fibromyalgia symptoms and health-related quality of life. *Orthopaedic Nursing, 22*(5), 353-360.

Wade, N. (2003). Autoimmune diseases share a genetic defect, scientists find. Accessed April 18, 2004, from http://www.immunesupport.com/library/showarticle.cfm/ID/1575.

Weinblatt, M.E., et al. (2003). Adalimumab, a fully human anti-tumor necrosis factor (monoclonal antibody, for the treatment of rheumatoid arthritis in patients taking concomitant methotrexate–the Armada Trial. *Arthritis & Rheumatism, 49*(1), 35-45.

Wenz, J.F., Gurkan, I., & Jibodh, S.R. (2002). Mini-incision total hip arthroplasty: A comparative assessment of perioperative outcomes. *Orthopedics, 25*(10), 1031-1043.

Windsor, R.E.M., & Insall, J.N. (2001). The knee. In W.N. Kelley, et al. (Eds.), *Textbook of rheumatology* (6th ed., pp. 1759-1769). Philadelphia: W.B. Saunders.

Wise, C. (2003). The rational use of steroid injections in arthritis and nonarticular musculoskeletal pain syndromes. *Bulletin on the Rheumatic Diseases, 52*(1), 1-4.

CHAPTER 25

Interventions for Clients with HIV/AIDS and Other Immunodeficiencies

JAMES G. SAMPSON

LEARNING OUTCOMES

After studying this chapter, you should be able to:

1. Compare primary and secondary immunodeficiencies for cause and onset of problems.
2. Explain the differences in nursing care required for a client with a pathogenic infection versus a client with an opportunistic infection.
3. Distinguish between the conditions of human immunodeficiency virus (HIV) infection and acquired immunodeficiency syndrome (AIDS) for clinical manifestations and risks for complications.
4. Describe the ways in which HIV is transmitted.
5. Identify techniques to reduce the risk for infection in an immunocompromised client.
6. Develop a teaching plan for condom use among sexually active, non–English-speaking adults.
7. Prioritize nursing care for the client with AIDS who has impaired gas exchange.
8. Identify teaching priorities for the HIV-positive client receiving highly active antiretroviral therapy.
9. Develop a community-based teaching plan for the client with immune deficiency living at home.
10. Plan a week of meals for the client who has protein-calorie malnutrition.
11. Identify drug therapy categories that have the potential to reduce immune function.
12. Describe the infections that adult clients with congenital immunodeficiencies are at greatest risk for developing.
13. Describe the nursing actions and responsibilities for administration of IV immunoglobulin.

Go to your Student CD-ROM for Review Questions for the NCLEX Examination keyed to these Learning Outcomes.

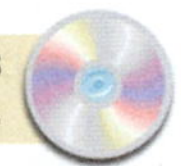

Immune system function is concerned with helping the body prevent infection. The immune system assists the body to monitor and maintain those cells and substances that are considered "self," belonging to the body. Such things as newly made cells and compatible blood transfusions are deemed self and safe by the immune system. However, when the immune system detects something that does not belong to the body and represents a potential threat, its job is then to attack and destroy the "non-self" or "foreign" substance. Infection is a major threat. We are exposed to many organisms every day. The efficiency of the immune system prevents disease despite this exposure.

When the immune system fails to recognize infectious threats, disaster can soon follow. Immune system failure can be the result of a primary (congenital) immunodeficiency in which one or more parts of the system are not functioning properly from birth. These problems are usually genetic mutations that are discovered in the infant or child who is repeatedly sick. Immune system failure can also be secondary (acquired after birth) as the result of viral infection, contact with a toxin, or medical therapy. These problems can cause a normal immune system to stop functioning. In either case, the immune system is no longer able to distinguish what should be in the body from a foreign invader. The consequences for the immunodeficient client can range from mild, localized health problems to total immune system failure, leaving the body open to attack from any foreign pathogen.

Acquired (Secondary) Immunodeficiencies

ACQUIRED IMMUNODEFICIENCY SYNDROME

PATHOPHYSIOLOGY

Acquired immunodeficiency syndrome (AIDS) is the most common secondary immunodeficiency disease in the world. First identified in 1981, HIV/AIDS is now a serious worldwide epidemic.

Etiology and Genetic Risk

The cause of HIV infection is a virus–the human immunodeficiency virus. Like most viruses, HIV is a parasite looking for a way into a cell, to take over the cell, and to force the cell into making more copies of itself. These new virus particles then look for additional cells to infect, repeating the cycle as long as there are new host cells to infect.

THE HIV INFECTIOUS PROCESS

VIRAL FEATURES. The virus particle has an outer envelope with special "docking proteins," known as gp41 and gp120, that assist in finding a host (Figure 25-1). Inside, the virus has two protein coatings and the genetic material with reverse transcriptase (RT) attached. The first challenge is for the HIV particle to get inside a host cell. HIV accomplishes this task by finding a way into the host's bloodstream. One of the cells that it "hijacks" is the CD4+ lymphocyte, also known as the CD4+ cell, helper/inducer T-cell, or T4-cell (see Chapter 23). This cell directs immune system defenses and regulates the activity of all immune system cells. If the HIV successfully enters a CD4+ cell, it can then create more virus particles.

VIRUS-HOST INTERACTIONS. When a person is infected with HIV, the virus randomly "bumps" into many cells. The docking proteins on the outside of the virus try to find special receptors on a host cell that will allow the virus to bind and then enter the cell. The CD4+ cell has receptors on its surface known as CD4 and CCR5 (Figure 25-2). Proteins on the HIV particle surface recognize the CD4 and CCR5 receptors on the CD4+ cell. These HIV proteins are gp120 and gp41. When the HIV gp120 binds to the CD4 receptor and the gp41 binds to the CCR5 receptor, the virus then enters CD4+ cell (Figure 25-3). *Viral binding to both receptors is needed to enter the cell.*

Viruses, like human cells, have genetic material. After entering a host cell, the HIV must get its genetic material into the host cell's DNA. HIV belongs to a family of viruses called **retroviruses.** Viruses, like human cells, have genetic material. The genetic material of the human cell is double-stranded DNA (ds-DNA). The genetic material of HIV is single-stranded RNA (ss-RNA). To infect and take over a human cell, the genetic material must be the same. HIV overcomes this problem by bringing along an enzyme at the time of infection, *reverse transcriptase (RT).* RT takes HIV's ss-RNA and converts it into ds-DNA, which makes the viral genetic material the same as human DNA. Then HIV must get its DNA into the nucleus of the CD4+ cell and place it within the human DNA. HIV also makes an enzyme called *integrase.* This enzyme allows the viral ds-DNA to be inserted into the host ds-DNA, which completes the infection of CD4+ cell.

HIV particles are made within the infected CD4+ cell, using all the metabolic machinery of the host. The new virus particle is made in the form of one long protein strand. The strand is clipped, using chemical scissors called HIV protease, into several small functional pieces. These pieces are formed into a new finished viral particle. (The drug class known as protease inhibitors work here to inhibit HIV protease.) Once the new virus particle is finished, it fuses with

Figure 25-1 ■ The human immunodeficiency virus (HIV).

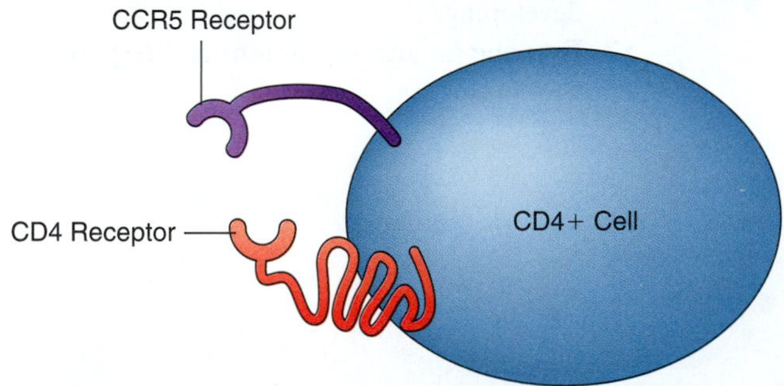

Figure 25-2 ■ The CD4+ cell receptors for the HIV "docking" proteins.

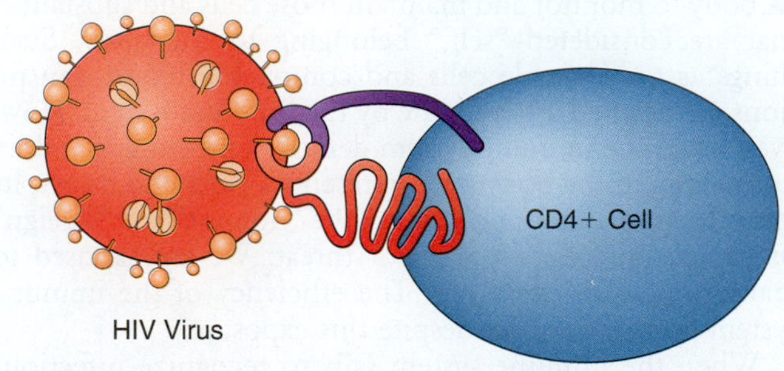

Figure 25-3 ■ The successful interaction of the HIV "docking" proteins with the CD4+ cell receptors.

the CD4+ cell membrane and buds off from the host cell in search of another CD4+ cell to infect (Figure 25-4).

EFFECTS OF HIV INFECTION. The new genetic instructions now direct CD4+ cells to change their role in immune system defenses. The new role is to be an "HIV factory." Not only is the immune system made weaker by removing some CD4+ cells from circulation, but also the most important cell in the immune system becomes an HIV factory. Up to 10 billion virus particles are made daily. In early HIV infection, the immune system can still attack and destroy most of the newly created virus particles. With time, however, the number of HIV particles overwhelms the immune system. Gradually, CD4+ cell counts fall, viral numbers (viral load) rise, and the client eventually dies of opportunistic infections or cancer.

Everyone who has AIDS has HIV infection; however, not everyone who has HIV infection has AIDS. The distinction rests with the number of CD4+ cells the client has and whether any opportunistic infections have occurred. A healthy adult usually has at least 800 to 1000 CD4+ cells/mm^3 of blood.

When a person is infected with HIV, the first manifestations are fever, night sweats, chills, headache and muscle aches. All of these problems can be caused by exposure to almost any virus, such as influenza–not just to HIV. With time, the symptoms go away, and the person feels well again. In actuality, there is a war going on in the body between HIV and the immune system.

As time passes, with more CD4+ cells infected and taken out of service, the CD4+ cell count drops to below normal levels and those that remain may not function normally. Poor CD4+ cell function as a result of HIV infection leads to the following immune system abnormalities:

- Lymphocytopenia (decreased numbers of lymphocytes)
- Increased production of incomplete and nonfunctional antibodies
- Abnormally functioning macrophages

As the CD4+ cell level drops, the client is at risk for bacterial, fungal, and viral infections, as well as for some opportunistic cancers (Figure 25-5). **Opportunistic infections** are those caused by organisms that are present as part of the normal environment and are kept in check by normal immune function.

Opportunistic infections occur because of the profound immune suppression of the person with AIDS. These infections may result from primary infection or reactivation of an old infection.

A diagnosis of AIDS requires that the person be HIV positive and have either a CD4+ cell count of less than 200 cells/mm^3 or an opportunistic infection. Once AIDS is diagnosed, even if the client's CD4+ cell count goes higher than 200 cells/mm^3 or if the infection is successfully treated, the AIDS diagnosis remains and the client never reverts to being just HIV positive.

HIV CLASSIFICATION

The Centers for Disease Control and Prevention (CDC) classifies HIV infection by combining clinical conditions that occur with HIV infection and three ranges of CD4+ cell counts (Table 25-1). The classification begins with acute HIV infection (clinical category A) and spans a continuum that ends with AIDS (clinical category C). The classifications are further divided into 1, 2, and 3 based on the client's CD4+ cell count. *The person with HIV infection can transmit the virus to others at all stages of disease.*

CLINICAL CATEGORY A. A person in clinical category A is HIV positive. The person might not have symptoms at this stage, may have persistently enlarged lymph nodes **(lymphadenopathy),** or may have acute but temporary "flu-like" symptoms as the only disease manifestations. Clients have the additional classification of A1, A2, or A3 depending on their CD4+ cell counts. When the count is at least 500/μL, the disease is classified as A1. When the count is between 200

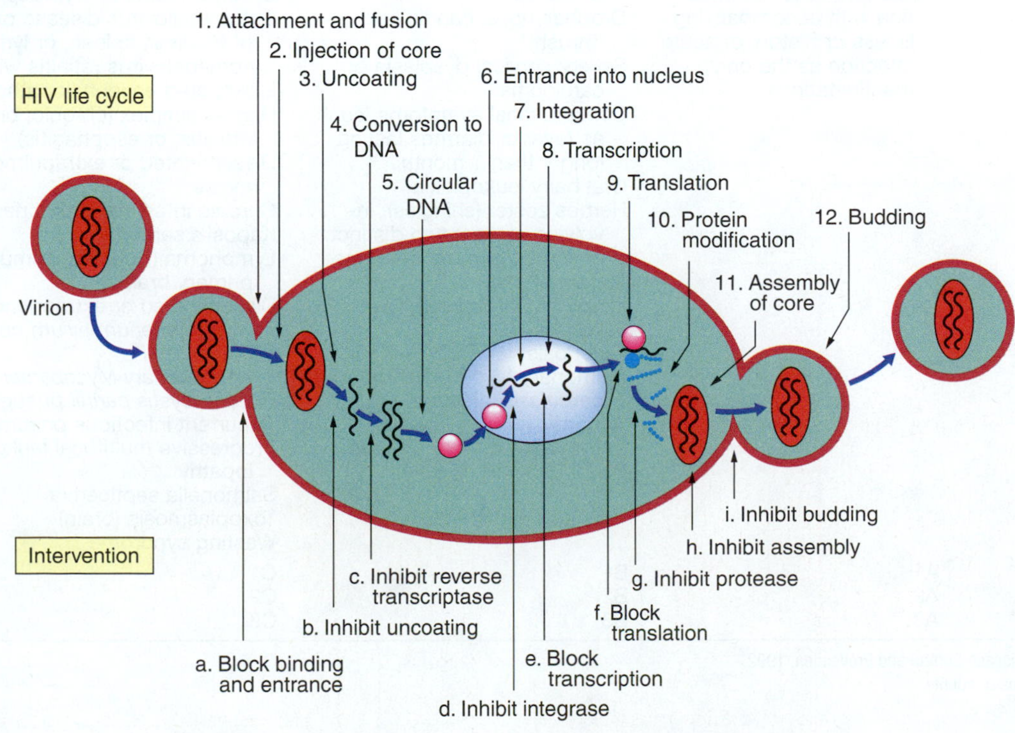

Figure 25-4 ■ The life cycle of HIV.

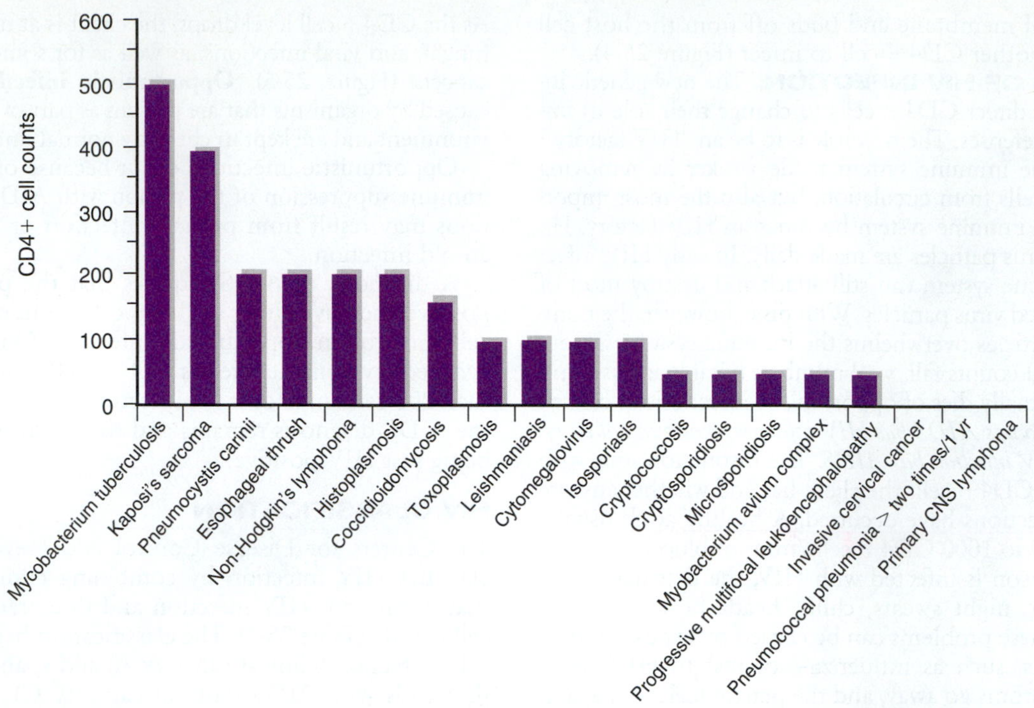

Figure 25-5 ■ Frequency of opportunistic infections among clients with AIDS.

TABLE 25-1 Centers for Disease Control and Prevention Classification System for HIV Infection and AIDS Case Definition

	Clinical Categories		
CD4+ Cell Categories	**A**	**B**	**C***
	HIV positive, asymptomatic *or* Persistent generalized lymphadenopathy *or* Acute (primary) HIV infection with accompanying illness or history of acute infection as the only manifestations	Bacterial endocarditis, meningitis, pneumonia, or sepsis Vulvovaginal candidiasis that is persistent for more than 1 month or poorly responsive to therapy Oropharyngeal candidiasis (thrush) Severe cervical dysplasia or carcinoma Constitutional symptoms, such as fever or diarrhea lasting longer than 1 month Oral hairy leukoplakia Herpes zoster (shingles), involving at least two distinct episodes or more than one dermatome Idiopathic thrombocytopenic purpura Listeriosis Pulmonary *Mycobacterium tuberculosis* infection Nocardiosis Pelvic inflammatory disease Peripheral neuropathy	Bronchial, tracheal, pulmonary, or esophageal candidiasis Invasive cervical cancer Disseminated or extrapulmonary coccidioidomycosis Chronic intestinal cryptosporidiosis Cytomegalovirus disease other than that of the liver, spleen, or lymph nodes Cytomegalovirus retinitis with vision loss HIV-related encephalopathy Herpes simplex (chronic; bronchitis, pneumonitis; or esophagitis) Disseminated or extrapulmonary histoplasmosis Chronic intestinal isosporiasis Kaposi's sarcoma Lymphoma (Burkitt's, immunoblastic, or primary brain) Disseminated or extrapulmonary *Mycobacterium avium* complex or *M. kansasii* Extrapulmonary *Mycobacterium tuberculosis* *Pneumocystis carinii* pneumonia Recurrent infectious pneumonia Progressive multifocal leukoencephalopathy Salmonella septicemia Toxoplasmosis (brain) Wasting syndrome
1 ≥ (500/μL	A1	B1	C1
2 200-499/μL	A2	B2	C2
3 <200/μL*	A3	B3	C3

Data from Centers for Disease Control and Prevention, 1992.
*AIDS indicator conditions or counts.

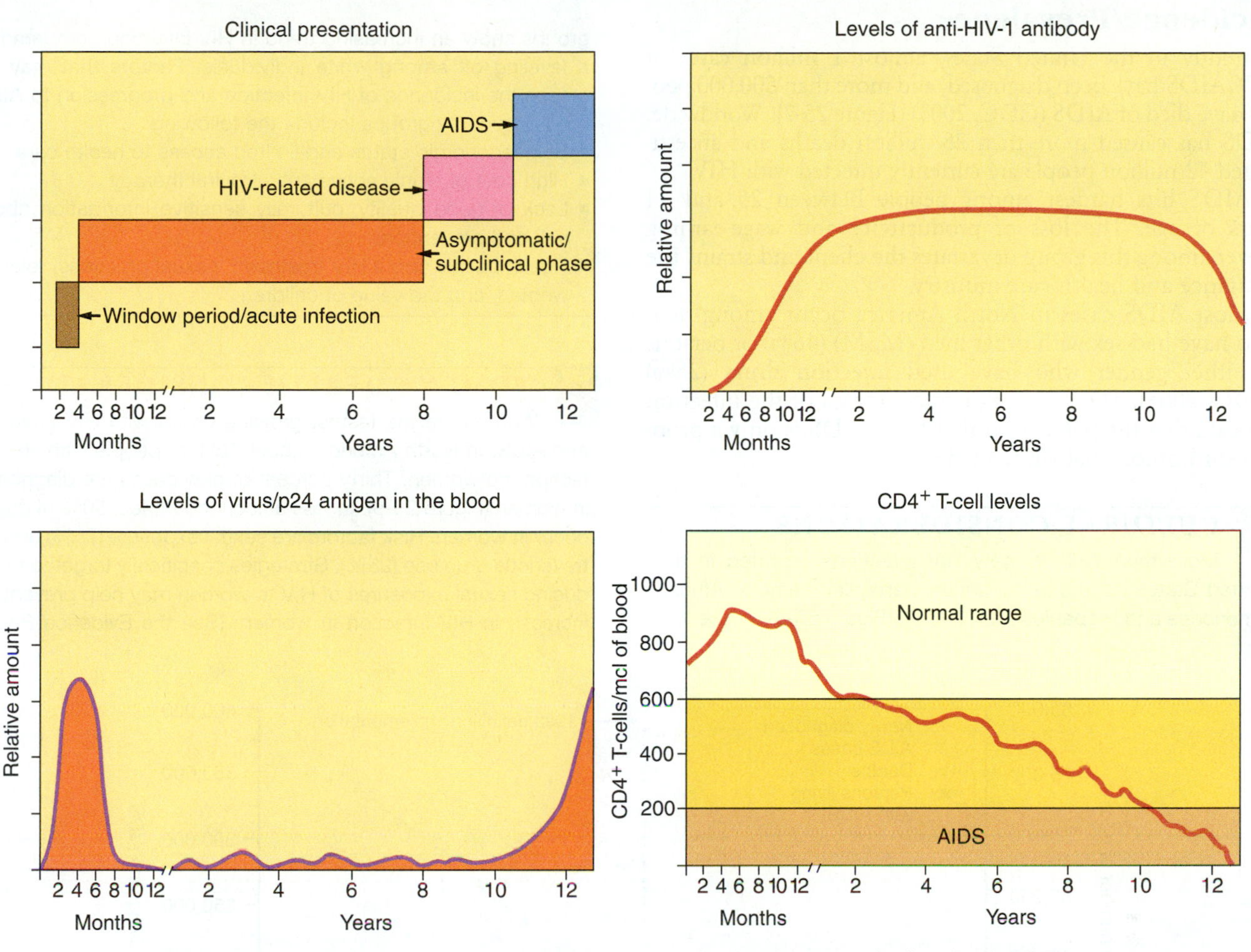

Figure 25-6 ■ Correlation of HIV infection stages, levels of HIV antibodies, levels of HIV, and levels of T4 (CD4+) cells over time.

and 499/μL, the disease is classified as A2. When the count is less than 200/μL, the disease is classified as A3.

CLINICAL CATEGORY B. The client with HIV infection is in clinical category B if one or more of the problems listed in Table 25-1, column B, are present and are (1) caused by HIV infection or indicate a deficiency in cell-mediated immunity, or (2) are complicated by HIV infection. The list gives examples of category B clinical conditions but is not comprehensive. Clients have the additional classification of B1, B2, or B3 depending on their CD4+ cell count. When the count is at least 500/μL, the disease is classified as B1. When the count is between 200 and 499/μL, the disease is classified as B2. When the count is less than 200/μL, the disease is classified as B3.

CLINICAL CATEGORY C. The HIV-positive client in clinical category C has AIDS if any one of the health problems listed on Table 25-1, column C, is present. These problems meet the CDC case definition for AIDS. Clients have the additional classification of C1, C2, or C3 depending on their CD4+ cell counts. When the count is at least 500/μL, the disease is classified as C1. When the count is between 200 and 499/μL, the disease is classified as C2. When the count is less than 200/μL, the disease is classified as C3.

HIV PROGRESSION

The time from the beginning HIV infection to development of AIDS ranges from months to years (Figure 25-6). The range depends on how HIV was acquired, personal factors, and interventions. For people who have been transfused with HIV-contaminated blood, for example, AIDS develops quickly. For those who become HIV positive as a result of a single sexual encounter, there is usually a longer period before progression to AIDS. Other personal factors that may influence progression to AIDS include frequency of re-exposure to HIV, presence of other sexually transmitted diseases (STDs), nutritional status, pregnancy, and stress.

Genetic Considerations

About 1% of people with HIV infection are **long-term nonprogressors (LTNPs).** These people have been infected with HIV for at least 10 years and have remained asymptomatic, with CD4+ cell counts within a normal range.

A genetic difference for this population is that their CCR5 receptors are abnormal and nonfunctional. Most LTNPs have mutations in both pairs of the CCR5 gene allele. The mutation creates a defective receptor called CCR5Δ32. This defective receptor does not bind to the HIV docking proteins. Cells with this defective receptor successfully resist the entrance of the HIV. People who have only one mutated CCR5 gene allele have fewer normal CCR5 receptors. Although these people can be infected with HIV, disease progression is slow compared with that in people who have normal CCR5 gene alleles.

Incidence/Prevalence

Currently in the United States, almost 1 million cases of HIV/AIDS have been diagnosed, and more than 500,000 people have died of AIDS (CDC, 2003) (Figure 25-7). Worldwide, AIDS has caused more than 28 million deaths and an estimated 42 million people are currently infected with HIV.

AIDS hits hardest among people between 25 and 44 years of age. The loss of productivity and wage-earning power among this group devastates the client and strains the insurance and health care industry.

Most AIDS cases in North America occur among men who have had sex with other men (MSM) (46%) or persons of either gender who have used injection drugs (25%) (CDC, 2003). The changing demographics of the infection indicate that the perception that HIV/AIDS is only a problem for homosexual white men is false.

CULTURAL CONSIDERATIONS

More than 73% of new HIV infections reported in the United States occurs in minorities, particularly among African Americans and Hispanics (CDC, 2003) (Figure 25-8). These two groups show an increasing trend in HIV infection compared to a leveling off among white individuals. Factors that may increase the incidence of HIV infection and progression to AIDS among minority groups include the following:

- Socioeconomic status and limited access to health care
- High cost of highly active antiretroviral therapy
- Lack of good quality, culturally sensitive information about risk and prevention
- Health beliefs about HIV treatment, sexual practices, roles of women, and the value of children

WOMEN'S HEALTH CONSIDERATIONS

Women are the fastest growing group with HIV infection and AIDS. In North America, about 16% of people with HIV infection are women. Thirty percent of new cases are diagnosed in women (Figure 25-9). In less affluent countries, 50% of cases occur in women. Risk factors are sexual exposure (75%) and intravenous drug use (25%). Strategies specifically targeted to reducing sexual exposures of HIV to women may help prevent an increase in HIV infection in women. (See the Evidence-Based

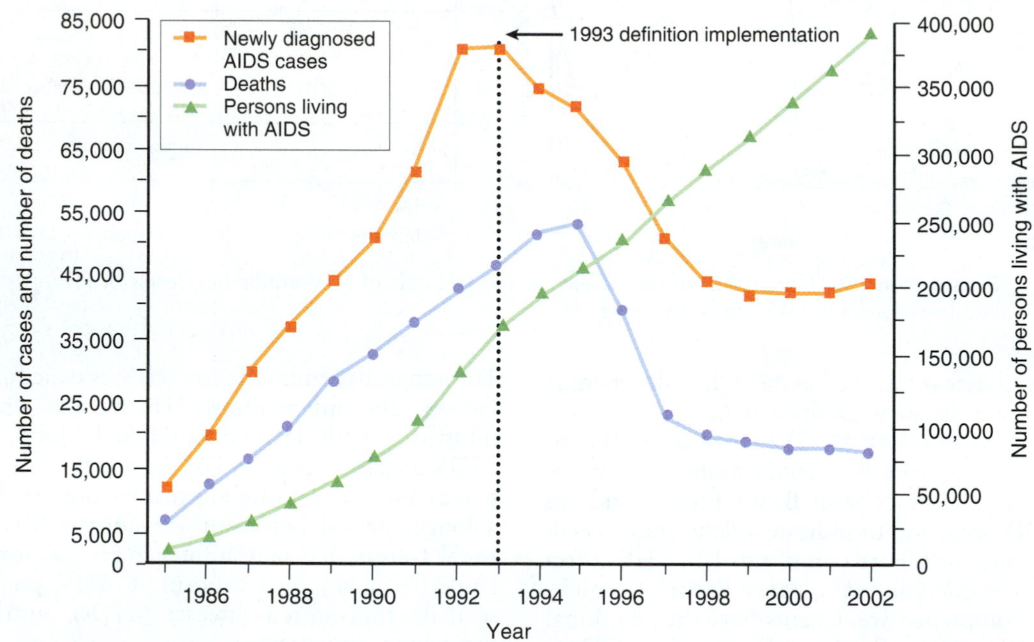

Figure 25-7 ■ AIDS cases, deaths, and persons living with AIDS by year, 1985-2002 (adjusted for reporting delays).

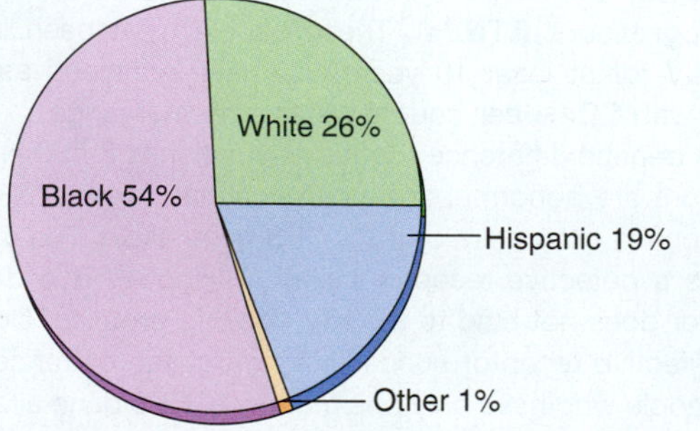

Figure 25-8 ■ Estimates of annual new HIV infections in the United States by ethnicity and race.

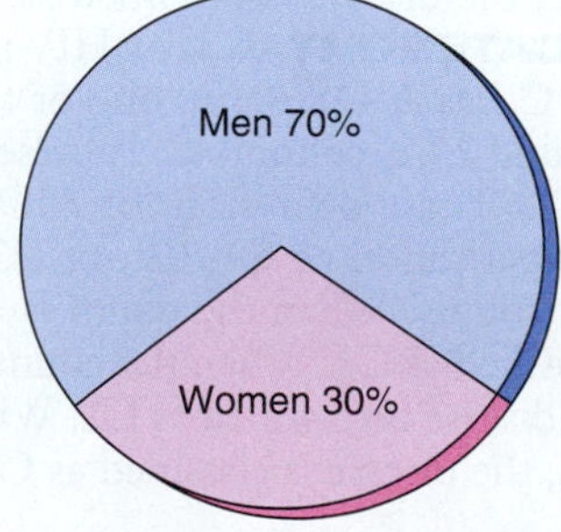

Figure 25-9 ■ Estimates of annual new HIV infections in the United States by gender.

Practice for Nursing box below.) Women with HIV infection have a poorer outcome with shorter mean survival time than men. This outcome may be the result of late diagnosis and social or economic factors that reduce access to medical care.

Gynecologic problems, especially persistent or recurrent vaginal candidiasis, may be the first signs of HIV infection in women. Other common problems include genital herpes, pelvic inflammatory disease, and cervical neoplasia.

Most women with HIV are of childbearing age. The effect of pregnancy on the course of HIV infection is not known. There is conflicting evidence that pregnancy may or may not speed up the progression of disease.

CONSIDERATIONS FOR OLDER ADULTS

Infection with HIV can occur at any age. Assess the older client for risk behaviors, including a sexual and drug use history. Decline in immune function increases the risk for HIV infection after exposure in this population. In the older woman, changes in vaginal tissue as a result of aging may increase susceptibility to sexually transmitted HIV infection.

AIDS is a disease with a high mortality rate. The fatality rate is at least 60% for adults and, to date, there is no cure. Thus a major focus for health care in North America and worldwide is prevention of HIV infection. The United States has defined several goals related to HIV and AIDS prevention, as shown in the Meeting Healthy People 2010 Objectives box on p. 430.

HEALTH PROMOTION/ILLNESS PREVENTION

The most important aspect for prevention of HIV transmission is education. All people, regardless of age, gender, ethnicity, or sexual orientation, are susceptible to HIV infection. HIV infection is preventable because of the modes of viral transmission and the fragile nature of the virus.

HIV has been found in most body fluids of infected clients, including blood, semen, vaginal secretions, breast milk, amniotic fluid, urine, feces, saliva, tears, cerebrospinal fluid, lymph nodes, cervical cells, corneal tissue, and brain tissue. HIV is transmitted most often in the following three ways:

- Sexual: genital, anal, or oral sexual contact with exposure of mucous membranes to infected semen or vaginal secretions
- Parenteral: sharing of needles or equipment contaminated with infected blood or receiving contaminated blood products
- Perinatal: from the placenta, from contact with maternal blood and body fluids during birth, or from breast milk from an infected mother to child

HIV is not transmitted by casual contact in the home, school, or workplace. Sharing household utensils, towels and linens, and toilet facilities does not transmit HIV. In addition, HIV is not spread by mosquitos or other insects.

Sexual Transmission

Abstinence and mutually monogamous sex with a noninfected partner are the only absolutely safe methods of preventing HIV infection through sexual contact. These practices may not be feasible because of personal, cultural, or economic factors.

Many forms of sexual expression can spread HIV infection if one partner is infected. The risk for becoming infected from a partner who is HIV positive is always present, although some sexual practices are more risky than others. The virus concentrates most heavily in blood and seminal fluid, although it is also present in vaginal secretions. Thus risk differs by gender, sexual act, and the viral load of the infected partner.

GENDER

HIV is most easily transmitted when infected body fluids come into contact with mucous membranes or nonintact skin. The vagina has much more mucous membrane than does the penis. Thus HIV, like all other sexually transmitted diseases (STDs), is more easily transmitted from infected male to uninfected female than vice versa.

EVIDENCE-BASED PRACTICE for Nursing

Gender-sensitive interventions are effective in changing behavior

Ehrhardt, A., et al. (2002). A gender-specific HIV/STD risk reduction intervention for women in a health care setting: Short- and long-term results of a randomized clinical trial. *AIDS Care, 14*(2), 147-161.

This study sought to determine whether a gender-specific group intervention had short-term and/or long-term effects in helping women to reduce their number of unsafe sexual encounters and enhance their implementation of sexual alternatives. The study included 360 subjects who received either an eight-session group intervention, a four-session group intervention, or no specific intervention. Subjects were followed up at 1 month, 6 months, and 12 months after intervention for an assessment of sexual practices/activities using a structured format with closed and open-ended items. The items assessed such variables as total number of sexual activities, activity by type, partner type, use of condoms, and other protection. Variables of age, work status, ethnicity, education levels, and number of children were similar for all three groups. The level of participation by the subjects in both intervention groups was similar and the percentage of participants who were available for follow-up at 12 months was high.

The results indicated that participants in the eight-session intervention were more than twice as likely to reduce unsafe sexual encounters as women in the control group. Women in the four-session intervention group overall had fewer unsafe sexual encounters compared with control subjects but the difference did not meet statistical significance.

Level of Evidence: 1—At least one properly designed randomized controlled clinical trial (RCT) of appropriate size (more than 100 subjects).

Critique. The study methods were appropriate for the purpose and study questions. The study limitations include that the subjects were drawn from a population that self-selected for a clinical trial on HIV/STD prevention, thus their overall motivation may have been different than that of the general population would be. Additionally, data regarding number of sexual encounters, safe or otherwise, was obtained by self-report and recall.

Implications for Nursing. With HIV infection increasing among American women and women worldwide, more interventions are needed that specifically target women. The results of this study indicate a positive "dose" effect, in that with each additional session attended, participants were better able to make changes in unsafe sexual practices. This finding may have represented an increasing level of confidence associated with more specific education on alternative sexual practices and means of protection.

Meeting HEALTHY PEOPLE 2010 Objectives

HIV/AIDS

Objective 21.10: Confine annual incidence of diagnosed AIDS cases among adolescents and adults to no more than 12 per 100,000 population.

- Include questions regarding sexual activity and use of safer sex practices whenever obtaining a health history from a client of any age, gender, occupation, socioeconomic status, religion, or educational background.
- Assess all clients for current and past exposures to blood-borne or sexually transmitted diseases.
- Encourage clients to know their own and their partners' HIV status.
- Teach clients safer sex practices.
- Direct clients who are IV drug users to drug rehabilitation programs and support groups.
- Direct clients who abuse alcohol to alcohol rehabilitation programs and support groups.
- Develop culturally sensitive and age-appropriate education materials of various literacy levels for HIV prevention.
- Enlist the assistance of educational, religious, and civic groups and institutions in the dissemination of information regarding prevention of HIV infection.
- Encourage people who are HIV positive to:
  - Avoid sharing toothbrushes, razors, or other items that could become contaminated with blood.
  - Not donate sperm, blood, plasma, or body organs or other body tissues.
  - Inform his or her physician, dentist, and eye doctor about the client's HIV status.
  - Clean blood or other body fluid spills on household or other surfaces with freshly diluted household bleach: 1 part bleach to 10 parts water. (Do not use bleach on wounds.)

Objective 21.11: Increase years of healthy life of an individual infected with HIV by extending the interval of time between an initial diagnosis of HIV infection and AIDS diagnosis and between AIDS diagnosis and death.

- Teach HIV-positive persons who have no signs or symptoms of immunodeficiency to seek regular medical evaluation and follow-up.
- Encourage HIV-positive persons to adhere to drug regimen, especially highly active antiretroviral therapy (HAART).
- Teach HIV-infected persons to begin or maintain behaviors known to assist in maintaining or improving immune function (e.g., diet appropriate in number of calories for the client's individual metabolic needs that is high in protein and vitamins and low in fat; regular exercise; adequate rest; and reduction of physical, emotional, or spiritual stress).
- Encourage HIV-positive persons to use safer sex practices for their own protection as well as for partner protection.
- Encourage HIV-positive women to avoid pregnancy.

SPECIFIC SEXUAL ACTS

Sexual acts or practices that permit infected seminal fluid to come into contact with mucous membranes or nonintact skin are the most risky for sexual transmission of HIV. Such practices include oral sex and anal intercourse.

In oral sex, the risk increases when the penis and seminal fluid of an infected person come into contact with the mucous membranes of the mouth and throat (fellatio) of a noninfected person. Oral sex in which the uninfected partner's oral mucous membranes and tongue come into contact with infected vaginal secretions (cunnilingus) also places the uninfected person at risk. This risk is increased if sores or other open areas are present in the mouth.

In anal intercourse, the risk increases when the penis and seminal fluid of an infected person come into contact with the mucous membranes of the uninfected partner's rectum. *Anal intercourse in which the semen depositor is infected is a risky sexual practice regardless of whether the semen receiver is male or female.* Anal intercourse not only allows seminal fluid contact with the mucous membranes of the rectum, but also causes tearing of the mucous membranes, making infection more likely.

CHART 25-1

CLIENT EDUCATION GUIDE

Condom Use to Prevent Sexually Transmitted Diseases

- Use latex condoms rather than natural membrane condoms.
- Store condoms in a cool, dry place.
- Do not use condoms that were in damaged packages or those that show signs of age, such as those that are brittle, sticky, or discolored.
- Handle condoms carefully to avoid puncturing them.
- Put a condom on before making any genital contact.
- Hold the tip of the condom and unroll it onto the erect penis, making sure that no air is trapped in the tip. Leave space at the tip to collect semen.
- Use adequate lubrication. Use water-based lubricants only. Petroleum or oil-based lubricants such as petroleum jelly, cooking oil, shortening, and lotions can damage the condom.
- Replace a broken condom immediately. If ejaculation occurs after the condom breaks, there may be some protection in the immediate use of a spermicide.
- After ejaculation, the condom must remain on until the penis is withdrawn. While the penis is still erect, hold the condom against the base of the penis while withdrawing.
- Never reuse condoms.

From Centers for Disease Control. (1988). Condoms for prevention of sexually transmitted diseases. *Morbidity and Mortality Weekly Report, 37*(9), 133-137.

VIRAL LOAD

The higher the blood level of HIV **(viremia),** the greater the risk for sexual and perinatal transmission. Current highly active antiretroviral therapy (HAART) has caused the viral load of some infected clients to drop below detectable levels. Although it is assumed that there is far less virus in seminal or vaginal fluids of these individuals, the risk for disease transmission is presumed to still exist.

Safer sex practices are those that reduce the risk of nonintact skin or mucous membranes coming in contact with infected body fluids and blood. Such practices include using the following:

- A latex condom for genital and anal intercourse (Chart 25-1)
- A condom or latex barrier (dental dam) over the genitals or anus during oral-genital or oral-anal sexual contact
- Latex gloves for finger or hand contact with the vagina or rectum

Parenteral Transmission

Preventive practices to reduce transmission among injection drug users include the use of proper cleaning of "works" (needles, syringes, and other drug paraphernalia). Instruct clients to clean a used needle and syringe by first filling and flushing with clear water. Next, the syringe should be filled with ordinary household bleach. The bleach-filled syringe should be shaken for 30 to 60 seconds. Advise drug users to carry a small container with this solution whenever sharing needles. Some communities have a needle exchange program in which needles and syringes are used only once and exchanged for clean ones.

CHART 25-2

BEST PRACTICE for
Postexposure Prophylaxis (PEP) for Occupational HIV Exposure

PEP is not recommended in the following scenarios:
- Percutaneous injury, source HIV negative
- Mucosal exposure, small volume (a few drops), source HIV negative

PEP should be considered in the following scenarios:
- Percutaneous injury or mucosal contact, source HIV status unknown, recommend two-drug PEP, until source client's HIV status is determined. If negative, discontinue PEP.
- Percutaneous injury, *source HIV positive, asymptomatic, viral load (VL) <1500*, solid needle, superficial injury, recommend two-drug PEP. Mucosal contact, small volume (a few drops), consider two-drug PEP.
- Percutaneous injury, *source HIV positive, symptomatic, AIDS or opportunistic infections (OIs), recent seroconverter, high VL*, solid needle, superficial injury, recommend three-drug PEP. Mucosal contact, small volume (a few drops), recommend two-drug PEP.
- Percutaneous injury, *source HIV positive, asymptomatic, VL <1500*, large-bore hollow needle, visible blood on device, needle used in source client's vein or artery, recommend three-drug PEP. Mucosal contact, large volume (major blood splash), recommend two-drug PEP.
- Percutaneous injury, *source HIV positive, symptomatic, AIDS or OIs, recent seroconverter, high VL*, large-bore hollow needle, visible blood on device, needle used in source client's vein or artery, recommend three-drug PEP. Mucosal contact, large volume (major blood splash), recommend three drug PEP.

PEP uses two or three drugs, generally from one, two, or three classes of antiretroviral agents:

NRTI Class
- ZVD + 3TC
- 3TC + d4T
- ddI + d4T

NNRTI Class
- Efavirenz

PI Class
- Indinavir
- Nelfinavir
- Lopinavir/ritonavir

Start PEP as soon as possible after exposure.
Standard therapy is to use these medications for 4 weeks.

NRTI, Nucleoside analog reverse transcriptase inhibitors; NNRTI, non-nucleoside analog reverse transcriptase inhibitors; PI, protease inhibitors.

The risk for AIDS transmission through blood and blood products has been reduced to a national average of 0.02%. Several measures are used to protect the nation's blood supply. All donated blood in North America is screened for the HIV antibody, and blood that is positive for HIV antibodies is discarded. Because of the time lag in antibody production (seroconversion) after exposure to HIV, infected blood can test negative for HIV antibodies. False-negative results also can occur. The small but real possibility of HIV transmission through blood and blood products has resulted in more stringent indications for transfusion and an increase in autologous transfusion.

Perinatal Transmission

The risk for perinatal transmission in pregnant clients with AIDS ranges between 14% and 45% for each pregnancy. Pregnant women who receive zidovudine have an 8.3% transmission rate to their babies compared with 25.5% in women who do not receive antiretroviral therapy. A single dose of nevirapine, given during labor to the mother, and a single dose given to the baby at 48 to 72 hours is an alternative therapy for infected women who have not received other antiretroviral therapy.

HIV transmission can occur across the placenta during pregnancy, with infant exposure to blood and vaginal secretions during birth or after birth through breast milk. Inform women of childbearing age with HIV infection about the risks for perinatal transmission. Consult a maternal-child textbook for more information about reducing perinatal transmission of HIV.

TABLE 25-2 Recommendations for Preventing HIV Transmission by Health Care Workers

- Workers should adhere to standard precautions.
- Workers with exudative lesions or weeping dermatitis should not perform direct client care or handle client care equipment and devices used in invasive procedures.
- Workers must follow guidelines for disinfection and sterilization of reusable equipment used in invasive procedures.
- Workers infected with HIV are not restricted from practice of non–exposure-prone procedures, as long as they comply with standard precautions and sterilization/disinfection recommendations.
- Workers should identify exposure-prone procedures by institutions where they are performed.
- Workers who perform exposure-prone procedures should know their HIV antibody status.
- Workers who are infected with HIV should seek advice from an expert review panel before performing exposure-prone procedures to determine under what circumstances they may continue to practice these procedures. These circumstances would include notification of prospective clients of HIV positivity.

Modified from Centers for Disease Control. (1991). Recommendations for preventing transmission of human immunodeficiency virus and hepatitis B virus to patients during exposure-prone invasive procedures. *Morbidity and Mortality Weekly Report, 40*(RR-8), 1-9.

Transmission and Health Care Workers

Needle stick or "sharps" injuries are the primary means of HIV infection for health care workers. In addition, health care workers can be infected through exposure of nonintact skin and mucous membranes to blood and body fluids. Because there is a time lag between the time of infection with HIV and the production of serum antibodies (seroconversion), infected people can test negative for HIV and still transmit the virus. *The best prevention for health care providers is the consistent use of standard precautions for all clients as recommended by the Centers for Disease Control and Prevention (CDC)* (see Chapter 29). Chart 25-2 lists the recommended actions for prevention of HIV infection after a needle stick or other occupational exposure (postexposure prophylaxis [PEP]).

The public may be alarmed about HIV transmission by health care workers. It is recommended that HIV-infected health care workers wear gloves when in contact with clients' mucous membranes or nonintact skin. Infected workers with weeping dermatitis or open lesions should not perform direct care activities. The CDC (1991) has recommended guidelines for preventing HIV transmission by health care workers during exposure-prone invasive procedures (Table 25-2). These include any procedure in which there is a risk for broken skin injury to the health care worker and the worker's blood is likely to make contact with

CHART 25-3

CLIENT EDUCATION GUIDE

CDC Recommendations for HIV Testing

You should be tested for AIDS if you fall within one or more of the following groups:

- People with sexually transmitted disease
- Injection drug users
- People who consider themselves at risk
- Women of childbearing age with identifiable risks, including the following:
  - Used injection drugs
  - Engaged in prostitution
  - Had sexual partners who were infected or at risk
  - Had contact with men from countries with high HIV prevalence
  - Received a transfusion between 1978 and 1985
- People planning to get married
- People undergoing medical evaluation or treatment for manifestations that may be HIV related
- People admitted to hospitals
- People in correctional institutions such as jails and prisons
- Prostitutes and their customers

Modified from Centers for Disease Control. (1987). Public Health Service guidelines for counseling and antibody testing to prevent HIV infection and AIDS. *Morbidity and Mortality Weekly Report, 36*(31), 509-515.

the client's body cavity, subcutaneous tissues, or mucous membranes. These recommendations aim to reduce the risk of HIV transmission to clients.

Testing

Testing for HIV antibodies or other features of the virus is complex, requiring interpretation, counseling, and confidentiality. Testing plays a role in prevention because tests are a way of diagnosing HIV infection before immune changes or symptoms develop. Those who test positive can be educated and encouraged to modify their behaviors to prevent transmission to others. Chart 25-3 lists conditions for which HIV antibody testing is advised.

Pretest and post-test counseling must be performed by trained personnel. Counseling helps the client make an informed decision about testing and provides an opportunity to teach risk reduction behaviors. Post-test counseling is needed to interpret the results, discuss risk reduction, and provide psychological support and health promotion information for the client with a positive test result. Testing methods, their accuracy, and indications are presented under the heading "Laboratory Assessment" on p. 436.

Recommendations for people who test positive for antibody to HIV are presented in the Meeting Healthy People 2010 Objectives box on p. 430. People who test positive should also be counseled on how to inform sexual partners and those with whom they have shared needles.

COLLABORATIVE MANAGEMENT

PHARM e REVIEW

The care of the client with HIV disease or AIDS is complex, affecting all body systems. The Concept Map on p. 433 addresses assessment and nursing care issues related to clients who have HIV disease or AIDS.

Assessment

The person who has HIV disease is monitored on a regular basis for changes in immune function or health status that indicate disease progression and warrant prophylaxis or intervention. Continuous, comprehensive assessment of the client with AIDS is crucial, because he or she may have problems related to disease in many organ systems. Assess subtle changes so that infections and other problems can be found early and treated.

HISTORY

Collect information about age, gender, occupation, and residence. Thoroughly assess the current illness, including its nature, when it started, the severity of symptoms, associated problems, and any interventions to date. Ask the client about when AIDS was diagnosed and what clinical symptoms led to that diagnosis. Ask the client to give a chronology of infections and clinical problems since the diagnosis. Assess the client's health history, including whether he or she received a blood transfusion between 1978 and 1985. (Since 1985, donated blood in the United States has been routinely tested for HIV contamination.)

Ask the client about sexual practices, any sexually transmitted diseases (STDs), and any major infectious diseases, including tuberculosis and hepatitis. If the client has hemophilia, ask about treatment with clotting factors. Determine whether the client has engaged in past or present injection drug use, including needle exposure and sharing. Assess the client's level of knowledge regarding the diagnosis, symptom management, diagnostic tests, treatments, community resources, and modes of HIV transmission. Also assess the client's understanding and use of safer sex practices.

PHYSICAL ASSESSMENT/CLINICAL MANIFESTATIONS

HIV disease and AIDS are a progression continuum. The client with HIV disease may either have few manifestations and problems or may have problems that are acute rather than chronically present. The client with AIDS, however, usually has more problems of long duration and greater severity. Look for many possible manifestations. These include shortness of breath or cough, fever, night sweats, fatigue, nausea and vomiting, weight loss, swollen lymph nodes, diarrhea, visual changes, headache, memory loss, confusion, seizures, personality changes, dry skin, rashes, skin lesions, and pain (Chart 25-4).

OPPORTUNISTIC INFECTIONS. The client with HIV/AIDS can develop pathogenic infections and opportunistic infections. Pathogenic infections are caused by virulent organisms and occur even among people whose immune systems are functioning normally. Opportunistic infections are those caused by organisms that are present as part of the normal environment and are kept in check by normal immune function. Only when immune function is depressed are such organisms capable of causing infection.

Opportunistic infections occur because of the profound immune suppression of the person with AIDS (see Figure 25-5). They may result from primary infection or reactivation of a latent infection. Opportunistic infections account for many of the clinical symptoms observed in AIDS and can be protozoan, fungal, bacterial, or viral. More than one infection may be present in a client with AIDS.

Opportunistic infections do not pose a threat to the immunocompetent health care worker caring for a client with HIV infection or AIDS. When the client with HIV infection or AIDS has a pathogenic infection, however, such as tuberculosis at a transmissi-

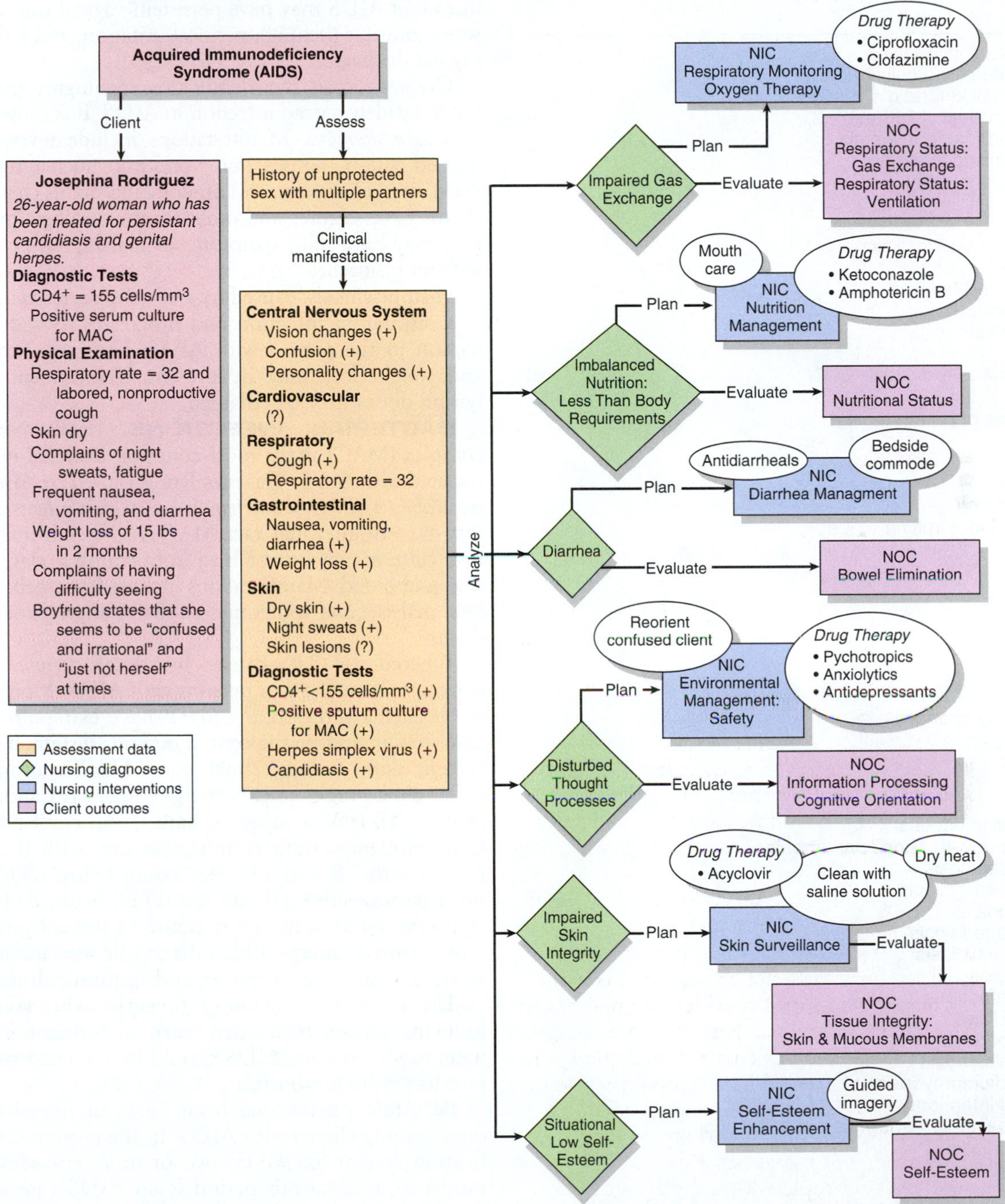

Concept Map by Elaine Bishop Kennedy, EdD, RN

ble stage, health care personnel must use appropriate precautions to prevent disease spread.

PROTOZOAL INFECTIONS. *Pneumocystis carinii* pneumonia (PCP) is the most common opportunistic infection in persons infected with HIV. Dyspnea on exertion, tachypnea, a persistent dry cough, and fever may be observed. The client with PCP has fatigue and weight loss. Crackles may be present on lung auscultation.

Toxoplasmosis encephalitis, caused by *Toxoplasma gondii,* is acquired through contact with contaminated cat feces or by ingesting infected, undercooked meat. The client may have subtle changes in mental status, neurologic deficits, headaches, and fever. Other symptoms include difficulties with speech, gait, and vision; seizures; lethargy; and confusion. Perform a comprehensive baseline mental status examination and monitor the client to detect subtle changes.

Cryptosporidiosis is an intestinal infection caused by *Cryptosporidium* organisms. In AIDS, this illness ranges from a mild diarrhea to a severe wasting with electrolyte imbalance. Diarrhea may result in fluid loss of up to 15 to 20 L/day.

FUNGAL INFECTIONS. *Candida albicans* is part of the natural flora of the gastrointestinal tract. In the person with AIDS, candidiasis (overgrowth of the *Candida* fungus) occurs because the weakened immune system can no longer

CHART 25-4

KEY FEATURES of AIDS

Immunologic Manifestations
- Low white blood cell counts:
  - CD4+/CD8+ ratio <2
  - CD4+ count <200/mm³
- Hypergammaglobulinemia
- Opportunistic infections
- Lymphadenopathy
- Fatigue

Integumentary Manifestations
- Dry skin
- Poor wound healing
- Skin lesions
- Night sweats

Respiratory Manifestations
- Cough
- Shortness of breath

Gastrointestinal Manifestations
- Diarrhea
- Weight loss
- Nausea and vomiting

Central Nervous System Manifestations
- Confusion
- Dementia
- Headache
- Fever
- Visual changes
- Memory loss
- Personality changes
- Pain
- Seizures

Opportunistic Infections
- Protozoal infections
  - *Pneumocystis carinii* pneumonia
  - Toxoplasmosis
  - Cryptosporidiosis
  - Isosporiasis
  - Microsporidiosis
  - Strongyloidiasis
  - Giardiasis
- Fungal infections
  - Candidiasis
  - Cryptococcosis
  - Histoplasmosis
  - Coccidioidomycosis
- Bacterial infections
  - *Mycobacterium avium* complex infection
  - Tuberculosis
  - Nocardiosis
- Viral infections
  - Cytomegalovirus infection
  - Herpes simplex virus infection
  - Varicella-zoster virus infection

Malignancies
- Kaposi's sarcoma
- Non-Hodgkin's lymphoma
- Hodgkin's lymphoma
- Invasive cervical carcinoma

control fungal growth. *Candida* stomatitis or esophagitis is a frequent finding in AIDS. Clients may report food tasting "funny," mouth pain, difficulty in swallowing, and retrosternal pain (pain behind the ribs). On examination of the mouth and the back of the throat, you may see cottage cheese–like, yellow-white plaques and inflammation. Esophagitis is diagnosed by endoscopic biopsy and culture. Women with HIV disease or AIDS may have persistent vaginal candidiasis with severe pruritus (itching), perineal irritation, and a thick, white vaginal discharge.

Cryptococcosis is a debilitating meningitis and is sometimes a widely spread infection in AIDS. It is caused by *Cryptococcus neoformans.* Manifestations include fever, headache, blurred vision, nausea and vomiting, nuchal rigidity (stiff neck), mild confusion, and other mental status changes. Some clients have seizures and other focal neurologic problems or they may have mild symptoms of malaise and fever with or without headaches.

Histoplasmosis, caused by *Histoplasma capsulatum,* begins as a respiratory infection and progresses to widespread infection in the person with AIDS. Dyspnea, fever, cough, and weight loss may be present. The spleen, liver, and lymph nodes may be enlarged.

BACTERIAL INFECTIONS. *Mycobacterium avium* complex (MAC) is the most common bacterial infection associated with AIDS. This problem is caused by *Mycobacterium intracellulare* or *Mycobacterium avium,* which infects the respiratory or gastrointestinal tract. MAC is a systemic infection. Positive cultures may be obtained from lymph nodes, bone marrow, and blood. Manifestations include fever, debility, weight loss, malaise, and sometimes swollen lymph glands or organ disease.

Tuberculosis (TB), caused by *Mycobacterium tuberculosis,* occurs in 2% to 10% of persons with AIDS. More than 50% of all clients with AIDS and TB have extrapulmonary disease sites, including the central nervous system, bones, liver, spleen, skin, and intestinal tract. Manifestations include fever, chills, night sweats, weight loss, and anorexia. Pulmonary TB causes cough, dyspnea, and chest pain. Symptoms of extrapulmonary infection vary with the site. The person with TB and a CD4+ count below 200/mm³ may not have a positive TB skin test (PPD) because of an inability to mount an immune response to the antigen, a condition known as **anergy.** Other diagnostic tests include a chest x-ray, acid-fast sputum smear, and sputum culture.

The nurse or respiratory therapist who gives cough-inducing aerosol treatments, such as pentamidine isethionate, to clients with AIDS should be screened with a PPD skin test every 6 months.

Recurrent pneumonia from bacterial infections occurs often among clients with AIDS. In the current CDC classification system for AIDS, two or more episodes of pneumonia in a 12-month period is an AIDS case definition. Manifestations include chest pain, productive cough, fever, and dyspnea.

VIRAL INFECTIONS. Cytomegalovirus (CMV) can infect many sites in persons with AIDS, including the eye (CMV retinitis), respiratory and gastrointestinal tracts, and central nervous system. CMV infection can also cause many nonspecific problems such as fever, malaise, weight loss, fatigue, and swollen lymph nodes. CMV retinitis impairs vision, ranging from slight to total blindness.

CMV infection also causes colitis, with diarrhea, abdominal bloating and discomfort, and weight loss. In addition, CMV can cause encephalitis, pneumonitis, adrenalitis, hepatitis, and disseminated infection.

Herpes simplex virus (HSV) infections in people with HIV disease or AIDS occur in the perirectal, oral, and genital areas. The manifestations are more widespread and of longer duration among clients with HIV/AIDS than among those who are immunocompetent. Numbness or tingling at the site of infection occur up to 24 hours before vesicle (blister) formation. Lesions are painful, with chronic ulcerative lesions after vesicle rupture. Clients may have fever, pain, bleeding, and lymph node enlargement in the affected area. Other manifestations include headache, myalgia, and malaise.

Varicella-zoster virus (VZV) infection (shingles) is usually not a new infection for people with AIDS. This virus, present in the nerve ganglia of many people, causes chickenpox. When people who have had the chickenpox previously are immunocompromised, VZV leaves the nerve ganglia and enters body fluids and other tissue areas, causing shingles. Manifestations begin with pain and burning along sensory nerve tracts. Large fluid-filled blisters form and crust over. Other problems include headache and low-grade fever.

MALIGNANCIES. The AIDS-weakened immune response increases the risk for cancer. Cancers occurring with AIDS include Kaposi's sarcoma, Hodgkin's lymphoma, non-Hodgkin's lymphoma, and invasive cervical cancer (CDC, 2003).

KAPOSI'S SARCOMA. Kaposi's sarcoma (KS) is the most common AIDS-related malignancy, occurring in 1% to 21% of clients with AIDS. The risk for KS appears to be related to co-infection with some types of herpes virus.

KS develops as small, purplish brown, raised lesions that are usually not painful or itchy. The lesions can occur anywhere on the body. Most clients with KS have skin or mucous membrane lesions. In some clients, lesions develop in the lymph nodes, intestinal tract, or lungs. KS is diagnosed by biopsy and histologic examination of the lesion. Assess KS lesions for number, size, and location, and monitor their progression.

MALIGNANT LYMPHOMAS. Malignant lymphomas occurring with AIDS are non-Hodgkin's B-cell lymphomas, such as Burkitt's lymphoma, immunoblastic lymphoma, and primary brain lymphoma. Manifestations include weight loss, fever, and night sweats.

ENDOCRINE COMPLICATIONS. Clients with HIV disease may have disease-related endocrine problems, such as gonadal dysfunction, body shape changes, adrenal insufficiency, diabetes mellitus, and elevated triglycerides and cholesterol (Table 25-3).

Many HIV-positive men have low testosterone levels and HIV-positive women often have irregular menstrual cycles. With this gonadal dysfunction comes a decrease in body muscle mass for both genders and a change in libido.

Body shape changes from fat redistribution or lipodystrophy are common in clients receiving antiretroviral therapies, especially protease inhibitors. Manifestations include "buffalo humps" or cervical (neck) fat development and large abdominal fat accumulations. Other body areas, such as the face, arms, and legs, have a wasted appearance.

Adrenal dysfunction can result from the glands being infected by opportunistic infections (cytomegalovirus, *Mycobacterium avium*, or tuberculosis), resulting in adrenal insufficiency. This problem manifests as fatigue, weight loss, nausea, vomiting, low blood pressure, and electrolyte disturbances, and can be life threatening.

Clients taking protease inhibitors have a higher than expected incidence of type 1 diabetes and hyperlipidemia.

TABLE 25-3 Endocrine Complications of HIV Infection or Treatment

Endocrine Gland	Problems/Dysfunction

Gonads	Decreased testosterone
	  Reduced libido
	  Reduced fertility
	  Decreased muscle mass
	Decreased estrogen
	  Reduced libido
	  Premature menopause
	  Decreased muscle mass

Adrenal cortex	Increased cortisol
	  Fat redistribution
	  Decreased muscle mass
	Decreased cortisol
	  Adrenal insufficiency
	    Hypoglycemia
	    Hyperkalemia
	    Hypotension
	    Fatigue
	    Weight loss

Pancreas	Reduced exocrine function
	  Fatty food intolerance
	  Cholelithiasis
	  Pancreatitis
	Reduced endocrine function
	  Diabetes mellitus
	  Hyperlipidemia

These problems are seen even among clients who have no other risks for these problems or the associated heart disease.

OTHER CLINICAL MANIFESTATIONS. All body systems are affected to some degree in AIDS.

AIDS DEMENTIA COMPLEX. HIV-associated dementia complex, or AIDS dementia complex (ADC), refers to the manifestations of central nervous system involvement. ADC occurs in about 70% of people with AIDS. It is a result of infection of cells within the central nervous system by HIV. ADC causes cognitive, motor, and behavioral impairments. Manifestations range from barely noticeable to severe dementia.

Some neurologic complications may be due to HIV infection or drug side effects, including peripheral neuropathies and myopathies. Symptoms of peripheral neuropathies include paresthesias and burning sensations, pain, and gait changes. Myopathies are accompanied by leg weakness, ataxia, and muscle pain.

WASTING SYNDROME. AIDS wasting syndrome is not due to any single factor. It may be a result of altered metabolism from malignancy or opportunistic infection. Diarrhea, malabsorption, anorexia, and oral and esophageal lesions can all contribute to persistent and sometimes extreme weight loss, and the client may appear quite emaciated.

SKIN CHANGES. Many clients have dry, itchy, irritated skin and many types of skin rashes. Folliculitis, eczema, or psoriasis may also be present. When the platelet count is low, petechiae or bleeding gums may be present.

PSYCHOSOCIAL ASSESSMENT

Psychosocial data collection for a client with AIDS is very important. Ask about the client's social support system, including family, significant others, and friends. To protect confidentiality, learn who in this support system is aware of the client's diagnosis so that it is not inadvertently mentioned.

Some clients, because of fear of discrimination, are quite selective about whom they tell. Health care professionals must respect the client's choices as much as possible without compromising care. Offer resources to help with disclosure to sexual partners or significant others.

The client may be closest to a lover or a friend who is not legally recognized as next of kin. Obtain the name and telephone number of that person and learn whether a health care proxy or durable power-of-attorney document has been signed.

Ask about the client's activities of daily living (ADLs), as well as any changes that may have occurred since the diagnosis. Also assess the client's employment status and occupation, social activities and hobbies, living arrangements, and financial resources, including health insurance.

To plan care and monitor changes, assess the client's anxiety level, mood, and cognitive ability. Ask about any experiences with discrimination and how they were handled. After assessing the client's level of self-esteem and changes in body image, work with him or her to identify strengths and coping strategies. Gather information about any suicidal ideation, depression, or other psychological problems. Also ask about the client's use of support groups or other community resources.

LABORATORY ASSESSMENT

LYMPHOCYTE COUNTS. A lymphocyte count is performed as part of a complete blood count (CBC) with differential (see Chapter 23). The normal white blood cell (WBC) count is between 4500 and 11,000 cells/mm^3, with a differential of about 30% to 40% lymphocytes (an absolute number of 1500 to 4500). Clients with AIDS are often leukopenic, with a WBC count of less than 3500 cells/mm^3, and lymphopenic (less than 1500 lymphocytes/mm^3).

CD4+/CD8+ COUNTS. The percentage and number of CD4+ (T4) and CD8+ (T8) cells are an important part of an immune profile. People with HIV disease usually have a lower than normal number of CD4+ cells. Some clients with AIDS have fewer than 100 cells/mm^3 (normal: 500 to 1600 cells/mm^3), whereas the number of CD8+ cells remains normal. The normal ratio of CD4+ to CD8+ cells is 2:1. In HIV disease and AIDS, because of a low number of CD4+ cells, this ratio is low. Low CD4+ cell counts and a low CD4+/CD8+ ratio are associated with increased manifestations of disease.

ANTIBODY TESTS. When the body is infected with HIV, the normal response is to make an antibody to the infecting agent. This antibody is usually made 3 weeks to 3 months after the infection first occurs, although in some people antibodies are not made until 36 months after initial infection.

Thus antibody tests measure the client's response to the virus (the antigen) rather than measuring parts of the virus. HIV antibody can be measured by enzyme-linked immunosorbent assay (ELISA) and Western blot analysis. False-negative results (incorrectly indicating the absence of HIV infection) have been reported early in the infection, in people with cancer, and in people receiving long-term immunosuppressive therapy.

ENZYME-LINKED IMMUNOSORBENT ASSAY (ELISA). The ELISA test is inexpensive and accurate. The client's serum is mixed with HIV grown in culture. If the client has antibodies to HIV, they bind to the HIV antigens and can be detected (a positive test). However, this test can be negative even when the person has HIV infection if the test is performed before antibodies are made in sufficient amounts. The period of time between when a person is first infected with the virus and when viral replication is occurring but the immune system has not yet started making antibodies is called the "window period." This means that if the client has an episode of unprotected sex with an HIV positive person one night and comes in for testing a week later, the ELISA will be negative even though the client may have active HIV. Thus testing during the window does not provide useful information

False-positive test results (incorrectly indicating HIV infection) occur in about 0.1% (1 of 1000) of those tested with ELISA. False-positive results sometimes occur in pregnant women and women who have had children, injection drug users, people who have had malaria, clients with lymphomas, and those with reactivity to the HLA-DR4 leukocyte antigen.

WESTERN BLOT. If the results of an ELISA are positive, they are confirmed by Western blot analysis. This test is more sophisticated and expensive than the ELISA. The Western blot detects serum antibodies to four specific major HIV antigens. A positive Western blot result is based on the presence of antibodies to at least two of the major HIV antigens.

The result is considered inconclusive if two of the major antibodies are not detected but other antibodies to HIV are. The person should then be retested. If a person has a positive test result for HIV antibodies, it does not mean that he or she has AIDS, only that he or she has been infected with the virus.

Both the ELISA and Western blot are blood-based tests. This means special equipment and trained personnel must be used to test for HIV infection. Some HIV testing is more simplified, using techniques that are not blood-based so that testing can be done anywhere, even at home. Two such tests involve oral testing for HIV antibody. The test uses a device that is placed against the gum and cheek for 2 minutes. Fluid (not saliva) is drawn into an absorbable pad, which, in an HIV-positive person, contains antibodies. The pad is placed in a solution, if the result is positive, a change is observed similar to a positive result in a urine pregnancy test. Total testing time is about 15 minutes. If results are positive for HIV, a blood test is needed to confirm the result. The oral tests have the same accuracy as blood testing, and can provide results quickly. A urine test to detect HIV antibodies is also available, but it is not a rapid test.

Home test kits require that a drop of blood be placed upon a test card with a special code number. The card is mailed to a laboratory where the blood is tested for HIV antibodies. A special telephone number is called and the code entered. Test results are then given.

VIRAL CULTURE. Virus cultures also can determine the presence of HIV. This test is rarely used because of the time involved.

VIRAL LOAD TESTING. Viral load testing (also called viral burden testing) measures the presence of HIV viral genetic material (ribonucleic acid [RNA]) or other viral proteins in the client's blood rather than the body's response to the virus. These tests are quantitative and indicate the level of viral burden or viral load. Such tests are useful in monitoring disease progression and treatment effectiveness.

QUANTITATIVE RNA ASSAYS. Currently, three quantitative assays are used for viral load testing: the reverse transcriptase-polymerase chain reaction (RT-PCR), the branched deoxyribonucleic acid method (bDNA), and the nucleic acid sequence–based assay (NASBA). All three assays use gene amplification to determine the amount of HIV RNA present in a client's serum, and all have a specificity of 100%. Even if only a few infected cells are present in a serum sample, tiny amounts of the HIV RNA are amplified by these methods to allow detection. Such tests are useful in the clinical management of disease and in diagnosing HIV infection in people who have no indication of infection. These tests are used to monitor therapy effectiveness and as indicators of the need to change drug regimens.

p24 ANTIGEN ASSAY. The p24 antigen assay quantifies the amount of p24 (HIV viral core protein) in the client's serum. Because this assay is not as sensitive as antibody tests or assays of viral genetic material, it is used mostly to determine treatment efficacy.

OTHER LABORATORY TESTS. Other laboratory tests monitor the overall health of the client and detect or diagnose any infections or other problems related to HIV disease. Such tests include blood chemistries, a complete blood count (CBC) with differential and platelets, prothrombin time and partial thromboplastin time, a serologic test for syphilis (STS), and antigens to hepatitis A, hepatitis B, and hepatitis C. Tests to further evaluate the immune profile of a client may include bone marrow aspiration with biopsy and cultures.

OTHER DIAGNOSTIC ASSESSMENTS

Other diagnostic tests are performed on the basis of the client's manifestations. Such tests may include testing stool for ova and parasites; biopsies of the skin, lymph nodes, lungs, liver, gastrointestinal tract, or brain; a chest x-ray; gallium scans; bronchoscopy, endoscopy, or colonoscopy; liver and spleen scans; computed tomography scans; pulmonary function tests; and arterial blood gas analysis.

Critical Thinking Challenge

Your client is a 32-year-old white man who is new to your outpatient clinic. He complains of fatigue, abdominal pain, mild fever, nausea, and anorexia for almost 2 months. His most worrisome symptoms are a yellowing of his eyes and a darkening of his urine for the past week. He has tried to eat right, take vitamins, and get more rest, but he feels that he is getting worse, not better. A social history reveals that he was in a monogamous gay relationship for 6 years, which recently broke up. He has been dating and occasionally has had unprotected sexual relations with his dates. His most recent HIV test was 1 year ago and was negative. His last episode of unprotected anal receptive intercourse was 2 weeks ago.

1. He asks if his current symptoms are related to his recent sexual encounters. How should you respond?
2. Would you counsel this man to have an HIV test? Why or why not?
3. Should you teach this client about safer sex practices? Why or why not?

evolve For suggested answer guidelines, go to http://evolve.elsevier.com/Iggy/.

Analysis

COMMON NURSING DIAGNOSES AND COLLABORATIVE PROBLEMS

The following are the most common nursing diagnoses for clients with AIDS:

1. Risk for Infection related to immunodeficiency
2. Impaired Gas Exchange related to anemia, respiratory infection (*Pneumocystis carinii* pneumonia [PCP], cytomegalovirus [CMV] pneumonitis, pulmonary Kaposi's sarcoma [KS]), anemia, fatigue, or pain
3. Acute Pain or Chronic Pain related to neuropathy, myelopathy, malignancy, or infection
4. Imbalanced Nutrition: Less Than Body Requirements related to high metabolic need, nausea and vomiting, diarrhea, difficulty chewing or swallowing, or anorexia
5. Diarrhea related to infection, food intolerance, or drugs
6. Impaired Skin Integrity related to KS, infection, altered nutritional state, incontinence, immobility, hyperthermia, or malignancy
7. Disturbed Thought Processes related to AIDS dementia complex (ADC), central nervous system infection, or malignancy
8. Chronic Low Self-Esteem related to changes in body image, decreased self-esteem, or helplessness
9. Social Isolation related to stigma, virus transmissibility, infection control practices, or fear

The primary collaborative problem is Potential for Infection (processed under Risk for Infection, below).

ADDITIONAL NURSING DIAGNOSES AND COLLABORATIVE PROBLEMS

In addition to the common nursing diagnoses and collaborative problems, clients with AIDS may have one or more of the following:

- Activity Intolerance related to fatigue, discomfort, central nervous system defect, weakness, or anemia
- Risk for Injury related to central nervous system defect, mental status changes, depression, or thrombocytopenia
- Disturbed Sensory Perception (Visual) related to CMV retinitis or blindness
- Disturbed Sleep Pattern related to pain, discomfort, anxiety, or depression
- Ineffective Coping related to the diagnosis of AIDS
- Disabled Family Coping related to the diagnosis of AIDS
- Anticipatory Grieving related to potential loss of role and function or impending death

Planning and Implementation

RISK FOR INFECTION

The client with AIDS is susceptible to opportunistic infections because of immunodeficiency secondary to HIV infection.

NOC **PLANNING: EXPECTED OUTCOMES.** The client is expected to remain free of opportunistic diseases. Indicators include the following:

- Absence of chills, fever, or temperature instability
- Absence of purulent drainage or sputum
- Absence of diarrhea
- Absence of chest x-ray infiltration
- Maintenance of white blood cell (WBC) count within the client's normal range

NIC **INTERVENTIONS.** NIC interventions that can help the client minimize the chances of acquiring an infection are provided in Chart 25-5. Chart 25-6 outlines best practices for prevention of infection in a hospitalized immunocompromised client. Some strategies are investigational, including drug therapy and immune function enhancement.

CHART 25-5

NIC INTERVENTION ACTIVITIES for
The Client at Risk for Infection

Infection Protection: *Prevention and early detection of infection in a client at risk*

- Monitor for systemic and localized signs and symptoms of infection.
- Monitor vulnerability to infection.
- Monitor absolute granulocyte count, WBC count, and differential results.
- Follow neutropenic precautions, as appropriate.
- Screen all visitors for communicable disease.
- Maintain asepsis for client at risk.
- Inspect skin and mucous membranes for redness, extreme warmth, or drainage.
- Obtain cultures, as needed.
- Promote sufficient nutritional intake.
- Monitor for change in energy level/malaise.
- Instruct client to take antibiotics as prescribed.
- Teach client and family members how to avoid infections.

NIC intervention activities selected from Dochterman, J.M., & Bulechek, G.M. (Eds.). (2004). *Nursing interventions classification (NIC)* (4th ed.). St. Louis: Mosby. No part of this work is to be altered without prior written permission from the Publisher.
WBC, White blood cell.

Drug Therapy. Chart 25-7 lists treatments for opportunistic infections. Some medications have demonstrated antiretroviral effects; however, *it is important to remember that antiretroviral therapy only inhibits viral replication and does not kill the virus.* Treatment with only one antiretroviral agent, known as monotherapy, promotes drug resistance and does not improve the duration or quality of life for the client with HIV/AIDS. Instead, multiple drugs are used together in regimens popularly called "cocktails." These regimens consist of combinations of different types of antiretroviral agents. Such a therapeutic approach is termed highly active antiretroviral therapy (HAART) and is showing good results as measured by reduced viral load and improved CD4+ lymphocyte counts.

The main actions of each drug category are explained below. The specific drugs, dosages, and nursing implications are presented in Chart 25-8. Drawbacks to HIV/AIDS drug therapy include the expense of the drugs, side effects, food and timing requirements, and the number of daily drugs. The daily regimen is lifelong and burdensome.

Nucleoside Analog Reverse Transcriptase Inhibitors. Nucleoside analogs have a similar structure to the four nucleoside bases of DNA. These drugs are converted in the virally infected cell into a "counterfeit" form of a nucleotide base and compete with the actual nucleotide for placement in DNA. Thus they suppress production of reverse transcriptase (RT) and inhibit viral DNA synthesis and replication. This class of anti-HIV agents includes zidovudine (Retrovir, AZT), didanosine (ddI, Videx), zalcitabine (ddC, HIVID), lamivudine (Epivir, 3TC✱), stavudine (d4T, Zerit), tenofovir (Viread), emtricitabine (Emtriva), and abacavir (Ziagen).

Non-Nucleoside Analog Reverse Transcriptase Inhibitors. Non-nucleoside analog reverse transcriptase inhibitors also inhibit synthesis of reverse transcriptase. These drugs suppress viral replication but do not kill the virus. These drugs include nevirapine (Viramune), delavirdine (Rescriptor), and efavirenz (Sustiva) (see Chart 25-8).

Protease Inhibitors. Protease inhibitors block the HIV protease enzyme, preventing viral replication and release of viral particles. The HIV initially produces all of its proteins, including the ones needed to move viral particles out of a cell, in one long strand. For the proteins to be active, this large protein must be broken down into separate smaller proteins through the action of the viral enzyme HIV protease. The protease inhibitor drugs, when taken into an HIV-infected cell, make the protease enzyme work on the drug rather than on the initial large protein. Thus active proteins are not produced and the viral particles cannot leave the cell to infect other cells. Drugs include ritonavir (Norvir), indinavir (Crixivan), saquinavir (Invirase), nelfinavir (Viracept), amprenavir (Agenerase), lopinavir (Kaletra), atazanavir (Reyataz), and fosamprenavir (Lexiva).

Fusion Inhibitors. Fusion inhibitors are the newest class of antiretroviral medications. Enfuvirtide (Fuzeon) was recently approved for treatment of advanced, drug-resistant HIV infection. After gp120 and the CD4+ cell interact, the next step is for gp41 to fuse HIV and the host cell together for transfer of genetic information. Enfuvirtide works by blocking the fusion of HIV with a host cell by blocking the ability of gp41 to fuse with the host cell. Without fusion, infection of new cells does not occur.

Immune Enhancement. Research is being conducted to evaluate treatments that may enhance or replenish the immune system of clients with AIDS. Some of these

CHART 25-6

BEST PRACTICE for
Prevention of Infection in an Immunocompromised Client

- Place the client in a private room whenever possible.
- Use good handwashing technique before touching the client or any of his or her belongings.
- Ensure that the client's room and bathroom are cleaned at least once each day.
- Do not use supplies from common areas for immunosuppressed clients. For example, keep a sleeve or box of paper cups in the client's room, and do not share this box with any other client. Other articles include drinking straws, plastic knives and forks, dressing materials, gloves, and bandages.
- Limit the number of health care personnel entering the client's room.
- Monitor vital signs every 4 hours; note minor temperature elevation, which may suggest early sepsis.
- Inspect the client's mouth at least every 8 hours.
- Inspect the client's skin and mucous membranes (especially the anal area) for the presence of fissures and abscesses at least every 8 hours.
- Inspect open areas, such as IV sites, every 4 hours for manifestations of infection.
- Change wound dressings daily.
- Obtain specimens of all suspicious areas for culture, and promptly notify physician.
- Assist the client in performing coughing and deep-breathing exercises.
- Encourage activity at appropriate level for the client's current health status.
- Change IV tubing daily.
- Keep frequently used equipment in the room for use by the client only (e.g., blood pressure cuff, stethoscope, thermometer).
- Limit visitors to healthy adults.
- Use strict aseptic technique for all invasive procedures.
- Monitor the white blood cell count, especially the absolute neutrophil count (ANC), daily.
- Avoid the use of indwelling urinary catheters.
- Keep fresh flowers and potted plants out of the client's room.

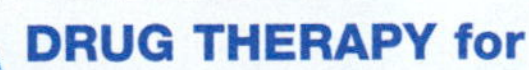

DRUG THERAPY for
AIDS-Related Opportunistic Infections

Drug	Indication	Usual Dosage	Nursing Interventions	Rationales
Trimethoprim (TMP)/ sulfamethoxazole (SMX) (Apo-Sulfatrim✱, Bactrim, Cotrim, Septra)	*Pneumocystis carinii* pneumonia	160 mg TMP and 800 mg SMX PO q12h	Monitor I&O. Encourage fluids. Monitor CBC, urinalysis, bilirubin, creatinine, alkaline phosphatase. Assess for sore throat, pallor, purpura, jaundice, weakness.	I&O are monitored because TMP/SMX is nephrotoxic. These values are monitored because TMP/SMX suppresses the immune system. These signs are assessed for because TMP/SMX is hepatotoxic.
Pentamidine isethionate (Pentam)	*P. carinii* pneumonia	4 mg/kg IM or IV once daily for 14-21 days	Monitor blood pressure, heart rate, and rhythm. Administer with client lying down. Monitor for hypoglycemia. Administer IV over 1 hr. Monitor liver function, CBC.	BP and heart rate are monitored because pentamidine causes hypotension when administered rapidly. Monitoring is necessary because pentamidine causes severe hypoglycemia that may be fatal. Liver function and CBC are monitored because pentamidine is hepatotoxic and immunosuppressive.
Pentamidine isethionate (Pentam, Pentacarinat✱)	*P. carinii* pneumonia	Inhalant 300 mg via nebulizer every 4 wk	See above.	See above.
Pyrimethamine (with sulfadoxine) (Daraprim)	Toxoplasmosis	50-75 mg PO daily for 1-3 wk, then 25 mg daily for 4-5 wk	Administer with food or milk. Monitor CBC and platelets.	Pyrimethamine irritates the GI tract. The CBC and platelets are monitored because pyrimethamine suppresses bone marrow activity.
Sulfadiazine	Toxoplasmosis Nocardiasis	500-2000 mg PO q6h daily for 3-4 wk	Monitor urine output, CBC. Encourage fluids. Advise client to avoid sun. Assess for sore throat, pallor, purpura, jaundice, weakness.	Urine output and the CBC are monitored because sulfadiazine causes renal toxicity. Fluids are necessary because sulfadiazine suppresses bone marrow activity. Clients should avoid the sun because sulfadiazine increases photosensitivity.
Dapsone (Avlosulfon✱, DDS)	Toxoplasmosis	50-100 mg PO daily	Monitor CBC. Assess for fever, sore throat, purpura, jaundice.	The CBC is monitored because dapsone suppresses bone marrow activity.
Metronidazole (Flagyl, Novonidazole✱)	Cryptosporidiosis Giardiasis	7.5 mg/kg PO q6h; 15 mg/kg IV initial dose, then 7.5 mg/kg PO q6h	Administer with food or milk. Teach client to avoid alcohol during treatment. Assess for dry mouth, dizziness, fungal infection.	Food or milk is recommended because metronidazole irritates the GI tract. Alcohol causes formation of acetaldehyde and headache, nausea, vomiting, and diarrhea.
[1] Ketoconazole (Nizoral) [1] *Med Error Alert! Do not confuse with Neoral, an immunosuppressant.*	Candidiasis Coccidioidomycosis Histoplasmosis	200-400 mg PO daily, single dose	Administer with food or milk. Avoid antacids for 2 hr. Teach client to avoid sun and alcohol during treatment. Monitor hepatic function.	Ketoconazole irritates the GI tract. Gastric acid is needed to activate drug. Ketoconazole increases photosensitivity. Hepatic function is monitored because ketoconazole is hepatotoxic.

I&O, Intake and output; *CBC*, complete blood count; *GI*, gastrointestinal; *MAO*, monoamine oxidase.

Continued

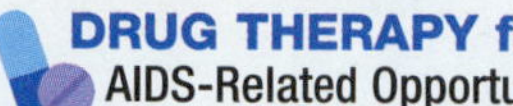

DRUG THERAPY for AIDS-Related Opportunistic Infections—*cont'd*

Drug	Indication	Usual Dosage	Nursing Interventions	Rationales
Fluconazole (Diflucan)	Candidiasis Cryptococcal meningitis	200-400 mg PO or IV initially, then 100-200 mg daily for 2-4 wk	Monitor hepatic function. Assess for abdominal pain, fever, diarrhea.	Hepatic function is monitored because fluconazole is hepatotoxic.
Rifampin (Rifadin, Rofact✱)	*Mycobacterium avium* complex Tuberculosis	10 mg/kg/day PO	Assess breath sounds, sputum.	Assessment of breath sounds and sputum determines treatment effectiveness.
			Monitor hepatic function, CBC. May turn body secretions orange.	Rifampin is hepatotoxic.
Ethambutol (Myambutol, Etibi✱)	*Mycobacterium avium* complex Tuberculosis	25-30 mg/kg PO 2-3 times/wk	Assess vision changes.	Vision changes are assessed because ethambutol causes retrobulbar neuritis and decreased visual acuity (reversible).
			Assess hepatic and renal function, CBC, urinalysis.	This assessment is necessary because ethambutol increases uric acid concentrations. Ethambutol suppresses bone marrow activity.
Amphotericin B (Fungizone)	Candidiasis Other fungal infections	0.3-1 mg/kg/day IV, maximum 50 mg daily	Assess renal function.	Renal function is assessed because amphotericin B is nephrotoxic.
			Assess infusion site.	Amphotericin B causes thrombophlebitis.
			Assess CBC.	The CBC is checked because amphotericin B suppresses bone marrow activity. Amphotericin B is *very* toxic.
Azithromycin (Zithromax)	*Mycobacterium avium* complex	600 mg PO daily plus ethambutol 15 mg/kg/day	Give with food.	Drug induces nausea and vomiting on an empty stomach.
			Assess for visual disturbances.	Azithromycin in combination with ethambutol can cause optic neuritis.
Ciprofloxacin (Cipro)	*Mycobacterium avium* complex Urinary tract infections	250-750 mg PO q12h; 200-400 mg IV q12h	Monitor I&O. Encourage fluids.	
			Administer on empty stomach (1 hr before or 2 hr after meals) if tolerated.	An empty stomach is recommended for best absorption.
			Teach client to avoid sun.	Client should avoid the sun because ciprofloxacin increases photosensitivity.
			Assess for dizziness, fungal infection. Infuse over 1 hr.	
Clarithromycin (Biaxin)	*Mycobacterium avium* complex	500 mg PO twice daily, given with 15 mg/kg/day ethambutol	Give with food.	Drug induces nausea and vomiting on an empty stomach.
			Assess for visual disturbances.	Clarithromycin in combination with ethambutol can cause optic neuritis.
Clofazimine (Lamprene)	*Mycobacterium avium* complex	50-300 mg PO daily	Assess vision changes, dizziness, drowsiness.	Vision changes and dizziness are assessed because clofazimine increases sedation.
			Instruct client to avoid sun.	Clofazimine increases photosensitivity (especially of eyes).
			Use lotions for dry skin. Monitor hepatic and renal function.	Clients should use lotions because clofazimine causes dry, scaly skin.

I&O, Intake and output; *CBC*, complete blood count; *GI*, gastrointestinal; *MAO*, monoamine oxidase.

CHART 25-7

DRUG THERAPY for AIDS-Related Opportunistic Infections—*cont'd*

Drug	Indication	Usual Dosage	Nursing Interventions	Rationales
Pyrazinamide (Tebrazid✱)	Tuberculosis	20-30 mg/kg/day PO	Monitor hepatic function, uric acid.	Pyrazinamide is hepatotoxic and increases uric acid concentration.
			Assess temperature q4h.	The client's temperature is assessed because pyrazinamide stimulates fever.
Isoniazid [2] (Laniazid, Isotamine)	Tuberculosis	5-10 mg/kg/day PO or IM, or 15 mg/kg PO or IM 2-3 times/wk	Administer on empty stomach.	Taking isoniazid on an empty stomach enhances absorption.
			Monitor hepatic function.	Isoniazid is hepatotoxic.
			Assess for vision changes.	Vision changes are assessed because isoniazid is neurotoxic.
			Instruct client to avoid alcohol and tyramine-containing foods.	Isoniazid is an MAO inhibitor.
Ganciclovir (Cytovene)	Cytomegalovirus retinitis	5 mg/kg IV q12h for 14-21 days 1000 mg PO q8h	Monitor neutrophil and platelet count. Infuse over 1 hr. Give with food.	Neutrophil and platelet counts are monitored because ganciclovir suppresses bone marrow activity.
Acyclovir (Zovirax)	Herpes simplex Herpes zoster Varicella zoster	200-800 mg PO five times daily; 5-10 mg/kg IV q8h for 7-10 days	Monitor renal function. Encourage fluids.	Acyclovir is nephrotoxic.
			Rotate infusion site.	Various infusion sites are used because acyclovir is a blood vessel irritant.

[2] *Med Error Alert! Do not confuse with Lamisil, an antifungal agent.*

CHART 25-8

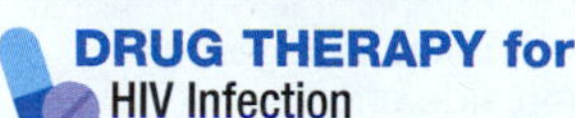

DRUG THERAPY for HIV Infection

Drug	Usual Dosage	Nursing Interventions	Rationales
Nucleoside Analog Reverse Transcriptase Inhibitors			
Zidovudine (Retrovir)	300 mg twice daily	Assess for dizziness.	Drug crosses the blood-brain barrier, causing dizziness.
		Monitor CBC, hepatic and renal function.	Zidovudine induces bone marrow suppression, hepatotoxicities, and nephrotoxicities.
Didanosine (ddI, Videx) (Videx EC)	125-300 mg twice daily 250-400 mg daily	Administer on an empty stomach.	Enhances drug absorption.
		Assess vision, hearing, touch, and balance.	Drug induces peripheral neuropathy.
		Monitor CBC.	Drug induces bone marrow suppression.
		Assess for abdominal pain.	Drug can cause severe pancreatitis.
Zalcitabine (ddC, HIVID)	0.75 mg PO q8h	Assess vision, hearing, touch, and balance.	Drug induces peripheral neuropathy.
		Tell client to avoid alcoholic beverages.	Elevates liver enzymes.
Lamivudine (Epivir, 3TC✱)	150 mg PO twice daily or 300 mg PO daily	Teach client to avoid fatty foods. Assess abdominal pain.	Can cause severe pancreatitis.
		Assess vision, hearing, touch, and balance.	Induces peripheral neuropathy.
Emtricitabine (Emtriva)	200 mg PO daily	Same as for lamivudine.	Same as for lamivudine.
Stavudine (d4T, Zerit)	40 mg twice daily	Assess vision, hearing, touch, and balance.	Induces peripheral neuropathy.
		Assess for generalized pain.	Induces arthralgias.

CNS, Central nervous system; *SC,* subcutaneous.
*Many drug interactions often occur with protease inhibitors.

Continued

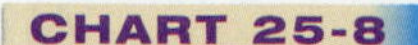
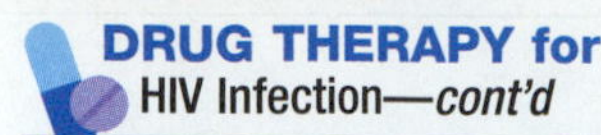

CHART 25-8 DRUG THERAPY for HIV Infection—*cont'd*

Drug	Usual Dosage	Nursing Interventions	Rationales
Nucleoside Analog Reverse Transcriptase Inhibitors—*cont'd*			
Abacavir (Ziagen)	300 mg twice daily	Assess for flu-like symptoms (fever, rash, headache, nausea, sore throat, fatigue, shortness of breath).	Manifestations of a hypersensitivity reaction.
		If flu-like symptoms are present, stop drug permanently.	Hypersensitivity can progress to life-threatening emergency.
Tenofovir (Viread)	250 mg PO daily	If also taking ddI, Videx, didanosine, must take these drugs at least 2 hr apart.	Can boost ddI levels into the toxic range in some people.
		Monitor liver and renal function.	Can cause high creatinine and transaminase levels.
Combivir (zidovudine 300 mg + lamivudine 150 mg)	1 tab PO twice daily	Same as with zidovudine and lamivudine individually.	A combination agent containing both drugs.
Trizivir (3 drugs in one) (zidovudine 300 mg + lamivudine 150 mg + abacavir 300 mg)	1 tab PO twice daily	Same as with zidovudine, lamivudine, and abacavir individually.	A combination agent containing all 3 drugs.
Epzicom (abacavir 600 mg + lamivudine 300 mg)	1 tab PO daily	Same as with abacavir and lamivudine individually.	A combination agent containing both drugs.
Truvada (tenofovir 300 mg + emtricitabine 200 mg)	1 tab PO daily	Same as with tenofovir and emtricitabine individually.	A combination agent containing both drugs.
Non-Nucleoside Analog Reverse Transcriptase Inhibitors			
Nevirapine (Viramune)	200 mg twice daily	Assess for rash. Assess for headache. Assess for abdominal pain.	Allergic reactions are common. Most common side effect. Drug may induce liver toxicity.
Efavirenz (Sustiva)	600 mg once daily	Assess for headaches, dysphoria, dizziness, insomnia, and nightmares.	Drug crosses blood-brain barrier and can induce CNS manifestations.
		Avoid contact with medication during pregnancy.	Drug is mutagenic and can induce birth defects.
Delavirdine (Rescriptor)	400 mg three times daily	Store at room temperature. Assess for headache or rash. Give 1 hr before or after antacids.	Recommended storage. Common side effects. Absorption is inhibited by antacids.
Protease Inhibitors*			
Saquinavir (Invirase)	600 mg q8h	Tell client to take with or just after a high-fat, high-calorie meal. Instruct client to wear sunscreen.	Drug is best absorbed with a fatty meal. Drug increases photosensitivity.
Indinavir (Crixivan)	800 mg q8h	Administer on an empty stomach. Assess for jaundice. Assess for flank or back pain or hematuria.	Enhances drug absorption. Induces hyperbilirubinemia. Induces nephrolithiasis.
Ritonavir (Norvir)	600 mg q12h	Administer with a light meal. Monitor serum lipid levels.	Enhances drug absorption. Can elevate serum lipid levels.
Nelfinavir (Viracept)	625 mg q12h	Administer with food.	Causes diarrhea, which is lessened when taken with food.
		Monitor blood glucose levels.	Can induce hyperglycemia.
Amprenavir (Agenerase)	200-800 mg daily	Monitor blood glucose levels.	Can induce hyperglycemia.
Lopinavir (Kaletra) (now available as combination: 133 mg lopinavir + 33 mg ritonavir)	3 capsules twice daily	Administer with food. Avoid giving to clients with known sulfonamide allergy.	Enhances drug absorption. Cross-reactivity possible.
Atazanavir (Reyataz)	400 mg PO daily	Monitor blood bilirubin levels. Administer with food. Check sclera and skin at each clinic visit.	Can induce hyperbilirubinemia. Enhances drug absorption. Icterus and jaundice are signs of high bilirubin levels.
Fosamprenavir (Lexiva)	1400 mg twice daily	Monitor serum lipid levels.	Can elevate serum lipid levels.
Fusion Inhibitors			
Enfuvirtide (Fuzeon)	90 mg SC twice daily	Monitor for skin reactions at injection site.	Infection risks and lipodystrophy if injection site is not rotated.

CNS, Central nervous system; *SC,* subcutaneous.
*Many drug interactions often occur with protease inhibitors.

TABLE 25-4 Complementary and Alternative Therapies for HIV/AIDS

Agents with Antiviral Effects	Immune-Enhancing Agents
▪ Shark cartilage	▪ Astragalus
▪ Curcumin	▪ Echinacea
▪ Hypercin	▪ Ascorbic acid
▪ Compound Q	
▪ SPV-30	
▪ Aloe vera	

methods include bone marrow transplantation, lymphocyte transfusion, and infusions of lymphokines, particularly interleukin-2, and other biological response modifiers.

Complementary and Alternative Therapies. Complementary therapies are often used by people with HIV/AIDS. Such therapies include vitamins, shark cartilage, and botanical products available at health food stores. The usefulness of these products has yet to be established through well-controlled clinical trials. In addition, some botanicals alter the effects of prescription drugs. Ask the client which botanicals are being used and check with the pharmacist to determine known drug interactions. Table 25-4 lists the botanical agents often used by clients to enhance immune function or slow viral replication.

Health Maintenance. HIV can remain latent inside a cell for long periods and only cause active infection when the cell is stimulated. The specific signals for the cell to become activated are not known, but concurrent viral or parasitic infections are suspected. Teach the client to avoid exposure to infection (Chart 25-9).

IMPAIRED GAS EXCHANGE

NOC **PLANNING: EXPECTED OUTCOMES.** The client is expected to maintain adequate oxygenation and perfusion and to experience minimal dyspnea. Indicators include the following:

- Rate and depth of respiration within the normal range
- Pulse oximetry within the normal range
- Absence of cyanosis or pallor

INTERVENTIONS. The nurse or respiratory therapist uses drug therapy, respiratory support and maintenance, comfort, and rest.

Drug Therapy. Appropriate drug therapy is started after identification of an infectious or other cause for respiratory difficulty (see Chart 25-7). A common respiratory infection among people with HIV disease or AIDS is *Pneumocystis carinii* pneumonia (PCP). The treatment of choice for PCP is trimethoprim/sulfamethoxazole (Apo-Sulfatrim✱, Bactrim, Cotrim, Septra), given intravenously or orally, depending on the severity of infection. Many clients with AIDS have adverse reactions to this medication, including nausea, vomiting, hyponatremia, rashes, fever, leukopenia, thrombocytopenia, and hepatitis.

Pentamidine isethionate (Pentacarinat✱, Pentam), usually given IV or IM, is also used to treat PCP. Aerosolized pentamidine isethionate is used for clients with CD4+ counts below 200 and for those who have already had PCP.

Other drug therapies include dapsone (Avlosulfon) and atovaquone (Mepron), which can be used as therapy for existing PCP or as prophylaxis. For moderate to severe PCP, steroids may be used to reduce the inflammation.

CHART 25-9

CLIENT EDUCATION GUIDE

Prevention of Infection Among Immunocompromised Clients

- Avoid crowds and other large gatherings of people who might be ill.
- Do not share personal toilet articles, such as toothbrushes, toothpaste, washcloths, or deodorant sticks, with others.
- If possible, bathe daily.
- Wash the armpits, groin, genitals, and anal area at least twice a day with an antimicrobial soap.
- Clean your toothbrush daily by either running it through the dishwasher or rinsing it in liquid laundry bleach.
- Wash your hands thoroughly with an antimicrobial soap before you eat or drink, after touching a pet, after shaking hands with anyone, as soon as you come home from any outing, and after using the toilet.
- Eat a low-bacteria diet, and avoid salads, raw fruit and vegetables, undercooked meat, pepper, and paprika.
- Wash dishes between use with hot, sudsy water or use a dishwasher.
- Do not drink water that has been standing for longer than 15 minutes.
- Do not reuse cups and glasses without washing.
- Avoid changing pet litter boxes. If unavoidable, use gloves or wash hands immediately.
- Avoid turtles and reptiles as pets.
- Do not feed pets raw or undercooked meat.
- Take your temperature at least once a day.
- Report any of the following signs or symptoms of infection to your physician immediately:
  - Temperature greater than 100° F (38° C)
  - Persistent cough (with or without sputum)
  - Pus or foul-smelling drainage from any open skin area or normal body opening
  - Presence of a boil or abscess
  - Urine that is cloudy or foul smelling or that causes burning on urination
- Take all prescribed medications as prescribed.
- Do not dig in the garden or work with houseplants.
- Avoid travel to areas of the world with poor sanitation or less-than-adequate health care facilities.

Respiratory Support and Maintenance. The client also needs care to maintain respiratory function and avoid complications. Assess the respiratory rate, rhythm, and depth; breath sounds; and vital signs and monitor for cyanosis at least every 8 hours. Apply oxygen and humidify the room as prescribed. Also monitor mechanical ventilation, perform suctioning and chest physical therapy as needed, and evaluate blood gas results.

Comfort. Assess the client's comfort. The client with respiratory difficulties may be more comfortable with the head of the bed elevated. Pace activities to reduce shortness of breath and exhaustion. Provide psychological support during periods of respiratory distress.

Rest and Activity. Most clients with HIV/AIDS have fatigue, especially when respiratory problems also are present. Fatigue can be made worse by certain therapies. Consult with the client to pace activities to conserve energy. Guide the client in active and passive range-of-motion (ROM) exercises. Schedule non–time-critical activities, such as bathing, so that he or she is not fatigued at mealtime.

PAIN

The client with severe HIV disease or AIDS often has pain from a variety of causes. Pain can result from enlarged organs stretching the viscera or compressing nerves. Tumor invasion of bone and other tissues can cause pain. Many clients with AIDS have peripheral neuropathy-induced pain from the disease or drug therapies. Many have generalized joint and muscle pain.

NOC **PLANNING: EXPECTED OUTCOMES.** The client is expected to achieve an acceptable level of comfort and pain reduction. Indicators include the following:

- Reporting that pain is controlled
- Absence of physiologic indicators of acute pain (increased heart rate and blood pressure)
- Absence of facial grimacing, teeth clenching
- Willingness to move and participate in self-care

INTERVENTIONS. Pharmacologic and nonpharmacologic approaches are used to manage pain in the client with HIV/AIDS, depending on the cause of the pain.

Comfort Measures. The use of pressure-relieving mattress pads, warm baths or other forms of hydrotherapy, massage, and applying heat or cold to painful areas may reduce pain levels, with or without drug therapy. Take care when moving or assisting the client. Use lift sheets to avoid pulling or grasping the client with joint pain. The client may be thin and have poor circulation, contributing to pain and discomfort. Help the client change positions often.

Drug Therapy. The type of drugs used depends on what is causing the pain. For arthralgia and myalgia, nonsteroidal anti-inflammatory drugs (NSAIDs) may reduce inflammation and increase comfort without inducing drowsiness. The neuropathic pain of peripheral neuropathy may respond best to tricyclic antidepressants such as amitriptyline (Elavil) or to anticonvulsant medication such as phenytoin (Dilantin) or carbamazepine (Tegretol). Drugs for neuropathic pain may take from several days to weeks before a full effect is seen. During this time, opioids may be needed to control pain.

When opioids are used, assess the client for pain intensity. Mild to moderate pain is treated with weaker opioids such as oxycodone or codeine. More intense pain is treated with stronger opioids such as morphine, hydromorphone (Dilaudid), or fentanyl transdermal (Duragesic). Combinations of weak and strong opioids along with non-opioid medications may be used to provide the best sustained pain relief and allow the client to participate in activities to the extent that he or she wishes.

Complementary and Alternative Therapies. Many clients with pain from HIV/AIDS use therapies such as guided imagery, distraction, progressive relaxation, body-talk, and biofeedback to help control pain. Such therapies can be used with more traditional and pharmacologic measures to improve comfort.

IMBALANCED NUTRITION: LESS THAN BODY REQUIREMENTS

Many clients with AIDS have difficulty maintaining their weight and nutritional status. This problem may be caused by fatigue, anorexia, nausea and vomiting, difficult or painful swallowing, diarrhea, or wasting syndrome.

NOC **PLANNING: EXPECTED OUTCOMES.** The client is expected to maintain optimal weight through adequate nutrition and hydration. Indicators include the following:

- Selecting foods high in calories and protein
- Maintaining current weight or gaining weight
- Drinking at least 3 L of oral fluids per day
- Maintaining blood levels of albumen, prealbumin, and hemoglobin within normal ranges

INTERVENTIONS. Because there are multiple factors for poor nutrition in AIDS, diagnostic procedures are needed to determine the cause. Once the cause is determined, appropriate therapy is initiated. For example, in the client who has candidal esophagitis, nutrition is affected because of swallowing difficulties.

Drug Therapy. Therapy can include ketoconazole (Nizoral) or fluconazole (Diflucan) orally, or intravenous (IV) amphotericin B (Fungizone). Administer the medication as prescribed and monitor for side effects such as nausea and vomiting, which further alter nutritional status. Provide mouth care and ice chips and keep unpleasant odors out of the client's environment. Antiemetics are used as needed.

Diet Therapy. Monitor the client's weight, intake and output, and calorie count. Assess food preferences and any dietary cultural or religious practices. Instruct the client about a high-calorie, high-protein, nutritionally sound diet. Encourage the client to avoid dietary fat, because fat intolerance often occurs as a result of the disease and as a side effect of some antiretroviral medications. In collaboration with the dietitian, provide an appropriate diet, including small, frequent meals (better tolerated than large meals). Supplemental vitamins and fluids are indicated in some cases. For the client who cannot achieve adequate nutrition through food, tube feedings or total parenteral nutrition may be needed.

Mouth Care. Provide frequent mouth care for clients susceptible to oral ulceration or infection. Rinses of sodium bicarbonate with normal saline every 2 hours or several times a day are helpful. Give the client a soft toothbrush and advise him or her to drink plenty of fluids. For oral pain, analgesics or viscous lidocaine may be needed.

DIARRHEA

Clients with AIDS often suffer from diarrhea. Sometimes an infectious cause (e.g., *Giardia* or amoeba) can be determined and treated, or the cause is determined but no effective therapy is available. Many clients are lactose intolerant, and HIV disease makes this condition worse. Diarrhea may occur as a side effect of therapy with protease inhibitors. In some cases, clients with AIDS have diarrhea and no cause can be identified.

NOC **PLANNING: EXPECTED OUTCOMES.** The client is expected to have decreased diarrhea; maintain fluid, electrolyte, and nutritional status; and reduce incontinence. Indicators include the following:

- Stool amount is appropriate for the diet
- Stools are formed and soft
- Recognizes urge to defecate
- Maintains control of stool passage

INTERVENTIONS. For most clients with AIDS and diarrhea, symptom management is all that is available. Antidiarrheals, such as diphenoxylate hydrochloride (Diarsed✱, Lomotil) or loperamide (Imodium), given on a regular schedule, provide some relief. Consult with the dietitian and offer dietary counseling about appropriate foods. Recommended dietary changes include less roughage; less fatty, spicy, and sweet food; and no alcohol or caffeine. Some clients obtain relief when they eliminate dairy products from the diet or eat smaller amounts of food more often and drink plenty of fluids, especially between meals.

Provide the client with a bedside commode or a bedpan if needed. Some clients cannot reach the bathroom in time because of immobility or anal sphincter weakness, others because of the urgency to defecate. Provide privacy, support, and understanding.

IMPAIRED SKIN INTEGRITY

The most common skin lesion in AIDS is Kaposi's sarcoma (KS). Lesions may be localized or widespread. Large lesions can cause pain and restrict movement. They can impede circulation, causing open, weeping, painful lesions. Another cause of impaired skin integrity is herpes simplex virus (HSV) infection.

NOC **PLANNING: EXPECTED OUTCOMES.** The client is expected to have healing of any existing lesions and avoid increased skin breakdown or secondary infection. Indicators include the following:

- Absence of new lesions or open skin areas
- Existing lesions become smaller in diameter
- Absence of purulent drainage, induration or redness in, from, or around skin lesions

INTERVENTIONS. KS can be treated with local radiation, intralesional chemotherapy, or cryotherapy. Systemic therapy is used in clients with rapidly progressive disease or with major involvement of the intestinal tract, lungs, or other organs. Therapies include chemotherapy (single agent or combination), interferon-alpha, and interferon-alpha plus zidovudine.

Treatment of painful KS lesions includes analgesics and comfort measures. Keep open, weeping KS lesions clean and dressed to reduce the risk for secondary infection. Many clients with skin KS are concerned about their appearance and the risk of being identified as HIV positive. Makeup (if lesions are not open), long-sleeved shirts, and hats may help in maintaining a normal appearance.

For the client with an HSV abscess, provide good skin care. Clean abscesses at least once per shift with normal saline and allow them to air-dry or dry with a heat lamp. This infection is painful and requires analgesics, assistance with position, and other comfort measures. Modified Burow's solution (Domeboro) soaks promote healing for some clients. HSV infection is treated with acyclovir (Zovirax) given intravenously, orally, or in some cases, topically, depending on the severity of the infection.

DISTURBED THOUGHT PROCESSES

Neurologic changes with disturbed thought processes are major areas of concern for clients with HIV infection or AIDS. These changes may be due to psychological stressors accompanying the disease or to organic disorders caused by opportunistic infections, cancer, or HIV encephalitis.

NOC **PLANNING: EXPECTED OUTCOMES.** The client is expected to show improved mental status. Indicators include that the client demonstates the following behaviors:

- Identifies self and significant others
- Identifies correct month and year
- Recalls immediate, recent, and remote information accurately

INTERVENTIONS. Clients with AIDS suffer from enormous loss and psychological stress, which complicates the assessment of any changes in behavior or affect. Assess baseline neurologic and mental status by using neurologic assessment tools (see Chapter 44) to compare any changes. Evaluate the client for subtle changes in memory, ability to concentrate, affect, and behavior. It is important to determine whether the cause of the neurologic changes is treatable.

Orientation. Reorient the confused client to person, time, and place as needed, reminding the client of your identity and explaining what is to be done at any given time. Using calendars, clocks, and radios and putting the bed close to a window also may help keep the client oriented. Give simple directions; use short, uncomplicated sentences; explain activities in simple language; and involve the client in planning the daily schedule. Ask relatives or significant others to bring in familiar items from home. Arrange all items in the client's environment in the same location as at home.

Drug Therapy. Various agents are used as appropriate for different conditions contributing to altered thought processes in the person with AIDS. Psychotropic drugs are used to treat ongoing behavioral problems or emotional disorders. Antidepressants and anxiolytics are often prescribed.

Safety Measures. Attention to safety is crucial to the well-being of the neurologically impaired client with AIDS. He or she may not be aware of activities or surroundings and may need help with bathing, dressing, eating, ambulating, and other activities of daily living (ADLs). Make the environment, whether a hospital room or long-term care facility, safe and comfortable.

Some clients are susceptible to seizures. Institute seizure precautions, including using padded siderails and having an artificial oral airway available. Anticonvulsants may be added to the medications.

Assess the client with neurologic manifestations for increased intracranial pressure. Report immediately any changes in level of consciousness, vital signs, pupil size or reactivity, or limb strength to the physician for appropriate intervention. Corticosteroids may be given to reduce intracranial pressure.

Support. Work closely with the family and significant others of the neurologically impaired client. There is great trauma in seeing a loved one unable to care for himself or herself or demonstrating unusual or childlike behavior. Answer questions honestly and sensitively. Teach the family and significant others how to reorient the client. Encourage them to continue to provide the client with news of family happenings or current events. Collaborate with the social worker to identify community resources for the client and family.

CHRONIC LOW SELF-ESTEEM

The client with AIDS may have changes in self-esteem and self-concept. Contributing to this are dramatic changes in appearance that alter the person's body image. Many clients also have abrupt, significant changes in their relationships with others and in day-to-day activities, including a job or other productive activities. All changes can disrupt the self-concept.

NOC **PLANNING: EXPECTED OUTCOMES.** The client is expected to identify positive aspects of himself or herself and accept himself or herself. Indicators include that the client often or consistently demonstrates the following behaviors:

- Verbalizes self-acceptance
- Maintains eye contact
- Accepts compliments from others
- Expresses feelings of self-worth

INTERVENTIONS. Provide a climate of acceptance for clients with AIDS by promoting a trusting relationship and by helping clients express feelings and identify positive aspects of themselves. Allow for privacy but do not avoid or isolate the client. Encourage self-care, independence, control, and decision making by helping the client set short-term, attainable goals and offering praise when these are achieved.

Complementary therapy in the form of guided imagery is used by many clients to increase their sense of control and enhance self-esteem. Imagery can focus on helping clients cope with distressing side effects or painful procedures. Other uses of imagery include picturing battle scenes in which the virus is killed by immune system cells.

SOCIAL ISOLATION

Many clients with AIDS face discrimination, rejection, and isolation. Friends or health care workers sometimes avoid or refuse to have anything to do with them. Misunderstanding and fear lead to misuse of proper infection control procedures, and clients are inappropriately isolated.

NOC **PLANNING: EXPECTED OUTCOMES.** The client is expected to identify behaviors that cause social isolation and demonstrate behaviors that reduce social isolation. Indicators include that the client often or consistently demonstrates the following behaviors:

- Interacts with close friends, significant others, and family members
- Demonstrates cooperation with others
- Uses assertive behaviors as appropriate

INTERVENTIONS. Interventions for social isolation focus on promoting interactions and on education to reduce fear of AIDS transmission.

Promotion of Interaction. Establish a therapeutic nurse-client relationship and do not isolate the client. Show understanding and concern while helping the client find ways to reduce feelings of rejection and isolation. Reduce barriers to social contact. Assess the client's social support resources. Teach family and significant others about HIV transmission and the use of standard precautions to reduce anxiety and increase contact with the client (see Chapter 29).

Encourage the client to verbalize feelings about self, coping skills, and a sense of control over the situation. Help the client to identify support systems, including those already in place and those that need to be arranged.

Education. The most important aspect for prevention of HIV transmission is education. All people, regardless of age, gender, ethnicity, or sexual orientation, are susceptible to HIV infection. HIV infection is preventable because of the mode of viral transmission and the fragile nature of the virus.

Critical Thinking Challenge

You are the new charge nurse on a busy medical-surgical floor at a community hospital. On a particularly busy day, one of the "new hires" tells you that she had a needle stick injury, at the start of shift, today. She was giving her 78-year-old diabetic client insulin and accidentally stuck herself, trying to put the needle into an overflowing sharps container. In talking with other nurses, she doubts that this is a high-risk needle stick since it was with an insulin syringe, and the client is an older woman, who is obviously at low risk for HIV. She washed off the blood thoroughly from her finger, applied Betadine, and covered it with a Band-Aid. Because it is almost change of shift, the nurse wants to fill out an incident report and go home.

1. How will you counsel this nurse about the needle stick injury?
2. What rights and obligations does she have?
3. For what other bloodborne diseases has this incident placed her at risk?
4. Should postexposure prophylaxis be started? Why or why not?
5. Should this nurse inform her sexual partner(s) of this incident? Why or why not?

evolve For suggested answer guidelines, go to http://evolve.elsevier.com/Iggy/.

Community-Based Care

The usual course of illness is one of intermittent acute infections and periods of relative wellness over months or years. Often, this period is followed by chronic, progressive debilitation. Because of the cyclic nature of HIV disease and AIDS, the client often spends long periods at home between hospital admissions or clinic visits. In some instances, especially as the illness becomes more severe, he or she may need referral to a long-term care facility, home care agency, or hospice. In collaboration with the social worker, dietitian, and other available resources, work with clients to plan what will be needed and how they will manage at home with self-care and activities of daily living (ADLs).

HOME CARE MANAGEMENT

When the client is discharged to home, assess the client's status, ability to function, and actual or potential needs for care. Some clients do not need home care but do need to maintain a link with primary care providers. Home care can range from help with ADLs for clients with weakness, debility, or limited function to around-the-clock nursing care, medications, and nutritional support for severely or terminally ill clients. Assess available resources, including family members and significant others willing and able to be caregivers. Help the family make arrangements for outside caregivers or respite care, if needed. Clients may need referrals or help in planning housing, finances, insurance, legal services, funeral arrangements, and spiritual counseling.

Home care aides may be involved in daily or weekly care of the client with AIDS in the home. Usually a home care nurse makes routine visits for assessment purposes, especially as the client becomes increasingly debilitated. Chart 25-10 lists focused assessment areas for the client with AIDS at home.

HEALTH TEACHING

Educating the client, family, and significant others is a high priority when preparing for discharge. Instruct about modes of transmission and preventive behaviors (guidelines for safer sex; not sharing toothbrushes, razors, and other potentially blood-contaminated articles). Caregivers also need instruction about best practices for infection control precautions to prevent transmission while caring for the client in the home (Chart 25-11), nursing techniques to use in the home, and coping or support strategies.

Teach the client, family, and significant others how to protect the client from infection, to identify manifestations of potential infections, and what to do if these appear. Teach

CHART 25-10

FOCUSED ASSESSMENT of
The Person with AIDS

Assess cardiovascular and respiratory status.
- Vital signs
- Presence of acute chest pain or dyspnea
- Presence of cough
- Presence of fever
- Activity tolerance

Assess nutritional status.
- Food intake
- Weight loss or gain
- General condition of skin
- Financial resources

Assess neurologic status.
- Cognitive changes
- Motor changes
- Sensory disturbances

Assess gastrointestinal status.
- Mouth and oropharynx
- Presence of dysphagia
- Presence of abdominal pain
- Presence of nausea, vomiting, diarrhea

Assess psychological status.
- Presence of anxiety
- Presence of depression

Assess activity and rest.
- Activities of daily living (ADLs)
- Mobility and ambulation
- Fatigue
- Sleep pattern
- Presence of pain

Assess home environment.
- Safety hazards
- Structural barriers affecting functional ability

Assess client's and caregiver's adherence and understanding of illness and treatment, including the following:
- Manifestations to report to nurse
- Medication schedule and side or toxic effects

Assess client's and caregiver's coping skills.

about the use of self-care strategies, such as good hygiene, balanced rest and exercise, skin care, mouth care, and safe administration of any prescribed drugs (including potential side effects). During dietary teaching, stress the following:
- Good nutrition
- Avoidance of raw or rare fish, fowl, or meat
- Thorough washing of fruits and vegetables
- Proper food handling and refrigeration practices

Teach the client to avoid large crowds, especially in enclosed areas, not to travel to countries with poor sanitation, and to avoid cleaning pet litter boxes.

PSYCHOSOCIAL PREPARATION

Clients with AIDS are often concerned about the possible social stigma and rejection. Be aware that this fear is realistic and help identify ways to avoid problems, as well as identify coping strategies for difficult situations. Support family members and significant others in efforts to help the client and provide protection from discrimination.

Encourage clients to continue as many usual activities as possible. Except when too ill or too weak, they can continue to work and participate in most social activities. Support clients in their selection of friends and relatives with whom to discuss the diagnosis. Stress that sexual partners and care providers should be informed; beyond that, it is up to the client. Some clients have severe depression or anxiety about the future. Almost all feel the burden of having a fatal disease widely considered unacceptable and feel compelled to maintain some secrecy about the illness. Referrals to community resources, mental health/behavioral health professionals, and support groups can help the client verbalize fears and frustrations and cope with the illness.

CHART 25-11

BEST PRACTICE for
Infection Control for Home Care of the Person with AIDS

Direct Care
- Follow standard precautions and good handwashing techniques.
- Do not share razors or toothbrushes.

Housekeeping
- Wipe up feces, vomitus, sputum, urine, or blood or other body fluids and the area with soap and water. Dispose of solid wastes and solutions used for cleaning by flushing them down the toilet. Disinfect the area by wiping with a 1:10 solution of household bleach (1 part bleach to 10 parts water). Wear gloves during cleaning.
- Soak rags, mops, and sponges used for cleaning in a 1:10 bleach solution for 5 minutes to disinfect them.
- Wash dishes and eating utensils in hot water and dishwashing soap or detergent.
- Clean bathroom surfaces with regular household cleaners, then disinfect them with a 1:10 solution of household bleach.

Laundry
- Rinse clothes, towels, or bedclothes if they become soiled with feces, vomitus, sputum, urine, or blood. Then dispose of the soiled water by flushing it down the toilet. Launder these clothes with hot water and detergent with 1 cup of bleach added per load of laundry.
- Keep soiled clothes in a plastic bag.

Waste Disposal
- Dispose of needles and other "sharps" in a labeled puncture-proof container such as a coffee can with a lid, using standard precautions to avoid needle stick injuries. Decontaminate full containers by adding a 1:10 bleach solution. Then seal the container with tape and place it in a paper bag. Dispose of the container in the regular trash.
- Remove solid waste from contaminated trash such as paper towels or tissues, dressings, disposable incontinence pads, and disposable gloves, then flush the waste down the toilet. Place these items in tied plastic bags and dispose of them in the regular trash.

HEALTH CARE RESOURCES

In many cities, community organizations have been set up to assist people with AIDS. Often composed of volunteers, they offer excellent services to the community. The types and number of services vary by agency and city, but many include HIV testing and counseling, clinic services, buddy systems, support groups, respite care, education and outreach, referral services, and even housing. Clients may also need referrals to other local resources, such as home care agencies, companies that provide home IV therapy, community mental health/behavioral health agencies, Meals on Wheels, and others. In addition, educational materials and support groups are available through Internet access.

Evaluation: Outcomes

The overall goals for care of clients with AIDS are to maintain the maximum possible level of function for as long as possible, minimize infections, and maintain quality of life and dignity during the course of progressive illness. Evaluate the care of the client with AIDS on the basis of the identified nursing diagnoses and collaborative problems. Expected outcomes include that the client should:

- Remain free from opportunistic infections
- Have adequate respiratory function
- Achieve an acceptable level of physical comfort
- Attain adequate weight, nutritional, and fluid status
- Maintain skin integrity
- Remain oriented
- Maintain self-esteem
- Maintain a support system and involvement with others
- Adhere to the prescribed therapy regimen

Specific indicators for these outcomes are listed for each nursing diagnosis and collaborative problem under the Planning and Implementation section (see earlier).

NUTRITION-RELATED IMMUNODEFICIENCIES

Good nutrition is needed for proper immune function. White blood cells (WBCs) are highly active cells that constantly shed surface proteins and need nutrients to remake these components. Immunodeficiency related to nutrition results from biologic, political, economic, and cultural factors. Immunodeficiency from poor nutrition can be prevented and treated.

Malnutrition is a major cause of global immunodeficiency, seen most often in less affluent countries, in the urban and rural poor of North America, and in the chronically ill. Hospitalized adult medical-surgical clients also are at high risk for malnutrition. Four points should be kept in mind:

- Anorexia occurring with chronic disease, acute infection, or treatment often leads to reduced oral intake.
- Absorption or utilization of nutrients is sometimes impaired because of gastrointestinal diseases or absorption problems.
- Host defenses during infection increase the demand for nutrients, which is met at the expense of the body's stores.
- Hospitalized clients are often undernourished because of many hours of nothing by mouth and because of IV fluid infusions that lack essential nutrients.

Malnutrition can impair any aspect of immune function. The degree of impairment is related to the severity of malnutrition. Nutrient excess, especially fats and carbohydrates, also have detrimental effects on immune function. Nutritional problems are often a complex of deficiency or excess of one or more nutrients.

Protein-Calorie Malnutrition

PATHOPHYSIOLOGY

Protein-calorie malnutrition (PCM) affects all aspects of immune function. The greatest impairment occurs in cell-mediated immunity, with decreased numbers of T-lymphocytes and thymic changes. The result is anergy and an increased risk for infection. The estimated incidence of PCM ranges from 25% to 50% of hospitalized clients. PCM causes reduced energy and protein synthesis. The following are manifestations of PCM in adults:

- Leanness and cachexia
- Decreased effort tolerance and lethargy
- Intolerance to cold
- Ankle and shin edema
- Dry, flaking skin and various types of dermatitis
- Poor wound healing
- A higher than usual incidence of postoperative infection

COLLABORATIVE MANAGEMENT

The management of clients with PCM is to treat the precipitating event and supply protein and calories, sometimes with nutrient supplements. In clients with severe PCM, any infection is treated first and then fluid and electrolyte imbalances are corrected. Then a gradual but steady replacement of protein and energy is undertaken. Often this refeeding begins parenterally, because a severely malnourished gut may be unable to absorb food. Replenishment of protein and calories is accompanied by vitamin supplementation as needed, nutrition education, and a progressive increase in physical activity.

PCM is easier to prevent than to treat. Be aware of hospitalized clients at risk for PCM. Chart 25-12 lists practices to reduce the risk for PCM in hospitalized clients.

Obesity

PATHOPHYSIOLOGY

The incidence and severity of infectious disease increase among obese people. Impaired cell-mediated immunity and decreased neutrophil activity occur with obesity, making obese people at greater risk for infection. Excess dietary fats suppress all aspects of immune function. The obese client also may have a coexisting PCM.

Often the obese client is not recognized as malnourished because of the excessive weight. For these clients, nutritional status is assessed by laboratory measurements and diet history.

COLLABORATIVE MANAGEMENT

Good nutrition is important to maintain and improve immune defenses. Consult with the physician and dietitian to provide a diet that is sufficient in calories and protein but is low in fat.

Protect the obese client by maintaining a safe environment. Use good handwashing before all contact with the

CHART 25-12

BEST PRACTICE for
Reducing the Risk for Protein-Calorie Malnutrition in the Hospitalized Client

- Measure height and weight when the client is admitted to the agency, reweighing at least weekly.
- Monitor the client's ability to eat the prescribed diet and the amounts eaten.
- Obtain dietary consultation when needed.
- Evaluate whether nutrients consumed are sufficient to meet basal and stress-related energy needs.
- Avoid prolonged use of standard IV fluids that provide less than 200 calories/L.
- Assess and monitor laboratory values for serum albumin, prealbumin, and leukocyte counts.
- Schedule tests and procedures so that the client spends minimal time fasting.

client. Ensure that strict aseptic techniques are used for all invasive procedures. Assess the client every shift for manifestations of local or systemic infection and notify the physician of any suspected infection.

THERAPY-INDUCED IMMUNODEFICIENCIES

PATHOPHYSIOLOGY

Some secondary immunodeficiencies may be related to other conditions that cause the loss of immunoglobulins or destruction of lymphocytes. The most common cause of secondary immunodeficiency is the use of drugs and other treatment modalities for various diseases. Sometimes immunosuppression is a desired effect, as in organ transplantation or for the treatment of autoimmune disorders. Often immunosuppression is an undesirable, complicating side effect of therapy that is used for another intent, such as cancer chemotherapy, and may even require changing the therapeutic regimen. Various therapies cause different types and degrees of immunosuppression. The challenge is to have maximal therapeutic effect without leaving the client overly immunosuppressed and susceptible to serious complications.

Drug-Induced Immunodeficiencies

Several drug classes have major immunosuppressive effects. Some induce general immunosuppression; others are more specific and target one part of the immune system more than another.

CYTOTOXIC DRUGS

Most cytotoxic drugs interfere with all rapidly dividing cells. White blood cells (WBCs), including lymphocytes and phagocytes, rapidly divide and are susceptible to this type of destruction. The result is a decrease in the number of lymphocytes and phagocytic cells. Cytotoxic drugs interfere with the ability of lymphocytes to produce and release products such as lymphokines and antibodies, causing general immunosuppression. Most cytotoxic drugs are used for cancer and autoimmune disorders.

CORTICOSTEROIDS

Corticosteroids are hormones used to treat many autoimmune diseases, neoplasms, and endocrine disorders. Corticosteroids have both anti-inflammatory and immunosuppressive effects. They inhibit inflammation by stabilizing blood vessel membranes and decreasing permeability, blocking the movement of neutrophils and monocytes. These drugs disrupt the synthesis of arachidonic acid, the main precursor for a variety of inflammatory chemicals.

Corticosteroids keep T-cells in the bone marrow, reducing the number of circulating T-cells and resulting in lymphopenia and suppressed cell-mediated immunity.

Corticosteroids interfere with immunoglobulin G (IgG) production and reduce antibody-antigen binding. These drugs have many effects that alter disease activity, and numerous side effects, including the following:

- Central nervous system changes, such as euphoria, insomnia, or psychosis
- Cardiovascular changes, such as hypertension or edema
- Gastrointestinal effects, such as gastric irritation, ulcers, and increased appetite (with weight gain)
- Other changes (e.g., hyperglycemia, muscle weakness, delayed wound healing, osteoporosis, and body fat redistribution)

CYCLOSPORINE

Cyclosporine (Sandimmune, Neoral) is a specific immunosuppressant that selectively suppresses the helper-inducer T-lymphocytes by blocking their growth and development. Cyclosporine is used to prevent organ transplant rejection and graft-versus-host disease. This drug is occasionally used for disorders, such as uveitis, rheumatoid arthritis, and other autoimmune diseases.

Radiation-Induced Immunodeficiencies

Radiation is toxic to dividing and resting cells. Because most lymphocytes are sensitive to radiation, exposure can induce profound lymphopenia, causing general immunosuppression. Whether or not immunodeficiency occurs after radiation therapy depends on the location and dose of radiation. Exposure to the iliac and femur in adults can cause generalized immunosuppression because these bone areas are the primary blood cell–producing sites.

◆COLLABORATIVE MANAGEMENT

Management of the client with treatment-induced immunodeficiency aims to improve immune function and protect him or her from infection. The most severe immunosuppression occurs while he or she is receiving the immunosuppressive drugs or during radiation treatment. The severity and duration of the immunosuppression are related to the dosage of specific drugs. Although this impairment is usually temporary, with good recovery of immune and inflammatory responses within weeks or months of therapy completion, the potential for severe infections makes this problem a major treatment concern. Common infections occurring during this period include those of fungal origin, yeast, residual viral breakthrough, and a variety of bacteria.

Work closely with clients and other health care professionals to provide safe care to those at risk for infection. Chart 25-6 lists specific nursing actions to prevent infection among clients with drug-induced or any type of immunosuppression. Good handwashing by all health care personnel before contact with the client is essential for infection prevention. Health care professionals must use aseptic technique with any invasive procedure.

In some instances, drug-induced immunosuppression can be reduced or avoided by giving biological response modifiers (BRMs) to stimulate bone marrow production of immune system cells. Although not appropriate for all types of disorders, this treatment can reduce the client's risk for infection during drug therapy. BRMs are expensive, however, and not consistently covered by insurance. See Chapters 28 and 43 for further discussion about this treatment.

Many clients remain at home during periods of immunosuppression. Teach the client and family best practices to reduce the client's risk for infection (see Chart 25-9).

For clients receiving chronic therapy with immunosuppressive drugs, drug dosages are altered according to their responses. The lowest dose that achieves the desired effect is given.

Congenital (Primary) Immunodeficiencies

Congenital, or primary, immunodeficiencies are disorders in which the immunodeficient person is born with a defect in the development or function of one or more immune components. As a result, the immune response does not adequately protect the client from infection, cancer, or other disease. Most congenital immunodeficiencies are rare.

Some congenital immunodeficiencies are inherited as an X-linked trait (such as Bruton's agammaglobulinemia or Wiskott-Aldrich syndrome), and some are recessive (such as ataxia-telangiectasia). For many congenital immunodeficiencies, however, the genetic defect and inheritance pattern have not been clearly identified. Examples of congenital immunodeficiencies are listed in Table 25-5.

Congenital immunodeficiencies are classified according to the type of immune function that is impaired: antibody mediated, cell mediated, or combined. Because cell-mediated and combined immunodeficiencies are so severe that the affected person usually does not survive childhood, only antibody-mediated problems (seen in adults) are discussed in this chapter.

BRUTON'S AGAMMAGLOBULINEMIA

PATHOPHYSIOLOGY

A classic congenital antibody-mediated immunodeficiency is Bruton's disease or Bruton's agammaglobulinemia. Boys born with this disease usually start to have problems at about 6 months of age, after maternal antibodies, transferred through the placenta, have been lost. The first manifestations are recurrent otitis, sinusitis, pneumonia, furunculosis, meningitis, and septicemia with organisms such as *Pneumococcus, Streptococcus,* and *Haemophilus.* Laboratory assessment shows an absence of circulating immunoglobulin (antibodies).

◆COLLABORATIVE MANAGEMENT

Except for clients with poliomyelitis, chronic echovirus infection, or a lymphoreticular malignancy, the overall prognosis for Bruton's disease is good if antibody replacement is started early. Immune serum globulin is regularly given to these clients, usually about 100 to 400 mg/kg IV every 3 to 4 weeks (Table 25-6). The dosage and schedule are individualized. Antibiotics are used for specific infections. Long-term prophylactic antibiotic therapy may also be used. Often, severe sinopulmonary disease later develops in some clients.

TABLE 25-5 Congenital Immunodeficiencies

Antibody-Mediated Immunodeficiencies
- X-linked agammaglobulinemia (Bruton's)
- Acquired hypogammaglobulinemia (common variable immunodeficiency)
- Selective IgA deficiency

Cell-Mediated Immunodeficiencies
- Congenital thymic aplasia (DiGeorge syndrome)
- Chronic mucocutaneous candidiasis

Combined Immunodeficiencies
- Severe combined immunodeficiencies
- Wiskott-Aldrich syndrome
- Immunodeficiency with ataxia-telangiectasia
- Nezelof syndrome

COMMON VARIABLE IMMUNODEFICIENCY

PATHOPHYSIOLOGY

The client with common variable immunodeficiency, or hypogammaglobulinemia, has recurrent bacterial infections similar to those seen with Bruton's disease. The client has low levels of circulating antibodies (immunoglobulins) of all classes.

Hypogammaglobulinemia differs from Bruton's disease in that it usually first appears later (in adolescence or young adulthood), occurs almost equally in males and females, and the infections are less severe. Common complications include giardiasis (intestinal infection with *Giardia lamblia*), gastric cancer, bronchiectasis, and cholelithiasis (gallbladder stones).

◆COLLABORATIVE MANAGEMENT

Treatment is similar to that for Bruton's disease. Regular infusions of immune serum globulin and regular or intermittent use of antibiotics protect the affected person against infection.

SELECTIVE IMMUNOGLOBULIN A DEFICIENCY

PATHOPHYSIOLOGY

Selective immunoglobulin A (IgA) deficiency is the most common congenital immunodeficiency seen in adults, occurring in 1 per 600 to 800 individuals (McCance & Huether, 2002). The client may be asymptomatic or have chronic recurrent upper respiratory tract infections, skin infections, urinary tract infections, vaginal infections, and diarrhea. Selective IgA deficiency does not reduce life span. Because IgA is the major antibody in secretions, bacterial infections are seen mostly in the respiratory, gastrointestinal, and urogenital tracts. Some clients with IgA deficiency also have malabsorption syndrome.

◆COLLABORATIVE MANAGEMENT

Therapy for IgA deficiency is limited to vigorous treatment of infections. *Unlike other immunoglobulin deficiencies, IgA deficiency should never be treated with exogenous immune globulin for two reasons. First, exogenous immune globulin contains very little IgA and would not help boost IgA levels. Second, because clients with IgA deficiency make normal amounts of all other antibodies, they are at high risk for severe allergic reactions to exogenous immune globulin.* If malabsorption syndrome occurs with IgA deficiency, the client needs nutritional supplements (e.g., partial or total enteral or parenteral nutrition).

TABLE 25-6 Administration of Intravenous Immune Serum Globulin

Indications	Dosage	Nursing Interventions	Rationales
B cell or humoral immunodeficiencies ▪ Bruton's hypogammaglobulinemia ▪ Common variable immunodeficiency ▪ Combined immunodeficiencies: severe combined immunodeficiencies	Gamimune 100-200 mg/kg or 2-4 mL/kg IV once monthly *or* Sandoglobulin 0.2-0.3 g/kg IV once monthly Gammagard 200-400 mg/kg IV once monthly Iveegam 200-800 mg/kg IV once monthly	Observe client closely and monitor vital signs during infusion and for 30-60 min thereafter. Slow the rate of infusion or stop it temporarily if side effects occur.	Monitoring detects signs of anaphylaxis and routine side effects. Side effects occur in 10% of clients and include skeletal pain, back pain, nausea, chills, headache, chest tightness, and abdominal cramps. Side effects appear to be related to the rate of infusion.

GET READY for the NCLEX Examination!

KEY POINTS

Safe Effective Care Environment

- Use standard precautions for all clients regardless of age, gender, race or ethnicity, sexual orientation, education level, and profession.
- Ask clients about Advance Directives and document the status.
- Use good handwashing techniques before providing any care to a client who is either immunocompromised or immunodeficient.

Health Promotion and Maintenance

- Identify clients at high risk for infection as a result of work environment or leisure activities.
- Encourage all clients who are HIV positive to use condoms and other precautions during sexual intimacy even if the partner is also HIV positive.
- Inform all clients who smoke that smoking decreases overall immune function.
- Assist clients interested in smoking cessation to find an appropriate smoking cessation program.
- Teach clients with protein-calorie malnutrition what foods to include in the diet.
- Teach the client and family about the clinical manifestations of infection and when to seek medical advice.

Psychosocial Integrity

- Treat all clients, regardless of diagnosis, with dignity.
- Do not assume that any visitor or family member knows the client's diagnosis.
- Pace your interview to match the learning needs and style of the individual client.
- Allow the client the opportunity to express fear or anxiety regarding a change in health status.
- Refer clients newly diagnosed with HIV infection to local resources and support groups.
- Encourage all clients who are HIV positive to inform their sexual partners of their HIV status.
- Explain all diagnostic procedures, restrictions, and follow-up care to the client scheduled for tests.
- Allow clients who experience a change in physical appearance to mourn this change.

Physiological Integrity

- Encourage clients to adhere to their antiviral drug regimen.
- Pace nonurgent health care activities to reduce the risk for fatigue among clients with AIDS.
- Teach clients the expected side effects and possible adverse reactions to prescribed drugs.
- Assess the immunodeficient client every shift for manifestations of infection.
- Assess the skin integrity of the perianal region of a client with AIDS-related diarrhea after every bowel movement.

ADDITIONAL STUDY RESOURCES

Go to your Student CD-ROM for Review Questions for the NCLEX Examination.

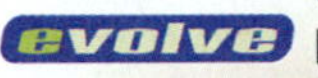

Go to http://evolve.elsevier.com/Iggy/ for Integrated Management of Care Questions for the NCLEX Examination.

SELECTED BIBLIOGRAPHY

Asterisk indicates a classic or definitive work on this subject.

*Abbas, A., Lichtman, A., & Pober, J. (1997). *Cellular and molecular immunology* (3rd ed.). Philadelphia: W.B. Saunders.

Ackley, B., & Ladwig, G. (2002). *Nursing diagnosis handbook: A guide to planning care* (5th ed.). St. Louis: Mosby.

AIDS: Its prevalence and treatment in the United States. (2001). *The American Journal for Nurse Practitioners, 5*(3), 58.

Barroso, J. (2002). HIV-related fatigue. *American Journal of Nursing, 102*(5), 83-85.

Bradley-Springer, L. (2001). HIV prevention: What works? *American Journal of Nursing, 101*(6) 45-50.

Brooke, P. (2001). The legal realities of HIV exposure. *RN, 64*(12), 71-73.

Bursaw, M., Keenan, K., & Ehrhart, M. (2001). HIV update. *Nursing 2001, 31*(2), 62-63.

*Centers for Disease Control. (1987). Public Health Service guidelines for counseling and antibody testing to prevent HIV infection and AIDS. *Morbidity and Mortality Weekly Report, 36*(31), 509-515.

*Centers for Disease Control. (1991). Recommendations for preventing transmission of human immunodeficiency virus and hepatitis B virus to clients during exposure-prone invasive procedures. *Morbidity and Mortality Weekly Report, 40*(RR-8), 1-9.

*Centers for Disease Control and Prevention. (1998a). Public Health Service guidelines for the management of health-care worker exposure to HIV and recommendations for postexposure prophylaxis. *Morbidity and Mortality Weekly Report, 47* (RR-7), 1-32.

*Centers for Disease Control and Prevention. (1998b). Public Health Service taskforce recommendations for the use of anti-retroviral drugs in pregnant women infected with HIV-1 for maternal health and reducing perinatal HIV-1 transmission in the U.S. *Morbidity and Mortality Weekly Report, 47*(RR-2), 1-30.

Centers for Disease Control and Prevention (2003). *HIV/AIDS surveillance report* 2002, *14*(10), 1-48. Rockville, MD: Author. Available at http://www.cdc.gov/hiv/stats/hasr1302.pdf.

Coyne, P., Lyne, M., & Watson, A. (2002). Symptom management in people with AIDS. *American Journal of Nursing, 102*(9), 48-57.

Daughtry, L., Bankston, J., & Deshotels, J. (2002). HIV meds: Keeping trouble at bay. *RN, 65*(2), 31-36.

Dochterman, J., & Bulechek, G. (Eds.). (2004). *Nursing interventions classification (NIC)* (4th ed.). St. Louis: Mosby.

Ebersole, P., Hess, P., & Luggen, A. (2004). *Toward healthy aging* (6th ed.). St. Louis: Mosby.

Ehrhardt, A., et al. (2002). A gender-specific HIV/STD risk reduction intervention for women in a health care setting: Short- and long-term results of a randomized clinical trial. *AIDS Care, 14*(2), 147-161.

Facts and Comparisons. (2004). *Drug facts and comparisons* (58th ed.). St. Louis: Author.

Godwin, C. (2004). What's new in the fight against AIDS? *RN, 67*(4), 46-52.

Goldrick, B. (2004). HIV advances. *American Journal of Nursing, 104*(5), 37-38.

Haddad, A. (2003). Ethics in action: HIV patient wants "natural therapy." *RN 66*(3), 27-30.

Holzemer, W. (2002). HIV and AIDS: The symptom experience. *American Journal of Nursing, 102*(4), 48-52.

Holzemer, W. (2002). The symptom experience: What cell counts and viral loads won't tell you. *American Journal of Nursing. 102*(4):48-52.

Holzemer, W., et al. (2000). The patient adherence profiling-intervention tailoring (CAP-IT) intervention for enhancing adherence to HIV/AIDS medications: A pilot study. *Journal of the Association of Nurses in AIDS Care, 11*(1) 36-44.

Jagger, J., & Perry, J. (2003). Lab workers: Small group, big risk. *Nursing2003, 33*(1), 72.

Jones, S. (2004). Taking HAART. *Nursing 2004, 34*(6), 6-11.

Kemppainen, J.K. (2001). Prediction of quality of life in AIDS patients. *Journal of the Association of Nurses in AIDS Care, 12*(1), 61-70.

Lactic acidosis a threat for HIV clients. (2002). *Nursing2002, 32*(7), 28.

McCance, K., & Huether, S. (2002). *Pathophysiology: The biologic basis for disease in adults and children* (4th ed.). St. Louis: Mosby.

New HIV test: Accurate results in 20 minutes flat. (2003). *Nursing 2003, 33*(1), 34.

Nussbaum, R., McInnes, R., & Willard, H. (2001). *Thompson & Thompson: Genetics in medicine* (6th ed.). Philadelphia: W.B. Saunders.

On-and-off therapy works and cuts costs too. (2002). *Nursing 2002, 32*(2), 33.

Pagana, K., & Pagana, T. (2002). *Mosby's manual of diagnostic and laboratory tests* (2nd ed.). St. Louis: Mosby.

Randolph, S. (2002). When candida turns deadly. *RN, 65*(3), 41-45.

Sande, M.A., & Volberding, P.A. (2002). *The medical management of AIDS* (6th ed.). Philadelphia: W.B. Saunders.

Sankar, A., et al. (2002). Adherence discourse among African-American women taking HAART. *AIDS Care, 14*(2), 203-218.

Sellers, C., & Angerame, M. (2002). HIV/AIDS in older adults: A case study and discussion. *AACN Clinical Issues, 13*(1), 5-21.

Trzcianowska, H., & Mortensen, E. (2001). HIV and AIDS: Separating fact from fiction. *American Journal of Nursing, 101*(6), 53-59.

Trzynka, S., & Erlen, J. (2004). HIV disease susceptibility in women and the barriers to adherence. *MEDSURG Nursing, 13*(2), 97-104.

Welch, K. (2002). Predictors of survival in older men with AIDS. *Geriatric Nursing, 23*(2), 62-68.

Williams, A. (2001). Adherence to HIV regimens: 10 vital lessons. *American Journal of Nursing, 101*(6), 37-44.

CHAPTER 26

Interventions for Clients with Immune Function Excess: Hypersensitivity (Allergy) and Autoimmunity

M. LINDA WORKMAN

LEARNING OUTCOMES

After studying this chapter, you should be able to:

1. Compare the bases and manifestations of allergy and autoimmunity.
2. Discuss anaphylaxis prevention measures.
3. Discuss the nursing responsibility for a client with anaphylaxis.
4. Identify the common drugs, dosages, and side effects used as therapy for anaphylaxis.
5. Describe allergy testing techniques.
6. List the defining characteristics of type I, type II, type III, type IV, and type V hypersensitivity reactions.
7. Explain the differences in mechanisms of action between antihistamines and mast cell stabilizers.
8. Develop a community-based teaching plan for the client who has severe allergic reactions.

Go to your Student CD-ROM for Review Questions for the NCLEX Examination keyed to these Learning Outcomes.

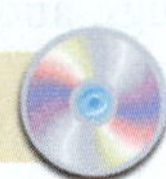

The inflammatory and immune responses are normally helpful, protecting the body against infection and cancer development. These responses also stimulate tissue growth and repair after injury. When inflammation or immune responses are prolonged, excessive, or occur at an inappropriate time, however, normal tissues are damaged. These responses are "overreactions" to invaders and foreign antigens, and are known as hypersensitivity or allergic responses. In addition, inflammatory and immune responses can fail to recognize self cells and attack normal body tissues. This type of reaction is known as an autoimmune response. Hypersensitivity and autoimmune responses can severely damage cells, tissues, and organs.

Hypersensitivities/Allergies

Hypersensitivity or allergy is an increased or excessive response to the presence of an **antigen** (foreign protein or allergen) to which the client has been previously exposed. These responses cause problems that range from uncomfortable (e.g., itchy, watery eyes or sneezing) to life-threatening (e.g., allergic asthma, anaphylaxis, bronchoconstriction, or circulatory collapse). The terms hypersensitivity and allergy are used interchangeably. Hypersensitivity reactions are classified into five basic types, determined by differences in timing, pathophysiology, and clinical manifestations (Table 26-1). Each type may occur alone or along with one or more other types.

TYPE I: RAPID HYPERSENSITIVITY REACTIONS

Type I, or rapid, hypersensitivity, also called *atopic allergy*, is the most common type of hypersensitivity. This type results from the increased production of the immunoglobulin E (IgE) antibody class. Acute inflammation occurs when IgE responds to an antigen, such as pollen, and causes the release of histamine and other vasoactive amines from basophils, eosinophils, and mast cells. Examples of type I reactions include anaphylaxis, allergic asthma (discussed in Chapter 33); atopic allergies such as hay fever, allergic rhinitis; and allergies to specific allergens such as latex, bee venom, peanut, iodine,

TABLE 26-1 Mechanisms and Examples of Types of Hypersensitivities

Mechanism	Clinical Examples
Type I: Immediate Reaction of IgE antibody on mast cells with antigen, which results in release of mediators, especially histamine	Hay fever Allergic asthma Anaphylaxis
Type II: Cytotoxic Reaction of IgG with host cell membrane or antigen adsorbed by host cell membrane	Autoimmune hemolytic anemia Goodpasture's syndrome Myasthenia gravis
Type III: Immune Complex–Mediated Formation of immune complex of antigen and antibody, which deposits in walls of blood vessels and results in complement release and inflammation	Serum sickness Vasculitis Systemic lupus erythematosus Rheumatoid arthritis
Type IV: Delayed Reaction of sensitized T-cells with antigen and release of lymphokines, which activate macrophages and induce inflammation	Poison ivy Graft rejection Positive TB skin tests Sarcoidosis
Type V: Stimulated Reaction of autoantibodies with normal cell-surface receptors, which stimulates a continual overreaction of the target cell	Graves' disease B-cell gammopathies

IgE, Immunoglobulin E; *IgG*, immunoglobulin G; *TB*, tuberculosis.

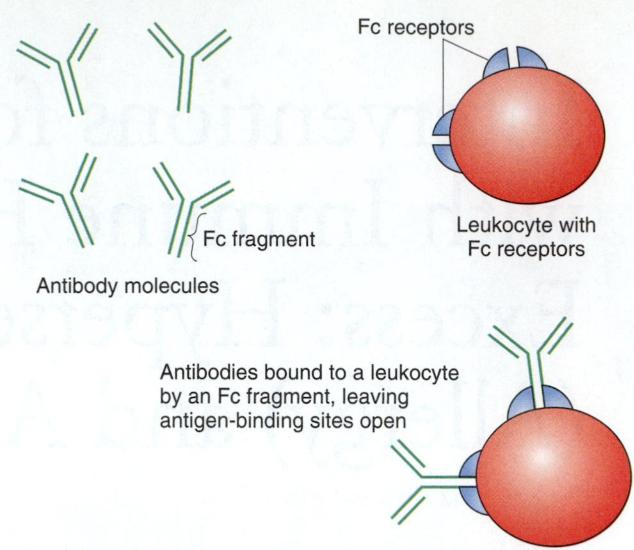

Figure 26-1 ■ Antibody Fc receptors on the basophils and mast cells.

shellfish, drugs, and thousands of other environmental antigens. Allergens can be contacted in the following ways:

- Inhaled (plant pollens, fungal spores, animal dander, house dust, grass, ragweed)
- Ingested (foods, food additives, drugs)
- Injected (bee venom, drugs, biologic substances such as contrast dyes and adrenocorticotropic hormone)
- Contacted (pollens, foods, environmental proteins)

Some reactions occur just in the areas exposed to the antigen, such as the mucous membranes of the nose and eyes, causing symptoms of rhinorrhea, sneezing, and itchy red, watery, eyes. Other reactions may involve all blood vessels and bronchiolar smooth muscle causing widespread blood vessel dilation, decreased cardiac output, and bronchoconstriction. This condition is known as **anaphylaxis.**

Allergic Rhinitis

PATHOPHYSIOLOGY

Allergic rhinitis, also called "hay fever," is triggered by reactions to airborne allergens, especially plant pollens, molds, dust, animal dander, wool, food, and air pollutants. Some acute episodes are "seasonal," tending to recur at the same time each year. They often coincide with the timing of large environmental exposure and last only a few weeks. Chronic rhinitis, or perennial rhinitis, tends to occur intermittently (with no predictable seasonal pattern) or continuously when a person is exposed to certain allergens. In "nonallergic rhinitis," the same manifestations are present although no allergic cause is identified and the immune system does not appear to be involved.

On first exposure to an **allergen** (an antigen that provokes allergic sensitization), the person responds by making antigen-specific IgE. This antigen-specific IgE binds to the surface of basophils and mast cells (Figure 26-1). These cells have many granules containing vasoactive amines (including histamine) that are released when stimulated. Once the antigen-specific IgE is formed, the person is sensitized to that allergen.

In a type I allergic reaction, the previously sensitized person is re-exposed to the provoking allergen. The resulting response has a primary phase and a secondary phase. In the primary phase, the allergen binds to two adjacent IgE molecules on the surface of a basophil or mast cell, which breaks or distorts the cell membrane. These membrane changes cause the cell to degranulate, releasing the vasoactive amines within the granules into the tissue fluids (Figure 26-2).

The most common vasoactive amine is *histamine,* a short-acting biochemical. Histamine causes capillary leak, nasal and conjunctival mucous secretion, and itching (pruritus), often occurring with erythema (redness). These symptoms last for about 10 minutes after histamine is first released. When the allergen is continuously present, mast cells continuously release histamine and other proteins, prolonging the response.

The secondary phase results from the release of other proteins. These other proteins draw more white blood cells to the area and stimulate a more general inflammatory reaction through actions of leukotriene and prostaglandins. This reaction occurs in addition to the allergic reaction stimulated in the primary phase. The resulting inflammation increases the clinical manifestations and is probably responsible for continuing the response.

Etiology and Genetic Risk

The tendency to produce IgE in response to antigen exposure is based on genetic inheritance, but no single gene has been found to be responsible. Specific allergies are *not* in-

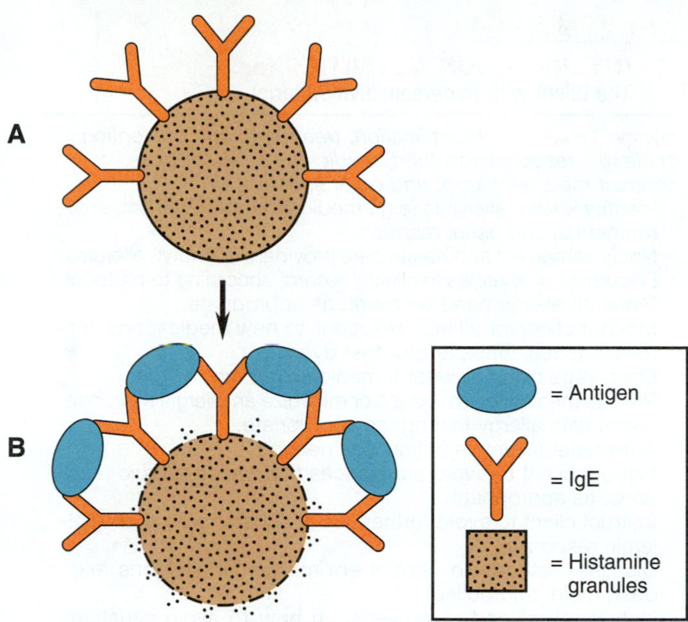

Figure 26-2 ■ Degranulation and histamine release. **A,** Mast cell with IgE. **B,** Mast cell degranulation and histamine release when allergen binds to IgE.

herited. About 50% of clients with allergic rhinitis have one parent with type I allergies.

Incidence/Prevalence

Atopic allergies, including allergic rhinitis, affect about 10% of the population in North America (McCance & Huether, 2002). Men and women are affected equally. Racial differences have not been documented.

COLLABORATIVE MANAGEMENT

Assessment

HISTORY

An accurate and detailed history may provide insight into the possibility of allergic rhinitis. Ask the client to describe the onset and duration of problems in relation to possible allergen exposure. Ask about work, school, and home environments, and possible exposures through hobbies, leisure time or sports activities. Because a tendency toward type I allergic responses can be inherited, ask about the presence of allergies among close relatives.

PHYSICAL ASSESSMENT/CLINICAL MANIFESTATIONS

The client with allergic rhinitis usually has **rhinorrhea** (a "runny" nose), a "stuffy" nose, and itchy, watery eyes. The client may breathe through his or her mouth and the voice has a nasal sound. Drainage from the nose is usually clear or white. The nasal mucosa appears swollen and pink. The client may have a headache or feel pressure over the frontal and maxillary sinuses. Transillumination of the sinuses may be decreased. If nasal secretions drip posteriorly, the client may have a dry, scratchy throat and pharyngitis. The client often feels as though he or she has a cold that has lasted longer than a week. Fever is rare unless an infection occurs with the rhinitis.

LABORATORY ASSESSMENT

A complete blood count and differential indicate the presence of an allergic response by an increase in eosinophils. A client with severe seasonal allergic rhinitis may have an eosinophil count as high as 12% (normal being 1 to 2%). Some clients have an increased total white blood count, but the percentage of neutrophils remains normal (55% to 70%). If an acute infection occurs with allergic rhinitis, both the total white blood cell count and the number of neutrophils increase.

Other laboratory tests that indicate the presence of an allergic reaction include serum immunoglobulin E (IgE) levels and the radioallergosorbent test (RAST). A normal level of IgE for adults is about 39 IU/mL (or less than 100 IU/mL). This level can increase greatly with allergies. The usual IgE test does not indicate the specific allergen, only the tendency to have allergic responses. The RAST test shows the blood level of IgE directed against a specific antigen and thus can determine specific allergies. However, the expense of this study limits its use in allergy testing.

ALLERGY TESTING

SKIN TESTING. With most type I reactions, skin testing can show which specific allergens are causing the reaction. Skin testing can be performed as scratch testing and intradermal testing. Patch testing is often reserved for contact dermatitis and other manifestations of type IV hypersensitivities.

Scratch Testing. A scratch or prick test can show an *immediate* hypersensitivity reaction to an allergen. Scratch tests are used in routine allergy testing to determine the cause of allergic rhinitis, asthma, urticaria (hives) or any other type I reactions. Allergens introduced through a scratch or prick cause a localized reaction (wheal) when the test result is positive. Results are usually determined after 15 to 20 minutes.

Client Preparation. For best results, systemic glucocorticoids and antihistamines are discontinued for 5 days before the test to avoid suppressing an allergic response during the test. Nasal sprays to reduce mucous membrane swelling are permitted, except for sprays that contain an antihistamine. Some allergists recommend that aspirin and other nonsteroidal anti-inflammatory agents be withheld before allergy testing.

Procedure. The best sites for scratch testing are the inside of the arm or on the back. Other sites are used if a rash or skin problem is present on the arms or back. Gently clean the skin with soap and water, and remove surface oils with alcohol.

Small drops of sera containing different known allergens are placed on the skin. The skin is scratched or pricked through the drop with a bifurcated skin testing needle. Control drops are also applied; normal saline drops are negative controls and histamine drops are positive controls. The reactions of the allergen-tested areas are examined for the presence and size of a reaction. These areas are then compared to the control areas. Areas showing erythema and wheal formation are considered positive for that antigen. Degree of sensitivity is estimated by the size of the response.

Serious reactions in response to scratch testing are rare. Ensure that emergency equipment is readily available during a scratch test.

Follow-up Care. After testing is completed for the day, wash the solution from the skin. Topical steroids and oral antihistamines may be given to reduce itching and increase client comfort. If an antihistamine that causes sedation is given, the client will need to have another person drive him or her home.

Intradermal Testing. Intradermal testing is reserved for substances that are strongly suspected of causing allergy but did not test positive with scratch testing. Intradermal testing increases the risk for an adverse reaction, including anaphylaxis, but it is usually a safe procedure. Ensure that emergency equipment is in the room with the client. Small amounts of testing sera (0.1 mL) are injected intradermally on the client's upper arm and the area is observed for erythema and wheal formation. The degree of allergy is estimated by the size of the response. Client preparation and follow-up care are the same as for scratch testing.

ORAL FOOD CHALLENGE. Some clients have allergic rhinitis even when the allergen does not come into contact with the nasal mucosa but is ingested orally. The oral food challenge is used to identify specific allergens if skin testing is not conclusive and if keeping a food diary has failed to determine the offending food items. This test requires the client to eliminate suspected foods for 7 to 14 days before testing. After this time, the client is directed to eat defined food for at least 1 day and to monitor for manifestations of allergy. When many food allergies are present, the client may have to eat only one food type per day of testing.

Interventions

Chart 26-1 lists NIC interventions for allergy management. Common interventions include avoidance therapy, desensitization therapy, and symptomatic therapy. Many clients use a combination of all three types of therapy for management of allergic rhinitis and other manifestations of type I allergy.

AVOIDANCE THERAPY. When specific allergens have been identified, urge the client to avoid direct or close contact with these agents. Some allergens, such as certain foods or drugs, may be easy to avoid. Other substances, such as pollen, mold, or dust mites, may require environmental changes.

Many airborne allergens can be reduced by air-conditioning and air-cleaning units. Removing cloth drapes, upholstered furniture, and carpeting reduces air-borne allergens. Covering mattresses and pillows with plastic or an ultra fine mesh cover also reduces exposure to dust mites and mold.

Pet-induced allergies pose special challenges. Sometimes simple interventions, such as keeping pets out of the bedroom and thorough cleaning of the room to remove animal hair and dander, may reduce symptoms. Frequent bathing of the pet or keeping the pet outdoors can decrease allergen exposure. Depending on the severity of the allergy and how well other methods provide relief, pets with fur, feathers, or dander may need to be removed from the household.

SYMPTOMATIC THERAPY. When avoidance therapy is impractical, symptomatic therapy can be effective in reducing the allergic response and making the client more comfortable.

CHART 26-1

NIC INTERVENTION ACTIVITIES for The Client with Hypersensitivity/Allergy

Allergy Management: *Identification, treatment, and prevention of allergic responses to food, medications, insect bites, contrast material, blood, and other substances*

- Identify known allergies (e.g., medication, food, insect, environmental) and usual reaction.
- Notify caregivers and health care providers of known allergies.
- Document all allergies in clinical record, according to protocol.
- Place an allergy band on client, as appropriate.
- Monitor client for allergic reactions to new medications, formulas, foods, latex, and/or test dyes.
- Encourage client to wear a medical alert tag.
- Provide medication to reduce or minimize an allergic response.
- Assist with allergy testing, as appropriate.
- Administer allergy injections, as needed.
- Instruct client to avoid substances that cause allergic reactions, as appropriate.
- Instruct client to avoid further use of substances causing allergic responses.
- Discuss methods to control environmental allergens (e.g., dust, mold, and pollen).
- Instruct client and caregiver(s) on how to avoid situations that put the client at risk and how to respond if an anaphylactic reaction should occur.
- Instruct client and caregiver on use of epinephrine pen.

Anaphylaxis Management: *Promotion of adequate ventilation and tissue perfusion for a client with a severe allergic (antigen-antibody) reaction*

- Place individual in a comfortable position.
- Apply tourniquet per protocol immediately proximal to the allergen point of entry (e.g., injection site, IV site, insect bite, etc.), when possible, as appropriate.
- Establish and maintain a patent airway.
- Administer oxygen at high flow rate (10-15 L/min).
- Start an IV infusion of normal saline, lactated Ringer's, or a plasma volume expander, as appropriate.
- Reassure the individual and family members.
- Monitor for signs of shock (e.g., respiratory difficulty, cardiac arrhythmias, seizures, and hypotension).
- Administer spasmolytics, antihistamines, or corticosteroids as indicated if urticaria, angioedema, or bronchspasm present.
- Monitor for recurrence of anaphylaxis within 24 hours.

NIC interventions selected from Dochterman, J.M., & Bulechek, G.M. (Eds.). (2004). *Nursing interventions classification (NIC)* (4th ed.). St. Louis: Mosby.

Drug Therapy. Drug therapy involves the use of steroidal and nonsteroidal agents (to reduce inflammation), vasoconstrictors, antihistamines, mast cell stabilizers, and drugs that inhibit the release or action of leukotrienes. Some drugs reduce the response and other drugs prevent the response. Chart 26-2 lists common drugs used for symptomatic relief of allergic rhinitis.

Decongestants. Decongestants are available as systemic oral drugs or nasal sprays. These drugs do not clear the allergen or prevent the release of mediators such as histamine. They have actions similar to adrenergic drugs and work by causing vasoconstriction in the inflamed tissue, thereby reducing the edema. Decongestants often contain ephedrine, phenylephrine, or pseudoephedrine. Secretions are reduced when vasoconstricting drugs are combined with an anticholinergic drug, such as scopolamine or atropine. Many combination decongestants are available by prescription and as over-the-counter cold and allergy drugs. Side ef-

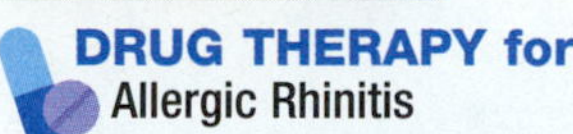

DRUG THERAPY for
Allergic Rhinitis

Drug	Usual Dosage	Nursing Implications	Rationales
Antihistamines			
Diphenhydramine (Benadryl, Allerdryl✱, Hyrexin)	25-50 mg q4-6h	Instruct client not to drive or operate heavy machinery. Do not give during an acute asthma attack.	Drug can cause significant sedation. Sedation decreases the voluntary muscle contractions needed for breathing.
Chlorpheniramine (Chlor-Trimeton, Telachlor, Teldrin, Phenetron)	2-8 mg 1-3 times daily	Avoid alcoholic beverages. Same as for diphenhydramine.	Drug potentiates the effects of alcohol.
Loratadine (Claritin)	10 mg daily	Give every other day to clients with renal or hepatic dysfunction.	Renal or hepatic dysfunction reduces drug clearance.
Desloratadine (Clarinex, Neoclarityn✱)	10 mg daily	Same as for loratadine.	Same as for loratadine.
Cetirizine (Zyrtec)	5-10 mg daily	Reduce dose for clients with renal or hepatic dysfunction.	Same as for loratadine.
Fexofenadine (Allegra)	60 mg twice daily or 180 mg daily	Same as for loratadine.	Same as for loratadine.
Ebastine (Ebastel)	5-10 mg daily	Instruct clients not to drive or operate heavy machinery. Do not take with erythromycin.	Induces drowsiness. Erythromycin inhibits elimination.
Mizolastine (Mistamine, Mizollen)	10 mg daily	Do not give to clients with cardiac disease, bradycardia, or dysrhythmias.	Increases the QT interval; may provoke fatal dysrhythmias.
Corticosteroids (Oral) *(may be given as a "taper" or "short-term burst")*			
Prednisolone (Cotolone, Delta-Cortef)	5-40 mg daily	Not recommended unless symptoms are severe or debilitating.	Systemic side effects are common and serious: ▪ GI ulceration ▪ Poor wound healing ▪ Decreased immune function ▪ Increased risk for infections ▪ Weight gain ▪ Hyperglycemia ▪ Personality changes ▪ Fluid retention
Prednisone (Deltasone, Prednicot, Orasone, Pred-Pak)	5-60 mg daily	Same as for prednisolone.	Same as for prednisolone.
Leukotriene Antagonists			
Zafirlukast (Accolate)	20 mg twice daily	Take 1 hr before or 2 hr after eating. There is an increased incidence of upper respiratory infections when co-administered with inhaled corticosteroids. Reduce dose in clients who are also taking aspirin.	Drug absorption is slowed by the presence of food. Drugs reduce local inflammatory and immune responses. Aspirin increases plasma concentration of drug.
Zileuton (Zyflo)	600 mg four times daily	Do not take with terfenadine or theophylline.	Drug increases plasma concentrations of terfenadine and theophylline.
Corticosteroids (Nasal)*			
Beclomethasone (Beconase)	1-2 metered sprays per nostril, 1-2 times daily (about 50 mcg/metered spray)	Use daily as directed. Symptoms may persist for 2-3 days after initial administration.	Effectiveness depends on regular use. Maximum effectiveness requires continued use for 48-72 hr.
Fluticasone (Flonase)	2 metered sprays per nostril daily (about 50 mcg/metered spray)	Same as for beclomethasone.	Same as for beclomethasone.

Med Error Alert! *Do not confuse with Zantac, a histamine blocker for gastric acidity.*

Data from Facts and Comparisons. (2004). *Drug facts and comparisons* (58th ed.). St. Louis: Author.
GI, Gastrointestinal.
*Additional drugs include Nasacort, Nasonex, and many others.

Continued

CHART 26-2

DRUG THERAPY for Allergic Rhinitis—*cont'd*

Drug	Usual Dosage	Nursing Interventions	Rationales
Mast Cell Stabilizers (Nasal)			
Cromolyn sodium (Nasalcrom)	1 spray/nostril 4-6 times daily	Use daily as directed.	Effectiveness depends on regular use.
		Start therapy 3-4 wk before expected allergy season.	Requires regular use for prophylactic effect.
Decongestants (Nasal)			
Phenylephrine (Neo-Synephrine, dozens of others)	1 spray/nostril 4-6 times daily	Caution client not to use more frequently than directed or for longer than 4 days.	Overuse or continued use causes a rebound nasal congestion and worsens symptoms.
Oxymetazoline (Afrin, many others)	1 spray/nostril twice daily	Same as for phenylephrine.	Same as for phenylephrine.

Data from Facts and Comparisons. (2004). *Drug facts and comparisons* (58th ed.). St. Louis: Author.

fects include dry mouth, increased blood pressure, and sleep difficulties. Because effects are systemic, instruct clients with high blood pressure, glaucoma, or urinary retention to consult with a health care professional before taking any decongestant.

Antihistamines. Antihistamines compete with histamine at its receptor site and block histamine from binding to the receptor. This action prevents vasodilation and capillary leak. Many antihistamines also decrease secretions. Older antihistamines, such as diphenhydramine (Allerdryl✱, Benadryl) and chlorpheniramine (Allergy, Aller-Chlor, Chlor-Trimeton), often induce sedation. Newer antihistamines, such as desloratadine (Clarinex), cetirizine (Zyrtec), and fexofenadine (Allegra), are less sedating. Not every client responds to each drug in the same way.

Corticosteroids. Corticosteroids decrease inflammatory and immune responses in many ways, one of which is by preventing the synthesis of mediators. Corticosteroid nasal sprays can prevent the symptoms of rhinitis. Systemic corticosteroids can produce severe side effects. These drugs are avoided for rhinitis and are used only on a short-term basis for other problems associated with type I reactions.

Mast Cell Stabilizers. Mast cell stabilizing nasal sprays, such as cromolyn sodium (Nasalcrom), prevent mast cell membranes from opening when an allergen binds to IgE. Thus these drugs prevent the symptoms of allergic rhinitis but are not useful during an acute episode.

Leukotriene Antagonists. Leukotriene antagonists may be used to treat allergic rhinitis. Zileuton (Zyflo) prevents leukotriene synthesis. Zafirlukast (Accolate) blocks the leukotriene receptor. Both are oral agents and work best in the prevention of allergic rhinitis.

Complementary and Alternative Therapies. Some clients with rhinitis obtain relief through the use of aromatherapy. Possible mechanisms of action include competition and desensitization. Clients with pollen allergies report decreased problems after eating unprocessed honey.

DESENSITIZATION THERAPY. Desensitization therapy, commonly called "allergy shots," may be needed when allergens are identified and cannot be avoided easily. Desensitization commonly involves subcutaneous injections of small amounts of the allergen. After the allergen has been identified, a very dilute injection solution (1:100,000 or 1:1,000,000) of the allergen is compounded. A 0.05-mL dose of this solution is injected subcutaneously. Usually an increasing dose is given weekly (or more often) until the client is receiving a 0.5-mL dose. The client is then started on the lowest dose of the next higher concentration of allergen solution. The process is repeated with increasing concentrations of allergen solutions until the client is receiving the maximum dose of the greatest concentration (usually 1:100), depending on his or her response. Injections are usually given at weekly intervals during the first year, every other week for the second year, and then every 3 to 4 weeks for the third year. The recommended course of treatment is about 5 years.

Desensitization appears to reduce allergic responses by competition. In theory, the very small amounts of allergen first injected are too low to bind to the IgE already present but are enough to induce immunoglobulin G (IgG) production against that allergen. Because IgG is not associated with either mast cells or basal cells, allergens that bind to IgG do not trigger allergic responses. IgG removes the allergen from the body by precipitation (see Chapter 23). By gradually increasing the allergen injection, large amounts of IgG are produced against the allergen. When the client is then exposed to the allergen in the environment, the IgG binds to it and clears it from the body before IgE can bind to it and trigger an allergic reaction. Because so much more IgG can be produced compared with IgE, IgG is successful in the competition to bind the allergen.

Desensitization can also be accomplished orally with sublingual immunotherapy (SLIT). Instead of injections, the allergen is introduced through sublingual absorption. The allergen is absorbed directly into the circulatory system through the blood vessels under the tongue. Two major drawbacks of SLIT are the difficulty of dose control and the expense. This method requires higher levels of the allergen (compared to subcutaneous injections), which increases the cost.

Anaphylaxis

PATHOPHYSIOLOGY

Anaphylaxis, the most dramatic and life-threatening example of a type I hypersensitivity reaction, occurs rapidly and systemically. It affects many organs within seconds to minutes after allergen exposure. Anaphylaxis is not common,

TABLE 26-2 Common Agents That Cause Anaphylaxis

Drugs/Foreign Proteins
Antibiotics (penicillin, cephalosporins, tetracycline, sulfonamides, streptomycin, vancomycin, chloramphenicol, amphotericin B, others)
Adrenocorticotropic hormone, insulin, vasopressin, protamine*
Allergen extracts, muscle relaxants, hydrocortisone, vaccines, local anesthetics (lidocaine, procaine)*
Whole blood, cryoprecipitate, immune serum globulin*
Radiocontrast media*
Opiates

Foods	Other Agents
Shellfish	Pollens
Eggs	Exercise
Legumes, nuts	Heat/cold
Grains	Other
Berries	
Preservatives	
Bananas	

Insects/Animals
Hymenoptera: bees, wasps, hornets
Fire ants
Snake venom

*Anaphylaxis caused by these substances is probably a result of direct mast cell degranulation rather than an IgE-mediated hypersensitivity event.

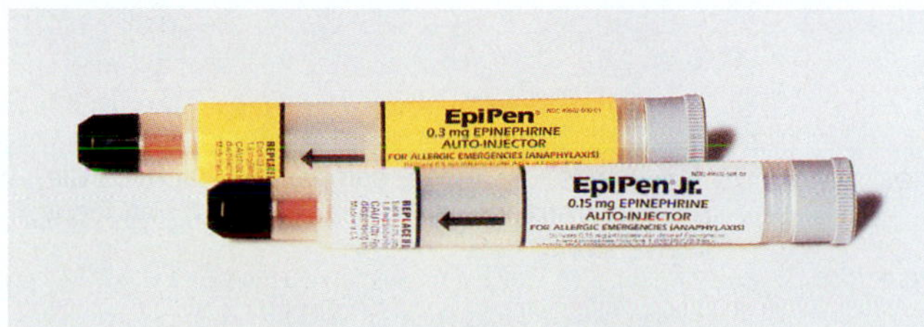

Figure 26-3 ■ EpiPen and EpiPen Jr. self-injectors for epinephrine (Courtesy of Dey, Napa, CA).

and the episodes can vary in severity. *It can be fatal.* Many substances can trigger anaphylaxis in a susceptible person (Table 26-2).

HEALTH PROMOTION/ILLNESS PREVENTION

Because anaphylaxis has a rapid onset and a potentially fatal outcome (even with appropriate medical intervention), prevention is critical. Teach the client with a history of allergic reactions to avoid allergens whenever possible, to wear a medical alert bracelet, and to alert health care personnel about specific allergies. Some clients must carry an emergency anaphylaxis kit (e.g., a bee sting kit with injectable epinephrine), or an epinephrine injector, such as the EpiPen automatic injector (Dey, Napa, CA). The EpiPen device is an easy-to-use, spring-loaded injector that delivers 0.3 mg of epinephrine per 2-mL dose (Figure 26-3).

The medical records of clients with a history of anaphylaxis should prominently display the list of specific allergens. Ask the client about drug allergies before giving any drug or therapeutic agent. Skin tests should be performed before giving any substance that has a high incidence of causing anaphylactic reactions, such as iodine-containing dyes. Be aware of common cross-reacting agents. For example, a client who is allergic to penicillin is also likely to react to cephalosporins because both have a similar chemical structure. People who have an allergy to bananas are likely to have a latex allergy.

Take precautionary measures if an agent must be used despite a history of allergic reactions. Start an IV solution and place intubation equipment and a tracheostomy set at the bedside. The client is often premedicated with diphenhydramine (Benadryl, Allerdryl✱). The substance is given first intradermally, then subcutaneously, and then intramuscularly in increasing doses at 20- to 30-minute intervals so the initial dose by the next route does not exceed the final dose by the previous route.

◆COLLABORATIVE MANAGEMENT

◆Assessment

A client having an anaphylactic reaction first has feelings of uneasiness, apprehension, weakness, and impending doom. Often the client is anxious and frightened. These feelings are followed, often quickly, by generalized itching and urticaria (hives). Erythema and sometimes **angioedema** (diffuse swelling) of the eyes, lips, or tongue occur next. Intensely itchy skin wheals or hives may appear and sometimes merge to form large, red blotches.

Histamine and other biochemicals cause bronchoconstriction, mucosal edema, and excess mucus production. Respiratory symptoms include congestion, rhinorrhea, dyspnea, and increasing respiratory distress with audible wheezing.

On auscultation, crackles, wheezing, and reduced breath sounds are heard. Clients may have laryngeal edema as a "lump in the throat," hoarseness, and stridor (a crowing sound). Distress increases as the tongue and larynx swell and more mucous is produced. Stridor and anxiety increase as the airway begins to close. Respiratory failure may follow from laryngeal edema, suffocation, or lower airway constriction causing hypoxemia (insufficient oxygenation of blood).

The client is usually hypotensive and has a rapid, weak, irregular pulse. These findings are due to vasodilation and extensive capillary leak. The client is faint and diaphoretic with increasing anxiety and confusion. If the client is not treated immediately, he or she may lose consciousness. Dysrhythmias, shock, and cardiac arrest may occur within minutes as intravascular volume is lost and the heart becomes hypoxic. Seventy percent of deaths are caused by respiratory failure or by shock and cardiac dysrhythmias.

◆Interventions

NIC interventions for clients with anaphylaxis are listed in Chart 26-1.

Assess respiratory function first. Emergency respiratory management is critical during an anaphylactic reaction, because the severity of the reaction increases with time. An airway must be established or stabilized immediately. Cardiopulmonary resuscitation may be needed. Epinephrine (1:1000) 0.3 to 0.5 mL is given subcutaneously as soon as symptoms of systemic anaphylaxis appear. This drug constricts blood vessels, improves cardiac contraction, and dilates the bronchioles. The same dose may be repeated every 15 to 20 minutes if needed. Other drugs used to treat anaphylaxis are listed in Chart 26-3.

Antihistamines, such as diphenhydramine (Allerdryl✱, Benadryl) 25 to 100 mg are usually given IV, IM, or orally to treat angioedema and urticaria. If needed, an endotracheal

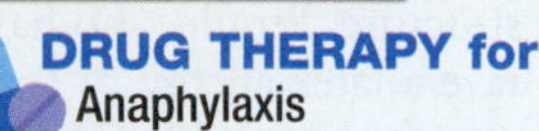

CHART 26-3

DRUG THERAPY for Anaphylaxis

Drug	Mechanism	Side Effects
Sympathomimetics		
Epinephrine (Adrenalin)	Rapidly stimulates alpha- and beta-adrenergic receptors of autonomic nervous system (alpha: vasoconstriction; beta: bronchodilation).	Pallor, tachycardia and palpitations, nervousness, muscle twitching, sweating, anxiety, insomnia, hypertension, headache, hyperglycemia.
Isoproterenol (Isuprel)	Stimulated beta-adrenergic receptors, relaxing bronchial muscle and dilating vessels.	Same as for epinephrine.
Ephedrine sulfate (Vatronol)	Similar to isoproterenol, but with longer duration of action.	Same as for epinephrine.
Antihistamines		
Diphenhydramine HCl (Allerdryl✱, Benadryl)	Competes with histamine for H_1 receptors on effector cells, thus blocking effects of histamine on bronchioles, gastrointestinal tract, and blood vessels.	Drowsiness, confusion, insomnia, headache, vertigo, photosensitivity, diplopia, nausea, vomiting, dry mouth.
CORTICOSTEROIDS		
Prednisone (PO) Hydrocortisone sodium succinate (Solu-Cortef) (IV/IM) Methylprednisolone sodium succinate (Solu-Medrol) (IV/IM) Beclomethasone (inhalant)	Anti-inflammatory; inhibits mast cell degranulation.	Fluid and sodium retention, hypertension, cushingoid state, gastric distress, adrenal suppression, psychosis, osteoporosis, susceptibility to infection.
Methylxanthines		
Aminophylline (Truphylline)	Relaxes bronchial smooth muscle.	Restlessness, dizziness, palpitations, tachycardia, nausea, vomiting, epigastric distress, headache, convulsions.
Vasopressors		
Norepinephrine (Levophed)	Raises blood pressure and cardiac output in severely decompensated states.	Headache, tachycardia, fibrillation, decreased urine output, hypertension, metabolic acidosis
Dopamine (Intropin)	Raises blood pressure and cardiac output in severely decompensated states.	Dysrhythmias, tachycardia, hypertension, dyspnea, nausea and vomiting, azotemia, headache.
Inhaled Beta-Adrenergic Agonists		
Metaproterenol (Alupent, Metaprel)	Rapidly stimulates $beta_2$-receptor sites in pulmonary smooth muscle, causing bronchodilation.	Palpitations, tachycardia, dysrhythmias, hypokalemia.
Albuterol (Proventil, Ventolin)	Same as for metaproterenol.	Same as for metaproterenol, plus painful urination, flushing of the face.

tube may be inserted or an emergency tracheostomy may be performed.

If the client can breathe independently, give oxygen to reduce hypoxemia. Start oxygen therapy via nasal cannula at 2 to 6 L/min or via face mask at 40% to 60% before arterial blood gas results are obtained. Monitor pulse oximetry to determine oxygenation adequacy, with the goal of maintaining oxygen saturation greater than 90%. Arterial blood gases may be ordered to determine therapy effectiveness. Use suction to remove excess mucous secretions, if indicated. Continually assess the client's respiratory rate and depth. Assess breath sounds continually for bronchospasm and other abnormal breath sounds. Elevate the bed to 45 degrees unless severe hypotension is also present.

For severe bronchospasm, the client is given theophylline 6 mg/kg IV over 20 to 30 minutes. If the client is taking aminophylline regularly, no more than 3 mg/kg is given. Maintenance aminophylline (0.3 to 0.5 mg/kg/hr) is initiated. The client may be given an inhaled beta-adrenergic agonist such as metaproterenol (Alupent) or albuterol (Proventil) via high-flow nebulizer every 2 to 4 hours. Corticosteroids are added to emergency interventions, but they are not effective immediately. Oral steroids are continued (at lower doses) after the anaphylaxis is under control to prevent the late recurrence of symptoms.

Continually assess for changes in any body system or for adverse effects of drug therapy. For severe anaphylaxis, the client is admitted to a critical care unit for cardiac, pulmonary arterial, and capillary wedge pressure monitoring. Observe the client for fluid overload from the rapid drug and IV fluid infusions and report changes to the physician immediately. The client is discharged from the hospital when respiratory and cardiovascular systems have returned to baseline.

Critical Thinking Challenge

The client is a 75-year-old woman with hypertension who comes to an urgent care center with a swollen lower face. Her lips and tongue are so swollen that she can hardly talk. She tells you (in response to your question about drugs) that she was started on a new blood pressure drug one week ago. When she gives you the drug bottle, you see that it is benazepril, an angiotensin-converting enzyme (ACE) inhibitor. She also tells you she has diabetes and did not take her insulin yet today.

1. What is your first action?
2. What additional assessment data should you obtain?
3. Is it likely that her new antihypertensive drug is responsible for this reaction since she has been taking it for a week?
4. Why should you or should you not start oxygen on this client?
5. Would epinephrine be helpful in this situation? Why or why not? Where, how much, and by what route would you administer it?
6. Would diphenhydramine (Benadryl) be helpful in this situation? Why or why not?
7. What other drugs should you be prepared to give?
8. Is this client's history of pollen allergies and diabetes an important factor in her immediate care?

evolve For suggested answer guidelines, go to http://evolve.elsevier.com/Iggy/.

Latex Allergy

PATHOPHYSIOLOGY

Latex allergy is a type I hypersensitivity reaction in which the specific allergen is a protein found in processed natural latex rubber products. When the allergen enters the body through inhalation or direct contact with blood vessels (such as might occur during surgery), interaction with IgE occurs, leading to a type I reaction. For some people, latex allergen contact is limited to the skin or mucous membranes, causing contact dermatitis, a type IV delayed hypersensitivity reaction (see p. 462). Others may have a "mixed" allergic response to latex, with symptoms of both type I and type IV hypersensitivities. Others may have only one or the other type of reaction.

The incidence of latex hypersensitivity is increasing (Becker, 2000; Floyd, 2000). People at greatest risk are those with a high exposure to natural latex products, such as health care workers, clients with spina bifida, and people who routinely use latex condoms.

COLLABORATIVE MANAGEMENT

Ask all clients about their use of and known reactions to natural latex products. In addition, consider your own exposure and risk for reactions to natural latex products.

Avoiding products that contain natural latex proteins can prevent reactions and initial sensitivity. More products, such as surgical gloves, tubing, and vial closures, are now being made from synthetic substances that do not contain latex proteins. One such product is the glove, ElastyLite. *It is essential to use latex-free products in the care of a client with a known latex allergy.* Interventions for the client who has a type I or a type IV reaction to latex are the same as for reactions caused by other allergens.

TYPE II: CYTOTOXIC REACTIONS

PATHOPHYSIOLOGY

In a type II (cytotoxic) reaction, the body makes special autoantibodies directed against self cells that have some form of foreign protein attached to them. The autoantibody binds to the self cell and forms an immune complex (Figure 26-4). The self cell is then destroyed along with the attached protein by phagocytosis or lysis (see Chapter 23). Clinical examples of type II reactions include hemolytic anemias, thrombocytopenic purpura, hemolytic transfusion reactions (when a client receives the wrong blood type during a transfusion), Goodpasture's syndrome, and drug-induced hemolytic anemia.

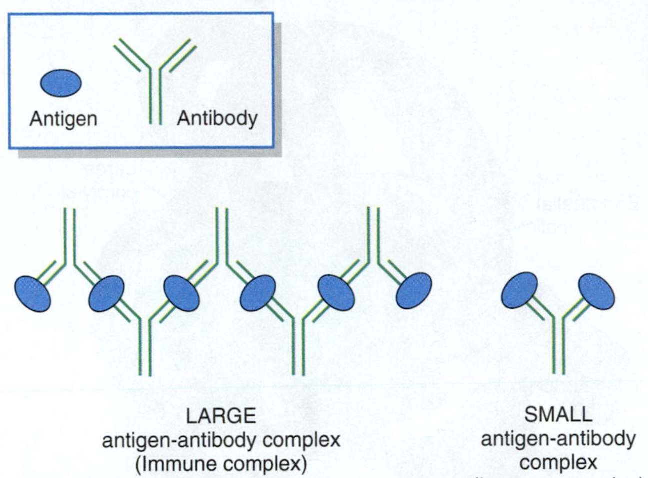

Figure 26-4 ■ Antibody-antigen complexes.

COLLABORATIVE MANAGEMENT

Treatment of type II cytotoxic reactions begins with discontinuation of the offending drug or blood product. Plasmapheresis (filtration of the plasma to remove specific substances) to remove autoantibodies may be beneficial. Otherwise, treatment is symptomatic. Complications such as hemolytic crisis and renal failure can be life threatening.

TYPE III: IMMUNE COMPLEX REACTIONS

PATHOPHYSIOLOGY

In a type III reaction, excess antigens cause immune complexes to form in the blood (Figure 26-5). These circulating complexes usually lodge in small blood vessel walls. Common sites include the kidneys, skin, joints, and other small blood vessels. The deposited complexes trigger inflammation, and tissue or vessel damage results.

There are many immune complex disorders (mostly connective tissue disorders) caused by type III reactions. For example, the manifestations of rheumatoid arthritis are caused by immune complexes that lodge in joint spaces followed by destruction of tissue and, later, scarring and fibrous changes. Systemic lupus erythematosus (SLE) has immune complexes lodged in the vessels (vasculitis), the glomeruli (nephritis), the joints (arthralgia, arthritis), and other organs and tissues. (See Chapter 24 for a discussion of SLE.)

Serum sickness is a group of symptoms that occurs after receiving serum or certain drugs. It is caused by a collection of immune complexes deposited in blood vessel walls of the skin, joints, and kidney. The most common causes of serum sickness today are penicillin, other antibiotics, and some animal serum-based drugs. Serum sickness is less common now

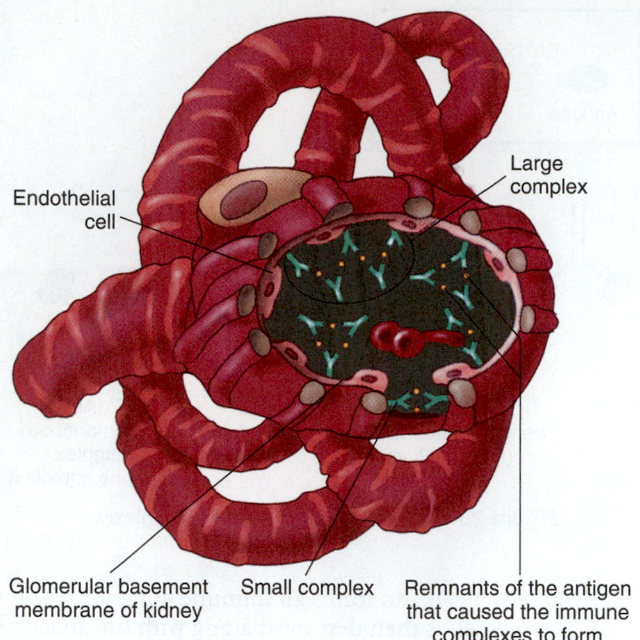

Figure 26-5 ■ An immune complex in a type III hypersensitivity reaction.

that vaccines are made with human proteins. Agents known to cause serum sickness include antilymphocyte globulin and antithymocyte globulin, used to treat organ transplant rejection.

COLLABORATIVE MANAGEMENT

The client with serum sickness has fever, **arthralgia** (achy joints), rash, lymphadenopathy (enlarged lymph nodes), malaise, and possibly polyarthritis and nephritis, about 7 to 12 days after receiving the causative agent. Alert the client to the possibility of serum sickness and what symptoms to look for whenever you give a foreign serum. Also keep emergency equipment and drugs close at hand in case the client has an anaphylactic reaction.

Serum sickness is usually self-limiting, and symptoms subside after several days. Treatment is usually symptomatic; antihistamines are given for itching and aspirin for arthralgias. Prednisone is given if symptoms are severe.

TYPE IV: DELAYED HYPERSENSITIVITY REACTIONS

PATHOPHYSIOLOGY

In a type IV reaction, the reactive cell is the T-lymphocyte (T-cell). Antibodies and complement are not involved. Sensitized T-cells (from a previous exposure) respond to an antigen by releasing chemical mediators and triggering macrophages to destroy the antigen. Unlike a type I reaction, which occurs immediately, a type IV response typically occurs hours to days after exposure. A type IV reaction consists of a local collection of lymphocytes and macrophages, causing edema, induration, ischemia, and tissue damage at the site.

An example of a small type IV reaction is a positive purified protein derivative (PPD) test for tuberculosis. In a client previously exposed to tuberculosis, an intradermal injection of this agent causes sensitized T-cells to clump at the injection site, release lymphokines, and activate macrophages. Induration and erythema at the site of the injection appear after about 24 to 72 hours.

Other examples of type IV reactions include contact dermatitis, poison ivy skin rashes, local response to insect stings, tissue transplant rejections, and sarcoidosis.

COLLABORATIVE MANAGEMENT

Interventions

Removal of the offending antigen is the major focus of management. The reaction is self-limiting in 5 to 7 days, and the client is treated symptomatically. Monitor the reaction site and sites distal to the reaction for circulation adequacy. Diphenhydramine (Benadryl) is of minimal benefit for type IV reactions because histamine is not the main mediator. In addition, IgE does not cause this type of reaction, and desensitization does not reduce the response. Corticosteroids or other anti-inflammatory agents can reduce the discomfort and help resolve the reaction more quickly.

Identification of Allergen. Patch testing can be used to identify the allergens. This type of testing involves skin contact with potential allergens. Contact with a specific allergen causes a delayed hypersensitivity reaction that develops in 48 to 96 hours.

Test chemicals are applied to intact skin under occlusive tape patches. After the patches are removed, the skin areas in contact with the chemical are examined closely for the presence of localized redness, swelling, and blisters. For a positive patch test result to have clinical relevance, the client must have a history of exposure to substances containing the allergen.

Client Preparation. To prevent suppression of a response to a potential allergen, systemic corticosteroids or antihistamines are discontinued for at least 48 hours before the test. Topical steroids may be used as long as the agent is not applied on the area to be tested. Explain that patch testing does not involve pricking the skin with needles. Inform the client that testing will involve three separate visits to the allergist or dermatologist; one to apply the test patches, a second for an initial reading, and a third for detection of delayed reactions.

Procedure. The upper back is the best site to apply test patches. After the client has undressed, inspect the back for a rash and the presence of hair. If rash is present, use other test sites such as the flanks, the lower back, or the upper arms. Shave any hair to prevent poor patch contact and false-negative results. Remove skin oils with alcohol to promote adhesion of the patches.

Small quantities of chemicals and solutions in standardized concentrations are placed in separate metal chambers that are backed with hypoallergenic adhesive tape. Carefully apply the tape to the skin so that each chemical is held in contact with the skin surface. Mark each chamber for later identification. As many as 60 or more chemicals may be tested at the same time.

Instruct the client to keep the test sites dry at all times. Baths are substituted for showers until testing is complete. Instruct the client to use caution when washing the hair to avoid getting the patches wet. Discourage the client from engaging in activity that will result in sweating. Tell the client not to reapply patches that come loose, because this interferes with interpretation of the test results. Reinforce the need to remove loose or nonadherent test patches for reapplication.

The initial reading is performed 2 days after application. The tape containing the chemical-filled chambers is peeled away from the skin, and each area of contact is marked with indelible ink for future reading. Document any initial allergic or irritant reactions in the client's medical record. The final reading of the test results is 2 to 5 days later.

Follow-up Care. If a potential allergen is identified, the client is given a list of items containing that chemical to be avoided.

Critical Thinking Challenge

The client is a 26-year-old man who crawled through poison ivy during a paint ball game 3 days ago. He now has poison ivy rash and blisters over his face, neck, hands, and arms. He said that he began itching yesterday and took oral Benadryl 25 mg six times yesterday. He is distressed that the rash is spreading even after using Benadryl. He is worried that the rash and blisters on his face and neck will make breathing difficult.

1. What additional assessment data should you obtain?
2. Why should you or should you not start oxygen on this client?
3. Would epinephrine be helpful in this situation? Why or why not? Where, how much, and by what route would you administer it?
4. Would more Benadryl be helpful in this situation? Why or why not?
5. What should you tell this client about potential respiratory problems?
6. What additional drugs should you be prepared to give and what should you teach this client about his medications?

evolve For suggested answer guidelines, go to http://evolve.elsevier.com/Iggy/.

TYPE V: STIMULATORY REACTIONS

PATHOPHYSIOLOGY

This type of reaction involves inappropriate stimulation of a normal cell surface receptor by an autoantibody, resulting in a continuous "turned-on" state for the cell. An example of this type of reaction is Graves' disease, a form of hyperthyroidism. In Graves' disease, an autoantibody binds to the thyroid-stimulating hormone (TSH) receptor sites on the thyroid gland. This binding continually stimulates thyroid cells to produce thyroid hormones, causing the client to have severe hyperthyroidism (see Chapter 67). The manifestations occur even though the thyroid gland itself is completely normal. In a sense, the tissue responding to the autoantibody is "out of control" from the body's normal feedback system of checks and balances.

COLLABORATIVE MANAGEMENT

For type V reactions involving only one organ, the management focuses on removing enough of the responding (stimulated) tissue to return the function to normal. With Graves' disease, thyroid tissue is either surgically removed or destroyed with radiation. For type V reactions in which antibody stimulation is more widespread, treatment focuses on reducing the production of autoantibodies through immunosuppression.

Autoimmunity

Autoimmunity is a process whereby a person develops an inappropriate immune response. In this response, antibodies and/or lymphocytes are directed against healthy normal cells and tissues. For unknown reasons, the immune system fails to recognize certain body cells or tissues as self and thus triggers immune reactions. The responses, both antibody- and cell-mediated, are similar to normal immune responses against invading organisms, but these reactions are now directed against normal body cells. Causes of loss of recognition of self cells are not known.

Examples of diseases that have an autoimmune cause include systemic lupus erythematosus (SLE), polyarteritis nodosa, scleroderma, rheumatoid arthritis, autoimmune hemolytic anemia, rheumatic fever, and Hashimoto's thyroiditis (Table 26-3). Other diseases, such as type 1 diabetes mellitus, may have multiple causes, one of which is autoimmune.

Management of autoimmunities depends on the organ or organs affected. Anti-inflammatory drugs and immunosuppressive drugs are commonly used along with symptomatic treatment.

TABLE 26-3 Known or Probable Autoimmune Disorders

Disorder	Autoantigen
Systemic Or Non-Organ Specific	
Systemic lupus erythematosus	DNA, DNA proteins
Rheumatoid arthritis	IgG, possibly cartilage
Progressive systemic sclerosis	DNA proteins
Mixed connective tissue disorder	DNA proteins
Organ Specific	
Autoimmune hemolytic anemia	Erythrocytes
Autoimmune thrombocytopenic purpura	Platelets
Diabetes mellitus, type I	Islet cells, insulin, insulin receptor
Dermatomyositis	Unknown
Glomerulonephritis	Glomerular basement membranes
Goodpasture's syndrome	Glomerular basement membranes, pulmonary basement membranes
Graves' disease	Thyroid-stimulating hormone receptor
Hashimoto's thyroiditis	Thyroid cell surface
Idiopathic Addison's disease	Adrenal cell
Myasthenia gravis	Acetylcholine receptor, acetylcholine
Pernicious anemia	Intrinsic factor, parietal cell, B_{12} complexes
Psoriasis	Stratum corneum
Reiter's syndrome	Possibly collagen, conjunctival cells
Sjögren's syndrome	Salivary gland cells, vaginal mucous cells, lacrimal gland cells
Uveitis	Uveal tract cells (eye)
Vasculitis	Unknown, possibly collagen or endothelial cells

IgG, Immunoglobulin G.

WOMEN'S HEALTH CONSIDERATIONS

Virtually all autoimmune disorders, especially rheumatic disorders, occur much more commonly among women than men (McCance & Huether, 2002; Workman, 2000). The risk for autoimmune disease among women compared to men ranges from 5:1 to 20:1. In addition, most autoimmune disorders occur more frequently among white women compared to women of any other ethnicity.

SJÖGREN'S SYNDROME

PATHOPHYSIOLOGY

Sjögren's syndrome (SS) is a group of problems that often appear with other autoimmune disorders. Problems include dry eyes, dry mucous membranes of the nose and mouth (xerostomia), and vaginal dryness. These problems are caused by autoimmune destruction of the lacrimal, salivary, and vaginal mucous producing glands. Often, the client with SS also has rheumatoid arthritis. Fibromyalgia often accompanies SS.

Most clients with SS are women between 35 and 45 years old. SS occurs more frequently among clients with certain tissue types, specifically HLA-DRW52, HLA-DR3, and HLA-B8. Although an exact triggering agent has not been identified, viral infection is strongly suspected. The three viruses thought to be triggers for the autoimmune changes leading to SS are the human immunodeficiency virus type 1 (HIV-1), human T-cell lymphotrophic virus type 1 (HTLV-1), and Epstein-Barr Virus (EBV).

Insufficient tears cause inflammation and ulceration of the cornea. Insufficient saliva decreases digestion of carbohydrates, promotes tooth decay, and increases the incidence of oral and nasal infections. Vaginal dryness increases the incidence of infection and may cause pain during sexual intercourse.

COLLABORATIVE MANAGEMENT

Assessment

The client with Sjögren's syndrome (SS) usually has blurred vision, burning and itching of the eyes, and thick mattering in the conjunctiva. Difficulty swallowing food is common and the client often has changes in taste sensation. Ask the client about nosebleeds **(epistaxis)** and frequent upper respiratory infections.

Physical examination reveals enlarged lymph nodes. If rheumatoid arthritis (RA) accompanies SS, the client has swollen, painful joints and limited joint mobility (see Chapter 24 for a complete discussion of RA). Laboratory assessment may show increased presence of general antinuclear antibodies, anti-SS-A or anti-SS-B antibodies, and elevated levels of IgM rheumatoid factor.

Interventions

IMMUNOMODULATION. Currently, there is no cure for SS. The intensity and the progression of the disorder can be slowed by suppressing immune and inflammatory responses. Drugs used to modulate the immune system in clients with SS include low-dose chemotherapy with methotrexate (Rheumatrex) or cyclophosphamide (Cytoxan). Both drugs have serious long-term side effects, especially on liver and bone marrow function. Other immunosuppressive drugs used to manage SS are corticosteroids, cyclosporine (Neoral, Sandimmune), and hydroxychloroquine (Plaquenil).

SYMPTOMATIC THERAPY. A variety of artificial tears and artificial saliva can help reduce the dry eye and dry mouth symptoms. Teach clients to use humidifiers in the home to increase environmental moisture. Use of water-soluble vaginal lubricants and moisturizers can increase client comfort and reduce the incidence of vaginitis. Some clients relieve dry mouth with systemic pilocarpine (Salagen). This agent mimics the effects of the parasympathetic nervous system, causing increased salivation.

Another intervention for dry eyes is to block the tear outflow channel (nasal punctum). The punctum can be blocked temporarily with small plugs or can be closed surgically. Either method allows the tears produced to remain in contact with the eye longer.

Pain control is an issue for clients who also have either rheumatoid arthritis or fibromyalgia. Nonsteroidal anti-inflammatory drugs (NSAIDs) rather than pure analgesics are commonly used to decrease the inflammation and reduce the associated pain. Many different types and strengths of NSAIDs are available by prescription and over-the-counter. The mechanism of action and side effects are similar for all NSAIDs although the duration of action and cost vary.

GOODPASTURE'S SYNDROME

PATHOPHYSIOLOGY

Goodpasture's syndrome is an autoimmune disorder in which autoantibodies are made against the glomerular basement membrane and neutrophils. The two organs with the most damage are the lungs and the kidney. Lung damage is manifested as pulmonary hemorrhage. Kidney damage manifests as glomerulonephritis that may rapidly progress to complete renal failure (see Chapters 74 and 75). Unlike other autoimmune disorders, Goodpasture's syndrome occurs most often in adolescent or young adult men (McCance & Huether, 2002). The exact cause or triggering agent is unknown.

COLLABORATIVE MANAGEMENT

Goodpasture's syndrome usually is not diagnosed until serious lung and/or kidney problems are present. Manifestations include shortness of breath, hemoptysis (bloody sputum), decreased urine output, weight gain, generalized nondependent edema, hypertension, and tachycardia. Chest x-rays show areas of consolidation. The most common cause of death is uremia as a result of renal failure.

Spontaneous resolution of Goodpasture's syndrome has occurred but is rare. Interventions focus on reducing the immune-mediated damage and performing some type of renal supportive therapy.

IMMUNOMODULATION

Drug Therapy. The mainstay of drug therapy for Goodpasture's syndrome is high-dose corticosteroids. Other drug therapy to suppress the autoimmune response is the same as that for Sjögren's syndrome (SS).

Other Therapy. Additional therapy to reduce immune responses involves plasmapheresis (filtration of the plasma to remove some proteins) to remove the autoantibodies. If the lungs and kidneys do not have permanent damage, clients undergoing plasmapheresis have shown clinical improvement. Some clients using plasmapheresis need infusions of intravenous immunoglobulin (IVIG) to maintain antibody protection against infection.

RENAL SUPPORT THERAPY. Depending upon the level of renal function remaining, the client may need ongoing dialysis. Therapy usually begins with hemodialysis. For long-term therapy, peritoneal or hemodialysis may be used depending on the client's health status, ability to self-manage the infusion and drainage systems, and lifestyle (see Chapter 75).

Renal transplantation is an option for some clients with Goodpasture's syndrome. After transplantation, renal function is normal. In rare instances, clients have been disease-free after transplantation. In others, the renal problems are improved but the lung destruction continues. Some of the drugs used to prevent kidney rejection also suppress the autoimmune response.

GET READY for the NCLEX Examination!

KEY POINTS

Safe Effective Care Environment

- Ensure that only latex-free products are used for a client who has a known latex allergy.
- Ensure that all allergies are documented in a prominent place in the client's medical record.
- Keep emergency equipment and drugs (epinephrine, Benadryl, and cortisol) in or near the room of a client with known severe allergies or a history of anaphylaxis.

Health Promotion and Maintenance

- Encourage all adult clients with severe allergies or those who have a history of anaphylaxis to wear a medical alert bracelet.
- Identify clients at high risk for allergic reactions as a result of home, work environment, or leisure activities.
- Teach the client and family about the clinical manifestations of allergic reactions and when to seek medical advice.

Psychosocial Integrity

- Stay with the client in anaphylaxis.
- Allow the client the opportunity to express fear or anxiety during an allergic response.
- Explain all diagnostic procedures, restrictions, and follow-up care to the client scheduled for tests.
- Reassure clients who are in anaphylaxis that the appropriate interventions are being instituted.

Physiological Integrity

- Assess the client receiving immunosuppressive drugs as treatment of an autoimmune disorder every shift for clinical manifestations of infection.
- Immediately assess the respiratory status and airway of clients who show any symptom of an allergic reaction.
- Immediately discontinue the IV medication of a client having an anaphylactic reaction to that medication. **Do not** discontinue the IV, but change the IV tubing and hang normal saline.
- Hold the dose of any prescribed medication when a client develops angioedema.
- Give oxygen to any client in anaphylaxis.
- Teach the client who has a known drug allergy, which other drugs are likely to stimulate the same reactions.
- Teach the client who carries an EpiPen, how to assemble and use the device. Obtain a return demonstration.

ADDITIONAL STUDY RESOURCES

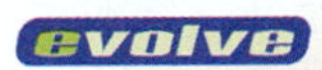

Go to your Student CD-ROM for Review Questions for the NCLEX Examination.

Go to http://evolve.elsevier.com/Iggy/ for Integrated Management of Care Questions for the NCLEX Examination.

SELECTED BIBLIOGRAPHY

Abbas, A., & Lichtman, A. (2003). *Cellular and molecular immunology* (5th ed.). Philadelphia: W. B. Saunders.

Ackley, B., & Ladwig, G. (2002). *Nursing diagnosis handbook: A guide to planning care* (5th ed.). St. Louis: Mosby.

Avella, P., & Walker, M. (2000). Goodpasture's syndrome: A nursing challenge. *Nursing2000, 30*(3), 32cc1-2, 32cc4, 32cc6.

Becker, H. (2000). An analysis of the epidemiology of latex allergy: Implications for primary prevention. *MEDSURG Nursing, 9*(3), 135-143.

Cohen, S. (2001). About latex allergy. *Nursing 2001, 31*(2), 76.

D'Epiro, N. (2000). Deciphering autoimmune disease in women. *Patient Care, 34*(7), 49-52, 54, 59, 63-66.

DeRaps, P., & Lynch, J. (2003). Focus on solutions for allergic rhinitis. *CE-Today for Nurse Practitioners, 2*(2), 15-23.

Dochterman, J., & Bulechek, G. (Eds.). (2004). *Nursing interventions classification (NIC)* (4th ed.). St. Louis: Mosby.

Facts and Comparisons. (2004). *Drug facts and comparisons* (58th ed.). St. Louis: Author.

Floyd, P. (2000). Latex allergy update. *Journal of Perianesthesia Nursing, 15*(1), 25-30.

Gelfand, E. (2000). The clinical use of intravenous immunoglobulin in immunodeficiency and allergic disorders. *Journal of Intravenous Nursing, 23*(5S), S14-S17.

Goldrick, B. (2003). Emerging infections: Allergic aspergillosis. *American Journal of Nursing, 103*(4), 89.

Gonzales, F. (2004). How will your patient respond to contrast media? *Nursing 2004, 34*(1), 32hn1-32hn3.

Green, S., & Martin, D. (2003). Is every sneeze an allergy? Diagnosing and treating allergic vs nonallergic rhinitis. *The American Journal for Nurse Practitioners, 7*(5), 9-18.

Hathaway, L. (2005). Patient-education guide: Anaphylaxis. *Nursing 2005, 35*(1), 46-47.

Hayden, M.L. (2003). Assessing and improving quality of life in allergic rhinitis. *CE-Today for Nurse Practitioners, 2*(2), 7-13.

Lenehan, G. (2002). Latex allergy: Separating fact from fiction. *Nursing2002, 32*(3), 58-63.

LoBuono, C. (2000). Eliminating allergy triggers. *Patient Care for the Nurse Practitioner, 3*(4), 45-52.

Lynch, J. (2003). An examination of severe, intractable, allergic rhinitis. *CE-Today for Nurse Practitioners, 2*(2), 25-28.

McCance, K., & Huether, S. (2002). *Pathophysiology: The biologic basis for disease in adults and children* (4th ed.). St. Louis: Mosby.

Moorhead, S., Johnson, M., & Maas, M. (Eds.). (2004). *Nursing outcomes classification (NOC)* (3rd ed.). St. Louis: Mosby.

Myers, J. (2000). Emergency: Chemotherapy-induced hypersensitivity reaction. *American Journal of Nursing, 100*(4), 53-54.

Nussbaum, R., McInnes, R., & Willard, H. (2001). *Thompson & Thompson: Genetics in medicine* (6th ed.). Philadelphia: W. B. Saunders.

Pagana, K., & Pagana, T. (2002). *Mosby's manual of diagnostic and laboratory tests* (2nd ed.). St. Louis: Mosby.

Pepper, G. (2000). Nonsteroidal anti-inflammatory drugs: New perspectives on a familiar drug class. *Nursing Clinics of North America, 35*(1), 223-244.

Swenson, M. (2000). Autoimmunity and immunotherapy. *Journal of Intravenous Nursing, 23*(5S), S8-S13.

Vale, D. (2000). Recognition and management of Sjögren's syndrome: Strategies for the advanced practice nurse. *Nursing Clinics of North America, 35*(1), 267-278.

van Steekelenburg, J., Clement, P., & Beel, M. (2002). Comparison of five new antihistamines (H1-receptor antagonists) in patients with allergic rhinitis using nasal provocation studies and skin tests. *Allergy, 57*(4), 346-350.

Wilburn, S. (2001). When latex allergies limit employment. *American Journal of Nursing, 101*(8), 88.

Workman, M.L. (2000). Immune mechanisms in rheumatic disease. *Nursing Clinics of North America, 35*(1), 175-188.

CHAPTER 27

Altered Cell Growth and Cancer Development

M. LINDA WORKMAN

LEARNING OUTCOMES

After studying this chapter, you should be able to:

1. Explain why causes of cancer can be hard to establish.
2. Compare the features of benign and malignant tumors.
3. List three cancer types associated with tobacco use.
4. Identify cancer types for which primary prevention is possible.
5. Compare the cancer development processes of initiation and promotion.
6. Describe the TNM system for cancer staging.
7. Explain the differences between a "low-grade" cancer and a "high-grade" cancer.
8. Discuss the roles of oncogenes and suppressor genes in cancer development.
9. Identify four common sites of distant metastasis for cancer.
10. Discuss the role of immunity in protection against cancer.
11. Identify which cancer types arise from connective tissues and which types arise from glandular tissues.
12. Describe how genetic predisposition can increase a person's risk for cancer development.
13. Identify behaviors that reduce the risk for cancer development and cancer death.
14. Identify specific issues about genetic testing for cancer predisposition.

Go to your Student CD-ROM for Review Questions for the NCLEX Examination keyed to these Learning Outcomes.

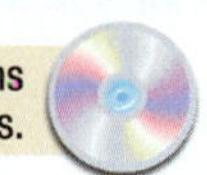

Many people have some type of altered cell growth such as a mole or a skin tag. Most types of altered cell growth are harmless (benign) and do not require intervention. Malignant cell growth or cancer, however, is serious and, without intervention, leads to death. Cancer is a common health problem in the United States and Canada. Nearly 1.5 million people are newly diagnosed with cancer each year (American Cancer Society, 2005). Some types of cancer can be prevented; others have better cure rates if diagnosed early. As a nurse, you can have a vital impact in educating the public about cancer prevention and early detection methods.

HISTORICAL PERSPECTIVE

Although cancer is common today, it is not a new disorder. Even prehistoric humans developed cancer. Some types of cancer are more common today, especially among more affluent societies, than in centuries past. Two reasons for this increase are the long life expectancy of people in more affluent countries and increased exposure to substances that cause cancer.

Cancer will occur in about 1 of every 3 persons currently living in North America (American Cancer Society, 2005), although cancer risk differs for each person. Cancer prevention is a major health focus for the United States (see the Meeting Healthy People 2010 Objectives box on p. 468). More than 10 million Americans with a history of cancer are alive today, nearly 5 million of whom are considered cured (American Cancer Society, 2005). Terms used to describe abnormal cell growth and cancer are listed in Table 27-1.

PATHOPHYSIOLOGY

Growth of cells and tissues is expected during infancy and childhood, and many human body cells continue to "grow" by cell division **(mitosis)** long after maturation is complete. Such cells are located in tissues where constant damage or wear is likely and continued cell growth is

Meeting HEALTHY PEOPLE 2010 Objectives

CANCER

Objective 17.1: Reduce cancer deaths to a rate of no more than 103 per 100,000 people.

- Assess all clients for current and past exposures to carcinogens.
- Assist clients to identify personal cancer risks.
- Assist clients to avoid known environmental carcinogens.
- Assess all clients for a family history of cancer to identify clients at genetic high risk for cancer.
- Refer identified clients at genetic high risk for cancer to an appropriate level genetic counselor.
- Teach clients to avoid excessive sun exposure and to use protective clothing, hats, and sun-screening agents when sun exposure is not avoidable.
- Teach client about tobacco-related cancers.
- Assist clients who smoke to reduce or quit smoking.
- Teach clients about alcohol-related cancers.
- Teach clients about the importance of limiting dietary fat, smoked meats, and red meats.
- Teach clients about the importance of increasing dietary fiber.
- Encourage clients to see a health care provider at least once per year for cancer screening.
- Teach clients the correct technique for breast self-examination or testicular self-examination.
- Encourage client to engage in self-screening measures, such as whole body skin examination, breast self-examination, or testicular self-examination, on a monthly basis.
- Instruct clients who have any of the seven warning signs of cancer to follow up with their primary care provider as soon as possible.
- Encourage female clients to follow American Cancer Society guidelines for cervical, breast, and colorectal cancer screening appropriate for age and risk categories.
- Encourage male clients to follow American Cancer Society guidelines for prostate and colorectal cancer screening appropriate for age and risk categories.

needed to replace dead tissues. Cells of the skin, hair, mucous membranes, bone marrow, and linings of organs such as the lungs, stomach, intestines, bladder, and uterus, among others, have the ability to divide throughout a person's life span. The growth of these cells is well controlled, ensuring that only the right number of cells is always present in any tissue or organ.

Some tissues and organs stop growing by cell division after development is complete. For example, heart muscle cells no longer divide after fetal life; the number of heart muscle cells is fixed at birth. The size of the heart increases as the person grows because each cell gets larger, but the number of heart muscle cells does not increase. Growth that causes tissue to increase in size by enlarging each cell is **hypertrophy.** Growth that causes tissue to increase in size by increasing the number of cells is **hyperplasia** (Figure 27-1).

Any new or continued cell growth not needed for normal development or replacement of dead and damaged tissues is called **neoplasia.** This cell growth is always abnormal even if it causes no harm. Whether the new cells are benign or malignant, neoplastic cells develop from normal cells (parent cells). Thus cancer cells were once normal cells but changed to no longer look, grow, or function normally. The strict processes controlling normal growth and function have been lost. To understand how cancer cells grow, it is helpful to first understand the regulation and function of normal cells.

Biology of Normal Cells

Many different normal cells work together to make the whole person function at an optimal level. For optimal function, each cell must perform in a predictable manner.

TABLE 27-1 Terminology Commonly Associated with Abnormal Cell Growth

anaplastic Without shape or differentiation, small and round
aneuploid More or less than the normal number of chromosomes
apoptosis The finite life span of normal cells; "programmed cell death"
benign New, nonmalignant cell growth not needed for normal growth or replacement
carcinogenesis The transformation of a normal cell into a cancer cell
doubling time The amount of time it takes for a tumor to double in size by mitotic cell divisions
euploid The normal chromosome number
fibronectin A large, extracellular, transformation-sensitive cell-surface protein present on normal cells that allows normal cells to adhere tightly together
gene expression The activation, or "turning on," of a specific gene to the extent that it synthesizes a specific protein that influences the activity of a cell or group of cells
gene suppression The deactivation, or "turning off," of a specific gene so that it is silent and does not synthesize a protein
generation time The period of time necessary for one cell to enter and complete one round of cell division by mitosis
initiation The damage of a normal cell's DNA by a carcinogen
latency The period of time between when a carcinogenic agent or substance damaged the DNA of a normal cell (initiated it) and when an overt cancer is present
malignant Cancerous, new growth of cells by invasion that is not needed for normal development or tissue replacement
metastasis Invasive growth of cancer cells from the original tumor into distant areas
mitosis Cell division by exact duplication
morphology Appearance or shape
multipotent An undifferentiated cell that has multiple potentials for maturation and differentiation (also called totipotent and pluripotent)
neoplasia New cell growth not needed for normal body growth or replacement of dead or missing tissue
oncogene A developmental gene (proto-oncogene) expressed at an inappropriate time, capable of transforming a normal cell into a cancer cell
ploidy The chromosome content of a cell
  aneuploid ploidy The chromosome content of a cell that is greater or lesser than the normal chromosome number for the species
  diploid (euploid) ploidy The normal chromosome content of a cell for the species (e.g., human cells have 46 chromosomes [23 pairs] per cell)
primary tumor A tumor formed in a specific tissue as a result of a carcinogenic agent or event
promotion Enhancement of cell division in a cell initiated by a carcinogen
proto-oncogene A developmental gene expressed during early embryonic development
secondary tumor A tumor formed as a result of breaking off from a primary tumor and spreading to distant sites (metastasis)
suppressor gene A gene that suppresses the expression of an oncogene
transformation The changing of a normal cell into a cancer cell by a carcinogenic agent or event

CHARACTERISTICS OF NORMAL CELLS

HAVE LIMITED CELL DIVISION. Normal cells divide (undergo mitosis) for one of two reasons: (1) to develop normal tissue or (2) to replace lost or damaged normal tissue. Even when they are capable of mitosis, normal cells divide only when body conditions and nutrition are just right.

UNDERGO APOPTOSIS. Normal cells have a finite life span. With each round of cell division, the telomeric DNA at the ends of the chromosomes shorten (see Chapter 11). When this DNA is gone, the cell responds to signals for programmed cell death, **apoptosis.** The purpose of apoptosis is to ensure each organ has adequate number of cells at their functional peak.

SHOW SPECIFIC MORPHOLOGY. Each normal cell type has a distinct and recognizable appearance, size, and shape, as shown in Figure 27-2.

HAVE A SMALL NUCLEAR-CYTOPLASMIC RATIO. As shown in Figure 27-2, the size of the normal cell nucleus is small compared with the size of the rest of the cell, including the cytoplasm.

PERFORM SPECIFIC DIFFERENTIATED FUNCTIONS. Every normal cell has at least one special function to contribute to whole-body homeostasis. For example, skin cells make keratin, liver cells make bile, cardiac muscle cells contract, nerve cells conduct impulses, and red blood cells make hemoglobin to carry oxygen.

ADHERE TIGHTLY TOGETHER. Normal cells make proteins that protrude from the cell surface, allowing cells to bind closely and tightly together. One such protein is fibronectin, which keeps most normal tissues bound tightly to each other. Exceptions are blood cells. Red blood cells and white blood cells produce no fibronectin and do not usually adhere together.

ARE NONMIGRATORY. Because normal cells are tightly bound together, they do not wander from one tissue into the next (with the exception of red blood cells and white blood cells).

GROW IN AN ORDERLY AND WELL-REGULATED MANNER. Normal cells do not divide unless body conditions are optimal for cell division. These conditions include the need for more cells, adequate space, and sufficient nutrients and other resources. Cell division, occurring in a well-recognized pattern, is described by the cell cycle. Figure 27-3 shows the phases of the cell cycle.

Living cells not actively reproducing are in a reproductive resting state termed G_0. During the G_0 period, cells actively carry out their functions but do not divide. Normal cells spend most of their lives in the G_0 state, just like most humans spend most of their lives in a nonpregnant state.

Mitotic cell division makes one cell divide into two cells. These two cells are identical to each other and to the original cell that started the mitotic cell division. The steps of entering and completing the cell cycle are tightly controlled.

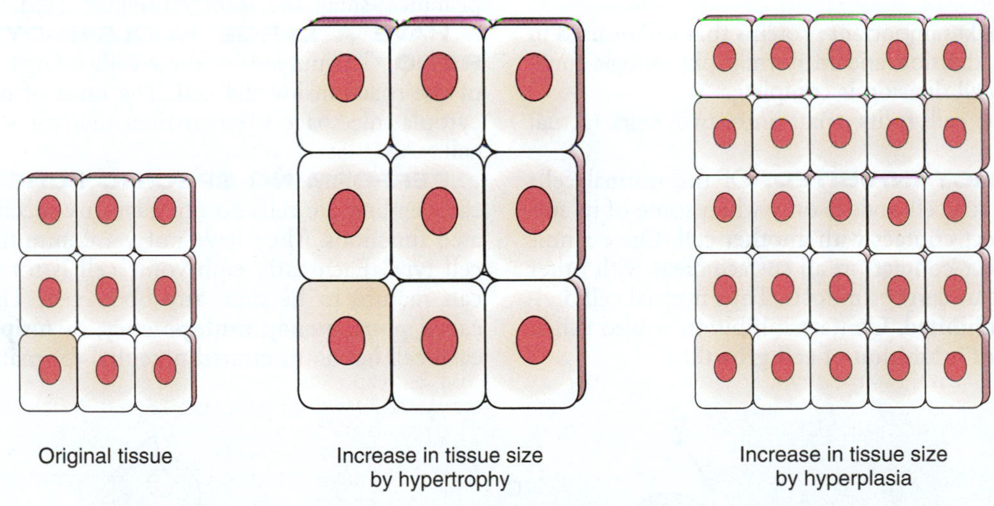

Figure 27-1 ■ Tissue growth by hypertrophy and hyperplasia.

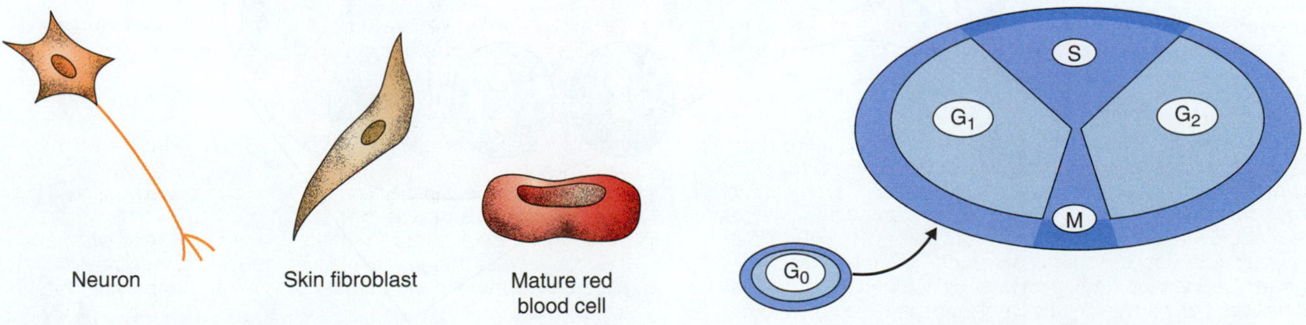

Figure 27-2 ■ Distinctive morphology of some normal cells.

Figure 27-3 ■ The cell cycle.

Much of this control is regulated by proteins produced by "suppressor genes."

Control of whether or not a cell enters the cell cycle and completes the cycle to form two new cells is dependent on the presence and absence of specific proteins. Proteins that promote cells to enter and complete cell division belong to a family of proteins known as "cyclins." When cyclins are activated, they first allow a cell to leave the G_0 state and enter the cycle. These activated cyclins then permit the cell to move through the different phases of the cell cycle and actually divide. The cyclins are the products of proto-oncogenes (see later discussion under Oncogene Activation on p. 476). Proteins produced by suppressor genes regulate the amount of cyclins present in a cell and ensure that cell division occurs only when it is needed. Thus normal cell division represents a balance between the proteins that promote cell division (cyclins) and the proteins that limit cell division (suppressor gene products).

Figure 27-4 shows the activities of the phases of the cell cycle:

- **G_1.** The cell is getting ready for division by taking on extra nutrients, making more energy, and growing extra membrane. The amount of cell fluid (cytoplasm) also increases.
- **S.** Because making one cell into two cells requires twice as much of everything, including deoxyribonucleic acid (DNA), the cell must double its DNA content through DNA synthesis. This process occurs in S phase.
- **G_2.** The cell makes important proteins that will be used in actual cell division and in normal physiologic function after cell division is complete.
- **M.** The single cell splits apart into two cells (actual mitosis).

ARE CONTACT INHIBITED. Of the normal cells that can divide, each cell divides only when some of its surface is not in direct contact with another cell. Once a normal cell is in direct contact on all surface areas with other cells, it no longer undergoes mitosis. Thus normal cell division is **contact inhibited.** Contact inhibition is also called **density-dependent inhibition of cell growth.**

ARE EUPLOID. Most normal human cells have 23 pairs of chromosomes, the correct number for human beings.

Each normal, mature cell has a specific structure and function. The fact that normal mature cells have many different shapes and functions is interesting, considering that all humans started life as a single cell. The function and behavior of that first single cell and its daughter cells are quite different from those of normal adult human cells. Knowledge about these differences has helped in understanding how cancer develops.

CHARACTERISTICS OF EARLY EMBRYONIC CELLS

HAVE RAPID AND CONTINUOUS CELL DIVISION. Early embryonic cells (from conception to the eighth day) spend most of their time within the cell cycle, actively reproducing. The time it takes one cell to divide into two cells **(generation time)** ranges from 2 to 8 hours.

DO NOT RESPOND TO SIGNALS FOR APOPTOSIS. Early embryonic cells have long telomeres that do not shorten with each cell division. Although some cells during fetal life undergo apoptosis for development of specific structures, this is not a feature of embryonic cells.

SHOW ANAPLASTIC MORPHOLOGY. Anaplasia means "without specific shape or differentiation." Early embryonic cells do not look like the mature cells they will eventually become. They all have the same anaplastic appearance–small and rounded (Figure 27-5).

HAVE A LARGE NUCLEAR-CYTOPLASMIC RATIO. The nucleus of these cells is large, taking up most of the space inside the cell. The ratio of nuclear space to cytoplasmic space is larger than that for a normal mature cell.

PERFORM NO SPECIFIC FUNCTIONS. These early embryonic cells do not have any specific or differentiated functions. They have not yet committed to a specific cell type. Each early embryonic cell is totally flexible and can mature to become any body cell. This flexibility is called **pluripotency, multipotency,** or **totipotency** because each cell has an unlimited potential for maturation.

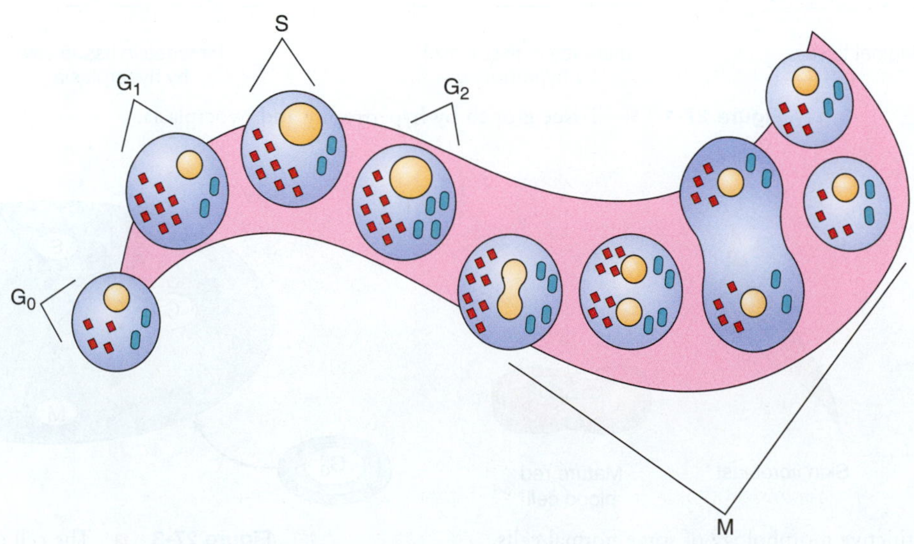

Figure 27-4 ■ Cellular events during mitotic cell division.

ADHERE LOOSELY TOGETHER. Early embryonic cells do not make fibronectin and are not tightly bound together.

ARE ABLE TO MIGRATE. Because early embryonic cells are not tightly bound together, they do not remain in one place within the embryo but migrate throughout the early embryo.

ARE NOT CONTACT INHIBITED. Having all sides of an early embryonic cell in continuous contact with the surfaces of other cells does not inhibit embryonic cell division.

ARE EUPLOID. Although early human embryonic cells differ from mature cells in many ways, they have 23 pairs of chromosomes.

COMMITMENT. At about day 8, early embryonic cells start changing into differentiated cells. In response to unknown signals, each cell commits itself to a specific outcome. The cell has not yet taken on any differentiated features; rather, it positions itself within a group of cells that will eventually become only one specific organ or tissue.

Commitment involves turning off specific early embryonic genes that controlled or regulated early rapid growth. These genes, called **proto-oncogenes,** remain as normal cellular genes but have limited function after early embryonic life. These genes are usually either "turned off," suppressed with little expression, or expressed but tightly controlled.

After the early embryonic regulatory genes are "turned off" **(suppressed),** other specific genes that control the expression of differentiated functions must be "turned on" **(expressed)** selectively in different cell types. For example, the gene for insulin is actively expressed only in pancreatic beta cells and is suppressed in all other cells. This selective gene expression directs the normal growth and differentiation of specific body cells.

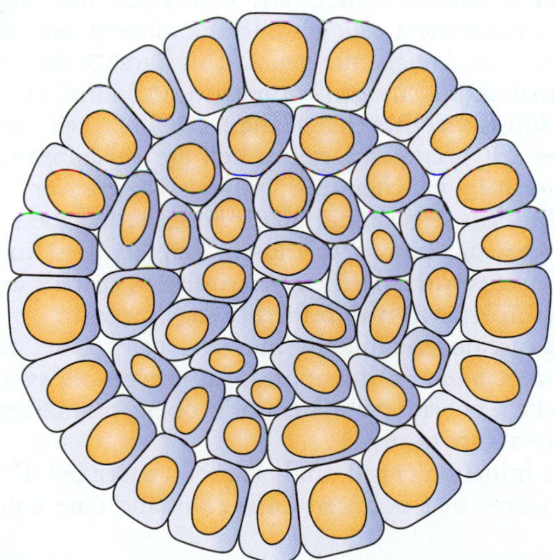

Figure 27-5 ■ Embryonic cells at about 5 days after conception.

Biology of Abnormal Cells

Body cells are exposed to personal and environmental conditions that can alter how the cells grow or function. When either cell growth or cell function is changed, the cells are considered abnormal. Table 27-2 compares features of normal, embryonic, benign tumor, and cancer cells.

CHARACTERISTICS OF BENIGN TUMOR CELLS

Benign tumor cells are normal cells growing in the wrong place or at the wrong time. Examples include moles, uterine fibroid tumors, skin tags, endometriosis, and nasal polyps. Benign tumor cells:

HAVE CONTINUOUS OR INAPPROPRIATE CELL GROWTH. Benign tumors are tissues not needed for normal function, growing too much or in the wrong place.

SHOW SPECIFIC MORPHOLOGY. Benign tumors look like the tissues they come from, retaining the specific morphology of parent cells.

HAVE A SMALL NUCLEAR-CYTOPLASMIC RATIO. Just like completely normal cells, benign tumor cells have a small nucleus compared with the rest of the cell.

PERFORM SPECIFIC DIFFERENTIATED FUNCTIONS. Not only do benign tumors look like their parent cells, but they also perform the same differentiated functions. For example, in endometriosis, one type of benign tumor, the normal lining of the uterus (endometrium) grows in an abnormal place (such as on an ovary, on the peritoneum, or in the chest cavity). This displaced endometrium acts just like normal endometrium by changing each month under the influence of estrogen. When the hormone level drops and the

TABLE 27-2 Characteristics of Normal and Abnormal Cells

Characteristic	Normal Cell	Embryonic Cell	Benign Tumor Cell	Malignant Cell
Cell division	None or slow	Rapid, continuous	Continuous or inappropriate	Rapid or continuous
Appearance	Specific morphologic features	Anaplastic	Specific morphologic features	Anaplastic
Nuclear-cytoplasmic ratio	Small	Large	Small	Large
Differentiated functions	Many	None	Many	Some or none
Adherence	Tight	Loose	Tight	Loose
Migratory	No	Yes	No	Yes
Growth	Well regulated	Well regulated	Expansion	Invasion
Chromosomes	Diploid (euploid)	Diploid (euploid)	Diploid (euploid)	Aneuploid*
Mitotic index	Low	High	Low	High*

*Depends on the degree of malignant transformation.

normal endometrium sheds from the uterus, the displaced endometrium, wherever it is, also sheds.

ADHERE TIGHTLY TOGETHER. Benign tumor cells make fibronectin and bind tightly to one another. In addition, many benign tissues are "encapsulated," or surrounded with fibrous connective tissue, helping to hold the benign tissue together.

ARE NONMIGRATORY. Benign tissues do not wander but remain tightly bound and do not invade other body tissues.

GROW IN AN ORDERLY MANNER. Benign tumor cells follow normal cell growth patterns even though their growth is not needed. Growth may continue beyond an appropriate time, but the rate of growth is normal. The benign tumor grows by hyperplastic expansion. *They do not invade.*

ARE EUPLOID. Benign tumor cells have 23 pairs of chromosomes, the correct number for human beings.

CHARACTERISTICS OF CANCER CELLS

Cancer (malignant) cells are abnormal, serve no useful function, and are harmful to normal body tissues. Malignant tumors commonly:

HAVE RAPID OR CONTINUOUS CELL DIVISION. Some cancer cells have a short generation time (2 to 4 hours), but most cancer cells have a generation time similar to that of the parent cells. Cancer cells divide nearly continuously. Almost as soon as one round of mitosis is complete, the daughter cells begin a new round.

DO NOT RESPOND TO SIGNALS FOR APOPTOSIS. Most cancer cells have long telomeres and a lot of the enzyme, telomerase, which maintains telomeric DNA. As a result, cancer cells do not respond to apoptotic signals and have an unlimited life span (are "immortal").

SHOW ANAPLASTIC MORPHOLOGY. Cancer cells lose the specific appearance of their parent cells, becoming **anaplastic.** As a cancer cell becomes even more malignant, it becomes smaller and rounded. This loss of specific appearance can make diagnosis of cancer type difficult, because many types of cancer cells look alike.

HAVE A LARGE NUCLEAR-CYTOPLASMIC RATIO. The nucleus of a cancer cell is larger than that of a normal cell, and the cancer cell is small. The nucleus occupies much of the space within the cancer cell, creating a large nuclear-cytoplasmic ratio.

LOSE SOME OR ALL DIFFERENTIATED FUNCTIONS. Along with losing the appearance of the parent cell, cancer cells lose some functions that the parent cells performed. *Cancer cells serve no useful purpose.*

ADHERE LOOSELY TOGETHER. Cancer cells do not make fibronectin. As a result, they adhere poorly to each other, and cancer cells easily break off from the main tumor.

ARE ABLE TO MIGRATE. Because cancer cells do not bind tightly together and have many enzymes on their cell surfaces, they are able to slip through blood vessels and tissues, spreading from the main tumor site to many other body sites. This ability to spread **(metastasize)** is a key feature of cancer cells and a major cause of death among people with cancer.

GROW BY INVASION. Cancer cells expand and extend into other tissues, both close by and more remote from the original tumor, by invasion. Invasion and persistent growth make untreated cancer deadly.

ARE NOT CONTACT INHIBITED. Cancer cells continue to divide even when touched on all surface areas by other cells; thus their growth is not contact inhibited. The persistence of cancer cell division is one factor making the disease so difficult to control.

ARE ANEUPLOID. As cancer cells become more malignant, they lose or gain chromosomes. Thus they can have more than 23 pairs or less than 23 pairs.

CANCER DEVELOPMENT

Carcinogenesis/Oncogenesis

Carcinogenesis and **oncogenesis** are other names for cancer development. Table 27-3 lists key concepts about cancer development. The process of changing a normal cell into a cancer cell is called **malignant transformation.** This process occurs through the steps of *initiation, promotion, progression,* and *metastasis.*

INITIATION

The first step in carcinogenesis is **initiation.** Normal cells can become cancer cells if their proto-oncogenes are turned back on at any time after early embryonic life. Anything that can penetrate a cell, get into the nucleus, and damage the DNA can damage the genes. This damage can turn on genes that should remain suppressed and turn off normal genes. Substances that change the activity of a cell's genes so that the cell becomes a cancer cell are **carcinogens.** Carcinogens may be chemicals, physical agents, or viruses. Table 27-4 lists a few common carcinogens and the types of cancer they are known to cause. Chapters presenting the care of clients with specific cancers discuss specific carcinogens (when known) within the Etiology sections.

Pure carcinogens initially mutate a cell's genes and are thus called *initiators.* Initiation is an irreversible event that can lead to cancer development if it does not interfere with the cell's ability to divide.

After initiation, a cell can become a cancer cell if the cellular changes that occurred during initiation are enhanced

TABLE 27-3 Key Concepts Related to Cancer Development

- Neoplastic cells originate from normal body cells.
- Transformation of a normal cell into a cancer cell involves mutation of the genes (DNA) of the normal cell.
- Early embryonic genes that are overexpressed can cause a cell to develop into a tumor.
- Only one cell has to undergo malignant transformation for cancer to begin.
- Benign tumors grow by expansion, whereas malignant tumors grow by invasion.
- Most tumors arise from cells that are capable of cell division.
- A key feature of cancer cells is the loss of apoptosis. These cells have an "infinite" life span.
- Primary prevention of cancer involves avoiding exposure to known causes of cancer.
- Secondary prevention of cancer involves screening for early detection.
- Tobacco use is a causative or permissive factor in 30% of all malignant neoplasms.
- Tumors that metastasize from the primary site into another organ are still designated as tumors of the originating tissue.

by **promotion.** A cancer cell is not a health threat unless it can divide. If it cannot divide, it cannot form a tumor. *If growth conditions are right, however, widespread metastatic disease can develop from just one cancer cell.*

PROMOTION

Once a normal cell has been initiated by a carcinogen and is a cancer cell, it can become a tumor if its growth is enhanced. The time between a cell's initiation and the development of an overt tumor is called the **latency period,** which can range from months to years.

Promoters are substances that promote or enhance growth of the initiated cancer cell. They can also shorten the latency period. Promoters may be hormones, drugs, or a wide variety of chemicals.

PROGRESSION

After cancer cells have grown to the point that a detectable tumor is formed (a 1-cm tumor has at least 1 billion cells in it), other events must occur for this tumor to become a health problem. First, the tumor must develop its own blood supply. In the early stages, the tumor receives nutrition only by diffusion. After the tumor reaches 1 cm, however, diffusion is not efficient, and cells in the center of the tumor become hypoxic and start to die. To continue to grow and survive, the tumor makes **tumor angiogenesis factor (TAF).** TAF triggers capillaries and other blood vessels in the area to grow new branches into the tumor. These blood vessels ensure the tumor's continued nourishment.

As tumor cells continue to divide, some of the new cells change features from the original, initiated cancer cell. Actual colonies or subpopulations within the tumor begin to appear. These cell groups differ from the original cancer cell. Some of the differences provide these cell groups with advantages that allow them to live and divide no matter how the conditions around them change; these differences are thus called "selection advantages." Changes that a tumor undergoes at this time can allow it to become more malignant. Over time, the tumor cells have fewer and fewer normal cell features.

The original tumor is called the **primary tumor.** It is usually identified by the tissue from which it arose (parent tissue), such as in breast cancer or lung cancer. When primary tumors are located in vital organs, such as the brain or lungs, they can grow excessively and either lethally damage the vital organ or "crowd out" healthy organ tissue and interfere with that organ's ability to perform its vital function. At other times, the primary tumor is located in soft tissue that can expand without damage as the tumor grows. One such site is the breast. The breast is not a vital organ, and even if it had a large tumor in it, the primary tumor alone would not cause the client's death. When the tumor spreads from the original site into vital areas, life functions can be disrupted.

TABLE 27-4 Known Environmental Carcinogens*

Carcinogen	Associated Cancer Site or Neoplasm
Alcoholic beverages	Liver, esophagus, mouth, pharynx, breast, colon, and rectum
Anabolic steroids	Liver
Arsenic	Lung, skin
Asbestos	Lung, pleura, peritoneum, pericardium
Benzene	Myelogenous leukemia
Chemotherapy drugs Alkylating agents Anthracycline antibiotics Antimetabolites	Acute leukemia, lymphoma
Cyclosporine	Non-Hodgkin's lymphoma
Diesel exhaust	Lung
Formaldehyde	Nasopharynx
Hair dyes	Bladder
Ionizing radiation	Bone marrow, thyroid, many organs
Mineral oils	Skin
Pesticides	Lung
Polycyclic hydrocarbons	Lung, skin, scrotum
Polychlorinated biphenyls	Liver, skin
Sunlight	Skin, eyes
Tobacco	Lung, esophagus, mouth, pharynx, larynx, pancreas, bladder, kidney, liver, stomach, colon, rectum, leukemia

Data from U.S. Department of Health and Human Services, Public Health Service, National Toxicology Program. (December 2002). *Report on Carcinogens* (10th ed.). Author.
*This is a partial list selected from over 200 substances listed by the above source.

METASTASIS

In metastasis, cancer cells move from the primary location by breaking off from the original group and establishing remote colonies. These additional tumors are called **metastatic** or **secondary tumors.** *Even though the tumor is now in another organ, it is still a cancer from the original altered tissue. For example, when breast cancer spreads to the lung and the bone, it is breast cancer in the lung and bone, not lung cancer and not bone cancer.* Metastasis occurs through many steps, as shown in Figure 27-6.

EXTENSION INTO SURROUNDING TISSUES. Tumors secrete enzymes that open up areas of surrounding tissue. Pressure, created as the tumor increases in size, forces tumor cells to invade new territory.

BLOOD VESSEL PENETRATION. Enzymes also make large pores in the client's blood vessels, allowing tumor cells to enter the blood and circulate throughout the body.

RELEASE OF TUMOR CELLS. Because tumor cells are loosely held together, clumps of cells break off of the primary tumor into blood vessels for transport.

INVASION. Tumor cells circulate through the blood and enter tissues at remote sites. When conditions in the remote site can support tumor cell growth, the cells stop circulating (arrest) and invade the surrounding tissues, creating secondary tumors. Table 27-5 lists the common sites of metastasis for specific tumor types. Three routes of spread are local seeding, bloodborne metastasis, and lymphatic spread.

Local Seeding. Local seeding is the shedding of cancer cells in the local area of the primary tumor. In ovarian cancer, for example, cells often spill from the primary tumor into the peritoneal cavity and set up multiple secondary sites.

Bloodborne Metastasis. Bloodborne metastasis (tumor cell release into the blood) is the most common cause of cancer spread. Clumps of cancer cells can become

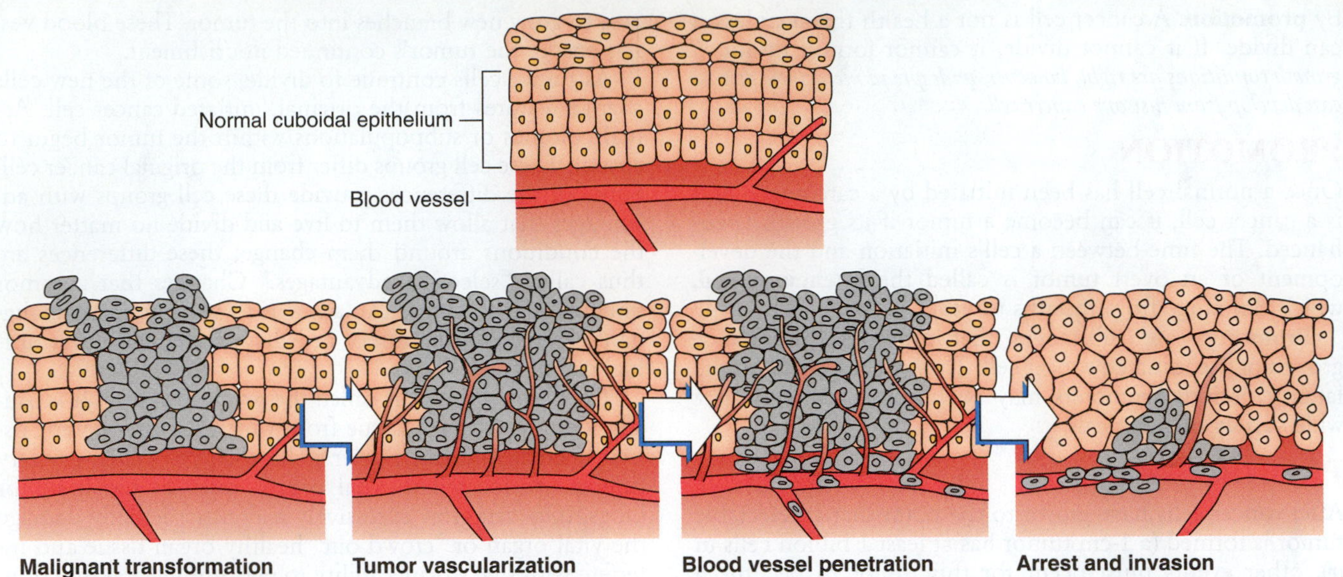

Malignant transformation
Some normal cuboidal cells have undergone malignant transformation and have divided enough times to form a tumorous area within the cuboidal epithelium.

Tumor vascularization
Cancer cells secrete tumor angiogenesis factor (TAF), stimulating the blood vessels to bud and form new channels that grow into the tumor.

Blood vessel penetration
Cancer cells have broken off from the main tumor. Enzymes on the surface of the tumor cells make holes in the blood vessels, allowing cancer cells to enter blood vessels and travel around the body.

Arrest and invasion
Cancer cells clump up in blood vessel walls and invade new tissue areas. If the new tissue areas have the right conditions to support continued growth of cancer cells, new tumors (metastatic tumors) will form at this site.

Figure 27-6 ■ The steps of metastasis.

TABLE 27-5 Common Sites of Metastasis for Different Cancer Types

Breast Cancer Bone* Lung* Liver Brain	**Prostate Cancer** Bone (especially spine and legs)* Pelvic nodes
Lung Cancer Brain* Bone Liver Lymph nodes Pancreas	**Melanoma** Gastrointestinal tract Lymph nodes Lung Brain
Colorectal Cancer Liver* Lymph nodes Adjacent structures	**Primary Brain Cancer** Central nervous system

*Most common site of metastasis for the specific malignant neoplasm.

trapped in capillaries. These clumps damage the capillary wall and allow cancer cells to enter the surrounding tissue.

Lymphatic Spread. Lymphatic spread is related to the number, structure, and location of lymph nodes and vessels. Primary sites that are rich in lymphatics have more early metastatic spread than areas with few lymphatics.

Cancer Classification

Cancers are classified by the type of tissue from which they arise (e.g., glandular, connective). Terms that describe cancer by tissue origin are listed in Table 27-6. Other ways to classify cancer include biologic behavior, anatomic site, and degree of differentiation.

About 100 different types of cancer arise from various tissues or organs. Figure 27-7 compares cancer distribution by site and gender. Cancers are divided into two major categories: solid and hematologic.

Solid tumors develop from specific tissues (e.g., breast cancer and lung cancer). Hematologic cancers (e.g., leukemias and lymphomas) arise from blood cell–forming tissues.

Cancer Grade and Stage

Systems of grading and staging have been developed to help standardize cancer diagnosis, prognosis, and treatment. Grading of a tumor classifies cellular aspects of the cancer. Staging classifies clinical aspects of the cancer.

GRADING

Some cancer cells are "more malignant" than others, varying in their aggressiveness and sensitivity to treatment. Some cancer cells barely resemble the tissue from which they arose, are aggressive, and spread rapidly. These cells are a "high-grade" cancer. On the basis of cell appearance and activity, grading compares the cancer cell with the normal parent tissue from which it arose.

Different clinical groups have established different grading systems for different types of cancer cells, but overall they resemble the standard system listed in Table 27-7. This system rates cancer cells with the lowest rating given to those cells that closely resemble normal cells, and the highest rating given to cancer cells that barely resemble normal cells.

TABLE 27-6 Classification of Tumors by Tissue of Origin

Prefix	Tissue of Origin	Benign Tumor	Malignant Tumor*
Adeno	Epithelial glands	Adenoma	Adenocarcinoma
Chondro	Cartilage	Chondroma	Chondrosarcoma
Fibro	Fibrous connective	Fibroma	Fibrosarcoma
Glio	Glial cells (brain)	Glioma	Glioblastoma
Hemangio	Blood vessel	Hemangioma	Hemangiosarcoma
Hepato	Liver	Hepatoma	Hepatocarcinoma Hepatoblastoma
Leiomyo	Smooth muscle	Leiomyoma	Leiomyosarcoma
Lipo	Fat/adipose	Lipoma	Liposarcoma
Lympho	Lymphoid tissues		Malignant lymphomas Hodgkin's lymphoma Non-Hodgkin's lymphoma Burkitt's lymphoma Cutaneous T-cell
Melano	Pigment-producing skin		Melanoma
Meningio	Meninges	Meningioma	Malignant meningioma Meningioblastoma
Neuro	Nerve tissue	Neuroma Neurofibroma	Neurosarcoma Neuroblastoma
Osteo	Bone	Osteoma	Osteosarcoma
Renal	Kidney		Renal cell carcinoma
Rhabdo	Skeletal muscle	Rhabdomyoma	Rhabdomyosarcoma
Squamous	Epithelial layer of skin, mucous membranes, and organ linings	Papilloma	Squamous cell carcinoma of skin, bladder, lungs, cervix

*Carcinomas are tumors of glandular tissue; sarcomas are tumors of connective tissue; blastomas are tumors of less differentiated, embryonal tissues.

Leading Sites of New Cancer Cases and Deaths – 2005 Estimates*

Estimated New Cases*: Male	Estimated New Cases*: Female	Estimated Deaths: Male	Estimated Deaths: Female
Prostate 232,090 (33%)	Breast 211,240 (32%)	Lung and bronchus 90,490 (31%)	Lung and bronchus 73,020 (27%)
Lung and bronchus 93,010 (13%)	Lung and bronchus 79,560 (12%)	Prostate 30,350 (10%)	Breast 40,410 (15%)
Colon and rectum 71,820 (10%)	Colon and rectum 73,470 (11%)	Colon and rectum 28,540 (10%)	Colon and rectum 27,750 (10%)
Urinary bladder 47,010 (7%)	Uterine corpus 40,880 (6%)	Pancreas 15,820 (5%)	Ovary 16,210 (6%)
Melanoma of the skin 33,580 (5%)	Non-Hodgkin lymphoma 27,320 (4%)	Leukemia 12,540 (4%)	Pancreas 15,980 (6%)
Non-Hodgkin lymphoma 29,070 (4%)	Melanoma of the skin 26,000 (4%)	Esophagus 10,530 (4%)	Leukemia 10,030 (4%)
Kidney and renal pelvis 22,490 (3%)	Ovary 22,220 (3%)	Liver and intrahepatic bile duct 10,330 (3%)	Non-Hodgkin lymphoma 9,050 (3%)
Leukemia 19,640 (3%)	Thyroid 19,190 (3%)	Non-Hodgkin lymphoma 10,150 (3%)	Uterine corpus 7,310 (3%)
Oral cavity and pharynx 19,100 (3%)	Urinary bladder 16,200 (2%)	Urinary bladder 8,970 (3%)	Multiple myeloma 5,640 (2%)
Pancreas 16,100 (2%)	Pancreas 16,080 (2%)	Kidney and renal pelvis 8,020 (3%)	Brain and other nervous system 5,480 (2%)
All sites 710,040 (100%)	All sites 662,870 (100%)	All sites 295,280 (100%)	All sites 275,000 (100%)

*Excludes basal and squamous cell skin cancers and in situ carcinoma except bladder.
Note: Percentages may not total 100% due to rounding.

Figure 27-7 ■ Cancer incidence and death by site and gender. (Courtesy American Cancer Society, Atlanta, GA.)

TABLE 27-7 Grading of Malignant Tumors

Grade	Cellular Characteristics
G_x	Grade cannot be determined.
G_1	Tumor cells are well differentiated and closely resemble the normal cells from which they arose. This grade is considered a low grade of malignant change. These tumors are malignant but are relatively slow growing.
G_2	Tumor cells are moderately differentiated; they still retain some of the characteristics of normal cells but also have more malignant characteristics than do G_1 tumor cells.
G_3	Tumor cells are poorly differentiated, but the tissue of origin can usually be established. The cells have few normal cell characteristics.
G_4	Tumor cells are poorly differentiated and retain no normal cell characteristics. Determination of the tissue of origin is difficult and perhaps impossible.

TABLE 27-8 Staging of Cancer—TNM Classification

	Primary Tumor (T)
T_x	Primary tumor cannot be assessed
T_0	No evidence of primary tumor
T_{is}	Carcinoma in situ
T_1, T_2, T_3, T_4	Increasing size and/or local extent of the primary tumor
	Regional Lymph Nodes (N)
N_x	Regional lymph nodes cannot be assessed
N_0	No regional lymph node metastasis
N_1, N_2, N_3	Increasing involvement of regional lymph nodes
	Distant Metastasis (M)
M_x	Presence of distant metastasis cannot be assessed
M_0	No distant metastasis
M_1	Distant metastasis

Modified from American Joint Committee on Cancer. (1988). In O.H. Beahrs, et al. (Eds.). *Manual for staging of cancer* (3rd ed., p. 7). Philadelphia: J. B. Lippincott.

Grading the cells is one of the first steps in confirming cancer. Grading is a means of evaluating the client with cancer for prognosis and appropriate therapy. It also allows health care professionals to evaluate the results of management and compare local, regional, national, and international statistics.

PLOIDY

Cancer cells can be described by chromosome number and appearance, or **ploidy.** Normal human cells have 46 chromosomes (23 pairs), the normal diploid number. When malignant transformation occurs, changes in the genes and chromosomes also occur. Some cancer cells gain or lose whole chromosomes and may have structural abnormalities of the remaining chromosomes. When a cancer cell has more or less than 23 pairs, it is said to be **aneuploid.** The degree of aneuploidy usually increases with the degree of malignancy.

STAGING

Staging determines the exact location of the cancer and its degree of metastasis at diagnosis. Staging is important because, for most cancers, the smaller the cancer is at diagnosis and the less it has spread, the greater the chances are that treatment will result in a cure. Cancer stage also influences selection of therapy. Staging is done in three ways:

1. *Clinical staging.* This staging assesses the client's clinical manifestations and evaluates clinical signs for tumor size and possible spread. Clinical tests are used, and cancer cells may be obtained for biopsy, but clinical staging does not include major surgery.
2. *Surgical staging.* This staging assesses the tumor size, number, sites, and spread by inspection at surgery.
3. *Pathologic staging.* This staging is the most definitive type. The tumor size, number, sites, and spread are determined by pathologic examination of tissues obtained at surgery.

Specific staging systems include Dukes' staging of colon and rectal cancer and Clark's levels method of staging skin cancer. The American Joint Committee on Cancer developed the **TNM (tumor, node, metastasis)** system to describe the anatomic extent of cancers. The stages guide treatment and are useful for prognosis and comparison of treatment results. The TNM staging systems have specific prognostic value for each solid tumor type. Table 27-8 shows a basic TNM staging system. TNM staging is not useful for leukemia or lymphomas. Staging for these cancers is discussed in Chapter 43.

Tumor growth is discussed in terms of **doubling time** (the amount of time it takes for a tumor to double in size) and **mitotic index** (the percentage of actively dividing cells within a tumor). The smallest detectable tumor is about 1 cm in diameter and contains 1 billion cells. To reach this size, a must undergo at least 30 doublings. A tumor with a mitotic index of less than 10% is a slow-growing tumor; a tumor with an index of 85% is fast growing. Tumors have a wide range of growth rates. Fast-growing tumors, such as lymphomas, may double in 4 weeks; an adenocarcinoma of the lung may double in 21 to 40 weeks.

Cancer Etiology and Genetic Risk

Carcinogenesis takes years and depends on several tumor and client factors. Three interacting factors influence cancer development: exposure to carcinogens, genetic predisposition, and immune function. These factors account for variation in cancer development from one person to another, even when each person is exposed to the same hazards.

ONCOGENE ACTIVATION

Regardless of specific cause, the mechanism of carcinogenesis appears to be the same: the activation of proto-oncogenes into oncogenes. These proto-oncogenes were the genes that directed early embryonic development. At about 8 days after conception, these genes should be controlled forever. They are turned off, controlled, or suppressed by "suppressor genes." Suppressor genes can act directly at the DNA level, preventing the proto-oncogene from being overexpressed. Another way that suppressor genes work is by preventing cells from dividing, or maintaining control over the cell cycle.

When a normal cell is exposed to any carcinogen (initiator), the normal cell's DNA can be damaged or mutated.

TABLE 27-9 Example Malignancies Associated with Altered Oncogene Activity

Oncogene	Malignancies
ABL1	Chronic myelogenous leukemia, other leukemias
BRAF	Gastric
CCND1	Breast
ERBB-1	Glioblastomas, squamous cell carcinoma
ERBB-2 (HER-2/neu)	Breast, salivary gland, ovarian carcinomas
FES	Acute promyelocytic leukemia, lung, bladder
HRAS	Breast, melanoma, lung, kidney, bladder, colon
JUN	Lung
Ki-RAS	Colorectal
MYC	Burkitt's lymphoma, T-cell and B-cell neoplasms, breast, gastric, lung
MYCL	Lung
MYCN	Small cell lung cancer
NRAS	Ovarian, thyroid, melanoma, leukemia
PRAD-1	Breast, squamous cell cancers
RET	Thyroid, multiple endocrine neoplasias
TRK	Colorectal, thyroid

The mutations damage suppressor genes, preventing them from controlling the expression of proto-oncogenes. As a result, the proto-oncogenes are turned on or overexpressed. When proto-oncogenes are turned on, they are then called **oncogenes** and can cause the cell to change from normal cells to cancer cells. When oncogenes are overexpressed in a cell, excessive amounts of cyclins are produced and upset the balance between cell growth enhancement and cell growth limitation. The effect of these excessive cyclins is greater than the effect of the suppressor gene products, thus allowing uncontrolled cell division.

About 70 different proto-oncogenes that can be activated into oncogenes have been identified. *These oncogenes are not abnormal genes but are part of every cell's normal makeup and were important in early development.* Oncogenes become a problem only if they are activated after development is complete, as a result of exposure to carcinogenic agents or events. Activation of some specific oncogenes causes specific cancers. Table 27-9 lists known oncogenes and the cancers they cause. External and personal factors are associated with oncogene activation.

EXTERNAL FACTORS CAUSING CANCER

Between 78% and 80% of cancer in North America may be the result of environmental, or external, factors (American Cancer Society, 2005). Environmental carcinogens are chemical, physical, or viral agents that cause cancer. Table 27-4 lists known environmental causes of human cancer.

Chemical Carcinogenesis

Many chemicals, drugs, and other products used in everyday life are known to be carcinogenic, and hundreds more are suspected of being carcinogenic.

TABLE 27-10 Malignancies Associated with Tobacco Use

- Lung
- Pharyngeal
- Esophagus
- Cervical
- Bladder
- Stomach
- Oral cavity
- Laryngeal
- Pancreatic
- Kidney
- Liver
- Myeloid leukemia

Data from American Cancer Society. (2005). *Cancer facts and figures—2005.* Report No. 00-300M-No. 5008.05. Atlanta: Author.

Some chemicals are complete carcinogens that can both initiate and promote cancer. Others are pure initiating agents, or incomplete carcinogens. Still others are only promoting agents. Some substances, such as tobacco and alcohol, appear to be only mildly carcinogenic; it takes long-term exposure to large amounts of these substances before a cancer develops. However, these two substances can act as co-carcinogens; when taken together, they enhance each other's carcinogenic activity.

Cells are not susceptible to chemical carcinogenesis to the same degree. Normal cells that have the ability to divide are at greater risk for cancer development than are normal cells that are not capable of cell division. For example, cancers commonly arise in bone marrow, skin, lining of the gastrointestinal tract, ductal cells of the breast, and lining of the lungs. All of these cells normally undergo cell division. Cancers of nerve tissue, cardiac muscle, and skeletal muscle are rare. These cells do not normally undergo cell division.

About 30% of cancers diagnosed in North America are related to tobacco use (American Cancer Society, 2005). Tobacco is the single most important source of preventable carcinogenesis. It contains many different carcinogens and co-carcinogens. Tobacco use both initiates and promotes cancer. The risk for cancer development from tobacco use depends on a person's immune function, amount of tobacco exposure, type of tobacco exposure, and tobacco tar content.

Tissues with the greatest risk for tobacco-induced cancer are those that have direct contact with tobacco or tobacco smoke. Cigarette smoking and tobacco use also promote the development of other cancers. Table 27-10 lists the specific cancers that appear to be associated with tobacco use.

Physical Carcinogenesis

Physical agents or events cause cancer by the same mechanism as for chemical carcinogens (i.e., DNA damage). Two physical agents that cause cancer are radiation and chronic irritation.

RADIATION

Even small doses of radiation affect cells. Some effects are temporary and can be repaired. Other effects cannot be repaired and either may be lethal to the damaged cell or induce cancer in the damaged cell. The two types of radiation that cause cancer are ionizing and ultraviolet (UV). Some ionizing radiation is found naturally in such elements as radon, uranium, and radium. Most rocks and soil contain various amounts of uranium and radium. Other sources of ionizing radiation include x-rays for diagnosis and treatment of disease, as well as cosmic radiation. UV radiation is a type of solar radiation, coming from the sun. Other sources of UV radiation include tanning beds and germicidal lights.

UV rays do not penetrate deeply and the most common cancer type caused by UV exposure is skin cancer.

Both ionizing and UV radiation mutate genes. Although radiation exposure induces cancers more often among cells that can divide, it can cause cancer among nondividing cells as well.

CHRONIC IRRITATION

Chronic irritation and tissue trauma are suspected to cause cancer. The incidence of skin cancer is higher in people with burn scars or other types of severe skin injury. Chronically irritated tissues undergo frequent cell division and thus are at an increased risk for spontaneous DNA mutation.

Viral Carcinogenesis

Few viruses have been proven to be carcinogenic to humans, although more are suspected to play major roles in cancer development. When viruses infect body cells, they break the DNA chain and insert their own genetic material into the human DNA chain. Breaking the DNA, along with viral gene insertion, mutates the normal cell's DNA and can either activate an oncogene or damage suppressor genes. Viruses that cause cancer are **oncoviruses.** Table 27-11 lists cancers of known viral origin.

Dietary Factors Related to Cancer Development

Cancer development may be related to many dietary practices. However, the relationship of diet to cancer is poorly understood. Because dietary factors are rarely independent of other possible carcinogenic agents, evidence of dietary contributions to cancer development is clouded. Suspected dietary factors include low fiber intake, high intake of red meat, and high animal fat intake. Preservatives, contaminants, preparation methods, and additives (dyes, flavorings, and sweeteners) may have cancer-promoting effects. Chart 27-1 lists foods that have carcinogenic potential.

PERSONAL FACTORS AND CANCER DEVELOPMENT

Personal factors, including immune function, age, and genetic risk, also affect whether a person is likely to develop cancer.

TABLE 27-11 Malignancies Associated with a Known Viral Origin

Virus	Malignancies
Epstein-Barr virus	Burkitt's lymphoma, B-cell lymphoma, nasopharyngeal carcinoma
Hepatitis B virus	Primary liver carcinoma
Human papillomavirus	Cervical carcinoma, vulvar carcinoma, and other anogenital carcinomas
Human lymphotrophic virus type I	Adult T-cell leukemia
Human lymphotrophic virus type II	Hairy cell leukemia

Data from Cooper, G. (1995). *Oncogenes* (2nd ed.). Boston: Jones & Bartlett.

Immune Function

The immune system protects the body from foreign invaders and non-self cells (see Chapter 23). Non-self cells include cells that are no longer normal, such as cancer cells. The part of the immune system that protects against cancer is cell-mediated immunity. Natural killer (NK) and helper T-cells provide immune surveillance.

The role of the immune system in protecting against cancer is supported by cancer incidence in immunosuppressed people. Adults older than 60 years of age have immune systems that function at less than optimal levels, and this group has a higher incidence of cancer compared with that of the general population. Organ transplant recipients taking immunosuppressive drugs to prevent organ rejection also have a higher incidence of cancer. In clients with acquired immunodeficiency syndrome (AIDS), incidence may be as high as 70%.

Age

Advancing age is the single most important risk factor for cancer (American Cancer Society, 2005).

CONSIDERATIONS FOR OLDER ADULTS

Seventy-seven percent of cancer occurs in people older than 55 years of age (American Cancer Society, 2005). This higher incidence reflects lifelong accumulation of DNA mutations that result in cell changes and cancer. Older adults may not be able to repair these mutations as they once did. Immune function, especially cell-mediated immunity, is also reduced in the older adult. Cancer assessment considerations for the older adult are listed in Chart 27-2.

Manifestations of cancer in older clients may be overlooked as changes of normal aging. Older adults must be aware of and report symptoms such as the seven warning signs of cancer (Table 27-12) to health care providers. Health care providers need to investigate all manifestations suggestive of disease.

Genetic Risk

As previously discussed, oncogenes are risk factors related to carcinogenesis. Proto-oncogenes, precursors of oncogenes, are passed on from generation to generation. The development of cancer, however, depends on more than these genes. The proto-oncogene must be overexpressed to an oncogene

CHART 27-1

CLIENT EDUCATION GUIDE
Dietary Habits to Reduce Cancer Risk

- Avoid excessive intake of animal fat.
- Avoid nitrites (prepared lunch meats, sausage, bacon).
- Minimize your intake of red meat.
- Keep your alcohol consumption to no more than one or two drinks per day.
- Eat more bran.
- Eat more cruciferous vegetables, such as broccoli, cauliflower, Brussels sprouts, and cabbage.
- Eat foods high in vitamin A (such as apricots, carrots, and leafy green and yellow vegetables) and vitamin C (such as fresh fruits and vegetables, especially citrus fruits).

for cancer to occur. In some people, the sequence of a specific proto-oncogene is different, which may allow it to be activated more easily. In other people, the proto-oncogene is normal, but the gene controlling proto-oncogene activity, the suppressor gene, may be abnormal.

These variations in gene sequence may be small single nucleotide polymorphisms (SNPs), or may be large areas of mutations. Both types of gene problems can be inherited or can occur as a result of exposure to carcinogens. Table 27-9 lists specific cancers associated with altered oncogene activity; Table 27-13 lists specific cancers associated with altered suppressor gene activity.

CHART 27-2

NURSING FOCUS on the OLDER ADULT
Cancer Assessment Considerations

Cancer Type	Assessment Consideration
Colorectal cancer	Ask the client whether bowel habits have changed over the past year (e.g., in consistency, frequency, or color). Is there any obvious blood in the stool? Test at least one stool specimen for occult blood during the client's hospitalization. Encourage the client to have a baseline colonoscopy. Encourage the client to reduce dietary intake of animal fats, red meat, and smoked meats. Encourage the client to increase dietary intake of bran, vegetables, and fruit.
Bladder cancer	Ask the client about the presence of: Pain on urination Blood in the urine Cloudy urine Increased frequency or urgency
Prostate cancer	Ask the client about: Hesitancy Change in the size of the urine stream Pain in the back or legs History of urinary tract infections
Skin cancer	Examine skin areas for moles or warts. Ask the client about changes in moles (e.g., color, edges, or sensation).
Leukemia	Observe the skin for color, petechiae, or ecchymosis. Ask the client about: Fatigue Bruising Bleeding tendency History of infections and illnesses Night sweats Unexplained fevers
Lung cancer	Observe the skin and mucous membranes for color. How many words can the client say between breaths? Ask the client about: Cough Hoarseness Smoking history Exposure to inhalation irritants Shortness of breath Activity tolerance Frothy or bloody sputum Pain in the arms or chest Difficulty swallowing

Patterns of genetic risk for cancer have also been identified, including the following:

- Inherited predisposition for specific cancers
- Inherited conditions associated with cancer
- Familial clustering
- Chromosomal aberrations

Table 27-14 lists conditions associated with an increased genetic risk for cancer development.

Genetic Testing for Cancer Predisposition

Genetic testing is available to confirm or rule out a person's genetic risk for a few specific cancers. Most tests are performed on peripheral blood. These tests are expensive and often not covered by insurance. Genetic testing should not

TABLE 27-12 The Seven Warning Signs of Cancer

C	Changes in bowel or bladder habits
A	A sore that does not heal
U	Unusual bleeding or discharge
T	Thickening or lump in the breast or elsewhere
I	Indigestion or difficulty swallowing
O	Obvious change in a wart or mole
N	Nagging cough or hoarseness

TABLE 27-13 Malignancies Associated with Altered Suppressor Gene Activity (Selected)

Suppressor Gene	Malignancies
APC	Colorectal, stomach, pancreatic
ATM	Leukemia, lymphoma, breast, ovarian
BRCA1	Breast, ovarian
BRCA2	Breast, ovarian
CDK4	Melanoma
CDKN2A	Mesothelioma, melanoma
DCC	Colorectal
DPC4	Pancreatic, colon
FUS1	Lung
Ink4a	Melanoma
MEN1	Parathyroid, pituitary, adrenal, carcinoid, pancreatic islet cell
MLH1	Colorectal
MSH2	Colorectal
MTS1	Melanoma, brain tumors, leukemia, sarcomas, breast, bladder, ovarian, lung, kidney
NF1	Neurofibroma, colon, astrocytoma
NF2	Neurofibroma, meningioma, schwannoma
NKX3.1	Prostate
PTEN	Breast, prostate, endometrial
RB1	Retinoblastoma, sarcomas, breast, bladder, esophageal, small cell lung
SMAD3	Prostate
Tp53	Breast, bladder, colorectal, esophageal, liver, lung, ovarian, brain tumors, sarcomas, leukemia, lymphoma
VHL	Renal cell carcinoma, pheochromocytoma, hemangioblastoma

TABLE 27-14 Conditions Associated with a Genetic Predisposition for Cancer

Condition	Specific Cancer Type
Inherited cancers*	Breast cancer Prostate cancer Ovarian cancer
Familial clustering	Breast cancer Melanoma
Bloom syndrome	Leukemia
Familial polyposis	Colorectal cancer
Chromosomal aberrations	
Down syndrome (47 chromosomes)	Leukemia
Klinefelter syndrome (47, XXY)	Breast cancer
Turner's syndrome (45, XO)	Leukemia Gonadal carcinoma Meningioma Colorectal cancer

*Not all breast, prostate, or ovarian cancers are inherited.

be performed unless a family history clearly indicates the possibility of increased genetic risk. *These tests do not diagnose the presence of cancer.*

A variety of issues and potential problems exist with genetic testing for cancer risk. Correct interpretation of the results is critical. Ideally, a genetic counselor is involved in giving the client information before, as well as after, testing is performed. *When a client tests positive for a cancer-causing gene mutation, his or her risk for cancer development is greatly increased, but the cancer may never develop.*

Other issues regarding genetic testing include who will have access to the information and whether or not to share the test results with family members. Many clients fear that if they test positive for a cancer-causing gene, they may face discrimination for insurance coverage or in the workplace. Some states have confidentiality safeguards and others do not. Genetic testing has implications for the entire family, not just the client being tested. For more information on genetic testing, see Chapter 11.

CULTURAL CONSIDERATIONS

The incidence of cancer varies among races. American Cancer Society data (2003a) show that African Americans have a higher incidence of cancer than white individuals do, and the death rate is higher for African Americans. Since 1960 the overall incidence among African Americans has increased 27%, whereas for white individuals it has increased 12%. Cancer sites and cancer-related mortality vary along racial lines as well. Table 27-15 shows common cancers among white, African American, Asian, and Hispanic populations. Understanding these variations can help in planning prevention and early detection strategies that are ethnically specific.

When risks for cancer development are assessed, however, ethnicity and genetic predisposition cannot be considered alone. Behavior and socioeconomic factors must also be assessed. The American Cancer Society (2005) reports that cancer incidence and survival are often related to socioeconomic factors. These factors include the availability of health

TABLE 27-15 Racial Differences in Cancer Development

White *Common Cancer Types*	Asian *Common Cancer Types*
1. Lung 2. Breast 3. Colorectal 4. Prostate	1. Breast 2. Colorectal 3. Prostate 4. Lung 5. Stomach
African American *Common Cancer Types*	**Hispanic** *Common Cancer Types*
1. Lung 2. Prostate 3. Breast 4. Colorectal 5. Uterine	1. Prostate 2. Breast 3. Colorectal 4. Lung

Data from American Cancer Society. (2005). *Cancer facts and figures—2005.* Report No. 00-300M-No. 5008.05. Atlanta: Author.

care services or the belief that seeking early health care has a positive effect on the outcome of cancer diagnosis. (See the Evidence-Based Practice for Nursing box on p. 481.)

CANCER PREVENTION

Cancer prevention activities can focus on primary prevention or secondary prevention. **Primary prevention** is the use of strategies to prevent the actual occurrence of cancer. This method of cancer prevention is most effective when there is a known cause for a cancer type. **Secondary prevention** is the use of screening strategies to detect cancer early, at a time when cure or control is more likely.

Primary Prevention

AVOIDANCE OF KNOWN OR POTENTIAL CARCINOGENS

An effective primary prevention strategy is to avoid known or potential carcinogens. This method is effective when a cause of cancer is known and avoidance is easily accomplished. Examples are using skin protection during sun exposure, avoiding tobacco, and eliminating environmental asbestos. As more cancer causes are identified, avoidance may become even more effective.

MODIFICATION OF ASSOCIATED FACTORS

Absolute causes are not known for many cancers, but some conditions appear to increase risk. Example are the increased incidence of cancer among people who consume alcohol; the association of a diet high in fat and low in fiber with colon cancer, breast cancer, and ovarian cancer; and a greater incidence of cervical cancer among women with many sexual partners. Modifying behavior to reduce the associated factor may decrease the risk for cancer development.

REMOVAL OF "AT RISK" TISSUES

When a person has a known high risk for developing a specific type of cancer, removal of the tissue reduces the risk. Examples include removing moles to prevent conversion to skin cancer,

EVIDENCE-BASED PRACTICE for Nursing

Limited access to health care is not the only factor in ethnicity-based differences in breast cancer outcomes

Bibb, S. (2001). The relationship between access and stage at diagnosis of breast cancer in African American and Caucasian women. *Oncology Nursing Forum, 28*(4), 711-719.

The purpose of this secondary analysis was to examine the influence of various factors on screening and early detection practices for breast cancer between African-American and Caucasian women using a Department of Defense military health system for primary care. The use of this health care system eliminated the bias of differences in consumer costs for preventive care.

The study examined the tumor registry records of 635 clients (62 African-American women and 573 Caucasian women) in whom breast cancer was diagnosed over a 10-year period at a specific military health system. Data were collected regarding stage at diagnosis, use of breast cancer screening techniques, age at diagnosis, means of discovery, and socioeconomic status.

Overall, diagnosis was made at later stages of the disease in African-American women than in Caucasian women. The age at diagnosis was younger among the African-American women and fewer tumors were discovered by mammography than for Caucasian women. Although socioeconomic status was different for the two groups, the health care consumer costs and access were not different. No significant difference between the time of disease diagnosis and the initiation of treatment was noted for the two groups.

The findings of an earlier age of disease onset and a higher stage of disease at diagnosis for African-American women are consistent with the findings from studies not confined to a military health system. The authors speculate that barriers to earlier diagnosis are personal rather than related to economic access to appropriate services. The investigators suggest that breast health care interventions for African-American women need to focus at least as much on increasing awareness of the need for adhering to recommended screening guidelines as it does on reducing economic access barriers.

Level of Evidence: 3—Well-designed trial without randomization (large cohort study).

Critique. The study examined differences in breast cancer diagnosis between African-American women and Caucasian women when equal economic access to health care was available. The study has some limitations based on the retrospective nature of a secondary analysis. Socioeconomic status was not directly measured in the initial data; instead, the surrogate of military rank was used as the economic indicator. The level of education for the individual women also was not collected. While the percentage of study participants who were African American (≈10%) reflects the national distribution, the small number (62) limits the generalizability of the study results.

Implications for Nursing. African-American women may have an average age of onset for breast cancer at an age younger than when annual mammography screenings are recommended. Therefore the importance of monthly breast self-examination (BSE) and yearly clinical breast examinations (CBE) must be stressed. The development and testing of culturally appropriate teaching tools for BSE are needed.

removing colon polyps to prevent colon cancer, and removing breasts to prevent breast cancer. Not all "at risk" tissues can be removed (e.g., those that are part of essential organs).

CHEMOPREVENTION

A newer form of cancer prevention, **chemoprevention,** is being tried. This strategy uses drugs, chemicals, natural nutrients, or other substances to disrupt one or more steps important to cancer development. These agents may be able to reverse existing gene damage or halt the progression of the transformation process. Chemopreventive agents work in one of the following ways to disrupt at least one step in the process of cancer:

- Blocking an inactive compound from becoming an active carcinogen
- Blocking the direct action of a carcinogen on DNA
- Enhancing the rate of elimination of a carcinogen from the body
- Suppressing the activity of a carcinogen
- Suppressing the promoting activity of a carcinogen
- Suppressing the progression of a premalignant or early-stage malignancy into a more malignant state

Table 27-16 lists agents under investigation for chemoprevention. At this time, only a few agents have been found effective and are commonly prescribed.

TABLE 27-16 Agents Under Investigation for Chemoprevention of Cancer

Category of Prevention	Specific Agents
Prevention of carcinogen formation	Ascorbic acid (vitamin C) Tocopherol (type of vitamin E) Selenium Caffeic acid
Blocking the action of a carcinogen on DNA ("antimutagens")	Carotenoids (vitamin A derivative) Retinoids (vitamin A derivative) Ellagic acid Flavones Oltipraz Butylated hydroxyanisole
Enhancing the elimination of a carcinogen	Isothiocyanate Indole-3-carbinol
Suppression of carcinogenic action	Aspirin Retinoids Indomethacin Selenium Steroidal anti-inflammatory agents Protease inhibitors
Antipromotion activity	Carotenoids Retinoids Selenium Coumarin Piroxicam Indomethacin Calciferol (vitamin D) Hormone antagonists Tamoxifen Finasteride Evista
Suppression of progression	Danazol Interferon Cysteamine Vorozole

The goal of chemopreventive strategies is prevention of cancer development. Target populations for whom chemoprevention might be effective include the following:

- Healthy people with no known specific cancer risk
- People at greater than normal risk because of increased environmental exposure or decreased immune function
- People with precancerous lesions
- People with a history of cancer

Secondary Prevention

SCREENING PROGRAMS

Regular screening for cancer does not reduce cancer incidence but can greatly reduce some types of cancer deaths. For most adults, specific routine screening techniques are encouraged annually as part of health maintenance. General screening recommendations are listed in chapters discussing cancers by organ system. The age and type of participation in specific screening tests are different for people who have an identified increased risk for a specific cancer type. Examples of recommended screenings include the following (American Cancer Society, 2003b):

- Yearly mammography for women older than age 40 years
- Yearly clinical breast examination for women older than age 40 years
- Colonoscopy at age 50 years and then every 10 years
- Yearly fecal occult blood in adults of all ages
- Yearly prostate specific antigen (PSA) test and digital rectal examination (DRE) for men over age 50 years

GENE THERAPY FOR CANCER PREVENTION

Because cancer development clearly involves gene changes (either inherited gene mutations or acquired gene damage), researchers have suggested that altering damaged genes could prevent cancer development. Currently, people can be screened for some gene mutations that increase the risk for cancer. Examples of these gene mutations include the BRCA-1 gene, which increases the risk for both breast and ovarian cancer; the BRCA-2 gene, which increases the risk for breast cancer; and the APC gene, which increases the risk for colon cancer. Screening can help a person at increased genetic risk for cancer to alter lifestyle factors, participate in early detection methods, or even have at-risk tissue removed. Although it is not yet possible to "fix" or remove an abnormal gene in humans, gene therapy in the future is not out of the realm of possibility.

GET READY for the NCLEX Examination!

KEY POINTS

Safe Effective Care Environment

- Ensure that clients in hospitals and other inpatient settings are not exposed to environmental chemicals.
- Position shields properly when clients in inpatient settings are having x-ray examinations taken at the bedside.

Health Promotion and Maintenance

- Teach clients to use sunscreen and to wear protective clothing during sun exposure.
- Encourage clients to participate in the recommended cancer screening activities for their age group and cancer risk category.
- Inform all clients who smoke that smoking increases the risk for development of many cancer types.
- Assist clients interested in smoking cessation to find an appropriate smoking cessation program.

Psychosocial Integrity

- Assess the client's knowledge about causes of cancer and his or her screening/prevention practices.
- Assist clients who fear a cancer diagnosis to understand that finding cancer at an early stage increases the chances for cure.
- Educate clients who undergo genetic testing for cancer predisposition about the risks to confidentiality of the test results.

Physiological Integrity

- Ask all clients about their exposures to environmental agents that are known or suspected to increase the risk for cancer.
- Obtain a detailed family history (at least three generations) to assess the client's risk for familial or inherited cancer.
- Teach clients the "seven warning signs of cancer" (see Table 27-12).

ADDITIONAL STUDY RESOURCES

Go to your Student CD-ROM for Review Questions for the NCLEX Examination.

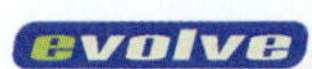

Go to http://evolve.elsevier.com/Iggy/ for Integrated Management of Care Questions for the NCLEX Examination.

SELECTED BIBLIOGRAPHY

Asterisk indicates a classic or definitive work on this subject.

American Cancer Society. (2003a). *Cancer facts and figures for African Americans-2003.* Report No. 8614.03. Atlanta: Author.

American Cancer Society. (2003b). *Cancer prevention and early detection. Facts & Figures-2003.* Report No. 8600.03. Atlanta: Author.

American Cancer Society. (2005). *Cancer facts and figures–2005.* Report No. 00-300M-No. 5008.05. Atlanta: Author.

Bargonetti, J., & Manfredi, J. (2002). Multiple roles of the tumor suppressor *p*53. *Current Opinion in Oncology, 14*(1), 86-91.

Bibb, S. (2001). The relationship between access and stage at diagnosis of breast cancer in African American and Caucasian women. *Oncology Nursing Forum, 28*(4), 711-719.

Calzone, K., & Biersecker, B. (2002). Genetic testing for cancer predisposition. *Cancer Nursing, 25*(1), 15-25.

Clark, P., & Gomez, E. (2001). Details on demand: Consumers, cancer information, and the internet. *Clinical Journal of Oncology Nursing, 5*(1), 19-24.

Frank-Stromborg, M., & Olsen, S. (2001). *Cancer prevention in diverse populations: Cultural implications for health care professionals.* Pittsburgh: Oncology Nursing Society.

Hanahan, D., & Weinberg, R. (2000). The hallmarks of cancer. *Cell, 100*(1), 57-70.

Hawkins, R. (2001). Mastering the intricate maze of metastasis. *Oncology Nursing Forum, 28*(6), 959-965.

Houftek, J., & Atwood, J. (2003). Genetic susceptibility to lung cancer: Implications for smoking cessation. *MEDSURG Nursing, 12*(1), 45-49.

Jegathesean, J. et al. (2005). Apoptosis: Understanding the new molecular pathway. *MEDSURG Nursing, 13*(6), 371-376.

Jennings-Dozier, K., & Lawrence, D. (2000). Sociodemographic predictors of adherence to annual cervical cancer screening in minority women. *Cancer Nursing, 23*(5), 350-356.

Lessick, M., et al. (2001). Advances in genetic testing for cancer risk. *MEDSURG Nursing, 10*(3), 123-127.

Likes, W., & Itano, J. (2003). Human papillomavirus and cervical cancer: Not just a sexually transmitted disease. *Clinical Journal of Oncology Nursing, 7*(3), 271-275.

Loescher, L. (2003). The biology of cancer. In A. Tranin, A. Masny, & J. Jenkins (Eds.). *Genetics in oncology practice: Cancer risk assessment.* Pittsburgh: Oncology Nursing Society.

Loud, J., et al. (2002). Applications of advances in molecular biology and genomics to clinical cancer care. *Cancer Nursing, 25*(2), 110-122.

Machia, J. (2001). Breast cancer: Risk, prevention, and tamoxifen. *American Journal of Nursing, 101*(4), 26-35.

Macleod, K. (2000). Tumor suppressor genes. *Current Opinion in Genetics and Development, 10*(1), 81-93.

Maes, S. (2004). Geriatric oncology comes of age. *ONS News, 19*(2), 1, 4-5, 7.

O'Rourke, J., & Mahon, S. (2003). A comprehensive look at the early detection of ovarian cancer. *Clinical Journal of Oncology Nursing, 7*(1), 41-47.

Peltomaki, P. (2003). Role of DNA mismatch repair defects in the pathogenesis of human cancer. *Journal of Clinical Oncology, 21*(6), 1174-1179.

Peters, J., et al. (2001). Cancer genetics fundamentals. *Cancer Nursing, 24*(6), 446-461.

*Singh, D., & Lippman, S. (1998). Cancer chemoprevention: Part 1. Retinoids, carotenoids and other classic antioxidants. *Oncology, 12*(11), 1643-1658.

Tranin, A., Masny, A., & Jenkins, J. *Genetics in oncology practice: Cancer risk assessment.* Pittsburgh: Oncology Nursing Society.

United States Preventive Services Task Force. (2003). Chemoprevention of breast cancer: Recommendations and rationale. *American Journal of Nursing, 103*(5), 107-113.

U.S. Department of Health and Human Services, Public Health Service, National Toxicology Program. (December 2002). *Report on Carcinogens* (10th ed.). Author.

Volker, D. (2001). Carcinogenesis: Application to clinical practice. *Clinical Journal of Oncology Nursing, 5*(5), 225-226, 229.

Workman, M.L. (2004). The biology of cancer. In C. Varrichio (Ed.). *A cancer source book for nurses* (8th ed., pp. 13-28). Boston: Jones & Bartlett.

Zimmerman, V. (2002). Gene mutations and cancer. *American Journal of Nursing, 1028*), 28-37.

CHAPTER

28 General Interventions for Clients with Cancer

M. LINDA WORKMAN

LEARNING OUTCOMES

After studying this chapter, you should be able to:

1. Identify the goals of cancer therapy.
2. Distinguish between cancer surgery for cure and cancer surgery for palliation.
3. Discuss how the nursing care needs for the client undergoing cancer surgery compare to those for the client undergoing any other type of surgery.
4. Compare the purposes and side effects of radiation therapy and chemotherapy for cancer.
5. Prioritize nursing care for the client with radiation-induced skin problems.
6. Develop a community-based teaching plan for the client receiving external beam radiation.
7. Compare the personnel safety issues for working with clients receiving teletherapy radiation versus those receiving brachytherapy radiation.
8. Identify nursing interventions to promote safety for the client experiencing chemotherapy-induced anemia or thrombocytopenia.
9. Develop a community-based teaching plan for the client receiving chemotherapy.
10. Prioritize nursing care for the client with chemotherapy-induced neutropenia.
11. Prioritize nursing care for the client with mucositis.
12. Explain the rationale for hormonal manipulation therapy.
13. Discuss the uses of biological response modifiers as supportive therapy in the treatment of cancer.
14. Explain the basis of targeted therapy for cancer.
15. Identify clients at risk for oncologic emergencies.
16. Prioritize nursing care needs for clients experiencing oncologic emergencies.

Go to your Student CD-ROM for Review Questions for the NCLEX Examination keyed to these Learning Outcomes.

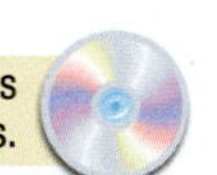

Most people fear cancer and consider a cancer diagnosis to involve suffering and death. In affluent countries, more than 50% of people diagnosed with cancer are cured, and thousands of others live 5 years or longer after the diagnosis (American Cancer Society, 2005). Regardless of treatment type, cancer always affects a person's physical and psychological functioning.

Providing care to clients and families experiencing cancer is complex and challenging. This chapter describes the general interventions for cancer and the problems associated with cancer treatment. For specific treatment regimens and client problems that occur with specific cancer types, consult the chapters in which the cancer is described. Table 28-1 lists common cancer types and the specific locations within this text where the interventions are presented.

GENERAL DISEASE-RELATED CONSEQUENCES OF CANCER

Cancer can develop in any organ or tissue but tends to occur more commonly in some tissues than in others. Cancer destroys normal tissue, decreasing function in that tissue or organ. Even when cancers occur in nonvital tissues or organs, they can cause death by **metastasizing** (spreading) into vital organs and disrupting critical physiologic processes (see Chapter 27). Cancers that are left untreated cause the following:

- Impaired immune and hematopoietic (blood-producing) function
- Altered gastrointestinal (GI) tract structure and function
- Motor and sensory deficits
- Decreased respiratory function

These impairments cause great physical and emotional distress. Without intervention, cancer invasion of normal tissues leads to death.

Impaired Immune and Hematopoietic Function

Impaired immune and hematopoietic function occurs most often in clients with leukemia and lymphoma, but also can occur with any cancer that invades the bone marrow. Tumor cells enter the bone marrow and reduce the production of healthy white blood cells, which are needed for normal immune function (see Chapter 23). Thus clients who have cancer, especially leukemia, are at an increased risk for infection.

When cancer invades the bone marrow, it also decreases the number of red blood cells **(anemia)** and platelets **(thrombocytopenia).** These changes may be caused by the cancer itself, such as in leukemia, or by the cancer treatment. In either case, the client is anemic and is at risk for excessive bleeding.

TABLE 28-1 Text Location of Specific Cancer Content

Cancer Type	Chapter	Patho/ Etiol	Treatment and Nursing Interventions
Bladder	73	1701	1702-1704
Brain	48	1055-1056	1056-1066
Breast	77	1794-1796	1802-1820
Cervical	78	1845-1846	1846-1849
Colorectal	60	1317-1319	1320-1325
Esophageal	58	1274	1276-1280
Head and Neck	32	571-572	573-580
Kidney	74	1722-1723	1723-1724
Leukemia	43	897-898	900-908
Lung	33	613-614	614-625
Lymphoma	43	908-909	909-910
Ovarian	78	1849	1850
Prostate	79	1864-1865	1865-1870
Skin	70	1608	1610
Stomach	59	1306	1308-1310

Altered Gastrointestinal Structure and Function

Cancer can alter gastrointestinal (GI) function and impair nutrition. For example, tumors may obstruct or compress structures anywhere along the GI tract, reducing the client's ability to absorb nutrients and eliminate wastes. Tumors also increase metabolic rate and increase the need for protein, carbohydrates, and fat at a time when the client has less energy for meal preparation or eating.

Many tumors spread to the liver, profoundly damaging this organ. The liver has many important functions in metabolism. Reduced liver function leads to malnutrition and death among clients with cancer.

Many clients with cancer have anorexia that often interferes with their ability to meet energy needs. **Cachexia** (extreme body wasting and malnutrition) develops from an imbalance between food intake and energy use. This problem may occur even when nutritional intake appears adequate. Changes in taste can result from the cancer or the treatment and reduce appetite. Cancer-related causes of malnutrition are listed in Table 28-2.

TABLE 28-2 Causes of Malnutrition in Clients with Cancer

Anorexia

Local causes
- Pelvic or abdominal tumors
- Hepatic metastases
- Intestinal compression or obstruction
- Others

Remote causes
- Food aversions
- Early satiety

Treatment-related causes
- Postsurgical small stomach or stasis
- Drugs, including chemotherapy
- Radiation—local and systemic effects

Systemic illness
- Infection
- Hepatitis or pancreatitis
- Endocrinopathies

Taste disorders
- Drugs (e.g., metronidazole)
- Remote effects of neoplasm and its treatment
- Local disease and its treatment (e.g., stomatitis, nasopharyngeal tumor, radiation, and surgery)
- Nausea and vomiting

Psychogenic causes
- Depression
- Anxiety
- Conditioned aversions

Intolerance of institutional food

Difficulty in Eating

Head and neck tumors and their treatment
Xerostomia
Stomatitis
Loss of teeth and dental problems
Dysphagia and odynophagia

Maldigestion or Malabsorption

Pancreatic insufficiency
Bile salt deficiency
Hypersecretory syndrome
- Zollinger-Ellison syndrome
- Pancreatic cholera
- Bowel infiltration
- Diffuse invasion (e.g., lymphoma)
- Local blockage
- Fistula

Postsurgical causes
- Esophageal surgery (with vagotomy, gastric statis, diarrhea, and steatorrhea)
- Gastrectomy—dumping, achlorhydria, or afferent loop syndrome
- Small intestine resections

Postirradiation causes
- Enteritis (may occur as late sequelae)
- Fistula
- Stenosis
- Obstruction

Protein-Losing Enteropathy Malutilization

Cancer cachexia
Steroids
- Nitrogen wasting
- Hyperglycemia
- Calcium loss

Nutritional support for the client with cancer, especially one undergoing cancer therapy, is complex and controversial. A diet high in protein and carbohydrates is often prescribed to help the client maintain weight and to provide the nutrients for energy and cellular repair. However, some scientists believe that an excessive intake of protein and vitamins increases the nutrition of the cancer cells and contributes to cancer progression. Clients often believe their cancers can be cured more easily if weight is gained or maintained. Currently no one nutritional plan meets the needs of all clients with cancer (Wilson, 2000).

Motor and Sensory Deficits

Motor (movement) and sensory deficits occur when cancers invade bone or the brain, or compress nerves. In clients with bone metastases, the primary cancer started in another organ (e.g., the prostate, breast, or lung). The bone sites most often affected are the vertebrae, ribs, pelvis, and femur. The humerus, scapula, sternum, skull, and clavicle are also common sites of cancer spread. Bone metastases cause fractures, spinal cord compression, and hypercalcemia, each of which reduces mobility.

The client may have sensory changes if the spinal cord is damaged by tumor pressure or if nerves are compressed. Sensory, motor, and cognitive functions are severely impaired when cancer spreads to the brain.

The client with cancer may also have pain. Pain does not always accompany cancer, but it can be a significant problem for clients with terminal cancer. Chapter 7 provides an in-depth discussion of the causes and management of cancer pain.

Decreased Respiratory Function

Cancer can disrupt gas exchange in several ways and often results in death. For example, tumors in the airways cause airway obstruction. If lung tissue is involved, lung capacity is decreased. Tumors can also press on blood and lymph vessels in the chest, blocking blood flow through the chest and lungs and resulting in pulmonary edema and dyspnea. Tumors also can thicken the alveolar membrane and damage pulmonary blood vessels, reducing gas exchange.

TREATMENT-RELATED CONSEQUENCES OF CANCER

The purpose of cancer treatment is to prolong survival time or improve quality of life (see the Meeting Healthy People 2010 Objectives box above). Although a few spontaneous regressions of cancer have been reported, most clients would die within months of diagnosis without cancer therapy. Therapies for cancer include surgery, radiation, chemotherapy, hormonal manipulation, immunotherapy, gene therapy, and targeted therapy. These therapies may be used separately or in combination to kill cancer cells. The type and amount of therapy depends on the specific type of cancer, whether or not the cancer has spread, and the health of the client. One or more regimens (protocols) have been established for most types of cancer. These regimens are based on experiments with cancer cells and animals and on experience with other clients with cancer.

Meeting HEALTHY PEOPLE 2010 Objectives

CANCER

Objective 17.16: Increase the number of cancer survivors who are living 5 years or longer after diagnosis.

- Encourage clients to seek early health care advice whenever one of the seven warning signs of cancer is present.
- Teach clients being treated for cancer the importance of compliance with the scheduled treatment regimen.
- Teach the client to follow up with health care visits after cancer treatment is completed.
- Teach the client with cancer to continue with recommended screening practices.
- Encourage the client who has been treated for cancer to avoid known environmental carcinogens.
- Assist clients who smoke to reduce or quit smoking.
- Teach clients about the importance of limiting dietary fat, smoked meats, and red meats.

Surgery

RATIONALE FOR CANCER TREATMENT

Surgery is the oldest form of cancer treatment and was the first method to cure cancer. Surgery for cancer involves the removal of diseased tissue. If cancer is confined to the removed tissue, surgery alone can result in a "cure" for that cancer. Although many cancers have spread too far at the time of diagnosis for surgery alone to cure, it may still be a useful part of diagnosis, treatment, follow-up, and rehabilitation.

MECHANISM OF ACTION

Cancer surgery may be used for any of the following purposes: prophylaxis, diagnosis, cure, control, palliation, determination of therapy effectiveness, and reconstruction.

PROPHYLAXIS. Prophylactic surgery is performed when a client has either an existing "premalignant" condition or a known family history that strongly predisposes the person to the development of cancer. The "at-risk" tissue or organ is removed to prevent cancer development. An example of prophylactic surgery for a premalignant condition is removing a benign mole from a location where continuous irritation or exposure to sunlight occurs.

DIAGNOSIS (BIOPSY). Diagnostic surgery provides proof of cancer. All or part of a suspected lesion is removed for examination and testing. Specific types of biopsies are listed Table 28-3.

CURE. Surgery alone can result in a cure rate of 27% to 30% when all visible and microscopic tumor is removed or destroyed. Types of curative surgeries are described in Table 28-4.

CONTROL (CYTOREDUCTIVE SURGERY). Cancer control, or cytoreductive surgery, "debulks" by removing part of the tumor and leaving a known amount of gross tumor. This type of surgery alone cannot result in a cure, but decreases the number of cancer cells and increases the chances that other therapies can be successful.

PALLIATION. The goal of palliative surgery is to improve quality of life during the survival time. Tumor tissue

TABLE 28-3 Diagnostic/Biopsy Surgeries for Cancer

Biopsy Type	Description	Problem/Limitations
Needle	Aspirating cells in a fluid or in very soft tissue Boring a "core" of solid tissue by using a long needle or making a punch, scrape, or bite	Sample error—may biopsy only noncancerous cells in a tissue or organ Sample size may not be adequate for accurate testing Procedure may spread cancer by seeding it into surrounding tissues Procedure may damage healthy tissue
Incisional	Removing a wedge of suspected tissue from a larger tissue mass, leaving some tumor cells in the tissue	Sample error Tumor seeding Damage to healthy tissue
Excisional	Completely removing an entire lesion without removing any adjacent normal tissues	Tumor seeding Leaving micrometastasis Damage to healthy tissue
Staging	Performing multiple needle or incisional biopsies in tissues where metastasis is suspected or likely	Tumor seeding Sample error Damage to healthy tissue

TABLE 28-4 Curative Surgeries for Cancer

Surgery Type	Description	Purpose/Use
Local excision	Removal of all identifiable tumor along with a small margin of normal tissues	Small, localized tumors
Wide local excision (radical)	Removal of identifiable tumor plus immediate tissue or adjacent tissue	Small tumors with only local tissue invasion
Wide excision	Removal of tumor, surrounding tissue, adjacent structures, and usual lymph channels draining the area	Small to moderate-size tumors with known local invasion
Extended radical excision	Removal of tumor, lymphatics, adjacent organs, and all tissues in the region	Tumor infiltrate in a wide area but with no known distant metastasis

that is causing pain, obstruction, or difficulty swallowing is removed. The specific procedure used depends on the client's specific problem.

DETERMINATION OF THERAPY EFFECTIVENESS ("SECOND LOOK"). Second-look surgery is a "rediagnosis" after treatment. The purpose is to assess the disease status in clients who have been treated and have no symptoms of remaining tumor. The results of this surgery are used to determine whether a specific therapy should be continued or discontinued.

RECONSTRUCTIVE OR REHABILITATIVE SURGERY. This type of surgery increases function, enhances appearance, or both. Examples include breast reconstruction after mastectomy, replacement of the esophagus after radiation damage, bowel reconstruction, revision of scars, release of contractures, and placement of penile implants.

SIDE EFFECTS OF SURGICAL THERAPY

Unlike surgery performed for many other reasons, cancer surgery involves the loss of a specific body part or its function. Sometimes whole organs are removed, such as the kidney, lung, breast, testes, arm, or tongue. Any organ loss reduces function. The amount of function lost and how much the loss affects clients depends on the location and extent of the surgery. Some cancer surgery results in major scarring or disfigurement. Clients may be anxious about the chances of surviving the cancer and may be grieving about a loss of body image or a change in lifestyle.

NURSING CARE OF CLIENTS UNDERGOING SURGICAL THERAPY

The physical care needs of the client having surgery for cancer are similar to those related to surgery for other reasons (see Chapters 20 to 22). Consider the client's ability (and the ability of family and significant others) to cope with the uncertainty of cancer and its treatment and with the changes in body image and role. For example, surgery involving the genitals, urinary tract, colon, and rectum may permanently damage these organs. Surgical procedures to create a urinary or fecal diversion (e.g., a colostomy) may damage nerves, causing erectile dysfunction in men and painful intercourse in women.

Radiation

RATIONALE FOR CANCER TREATMENT

The purpose of radiation therapy for cancer is to destroy cancer cells with minimal exposure of the normal cells to the damaging actions of radiation. The effects of radiation are seen only in the tissues in the path of the radiation beam. Some effects are apparent within days or weeks, whereas other effects may not be apparent for months to years after radiation therapy is completed.

MECHANISM OF ACTION

Most radiation therapy for cancer is ionizing radiation. When cells are exposed to this type of radiation, atoms within the cell are "kicked out" of orbit, resulting in a tremendous release of intracellular energy. Ionizing radiation is given off naturally by radium and cobalt, and can also be generated by linear accelerators. Naturally occurring radiation is called **gamma radiation;** radiation that is generated by machine is called **roentgen radiation.** Their effect on cells is the same.

Cells damaged by radiation either die outright or become unable to divide. Radiation damage can occur any time a cell is exposed to radiation and is not confined to cells actively dividing. However, cells in the cell cycle have more damage when exposed to radiation than do nondividing cells.

Three different types of energy, or rays, are produced by gamma radiation: gamma, beta, and alpha rays. These rays vary in their ability to penetrate tissues and damage cells. Table 28-5 lists the features of these three types of gamma radiation, and Figure 28-1 shows the penetrating ability of each.

TABLE 28-5 Characteristics of Different Types of Gamma Radiation

Gamma Ray

Gamma rays are very light and have a low energy-transfer potential. They travel at the speed of light, allowing them to be concentrated and penetrate deeply into tissues.

This is the most common type of radiation used for the treatment of cancer.

This type of radiation can also cause serious, irreversible harm to tissues.

Exposure to this type of radiation must be avoided or severely limited.

Beta Ray

Beta rays are heavier and travel at a moderate to high speed. They have a high linear energy-transfer potential and do not penetrate tissues or other substances well.

Some beta rays are used inside the body for specific radiation therapy.

Beta rays are used in some diagnostic tests.

Beta rays pose health hazards to humans exposed to them, but exposure must be considerable for damage to occur.

Alpha Ray

Alpha rays are very heavy and slow. They easily transfer energy to their surroundings and quickly lose their ability to penetrate tissues (0.04 mm into tissue).

Currently, alpha rays are used in laboratory tests rather than as treatment for cancer.

This type of radiation is harmful to humans only if it is ingested chronically.

The amount of radiation delivered to a tissue is called the **exposure;** the amount of radiation absorbed by the recipient tissue is called the **dose.** The dose is always less than the exposure. Three factors determine the absorbed dose: intensity of exposure, duration of exposure, and closeness of the radiation source to the cells.

The intensity of the radiation decreases with the distance from the radiation source (Figure 28-2). This factor is known as the **inverse square law.** For example, the radiation dose received at a distance of 2 feet from the radiation source is only one fourth of the dose received at a distance of 1 foot from the radiation source; the dose of radiation received at 3 feet is only one ninth of the dose received at 1 foot.

KILLING EFFECTS OF RADIATION. If the dose of radiation is high enough, all cells are killed immediately. This does not usually happen because all cells within a tumor absorb the radiation dose slightly differently. Therefore their overall response to the radiation is slightly different. A few cells die immediately, and more die within the next 24 hours as they attempt to divide. Some cells become sterile as a result of this single treatment. Still other cells repair the radiation-induced damage and recover.

Because of the varying responses of all cancer cells within a given tumor, radiation is given as a series of divided doses. Small doses of radiation are given on a daily basis for a set period of time to allow greater destruction of cancer cells while reducing the damage to normal tissues. This dose division is called **fractionation.** Standard radiotherapy is usually fractionated between 180 and 280 rad/day, multiplied by as many days as needed to achieve the total prescribed dose (rad is an acronym meaning "radiation absorbed dose").

The total dose of radiation needed depends on the size and location of the tumor and on the radiation sensitivity of the tumor and surrounding normal tissues. Some normal tissues are more sensitive than others to radiation. For example, healthy breast tissue can tolerate much higher doses of radiation than can the liver. A total dose of 1200 rad might be prescribed for a primary liver tumor, but a total dose of 5000 to 6000 rad might be needed for a breast cancer (delivered over 28 to 30 separate days). A 6000-rad dose delivered to the liver would destroy the liver as well as the tumor.

Two types of radiation delivery are usually used for cancer therapy: teletherapy and brachytherapy. The type used depends on the client's general health and on the site, size, and location of the tumor to be irradiated. The optimum

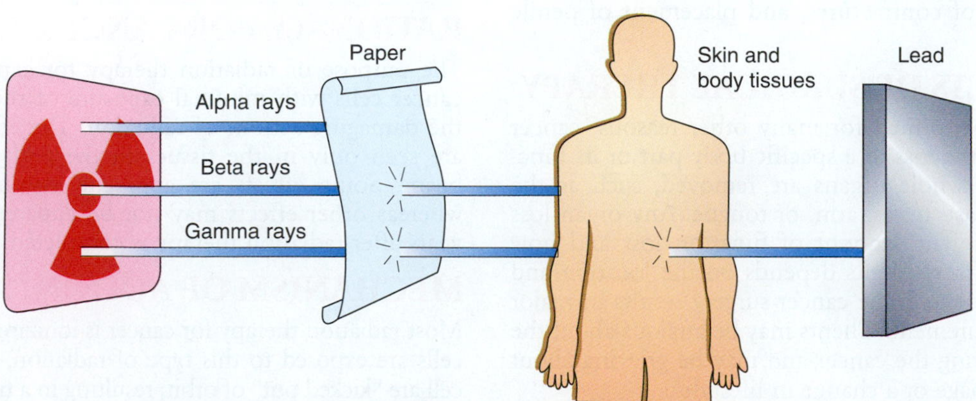

Figure 28-1 ■ Penetrating capacity of different types of radiation.

dose of radiation is one that can kill the cancer cells with an acceptable level of damage to normal tissues (some damage to normal tissues cannot be avoided).

TELETHERAPY. Teletherapy means distant treatment. In teletherapy, the radiation source is external to the client. Because the source is external, the client is not radioactive and poses no hazard to anyone. This type of therapy is also called **beam radiation.**

The exact location of the tumor is determined for greater accuracy of radiation therapy. Once the pattern of radiation delivery is determined, the client must always be in exactly the same position for all treatments. Ensure that the client can get into and maintain this position. Position-fixing devices and markings, either on the client's body or on the devices, ensure the proper position each day of treatment.

BRACHYTHERAPY. Brachytherapy means "short" or "close" therapy. With brachytherapy, the radiation source comes into direct, continuous contact with the tumor tissues for a specific period of time. This method provides a high dose of radiation in tumor tissues and a limited dose in surrounding normal tissues. Brachytherapy radiation has the same tissue effects as radiation delivered by external sources.

Brachytherapy uses radioactive isotopes either in solid form or within body fluids. Isotopes can be delivered to the tumor tissues in several ways. *With all types of brachytherapy, the radiation source is within the client. Therefore the client emits radiation for a period of time and is a hazard to others.*

Unsealed Radiation Sources. Isotopes that can be suspended in a fluid are unsealed and given via the oral or intravenous (IV) routes or as an instillation into body cavities, such as the peritoneal cavity and the spinal fluid space. Because the isotopes are unsealed, they are not completely confined to any one body area. Usually, they concentrate more in some body tissues than in others. These soluble isotopes enter body fluids and eventually are eliminated in waste products, which are radioactive and can be harmful to other people.

An example of brachytherapy with soluble isotopes is the ingestion or injection of the radionuclide iodine^{131} (an iodine base with a half-life of 8.05 days) to treat some thyroid cancers. The radioactive iodine concentrates in the thyroid gland and destroys the thyroid cancer cells. Most of this isotope is eliminated within 48 hours. Once the isotope is eliminated, neither the client nor the body wastes are radioactive.

Sealed Radiation Sources. Solid or sealed radiation sources are implanted within or very near the tumor. These radiation sources can be temporary or permanent. Most of the implants emit continuous, low-energy radiation to tumor tissues. Some devices (e.g., seeds or needles) can be placed into the tissues and stay in place by themselves. Other sources must be held in place with special applicators. Needles and seeds are preloaded with the radioactive isotope and are radioactive at the time of insertion into the tumor ("hot implantation"). Some of these devices are so small and the half-life of the isotope so short that the device is permanently left in place (most often for prostate cancer). Other devices are removed and reused in other clients.

In "afterloading," the implant is placed within the cavity without the radioactive isotope. Special applicators hold the implant in position. When placement is correct and the client is in the proper environment, the implant is loaded with the radioisotope. After the prescribed dose has been delivered, the implant, radioisotopes, and position-holding applicators are removed. *With solid implants, the client emits radiation while the implant is in place, but the excreta are not radioactive.*

Traditional implants deliver "low-dose rates" (LDR) of radiation continuously and clients are hospitalized for several days. A new variation on this therapy is radiation delivery at "high-dose rates" (HDR). For this type of delivery, the client comes into the radiation therapy department several times a week and the stronger radiation device is placed for only an hour or so each time. The client goes home between treatments and is only radioactive when the implant is in place. Chart 28-1 lists the best practices for care of the client with sealed implant radiation sources.

SIDE EFFECTS OF RADIATION THERAPY

The immediate and long-term side effects of all types of radiation are limited to the tissues exposed to the radiation. Therefore the side effects vary according to the site. Skin

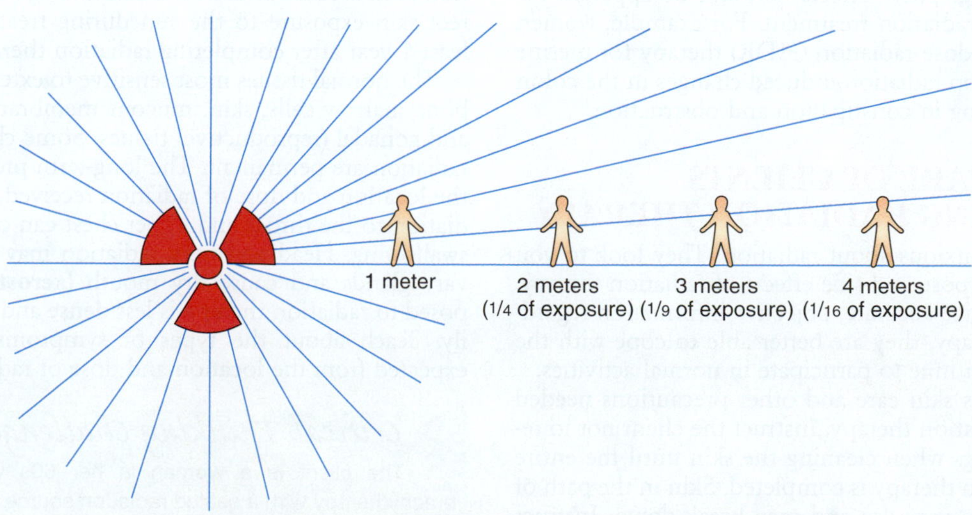

Figure 28-2 ■ The inverse square law of radiation exposure.

CHART 28-1

BEST PRACTICE for
Care of the Client with Sealed Implants of Radioactive Sources

- Assign the client to a private room with a private bath.
- Place a "Caution: Radioactive Material" sign on the door of the client's room.
- Wear a dosimeter film badge at all times while caring for clients with radioactive implants. The badge offers no protection but measures an individual's exposure to radiation and should be used by only one individual.
- Pregnant nurses should not care for these clients; do not allow pregnant women or children younger than 16 years of age to visit.
- Limit each visitor to one-half hour per day. Be sure visitors are at least 6 feet from the source.
- Never touch the radioactive source with bare hands. In the rare instance that it is dislodged, use a long-handled forceps to retrieve it. Deposit the radioactive source in the lead container kept in the client's room.
- Save all dressings and bed linens until after the radioactive source is removed. After the source is removed, dispose of dressings and linens in the usual manner. Other equipment can be removed from the room at any time.

changes and hair loss are local but are likely to be permanent depending on the total absorbed dose.

Depending on the dose, altered taste sensations and fatigue are two systemic side effects often noted by clients receiving external beam radiation, regardless of the radiation site. Taste changes are thought to be caused by metabolites released from dead and dying cells. Many clients develop an aversion to the taste of red meats. Fatigue may be related to the increased energy demands needed to repair damaged cells. Regardless of the cause, radiation-induced fatigue can be debilitating and may last for weeks to months. Many clients are surprised by the degree of fatigue they have and adjust their lifestyle to manage this symptom. Although clinicians have suggested that clients increase rest time to reduce fatigue, early research indicates exercise may help reduce radiation-related fatigue (see the Evidence-Based Practice for Nursing box at right).

Radiation damage to normal tissues during cancer therapy can start the inflammatory responses that cause tissue fibrosis and scarring. These effects may not be apparent for many years after radiation treatment. For example, women who receive high-dose radiation (HDR) therapy for uterine cancer may develop radiation-induced changes in the colon years later, resulting in constipation and obstruction.

NURSING CARE OF CLIENTS UNDERGOING RADIATION THERAPY

Most clients are anxious about radiation. They look to you to explain the purpose and side effects of radiation therapy. When clients receive accurate, objective information regarding radiation therapy, they are better able to cope with the treatment and continue to participate in normal activities.

Chart 28-2 lists skin care and other precautions needed with external radiation therapy. Instruct the client not to remove the markings when cleaning the skin until the entire course of radiation therapy is completed. Skin in the path of radiation becomes very dry and may break down. Instruct clients not to use lotions or ointments in these areas unless the radiologist prescribes them. Because skin in the radiation path is more sensitive to sun damage, advise against direct skin exposure to the sun during treatment and for at least 1 year after completing radiation therapy.

The normal tissues most sensitive to external radiation are bone marrow cells, skin, mucous membranes, hair follicles, and gonadal (reproductive) tissues. Some changes caused by radiation are permanent. The long-term problems vary with the location and dose of radiation received. For example, radiation to the throat and upper chest can cause difficulty in swallowing. Head and neck radiation may damage the salivary glands and cause dry mouth **(xerostomia).** Bone exposed to radiation therapy is less dense and breaks more easily. Teach about the types of symptoms that might be expected from the location and dose of radiation received.

EVIDENCE-BASED PRACTICE for Nursing

Exercise may reduce radiation-related fatigue

Sarna, L., & Conde, F. (2001). Physical activity and fatigue during radiation therapy: A pilot study using Actigraph monitors. *Oncology Nursing Forum, 28*(6), 1043-1046.

This prospective, descriptive pilot study sought to explore the effect of purposeful exercise on the experience of radiation-induced fatigue. Seven subjects who were receiving a 5-week course of external beam radiation therapy for cancer participated in this repeated measures study. Activity and fatigue were measured at the beginning and end of the second and fifth weeks of therapy. Activity was determined by Actigraph watch recordings and self-reports with the use of activity diaries. Fatigue was measured using the Profile of Mood States (POMS) vigor-activity and fatigue-inertia subscales, a Linear Analogue Scales for Fatigue (LAS-F), and the Symptom Distress Scale (SDS).

The data indicated that subjects who participated in purposeful exercise had an overall increase in activity at the end of the second and fifth weeks of therapy compared to the beginnings of the same weeks of therapy. Fatigue scores decreased at the ends of the same weeks compared to the beginnings of those weeks. Additionally, the subjects reported less fatigue by the fifth week of therapy compared to the second week of therapy. These findings are different from the levels of activity and perceptions of fatigue typically reported by clients receiving radiation therapy who do not participate in purposeful exercise activity. The findings do, however, support those of recent research examining the effects of exercise in clients receiving chemotherapy for cancer.

Level of Evidence: 6—Uncontrolled case series.

Critique. The study represented pilot work in the area of the effects of exercise on side effects for clients receiving radiation therapy for cancer. The sample size was small and no control group was used for comparison. The investigators used appropriate data collection techniques. Although the results of this study cannot be generalized at this time, they indicate that more study of an exercise intervention for ameliorating side effects of radiation therapy is needed.

Implications for Nursing. Fatigue is a distressing and often debilitating side effect of radiation therapy. Current interventions have included more frequent rest periods and reduction of nonessential activity. The results of this study suggest that activity not only may not worsen the perception of fatigue among clients undergoing radiation therapy, but might actually decrease the fatigue.

Critical Thinking Challenge

The client is a woman in her 60s who is receiving brachytherapy with a sealed radiation source for 49 hours. She is concerned about being radioactive and the side effects of therapy, especially alopecia.

1. What precautions will you teach this client to prevent radiation exposure to others?
2. What precautions should you take when you provide direct care to this client?
3. How should you handle her excrement?
4. What should you tell her about the possibility of alopecia?
5. What immediate and long-term side effects of therapy could this client expect to have?

evolve For suggested answer guidelines, go to http://evolve.elsevier.com/Iggy/.

Chemotherapy

Chemotherapy, the treatment of cancer with chemical agents, has a major role in cancer therapy. Chemotherapy is used to cure and to increase survival time.

RATIONALE FOR CANCER THERAPY

As described in Chapter 27, cancer cells are able to separate from the original tumor, spread to new areas, and establish new cancers at distant sites **(metastasize).** Clients with metastatic cancer will die unless treatment eliminates the metastatic cancer cells and the original cancer cells.

Chemotherapy is useful in treating cancer because its effects are systemic, providing the opportunity to kill metastatic cancer cells that may have escaped local treatment. Chemotherapy used along with surgery or radiation is termed **adjuvant** therapy.

MECHANISM OF ACTION

Chemotherapy is used as cancer treatment because it has some selectivity for killing cancer cells over normal cells. This killing effect on cancer cells is related to the ability of chemotherapy to damage DNA and interfere with cell division. Thus the tumors most sensitive to chemotherapy are those that have rapid growth.

Chemotherapy drugs usually are given systemically and exert their cell-damaging **(cytotoxic)** effects against healthy cells as well as cancer cells. The normal cells most affected by chemotherapy are those that divide rapidly, including skin, hair, intestinal tissues, spermatocytes, and blood-forming cells.

Chemotherapy drugs are classified by the specific types of action they exert in the cancer cell. Table 28-6 lists categories and specific agents.

ANTIMETABOLITES. Antimetabolites are similar to normal metabolites needed for vital cell processes. Most cell reactions require metabolites in order to begin or continue the reaction. Antimetabolites closely resemble normal metabolites and are "counterfeit" metabolites that fool cancer cells into using the antimetabolites in cellular reactions. Because antimetabolites cannot function as proper metabolites, their presence impairs cell division.

ANTITUMOR ANTIBIOTICS. Antitumor antibiotics damage the cell's DNA and interrupt DNA or ribonucleic acid (RNA) synthesis. Exactly how the interruptions occur varies with each agent.

ALKYLATING AGENTS. All alkylating agents cross-link DNA, making the two DNA strands bind tightly together. This tight binding prevents proper DNA and RNA synthesis, inhibiting cell division.

ANTIMITOTIC AGENTS. Antimitotic agents are usually made from plant sources. They interfere with the formation of microtubules so cells cannot complete mitosis during cell division. As a result, the cancer cell either does not divide at all or divides only once, resulting in two daughter cells that cannot continue to divide.

CHART 28-2

CLIENT EDUCATION GUIDE

Radiation Therapy for Cancer

- Wash the irradiated area gently each day with either water alone or with a mild soap and water.
- Use your hand rather than a washcloth to be more gentle.
- Rinse soap thoroughly from your skin.
- Take care not to remove the markings that indicate exactly where the beam of radiation is to be focused.
- Dry the irradiated area with patting motions rather than rubbing motions; use a clean, soft towel or cloth.
- Use no powders, ointments, lotions, or creams on your skin at the radiation site unless they are prescribed by your *radiologist*.
- Wear soft clothing over the skin at the radiation site.
- Avoid wearing belts, buckles, straps, or any type of clothing that binds or rubs the skin at the radiation site.
- Avoid exposure of the irradiated area to the sun.
- Avoid heat exposure.

TOPOISOMERASE INHIBITORS. Topoisomerase is an enzyme needed for DNA synthesis and cell division. It nicks and straightens the DNA helix, allowing the DNA to be copied, and then reattaches the DNA together. Topoisomerase inhibitors prevent these processes, causing DNA breakage and cell death.

MISCELLANEOUS CHEMOTHERAPEUTIC AGENTS. The actions of other chemotherapeutic agents do not fit any of the chemotherapy categories and include the following:

- Inhibition of important enzyme systems
- Competition for important substances in metabolic pathways

COMBINATION CHEMOTHERAPY. Successful cancer chemotherapy involves giving more than one specific anticancer drug in a timed manner. This technique is called **combination chemotherapy.** Using more than one drug is much more effective in killing cancer cells than using a single agent. However, the damage caused to normal tissues also increases with combination chemotherapy.

The selection of drugs is based on known tumor sensitivity to the drugs and the degree of side effects expected. For example, most chemotherapy drugs suppress bone marrow activity and immune function to some degree, but some agents cause more immunosuppression than others. There is also variation in the timing of drug-induced immunosuppression.

The time when bone marrow activity and white blood cell counts are at their lowest levels after chemotherapy is the **nadir.** The nadir occurs at different times for different drugs (see Table 28-6). For instance, the expected nadir for cytarabine is 5 to 7 days and for mitomycin C is about 4 weeks. To reduce immunosuppression, combination chemotherapy avoids using drugs with nadirs that occur at or near the same time.

TREATMENT ISSUES

DRUG DOSAGE. The doses of most chemotherapy agents are calculated according to the type of cancer and the client's size. Most commonly, calculations are based on milligrams per square meter of total body surface area (TBSA). This measure uses the client's height and weight

TABLE 28-6 Categories of Chemotherapeutic Agents

Generic Name	Usual Dose	Nadir
Antimetabolites		
Capecitabine (Xeloda)	2500 mg/m²	Not reported
Cladribine (Leustatin)	0.09 mg/kg/day	10-14 days
**Cytarabine (Cytosar, ara-C)	100-300 mg/m²	4-7 days
Floxuridine (FUDR)	0.1-0.6 mg/kg	4-7 days
*5-Fluorouracil (Adrucil, Efudex, Fluoroplex)	300-750 mg/m²	9-14 days
Fludarabine (Fludara)	25 mg/m²	3-25 days
*Gemcitabine (Gemzar)	1000-1250 mg/m²	7-12 days
6-Mercaptopurine (Purinethol)	80-100 mg/m²	5-40 days
**Methotrexate (Mexate, Folex)	3.3 mg/m²	10-14 days
Pentostatin (Nipent)	4 mg/m²	3-10 days
Raltitrexed (Tomudex)	3 mg/m²	7-10 days
6-Thioguanine (Lanvis)	2-3 mg/kg	1-4 wk
Trimetrexate (Neutrexin)	45 mg/m²	10-14 days
Antitumor Antibiotics		
Bleomycin (Blenoxane)	10-20 units/m²	7-14 days
**Dactinomycin (Cosmegen)	0.4-0.6 mg/m²	14-21 days
**Daunorubicin (Cerubidine)	30-60 mg/m²	10-14 days
**Doxorubicin (Adriamycin, Rubex)	50-80 mg/m²	10-15 days
**Epirubicin (Ellence)	100-120 mg/m²	10-14 days
**Idarubicin (Idamycin)	12-25 mg/m²	10-14 days
*Mitomycin C (Mutamycin)	10-20 mg/m²	21-50 days
*Mitoxantrone (Novantrone)	12-14 mg/m²	7-10 days
**Plicamycin (Mithracin)	0.025-0.03 mg/m²	10-12 days
Alkylating Agents		
Altretamine (Hexalen)	260 mg/m²	3-4 weeks
**Busulfan (Myleran)	1-8 mg	14-21 days
**Carboplatin (Paraplatin)	360 mg/m²	21-28 days
**Carmustine (BiCNU)	200-250 mg/m²	4-6 weeks
Chlorambucil (Leukeran)	1-4 mg/m²	28 days
**Cisplatin (Platinol)	25-120 mg/m²	10-20 days
Cyclophosphamide (Cytoxan, Procytox)	50-500 mg/m²	7-14 days

Generic Name	Usual Dose	Nadir
Alkylating Agents—*cont'd*		
Estramustine (Emcyt)	14 mg/kg/day	≈4 wk
**Ifosfamide (IFEX)	1.2 g/m²	10 days
**Lomustine (CCNU, CeeNU)	130 mg/m²	4-6 wk
**Mechlorethamine (Mustargen)	0.2-0.3 mg/kg	10-14 days
**Melphalan (Alkeran)	1-6 mg/m²	14-21 days
Oxaliplatin (Eloxatin)	50-85 mg/m²	5-14 days
**Streptozocin (Zanosar)	500-1500 mg/m²	14 days
Temozolomide (Temodar)	150-200 mg/m²	21-28 days
Thiotepa (Thioplex)	0.3-0.8 mg/kg	15-30 days
Antimitotics		
*Docetaxel (Taxotere)	60-100 mg/m²	8-10 days
*Paclitaxel (Taxol)	100-250 mg/m²	8-11 days
Vinblastine (Velban, Velbe, Velsar)	5-10 mg/m²	5-11 days
Vincristine (Oncovin, leurocristine, VCR)	0.5-2 mg/m²	7 days
Vindesine (DAVA, Eldisine)	2 mg/m²	2-7 days
Vinorelbine (Navelbine)	30 mg/m²	7-10 days
Topoisomerase Inhibitors		
*Etoposide (VP16, VePesid)	50-100 mg/m²	8-10 days
*Irinotecan (Camptosar)	125-150 mg/m²	18-25 days
*Teniposide (Vumon, VM-26)	100-180 mg/m²	8-10 days
*Topotecan (Hycamtin)	1.5 mg/m²	7-14 days
Other Agents		
*Asparaginase (Elspar, Kidrolase)	200-1000 International Units/kg	4-10 days
Bexarotene (Targretin)	300 mg/m²	4-8 wk
Dacarbazine (DTIC)	75-250 mg/m²	10-14 days
Hydroxyurea (Hydrea)	25 mg/kg	4-7 days
Leucovorin (Wellcovorin)	10 mg/m²	N/A
Levamisole (Ergamisol)	50 mg	N/A
**Procarbazine (Matulane, Natulan✱)	100-300 mg	14-28 days
Thalidomide (Thalomid)	100-300 mg	N/A

Facts and Comparisons. (2004). *Drug facts and comparisons* (58th ed.). St. Louis: Author.
*, Moderately emetogenic; **, highly emetogenic

and is calculated as follows: the height of the client (in centimeters) is multiplied by his or her weight (in kilograms), and the result is divided by 10,000 (moving the decimal point four spaces to the left). For example, a woman who is 68 inches tall (173 cm) and weighs 143 pounds (65 kg) has a TBSA of 11,245 cm^2, or 1.12 m^2.

DRUG SCHEDULE. Chemotherapy drugs are given on a regular basis and are timed to maximize cancer cell kill and minimize damage to normal cells. The schedule may vary somewhat to accommodate a client's response to therapy, but chemotherapy is usually scheduled every 3 to 4 weeks for a specified number of times (on average, 6 to 12 times). The entire planned schedule is the *course* of chemotherapy.

DRUG ADMINISTRATION. Most chemotherapy drugs are given IV, although other routes may be used for specific cancers (Table 28-7). The techniques and care needs for different routes are described with the specific cancer type most commonly associated with the specific administration route. Chapter 17 describes the types of venous access devices, many of which are used for chemotherapy.

TABLE 28-7 Routes of Chemotherapy Administration

Route	Typical Cancer
Oral	Hodgkin's lymphoma Leukemia (maintenance phase) Small cell lung cancer
Intravenous	Most solid tumors, leukemias Lymphomas
Intra-arterial	Hepatic tumors (primary and metastatic) Head and neck cancers
Isolated limb perfusion	Cancers confined to a limb ▪ Osteogenic sarcoma ▪ Ewing's sarcoma ▪ Rhabdomyosarcoma ▪ Regional melanoma
Intracavitary	
▪ Intraperitoneal	Ovarian cancer
▪ Intraventricular	Brain tumors
▪ Intrathecal	Brain tumors Prophylaxis for acute lymphocytic leukemia
▪ Intravesical	Bladder tumors

TABLE 28-8 Chemotherapy Tissue Vesicants and Irritants

Vesicants	Irritants
Amsacrine	Bleomycin
Dactinomycin	Carmustine
Daunorubicin	Cisplatin
Doxorubicin	Dacarbazine
Epirubicin	Etoposide
Esorubicin	Fluorouracil
Idarubicin	Mitoxantrone
Mechlorethamine	Paclitaxel
Menogaril	Plicamycin
Mitomycin C	Streptozocin
Pyrazofurin	Teniposide
Vinblastine	
Vincristine	
Vindesine	
Vinorelbine	

The IV route is the most preferred route for chemotherapy because the effects of the drugs are rapid and because many of these agents are irritating or damaging to tissues. A major complication of IV infusion is **extravasation,** or the movement of the IV needle so the drug leaks into the surrounding tissues. When the drugs given are **vesicants** (chemicals that cause tissue damage on direct contact), the results of extravasation can include pain, infection, and tissue loss. Surgical intervention is sometimes needed. Table 28-8 lists known vesicant and irritant chemotherapy drugs.

The most important nursing intervention for extravasation is prevention. Small extravasations resolve without extensive treatment if less than 0.5 mL of the drug has leaked into the tissues. If a larger amount has leaked, extensive tissue damage occurs and surgical intervention may be necessary. Immediate treatment depends on the specific drug. With some drugs, cold compresses to the area are prescribed; for other agents, warm compresses are used. Antidotes may be injected into the site of extravasation. Consult with the oncologist and pharmacist to determine the specific antidote needed for the extravasated drug. Chart 28-3 outlines the best practices for documenting an extravasation event.

Most chemotherapy drugs are absorbed through the skin and mucous membranes. As a result, the health care workers who prepare or give these drugs (especially nurses and pharmacists) are at risk for absorbing them. Even at low doses, long-term exposure to chemotherapy drugs can affect health. Use extreme caution and wear protective clothing whenever preparing, giving, or disposing of chemotherapy drugs. The Occupational Safety and Health Administration (OSHA) and the Oncology Nursing Society have established practice guidelines and protective standards.

CHART 28-3

BEST PRACTICE for
Documentation of Extravasation

- Document the date and time when extravasation was suspected or identified.
- Document the date and time when the infusion was started.
- Record the time when the infusion was stopped.
- Document the exact contents of the infusion fluid and the volume of fluid infused.
- Document the estimated amount of fluid extravasated.
- Document the needle type and size.
- Diagram the exact insertion site.
- Indicate on the diagram the location and number of venipuncture attempts.
- Record the time between the extravasation and the last full blood return.
- Identify all agents administered in the previous 24 hours through this site (list agent administered, dosage and volume, and order of administration).
- Take and record the client's vital signs.
- Take a photograph of the site.
- Document the administration of neutralizing or antidote agents.
- Document the application of compresses.
- Document other nursing interventions.
- Record the client's responses to nursing interventions.
- Document the physician notification (including the time).
- Document the written and oral instructions given to the client about follow-up care.
- Document any consultation request.
- Sign the documentation.

SIDE EFFECTS OF CHEMOTHERAPY

Serious side effects occur with aggressive chemotherapy, including **alopecia** (hair loss), nausea and vomiting, open sores on mucous membranes **(mucositis),** and many skin changes. Other distressing side effects include anxiety, sleep disturbance, altered bowel elimination, and decreased mobility.

Drug therapy is used to reduce the severity of these symptoms. Nonpharmacologic nursing interventions include massage, guided imagery, Reiki, aromatherapy, and other forms of complementary therapy. Many clients have found these interventions to be helpful in reducing distressing side effects (see the Evidence-Based Practice for Nursing Box below).

EVIDENCE-BASED PRACTICE for Nursing

Massage helps manage cancer treatment symptoms

Smith, M., et al. (2002). Outcomes of therapeutic massage for hospitalized cancer patients. *Journal of Nursing Scholarship, 34*(3), 257-263.

This prospective, quasiexperimental study examined the effect of therapeutic massage on the perception of pain, sleep quality, anxiety, and treatment-related symptom distress among clients hospitalized for cancer treatment. The study used a two-group design with one group of 20 subjects receiving the therapeutic massage intervention of 15 to 30 minutes of light Swedish massage techniques performed by a registered nurse who was also a certified massage therapist. Each subject in the intervention group received three massages during 1 week of hospitalization. The control group of 21 subjects received a nurse interaction of 20 minutes of deliberate focused communication with the same nurse who provided massage to the treatment group. Pre- and post-testing of the subjects' perceptions of pain (numerical rating scale; 4-point Likert-type scale), sleep patterns (Verran and Snyder-Halpern Sleep Scale), symptom distress (Symptom Distress Scale), and anxiety (State-Trait Anxiety Inventory) were performed for all subjects and analyzed using a repeated measures factorial analysis of variance.

The mean scores for pain, symptom distress, and anxiety improved from baseline for subjects in the treatment group. Only anxiety improved over baseline for subjects in the nursing interaction group. Neither group experienced improvement in sleep quality.

Level of Evidence: 5—Well-conducted case control study.

Critique. The study provides data to support nonpharmacologic interventions to improve the comfort of clients undergoing cancer therapy. The sample was small, nonrandomized, and mostly male (95%), limiting generalizability. Except for the dimension of pain, the measurement instruments used had well-established validity and reliability. Several strengths of the study included that the intervention was performed by one individual and the study controlled for the issue of attention.

Nursing Implications. The nursing shortage has reduced the amount of time available for nurses to use massage as an intervention. Few well-designed studies have been performed to examine the benefit of therapeutic massage as an intervention for clients with cancer. This study supports the use of this intervention by nurses in the hospital setting.

TABLE 28-9 Agents Used for Chemoprotection

Agent	Cytotoxic Problem Prevented
Amifostine (Ethyol)	Xerostomia
Dexrazoxane (Zinecard)	Cardiomyopathy
Mesna (MESNEX)	Hemorrhagic cystitis
Pamidronate (Aredia)	Skeletal complications

The side effects on the hematopoietic (blood-producing) system can be life threatening and are the most common reason for changing the dosage or schedule. The suppressive effects on the blood-forming cells of bone marrow cause anemia, immunosuppression, and **thrombocytopenia** (decreased numbers of platelets).

One approach to decrease the impact of chemotherapy on normal tissues is to give the agents with drugs that protect specific healthy cells. These drugs, called **cytoprotectants,** have little effect on cancer cells but do protect some normal cells (Table 28-9).

NURSING CARE OF CLIENTS UNDERGOING CHEMOTHERAPY

The major care issue during chemotherapy is managing the distressing symptoms occurring with therapy. For some clients, the symptoms are so unpleasant that they stop treatment. Chart 28-4 lists NIC interventions for clients undergoing chemotherapy.

ALOPECIA. Clients receiving cancer chemotherapy often have whole-body hair loss. Some drugs may cause only thinning of the scalp hair. Others cause a more complete hair loss.

Reassure clients that hair loss is temporary. Hair regrowth usually begins about 1 month after completion of chemother-

CHART 28-4

NIC INTERVENTION ACTIVITIES for The Client with Cancer

Chemotherapy Management: *Assisting the client and family to understand the action and minimize side effects of antineoplastic agents*

- Monitor for side effects and toxic effects of chemotherapeutic agents.
- Provide information to client and family on how antineoplastic drugs work on cancer cells.
- Instruct client and family on ways to prevent infection, such as avoiding crowds and using good hygiene and handwashing techniques.
- Instruct client to promptly report fever, chills, nosebleeds, excessive bruising, and tarry stools.
- Instruct client and family to avoid the use of aspirin products.
- Administer antiemetic drugs for nausea and vomiting.
- Teach the client relaxation and imagery techniques to use before, during, and after treatments, as appropriate.
- Ensure adequate fluid intake to prevent dehydration and electrolyte imbalance.
- Monitor the effectiveness of measures to control nausea and vomiting.
- Teach client and family to monitor for signs and symptoms of stomatitis.
- Instruct client on proper oral hygiene techniques.
- Inform client that hair loss is expected, as determined by type of chemotherapeutic agent used.
- Assist client in obtaining a wig or other head-covering device, as appropriate.
- Provide nutritious, appetizing foods of client's choice.
- Monitor nutritional status and weight.
- Discuss with client the possibility of sterility and other reproductive system impairments, as appropriate.
- Instruct long-term survivors and their families of the possibility of second malignancies and the importance of reporting increased susceptibility to infection, fatigue, or bleeding.

NIC intervention activities selected from Dochterman, J.M., & Bulechek, G.M. (Eds.). (2004). *Nursing interventions classification (NIC)* (4th ed.). St. Louis: Mosby.

apy. Inform the client that the new hair may differ from the original hair in color, texture, and thickness. No known treatment completely prevents alopecia.

Assist clients in selecting a type of head covering that suits their income and lifestyle. High-quality wigs are expensive but can look very much like the client's own hair. Many local units of the American Cancer Society offer wigs that other clients have used and then donated to be lent to other clients with cancer. Clients can disguise hair loss with caps, scarves, and turbans.

NAUSEA AND VOMITING. Chemotherapy-induced nausea and vomiting arises from a variety of local and central nervous system mechanisms. Most chemotherapy drugs are **emetogenic** (vomiting inducing) to some degree, depending on the dose. Most drugs induce nausea and vomiting when the drug is given and for 1 to 2 days afterward. Some drugs, such as cisplatin, induce delayed nausea and vomiting that can continue as long as 5 to 7 days after receiving it. Clients who have chemotherapy-related nausea and vomiting during one round of chemotherapy may begin to have the same symptoms before the next round as a result of sheer anticipation.

CONSIDERATION FOR OLDER ADULTS

At times, older clients have received lower doses of chemotherapy drugs because it was thought the older person would not be able to tolerate the side effects of nausea and vomiting. Research indicates that older clients do not have greater nausea and vomiting than do younger clients. Therefore their chemotherapy regimens should not be altered on this basis alone.

Drug Therapy. Many antiemetics are available to relieve nausea and vomiting. These drugs vary in the side effects they produce and how well they control chemotherapy-induced nausea and vomiting. One or more antiemetics are usually given before and after chemotherapy. Antiemetic drugs commonly used to control chemotherapy-induced nausea and vomiting are listed in Chart 28-5. Client response to antiemetic therapy is highly variable, and the drug combinations must be individualized for best effect. Antiemetic drugs vary in cost.

CHART 28-5

DRUG THERAPY for Chemotherapy-Induced Nausea and Vomiting

Drug	Usual Dosage	Side Effects
Serotonin Antagonists		
Ondansetron (Zofran)	8 mg q8h	Constipation, diarrhea, fever, light-headedness, drowsiness
Granisetron Kytril)	1 mg q12h	Fever, dysrhythmias, chest pain, fainting
Dolasetron (Anzemet)	1.8 mg/kg	
Palonosetron (Aloxi)	0.25 mg	
CNS Depressants		
Trimethobenzamide (Tigan, Benzacot, Arrestin, T-Gen)	200 mg three or four times daily	Drowsiness, blurred vision, dizziness, diarrhea, headache, mental depression, tremors
Benzodiazepines		
Lorazepam (Ativan)	1-3 mg twice or three times daily	Amnesia, bradycardia, hypotension, muscle weakness, anemia
Phenothiazines		
Prochlorperazine (Compazine, Stemetil✱)	10-20 mg four times daily	Hypotension, CNS depression, extrapyramidal reactions, dry mouth, blurred vision
Chlorpromazine (Thorazine, Ormazine)	25-50 mg four times daily	Hypotension, CNS depression, extrapyramidal reactions, dry mouth, blurred vision
Antihistamines		
Diphenhydramine (Benadryl)	25-50 mg four times daily	Drowsiness, dry mouth, hypotension
Corticosteroids		
Dexamethasone (Decadron)	5-10 mg daily	Fluid and electrolyte imbalances, immunosuppression, GI bleeding, bruising, cushingoid symptoms
Prokinetic Agents		
Metoclopramide (Reglan)	20-40 mg four times daily	Drowsiness, dry mouth, diarrhea, depression, dysrhythmias
Cannabinoids		
Dronabinol (Marinol)	2.5-10 mg twice or three times daily	Potential dependency mood changes, drowsiness, tachycardia, increased appetite

CNS, Central nervous system; *GI*, gastrointestinal.

Complementary and Alternative Therapies. Assist the client with nausea and vomiting to achieve comfort through nonpharmacologic means along with antiemetics. Music, progressive muscle relaxation, guided imagery, acupressure, or distraction may help reduce anxiety and relieve nausea and vomiting. Assess the client for complications resulting from excessive vomiting, such as dehydration and electrolyte imbalances.

MUCOSITIS. Clients undergoing chemotherapy often develop *mucositis* (sores in mucous membranes) of the entire gastrointestinal (GI) tract, especially in the mouth (stomatitis). Normally, the lining of the GI tract undergoes rapid cell division and quickly replaces cells. In chemotherapy, mucous membrane cells are killed more rapidly than they are replaced, resulting in sore formation. Mouth sores are painful and interfere with eating. Chart 28-6 lists the best practices for clients with mucositis.

Frequent mouth assessment and oral hygiene are key in managing stomatitis and mucositis. Stress the importance of good and frequent oral hygiene, including tooth cleaning and mouth rinsing. Because most clients with mucositis also have bone marrow suppression and are at risk for bleeding, they must take care to avoid traumatizing the oral mucosa. Instruct clients to use a soft-bristled toothbrush or disposable mouth sponges and to avoid using dental floss and water pressure gum cleaners (e.g., a WaterPik). Encourage clients to rinse the mouth with plain water or saline every hour while awake. Teach them to avoid mouthwashes that contain alcohol or other drying agents that may further irritate the mucosa.

Oral hygiene equipment must be kept clean. Remind clients not to share toothbrushes with anyone. Toothbrushes can be cleaned daily by running them through a home dishwasher or by rinsing them with a concentrated solution of liquid bleach or hydrogen peroxide.

Many compounds are available for pain relief from stomatitis or mucositis. Many hospitals offer their own special "swish and spit" mixtures, which contain a local anesthetic combined with anti-inflammatory agents. Tell the client that these mixtures are not to be swallowed.

CHART 28-6

BEST PRACTICE for
Mouth Care for Clients with Mucositis

- Examine the client's mouth (including the roof, under the tongue, and between the teeth and cheek) every 4 hours.
- Document the location, size, and character of fissures, blisters, sores, or drainage.
- Get an order to obtain specimens of sores or drainage for culture.
- Brush the teeth and tongue with a soft-bristled brush or sponges every 8 hours.
- Rinse the mouth with a solution of one-half peroxide and one-half normal saline every 12 hours.
- Avoid the use of alcohol or glycerin-based mouthwashes.
- Administer antimicrobial medications as prescribed.
- Administer topical analgesic medications as prescribed or as needed.
- Help the conscious client to "swish and spit" room-temperature tap water or normal saline as needed.
- Apply petrolatum jelly to the client's lips after each episode of mouth care and as needed.
- Assist the client in using "artificial saliva" as needed, if prescribed.
- Assist the client in menu choices to avoid spicy or hard food.
- Offer complete mouth care before and after every meal.

BONE MARROW SUPPRESSION. Bone marrow suppression reduces the circulating number of leukocytes, erythrocytes, and platelets. Decreased leukocyte numbers, especially neutrophils **(neutropenia),** cause immunosuppression. Decreased erythrocytes and platelets cause hypoxia, fatigue, and an increased tendency to bleed.

Immunosuppression places the client at extreme risk for infection and is the major dose-limiting side effect of cancer chemotherapy. Most chemotherapy drugs suppress bone marrow function to some degree and contribute to the life-threatening complication of neutropenia. This problem decreases the client's protective responses to organism invasion. The severity and duration of the impairment are related directly to the dosage of specific chemotherapeutic agents. This impairment is temporary, with good recovery of protection within weeks after therapy completion. However, the seriousness of potential infection complications makes this problem a major treatment concern. The infectious processes that occur most commonly are fungal, bacterial, and some residual viral breakthrough. *Most of the infections that develop in a client with neutropenia result from overgrowth of the client's own normal flora.*

Decreased numbers of circulating erythrocytes **(anemia)** and platelets **(thrombocytopenia)** also result from the bone marrow suppression caused by some chemotherapy drugs. Anemia causes clients to feel fatigued, and some tissues are hypoxic. The cardiac and respiratory systems may not be able to maintain adequate oxygenation. Thrombocytopenia increases the risk for excessive bleeding. When the platelet count is less than 50,000/mm^3, any small trauma can lead to prolonged bleeding. Clients with fewer than 20,000 platelets/mm^3 may have spontaneous and uncontrollable bleeding requiring transfusion therapy.

Drug Therapy. Immunosuppression can be managed with the use of biological response modifiers (BRMs) to stimulate bone marrow production of immune system cells. Although not appropriate for all types of cancer, this supportive treatment can reduce the risk for infection during chemotherapy. However, BRMs are expensive and not consistently covered by insurance. This treatment is discussed under Immunotherapy on p. 499.

Complementary and Alternative Therapies. Many clients with cancer use complementary and alternative therapies to boost immune function and prevent infection. Common therapies include shark cartilage, Echinacea, and megadoses of vitamin C. Although benefit has not yet been determined in clinical trials, the use of these therapies does not appear to have harmful effects.

Protection from Infection. Chart 28-7 lists the best practices for infection prevention among immunosuppressed clients. Good handwashing before contact with the client is essential for prevention of infection. Health care workers must use aseptic technique when performing any invasive procedure.

Many clients remain at home during periods of immunosuppression. Teach clients and family members precautions to reduce the risk for infection (Chart 28-8).

Provide a safe hospital environment for clients with thrombocytopenia. Teach them how to avoid excessive bleeding when they are discharged before the platelet count has returned to normal. Chart 28-9 lists the best practices for bleeding precautions during hospitalization. Teach clients how to prevent bleeding and what to do if bleeding occurs (Chart 28-10).

Critical Thinking Challenge

The client is a 65-year-old man receiving combination chemotherapy for cancer. He is a very active man who works in his garden daily, plays tennis three times each week, bowls weekly, works at his church as a counselor, and tutors second graders in reading. He will receive six rounds of cyclophosphamide, doxorubicin, vincristine, and prednisone. He is concerned about his appearance, especially alopecia, and what activities he can continue to perform throughout his course of chemotherapy. He also wants to know if he can still have sex with his wife during the months he will be receiving treatment.

1. What will you tell this client about hair loss?
2. Which activities should this client **not** perform during the week of nadir? Why?
3. Which activities are safe for this client to perform during the week in which nadir is reached? Why?
4. What modifications should this client make (if any) for sexual intercourse? Why?

evolve For suggested answer guidelines, go to http://evolve.elsevier.com/Iggy/.

CHART 28-7

BEST PRACTICE for
Care of the Client with Neutropenia

- Place the client in a private room whenever possible.
- Use good handwashing technique before touching the client or any of the client's belongings.
- Ensure that the client's room and bathroom are cleaned at least once each day.
- Do not use supplies from common areas for immunosuppressed clients. For example, keep a sleeve or box of paper cups in the client's room, and do not share this box with any other client. Other articles include drinking straws, plastic knives and forks, dressing materials, gloves, and bandages.
- Limit the number of health care personnel entering the client's room.
- Monitor vital signs every 4 hours; note minor temperature elevation, which may suggest early sepsis.
- Inspect the client's mouth at least every 8 hours.
- Inspect the client's skin and mucous membranes (especially the anal area) for the presence of fissures and abscesses at least every 8 hours.
- Inspect open areas, such as IV sites, every 4 hours for manifestations of infection.
- Change wound dressings daily.
- Obtain specimens of all suspicious areas for culture, and promptly notify the physician.
- Assist the client in performing coughing and deep-breathing exercises.
- Encourage activity at a level appropriate for the client's current health status.
- Change IV tubing daily.
- Keep frequently used equipment in the room for use with this client only (e.g., blood pressure cuff, stethoscope, thermometer).
- Limit visitors to healthy adults.
- Use strict aseptic technique for all invasive procedures.
- Monitor the white blood cell count, especially the absolute neutrophil count (ANC), daily.
- Avoid the use of indwelling urinary catheters.
- Keep fresh flowers and potted plants out of the client's room.
- Teach the client to eat a low-bacteria diet.

CHART 28-8

CLIENT EDUCATION GUIDE
Prevention of Infection

- Avoid crowds and other large gatherings of people who might be ill.
- Do not share personal toilet articles, such as toothbrushes, toothpaste, washcloths, or deodorant sticks, with others.
- If possible, bathe daily.
- Wash the armpits, groin, genitals, and anal area at least twice a day with an antimicrobial soap.
- Clean your toothbrush daily by either running it through the dishwasher or rinsing it in liquid laundry bleach.
- Wash your hands thoroughly with an antimicrobial soap before you eat or drink, after touching a pet, after shaking hands with anyone, as soon as you come home from any outing, and after using the toilet.
- Eat a low-bacteria diet, and avoid salads, raw fruit and vegetables, undercooked meat, pepper, and paprika.
- Wash dishes between use with hot, sudsy water, or use a dishwasher.
- Do not drink water that has been standing for longer than 15 minutes.
- Do not reuse cups and glasses without washing.
- Do not change pet litter boxes.
- Take your temperature at least once a day.
- Report any of the following signs or symptoms of infection to your physician immediately:
  - Temperature greater than 100° F (38° C)
  - Persistent cough (with or without sputum)
  - Pus or foul-smelling drainage from any open skin area or normal body opening
  - Presence of a boil or abscess
  - Urine that is cloudy or foul smelling or that causes burning on urination
- Take all prescribed medications.
- Do not dig in the garden or work with houseplants.

CHART 28-9

BEST PRACTICE for
Care of the Client with Thrombocytopenia

- Handle the client gently.
- Use a lift sheet when moving and positioning the client in bed.
- Avoid intramuscular injections and venipunctures.
- When injections or venipunctures are necessary, use the smallest-gauge needle for the task.
- Apply firm pressure to the needle stick site for 10 minutes or until the site no longer oozes blood.
- Apply ice to areas of trauma.
- Test all urine and stool for the presence of occult blood.
- Observe IV sites every 2 hours for bleeding.
- Avoid trauma to rectal tissues:
  - Do not take temperatures rectally.
  - Do not administer enemas.
  - Administer well-lubricated suppositories and with caution.
  - Advise the client not to have anal intercourse.
- Measure the client's abdominal girth daily.
- Use an electric razor.
- Teach the client to avoid mouth trauma by:
  - Using soft-bristled toothbrush or tooth sponges
  - Not flossing
  - Avoiding dental work, especially extractions
  - Avoiding hard foods
  - Making certain that dentures fit and do not rub
- Encourage the client not to blow the nose or insert objects into the nose.
- Instruct the client to avoid contact sports.
- Advise the client to wear shoes with firm soles whenever he or she is ambulating.

CHART 28-10

CLIENT EDUCATION GUIDE

The Client at Risk for Bleeding

- Use an electric razor.
- Use a soft-bristled toothbrush, and do not floss.
- Do not have dental work performed without consulting your doctor.
- Do not take aspirin or any aspirin-containing products. Read the label to be sure that the product does not contain aspirin or salicylates.
- Do not participate in contact sports or any activity likely to result in your being bumped, scratched, or scraped.
- If you are bumped, apply ice to the site for at least 1 hour.
- Notify your doctor if you:
  - Experience an injury and persistent bleeding results
  - Have excessive menstrual bleeding
  - See blood in your urine or bowel movement
- Avoid anal intercourse.
- Take a stool softener to prevent straining during a bowel movement.
- Do not use enemas or rectal suppositories.
- Avoid bending over at the waist.
- Do not wear clothing or shoes that are tight or that rub.
- Avoid blowing your nose or placing objects in your nose. If you must blow your nose, do so gently without blocking either nasal passage.

Hormonal Manipulation

RATIONALE FOR CANCER TREATMENT

Hormones are naturally occurring chemicals secreted by endocrine (ductless) glands and picked up by capillaries. Once in the bloodstream, hormones circulate to all body areas but exert their effects only on their specific target tissues. Some hormones make hormone-sensitive tumors grow more rapidly. Some tumors require specific hormones to divide. Thus decreasing the amount of these hormones to hormone-sensitive tumors can slow the cancer growth rate.

MECHANISM OF ACTION

HORMONE AGONISTS. Hormonal manipulation can help control some types of cancer for many years. Usually, this therapy does not lead to a cure. The endocrine system usually maintains a delicate hormone balance. When a large amount of one hormone is given, it upsets the balance and disturbs the uptake of other hormones. If a tumor depends on hormone A for growth and a large quantity of hormone B (similar to A) is given to the client, hormone B will interfere with the tumor's uptake of hormone A or will limit the amount of hormone A produced. As a result, tumor growth is slowed and survival time increases. Table 28-10 lists the drugs commonly used in hormonal manipulation for cancer therapy.

HORMONE ANTAGONISTS. Some drugs are hormone antagonists that compete with natural hormones at the receptor sites. Often, they are antibodies specific to the receptor. When hormone antagonists are given, they bind to the specific hormone receptor on or in the tumor cell and prevent the needed hormone from binding to the receptor. If a tumor needs a certain hormone to grow and the hormone can enter or activate the cell only through a receptor, hormone antagonists can slow down tumor growth.

TABLE 28-10 Common Agents Used for Hormonal Manipulation of Cancer

Type of Agent	Example
Hormone Agonists	
Androgen	Calusterone Danocrine Fluoxymesterone Testosterone Testolactone
Estrogen	Conjugated estrogens Diethylstilbestrol Ethinyl estradiol
Progestin	Medroxyprogesterone Megestrol
Luteinizing-hormone releasing hormone (LHRH)	Leuprolide Goserelin
Hormone Antagonists	
Antiandrogens	Bicalutamide Nilutamide Fluoxymesterone Flutamide Cyproterone acetate
Antiprogestins	Mifepristone
Antiestrogens	Droloxifene Idoxifene Tamoxifen Toremifene Trioxifene mesylate Zindoxifene
Gonadotropin-releasing hormone (GnRH)	Abarelix
Aromatase Inhibitors	Anastrozole Exemestane Fulvestrant Letrozole

HORMONE INHIBITORS. A new class of drugs used for hormonal therapy in breast cancer is the aromatase inhibitors. Aromatase is an enzyme that leads to the production of estrogen in the adrenal gland. Aromatase inhibitors prevent this production and reduce blood levels of estrogens (see Table 28-10).

SIDE EFFECTS OF HORMONE THERAPY

Androgens and the antiestrogen receptor drugs cause masculinizing effects in women. Chest and facial hair may develop, menstrual periods stop, and breast tissue shrinks. Clients may have some fluid retention. For men and women receiving androgens, acne may develop, hypercalcemia is common, and liver dysfunction may occur with prolonged therapy. Women receiving estrogens or progestins have irregular but heavy menses, fluid retention, and breast tenderness. Male and female clients who take estrogen or progestins are at increased risk for deep vein thrombosis.

Feminine manifestations often appear in men who take estrogens, progestins, or antiandrogen receptor drugs. Facial hair thins or disappears, facial skin becomes smoother, body fat is redistributed, and **gynecomastia** (breast development in men) can occur. Testicular and penile atrophy also occurs to some degree. Although sexual function may continue, achieving and maintaining an erection is much more difficult.

Immunotherapy: Biological Response Modifiers

Biological response modifiers (BRMs) modify the client's biologic responses to tumor cells. The BRMs in current use as cancer therapy are cytokines, which are small protein hormones made by white blood cells. Cytokines made by macrophages, neutrophils, eosinophils, and monocytes are *monokines*; cytokines produced by lymphocytes (especially the T-lymphocytes) are *lymphokines*. Cytokines generally make the immune system work better (see Chapter 23).

RATIONALE FOR CANCER TREATMENT

Cytokines enhance the immune system. Immune function plays an important role in cancer prevention (see Chapters 23 and 27). Cytokines and other BRMs work as a cancer treatment by stimulating the immune system to recognize cancer cells and take actions to eliminate or destroy them. Some BRMs may also be useful in a supporting role. Other BRMs (colony-stimulating factors) stimulate faster recovery of bone marrow function after treatment-induced suppression.

MECHANISM OF ACTION

The activity of cytokines is similar to that of any other peptide hormone in that one cell produces and secretes a cytokine, which then exerts its effects on other cells of the immune system. The cells responding to the cytokine may be right next to the cytokine-secreting cell or quite remote from it. Cells that change their activity in response to the cytokine are *responder* cells. For a responder cell to respond to a cytokine, the membrane of the responder cell must have a specific receptor for the cytokine. The cytokine binds to this receptor and changes the activity of the responder cell.

BIOLOGICAL RESPONSE MODIFIERS FOR CANCER THERAPY. Two types of BRMs are used as cancer therapy: interleukins (ILs) and interferons (INFs). Some agents can stimulate specific immune system cells to attack and destroy cancer cells; other agents block cancer cell access to an essential function or nutrient.

Interleukins. More than 25 ILs have been identified. Some are produced through recombinant DNA technology. ILs help different immune system cells recognize and destroy abnormal body cells. In particular, IL-1, -2, and -6 appear to "charge up" the immune system and enhance attacks on cancer cells by macrophages, natural killer (NK) cells, and tumor-infiltrating lymphocytes.

Interferons. Interferons are cell-produced proteins that can protect noninfected cells from viral infection and replication. There are many types of INFs. Although all of them are similar, each type has unique functions. The most completely characterized INF is INF alfa-2b.

Different body cells can produce INF, with leukocytes producing the most. INFs also are commercially produced by recombinant DNA technology. Cancer-related functions of INF include the ability to do the following:

- Slow down tumor cell division
- Stimulate the growth and activation of NK cells

TABLE 28-11 Colony-Stimulating Factors

Agent	Cell Type Affected	Indications
Sargramostim (Leukine, Prokine)	All granulocytes ▪ Neutrophils ▪ Eosinophils Monocytes Macrophages	Chemotherapy-induced leukopenia
Filgrastim (Neupogen) Pegfilgrastim (Neulasta)	Neutrophils	Chemotherapy-induced neutropenia
Epoetin alfa (Epogen, Procrit) Darbepoetin alfa (Aranesp)	Erythrocytes	Chemotherapy-induced anemia Chemotherapy-induced fatigue Anemia induced by renal failure
Oprelvekin (Neumega)	Platelets	Chemotherapy-induced thrombocytopenia

- Help cancer cells resume a more normal appearance and revert to their previous normal cell features
- Inhibit the expression of oncogenes

INFs have been effective to some degree in the treatment of malignant melanoma, hairy cell leukemia, renal cell carcinoma, ovarian cancer, and cutaneous T-cell lymphoma.

BIOLOGICAL RESPONSE MODIFIERS FOR CANCER SUPPORT. BRMs used for supportive therapy during cancer treatment are the colony-stimulating factors (Table 28-11). These factors induce more rapid recovery of the bone marrow after suppression by chemotherapy. This effect has two benefits. First, when bone marrow suppression is shortened or less severe, clients are less at risk for life-threatening infections and anemia. Second, because the colony-stimulating factors allow more rapid bone marrow recovery, clients can receive their chemotherapy on time and may even be able to tolerate higher doses, improving the curative outcome of chemotherapy. These agents must be used cautiously in clients with leukemia or lymphoma.

SIDE EFFECTS OF BIOLOGICAL RESPONSE MODIFIER THERAPY

Clients receiving interleukins have generalized and sometimes severe inflammatory reactions. Fluid shifts and capillary leak are widespread with edema forming in most tissues. Tissue swelling affects the function of all organs and can be life threatening. Clients receiving high-dose BRM therapy should receive care in an intensive care or monitoring unit. The effects of BRM therapy are limited to the period of acute drug infusion and resolve when treatment is completed.

Many BRMs induce symptoms of mild inflammation during and immediately after receiving the drug, including fever, chills, rigors, and flu-like general malaise. Problems are worse when higher doses are given, and they seem to become less severe over time. Fever is treated with acetaminophen. Clients with severe rigors are managed with meperidine (Demerol).

Interferon therapy causes peripheral neuropathy similar to that found in clients who have long-standing diabetes mellitus. Some of the problems resulting from the neuropathy include decreased sensory perception, visual disturbances, decreased hearing, unsteady balance and gait, and orthostatic hypotension. It is not known whether the neuropathy is temporary or permanent.

Skin rashes, dryness, itching, and peeling occur with many types of BRM therapy. The skin problems are more severe at higher doses and when more than one type of BRM is used at the same time. These reactions are temporary but can cause much discomfort and distress to the client. Advise clients to apply moisturizers (perfume-free) to the skin and to use mild soap to clean the skin. Involved areas must be protected from the sun with clothing or the use of sunscreen agents. Inform clients to avoid swimming and to refrain from using topical steroid creams on affected areas.

Interferon therapy has been reported to increase depression. It is not known whether this symptom is more intense among clients who have pre-existing depression.

Gene Therapy

Gene therapy as a cancer treatment is experimental. Although response rates have been limited, these successes indicate the potential for gene therapy as a form of cancer treatment.

MECHANISM OF ACTION

INCREASED TUMOR CELL SUSCEPTIBILITY. One method of using gene therapy for cancer is to render the tumor cells more susceptible to damage or death by other treatments. Inserting a viral enzyme gene into brain tumor cells makes them more susceptible to being killed by antiviral agents. Other techniques involve inserting human leukocyte antigen (HLA) genes different from the client's own HLAs into the tumor cells. This technique makes the client's immune system cells better able to recognize the cancer cells as foreign and take steps to eliminate or destroy them. Both methods of gene therapy for cancer have shown some success in early-phase clinical trials.

INCREASED IMMUNE SYSTEM CELL ACTIVITY. Some immune system cells are capable of attacking and killing cancer cells (see Chapter 23). This ability is increased when more of certain cytokines, such as IL-2, are present. Some gene therapy involves inserting additional genes for cytokines into the client's own immune system cells. These "charged-up" cancer-fighting immune system cells remain active for up to 6 months and can participate in cancer cell–killing episodes.

POTENTIAL USES OF GENE THERAPY FOR CANCER TREATMENT. Because cancer is caused by one or more changes in the genes of a normal cell, it is reasonable to think that planned gene changes could influence a cancer cell to become normal. Research for gene therapy against cancer includes the following areas:

- Inserting additional or healthy suppressor genes into cancer cells
- Inserting chemotherapy resistance genes into normal cells so higher doses of chemotherapy can be given without affecting normal cells
- Removing damaged, mutated, or activated oncogenes
- Inserting multiple genes into cancer cells to make them more easily recognized by immune system cells and more susceptible to other treatment modalities

TABLE 28-12 Agents Used for Targeted Cancer Therapy

Agent	Cancer Type
Antibodies	
Alemtuzumab (MabCampath)	Chronic myelogenous leukemia
Campath-1H	Chronic lymphocytic leukemia
CD22 (LymphoCide)	B-cell leukemia
Cetuximab (Erbitux)	Colorectal cancer, non–small cell lung cancer
Gemtuzumab ozogamicin (Mylotarg)	Acute myelocytic leukemia
Imatinib mesylate (Gleevec)	Chronic myelogenous leukemia
Lym-1 (Oncolym)	Lymphoma
Rituximab (Rituxan)	Non-Hodgkin's lymphoma
Tositumomab (Bexxar)	Non-Hodgkin's lymphoma
Trastuzumab (Herceptin)	Breast cancer
Antisense Agents	
AP 12009	Brain tumors
GEM 231	Multiple types of cancer
ISIS 2503	Lymphomas; multiple types of cancer
ISIS 3521/LY900003	Lung cancer
MG98	Bladder cancer; head and neck cancer
Oblimersen sodium (Genasense)	Pancreatic cancer

Targeted Therapy

Targeted therapies combine biologic therapy and gene therapy. These therapies take advantage of one or more differences in a cancer cell that is either not present or only slightly present in normal cells. Agents used as targeted therapies are either antibodies that "target" a cellular element of the cancer cell or "antisense" drugs that work at the gene level. These differences are a result of specific gene expression in cancer cells. Table 28-12 lists some agents used for targeted therapy.

MECHANISM OF ACTION

MONOCLONAL ANTIBODIES. Usually, antibodies are specific to a protein, receptor, or a cellular substance needed by the cancer cell for growth. When the antibody binds to the target within a cancer cell, some process important to cancer cell survival does not take place.

Many antibodies for cancer treatment have recently been approved and are currently in use. Trastuzumab (Herceptin) binds to a receptor for a protein made by some breast cancer cells. Binding this receptor prevents the division of cancer cells and makes them more easily killed by immune system cells. Another monoclonal antibody, rituximab (Rituxan) has a similar effect in some types of lymphoma.

In certain types of colorectal carcinoma, epidermal growth factor binds to the epidermal growth factor receptor (EGFR) site and activates it, leading to the generation of signals that increase the growth potential of the cancer cell. Blocking the EGFR reduces this potential. Anti-EGFR antibodies are a targeted therapy that bind to the EGFR receptor and prevent it from binding to epidermal growth factor. Another approach that targets the EGFR is a chemical that inhibits an enzyme, tyrosine kinase, which is important in the signaling pathway. Another targeted therapy drug is imatinib mesylate (Gleevec). This drug binds to the energy site of tyrosine kinase and prevents its activation. The drug is most useful in cancers that over-express the ABL1 oncogene, such as Philadelphia-chromosome positive chronic myeloid leukemia.

ANTISENSE DRUGS. Antisense drugs are a new form of cancer therapy that targets the process of making proteins important to the cancer development pathway. Genes for these proteins first make messenger RNA (mRNA). See Chapter 11 for a discussion of the steps of protein synthesis. Normally, the mRNA is then translated into protein. Some of these proteins then either enhance the growth of tumor cells or convert normal cell into cancer cells. The antisense drugs bind to the mRNA made by specific cancer genes, preventing them from making the cancer causing protein.

Currently, most antisense drugs are in the experimental stage but have the potential for great future benefit. They are given by continuous IV infusion.

SIDE EFFECTS OF TARGETED THERAPY

Allergic reactions are an issue in clients receiving monoclonal antibodies. Most of these antibodies were developed in animals and may express some animal proteins. More recently, much of the animal portion of these antibodies was removed. Thus the risk for allergic reactions is reduced but not eliminated. Clients receiving antibodies over time may develop their own antibodies to the drugs, making them less effective and possibly causing severe inflammatory or allergic reactions.

ONCOLOGIC EMERGENCIES

Cancer is a chronic disease. However, a number of acute conditions associated with cancer and its treatment can occur. These conditions, or complications, often require immediate intervention and are thus *oncologic emergencies.* Early diagnosis of such conditions is essential to avoid life-threatening situations.

Sepsis and Disseminated Intravascular Coagulation

PATHOPHYSIOLOGY

Sepsis, or septicemia, is a condition in which organisms enter the bloodstream. Septic shock is a life-threatening result of sepsis and a common cause of death in clients with cancer. Clients with cancer are at risk for infection and sepsis because their white blood cell counts are often low and their immune function is usually impaired. Chapter 40 describes the pathophysiology of sepsis and septic shock.

Disseminated intravascular coagulation (DIC) is a problem with the blood-clotting process. DIC is triggered by many severe illnesses, including cancer. In clients with cancer, DIC is caused by sepsis (often a gram-negative infection), by the release of thrombin or thromboplastin (clotting factors) from cancer cells, or by blood transfusions. DIC is most often seen in leukemia and in adenocarcinomas of the lung, pancreas, stomach, and prostate.

Extensive, abnormal clotting occurs throughout the small blood vessels of clients with DIC. This widespread clotting uses up the existing clotting factors and platelets. This process is followed by extensive bleeding. Bleeding from many sites is the most common problem and ranges from minimal to fatal hemorrhage. Clots block blood vessels and decrease blood flow to major body organs and results in pain, strokelike manifestations, dyspnea, tachycardia, oliguria (decreased urine output), and bowel necrosis (tissue death). Chapter 40 describes in-depth the collaborative management of sepsis-induced DIC.

◆COLLABORATIVE MANAGEMENT

DIC is a life-threatening problem and has a mortality rate greater than 70% even when proper therapies are instituted. Thus the best treatment plan for sepsis and DIC is prevention. Identify those clients at greatest risk for sepsis and DIC. Practice strict adherence to aseptic technique during invasive procedures and during contact with nonintact skin and mucous membranes in immunocompromised clients. Teach clients and family members the early manifestations of infection and sepsis and when to seek medical assistance.

When sepsis is present and DIC is likely, treatment focuses on reducing the infection and halting the DIC process. IV antibiotic therapy is initiated. During the early phase of DIC, anticoagulants (especially heparin) are given to limit clotting and prevent the rapid consumption of circulating clotting factors. Cryoprecipitated clotting factors are given when DIC has progressed and hemorrhage is the primary problem.

Syndrome of Inappropriate Antidiuretic Hormone

PATHOPHYSIOLOGY

In healthy people, antidiuretic hormone (ADH) is secreted by the posterior pituitary gland only when more fluid (water) is needed in the body, such as when plasma volume is decreased (see Chapter 14). Certain health problems induce ADH secretion when not needed by the body.

Cancer is the most common cause of the syndrome of inappropriate antidiuretic hormone (SIADH). The cancer most commonly causing SIADH is carcinoma of the lung (especially small cell lung cancer), but SIADH may occur in other types of cancer, especially when tumors are present in the brain. Some tumors actually make and secrete ADH, whereas others stimulate the brain to make and secrete ADH. Drugs often used in clients with cancer also can cause SIADH (e.g., morphine sulfate, cyclophosphamide).

In SIADH, water is reabsorbed to excess by the kidney and put into systemic circulation. The increased water causes hyponatremia (decreased serum sodium levels) and fluid retention. Mild manifestations include weakness, muscle cramps, loss of appetite, and fatigue. Serum sodium levels range from 115 to 120 mEq/L (normal range is 135 to 145 mEq/L). More serious problems occur when even more water is retained, including weight gain, nervous system changes, personality changes, confusion, and extreme muscle weakness. As the sodium level drops toward 110 mEq/L, seizures, coma and death may follow.

◆COLLABORATIVE MANAGEMENT

SIADH is managed by treating the condition and the cause. Treatment includes fluid restriction (sometimes total fluid intake is reduced to 1 L/day), increased sodium intake, and drug therapy. The drug most often used is demeclocycline, which is taken orally. This drug, an antibiotic, works in opposition to ADH. Monitor serum sodium levels closely, because hypernatremia can develop suddenly as a result of this treatment.

A second method for managing SIADH is to reduce or eliminate the underlying cause. Immediate cancer therapy, usually either radiation or chemotherapy, can cause such tumor regression that ADH production returns to normal.

Spinal Cord Compression

PATHOPHYSIOLOGY

Spinal cord compression and damage occur either when a tumor directly enters the spinal cord or when the vertebrae collapse from tumor degradation of the bone. Tumors may begin in the spinal cord but more often spread from other areas of the body, such as the lung, prostate, breast, and colon. Spinal cord compression often causes back pain before neurologic deficits occur. Neurologic problems are specific to the level of spinal compression and include numbness; tingling; loss of urethral, vaginal, and rectal sensation; and muscle weakness. If paralysis occurs, it is usually permanent.

COLLABORATIVE MANAGEMENT

Early recognition and treatment of spinal cord compression are key to a good outcome. Assess the client for neurologic changes consistent with spinal cord compression. Teach clients and families to recognize the manifestations of early spinal cord compression and to seek help as soon as problems are apparent.

Treatment is often palliative. Usually, high-dose corticosteroids are given first to reduce swelling around the spinal cord and relieve symptoms. High-dose radiation may be given to reduce the size of the tumor in the area and relieve compression. Radiation also may be used along with chemotherapy to treat the total disease. Surgery may be performed to remove the tumor from the area and rearrange the bony tissue so less pressure is placed on the spinal cord. External back or neck braces may be used to reduce the weight borne by the spinal column and to reduce pressure on the spinal cord or spinal nerves.

Hypercalcemia

PATHOPHYSIOLOGY

Hypercalcemia (increased serum calcium level) occurs most often in clients with bone metastasis. Cancer in bone causes the bone to release calcium into the bloodstream. In clients with cancer in other parts of the body (especially the lung, head and neck, kidney, or lymph nodes), the tumor secretes parathyroid hormone, causing bone to release calcium. Decreased mobility and dehydration worsen hypercalcemia.

Early manifestations of hypercalcemia include fatigue, loss of appetite, nausea, vomiting, constipation, and polyuria (increased urine output). More serious problems include severe muscle weakness, loss of deep tendon reflexes, paralytic ileus, dehydration, and electrocardiographic (ECG) changes. The severity of manifestations depends on how high the serum calcium level is and how quickly it developed (see also Chapter 16).

COLLABORATIVE MANAGEMENT

Cancer-induced hypercalcemia develops very slowly for many clients, which allows the body time to adapt to this electrolyte change. As a result, symptoms of hypercalcemia may not be evident until the serum calcium level is greatly elevated. Because adaptation does occur, cancer-induced hypercalcemia is treated only when manifestations are present.

Oral hydration alone may be enough to reduce the serum calcium and relieve symptoms. Normal saline is used when parenteral hydration is needed.

Many drugs lower serum calcium levels. Some agents, such oral glucocorticoids, calcitonin, diphosphonate, gallium nitrate, and mithramycin, lower levels quite dramatically. These drugs do not cure hypercalcemia but instead reduce serum calcium levels temporarily. When cancer-induced hypercalcemia is life threatening or occurs with renal impairment, dialysis can temporarily reduce serum calcium levels.

Superior Vena Cava Syndrome

PATHOPHYSIOLOGY

Superior vena cava (SVC) syndrome occurs when the SVC is compressed or obstructed by tumor growth (Figure 28-3). SVC compression can lead to a painful and life-threatening emergency, most often in clients with lymphomas and lung cancer. Clients with cancer of the breast, esophagus, colon, and testes may also be affected.

The manifestations of SVC syndrome result from the blockage of blood flow in the venous system of the head, neck, and upper trunk. Early manifestations occur when the client arises after a night's sleep and include edema of the face, especially around the eyes, and tightness of the shirt or blouse collar (Stokes' sign). As the compression worsens, the client develops edema in the arms and hands, dyspnea, erythema of the upper body, and epistaxis (nosebleeds). Late manifestations include hemorrhage, cyanosis, mental status changes from lack of blood to the brain, decreased cardiac output, and hypotension. Death results if compression is not relieved.

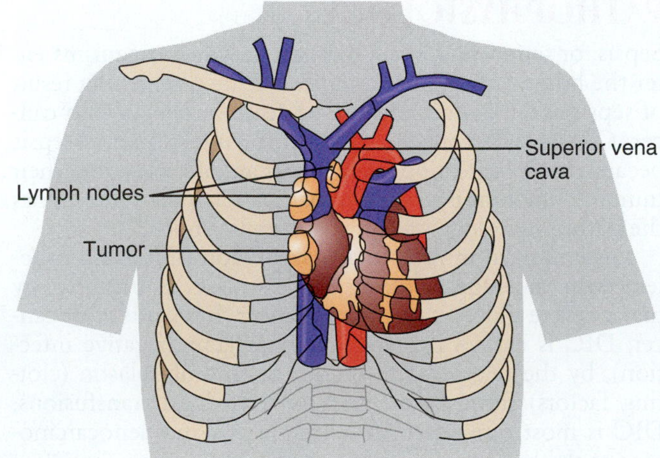

Figure 28-3 ■ Compression of the superior vena cava in SVC syndrome.

COLLABORATIVE MANAGEMENT

SVC syndrome is a late-stage manifestation; the tumor is usually widespread. High-dose radiation therapy to the mediastinal area may be used to provide temporary relief. Surgery is rarely performed for this condition because the tumor may have increased intrathoracic pressure to such a level that it may be impossible to close the chest after the procedure. A metal stent can be placed in the vena cava in an interventional radiation department to relieve swelling. Follow-up angioplasty can keep this stent open for a longer period of time. (See Chapter 39 for more information on stenting procedures.)

The best treatment results occur when SVC syndrome is in the early stages. Assess each client for manifestations of SVC syndrome and notify the physician.

Tumor Lysis Syndrome

PATHOPHYSIOLOGY

In tumor lysis syndrome (TLS), large numbers of tumor cells are destroyed rapidly. Their intracellular contents, including potassium and purines (DNA components), are released into the bloodstream faster than the body can eliminate them (Figure 28-4). Unlike other oncologic emergencies, TLS is a positive sign that cancer treatment is effective.

Severe or untreated TLS can cause severe tissue damage and death. Serum potassium levels can increase to the point of hyperkalemia, causing severe cardiac dysfunction (see Chapter 16). The large amounts of released purines are converted in the liver to uric acid and released into the blood, causing hyperuricemia. These uric acid crystals precipitate in the kidney, forming a sludge in the kidney tubules; this effect blocks the tubules and leads to acute renal failure.

TLS is most often seen in clients receiving radiation or chemotherapy for cancers that are very sensitive to these therapies, including leukemia, lymphoma, small cell lung cancer, and multiple myeloma.

COLLABORATIVE MANAGEMENT

Prevention through hydration is the best management for TLS. Hydration alone can dilute the serum potassium level and increases the kidney filtration rate. As a result, urine flows through the kidney at a greatly increased rate. This action prevents the precipitation of uric acid crystals, increases the excretion of potassium, and mechanically flushes any renal tubular sludge.

With tumors known to be very sensitive to cancer therapy, instruct clients to drink at least 3000 mL (5000 mL is more desirable) of fluid the day before, the day of, and for 3 days after treatment. Some fluids should be alkaline (sodium bicarbonate) to help prevent uric acid precipitation. Stress the importance of keeping fluid intake consistent throughout the 24-hour day and help clients draw up a schedule of fluid intake.

Because some clients have nausea and vomiting after cancer therapy and may not feel like drinking fluids, stress the importance of following the antiemetic regimen. Instruct clients to contact their health care provider or cancer clinic immediately if nausea and vomiting prevent adequate fluid intake so they can be started on parenteral fluids.

Treatment becomes more aggressive for clients who become hyperkalemic or hyperuricemic. In addition to increased fluid intake (oral or parenteral), diuretics (especially osmotic types) are given to increase urine flow through the kidney. These agents are given with caution because clients must not become dehydrated. Drugs that increase the excretion of purines, such as allopurinol (Aloprim, Zyloprim) or rasburicase (Elitek), are given. To reduce serum potassium levels for mild to moderate hyperkalemia, sodium polystyrene sulfonate can be given orally or as a retention enema. This treatment does not immediately reduce serum potassium level. For more severe hyperkalemia, IV infusions containing glucose and insulin may be given. Clients who have severe hyperkalemia and hyperuricemia may need dialysis.

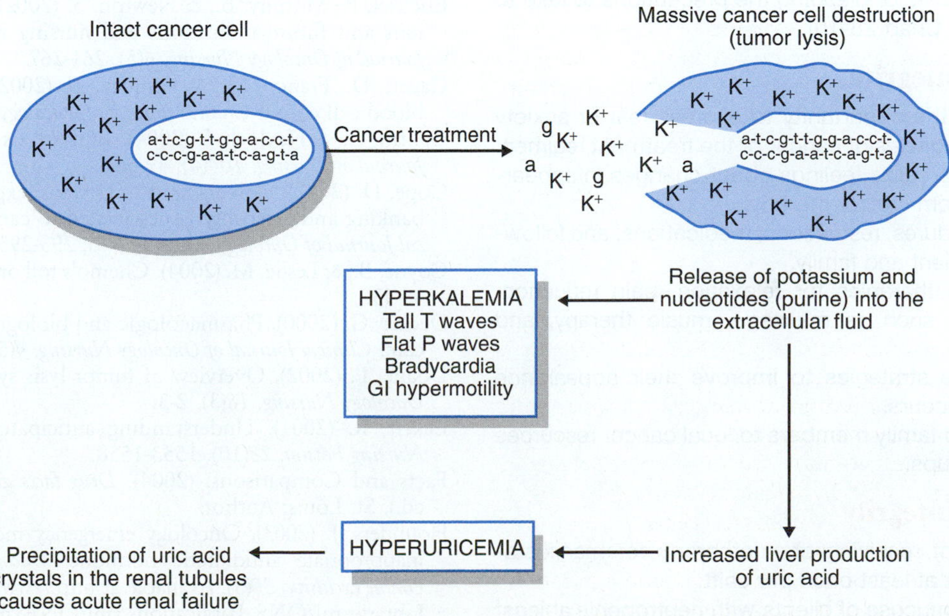

Figure 28-4 ■ Pathology of tumor lysis syndrome.

CANCER TREATMENT FAILURE

More than 50% of people diagnosed with cancer in North America each year are cured of their disease, and many others live 5 years or longer. However, some will have cancer treatment failure and die. With cancer, the process of dying is usually long, lasting weeks or months. Clients and families need special support and assistance during this time. Chapter 9 addresses hospice care and important physical, emotional, social, and spiritual needs of clients and families during and after the dying process.

GET READY for the NCLEX Examination!

KEY POINTS

Safe Effective Care Environment

- Use aseptic technique during all central line dressing changes or any invasive procedure.
- Ask all clients about Advance Directives and document their status.
- Use good handwashing techniques before providing any care to a client who is immunosuppressed.
- Use bleeding precautions for any client with thrombocytopenia or pancytopenia (see Chart 28-9).
- Position shields properly when clients in inpatient settings are receiving brachytherapy.
- Use appropriate personal protection (gowns, gloves, masks) when mixing or administering chemotherapeutic agents.

Health Promotion and Maintenance

- Teach clients receiving radiation therapy how to care for the skin in the radiation path (see Chart 28-2).
- Identify clients at high risk for infection because of disease or therapy.
- Teach the client and family about the clinical manifestations of infection and when to seek medical advice.
- Teach clients at risk for bleeding the precautions to take to avoid injury (see Chart 28-10).

Psychosocial Integrity

- Allow the client the opportunity to express fear or anxiety regarding the diagnosis of cancer or the treatment regimen.
- Allow client to verbalize feelings about changes in appearance resulting from cancer therapy.
- Explain all procedures, restrictions, medications, and follow-up care to the client and family.
- Offer alternative therapies for relaxation, pain reduction, and distraction, such as massage, music therapy, and guided imagery.
- Help clients use strategies to improve their appearance when alopecia occurs.
- Refer clients and family members to local cancer resources and support groups.

Physiological Integrity

- Assess the client receiving chemotherapy for manifestations of infection at least once per shift.
- Inspect the oral mucosa of clients with neutropenia at least once per shift.
- Report any temperature over 100° F in a client with neutropenia.
- Teach the client about any medications to be continued after discharge from the hospital.
- Instruct the client and family in the clinical manifestations of complications and when to seek assistance.
- Pace nonurgent health care activities to reduce the risk for fatigue among clients with anemia or pancytopenia.

ADDITIONAL STUDY RESOURCES

Go to your Student CD-ROM for Review Questions for the NCLEX Examination.

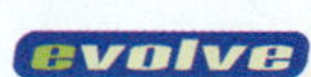

Go to http://evolve.elsevier.com/Iggy/ for Integrated Management of Care Questions for the NCLEX Examination.

SELECTED BIBLIOGRAPHY

American Cancer Society. (2005). *Cancer facts and figures–2005.* Report No. 00-300M-No. 5008.05. Atlanta: Author.

Anastasia, P. (2001). Nursing considerations for managing topotecan-related hematologic side effects. *Clinical Journal of Oncology Nursing, 5*(1), 9-13.

Bedell, C. (2003) Pegfilgrastim for chemotherapy-induced neutropenia. *Clinical Journal of Oncology Nursing, 7*(1),55-64.

Bender, C., et al. (2002). Chemotherapy-induced nausea and vomiting. *Clinical Journal of Oncology Nursing, 6*(2), 94-102.

Birner, A. (2003). Safe administration of oral chemotherapy. *Clinical Journal of Oncology Nursing, 7*(2), 158-162.

Brandt, J. (2002). Rasburicase: An innovative new treatment for hyperuricemia associated with tumor lysis syndrome. *Clinical Journal of Oncology Nursing, 6*(1), 12-16.

Bremerkamp, M. (2000). Mechanism of action of 5-HT3 receptor antagonists: Clinical overview and nursing implications. *Clinical Journal of Oncology Nursing, 4*(5), 201-207.

Brown, C., & Yoder, L. (2002). Stomatitis: An overview. *American Journal of Nursing, 102*(4), 20-23.

Bruce, S. (2004). Radiation-induced xerostomia: How dry is your patient? *Clinical Journal of Oncology Nursing, 8*(1), 61-67.

Buchsel, P. (2003). Gelclair7 oral gel. *Clinical Journal of Oncology Nursing, 7*(1), 109-112.

Buchsel, P., Murphy, B., & Newton, S. (2002). Epoetin Alfa: Current and future indications and nursing implications. *Clinical Journal of Oncology Nursing, 6*(5), 261-267.

Cagen, D., Franco, M., & Vasquez, D. (2002). The ABCs of low blood cell count. *Clinical Journal of Oncology Nursing, 6*(1), 34-36.

Cantril, C., & Haylock, P. (2004). Tumor lysis syndrome. *American Journal of Nursing, 104*(4), 49-56.

Cope, D. (2002). Patients' and physicians' experiences with sperm banking and infertility issues related to cancer treatment. *Clinical Journal of Oncology Nursing, 6*(5), 293-295, 309.

Coyne, B., & Leslie, M. (2004). Chemo's toll on memory. *RN, 67*(4), 40-43.

Decker, G. (2000). Pharmacologic and biologic therapies in cancer care. *Clinical Journal of Oncology Nursing, 4*(5), 242-244.

Doane, L. (2002). Overview of tumor lysis syndrome. *Seminars in Oncology Nursing, 18*(3), 2-3.

Eckert, R. (2001). Understanding anticipatory nausea. *Oncology Nursing Forum, 28*(10), 1553-1558.

Facts and Comparisons. (2004). *Drug facts and comparisons* (58th ed.). St. Louis: Author.

Flounders, J. (2003). Oncology emergency modules: Syndrome of inappropriate antidiuretic hormone. *Oncology Nursing Forum–Online exclusive, 30*(3). Available at http://www.ons.org/xp6/ONS/Library.xml/ONS_Publications.xml/ONF.xml Digital object identifier is 10.1188/03.ONF.E63-E70

Flounders, J., & Ott, B. (2003). Oncology emergency modules: Spinal cord compression. *Oncology Nursing Forum–Online exclusive, 30*(1). Available at http://www.ons.org/xp6/ONS/Library.xml/ONS_Publications.xml/ONF.xml Digital object identifier is 10.1188/03.ONF.E17-E23

Gillespie, T. (2003). Anemia in cancer: Therapeutic implications and interventions. *Cancer Nursing, 26*(2), 119-128.

Gobel, B. (2002). Management of tumor lysis syndrome: Prevention and treatment. *Seminars in Oncology Nursing, 18*(3), 12-16.

Golant, M., Altman, T., & Martin, C. (2003). Managing cancer side effects to improve quality of life. *Cancer Nursing, 26*(1), 37-43.

Gosselin, T., & Waring, J. (2001) Nursing management of patients receiving brachytherapy for gynecologic malignancies. *Clinical Journal of Oncology Nursing, 5*(2), 59-63.

Held-Warmkessel, J. (2005). Managing 3 critical cancer complications. *Nursing 2005, 35*(1), 58-63.

Hellerstedt, B., & Pienta, K. (2002). The current state of hormonal therapy for prostate cancer. *CA A Cancer Journal for Clinicians, 52*(3), 154-179.

Hendrix, C., deLeon, C., & Dillman, R. (2002). Radioimmunotherapy for non-Hodgkin's lymphoma with yttrium 90 ibritumomab tiuxetan. *Clinical Journal of Oncology Nursing, 6*(3), 144-148.

Hodgson, N., & Given, C. (2004). Determinants of functional recovery in older adults surgically treated for cancer. *Cancer Nursing, 27*(1), 10-16.

Hood, L. (2003). Chemotherapy in the elderly: Supportive therapy for chemotherapy-induced myelotoxicity. *Clinical Journal of Oncology Nursing, 7*(2), 185-190.

Jenkins, M., & Ashley, J. (2002). Sex and the oncology patient. *American Journal of Nursing, 102*(4 Suppl.), 13-15.

Kaplow, R. (2002). Pathophysiology, signs, and symptoms of acute tumor lysis syndrome. *Seminars in Oncology Nursing, 18*(3), 6-11.

Lengacher, C., et al. (2002). Frequency of use of complementary and alternative medicine in women with breast cancer. *Oncology Nursing Forum, 29*(10), 1445-1452.

Marek, C. (2003). Antiemetic therapy in patients receiving cancer chemotherapy. *Oncology Nursing Forum, 30*(2), 259-269.

McCance, K., & Huether, S. (2002). Pathophysiology: The biologic basis for disease in adults and children (4th ed.). St. Louis: Mosby.

McGrath, P. (2002). Reflections on nutritional issues associated with cancer therapy. *Cancer Practice, 10*(2), 94-101.

McGuire, D. Mucosal tissue injury in cancer therapy. (2002) *Cancer Practice, 10*(4), 179-191.

Moran, A., & Camp-Sorrell, D. (2002). Maintenance of venous access devices in patients with neutropenia. *Clinical Journal of Oncology Nursing, 6*(3), 126-130.

Ott, M. (2002). Complementary and alternative therapies in cancer symptom management. *Cancer Practice, 10*(3), 162-166.

Peterson, K. (2003). Central line sepsis. *Clinical Journal of Oncology Nursing, 7*(2), 218-221.

Phillips, M. (2003). Pegfilgrastim. *Clinical Journal of Oncology Nursing, 7*(2), 238-239.

Plaisance, L., & Ellis, J. (2002). Opioid-induced constipation. *American Journal of Nursing, 102*(3), 72-73.

Rittenberg, C. (2002). A new class of antiemetic agents on the horizon. *Clinical Journal of Oncology Nursing, 6*(2), 103-104.

Robbins, M., & Gosselin, T. (2002). Symptom management in radiation oncology. *American Journal of Nursing, 102*(4 Suppl.), 32-36.

Sarna, L., & Conde, F. (2001). Physical activity and fatigue during radiation therapy: A pilot study using Actigraph monitors. *Oncology Nursing Forum, 28*(6), 1043-1046.

Schneider, S., Prince-Paul, M., & Allen, M. (2004). Virtual reality as a distraction intervention for women with breast cancer. *Oncology Nursing Forum, 31*(1), 81-88.

Seeley, K., & DeMeyer, E. (2002). Nursing care of patients receiving Campath. *Clinical Journal of Oncology Nursing, 6*(3), 138-143.

Shih, A., et al. (2003). Mechanisms for radiation-induced oral mucositis and the consequences. *Cancer Nursing, 26*(3), 222-229.

Smith, M., et al. (2002). Outcomes of therapeutic massage for hospitalized cancer patients. *Journal of Nursing Scholarship, 34*(3), 257-263.

Sorokin, P. (2002). New agents and future directions in biotherapy. *Clinical Journal of Oncology Nursing, 6*(1), 19-26.

Spencer-Cisek, P. (2002). The role of growth factors in malignancy: A focus on the epidermal growth factor receptor. *Seminars in Oncology Nursing, 18*(2, Suppl. 2), 13-19.

Sweeney, C. (2002). Understanding peripheral neuropathy in patients with cancer: Background and patient assessment. *Clinical Journal of Oncology Nursing, 6*(3), 163-167.

Tan, S. (2002). Recognition and treatment of oncologic emergencies. *Journal of Infusion Nursing, 25*(3), 182-188.

Tariman, J. (2003). Thalidomide: Current therapeutic uses and management of its toxicities. *Clinical Journal of Oncology Nursing, 7*(2), 143-147.

Tasota, F., & Tate, J. (2001). Interpreting the highs and lows of platelet counts. *Nursing2001, 31*(2), 25.

Tuinstra, N. (2003). Outpatient administration of radiolabeled monoclonal antibodies. *Clinical Journal of Oncology Nursing, 7*(1), 106.

Viele, C. (2002). Gemtuzumab ozogamicin. *Clinical Journal of Oncology Nursing, 6*(5), 298-299, 304.

Waxman, E., & Herbst, R. (2002). The role of the epidermal growth factor receptor in the treatment of colorectal carcinoma. *Seminars in Oncology Nursing, 18*(2, Suppl. 2), 20-29.

West, C., et al. (2003). The PRO-SELF: Pain control program–An effective approach for cancer pain management. *Oncology Nursing Forum, 30*(1), 65-73.

White, C. (2002). Painful lesions in a pancytopenic patient. *Clinical Journal of Oncology Nursing, 6*(1), 47-49, 51.

Whitman, M. (2001). Understanding the perceived need for complementary and alternative nutraceuticals: Lifestyle issues. *Clinical Journal of Oncology Nursing, 5*(5), 190-194.

Wilkes, G. (2002). New therapeutic options in colon cancer: Focus on oxaliplatin. *Clinical Journal of Oncology Nursing, 6*(3), 131-137.

Wilson, R. (2000). Optimizing nutrition for patients with cancer. *Clinical Journal of Oncology Nursing, 4*(1), 23-28.

Witt, J. (2002). Living with fatigue. *American Journal of Nursing, 102*(4), 28-31.

Workman, M.L. (2002). Breast cancer: New strategies to beat an old enemy. *Nursing2002, 32*(10), 58-63.

CHAPTER

29

Interventions for Clients with Infection

FRANK EDWARDS MYERS • GAYLE K. GILMORE

LEARNING OUTCOMES

After studying this chapter, you should be able to:

1. Explain the chain of infection.
2. Describe the principles of infection control in inpatient and community-based settings.
3. Identify the Centers for Disease Control and Prevention (CDC) hand hygiene recommendations for health care workers.
4. Differentiate the four types of transmission-based precautions.
5. Identify the major causes and results of inadequate antimicrobial therapy.
6. Assess the common clinical manifestations of infection.
7. Interpret laboratory test findings related to infections and infectious diseases.
8. Evaluate nursing interventions for management of the client with an infection.
9. Develop a teaching plan for clients who have an infection or infectious disease.

Go to your Student CD-ROM for Review Questions for the NCLEX Examination keyed to these Learning Outcomes.

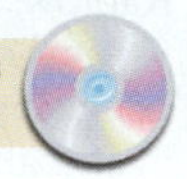

Infections and infectious diseases have been the major cause of millions of deaths worldwide for centuries. Today threats of bioterrorism have been added to the concerns about drug-resistant and re-emerging infections. Appropriately used, antibiotics and vaccines prevent many types of infection, but their utility is limited by misuse, cost, and distribution issues. World trade and people traveling and interacting with each other and their diversified environments cause exposure to a wider variety of infectious agents than in the past. Advancing technology and invasive procedures introduce microorganisms into the body, resulting in infection, even though in other environments these microorganisms are harmless. This chapter provides an overview of infection and general principles for prevention and management. Specific infections are described throughout this text.

OVERVIEW

Definitions

The infection process requires the following:

- Pathogen (agent)
- Portal of exit for the agent
- Means of transmission
- Portal of entry to the host
- Susceptible **host** (infection recipient)

A **pathogen** is any microorganism capable of producing disease. Infections can be **communicable** (transmitted from person to person, such as influenza) or not communicable (e.g., peritonitis). Microorganisms with differing levels of **pathogenicity** (ability to cause disease) surround everyone. **Virulence** is a term often used as a synonym for pathogenicity; however, virulence is related more to the frequency with which a pathogen causes disease (degree of communicability) and its ability to invade and damage a host. Virulence can also indicate the severity of the disease.

Many microorganisms live in or on the human host without causing disease. Some microbes are beneficial. Each body location harbors its own characteristic bacteria, or **normal flora.** Normal flora often functions to compete with and prevent infection from unfamiliar microorganisms attempting to invade a body site. In some instances, microorganisms that are often pathogenic may be present in the tissues of the host and yet not cause symptomatic disease; this process is called **colonization.**

In the United States, the Centers for Disease Control and Prevention (CDC) collect epidemiologic information about the occurrence and nature of infectious diseases. The CDC then makes recommendations to health care agencies for infection control and prevention. Certain diseases, such as tuberculosis, must be reported to health departments and the CDC. The Infection Control (IC) Officer for each health care agency is responsible for tracking infections and ensuring compliance with federal and local requirements.

Chain of Infection

The development of infection depends on a series of factors noted as the **chain of infection** (Figure 29-1). To prevent the spread of infection, the chain of infection must be broken at any point. Eliminating microorganisms, establishing host immunity, and interrupting transmission are examples of ways to break this chain.

RESERVOIR

Reservoirs (sources of infectious agents) are numerous. Animate reservoirs include people, animals, and insects. Inanimate reservoirs include soil, water, other environmental sources, or medical equipment (e.g., intravenous [IV] solutions and urine collection devices). The host's body can be a reservoir; pathogens colonize skin and body substances (e.g., feces, sputum, saliva, wound drainage). A person with an active infection or an asymptomatic **carrier** (one who harbors an infectious agent without active disease) is a reservoir. Examples of community reservoirs include sewage, stagnant or contaminated water, and improperly handled foods.

PATHOGEN

Several classes of microorganisms produce infection (Table 29-1). Bacteria like *Neisseria meningitidis* can exist in the respiratory tract while causing no illness, but if the bacteria invade the bloodstream or cerebrospinal fluid, the bacteria become extremely pathogenic. Another example is *Enterococcus,* which lives as normal flora in our gastrointestinal system, where it is nonpathogenic and assists in the digestive process; but if it enters the bloodstream, *Enterococcus* can cause disease.

Continued multiplication of a pathogen is sometimes accompanied by toxin production. **Toxins** are protein molecules released by bacteria to affect host cells at a distant site. **Exotoxins** are produced and released by certain bacteria into the surrounding environment. Botulism, tetanus, diphtheria, and *Escherichia coli* 0157:H7–related systemic diseases are attributed to exotoxins. **Endotoxins** are produced in the cell walls of certain bacteria and released only with cell lysis. Typhoid and meningococcal diseases are caused by endotoxins.

HOST

Host factors influence the development of infection (Table 29-2). Host defenses provide the body with an efficient system for protection against pathogens. Breakdown of these defense mechanisms may increase the **susceptibility** (risk) of the host to infection.

IMMUNITY. The client's immune status plays a large role in determining risk for infection. Congenital abnormalities, as well as acquired health problems (e.g., renal failure, steroid dependence, cancer, acquired immunodeficiency syndrome [AIDS]), can result in numerous immunologic deficiencies. Depression of the immune system may render the host more susceptible to infection or cripple the host's ability to combat organisms that have gained entry.

Immunity is resistance to infection; it is usually associated with the presence of antibodies or cells that act on specific microorganisms. **Passive immunity** is of short duration (days or months) and either natural by transplacental transfer from the mother or artificial by injection of antibodies (e.g., immune globulin). **Active immunity** lasts for years and is natural by infection or artificial by stimulation (e.g., vaccine) of the body's immune defenses. Chapter 23 discusses the immune system and immunity in detail.

Environmental factors can also influence clients' immune status and thus their susceptibility to or ability to fight infection. Examples include alcohol consumption, nicotine use, inhalation of bone marrow–suppressing toxic chemicals, and certain vitamin deficiencies. Malnutrition, especially protein-calorie malnutrition, places clients at increased risk for infection.

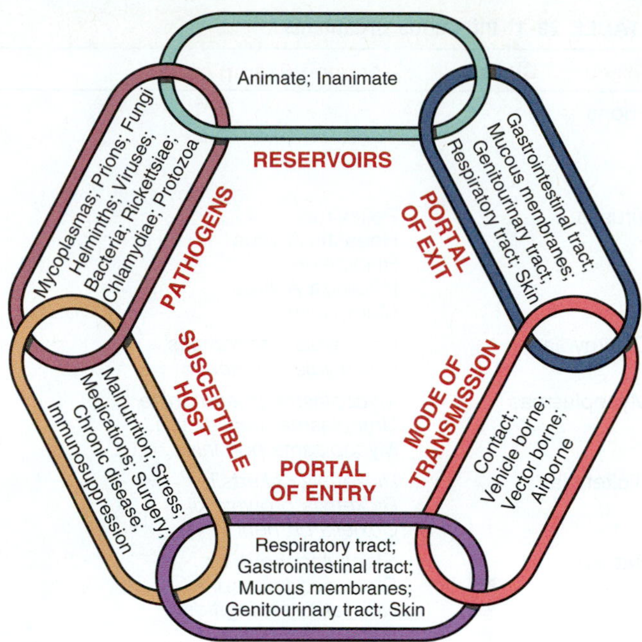

Figure 29-1 ■ The chain of infection: the process by which pathogens are transmitted from the environment to a host, invade the host, and cause infection.

Medical and surgical interventions may impair normal immune response. Steroid therapy, chemotherapy for malignant neoplasms, and cytotoxic therapy intended to suppress the immune response (e.g., cyclosporine in organ transplant recipients) increase the risk of infection. Medical devices (e.g., intravascular or urinary catheters, endotracheal tubes) may also interfere with normal host defense mechanisms. Surgery, trauma, and burns result in non-intact skin. *The body's skin is the best barrier or defense against infection.* When this barrier is broken, infection often results.

OTHER FACTORS. Hormonal factors play a role in the incidence and mortality rate of many infectious diseases. People with diabetes mellitus and adrenal insufficiency experience increased numbers of acute and chronic bacterial infections.

PORTAL OF ENTRY

Microorganisms may enter the body in a variety of ways (Table 29-3), and some specific sites of infection have key features.

RESPIRATORY TRACT. Pathogens may enter the body through the respiratory tract. Microbes in droplets are sprayed into the air when people with infected oral or nasal tissue talk, cough, or sneeze. A susceptible host then inhales droplets, and pathogens localize in the lungs or are distributed via the lymphatic system or bloodstream to other areas of the body. Microorganisms that enter the body by the respiratory tract and produce distant infection include influenza virus, *Mycobacterium tuberculosis,* and *Streptococcus pneumoniae.*

GASTROINTESTINAL TRACT. Some pathogens enter the body by ingestion through the gastrointestinal

TABLE 29-1 Infectious Organisms*

Organism Class	Common Examples	Common Disease Manifestations
Prions		Bovine spongiform encephalitis (BSE),† Creutzfeldt-Jakob disease, Kuru†
		Possible role in Alzheimer's disease, Parkinson disease, and amyotrophic lateral sclerosis (ALS)‡
Viruses	Poliovirus	Poliomyelitis
	Hepatitis A virus	Hepatitis
	Rhinovirus	Common cold
	Influenza A virus	Influenza
	Mumps virus	Mumps
Chlamydiae	*Chlamydia trachomatis*	Trachoma, lymphogranuloma venereum, conjunctivitis
	Chlamydia psittaci	Psittacosis (parrot fever)
Mycoplasmas	*Mycoplasma pneumoniae*	Pneumonia
	Ureaplasma urealyticum	Urethritis
	Mycoplasma hominis	Pyelonephritis, pelvic inflammatory disease
Rickettsiae	*Rickettsia rickettsii*	Rocky Mountain spotted fever
	Rickettsia prowazekii	Typhus
	Coxiella burnetii	Q fever
Bacteria	*Staphylococcus* sp.	Superficial skin infections, osteomyelitis, pneumonia, bacteremia
	Streptococcus sp.	Pharyngitis, skin infections, pneumonia
	Neisseria meningitidis	Meningitis
	Escherichia coli	Urinary tract infection
	Pseudomonas aeruginosa	Skin infection, otitis, urinary tract infection
Fungi	*Candida albicans*	Thrush, vaginitis
	Aspergillus sp.	Sinusitis, brain abscess
	Cryptococcus neoformans	Meningitis, pneumonia
	Histoplasma capsulatum	Pneumonia
	Coccidioides immitis	Pneumonia
Protozoa	*Entamoeba histolytica*	Diarrhea, colitis
	Plasmodium sp.	Malaria
	Leishmania sp.	Fever, weight loss, cutaneous lesions
	Toxoplasma gondii	Chorioretinitis, encephalitis
	Pneumocystis carinii	Pneumonia
Helminths	*Ancylostoma duodenale* (hookworm)	Anemia
	Ascaris lumbricoides (roundworm)	Intestinal obstruction
	Enterobius vermicularis (pinworm)	Anal pruritus
	Schistosoma sp. (blood flukes)	Hydronephrosis
	Taenia solium (pork tapeworm)	Epilepsy from cysticercosis

*Organisms are presented in order of increasing complexity.
†Prusiner, S. Nobelist believes prions may be at root of Alzheimer's, Parkinson's, ALS. *Reuter's health*, October 20, 1999; available at http://www.reutershealth.com. (Dr. Stanley Prusiner is a 1997 Nobel Prize winner for the discovery of prions.)
‡Mastrianni, J.A., & Roos, R.P. (2000). The prion diseases. *Seminars in Neurology*, *20*(3), 337-352.

TABLE 29-2 Host Factors That Influence the Development of Infection

Host Factor	Increased Risk of Infection
Natural immunity	Congenital or acquired immunodeficiencies
Normal flora	Alteration of normal flora by antibiotic therapy
Age	Infants and older clients
Hormonal factors	Pregnancy, diabetes, corticosteroid therapy, and adrenal insufficiency
Phagocytosis	Defective phagocytic function, circulatory disturbances, and neutropenia
Skin/mucous membranes/ normal excretory secretions	Break in skin or mucous membrane integrity; interference with flow of urine, tears, or saliva; interference with cough reflex or ciliary action; changes in gastric secretions
Nutrition	Malnutrition or dehydration
Environmental factors	Smoking, alcohol consumption, and inhalation of toxic chemicals
Medical interventions	Invasive therapy, chemotherapy, radiation therapy, and steroid therapy; surgery

(GI) tract. Some stay in the GI tract and produce disease (e.g., *Shigella* causing self-limited disease). Others invade the GI tract to produce local and distant infection (e.g., *Salmonella enteritidis*). Some produce limited GI symptoms, causing systemic infection (e.g., *Salmonella typhi*) or profound involvement of organs (e.g., hepatitis A virus). An estimated 76 million cases of foodborne illness in the United States occur each year. This type of illness results in 325,000 hospitalizations and 1,800 deaths every year (Centers for Disease Control and Prevention [CDC], 2003).

TABLE 29-3 Portals of Entry of Selected Disease-Producing Organisms

Infecting Organisms	Resultant Diseases
Respiratory Tract	
Neisseria meningitidis	Meningococcal pneumonia, meningococcal meningitis, meningococcemia
Cryptococcus neoformans	Cryptococcal meningitis, cryptococcal pneumonia
Mycobacterium tuberculosis	Tuberculosis
Influenza A virus	Influenza
Streptococcus pneumoniae	Pneumococcal pneumonia
Measles virus (rubeola)	Measles
Legionella pneumophila	Legionnaires' disease
Varicella-zoster virus	Chickenpox
Gastrointestinal Tract	
Salmonella enteritidis	Gastroenteritis
Salmonella typhi	Typhoid fever
Clostridium botulinum	Botulism
Poliovirus	Poliomyelitis
Hepatitis A virus	Hepatitis A
Escherichia coli 0157:H7	Possibly, hemolytic uremic syndrome
Genitourinary Tract	
Neisseria gonorrhoeae	Gonorrhea
Chlamydia trachomatis	Lymphogranuloma venereum, cervicitis, urethritis, endometritis
Enterobacteriaceae (*E. coli, Klebsiella sp., Serratia sp., Proteus sp.)*	Urinary tract infections
Intact Skin or Mucous Membranes	
Rhinovirus	Common cold
Respiratory syncytial virus	Pneumonia, bronchiolitis, tracheobronchitis
Schistosoma sp.	Schistosome dermatitis (swimmer's disease)
Herpes simplex virus	Oral or genital herpes
Bloodstream	
Hepatitis B or C viruses	Hepatitis B or C
Plasmodium sp.	Malaria
Clostridium tetani	Tetanus
Human immunodeficiency virus	Acquired immunodeficiency syndrome

GENITOURINARY TRACT. Microorganisms also enter through the genitourinary tract. Urinary tract infection (UTI) is one of the most common **health care–associated infections** (HAIs). More than 55% of clients in adult intensive care units (ICU) have urinary catheters in place. Indwelling urinary catheters are a primary cause of UTIs (National Nosocomial Infectious Surveillance, 2002a). The use of urinary catheters coated with silver alloy may reduce the risk of urinary tract infections (Saint et al., 2000).

WOMEN'S HEALTH CONSIDERATIONS

Women have a higher risk for UTIs than men because they have shorter urethras. Microorganisms (often colonic flora) colonize the perineal area, the urethral meatus and, potentially, the bladder. Older women are at even a greater risk because of decreased resistance to infection, stress incontinence, decreased thirst (causing dehydration), and in some cases the inability to use proper hygiene.

SKIN/MUCOUS MEMBRANES. While intact skin is the best barrier to prevent most infections, some pathogens, such as *Treponema pallidum,* can enter the body through intact skin or mucous membranes. Most enter through breaks in these normally effective surface barriers. Sometimes a medical procedure creates a break in cutaneous or mucocutaneous barriers, as in catheter-acquired **bacteremia** (bacteria in the bloodstream) and surgical-wound infections. Fragile skin of older clients and of those receiving prolonged steroid therapy increases infection risk.

BLOODSTREAM. Microorganisms can gain direct access to the bloodstream, especially when invasive devices or tubes are used. The National Nosocomial Infection Surveillance (NNIS) reported that for every 1000 days that central venous catheters are in place in medical/surgical and intensive care unit (ICU) clients, 4.8 infections result (NNIS, 2002b). As technology changes, improvements such as new materials for catheters reduce the risk of acquiring bloodstream infections. In the community setting, biting insects can inject organisms into the bloodstream, causing infection (e.g., Lyme disease and West Nile viral encephalitis).

MODE OF TRANSMISSION

For infection to be transmitted from an infected source to a susceptible host, a transport mechanism is required. Microorganisms are transmitted by several routes. The following are four common routes:

- Contact transmission
- Droplet transmission
- Airborne transmission
- Vector-borne transmission

CONTACT TRANSMISSION. Contact transmission is the usual mode of transmission of all infections. Many infections are spread by direct or indirect contact. With **direct contact,** the source and host have physical contact; microorganisms are transferred directly from skin to skin or from mucous membrane to mucous membrane. Often called person-to-person transmission, direct contact is best illustrated by the spread of the "common cold."

Indirect contact transmission involves the transfer of microorganisms from a source to a host by passive transfer from an inanimate object (a fomite). Contaminated articles may serve as sources of infection (e.g., the transfer of hepatitis B virus to a susceptible via a shared contaminated glucometer). **Fecal-oral transmission** is another route of transmitting infection. Ingestion of enteric pathogens (e.g., eating food prepared by a hepatitis A–infected person with unwashed hands) can result in disease transmission.

DROPLET TRANSMISSION. Indirect transmission may involve contact with infected secretions or **droplets.** Droplets are produced when a person talks or sneezes. These droplets travel short distances (less than 1 m). Susceptible hosts may acquire infection by contact with droplets deposited on the nasal, oral, or conjunctival membranes. An example of droplet-spread infection is influenza. Droplets, unlike airborne droplet nuclei, discussed below, do not stay suspended in the air.

AIRBORNE TRANSMISSION. Airborne transmission occurs when small airborne particles containing pathogens leave the infected source and enter a susceptible host. These pathogens can be suspended in the air for a prolonged time. The particles carrying pathogens are usually contained in droplet nuclei or dust; they are most often propelled from the respiratory tract by coughing or sneezing. A susceptible person then inhales the particles directly into the respiratory tract. Tuberculosis is communicated via airborne transmission.

VECTOR-BORNE TRANSMISSION. Vector-borne transmission of infection involves insects and animals as intermediaries between two or more hosts (e.g., ticks transmit Rocky Mountain spotted fever and Lyme disease; mosquitoes spread malaria). In these cases, the vector usually bites an infected source that has the pathogen. The vector then carries the pathogen and injects it into its new host.

PORTAL OF EXIT

The portal of exit completes the chain of infection. Exit of the microbe from the host often occurs through the portal of entry. An organism, such as *Mycobacterium tuberculosis,* enters the respiratory tract and then exits the respiratory tract as the infected host coughs. Some organisms can exit from the infected host by several routes. For example, varicella-zoster virus can spread through direct contact with infective fluid in vesicles and by airborne transmission.

Physiologic Defenses Against Infection

Strong and intact host defenses can prevent microbes from entering the body or destroy a pathogen that has entered. Conversely, impaired host defenses may be unable to defend against microbial invasion, allowing entry of microbes that can destroy cells and cause infection. Host defense mechanisms may be classified as nonspecific or specific.

NONSPECIFIC DEFENSES

Nonspecific mechanisms, usually representing the first encounter an invading pathogen has with its human host, include invasion of body tissues, such as skin and mucous membranes; phagocytosis; and inflammation.

BODY TISSUES. Intact skin forms the first and most important physical barrier to the entry of microorganisms. In addition to providing a mechanical barrier, the skin's slightly acidic pH (resulting from breakdown of lipids into fatty acids), together with normal skin flora, creates an unfriendly environment for many bacteria.

Mucous membranes' mucociliary action provides some mechanical protection against pathogenic invasion. More important, however, mucous membranes are bathed in secretions that inactivate many microorganisms. **Lysozymes,** which dissolve the cell walls of some bacteria, are present in large quantities in many body secretions, particularly in tears and nasal mucus.

Other body systems provide natural barriers to infection. The healthy respiratory tract clears about 90% of all inhaled material by upper airway filtration, humidification, mucociliary transport, and expulsion by coughing. Peristaltic action mechanically empties the gastrointestinal (GI) tract of pathogenic organisms. Stomach acid, intestinal secretions, pancreatic enzymes, and bile, together with the competition from normal bowel flora, provide an environment that protects the GI tract from invasion by harmful organisms. In the genitourinary tract, the flushing action of urine eliminates pathogenic organisms. The low pH of urine also maintains a sterile environment, although some microorganisms, such as *E. coli,* thrive in an acid medium.

PHAGOCYTOSIS. Phagocytosis occurs when a foreign substance evades the first-line mechanical barriers and enters the body. Various leukocyte types function differently in the immune reaction, but neutrophils bear primary responsibility for phagocytosis. This process of engulfing, ingesting, killing, and disposing of an invading organism is an essential mechanism in host defense. Phagocytic dysfunction dramatically increases a client's risk for infection.

INFLAMMATION. Inflammation is another important nonspecific defense mechanism in preventing the spread of infection. Inflammation occurs when tissue becomes damaged. Damaged cells release enzymes, and polymorphonuclear leukocytes are attracted to the infected site from the bloodstream. One important enzyme, histamine, increases the permeability of the capillaries in inflamed tissues, thus allowing fluid, proteins, and white blood cells to enter an inflamed area. Other enzymes activate fibrinogen, which causes leaked fluid to clot and prevents its flow away from the damaged site into unaffected tissue, essentially "walling off" the inflamed tissue. The process of phagocytosis disposes of the invading microorganism and often dead tissue. If inflammation is caused by infection, the end products of inflammation form pus, which is subsequently absorbed or exits the body through a break in the skin. Chapter 23 discusses the process of inflammation in more detail.

SPECIFIC DEFENSES

Specific defense responses to specific microorganisms are provided by the antibody- and cell-mediated immune systems. The **antibody-mediated immune system** produces antibodies directed against certain pathogens. These antibodies inactivate or destroy invading microorganisms as well as protect against future infection from that microorganism. Resistance to other microorganisms is mediated by the action of specifically sensitized T-lymphocytes and is called **cell-mediated immunity.** The components of the immune system work both independently and together to protect against infection. Chapter 23 describes the function of the immune system in detail.

HEALTH PROMOTION/ILLNESS PREVENTION

Infection Control in Inpatient Health Care Agencies

Infections occur most often in high-risk clients, such as older adults and those who have inadequate immune systems (immunocompromised). Physiologic and other factors contribute to infection risk in older adults (Chart 29-1). Implement interventions to prevent infection and detect signs and symptoms as early as possible. Chart 29-2 summarizes nursing interventions for Infection Protection.

Infection acquired in the inpatient health care setting (not present or incubating at admission) is termed **nosocomial,** or **health care–associated infection (HAI).** HAIs can be **endogenous** (from a client's flora) or **exogenous** (from outside the client, often from the hands of health care workers). Therefore, use of the term *nosocomial infection* does

CHART 29-1

NURSING FOCUS on the OLDER ADULT

Factors That May Increase Risk of Infection in the Older Client

Factor	Aging-Associated Changes or Conditions
Immune system	Decreased antibody production, lymphocytes, and fever response
Integumentary system	Thinning skin, decreased subcutaneous tissue, decreased vascularity, slower wound healing
Respiratory system	Decreased cough and gag reflexes
Gastrointestinal system	Decreased gastric acid and intestinal motility
Chronic illness	Diabetes mellitus, chronic obstructive pulmonary disease, neurologic impairments
Functional/cognitive impairments	Immobility, incontinence, dementia
Invasive devices	Urinary catheters, feeding tubes, IV devices, tracheostomies
Institutionalization	Increased person-to-person contact and transmission

CHART 29-2

NIC INTERVENTION ACTIVITIES for

The Client at Risk for Infection

Infection Protection: *Prevention and early detection of infection in a client at risk*

- Monitor for systemic and localized signs and symptoms of infection.
- Monitor vulnerability to infection.
- Monitor absolute granulocyte count, WBC count, and differential results.
- Screen all visitors for communicable disease.
- Inspect skin and mucous membranes for redness, extreme warmth, or drainage.
- Obtain cultures, as needed.
- Promote sufficient nutritional intake.
- Encourage fluid intake, as appropriate.
- Teach the client and family about signs and symptoms of infections and when to report them to the health care provider.
- Teach client and family members how to avoid infections.

NIC intervention activities selected from Dochterman, J.M., & Bulechek, G.M. (Eds.). (2004). *Nursing interventions classification (NIC)* (4th ed.). St. Louis: Mosby. No part of this work is to be altered without prior written permission from the Publisher.
WBC, White blood cell.

not imply that an infection was caused by health care (or poor health care delivery) but only that it occurred while receiving health care. HAIs are acquired by about two million inpatients yearly, causing 88,000 deaths with a cost of about $4.6 billion annually (CDC, 2000). Clients who develop nosocomial surgical site infection (SSI) have longer and more costly hospitalizations, are 60% more likely to spend time in an intensive care unit (ICU) and are twice as likely to die as those who do not have an SSI (Kirkland et al., 1999). Although the exact causes of HAIs are difficult to identify, it is estimated that about one third of them could be prevented using the recommended CDC infection control interventions (Harbarth, Sax, & Gastmeier, 2003).

Infection control within a health care facility is designed to reduce the risk of HAIs and thus reduce morbidity and mortality. Infection control and prevention programs include the following:

- Facility- and department-specific infection control policies and procedures
- Surveillance and analysis
- Client and staff education
- Community and multidisciplinary networking
- Product evaluation with an emphasis on quality and cost savings

Monitoring HAIs promotes client safety, as evidenced by the decreased rate in ICUs during 1990 and 1999 (CDC, 2000). The program is usually coordinated and implemented by a health care professional certified in infection control (CIC) who has varied clinical and administrative experience.

Infection Control in Community-Based Settings

The Association for Professionals in Infection Control and Epidemiology (APIC) and the Society for Healthcare Epidemiology of America (SHEA) consensus panel have published requirements for activities of infection control and epidemiology in community-based settings (Friedman et al., 1999). Three primary goals were noted:

- To protect the client
- To protect health care providers, visitors, and others in the health care environment
- To accomplish these goals in a timely, efficient, and cost-effective manner

Of special note are the CDC guidelines for pregnant health care personnel.

The goals for infection control and epidemiology are the same for all health care settings. Functions of infection control and epidemiology, including the following principal functions, were summarized by the APIC and SHEA consensus report:

- To obtain and manage critical data, including infection surveillance
- To develop and recommend policies and procedures
- To intervene directly to prevent infections
- To educate and train health care workers, clients, and nonmedical caregivers

Methods of Infection Control

All health care workers who come in contact with clients or care areas are involved in some aspect of the infection control program of the agency. Infections can be prevented or controlled in at least three ways:

- Hand hygiene
- Disinfection/sterilization
- Barriers (e.g., gloves; see discussion of transmission precautions)

HAND HYGIENE

Health care workers' hands are the primary way in which disease is transmitted from client to client. In 2002 the Centers for Disease Control and Prevention (CDC) released a document entitled "CDC Hand Hygiene Recommendations." These recommendations are summarized in Chart

29-3. Handwashing is still an important part of hand hygiene, but it is recognized that in some health care settings, sinks may not be readily available. Despite years of education, health care workers often find it difficult to leave the client care setting to wash their hands. Effective **handwashing** includes wetting, soaping, lathering, applying friction under running water for at least 15 seconds, rinsing, and adequate drying. Friction is essential to emulsify skin oils and to disperse transient bacteria and soil from hand surfaces. The time it takes for health care workers to leave the client care area, find a sink, get the water temperature correct, wash their hands, and dry them was one reason why poor hand hygiene existed long after definitive evidence showed that it was essential to quality care. Handwashing can also cause dry skin, and therefore hand lotions are essential to maintain good hand health and hygiene.

Alcohol-based hand rubs have allowed care providers to spend less time seeking out sinks and more time delivering care. Nevertheless, hand rubs have their limitations. If your hands are visibly dirty, soiled, or feel sticky or you have just toileted, wash your hands instead of using alcohol-based rubs. Alcohol-based hands rubs are also ineffective against spore-forming organisms such as *Clostridium difficile,* a common cause of health care–associated diarrhea, especially in older adults taking antibiotics.

The CDC recommends the use of antiseptic solutions such as chlorhexidine, povidone-iodine, or PCMX, for handwashing in the care of clients who are at high risk (e.g., immunocompromised clients). The use of these solutions is also recommended after caring for clients who are infected with multiply resistant or other virulent organisms.

ARTIFICIAL FINGERNAILS. The CDC guidelines (2002) also addressed the issue of artificial fingernails, which have been linked to a number of outbreaks due to poor fingernail health and hygiene. The guidelines recommended that artificial fingernails and extenders not be worn during the provision of caring for clients at high risk for infections, such as those in ICUs or operating suites. Some health care agencies have banned artificial nails for all health care workers in any client care unit or clinical department. The Joint Commission on Accreditation of Healthcare Organizations has incorporated the CDC guidelines into their 2004 National Patient Safety Goals.

GLOVES. Gloves are an essential part of infection control and should be worn as part of Standard Precautions. However, gloves are not impervious barriers. Either handwashing or use of alcohol-based hand rubs should be done after removing gloves.

Most health care settings in the United States and Canada have switched from latex to non-latex gloves. The National Institute of Occupational Safety and Health (NIOSH) issued a public warning about potential allergic reactions to those exposed to latex in gloves and other medical products. Reactions include rashes, nasal or eye symptoms, asthma, and (rarely) shock (NIOSH, 1998). People with **latex allergy** usually have an allergy to foods such as bananas, kiwis, and avocados. Hands should be washed after removal of latex gloves to minimize contact time between the skin and proteins in the gloves that may cause allergic reactions.

CHART 29-3

BEST PRACTICE for Hand Hygiene

- When hands are visibly soiled or contaminated with proteinaceous material or are visibly soiled with blood or other body fluids, wash hands with soap and water.
- If hands are not visibly soiled, use an alcohol-based hand rub for decontaminating hands or wash hands with soap and water.
- Use either alcohol-based hand rub or wash with soap and water (decontaminate hands) before having direct contact with clients.
- Decontaminate hands before donning sterile gloves to perform a procedure, such as inserting an invasive device (e.g., indwelling urinary catheter).
- Decontaminate hands after contact with a client's intact skin (e.g., taking a pulse) or with body fluids or excretions/ secretions.
- Decontaminate hands after removing gloves.
- Decontaminate hands after contact with inanimate objects (including medical equipment) in the immediate vicinity of the client.

Data from CDC Hand Hygiene Recommendations (2002).

DISINFECTION/STERILIZATION

Sterilization and disinfection have allowed invasive procedures to become much more common and safe. **Sterilization** means destroying all living organisms and bacterial spores. All items that invade human tissue where bacteria are not commonly found should be sterilized. **Disinfection** does not kill spores and only ensures a reduction in the level of disease-causing organisms. High-level disinfection is adequate when an item is going into an internal area of the body where the client has resident bacteria or normal flora (e.g., GI and respiratory tracts). As with sterilization, no high-level disinfection can occur without first cleaning the item. This can be especially difficult with items that have narrow lumens where organic debris can become trapped and are not easily visible. For example, endoscopes have been especially challenging to clean and have been linked to a number of infectious outbreaks.

CENTERS FOR DISEASE CONTROL AND PREVENTION TRANSMISSION-BASED GUIDELINES

PRECAUTIONS. The isolation guidelines from the Centers for Disease Control and Prevention (CDC) focus on transmission mechanisms and combine the best aspects of previous guidelines. Included in these guidelines are standard, airborne, droplet, and contact precautions.

Standard precautions acknowledge that all body excretions, secretions, and moist membranes and tissues, excluding perspiration, are potentially infectious. The protective measures from universal precautions and body-substance isolation are combined. Table 29-4 outlines the guidelines for standard precautions. Table 29-5 notes which body fluids have the highest risk for transmission of bloodborne disease.

Airborne precautions are used for clients known or suspected to have infections transmitted by the airborne transmission route; such infections are caused by organisms that can be suspended in air for prolonged periods. Negative airflow rooms are required to prevent airborne spread of microbes. Enclosed booths with high-efficiency particulate air (HEPA) filtration or ultraviolet light may be used for sputum induction procedures. Tuberculosis, measles (rubeola), and chickenpox (varicella) are examples of airborne diseases (Table 29-6).

Droplet precautions are used for clients known or suspected to have infections transmitted by the droplet transmission route. Such infections are caused by organisms in droplets that may travel 3 feet but are not suspended for long time periods. Examples of infectious conditions requiring droplet precautions include influenza, mumps, pertussis, and meningitis caused by either *Neisseria meningitidis* or *Haemophilus influenzae* type B (see Table 29-6).

Contact precautions are used for clients known or suspected to have infections transmitted by direct contact or contact with items in the client's environment. Clients with significant multidrug-resistant organism infection or colonization, such as methicillin-resistant *Staphylococcus aureus* [MRSA] or vancomycin-resistant *Enterococcus* [VRE], are placed on contact precautions. Other infections requiring contact precautions include pediculosis, scabies, respiratory syncytial virus (RSV), and *Clostridium difficile* (see Table 29-6).

MULTIDRUG-RESISTANT INFECTIONS. It is important to note that MRSA and VRE are no more transmissible than their drug-sensitive counterparts, *S. aureus* and *Enterococcus* organisms. The precautions in these cases are due to the implications for clients if they acquire these infections. Containment of drug-resistant organisms is an area in which there is currently much debate.

The CDC suggests a 12-step program to control antimicrobial resistance in health care settings. Those steps are based on preventing infections, diagnosing and treating infections effectively, using antimicrobials wisely, and preventing transmission of these microbes. In addition to infection control measures to prevent infection transmission, the CDC recommends that nurses educate clients about protection against influenza and pneumonia through immunization. Specific interventions for caring for clients with indwelling urinary catheters were also included in the 12-step program.

TABLE 29-4 Standard Precautions

These precautions are to be used with all clients to protect all health care workers from contracting or transmitting communicable disease:

- *Gloves* should be worn for contact with all body fluids, moist body tissues and mucous membranes, and nonintact skin of all clients; for handling *o*ther *p*otentially *i*nfectious *m*aterials (OPIM), items, or surfaces; and for performing venipuncture and other vascular access procedures. Gloves should be changed after each client contact.
- *Masks and/or protective eyewear* should be worn during procedures that are likely to cause splashes of body fluids.
- *Gowns or aprons* should be worn during procedures likely to result in splashes of blood or body fluids.
- *Handwashing* should be done immediately on contact with body fluids or OPIM. Hands should be washed as soon as gloves are removed.
- *Needles and sharp instruments* should be placed in puncture-resistant containers for disposal to prevent injuries from needles or other sharp items. Needles should not be recapped, bent, or removed from syringe.
- *Mouth-to-mouth resuscitation* should be performed with use of mouthpieces or other ventilation devices.

Modified from Garner, J.S., & Hospital Infection Control Practices Advisory Committee (HICPAC). (1996). Guidelines for isolation precautions in hospitals. *American Journal of Infection Control, 24*, 24-52.

TABLE 29-5 Transmission of Bloodborne Disease by Various Body Fluids

Body Fluids Likely to Transmit Bloodborne Disease

- Blood and other body fluids containing visible blood
- Semen and vaginal/cervical secretions
- Tissues
- Cerebrospinal fluid
- Amniotic fluid
- Synovial fluid
- Pleural fluid
- Peritoneal fluid
- Pericardial fluid
- Breast milk—from mother to child

Body Fluids Not Likely to Transmit Bloodborne Disease Unless Blood is Visible

- Feces
- Nasal secretions
- Sputum
- Vomitus
- Sweat
- Tears
- Urine
- Saliva, except in oral surgery or dentistry

Occupational Exposure to Sources of Infection

The Occupational Safety and Health Administration (OSHA) is a federal agency that protects workers from injury or illness at their place of employment. Unlike the voluntary guidelines developed by the CDC, OSHA regulations are law. Employers can be fined or disciplined for noncompliance with OSHA regulations. The regulation for prevention of exposure to bloodborne pathogens, such as hepatitis B and C or the human immunodeficiency virus (HIV), is one example of an OSHA regulation.

Reduction of skin and soft tissue injuries (e.g., needle sticks) is of utmost importance to reduce bloodborne pathogen transmission to health care personnel. OSHA mandates that sharp objects ("sharps") and needles be handled with care. Availability and consistency in the use of protective devices are vital. Almost half of contaminated sharp-object exposures involve nurses. Needleless devices have helped to decrease these exposures, especially when caring for clients receiving infusion therapy (see Chapter 17).

Problems from Inadequate Antimicrobial Therapy

Inadequate antimicrobial therapy may range from an incorrect choice of antibiotics to poor compliance. Some infections relapse in a subtle fashion. Drug regimen **noncompliance** (deliberate failure to take medication) or **nonadherence** (accidental failure to take medication) prevents contact of harmful microorganisms with sufficient concentrations of antibiotics and contributes to resistant-organism development.

Some diseases have legal sanctions that compel a client to complete treatment. Tuberculosis (TB) is the most common disease that has such a requirement. Clients who are at risk for noncompliance with an anti-TB drug regimen may be placed on **directly observed therapy** (DOT). This means that a health care worker must observe and validate client compliance with the drug regimen. DOT has been very effective at reducing the spread of multidrug resistant TB.

TABLE 29-6 Transmission-Based Infection Control Precautions*

Precautions (In Addition to Standard Precautions)	Examples of Diseases in Category
Airborne Precautions 1. Private room with monitored negative airflow (with appropriate number of air exchanges and air discharge to outside or through HEPA); keep door(s) closed 2. Special respiratory protection: N-95† or HEPA† respirator for known or suspected TB Susceptible persons not to enter room of client with known or suspected measles or varicella unless immune caregivers are not available Susceptible persons who must enter room must wear N-95 or HEPA 3. Transport: client to leave room only for essential clinical reasons, wearing surgical mask	Diseases that are known or suspected to be transmitted by air: Measles (rubeola) *M. tuberculosis*, including multidrug-resistant TB (MDRTB) Varicella (chickenpox)‡; disseminated zoster (shingles)‡
Droplet Precautions 1. Private room: if not available, may cohort with client with same active infection with same microorganisms if no other infection present; maintain distance of at least 3 feet from other clients if private room not available 2. Mask: required when working within 3 feet of client 3. Transport: as above	Diseases that are known or suspected to be transmitted by droplets: Diphtheria (pharyngeal) Streptococcal pharyngitis Pneumonia Scarlet fever (in infants or young children) Influenza Rubella Invasive disease (meningitis, pneumonia, sepsis) caused by *Haemophilus influenzae* type B or *Neisseria meningitidis* Mumps Pertussis
Contact Precautions 1. Private room: if not available, may cohort with client with same active infection with same microorganisms if no other infection present 2. Wear gloves when entering room 3. Wash hands with antimicrobial soap before leaving client's room 4. Wear gown to prevent contact with client or client-contaminated items or if client has uncontrolled body fluids; remove gown before leaving room 5. Transport: client to leave room only for essential clinical reasons; during transport, use needed precautions to prevent disease transmission 6. Dedicated equipment for this client only (or disinfect after use before taking from room)	Diseases that are known or suspected to be transmitted by direct contact: *Clostridium difficile* Colonization or infection caused by multidrug-resistant organisms (e.g., MRSA, VRE) Pediculosis Respiratory syncytial virus Scabies Viral hemorrhagic infections (Ebola, Lassa, or Marburg)

Modified from Garner, J.S., & Hospital Infection Control Practices Advisory Committee (HICPAC). (1996). Guidelines for isolation precautions in hospitals. *American Journal of Infection Control, 24*, 24-52.
HEPA, High-efficiency particulate air filter; *MRSA*, methicillin-resistant *Staphylococcus aureus; TB*, tuberculosis; *VRE*, vancomycin-resistant *Enterococcus*.
*Modification by facilities: The Centers for Disease Control and Prevention encourages facilities to adapt these guidelines, still following sound epidemiologic principles (e.g., some have removed TB transmission prevention guidelines from the airborne precautions category and added a separate category).
†Before use: training and fit testing required for personnel.
‡Add contact precautions for draining lesions.

Serious complications of infection may also result from incomplete or inadequate antibiotic therapy. Local infections that could be cured without complications, such as cellulitis and pneumonia, may progress to abscess formation if appropriate drug therapy is not continued. Although antibiotics do not always prevent abscess, early therapy may prevent or limit the size of an abscess.

In addition to abscess formation, inadequate therapy may promote systemic complications. If the infection is not resolved, or if it is treated with drugs that are ineffective for the offending microorganism, the pathogen may enter the bloodstream. Inadequately treated small local infections may also spread to produce complications, such as **septicemia** (systemic sepsis) with leukocytosis (increased white blood cell count) or leukopenia (decreased white blood cell count) and disseminated intravascular coagulation (DIC). After pathogens invade the bloodstream, no site is protected from invasion.

Systemic sepsis may progress to **septic shock,** more accurately called sepsis-induced distributive shock. In septic shock, insufficient cardiac output is compounded by hypovolemia; inadequate blood supply to vital organs leads to hypoxia (lack of oxygen) and metabolic failure. Chapter 40 describes this type of shock and its management in detail.

COLLABORATIVE MANAGEMENT

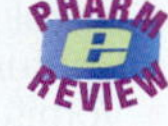

Assessment

HISTORY

Careful attention to the history of a client with a possible infectious disease will help you determine risk factors for infection. The age of the client, a history of cigarette smoking or alcohol use, current illness or disease (such as diabetes), past and current medication use (such as steroids), familial predisposition, and poor nutritional status may place him or her at increased risk for a number of infectious diseases. Ask the client about previous vaccinations or immunizations, including the dates of administration.

Determine whether the client has been exposed to infectious agents. A history of recent exposure to someone with similar clinical symptoms or to contaminated food or water, as well as the time of exposure, assists in identifying a possible source of infection. This information will be helpful in determining the incubation period for the disease and thus for providing a clue to its cause.

Contact with animals, including pets, may facilitate exposure to infection. Question the client about recent animal contact at home or work or in leisure activities (e.g., hunting). Insect bites should be documented.

A travel history should also be obtained. Travel to areas both within and outside the client's home country may expose a susceptible client to infectious organisms not encountered in the local community.

A thorough sexual history may reveal behavior associated with an increased risk of sexually transmitted diseases. Obtain a history of IV drug use and a transfusion history to assess the client's risk for hepatitis B, hepatitis C, and HIV infections.

Identifying the type and location of symptoms may point to affected organ systems. The onset order of symptoms gives clues to the specific problem. Gathering a history of past infection or colonization with multidrug-resistant organisms will allow for proper initiation of isolation.

PHYSICAL ASSESSMENT/CLINICAL MANIFESTATIONS

Disorders caused by pathogens vary, depending on the infection cause and site. Common clinical manifestations are associated with specific sites of infection. Carefully inspect the skin for symptoms of local infection at any site (pain, swelling, heat, redness, or pus). Wounds can become infected because the integrity of the skin is violated.

Fever (generally a temperature above 101° F [38° C]), chills, and malaise are primary indicators of a systemic infection. Fever may accompany other noninfectious disorders, and infection can be present without fever. The older adult, whose normal temperature may be 1° to 2° lower than the normal temperature in younger adults, may manifest fever at 99° F (37° C). In a client with an infection, fever (hyperthermia) is a normal immune response that can help eliminate the pathogen. Assess the client for these symptoms and carefully ask about the history and pattern of symptoms.

Lymphadenopathy, photophobia, pharyngitis, and gastrointestinal (GI) disturbance (usually diarrhea or vomiting) are often associated with infection. To detect enlargement, palpate the cervical, axillary, and other lymph nodes; examine the throat for redness.

PSYCHOSOCIAL ASSESSMENT

The client with an infectious disease often has psychosocial concerns. Delay in diagnosis because of the need to await clinical test results produces anxiety. Assess the client's level of understanding about various diagnostic procedures and the time required to obtain test results. Plan education on risk reduction or harm minimization for a time in which the client is receptive to education and motivated.

Feelings of malaise and fatigue often accompany infection. Assess the client's current level of activity and the impact of these symptoms on family, occupational, and recreational activities.

The potential spread of infection to others is an additional stress associated with the diagnosis of infection. The client may curtail family and social interactions for fear of spreading the illness. Determine the client's and family's understanding of the infection, the mode of transmission, and mechanisms that may limit or prevent transmission. Isolation, although sometimes necessary for preventing transmission of the organism, can be emotionally difficult for the client and family. Loss of contact with job and social gatherings can lead to depression, which may result in a weakening of the immune system.

Finally, a number of transmissible infectious diseases, especially those identified with socially stigmatized behaviors (such as IV drug abuse), are associated with some degree of social labeling. The client may feel socially isolated and may experience guilt related to behavior that increased the risk for infection. Observe the client carefully for signs of the client's reaction to social labels and how these feelings further affect socialization.

LABORATORY ASSESSMENT

The definitive diagnosis of an infectious disease requires identification of a microorganism in the tissues of an infected client in the presence of symptoms of the disease caused by that organism. Direct examination of blood, body fluids, and tissues under a microscope in the laboratory may not yield a definitive identification; however, laboratory assessment usually provides helpful information about microorganisms, such as shape, motility, and reaction to staining agents. Even when direct microscopy does not provide a conclusive specific diagnosis, often enough information is gathered for initiating appropriate antibiotic therapy.

CULTURE AND SENSITIVITY. The most definitive procedure for identification of a microorganism is **culture,** or isolation of the pathogen by cultivation in tissue cultures or artificial media. Specimens for culture can be obtained from almost any body fluid or tissue. The health care provider usually decides when and where the specimen for culture is taken. It is important to note, however, that sometimes a well-intentioned specimen acquisition can result in poor client care.

Proper collection and handling of specimens for culture, following standard precautions, are essential for obtaining accurate results. Specimens collected must be appropriate for the suspected infection. Material must be of adequate quantity, freshly obtained and placed in a sterile container to preserve the specimen and microorganism, and properly labeled.

After isolation of a microorganism in culture, antibiotic **sensitivity** testing is usually performed to determine the effects of various antibiotics on that particular microorganism. A microorganism that is killed by acceptable levels of an antibiotic is considered sensitive to that drug. An organism that is not killed by tolerable levels of an antibiotic is considered resistant to that drug. Preliminary results are usually available in 24 to 48 hours, but the final results generally take 72 hours. Antibiotic therapy should not begin until after the culture specimen is obtained.

COMPLETE BLOOD COUNT. A complete blood count (CBC) is often done for the client with a suspected infection. Five types of leukocytes (white blood cells) have been identified:

- Neutrophils
- Lymphocytes
- Monocytes
- Eosinophils
- Basophils

In most active infections, especially those caused by bacteria, the total leukocyte count is elevated. Various diseases are characterized by changes in the percentages of the different types of leukocytes. The differential count most often shows an increased number of immature neutrophils, or a **shift to the left.** A few infectious diseases, however, such as malaria and infectious mononucleosis, are associated with neutropenia (decreased neutrophils).

ERYTHROCYTE SEDIMENTATION RATE. The erythrocyte sedimentation rate (ESR) measures the rate at which red blood cells fall through plasma. This rate is most significantly affected by an increased number of acute-phase reactants, which occurs with inflammation. Thus an elevated ESR (>20 mm/hr) indicates inflammation or infection somewhere in the body. Chronic infection, most notably osteomyelitis, and chronic abscesses are commonly associated with an elevated ESR. The ESR is chronically elevated with arthritis as well. The effectiveness of therapy is often monitored by a decrease in this value.

SEROLOGIC TESTING. Serologic testing is performed to identify pathogens by detecting antibodies to the organism. The antibody titer tends to increase during the acute phase of infectious diseases such as hepatitis B. The titer decreases as the client improves.

RADIOGRAPHIC ASSESSMENT

X-ray films are often obtained to determine activity or destruction by an infectious microorganism. Radiologic studies (such as chest films, sinus films, joint films, GI studies, and renal films) are typically done for diagnosis of infection in a specific body site.

OTHER DIAGNOSTIC ASSESSMENTS

More sophisticated techniques for infection diagnosis include computed tomography (CT) scans and magnetic resonance imaging (MRI). Tomography is helpful in assessing for abscesses. CT scans help identify suspected osteomyelitis and fluid collections that point to possible infection. MRI scans provide a cross-sectional assessment for infection.

Another diagnostic tool for the evaluation of a client with an infectious disease is ultrasonography. This noninvasive procedure is particularly helpful in detecting infection involving the heart valves.

Scanning techniques using radioactive substances, such as gallium, can determine the presence of inflammation. Inflammatory tissue is identified by its increased uptake of the injected radioactive material.

Biopsy of the infected site may be needed for tissue culture. Biopsy sites may include the liver, bone marrow, skin, pleura, lymph nodes, kidney, bone, or even the brain. To obtain specimens, invasive procedures (e.g., bronchoscopy or endoscopy) or surgery (e.g., open lung biopsy or laparotomy) may be necessary.

Analysis

COMMON NURSING DIAGNOSES AND COLLABORATIVE PROBLEMS

The following are priority nursing diagnoses for clients with an infection or infectious disease:

1. Hyperthermia related to an increased metabolic state
2. Risk for Social Isolation related to altered state of wellness

The inclusion of other nursing diagnoses depends on the type and extent of the infection. For example, a client with pneumonia might experience Ineffective Airway Clearance and Fatigue; a client with a sexually transmitted disease may have Altered Sexuality Patterns.

ADDITIONAL NURSING DIAGNOSES AND COLLABORATIVE PROBLEMS

In addition to the priority nursing diagnoses, clients with an infection or infectious disease may have one or more of the following:

- Acute Pain related to physical injury
- Fatigue related to disease state
- Risk for Deficient Fluid Volume related to hypermetabolic state

The primary additional collaborative problem is Risk for Sepsis, Septic Shock, and Disseminated Intravascular Coagulation (DIC).

Planning and Implementation

HYPERTHERMIA

NOC **PLANNING: EXPECTED OUTCOMES.** The client with an infection or infectious disease is expected to have a balance of heat production, heat gain, and heat loss. Indicators include that the client will have noncompromised:

- Sweating when hot
- Shivering when cold
- Apical heart rate
- Respiratory rate
- Reported thermal comfort

INTERVENTIONS. The primary concern is to provide measures to eliminate the underlying cause of hyperthermia (fever) and to destroy the causative microorganism. In collaboration with the health care team, nurses use a variety of methods to manage fever.

Drug Therapy. Drug therapy plays a major role in collaborative management of clients with infection. Antimicrobials, also called anti-infective agents, are the cornerstone of drug therapy. Antipyretics are used to decrease client discomfort and prevent fever from worsening.

Antimicrobial Therapy. Antibiotics, antiviral agents, and antifungals are common types of antimicrobials. The sulfonamides, the first antibiotic group, were used in the mid-1930s. Shortly thereafter, in the 1940s, penicillin became the primary antibiotic used systemically. Since then, a wide variety of antimicrobial drugs have been developed for treatment, as well as prevention, of infection associated with virtually every class of microorganism. Effective antibiotics are available to treat nearly all bacterial infections, but misuse of antibiotics has contributed to the development of antibiotic-resistant bacteria. A few effective antifungal agents have been developed, but these drugs generally exhibit more toxicity than antibacterial agents. Effective agents are currently available for the treatment of influenza type A virus infection and HIV, but some viruses, such as HIV, mutate rapidly; thus these agents have a limited duration of effectiveness.

Effective antimicrobial therapy requires delivery of an appropriate agent, sufficient dosage, proper administration route, and sufficient therapy duration. These four requirements ensure delivery of a concentration of drug sufficient to inhibit or kill infecting microorganisms. Health care providers collaborate on selecting drugs and dosing. Teach the drug's actions, side effects, and toxic effects to your clients. Antimicrobials act on susceptible pathogens by doing the following:

- Inhibiting cell wall synthesis (penicillins and cephalosporins)
- Injuring the cytoplasmic membrane (antifungal agents)
- Inhibiting biosynthesis, or reproduction (erythromycin, tetracycline, and gentamicin)
- Inhibiting nucleic acid synthesis (actinomycin)

Observe and report side effects and toxic effects. These adverse reactions vary according to the specific classification of the drug. Most antibiotics can cause nausea, vomiting, and rashes. Before administering an antimicrobial agent, check to see that the prescribed drug is not one to which the client is allergic (Table 29-7). An accurate allergy history before drug therapy begins is essential.

Antipyretic Therapy. Antipyretic drugs, such as aspirin (ASA, Ancasal✱) and acetaminophen (Tylenol, Ace-Tabs✱), are given to reduce hyperthermia. Because antipyretics mask fever, monitoring the course of the disease may be difficult. Therefore, unless the client is extremely uncomfortable or if hyperthermia presents a significant risk (e.g., in the client with heart failure, febrile seizures, or head injury), antipyretics are not always prescribed.

Be alert for waves of sweating after each dose. Sweating may be accompanied by a fall in blood pressure followed by return of fever. These unpleasant side effects of antipyretic therapy can often be alleviated by liberal administration of fluids and by regular scheduling of drug administration.

NIC ***Fever Treatment.*** Other interventions to reduce fever may include external cooling and fluid administration. Performing a thorough assessment before and after interventions are implemented is essential (Chart 29-4).

External Cooling. Cooling or hypothermia blankets, or ice bags and packs, can be effective external mechanisms for reducing fever. Alternative cooling methods may be used. Sponging the client's body with tepid water or saline solution or applying cool compresses to the skin and pulse points to reduce body temperature is sometimes helpful. Observe the client for shivering during any form of external cooling. Shivering may indicate that the client is being cooled too quickly.

The use of fans is discouraged because they can disperse airborne- or droplet-transmitted pathogens. Fans can also disturb air balance in negative pressure rooms, making them positive pressure rooms and allowing possible transmission of the agent to those outside the room.

Fluid Administration. In clients with fever, fluid volume loss is increased from rapid evaporation of body fluids and increased perspiration. As body temperature increases, fluid volume loss increases. Therefore the client may be at risk for deficient fluid volume, or *dehydration.* Monitor carefully for signs of dehydration, such as increased thirst, decreased skin turgor, dry mucous membranes, and disorientation, especially in older adults. Increase oral fluid intake and provide IV fluids as prescribed. Chapter 15 discusses interventions for dehydration in detail.

TABLE 29-7 Allergic Reactions to Antibiotic Therapy

- Flushing
- Wheezing
- Sneezing
- Pruritus
- Urticaria
- Rashes
- Maculopapular to exfoliative dermatitis
- Vascular eruptions
- Erythema multiforme (Stevens-Johnson syndrome)
- Angioneurotic edema
- Serum sickness (headache, fever, chills, hives, malaise, and conjunctivitis)
- Anaphylaxis (laryngeal edema, bronchospasm, hypotension, vascular collapse, and cardiac arrest)
- Death

RISK FOR SOCIAL ISOLATION

PLANNING: EXPECTED OUTCOMES. The client with an infection or infectious disease is expected to cope with feelings of social isolation and to interact with others.

INTERVENTIONS. Education is the major intervention for meeting this goal. Develop an educational program to instruct the client and family about the mode of transmission of infection and mechanisms that prevent spread to others. Assess coping mechanisms that the client has used in the past.

As part of the health care team, ensure that the client and family understand the disease process and its cause. Explain the mode of transmission of the infecting microorganism, risk for transmission to others, and mechanisms that may prevent transmission. If necessary, ensure that the client and

CHART 29-4

NIC INTERVENTION ACTIVITIES for The Client with Infection

Fever Treatment: *Management of a client with hyperpyrexia caused by nonenvironmental factors*

- Monitor temperature as frequently as is appropriate.
- Monitor blood pressure, pulse, and respiration, as appropriate.
- Monitor skin color and temperature.
- Monitor for decreasing levels of consciousness.
- Monitor for intake and output.
- Monitor for seizure activity.
- Monitor WBC, hemoglobin, and hematocrit values.
- Administer antipyretic medication, as appropriate.
- Cover the client with a sheet only, as appropriate.
- Administer a tepid sponge bath, as appropriate.
- Encourage increased intake of oral fluids, as appropriate.
- Administer IV fluids, as appropriate.
- Encourage or administer oral hygiene, as appropriate.
- Place client on hypothermia blanket, as appropriate.
- Monitor temperature closely to prevent treatment-induced hypothermia.

NIC intervention activities selected from Dochterman, J.M., & Bulechek, G.M. (Eds.). (2004). *Nursing interventions classification (NIC)* (4th ed.). St. Louis: Mosby. No part of this work is to be altered without prior written permission from the Publisher.
WBC, White blood cell.

family can state specific ways in which precautions will be instituted in the home after discharge from the hospital.

Because the client requiring precautions may feel secluded, health care workers, as well as family members and friends, are encouraged to maintain contact with the client. Personnel caring for the client are reminded that the pathogen, not the client, requires isolation. Encourage family members and friends to visit and to use appropriate infection control measures. Communication by telephone or Internet is often effective for continuing contact with loved ones. Television, Internet, and radio help bring the outside world into the life of the client confined to the room.

In the long-term care setting, an outbreak of respiratory or gastrointestinal (GI) infection usually requires limiting visitors, activities, and admissions to the facility. Nurses working in a nursing home need to be familiar with state regulations regarding managing infections in this type of setting.

Community-Based Care

Clients with infections may be cared for in the home, hospital, nursing home, or an ambulatory setting, depending on the type and severity of the infection. Infections among older adults in nursing homes are common. Residents often have meals together in a communal dining room and participate in group activities. Immunizing residents against respiratory infections is highly recommended because these illnesses can cause severe complications or death in older adults. Other sources of infection, such as indwelling urinary catheters, are removed when possible to prevent urinary tract infections.

HOME CARE MANAGEMENT

The client with an infectious disease, such as osteomyelitis, who is discharged from the hospital to home may require continued, long-term antibiotic therapy. Emphasizing the importance of a clean home environment, especially for the client who continues to be immunocompromised or who is uniquely susceptible to **superinfection** (i.e., reinfection or a second infection of the same kind) helps to reduce the chance of infection. Medications often need to be refrigerated. Ensure that the client has access to proper storage facilities and instruct him or her to check for signs of improper storage, such as discoloration of the medication.

Inquire about the availability of handwashing facilities in the home, and check that supplies and instructions are provided as needed. Most individuals do not know how to wash hands correctly, so demonstration with the client and requesting a repeat demonstration may be necessary.

HEALTH TEACHING

INFECTION CONTROL. Explaining the disease and making certain that the client understands what is causing the illness is the primary goal of health teaching. Discuss whether the pathogen causing the infection can be spread to others and the modes of transmission.

If the client has an infectious disease that is potentially transmissible, teach the client, family, or home caregivers transmission prevention precautions. Explain whether any special household cleaning is necessary and, if so, what those special steps include. If syringes with needles are used to administer medication, explain how to dispose safely and legally of needles in the community. Clothing soiled with blood or other body fluids can be washed with bleach or disinfectant (e.g., Lysol). Recommended cleaning measures should be based on actual available equipment and facilities.

DRUG THERAPY. For the client who is discharged to the home setting to complete a course of antibiotic therapy, the importance of compliance with the planned drug regimen needs to be stressed. Explain the importance of both the timing of doses and the completion of the planned number of days of therapy. The client (and family as appropriate) should also be taught how the agents need to be taken (e.g., before meals, with meals, and without other agents) and the possible side effects. Side effects include those that are expected (such as gastric distress after oral administration of erythromycin) as well as more severe adverse reactions (such as rash, fever, or other systemic signs and symptoms of an acute adverse drug reaction). Emphasis should be placed on teaching about allergic manifestations and the need for notifying a health care provider if an adverse reaction occurs (see Table 29-7). Also discuss what to do if a drug dose is missed (e.g., doubling the dosage, waiting until the next dose time).

In the past, many clients with severe infection were hospitalized for several weeks or longer, simply to receive IV antibiotic therapy. Since the implementation of managed care, many clients have been discharged with an IV device to continue parenteral antibiotics at home or in the nursing home. The client, family member, or home care nurse administers the drugs. Chapter 17 describes infusion therapy in the community setting.

PSYCHOSOCIAL SUPPORT. The client with an infection is often anxious and fearful that the infection will be transmitted to family members or friends. Teaching the client and the family ways of preventing the spread of disease allays these fears. Careful attention is paid to the client's concerns. Making concrete suggestions (e.g., "Your wife can wear gloves when changing your dressing") to address specific concerns reduces these fears.

The client with an infectious disease associated with lifestyle behaviors, such as sexual activity or IV drug abuse, may experience guilt related to the disease. Encourage verbalization of feelings associated with the illness, and assist in locating support systems that may help alleviate these feelings.

HEALTH CARE RESOURCES

In unusual instances, a client who has been hospitalized for an infectious disease may not be able to return to the home setting immediately. In such circumstances, temporary placement in a long-term care facility may be advantageous. Care requirements, client history of infection or colonization with multidrug-resistant organisms, medication schedules, and personal needs and preferences are carefully noted on transfer documents. When possible, person-to-person communication between the two facilities will facilitate a smooth transition from the hospital to the intermediate care setting.

Home care services are often used to ensure appropriate administration of antibiotics in the client's home. Health teaching and wound care may also be needed. These services have proved efficient, effective, psychologically supportive, and less expensive than hospitalization or intermediate care facilities.

◆Evaluation: Outcomes

Evaluating the care of the client with an infection or infectious disease on the basis of the identified nursing diagnoses

TABLE 29-8 Sample Bioterrorism Agents and Clinical Management

Pathogen or Agent and Disease Information	Clinical Management*
Anthrax (Bacillus anthracis) ▪ **Cutaneous:** 1-7 days after contact, exposed skin itching progressing to papular and vesicular lesions, eschar, edema, ulceration, and sloughing. If untreated, may spread to lymph nodes and bloodstream. Fatality 5%-20%. ▪ **Inhalation:** 48 hr after organism or spore inhalation, flu-like illness with possible brief improvement. 2-4 days from initial symptoms, abrupt onset of severe cardiopulmonary illness (dyspnea, tachycardia, fever, diaphoresis, thoracic edema, shock, and respiratory failure). If antibiotics delayed until onset of cardiopulmonary symptoms, mortality high. May be confused with common upper respiratory infection (URI). ▪ **Other forms:** Gastrointestinal, meningeal, and sepsis.	**For cutaneous and inhaled anthrax:** No person-to-person spread. Contact precautions are not needed unless client presents directly from exposure. Standard precautions for: ▪ Prescribed wound cleansing and management of lesions ▪ Ventilator support for respiratory failure ▪ Postmortem care
Botulism (*Clostridium botulinum* and Neurotoxin) ▪ Toxin ingestion results in dysphasia, dry mouth, drooping eyelids, and blurred or double vision. Vomiting and constipation or diarrhea may be present initially, extending to symmetric flaccid paralysis in an alert person. Acute bilateral cranial nerve impairment and descending weakness or paralysis follow. ▪ Neurologic symptoms after 12-36 hr for foodborne botulism and in 24-72 hr after aerosol exposure. Case fatality up to 10%. Recovery may take months.	Standard precautions: decontamination of client is not required. No person-to-person spread. Consider outbreak with suspicion of a single case. Consult with Centers for Disease Control and Prevention (CDC) and health departments. Advise careful cleanup and disposal of suspected contaminated food source *after* consultation with health department about any needed laboratory sampling. Interdisciplinary planning for nutrition and rehabilitation support during lengthy neuromuscular and respiratory recovery.
Plague *(Yersinia pestis)* ▪ **Lymphatic infection:** 2-8 days after bites from fleas of an infected rodent (rarely after infected tissue or body fluid contact), onset of fever and chills, painful lymphadenopathy (or bubo—usually inguinal, axillary, or cervical lymph nodes), headache, gastrointestinal (GI) symptoms, and rapidly progressive weakness. 50%-60% fatality if untreated. ▪ **Pneumonic:** 1-3 days after aerosolized organism inhalation, fever and chills, productive cough, hemoptysis, rapidly progressive weakness. GI symptoms and bronchopneumonia. Survival unlikely if not treated within 18 hr of symptom onset. ▪ **Other forms:** Sepsis with coagulopathy, rarely meningitis.	Droplet precautions: required for pneumonic plague (until 72 hr of antibiotic therapy). Contact precautions until decontamination is complete: ▪ For any suspected gross contamination. See documentation information listed under Anthrax—above. Standard precautions: ▪ For prescribed management of bubo(s) if incised to drain. Community and other environmental modifications: ▪ Apply insecticide to infested environment and pets (to kill fleas). ▪ Reduce food and water supply for rodents. ▪ Avoid sick or dead animals.
Smallpox (Variola Virus) (Variola Major and Minor) ▪ 10-17 days after droplet or airborne virus inhalation or contact with bleeding lesions, onset of severe myalgias, headache, and high fever. 2-3 days later, a papular rash appears on face and spreads to extremities (and palms and soles). The rash quickly (simultaneously) becomes vesicular, then painful and pustular (contrasted to varicella rash that crops and concentrates more on trunk with various stages of macules to vesicles seen at one time). Clients are infectious at onset of rash until scabs separate (3 wk). Historically, variola major kills 20%. ▪ May be confused with varicella.	Standard, contact, and airborne precautions for clients with vesicular rash pending diagnosis. Same for varicella and variola. ▪ Also, avoid contact with organism while handling contaminated clothes and bedding. Wear protective attire (gloves, gown, and N-95 respirator). One case is a public health emergency—highly communicable. Consult CDC and health departments at earliest suspicion. Vaccine does not give reliable lifelong immunity. Previously vaccinated persons are considered susceptible. *Following exposure:* Initiate airborne precautions and observe for unprotected contacts (from days 10-17). Vaccinate within 2-3 days of exposure.

Other Key Points

Other agents besides the preceding may be used (e.g., salmonella, shigella, tularemia, brucellosis, and various bacterial toxins).

Assessment: Include account of symptoms, client's incident (what, where, when, how, others exposed or ill, and officials aware).

Treatment: Antibiotic-resistance possible. Vaccine and postexposure prophylaxis are subject to change. If any of the above diseases are suspected, consult infection control practitioner for coordination with community health officials and CDC about current recommendations and specimen collection. *If terrorism suspected*, Federal Bureau of Investigation (FBI) will coordinate evidence collection and delivery.

Multiple exposures planning: Emergency and critical care managers must address availability and acquisition of stocks of medications, vaccines, equipment (e.g., ventilators), and communications with officials, as well as public information needs.

Data from *CDC Emerging Infectious Diseases Journal, 5*(4), July-August 1999, available at http://www.cdc.gov/ncidod/eid/; and English, J., et al. (1999). *Bioterrorism readiness plan: A template for healthcare facilities* (pp. 11-26). APIC Bioterrorism Task Force and CDC Hospital Infections Program Bioterrorism Working Group (http://www.apic.org/bioterror/).

*See CDC transmission precautions.

and collaborative problems is important. The expected outcomes include that the client:

- Have a balance of heat production, heat gain, and heat loss
- Copes with feelings of social isolation
- Interacts with others as appropriate

Specific indicators for these outcomes are listed for each nursing diagnosis under the Planning and Implementation section (see earlier).

CRITICAL ISSUES FOR THE NEXT DECADE

In 1969 the U.S. Surgeon General, testifying to the U.S. Congress, made the following historic statement, "The time has come to close the book on infectious disease." Thirty-five years later, infections and infectious diseases are stronger than any time in the past 40 years. Predicting the critical issues for the next decade can be difficult, but certain critical issues internationally, nationally, and locally in some cases stand out. Critical issues for the next 5 to 10 years include bioterrorism (Table 29-8), pandemic influenza, emerging and re-emerging infectious diseases, and multidrug-resistant pathogens.

If left unchecked, multidrug resistance may bring us to a post-antibiotic era. Some microbes formerly treatable with antibiotics have become resistant to all but rarely used antibiotics. *Enterococcus, Yersinia pestis, Mycobacterium tuberculosis, and Staphylococcus aureus* are among these organisms. More information can be obtained on these critical issues from the *Emerging Infectious Diseases Journal* (see http://www.cdc.gov/ncidod/eid/).

GET READY for the NCLEX Examination!

KEY POINTS

- The chain of infection includes pathogen, portal of exit for the pathogen, means of transmission, portal of entry to the host, and susceptible host.
- Nonspecific defenses against infection include body tissues, phagocytosis, and inflammation; specific defenses rely on the immune system.
- Health care–associated infection, also called nosocomial infection, is acquired in a health care setting and is not present or incubating on admission to the facility.
- Infections can be prevented or controlled through hand hygiene, disinfection/sterilization, and barriers; proper hand hygiene is the most important intervention because health care workers' hands are the primary way in which disease is transmitted from client to client.
- Handwashing and alcohol-based hand rubs are two methods of hand hygiene (see Chart 29-3).
- The Centers for Disease Control and Prevention (CDC) recommend a ban on artificial fingernails for health care professionals when they are caring for clients at high risk for infection.
- Standard precautions are used with all clients in health care settings, assuming that all body excretions and secretions are potentially infectious.
- Airborne precautions are used for clients who have infections transmitted through the air, such as tuberculosis.
- Droplet precautions are used for clients who have infections transmitted by droplets, such as influenza and certain types of meningitis.
- Contact precautions are used for clients who have infections transmitted by direct contact or contact with items in the client's environment.
- Examples of multiple-resistant organisms include methicillin-resistant *Staphylococcus aureus* (MRSA) and vancomycin-resistant *Enterococcus* organisms.
- If infections are not treated or are inadequately treated, systemic sepsis (septicemia), septic shock, and disseminated intravascular coagulation (DIC) may result.
- A culture is the most definitive way to confirm and identify microorganisms; sensitivity testing determines which antibiotics will destroy the identified microbes.
- The differential count usually shows a shift to the left (increased number of immature neutrophils) during active infections.
- Antimicrobials and antipyretics are the most common types of drugs used when infection is accompanied by hyperthermia (fever).
- Antipyretics are used only when the fever presents a significant risk or the client is extremely uncomfortable because they may mask the disease.
- Nursing interventions for fever management are listed in Chart 29-4.
- Health teaching about clinical manifestations of infection and drug therapy is important for the client with an infection being managed at home; some clients may need health care nursing services for IV antibiotic therapy.
- Critical issues for the next decade include bioterrorism, pandemic influenza, emerging and re-emerging infectious diseases, and multidrug-resistant pathogens.

ADDITIONAL STUDY RESOURCES

Go to your Student CD-ROM for Review Questions for the NCLEX Examination.

evolve Go to http://evolve.elsevier.com/Iggy/ for Integrated Management of Care Questions for the NCLEX Examination.

SELECTED BIBLIOGRAPHY

Asterisk indicates a classic or definitive work on this subject.

Antimicrobial Resistance Interagency Task Force. (2002). Antimicrobial Resistance Interagency Task Force 2002 annual report on a public health action plan to combat antimicrobial resistance. Available at http://www.cdc.gov/drugresistance/actionplan/index.htm.

*Binder, S., & Levitt, A. Centers for Disease Control and Prevention (CDC). (1998). *Preventing emerging infectious diseases: A strategy for the 21st century.* Atlanta: Author.

Celia, F. (2002). Cutaneous anthrax: An overview. *Dermatology Nurse, 14*(2), 89-92.

*Centers for Disease Control and Prevention. (1994). Guidelines for preventing the transmission of *Mycobacterium tuberculosis* in health-care facilities, 1994. *Morbidity and Mortality Weekly Report, 43*(RR-13), 1-132.

*Centers for Disease Control and Prevention. (1998). Guidelines for infection control in health care personnel, 1998. *American Journal of Infection Control, 26,* 322.

Centers for Disease Control and Prevention. (2000). Monitoring hospital-acquired infections to promote patient safety, 1990-1999. *Morbidity and Mortality Weekly Report, 49*(8), 149-153.

Centers for Disease Control and Prevention. (2001). Management of occupational exposures to hepatitis B, hepatitis C, and HIV and recommendations for postexposure prophylaxis. *Morbidity and Mortality Weekly Report,* 50 (RR-11), 1-42.

Centers for Disease Control and Prevention. (2001). Recognition of illness associated with the intentional release of biologic agent. *Morbidity and Mortality Weekly Report, 50*(41), 893-897.

Centers for Disease Control and Prevention (CDC). (2002). Guideline for hand hygiene in health-care settings: recommendations of the Healthcare Infection Control Practices Advisory Committee and the HICPAC/SHEA/APIC/IDSA Hand Hygiene Task Force. *Morbidity and Mortality Weekly Report, 51*(RR-16), 1-44.

Centers for Disease Control and Prevention (2002). Guidelines for the prevention of intravascular catheter-related infections, 2002. *Morbidity and Mortality Weekly Report, 51*(RR-10), 1-36.

Centers for Disease Control and Prevention (2002). Smallpox response plan and guidelines, Draft 3.0 available at http://www.bt.cdc.gov/agent/smallpox/response-plan/index.asp#guidec.

Centers for Disease Control and Prevention. Food Safety Office (2003). Available at http://www.cdc.gov/foodsafety/.

Centers for Disease Control and Prevention (2003). Guideline for environmental infection control in health-care facilities: 2003 recommendations of CDC and the Healthcare Infection Control Practices Advisory Committee (HICPAC). *Morbidity and Mortality Weekly Report, 52* (RR-10), 1-48.

*Centers for Disease Control and Prevention & Hospital Infection Control Practices Advisory Committee (HICPAC). (1999). Guidelines for prevention of surgical site infection. *Infection Control and Hospital Epidemiology, 20*(4), 254-255, 257.

Chin, J. (Ed.) (2000). *Control of communicable diseases manual* (17th ed.). Washington, DC: American Public Health Association.

*Crabtree, T.D., et al. (1999). Gender-dependent differences in outcome after the treatment of infection in hospitalized patients. *Journal of the American Medical Association, 282*(22), 2143-2148.

*English, J., et al. (1999). *Bioterrorism readiness plan: A template for healthcare facilities* (pp. 11-26). APIC Bioterrorism Task Force and CDC Hospital Infections Program Bioterrorism Working Group; available at http://www.cdc.gov/ncidod/hip/Bio/13apr99APIC-CDC Bioterrorism PDF.

*Friedman, C., et al. (1999). Requirements for infrastructure and essential activities of infection control and epidemiology in out-of-hospital settings: A Consensus Panel report. *American Journal of Infection Control, 27*(5), 418-430.

*Garner, J.S., & Hospital Infection Control Practices Advisory Committee (HICPAC). (1996). Guidelines for isolation precautions in hospitals. *American Journal of Infection Control, 24,* 24-52.

*Gehring, L.L., & Ring, P. (1999). Latex allergy: Creating a safe environment. *MEDSURG Nursing, 8*(6), 358-362.

Harbarth, S., Sax, H., & Gastmeier, P. (2003). The preventable proportion of nosocomial infections. *Journal of Hospital Infections, 54,* 258-266.

*Henderson, D.A. (1999). Consensus statement of smallpox: Clinical and epidemiologic features. *Emerging Infectious Diseases Journal, 5*(4), 2127-2137.

*Herwaldt, L.A., Smith, S.D., & Carter, C.D. (1998). Infection control in the outpatient setting. *Infection Control and Hospital Epidemiology, 19*(1), 41-73.

Kahn, A.S., et al. (2000). Biological and chemical terrorism: Strategic plan for preparedness and response: Recommendations of the CDC Strategic Planning Workgroup. *Morbidity and Mortality Weekly Report, 49*(RR-4), 1-14.

*Kaufmann, A.F., Meltzer, M.I., & Schmid, G.P. (1997). The economic impact of a bioterrorism attack: Are prevention and postattack intervention programs justifiable? *Emerging Infectious Diseases Journal, 3*(2), 4.

*Kirkland, K.B., et al. (1999). The impact of surgical site infections in the 1990's: Attributable mortality, excess length of hospitalization, and extra costs. *Infection Control and Hospital Epidemiology, 20*(11), 725-730.

*McGuckin, M., et al. (1999). Patient education model for increasing hand washing compliance. *American Journal of Infection Control, 27*(4), 309-314.

*Meltzer, M.I., Cox, N.J., & Fukuda, K. (1999). The economic impact of pandemic influenza in the United States: Priorities for intervention. *Emerging Infectious Diseases Journal, 5*(5), 659-670.

*Miller, J.M. (1998) *A guide to specimen management in clinical microbiology* (2nd ed.). Washington, DC: American Society for Microbiology.

Muto, C.A., et al. (2003). SHEA guideline for preventing nosocomial transmission of multidrug-resistant strains of *Staphylococcus aureus* and *Enterococcus. Infection Control and Hospital Epidemiology 24*(5), 362-386

*National Institute for Occupational Safety and Health. (1998). *NISOH alert: Preventing allergic reactions to natural rubber latex in the workplace* (updated September 1998, pp. 1, 3, 5-7). Atlanta: U.S. Government Printing Office. No. 97-135. Available at http://www.cdc.gov/niosh/latexalt.html.

National Nosocomial Infections Surveillance System. (2002a). *National nosocomial infections surveillance (NNIS) system report, data summary from January 2002-June 2002, issued August 2002.* Atlanta: Hospital Infection Program, National Center for Infectious Diseases, Centers for Disease Control and Prevention.

National Nosocomial Infections Surveillance System. (2002b). *NNIS antimicrobial resistance report of selected antimicrobial resistant pathogens associated with nosocomial infections in intensive care unit patients.* Atlanta: Hospital Infection Program, National Center for Infectious Diseases, Centers for Disease Control and Prevention; available at http://www.cdc.gov/ncidod/hip/surveill/nnis.htm.

Osterholm, M.T. (2000). Emerging infections–Another warning. *New England Journal of Medicine, 342*(17), 1280-1281.

Parker, P.J., & Jagger, G.J. (2003). 2001 Percutaneous injury rates. *Advances in Exposure Prevention, 6*(3), 32-36.

*Rhinehart, E., & Friedman, M. (1999) Infection control in home care. Gaithersburg, MD: Association for Professionals of Infection Control and Epidemiology.

Saint S., et al (2000a). Are physicians aware of which of their patients have indwelling urinary catheters? *American Journal of Medicine 109*(6) 476-480.

Saint, S., et al. (2000b). The potential clinical and economic benefits of silver alloy urinary catheters in preventing urinary tract infections. *Archives of Internal Medicine, 160,* 2670-2675.

*Smith, P.W., & Rusnak, P.G. (1997). Infection prevention and control in the long-term-care facility. *American Journal of Infection Control, 25*(6), 488-512.

*Steed, C.J. (1999). Common infections in the hospital: The nurse's role in prevention. *Nursing Clinics of North America, 34*(2), 443-461.

UNIT **SEVEN**

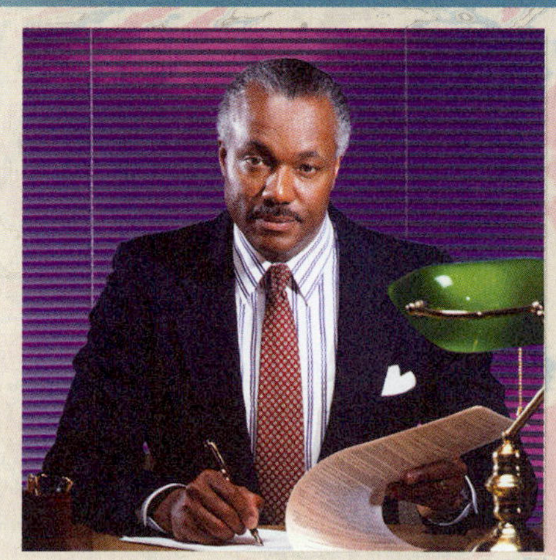

PROBLEMS of OXYGENATION

Management of Clients with Problems of the Respiratory Tract

CHAPTER 30

Assessment of the Respiratory System

CHRISTINE A. GATES • M. LINDA WORKMAN

LEARNING OUTCOMES

After studying this chapter, you should be able to:

1. Compare the structures and functions of the upper airways to those of the lower airways.
2. Distinguish between normal and abnormal (adventitious) breath sounds.
3. Describe the respiratory changes associated with aging.
4. Calculate the pack-year smoking history for the client who smokes or who has ever smoked cigarettes.
5. Demonstrate proper technique when using observation and auscultation to assess the respiratory system.
6. Demonstrate proper technique when using palpation and percussion to assess the respiratory system.
7. Interpret arterial blood gas values to assess the client's respiratory status.
8. Prioritize educational needs for the client undergoing pulmonary function tests.
9. Prioritize nursing care needs for the client after bronchoscopy or open lung biopsy.

Go to your Student CD-ROM for Review Questions for the NCLEX Examination keyed to these Learning Outcomes.

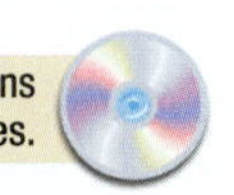

Respiratory problems are common and are the fifth leading cause of death in the United States. Some respiratory problems are chronic, and the client has physical and lifestyle limitations. Many acute health problems, medical therapies, and surgeries adversely affect respiratory function temporarily or permanently. Knowledge of anatomy, physiology, pathophysiology, and pulmonary diagnostic tests is needed to assess the client with respiratory problems.

ANATOMY AND PHYSIOLOGY REVIEW

The two purposes of breathing are to provide oxygen for tissue metabolism and to remove carbon dioxide, the major waste product of metabolism. The respiratory system also influences the following functions:

- Acid-base balance
- Speech
- Sense of smell
- Fluid balance
- Temperature control

Upper Respiratory Tract

The upper airways consist of the nose, the sinuses, the **pharynx** (throat), and the **larynx** ("voice box") (Figure 30-1).

NOSE AND SINUSES

The nose is the organ of smell, with receptors from cranial nerve I (olfactory) located in the upper areas. This organ is rigid and contains two passages separated in the middle by the **septum.** The upper one third of the nose is composed of bone; the lower two thirds is composed of cartilage, allowing limited movement. The septum and interior walls of the nasal cavity are lined with mucous membranes that have a rich blood supply. The **anterior nares** (nostrils or external openings into the nasal cavities) are lined with skin and hair, which help keep foreign particles or organisms from entering the lungs. The posterior nares are openings from the nasal cavity into the nasopharynx.

Three bony projections **(turbinates)** protrude into the nasal cavities from the walls of the internal portion of the nose (see Figure 30-1). Turbinates increase the total surface area for filtering, heating, and humidifying inspired air before it passes into the nasopharynx. Inspired air entering the nose is first filtered in the nares. Particles not filtered out in the nares are trapped in the mucous layer of the turbinates. These particles are moved by **cilia** (hairlike projections) to the oropharynx, where they are either swallowed or expectorated. Inspired air is humidified by contact with the mucous membrane and is warmed by heat from the vascular network.

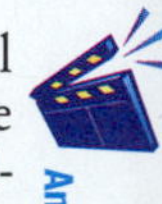

Animation: Location of Sinuses

The **paranasal sinuses** are air-filled cavities within the bones that surround the nasal passages (Figure 30-2). Lined with ciliated membrane, the purposes of the sinuses are to

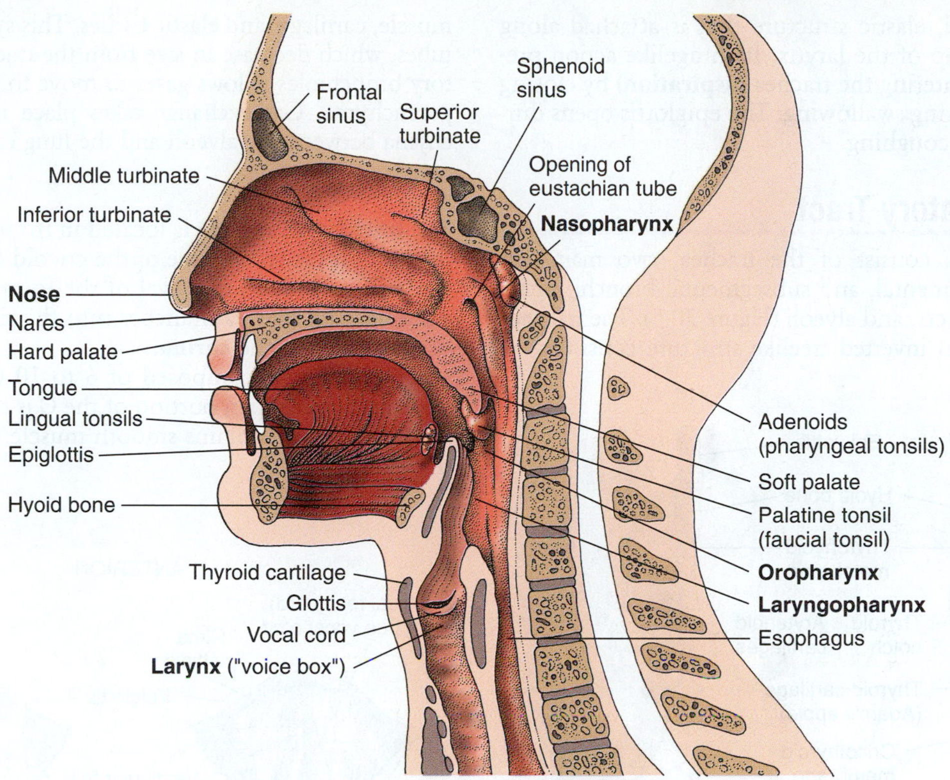

Figure 30-1 ■ Structures of the upper respiratory tract.

provide resonance during speech and to decrease the weight of the skull.

PHARYNX

The **pharynx,** or throat, is a passageway for both the respiratory and digestive tracts. It is located behind the oral and nasal cavities. The throat is divided into the nasopharynx, the oropharynx, and the laryngopharynx (see Figure 30-1).

The **nasopharynx** is located behind the nose, above the soft palate. It contains the adenoids and the opening of the eustachian tube. The **adenoids** (pharyngeal tonsils) trap organisms that enter the nose or mouth. The *eustachian tube* connects the nasopharynx with the middle ear and opens during swallowing to equalize pressure within the middle ear.

The oropharynx is located behind the mouth, below the nasopharynx. It extends from the soft palate to the base of the tongue and is used for breathing and swallowing. The *palatine tonsils* (also known as *faucial tonsils*) are located on the side borders of the oropharynx. These tonsils also guard the body against invading organisms.

The laryngopharynx is located behind the larynx and extends from the base of the tongue to the esophagus. It is the critical dividing point where solid foods and fluids are separated from air. At this point, the passageway divides into the larynx and the esophagus.

LARYNX

The **larynx** is located above the trachea, just below the throat at the base of the tongue. It is innervated by the recurrent laryngeal nerves. The larynx is composed of several cartilages (Figure 30-3). The *thyroid cartilage* is the largest and is commonly called the "Adam's apple." The *cricoid cartilage,* which contains the vocal cords, lies below the thyroid cartilage. The *cricothyroid membrane* is located below the level of the vocal cords and joins the thyroid and cricoid cartilages. This site is used in an emergency for access to the lower airways. In this procedure, called a **cricothyroidotomy** (or cricothyrotomy), an opening is made between the thyroid and cricoid cartilage and results in a tracheostomy. The two *arytenoid cartilages,* which attach at the back ends of the vocal cords, work with the thyroid cartilage in vocal cord movement.

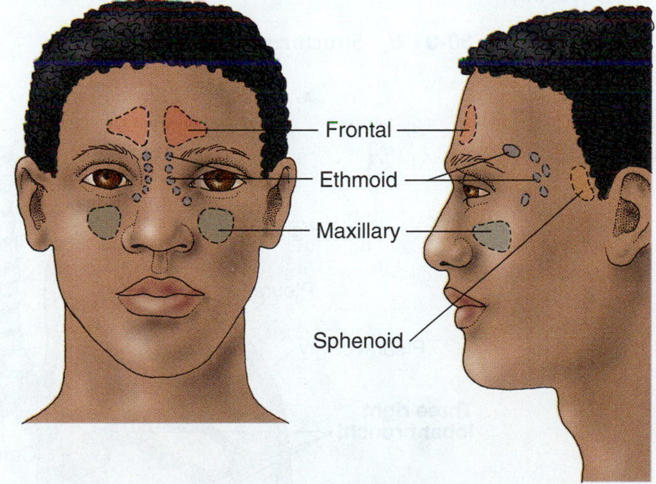

Figure 30-2 ■ The paranasal sinuses.

Inside the larynx are two pairs of vocal cords: the false vocal cords and the true vocal cords. The opening between the true vocal cords is the **glottis** (Figure 30-4). The **epiglot-**

tis is a leaf-shaped, elastic structure that is attached along one edge to the top of the larynx. Its hingelike action prevents food from entering the trachea **(aspiration)** by closing over the glottis during swallowing. The epiglottis opens during breathing and coughing.

Lower Respiratory Tract

The lower airways consist of the trachea; two mainstem bronchi; lobar, segmental, and subsegmental bronchi; bronchioles; alveolar ducts; and alveoli (Figure 30-5). The tracheobronchial tree is an inverted treelike structure consisting of muscle, cartilage, and elastic tissues. This system of branching tubes, which decrease in size from the trachea to the respiratory bronchioles, allows gases to move to and from the lung parenchyma. Gas exchange takes place in the lung parenchyma between the alveoli and the lung capillaries.

TRACHEA

The **trachea** (windpipe) is located in front of the esophagus. It begins at the lower edge of the cricoid cartilage of the larynx and extends to the level of the fourth or fifth thoracic vertebra. The trachea branches into the right and left mainstem bronchi at the **carina.**

The trachea is composed of 6 to 10 C-shaped cartilaginous rings. The open portion of the C is the back portion of the trachea and contains smooth muscle that is shared with the esophagus.

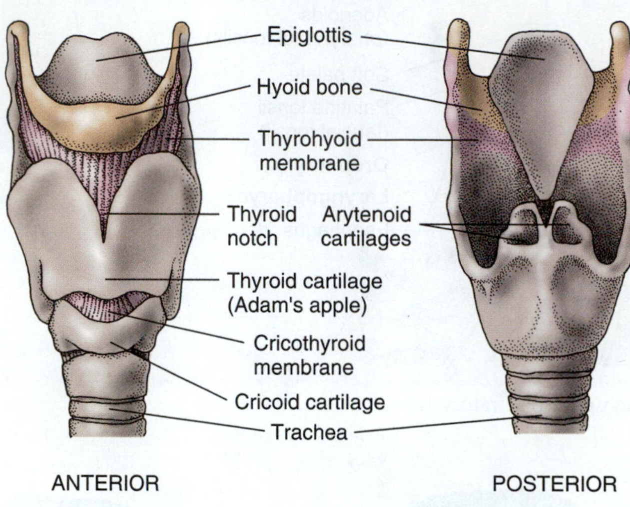

Figure 30-3 ■ Structures of the larynx.

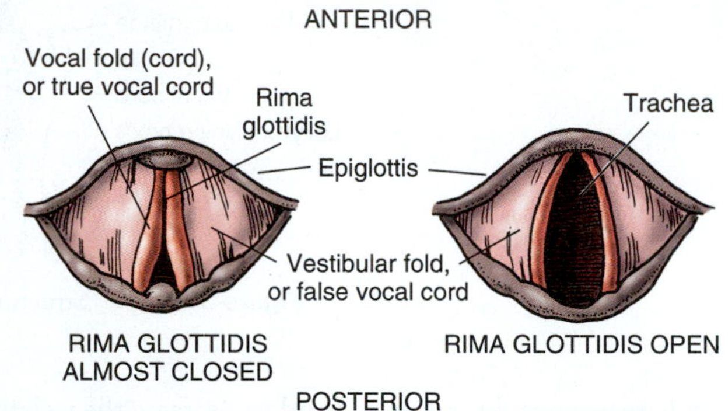

Figure 30-4 ■ Detail of the glottis (two vocal folds and the intervening space, the rima glottidis).

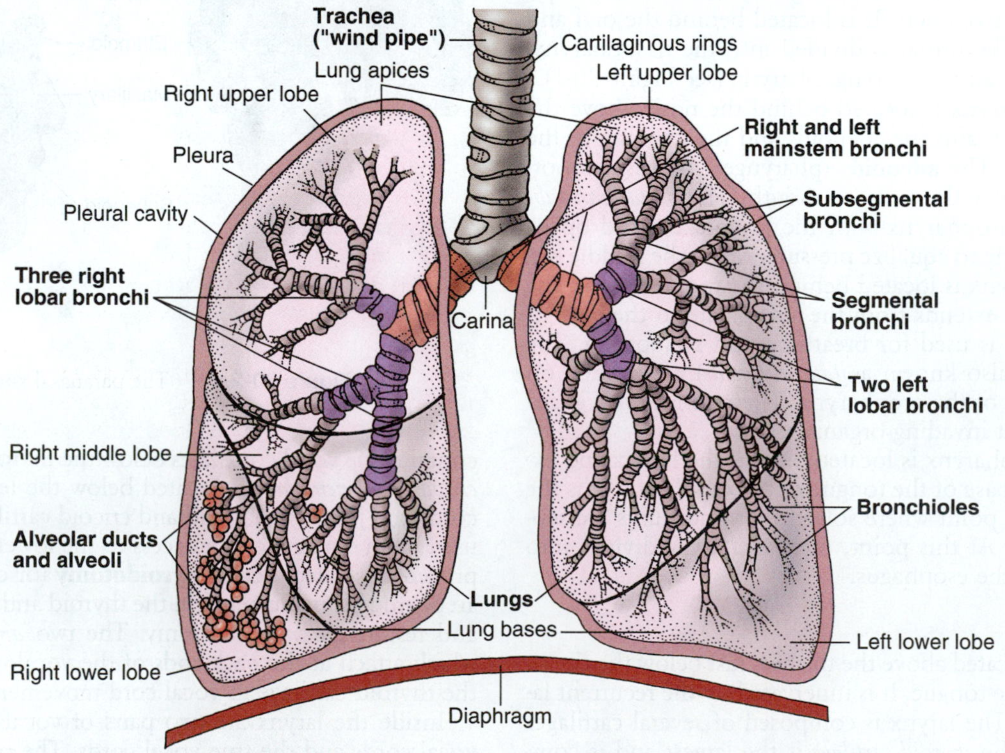

Figure 30-5 ■ Structures of the lower respiratory tract (structural size and proportions not drawn to scale).

MAINSTEM BRONCHI

The mainstem, or primary, bronchi begin at the carina. The bronchus is similar in structure to the trachea. The right bronchus is slightly wider, shorter, and more vertical than the left bronchus. Because of the more vertical line of the right bronchus, it can be accidentally intubated when an endotracheal tube is passed. Similarly, when a foreign object is aspirated from the throat, it most often enters the right bronchus.

LOBAR, SEGMENTAL, AND SUBSEGMENTAL BRONCHI

The mainstem bronchi each branch into the five secondary (lobar) bronchi that enter each of the five lobes of the lung. Each lobar bronchus is surrounded by connective tissue, blood vessels, nerves, and lymphatics, and each branches into segmental and subsegmental divisions. The cartilage of these lobar bronchi is ring-shaped and resists collapse. The bronchi are lined with a ciliated, mucus-secreting membrane. The cilia move mucus up and away from the lower airway to the trachea, where the mucus is either spit out or swallowed.

BRONCHIOLES

The bronchioles branch from the secondary bronchi and divide into smaller and smaller tubes: the terminal and respiratory bronchioles (Figure 30-6). These tubes are less than 1 mm in diameter. They have no cartilage and depend entirely on the elastic recoil of the lung to remain open **(patent).** The terminal bronchioles do not participate in gas exchange.

ALVEOLAR DUCTS AND ALVEOLI

Alveolar ducts branch from the respiratory bronchioles and resemble a bunch of grapes. Alveolar sacs arise from these ducts. The alveolar sacs contain groups of alveoli, which are the basic units of gas exchange (see Figure 30-6). A pair of healthy adult lungs has about 300 million alveoli, which are surrounded by lung capillaries. These small alveoli are numerous and share common walls, making a large surface area for gas exchange. In a healthy adult, this surface area is about the size of a tennis court. **Acinus** is a term for the structural unit consisting of a respiratory bronchiole, an alveolar duct, and an alveolar sac.

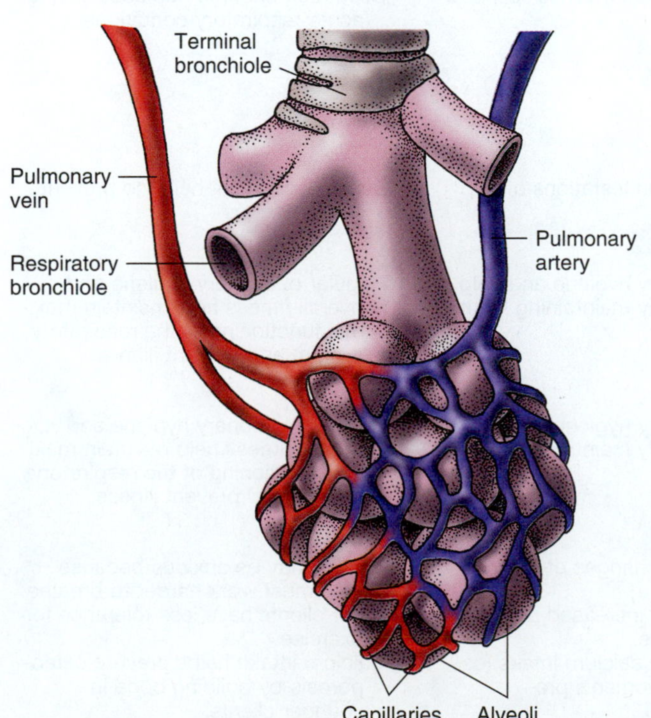

Figure 30-6 ■ The terminal bronchioles and the acinus.

In the walls of the alveoli, specific cells **(type II pneumocytes)** secrete **surfactant,** a fatty protein that reduces surface tension in the alveoli. Without surfactant, **atelectasis** (collapse of the alveoli) occurs. In atelectasis, gas exchange is reduced because the alveolar surface area is reduced.

LUNGS

The lungs are spongelike, elastic, cone-shaped organs located in the pleural cavity in the chest. The apex (top) of each lung extends above the clavicle; the base (bottom) of each lung lies just above the **diaphragm** (the major muscle of inspiration). The lungs are composed of millions of alveoli and their related ducts, bronchioles, and bronchi. The right lung, which is larger than the left, is divided into three lobes: upper, middle, and lower. The left lung, which is somewhat narrower than the right lung to make room for the heart, is divided into two lobes.

The hilum is the point at which the primary bronchus, blood vessels, nerves, and lymphatics enter each lung. The chest wall is innervated by the phrenic (diaphragm) and intercostal (pleura, ribs, and muscles) nerves. The bronchi are innervated by the vagus nerve. The lung parenchyma is not innervated.

Animation: Pulmonary Circulation ◀

The **pleura** is a continuous smooth membrane composed of two surfaces that totally enclose the lungs. The **parietal pleura** lines the inside of the chest cavity and the upper surface of the diaphragm. The **visceral pleura** covers the lung surfaces. These two surfaces are lubricated by a thin fluid that is produced by the cells lining the pleura. This fluid allows the surfaces to glide smoothly and painlessly during respirations.

Blood flow in the lungs occurs through two separate systems: bronchial and pulmonary. The bronchial system carries the blood needed to meet the metabolic demands of the lungs. The bronchial arteries, which arise from the thoracic aorta, are part of the systemic circulation and do not participate in gas exchange.

The pulmonary circulation is a highly vascular capillary network. Oxygen-poor blood travels from the right ventricle of the heart into the pulmonary artery, which eventually branches into arterioles that form the capillary networks. The capillaries are meshed around and through the alveoli, the site of gas exchange (see Figure 30-6). Freshly oxygenated blood travels from the capillaries and through the venules to the pulmonary veins and then to the left atrium. From the left atrium, oxygenated blood flows into the left ventricle, where it is pumped throughout the systemic circulation.

Accessory Muscles of Respiration

Breathing occurs through changes in the size of and pressure within the chest cavity. Contraction and relaxation of specific skeletal muscles (and the diaphragm) cause changes in the size and pressure of the chest cavity. Accessory muscles that help in this process include the scalene muscles, which lift the first two ribs; the sternocleidomastoid muscles, which raise the sternum; and the trapezius and pectoralis muscles, which fix the shoulders. At times, various back and abdominal muscles are used when the work of breathing is increased.

Respiratory Changes Associated with Aging

The respiratory changes that occur with aging are described in Chart 30-1. Many changes in older clients result from heredity and a lifetime of exposure to environmental stimuli (e.g., cigarette smoke, bacteria, air pollutants, and industrial fumes and irritants). Table 30-1 shows the age-related changes in the partial pressure of arterial oxygen (PaO_2).

Respiratory disease is a major cause of illness and chronic disability in older clients. Although respiratory function normally declines with age, there is usually no problem keeping pace with the demands of ordinary activ-

CHART 30-1

NURSING FOCUS on the OLDER ADULT

Changes in the Respiratory System Related to Aging

Physiologic Change	Nursing Interventions	Rationales
Alveoli		
Alveolar surface area decreases. Diffusion capacity decreases. Elastic recoil decreases. Bronchioles and alveolar ducts dilate. Ability to cough decreases. Airways close early.	Encourage vigorous pulmonary hygiene (i.e., encourage the client to turn, cough, and deep breathe), especially if he or she is confined to bed or has had surgery. Encourage upright position.	There is increased potential for mechanical or infectious respiratory complications in these situations. The upright position minimizes ventilation-perfusion mismatching.
Lungs		
Residual volume increases. Vital capacity decreases. Efficiency of oxygen and carbon dioxide exchange decreases. Elasticity decreases.	Include inspection, palpation, percussion, and auscultation in lung assessments. Help client in actively maintaining health and fitness. Assess the client's respirations for abnormal breathing patterns. Encourage frequent oral hygiene.	Inspection, palpation, percussion, and auscultation are needed to detect normal age-related changes. Health and fitness helps to keep losses in respiratory functioning to a minimum. Periodic breathing patterns (e.g., Cheyne-Stokes) can occur. Oral hygiene aids in the removal of secretions.
Pharynx and Larynx		
Muscles atrophy. Vocal cords become slack. Laryngeal muscles lose elasticity and cartilage.	Have face-to-face conversations with client when possible.	Client's voice may be soft and difficult to understand.
Pulmonary Vasculature		
Increased vascular resistance to blood flow through pulmonary vascular system occurs. Pulmonary capillary blood volume decreases. Risk of hypoxia increases.	Assess the client's level of consciousness.	Client can become confused during acute respiratory conditions.
Exercise Tolerance		
Body's response to hypoxia and hypercarbia decreases.	Assess for subtle manifestations of hypoxia.	Early assessment helps to prevent complications.
Muscle Strength		
Respiratory muscle strength, especially the diaphragm and the intercostals, decreases.	Encourage pulmonary hygiene and help the client in actively maintaining health and fitness.	Regular pulmonary hygiene and overall fitness help maintain maximal functioning of the respiratory system and prevent illness.
Susceptibility to Infection		
Effectiveness of the cilia decreases. Immunoglobulin A decreases. Alveolar macrophages are altered.	Encourage pulmonary hygiene, and help the client in actively maintaining health and fitness.	Regular pulmonary hygiene and overall fitness help maintain maximal functioning of the respiratory system and prevent illness.
Chest Wall		
Anteroposterior diameter increases. Thorax becomes shorter. Progressive kyphoscoliosis occurs. Chest wall compliance (elasticity) decreases. Mobility may decrease. Osteoporosis is possible.	Discuss the normal changes of aging. Discuss the need for increased rest periods during exercise. Encourage adequate calcium intake (especially during a woman's premenopause phase).	Clients may be anxious because they must work harder to breathe. Older clients have less tolerance for exercise. Calcium intake helps prevent osteoporosis by building bone in younger clients.

ity. The sedentary older adult, however, often feels breathless during exercise.

It is difficult to determine which respiratory changes in older adults are related to normal aging and which changes are caused by respiratory disease or exposure to pollutants. Age-related neuromuscular and cardiovascular changes also may cause abnormal breathing, even if the lungs are normal.

ASSESSMENT TECHNIQUES

History

Obtaining accurate information from the client is important for identifying the type and severity of breathing problems. Chart 30-2 lists questions to ask clients (based on Gordon's Functional Health Patterns) to assess the impact of pulmonary function.

DEMOGRAPHIC DATA

Age, gender, and race can affect the physical and diagnostic findings related to breathing. Many of the diagnostic studies for respiratory disorders (e.g., pulmonary function tests) use these data for determining predicted normal values.

WOMEN'S HEALTH CONSIDERATIONS

Women, especially smokers, have greater bronchial responsiveness (i.e., bronchial hyperreactivity) and larger airways than men. This factor increases the risk for a more rapid decline in lung function as an older adult, especially in people who were or are smokers.

CULTURAL CONSIDERATIONS

The largest chest volumes are found in white individuals; the smallest volumes are found in Native Americans/American Indians. The chest volumes of black individuals are significantly larger than those of Asian Americans but not as large as those of whites (Jarvis, 2004). Compared with whites, black individuals and other people with dark skin usually show a lower oxygen saturation rate (3% to 5% lower) as measured by pulse oximetry; this results from deeper coloration of the nail bed and does not reflect true oxygen status.

TABLE 30-1 Age Distributions and Partial Pressure of Arterial Oxygen (Pa_{O_2}) Values (Mean)

Age (yr)	Pa_{O_2} (mm Hg)
40-44	95
45-49	88.6
50-54	87.1
55-59	85.1
60-64	84.8
65-69	82.3
70-74	79.1
75-79	82.9
80-84	83.4
85-90	83.2

Modified with permission from Cerveri, I., et al. (1995). Reference values of arterial oxygen tension in the middle-aged and elderly. *American Journal of Respiratory and Critical Care Medicine, 152*, 934-941.

FAMILY HISTORY AND GENETIC RISK

Obtain a family history to assess for respiratory disorders with a genetic component, such as cystic fibrosis, some lung cancers, and alpha$_1$-antitrypsin deficiency (one risk factor for emphysema). Clients with asthma often have a family history of allergic symptoms and reactive airways. Ask about a history of infectious disease, such as tuberculosis, because family members may have similar environmental or occupational exposures.

PERSONAL HISTORY

Ask clients about their own respiratory history (Table 30-2).

Smoking History

Ask the client about the use of cigarettes, cigars, pipe tobacco, marijuana, and other controlled substances. Assess whether the client has passive exposure to smoke in the home or workplace. If the client smokes, ask for how long, how many packs a day, and whether the client has quit smoking (and how long ago). Document the smoking history in **pack-years** (number of packs smoked per day multiplied by number of years). Because the client may have guilt or denial about this habit, assume a nonjudgmental attitude during the interview.

Smoking induces changes in the airways, and these changes lead to varying degrees of airway obstruction. Men who continue to smoke have a more rapid decline in their pulmonary function than do nonsmokers. The pulmonary function of clients who have quit smoking for 2 or more

CHART 30-2

Respiratory Assessment USING GORDON'S FUNCTIONAL HEALTH PATTERNS

Health Perception–Health Management Pattern

- How has your general health been?
- Have you had any colds this past year?
- Have you missed work or school because of illness this past year?
- Do you use cigarettes? For how many years? How many packs per day?

Activity-Exercise Pattern

- Do you feel you have sufficient energy to perform tasks or routines that are required of you?
- Do you feel you have sufficient energy to do what you would like to do?
- Do you exercise? How often? For how long each time? What type(s) of exercise do you perform?
- What activities do you perform in your spare time?
- What is your ability to perform the following tasks?

Feeding ________	Grooming ________
Bathing ________	General mobility ________
Toileting ________	Cooking ________
Bed mobility ________	Home maintenance ________
Dressing ________	Shopping ________

Functional Levels Code

Level 0: Full self-care
Level I: Requires use of equipment or device
Level II: Requires assistance or supervision of another person
Level III: Requires assistance or supervision of another person and the use of equipment or devices
Level IV: Is dependent and does not participate

Based on Gordon, M. (2002). *Manual of nursing diagnosis* (10th ed.). St. Louis: Mosby.

TABLE 30-2 Important Aspects to Assess in a Respiratory System History

Smoking history
Childhood illnesses
- Asthma
- Pneumonia
- Communicable diseases
- Hay fever
- Allergies
- Eczema
- Frequent colds
- Croup
- Cystic fibrosis

Adult illnesses
- Pneumonia
- Sinusitis
- Tuberculosis
- HIV and AIDS
- Lung disease such as emphysema and sarcoidosis
- Diabetes
- Hypertension
- Heart disease

Influenza, pneumococcal (Pneumovax) and BCG vaccinations
Surgeries of the upper or lower respiratory system
Injuries to the upper or lower respiratory system
Hospitalizations
Date of last chest x-ray, pulmonary function test, tuberculin test, or other diagnostic tests and results
Recent weight loss
Night sweats
Sleep disturbances
Lung disease and condition of family members
Geographic areas of recent travel
Occupation and leisure activities

AIDS, Acquired immunodeficiency syndrome; *BCG,* bacille Calmette-Guérin; *HIV,* human immunodeficiency virus.

years appears to decline less rapidly than in clients who continue to smoke.

Drug Use

Ask about drugs taken for breathing problems and about drugs taken for other conditions. For example, a cough can be a side effect of some antihypertensive drugs (angiotensin-converting enzyme [ACE] inhibitors). Determine which over-the-counter drugs (e.g., cough syrups, antihistamines, decongestants, inhalants, nasal sprays) the client is using. Also assess the use of home remedies. Ask about past drug use and the reason for its discontinuation. For example, the client may have used many bronchodilator inhalers but may prefer one particular drug for relieving breathlessness. Some drugs for other conditions can cause permanent changes in lung function. For example, clients may have pulmonary fibrosis if they received bleomycin (Blenoxane) as chemotherapy for cancer or amiodarone (Cordarone) for cardiac problems.

Allergies

Information about allergies is important to the respiratory history. Ask whether the client has any known allergies to substances such as foods, dust, molds, pollen, bee stings, trees, grass, animal dander and saliva, or any drugs. Ask the client to describe specific allergic responses. For example, does he or she wheeze, have trouble breathing, cough, sneeze, or have rhinitis after exposure to the allergen? Has he or she ever been treated for an allergic response? If the client has received treatment for allergies, ask about what caused the need for treatment, the type of treatment, and the response to treatment.

Document any known allergies and the specific type of allergic response in a prominent place in the client's medical record.

Travel and Area of Residence

Travel and area of residence may be relevant for a history of exposure to certain diseases. For example, *histoplasmosis,* a fungal disease caused by inhalation of contaminated dust, is found in the central United States and Central America. *Coccidioidomycosis,* another fungal disease, is found mostly in the western and southwestern United States, Mexico, and portions of Central America.

DIET HISTORY

Assess the client's diet history to determine allergic reactions to certain foods or preservatives. Manifestations range from rhinitis, chest tightness, weakness, shortness of breath **(dyspnea),** urticaria, and severe wheezing to loss of consciousness. Ask about his or her usual food intake and whether any breathing problems occur with eating. Malnutrition may occur if the client has difficulty breathing during eating or while preparing food.

OCCUPATIONAL HISTORY AND SOCIOECONOMIC STATUS

Explore the home, community, and workplace for environmental factors that could cause or worsen lung disease. Occupational lung diseases include pneumoconiosis, which results from the inhalation of dust (e.g., coal dust, stone dust, silicone dust); toxic lung injury; and hypersensitivity disease (e.g., hypersensitivity to latex). The occupational history includes the exact dates of employment and a brief job description. Exposure to industrial dusts of any type or to the chemicals found in smoke and fumes may cause breathing disorders. Bakers, coal miners, stone masons, cotton handlers, woodworkers, welders, potters, plastic and rubber manufacturers, printers, farm workers, and steel foundry workers are at risk for breathing problems.

Ask the client about the home and living conditions, such as the type of heat used (e.g., gas heater, wood-burning stove, fireplace, kerosene heater). Determine exposure to environmental irritants (e.g., noxious fumes, chemicals, animals, birds, air pollutants). Ask about hobbies and leisure activities. Pastimes such as painting, working with ceramics, model airplane building, furniture refinishing, or woodworking may have exposed the client to harmful chemical irritants.

CURRENT HEALTH PROBLEMS

Whether the breathing problem is acute or chronic, the current health problem usually includes cough, sputum production, chest pain, and shortness of breath at rest or on exertion. During the interview, explore the present illness in chronologic order. This analysis of the problem(s) includes the following:

- Onset
- Duration
- Location
- Frequency
- Progressing and radiating patterns

- Quality and number of symptoms
- Aggravating and relieving factors
- Associated manifestations
- Treatments

Cough

Cough is the main sign of lung disease. Ask the client how long the cough has been present (e.g., 1 week, 3 months) and whether it occurs at a specific time of day (e.g., on awakening in the morning, which is common in smokers) or in relation to any physical activity. Determine whether the cough is productive or nonproductive, congested, dry, tickling, or hacking.

Sputum Production

Sputum production is an important symptom associated with coughing. Check the duration, color, consistency, odor, and amount of sputum. Sputum may be clear, white, tan, gray or, if infection is present, yellow or green.

Describe the consistency of sputum as thin, thick, watery, or frothy. Smokers with chronic bronchitis have mucoid sputum. Excessive pink, frothy sputum common occurs with pulmonary edema. Pneumococcal pneumonia often produces rust-colored sputum, and foul-smelling sputum often occurs with a lung abscess. Blood in the sputum **(hemoptysis)** is most often seen in clients with chronic bronchitis or lung cancer. Clients with tuberculosis, pulmonary infarction, bronchial adenoma, or lung abscess may have grossly bloody sputum.

Quantify sputum by describing its volume in terms such as teaspoon, tablespoon, and cups or fractions of cups. Normally, the bronchial tree can produce up to 3 ounces (90 mL) of sputum per day. Determine whether sputum production is increasing, possibly from external stimuli (e.g., an irritant in the work setting) or an internal cause (e.g., chronic bronchitis or a pulmonary abscess).

Chest Pain

A detailed description of chest pain helps distinguish whether pain is pleural, musculoskeletal, cardiac, or gastrointestinal in origin. Ask the client whether the pain is continuous or made worse by coughing, deep breathing, or swallowing.

Dyspnea

The perception of **dyspnea** (difficulty in breathing or breathlessness) is subjective and varies among clients. A client's feeling of dyspnea may not be consistent with the severity of the presenting problem. Determine the type of onset (slow or abrupt); the duration (number of hours, time of day); relieving factors (changes of position, drug use, activity cessation); and whether wheezing, crackles, or stridor occurs with the breathlessness.

Try to quantify dyspnea by asking whether this symptom interferes with **activities of daily living (ADLs)** and, if so, how severely. For example, is the client breathless while dressing, showering, shaving, or eating? Does dyspnea occur after walking one block or climbing one flight of stairs? Table 30-3 classifies dyspnea with changes in ADL performance. A dyspnea assessment scale may be used to assess dyspnea (see Chapter 33).

Ask about **paroxysmal nocturnal dyspnea (PND),** which is intermittent dyspnea during sleep, and about **orthopnea,** which is a shortness of breath that occurs when lying down but is relieved by sitting up. These two conditions often occur with chronic lung disease and left-sided heart failure. In PND, the client has a sudden onset of breathing difficulty that is severe enough to awaken the client from sleep.

TABLE 30-3 Correlation of Dyspnea Classification with Performance of Activities of Daily Living

Classification	Activities of Daily Living Key
Class I: No significant restrictions in normal activity. Employable. Dyspnea occurs only on more than normal or strenuous exertion.	*4:* No breathlessness, normal.
Class II: Independent in essential ADLs but restricted in some other activities. Dyspneic on climbing stairs or on walking on an incline but not on level walking. Employable only for sedentary job or under special circumstances.	*3:* Satisfactory, mild breathlessness. Complete performance is possible without pause or assistance but not entirely normal.
Class III: Dyspnea commonly occurs during usual activities, such as showering or dressing, but the client can manage without assistance from others. Not dyspneic at rest; can walk for more than a city block at own pace but cannot keep up with others of own age. May stop to catch breath partway up a flight of stairs. Is probably not employable in any occupation.	*2:* Fair, moderate breathlessness. Must stop during activity. Complete performance is possible without assistance, but performance may be too debilitating or time consuming.
Class IV: Dyspnea produces dependence on help in some essential ADLs such as dressing and bathing. Not usually dyspneic at rest. Dyspneic on minimal exertion; must pause on climbing one flight, walking more than 100 yards, or dressing. Often restricted to home if lives alone. Has minimal or no activities outside of home.	*1:* Poor, marked breathlessness. Incomplete performance; assistance is necessary.
Class V: Entirely restricted to home and often limited to bed or chair. Dyspneic at rest. Dependent on help for most needs.	*0:* Performance not indicated or recommended; too difficult.

ADLs, Activities of daily living.

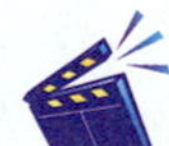
Video Clip: Inspection of the Nose ◀

Physical Assessment

ASSESSMENT OF THE NOSE AND SINUSES

Inspect the client's external nose for deformities or tumors, and inspect the nostrils for symmetry of size and shape. Nasal flaring may indicate increased respiratory effort. To observe the interior nose, ask the client to tilt the head back for a penlight examination. Use a nasal speculum and nasopharyngeal mirror for a more thorough inspection of the nasal cavity.

Inspect for color, swelling, drainage, and bleeding. The mucous membrane of the nose normally appears redder than the oral mucosa, but it is usually pale, engorged, and bluish-gray

Figure 30-7 ■ Anterior and posterior thoracic landmarks.

in clients with allergic rhinitis. Check the nasal septum for bleeding, perforation, or deviation. Some degree of septal deviation is common in most adults and appears as an S shape, inclining toward one side or the other. A perforated septum is present if the light shines through the perforation into the opposite nostril; this condition is often found in cocaine users. Nasal polyps, a common cause of obstruction, are pale, shiny, gelatinous lumps or "bags" attached to the turbinates.

Occlude one naris at a time to check whether air moves through the nonoccluded side easily. Palpate the nose and paranasal sinuses to detect tenderness or swelling. Only the frontal and maxillary sinuses are easily examined because the ethmoid and sphenoid sinuses lie deep within the skull (see Figure 30-2). Using your thumbs, check for sinus tenderness by pressing upward on the frontal and maxillary areas. Assess both sides at the same time. Tenderness in these areas suggests inflammation or acute sinusitis. Tenderness in response to tapping a finger over these areas also indicates inflammation.

Transillumination of the sinuses may be used to detect sinusitis. In a darkened room, place the bulb of a penlight on the client's cheek (just under the corner of the eye) and observe for light penetration through the roof of the mouth. Normally a faint glow of light through the bone outlines the sinus. Transillumination is absent or decreased in sinusitis; however, this test is not conclusive for sinusitis.

ASSESSMENT OF THE PHARYNX, TRACHEA, AND LARYNX

Assessment of the pharynx begins with inspection of the external structures of the mouth. To examine the posterior pharynx, use a tongue depressor to press down one side of the tongue at a time (to avoid stimulating the gag reflex). As the client says "ah," observe the rise and fall of the soft palate and uvula and inspect for color and symmetry, evidence of discharge (postnasal drainage), edema or ulceration, and tonsillar enlargement or inflammation.

Inspect the neck for symmetry, alignment, masses, swelling, bruises, and the use of accessory neck muscles in breathing. Palpate lymph nodes for size, shape, mobility, consistency, and tenderness. Tender nodes are usually movable and suggest inflammation. Malignant nodes are often hard and are fixed to the surrounding tissue.

Gently palpate the trachea for position, mobility, tenderness, and masses. Firm palpation may trigger coughing or gagging. The space on either side of the trachea should be equal. Many lung disorders cause the trachea to deviate from the midline. Tension pneumothorax, large pleural effusion, mediastinal mass, and neck tumors push the trachea away from the affected area. Pneumonectomy, fibrosis, and atelectasis pull the trachea toward the affected area. Decreased tracheal mobility may occur with cancer or fibrosis of the mediastinum.

The larynx is usually examined by a specialist with a laryngoscope. An abnormal voice, especially hoarseness, may be heard when there are problems of the larynx.

ASSESSMENT OF THE LUNGS AND THORAX

Inspection

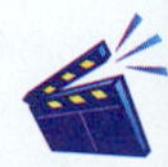

Begin inspection of the chest by assessing the anterior and posterior thorax. Normal landmarks of the chest and thorax are shown in Figure 30-7. If possible, have the client sit up during the assessment. He or she should be undressed to the waist and draped for privacy and warmth. Observe the chest and compare one side with the other. Work from the top (apex) and move downward toward the base while inspecting for discoloration, scars, lesions, masses, and spinal deformities such as kyphosis, scoliosis, and lordosis.

Observe the rate, rhythm, and depth of inspirations as well as the symmetry of chest movement. Impaired movement or unequal expansion may indicate disease of the lung or the pleura. Observe the type of breathing (e.g., pursed-lip or diaphragmatic breathing) and the use of accessory muscles. While observing respiration, document the duration of the inspiratory (I) and expiratory (E) phases. The ratio of these phases (the I-E ratio) is normally 1:2. A prolonged expiratory phase indicates an obstruction of air outflow and is often seen in clients with asthma or chronic obstructive pulmonary disease (COPD).

Animation: Patterns of Respiration

Examine the shape of the client's chest and compare the anteroposterior (AP) diameter with the lateral diameter. This ratio normally ranges from 1:2 to about 5:7, depending on body build. The ratio increases to 1:1 in clients with emphysema, which results in the typical barrel-chest appearance.

Normally the ribs slope downward. Clients with air trapping in the lungs caused by chronic asthma or emphysema, however, have little or no slope to the ribs (i.e., the ribs are more horizontal).

Check for abnormal retractions of the intercostal spaces during inspiration, which indicate airflow obstruction. These retractions may be due to lung fibrosis, severe acute asthma, emphysema, or tracheal or laryngeal obstruction.

Palpation

Video Clip: Respiratory Excursion, Tactile Fremitus

Palpate the chest after inspection. Palpation is performed to assess respiratory movement symmetry and observable abnormalities, to identify areas of tenderness, and to check vocal or tactile **fremitus** (vibration).

Assess chest expansion by placing your thumbs on the client's spine at the level of the ninth ribs and extending the fingers laterally around the rib cage. As the client inhales, both sides of the chest should move upward and outward together in one symmetric movement and move your thumbs apart. On exhalation, the thumbs should come back together as they return to the midline. Decreased movement on one side (unilateral or unequal expansion) may be a result of pain, trauma, or **pneumothorax** (air in the pleural cavity). Respiratory lag or slowed movement on one side occurs with the presence of a pulmonary mass, pleural fibrosis, atelectasis, pneumonia, or a lung abscess.

Palpate any abnormalities found on inspection (e.g., masses, lesions, bruises, swelling). Also palpate for tenderness, particularly if the client has reported pain. **Crepitus** (subcutaneous emphysema) is felt as a crackling sensation beneath the fingertips. Document this finding, especially if it occurs around a wound site or if a pneumothorax is suspected. Crepitus indicates that air is trapped within the tissues.

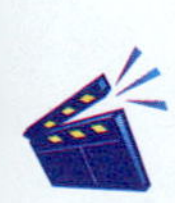

Video Clip: Tactile Fremitus

Tactile (vocal) fremitus is a vibration of the chest wall produced when the client speaks. This vibration can be palpated on the chest wall. To check tactile fremitus, place the palm or the base of your fingers against the client's chest wall and instruct him or her to say the number *99*. Using the same hand and moving from the apices to the bases, compare vibrations from one side of the chest with those from the other side. Palpable vibrations are transmitted from the tracheobronchial tree, along the solid surface of chest wall, to your hand.

Check the symmetry of the vibrations and areas of enhanced, diminished, or absent fremitus. Fremitus is decreased if the transmission of sound waves from the larynx to the chest wall is slowed. This situation can occur when the pleural space is filled with air **(pneumothorax)** or fluid **(pleural effusion)** or when the bronchus is obstructed.

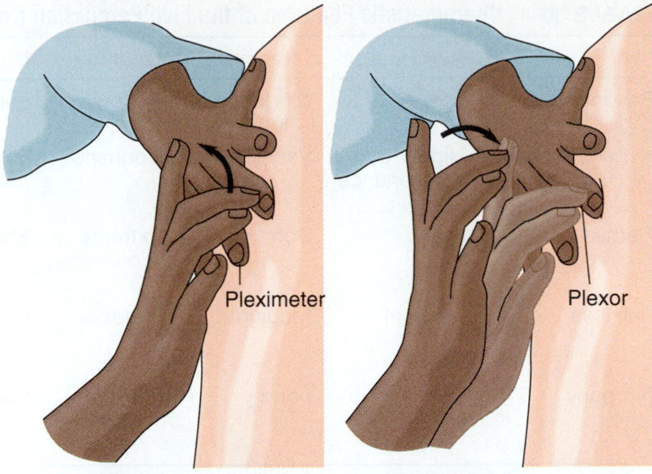

Figure 30-8 ■ Percussion technique.

Fremitus is increased over large bronchi because of their proximity to the chest wall. Diseases such as pneumonia and abscesses increase the density of the thorax and enhance transmission of the vibrations.

Percussion

Video Clip: Diaphragmatic Excursion

Use percussion to assess for pulmonary resonance, the boundaries of organs, and diaphragmatic excursion. Percussion involves tapping the chest wall, which sets the underlying tissues into motion and produces audible sounds. Place the distal joint of the middle finger of the less dominant hand firmly over the intercostal space to be percussed. No other part of your hand should touch the client's chest wall because doing so will absorb the vibrations. Then deliver a quick, sharp strike with the middle finger of your dominant hand to the distal joint of the positioned finger (Figure 30-8). Maintain a loose, relaxed wrist while delivering the taps with the tip of your finger, not the finger pad. Repeat this technique two or three times to determine the intensity, pitch, quality, and duration of the sound produced. Long fingernails limit the ability to percuss.

Animation: Percussion Tones

Percussion produces five distinguishable notes (Table 30-4). These sounds assist in determining the density of the underlying structures (i.e., whether the lung tissue contains air or fluid or is solid). Percuss over the intercostal spaces only because percussing the sternum, ribs, or scapulae yields bone sound. Percussion penetrates only 2 to 3 inches (5 to 7 cm), and therefore deeper lesions are not detected using this technique.

Begin percussion with the client sitting in an upright position. Assess the posterior thorax first and proceed systematically, beginning at the apex and working toward the base. The apex of the lung extends about $\frac{3}{4}$ to $1\frac{1}{2}$ inches (2 to 4 cm) above the clavicle. Posteriorly there is about a 2-inch (5-cm) width of lung tissue at the apex.

Assess diaphragmatic excursion by instructing the client to "take a deep breath and hold it" while you percuss downward until dullness is heard at the lower lung border. Normal resonance of the lung stops at the diaphragm, where the sound becomes dull; mark this site. Repeat the process after instructing the client to "let out all your breath and hold." The difference between the two markings or sounds is the **diaphragmatic excursion.** Normal excursion ranges from 1 to 2 inches (3 to 5 cm). The diaphragm is normally higher on the right because of the location of the liver. Diaphragmatic

TABLE 30-4 Characteristic Features of the Five Percussion Notes

Note	Pitch	Intensity	Quality	Duration	Findings
Resonance	Low	Moderate to loud	Hollow	Long	Resonance is characteristic of normal lung tissue.
Hyperresonance	Higher than resonance	Very loud	Booming	Longer than resonance	Hyperresonance indicates the presence of trapped air, so it is commonly heard over an emphysematous or asthmatic lung and occasionally over a pneumothorax.
Flatness	High	Soft	Extreme dullness	Short	An example location is the sternum. Flatness percussed over the lung fields may indicate a massive pleural effusion.
Dullness	Medium	Medium	Thudlike	Medium	An example location is over the liver and the kidneys. Dullness can be percussed over an atelectatic lung or a consolidated lung.
Tympany	High	Loud	Musical, drumlike	Short	Examples are the cheek filled with air and the abdomen distended with air. Over the lung, a tympanic note usually indicates a large pneumothorax.

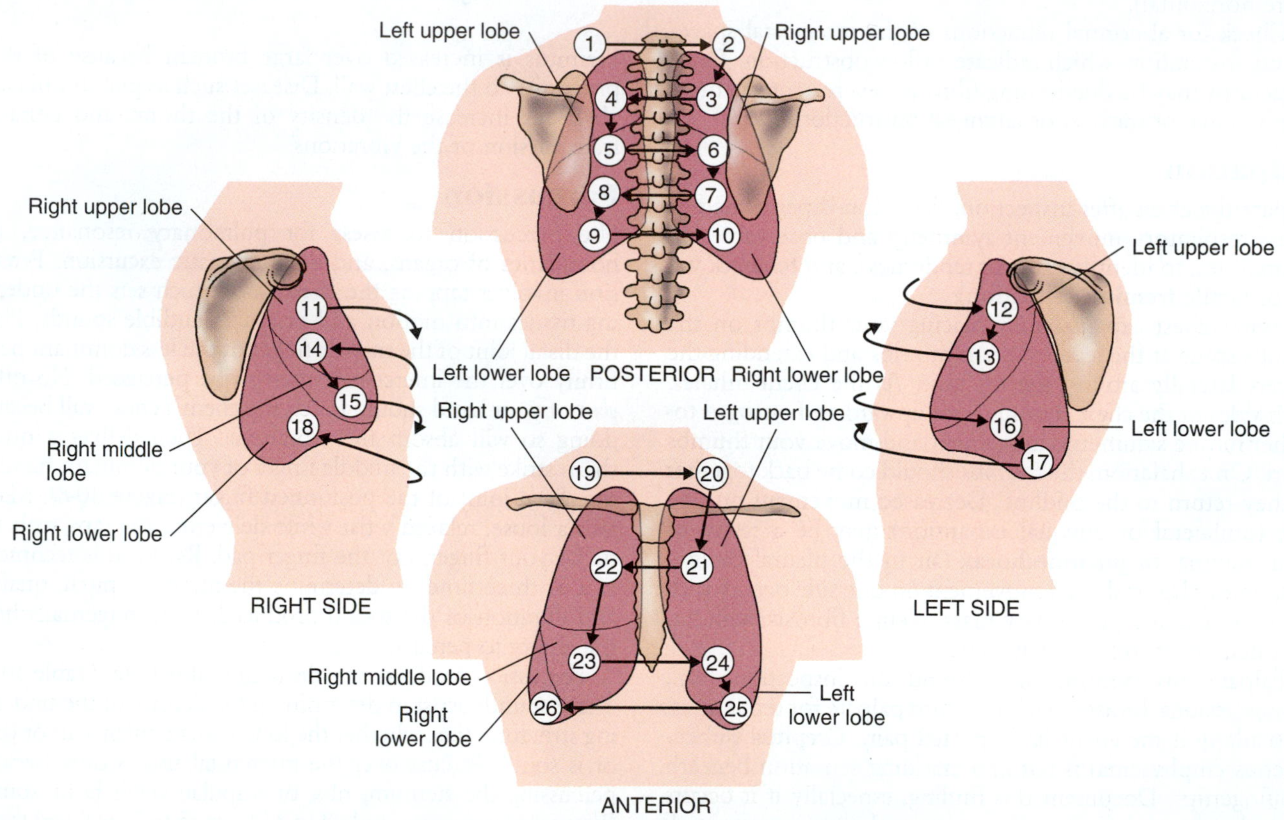

Figure 30-9 ■ Sequence for percussion and auscultation.

excursion may be decreased or absent in clients with pleurisy, diaphragm paralysis, or emphysema.

Video Clip: Anterior Thorax

Continue to assess the thorax with percussion of the anterior and lateral chest. The percussion note changes from resonance of the normal lung to dullness at the borders of the heart and liver. The presence of fluid or solid material (e.g., pneumonia, pleural effusion, fibrosis, atelectasis, and tumors) is indicated by a dull percussion note over lung tissue.

Auscultation

Auscultation includes listening for normal breath sounds, adventitious sounds, and voice sounds. This technique provides information about the flow of air through the tracheobronchial tree and helps to identify fluid, mucus, or obstruction in the respiratory system. The diaphragm of the stethoscope is designed to detect high-pitched sounds.

Begin auscultation with the client sitting in an upright position. With the stethoscope pressed firmly against the chest wall (clothing can distort or muffle sounds), instruct the client to breathe slowly and deeply through an open mouth. (Breathing through the nose would set up turbulent sounds that are transmitted to the lungs.) Use a systematic approach, beginning at the apices and moving down through the intercostal spaces to the bases (Figure 30-9). Avoid listening over bony structures while auscultating the thorax posteriorly, laterally, and anteriorly. Listen to a full respiratory cycle, noting the quality and intensity of the breath sounds. Observe the client for dizziness caused by

TABLE 30-5 Characteristics of Normal Breath Sounds

	Pitch	Amplitude	Duration	Quality	Normal Location
Bronchial (tubular, tracheal)	High	Loud	Inspiration < expiration	Harsh, hollow, tubular, blowing	Trachea and larynx
Bronchovesicular	Moderate	Moderate	Inspiration = expiration	Mixed	Over major bronchi where fewer alveoli are located; posterior, between scapulae (especially on right); anterior, around upper sternum in first and second intercostal spaces
Vesicular	Low	Soft	Inspiration > expiration	Rustling, like the sound of the wind in the trees	Over peripheral lung fields where air flows through smaller bronchioles and alveoli

From Jarvis, C. (2000). *Physical examination and health assessment* (3rd ed.). Philadelphia: W.B. Saunders. Used with permission.

hyperventilation during auscultation. If dizziness occurs, tell the client to breathe normally for a few minutes.

NORMAL BREATH SOUNDS

Normal breath sounds are produced as air vibrates while moving through the respiratory passages from the larynx to the alveoli. Breath sounds are identified by their location, intensity, pitch, and duration within the respiratory cycle (e.g., early or late inspiration and expiration). Normal breath sounds are known as **bronchial** or tubular (harsh hollow sounds heard over the trachea and mainstem bronchi), **bronchovesicular** (heard over the branching bronchi), and **vesicular** (a soft rustling sound heard in the periphery over small bronchioles) (Table 30-5). Describe these sounds as normal, increased, decreased (diminished), or absent.

When bronchial breath sounds are heard peripherally, they are abnormal. This increased sound occurs when the bronchial sounds are transmitted to an area of increased density, such as in clients with atelectasis, tumor, or pneumonia. When audible in an abnormal location, bronchovesicular breath sounds may indicate normal aging or an abnormality such as pulmonary consolidation and chronic airway disease.

ADVENTITIOUS BREATH SOUNDS

Adventitious sounds are additional breath sounds superimposed on normal sounds, and they indicate pathologic changes in the lung. Table 30-6 describes adventitious sounds: crackle, wheeze, rhonchus, and pleural friction rub. Adventitious sounds vary in pitch, intensity, duration, and the phase of the respiratory cycle in which they occur. Document exactly what you hear on auscultation.

VOICE SOUNDS

If abnormalities are found during the physical assessment of the lungs and thorax, assess the client for vocal resonance. Voice sounds through the normally air-filled lung produce a muffled, unclear sound because sound vibrations travel poorly through air. Vocal resonance is increased when the sound travels through a solid or liquid medium. The presence of a consolidated area of the lung, pneumonia, atelectasis, pleural effusion, tumor, or abscess causes increased vocal resonance.

BRONCHOPHONY. **Bronchophony** is the abnormally loud and clear transmission of voice sounds through an area of increased density. To assess bronchophony, ask the client to repeat the number *99* while you systematically auscultate the thorax.

WHISPERED PECTORILOQUY. **Whispered pectoriloquy** is the enhanced voice heard through the chest wall. It is much more sensitive than bronchophony. Ask the client to whisper the number sequence *one, two, three* while you listen with a stethoscope. Whispered words normally sound faint and indistinct. If they are heard loudly and distinctly, consolidation of lung tissue may be present.

EGOPHONY. **Egophony** is another abnormally enhanced vocal resonance and has a high-pitched, bleating, nasal quality. Auscultate the thorax while the client repeats the letter *E*. Egophony exists when this letter is heard as a flat, nasal sound of *A* through the stethoscope. This abnormal sound occurs in areas of consolidation, pleural effusion, or abscess.

OTHER INDICATORS OF RESPIRATORY ADEQUACY

Assess other indicators of respiratory adequacy because gas exchange affects all body systems. Some indicators (e.g., cyanosis) indicate immediate oxygenation problems. Other changes (e.g., clubbing, weight loss, unevenly developed muscles) reflect long-term oxygenation problems.

Skin and Mucous Membranes

Assess the skin and mucous membranes for the presence of pallor or cyanosis, which could indicate inadequate oxygenation. Areas to assess include the nail beds and the mu-

TABLE 30-6 Characteristic Features of Adventitious Breath Sounds

Adventitious Sound	Occurrence in the Respiratory Cycle	Character	Association
Discontinuous			
Fine crackles Fine rales High-pitched rales	Either early or late inspiration	Popping, discontinuous sounds caused by air moving into previously deflated airways; sounds like hair being rolled between fingers near the ear "Velcro" sounds late in inspiration usually associated with restrictive disorders	Asbestosis Atelectasis Interstitial fibrosis Bronchitis Pneumonia Chronic pulmonary diseases
Coarse crackles Low-pitched crackles	More common on expiration but may be present early in inspiration	Lower pitched, coarse, discontinuous rattling sounds caused by fluid or secretions in large airways; likely to change with coughing or suctioning	Bronchitis Pneumonia Tumors Pulmonary edema
Continuous			
Wheeze	Audible during either inspiration, expiration, or both	Squeaky, musical, continuous sounds associated with air rushing through narrowed airways; may be heard without a stethoscope Arise from the small airways Usually do not clear with coughing	Inflammation Bronchospasm Edema Secretions Pulmonary vessel engorgement (as in cardiac "asthma")
Rhonchus (rhonchi)	Audible during both inspiration and expiration but commonly more prominent on expiration	Lower-pitched, coarse, continuous snoring sounds Arise from the large airways	Thick, tenacious secretions Sputum production Obstruction by foreign body Tumors
Pleural Friction Rub	Heard during both inspiration and expiration, generally at the end of inspiration and the beginning of expiration	Loud, rough, grating, scratching sounds caused by the inflamed surfaces of the pleura rubbing together; often associated with pain on deep inspirations Heard in lateral lung fields	Pleurisy Tuberculosis Pulmonary infarction Pneumonia Lung cancer

cous membranes of the oral cavity. Examine the fingers for clubbing (see Figure 33-10), which indicates hypoxia of long duration.

General Appearance

Observe the client for muscle development and general body build. Long-term respiratory problems limit the ability to maintain body weight and lead to a loss of general muscle mass. Arms and legs may appear thin or poorly muscled. The muscles of the neck and chest may be hypertrophied, especially in the client with chronic obstructive pulmonary disease (COPD).

Endurance

Observe how easily the client moves and whether he or she is short of breath while resting or becomes short of breath when walking 10 to 20 steps. As the client speaks, note how often he or she pauses for breath between words.

Psychosocial Assessment

Assess those aspects of the client's lifestyle that either can affect respiratory function or are affected by it. Some respiratory problems may be worsened by stress. Ask about present life stresses and usual coping mechanisms.

Chronic respiratory disease may cause changes in family roles and relationships, social isolation, financial problems, and unemployment or disability. Discuss coping mechanisms to assess the client's reaction to these psychosocial stressors and discover strengths and ineffective behaviors. For example, the client may react to stress with dependence on family members, withdrawal, or nonadherence with interventions. After completing the psychosocial assessment, assist the client in determining the support systems available to help cope with changes resulting from breathing problems.

Critical Thinking Challenge

The client is a 68-year-old female homemaker who comes to the emergency department with shortness of breath and cough. She had been a smoker for 45 years until the last 5 years, when she quit successfully with family support. She is anxious, as are her daughter and husband, who have accompanied her.

1. What specific family information should you obtain?
2. Is the client's socioeconomic status relevant? Why or why not?
3. What other assessment questions should you ask?

evolve For suggested answer guidelines, go to http://evolve.elsevier.com/Iggy/.

Diagnostic Assessment

LABORATORY TESTS

Blood Tests

Several laboratory tests (Chart 30-3) are useful in assessing respiratory problems. A red blood cell (RBC) count provides data about the transport of oxygen. The hemoglobin molecule, found in RBCs, transports oxygen to the tissues. A deficiency of hemoglobin could cause hypoxemia.

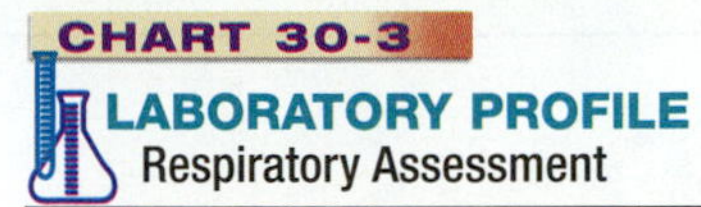

CHART 30-3

LABORATORY PROFILE

Respiratory Assessment

Test	Normal Range for Adults	Significance of Abnormal Findings
Blood Studies		
Complete Blood Count		
Red blood cells	*Females:* 18-44 yr: 3.8-5.1 million/mm^3 45-64 yr: 3.8-5.3 million/mm^3 65-74 yr: 3.8-5.2 million/mm^3 *Males:* 18-44 yr: 4.3-5.7 million/mm^3 45-64 yr: 4.2-5.6 million/mm^3 65-74 yr: 3.8-5.8 million/mm^3	*Elevated levels* (polycythemia) may be due to the excessive production of erythropoietin, which occurs in response to a hypoxic stimulus, as in COPD, and from living at a high altitude. *Decreased levels* indicate possible anemia, hemorrhage, or hemolysis.
Hemoglobin, total	*Females:* 18-44 yr: 11.7-15.5 g/dL, or 117-155 g/L 45-64 yr: 11.7-16 g/dL, or 117-160 g/L 65-74 yr: 11.7-16.1 g/dL, or 117-161 g/L *Males:* 18-44 yr: 13.2-17.3 g/dL, or 132-173 g/L 45-64 yr: 13.1-17.2 g/dL, or 131-172 g/L	Same as for red blood cells.
Hematocrit	*Females:* 18-44 yr: 35%-45% 45-74 yr: 35%-47% *Males:* 18-44 yr: 39%-49% 45-64 yr: 39%-50% 65-74 yr: 37%-51%	Same as for red blood cells.
White blood cell count (leukocyte count, WBC count)	*Total:* 4.5-11.0 × 10^3 cells/μL, or 7.4 IRU *Black clients:* 3.6-10.2 × 10^3 cells/μL	*Elevations* indicate possible acute infections or inflammations, pneumonia, meningitis, tonsillitis, or emphysema. *Decreased levels* may indicate an overwhelming infection, an autoimmune disorder, or immunosuppressant therapy.
Differential White Blood Cell (Leukocyte) Count		
Neutrophils	1.8-7.7 × 10^3 cells/μL; 18%-77% of total *Black clients:* slightly lower	*Elevations* indicate possible acute bacterial infection (pneumonia), COPD, or inflammatory conditions (smoking). *Decreased levels* indicate possible viral disease (influenza).
Eosinophils	0-0.7 × 10^3 cells/μL; 0%-7% of total	*Elevations* indicate possible COPD, asthma, or allergies. *Decreased levels* indicate pyogenic infections.
Basophils	0-0.15 × 10^3 cells/μL; 0%-1.5% of total	*Elevations* indicate possible inflammation; seen in chronic sinusitis, hypersensitivity reactions. *Decreased levels* may be seen in an acute infection.
Lymphocytes	1.5-4.0 × 10^3 cells/μL; 15%-40% of total	*Elevations* indicate possible viral infection, pertussis, and infectious mononucleosis. *Decreased levels* may be seen during corticosteroid therapy.
Monocytes	0-0.8 × 10^3 cells/μL; 0%-8% of total	*Elevations:* see Lymphocytes; also may indicate active tuberculosis. *Decreased levels:* see Lymphocytes.
Arterial Blood Gases		
Pao_2	83-100 mm Hg *Older adults:* values may be lower	*Elevations* indicate possible excessive oxygen administration. *Decreased levels* indicate possible COPD, asthma, chronic bronchitis, cancer of the bronchi and lungs, cystic fibrosis, respiratory distress syndrome, anemias, atelectasis, or any other cause of hypoxia.
$Paco_2$	*Females:* 32-45 mm Hg *Males:* 35-48 mm Hg	*Elevations* indicate possible COPD, asthma, pneumonia, anesthesia effects, or use of opioids (respiratory acidosis). *Decreased levels* indicate hyperventilation/respiratory alkalosis.
pH	Up to 60 yr: 7.35-7.45 60-90 yr: 7.31-7.42 >90 yr: 7.26-7.43	*Elevations* indicate metabolic or respiratory alkalosis. *Decreased levels* indicate metabolic or respiratory acidosis.
HCO_3^-	22-26 mEq/L	*Elevations* indicate possible respiratory acidosis as compensation for a primary metabolic alkalosis. *Decreased levels* indicate possible respiratory alkalosis as compensation for a primary metabolic acidosis.
Sao_2	94%-98% *Older adults:* values may be slightly lower	*Decreased levels* indicate possible impaired ability of hemoglobin to release oxygen to tissues.

COPD, Chronic obstructive pulmonary disease; *HCO_3^-,* bicarbonate ion; *IRU,* international recommended unit; *$Paco_2$,* partial pressure of arterial carbon dioxide; *Pao_2,* partial pressure of arterial oxygen; *Sao_2,* arterial oxygen saturation; *WBC,* white blood cell count.

Continued

CHART 30-3

LABORATORY PROFILE
Respiratory Assessment—*cont'd*

Test	Normal Range for Adults	Significance of Abnormal Findings
Sputum Studies		
Gram stain	Negative	Presence of gram-positive or gram-negative bacteria indicates the type of microorganism causing the respiratory infection.
Culture and sensitivity	Negative	Presence of microorganisms indicates possible respiratory infections (e.g., pneumonia or bronchitis).
Acid-fast stain	No acid-fast bacilli	Presence of bacilli indicates possible tuberculosis.
Cytologic tests	Negative	Presence of abnormal cells indicates possible malignancy.

Arterial blood gas (ABG) analysis assesses oxygenation (partial pressure of arterial oxygen [PaO_2]), alveolar ventilation (partial pressure of arterial carbon dioxide [$PaCO_2$]), and acid-base balance. Blood gas studies provide information for monitoring treatment results, adjusting oxygen therapy, and evaluating the client's responses.

Sputum Tests

Sputum specimens obtained by expectoration or tracheal suctioning assist in the identification of organisms or abnormal cells, such as in cancer or an allergy. Sputum culture and sensitivity analyses identify bacterial infection and determine which specific antibiotics will be most effective. Sputum cytologic examination helps diagnose malignant lesions by identifying cancer cells. Benign conditions, such as allergy or autoimmunity, may also be identified by cytologic testing. Eosinophils and Curschmann's spirals (a mucous form) are often found by cytologic study in clients with allergic asthma.

RADIOGRAPHIC EXAMINATIONS

Standard X-rays

Chest x-rays are used for clients with respiratory tract disorders to evaluate the status of the chest and to provide a baseline for comparison with future changes. Standard chest x-rays are performed from **posteroanterior** (PA; back to front) and left lateral (LL) positions. Portable chest x-rays (taken anteroposterior [AP], front to back) cost more, and the films are of lower quality and are more difficult to interpret.

Chest x-rays are used to assess pathologic changes in the lung, such as with pneumonia, atelectasis, pneumothorax, and tumor. Chest x-rays also can be used to detect the presence of pleural fluid and the position and placement of an endotracheal tube or other invasive catheters. These films have limitations, however, and may appear normal, even when severe chronic bronchitis, asthma, or emphysema is present.

Sinus and facial x-rays are used to assess fluid levels in the sinus cavities to assist in the diagnosis of acute or chronic sinusitis.

Digital Chest Radiography

Digital imaging, which uses less radiation, has started to replace most film images. Digital imaging is especially useful to assess lung and chest lesions. A computer enhances the image to give the greatest amount of detail. The image can be adjusted to emphasize a specific area.

Computed Tomography

When an x-ray reveals a suspicious lesion, computed tomography (CT) is useful because pulmonary soft tissue densities, tumors, and blood clots can be seen. Chest CT is usually performed with consecutive 5- to 10-mm cross-sectional views of the entire thorax. Then, using higher resolution, 1-mm scans are taken of suspicious areas.

Usually CT scans require a contrast agent injected intravenously. The contrast enhances the visibility of structures such as tumors, blood vessels, and chambers of the heart. These scans assist in making a diagnosis. Your role in this diagnostic test is to provide information to the client and to determine whether the client has any sensitivity to the contrast material. Ask the client whether he or she has a known allergy to iodine or shellfish.

Ventilation and Perfusion Scanning

A ventilation and perfusion scan ($\dot{V}/\dot{Q}$ scan) identifies the areas of the lung being ventilated and the distribution of blood within the lungs. It is one of the tests used to support or rule out a diagnosis of pulmonary embolism.

The physician first injects a radionuclide with the client in a supine position and then takes six perfusion views: anterior, posterior, right and left lateral, and two obliques. If the perfusion scan is normal, there is no reason to continue with the ventilation scan. Otherwise, the client inhales a radioactive gas or radioaerosol, and the lung is scanned continuously as the gas makes its way into the lungs (the "wash-in" phase) once the gas has reached equilibrium within the lungs, and then while the gas is leaving the lungs (the "wash-out" phase).

Teach the client about the procedure, and explain that the radioactive substance clears from the body in about 8 hours.

OTHER NONINVASIVE DIAGNOSTIC TESTS

Pulse Oximetry

Pulse oximetry identifies hemoglobin saturation. Usually hemoglobin is almost 100% saturated with oxygen. The pulse oximeter uses a wave of infrared light and a sensor placed on the client's finger, toe, nose, earlobe, or forehead. Ideal normal pulse oximetry values are 95% to 100%. Normal values are a little lower in older clients and in clients with dark skin. To avoid confusion with the PaO_2 values from arterial blood gases, pulse oximetry readings are recorded as the SaO_2 (arterial oxygen saturation), or SpO_2.

Pulse oximetry can detect desaturation before manifestations (e.g., dusky skin, pale mucosa, nail beds) occur. Causes for low readings include client movement, hypothermia, decreased peripheral blood flow, ambient light (sunlight, infrared lamps), decreased hemoglobin, edema, and fingernail polish. Covering the sensor or changing its position may help accuracy if too much ambient light is present.

Results lower than 91% (and certainly below 86%) are an emergency and require immediate treatment. When the SaO_2 is below 85%, body tissues have a difficult time becoming oxygenated. An SaO_2 less than 70% is usually life threatening, but in some cases values below 80% may be life threatening. *Pulse oximetry is less accurate at lower values.*

Pulmonary Function Tests

Pulmonary function tests (PFTs) evaluate lung function and breathing problems. These studies include lung volumes and capacities, flow rates, diffusion capacity, gas exchange, airway resistance, and distribution of ventilation. The results are interpreted by comparing the client's data with expected findings for age, gender, race, height, weight, and smoking status.

The PFTs are useful in screening clients for lung disease even before the onset of manifestations. Serial testing provides objective data that may be used as a guide to treatment (e.g., changes in lung function can support a decision to continue, change, or discontinue a specific therapy). PFTs performed before surgery may identify the client at risk for lung complications after surgery. One of the most common reasons for performing such tests is to determine the cause of dyspnea. When performed while the client exercises, PFTs help to determine whether dyspnea is caused by lung or cardiac dysfunction or by muscle weakness. These tests are also useful for determining the effect of occupation on lung function and any related disability.

CLIENT PREPARATION. Explain the purpose of the tests for planning care. Advise the client not to smoke for 6 to 8 hours before testing. According to institutional policy and procedure, bronchodilator drugs may be withheld for 4 to 6 hours before the test. The client with breathing problems often fears further breathlessness and is anxious before these "breathing" tests. Help reduce anxiety by describing what will happen during and after the testing.

PROCEDURE. Pulmonary function tests (PFTs) can be performed at the bedside or in the respiratory laboratory. The client is asked to breathe through the mouth only. A nose clip may be used to prevent air from escaping. The client performs different breathing maneuvers while measurements are obtained (Figure 30-10). Table 30-7 describes the most commonly used PFTs and their purpose.

FOLLOW-UP CARE. Because many breathing maneuvers are performed during PFTs, observe the client for increased dyspnea or bronchospasm after these studies. Document whether drugs were given during testing.

Exercise Testing

Exercise increases metabolism and gas transport as energy is used. Reasons for exercise testing are listed in Table 30-8. These tests are performed on a treadmill or bicycle or by a self-paced 12-minute walking test. The normal client's exercise is limited by hemodynamic factors, whereas the pulmonary client is limited by breathing capacity, gas exchange compromise, or both. Explain exercise testing and assure the client of close monitoring by trained professionals throughout the test.

Skin Tests

Skin tests are used with other diagnostic data to identify various infectious diseases (e.g., tuberculosis), viral diseases (e.g., mononucleosis and mumps), and fungal diseases (e.g., coccidioidomycosis and histoplasmosis). Allergies and the status of the immune system also can be demonstrated through skin

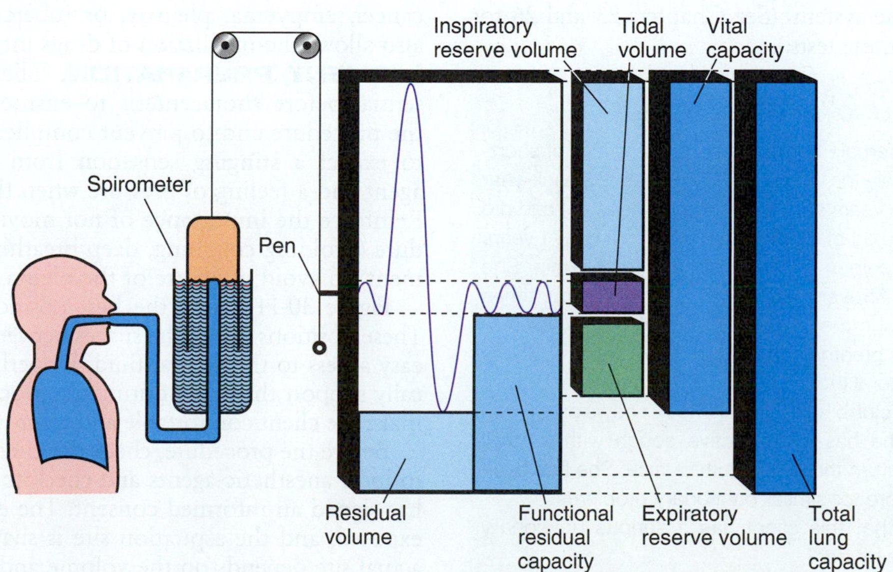

Figure 30-10 ■ Common measurements in pulmonary function testing. (Modified from Luce, J.M., Pierson, D.J., & Tyler, M.L. [1993]. *Intensive respiratory care* [2nd ed.]. Philadelphia: W.B. Saunders.)

TABLE 30-7 Characteristics and Purposes of Pulmonary Function Tests

Test	Purpose
FVC (forced vital capacity) records the maximum amount of air that can be exhaled as quickly as possible after maximum inspiration.	*FVC* gives an indication of respiratory muscle strength and ventilatory reserve. FVC is often reduced in obstructive disease (because of air trapping) and in restrictive disease.
FEV_1 (forced expiratory volume in 1 sec) records the maximal amount of air that can be exhaled in the first second of expiration.	*FEV_1* is effort dependent and declines normally with age. It is reduced in certain obstructive and restrictive disorders.
FEV_1/FVC is the ratio of expiratory volume in 1 sec to FVC.	This ratio provides a much more sensitive indication of obstruction to airflow. This ratio is the hallmark of obstructive pulmonary disease. It is normal or increased in restrictive disease.
$FEF_{25\%-75\%}$ records the forced expiratory flow over the 25%-75% volume (middle half) of the FVC.	This measure provides a more sensitive index of obstruction in the smaller airways.
FRC (functional residual capacity) is the amount of air remaining in the lungs after normal expiration. FRC test requires use of the helium dilution, nitrogen washout, or body plethysmography technique.	Increased FRC indicates hyperinflation or air trapping, which may result from obstructive pulmonary disease. FRC is normal or decreased in restrictive pulmonary diseases.
TLC (total lung capacity) is the amount of air in the lungs at the end of maximum inhalation.	Increased TLC indicates air trapping associated with obstructive pulmonary disease. Decreased TLC indicates restrictive disease.
RV (residual volume) is the amount of air remaining in the lungs at the end of a full, forced exhalation.	RV is increased in obstructive pulmonary disease such as emphysema.
DLCO (diffusion capacity of carbon monoxide) reflects the surface area of the alveolocapillary membrane. The client inhales a small amount of CO, holds for 10 sec, and then exhales. The amount inhaled is compared with the amount exhaled.	DLCO is reduced whenever the alveolocapillary membrane is diminished, such as occurs in emphysema, pulmonary hypertension, and pulmonary fibrosis. It is increased with exercise and in conditions such as polycythemia and congestive heart disease.

TABLE 30-8 Indications for Exercise Testing

- To assess a client's functional capacity (ability to work and perform activities of daily living)
- To determine the reason for exercise limitation: cardiac, pulmonary, or poor conditioning
- To evaluate changes in exercise capacity related to disease or treatment
- To determine the basis for the development of a pulmonary rehabilitation program
- To determine whether supplemental oxygen is required during exercise

testing. Exposure to the allergen or organism used in testing produces a specific reaction (delayed hypersensitivity reaction) of the client's immune system. (See Chapters 23 and 26 for further discussion of these tests.)

Critical Thinking Challenge

The 68-year-old female homemaker has a history of shortness of breath, especially on exertion. She was an 80 pack-year smoker until she quit 5 years ago. Her husband does not and did not smoke. Her father died of emphysema when he was 71 years old. She is on home oxygen continuously at 2 to 3 L/min. She uses an albuterol and Atrovent solution in a nebulizer four times daily and PRN to treat shortness of breath and wheezing. Her respiratory rate (RR) is 24 breaths/min, labored, and shallow. She is pale, anxious, has bilateral though limited chest movement, slight retractions, and digital clubbing. Pulse oximetry shows an oxygen saturation of 87%. She has a productive cough with a small amount of mucoid sputum that is difficult to raise. She has been hospitalized twice before for similar pulmonary problems.

1. Can you assume that this client has a serious pulmonary problem? Why or why not?
2. What additional, noninvasive physical data should you obtain?
3. How could you determine whether the data you have already obtained accurately reflect the client's respiratory status?

evolve For suggested answer guidelines, go to http://evolve.elsevier.com/Iggy/.

OTHER INVASIVE DIAGNOSTIC TESTS

Endoscopic Examinations

Endoscopic studies to assess breathing problems include bronchoscopy, laryngoscopy, and mediastinoscopy (Table 30-9). The most common complications are related to the anesthetic agents and bleeding.

Thoracentesis

Thoracentesis is the aspiration of pleural fluid or air from the pleural space. It can be used for diagnosis or treatment. Microscopic examination of the pleural fluid helps in making a diagnosis. Pleural fluid may be drained to relieve pulmonary compression and the respiratory distress caused by cancer, empyema, pleurisy, or tuberculosis. Thoracentesis also allows the instillation of drugs into the pleural space.

CLIENT PREPARATION. Client preparation is essential before thoracentesis to ensure cooperation during the procedure and to prevent complications. Tell the client to expect a stinging sensation from the local anesthetic agent and a feeling of pressure when the needle is inserted. Reinforce the importance of not moving during the procedure (avoiding coughing, deep breathing, or sudden movement) to avoid puncture of the pleura or lung.

Figure 30-11 shows the best positions for thoracentesis. These positions widen the spaces between the ribs and permit easy access to the pleural fluid. Properly position and physically support the client during the procedure. Use pillows to make the client comfortable and to provide physical support.

Before the procedure, check the client's history for allergy to local anesthetic agents and check to make sure the client has signed an informed consent. The entire chest or back is exposed, and the aspiration site is shaved if necessary. The actual site depends on the volume and location of the effusion (determined by x-rays, sonography, and percussion).

PROCEDURE. Thoracentesis is often performed at the bedside, although sonography or computed tomography may be used to guide it. After draping the client and

TABLE 30-9 Care of the Client Undergoing Endoscopic Tests for Respiratory Disorders

Purpose and Description	Nursing Interventions	Rationales
Bronchoscopy		
To assess airway anatomy for tumors, obstruction, and atelectasis.	Allow the client nothing by mouth for several hours before the test.	The client may aspirate gastric contents if vomiting occurs.
To assist in the diagnosis of infection or cancer by biopsy of lesions; biopsy techniques include the brush biopsy and needle aspiration.	Assess for allergies to iodine, local anesthetics, or pretest medications.	A knowledge of allergies helps prevent allergic reactions.
	Place pulse oximeter.	Pulse oximetry allows continuous monitoring throughout the procedure.
To remove thick secretions, mucus plugs, or foreign bodies.	Administer pretest medications (atropine, diazepam) as prescribed.	Pretest medications help decrease secretions, prevent bradycardia, and reduce anxiety.
A flexible fiberoptic bronchoscope is inserted through the mouth, nose, endotracheal tube, or tracheostomy tube. The procedure may be performed in the operating room or radiology department. Oxygen administration and blood pressure monitoring are standard procedures.	Prepare the client for topical anesthetic administration into the oropharynx.	Explanations about the effects of the anesthetic agent (numbness and gagging) help to decrease anxiety.
	Remove the client's dentures if present.	Injury may occur if dentures are left in place.
	After the procedure, monitor the client's vital signs for 15 min until stable, and monitor for hemoptysis.	Assessment helps detect respiratory distress and signs of complications related to the procedure.
	After the procedure, allow the client nothing by mouth until the gag reflex returns.	Allowing the client nothing by mouth reduces the possibility of aspiration.
	Discourage smoking, talking, and coughing for several hours.	Throat irritation is decreased by avoiding these activities.
Laryngoscopy		
Direct: To detect or remove lesions or foreign bodies in the larynx or to diagnose cancer by removing tissue for biopsy or samples for culture. A fiberoptic laryngoscope is used.	Allow the client nothing by mouth for several hours before the test.	Aspiration is possible if vomiting occurs.
	Assess the client for allergies to iodine, contrast media, or local anesthetics.	A knowledge of allergies helps prevent allergic reactions.
	Administer pretest medications (atropine, diazepam) as prescribed.	Pretest medications help decrease secretions, prevent bradycardia, and reduce anxiety.
Indirect: To assess the function of the vocal cords or to obtain tissue for biopsy. Observations are made during rest and phonation by using a laryngeal mirror, head mirror, and light source.	Assess the client for fears concerning the procedure. Assure the client that he or she will be monitored for any respiratory problems.	Reassurance helps decrease fears about not being able to breathe during the procedure.
	For indirect laryngoscopy, assist the client to sit in an upright position, and encourage normal breathing.	An upright sitting position facilitates the passage of the laryngeal mirror into the mouth.
	After the procedure, allow the client nothing by mouth until the gag reflex returns.	The client may aspirate gastric contents if vomiting occurs.
	Encourage coughing and fluid intake.	Hydration and coughing promote the expectoration of secretions.
	Assess vital signs every 15 min for at least 2 hr after procedure and then every 2 hr for the first 24 hr. Assess the client for bleeding.	Frequent monitoring of vital signs enables the nurse to detect changes such as dyspnea.
	After the procedure, administer lozenges or gargles as prescribed.	Lozenges and gargles help to relieve a sore throat.
Mediastinoscopy		
To inspect and remove samples for biopsy of lymph nodes that drain the lung.	Explain preoperative measures and the procedure to the client.	Explanations about the anticipated procedure help to decrease anxiety.
To detect metastasis of lung cancer.	Assess the client postoperatively for bleeding, pneumothorax, and vocal cord paralysis.	Ongoing assessment for complications helps to ensure prompt treatment.
To obtain tissue for biopsy for diagnosis of tuberculosis or sarcoidosis.	Assess the client for pain, and administer analgesics as prescribed.	Medication decreases the discomfort associated with the procedure.
The procedure is performed in the operating room with the client under local or general anesthesia; a suprasternal incision is used.	Assess vital signs every 15 min for at least 2 hr after procedure and then every 2 hr for the first 24 hr.	Frequent monitoring of vital signs helps to detect changes such as dyspnea.

cleaning the skin with an antiseptic agent, a local anesthetic is injected into the selected site. Keep the client informed of the procedure while observing for shock, pain, nausea, pallor, diaphoresis, cyanosis, tachypnea, and dyspnea.

The short 18- to 25-gauge thoracentesis needle (with an attached syringe) is advanced into the pleural space. Gentle suction is applied as the fluid in the pleural space is slowly aspirated. A vacuum collection bottle is sometimes needed to remove larger volumes of fluid. To prevent re-expansion pulmonary edema, usually no more than 1000 mL of fluid is removed at one time. If a pleural biopsy is to be performed, a second, larger needle with a cutting edge and collection chamber is used. After the needle is withdrawn, pressure is applied to the puncture site, and a small sterile dressing is applied.

FOLLOW-UP CARE. After thoracentesis, a chest x-ray is performed to rule out possible pneumothorax and subsequent **mediastinal shift** (shift of center thoracic structure toward one side). Monitor vital signs and auscultate breath

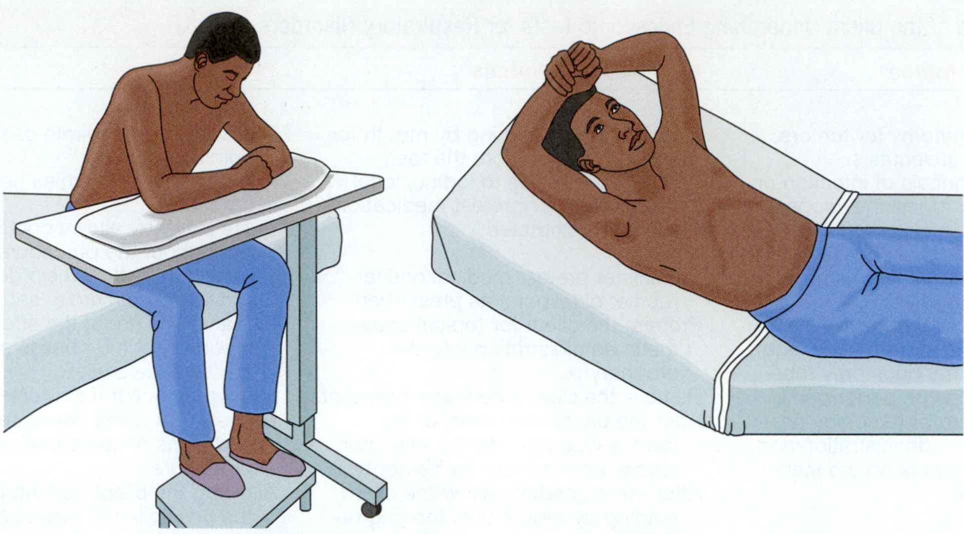

Figure 30-11 ■ Positions for thoracentesis.

sounds for absent or reduced sounds on the affected side. Observe the puncture site and dressing for leakage or bleeding. Also assess for complications, such as reaccumulation of fluid in the pleural space, subcutaneous emphysema, infection, and tension pneumothorax. Encourage the client to breathe deeply to promote re-expansion of the lung. Document the procedure, including the client's response; the volume and character of the fluid removed; any specimens sent to the laboratory; the location of the puncture site; and respiratory assessment findings before, during, and after the procedure.

Lung Biopsy

A lung biopsy is performed to obtain tissue for histologic analysis, culture, or cytologic examination. The tissue samples are used to make a definite diagnosis about the type of cancer, infection, inflammation, or lung disease. There are several types of lung biopsies. The site and extent of the lesion determine which one is used. Transbronchial biopsy (TBB) and transbronchial needle aspiration (TBNA) are performed during bronchoscopy. Transthoracic needle aspiration is a percutaneous approach for areas not accessible by bronchoscopy. An open lung biopsy is performed in the operating room.

CLIENT PREPARATION. The client may worry about the outcome of the biopsy and may associate the term *biopsy* with *cancer.* Explain what to expect before and after the procedure and explore the client's feelings and fears. To reduce discomfort and anxiety, an analgesic or sedative may be prescribed before the procedure. Inform the client undergoing percutaneous biopsy that discomfort is reduced with a local anesthetic agent but that pressure may be felt during needle insertion and tissue aspiration. Open lung biopsy is performed in the operating room with the client under general anesthesia, and the usual preoperative preparations apply (see Chapter 20).

PROCEDURE. Percutaneous lung biopsy may be performed in the client's room or in the radiology department after an informed consent has been obtained. Fluoroscopy, CT, or ultrasonography is often used to visualize more clearly the area undergoing biopsy and to guide the procedure. Positioning of the client is similar to that for thoracentesis. The skin is cleansed with an antiseptic agent and a local anesthetic is given. Under sterile conditions, a spinal-type 18- to 22-gauge needle is inserted through the skin into the desired area (e.g., tissue, nodule, lymph node) and tissue needed for microscopic examination is obtained. Apply a dressing after the procedure.

An open lung biopsy is performed in the operating room. The client undergoes a thoracotomy where lung tissue is exposed. At least two tissue specimens are taken (usually from an upper lobe and a lower lobe site). A chest tube is placed to remove air and fluid so the lung can reinflate, and then the chest is closed.

FOLLOW-UP CARE. Monitor the client's vital signs and breath sounds at least every 4 hours for 24 hours, and assess for signs of respiratory distress (e.g., dyspnea, pallor, diaphoresis, tachypnea). Pneumothorax is a serious complication of needle biopsy and open lung biopsy. Report reduced or absent breath sounds immediately. Monitor for hemoptysis (which may be scant and transient) or, in rare cases, for frank bleeding from vascular or lung trauma.

GET READY for the NCLEX Examination!

KEY POINTS

Safe Effective Care Environment

- When using aerosolized drugs or other chemicals, close the door to the room where they are being used.
- Use gloves when obtaining a sputum specimen.

Health Promotion and Maintenance

- Teach clients who come into contact with inhalation irritants in their workplaces or for leisure time activities to use a mask to avoid respiratory contact with these substances.
- Inform all clients who smoke that smoking increases the risk for development of many pulmonary problems.
- Assist clients interested in smoking cessation in finding an appropriate smoking cessation program.

- Encourage older adults who are confined to bed for any reason or who are recovering from surgery to turn, cough, and deep breathe at least every 2 hours.
- Encourage all clients over 50 years of age and anyone with a respiratory problem to receive a yearly influenza vaccination.

Psychosocial Integrity

- Assess the degree to which breathing problems interfere with the client's ability to perform activities of daily living.
- Pace your interview to match the learning needs and style of the individual client.
- Explain all diagnostic procedures, restrictions, and follow-up care to the client scheduled for tests.

Physiological Integrity

- Document any known specific allergies that have respiratory manifestations.
- Ask the client about recent travel.
- Assess the airway and breathing effectiveness for any client who experiences shortness of breath or any change in mental status.
- Assess the client's respiratory status every 15 minutes for at least the first 2 hours after undergoing an endoscopic test for respiratory disorders.

ADDITIONAL STUDY RESOURCES

Go to your Student CD-ROM for Review Questions for the NCLEX Examination.

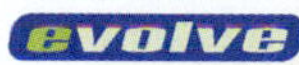

Go to http://evolve.elsevier.com/Iggy/ for Integrated Management of Care Questions for the NCLEX Examination.

SELECTED BIBLIOGRAPHY

Berne, R., et al. (2004). *Physiology* (5th ed.). St. Louis: Mosby.

Carroll, P. (2002). Procedural sedation: Capnography's heightened role. *RN, 65*(10), 54-62.

Ebersole, P., Hess, P., & Luggen, A. (2004). *Toward healthy aging: Human needs and nursing response* (6th ed.). St. Louis: Mosby.

Finesilver, C. (2001). Perfecting your skills: Respiratory assessment. *RN,* April suppl., 16-28.

Frakes, M. (2001). Measuring end-tidal carbon dioxide: Clinical applications and usefulness. *Critical Care Nurse, 21*(5), 23-35.

Gordon, M. (2002). *Manual of nursing diagnosis* (10th ed.). St. Louis: Mosby.

Hess, D. (2000). Detection and monitoring of hypoxemia and oxygen therapy. *Respiratory Care, 45*(1), 65-83.

Interpreting pulmonary function test results. (2002). *Nursing2002, 32*(2), 78.

Jarvis, C. (2004). *Physical examination and health assessment* (4th ed.). Philadelphia: W.B. Saunders.

Mahler, D., Fierro-Carrion, G., & Baird, J. (2003). Evaluation of dyspnea in the elderly. *Clinics in Geriatric Medicine, 19*(1), 19-33.

Moore, A. (2000). Tips for getting a more reliable O_2 sat reading. *RN, 63*(2), 73.

Nussbaum, R., McInnes, R., & Willard, H. (2001). *Thompson & Thompson: Genetics in medicine* (6th ed.). Philadelphia: W.B. Saunders.

Pagana, K., & Pagana, T. (2002). *Mosby's manual of diagnostic and laboratory tests* (2nd ed.). St. Louis: Mosby.

Petty, T. (2002). Spirometry: A key tool for every office. *Consultant, 42*(14), 1753.

Pruitt, W., & Jacobs, M. (2004). Interpreting arterial blood gases: Easy as ABC. *Nursing 2004, 34*(8), 50-53.

Schallom, L., & Aherns, T. (2002). Will my patient survive this cardiac arrest? *Nursing2002, 32*(2), 32cc1-32cc2.

Villars, P., Kanusky, J., & Levitzky, M. (2002). Functional residual capacity: The human windbag. *American Association of Nurse Anesthetist Journal, 70*(5), 399-407.

Zeleznik, J., (2003). Normative aging of the respiratory system. *Clinics in Geriatric Medicine, 19*(1), 1-18.

CHAPTER 31

Interventions for Clients Requiring Oxygen Therapy or Tracheostomy

CHRISTINE A. GATES • M. LINDA WORKMAN

LEARNING OUTCOMES

After studying this chapter, you should be able to:

1. Compare the uses and nursing care issues of oxygen delivery by nasal cannula with oxygen delivery by mask.
2. Explain the problems of oxygen therapy for those clients whose respiratory efforts are controlled by the hypoxic drive.
3. Analyze changes in clinical manifestations to determine the effectiveness of therapy for the client receiving oxygen.
4. Use laboratory data and clinical manifestations to determine the presence of hypoxemia or hypercarbia.
5. Develop a community-based teaching plan for the client receiving supportive oxygen therapy at home.
6. Prioritize nursing care needs for the client with a new tracheostomy.
7. Identify techniques to reduce the risk for aspiration when helping the client with a tracheostomy to eat.
8. Develop a community-based teaching plan for the client with a tracheostomy living at home.

Go to your Student CD-ROM for Review Questions for the NCLEX Examination keyed to these Learning Outcomes.

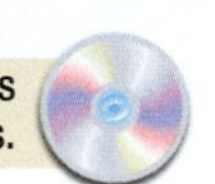

OXYGEN THERAPY

OVERVIEW

Oxygen (O_2) is a gas that is essential for life, as well as a potent drug used for relief of **hypoxemia** (low levels of oxygen in the blood) and **hypoxia** (decreased tissue oxygenation). The oxygen content of atmospheric air is about 21%. Therapeutic oxygen is prescribed when the oxygen needs of the client cannot be met by atmospheric or "room air" alone. Oxygen is used for both acute and chronic breathing problems that cause decreased blood and tissue oxygen levels as indicated by decreased partial pressure of arterial oxygen (PaO_2) levels or by decreased arterial oxygen saturation (SaO_2). Conditions outside the respiratory system that increase oxygen demand, decrease oxygen-carrying capability of the blood, or decrease cardiac output also are indications for oxygen therapy. Such conditions include sepsis, fever, some poisons, and decreased hemoglobin levels or poor hemoglobin quality.

The goal of oxygen therapy is to use the lowest *fraction of inspired oxygen (FIO_2)* to have an acceptable blood oxygen level without causing harmful side effects. Although oxygen improves the PaO_2 level, it does not cure the problem or stop the disease process. The average client requires an oxygen flow of 2 to 4 L/min via nasal cannula or up to 40% via Venturi mask. The client who is hypoxemic and has chronic **hypercarbia** (increased partial pressure of arterial carbon dioxide [$PaCO_2$] levels) needs lower levels of oxygen delivery, usually 1 to 2 L/min via nasal cannula, to prevent decreased respiratory effort. (A low PaO_2 level is this client's primary drive for breathing.)

◆COLLABORATIVE MANAGEMENT

◆Assessment

Arterial blood gas (ABG) analysis is the best measure for determining the need for oxygen therapy and for evaluating its effects. Oxygen need can also be determined by noninvasive monitoring, such as pulse oximetry.

Common Nursing Diagnoses and Collaborative Problems

Nursing diagnoses and collaborative problems that may apply to clients requiring oxygen therapy include the following:

- Anxiety related to hypoxemia
- Acute Confusion related to hypoxemia
- Risk for Impaired Spontaneous Ventilation related to oxygen therapy.

Critical Thinking Challenge

The client is an 87-year-old man who is currently in the ICU after a CABG repair. He has been weaned from the ventilator and is currently using a 40% Venturi mask for O_2 delivery. You note that his $Sa{O_2}$ is dropping gradually from 98% to 90% over the last 30 minutes and he appears short of breath. The physician and respiratory therapist have been notified.

1. What additional assessment data should you obtain?
2. What interventions might you initiate until the doctor or RT arrives?

evolve For suggested answer guidelines, go to http://evolve.elsevier.com/Iggy/.

Interventions

Before starting oxygen therapy and while caring for a client receiving oxygen therapy, you must be knowledgeable about oxygen hazards and complications. You should also know the rationale and the expected outcome related to oxygen therapy for each client receiving oxygen. Chart 31-1 lists NIC interventions for clients using oxygen therapy.

HAZARDS AND COMPLICATIONS OF OXYGEN THERAPY

COMBUSTION. Oxygen itself does not burn, but it supports and enhances combustion. Therefore a fire burns more readily in the presence of oxygen. Take special precautions during oxygen delivery, including posting a sign on the door of the client's room. Smoking is prohibited in the client's room, including at home, when oxygen is in use. All electrical equipment must be grounded (i.e., with three prongs having a green or red dot on the plate). Frayed cords must be repaired because they can cause a spark that can ignite a flame. Flammable solutions (containing alcohol or oil) are not used in rooms where oxygen is in use.

OXYGEN-INDUCED HYPOVENTILATION. Assess for oxygen-induced hypoventilation in the client whose main respiratory drive is hypoxia (hypoxic drive), such as in the client with chronic lung disease who also has hypercarbia. The arterial carbon dioxide ($Pa{CO_2}$) level for these clients gradually rises over time. The central chemoreceptors in the brain (medulla) are normally sensitive to increased $Pa{CO_2}$ levels. When these receptors are active, they stimulate breathing and cause an increased respiratory rate. When the $Pa{CO_2}$ increases gradually to above 60 to 65 mm Hg, this normal mechanism no longer functions. The central chemoreceptors lose sensitivity to increased levels of $Pa{CO_2}$ and do not respond by increasing the rate and depth of respiration. This loss of sensitivity to high levels of $Pa{CO_2}$ is called **CO_2 narcosis**. For these

CHART 31-1

NIC INTERVENTION ACTIVITIES for The Client with Respiratory Problems

Oxygen Therapy: *Administration of oxygen and monitoring of its effectiveness*

- Clear oral, nasal, and tracheal secretions, as appropriate.
- Maintain airway patency.
- Set up oxygen equipment and administer through a heated, humidified system.
- Monitor the oxygen liter flow.
- Monitor position of oxygen delivery device.
- Periodically check oxygen delivery device to ensure that the prescribed concentration is being delivered.
- Monitor the effectiveness of oxygen therapy (e.g., pulse oximetry, ABGs), as appropriate.
- Ensure replacement of oxygen mask/cannula whenever the device is removed.
- Observe for signs of oxygen-induced hypoventilation.
- Monitor for signs of oxygen toxicity and absorption atelectasis.
- Monitor oxygen equipment to ensure that it is not interfering with the client's attempts to breathe.
- Monitor client's anxiety related to need for oxygen therapy.
- Monitor for skin breakdown from friction of oxygen device.
- Provide for oxygen when client is transported.
- Instruct client and family about use of oxygen at home.
- Arrange for use of oxygen devices that facilitate mobility and teach client accordingly.

Artificial Airway Management: *Maintenance of endotracheal and tracheostomy tubes and prevention of complications associated with their use*

- Provide 100% humidification of inspired gas/air.
- Provide adequate systemic hydration via oral or intravenous fluid administration.
- Inflate endotracheal/tracheostomy cuff using minimal occlusive volume technique or minimal leak technique.
- Suction the oropharynx and secretions from the top of the tube cuff before deflating cuff.
- Monitor cuff pressures every 4 to 8 hours during expiration using a three-way stopcock, calibrated syringe, and mercury manometer.
- Change endotracheal tapes/ties every 24 hours, inspect the skin and oral mucosa, and move ET tube to the other side of the mouth.
- Monitor for presence of crackles and rhonchi over large airways.
- Institute measures to prevent spontaneous decannulation: secure artificial airway with tape/ties; administer sedation and muscle paralyzing agent, as appropriate, and use arm restraints, as appropriate.
- Provide additional intubation equipment and Ambu bag in a readily available location.
- Provide trachea care every 4 to 8 hours as appropriate: clean the inner cannula, clean and dry the area around the stoma, and change tracheostomy ties.
- Inspect skin around tracheal stoma for drainage, redness, and irritation.
- Maintain sterile technique when suctioning and providing tracheostomy care.
- Shield the tracheostomy from water.
- Tape the tracheostomy obturator to head of bed.
- Tape a second tracheostomy tube (same type and size) and forceps to head of bed.
- Institute chest physiotherapy, as appropriate.
- Elevate head of the bed or assist client to a sitting position in a chair during feedings, as appropriate.
- Add food coloring to enteral feedings as appropriate.

NIC intervention activities selected from Dochterman, J.M., & Bulechek, G.M. (Eds.). (2004). *Nursing interventions classification (NIC)* (4th ed.). St. Louis: Mosby.

ABG, Arterial blood gas.

clients, the stimulus to breathe is a decreased arterial oxygen level. The low oxygen levels are sensed by peripheral chemoreceptors in the carotid sinus areas and aortic arch. When arterial oxygen ($Pa{O_2}$) levels drop (hypoxemia), these receptors signal the brain to increase the respiratory rate and depth—this is known as the **hypoxic drive** to breathe.

The hypoxic drive occurs only in the presence of severely elevated $Pa{CO_2}$ *levels (i.e., in the client who has hypoxemia and hypercarbia).* When the client with low $Pa{O_2}$ levels and high $Pa{CO_2}$ levels receives oxygen therapy, the $Pa{O_2}$ level increases, removing the stimulation for breathing, and the client has respiratory depression. (The client being ventilated mechanically is not at risk for this complication.)

Oxygen therapy is prescribed at the lowest liter flow (usually 1, 2, or 3 L/min) needed to treat the hypoxemia. A system that delivers precise oxygen levels (e.g., a Venturi mask) is preferred for this client. However, a client with chronic obstructive pulmonary disease may not tolerate a face mask.

Closely monitor the respiratory rate and depth while the client is receiving oxygen. This monitoring is especially important when it is the first time the client receives oxygen or when the $Pa{CO_2}$ levels are not known. Manifestations of hypoventilation are seen during the first 30 minutes of oxygen therapy. The client's color improves (from ashen or gray to pink) because of an increase in the $Pa{O_2}$ level before the apnea or respiratory arrest occurs from loss of the hypoxic drive. Therefore carefully monitor the level of consciousness, respiratory pattern and rate, and pulse oximetry for clients at risk for oxygen-induced hypoventilation, apnea, and respiratory arrest. *Although oxygen-induced hypoventilation is a serious concern, untreated or inadequately treated hypoxemia is a greater threat to life.*

OXYGEN TOXICITY. Oxygen toxicity is related to the concentration of oxygen delivered, duration of oxygen therapy, and degree of lung disease present. In general, an oxygen level greater than 50% given continuously for more than 24 to 48 hours may damage the lungs. *Although oxygen toxicity is a serious concern, inadequately treated hypoxemia is a greater threat to life.*

The causes and manifestations of lung injury from oxygen toxicity are the same as those for acute respiratory distress syndrome (ARDS) (see Chapter 35). Initial symptoms include nonproductive cough, substernal chest pain, gastrointestinal (GI) upset, and dyspnea. As exposure to high levels of oxygen continues, the symptoms become more severe with decreased vital capacity, decreased compliance (which results in more dyspnea), crackles, and hypoxemia. Prolonged exposure to high oxygen levels damages lung tissues. Atelectasis, pulmonary edema, hemorrhage, and hyaline membrane formation result. Surviving this critical condition depends on correcting the underlying disease process and decreasing the oxygen amount delivered.

The toxic effects of oxygen are difficult to treat, making prevention a priority. The lowest level of oxygen needed to maintain oxygenation and prevent oxygen toxicity is prescribed. Closely monitor arterial blood gases (ABGs) during oxygen therapy and notify the physician of $Pa{O_2}$ levels greater than 90 mm Hg. Also monitor the prescribed oxygen level and length of therapy to identify the client at higher risk. High oxygen levels are avoided unless absolutely necessary. The use of continuous positive airway pressure (CPAP) with an oxygen mask, bilevel positive airway pressure (BiPAP), or positive end-expiratory pressure (PEEP) on the mechanical ventilator (see Chapter 35) may reduce the amount of oxygen needed. As soon as the client's condition allows, the prescribed amount of oxygen is decreased.

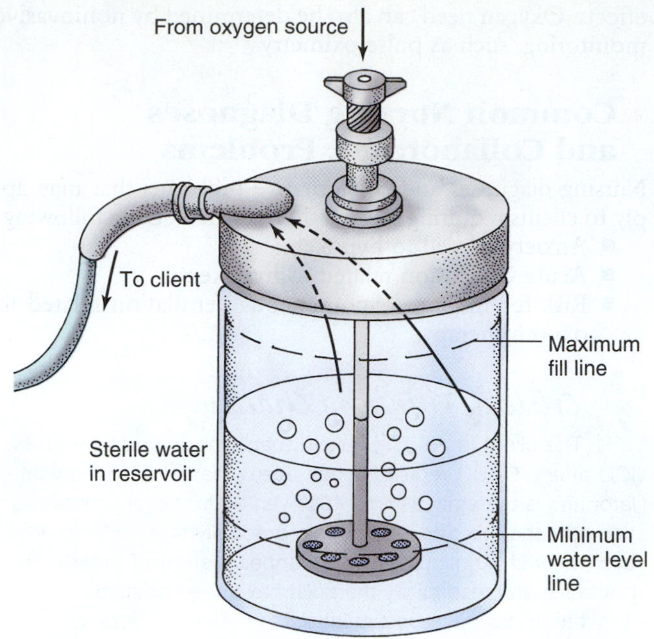

Figure 31-1 ■ A bubble humidifier bottle used with oxygen therapy.

ABSORPTION ATELECTASIS. Nitrogen in the air normally helps maintain patent airways and alveoli. Making up 79% of room air, nitrogen prevents alveolar collapse. When high oxygen levels are delivered, nitrogen is diluted, oxygen diffuses from the alveoli into the circulation, and the alveoli collapse. Collapsed alveoli cause atelectasis (called absorption atelectasis), which is detected by auscultation. Monitor the client closely for crackles and decreased breath sounds every 1 to 2 hours when oxygen therapy is started and as often as needed thereafter.

DRYING OF MUCOUS MEMBRANES. When an oxygen flow rate higher than 4 L/min is needed, humidity is added to the delivery system (Figure 31-1). Ensure that oxygen can be seen bubbling through the water in the humidifier.

Oxygen can also be humidified via a large-volume jet nebulizer (LVN) in mist form (aerosol) (Figure 31-2). A heated nebulizer raises the humidity even more and is used when oxygen is delivered through an artificial airway. Usually the upper airway passages warm the air during breathing, but these passages are bypassed when an artificial airway is in use.

For the client to receive properly humidified oxygen, the humidifier or LVN must have a sufficient amount of sterile water and the flow rate must be adequate. Condensation often forms in the tubing. Remove this condensation as it collects by disconnecting the tubing and emptying the water. Some humidifiers and LVNs have a water trap that hangs from the tubing so that the condensation can be drained without disconnecting. *To prevent bacterial contamination, never drain the fluid back into the humidifier or LVN.* Check the water level and change the humidifier as needed.

INFECTION. The humidifier or LVN may be a source of bacteria, especially if it is heated. The LVN is more likely to be a bacterial source because it uses room air. *Pseudomonas aeruginosa* is often the organism involved. Oxygen delivery

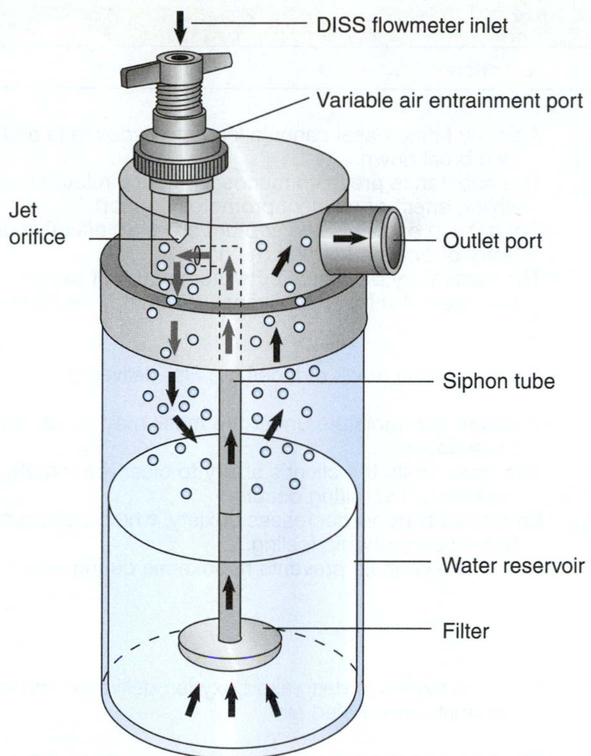

Figure 31-2 ■ An all-purpose large-volume jet nebulizer (LVN).

CHART 31-2

BEST PRACTICE for
Oxygen Therapy

- Check the physician's order with the type of delivery system and liter flow or percentage of oxygen actually in use.
- Obtain an order for humidification if oxygen is being delivered at 4 L/min or more.
- Be sure the oxygen and humidification equipment is functioning properly.
- Check the skin around the client's ears, back of the neck, and face every 4 to 8 hours for pressure points and signs of irritation.
- Provide mouth care every 8 hours and as needed; assess nasal and oral mucous membranes for cracks or other signs of dryness.
- Pad the elastic band and change its position frequently to prevent skin breakdown.
- Pad tubing in areas that put pressure on the skin.
- Cleanse the cannula or mask by rinsing with clear, warm water every 4 to 8 hours or as needed.
- Cleanse skin under the tubing, straps, and mask every 4 to 8 hours or as needed.
- Lubricate the client's nostrils, face, and lips with nonpetroleum cream to relieve the drying effects of oxygen.
- Position the tubing so it does not pull on the client's face, nose, or artificial airway.
- Ensure that there is no smoking and that no candles or matches are lit in the immediate area.
- Assess and document the client's response to oxygen therapy.
- Provide the client with ongoing teaching and reassurance to enhance the client's adherence with oxygen therapy.

equipment such as cannulas and masks can also harbor organisms. Change equipment as per policy or protocol, which ranges from every 24 hours for humidification systems to every 7 days or whenever necessary for cannulas and masks.

OXYGEN DELIVERY SYSTEMS

Oxygen can be delivered by many systems. Regardless of the type of delivery system used, it is important to understand its indications, advantages, and disadvantages. Use the equipment properly and ensure appropriate equipment maintenance. Consult a respiratory therapist whenever there is a question or concern about an oxygen delivery system.

The type of delivery system used depends on the following:

- Oxygen concentration required by the client
- Oxygen concentration achieved by a delivery system
- Importance of accuracy and control of the oxygen concentration
- Client comfort
- Expense to the client
- Importance of humidity
- Client mobility

Oxygen delivery systems are classified by the rate of oxygen delivery. There are two systems: low-flow systems and high-flow systems. Low-flow systems do not provide enough flow of oxygen to meet the total oxygen need and air volume of the client. Part of the tidal volume is supplied by breathing room air. The total level of oxygen received depends on the respiratory rate and tidal volume. High-flow systems have a flow rate that meets the entire oxygen need and tidal volume regardless of the client's breathing pattern. High-flow systems are used for critically ill clients and when delivery of precise levels of oxygen is needed.

If the client needs a mask but is able to eat, request a prescription for a nasal cannula to be used at mealtimes only. Reapply the mask after the meal is completed. To increase mobility, up to 50 feet of connecting tubing can be used with connecting pieces. Best nursing practices for clients receiving oxygen therapy are listed in Chart 31-2.

LOW-FLOW OXYGEN DELIVERY SYSTEMS.

Low-flow delivery systems include the nasal cannula, simple face mask, partial rebreather mask, and non-rebreather mask (Table 31-1). These systems are inexpensive, easy to use, and fairly comfortable. A disadvantage is that the actual amount of oxygen delivered is variable and depends on the client's breathing pattern. The oxygen is diluted with room air (21% oxygen), which lowers the amount of oxygen actually received.

NASAL CANNULA. The nasal cannula, or nasal prongs (Figure 31-3), is used at flow rates of 1 to 6 L/min. Oxygen concentrations of 24% (at 1 L/min) to 44% (at 6 L/min) can be achieved. Flow rates greater than 6 L/min do not increase oxygenation because the **anatomic dead space** (places where air flows but the structures are too thick for gas exchange) is full. In addition, high flow rates increase mucosal irritation. With the use of a nasal cannula, an effective oxygen level can be delivered to clients who are nose breathers and those who are mouth breathers.

The nasal cannula is often used for clients with chronic lung disease and for any client requiring long-term oxygen therapy. The client who retains carbon dioxide rarely receives oxygen at a rate higher than 2 to 3 L/min because of the risk for losing the drive to breathe, thereby increasing the risk for apnea or respiratory arrest. Place the nasal prongs in the nostrils, with the openings facing the client.

SIMPLE FACE MASK. A simple face mask is used to deliver oxygen concentrations of 40% to 60% for short-term oxygen therapy or in an emergency (Figure 31-4). A minimum flow rate of 5 L/min is needed to prevent the re-

TABLE 31-1 Comparison of Low-Flow Oxygen Delivery Systems

FiO_2 Delivered	Nursing Interventions	Rationales
Nasal Cannula		
24%-40% FiO_2 at 1-6 L/min ≈24% at 1 L/min ≈28% at 2 L/min ≈32% at 3 L/min ≈36% at 4 L/min ≈40% at 5 L/min ≈44% at 6 L/min	Ensure that prongs are in the nares properly. Provide water-soluble jelly to nares PRN. Assess the patency of the nostrils. Assess the client for changes in respiratory rate or depth.	A poorly fitting nasal cannula leads to hypoxemia and skin breakdown. This substance prevents mucosal irritation related to the drying effect of oxygen; promotes comfort. Congestion or a deviated septum prevents effective delivery of oxygen through the nares. The respiratory pattern affects the amount of oxygen delivered. A different delivery system may be needed.
Simple Face Mask		
40%-60% FiO_2 at 5-8 L/min; flow rate must be set at least at 5 L/min to flush mask of carbon dioxide ≈40% at 5 L/min ≈45%-50% at 6 L/min ≈55%-60% at 8 L/min	Be sure mask fits securely over nose and mouth. Assess skin and provide skin care to the area covered by the mask. Monitor the client closely for risk of aspiration. Provide emotional support to the client who feels claustrophobic. Suggest to the physician to switch the client from a mask to the nasal cannula during eating.	A poorly fitting mask reduces the FiO_2 delivered. Pressure and moisture under the mask may cause skin breakdown. The mask limits the client's ability to clear the mouth, especially if vomiting occurs. Emotional support decreases anxiety, which contributes to a claustrophobic feeling. Use of the cannula prevents hypoxemia during eating.
Partial Rebreather Mask		
60%-75% at 6-11 L/min, a liter flow rate high enough to maintain reservoir bag two thirds full during inspiration and expiration	Make sure that the reservoir does not twist or kink, which results in a deflated bag. Adjust the flow rate to keep the reservoir bag inflated.	Deflation results in decreased oxygen delivered and rebreathing of exhaled air. The flow rate is adjusted to meet the pattern of the client.
Non-Rebreather Mask		
80%-95% FiO_2 at liter flow to maintain reservoir bag two-thirds full	Interventions as for partial rebreather mask; this client requires close monitoring. Make sure that valves and rubber flaps are patent, functional, and not stuck. Remove mucus or saliva. Closely assess the client on increased FiO_2 via non-rebreather mask. Intubation is the only way to provide more precise FiO_2.	Rationales as for partial rebreather mask. Monitoring ensures proper functioning and prevents harm. Valves should open during expiration and close during inhalation to prevent dramatic decrease in FiO_2. Suffocation can occur if the reservoir bag kinks or if the oxygen source disconnects. The client may require intubation.

FiO_2, Fraction of inspired oxygen.

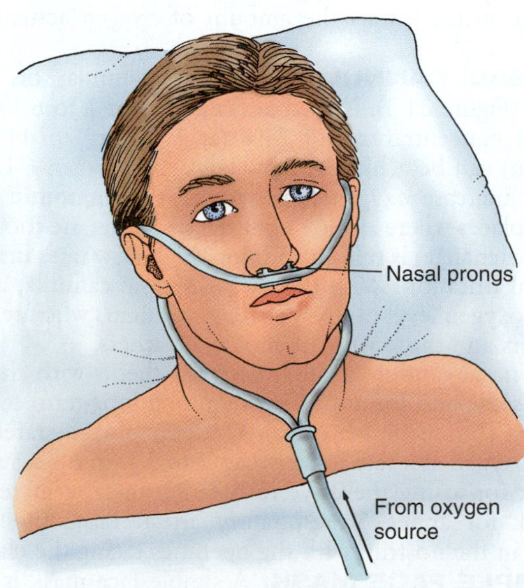

Figure 31-3 ■ A nasal cannula (prongs).

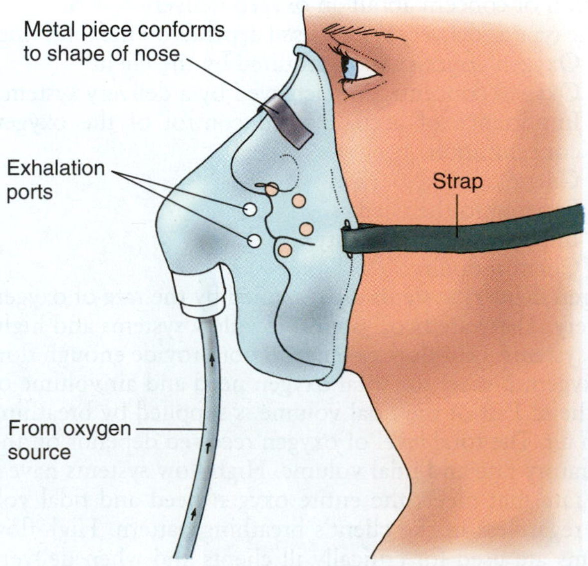

Figure 31-4 ■ A simple face mask used to deliver oxygen.

breathing of exhaled air. Give special attention to skin care and to the proper fitting of the mask so that inspired oxygen levels are maintained.

PARTIAL REBREATHER MASK. A partial rebreather mask provides oxygen concentrations of 60% to 75%, with flow rates of 6 to 11 L/min. It is a mask with a reservoir bag but no flaps (Figure 31-5). The client first rebreathes with each breath, one third of the exhaled tidal volume, which is high in oxygen and provides a high fraction of inspired oxygen (FIO_2). Ensure that the bag remains slightly inflated at the end of inspiration; otherwise, the client will not be getting the desired amount of oxygen. If needed, call the respiratory therapist for assistance.

NON-REBREATHER MASK. A non-rebreather mask provides the highest oxygen level of the low-flow systems and can deliver an FIO_2 greater than 90%, depending on the client's breathing pattern. This type of mask is often used with clients whose respiratory status is unstable and who may require intubation.

The non-rebreather mask has a one-way valve between the mask and the reservoir and two flaps over the exhalation ports (Figure 31-6). The valve allows the client to draw all needed oxygen from the reservoir bag, and the flaps prevent room air from entering through the exhalation ports. During exhalation, air leaves through these exhalation ports while the one-way valve prevents exhaled air from re-entering the reservoir bag. *It is crucial to ensure that the valve and flaps are intact and functional during each breath.* Some models include only one flap on the mask, or one of the exhalation flaps may be removed for safety purposes. *If the oxygen source should fail or be depleted when both flaps are in place, the client would not be able to inhale room air.* The flow rate is kept at a level high enough to keep the bag inflated during inhalation, usually 10 to 15 L/min. Assess for this safety feature at least hourly.

HIGH-FLOW OXYGEN DELIVERY SYSTEMS. High-flow systems (Table 31-2) include the Venturi mask, aerosol mask, face tent, tracheostomy collar, and T-piece. These devices deliver an accurate oxygen level that meets the client's oxygen needs when properly fitted. A high-flow system provides oxygen concentrations of 24% to 100% at 8 to 15 L/min.

VENTURI MASK. The Venturi mask (commonly called Venti mask) delivers the most accurate oxygen concentration. It works by pulling in a proportional amount of room air for each liter flow of oxygen. An adaptor is located between the bottom of the mask and the oxygen source (Figure 31-7). Adaptors with holes of different sizes allow specific amounts of air to mix with the oxygen. Precise delivery of oxygen results. Each adaptor also determines the needed flow rate. For example, to deliver 24% of oxygen, the flow rate must be 4 L/min. Another type of Venturi mask has one adaptor with a dial that is used to select the amount of oxygen desired. Humidification is not needed with the Venturi mask. This system is best for the client with chronic lung disease because it delivers a precise oxygen concentration.

OTHER HIGH-FLOW SYSTEMS. The face tent, aerosol mask, tracheostomy collar, and T-piece are often used to provide high humidity with oxygen delivery. A dial on the humidification source regulates the oxygen level being delivered. A face tent fits over the chin, with the top extending halfway across the face. The oxygen level delivered varies, but the face tent, instead of a tight-fitting mask, is useful for facial trauma or burns. An aerosol mask is used when high humidity is needed after extubation or upper airway surgery, or for thick secretions. The tracheostomy collar is used to deliver high humidity and the desired oxygen to the client with a tracheostomy. A special adaptor, called the T-piece, is used to deliver any desired FIO_2 to the client with a tracheostomy, laryngectomy, or endotracheal tube (Figure 31-8). Adjust the

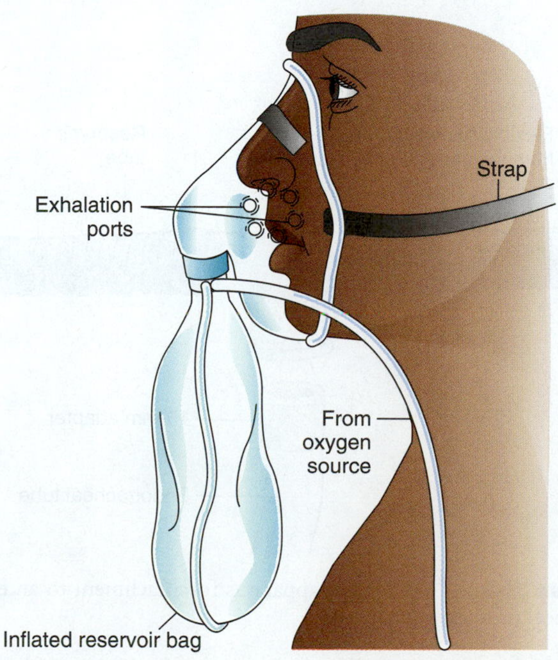

Figure 31-5 ■ A partial rebreather mask.

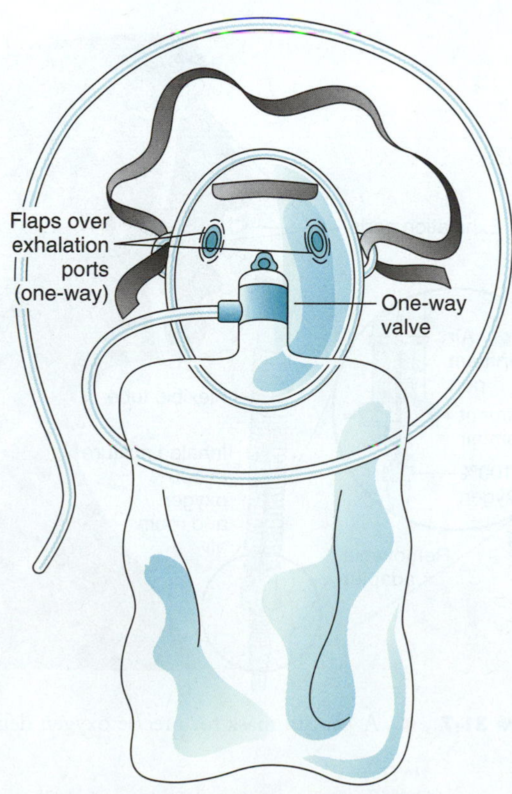

Figure 31-6 ■ A non-rebreather mask.

TABLE 31-2 Comparison of High-Flow Oxygen Delivery Systems

FIO_2 Delivered	Nursing Interventions	Rationales
Venturi Mask (Venti Mask)		
24%-55% FIO_2 with flow rates as recommended by the manufacturer, usually 4-10 L/min; provides high humidity	Perform constant surveillance to ensure an accurate flow rate for the specific FIO_2.	An accurate flow rate ensures FIO_2 delivery.
	Keep the orifice for the Venturi adaptor open and uncovered.	If the Venturi orifice is covered, the adaptor does not function and oxygen delivery varies.
	Provide a mask that fits snugly and tubing that is free of kinks.	FIO_2 is altered if kinking occurs or if the mask fits poorly.
	Assess the client for dry mucous membranes.	Comfort measures may be indicated.
	Change to a nasal cannula during mealtimes.	Oxygen is a drug that needs to be given continuously.
Aerosol Mask, Face Tent, Tracheostomy Collar		
24%-100% FIO_2 with flow rates of at least 10 L/min; provides high humidity	Assess that aerosol mist escapes from the vents of the delivery system during inspiration and expiration.	Humidification should be delivered to the client.
	Empty condensation from the tubing.	Emptying prevents the client from being lavaged with water, promotes an adequate flow rate, and assures a continued prescribed FIO_2.
	Change the aerosol water container as needed.	Adequate humidification is ensured only when there is sufficient water in the canister.
T-Piece		
24%-100% FIO_2 with flow rates of at least 10 L/min; provides high humidity	Empty condensation from the tubing.	Condensation interferes with flow rate delivery of FIO_2 and may drain into the tracheostomy if not emptied.
	Keep the exhalation port open and uncovered.	If the port is occluded, the client can suffocate.
	Position the T-piece so that it does not pull on the tracheostomy or endotracheal tube.	The weight of the T-piece pulls on the tracheostomy and causes pain or erosion of skin at the insertion site.
	Make sure the humidifier creates enough mist. A mist should be seen during inspiration and expiration.	An adequate flow rate is needed to meet the inspiration effort of the client. If not, the client will be "air-hungry."

FIO_2, Fraction of inspired oxygen.

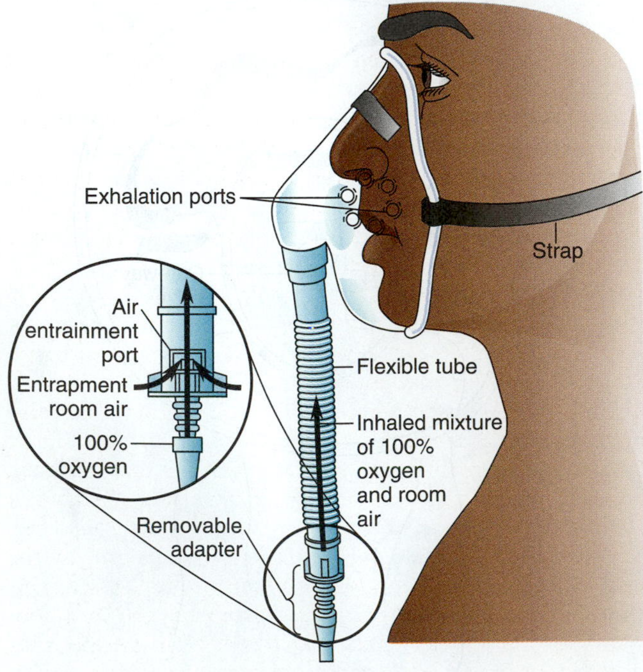

Figure 31-7 ■ A Venturi mask for precise oxygen delivery.

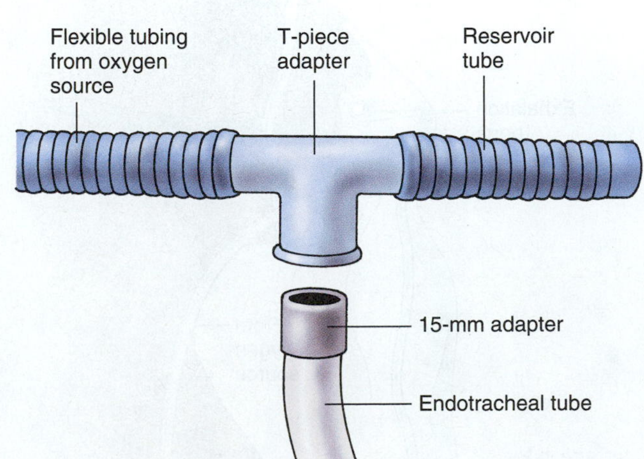

Figure 31-8 ■ A T-piece apparatus for attachment to an endotracheal or tracheostomy tube.

flow rate so that the aerosol appears on the exhalation side of the T-piece.

NONINVASIVE POSITIVE-PRESSURE VENTILATION. Noninvasive positive-pressure ventilation (NPPV) is a technique using positive pressure to keep alveoli open and improve gas exchange without the need for airway intubation. This type of ventilation can deliver oxygen or may just use room air. A nasal mask or full face mask delivery system allows mechanical delivery of either bi-level positive airway pressure (BiPAP) or continuous nasal positive airway pressure (CPAP).

For BiPAP, a cycling machine delivers a set inspiratory positive airway pressure each time the client begins to inspire. As the client begins to exhale, the machine delivers a lower set end-expiratory pressure. Together, these two pressures improve tidal volume.

Nasal continuous positive airway pressure delivers a set positive airway pressure throughout each cycle of inhalation and exhalation. The effect is to open collapsed alveoli. Clients who may benefit from this form of oxygen or air delivery include those with atelectasis after surgery or cardiac-induced pulmonary edema. This technique is also used for sleep apnea. The effect of this use is to hold open the upper airways.

TRANSTRACHEAL OXYGEN THERAPY. Transtracheal oxygen (TTO) is a long-term method of delivering oxygen directly into the lungs. A small, flexible catheter is passed into the trachea via a small incision (Figure 31-9) under local anesthesia. TTO avoids the irritation that nasal prongs cause. Clients also report it to be more cosmetically acceptable. A TTO team provides formal client education, including the purpose of TTO and care of the catheter. A TTO flow rate is prescribed for rest and for activity. A flow rate also is prescribed for the nasal cannula, which is to be used when the TTO catheter is being cleaned. Most clients using this delivery method have a 55% reduction in required oxygen flow at rest and a 31% decrease with activity.

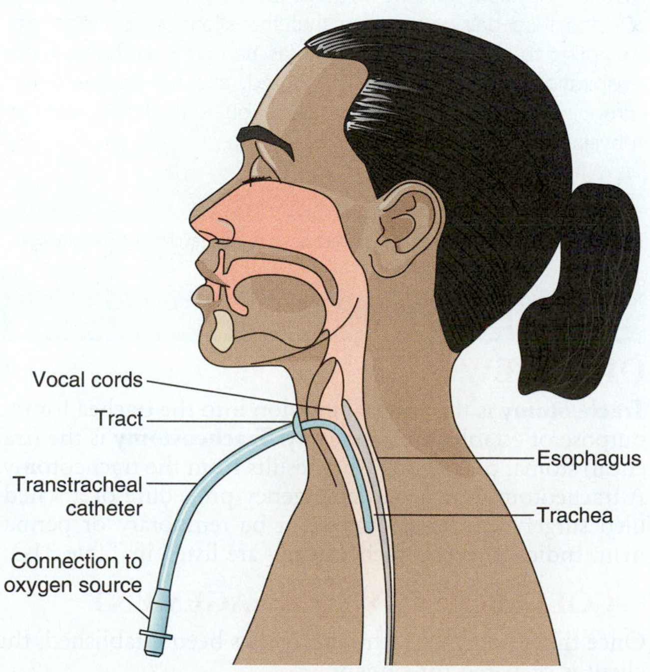

Figure 31-9 ■ Example of transtracheal oxygen delivery.

Community-Based Care

HOME CARE MANAGEMENT

CRITERIA FOR HOME OXYGEN THERAPY. The client must be stable and optimally treated before the need for home oxygen is considered. For Medicare to cover the cost of continuous oxygen therapy, the client must have severe hypoxemia defined as a partial pressure of arterial oxygen ($Pa{O_2}$) level of less than 55 mm Hg or an arterial oxygen saturation ($Sa{O_2}$) of less than 88% on room air and at rest. The criteria vary when hypoxemia is caused by cardiac rather than pulmonary problems, or when oxygen is needed only at night or with exercise.

CLIENT EDUCATION. After the need for home oxygen therapy is verified, begin a teaching plan about oxygen therapy. Assist the client to select a durable medical equipment (DME) company to deliver oxygen equipment and a community health nursing agency for follow-up care in the home. The client is re-evaluated for the need for oxygen therapy about 6 months after discharge from the health care facility and yearly thereafter.

While providing discharge planning and teaching, be sensitive to the client's psychological adjustment to oxygen therapy. Encourage the client to share feelings and concerns. The client may be concerned about social acceptance. Help the client realize that adherence to oxygen therapy is important for being able to participate in activities of daily living (ADLs) and other events that bring enjoyment.

HOME CARE PREPARATION

EQUIPMENT FOR HOME OXYGEN THERAPY. The nurse or respiratory therapist teaches the client about the equipment needed for home oxygen therapy:

- Oxygen source
- Oxygen delivery device
- Humidification source
- Safety aspects of using and maintaining the equipment

Home oxygen therapy is provided in one of three ways: compressed gas in a tank or a cylinder, liquid oxygen in a reservoir, or an oxygen concentrator. Compressed gas in an oxygen tank (green) is the most often used oxygen source. An oxygen tank is economical, and pure oxygen can be delivered at a wide range of flow rates. The large H cylinder may be used as a stationary source and the small E tank is available for transporting the client (Figure 31-10). As a safety precaution, the tanks must always be in a stand or rack. A tank that is accidentally knocked over could suddenly decompress and move around in an uncontrolled manner. Smaller (and lighter) D or C cylinders are also available for the client to carry.

Liquid oxygen for home use is oxygen gas that has been liquefied. A concentrated amount of oxygen is available in a lightweight and easy-to-carry container similar to a Thermos bottle (Figure 31-11). The client is able to fill the portable tank from the large stationary liquid vessel. This type of oxygen lasts longer than gaseous oxygen in a conventional tank of the same size; however, it is expensive, and the oxygen evaporates if it is not used continuously.

The oxygen concentrator is a machine that removes nitrogen, water vapor, and hydrocarbons from room air. It is sometimes referred to as an *oxygen extractor*. Oxygen is concentrated from room air and is delivered at more than 90%.

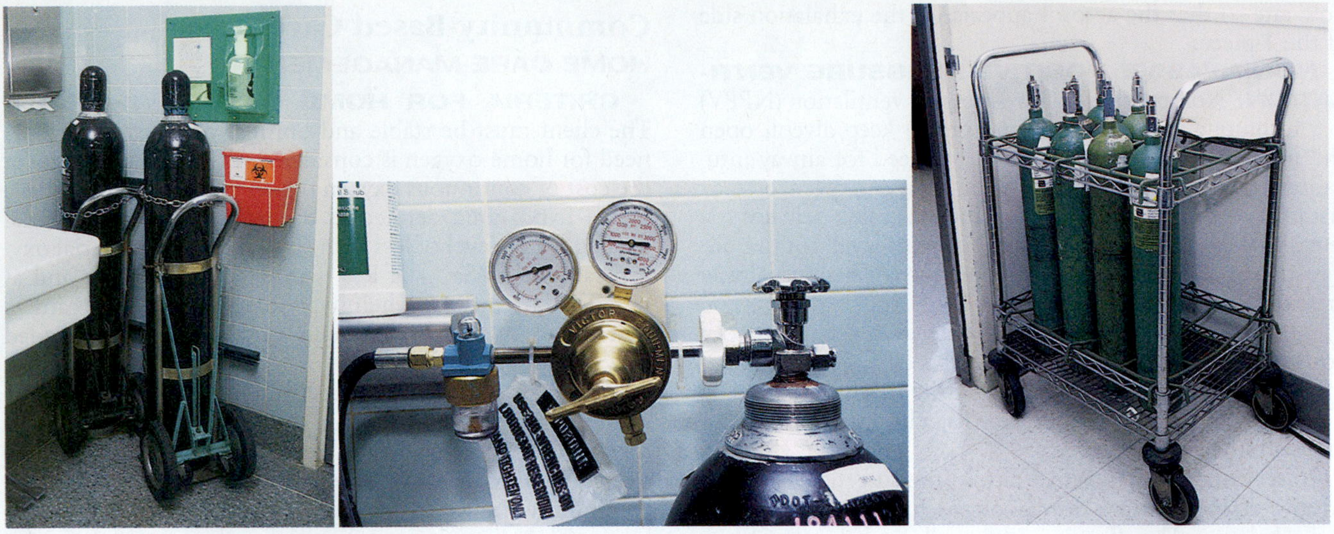

Figure 31-10 ■ Comparison of a large H oxygen cylinder, with a stand *(left)*, regulator, and flowmeter *(middle)*, and several small E cylinders *(right)*.

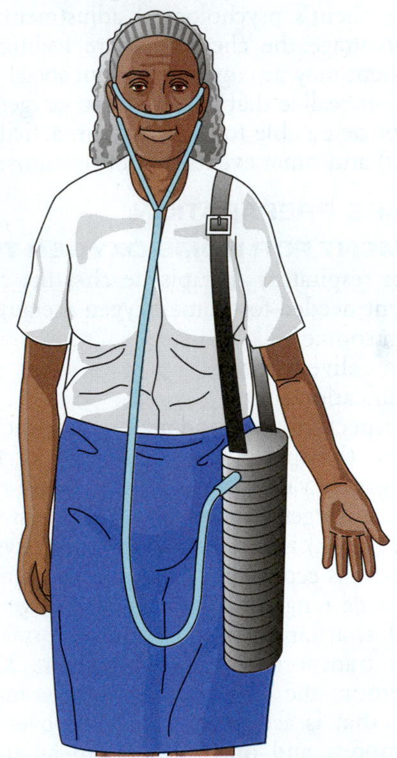

Figure 31-11 ■ Liquid oxygen.

The concentrator, although noisy and not portable, is often used in the home as a stationary system. Portable tanks are used when the client leaves home. The system is the least expensive and does not need to be filled.

Humidification is rarely needed for any of these oxygen systems. Humidification may be helpful, however, when the flow rate is higher than 4 L/min.

In any of the three home oxygen systems, an oxygen-conserving reservoir-type nasal cannula can be used to reduce oxygen flow needs by about 50%. Two types available are the mustache type and the pendant type. A reservoir for storage of exhaled oxygen is attached to the tubing. The stored oxygen is then delivered back to the client on the next inhalation. The reservoir sits on top of the upper lip (mustache type) or hangs around the neck (pendant type).

Critical Thinking Challenge

The 87-year-old, post-CABG repair male client is in the ICU. His respiratory rate is 28, heart rate is 100 to 110, BP is slightly elevated, and ABG shows hypoxemia and mild hypercarbia. Lungs have wheezes and mild crackles bilaterally with reduced breath sounds at the bases. The physician orders BiPAP started. The RT starts the client on the machine at the prescribed settings, with an 8 L/min bleed-in of oxygen to the circuit. The client remains on these settings for the next 2 days. On the third day, you notice that the client is no longer attempting to cough up secretions (as he had been before), his respirations are 36 to 40 and labored, and his Sa_{O_2} is again dropping to between 89% and 90%. You notify the RT and the physician.

1. What assessments should be made?
2. What interventions could be initiated?

evolve For suggested answer guidelines, go to http://evolve.elsevier.com/Iggy/.

TRACHEOSTOMY

OVERVIEW

Tracheotomy is the surgical incision into the trachea for the purpose of establishing an airway. **Tracheostomy** is the (tracheal) stoma, or opening, that results from the tracheotomy. A tracheotomy can be an emergency procedure or a scheduled surgery. Tracheostomies can be temporary or permanent. Indications for tracheostomy are listed in Table 31-3.

COLLABORATIVE MANAGEMENT

Once the need for a tracheostomy has been established, the client is prepared for surgery.

TABLE 31-3 Indications for Tracheostomy

- Acute airway obstruction when oral or nasal intubation is not feasible
- Airway protection (e.g., after head and neck cancer surgery)
- Prolonged intubation or need for mechanical ventilation
- Decreased airway dead space in combination with other indicators
- Control of pulmonary secretions refractory to conventional methods
- Airway reconstruction after laryngeal trauma or laryngeal cancer surgery
- Obstructive sleep apnea refractory to conventional therapy

Common Nursing Diagnoses and Collaborative Problems

Nursing diagnoses and collaborative problems that may apply to clients requiring tracheostomy include the following:

- Impaired Verbal Communication related to physical barrier (tracheostomy; intubation)
- Imbalanced Nutrition: Less Than Body Requirements related to presence of endotracheal tube
- Risk for Infection related to invasive procedures
- Impaired Oral Mucous Membrane related to mechanical factors (endotracheal tube)
- Impaired Social Interaction related to communication barriers

Interventions

PREOPERATIVE CARE

The care for the client having a tracheostomy is similar to that for a laryngectomy (see Chapter 32). Focus on the client's knowledge deficits through teaching, and discuss tracheostomy care, communication, and speech.

OPERATIVE PROCEDURES

Initially, the neck is extended and an endotracheal (ET) tube is placed by the anesthesia provider to maintain the airway. An incision is then made through the anterior skin of the neck, exposing the tracheal rings and moving other tissues out of the surgical path. A second incision is made through the tracheal rings to enter the trachea (Figure 31-12). The types of incisions and specific techniques vary, depending on the surgeon's preference and the reason for the surgery.

After the trachea is entered, the ET tube is removed while the tracheostomy tube is inserted. The tracheostomy tube is secured in place with sutures and tracheostomy ties (or Velcro tube holders). A chest x-ray is obtained to ensure proper placement of the tube. If intubation is not possible, a tracheotomy can be done with the client awake under local anesthesia.

POSTOPERATIVE CARE

Immediately after surgery, focus care on ensuring a patent airway. Confirm the presence of bilateral breath sounds. Assess the client for complications from the procedure.

COMPLICATIONS

Major complications can arise after surgery. Table 31-4 lists the manifestations, management, and prevention of other serious complications of tracheostomy.

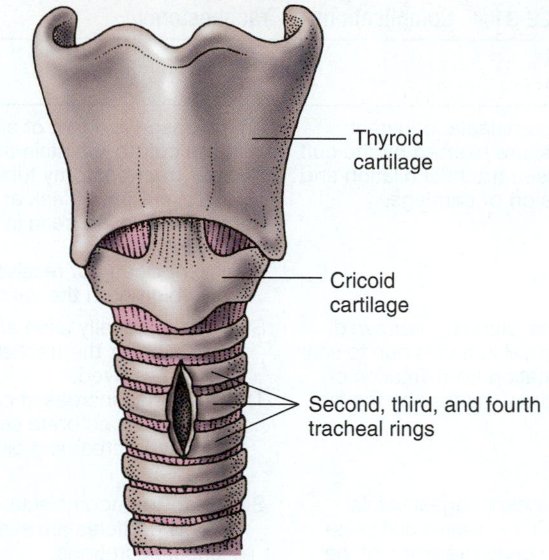

Figure 31-12 ■ A vertical tracheal incision for a tracheostomy.

TUBE OBSTRUCTION. The tube can be obstructed by secretions or by cuff displacement. Indicators of obstruction include difficulty breathing; noisy respirations; difficulty inserting a suction catheter; thick, dry secretions; and unexplained peak pressures (if a mechanical ventilator is in use). Assess the client at least hourly for tube patency. Prevent obstruction by helping the client to cough and deep breathe, providing inner cannula care, humidifying the oxygen source, and suctioning. If tube obstruction occurs as a result of cuff prolapse over the end of the tracheostomy tube, the physician repositions or replaces the tube.

TUBE DISLODGMENT AND ACCIDENTAL DECANNULATION. Prevent tube dislodgment and decannulation by securing the tube in place. This intervention reduces movement and traction on the tube from oxygen or ventilator tubing or accidental pulling by the client. *Tube dislodgment in the first 72 hours after surgery is an emergency because the tracheostomy tract has not matured and replacement is difficult.* The tube may end up in the subcutaneous tissue instead of in the trachea. If this occurs, first ventilate the client using a manual resuscitation bag and face mask while another nurse calls for help.

Ensure that a tracheostomy tube of the same type (including an obturator) and size (or one size smaller) is at the bedside at all times, along with a tracheostomy insertion tray. If decannulation occurs after 72 hours, extend the client's neck and open the tissues of the stoma to secure the airway. With the obturator inserted into the tracheostomy tube, quickly and gently replace the tube and remove the obturator. Check for airflow through the tube and for bilateral breath sounds. If you are unable to secure the airway, notify a more experienced nurse, respiratory therapist, or physician for assistance. Ventilate via a bag-valve mask. If the client is in distress and further attempts to secure the airway fail, call the resuscitation team, including an anesthesiologist, for assistance.

PNEUMOTHORAX. **Pneumothorax** (air in the chest cavity) can develop during the tracheotomy procedure if the thoracic cavity is accidentally entered. When pneumothorax

TABLE 31-4 Complications of Tracheostomy

Complications and Description	Manifestations	Management	Prevention
Tracheomalacia: constant pressure exerted by the cuff causes tracheal dilation and erosion of cartilage.	An increased amount of air is required in the cuff to maintain the seal. A larger tracheostomy tube is required to prevent an air leak at the stoma. Food particles are seen in tracheal secretions. The client does not receive the set tidal volume on the ventilator.	No special management is needed unless bleeding occurs.	Use an uncuffed tube as soon as possible. Monitor cuff pressure and air volumes closely and detect changes.
Tracheal stenosis: narrowed tracheal lumen is due to scar formation from irritation of tracheal mucosa by the cuff.	Stenosis is usually seen after the cuff is deflated or the tracheostomy tube is removed. The client has increased coughing, inability to expectorate secretions, or difficulty in breathing or talking.	Tracheal dilation or surgical intervention is used.	Prevent pulling of and traction on the tracheostomy tube. Properly secure the tube in the midline position. Maintain proper cuff pressure. Minimize oronasal intubation time.
Tracheoesophageal fistula (TEF): excessive cuff pressure causes erosion of the posterior wall of the trachea. A hole is created between the trachea and the anterior esophagus. The client at highest risk also has a nasogastric tube present.	Similar to tracheomalacia: ▪ Food particles are seen in tracheal secretions. ▪ Increased air in cuff is needed to achieve a seal. ▪ The client has increased coughing and choking while eating. ▪ The client does not receive the set tidal volume on the ventilator.	Manually administer oxygen by mask to prevent hypoxemia. Use a small soft feeding tube instead of a nasogastric tube for tube feedings. A gastrostomy or jejunostomy may be performed. Monitor the client with a nasogastric tube closely; assess for TEF and aspiration.	Maintain cuff pressure. Monitor the amount of air needed for inflation and detect changes. Progress to a deflated cuff or cuffless tube as soon as possible.
Trachea-innominate artery fistula: a malpositioned tube causes its distal tip to push against the lateral wall of the tracheostomy. Continued pressure causes necrosis and erosion of the innominate artery. ***This is a medical emergency.***	The tracheostomy tube pulsates in synchrony with the heartbeat. There is heavy bleeding from the stoma. ***This is a life-threatening complication.***	Remove the tracheostomy tube immediately. Apply direct pressure to the innominate artery at the stoma site. Prepare the client for immediate repair surgery.	Correct the tube size, length, and midline position. Prevent pulling or tugging on the tracheostomy tube. Immediately notify the physician of the pulsating tube.

occurs during tracheotomy, it usually does so at the apex of the lung. Chest x-rays after placement are used to assess for pneumothorax.

SUBCUTANEOUS EMPHYSEMA. When there is an opening (rent) in the trachea, air escapes into fresh tissue planes of the neck, causing subcutaneous emphysema. Air can also progress throughout the chest and axillary tissues into the face. Inspect and palpate for air under the skin around the new tracheostomy.

BLEEDING. A small amount of bleeding from the tracheotomy incision can be expected for the first few days, but constant oozing is abnormal. Wrap gauze around the tube and pack gauze gently into the wound to apply pressure to the bleeding sites.

INFECTION. In the hospital, use sterile technique to prevent infection during suctioning and tracheostomy care. Assess the stoma site at least once per shift for purulent drainage, redness, pain, or swelling. Tracheostomy dressings may be used to keep the stoma clean and dry. Change these dressings often because moist dressings provide a medium for bacterial growth. Careful wound care prevents most local infections.

TRACHEOSTOMY TUBES

Many types of tracheostomy tubes are available (Table 31-5 and Figure 31-13). The one chosen depends on the specific needs of the client. Tracheostomy tubes are available in many sizes and are made of various types of materials, such as plastic or metal. The tubes may be disposable or reusable. A tracheostomy tube may or may not have a cuff. It also may have an inner cannula that can be either disposable or reusable. For clients receiving mechanical ventilation, a cuffed tube is used in acute care settings. A noncuffed tube is used for airway maintenance when mechanical ventilation is not required.

For tubes with a reusable inner cannula, inspect, suction, and clean the inner cannula. During the first 24 hours after surgery, perform cannula care as often as needed, perhaps every 30 to 60 minutes. Thereafter, care is determined by the client's needs and agency policy. In planning for self-care, teach the client to remove the inner cannula and check for cleanliness. Also instruct the client about suctioning and tracheostomy cleaning.

Because breathing and swallowing move the tube, a cuffed tube is not protective against aspiration. Having a cuffed tube inflated may give a false sense of security that aspiration cannot occur during feeding or mouth care. In addition, the pilot balloon does not reflect whether the correct amount of air is present in the cuff.

A fenestrated tube can function in many different ways. When the inner cannula is in place, the fenestration is covered over (closed), and the tube functions as a double-lumen tube. With the inner cannula removed and the plug or red de-

TABLE 31-5 Types of Tracheostomy Tubes

Double-Lumen Tube
The double-lumen tube has three major parts:

- Outer cannula—fits into the stoma and keeps the airway open. The faceplate indicates the size and type of tube and has small holes on both sides for securing the tube with tracheostomy ties.
- Inner cannula—fits snugly into the outer cannula and locks into place. Provides the universal adaptor for use with the ventilator and other respiratory therapy equipment. Some may be removed, cleaned, and reused; others are disposable.
- Obturator—is a stylet with a blunt end used to facilitate the direction of the tube when inserting or changing a tracheostomy tube. It is removed immediately after tube placement and is always kept with the client and at the bedside in case of accidental decannulation.

Single-Lumen Tube
The single-lumen tube is a long tube used for clients with long or extra-thick necks. Often called a "bull neck trach" because of the long distance from the skin to the trachea or the longer length of the trachea in large people. More intensive nursing care is required with this tube because there is no inner cannula to ensure a patent lumen.

Cuffed Tube
A cuff, when inflated, seals the airway. Used with mechanical ventilation to prevent aspiration of oral or gastric secretions, or for tube feeding. A pilot balloon attached to the outside of the tube indicates the presence or absence of air in the cuff.

Cuffless Tube
The cuffless tube is a plastic, silicone-like (Silastic) tube or a metal tube, usually double lumen, used for long-term airway management in clients who require a tracheostomy, who can protect themselves from aspiration, and who do not require mechanical ventilation. Many people can speak with this tube in place.

Fenestrated Tube
The fenestrated tube has a precut opening (fenestration) in the upper posterior wall of the outer cannula. It is used to wean the client from a tracheostomy by ensuring that the client can tolerate breathing through his or her natural airway before the entire tube is removed. This tube allows the client to speak.

Cuffed Fenestrated Tube
The cuffed fenestrated tube facilitates mechanical ventilation and speech. It is often used for clients with spinal cord paralysis or neuromuscular disease who do not require ventilation all the time. When not being mechanically ventilated, the client can have the cuff deflated and the tube capped for speech. A cuffed fenestrated tube is never used in weaning from a tracheostomy because the cuff, even fully deflated, may partially obstruct the airway.

Metal Tracheostomy Tube
The metal tracheostomy tube is used for permanent tracheostomy. It is a cuffless double-lumen tube and can be cleaned and reused indefinitely. A special adaptor attaches a manual resuscitation bag. Popular types are the Jackson and Holinger tubes.

Talking Tracheostomy Tube
The talking tracheostomy tube provides a means of communication for the client who is using a ventilator on a long-term basis. An extra air channel allows air to flow up through the vocal cords so that the client can speak with the cuff inflated. The air can cause drying of the vocal cords from constant dry airflow. Examples are the Pitt Trach Speaking Tube (National Catheter Corporation) and Communitrach (Implant Technologies, Inc.).

cannulation stopper locked in place, air can pass through the fenestration, as well as around the tube and up through the natural airway. The client can cough and speak, adjusting to breathing through the upper air passages. If the client has trouble with any of these actions, he or she should be evaluated for proper tube placement, patency, size, and fenestration. *Do not cap the tube until the problem is identified and corrected.* A fenestrated tube may or may not have a cuff.

With a cuffed fenestrated tube, some air flows through the natural airway when the client is not being mechanically ventilated. *Always deflate the cuff before capping the tube with the decannulation cap; otherwise, the client has no airway* (Figure 31-14).

Clients with metal tracheostomy tubes scheduled for magnetic resonance imaging (MRI) need to change to a plastic tube. Metal tubes could be dislodged or heat up with exposure to the magnetic field during the scan.

Care Issues for the Client with a Tracheostomy

PREVENTION OF TISSUE DAMAGE

Tissue damage can occur at the point where the inflated cuff presses against the tracheal mucosa. Mucosal ischemia occurs when the pressure exerted by the cuff on the mucosa exceeds the capillary perfusion pressure. To reduce the risk for tracheal damage, keep the cuff pressure between 14 and 20 mm Hg or 20 and 28 cm H_2O (ideally, 25 cm H_2O or less).

Most cuffs are designed to use a high volume of air while maintaining a low pressure on the tracheal mucosa. Inflate the cuff to form a seal between the trachea and the cuff while creating the least amount of pressure. If the cuff cannot be inflated to seal well enough, a larger-diameter tube may be needed. The two methods of cuff inflation are (1) the *minimal leak technique* (for cuffs without pressure relief valves) and (2) the *occlusive technique* (for cuffs with pressure relief valves). A pressure cuff inflator can be used to inflate the cuff to a specified pressure or to check the cuff pressure (Figure 31-15).

Check the cuff pressure at least once during each shift, especially with the minimal leak technique, and keep the pressure at 14 to 20 mm Hg or 20 to 28 cm H_2O. In rare situations, the cuff pressure is increased to maintain ventilator volumes when peak pressures are greater than 50 mm Hg (65 cm H_2O) and positive end-expiratory pressure (PEEP) is greater than 10 mm Hg (14 cm H_2O). High PEEP values can deflate the cuff over time and more air may need to be added periodically to maintain a proper seal. Manufacturers provide guidelines for the recommended volumes for each tracheostomy cuff size. Most cuffs are adequately inflated with less than 10 mL of air.

Although a high cuff pressure causes tracheal damage, other factors may make the damage worse. The client who is malnourished, hypotensive, dehydrated, hypoxic, older, or receiving corticosteroids has poor tissue healing and is at risk for greater tissue damage. Tube friction and movement are important factors that contribute to tracheal mucosa damage. Reduce local airway damage by maintaining proper cuff pressures, stabilizing the tube, suctioning judiciously, and preventing and treating malnutrition, hemodynamic instability, or hypoxia.

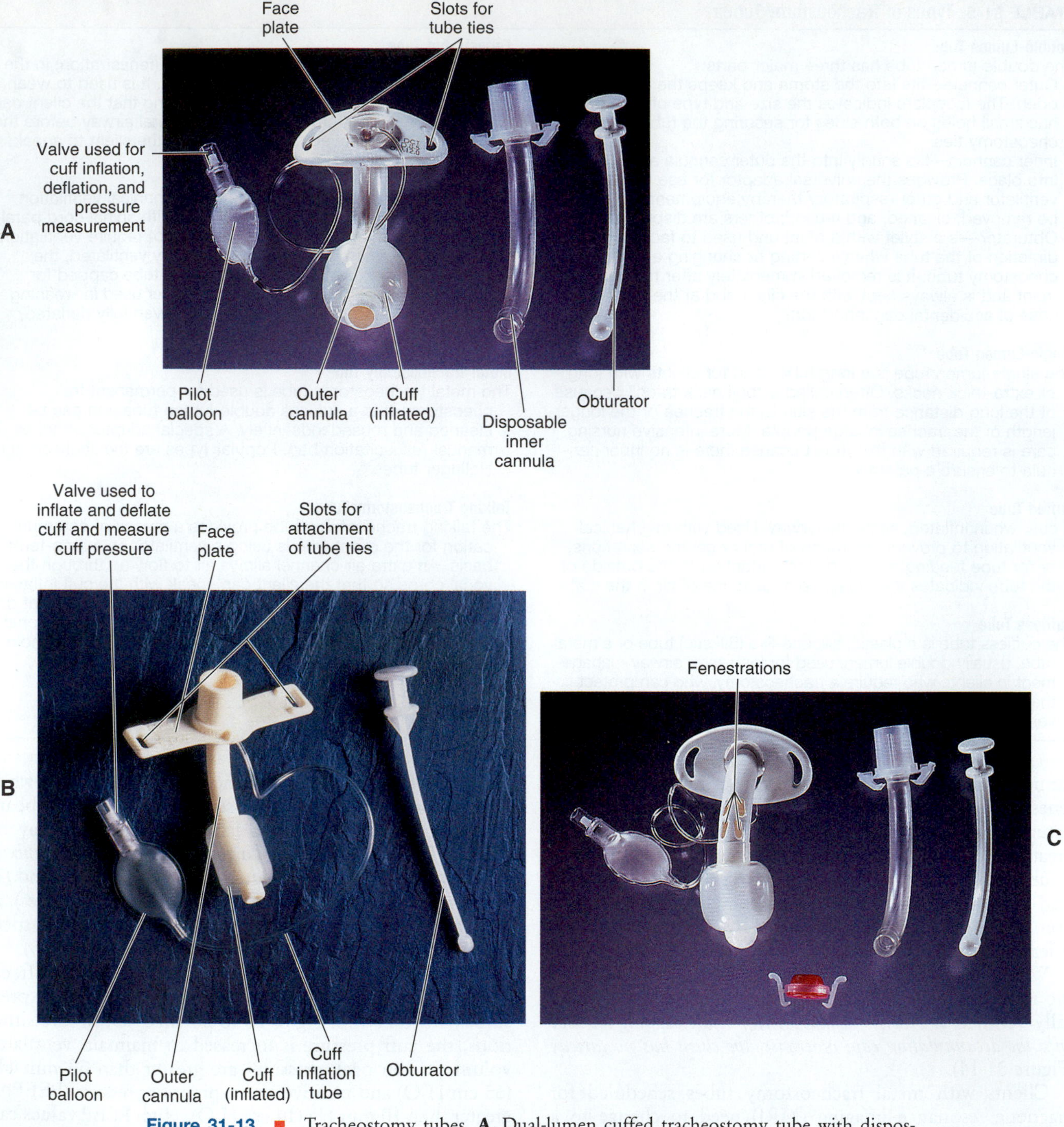

Figure 31-13 ■ Tracheostomy tubes. **A,** Dual-lumen cuffed tracheostomy tube with disposable inner cannula. **B,** Single-lumen cannula cuffed tracheostomy tube. **C,** Dual-lumen cuffed fenestrated tracheostomy tube. (Courtesy of Mallinckrodt, Inc., Shiley Tracheostomy Products, St. Louis, MO.)

AIR WARMING AND HUMIDIFICATION

The tracheostomy tube bypasses the nose and mouth, which normally humidify, warm, and filter the air before it reaches the lower respiratory tract. If humidification and warming are not adequate, tracheal damage can occur. Thick, dried secretions can occlude the airways.

To prevent these complications, humidify the air as prescribed. On an ongoing basis, assess for a fine mist emerging from the tracheostomy collar or T-piece during inspiration and expiration. To increase the amount of humidity delivered, a warming device can be attached to the humidification source. At the same time, a temperature probe is placed in the tubing circuit. *The temperature is kept between 98.6° and 100.4° F (37° and 38° C). It should never exceed 104° F (40° C).* Monitor the circuit temperature at least hourly by feeling the tubing and by checking the temperature probe. Ensure adequate hydration, which also helps to liquefy secretions. Increasing the flow rate at the flowmeter also increases the amount of delivered humidity.

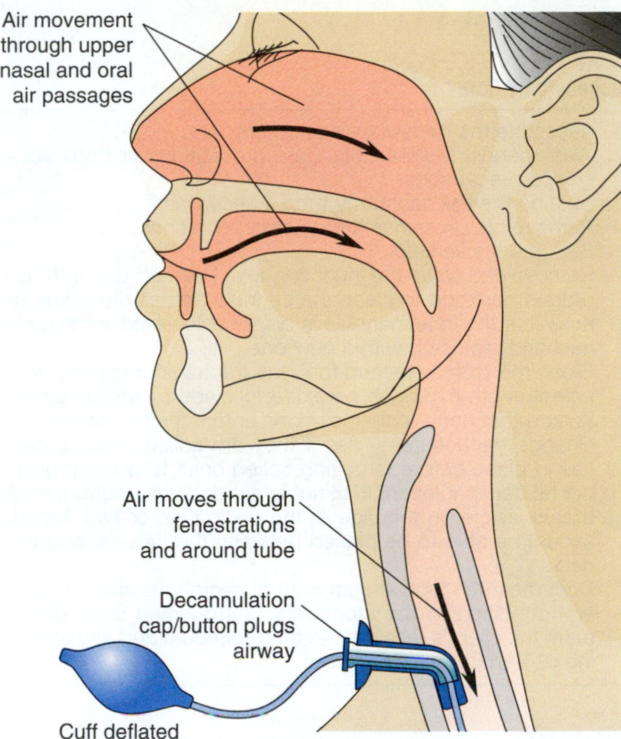

Figure 31-14 ■ Breathing through a fenestrated tracheostomy tube with a cap in place and the cuff deflated.

CHART 31-3

BEST PRACTICE for
Suctioning the Artificial Airway

1. Assess the need for suctioning (routine unnecessary suctioning causes mucosal damage, bleeding, and bronchospasm).
2. Wash hands. Don protective eyewear. Maintain standard precautions or body substance precautions.
3. Explain to the client that sensations such as shortness of breath and coughing are to be expected but that any discomfort will be very short in duration.
4. Check the suction source. Occlude the suction source, and adjust the pressure dial to between 80 and 120 mm Hg to prevent hypoxemia and trauma to the mucosa.
5. Set up a sterile field.
6. Preoxygenate the client with 100% oxygen for 30 seconds to 3 minutes (at least three hyperinflations) to prevent hypoxemia. Keep hyperinflations synchronized with inhalation.
7. Quickly insert the suction catheter until resistance is met. *Do not apply suction during insertion.*
8. Withdraw the catheter 0.4 to 0.8 inch (1 to 2 cm), and begin to apply suction. Use intermittent suction and a twirling motion of the catheter during withdrawal. *Never suction longer than 10 to 15 seconds.*
9. Hyperoxygenate for 1 to 5 minutes or until the client's baseline heart rate and oxygen saturation are within normal limits.
10. Repeat as needed for up to three total suction passes.
11. Suction mouth as needed, and provide mouth care.
12. Describe secretions, and document client's responses.

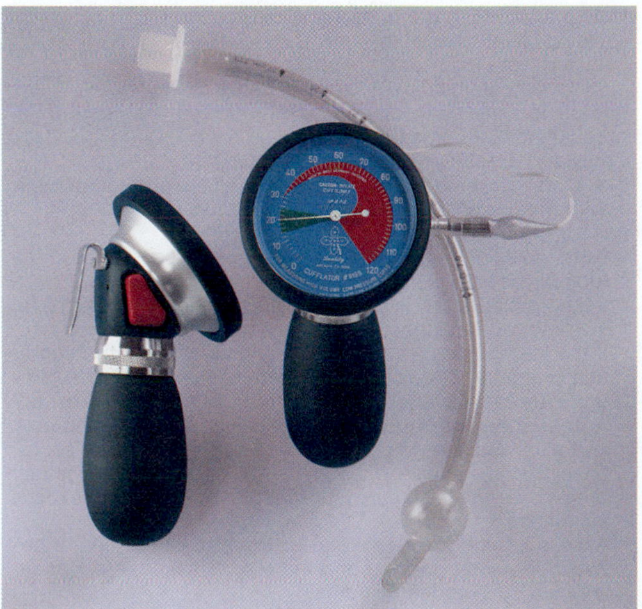

Figure 31-15 ■ An aneroid pressure manometer for cuff inflation and measuring cuff pressures. (Courtesy of J.T. Posey Company, Arcadia, CA.)

SUCTIONING

Suctioning maintains a patent airway and promotes gas exchange by removing secretions from the client who cannot cough adequately. Chart 31-3 lists best practices for suctioning. Assess the client's need for suctioning. Suctioning is indicated when audible or noisy secretions, crackles or wheezes on auscultation, restlessness, increased pulse or respiratory rates, or mucus in the artificial airway is present. Other indications include client requests for suctioning or an increase in the peak airway pressure on the ventilator.

Suctioning is performed most often through an artificial airway but can be accomplished either through the nose or the mouth. Suctioning of both routes is considered routine for the client with retained secretions.

Suctioning through the nose has similar complications as suctioning through an artificial airway. Entry through the nasal vault into the throat can be painful. Slow, careful placement of the catheter, with a good understanding of the nasopharyngeal anatomy, can make the procedure less traumatic. Placing a nasopharyngeal airway and suctioning through it helps prevent trauma to the nasal mucosa. Advance the catheter through the nasopharynx and into the laryngopharynx while the client receives oxygen by mask or nasal cannula. Once the catheter enters the larynx, the client may cough. On inhalation, insert the catheter through the vocal cords and into the trachea. Occasionally, the catheter can be disconnected from suction and attached to an oxygen source, with the client receiving oxygen via the catheter.

Suctioning can cause hypoxia, tissue (mucosal) trauma, infection, vagal stimulation, bronchospasm, and cardiac dysrhythmias.

HYPOXIA. The following are causes of hypoxia in the client with a tracheostomy:

- Ineffective oxygenation before, during, and after suctioning
- Use of a catheter that is too large for the artificial airway
- Prolonged suctioning time
- Excessive suction pressure
- Too frequent suctioning

Prevent hypoxia by hyperoxygenating the client with 100% oxygen with a manual resuscitation bag attached to an oxygen source. If the client is able to take deep breaths, instruct him or her to do so three or four times with the existing oxygen delivery system before suctioning. If possible, monitor the heart rate or use a pulse oximeter while suctioning to assess tolerance of the procedure. Assess for hypoxia (e.g., increased heart rate and blood pressure, oxygen desaturation, cyanosis, restlessness, anxiety, and cardiac dysrhythmias). Oxygen saturation below 90% by pulse oximetry indicates hypoxemia. If hypoxia occurs, stop the suctioning procedure. Using the 100% oxygen delivery system, reoxygenate the client until baseline parameters are achieved.

Use a catheter of the correct size to reduce the risk for hypoxia. The size should not exceed half of the size of the tracheal lumen. In adults, the standard catheter size is 12 Fr or 14 Fr. Correct catheter size allows efficient removal of secretions without causing hypoxemia.

TISSUE TRAUMA. The respiratory tract mucosa is fragile, and frequent suctioning, prolonged suctioning time, excessive suction pressure, and nonrotation of the catheter cause damage. Prevent trauma by suctioning only when needed. Lubricate the catheter with sterile water or saline before insertion. *Apply suction only during the withdrawal of the catheter.* Use a twirling motion during withdrawal to prevent grabbing of the mucosa.

Apply suction intermittently for only 10 to 15 seconds. Estimate this time frame by holding your own breath and counting to 10 or 15 during suctioning. At the end of the 15 seconds, end the suctioning procedure. Fifteen seconds does not seem long to a healthy person, but most clients who need suctioning have respiratory compromise and cannot tolerate more than 15 seconds of suctioning.

INFECTION. Each catheter pass introduces bacteria into the trachea. In the hospital, use sterile technique for suctioning and for all suctioning equipment, including suction catheters, gloves, and saline or water. Suction the mouth after suctioning the artificial airway. *Never use oral suction equipment for suctioning an artificial airway, because the mouth contains bacteria, which could be introduced into the lungs.* Use clean technique with home suctioning procedures because the number of virulent organisms in the home environment is lower than in the hospital.

VAGAL STIMULATION AND BRONCHOSPASM. Vagal stimulation results in severe bradycardia, hypotension, heart block, ventricular tachycardia, asystole, or other dysrhythmias. *If vagal stimulation occurs, stop suctioning immediately and oxygenate the client manually with 100% oxygen.* Bronchospasm sometimes occurs when the catheter passes into the airway. The client may need a bronchodilator to relieve bronchospasm and respiratory distress. In addition, hypoxia caused by suctioning can stimulate a variety of cardiac dysrhythmias. If the client has cardiac monitoring in place, check the monitor during suctioning.

TRACHEOSTOMY CARE

Tracheostomy care keeps the tube free of secretions, maintains a patent airway, and provides wound care. This procedure is performed whether or not the client is able to clear secretions. Perform tracheostomy care according to agency policy, usually every shift and as needed. Charts 31-3 and 31-4 outline best practices for tracheostomy care.

CHART 31-4

BEST PRACTICE for
Tracheostomy Care

1. Assemble the necessary equipment.
2. Wash hands. Maintain standard precautions or body substance precautions.
3. Suction the tracheostomy tube if necessary.
4. Remove old dressings and excess secretions.
5. Set up a sterile field.
6. Remove and clean the inner cannula. Use half-strength hydrogen peroxide to clean the cannula and sterile saline to rinse it. If the inner cannula is disposable, remove the cannula and replace it with a new one.
7. Clean the stoma site and then the tracheostomy plate with half-strength hydrogen peroxide followed by sterile saline. Ensure that none of the solutions enters the tracheostomy.
8. Change tracheostomy ties if they are soiled. Secure new ties in place before removing soiled ones to prevent accidental decannulation. If a knot is needed, tie a square knot that is visible on the side of the neck. One or two fingers should be able to be placed between the tie tape and the neck.
9. Document the type and amount of secretions and the general condition of the stoma and surrounding skin. Document the client's response to the procedure and any teaching or learning that occurred.

CHART 31-5

FOCUSED ASSESSMENT of
The Client with a Tracheostomy

Note the quality, pattern, and rate of breathing:
- Within client's baseline?
  Tachypnea can indicate hypoxia.
  Dyspnea can indicate secretions in the airway.

Assess for any cyanosis, especially around the lips, which could indicate hypoxia.
Check the client's pulse oximetry reading.
If oxygen is ordered, is the client receiving the correct amount, with the correct equipment and humidification?
Assess the tracheostomy site:
- Note the color, consistency, and amount of secretions in the tube or externally.
- If the tracheostomy is sutured in place, is there any redness, swelling, or drainage from suture sites?
- If the tracheostomy is secured with ties, what is the condition of the ties? Are they moist with secretions or perspiration? Are the secretions dried on the ties? Is the tie secure?
- Assess the condition of the skin around the tracheostomy and neck. Be sure to check underneath the neck for secretions that may have drained to the back. Check for any breakdown related to pressure from the ties or from excess secretions.
- Assess behind the faceplate for the size of the space between the outer cannula and the client's tissue. Are any secretions collected in this area?

If the tube is cuffed, check cuff pressure.
Auscultate the lungs.
Is a second (emergency) tracheostomy tube and obturator available?

Before proceeding with tracheostomy care, assess the client as shown in Chart 31-5. The need for suctioning and tracheostomy care is determined by the amount and consistency of secretions, medical diagnosis (specifically pulmonary diseases), ability of the client to cough and deep breathe, need for mechanical ventilation, and wound care required. Inspect the inner lumen of a single-lumen tube

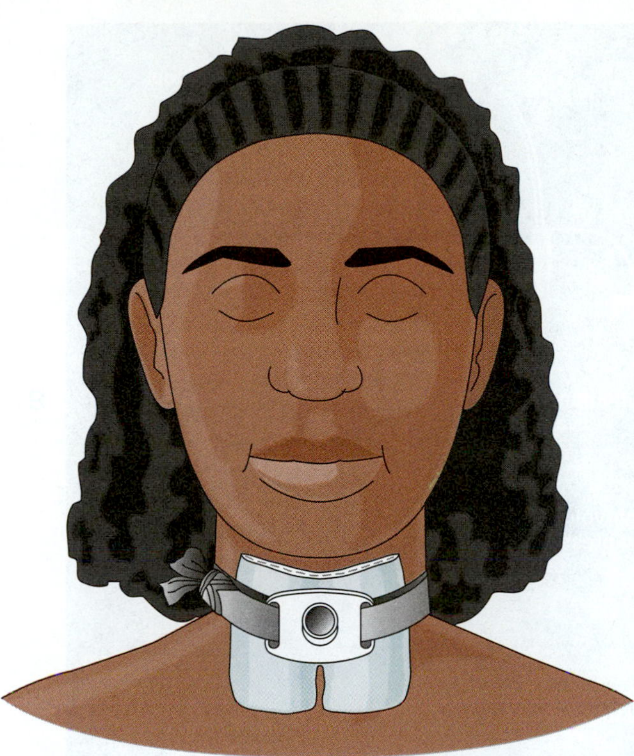

Figure 31-16 ■ Placement of precut gauze and tie around a tracheostomy tube.

with a flashlight or penlight to assess for the presence of secretions.

Secure tracheostomy tubes in place using either twill tape ties or Velcro tracheostomy tube holders. Both devices require changing when soiled to keep them clean and to avoid having them act as a medium for infection. A properly secured tie or holder allows space for only one or two fingers to be placed between the tie or holder and the neck. Tube movement causes irritation and coughing, which in turn may cause decannulation. *Keeping the tube secure while changing the ties or holder to prevent accidental decannulation is critical.* One way to accomplish this safely is to keep the old ties or holder on the tube while changing tubes, but a secure hand on the tube is the most reliable method of tube stabilization. Include the client in this process as a step toward self-care. Figure 31-16 shows correct technique for applying a tracheostomy dressing. Figure 31-17 shows the use of Velcro tracheostomy tube holders.

BRONCHIAL AND ORAL HYGIENE

Bronchial hygiene promotes a patent airway and prevents infection. Turn and reposition the client every 1 to 2 hours, support out-of-bed activities, and encourage ambulation. These actions promote lung expansion and gas exchange, and help remove secretions. Coughing and deep breathing, combined with the chest percussion, vibration, and postural drainage, promote pulmonary care (see Chapter 33).

Oral hygiene is important to ensure a patent airway, prevent bacterial overgrowth and dental caries, and to promote comfort. Maintain standard or body substance precautions during the procedure. Avoid using glycerin swabs or mouthwash that contains alcohol to clean the mouth because these products dry the mouth, change its pH, and promote

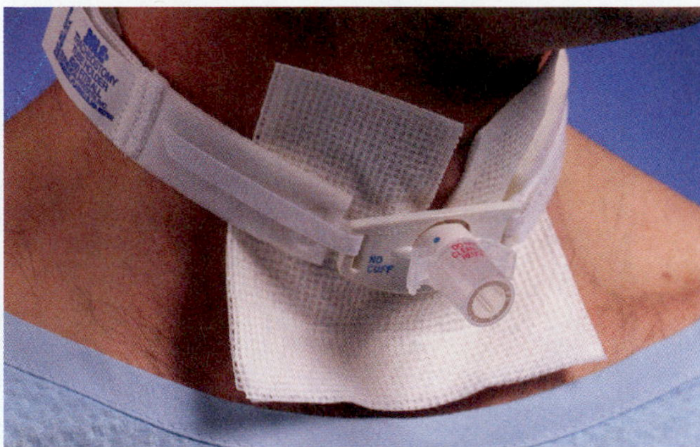

Figure 31-17 ■ Velcro tracheostomy tube holder. (Courtesy of Dale Medical Products, Inc., Plainville, MA.)

bacterial growth. Instead, use a toothette or soft-bristled toothbrush moistened in water for mouth care. Hydrogen peroxide solutions can help remove crusted matter but may break down healing tissue. Use these agents only with a physician's prescription.

During oral care, examine the mouth for any change in mucosal integrity or dental problems. Ulcers, bacterial or fungal *(Candida)* growth, and other infections are treated medically. Apply lip balm or water-soluble jelly to prevent cracked lips or skin breakdown and to promote client comfort. Mouth care is a simple method of promoting oral health, comfort, and aesthetic appearance. Offering an opportunity for the client or family member to perform mouth care encourages participation in care and increases self-esteem.

Oral secretions can move down the trachea and collect above the inflated cuff of the endotracheal tube. When the cuff is deflated, the secretions can move into the lungs. The Hi-Lo Evac endotracheal tube has an additional lumen open to the area above the cuff and can help prevent aspiration of oral secretions (Figure 31-18). The additional lumen allows suctioning of the airway above the cuff before deflating, thus preventing movement of oral secretions deeper into the airway.

NUTRITION

Swallowing can be a major problem for the client with a tracheostomy tube in place. In a normal swallow, the larynx lifts and moves forward to protect itself from the passing stream of food and saliva. Laryngeal lift also opens the upper esophageal sphincter. The tracheostomy tube sometimes tethers the larynx in place, making it unable to move efficiently. The result is difficulty in swallowing. Also, when the tracheostomy tube cuff is inflated, it can balloon backward and interfere with the passage of food through the esophagus. The common wall of the posterior trachea and the anterior esophagus is very thin, allowing this pushing problem. Instruct the client to keep the head of the bed elevated for at least 30 minutes after eating. Chart 31-6 outlines best practices to prevent aspiration during swallowing.

SPEECH AND COMMUNICATION

The client can speak when there is a cuffless tube, when a fenestrated tracheostomy tube is in place, and when the fenestrated tube is capped or covered. Until natural speech is fea-

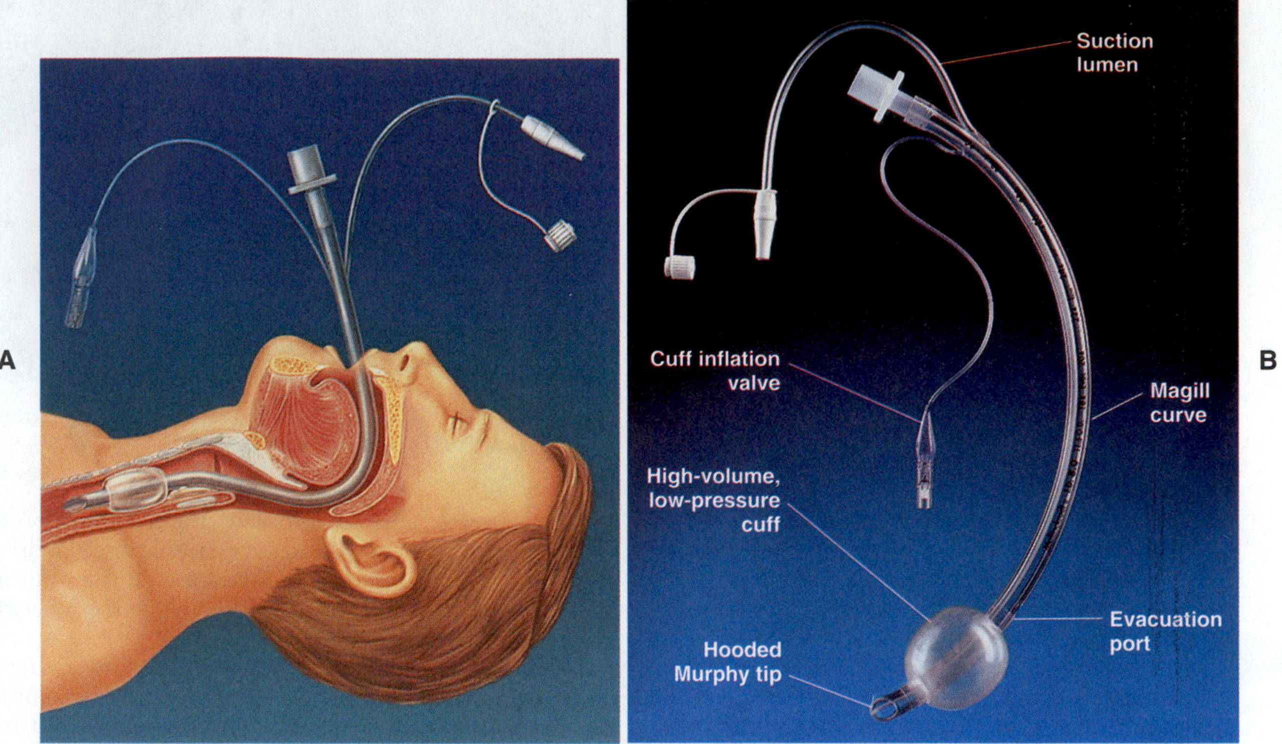

Figure 31-18 ■ The Hi-Lo Evac endotracheal tube system. **A,** The system positioned within a client. **B,** The Hi-Lo Evac tube. (Courtesy of Mallinckrodt, Inc., Shiley Tracheostomy Products, St. Louis, MO.)

sible, teach the client and family about other communication means. A writing tablet, Magic Slate, communication board with pictures and letters, hand signals, or a computer, as well as a call light within reach, are used to promote communication and decrease frustration from not being able to speak or be understood. Phrase questions for "yes" or "no" answers to help the client respond efficiently. Move the client closer to the nurses' station and mark the central call light system to indicate that the client cannot speak.

The inability to talk is a major stressor for the client. Helping communication is an important nursing function. When the client can tolerate cuff deflation, he or she places a finger over the tracheostomy tube on exhalation. This forces air up through the larynx, vocal cords, and mouth and allows speech. During the process of decannulation, when the fenestrated tube is "capped," the client has the benefit of speech without the need to cover the tube.

A device to increase speech for the client with a tracheostomy is a special one-way valve that fits over the tube and replaces the need for finger occlusion (Figure 31-19). The valve allows the client to breathe in through the tracheostomy tube. On exhalation, the valve closes so that air is forced through the vocal cords, allowing speech. For this valve to assist in speech, the client must not be connected to a ventilator, must have the cuff deflated, and must be able to breathe around the tube. Some valves have an extra port for supplemental oxygen without impairing the ability to speak.

EMOTIONAL CARE

Addressing psychological concerns is an important aspect of nursing care of clients recovering from a tracheostomy. While providing physical care, keep in mind the emotional impact of an artificial airway. Acknowledge the client's frustration in communication and allow sufficient time for communication. When speaking to the client, use a normal tone of voice. The tracheostomy tube does not alter hearing or comprehension.

BODY IMAGE

The client may have a change in body image because of deformity, the presence of a stoma or artificial airway, speech changes, a change in the method of eating, or difficulty with speech. Help the client set realistic goals, starting with involvement in self-care.

Work with the family to ease the client into a more normal social environment. Provide encouragement and positive reinforcement while demonstrating acceptance and caring behaviors. Assess the family for the need for counseling.

After surgery, the client may feel shy and socially isolated. He or she can wear loose-fitting shirts, decorative collars, or scarves to cover the tracheostomy tube.

WEANING

Weaning the client from a tracheostomy tube entails a gradual decrease in the tube size and ultimate removal of the tube. Carefully monitor this process, especially after each change. The physician, nurse practitioner, or respiratory advanced-practice nurse performs the steps in the process.

CHART 31-6

BEST PRACTICE for
Preventing Aspiration During Swallowing

- Avoid having meals when the client is fatigued.
- Provide smaller and more frequent meals.
- Provide adequate time; do not "hurry" the client.
- Provide close supervision if the client is self-feeding.
- Keep emergency suctioning equipment close at hand.
- Avoid water and other "thin" liquids.
- Thicken liquids.
- Avoid foods that generate thin liquids during the chewing process, such as fruit.
- Position the client in the most upright position possible.
- When possible, completely (or at least partially) deflate the tube cuff during meals.
- Suction after initial cuff deflation to clear the airway and allow maximal comfort during the meal.
- Feed each bite or encourage the client to take each bite slowly.
- Encourage the client to "dry swallow" after each bite to clear residue from the throat.
- Avoid consecutive swallows by cup or straw.
- Provide controlled small volumes of liquids, using a spoon.
- Encourage the client to "tuck" his or her chin down and forward while swallowing.
- Allow the client to indicate when he or she is ready for the next bite.
- If the client coughs, stop the feeding until the client indicates that the airway has been cleared.
- Continuously monitor tolerance to oral food intake by assessing respiratory rate, ease, pulse oximetry, and heart rate.

First, the cuff is deflated as soon as the client can manage secretions and does not need mechanical ventilation. This change allows him or her to breathe through the tube and through the upper airway. Next, the tube is changed to an uncuffed tube. If this is tolerated, the size of the tube is gradually decreased. When a small fenestrated tube is placed (No. 4 or 6, depending on the size of the airway), the tube is capped so that all air passes through the upper airway and the fenestra, with none passing through the tube. Assess the client to ensure adequate airflow around the tube when it is capped. The tube may be removed after he or she tolerates more than 24 hours of capping. Place a dry dressing over the stoma (which gradually heals on its own). Usually, a small scar remains.

Another device used for the transition from tracheostomy to natural breathing is a *tracheostomy button*. The button maintains stoma patency and assists spontaneous breathing. The Kistner tracheostomy tube and Olympic tracheostomy button are examples of this type of device. To function, they must fit properly. A disadvantage is the possibility of decannulation: the tube can dislodge from the trachea but remain in the neck tissues.

Critical Thinking Challenge

The 87-year-old post-CABG repair client has been reintubated due to respiratory failure. The client went to surgery 7 days later for a tracheotomy and returned to the ICU, where he remained on the ventilator.

1. What indications for a tracheotomy did this client meet?
2. What factor is foremost in determining this client's ability to be weaned from the ventilator?

evolve For suggested answer guidelines, go to http://evolve.elsevier.com/Iggy/.

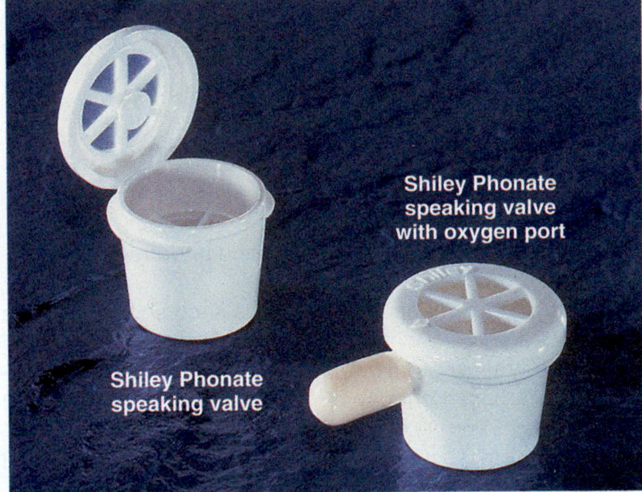

Figure 31-19 ■ The Shiley Phonate Speaking Valve. (Courtesy of Mallinckrodt, Inc., Shiley Tracheostomy Products, St. Louis, MO.)

Community-Based Care

By the time of discharge from the hospital, the client should be able to provide self-care, which may include tracheostomy care, nutritional care, suctioning, and methods of communication. Although education begins before surgery, most self-care is taught in the hospital. Teach the client and family how to care for the tracheostomy tube. Review airway care, including cleaning and inspecting for signs of infection. Teach clean suction technique and review the plan of care.

Instruct the client to use a shower shield over the tracheostomy tube when bathing to prevent water from entering the airway. Teach the client to cover the airway with cotton or foam to protect it during the day. Covering the permanent opening filters the air entering the stoma, keeps humidity in the airway, and enhances appearance. Attractive coverings are available in the form of cotton scarves, decorative collars, crocheted bibs, and jewelry. Using colored seam binding for tracheostomy ties after the stoma has matured may enhance overall body image. Shirt or dress color can be matched or coordinated with seam bindings.

Teach the client to increase humidity in the home. Instruct him or her to instill normal saline into the artificial airway 10 to 15 times a day, as prescribed. The client should continue the selected method of communication that began in the hospital and should wear a medical alert bracelet.

The health care team assesses specific discharge needs and makes referrals to home care agencies and durable medical equipment (DME) companies (for suction equipment and tracheostomy supplies). Clinic or physician follow-up visits occur early after discharge, but the home care nurse also is an important resource for the client and family. The home care nurse initiates (with a physician's prescription) and coordinates the services of nutritionists, nurses, speech pathologists, and social workers. The home care or hospital nurse informs the client and family of community resources that can offer support and friendships.

GET READY for the NCLEX Examination!

KEY POINTS

Safe Effective Care Environment

- Never allow water condensation in an oxygen delivery system to drain back into the system.
- Use sterile technique when performing endotracheal or tracheal suctioning.
- Inspect the oral mucous membranes each shift for anyone who has an endotracheal tube.
- Keep a tracheostomy tube (and obturator) and tracheostomy insertion tray at the bedside for the first 72 hours after a tracheostomy has been performed.
- Never use oral suctioning equipment to suction an artificial airway.

Health Promotion and Maintenance

- Monitor the rate and depth of respiration at least every hour for any client with hypercarbia and CO_2 narcosis who is receiving oxygen by mask or nasal cannula.
- Use aspiration precautions for any client with an altered level of consciousness or who has an endotracheal tube (see Chart 31-6).
- Teach the client and family how to perform tracheostomy care (see Chart 31-4).

Psychosocial Integrity

- Allow the client and family members the opportunity to express fear or anxiety regarding a change in breathing status or the possibility of intubation and mechanical ventilation.
- Teach family members ways to communicate with a client who is intubated or being mechanically ventilated.
- Reassure clients who are intubated that the loss of speech is temporary.
- Encourage clients with permanent tracheostomies to become involved in self care.

Physiological Integrity

- Apply oxygen to anyone who is hypoxemic.
- Ensure that all oxygen therapy delivered to the client is humidified (and warmed, when possible).
- Monitor arterial blood gases (ABGs) and oxygen saturation of all clients receiving oxygen therapy.
- Assess the skin under the mask and under the plastic tubing every shift for clients receiving oxygen by mask.
- Assess the skin of the nares and under the elastic band every shift for clients receiving oxygen by nasal cannula.
- Observe any client receiving oxygen at greater than a 50% concentration for early symptoms of oxygen toxicity (i.e., nonproductive cough, substernal chest pain, gastrointestinal [GI] upset, and dyspnea).
- Use a manual resuscitation bag to ventilate the client if the tracheostomy tube has dislodged or been decannulated.
- Assess the new tracheostomy stoma site at least once per shift for purulent drainage, redness, pain, and swelling as indicators of infection.
- Keep the tracheal cuff pressure between 14 and 20 mm Hg to prevent tissue injury.
- Secure new tracheostomy ties or tube holders in place before removing the soiled ones to prevent accidental decannulation.

ADDITIONAL STUDY RESOURCES

Go to your Student CD-ROM for Review Questions for the NCLEX Examination.

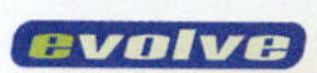

Go to http://evolve.elsevier.com/Iggy/ for Integrated Management of Care Questions for the NCLEX Examination.

SELECTED BIBLIOGRAPHY

Asterisk indicates a classic or definitive work on this subject.

Brook, A., et al. (2000). Early versus late tracheostomy in patients who require prolonged mechanical ventilation. *American Journal of Critical Care, 9*(5), 352-359.

Dixon, B., & Tasota, F. (2003). Action stat: Inadvertent tracheal decannulation. *Nursing2003, 33*(1), 96.

Frakes, M. (2001). Measuring end-tidal carbon dioxide: Clinical applications and usefulness. *Critical Care Nurse, 21*(5), 23-35.

Francois, B., et al. (2003). Complications of tracheostomy performed in the ICU: Subthyroid tracheostomy vs surgical cricothyroidotomy. *Chest, 123*(1), 151-158.

Harkin, H., & Russell, C. (2001a). Preparing the patient for tracheostomy tube removal. *Nursing Times, 97*(26), 34-36.

Harkin, H., & Russell, C. (2001b). Tracheostomy patient care. *Nursing Times, 97*(25), 34-36.

Hess, D. (2000). Detection and monitoring of hypoxemia and oxygen therapy. *Respiratory Care, 45*(1), 65-83.

McConnell, E. (2002). Clinical dos & don'ts: Providing tracheostomy care. *Nursing2002, 32*(1), 17.

Mahler, D., Fierro-Carrion, G., & Baird, J. (2003). Evaluation of dyspnea in the elderly. *Clinics in Geriatric Medicine, 19*(1), 19-33.

Moore, A. (2000). Tips for getting a more reliable O_2 sat reading. *RN, 63*(2), 73.

Pagana, K., & Pagana, T. (2002). *Mosby's manual of diagnostic and laboratory tests* (2nd ed.). St. Louis: Mosby.

Paul-Allen, J., & Ostrow, L. (2000). Survey of nursing practices with closed-system suctioning. *American Journal of Critical Care, 9*(1), 9-19.

Perkins, L., & Shortall, S. (2000). Ventilation without intubation. *RN, 63*(1), 34-38.

Pruitt, W., & Jacobs, M. (2003). Basics of oxygen therapy. *Nursing 2003, 33*(10), 43-45.

Richmond, A., Jarog, D., & Hanson, V. (2004). Unplanned extubation in adult critical care. *Critical Care Nurse, 24*(1), 32-37.

Schreiber, D. (2001). Trach care at home: A how-to guide. *RN, 64*(7), 43-46.

Seay, S., Gay, S., & Strauss, M. (2002). Emergency: Tracheostomy emergencies: Correcting accidental decannulation or displaced tracheostomy tube. *American Journal of Nursing, 102*(3), 61-63.

Sell, S., & Tasota, F. (2004). Action stat: Tracheostomy mucus plug. *Nursing 2004, 34*(10), 88.

Simmons, P., & Simmons, M. (2004). Informed nursing practice: The administration of oxygen to patients with COPD. *MEDSURG Nursing, 13*(2), 82-85.

*St. John, R. (1999). Advances in artificial airway management. *Critical Care Clinics of North America, 11*(1), 7-17.

St. John, R. (2004). Airway management. *Critical Care Nurse, 24*(2), 93-96.

Woodrow, P. (2002). Managing patients with a tracheostomy in acute care. *Nursing Standard, 16*(44), 17-23.

CHAPTER 32

Interventions for Clients with Noninfectious Problems of the Upper Respiratory Tract

M. LINDA WORKMAN

LEARNING OUTCOMES

After studying this chapter, you should be able to:

1. Prioritize nursing care needs for the client after a nasoseptoplasty.
2. Compare the manifestations and care needs of a client with an anterior nosebleed with those of a client with a posterior nosebleed.
3. Prioritize nursing care needs for a client with facial trauma.
4. Describe the pathophysiology and the potential complications of sleep apnea.
5. Develop a plan of communication for a client who has a disruption of speech and cannot read.
6. Use clinical manifestations and laboratory data to determine airway adequacy in a client with laryngeal or neck injury.
7. Identify the risk factors for head and neck cancer.
8. Explain the psychosocial consequences of surgery for head and neck cancer.
9. Develop a community-based teaching plan for the client who is getting ready to go home after undergoing a complete laryngectomy.

Go to your Student CD-ROM for Review Questions for the NCLEX Examination keyed to these Learning Outcomes.

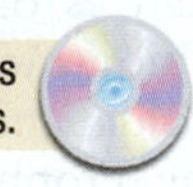

The upper airway structures include the nose, sinuses, oropharynx, larynx, and trachea. These areas may have specific health problems and also may be affected by other common acute and chronic disorders. Clients with upper respiratory problems are found in the community and many health care settings. The major nursing priority with disorders of the upper respiratory tract is maintaining a patent airway.

NONINFECTIOUS DISORDERS OF THE NOSE AND SINUSES

Fracture of the Nose

PATHOPHYSIOLOGY

Nasal fractures often result from injuries received during falls, sports activities, motor vehicle accidents, or physical assaults. If the bone or cartilage is not displaced, serious complications usually do not result from the fracture, and treatment may not be needed. Displacement of either the bone or cartilage, however, can cause airway obstruction or cosmetic deformity and is a potential source of infection.

COLLABORATIVE MANAGEMENT

Assessment

Document any nasal problem, including deviation, malaligned nasal bridge, a change in nasal breathing, crepitus on palpation, midface bruising, and pain. Blood or clear (cerebrospinal) fluid rarely drains from one or both nares. The presence of drainage could indicate a skull fracture. Although important in evaluating general facial fractures, x-rays are not always useful in the diagnosis of nasal fractures.

Interventions

The physician performs a simple closed reduction of the nasal fracture (using local or general anesthesia) within the first 24 hours after injury. After 24 hours the fracture is more difficult to reduce because of edema and scar formation. Simple closed fractures need not be surgically treated. Treatment focuses on pain relief and local cold compresses to decrease swelling.

Rhinoplasty. Reduction and surgery may be needed for severe fractures or for those that do not heal properly. **Rhinoplasty** is a surgical reconstruction of the nose for cosmetic purposes and to improve airflow. The client returns from surgery with packing in both nostrils; this packing prevents bleeding and provides support for the reconstructed nose. The gauze packing is usually treated with an antibiotic ointment, such as bacitracin (Bacitin✱) to reduce the risk for infection. A "moustache" dressing (or drip pad), often a folded 2 × 2 gauze pad, is usually placed under the nose (Figure 32-1). A splint or cast may cover the nose for additional alignment and protection. The nurse or client changes the drip pad as necessary.

After surgery, observe for edema and bleeding. Check vital signs every 4 hours until the client is discharged. Assessing how often the client swallows is a priority. Repeated swallowing may indicate posterior nasal bleeding. Use a penlight to examine the throat for bleeding, and notify the surgeon if bleeding is present. The client with uncomplicated rhinoplasty is usually discharged the day of surgery. Instruct the client and family about routine care.

Place the client in a semi-Fowler's position and instruct him or her to move slowly and to rest as much as possible. Apply cool compresses to the nose, eyes, or face to reduce swelling and discoloration. If a general anesthetic was used, the client may eat soft foods once he or she is alert and the gag reflex has returned. Urge the client to drink at least 2500 mL/day.

To prevent bleeding, teach the client to limit Valsalva maneuvers (e.g., forceful coughing or straining during a bowel movement) for the first few days after the packing is removed. Laxatives or stool softeners may be prescribed to ease bowel movement. Instruct the client to avoid aspirin and nonsteroidal anti-inflammatory drugs (NSAIDs) to prevent bleeding. Prophylactic antibiotics may be prescribed to prevent infection. Recommend the use of a humidifier at home to prevent excessive drying of the mucosa. Explain that edema and discoloration may last for weeks and that the final surgical result will be evident in 6 to 12 months.

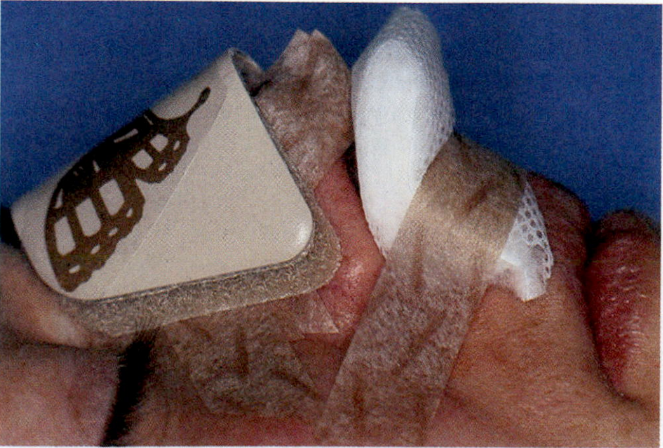

Figure 32-1 ■ Immediate postoperative appearance of a client who has undergone rhinoplasty. Note the splint and gauze drip pad (moustache dressing). (From Tardy, M.E. [1997]. *Rhinoplasty: The art and science* [p. 207]. Philadelphia: W.B. Saunders. Used with permission.)

Nasoseptoplasty. Nasoseptoplasty, or **submucous resection (SMR),** may be needed to straighten a deviated septum when chronic symptoms (e.g., a "stuffy" nose) or discomfort occur. Most adults have a slight nasal septum deviation with no symptoms. Major deviations, however, may obstruct the nasal passages or interfere with airflow and sinus drainage. The deviated section of the cartilage and bone is removed as an outpatient surgical procedure. The amount resected depends on the type and degree of deformity. Nursing care is similar to that for a rhinoplasty.

Epistaxis

PATHOPHYSIOLOGY

Epistaxis (nosebleed) is a common problem because of the rich capillary network within the nose. Nosebleeds may occur as a result of trauma, hypertension, blood dyscrasia (e.g., leukemias), inflammation, tumor, decreased humidity, nose blowing, nose picking, chronic cocaine use, and procedures such as nasogastric suctioning. Men are usually affected more often than women. Older adults tend to bleed most often from the posterior portion of the nose.

◆COLLABORATIVE MANAGEMENT

◆Assessment

The client often reports that the bleeding started after sneezing or blowing the nose. Document the amount and color of the blood and take the vital signs. Ask the client about the number, duration, and causes of previous bleeding episodes. Record this information in the client's medical record.

◆Interventions

Chart 32-1 lists the best practices for emergency care of the client with a nosebleed. Medical attention is needed if the nosebleed does not respond to these interventions. In such cases the affected capillaries may be cauterized with silver nitrate or electrocautery and the nose packed. Anterior packing controls bleeding from the anterior nasal cavity.

Posterior nasal bleeding is an emergency. Posterior packing or nasal pressure tubes are used to stop bleeding that originates in the posterior nasal region. With packing, a string is attached to a large gauze pack and then threaded through the nose and out the mouth. The physician positions the pack in the posterior nasal cavity above the pharynx and then tapes the string to the client's cheek to prevent movement of the pack. Balloon pressure catheter tubes or stents look like very short (about 6 inches) urinary catheters. These tubes have an exterior balloon along the tube length in addition to an anchoring balloon on the end. The tubes are inserted into both nares. The physician first inflates the anchoring balloon to keep the tubes in place. Then the pressure balloons are inflated carefully for both tubes at the same time to compress bleeding vessels (Figure 32-2). Placement of posterior packing or pressure tubes is uncomfortable, and the airway may be obstructed if the pack slips. Most clients who have posterior nasal bleeding are hospitalized.

Observe the client for respiratory distress and for tolerance of the packing or tubes. Humidification, oxygen, bedrest, and antibiotics may be prescribed. Opioid pain medication may be prescribed. Assess clients receiving opioids at least hourly for gag and cough reflexes. Oral care and adequate hydration are important because of mouth breathing. Use pulse oximetry to monitor for hypoxemia. The tubes or packing are usually removed after 1 to 5 days.

After the tubes or packing are removed, teach the client interventions to use at home for comfort and safety. Petroleum jelly can be applied to the nares for lubrication and comfort. Nasal saline sprays and humidification add moisture and prevent rebleeding. Instruct the client to avoid vigorous nose blowing, the use of aspirin or other NSAIDs, and strenuous activities such as heavy lifting.

Nasal Polyps

PATHOPHYSIOLOGY

Nasal polyps are benign grapelike clusters of mucous membrane and connective tissue. They often occur bilaterally and are caused by irritation to the nasal mucosa or sinuses, allergies, or infection (chronic sinusitis). If polyps become too large, airway obstruction may result.

CHART 32-1

BEST PRACTICE for
Emergency Care of a Client with an Anterior Nosebleed

EMERGENCY CARE

- Position the client upright and leaning forward to prevent blood from entering the stomach and possible aspiration.
- Reassure the client and attempt to keep him or her quiet to reduce anxiety and blood pressure.
- Apply direct lateral pressure to the nose for 5 minutes, and apply ice or cool compresses to the nose and face if possible.
- Maintain standard or body substance precautions.
- If nasal packing is necessary, loosely pack both nares with gauze or nasal tampons.
- To prevent rebleeding from dislodging clots, instruct the client not to blow the nose for several hours after the bleeding stops.
- Seek medical assistance if these measures are ineffective or if the bleeding occurs frequently.

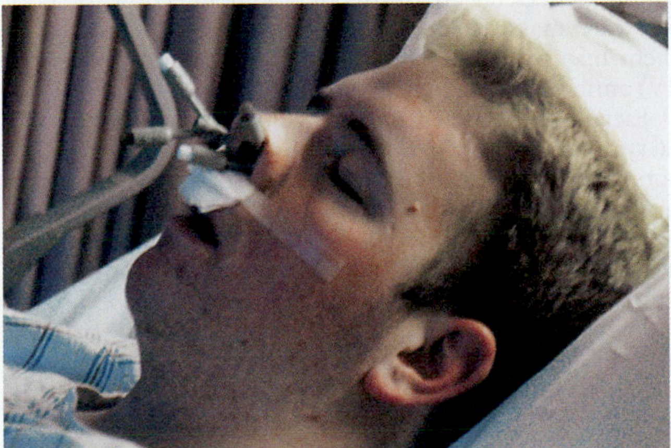

Figure 32-2 ■ Client with balloon stents in place to control a posterior nasal bleed.

COLLABORATIVE MANAGEMENT

Assessment

Manifestations of nasal polyps include obstructed nasal breathing, a change in the character of nasal discharge, and a change in speech quality. Clients who have had polyps are at risk for recurrence.

Interventions

Surgery is the treatment of choice for nasal polyps. The extent of the surgery required depends on the location and type of polyp present.

Benign nasal polyps are treated with nasally inhaled steroids and surgical removal **(polypectomy).** A polypectomy can be performed using either local or general anesthesia. Observe the client for bleeding after surgery. The nostrils are usually packed with gauze for 24 hours after surgery. Nasal polyps often recur if they are not completely removed.

Inverting papilloma is a rare, benign lesion that erodes nasal and facial bones and is often first diagnosed as a benign polyp. Inverting papillomas grow by pressure into adjacent structures. Extensive sinus and nasal surgery is needed for complete removal and prevention of regrowth.

Juvenile angiofibromas are cellularly different from other polyps. These tumors often occur in adolescent males and may resolve spontaneously when adulthood is reached. When the lesions are local, they can be removed by nasal surgery. Invasive tumors may require removal by skull-base resection.

Cancer of the Nose and Sinuses

PATHOPHYSIOLOGY

Tumors of the nasal cavities and sinuses are rare and may be either benign or malignant. Malignant tumors can occur at all ages, but the peak incidence is 40 to 45 years of age in men and 60 to 65 years of age in women. Asian Americans have a higher incidence of nasopharyngeal cancer.

COLLABORATIVE MANAGEMENT

Assessment

The onset of sinus cancer is slow, and manifestations resemble sinusitis. Thus the client may have advanced disease at diagnosis. Manifestations of nasal or sinus cancer include persistent nasal obstruction, drainage, bloody discharge, and pain that does not improve after treatment of sinusitis. Local lymph node enlargement often occurs on the side with tumor mass.

Interventions

Radiation therapy is the main treatment for nasopharyngeal cancers. Chart 32-2 lists some NIC interventions for clients having radiation therapy. Surgical removal is performed if radiation therapy is not successful.

The specific surgery depends on tumor size and location and the degree of invasion. Problems after surgery include a change in body image or speech and altered nutrition. These problems are most common when the maxilla and floor of the nose are involved in the surgery. Clients often also have changes in taste and smell.

CHART 32-2

NIC **INTERVENTION ACTIVITIES for**
The Client with Noninfectious Disorders of the Nose and Sinus

Radiation Therapy Management: *Assisting the client to understand and minimize the side effects of radiation treatments*

- Monitor for alterations in skin integrity and treat appropriately.
- Avoid use of adhesive tapes and other skin-irritating substances.
- Avoid application of deodorants and aftershave lotion to treated area.
- Discuss the need for skin care, such as maintenance of dye markings, avoidance of soap and other ointments, and protection during sunbathing or heat application.
- Monitor for indications of infection of oral mucous membranes.
- Encourage good oral hygiene with use of dental floss or WaterPik, as appropriate.
- Initiate oral health restoration activities, such as use of artificial saliva, mouth sprays, and use of sugarless mints, as appropriate.
- Monitor client for anorexia, nausea, vomiting, changes in taste, esophagitis, and diarrhea, as appropriate.
- Promote adequate fluid and nutritional intake.
- Assist client in managing fatigue by planning frequent rest periods, spacing activities, and limiting daily demands, as appropriate.
- Encourage rest immediately after radiation treatment.
- Facilitate expression of fears about prognosis or success of radiation treatments.

Communication Enhancement: *Speech Deficit: Assistance in accepting and learning alternate methods for living with impaired speech*

- Provide verbal prompts/reminders.
- Listen attentively.
- Refrain from shouting at the client with communication disorders.
- Use picture board, if appropriate.
- Use hand gestures, as appropriate.
- Perform prescriptive speech-language therapies during informal interactions with client.
- Teach esophageal speech, as appropriate.
- Instruct client and family on use of speech aids (e.g., tracheal-esophageal prosthesis and artificial larynx).
- Encourage client to repeat words.
- Provide positive reinforcement and praise, as appropriate.
- Carry on one-way conversations, as appropriate.
- Reinforce need for follow-up with speech pathologist after discharge.

NIC intervention activities selected from Dochterman, J.M., & Bulechek, G.M. (Eds.). (2004). *Nursing interventions classification (NIC)* (4th ed.). St. Louis: Mosby.

Provide general postoperative care (see Chapter 22), including maintaining a patent airway, monitoring for hemorrhage, providing wound care, assessing nutritional status, and performing tracheostomy care (if needed). (See Chapter 31 for tracheostomy care.) Perform meticulous mouth and maxillary cavity care with saline irrigations using a water pick (e.g., WaterPik) or a syringe. Assess the client for pain and infection. Optimal nutrition is essential after surgery to promote healing.

Facial Trauma

PATHOPHYSIOLOGY

Facial trauma is described by the specific bones (e.g., mandibular, maxillary, orbital, or nasal fractures) and the side of the face involved. Mandibular (lower jaw) fractures can occur at any point on the mandible and are the most common facial fractures. **Le Fort I** is a nasoethmoid complex fracture. **Le Fort II** is a maxillary *and* nasoethmoid complex fracture. **Le Fort III** is a combination of I and II plus an orbital-zygoma fracture, often called "craniofacial disjunction" because it leaves the midface with no connection to the skull. The rich blood supply of the face leads to extensive bleeding with facial trauma.

COLLABORATIVE MANAGEMENT

Assessment

The first action to take with facial trauma is airway assessment. Manifestations of an airway obstruction include stridor, shortness of breath, dyspnea, anxiety, restlessness, hypoxia, hypercarbia, decreased oxygen saturation, cyanosis, and loss of consciousness. After establishing the airway, assess the amount and site of soft-tissue trauma, bleeding, and possible fractures. Check for soft-tissue edema, facial asymmetry, pain, or leakage of spinal fluid through the ears or nose, indicating a temporal bone or basilar skull fracture. Assess vision and eye movement because orbital and maxillary fractures can entrap the eye. Because facial trauma can occur with spinal cord trauma and skull fractures, cranial computed tomography, facial series, and cervical spine films also are obtained.

Interventions

The priority action is to establish and maintain a patent airway. Anticipate the need for emergency intubation, tracheotomy, or cricothyroidotomy. When the client arrives at a trauma center, care focuses on establishing an airway, controlling hemorrhage, and assessing for the extent of injury. If shock is present, fluid resuscitation and identification of bleeding sites are started immediately.

Time is critical in stabilizing the client who has head and neck trauma. Early response and treatment by the following appropriate services, including the trauma team, maxillofacial surgeon, general surgeon, otolaryngologist, plastic surgeon, and dentist, optimize the client's recovery.

Stabilization of the fractured segment of a *mandibular fracture* allows the teeth to heal in proper alignment. The client remains in fixed occlusion for 6 to 10 weeks. Antibiotic therapy may be prescribed because of oral wound contamination. Delay in treatment, tooth infection, or poor oral care may result in mandibular bone infection. The client may then require surgical debridement, intravenous (IV) antibiotic therapy, and an extended period in fixation.

Facial fractures often are repaired with microplating surgical systems such as BoneSource. These shaping plates hold the bone fragments in place until **osteoneogenesis** (new bone growth) occurs. Large areas of skull can be replaced with BoneSource. Bone cells grow into the BoneSource and rematrix into a stable bone support. The plates may remain in place permanently or may be removed after healing has occurred.

If the mandibular fracture is repaired with titanium plates, teach the client about oral care, soft-diet restrictions, and follow-up care with a dentist. These plates are permanent and do not interfere with magnetic resonance imaging (MRI) studies.

Fixation methods may use resorbable devices (plates and screws) to hold tissues in place. These devices are made from a plastic-like material that retains its integrity for about

8 weeks and then slowly biodegrades. Resorbable devices are not used when the area has previously been irradiated or for clients who smoke, have drug or alcohol dependence, uncontrolled diabetes mellitus, immunosuppression, or impaired cardiac function.

Inner maxillary fixation (IMF) is another common method of securing a mandibular fracture. The bones are realigned and then wired in place with the bite closed. The physician can repair nondisplaced aligned fractures in a clinic or office using local dental anesthesia. General anesthesia is used to repair displaced or complex fractures or fractures that occur with other facial bone fractures.

After surgery teach the client about oral care with an irrigating device, such as a WaterPik. If the client is undergoing inner maxillary fixation, teach self-care with wires in place, including a dental liquid diet. There is a risk for aspiration if vomiting occurs because of the inability to open the jaws to allow ejection of the emesis. Teach the client how to cut the wires if emesis occurs. *Instruct the client to keep wire cutters with him or her at all times in case this emergency arises.* If the wires are cut, instruct the client to return to the physician for rewiring as soon as possible to reinstitute fixation.

Nutrition is important for any client with fractures. Oral needs may be difficult to meet because of oral fixation, pain, and surgery. Consult with the dietitian for client teaching and support.

NONINFECTIOUS DISORDERS OF THE ORAL PHARYNX AND TONSILS

Obstructive Sleep Apnea

PATHOPHYSIOLOGY

Sleep apnea is a breathing disruption during sleep that lasts at least 10 seconds and occurs a minimum of 5 times in an hour. Although sleep apnea can have a neurologic origin, the most common form occurs as a result of upper-airway obstruction by the soft palate or tongue. Factors that contribute to sleep apnea include obesity, a large uvula, a short neck, smoking, enlarged tonsils or adenoids, and oropharyngeal edema. Men are affected more often than women, and the risk increases with age.

During sleep, the muscles relax and the tongue and neck structures are displaced. As a result, the upper airway is obstructed even though chest-wall movement is unimpaired. The apnea increases the arterial carbon dioxide level and decreases the pH. These blood-gas changes stimulate neural activity. The sleeper is aroused spontaneously after 10 seconds or longer of apnea and corrects the obstruction, and respiration resumes. After the client goes back to sleep, the cycle begins again, sometimes as often as every 5 minutes.

This cyclic pattern of disrupted sleep prevents the state of deep sleep needed for maximum rest. As a result, the person may have excessive daytime sleepiness, an inability to concentrate, and irritability.

◆COLLABORATIVE MANAGEMENT

◆Assessment

Clients are often unaware that they have sleep apnea. The disorder should be suspected for any person who has persistent daytime sleepiness or complains of "waking up tired," particularly if he or she snores heavily. Other manifestations include irritability and personality changes. In some cases sleep apnea is diagnosed by family members who observe the problem while the client sleeps in a supine position. A complete health assessment should be performed when excessive daytime sleepiness is a problem.

The most accurate test for sleep apnea is polysomnography (PSG) performed during an overnight sleep study. The client is directly observed while wearing a variety of monitoring equipment, including an electroencephalograph (EEG), an electrocardiograph (ECG), a pulse oximeter, and an electromyograph (EMG). This test determines the depth of sleep, type of sleep, respiratory effort, oxygen saturation adequacy, and muscle movement. Nursing diagnoses that may apply to clients with sleep apnea include the following:

- Sleep Deprivation related to disrupted sleep cycle
- Ineffective Breathing pattern related to obesity, musculoskeletal issues, and soft tissue position
- Fatigue related to sleep deprivation
- Risk for Injury related to decreased mental awareness

◆Interventions

NONSURGICAL MANAGEMENT. A change in sleeping position or weight loss may be all that is needed to reduce or correct mild sleep apnea. Position-fixing devices that prevent subluxation of the tongue and neck structures also may be effective in preventing obstruction. For more severe sleep apnea, nonsurgical or surgical methods to prevent obstruction may be needed.

A common nonsurgical method to prevent airway collapse is the use of noninvasive positive-pressure ventilation (NPPV) to hold open the upper airways. A nasal mask or full-face mask delivery system allows mechanical delivery of either bilevel positive airway pressure (BiPAP) or nasal continuous positive airway pressure. With BiPAP, a cycling machine delivers a set inspiratory positive airway pressure at the beginning of each inspiration. As the client begins to exhale, the machine delivers a lower set end expiratory pressure. These two pressures improve tidal volume and hold open the upper airways.

Nasal continuous positive airway pressure (CPAP) delivers a set positive airway pressure continually during each cycle of inhalation and exhalation. For CPAP ventilation through a face mask during sleep, a small electric compressor delivers positive pressure at an individually determined setting. Proper fit of the mask over the nose and mouth is key to successful treatment. Although intrusive, these methods are well accepted by most clients after an initial adjustment period.

Two drugs have been approved to treat sleep apnea. One drug, Xyrem (sodium oxybate), a CNS depressant, induces a deep sleep state. This action does not treat the cause of sleep apnea but works by improving the sleep cycle and thus increasing daytime wakefulness. This drug has been widely abused as a "date rape" agent, and many health care providers are reluctant to prescribe it. Provigil (modafinil) is helpful for clients who have *narcolepsy* (uncontrolled daytime sleep) from sleep apnea by promoting daytime wakefulness.

SURGICAL MANAGEMENT. Surgical intervention for sleep apnea may involve a simple adenoidectomy, uvulectomy, or remodeling of the entire posterior oropharynx **(uvulopalatopharyngoplasty [UPP]).** Both conventional and laser surgeries are used for this purpose. A tracheostomy may be needed for very severe sleep apnea that is not relieved by more moderate interventions.

Oropharyngeal Cancer

Clients with cancer of the mouth, tongue, tonsils, and pharynx have many nursing needs related to airway maintenance, communication, nutrition, and self-image. Chapter 57 provides an in-depth discussion of the management of clients with oropharyngeal cancer.

NONINFECTIOUS DISORDERS OF THE LARYNX

Vocal Cord Paralysis

PATHOPHYSIOLOGY

Vocal fold (cord) paralysis may result from injury, trauma, or disease that affects the larynx, laryngeal nerves, or vagus nerve. Prolonged intubation with an endotracheal (ET) tube may cause temporary or, rarely, permanent paralysis. Laryngeal paralysis may occur in clients with neurologic disorders. Damage to the vagus nerve (by chest injury) or brainstem may lead to nerve dysfunction. The laryngeal nerves may be damaged from trauma or disorders that involve the chest, esophagus, or thyroid. Paralysis of both vocal cords may result from direct injury, stroke involving the brainstem, or total thyroidectomy.

COLLABORATIVE MANAGEMENT

Assessment

Vocal fold paralysis may be unilateral or bilateral. When only one vocal cord is involved (most common), the airway remains patent but the voice is affected. Manifestations of **abducted** (open) bilateral vocal cord paralysis include hoarseness; a breathy, weak voice; and aspiration of food. Bilateral **adducted** (closed) vocal cord paralysis causes airway obstruction and is a medical emergency if the symptoms are severe and the client is unable to compensate. Stridor is the major manifestation. The client with vocal cord paralysis is at risk for aspiration because airway may not close during swallowing.

Interventions

Securing a patent airway is the primary intervention. Place the client in a high Fowler's position to aid in breathing and proper alignment of airway structures. Assess for upper airway obstruction. *Immediately notify the physician if dyspnea with stridor occurs.* Emergency endotracheal intubation or tracheostomy may be needed.

Various surgical procedures can improve the voice. One procedure for abducted vocal cord paresis involves injecting polytef (Teflon) into the affected cord so it enlarges toward the unaffected cord. This technique improves closure during speaking and eating.

Teach the client to hold his or her breath during swallowing. This action allows the larynx to rise, close, and divert food back into the esophagus during swallowing. Also teach the client to tuck his or her chin down and forward during swallowing to prevent aspiration. Indications of aspiration include immediate coughing on swallowing of liquids or solids, a "wet"-sounding voice, and "tearing up" or watery eyes on swallowing. Chest x-rays and laryngeal and chest auscultation are also useful to diagnose aspiration pneumonia.

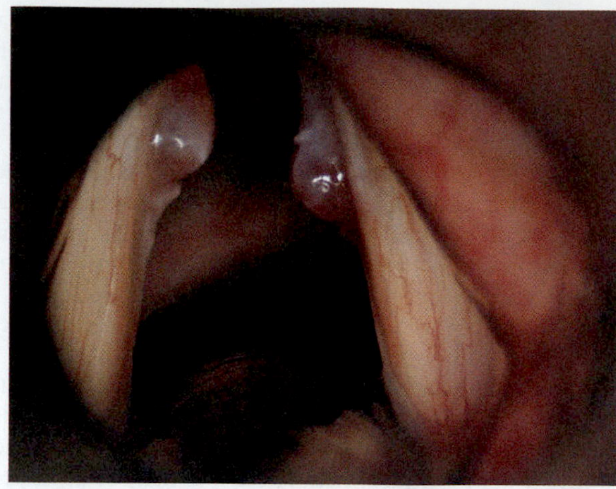

Figure 32-3 ■ Unilateral left vocal cord nodule caused by contact and voice abuse, often seen after viral illnesses. Differential diagnosis includes cancer and trauma. The origin of the nodule may be scar tissue, bacteria, or viruses.

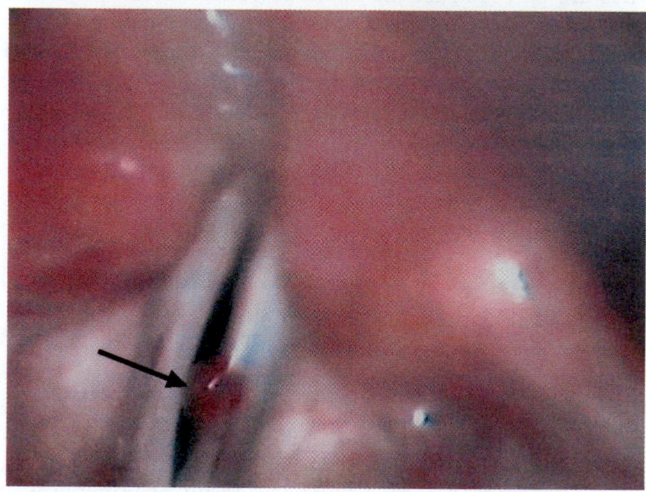

Figure 32-4 ■ A hemorrhagic vocal cord polyp.

Vocal Cord Nodules and Polyps

PATHOPHYSIOLOGY

Nodules often appear at the point at which the vocal cords touch during speech. **Nodules** are enlarged fibrous tissues (Figure 32-3) caused by infectious processes or overuse of the voice. People most affected are teachers, coaches, sports fans, singers, and those who use their voices in noisy environments.

Vocal cord polyps (Figure 32-4) are chronic, edematous masses. They occur most often in smokers, people with allergies, or those who live in dry climates. Vocal cysts also may occur.

COLLABORATIVE MANAGEMENT

Nodules and polyps are painless. The main manifestation is hoarseness because of the loss of coordinated closure of the vocal cords and vocal wave (Figure 32-5).

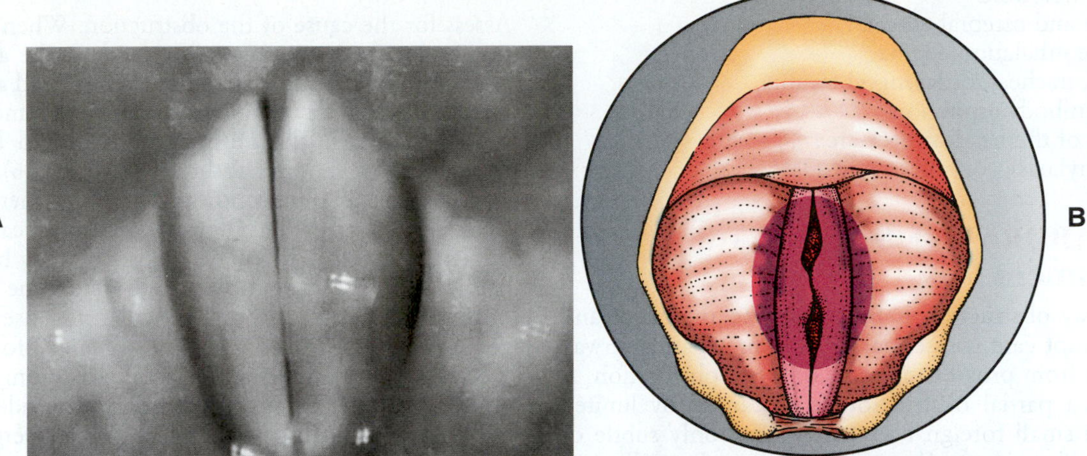

Figure 32-5 ■ **A,** Close-up view of normal vocal cords in phonation. Saying the letter *E* in a high pitch allows the examiner to evaluate the total movement of the cords in all pitch ranges and evaluate the membrane contact. **B,** Vocal cord nodules and polyps prevent approximation of the vocal cords. Hoarseness results.

Management of cord nodules or polyps is aimed at educating the client and family. Instruct the client about tobacco use hazards, smoking-cessation programs, and the importance of voice rest. Treatment includes not whispering and avoiding heavy lifting. Stool softeners are used to avoid bearing down during elimination **(Valsalva maneuvers),** which would cause the glottis to close. Humidifying inspired air may soothe the vocal cords and prevent overdrying.

Speech therapy is used for behavioral voice changes and helps the client learn to reduce speech intensity. Speech therapy may make surgery unnecessary.

If hoarseness is not relieved by voice rest or speech therapy, the surgeon may remove the nodules or polyps under direct laryngoscopy. Laser and surgical resection are used to remove the mucous membrane of the affected cord. If both cords are involved, one cord is usually allowed to heal before surgery is performed on the other cord. These procedures are often performed as outpatient surgery. Thus, client education must be performed before surgery and before the client goes home.

After surgery the client must maintain complete voice rest for about 14 days to promote healing. Chart 32-2 on p. 566 lists NIC interventions for communication enhancement. Teach about alternative methods of communication such as a slate board, pen and paper, "magic slate," or alphabet board. While the client is an inpatient, place a sign on the client's door, over the bed, and on the intercom system to help implement voice rest.

Laryngeal Trauma

PATHOPHYSIOLOGY

Laryngeal trauma occurs with a crushing or direct blow injury, fracture, or injury such as that induced by prolonged endotracheal intubation.

◆COLLABORATIVE MANAGEMENT

Manifestations of laryngeal trauma include **dyspnea** (difficulty breathing), **aphonia** (inability to produce sound), hoarseness, and **subcutaneous emphysema** (air present in the subcutaneous tissue). Bleeding from the airway **(hemoptysis)** may, occur depending on the location of the trauma. The physician performs a direct visual examination by laryngoscopy or fiberoptic laryngoscopy of the larynx to determine the nature and extent of the injury.

Management of clients with laryngeal injuries consists of airway assessment and monitoring vital signs (including respiratory status and pulse oximetry) every 15 to 30 minutes. *Maintaining a patent airway is a priority.* Apply oxygen and humidification as prescribed to maintain adequate oxygen saturation. If the client is experiencing respiratory difficulty, stay with him or her and instruct other trauma team members to prepare for an emergency intubation or tracheostomy. Manifestations of respiratory difficulty include increasing tachypnea, nasal flaring, anxiety, sternal retraction, shortness of breath, dyspnea, restlessness, decreased oxygen saturation, decreased level of consciousness, and stridor.

Surgical intervention is necessary for lacerations of the mucous membranes, cartilage exposure, and paralysis of the cords. Laryngeal repair is performed as soon as possible to prevent laryngeal stenosis and to cover any exposed cartilage. An artificial airway may be needed.

OTHER UPPER AIRWAY DISORDERS

Upper Airway Obstruction

PATHOPHYSIOLOGY

Upper airway obstruction is a life-threatening emergency in which there is an interruption in airflow through the nose, mouth, pharynx, or larynx. Early recognition is essential to prevent further complications, including respiratory arrest. Causes of upper airway obstruction include the following:

- Tongue edema (surgery, trauma)
- Occlusion by the tongue (e.g., with loss of gag reflex, loss of pharyngeal muscle tone, unconsciousness, and coma)
- Laryngeal edema
- Peritonsillar and pharyngeal abscess
- Head and neck cancer

- Thick secretions
- Stroke and cerebral edema
- Smoke inhalation edema
- Facial, tracheal, or laryngeal trauma
- Foreign-body aspiration
- Burns of the head or neck area
- Anaphylaxis

COLLABORATIVE MANAGEMENT

Assessment

Upper airway obstruction is frightening to the client and family. Prompt care is essential to prevent a partial airway obstruction from progressing to a complete obstruction. A client with a partial obstruction (e.g., caused by limited edema or a small foreign body) may have only subtle or general manifestations such as diaphoresis, tachycardia, and elevated blood pressure. Unexplained or persistent recurrent symptoms warrant evaluation even though the symptoms are vague. To rule out any potentially life-threatening condition (e.g., tumor, foreign body, or infection), diagnostic procedures, such as a chest x-ray, lateral neck films, direct laryngoscopic examination, and computed tomography, are performed.

Observe for hypoxia and hypercarbia, restlessness, increasing anxiety, sternal retractions, a "seesawing" chest, abdominal movements, or a feeling of impending doom related to actual air hunger. Use pulse oximetry for ongoing monitoring of oxygen saturation. Continually assess for stridor, cyanosis, and changes in level of consciousness.

Interventions

Assess for the cause of the obstruction. When the obstruction is due to the tongue falling back or the accumulation of secretions, slightly extend the client's head and neck and insert a nasal or an oral airway. Suction to remove obstructing secretions. If the obstruction is caused by a foreign body, perform abdominal thrusts (Figure 32-6).

Upper airway obstruction may require emergency procedures such as cricothyroidotomy, endotracheal intubation, or a tracheostomy. Direct laryngoscopy may be performed before or with these procedures to determine the cause of obstruction. The health care provider may use direct laryngoscopy in a controlled situation to remove foreign bodies.

Cricothyroidotomy. Cricothyroidotomy is an emergency procedure that is often performed outside the hospital by emergency medical personnel or in the emergency department by a physician. A **cricothyroidotomy** is a stab wound at the cricothyroid membrane between the thyroid cartilage and the cricoid cartilage ring (see Figure 30-3). Any hollow tube–but preferably a tracheostomy tube–can be placed through this opening to keep the new airway open until a formal tracheotomy can be performed. This procedure is used when it is the *only* way to secure an airway. Another emergency procedure to bypass an obstruction involves the physician inserting a 14-gauge needle directly into the cricoid space to allow air into and out of the lungs.

Endotracheal Intubation. Endotracheal intubation is performed by inserting a tube into the trachea via the nose **(nasotracheal)** or mouth **(orotracheal)** by a physician, nurse anesthetist, or other specially trained personnel.

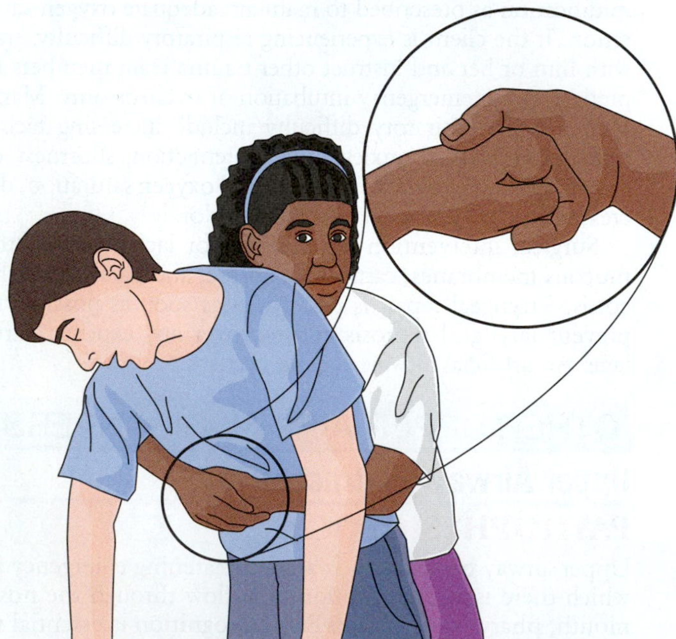

With the conscious victim standing or sitting, place your fist between the victim's lower rib cage and navel. Wrap the palm of your hand around your fist. A quick inward, upward thrust expels the air remaining in the victim's lungs, and with it the foreign body. If the first thrust is unsuccessful, repeat several thrusts in rapid succession until the foreign body is expelled or until the victim loses consciousness.

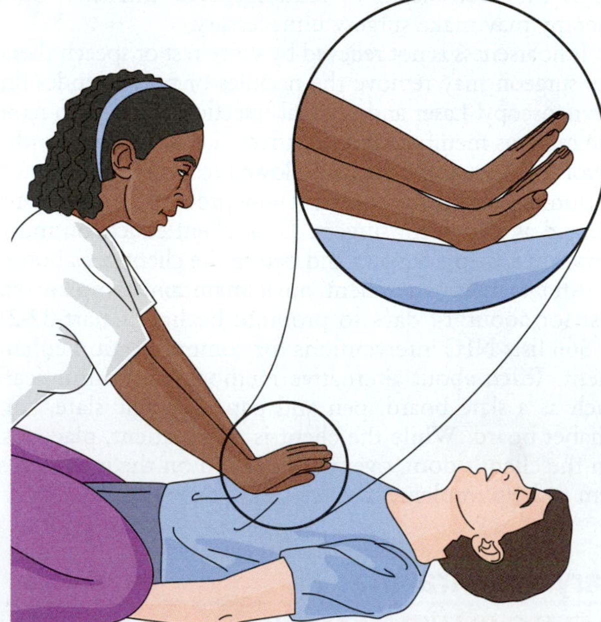

With the unconscious victim lying supine, straddle the victim's thighs. Place one hand on top of the other as shown, with the heel of the bottom hand just above the victim's navel. Quickly thrust inward and upward, toward the victim's head.

Figure 32-6 ■ The abdominal thrust maneuver (formerly known as the Heimlich maneuver) for relief of upper airway obstruction caused by a foreign body.

Tracheostomy. A tracheostomy is a surgical procedure that takes about 5 to 10 minutes to perform. Ideally it is performed in the operating room with the client under local or general anesthesia. It can be performed at the bedside. A tracheostomy can be performed with the client under local anesthesia if there is concern that the airway will be lost during the induction of anesthesia. An emergency tracheostomy is reserved for the client who cannot be easily intubated with an endotracheal tube. The emergency tracheostomy can establish an airway in less than 2 minutes. Care of the client with a tracheostomy is discussed in detail in Chapter 31.

Clients receiving mechanical ventilation as part of the treatment for upper airway obstruction or respiratory failure may require a tracheostomy after 7 or more days of continuous oral or nasal intubation. In such cases the procedure is performed to prevent laryngeal injury by the endotracheal tube.

Neck Trauma

PATHOPHYSIOLOGY

Neck injuries may be caused by a knife, gunshot, or traumatic accident. The client with neck trauma may have more than one injury, including cardiovascular, respiratory, intestinal, and neurologic damage. The final outcome of this type of injury depends on the initial assessment and care. Consult a critical care or emergency textbook and see Chapter 48 for more in-depth information.

COLLABORATIVE MANAGEMENT

Assessment

The priority in caring for a client with neck trauma is assessment for a patent airway. After airway patency is assured, then assess for manifestations of bleeding or impending shock.

Perform a baseline neurologic assessment for mental status, sensory level, and motor function. Injury to the carotid artery may result in death, stroke, or paralysis related to disruption of blood flow to the brain (see Chapter 44). A carotid angiogram may be performed to rule out vascular injuries.

Esophagus injury may occur with neck trauma. Assess for chest pain and tenderness, oral bleeding, and **crepitus** (crackling sounds when palpating the skin). A barium or meglumine diatrizoate (Gastrografin) swallow may be needed to rule out an esophageal perforation injury.

Interventions

Cervical spine injuries often occur at the same time as a neck injury (see Chapter 46). Health care personnel must take great care not to make these injuries worse by causing neck movement while establishing the airway. Prepare to assist in emergency intubation, cricothyrotomy, or tracheostomy to establish a patent airway. Interventions for clients in shock are detailed in Chapter 40.

Head and Neck Cancer

PATHOPHYSIOLOGY

Head and neck cancer can disrupt breathing, eating, facial appearance, self-image, speech, and communication. This form of cancer can be devastating, even when treated successfully. The care needs for clients with these problems are complex, requiring a comprehensive team approach. The client can receive appropriate care only after the location and size of the tumor are accurately identified.

Head and neck cancer is curable when treated early. The prognosis for those who have more advanced disease at diagnosis depends on the extent and location of the tumor. Untreated cancer of the head and neck is a fatal disease within 2 years of diagnosis.

Most head and neck cancers (80%) are squamous cell (mucosal epithelial) carcinomas that are slow growing, usually requiring several years to develop (Figure 32-7). Many head and neck tumors first appear as infiltrating ulcerations.

The cancer begins when the mucosa is chronically irritated and changes into a tougher mucosa **(squamous metaplasia)**. This tougher mucosa occurs by increasing the mucosal thickness (**acanthosis** or hyperplasia) or by developing a keratin layer **(keratosis).** At the same time, changes at the gene level enhance the growth of abnormal epithelial cells that eventually become malignant. These lesions may then take the form of white, patchy lesions **(leukoplakia)** or red, velvety patches **(erythroplasia).**

The growth and spread **(metastasis)** of head and neck cancer first occur into nearby structures, such as mucosa, muscle, and bone. Systemic spread through the blood and lymphatic systems may also occur. Distant metastasis occurs most often to the lungs or liver.

At diagnosis, the degree of malignancy is determined by cellular analysis. Earlier stage cancers are described as *carcinoma in situ* and *well differentiated.* Without treatment, cancers progress to be *moderately differentiated* and, finally, *poorly differentiated.* Most head and neck cancers arise from squamous tissue, but they also can start from salivary glands or

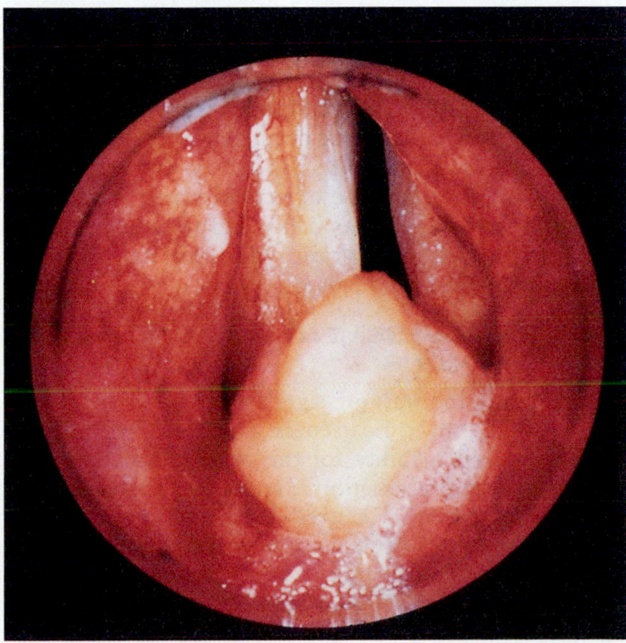

Figure 32-7 ■ Laryngeal cancer is frequently caused by the combination of alcohol and tobacco. This laryngoscopic photograph shows a large granular cell tumor of the true vocal cord. (From Wenig, B.M. [1993]. *Atlas of the head and neck pathology.* Philadelphia: W.B. Saunders. Used with permission.)

thyroid cells. Less common head and neck tumors are malignant melanomas and adenocarcinomas. Treatment is based on tumor cell type and degree of spread at diagnosis.

Etiology

Many risk factors contribute to the development of head and neck cancer, but the actual cause is unknown. The two most important risk factors are tobacco and alcohol use, especially in combination. Other risk factors include chewing tobacco, pipe smoking, marijuana, voice abuse, chronic laryngitis, exposure to industrial chemicals or hardwood dust, and poor oral hygiene.

Incidence/Prevalence

The frequency of occurrence of head and neck carcinoma is increasing. The American Cancer Society (ACS) estimates 47,000 newly diagnosed cases of *oral* and *laryngeal* cancers occur in the United States each year. This cancer type accounts for more than 4% of all carcinomas and more than 11,000 deaths per year (ACS, 2005). Men are affected three times more often than women. Most head and neck cancers occur in people over 60 years of age.

COLLABORATIVE MANAGEMENT

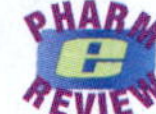

Assessment

HISTORY

The client with head and neck cancer may have difficulty speaking because of hoarseness, shortness of breath, tumor bulk, and pain. It is important to be sensitive to these difficulties during the interview.

Ask about tobacco and alcohol use, history of recurrent acute or chronic laryngitis or pharyngitis, oral sores, and lumps in the neck. Calculate the client's smoking history in **pack-years** (the number of packs smoked per day times the number of years the client has smoked). Ask about alcohol intake (how many drinks per day and for how many years). These questions may be uncomfortable for both you and the client but are an important part of the history. Also ask about exposure to environmental or occupational pollutants.

Assess problems related to risk factors. For example, nutrition may be poor because of alcohol intake and impaired liver function. Assess dietary habits and any weight loss. Ask about any chronic lung disease, which may have an impact on the client's breathing pattern.

PHYSICAL ASSESSMENT/CLINICAL MANIFESTATIONS

Table 32-1 lists the warning signs of head and neck cancer. With *laryngeal* cancer, hoarseness may occur because of tumor size and an inability for the vocal cords to come together for normal phonation. Figure 32-8 shows the common sites of laryngeal cancer. Lesions of the true vocal cords are the earliest form of laryngeal cancer. Any person who has a history of hoarseness, mouth sores, or a lump in the neck for 3 to 4 weeks or longer should be evaluated for laryngeal cancer.

Inspection and palpation of the head and neck are important parts of the physical examination. A nurse practitioner may perform a laryngeal examination using a laryngeal mirror or fiberoptic laryngoscope. Lesions may be seen on inspection. The neck is palpated to assess for enlarged lymph nodes.

TABLE 32-1 Warning Signs of Head and Neck Cancer

- Pain
- Lump in the mouth, throat, or neck
- Difficulty swallowing
- Color changes in the mouth or tongue to red, white, gray, dark brown, or black
- Oral lesion or sore that does not heal in 2 weeks
- Persistent or unexplained oral bleeding
- Numbness of the mouth, lips, or face
- Change in the fit of dentures
- Burning sensation when drinking citrus juices or hot liquids
- Persistent, unilateral ear pain
- Hoarseness or change in voice quality
- Persistent or recurrent sore throat
- Shortness of breath
- Anorexia and weight loss

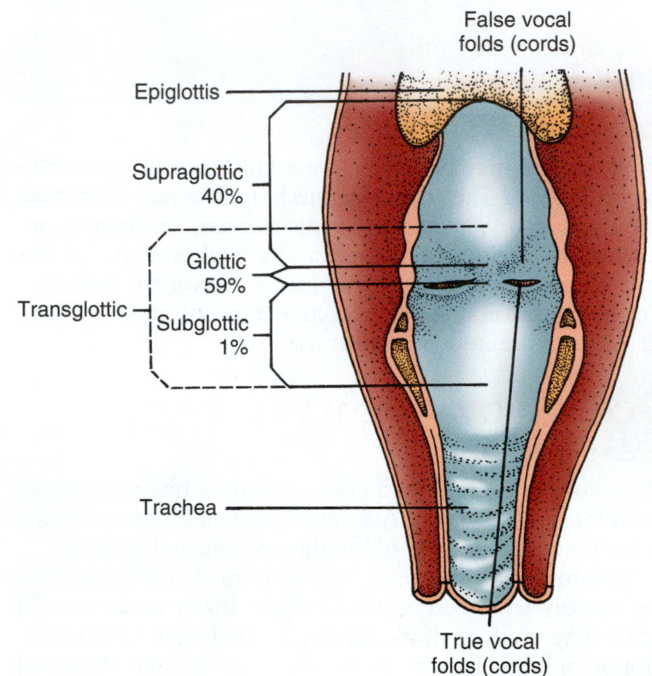

Figure 32-8 ■ Sites and incidence of primary laryngeal tumors.

PSYCHOSOCIAL ASSESSMENT

Often the client with head and neck cancer has a longstanding history of cigarette or alcohol use or both. The client or family may feel denial, guilt, blame, or shame once the diagnosis is suspected. Assess the adequacy of support systems and coping mechanisms. Documentation of social and family support is needed because the client often needs extensive assistance at home after treatment. Consult with a social worker as needed. Evaluate the cognitive functioning (see Chapter 44) and the level of education or literacy of the client and family to plan important teaching before and after surgery.

Document any family history of cancer as well as the client's age, gender, occupation, and ability to perform the activities of daily living (ADLs). Ask the client whether his or her occupation requires continual oral communication. Job retraining may be needed if treatment affects speech.

LABORATORY ASSESSMENT

Diagnostic laboratory tests include a complete blood count, bleeding times, urinalysis, and blood chemistries. The client with chronic alcoholism may have low protein and albumin levels from poor nutrition. Renal and liver function tests are performed to rule out cancer spread and to evaluate the client's ability to metabolize drugs and chemotherapeutic agents.

RADIOGRAPHIC ASSESSMENT

Many types of radiographic studies, including x-rays of the skull, sinuses, neck, and chest, are useful in diagnosing cancer spread, second primary tumors, and the extent of tumor invasion. Computed tomography (CT) of the head and neck, with or without contrast media, helps to evaluate the tumor's exact location.

OTHER DIAGNOSTIC ASSESSMENTS

Magnetic resonance imaging (MRI) can help differentiate normal from diseased tissue. An MRI is more sensitive than a CT in defining the extent of soft-tissue invasion.

The brain, bone, and liver are evaluated with nuclear imaging, bone scans, SPECT (single-photon emission computerized tomography) scans, and PET (positron emission tomography) scans. These tests help locate additional tumor sites.

Other helpful tests include direct and indirect laryngoscopy, tumor mapping, and biopsy. Panendoscopy is performed with general anesthesia to define the extent of the tumor. This procedure includes laryngoscopy, nasopharyngoscopy, esophagoscopy, and bronchoscopy. Tumor-mapping biopsies are performed to identify tumor location. Biopsy tissues taken at the time of the panendoscopy confirm the diagnosis and determine the tumor type, cell features, and location. Tumor staging by the TNM (tumor, nodes, metastasis) method (see Chapter 27) is performed at this time.

Analysis

COMMON NURSING DIAGNOSES AND COLLABORATIVE PROBLEMS

The primary collaborative problem is Potential for Respiratory Obstruction.

The following are priority nursing diagnoses for clients with head and neck carcinomas:

1. Risk for Aspiration related to edema, anatomic changes, or alteration of protective oropharyngeal reflexes
2. Anxiety related to threat of death, change in role status, change in economic status
3. Disturbed Body Image related to tumor and treatment modalities

ADDITIONAL NURSING DIAGNOSES AND COLLABORATIVE PROBLEMS

In addition to the common nursing diagnoses and collaborative problems, clients with head and neck carcinomas may have one or more of the following:

- Acute Pain or Chronic Pain related to tumor invasion of tissues and nerves and surgical intervention
- Imbalanced Nutrition: Less Than Body Requirements related to dysphagia, anxiety, tumor process, surgical resection, or chronic alcohol intake
- Impaired Verbal Communication related to tumor invasion, hoarseness, pain, or surgical resection
- Impaired Skin Integrity related to altered circulation, nutritional deficit, tumor invasion, radiation, chemical factors (body secretions or substances), or surgical wound
- Ineffective Coping related to altered body image, communication method, or ineffective social support
- Impaired Social Interaction related to body image disturbance and lifestyle practices
- Impaired Adjustment related to self-care of the tracheostomy and nasogastric tubes, alternative communication methods, and body-image disturbance
- Deficient Knowledge (treatment regimen and resources) related to lack of exposure to or lack of interest in learning

Critical Thinking Challenge

The client is a 65-year-old man who recently retired from his job as a laborer in a steel mill for 47 years. He has just been diagnosed with laryngeal cancer. He started smoking at 15 years of age and smoked three packs per day until he was 60 years of age, when he was able to quit successfully. He drinks two beers every evening. His hobbies include bowling, playing poker with his friends weekly, refinishing furniture, and singing in his church choir. His other health problems include seasonal asthma and hypertension. He once had a deep vein thrombosis in his right calf. His current over-the-counter and prescribed drugs include aspirin 81 mg daily, hydrochlorothiazide, and Primatene Mist oral inhaler. He is angry about the diagnosis, saying that he might as well take up smoking again for all the good it did him to quit.

1. Calculate this client's smoking history in pack-years.
2. What risk factors does this client have for head and neck cancer?
3. Should you encourage him to refrain from smoking now? Why or why not?
4. What activities are likely to be affected by the disease or its treatment?

evolve For suggested answer guidelines, go to http://evolve.elsevier.com/Iggy/.

Planning and Implementation

POTENTIAL FOR RESPIRATORY OBSTRUCTION

NOC PLANNING: EXPECTED OUTCOMES. The client with head and neck cancer is expected to attain and maintain adequate tissue oxygenation. Indicators include the following:

- Arterial blood gas values within the normal range
- Rate and depth of respiration within the normal range
- Pulse oximetry within the normal range
- Absence of cyanosis or pallor

INTERVENTIONS. The goal of treatment is to remove or eradicate the cancer while preserving as much normal function as possible. The physician presents the available treatment options. Surgery, radiation, or chemotherapy may each be used alone or in combination. In planning treatment options, the client's general physical condition, nutritional status, and age; the effects of the tumor on body function; and the client's personal choice are all considered. Treatment for laryngeal cancer may range from radiation therapy (for a small specific area or tumor) to total laryngopharyngectomy, with bilateral neck dissections followed by radiation therapy. The specific treatment depends on the extent and location of the lesion. Voice-conservation procedures are used only if they do not risk incomplete removal of the tumor. Nursing care focuses on the client's total needs, including preoperative preparation, competent in-hospital care, discharge planning and teaching, and extensive outpatient rehabilitation.

NONSURGICAL MANAGEMENT. Monitor the respiratory system by assessing respiratory rate, breath sounds, pulse oximetry, arterial blood gas values, and the results of pulmonary function tests. Respiratory distress may indicate narrowing of the airway related to tumor growth, edema, or both. Position the client for optimal air exchange. Teach client and family about the use of Fowler's and semi-Fowler's positions. Sitting upright in a reclining chair may promote more comfortable breathing. Chapters 7 and 9 provide additional information on palliation and pain control for clients who elect not to have therapy and for those whose therapy has not been effective.

Radiation Therapy. Radiation treatment of small cancers in specific locations has a cure rate of at least 80%. The cure rate for larger cancers is lower when radiation is used as the only therapy. Standard therapy uses 5000 to 7500 rad (radiation absorbed dose), usually over 6 weeks and in daily or twice-daily doses. The physician may recommend radiation alone or in combination with surgery. Because radiation therapy slows tissue healing, it might *not* be recommended before surgery. Radiation therapy is an outpatient treatment (see Chapter 28). Most clients have uncomfortable side effects during and for a few weeks following radiation therapy (see Chart 32-2).

Hoarseness may become worse. Reassure the client and family that voice improves within 4 to 6 weeks after completion of radiation therapy. Urge the client to use voice rest and alternate means of communication until the effects of radiation therapy have passed.

Most clients have a sore throat and difficulty swallowing during radiation therapy to the neck. Gargling with saline or sucking ice may decrease discomfort. Mouthwashes and throat sprays containing a local anesthetic agent such as lidocaine or diphenhydramine can provide temporary relief. Alert the physician to the client's pain so that analgesic drugs can be prescribed.

The skin at the site of irradiation becomes red and tender and may peel during therapy. Instruct the client to avoid exposing this area to sun, heat, cold, and abrasive treatments such as shaving. Teach the client to wear protective clothing made of soft cotton and to wash this area gently with a mild soap, such as Dove. Stress that only the lotions or powders prescribed by the radiologist should be used until the area has healed.

If the salivary glands are in the path of irradiation, the client has a dry mouth **(xerostomia)**. This side effect is long-term and may be permanent. Some of the consequences of reduced saliva include increased risk for dental caries, increased risk for oral infections, halitosis (bad breath), and changes in taste sensation. Although there is no cure for xerostomia, interventions can help reduce the discomfort. Heavy fluid intake, particularly water, and humidification can help ease the discomfort. Some clients benefit from the use of artificial saliva, such as Salivart, or saliva stimulants, such as Salagen and cevimeline (pilocarpine-based cholinergic drugs). Additional interventions for dry mouth include chewing gum and sucking hard candy.

Chemotherapy. Chemotherapy can be used alone or in addition to surgery or radiation for head and neck cancer. Chapter 28 discusses the general care needs of clients receiving chemotherapy.

SURGICAL MANAGEMENT. Tumor size and location (TNM classification) determines the type of surgery needed for the specific head and neck cancer. Reconstruction is also determined by the tumor size and amount of tissue to be resected and reconstructed. Surgical procedures for head and neck cancers include laryngectomy (total and partial), tracheostomy, and oropharyngeal cancer resections.

Laryngectomy and Related Surgery. The major types of surgery for laryngeal cancer include cordal stripping, **cordectomy** (excision of a vocal cord), partial laryngectomy, and total laryngectomy. If cancer is in the lymph nodes in the neck or if the tumor has a high rate of nodal spread, the surgeon performs a nodal neck dissection along with removal of the primary tumor ("radical neck"). A pathologist evaluates the resected lymph nodes for tumor invasion.

Preoperative Care. Teach the client and family about the tumor. The surgeon explains the surgical procedure and obtains informed consent. Discuss and interpret the implications of such consent with the client and family.

Explain about self-care of the airway, alternate methods of communication, suctioning, pain control methods, the critical care environment (including ventilators and critical care routines), nutritional support, feeding tubes, and goals for discharge. The client will need to learn new methods of speech. Help the client prepare for this change through preoperative teaching and the use of an alternate form of communication (e.g., pen and pencil, "magic slate," picture or alphabet board). Assess which communication method is most preferred by the client before surgery.

A team approach for planning care and rehabilitation is critical for the best outcome. The team should include nurses, physicians, speech pathologists, social workers, dietitians, respiratory therapists, and occupational and physical therapists. Professionals from all these disciplines help to evaluate and prepare the client who has head and neck cancer. Chapter 20 describes general preoperative assessment and education in detail.

Operative Procedures. Hemilaryngectomy (vertical or horizontal) and supraglottic laryngectomy are types of partial voice conservation laryngectomies. Table 32-2 lists specific information about the various surgical procedures for laryngeal cancer.

To protect the airway, a tracheostomy is needed. With a partial laryngectomy, the tracheostomy is usually temporary. With a total laryngectomy, the upper airway is separated from the pharynx and esophagus, and the trachea is brought out through the skin in the neck and sutured in place, creating a stoma. This airway opening is *always* permanent and is referred to as a laryngectomy stoma.

Neck dissection includes the removal of lymph nodes, the sternocleidomastoid muscle, the jugular vein, the 11th cranial nerve, and surrounding soft tissue. Because the 11th cranial nerve (spinal accessory nerve) is cut during this procedure, shoulder drop will be present after surgery. Physical therapy exercises are needed after surgery to help the client ease the shoulder drop by using other muscle groups.

Postoperative Care. Head and neck surgery often lasts 8 hours or longer. Usually the client spends the immediate period after surgery in the surgical intensive care unit. Monitor airway patency, vital signs, hemodynamic status,

TABLE 32-2 Surgical Procedures for Laryngeal Cancer and Their Effect on Voice Quality

Procedure	Description	Resulting Voice Quality
Laser surgery	Tumor reduced or destroyed by laser beam through laryngoscope	Normal/hoarse
Transoral cordectomy	Tumor (early lesion) resected through laryngoscope	Normal/hoarse (high cure rate)
Laryngofissure	No cord removed (early lesion)	Normal (high cure rate)
Supraglottic partial laryngectomy	Hyoid bone, false cords, and epiglottis removed Neck dissection on affected side performed if nodes involved	Normal/hoarse
Hemilaryngectomy or vertical laryngectomy	One true cord, one false cord, and one half of thyroid cartilage removed	Hoarse voice
Total laryngectomy	Entire larynx, hyoid bone, strap muscles, one or two tracheal rings removed Nodal neck dissection if nodes involved	No natural voice

and comfort level. Monitor for hemorrhage and other general complications of anesthesia and surgery (see Chapter 22). Take vital signs hourly for the first 24 hours and then every 2 hours until the client is stable. After the client is transferred from the critical care unit, monitor vital signs every 4 hours or according to agency policy. The client is generally out of bed by the second postoperative day.

Complications after head and neck cancer surgery include airway obstruction, hemorrhage, wound breakdown, and tumor recurrence. The first priorities after head and neck surgery are airway maintenance and ventilation. Other priorities include wound, flap, and reconstructive tissue care; pain management; nutrition; and psychological adjustment, including speech therapy.

Airway Maintenance and Ventilation. Immediately after surgery, the client may need ventilatory assistance because of a long-term smoking history, chronic lung disease, and a long duration of anesthesia. Most clients wean easily from the ventilator after this type of surgery because the thoracic and abdominal cavities are not entered. When weaned from the ventilator, the client usually uses a tracheostomy collar (over the artificial airway or open stoma) with oxygen and humidification to help mobilize mucus secretions. Secretions may remain blood-tinged for 1 to 2 days. Use body substance precautions, and report any increase in bleeding to the surgeon. Humidifying the air helps to remove crusts and prevent obstruction of the tube with secretions. Some surgeons prescribe instillations of 5 to 10 mL of sterile saline into the airway every 2 hours; however, this practice is controversial.

A laryngectomy tube is used for clients who have undergone a *total laryngectomy* and need an appliance to prevent scar tissue contracture at the skin-tracheal border. This tube is similar to a standard tracheostomy tube but is shorter and fatter with a larger lumen and more acute angle (Figure 32-9). Laryngectomy tube care is similar to tracheostomy tube care (see Chapter 31) except that the client can change the laryngectomy tube daily or as needed. A laryngectomy button is similar to a laryngectomy tube but is made of Silastic, has a single lumen, and is very short. A button is comfortable for the client, is easily removed for cleaning, and is available in various sizes and lengths for a custom fit. Provide a "magic slate" or paper and pencil for communication because the client cannot create speech other than mouthing words.

Coughing, deep breathing, and saline instillation are usually effective in clearing secretions. The lack of a surgical incision in the chest or abdomen improves the ability

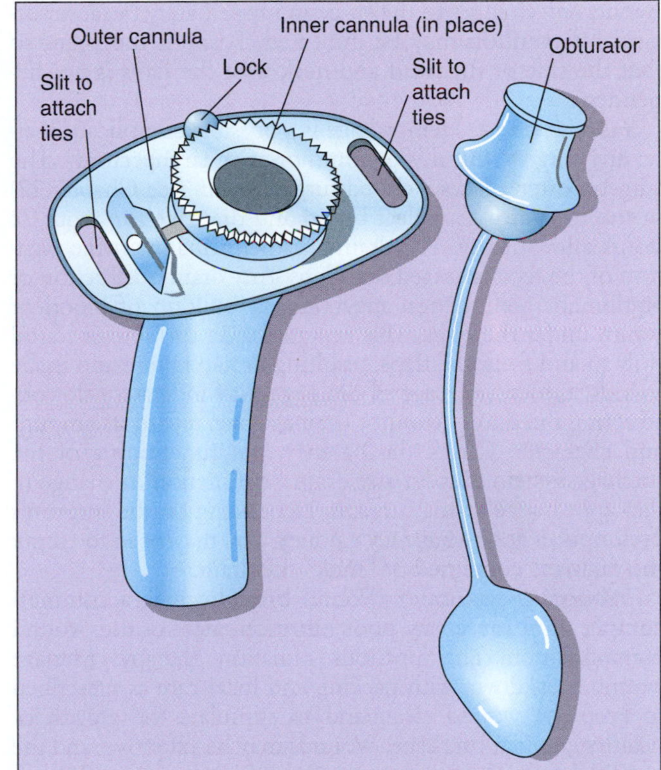

Figure 32-9 ■ A laryngectomy tube. Note that the outer cannula is shorter and has a diameter wider than that of a tracheostomy tube.

to cough. Instruct the client in the proper techniques for coughing and deep breathing to clear secretions (see Chapter 22).

Oral secretions can be suctioned by the client using a Yankauer or tonsillar suction or with a soft red latex catheter. Teach the client to suction away from the side of the surgery to prevent wound opening immediately after surgery. Clients can participate in their own care by using a table mirror for visibility. Provide a clean environment for the catheter.

Stoma care following a total laryngectomy is a combination of wound care and airway care. Inspect the stoma with a flashlight. Clean the suture line with half-strength hydrogen peroxide to prevent secretions from forming crusts and obstructing the airway. Perform suture line care every 1 to 2 hours during the first few days after surgery and then every 4 hours thereafter. The mucosa of the stoma and trachea should be bright and shiny and without crusts, similar to the appearance of the oral mucosa.

Wound, Flap, and Reconstructive Tissue Care. Tissue "flaps" may be used to close the wound and improve appearance. Commonly used reconstructive flaps are pectoralis major myocutaneous flaps, island flaps, rotation flaps, trapezius flaps, split-thickness skin grafts (STSGs), and free flaps with microvascular anastomosis (scapula, fibula, or radial forearm free flaps). These flaps may be used for reconstruction after any type of head and neck resection. After neck dissection, the surgeon places an STSG over the exposed carotid artery before covering it with skin flaps or reconstructive flaps.

The first 24 hours after surgery are critical. Evaluate all flaps every hour for the first 72 hours. Monitor capillary refill, color, and Doppler activity of the major feeding vessel. Report any changes to the surgeon immediately because surgical intervention may be indicated. Position the client so that the side of the head and neck with the flaps is not dependent.

Hemorrhage. Hemorrhage is a possible complication after any surgery, but it is uncommon with laryngectomy. The surgeon often places a closed surgical drain (see Chapter 22) in the neck area to collect blood and drainage for about 72 hours after surgery. The drain also helps maintain the position of the reconstructed skin flaps. Any drain obstruction or equipment malfunction may cause a buildup of blood or serum under the flaps. This accumulation can impair blood flow to and from the flaps, resulting in flap failure and tissue loss. A sudden stoppage of drainage may indicate a clot obstructing the drain. Monitor drainage and record its amount and character. Check the patency and functioning of the drainage system. Report any drain malfunction or change in flap appearance to the surgeon. Depending on the surgeon's prescription and the agency's policy, you may need to empty the drainage contained or "milk" the drain.

Wound Breakdown. Wound breakdown is a common complication caused by poor nutrition, alcohol use, wound contamination, and previous radiation therapy. Manage wound breakdown with packing and local care as prescribed to keep the wound clean and to stimulate the growth of healthy granulation tissue. Wounds may be extensive, and the carotid artery may be exposed. Split-thickness skin grafts often are placed over the carotid artery for protection in the event of wound dehiscence. As the wound heals, granulation tissue covers the artery and prevents rupture. If granulation is slow and the carotid artery is at risk, another surgical flap may be made to cover the carotid artery and close the wound.

If the carotid artery ruptures because of drying or infection, place *immediate constant pressure* over the site and secure the airway. Maintain direct manual pressure on the carotid artery and *immediately* transport the client to the operating room for carotid resection. *Carotid artery rupture has a high risk of stroke and death.* An immediate nursing response can save the client's life.

Pain Management. After surgery, pain should be controlled and the client should still be able to participate in his or her care. Morphine (Statex✱) often is given by IV bolus and continuously for the first days after surgery. As the client progresses, acetaminophen with codeine, then acetaminophen alone, can be given by feeding tube. Oral drugs for pain and discomfort are started only after the client can tolerate oral nutrition. After discharge, the client still requires pain management, especially if he or she is receiving radiation therapy. An adjunct to the pain regimen may be liquid nonsteroidal anti-inflammatory drugs (NSAIDs). These drugs provide excellent pain relief and can be used along with opioid analgesics (see also Chapter 7). Amitriptyline (Elavil) or other tricyclic antidepressants may also be used for the lancinating pain of nerve-root involvement.

Nutrition. A nasogastric, gastrostomy, or jejunostomy tube is placed during surgery for nutritional support while the head and neck heal. Initially the client receives IV fluids or parenteral nutrition until the intestinal tract has recovered from the effects of anesthesia. After that, nutrients can be given via the feeding tube. The nutritional support team or dietitian assesses the client before surgery and is available for consultation after surgery. The common nutrition goal is to provide 35 to 40 kcal/kg of body weight. Replacement of protein and water loss is calculated carefully.

The nasogastric tube (the most commonly used type of tube) usually remains in place for 7 to 10 days after surgery. Before removing the tube, assess the client's ability to swallow if nutrition is to be given by mouth. Aspiration *cannot* occur following a total laryngectomy because the airway and esophagus have been completely separated. Reassure the client that aspiration will not occur, and stay with him or her during the first few swallowing attempts. Swallowing may be uncomfortable at first, and the prescribed analgesics may be needed.

Speech Rehabilitation. The client's voice quality and speech are altered after surgery. Although this problem has enormous effects on the client's ability to maintain social interactions, continue employment, and maintain a desired quality of life, it is often poorly addressed while he or she is hospitalized (see the Evidence-Based Practice for Nursing box on p. 577). Working with the client and family toward developing an acceptable communication method during the inpatient period is essential for a satisfactory outcome.

Together with the speech pathologist, discuss the principles of speech therapy with the client and family early in the course of the treatment plan (see Chart 32-2). Voice and speech differences depend on the type of surgical resection (see Table 32-2). Speech production varies with client practice, amount of tissue removed, and radiation effects, but the speech can be very understandable.

The speech rehabilitation plan for clients who have a total laryngectomy at first consists of writing or using a picture board. The client then uses an artificial larynx and eventually learns esophageal speech. For success, the client needs support and encouragement from the speech pathologist, hospital team, and family while relearning to speak. This process can be time consuming and requires concentration each time the client speaks. Having a **laryngectomee** (person who has had a laryngectomy) from one of the local self-help organizations visit the client and family is often beneficial. The International Association of Laryngectomees is very active and supportive, as is the American Cancer Society (ACS) Visitor Program.

Common means of speech communication after laryngectomy include esophageal speech, the use of mechanical devices, and the use of a tracheoesophageal fistula (TEF).

ESOPHAGEAL SPEECH. Most clients who have a total laryngectomy attempt esophageal speech. Sound can be produced this way by "burping" the air swallowed or injected into

EVIDENCE-BASED PRACTICE for Nursing

Silence is not golden

Happ, M.B., Roesch, T., & Kagan, S. (2004). Communication needs, methods, and perceived voice quality following head and neck surgery: A literature review. *Cancer Nursing, 27*(1), 1-9.

The authors sought to examine the problems associated with loss of speech as a result of temporary or permanent changes induced by medical or surgical intervention for head and neck cancer. Although numerous articles in both the nursing and medical literature discussed issues related to temporary speech loss through intubation, mechanical ventilation, and chemical paralysis in the critical care setting, only one study targeted the inpatient postoperative recovery period for clients with head and neck cancer. The authors then expanded their search to include the first 12 months after head and neck surgery. The search of relevant literature from 1968 through 2002 revealed a total of only 10 published studies and one clinical case report specifically addressing the communication needs, methods, or perceived voice quality of clients with head and neck cancer surgery during the postoperative period.

The 11 studies varied considerably in sample size, timing of data collection (postoperative stage of clients), and study design, but three common themes consistently emerged. These themes were information needs (of the client and family), communication methods and perceived voice quality, and quality-of-life perceptions that included disfigurement and socialization. Overwhelmingly, the studies indicated that the education needs and preparation for postoperative communication impairment were unaddressed or poorly addressed for this client population.

Level of Evidence: 4—Well-conducted qualitative systematic review (integrative review on nonexperimental design studies).

Critique. The authors used the appropriate methods of searching the literature for an exhaustive review on the topic. This review highlights the need for additional studies to understand the dimensions of information needed among these clients and their families.

Implications for Nursing. Whereas all cancer surgeries result in some degree of tissue loss and potential function reduction, surgery for head and neck cancer is the most obviously disfiguring and often results in a permanent speech change or loss. These results are obvious to anyone who interacts with the client and are a constant reminder to the client of the cancer diagnosis.

Adjustment to the changes require much time and work. Nursing care can be key to this adjustment but must begin during the perioperative time. Nurses need to help the client and family learn exactly what to expect after surgery. Presenting accurate information in a matter-of-fact but sensitive way before surgery can reduce anxiety and help the client and family to have realistic and optimistic expectations. Working with a client for whom speech has been lost is frustrating to the client, nurse, and family. Talking for the client does not help, nor does pretending to understand what the client is trying to communicate. Nurses must allow whatever time it takes to ensure that the client's needs and wishes are accurately understood. The in-hospital time for these clients after surgery is longer than are most other hospital stays and therefore represents an opportune time for nurses to implement interventions for symptom management, client education for self-care and communication, stress and anxiety reduction, and resocialization.

the esophageal pharynx and shaping the words in the mouth. The voice produced is a monotone; it cannot be raised or lowered and carries no pitch. In the English language, the vocal cords are necessary for 15 consonants; the remaining 10 consonants can be formed by shaping the mouth. Clients must have adequate hearing, or esophageal speech will be difficult because they will use their mouth to shape the words as they hear them. Hearing-impaired clients may require hearing aids.

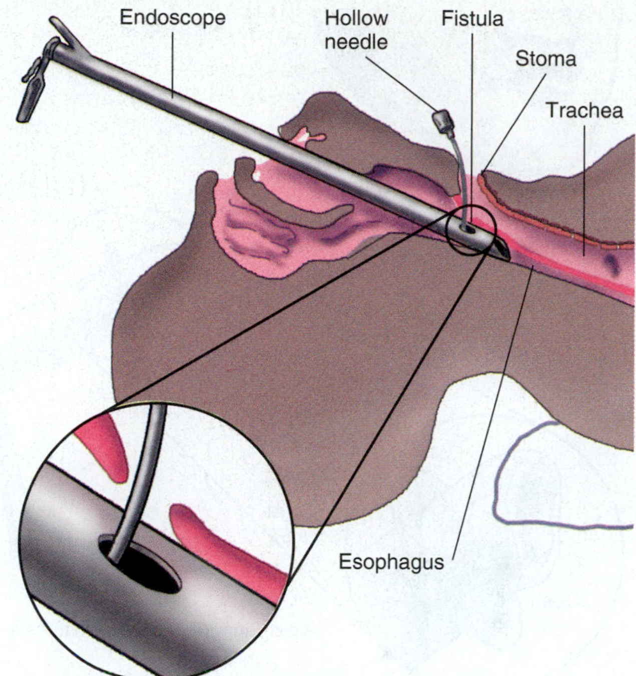

Figure 32-10 ■ One method of creating a tracheoesophageal fistula.

Some clients have intestinal bloating as a result of swallowing air for esophageal speech. Antacids may help to reduce bloating sensations. Esophageal speech also helps to strengthen the respiratory and abdominal muscles, which aids in clearing secretions and in breathing.

MECHANICAL DEVICES. The client who cannot attain esophageal speech can use mechanical devices called **electrolarynges.** Most are battery-powered devices placed against the side of the neck or cheek. The air inside the mouth and throat is vibrated, and the client moves his or her lips and tongue as usual. Another external device (Cooper-Rand), also battery powered, consists of a plastic tube that is placed in the client's mouth and vibrates during speech. The quality of speech generated with these devices is robot-like and does not sound natural.

TRACHEOESOPHAGEAL FISTULA. A tracheoesophageal fistula (TEF) may be used if esophageal speech is ineffective and if the client meets strict criteria. A surgical fistula is created between the trachea and the esophagus either at the time of the laryngectomy or later (Figure 32-10). The surgeon places a catheter into the laryngectomy stoma and surgically creates a fistula into the esophagus. The catheter is usually sutured to the neck to prevent accidental dislodgment. After the fistula heals, a silicone prosthesis (e.g., the Blom-Singer prosthesis) is inserted in place of the catheter (Figure 32-11). The client covers the stoma and the opening of the prosthesis with a finger or opens and closes the opening with a special valve to divert air from the lungs, through the trachea, into the esophagus, and out of the mouth. Lip and tongue movement, not the prosthesis itself, produces speech.

Surgical Procedures for Other Head and Neck Cancers. The major types of resections, defined by the tumor location of the *oropharyngeal cancer,* are called composite resections. **Composite resections** are a combina-

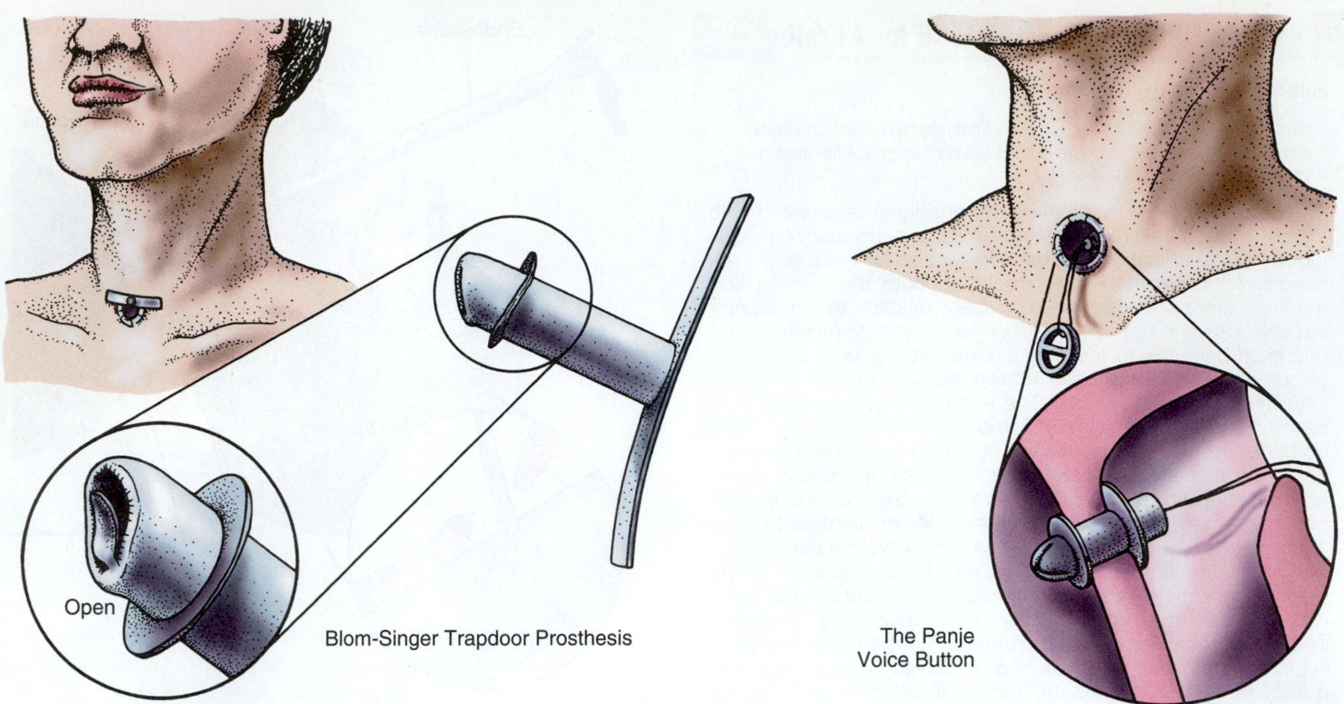

Figure 32-11 ■ Examples of tracheoesophageal prostheses.

tion of surgical procedures that include partial or total glossectomies, partial mandibulectomies and, if needed, nodal neck dissections. Tracheostomy may be planned to provide an adequate airway. (See Chapter 57 for more information about oral cancer.)

Tracheotomy. A **tracheotomy** is a surgical incision into the trachea for the purpose of establishing an airway (tracheostomy). It can be performed as an emergency procedure or as a scheduled surgical procedure. A tracheostomy can be temporary or permanent. Chapter 31 discusses the nursing care of a client with a tracheostomy.

RISK FOR ASPIRATION

NOC **PLANNING: EXPECTED OUTCOMES.** The client with head and neck cancer is expected not to aspirate food, gastric contents, or oral secretions into the lungs. Indicators include that the client often or consistently demonstrates the following behaviors:

- Positions self upright for eating or drinking
- Selects foods according to swallowing ability
- Chooses liquids and foods of proper consistency

INTERVENTIONS. The surgical changes in the upper respiratory tract and altered swallowing mechanisms increase the client's risk for aspiration. Aspiration can result in life-threatening pneumonia, weight loss, prolonged hospitalization, and increased costs. Chart 32-3 lists NIC interventions for aspiration prevention.

The presence of a nasogastric (NG) feeding tube may further increase the potential for aspiration because of the incompetent lower esophageal sphincter (LES). The one exception is the client who has undergone a total laryngectomy. In these cases the airway is separated from the esophagus, making aspiration impossible; such a client is *not* at risk.

A dynamic swallow study, such as a barium swallow under fluoroscopy, evaluates a client's ability to protect the airway from aspiration and helps determine the appropriate method of swallow rehabilitation. In many cases enteral feedings are used either because of the client's inability to swallow or because of continued aspiration potential.

When an NG tube is in place, help prevent aspiration through the use of routine reflux precautions. These precautions include elevating the head of the bed and strictly adhering to tube feeding regimens, including no bolus feedings at night. Check residual feeding before each bolus feeding (or every 4 to 6 hours with continuous feeding), and evaluate the client's tolerance of the tube feeding. If the residual volume is too high (above 100 mL or as otherwise prescribed by the physician), withhold the feeding and notify the physician. Check the pH of pulmonary secretions. Because residual volume cannot be checked with micropore feeding tubes, use other techniques to assess tube placement. (See Chapter 64 for other interventions related to NG tubes and tube feedings.)

Swallowing can be a major problem for the client who has a tracheostomy tube. Swallowing can be normal if the cranial nerves and anatomic structures are intact. In a normal swallow, the larynx elevates and moves forward to protect itself from the passing stream of food and saliva. Laryngeal elevation also assists in opening the upper esophageal sphincter. The tracheostomy tube sometimes fixes the larynx in place, making it unable to perform this motion efficiently. The result is difficulty in swallowing.

The tracheostomy tube cuff can balloon backward when inflated and interfere with the passage of food through the esophagus. The common wall of the posterior trachea and the anterior esophagus is very thin, which allows this pushing phenomenon. The client with head and neck cancer who

CHART 32-3

NIC INTERVENTION ACTIVITIES for The Client with Head and Neck Cancer

Aspiration Precautions: *Prevention or minimization of risk factors in the client at risk for aspiration*

- Monitor level of consciousness, cough reflex, gag reflex, and swallowing ability.
- Monitor pulmonary status.
- Maintain an airway.
- Position upright 90 degrees or as far as possible.
- Keep suction setup available.
- Feed in small amounts.
- Check NG or gastrostomy tube placement before feeding.
- Check NG or gastrostomy tube residual before feeding.
- Avoid liquids or use thickening agent.
- Offer foods or liquids that can be formed into a bolus before swallowing.
- Cut food into small pieces.
- Request medication in elixir form.
- Break or crush pills before administration.
- Keep head of bed elevated 30 to 45 minutes after feeding.

Smoking Cessation Assistance: *Helping another to stop smoking*

- Give smoker clear, consistent advice to quit smoking.
- Help choose best method for giving up cigarettes, when client is ready to quit.
- Refer to group programs or individual therapists, as appropriate.
- Assist client with any self-help methods.
- Help client plan specific coping strategies and resolve problems that result from quitting.
- Inform client that dry mouth, cough, scratchy throat, and feeling on edge are symptoms that may occur after quitting; the patch or gum may help with cravings.
- Advise client to keep a list of "slips" or near-slips, what causes them, and what he or she learned from them.
- Advise client to avoid smokeless tobacco, dipping, and chewing as these can lead to addiction and/or health problems including oral cancer, gum problems, loss of teeth, and heart disease
- Manage nicotine replacement therapy.
- Contact national and local resource organizations for resource materials.
- Follow client for 2 years after quitting, if possible, to provide encouragement.
- Help client deal with any lapses (e.g., reassure client that he or she is not a "failure," reassure that much can be learned from this temporary regression, assist client in identifying reasons for the relapse).
- Support client who begins smoking again by helping to identify what has been learned.
- Encourage the relapsed client to try again.
- Serve as a nonsmoking role model.

NIC intervention activities selected from Dochterman, J.M., & Bulechek, G.M. (Eds.). (2004). *Nursing interventions classification (NIC)* (4th ed.). St. Louis: Mosby. No part of this work is to be altered without prior written permission from the Publisher.

is cognitively intact may adapt to eating normal food when the tracheostomy tube is small and the cuff is not inflated.

The client who has had a subtotal, vertical, or supraglottic laryngectomy *must* be observed for aspiration. It is critical to teach the client to use alternate methods of swallowing without aspirating. The "supraglottic" method of swallowing is especially effective after a partial laryngectomy or base-of-tongue resection (Chart 32-4). To reinforce teaching and learning, place a chart in the client's room detailing the steps. A dynamic swallow study is performed to guide rehabilitation therapy for swallowing and to evaluate the client's ability to protect the airway.

CHART 32-4

CLIENT EDUCATION GUIDE
The Supraglottic Method of Swallowing

1. Place yourself in an upright, preferably out-of-bed, position.
2. Clear your throat.
3. Take a deep breath.
4. Place ½ to 1 teaspoon of food into your mouth.
5. Hold your breath or "bear down" (Valsalva maneuver).
6. Swallow twice.
7. Release your breath, and clear your throat.
8. Swallow twice again.
9. Breathe normally.

This method exaggerates the normal protective mechanisms of cessation of respiration during the swallow. The double swallow attempts to clear food that may be pooling in the pharynx, vallecula, and piriform sinuses. This method is used only after a dynamic radiographic swallow study has demonstrated that it is appropriate and safe for the client.

ANXIETY

NOC **PLANNING: EXPECTED OUTCOMES.** The client with head and neck cancer is expected to have decreased anxiety. Indicators include that the client often or consistently demonstrates the following behaviors:

- Verbalization of reduced anxiety
- Absence of distress, irritability, and facial tension
- Effective use of coping strategies

INTERVENTIONS. Conferences with the physician, clinical nurse specialist, dietitian, speech pathologist, physical therapist, psychologist, social worker, and general nursing staff may be beneficial. Explore the reason for anxiety (e.g., fear of the unknown, lack of preoperative teaching, fear of pain, fear of airway compromise, fear of hospitalization, loss of control). The client and family often benefit from further information. Before the client is scheduled for surgery (and while still at home), home care nurses or community-sponsored associations (e.g., ACS) may be able to decrease fears about the disease process and surgical interventions.

Give prescribed antianxiety drugs, such as diazepam (Valium, Meval✱), with caution because of the possibility of respiratory depression. The location of the tumor and the presence of any other lung disease may cause some degree of airway obstruction. For anxiety in these clients, the physician prescribes drug therapy judiciously and may choose lorazepam (Ativan, Novo-Lorazem✱) rather than a sedating agent.

DISTURBED BODY IMAGE

NOC **PLANNING: EXPECTED OUTCOMES.** The client with head and neck cancer is expected to accept body image changes. Indicators include that the client often or consistently demonstrates the following behaviors:

- Willingness to touch the affected body part
- Willingness to use strategies to enhance appearance
- Participation in self-care
- Interaction with visitors, staff, and family members

INTERVENTIONS. The client with head and neck cancer may have a permanent change in body image because of deformity, the presence of a stoma or artificial airway, speech changes, and a change in the method of eating.

The client may not be able to speak at all or have permanent hoarseness or speech deficits. Help the client set realistic goals, starting with involvement in self-care. Teach the client alternate communication methods so he or she can functionally communicate in the hospital and after discharge.

Teach the family to ease the client into a more normal social environment. Provide encouragement and positive reinforcement while demonstrating acceptance and caring behaviors. The family also may benefit from counseling sessions initiated while the client is still in the hospital.

After surgery the client may feel reserved and socially isolated because of the change in voice and facial appearance. Loose-fitting, high-collar shirts or sweaters (e.g., turtleneck), scarves, and jewelry can be worn to cover the laryngectomy stoma, tracheostomy tube, and physical changes related to surgery. Cosmetics may aid in covering any disfigurement. Most surgeons try to place the surgical incisions in the natural skin fold lines if doing so does not pose a risk for cancer recurrence.

Critical Thinking Challenge

The client, a 65-year-old man 7 days postoperative after a laryngectomy and radical neck dissection, is being discharged to home. After hearing the discharge order, he starts to cry and shake his head in a "no" gesture. His wife, who has been saying throughout the postoperative period that "everything will be all right," is amazed that he does not want to come home today, especially because she has planned a little get-together with their grown children, minister, and the neighbors to welcome him back.

1. Should you try to get this client's discharge orders changed?
2. What question(s) should you ask the wife? The client?
3. What might be causing the client's anxiety?
4. What teaching priorities are needed?

evolve For suggested answer guidelines, go to http://evolve.elsevier.com/Iggy/.

CHART 32-5

HOME CARE ASSESSMENT of Clients After Laryngectomy

Assess respiratory status.
- Observe rate and depth of respiration.
- Auscultate lungs.
- Check patency of airway.
- Examine the tracheostomy exudate for amount, color, and character.
- Examine nail beds and mucous membranes for evidence of cyanosis.
- Obtain a pulse oximetry reading.

Assess condition of wound.
- Remove dressings (noting condition of dressings).
- Cleanse the wound.
- Compare with previous notations of wound condition:
  - Presence, amount, and nature of exudate
  - Presence/absence of cellulitis
  - Presence/absence of odor

Assess client's psychosocial functioning.
- Ask the client about passing the time, visitors, and trips outside the house.
- Observe whether the client communicates responses directly or whether a family member speaks for the client.
- Observe client and family member interactions.
- Determine what method of communication the client has selected, and observe the client's skill with it.
- Is the client wearing pajamas, or is the client dressed?

Take the client's temperature.

Assess the client's understanding of illness and compliance with treatment.
- Manifestations to report to the health care provider
- Medication plan (correct timing and dose)
- Ambulation or positioning schedule
- Dressing changes/skin care
- Diet modifications (24-hour diet recall)
- Skill in tracheostomy or dressing care

Assess client's nutritional status.
- Change in muscle mass
- Lackluster nails/sparse hair
- Recent weight loss greater than 10% of usual weight
- Impaired oral intake
- Difficulty swallowing
- Generalized edema

Community-Based Care

If no complications occur, the client is usually ready to be discharged home or to an extended care facility within 2 weeks. At the time of discharge, he or she should be able to provide self-care, which may include tracheostomy or stoma care, nutrition, wound care, and methods of communication.

The client and family may feel more secure about discharge if they receive a referral to selected support groups or a community health agency familiar with the care of clients recovering from head and neck cancer. The health care team assesses the specific discharge needs and makes the appropriate referrals to home care agencies, including professionals such as nutritionists, nurses, physical therapists, speech pathologists, and social workers. Coordinate the scheduling for chemotherapy or radiation therapy with the client and family.

HOME CARE MANAGEMENT

Extensive home care preparation is needed after a laryngectomy for cancer. The convalescent period is long, and airway management is complicated. The client or family must be able to take an active role in care.

General cleanliness of the home is assessed. If the client has severe or long-standing respiratory problems, adjustments in the home to allow for one-floor living may be needed. Increased humidification is needed. A humidifier add-on to a forced-air furnace can be obtained. If the cost of this add-on is not manageable or if the home is heated by radiators, a room humidifier or vaporizer may be appropriate.

A home care nurse is involved with care after discharge and is an important resource for the client and family. The home care nurse assesses the client and home situation for problems in self-care, complications, adjustment, and adherence to the medical regimen. Chart 32-5 lists assessment areas for the client in the home following a laryngectomy. This nurse reinforces health care teaching, self-care teaching, and smoking-cessation regimens.

HEALTH TEACHING

Although education begins before surgery, most self-care is taught in the hospital. Teach the client and family how to care for the stoma or tracheostomy or laryngectomy tube, depending on the type of surgery performed. Review incision and airway care, including cleaning and inspecting for signs of infection. Chart 32-6 lists the highlights of self-care for the client who is discharged after laryngeal cancer surgery. Many of these actions also apply to any surgery for head and neck cancer.

CHART 32-6

CLIENT EDUCATION GUIDE

Home Laryngectomy Care

- Avoid swimming, and use care when showering or shaving.
- Lean slightly forward and cover the stoma when coughing or sneezing.
- Wear a stoma guard or loose clothing to cover the stoma.
- Clean the stoma with mild soap and water. Lubricate the stoma with a non–oil-based ointment as needed.
- Increase humidity by using saline in the stoma as instructed, a bedside humidifier, pans of water, and houseplants.
- Obtain and wear a MedicAlert bracelet and emergency care card for life-threatening situations.

STOMA CARE. Instruct the client to use a shower shield over the tracheostomy tube or laryngectomy stoma when bathing to prevent water from entering the airway. Suggest that the client wear a protective cover or stoma guard to protect the stoma during the day. For clients with permanent stomas following laryngectomy or for those with permanent tracheostomies, covering the permanent opening has a double benefit: (1) filtering the air entering the stoma while keeping humidity in the airway and (2) enhancing aesthetic appearance. Attractive coverings are available in the form of cotton scarves, crocheted bibs, and jewelry. Using colored seam binding for tracheostomy ties after the stoma has matured may enhance overall body image. Shirt or dress color can be matched or coordinated with seam bindings of various colors.

Instruct the client how to increase humidity in the home. If prescribed, teach the client to instill normal saline into the artificial airway 10 to 15 times a day.

COMMUNICATION. The client continues the selected method of alternate communication that began in the hospital. Instruct him or her to wear a medical alert (MedicAlert) bracelet and carry a special identification card (Figure 32-12). For clients who have a laryngectomy, this card is available from the local chapters of the International Association of Laryngectomees. The card instructs the reader about providing an emergency airway or resuscitating someone who has a stoma.

SMOKING CESSATION. A difficult but important issue after head and neck cancer surgery is smoking cessation. Smoking is a major risk factor for head and neck cancer. Stress that smoking cessation can reduce the risk for developing other cancers and can increase the rate of healing from surgery.

Smoking cessation is not an easy task, and most clients require continuing support and reinforcement to sustain this action. Chemical and psychological assistance are available for smoking cessation (see Chart 32-3).

PSYCHOSOCIAL PREPARATION

The many changes resulting from a laryngectomy influence physical, social, and emotional functioning. Many clients perceive changes in their quality of life. Begin preparing the client and family for these changes by scheduling a visit from a person who has adjusted to these changes.

The client who is discharged to home with a permanent stoma, tracheostomy tube, nasogastric (NG) tube, and wounds has an altered body image. Stress the importance of returning to as normal a lifestyle as possible. Most clients can resume many of their usual activities within 4 to 6 weeks after surgery. A longer time is required after a combination of radiation therapy and surgery. The client may be frustrated at times while trying to adjust to changes in smell, taste, and communication.

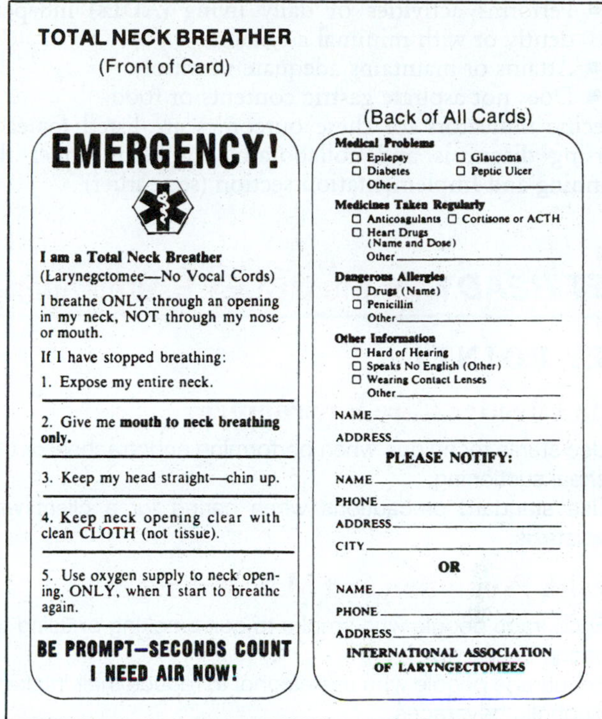
TOTAL NECK BREATHER

(Front of Card)

EMERGENCY!

I am a Total Neck Breather
(Larynegctomee—No Vocal Cords)

I breathe ONLY through an opening in my neck, NOT through my nose or mouth.

If I have stopped breathing:

1. Expose my entire neck.
2. Give me **mouth to neck breathing only.**
3. Keep my head straight—chin up.
4. Keep neck opening clear with clean CLOTH (not tissue).
5. Use oxygen supply to neck opening, ONLY, when I start to breathe again.

BE PROMPT—SECONDS COUNT
I NEED AIR NOW!

(Back of All Cards)

Medical Problems
☐ Epilepsy ☐ Glaucoma
☐ Diabetes ☐ Peptic Ulcer
Other_____

Medicines Taken Regularly
☐ Anticoagulants ☐ Cortisone or ACTH
☐ Heart Drugs (Name and Dose)
Other_____

Dangerous Allergies
☐ Drugs (Name)
☐ Penicillin
Other_____

Other Information
☐ Hard of Hearing
☐ Speaks No English (Other)
☐ Wearing Contact Lenses
Other_____

NAME_____
ADDRESS_____

PLEASE NOTIFY:

NAME_____
PHONE_____
ADDRESS_____
CITY_____

OR

NAME_____
PHONE_____
ADDRESS_____

INTERNATIONAL ASSOCIATION OF LARYNGECTOMEES

Figure 32-12 ■ Emergency wallet card for identification of laryngectomy.

The client with a total laryngectomy cannot produce sounds during laughing and crying, and mucous secretions may appear unexpectedly when these emotions arise or when coughing or sneezing occur. The mucus can be embarrassing, and the client needs to be prepared to cover the stoma with a handkerchief or gauze. The client who has undergone composite resections has difficulty with speech *and* swallowing. He or she may need to deal with tracheostomy and feeding tubes in public places.

HEALTH CARE RESOURCES

Inform the client and family of community organizations (e.g., ACS) and local laryngectomee clubs, which can offer support, information, and friendships. When the client has problems paying for health care services, equipment, and prescriptions, a visiting nurse agency may be helpful in directing him or her to available resources.

In many areas the local unit of the ACS or Canadian Cancer Society can help provide dressing materials and nutritional supplements to clients in need. This organization may also provide transportation to and from follow-up visits or radiation therapy.

Evaluation: Outcomes

Evaluate the care of the client with head and neck carcinomas on the basis of the identified nursing diagnoses and collaborative problems. The expected outcomes are that the client:

- Maintains a patent airway
- Performs self-care of the artificial airway and wound

- Performs activities of daily living (ADLs) independently or with minimal assistance
- Attains or maintains adequate nutrition
- Does not aspirate gastric contents or food

Specific indicators for these outcomes are listed for each nursing diagnosis and collaborative problem under the Planning and Implementation section (see earlier).

GET READY for the NCLEX Examination!

KEY POINTS

Safe Effective Care Environment

- Use sterile technique when performing endotracheal or tracheal suctioning.
- Use standard precautions when caring for a client with epistaxis.

Health Promotion and Maintenance

- Encourage people who smoke to quit smoking or using tobacco in any way.
- Encourage people who use alcohol to reduce their intake of alcoholic beverages.
- Teach clients how to blow the nose without closing off one nostril.
- Use aspiration precautions for any client with an altered level of consciousness or who has an endotracheal tube (see Chart 31-6).
- Teach the client and family how to perform tracheostomy care (see Chart 31-4)
- Teach clients who have had radiation therapy to the neck or oral cavity to have dental examinations at least every 6 months.

Psychosocial Integrity

- Allow the client and family members the opportunity to express fear or anxiety regarding a cancer diagnosis or a change in breathing status.
- Teach family members ways to communicate with a client who is unable to speak after surgery for head and neck cancer.
- Encourage clients with permanent tracheostomies to become involved in self-care.
- Encourage the client who has had head and neck surgery for cancer to look at the wound and touch the affected area.
- Allow the client and family to grieve about the loss of function and change in body image.
- Allow time to communicate with the client who has voice loss as a result of disease or treatment.
- Refer clients and families to the ACS after surgery for head and neck cancer.

Physiological Integrity

- Assess airway patency for any client who experiences facial or nasal trauma.
- Notify the emergency team when a client experiences a posterior nasal bleed.
- Check the airway and packing at least every hour for a client who has posterior nasal packing placed after nasal surgery or posterior nasal epistaxis.
- Instruct clients who have had mandibular immobilization or fixation after a mandibular fracture to keep wire cutters with them at all times.
- Apply oxygen to any client who develops stridor.
- Ensure that oxygen therapy delivered to the client is humidified (and warmed, when possible).
- Use a manual resuscitation bag to ventilate the client if the tracheostomy tube has dislodged or been decannulated.
- Assess the new tracheostomy stoma site at least once per shift for purulent drainage, redness, pain, and swelling, as indicators of infection.
- Keep the tracheal cuff pressure between 14 and 20 mm Hg to prevent tissue injury.
- Teach clients receiving radiation therapy how to care for the skin in the radiation path (see Chart 28-2).

ADDITIONAL STUDY RESOURCES

Go to your Student CD-ROM for Review Questions for the NCLEX Examination.

evolve Go to http://evolve.elsevier.com/Iggy/ for Integrated Management of Care Questions for the NCLEX Examination.

SELECTED BIBLIOGRAPHY

Abernathy, W., et al. (2000). Nonmetallic fixation in elective maxillofacial surgery. *AORN Journal, 71*(1), 193-198.

American Cancer Society. (2005). *Cancer facts and figures, 2005.* 01-300M-No.5008.05. Atlanta: Author.

Astle, A., & Caufield, E. (2003). Bedside tracheostomy: A step by step guide. *RN, 66*(10), 41-45.

Bhattacharyya, N. (2002). Cancer of the nasal cavity. *Archives of Otolaryngology Head and Neck Surgery, 128,* 1079-1083.

Bruce, S. (2004). Radiation-induced xerostomia: How dry is your patient? *Clinical Journal of Oncology Nursing 8*(1), 61-67.

Cady. J. (2002). Laryngectomy: Beyond loss of voice–caring for the patient as a whole. *Clinical Journal of Oncology Nursing, 6*(6), 347-353.

Carr, M., et al. (2000). Communication after laryngectomy: An assessment of quality of life. *Otolaryngology C Head and Neck Surgery, 122*(1), 39-43.

Chasens, E., & Umlauf, M. (2003). Nocturia: A problem that disrupts sleep and predicts obstructive sleep apnea. *Geriatric Nursing, 24*(2), 76-81, 105.

Dochterman, J., & Bulechek, G. (Eds.). (2004). *Nursing interventions classification (NIC)* (4th ed.). St. Louis: Mosby.

Ebersole, P., Hess, P., & Luggen, A. (2004). *Toward healthy aging: Human needs and nursing response* (6th ed.). St. Louis: Mosby.

Edwards, S., & Metheny, N. (2000). Measurement of gastric residual volume: State of the science. *MEDSURG Nursing, 9*(3), 125-128.

Facts and Comparisons. (2004). *Drug facts and comparisons* (58th ed.). St. Louis: Author.

Happ, M.B., Roesch, T., & Kagan, S. (2004). Communication needs, methods, and perceived voice quality following head and neck surgery: A literature review. *Cancer Nursing, 27*(1), 1-9.

Harrahill, M. (2002). Tracheobronchial injuries. *Journal of Emergency Nursing, 28*(3), 265-266.

Jagim, M. (2003). Airway management: Rapid-sequence intubation in trauma patients. *American Journal of Nursing, 103*(10), 32-35.

Koliha, C. (2003). Obstructive sleep apnea in head and neck cancer patients post-treatment...Something to consider? *ORL Head and Neck Nursing, 21*(1), 10-14.

Lennie, T., Christman, S., & Jadack, R. (2001). Educational needs and altered eating habits following a total laryngectomy. *Oncology Nursing Forum, 28*(4), 667-674.

Levin, W., & Parraga, M. (2002). The current management of epistaxis. *The Clinical Advisor. November/December 2002,* 33-40.

Marchiondo, K. (2000). Pickwickian syndrome: The challenge of severe sleep apnea. *MEDSURG Nursing, 9*(4), 183-188.

McCance, K., & Huether, S. (2002). *Pathophysiology: The biologic basis for disease in adults and children* (4th ed.). St. Louis: Mosby.

Merritt, S., & Berger, B. (2004). Obstructive sleep apnea-hypopnea syndrome. *American Journal of Nursing, 104*(7), 49-52.

Metheny, N., & Titler, M. (2001). Assessing placement of feeding tubes. *American Journal of Nursing, 101*(5), 36-45.

Moorhead, S., Johnson, M., & Maas, M. (Eds.). (2004). *Nursing outcomes classification (NOC)* (3rd ed.). St. Louis: Mosby.

Pagana, K., & Pagana, T. (2002). *Mosby's manual of diagnostic and laboratory tests* (2nd ed.). St. Louis: Mosby.

Perkins, L., & Shortall, S. (2000). Ventilation without intubation. *RN, 63*(1), 34-38.

Prettyman, A. (2001). Obstructive sleep apnea: Diagnosis and management. *The American Journal for Nurse Practitioners, 5*(8), 27-32.

Pruitt, W., & Jacobs, M. (2003). Basics of oxygen therapy. *Nursing 2003, 33*(10), 43-45.

Pullen, R. (2003). Caring for a patient on pulse oximetry. *Nursing 2003, 33*(9), 30.

Pullen, R. (2004). Measuring gastric residual volume. *Nursing 2004, 34*(4), 18.

Schoem, S. (2000). Oral appliances for the treatment of snoring and obstructive sleep apnea. *Otolaryngology C Head and Neck Surgery, 122*(2), 259-262.

Shellenbarger, T. (2000). Nosebleeds: Not just kids = stuff. *RN, 63*(2), 50-54, 56.

Stansberry, T. (2001). Narcolepsy: Unveiling a mystery. *American Journal of Nursing, 101*(8), 50-53.

St. John, R. (2004). Airway management. *Critical Care Nursing,* 24(2), 93-96.

Tate, J., & Tasota, F. (2002). More than a snore: Recognizing the danger of sleep apnea. *Nursing2002, 32*(8), 46-49.

Yantis, M. (2002). Obstructive sleep apnea syndrome. *American Journal of Nursing, 102*(6), 83-85.

CHAPTER

33 Interventions for Clients with Noninfectious Problems of the Lower Respiratory Tract

M. LINDA WORKMAN

LEARNING OUTCOMES

After studying this chapter, you should be able to:

1. Explain the differences in pathophysiology between asthma from bronchospasm, and asthma from inflammation.
2. Prioritize educational needs for the client at step III of stepped therapy for asthma.
3. Interpret peak expiratory rate flow (PERF) readings for the need for intervention.
4. Discuss the complications of chronic oral steroid therapy for treatment of chronic airflow limitation (CAL).
5. Compare the pathophysiology and clinical manifestations of asthma, bronchitis, and emphysema.
6. Identify risk factors for chronic obstructive pulmonary disease (COPD).
7. Prioritize educational needs for the client with COPD who is receiving oxygen therapy at home.
8. Describe the mechanisms of action, side effects, and nursing implications for pharmacologic management of COPD.
9. Describe interventions for energy conservation for the client with COPD.
10. Prioritize nursing care needs for the client immediately following lung volume reduction surgery.
11. Explain the nutritional needs for the client with COPD.
12. Use laboratory data and clinical manifestations to determine the effectiveness of therapy for impaired gas exchange in a client with obstructive or restrictive breathing problems.
13. Identify the risk factors for lung cancer.
14. Compare the side effects of radiation treatment for lung cancer with those of chemotherapy for lung cancer.
15. Explain how to troubleshoot the chest tube drainage system in a client 1 day after a thoracotomy.
16. Develop a community-based teaching plan for a client getting ready to go home after a pneumonectomy.

Go to your Student CD-ROM for Review Questions for the NCLEX Examination keyed to these Learning Outcomes.

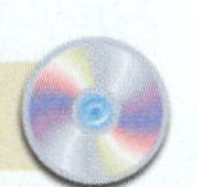

Lower airway problems directly affect gas exchange and have serious consequences. Many of these problems are chronic and progressive, requiring major changes in a person's lifestyle. The older client with an airway problem may need special help even before the disorder becomes severe. Chart 33-1 lists nursing issues for the older client with a respiratory problem.

CHRONIC AIRFLOW LIMITATION

Chronic airflow limitation (CAL) is group of chronic lung diseases that includes asthma, chronic bronchitis, and pulmonary emphysema. Emphysema and chronic bronchitis, termed **chronic obstructive pulmonary disease (COPD),** are characterized by bronchospasm and dyspnea (Figure 33-1).

CHART 33-1

NURSING FOCUS on the OLDER ADULT

Respiratory Disorders

- Provide rest periods between such activities as bathing, meals, and ambulation.
- Place the client in an upright position for meals to prevent aspiration.
- Encourage nutritional fluid intake after the meal to promote increased calorie intake.
- Schedule medications around routine activities to increase medication adherence.
- Arrange chairs in strategic locations to allow the client with dyspnea to walk and rest as needed.
- Encourage prompt access to a health care facility for any manifestation of infection.
- Ensure that the client has received the pneumococcal vaccine.
- Encourage the client to have an annual flu vaccination.

The tissue damage is not reversible and increases in severity, eventually leading to respiratory failure. Asthma, unlike COPD, is an intermittent disease with *reversible* airflow obstruction and wheezing.

More than 40 million Americans suffer from some form of CAL, and 1 million people between the ages of 40 and 65 years have moderate to severe disability from CAL. Although some problems are not reversible, good management strategies can help maintain optimal functioning and improve overall health (see the Meeting Healthy People 2010 Objectives box at right).

Meeting HEALTHY PEOPLE 2010 Objectives

RESPIRATORY DISEASES

Objective 24.2: Reduce the overall asthma morbidity, as measured by a reduction in asthma hospitalization rates to 10 per 10,000 people.

- Teach the client with asthma to develop an asthma action plan in conjunction with their primary health care provider.
- Assist clients with asthma who smoke to reduce or quit smoking.
- Instruct the client with asthma in the correct technique for use of an inhaler.
- Educate clients with asthma that taking asthma medications as prescribed can reduce asthma exacerbations and morbidity.
- Teach the client with asthma to correctly use a peak flow meter.
- Assist the client with asthma to identify personal triggers for asthma attacks.
- Instruct the client with asthma how to adjust medications based on peak flow readings and expected exposures to environments or activities likely to trigger an asthma attack.
- Instruct clients with asthma to obtain annual vaccinations against influenza
- Remind clients to avoid secondhand smoke.

Objective 24.14: Reduce to no more than 3% the proportion of adults 45+ with chronic obstructive pulmonary disease.

- Educate clients who smoke cigarettes to reduce or quit smoking.
- Teach clients who have occupations or hobbies that cause exposure to inhalation irritants to use respiratory protection.
- Encourage clients with a family history of emphysema to be tested for alpha$_1$ antitrypsin deficiency.
- Teach clients the importance of seeing a health care provider promptly for any new or persistent respiratory symptoms.

Asthma

PATHOPHYSIOLOGY

Bronchial asthma is an intermittent and reversible airflow obstruction affecting only the airways, not the alveoli (see Figure 33-1). Airway obstruction can occur in two ways: (1) inflammation, and (2) airway hyperresponsiveness (sometimes called "twitchy airways"). Inflammation obstructs the **lumen** (i.e., the inside) of airways. Airway hyperresponsiveness obstructs airways by constricting bronchial smooth muscle causing a narrowing of the airway from the outside. Airway inflammation can trigger bronchiolar hyperresponsiveness, and many people with asthma have both problems at the same time. Severe airway obstruction can be fatal. More than 5000 deaths from acute asthma occur in the United States each year (Centers for Disease Control and Prevention, 2003).

Etiology and Genetic Risk

Asthma may be classified into different types based on the events known to trigger the attacks; however, the pathophysiology is similar for all types of asthma. Inflammation of the mucous membranes lining the airways is a key event in triggering an asthma attack. Inflammation occurs in response to the presence of specific allergens; nonallergenic general irritants such as cold air, dry air, or fine airborne particles; microorganisms; and aspirin. Airway hyperresponsiveness can occur with exercise, an upper respiratory illness, and for unknown reasons. Asthma from inflammation or hyperresponsive airways may have a genetic component, although a specific gene or mutation has not yet been identified.

When asthma is well controlled, the airway changes are temporary and reversible. With poor control, chronic inflammation can lead to damage and hyperplasia of the bronchial epithelial cells and of the bronchial smooth muscle. When asthma attacks are frequent, even exposure to low levels of the triggering agent or event may stimulate an attack.

INFLAMMATION

For some people, allergens bind to specific antibody molecules (especially immunoglobulin E [IgE]). These molecules are attached to tissue cells called mast cells and white blood cells called basophils. These cells are filled with granules containing chemicals that can start local inflammatory responses (see Chapters 23 and 26). Some of these chemicals, such as histamine, start an immediate inflammatory response. Others, such as leukotriene, interleukin-4, and eotaxin, are slower and cause later, prolonged inflammatory responses. These chemicals also attract more white blood cells (eosinophils, macrophages, and basophils) to the area, which then release even more inflammatory-inducing chemicals **(mediators).**

When allergens bind to the IgE molecules on mast cells, chemicals are released that start inflammatory responses in the airway mucous membranes (see Figure 26-2). Responses include blood vessel dilation and capillary leak, leading to tissue swelling with increased secretions and mucus production. This is the most common cause of asthma and is termed **atopic asthma** (McCance & Huether, 2002).

Inflammation can also occur through general irritation rather than allergic responses. Although some of the same

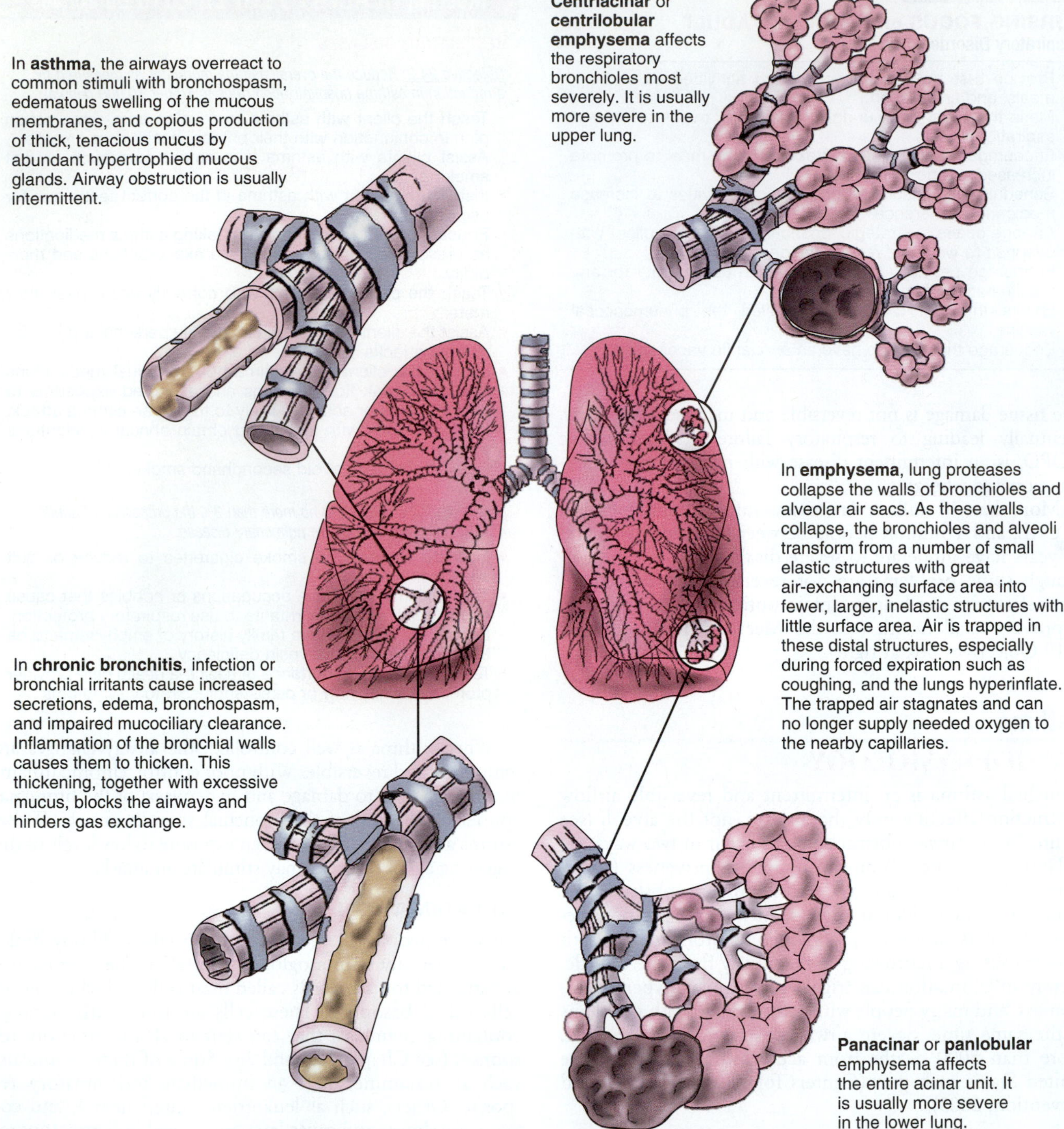

Figure 33-1 ■ The pathophysiology of chronic airflow limitation (CAL).

cells and chemicals cause this response, allergy therapy is not useful for general irritation-induced asthma.

BRONCHOSPASM

Hyperresponsive airways cause **bronchospasms,** narrowing of the bronchial tubes through constriction of the smooth muscle around and within the bronchial walls. In some people, small amounts of pollutants or respiratory viruses stimulate nerve fibers, causing constriction of bronchial smooth muscle. If these substances also stimulate an inflammatory response at the same time, the chemicals released during inflammation bind to smooth muscle receptors and cause constriction. Severe bronchospasm alone, especially in smaller bronchioles, can profoundly limit airflow to the alveoli.

ASPIRIN AND OTHER NONSTEROIDAL ANTI-INFLAMMATORY DRUGS

Some clients have asthma after taking aspirin and other nonsteroidal anti-inflammatory drugs (NSAIDs). This response is not a true allergy. It results from increased production of

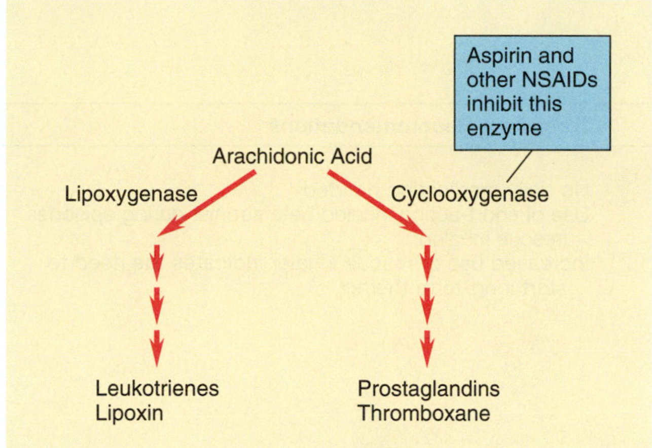

Figure 33-2 ■ Production pathways of inflammatory biochemicals.

leukotriene when other inflammatory pathways are suppressed. One chemical, arachidonic acid, can be converted into different substances when it is acted on by different enzymes. Aspirin and other NSAIDs inhibit the cyclooxygenase enzyme pathway. When this pathway is blocked, more arachidonic acid is available to be acted on by another enzyme, lipoxygenase, and changed to leukotriene (Figure 33-2).

Incidence/Prevalence

Asthma can occur at any age. About half of adults with asthma also had the disease in childhood. Asthma is more common in urban settings than in rural settings.

> **CONSIDERATIONS FOR OLDER ADULTS**
>
> Asthma occurs as a new disorder in about 3% of people older than 55 years of age. Another 3% of people older than 60 years of age have asthma as a continuing chronic disorder. Lung and airway changes as a part of aging make any breathing problem more serious in the older adult. One problem related to aging is a change in the sensitivity of beta-adrenergic receptors. When stimulated, these receptors relax smooth muscle and cause bronchodilation. As these receptors become less sensitive, they no longer respond as quickly or as strongly to agonists (epinephrine, dopamine) and beta-adrenergic drugs.

COLLABORATIVE MANAGEMENT

Assessment

Asthma is diagnosed and classified on the basis of the frequency and severity of the manifestations, as well as on the client's response to asthma drugs. These classes are the basis for current asthma therapy (Chart 33-2).

HISTORY

The client with asthma usually has a pattern of episodes of shortness of breath **(dyspnea),** chest tightness, coughing, wheezing, and increased mucus production. Ask whether the manifestations occur continuously, seasonally, in association with specific activities or exposures, or more frequently at night. Some clients notice these manifestations lasting 4 to 8 weeks after a chest cold or other upper respiratory tract infection. The client with atopic or allergic asthma may also have other allergic symptoms such as rhinitis, skin rash, or pruritus. Ask whether any other family members have asthma or respiratory problems. Ask about the client's current or previous smoking habits. Wheezing in nonsmokers is an important symptom in the diagnosis of asthma.

PHYSICAL ASSESSMENT/CLINICAL MANIFESTATIONS

The client with mild to moderate asthma may have no manifestations between asthma attacks. During an acute episode the most common manifestations are an audible wheeze and increased respiratory rate. The wheeze is louder on exhalation. When inflammation occurs with asthma, coughing may increase.

The client may use accessory muscles to help breathe during an attack. Observe for muscle retraction at the sternum, the suprasternal notch, and between the ribs. The client with long-standing, severe asthma may have a "barrel chest," caused by air trapping (Figure 33-3). The anteroposterior (AP) diameter (diameter between the front and the back of the chest) increases with air trapping, giving the chest a rounded rather than an oval shape. The normal chest is nearly twice as wide as it is thick. In the client with severe, chronic asthma, the AP diameter may equal or exceed the lateral diameter. Compare the AP diameter of the chest with the lateral diameter. Air trapping also increases the space between the ribs.

Along with an audible wheeze, the breathing cycle is longer and requires more effort. The client may be unable to complete a sentence of more than five words between breaths. Examine the oral mucosa and nail beds for cyanosis. Pulse oximetry shows poor oxygen saturation related to the degree of dyspnea. Other indicators of hypoxemia include changes in the level of consciousness and tachycardia.

LABORATORY ASSESSMENT

Laboratory tests can help determine the type of asthma and the degree of breathing impairment. Arterial blood gas (ABG) levels show how well the client is obtaining oxygen (see Chapter 19 for discussion of ABGs). The arterial oxygen level (PaO_2) may decrease during an asthma attack. Early in the attack, the arterial carbon dioxide level ($PaCO_2$) may be decreased as the client increases respiratory effort. Later in an asthma episode, $PaCO_2$ rises, indicating carbon dioxide retention and poor gas exchange. Atopic asthma often occurs with an elevated serum eosinophil count and immunoglobulin E (IgE) levels. The sputum may contain eosinophils and mucous plugs with shed epithelial cells (Curschmann spirals).

PULMONARY FUNCTION TESTS

The most accurate tests for asthma are the pulmonary function tests (PFTs) measured using spirometry. Baseline PFTs are obtained for all clients diagnosed with asthma. The most important PFTs for a client with asthma are the **forced vital capacity (FVC)** (volume of air exhaled from full inhalation to full exhalation), **forced expiratory volume in the first second (FEV_1)** (volume of air blown out as hard and fast as possible during the first second of the most forceful exhalation after the greatest full inhalation), and **peak expiratory**

CHART 33-2

KEY FEATURES of
Asthma: The Step System

Clinical Manifestations	Treatment Recommendations
I. Mild Intermittent Symptoms or episodes occur twice per week or less. Client is symptom free between episodes/exacerbations. Episodes/exacerbations are short, lasting only a few hours. Symptoms are present at night no more frequently than twice per month. PFTs are normal between episodes. During episodes/exacerbations, FEV_1 or PEF is at least 80% of normal. PEF variability is less than 20%.	No daily medication needed Use of short-acting inhaled beta agonist during episodes (rescue inhaler) Increased use of rescue inhaler indicates the need to start long-term therapy
II. Mild Persistent Symptoms or episodes occur more than twice per week but not daily. Symptoms are present at night more than twice per month. During episodes/exacerbations, FEV_1 or PEF is at least 80% of normal. PEF variability is 20% to 30%. Activity is affected during episodes/exacerbations.	Use of a daily anti-inflammatory: Inhaled corticosteroid (CSC) Inhaled cromolyn Leukotriene antagonist Use of a rescue inhaler for relief during episodes
III. Moderate Persistent Symptoms occur daily. Symptoms or episodes occur more than twice per week and may persist for days. Client uses short-acting inhaled bronchodilator daily. Symptoms are present at night at least once per week. PEF variability is greater than 30%.	Daily use of inhaled CSC (low to moderate dose) Use of long-acting inhaled beta agonist (bronchodilator) Use of a rescue inhaler for relief during episodes (daily use means the client should be evaluated for progression to step IV)
IV. Severe Persistent Symptoms are continuously present. Episodes/exacerbations are frequent. During episodes/exacerbations, FEV_1 or PEF is less than 60% of normal. Physical activity is limited. Symptoms are frequently present at night. PEF variability is greater than 30%.	Daily use of inhaled CSC (high dose) Daily use of long-acting inhaled bronchodilator Frequent courses of systemic corticosteroids May include systemic methylxanthines

Modified from National Institutes of Health. (1997). *Guidelines for the diagnosis and management of asthma.* Expert panel report 2(97 4051). Bethesda, MD: U.S. Department of Health and Human Services.

PFTs, Pulmonary function tests; *PEF*, peak expiratory flow; *FEV_1*, volume of air blown out as hard and fast as possible during the first second of the most forceful exhalation after the greatest full inhalation.

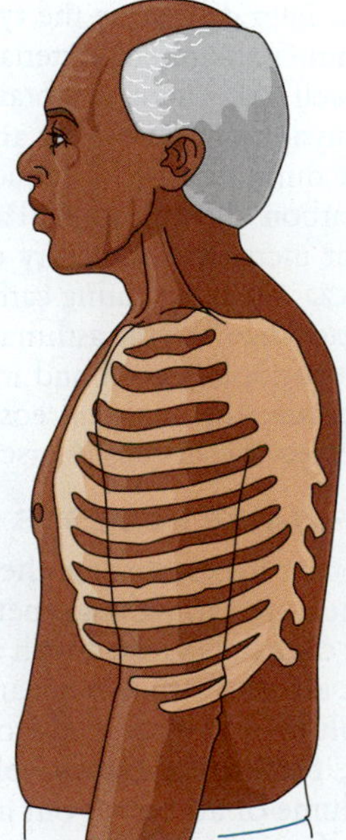

Figure 33-3 ■ Typical barrel chest in a client with chronic airflow limitation (CAL).

rate flow (PERF) (fastest airflow rate reached at any time during exhalation). A decrease in either the FEV_1 or the PERF of 15% to 20% below the expected value for age, gender, and size is common for the client with asthma. An increase of 12% in these values after treatment with bronchodilators is diagnostic for asthma. Airway responsiveness is tested by measuring the PERF and FEV_1 before and after the client inhales the drug methacholine, which induces bronchospasm in susceptible people.

OTHER DIAGNOSTIC ASSESSMENTS

Chest x-rays may be used to rule out other causes of dyspnea or to track changes in chest structure over time. For the client taking theophylline, blood drug levels are used to determine whether a therapeutic level is being maintained.

Interventions

The goals of asthma therapy are to improve airflow, relieve symptoms, and prevent episodes. Adult asthma is best managed when the client is an active partner in the management plan. The successful management plan includes client education, drug therapy, and lifestyle management, including exercise. Chart 33-3 lists NIC intervention activities for the client with asthma.

CHART 33-3

NIC **INTERVENTION ACTIVITIES for**
The Client with Asthma

Asthma Management: *Identification, treatment, and prevention of reactions to inflammation/constriction in the airway passages.*

- Determine baseline respiratory status to use as a comparison point.
- Document baseline measurements in clinical record.
- Compare current status with previous status to detect changes in respiratory status.
- Monitor peak expiratory flow rate (PERF), as appropriate.
- Educate client about the use of PERF meter at home.
- Determine client/family understanding of disease and management.
- Instruct client/family on antiinflammatory and bronchodilator medications and their appropriate use.
- Teach proper techniques for using medication and equipment (e.g., inhaler, nebulizer, peak flow meter).
- Determine compliance with prescribed treatments.
- Assist in the recognition of signs/symptoms of impending asthmatic reaction and implementation of appropriate response measures.
- Monitor rate, rhythm, depth, and effort of respiration.
- Observe chest movement, including symmetry, use of accessory muscles, and supraclavicular and intercostal muscle retractions.
- Administer medications as appropriate and/or per policy and procedural guidelines.
- Auscultate lung sounds after treatment to determine results.
- Use a calm reassuring approach during asthma attack.

NIC intervention activities selected from Dochterman, J.M., & Bulechek, G.M. (Eds.). (2004). *Nursing interventions classification (NIC)* (4th ed.). St. Louis: Mosby. No part of this work is to be altered without prior written permission from the Publisher.

CHART 33-4

CLIENT EDUCATION GUIDE
Asthma

- Avoid potential environmental asthma triggers, such as smoke, fireplaces, dust, mold, and weather changes (especially warm to cold or sudden barometric changes).
- Avoid medications that could trigger asthma (e.g., aspirin, nonsteroidal anti-inflammatory drugs [NSAIDs], and beta blockers).
- Avoid food that has been prepared with monosodium glutamate (MSG) or metabisulfite.
- If you experience symptoms of exercise-induced asthma, use your bronchodilator inhaler 30 minutes before exercise to prevent or reduce bronchospasm.
- Be sure you know the proper technique and correct sequence when you use metered dose inhalers.
- Be sure to get adequate rest and sleep.
- Reduce stress and anxiety; learn relaxation techniques; adopt coping mechanisms that have worked for you in the past.
- Wash all bedding with hot water to destroy dust mites.
- Monitor your peak expiratory flow rates as you were instructed.
- Seek immediate emergency care if you experience any of the following:
  - Gray or blue fingertips or lips
  - Difficulty breathing, walking, or talking
  - Retractions of the neck, chest, or ribs
  - Nasal flaring
  - Failure of medications to control worsening symptoms
  - Peak expiratory rate flow declining steadily after treatment, or a flow rate 50% below your usual flow rate

Client Education. Asthma is often an intermittent disease. With guided self-care, clients can co-manage this disease, increasing symptom-free periods and decreasing the number and severity of attacks. Such management decreases the number of hospital admissions and increases participation in client-chosen pleasure, work, and family activities. Overall improved management through guided self-care has been shown to decrease health care costs. Self-care requires extensive education for the client to be able to self-treat (including adjusting the frequency and dosage of prescribed drugs) and determine when to consult the health care provider. Teach the client to assess symptom severity at least twice daily with a peak flow meter and adjust drugs to manage inflammation and bronchospasms to prevent or relieve symptoms. Education involves a specified drug therapy plan that is tailored to meet the personal pattern of asthma for the client. The client keeps a symptom and intervention diary to learn his or her triggers of asthma symptoms, early cues for impending attacks, and personal response to drugs. Proper use of an asthma action plan is helpful for any severity of asthma. Chart 33-4 lists areas to emphasize when teaching the client with asthma.

Drug Therapy. Pharmacologic management of adult clients with asthma is based on the step category for severity and treatment (see Chart 33-2). Some may need drug therapy only during an asthma episode. For others, daily drugs are needed to keep asthma episodic rather than a more frequent problem. This therapy involves the use of bronchodilators, steroidal and nonsteroidal agents to reduce inflammation, mast cell stabilizers, monoclonal antibodies, and drugs that inhibit the release or action of leukotrienes. Thus some drugs reduce the response, and other drugs actually prevent the response. Some drugs combine two agents from different classes for better response. Chart 33-5 lists common agents used for preventive and symptomatic therapy of asthma.

Bronchodilators. Bronchodilators increase bronchiolar smooth muscle relaxation. They have no effect on inflammatory processes. Thus when a client with asthma has airflow obstruction by both bronchospasm and inflammation, at least two types of drug therapy are needed. Bronchodilators work by stimulating the beta$_2$-adrenergic receptors on bronchial smooth muscle in the same way that the sympathetic nervous system transmitters, epinephrine and norepinephrine, do. These drugs include beta$_2$ agonists, cholinergic antagonists, and methylxanthines

Beta$_2$ Agonists. Beta$_2$ agonists bind to the beta$_2$-adrenergic receptors and cause an increase in the intracellular level of a substance called cyclic adenosine monophosphate (cAMP). This substance triggers smooth muscle relaxation.

SHORT-ACTING BETA$_2$ AGONISTS. Short-acting beta$_2$ agents provide rapid but short-term relief. These inhaled drugs are most useful when an attack begins or as premedication when the client is about to begin an activity that is likely to induce an asthma attack. Such agents include albuterol (Proventil, Ventolin), bitolterol (Tornalate), and pirbuterol (Maxair). When inhaled from either a metered dose inhaler (MDI) or a dry powder inhaler (DPI), the drug is delivered directly to the site of action and systemic effects are minimal (unless the agent is overused or abused). Teach the client the correct technique to use with an inhaled drug to

CHART 33-5

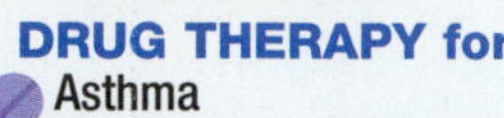

DRUG THERAPY for Asthma

Drug	Usual Dosage	Nursing Interventions	Rationales
Bronchodilators			
Short-Acting Beta$_2$ Agonists Albuterol (Proventil, Ventolin)	1-2 inhalations q4-6h (90 mcg/inhaled dose)	Teach client to monitor heart rate.	Excessive use causes systemic symptoms, especially tachycardia.
		Increase water/fluid intake.	Chronic use increases mouth and throat dryness.
		Instruct client to use bronchodilator at least 5 min before other inhaled drugs.	Bronchodilation allows better penetration of other inhaled drugs.
		Teach client the correct technique for using the inhaler and obtain a return demonstration.	Correct technique is essential in getting the medication to the site of action. If the client does not inhale during medication delivery, drug exits the nose or is swallowed.
Bitolterol (Tornalate)	2 inhalations q8h (370 mcg/inhalation)	Same as for albuterol.	Same as for albuterol.
Pirbuterol (Maxair)	1-2 inhalations q4-6h (200 mcg/inhalation)	Same as for albuterol.	Same as for albuterol.
Long-Acting Beta$_2$ Agonists Salmeterol (Serevent)	2 inhalations q12h (≈25 mcg/inhalation with an aerosol inhaler) (50 mcg/inhalation with a dry powder inhaler)	Do not use to relieve acute symptoms.	Drug has slow onset of action.
		Shake inhaler well before using.	Drug separates easily.
		Teach client not to exhale into device.	Exhaling into device moistens the drug and causes clumping.
Formoterol fumarate (Foradil Aerolizer)	1 inhalation q12h (12 mcg/inhalation with dry powder inhaler)	Same as for salmeterol.	Same as for salmeterol.
Methylxanthines			
Theophylline (Theo-Dur, Uniphyl, Theolair, Bronkodyl)	10-12 mg/kg/day PO (loading dose)	Monitor drug levels.	Drug has narrow therapeutic range and many toxicities.
	Maintenance dose is usually 200-800 mg daily	Space doses equally throughout the 24-hr day.	Maintains more even blood drug levels.
		Observe client for nausea, vomiting, diarrhea, tachycardia, dysrhythmias, restlessness.	These are symptoms of toxicity.
		Teach client to avoid caffeine intake while on this drug.	Caffeine potentiates side effects.
		Encourage client to take as prescribed daily.	Efficacy is related to continued correct use.
		Teach client to take oral dose with meals.	Food reduces GI irritation.
		Administer IV doses using a pump or controller.	A pump or controller prevents accidental overdose.
Aminophylline (Truphylline)	Loading dose: 5-7 mg/kg IV Maintenance dose: 0.5-1.2 mg/kg/hr	Observe for skin rash or sloughing.	A drug component, ethylenediamine, can cause severe skin reactions.
		Same as for theophylline.	Drug is 80% theophylline.
Oxtriphylline (Apo-Oxtriphylline✱, Choledyl)	75-150 mg PO four times daily	Same as for theophylline.	Drug contains significant amounts of theophylline.
Cholinergic Antagonists			
Ipratropium (Atrovent, Apo-Ipravent✱)	2-4 inhalations 4-6 times daily 18 mcg/inhalation	Shake container well.	Drug separates on standing.
		Increase water/fluid intake.	Drug causes mouth dryness.
		Teach client to observe for blurred vision, eye pain, headache, nausea, nervousness, palpitations.	These are systemic symptoms of overdose.

Data from Facts and Comparisons. (2004). *Drug facts and comparisons* (58th ed.). St. Louis: Wolters Kluwer.
SC, Subcutaneous.

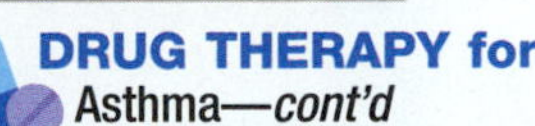

DRUG THERAPY for Asthma—*cont'd*

Drug	Usual Dosage	Nursing Interventions	Rationales
Anti-Inflammatories			
Corticosteroids—Oral			
Prednisolone (Cotolone, Delta-Cortef)	5-40 mg daily	Not recommended unless symptoms are severe or debilitating.	Systemic side effects are common and serious: ▪ GI ulceration ▪ Poor wound healing ▪ Decreased immune function ▪ Increased risk for infections ▪ Weight gain ▪ Hyperglycemia ▪ Personality changes ▪ Fluid retention
Prednisone (Deltasone, Prednicot, Orasone, Pred-Pak)	5-60 mg daily	Same as for prednisolone.	Same as for prednisolone.
Corticosteroids—Inhaler			
Budesonide (Pulmicort)	200 mcg/inhalation (dry powder inhaler)	Use daily as directed.	Effectiveness depends on regular use.
		Symptoms may persist for 2-3 days after initial administration.	Maximum effectiveness requires continued use for 48-72 hr.
		Observe mouth and throat for lesions.	Excessive use decreases local immune response and increases susceptibility to oral infections, especially candidiasis.
Fluticasone (Flovent)	2 metered sprays daily (50 mcg/metered spray) (100-250 mcg per Rotadisk dry powder inhaler)	Same as for budesonide.	Same as for budesonide.
Beclomethasone (Vanceril, Beclovent, Qvar✱, Becloforte✱)	2-4 inhalations three to four times daily (42 mcg/inhalation)	Same as for budesonide.	Same as for budesonide.
Triamcinolone (Azmacort)	2 inhalations three to four times daily (100 mcg/inhalation)	Same as for budesonide.	Same as for budesonide.
Flunisolide (AeroBid, Bronalide✱)	2 inhalations twice daily (250 mcg/inhalation)	Same as for budesonide.	Same as for budesonide.
Leukotriene Antagonists			
Zafirlukast (Accolate)	20 mg twice daily	Take 1 hr before or 2 hr after eating.	Drug absorption is slowed by presence of food.
		Incidence of upper respiratory infections is increased when co-administered with inhaled corticosteroids.	Drugs reduce local inflammatory and immune responses.
		Reduce dose in clients also taking aspirin.	Aspirin increases plasma concentration of drug.
Zileuton (Zyflo)	600 mg four times daily	Do not take with terfenadine or theophylline.	Drug increases plasma concentrations of terfenadine and theophylline.
Montelukast (Singulair)	10 mg daily	Do not abruptly substitute for oral or inhaled steroids.	Drug requires time to peak action.
		Reduce dose in clients with hepatic impairment.	Hepatic impairment prolongs blood levels of drug.
Inhaled Anti-Inflammatory			
Nedocromil (Tilade)	2 inhalations q6h (2 mg/inhalation)	Not for use during acute attack.	Drug has slow onset to peak action.
		Instruct client to use daily even when no symptoms are present.	Efficacy is related to continued correct use.
		Discontinue use if symptoms worsen with drug.	Client may be sensitive to propellants.

Continued

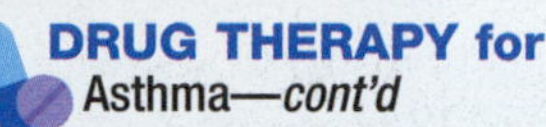

CHART 33-5

DRUG THERAPY for Asthma—*cont'd*

Drug	Usual Dosage	Nursing Interventions	Rationales
Combination Agents			
Fluticasone and salmeterol (Advair Diskus)	1 inhalation q12h 250/50 (250 mcg of fluticasone with 50 mcg of salmeterol) 500/50 (500 mcg of fluticasone with 50 mcg of salmeterol)	Same as for each agent alone.	Same as for each agent alone.
Ipratropium and albuterol (Combivent)	2 inhalations four times daily (18 mcg ipratropium with 103 mcg albuterol)	Same as for each agent alone.	Same as for each agent alone.
Mast Cell Stabilizers			
Cromolyn sodium (Intal)	1-2 inhalations four times daily	Use daily as directed. Start therapy 3-4 wk before expected allergy season.	Effectiveness depends on regular use. Requires regular use for prophylactic effect.
Monoclonal Antibodies			
Omalizumab (Xolair)	150-375 mg SC every 3-4 wk	Assess client for anaphylaxis for the first 2 hr after injection. Not for use during acute attack. Roll vial gently for 10-20 min until drug is no longer gel-like.	Some clients have allergies to the mouse parts of the antibody. Drug has slow onset to peak action. Drug is slow to dissolve.

Data from Facts and Comparisons. (2004). *Drug facts and comparisons* (58th ed.). St. Louis: Author.
SC, Subcutaneous.

achieve the greatest benefit from the drug. Chart 33-6 describes the proper way to use an MDI. Figure 33-4 shows a client using a "spacer" with an MDI inhaler. Chart 33-7 describes the proper care and use of a DPI. Figure 33-5 shows a client using a DPI.

LONG-ACTING BETA$_2$ AGONISTS. Long-acting beta$_2$ agonists are also delivered by inhaler directly to the site of action: the bronchioles. Unlike short-acting agonists, long-acting drugs need time to build up an effect, but the effects are longer lasting. Thus these drugs are useful in preventing an asthma attack but have no value during an acute attack. Proper use of the long-acting agonists can decrease reliance on short-acting agonists.

Cholinergic Antagonists. Cholinergic antagonists, sometimes called anticholinergic drugs, are similar to atropine and block the parasympathetic nervous system. This blockade allows the sympathetic nervous system to dominate, resulting in increased bronchodilation and decreased pulmonary secretions. The most common drug in this class is ipratropium (Atrovent), which is used as an inhalant. Most cholinergic antagonists are short acting and must be used several times a day. Tiotropium is a new long-acting drug for use once a day (Boyle & Locke, 2004).

Methylxanthines. Methylxanthines are used when other types of management are ineffective. The classic drug in this class is theophylline (Theo-Dur). Other drugs include aminophylline (Truphylline), oxtriphylline (Choledyl✱), and dyphylline (Dilor, Lufyllin). These drugs are given systemically, have narrow therapeutic ranges, and have many side effects. Blood levels of these drugs need to be monitored closely because the drug level that causes dangerous side effects is not much higher than the level needed to dilate the bronchioles. The most dangerous side effects result from excessive cardiac and central nervous system stimulation.

Anti-Inflammatory Agents. Anti-inflammatory agents decrease the inflammatory responses in the airways. Some are given systemically and have more side effects. Others are used as inhalants and have few systemic side effects.

Corticosteroids. Corticosteroids decrease inflammatory and immune responses in many ways, including by preventing the synthesis of mediators. Local corticosteroids in inhaled sprays can be helpful in preventing the manifestations of asthma. Newer high-potency steroid inhalers, such as fluticasone (Flovent) and budesonide (Pulmicort), may be used once per day for maintenance. Systemic corticosteroids, because of severe side effects, are avoided for mild to moderate asthma and are used on a short-term basis for moderate asthma. For some clients with severe asthma, daily systemic corticosteroids may be needed.

Inhaled Anti-Inflammatory Agents. A newer category of nonsteroidal inhaled anti-inflammatory agent is nedocromil (Tilade). This agent inhibits the release of inflammatory mediators from respiratory cells and white blood cells. In addition, it reduces nerve stimulation in the lung. These actions prevent asthma episodes rather than reversing an episode.

Mast Cell Stabilizers. Inhaled sprays containing mast cell stabilizers, such as cromolyn sodium (Intal), prevent mast cell membranes from opening when an allergen binds to IgE. Thus these drugs help prevent atopic asthma attacks but are not useful during an acute episode.

Monoclonal Antibodies. This new drug class was approved in 2003. Omalizumab (Xolair) binds to the IgE re-

CHART 33-6

CLIENT EDUCATION GUIDE
How to Use an Inhaler Correctly*

Without a Spacer (Preferred Technique)
1. Before each use, remove the cap and shake the inhaler according to the instructions in the package insert.
2. Tilt your head back slightly and breathe out fully.
3. Open your mouth and place the mouthpiece 1 to 2 inches away.
4. As you begin to breathe in deeply through your mouth, press down firmly on the canister of the inhaler to release one dose of medication.
5. Continue to breathe in slowly and deeply (usually over 3 to 5 seconds).
6. Hold your breath for at least 10 seconds to allow the medication to reach deep into the lungs, then breathe out slowly.
7. Wait at least 1 minute between puffs.
8. Replace the cap on the inhaler.
9. At least once a day, remove the canister and clean the plastic case and cap of the inhaler by thoroughly rinsing in warm, running tap water.

Without a Spacer (Alternative Method)
1. Follow steps 1 and 2 above.
2. Place the mouthpiece into your mouth, over your tongue, and seal your lips tightly around it.
3. Follow steps 4 to 9 above.

With a Spacer
1. Before each use, remove the caps from the inhaler and the spacer.
2. Insert the mouthpiece of the inhaler into the non-mouthpiece end of the spacer.
3. Shake the whole unit vigorously three or four times.
4. Place the mouthpiece into your mouth, over your tongue, and seal your lips tightly around it.
5. Press down firmly on the canister of the inhaler to release one dose of medication into the spacer.
6. Breathe in slowly and deeply. If the spacer makes a whistling sound, you are breathing in too rapidly.
7. Remove the mouthpiece from your mouth and, keeping your lips closed, hold your breath for at least 10 seconds, then breathe out slowly.
8. Wait at least 1 minute between puffs.
9. Replace the caps on the inhaler and the spacer.
10. At least once a day, clean the plastic case and cap of the inhaler by thoroughly rinsing in warm, running tap water; at least once a week, clean the spacer in the same manner.

*Avoid spraying in the direction of the eyes.

ceptor sites on mast cells and basophils. This action prevents allergens from triggering the release of mediators from mast cells and basophils. Thus these drugs help prevent atopic asthma attacks but are not useful during an acute episode.

Leukotriene Antagonists. Leukotriene antagonists work in several ways to prevent an asthma episode. Zileuton (Zyflo) prevents leukotriene synthesis. Zafirlukast (Accolate) and montelukast (Singulair) block the leukotriene receptor. All are oral drugs.

Exercise/Activity. Regular exercise, including aerobic exercise, is a recommended part of asthma therapy. Aerobic exercise assists in maintaining cardiac health, enhancing skeletal muscle strength, and promoting ventilation and perfusion. Clients with asthma need to examine the conditions that trigger an attack and adjust the exercise routine as needed. Some may need to premedicate with inhaled beta agonists before beginning activity. For others, adjusting the environment may be needed. For example, outdoor ice-skating

CHART 33-7

CLIENT EDUCATION GUIDE
How to Use a Dry Powder Inhaler (DPI)

For Inhalers Requiring Loading
First load the drug by:
- Turning the device to the next dose of drug, or
- Inserting the capsule into the device, or
- Inserting the disk or compartment into the device.

After Loading the Drug and for Inhalers That Do Not Require Drug Loading
- Read your doctor's instructions for how fast you should breathe for your particular inhaler.
- Place your lips over the mouthpiece and breathe in forcefully. (There is no propellant in the inhaler; only your breath pulls the drug in.)
- Remove the inhaler from your mouth as soon as you have breathed in.
- Never exhale (breathe out) into your inhaler. Your breath will moisten the powder, causing it to clump and not be delivered accurately.
- Never wash or place the inhaler in water.
- Never shake your inhaler.
- Keep your inhaler in a dry place at room temperature.
- If the inhaler is preloaded, discard the inhaler after it is empty.
- Because the drug is a dry powder and there is no propellant, you may not feel, smell, or taste it as you inhale.

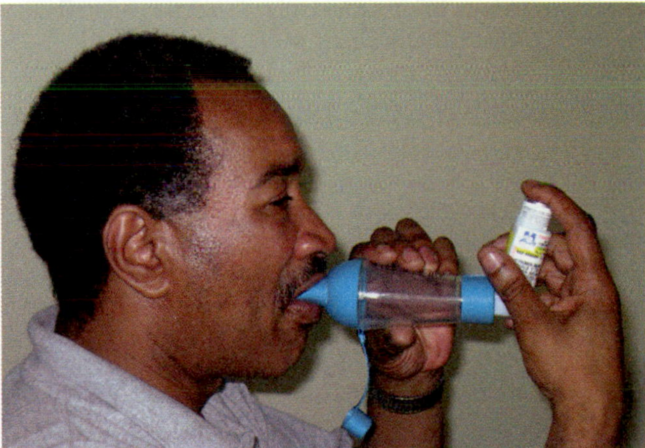

Figure 33-4 ■ Client using an aerosol inhaler with a spacer.

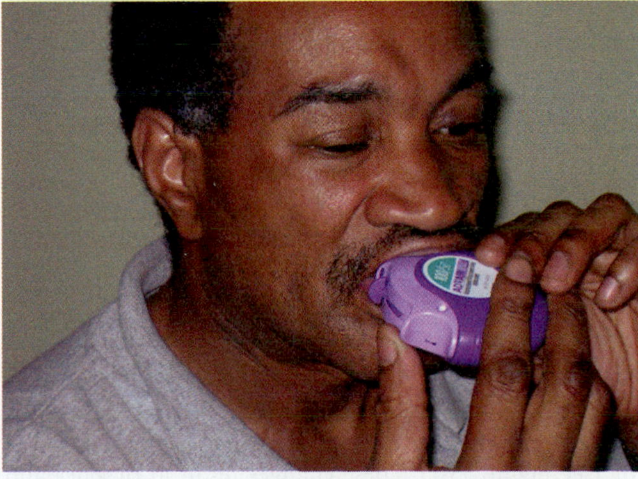

Figure 33-5 ■ Client using a dry powder inhaler (DPI).

in cold, dry air can trigger an attack; indoor ice-skating may be less of a problem. Sports that involve more "rest" action, such as baseball, are less likely to trigger symptoms than "nonrest" action sports, such as basketball.

Oxygen Therapy. Supplemental oxygen is often used during an acute asthma attack. Oxygen is delivered by mask, nasal cannula, or endotracheal tube. High flow rates or concentrations may be needed when bronchospasms are severe and limit flow of oxygen through the bronchiole tubes. Heliox, a mixture of helium and oxygen (often 50% helium and 50% oxygen) can help improve oxygen delivery to the alveoli. This gas mixture is lower in density than oxygen alone or oxygen with atmospheric air (which contains nitrogen) and flows even when airway resistance is high.

Status Asthmaticus. Status asthmaticus is a severe, life-threatening acute episode of airway obstruction that intensifies once it begins and often does not respond to common therapy. The client arrives in the emergency department with extremely labored breathing and wheezing. Use of accessory muscles for breathing and distention of neck veins are observed. If the condition is not reversed, the client may develop pneumothorax, and cardiac or respiratory arrest. The physician immediately prescribes intravenous (IV) fluids, potent systemic bronchodilators, steroids (to decrease inflammation), epinephrine, and oxygen in an attempt to reverse the acute condition. Prepare for emergency intubation. When wheezing decreases, management is similar to that for any client with asthma.

Critical Thinking Challenge

It is March in Minnesota. The client is a 22-year-old female college athlete who comes to the health clinic with audible wheezes on exhalation. She explains, between breaths, that she was running her normal 5 miles on the outdoor track when she started wheezing. She does have asthma and usually carries an albuterol inhaler with her when she runs. Today, she forgot her "rescue" inhaler but did take Advair one puff by DPI, 2 hours ago. Her vital signs are as follows: BP 132/92, P 68, R 34.

1. What additional assessment data should you obtain?
2. Should you start oxygen on this client? Why or why not?
3. Should she take another dose of Advair? Why or why not?
4. What is the probable cause of this client's asthma attack?
5. What should you teach her to help her avoid another episode?

evolve For suggested answer guidelines, go to http://evolve.elsevier.com/Iggy/.

Chronic Obstructive Pulmonary Disease

PATHOPHYSIOLOGY

Most clients with emphysema have chronic bronchitis at the same time, but each condition has its own pathophysiologic process (Figure 33-6).

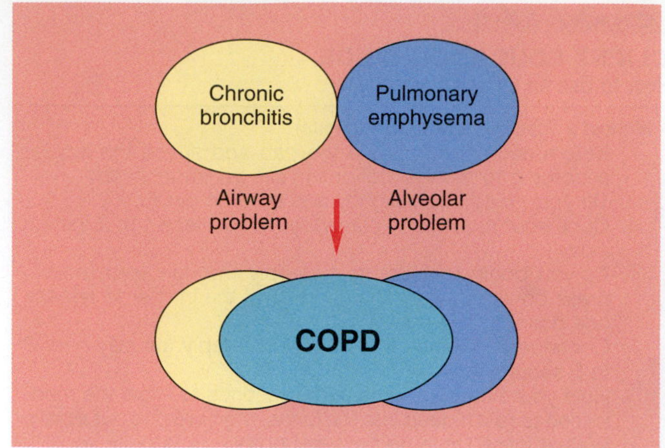

Figure 33-6 ■ The interaction of chronic bronchitis and emphysema in COPD.

Emphysema

ANATOMIC AND FUNCTIONAL CHANGES

The two major changes that occur with pulmonary emphysema are loss of lung elasticity and hyperinflation of the lung (see Figure 33-1). These changes result in dyspnea and the need for an increased respiratory rate.

Enzymes that degrade protein (proteases) damage the alveoli and the small airways by breaking down elastin. This causes the alveolar sacs to lose their elasticity and the small airways to collapse or narrow. Some alveoli are destroyed, and others become large and flabby, with decreased area for gas exchange.

An increased amount of air becomes trapped in the lungs. Causes of air trapping are loss of elastic recoil in the alveolar walls, overstretching and enlargement of the alveoli into air-filled spaces called bullae, and collapse of small airways (bronchioles). These changes greatly increase the work of breathing. The hyperinflated lung flattens the diaphragm (Figure 33-7), weakening the effect of this muscle. As a result, the client with emphysema needs to use additional muscles (accessory muscles) in the neck, chest wall, and abdomen to inhale and exhale. This increased effort increases the need for oxygen, making the client work harder and have an "air hunger" sensation. Often, inhalation starts before exhalation is completed, resulting in an uncoordinated pattern of breathing.

Gas exchange is affected by the increased work of breathing and the loss of alveolar tissue. Although some alveoli enlarge, the curves of alveolar walls decrease and there is less surface area available for gas exchange. Often the client adjusts by increasing the respiratory rate, so arterial blood gas (ABG) values may not show gas exchange problems until the client has advanced disease. Then carbon dioxide is produced faster than it can be eliminated, resulting in carbon dioxide retention and chronic respiratory acidosis (see Chapter 19). The client with late-stage emphysema also has a low arterial oxygen (PaO_2) level, because it is difficult for oxygen to move from diseased lung tissue into the bloodstream.

EMPHYSEMA CLASSIFICATION

Emphysema is classified as panlobular, centrilobular, or paraseptal depending on the pattern of destruction and dilation of the gas-exchanging units (acini) (see Figure 33-1). Each type can occur alone or in combination in the same lung.

Panlobular (panacinar) emphysema (PLE) has destruction of the entire alveolus uniformly. This type is diffuse and more severe in the lower lung areas.

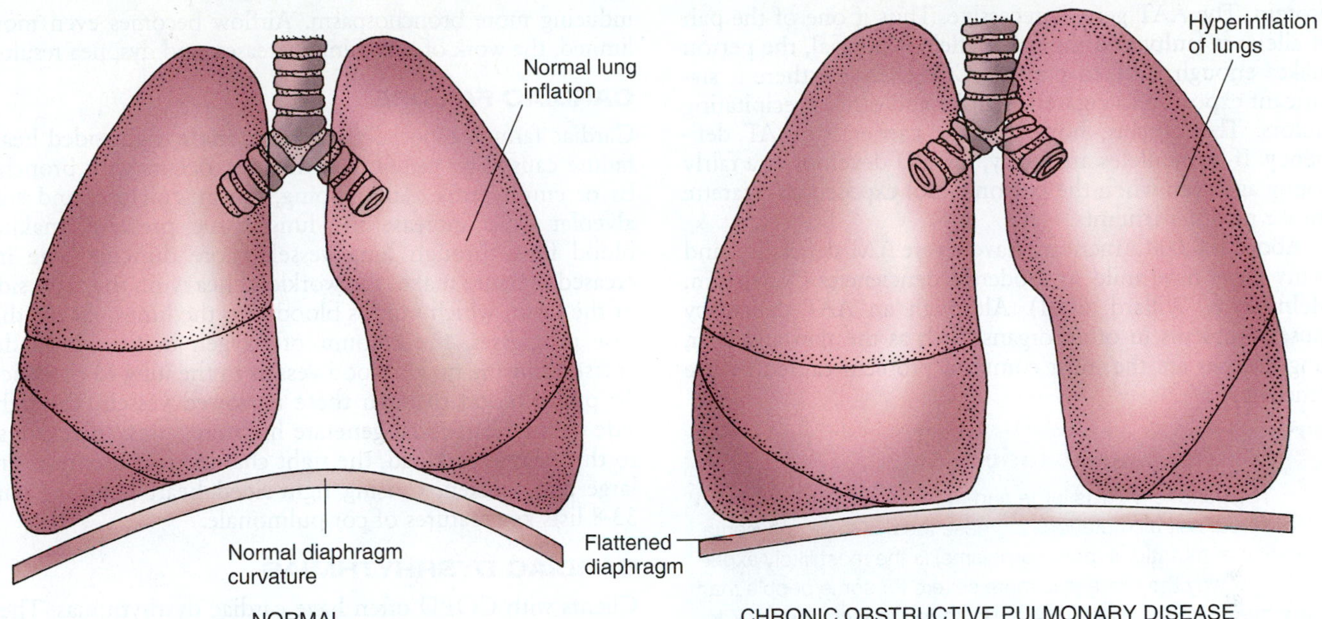

Figure 33-7 ■ Diaphragm shape and lung inflation in the normal client and in the client with chronic airflow limitation (CAL).

In centrilobular (centriacinar) emphysema (CLE), openings occur in the bronchioles and allow spaces to develop as tissue walls break down. Although this is a diffuse disease, the upper lung sections are most severely affected. This type of emphysema is often seen in long-standing cigarette smokers.

In paraseptal or distal acinar emphysema, the disease is confined to only the alveolar ducts and alveolar sacs. This type forms bullae and often affects the upper half of the lungs.

Chronic Bronchitis

Bronchitis is an inflammation of the bronchi and bronchioles caused by chronic exposure to irritants, especially tobacco smoke. The irritant triggers inflammation, with vasodilation, congestion, mucosal edema, and bronchospasm. Unlike emphysema, bronchitis affects only the airways rather than the alveoli.

Chronic inflammation causes an increase in the number and size of mucous glands, which produce large amounts of thick mucus. The bronchial walls thicken (often to twice the normal thickness) and impair airflow. This thickening, along with excessive mucus, blocks some of the smaller airways and narrows larger ones. Small airways are affected before large airways become involved.

Chronic bronchitis hinders airflow and gas exchange because of mucous plugs and infection narrowing the airways. As a result, the PaO_2 decreases (hypoxemia) and the arterial blood carbon dioxide level ($PaCO_2$) increases (respiratory acidosis).

Etiology and Genetic Risk

CIGARETTE SMOKING

Smoking is the most important risk factor for COPD. The client with an 8-pack-year history usually has obstructive lung changes but no manifestations of disease. The client with a 20-pack-year history or longer often has early stage COPD found as changes in pulmonary function tests (PFTs).

The harmful effects of tobacco result in part because inhaled smoke triggers the release of excessive amounts of the enzyme elastase protease from cells in the lungs. The elastase protease breaks down elastin, the major component of alveoli. By impairing the action of cilia, smoking also inhibits the cilia from clearing the bronchi of mucus, cellular debris, and fluid.

In addition to the increased risk for COPD from active smoking, passive smoking (or secondhand smoke) contributes to upper and lower respiratory problems. The risk is greater when exposure occurs in small, confined spaces.

CULTURAL CONSIDERATIONS

The prevalence of smoking remains higher among African-Americans, blue-collar workers, and less educated people than in the overall population of the United States. Smoking prevalence is highest among Northern Plains American Indians/Native Americans and Alaskan Natives. The overall prevalence of smoking for both men and women has decreased over the past two decades, but the decrease for women has been less than it has for men (American Cancer Society, 2005). Development of culturally appropriate smoking cessation programs as well as research examining barriers to cessation in these populations may help reduce this disparity.

ALPHA$_1$-ANTITRYPSIN DEFICIENCY

A special enzyme, alpha$_1$-antitrypsin (AAT), is made by the liver and is normally present in the lungs. One purpose of AAT is to regulate the other enzymes (proteases) that are present to break down inhaled pollutants and microorganisms. AAT prevents the proteases from working on lung structures.

The production of normal amounts of AAT is dependent on the inheritance of a pair of normal gene alleles for this protein. The AAT gene is recessive. Thus if one of the pair of alleles is faulty and the other allele is normal, the person makes enough AAT to prevent COPD unless there is significant exposure to cigarette smoke and other precipitating factors. This person, however, is a carrier for AAT deficiency. If both alleles are faulty, COPD develops at a fairly young age even when the person is not exposed to cigarette smoke or other irritants.

About 100,000 Americans have severe AAT deficiency, and many more have mild to moderate deficiencies (Nussbaum, McInnes, & Willard, 2001). Although an AAT deficiency causes problems in other organs, such as the skin and liver, lung diseases are the most common problem caused by the deficiency.

Genetic Considerations

The gene for AAT is large and many mutations have been discovered. Not all mutations increase the risk for emphysema. Variation of mutations (polymorphisms) is the most likely explanation for why the disease is more severe for some people than for others. The most serious mutation for an increased risk for emphysema is at the Z allele, although other mutations also increases the risk but to a lesser degree.

Replacement of the deficient enzyme is a promising new treatment. Currently, the enzyme can be replaced intravenously, with one dose maintaining blood levels for about a week. Delivery of the enzyme by aerosol inhaler is also being tried.

AIR POLLUTION

Air pollution alone plays only a relatively small role in the client with emphysema and chronic bronchitis. The effect of air pollution is additive to tobacco exposure.

Incidence/Prevalence

The prevalence of chronic bronchitis and emphysema in the United States has been estimated at about 13.5 million (for chronic bronchitis) and 2 million (for emphysema). Chronic obstructive pulmonary disease/chronic airflow limitation (COPD/CAL) is the fourth leading cause of death for women of all ages and is the fifth for men (Centers for Disease Control and Prevention, 2002).

Complications

COPD affects the delivery of oxygen to all tissues. Complications of the disorder can result in organ anoxia and tissue death. Major problems occur, such as hypoxemia, acidosis, respiratory infection, cardiac failure, and dysrhythmias.

HYPOXEMIA AND ACIDOSIS

As the client with COPD is less able to exchange gas, oxygenation decreases and carbon dioxide levels increase, leading to hypoxemia and acidosis. Thus most tissues have decreased function.

RESPIRATORY INFECTIONS

The client with COPD is at risk for respiratory infections from the increased mucus and poor oxygenation. The organisms most often causing bacterial infections include *Streptococcus pneumoniae, Haemophilus influenzae,* and *Moraxella catarrhalis.* Acute respiratory infections make COPD manifestations worse by increasing inflammation and mucus production, and inducing more bronchospasm. Airflow becomes even more limited, the work of breathing increases, and dyspnea results.

CARDIAC FAILURE

Cardiac failure, especially **cor pulmonale** (right-sided heart failure caused by pulmonary disease), occurs with bronchitis or emphysema. Air trapping, airway collapse, and stiff alveolar walls increase the lung tissue pressure, making blood flow through lung vessels more difficult. The increased pressure makes the workload heavy on the right side of the heart, which pumps blood into the lungs. As the disease progresses, the amount of oxygen in the blood decreases, causing major blood vessels in the lung to constrict. To pump blood through these narrowed vessels, the right side of the heart must generate high pressures. In response to this heavy workload, the right chambers of the heart enlarge and thicken, causing right-sided heart failure. Chart 33-8 lists key features of cor pulmonale.

CARDIAC DYSRHYTHMIAS

Clients with COPD often have cardiac dysrhythmias. They may be a result of hypoxemia (from decreased oxygen to the heart muscle), other cardiac disease, drug effects, or acidosis.

HEALTH PROMOTION/ILLNESS PREVENTION

Health experts agree that the incidence and severity of COPD would be drastically reduced by smoking cessation. COPD is rare among people who have never smoked cigarettes. Disease progression can be slowed by smoking cessation. Other measures to reduce the incidence of COPD are to avoid inhalation irritants in all environments. Using masks when working in areas with high levels of particulate matter can reduce individual exposure. Proper venting of workplaces and recreation areas that have airborne or particulate matter also reduces exposure.

◆COLLABORATIVE MANAGEMENT

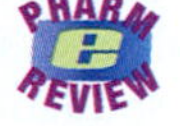

◆Assessment

HISTORY

RISK FACTORS. Consider age, gender, occupational history, and ethnic-cultural background when taking a history from a client who may have chronic obstructive pul-

CHART 33-8

KEY FEATURES of
Cor Pulmonale

- Hypoxia and hypoxemia
- Increasing dyspnea
- Fatigue
- Weakness
- Enlarged and tender liver
- Warm, cyanotic extremities with bounding pulses
- Cyanotic lips
- Distended neck veins
- Right ventricular enlargement (hypertrophy)
- Lower sternal or epigastric pulsations
- Gastrointestinal disturbances, such as nausea or anorexia
- Dependent edema
- Metabolic and respiratory acidosis
- Pulmonary hypertension

monary disease (COPD). COPD is seen more often in older men. Some types of COPD, particularly panlobular emphysema, occur in families, especially those with alpha$_1$ antitrypsin (AAT) deficiency.

Obtain a thorough smoking history, because tobacco use is a major risk factor. Ask about the length of time the client has smoked and the number of packs smoked daily. Use these data to determine the pack-year smoking history.

CURRENT PROBLEM. Ask the client to describe his or her breathing problems. Assess whether the client has any difficulty breathing while talking. Can he or she speak in complete sentences, or is it necessary to take a breath between every one or two words? Ask about the presence, duration, or worsening of wheezing, coughing, and shortness of breath. Determine what activities trigger these problems. Assess the client's cough pattern. If the cough is productive, ask whether sputum is clear or colored and how much is produced each day. Ask the client to recall the time of day when the sputum production is greatest. Smokers often have a productive cough when they get up in the morning; nonsmokers generally do not. Ask whether sputum production has increased or changed during the past year.

Check the relationship between activity tolerance and dyspnea by asking the client to compare his or her activity level and shortness of breath now with those of a month ago and a year ago. Likewise, ask about any difficulty with eating and sleeping. Many clients sleep in a semi-sitting position because breathlessness is worse when lying down **(orthopnea).** Ask about usual daily activities and any difficulty with sleeping, bathing, dressing, or sexual activity.

WEIGHT AND DIET. Weigh the client and compare this weight with previous weights. Unplanned weight loss occurs with an increase in COPD severity. The client with COPD has increased metabolic needs as a result of the increased work of breathing. Dyspnea and mucus production often result in poor food intake and inadequate nutrition. Ask the client to recall a typical day's meals and fluid intake.

PHYSICAL ASSESSMENT/CLINICAL MANIFESTATIONS

GENERAL APPEARANCE. Observe the client's general appearance, including weight in proportion to height, posture, mobility, muscle mass, and overall hygiene. The client with increasingly severe COPD is thin, with loss of muscle mass in the extremities, although the neck muscles may be enlarged. The client tends to be slow moving and slightly stooped. Usually he or she will sit with a forward-bending posture, sometimes with the arms held forward (Figure 33-8). When dyspnea becomes severe, the client may have such activity intolerance that bathing and general grooming are neglected.

RESPIRATORY CHANGES. Inspect the chest to assess the breathing rate and pattern. The client with respiratory muscle fatigue breathes with rapid, shallow respirations and may have paradoxical respirations or use accessory muscles in the abdomen or neck. The respiratory rate could be as high as 40 to 50 breaths/min. Three breathing patterns often seen with respiratory muscle fatigue are abdominal paradox, respiratory alternans, and asynchronous breathing (Table 33-1).

Palpate the client's chest for areas of tenderness and abnormal retractions and for symmetric chest expansion. The client with emphysema has limited diaphragmatic movement (excursion) because the diaphragm is flattened and below its usual resting state. Decreased vibration (fremitus) may be felt when the client says "ninety-nine" because vibrations are not transmitted through obstructed airways. On percussion the chest is hyperresonant because of the presence of trapped air.

Auscultate the chest to assess the depth of inspiration and any abnormal breath sounds. Crackles occur with emphysema and chronic bronchitis. Note the pitch and location of the sound, and the point in the respiratory cycle at which the sound is heard. A silent chest may indicate obstruction or pneumothorax.

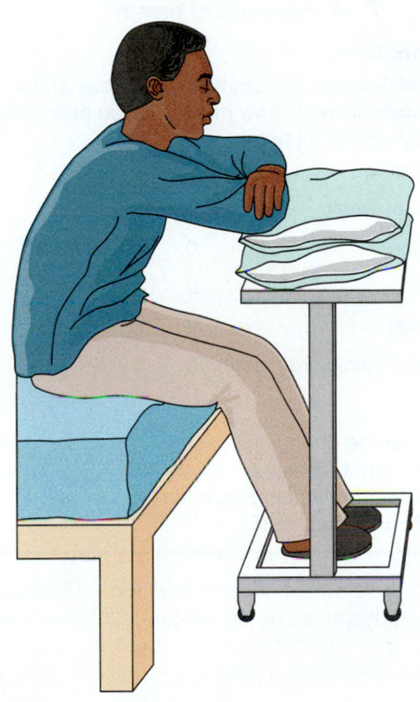

Sitting on the edge of a bed with the arms folded and placed on two or three pillows positioned over a nightstand.

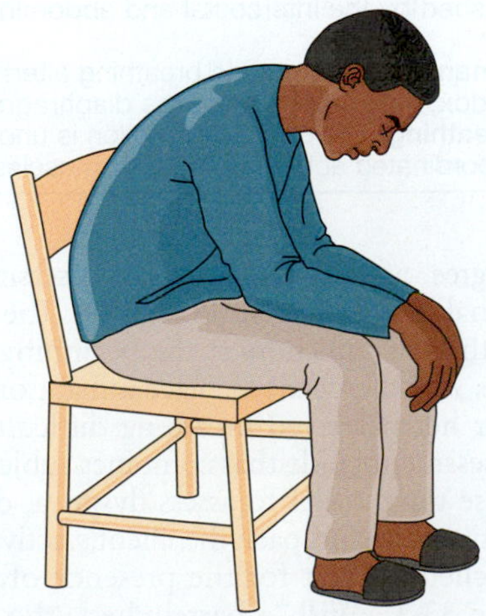

Sitting in a chair with the feet spread shoulder-width apart and leaning forward with the elbows on the knees. Arms and hands are relaxed.

Figure 33-8 ■ Orthopnea positions that clients with chronic airflow limitation (CAL) can assume to ease the work of breathing.

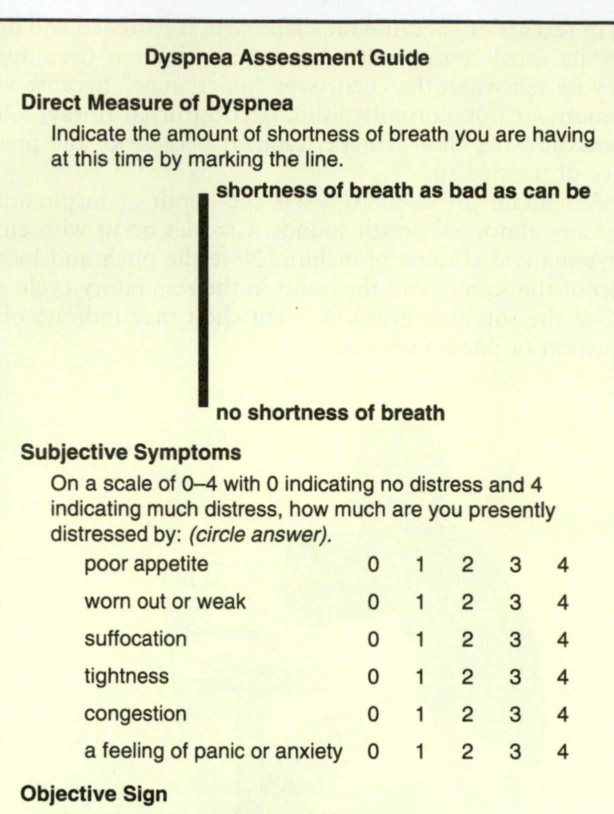

Dyspnea Assessment Guide

Direct Measure of Dyspnea

Indicate the amount of shortness of breath you are having at this time by marking the line.

shortness of breath as bad as can be

no shortness of breath

Subjective Symptoms

On a scale of 0–4 with 0 indicating no distress and 4 indicating much distress, how much are you presently distressed by: *(circle answer)*.

poor appetite	0	1	2	3	4
worn out or weak	0	1	2	3	4
suffocation	0	1	2	3	4
tightness	0	1	2	3	4
congestion	0	1	2	3	4
a feeling of panic or anxiety	0	1	2	3	4

Objective Sign

Rise of the clavicle during inspiration:

ABSENT = not detected
MILD = seen but not pronounced
SEVERE = pronounced

Figure 33-9 ■ A dyspnea assessment tool. (Redrawn from Gift, A.G. [1989]. A dyspnea assessment guide. *Critical Care Nurse, 9*[8], 79.)

TABLE 33-1 Breathing Patterns Commonly Seen in Clients with Respiratory Muscle Fatigue

Abdominal paradox. The diaphragm is nonfunctional; inspiration is accomplished by the intercostal and abdominal accessory muscles.
Respiratory alternans. Diaphragmatic breathing alternates with abdominal paradox; may serve to rest the diaphragm.
Asynchronous breathing. The chest wall motion is unorganized; reflects the uncoordinated activity of fatigued muscles.

Assess the degree of dyspnea using an assessment tool called a Visual Analog Dyspnea Scale (VADS). The VADS is a straight line with verbal anchors at the beginning and end of a 100-mm line. Ask the client to place a mark on the line to indicate his or her perceived breathing difficulty. Figure 33-9 shows an assessment guide that combines subjective and objective data. Use these scales to assess dyspnea, determine the therapy effectiveness, and pace the client's activities.

Examine the client's chest for the presence of a "barrel chest" (see Figure 33-3). With a barrel chest, the ratio between the anteroposterior (AP) diameter of the chest and its lateral diameter is 2:2 rather than the normal ratio of 1:2. This shape change results from lung overinflation and diaphragm flattening.

The client with chronic bronchitis often has a cyanotic, or blue-tinged, dusky appearance and has excessive sputum

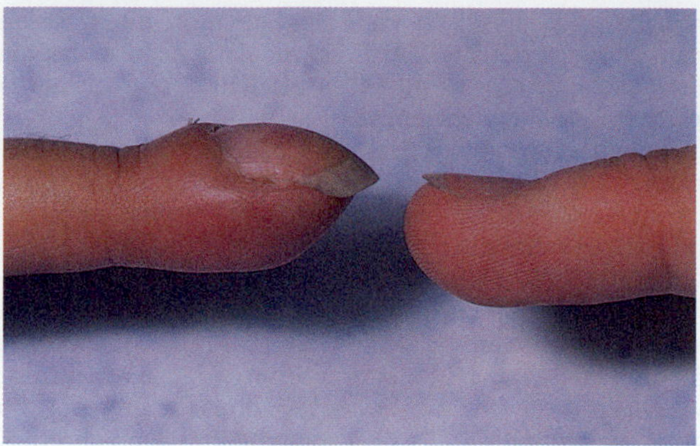

Figure 33-10 ■ Late digital clubbing *(left)* compared to a normal digit *(right)*. (From Swartz, M.H. [1998]. *Textbook of physical diagnosis: History and examination.* Philadelphia: W.B. Saunders.)

production. Assess the client for cyanosis, delayed capillary refill, and clubbing of the fingers (Figure 33-10), which indicate chronically decreased arterial oxygen levels.

CARDIAC CHANGES. Assess the client's heart rate and rhythm. Check for swelling of the feet and ankles (dependent edema) or other manifestations of right-sided heart failure. Examine nail beds and oral mucous membranes. The client with later-stage emphysema may have pallor or frank cyanosis.

PSYCHOSOCIAL ASSESSMENT

COPD affects all aspects of a person's life. Socialization may be reduced when friends avoid the client with COPD because of annoying coughs, excessive sputum, or dyspnea. The client may choose to be isolated because dyspnea causes fatigue or because of embarrassment from coughing and excessive sputum production. In addition, because of the association with cigarette smoking and disease development, the client may feel a social stigma (see the Evidence-Based Practice for Nursing box on p. 599).

Ask the client about interests and hobbies to assess whether socialization has decreased or whether hobbies cause exposure to inhalation irritants. Ask about home conditions for exposure to smoke or crowded living conditions that promote transmission of respiratory infections.

The client's economic status may be affected by the disease through changes in income and health insurance coverage. If the client is the head of the household, severe COPD may require role changes that have a negative impact on self-image. Drugs, especially the metered dose inhalers (MDIs) and dry powder inhalers (DPI), are expensive, and many clients with limited incomes may use them only during exacerbations and not as prescribed on a scheduled basis.

Anxiety and fear related to dyspnea and feelings of breathlessness may reduce the client's ability to participate in a full life. Work, family, social, and sexual roles can be affected. Assess the client's awareness and use of support groups and services.

LABORATORY ASSESSMENT

Arterial blood gas (ABG) values identify abnormal oxygenation, ventilation, and acid-base status. Compare serial or repeated ABG values to assess changes in the client's respiratory status. Once baseline ABG values are obtained, pulse oximetry

EVIDENCE-BASED PRACTICE for Nursing

Women with COPD need social support and specific guidelines for management of dyspnea and fatigue to cope well with the disease.

O'Neill, E. (2002). Illness representations and coping of women with chronic obstructive pulmonary disease: A pilot study. *Heart & Lung, 31*(4), 295-302.

The purpose of this qualitative study was to determine how women with chronic obstructive pulmonary disease (COPD) recognize and respond to symptoms. A total of 21 participants were interviewed and kept symptom diaries.

The most difficult physical problems for the subjects were fatigue and dyspnea. Other important findings included the high level of depression and stigma felt by the subjects. They also perceived a loss of social support and intimacy.

Level of Evidence: 6—Uncontrolled descriptive qualitative study.

Critique. The study designed followed acceptable procedures for qualitative research. Data were collected until redundancy was apparent. Information was obtained by audiotaping direct interviews using an open guide with questions and probes to allow for flexibility of response. The interviewer also took notes. A professional transcriptionist transcribed the tapes. Feedback from participants was used to verify the data. An independent researcher analyzed selective portions of the transcripts for reliability. A drawback of the study was that all participants were also participating in a pulmonary rehabilitation program. Thus the sample may have different motivations and perceptions compared to women with COPD who do not choose or are unable to participate in a pulmonary rehabilitation program.

Implications for Nursing. Nurses must provide more practical information on ways to manage dyspnea and fatigue. These physical problems have a large impact on the client's quality of life and degree of continued socialization. Nurses must individualize energy conservation plans to meet each client's needs rather than just provide a general listing of energy conservation measures.

can gauge the response to treatment. As COPD worsens, the amount of oxygen in the blood decreases **(hypoxemia)** and the amount of carbon dioxide in the blood increases **(hypercarbia).** Chronic respiratory acidosis (increased arterial carbon dioxide [$Pa{CO_2}$]) then results; metabolic alkalosis (increased arterial bicarbonate) occurs as compensation. Not all clients with COPD are carbon dioxide retainers, even when hypoxemia is present. Carbon dioxide diffuses more easily across lung membranes than does oxygen. Hypercarbia is a problem in advanced emphysema (because the alveoli are affected) rather than in bronchitis (wherein the airways are affected).

Sputum samples are obtained for culture from hospitalized clients with an acute respiratory infection. In the community, sputum cultures are rarely obtained. The infection is treated on the basis of manifestations and the common bacterial organisms. A white blood cell count helps to confirm the presence of infection.

Other blood tests include hemoglobin and hematocrit to determine polycythemia (a compensatory increase in red blood cells in the chronically hypoxic client). Serum electrolyte levels are examined because hypophosphatemia, hyperkalemia, hypocalcemia, and hypomagnesemia reduce muscle strength. In clients suspected of alpha$_1$-antitrypsin (AAT) deficiency, serum AAT levels are drawn.

RADIOGRAPHIC ASSESSMENT

Chest x-rays are obtained to rule out other chest diseases and to check the progress of clients with respiratory infections or chronic disease. With advanced emphysema, chest x-rays show hyperinflation and a flattened diaphragm. Chest x-rays may not be helpful in the diagnosis of early or moderate disease.

TABLE 33-2 Classification of COPD Severity

Stage	Manifestations	Pulmonary Function Test Results
0 (At risk)	Chronic cough Chronic sputum production Exposure to environmental risk factors	Normal
I (Mild)	±Chronic cough ±Sputum production	FEV_1/FVC <70% FEV_1 <80% of predicted
II (Moderate)	±Dyspnea ±Chronic cough ±Sputum production	FEV_1/FVC <70% FEV_1 <80% but at least 50% of predicted
III (Severe)	±Dyspnea ±Chronic cough ±Sputum production	FEV_1/FVC <70% FEV_1 <50% but at least 30% of predicted
IV (Very severe)	±Dyspnea ±Chronic cough ±Sputum production	FEV_1/FVC <70% FEV_1 <30% of predicted OR FEV_1 <50% of predicted **with either** respiratory failure or heart failure

Data from National Heart, Lung, and Blood Institute. (2003). *Global initiative for chronic obstructive pulmonary disease: Global strategy for the diagnosis, management, and prevention of chronic obstructive pulmonary disease.* (NIH Publication No. 2701A.) Rockville, MD. Author.

OTHER DIAGNOSTIC ASSESSMENTS

COPD is classified from mild to severe on the basis of manifestations and pulmonary function test (PFT) changes (Table 33-2; see Table 30-7). Airflow rates and lung volume measurements help distinguish airway disease (obstructive disease) from interstitial lung disease (restrictive diseases). PFTs determine lung volumes, flow volume curves, and diffusion capacity. Each test is performed before and after the client inhales a bronchodilator agent.

The lung volumes measured for COPD are vital capacity (VC), residual volume (RV), and total lung capacity (TLC). RV is most profoundly affected, although all volumes and capacities change to some degree in COPD. The RV increase reflects the trapped, stale air remaining in the lungs.

Flow volume curves measure the client's ability to move air into and out of the lung. The rate of airflow out of the lungs during a rapid, forceful, and complete exhalation from TLC to RV (forced expiratory volume [FEV]) indirectly measures the flow resistance of the lung. A diagnosis of COPD is based mostly on the FEV_1 (the FEV in the first second of exhalation). FEV_1 can also be expressed as a percentage of the forced vital capacity (FVC). As the disease progresses, the ratio of FEV_1 to FVC becomes smaller.

The diffusion test measures how well a test gas (carbon monoxide) diffuses across the alveolar-capillary membrane and combines with the hemoglobin of red blood cells. In emphysema, alveolar wall destruction causes a large decrease in surface area for diffusion of gas into the blood, leading to a decreased diffusion capacity. In bronchitis, even though lung volumes are increased, the diffusion capacity is usually normal.

The client with COPD has decreased oxygen saturation, often as low as 91%. Pulse oximetry results lower than 90% require medical attention.

Peak expiratory flow meters are used to monitor the effectiveness of the prescribed drugs to relieve obstruction. Peak flow rates increase as obstruction resolves. Teach the client to self-monitor the peak expiratory flow rates at home and adjust drugs as needed.

Analysis

COMMON NURSING DIAGNOSES AND COLLABORATIVE PROBLEMS

The following are priority nursing diagnoses for clients with chronic obstructive pulmonary disease (COPD):

1. Impaired Gas Exchange related to alveolar-capillary membrane changes, reduced airway size, ventilatory muscle fatigue, and excessive mucus production
2. Ineffective Breathing Pattern related to airway obstruction, diaphragm flattening, fatigue, and decreased energy
3. Ineffective Airway Clearance related to excessive secretions, fatigue, decreased energy, and ineffective cough
4. Imbalanced Nutrition: Less Than Body Requirements related to dyspnea, excessive secretions, anorexia, and fatigue
5. Anxiety related to dyspnea, a change in health status, and situational crisis
6. Activity Intolerance related to fatigue, dyspnea, and an imbalance between oxygen supply and demand

A primary collaborative problem for clients with COPD is Potential for Pneumonia or Other Respiratory Infections.

ADDITIONAL NURSING DIAGNOSES AND COLLABORATIVE PROBLEMS

In addition to the common nursing diagnoses and collaborative problems, clients with COPD may have one or more of the following:

- Fatigue related to a change in metabolic energy or hypoxemia
- Deficient Knowledge (disease process, prescribed treatments, activity limitations) related to unfamiliarity with information resources
- Sexual Dysfunction related to extreme fatigue
- Impaired Spontaneous Ventilation related to ventilatory muscle fatigue
- Disturbed Sleep Pattern related to dyspnea or an unfamiliar environment (hospitalization)
- Disturbed Thought Processes related to hypoxemia or sleep deprivation
- Ineffective Coping related to high degree of threat, inadequate level of perception of control, changes in lifestyle, situational crisis, or knowledge deficit
- Ineffective Role Performance related to a change in health status or role loss

Other collaborative problems for clients with COPD include Potential for Respiratory Failure and Potential for Right-Sided Heart Failure.

Critical Thinking Challenge

The client is a 54-year-old secretary who is newly diagnosed with emphysema after having two episodes of pneumonia this year. She is currently a smoker and has smoked two packs of cigarettes per day since age 16 years. She is divorced and lives in an apartment in the same city as her three grown children. Her COPD is classified as II—moderate (see Table 33-2). She is crying and blaming herself for this disease. Although she says she would like to quit smoking, she thinks it will not help because "the damage has already been done." She also tells you that her father died with COPD at the age of 62. She worries that her smoking may have harmed her children.

1. What is the priority nursing responsibility for this client?
2. Explain your rationale for its priority.
3. Calculate this client's smoking history in pack-years.
4. Would smoking cessation at this time help this client? Why or why not?

evolve For suggested answer guidelines, go to http://evolve.elsevier.com/Iggy/.

Planning and Implementation

IMPAIRED GAS EXCHANGE

NOC **PLANNING: EXPECTED OUTCOMES.** The client with COPD is expected to attain and maintain gas exchange at a level within his or her chronic baseline values. Indicators include the following:

- Maintenance of SpO_2 of at least 88%
- Absence of cyanosis
- Maintenance of cognitive orientation

INTERVENTIONS. NIC interventions for the client with COPD are listed in Chart 33-9. Most clients with COPD use nonsurgical management to improve or maintain gas exchange. Surgical management requires that the client meet strict criteria.

NONSURGICAL MANAGEMENT. The mainstays of COPD management include airway maintenance, monitoring, drug therapy, and oxygen therapy.

Airway Maintenance. The most important intervention to improve gas exchange is to maintain a patent airway. Keep the client's head, neck, and chest in alignment. Assist him or her to liquefy secretions and clear the airway of secretions.

Monitoring. Assess the hospitalized client with COPD at least every 2 hours, even when the purpose of hospitalization is not COPD management. Provide the prescribed oxygen, assess the client's response to treatment, and prevent complications.

If the client's condition continues to worsen despite treatment, more aggressive therapy is needed. Intubation and mechanical ventilation may be needed for clients in respiratory failure, including those who are unable to sustain spontaneous breathing patterns.

NIC **Oxygen Therapy.** Oxygen is prescribed for relief of hypoxemia (decreased blood oxygen levels) and hypoxia (decreased tissue oxygenation). The need for oxygen therapy and its effectiveness can be determined by arterial blood gas values and oxygen saturation by pulse oximetry. The client with COPD may need an oxygen flow of 2 to 4 L/min via nasal cannula or up to 40% via Venturi mask. The client who is hypoxemic and also has chronic hypercarbia requires lower levels of oxygen delivery, usually 1 to 2 L/min via nasal cannula.

CHART 33-9

NIC INTERVENTION ACTIVITIES for The Client with Chronic Obstructive Pulmonary Disease

Airway Management: *Facilitation of patency of air passages*

- Position client to maximize ventilation potential.
- Perform chest physical therapy, as appropriate.
- Remove secretions by encouraging coughing or by suctioning.
- Instruct how to cough effectively.
- Assist with incentive spirometer, as appropriate.
- Auscultate breath sounds, noting areas of decreased or absent ventilation and presence of adventitious sounds.
- Administer bronchodilators, as appropriate.
- Teach client how to use prescribed inhalers, as appropriate.
- Administer aerosol treatments, as appropriate.
- Administer ultrasonic nebulizer treatments, as appropriate.
- Administer humidified air or oxygen, as appropriate.
- Regulate fluid intake to optimize fluid balance.
- Position to alleviate dyspnea.
- Monitor respiratory and oxygenation status, as appropriate.

Cough Enhancement: *Promotion of deep inhalation by the client with subsequent generation of high intrathoracic pressures and compression of underlying lung parenchyma for the forceful expulsion of air*

- Monitor results of pulmonary function tests, particularly vital capacity, maximal inspiratory force, forced expiratory volume in 1 second (FEV_1), and FEV_1/FVC, as appropriate.
- Assist client to a sitting position with head slightly flexed, shoulders relaxed, and knees flexed.
- Encourage client to take several deep breaths.
- Encourage client to take a deep breath, hold it for 2 seconds, and cough two or three times in succession.
- Instruct client to inhale deeply several times, to exhale slowly, and to cough at the end of exhalation.

Oxygen Therapy: *Administration of oxygen and monitoring of its effectiveness*

- Clear oral, nasal, and tracheal secretions, as appropriate.
- Maintain airway patency.
- Set up oxygen equipment and administer through a heated, humidified system.
- Monitor the oxygen liter flow.
- Monitor position of oxygen delivery device.
- Periodically check oxygen delivery device to ensure that the prescribed concentration is being delivered.
- Monitor the effectiveness of oxygen therapy (e.g., pulse oximetry, ABGs), as appropriate.
- Ensure replacement of oxygen mask/cannula whenever the device is removed.
- Monitor client's ability to tolerate removal of oxygen while eating.
- Observe for signs of oxygen-induced hypoventilation.
- Monitor for signs of oxygen toxicity and absorption atelectasis.
- Monitor oxygen equipment to ensure that it is not interfering with the client's attempts to breathe.
- Monitor client's anxiety related to need for oxygen therapy.
- Monitor for skin breakdown from friction of oxygen device.
- Provide for oxygen when client is transported.
- Instruct client and family about use of oxygen at home.
- Arrange for use of oxygen devices that facilitate mobility and teach client accordingly.

Energy Management: *Regulating energy use to treat or prevent fatigue and optimize function*

- Determine client's physical limitations.
- Encourage verbalization of feelings about limitations.
- Monitor nutritional intake to ensure adequate energy resources.
- Consult with dietitian about ways to increase intake of high-energy foods.
- Monitor cardiorespiratory response to activity (e.g., tachycardia, other dysrhythmias, dyspnea, diaphoresis, pallor, hemodynamic pressures, and respiratory rate).
- Limit environmental stimuli (e.g., light and noise) to facilitate relaxation.
- Promote bedrest/activity limitation (e.g., increase number of rest periods).
- Arrange physical activities to reduce competition for oxygen supply to vital body functions (e.g., avoid activity immediately after meals).
- Assist client to schedule rest periods.
- Avoid care activities during scheduled rest periods.
- Plan activities for periods when the client has the most energy.
- Assist with regular physical activities (e.g., ambulation, transfers, turning, and personal care), as needed.
- Monitor client's oxygen response (e.g., pulse rate, cardiac rhythm, and respiratory rate) to self-care or nursing activities.
- Teach client and significant other techniques of self-care that will minimize oxygen consumption (e.g., self-monitoring and pacing techniques for performance of activities of daily living).
- Assist the client to identify tasks that family and friends can perform in the home to prevent/relieve fatigue.
- Assist the client in assigning priority to activities to accommodate energy levels.
- Assist client to identify preferences for activity.
- Evaluate programmed increases in levels of activities.

NIC intervention activities selected from Dochterman, J.M., & Bulechek, G.M. (Eds.). (2004). *Nursing interventions classification (NIC)* (4th ed.). St. Louis: Mosby.
ABG, Arterial blood gas.

A low arterial oxygen level is this client's primary drive for breathing. The use of continuous low-flow oxygen for the client with stage III or IV COPD has been shown to increase life span (Boyle & Locke, 2004; Wong, 2001). More information on oxygen therapy is found in Chapter 31.

Drug Therapy. Drug therapy for COPD involves the same inhaled and systemic drugs as for asthma. These drugs include beta-adrenergic agents, cholinergic antagonists, methylxanthines, corticosteroids, cromolyn sodium/nedocromil, and leukotriene modifiers (see Chart 33-5). The client with COPD is more likely to be taking systemic agents (in addition to inhaled drugs) than is the client with asthma. An additional drug class for COPD is the mucolytics, which thin secretions, making them easier to expectorate.

Mucolytic agents are prescribed for the client with thick, tenacious (sticky) mucous secretions. Nebulizer treatments with normal saline or with a mucolytic agent such as acetylcysteine (Mucosil, Mucomyst✱) or dornase alfa (Pulmozyme) and normal saline help thin secretions and facilitate expectoration. Guaifenesin (Organidin, Naldecon Senior EX) is a systemic mucolytic that is taken orally.

Stepped therapy is recommended for clients with chronic bronchitis or emphysema (Table 33-3). The key elements of stepped therapy include drug therapy, monitoring, and control of environmental irritants and allergens. The expected outcomes of stepped therapy are for the client to have more awareness of the disease and to participate in symptom management.

SURGICAL MANAGEMENT. Lung transplantation is performed for select clients with end-stage COPD. (See the lung transplantation section under Surgical Management [Cystic Fibrosis] on p. 608.) The more common surgical procedure for clients with COPD is lung reduction surgery.

TABLE 33-3 The Stepped Approach of Drug Therapy for COPD

Step	COPD Stage*	Drug Recommendations
1	I	Ipratropium 3-6 puffs four times daily by MDI with spacer. Beta$_2$ agonist for rescue as needed by MDI with spacer. (If symptoms are not well controlled, proceed to next step.)
2	II	Add beta$_2$ agonist (short-acting) 2-6 puffs q3-6h by MDI with spacer. Consider use of long-acting beta$_2$ agonist once daily. (If symptoms are not well controlled, proceed to next step.)
3	III	Add long-acting theophylline 200-400 mg PO twice daily for a therapeutic blood level of 8 to 12 mcg/mL. (If response is unsatisfactory, discontinue theophylline and proceed to the next step.)
4	IV	Add prednisone 40 mg PO daily. If client improves, taper dose to the lowest dose that manages symptoms. At lowest prednisone dose, consider an inhaled steroid.

MDI, Metered dose inhaler.
*Although the steps of therapy are correlated to COPD stage, client response is the best indicator for maintaining or changing steps.

Lung reduction surgery can improve gas exchange in the client with COPD. The goal of this surgery is improvement of gas exchange through removal of hyperinflated lung tissue. These areas of the lungs are filled with stagnant air that is not renewed with some atmospheric air (containing oxygen) during each respiratory cycle. Instead, this stagnant air continues to receive carbon dioxide until the level of carbon dioxide in the hyperinflated alveolus is the same as that in the capillary. Hyperinflated lung areas are useless for gas exchange. After successful lung reduction, most clients have at least a 75% improvement in FEV_1, decreased TLC and RV, and increased activity tolerance. Oxygen therapy may no longer be needed.

Preoperative Care. Clients are selected for this procedure on the basis of having end-stage emphysema, minimal chronic bronchitis, and stable cardiac function; being ambulatory and not dependent on a ventilator; not having pulmonary fibrosis, asthma, or late-stage cancer; and having been a nonsmoker for at least 6 months. The client must complete pulmonary rehabilitation before surgery to maximize lung and muscle function. The client must reach a state in which he or she is able to walk, without stopping, for 30 minutes at 1 mile/hr and maintain a 90% or better oxygen saturation level.

In addition to standard preoperative testing, the client having lung reduction surgery has tests to determine the location of greatest lung hyperinflation and poorest lung blood flow. These tests include pulmonary plethysmography, gas dilution, and perfusion scans.

Operative Procedures. Usually, lung reduction is performed on both lungs through either a large midline incision or a transverse anterior thoracotomy. Each lung is deflated separately and examined for color and texture differences. Normal lung tissue darkens to purple or gray when deflated and becomes more dense or rubbery in texture. Hyperinflated areas do not deflate, and they remain pink with a spongy texture. After areas to remove have been identified, the surgeon removes as much of this tissue as possible, sealing off and reinforcing the remaining normal lung tissue.

Postoperative Care. After lung reduction surgery, the client needs close monitoring for continuing respiratory problems as well as for usual postoperative complications. In addition to the usual care required after thoracotomy (see Surgical Management [Lung Cancer], p. 617), bronchodilator and mucolytic therapies are maintained initially. Pulmonary hygiene includes incentive spirometry 10 times per hour while awake, chest physiotherapy starting on the first day after surgery, and hourly pulmonary assessment.

Pain is usually managed by epidural delivery of opioids during the early period after surgery. This type of analgesic delivery reduces pain, limits sedation and cognitive dysfunction, and allows the client to more fully participate in pulmonary hygiene measures.

INEFFECTIVE BREATHING PATTERN

NOC **PLANNING: EXPECTED OUTCOMES.** The client with COPD is expected to achieve an effective breathing pattern that decreases the work of breathing. Indicators include the following:

- Respiratory rhythm within normal limits for the client's age
- Presence of synchronous thoracoabdominal movement
- Use of accessory muscles appropriate to the client's activity level
- Increased activity tolerance

INTERVENTIONS. Before any intervention, assess the client to determine the breathing pattern, especially the rate, rhythm, depth, and use of accessory muscles. The client with COPD relies more on accessory muscles than on the diaphragm for breathing. These muscles, however, are less efficient than the diaphragm, and the work of breathing increases. Determine whether there are any contributing factors to the increased work of breathing, such as respiratory infection. Most clients with COPD can benefit from some degree of pulmonary rehabilitation therapy. These interventions aim to improve the client's breathing efforts and decrease the work of breathing through the use of specific breathing techniques, positioning, exercise conditioning, and energy conservation.

Breathing Techniques. Diaphragmatic or abdominal and pursed-lip breathing techniques may be helpful for managing dyspneic episodes. The client uses these techniques, shown in Chart 33-10, during all activities. The amount of stale air in the lungs is reduced, and the client gains confidence and control in managing dyspnea. Teach these techniques when the client is free of dyspnea.

Diaphragmatic or Abdominal Breathing. In diaphragmatic breathing, the client consciously increases movement of the diaphragm. Lying on the back allows the abdomen to relax.

Pursed-Lip Breathing. Breathing through pursed lips uses the mild resistance of partially closed lips to prolong exhalation and to increase airway pressure. This technique delays airway compression and reduces air trapping.

CHART 33-10

CLIENT EDUCATION GUIDE

Breathing Exercises

Diaphragmatic or Abdominal Breathing

- Lie on your back with your knees bent.
- Place your hands or a book on your abdomen to create resistance.
- Begin breathing from your abdomen while keeping your chest still. You can tell if you are breathing correctly if your hands or the book rises and falls accordingly.

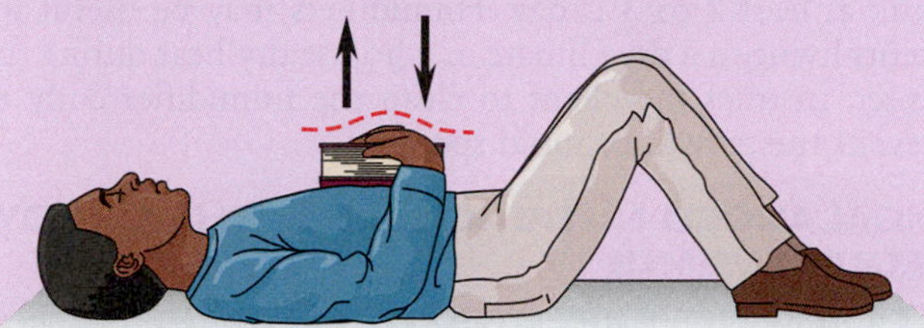

Pursed-Lip Breathing

- Close your mouth and breathe in through your nose.
- Purse your lips as you would to whistle. Breathe out slowly through your mouth, without puffing your cheeks. Spend at least twice the amount of time it took you to breathe in. Use your abdominal muscles to squeeze out every bit of air you can.
- Remember to use pursed-lip breathing during any physical activity. Always inhale before beginning the activity and exhale while performing the activity. Never hold your breath.

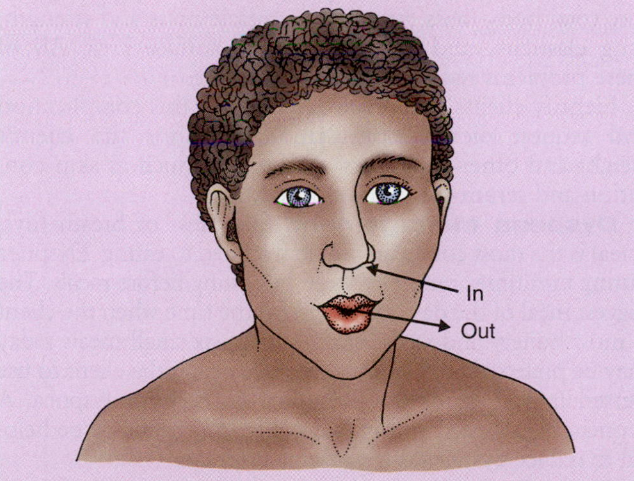

Pursed-lip breathing can be used during diaphragmatic or abdominal breathing.

Positioning. Assist the client to an upright position, with the head of the bed elevated. Various positions help alleviate dyspnea by increasing chest expansion, relaxing the chest muscles, and placing the diaphragm in the proper position to contract. These positions conserve energy by supporting the client's arms and upper body.

The client uses the standing position when there is no place to sit (Figure 33-11). Clients with COPD rely on use of accessory muscles for breathing. Supporting the thorax allows these muscles to work better.

Exercise Conditioning. Clients with exercise-induced shortness of breath respond to dyspnea by limiting their activity, even basic activities of daily living (ADLs). Over time, the muscles of ventilation and other large muscle groups weaken and are less efficient in the use of oxygen. The result is increased dyspnea with lower activity levels.

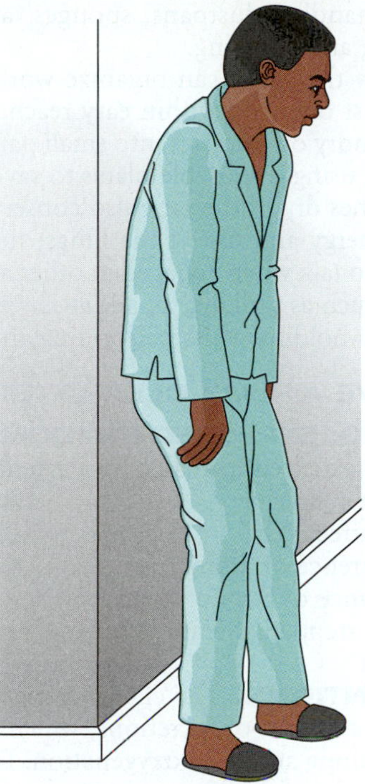

Figure 33-11 ■ The standing position that is used to help clients with chronic airflow limitation (CAL) to breathe. The client stands with back and hips against a wall and with the feet about 30 cm (12 inches) from the wall. The shoulders are relaxed and bent slightly forward.

Exercise conditioning of the large muscle groups or retraining of the ventilatory muscles may be part of a pulmonary rehabilitation program. Two techniques are isocapneic hyperventilation and resistive breathing. Isocapneic hyperventilation increases endurance. The client hyperventilates into a machine that controls the levels of oxygen and carbon dioxide. In resistive breathing, the client breathes against a set resistance. Resistive breathing increases ventilatory muscle strength and endurance.

Energy Conservation. Energy conservation is the planning and pacing of activities for maximal tolerance and minimal discomfort. Once the FEV_1 falls below 50% predicted, the client's ability to perform ADLs is limited. Ask the client to describe a typical daily schedule. Each activity is divided into its smaller parts to determine whether that task can be performed in a different way or at a different time of the day. Assist the client to plan and pace daily activities. Rest periods are paced between activities. Development of a personal chart outlining the day's activities and planned rest periods is helpful (see Chart 33-9).

Instruct the client to avoid working with the arms raised. Activities involving the arms decrease exercise tolerance because the accessory muscles of ventilation are then used to stabilize the arms and shoulders. Many activities involving the arms can be done sitting at a table leaning on the elbows. Teach the client to adjust work heights to reduce back strain and fatigue. Remind him or her to keep arm motions smooth and flowing to prevent jerky motions that waste energy. The use of adaptive tools for housework, such as long-handled dustpans, sponges, and dusters, reduces bending and reaching.

Suggest how the client can organize work spaces so that items used most often are within easy reach. Measures such as dividing laundry or groceries into small parcels that can be handled easily, using disposable plates to save washing time, and letting dishes dry in the rack also conserve energy. Talking requires energy and use of the lungs; therefore instruct the client not to talk when engaged in other activities that require energy, such as walking. In addition, teach him or her to avoid breath-holding while performing any activity.

INEFFECTIVE AIRWAY CLEARANCE

NOC **PLANNING: EXPECTED OUTCOMES.** The client with COPD is expected to maintain a patent airway. Indicators include the following:

- Coughs effectively
- No occurrence of aspiration
- Maintenance of SpO_2 of at least 88%
- Uses the stepped therapy approach to control manifestations

INTERVENTIONS. The client with COPD often has difficulty with removal of secretions, which results in compromised breathing and poor oxygenation. Excessive mucus also increases the risk for respiratory infections. Assess breath sounds routinely as part of physical assessment and before and after interventions. Careful use of drugs combined with controlled coughing, hydration, and postural drainage may help in airway clearance. If these measures fail, a tracheostomy may be needed on a temporary or permanent basis.

Controlled Coughing. Because the client with COPD has excessive mucus, coughing at specific times of the day is helpful. Teach the client to cough on arising in the morning to eliminate mucus that collected during the night. Coughing to clear mucous before mealtimes may facilitate a more pleasant meal. Coughing before bedtime may ensure clear lungs for a less interrupted night's sleep.

To cough effectively, the client sits in a chair or on the side of a bed with feet placed firmly on the floor. Instruct him or her to turn the shoulders inward and to bend the head slightly downward, hugging a pillow against the stomach. The client then takes a few deep breaths. After the third to fifth deep breath (in through the nose, out through pursed lips), instruct the client to bend forward slowly while coughing two or three times from the same breath. Observe the color, consistency, odor, and amount of secretions. On return to a sitting position, the client takes a comfortable deep breath. The entire coughing procedure is repeated at least twice. After coughing exercises, allow the client to rest; provide mouth care.

Chest Physiotherapy and Postural Drainage. Chest physiotherapy (PT) with postural drainage (Figure 33-12) helps move secretions into central airways, re-expand lung tissue, and promote efficient use of the ventilatory muscles. Chest PT combines chest percussion with vibration to loosen secretions. Postural drainage uses specific positions and gravity to help remove secretions. Postural drainage with chest PT, although helpful for some clients, is not used routinely on all clients with COPD.

Suctioning. Suctioning is performed only when abnormal breath sounds are present, not on a routine schedule. For the client with a weak cough, weak pulmonary muscles, and inability to expectorate effectively, the nurse or respiratory therapist performs nasotracheal suctioning. Assess the client for dyspnea, tachycardia, and dysrhythmias during the procedure. Assess for improved breath sounds after suctioning. Suctioning is discussed in detail in Chapter 31.

Positioning. Assist the client who can tolerate sitting in a chair out of bed for 1-hour periods two to three times a day. This position helps move secretions and keeps the diaphragm in a better position for ventilation.

Hydration. Unless hydration needs to be avoided for other health problems, instruct the client with COPD to drink at least 2 to 3 L/day. Humidifiers may be useful for clients living in a dry climate or who use dry heat during the winter. Instruct the client to clean the humidifier daily to prevent the growth of mold spores.

IMBALANCED NUTRITION: LESS THAN BODY REQUIREMENTS

NOC **PLANNING: EXPECTED OUTCOMES.** The client with COPD is expected to achieve and maintain a body weight within 10% of ideal. Indicators include the following:

- Maintains an appropriate weight/height ratio
- Maintains serum albumin or prealbumin within the normal range

INTERVENTIONS. The client with COPD often has food intolerance, nausea, early satiety, loss of appetite, and meal-related dyspnea. The increased work of breathing raises calorie and protein needs. These conditions lead to protein-calorie malnutrition for many clients. Malnourished clients lose total body mass, ventilatory muscle mass and strength, lung elasticity, and alveolar-capillary surface area. All of these problems reduce effective breathing.

Identify clients at risk for or who have this complication and request dietary consultation. Monitor the client's weight and other indicators of nutrition, such as skin condition and serum prealbumin levels.

Dyspnea Management. Shortness of breath (dyspnea) is the most common problem related to eating. Dyspnea during mealtimes can be reduced by resting before meals. The biggest meal of the day is planned for the time when the client is most hungry and well rested. Four to six small meals a day may be preferred to three larger ones. Instruct the client to use pursed-lip and abdominal breathing to alleviate dyspnea. A bronchodilator used 30 minutes before the meal may be helpful to reduce dyspnea due to bronchospasm.

Food Selection. Abdominal bloating and a feeling of fullness often prevent the client from eating a complete meal. Teach about foods that are easy to chew and not gas forming. Dry foods stimulate coughing, and foods such as milk and chocolate may increase the thickness of saliva and secretions. Advise the client to avoid these foods when symptomatic. Inform the client that caffeinated beverages should be avoided because they increase urine output and may lead to dehydration.

Urge the client to eat high-calorie, high-protein foods. Dietary supplements, such as Pulmocare, provide nutrition with reduced carbon dioxide production. If early satiety (feeling too "full" to eat) is a problem, advise the client to avoid drinking fluids before and during the meal.

Assistance with Feeding. Help the client who tires easily. Many clients do not have the energy to feed themselves when they are working hard to breathe and may not have the urge to eat. Oral hygiene before meals may increase appetite.

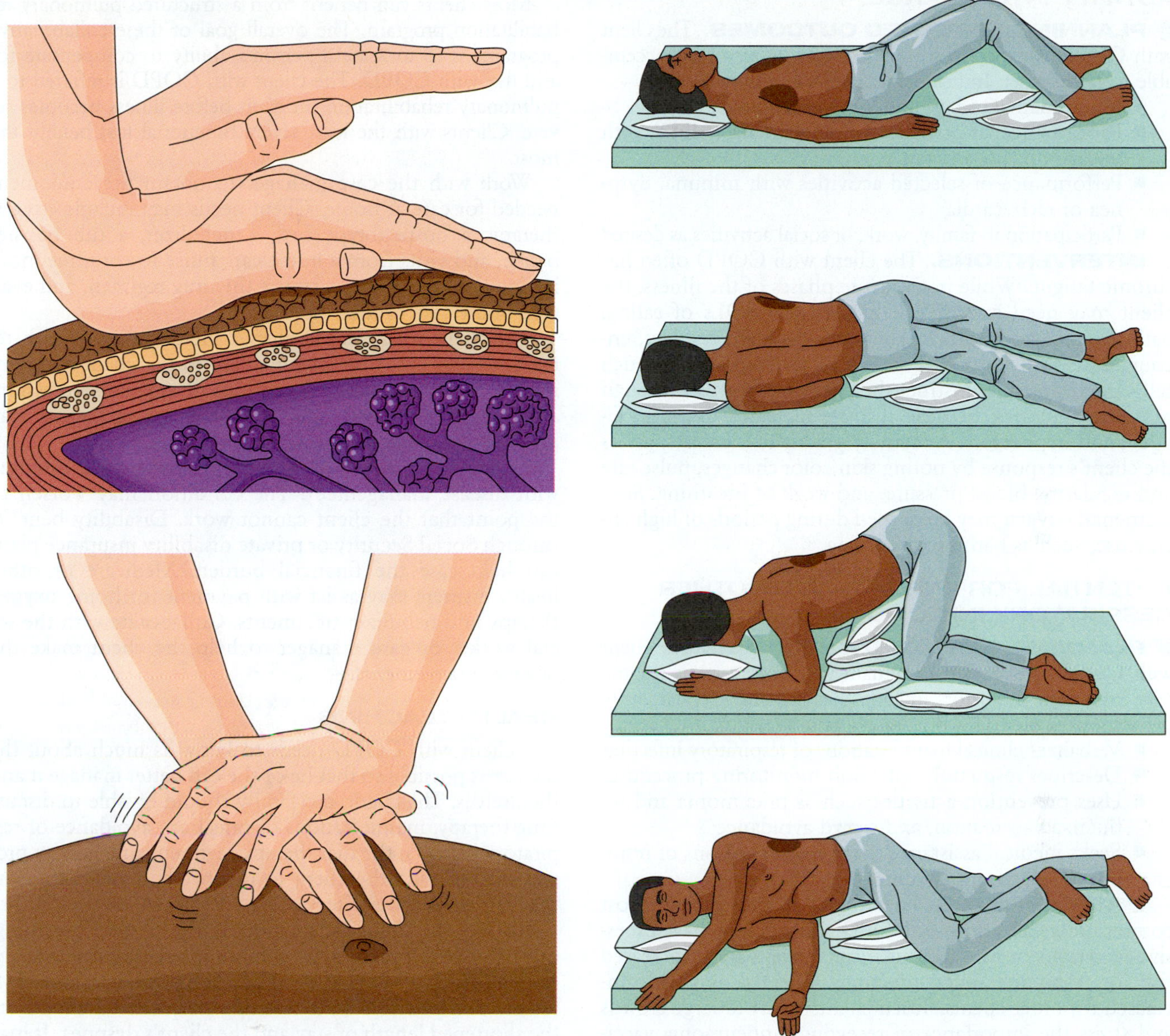

Figure 33-12 ■ Chest physiotherapy (chest PT) and postural drainage. *Left,* Percussion and vibration techniques. The nurse may use one or two hands with vibration, which is performed when the client exhales or coughs. *Right,* Positions for postural drainage of respiratory secretions.

ANXIETY

NOC PLANNING: EXPECTED OUTCOMES. The client with COPD is expected to have decreased anxiety. Indicators include that the client consistently demonstrates the following behaviors:

- Identifying factors that contribute to anxiety
- Identifying activities to decrease anxiety
- Verbalizing anxiety is reduced or absent

INTERVENTIONS. Clients with COPD often have increased anxiety during acute dyspneic episodes, especially if they feel as though they are choking on excessive secretions. Also, anxiety has been shown to cause dyspnea.

Psychological Interventions. If symptoms are worsened because of anxiety, it is important that the client understand this effect and has a plan for dealing with anxiety. Together with the client, develop a written plan that states exactly what the client should do if symptoms flare. Having a plan provides confidence and control in knowing what to do, which often helps reduce anxiety. Stress the use of pursed-lip and diaphragmatic breathing techniques during periods of anxiety or panic.

Family, friends, and support groups can be helpful. Recommend professional counseling, if needed, as a positive suggestion and in no way suggest that this need represents a failure of the client to cope. Stress that talking with a counselor can help identify techniques to maintain control over the dyspnea and feelings of panic.

Complementary and Alternative Therapy. Explore other approaches to help the client control dyspneic episodes and panic attacks. Examples include progressive relaxation, hypnosis therapy, and biofeedback. Biofeedback helps the client determine the impact of various stimuli on symptoms. Ultimately the client learns to relax and control these stimuli to avoid the aggravating symptoms.

ACTIVITY INTOLERANCE

NOC **PLANNING: EXPECTED OUTCOMES.** The client with COPD is expected to increase activity to a level acceptable to him or her. Indicators include the following:

- Maintenance of baseline SaO_2 with activity
- Performance of activities of daily living (ADLs) with no or minimal assistance
- Performance of selected activities with minimal dyspnea or tachycardia
- Participation in family, work, or social activities as desired

INTERVENTIONS. The client with COPD often has chronic fatigue. While in the acute phases of the illness, the client may need extensive help with the ADLs of eating, bathing, and grooming. As the acute problem resolves, encourage the client to pace activities and provide as much self-care as possible. Instruct the client not to rush through morning activities, because rushing increases dyspnea, fatigue, and hypoxemia. As activity gradually increases, assess the client's response by noting skin color changes, pulse rate and regularity, blood pressure, and work of breathing. Supplemental oxygen may be needed during periods of high energy use, such as bathing or walking.

POTENTIAL FOR PNEUMONIA OR OTHER RESPIRATORY INFECTIONS

NOC **PLANNING: EXPECTED OUTCOMES.** The client with COPD is expected to remain free from serious respiratory infection. Indicators include that the client consistently demonstrates the following behaviors:

- Verbalizes clinical manifestations of respiratory infection
- Describes respiratory infection monitoring procedures
- Uses prevention activities such as pneumonia and influenza vaccination, and crowd avoidance
- Seeks medical assistance when manifestations of respiratory infection first appear

INTERVENTIONS. Pneumonia is one of the most common complications of COPD. Clients who have excessive secretions or who have artificial airways are at increased risk for respiratory tract infections. The risk is greatly increased for older clients. Teach clients to avoid large crowds and stress the importance of receiving a pneumonia vaccination and a yearly influenza vaccine ("flu shot").

Community-Based Care

HOME CARE MANAGEMENT

Most clients with chronic obstructive pulmonary disease (COPD) are treated in the ambulatory care setting and cared for at home. When pneumonia or a severe exacerbation of the disease develops, the client usually returns home after treatment. For clients with advanced disease, however, 24-hour care may be needed for ADLs and for monitoring for acute episodes or progression of the illness. Clients may not be able to enjoy work or recreational activities because of severe dyspnea and fatigue. If home care is not possible, placement in a long-term care setting may be needed.

Hypoxemic clients can benefit from long-term use of oxygen at home. Home oxygen may be needed only during periods of exercise or sleep if hypoxemia occurs only during these times. Continuous, long-term oxygen therapy can reverse tissue hypoxia and decrease pulmonary vascular resistance. It can also improve cognitive ability and well-being. For more information on oxygen therapy, see Chapter 31.

Most clients can benefit from a structured pulmonary rehabilitation program. The overall goal of these collaborative programs is to increase a person's ability to compensate for and live with COPD. The client with COPD is referred to a pulmonary rehabilitation program before illness becomes severe. Clients with the least severe functional loss benefit the most.

Work with the case manager to obtain the equipment needed for care at home. Client needs may include oxygen therapy, a hospital-type bed, a nebulizer, a tub transfer bench, and visits from a home care nurse to continue monitoring the health status, review the drug regimen, and evaluate home care needs.

The client with COPD faces a lifelong disease with remissions and exacerbations. Explain to the client and family that he or she may have periods of anxiety, depression, and ineffective coping. The client who was a smoker may also have self-directed anger.

Financial concerns often increase anxiety and interfere with disease management. The condition may worsen to the point that the client cannot work. Disability benefits through Social Security or private disability insurance plans can help ease the financial burden. Medicare or other health insurers may assist with payment for home oxygen therapy and nebulizer treatments. Collaborate with the social worker or case manager to help the client make the needed arrangements.

HEALTH TEACHING

The client with COPD needs to know as much about the disease as possible so that he or she can better manage it and themselves. The client and family should be able to discuss drug therapy, manifestations of infection, avoidance of respiratory irritants, the diet therapy regimen, and activity progression. Instruct the client to identify and avoid stressors that can worsen the disease.

Instruct the client in techniques of pursed-lip breathing, diaphragmatic breathing, positioning, relaxation therapy, energy conservation, and coughing and deep breathing. Two factors that interfere with teaching hospitalized clients are the shortened length of stay and the client's dyspnea. It may be unrealistic to cover all of the topics in the education checklist during a single hospitalization. The primary nurse or case manager must coordinate teaching with the home care or clinic staff.

HEALTH CARE RESOURCES

Provide appropriate referrals as needed. Home care visits may be warranted, particularly if the client must use home oxygen therapy for the first time. Chart 33-11 lists assessment areas for the client with COPD at home. Referral to assistance programs, such as Meals on Wheels, can be helpful. Provide a list of support groups, as well as Better Breathing groups sponsored by the American Lung Association. If the client is having difficulty with smoking cessation and indicates the desire for assistance, make the referrals.

Critical Thinking Challenge

The client is a 68-year-old man with stage III COPD. He is being discharged to home on newly prescribed supplemental oxygen and is to start using a spacer with his inhaled drugs. He has concerns that the use of oxygen means that he is dying and that he will no longer be able to leave the house. He asks you if he should try to use the oxygen only when he feels severely breathless. Upon hearing that her husband is about to be discharged, his wife says "Not today. Home isn't ready for him yet."

1. What is your priority nursing interventions for this client and his wife?
2. Are this client's fears justified? Why or why not?
3. What will you teach this client about the use of oxygen therapy?
4. How will you address the wife's concerns?

evolve For suggested answer guidelines, go to http://evolve.elsevier.com/Iggy/.

Evaluation: Outcomes

Evaluate the care of the client with COPD on the basis of the identified nursing diagnoses and collaborative problems. The expected outcomes are that the client should:

- Attain and maintain gas exchange at a level within his or her chronic baseline values
- Achieve an effective breathing pattern that decreases the work of breathing.
- Maintain a patent airway
- Achieve and maintain a body weight within 10% of his or her ideal weight
- Have decreased anxiety

CHART 33-11

HOME CARE ASSESSMENT of
The Client with Chronic Obstructive Pulmonary Disease

Assess respiratory status and adequacy of ventilation.
- Measure rate, depth, and rhythm of respirations.
- Examine mucous membranes and nail beds for evidence of hypoxia.
- Determine use of accessory muscles.
- Examine chest and abdomen for paradoxical breathing.
- Count number of words client can speak between breaths.
- Determine need and use of supplemental oxygen. (How many liters per minute is the client using?)
- Determine level of consciousness and presence/absence of confusion.
- Auscultate lungs for abnormal breath sounds.
- Measure oxygen saturation by pulse oximetry.
- Determine sputum production, color, and amount.
- Ask about activity level.
- Observe general hygiene.
- Measure body temperature.

Assess cardiac status.
- Measure rate, quality, and rhythm of pulse.
- Check dependent areas for edema.
- Check neck veins for distention with the client in a sitting position.
- Measure capillary refill.

Assess nutritional status.
- Weight maintenance, loss, or gain
- Food and fluid intake
- Use of nutritional supplements
- General condition of the skin

Assess client's and caregiver's adherence and understanding of illness and treatment, including the following:
- Correct use of supplemental oxygen
- Correct use of inhalers
- Medication schedule and side effects
- Manifestations to report to the health care provider
- Use of pursed-lip and diaphragmatic breathing techniques
- Scheduling of rest periods and priority activities
- Participation in rehabilitation activities

- Increase activity to a level acceptable to him or her
- Avoid serious respiratory infections

Specific indicators for these outcomes are listed for each nursing diagnosis and collaborative problem under the Planning and Implementation section (see earlier).

CYSTIC FIBROSIS

PATHOPHYSIOLOGY

Cystic fibrosis (CF) is a genetic disease that affects many organs and lethally impairs pulmonary function. Although this disorder is present from birth and is first seen in early childhood, many clients now live into adulthood.

The underlying problem of CF is blocked chloride transport in the cell membranes. The error in chloride transport causes the formation of mucus that has little water content. The thick, sticky mucus causes problems in the lungs, pancreas, liver, salivary glands, and testes. The mucus plugs up glands in these organs, causing atrophy and organ dysfunction. Nonpulmonary problems include pancreatic insufficiency with malnutrition and intestinal obstruction, poor growth, male sterility, and cirrhosis of the liver. These primary problems cause a multitude of secondary problems. The primary cause of death in the client with CF is respiratory failure.

The pulmonary problems of CF result from the constant presence of thick, sticky mucus and are the most serious complications of the disease. The mucus narrows airways, reducing airflow. The constant presence of mucus results in chronic respiratory tract infections, chronic bronchitis, and chronic dilation of the bronchioles (bronchiectasis). Lung abscesses are common. Over time, the bronchioles distend and have increased numbers (hyperplasia) of mucus-producing cells and increased mucus-producing cell size (hypertrophy). Complications include pneumothorax, arterial erosion and hemorrhage, and respiratory failure.

Etiology and Genetic Risk

CF is an autosomal recessive disorder in which both gene alleles must be mutated for the disease to be expressed. The CF gene is located on chromosome 7 and produces a protein that controls chloride movement across cell membranes. There is great variation in the severity of CF; however, life expectancy is always considerably reduced, with an average of 33 years. People with one mutated allele are carriers and have few or no symptoms of CF but can pass the abnormal allele on to their children. Currently, more than 1000 different mutations have been identified. The inheritance of different mutations is thought to be responsible for the wide variation in disease severity.

Incidence/Prevalence

The disorder is most common among white individuals, and about 4% are carriers. CF is very rare among African Americans or Asians. Males and females are affected equally.

COLLABORATIVE MANAGEMENT

Assessment

Usually cystic fibrosis (CF) is diagnosed in childhood. The major diagnostic test is sweat chloride analysis. The defect in chloride movement prevents absorption of sodium chloride in the sweat glands; thus more chloride than normal is present in the sweat. The sweat chloride test is positive for CF when the chloride level in the sweat ranges between 60 and 200 mEq/L (mmol/L), compared with the normal value of 5 to 35 mEq/L.

NONPULMONARY MANIFESTATIONS

The adult client with CF is usually smaller and thinner than average. Other manifestations include abdominal distention, gastroesophageal reflux, rectal prolapse, foul-smelling stools, and **steatorrhea** (excessive fat in stools). The client may be malnourished and have many vitamin deficiencies. As pancreatic function decreases, the client has symptoms of diabetes mellitus from loss of insulin production.

PULMONARY MANIFESTATIONS

The pulmonary problems caused by CF are progressive. The respiratory infections are frequent or chronic with periods of exacerbations. Clients usually have chest congestion, limited exercise tolerance, cough, sputum production, use of accessory muscles, and decreased pulmonary function (especially FVC and FEV_1). Chest x-rays show persistent infiltrate and an increased anteroposterior (AP) diameter.

During an acute exacerbation or when the disease progresses to end stage, the client has increased chest congestion, reduced activity tolerance, increased crackles, increased cough, increased sputum production (often with hemoptysis), and severe dyspnea. Fatigue increases in proportion with the dyspnea. Arterial blood gas (ABG) studies show acidosis with greatly reduced partial pressure of arterial oxygen (PaO_2), increased partial pressure of arterial carbon dioxide ($PaCO_2$), increased bicarbonate levels, and low pH.

When infection is present, the client has fever, an elevated white blood cell count, and decreased oxygen saturation. Other manifestations of infection include tachypnea, tachycardia, intercostal retractions, weight loss, and increased fatigue.

Interventions

The client with CF needs daily therapy to slow disease progress and enhance gas exchange. There is no cure for CF.

NONSURGICAL MANAGEMENT. The management of the client with CF is complex and lifelong. Nutritional management focuses on weight maintenance, vitamin supplementation, diabetes management, and pancreatic enzyme replacement. Pulmonary management is focused on preventive maintenance and management of pulmonary exacerbation.

Preventive/Maintenance Therapy. The client with CF uses a regimen of chest physiotherapy, positive expiratory pressure, active cycle breathing technique, and an individualized regular exercise program. Pulmonary function tests (PFTs), especially FEV_1, are monitored regularly. Maintenance drugs include bronchodilators, anti-inflammatory agents, mucolytics, and antibiotics.

Exacerbation Therapy. Exacerbation therapy is needed when the client with CF has a change in manifestations from baseline. Such changes include increased chest congestion, decreased activity tolerance, increased or new-onset crackles, and at least a 10% decrease in FEV_1. Other manifestations occurring with exacerbation include increased sputum production with bloody or purulent sputum, increased frequency and duration of coughing, decreased appetite, weight loss, fatigue, decreased SaO_2, and ventilatory muscle retractions. Often infection is present and the client also has fever, increased lung infiltrate on chest x-ray, and an elevated white blood cell count.

Every attempt is made to avoid having the client with CF mechanically ventilated. Treatment focuses on airway clearance, increased oxygenation, and antibiotic therapy. Supplemental oxygen is prescribed on the basis of SaO_2 levels. Heliox delivery of 50% oxygen and 50% helium may improve gas exchange and oxygen saturation. The respiratory therapist initiates airway clearance techniques (ACTs) four times a day. Bronchodilator and mucolytic therapies are intensified (higher doses given more frequently than for maintenance). Steroidal anti-inflammatory agents are started or increased.

Depending on the severity of the exacerbation, a 10- to 14-day course of oral antibiotics may be prescribed. If the exacerbation is more severe, aerosolized tobramycin is prescribed. If oral/inhaled antibiotics are not effective, or if the exacerbation is very severe, IV antibiotics are used, usually an aminoglycoside, such as tobramycin and colistin or meropenem (Merrem).

As specialized treatment for CF improves and life span increases, other problems may occur. Clients may have bronchiole bleeding from lung arteries. Interventional radiology may be needed to embolize the bleeding arterial branches. Clients with CF may undergo this procedure repeatedly to control hemoptysis. See Chapter 39 for information on interventional radiology vascular procedures.

SURGICAL MANAGEMENT. The surgical management of the client with CF involves lung and/or pancreatic transplantation. *These procedures do not cure the disease, because the genetic defect in chloride transport and production of thick, sticky mucus remains.* Rather, the client has reduced manifestations initially and then has gradual progression of the disease. Transplantation extends life by 10 to 20 years, depending on other factors.

Fewer lung transplants are performed compared with transplantation of other solid organs. The problem is related to the scarcity of available lungs. In addition, many of the people who could benefit from lung transplantation have serious problems in other organs that make extended surgical procedures dangerous.

Lung transplant procedures include a lobe or a single lung transplantation, as well as double-lung transplantation. The type of procedure is determined by the client's age and overall condition, the cause of the lung problem, and the life expectancy after transplantation. Usually, the client with CF has a unilateral or bilateral lobe transplant from a living-related donor.

Preoperative Care. Many factors are considered before lung transplantation surgery. Recipient and donor criteria vary from one program to another, but some criteria are universal.

Recipient Criteria. The person who will receive the transplant, the **recipient,** must have severe, irreversible lung damage. It is important, however, that the client be well enough to survive the surgery. Usually clients must be younger than 55 years of age, although transplantation is considered on an individual basis. The following are exclusion criteria:

- Severe psychiatric disorders or self-destructive tendency
- Proven history of noncompliance or poor compliance with medical regimens

- Current cancer or cancer within the last 5 years
- Systemic infection
- Irreversible heart, kidney, or liver damage/disease
- Presence of any problem that would be made worse by immunosuppression

Donor Criteria. The following are donor criteria, regardless of whether the lung tissue is obtained from a cadaver or from a living-related donor:

- Infection free
- Cancer free
- Healthy lung tissue
- Close tissue match with the recipient
- Same blood type as the recipient

When the donor is living-related, the following are additional criteria:

- Age is younger than 55 years.
- Donor has normal cardiac function.
- Pulmonary function will remain adequate after tissue removal.
- The donor has had no previous chest surgery.
- Donor is psychologically stable.
- Donor has not been coerced into this situation.

Teaching. Regardless of the disease process that led to the need for lung transplantation, two activities are important before surgery. These activities are teaching the client the expected regimen of pulmonary hygiene to be used in the period immediately after surgery and assisting the client in a pulmonary muscle strengthening/conditioning regimen.

Operative Procedures. The client may or may not need to be placed on cardiopulmonary bypass, depending on the exact procedure. The client having single-lung or lobe transplantation usually does not need bypass. The client having double-lung transplantation needs cardiopulmonary bypass.

The most common incision used for lung transplantation is a transverse thoracotomy ("clamshell") for best access. The diseased lung or lungs are removed. The new lobes, lung, or lungs are placed in the chest cavity with **anastomoses** (connections) made to the proper airways (trachea, mainstem bronchus, or secondary bronchus) and blood vessels. Usually, lung transplantation surgery is completed within 4 to 6 hours.

Postoperative Care. The client is intubated for at least 48 hours. In addition, chest tubes and arterial lines are in place. Much of the care needed is the same as that for any thoracic surgery.

Major problem areas after lung transplantation are bleeding, infection, and transplant rejection. Bleeding is most common in clients who had cardiopulmonary bypass with anticoagulation. Usually the client remains in the intensive care unit for several days following transplantation.

Immunosuppressive drug regimens must be started immediately after surgery, which increases the risk for infection. The drugs generally used for routine long-term immunosuppressive therapy after organ transplantation are combinations of very specific immunosuppressants (cyclosporine [Sandimmune]), less specific immunosuppressants (azathioprine [Imuran] or mycophenolate mofetil [CellCept]), and one of the corticosteroids, such as prednisone (Apo-Prednisone✱, Deltasone✱) or prednisolone (Delta-Cortef). Corticosteroids are avoided in the first 10 to 14 days after surgery because of their negative impact on the healing process. (See Chapter 23 for more information on antirejection therapy.)

PRIMARY PULMONARY HYPERTENSION

PATHOPHYSIOLOGY

Pulmonary hypertension can occur as a complication of other lung disorders. Primary pulmonary hypertension (PPH) occurs in the absence of other lung disorders, and its cause is unknown although exposure to some drugs increases the risk. This disorder is rare and occurs mostly in women between the ages of 20 and 40 years.

The pathologic problem in PPH is blood vessel constriction with increasing vascular resistance in the lung. Pulmonary blood pressure rises and blood flow decreases, leading to poor perfusion and hypoxemia. Eventually, the right side of the heart fails **(cor pulmonale)** from the continuous workload of pumping against the high pulmonary pressures. Without treatment, death usually occurs within 2 years after diagnosis.

Genetic Considerations

Although most cases of primary pulmonary hypertension (PPH) are sporadic with no known cause, about 6% of people who develop PPH also have a close relative with the disorder. This type of PPH is considered to be "familial," in that genetics probably play a role but no single gene has been identified. In performing a pulmonary assessment for any client with breathing problems, especially young women, ask whether any family members have PPH. It is suggested that these relatives have baseline pulmonary function tests performed.

◆COLLABORATIVE MANAGEMENT

◆Assessment

The most common early manifestations are dyspnea and fatigue in an otherwise healthy adult. Some clients also have angina-like chest pain. Table 33-4 lists the classification of PPH.

Diagnosis is made from the results of right-sided heart catheterization showing elevated pulmonary pressures. Other test results suggesting pulmonary hypertension include abnormal ventilation-perfusion scans and pulmonary function tests (PFTs) showing reduced functional pulmonary volumes with reduced diffusion capacity, and spiral computed tomography (CT).

◆Interventions

Nonsurgical interventions that reduce pulmonary pressures and slow the development of cor pulmonale involve drugs that dilate pulmonary vessels and prevent clot formation. Warfarin (Coumadin) therapy is taken daily to achieve an International Normalized Ratio (INR) of 1.5 to 2.0. Calcium channel blockers, such as nifedipine (Procardia) and diltiazem (Cardizem) have been used to dilate blood vessels. These agents, however, cause general vessel dilation and some degree of hypotension. Prostacyclin agents provide the best specific dilation of pulmonary

TABLE 33-4 Severity Classification for Pulmonary Hypertension

Class	Manifestations
I	Pulmonary hypertension diagnosed by pulmonary function tests and right-sided cardiac catheterization No limitation of physical activity Moderate physical activity does not induce dyspnea, fatigue, chest pain, or light-headedness
II	No manifestations at rest Mild to moderate physical activity induces dyspnea, fatigue, chest pain, or light-headedness
III	No or slight manifestations at rest Mild (less than ordinary) activity induces dyspnea, fatigue, chest pain, or light-headedness
IV	Dyspnea and fatigue present at rest Unable to carry out any level of physical activity without manifestations Manifestations of right-sided heart failure apparent (dependent edema, engorged neck veins, enlarged liver)

Data from Eells, P. (2004). Advances in prostacyclin therapy for pulmonary arterial hypertension. *Critical Care Nurse, 24*(2), 42-54.

blood vessels. Continuous infusion of a naturally occurring prostacyclin agent, epoprostenol (Flolan), through a small IV pump reduces pulmonary pressures and increases lung blood flow. An alternate therapy is the delivery of a synthetic prostacyclin, treprostinil (Remodulin) by subcutaneous infusion through a microinfusion pump is also effective.

When the heart has undergone some hypertrophy and cardiac output has fallen, the client may be started on a regimen of digoxin (Lanoxin) and diuretics. Oxygen therapy is used when dyspnea is continuous or uncomfortable. These therapies do not cure the disorder; they just improve function and reduce symptoms.

Surgical management of primary pulmonary hypertension involves whole-lung transplantation. When cor pulmonale also is present, the client may need a combined heart-lung transplantation. It is not known whether the process of pulmonary vasoconstriction can begin again in the transplanted lungs or if the transplant is a "cure."

INTERSTITIAL PULMONARY DISEASES

The category of interstitial pulmonary diseases contains a variety of lung disorders, also called **fibrotic lung** diseases, that have some features in common. All affect the alveoli, blood vessels, and surrounding support tissue of the lungs rather than the airways. Thus these disorders are **restrictive** (preventing good expansion and recoil of the gas exchange unit) rather than obstructive. With restrictive disease, the lung tissues thicken, causing reduced gas exchange and "stiff" lungs that do not expand well. Unlike obstructive problems, air trapping does not occur and the client does not develop a "barrel chest." Often the onset of these disorders is slow and dyspnea is the most common manifestation.

Sarcoidosis

PATHOPHYSIOLOGY

Sarcoidosis is a granulomatous disorder of unknown cause that can affect any organ, but the lung is involved most often. Sarcoidosis develops over time with growths called **granulomas** forming in the lungs. Granulomas contain lymphocytes, macrophages, epithelioid cells, and giant cells.

Pulmonary sarcoidosis involves autoimmune responses in which the normally protective T-lymphocytes increase and cause damaging actions in lung tissue. Alveolar cells are the targets of the damaging actions. No single cause for T-lymphocyte activation has been identified, although infection and genetic predisposition appear to play a role. Alveolar inflammation **(alveolitis)** occurs from the presence of immune cells in the alveoli. Chronic inflammation causes **fibrosis** (scar tissue formation in the lungs). The fibrosis reduces **lung compliance** (elasticity) and the ability to exchange gases. **Cor pulmonale** (right-sided cardiac failure) is often present, because the heart can no longer pump effectively against the stiff, fibrotic lung.

The disease usually affects young adults. Manifestations include enlarged lymph nodes in the hilar area of the lungs, lung infiltrate on chest x-ray, skin lesions, and eye lesions. The first indication of disease may be an abnormal chest x-ray in an otherwise healthy client. The most common symptoms include cough, dyspnea, hemoptysis, and chest discomfort. In many clients, the illness resolves permanently. Others may have progressive pulmonary fibrosis and severe systemic disease.

COLLABORATIVE MANAGEMENT

Assessment

Sarcoidosis is suspected in the client who has a cough, dyspnea, and abnormal chest x-ray but is otherwise asymptomatic. Other conditions to rule out before diagnosing sarcoidosis are lung infections and cancer. Fiberoptic bronchoscopy may also be used in the diagnosis of this disorder (see Chapter 30).

Sarcoidosis is staged on the basis of x-ray findings. Higher stages have greater damage and more widespread disease. Pulmonary function studies often show a restrictive pattern of decreased lung volumes and impaired diffusing capacity. Irreversible lung changes develop in 10% to 15% of clients. Clients who develop severe restrictive disease may also develop secondary pulmonary hypertension.

Interventions

The goal of therapy is to lessen symptoms and prevent fibrosis. Management varies. If the client is asymptomatic and has normal pulmonary function, no treatment is given. The presence of manifestations; decreased total lung capacity (TLC), diffusing capacity, or forced vital capacity (FVC); involvement of other organs; and hypercalcemia are indicators for treatment.

Corticosteroids are the main type of therapy. Dosages vary from 40 to 60 mg daily with tapering doses over 6 to 8 weeks, to a maintenance dose of 10 to 15 mg for 6 months. Further therapy may occur over 12 months. Follow-up and monitoring include assessment of symptom severity, pulmonary function studies, chest x-rays, a complete blood count, serum creatinine, serum calcium, and urinalysis. Teach the client about side effects of steroid therapy and other aspects of physical care as indicated.

Idiopathic Pulmonary Fibrosis

PATHOPHYSIOLOGY

Idiopathic pulmonary fibrosis is a common restrictive lung disease. The typical client is an older adult with a history of cigarette smoking or chronic exposure to inhalation irritants such as metal particles, dust, organic chemicals, and wood fires. Unlike sarcoidosis, pulmonary fibrosis is highly lethal. Most clients have progressive disease with few remission periods. Even with proper treatment, clients usually survive less than 5 years after diagnosis.

Pulmonary fibrosis is an example of excessive wound healing. Once lung injury occurs, an inflammatory process begins tissue repair. The inflammation continues beyond normal healing time, causing extensive fibrosis and scarring. These changes thicken alveolar tissues, making gas exchange difficult.

COLLABORATIVE MANAGEMENT

Assessment

The onset of disease is slow, with early symptoms of mild dyspnea on exertion. Pulmonary function tests show decreased FVC. As the fibrosis progresses, the client becomes more dyspneic and hypoxemia becomes severe. Eventually, the client needs high levels of oxygen and often is still hypoxemic. Respirations are rapid and shallow.

Interventions

The goal of therapy is to slow the fibrotic process and manage dyspnea. Corticosteroids and other immunosuppressants are the mainstays of therapy. Immunosuppressant drugs include cytotoxic drugs such as cyclophosphamide (Cytoxan, Neosar, Procytox✱), azathioprine (Imuran), chlorambucil (Leukeran), or methotrexate (Folex). These drugs have many side effects, including immunosuppression, nausea, and lung and liver damage. Starting drug therapy early is critical, even though not all clients respond to therapy. Even among those who have a response to therapy, the disease continues to progress and leads to death by respiratory failure.

Lung transplantation is a curative therapy; however, the selection criteria, cost, and availability of organs make this option unlikely for most clients.

The client and family need support and help with community resources after diagnosis. The health care team assists the client and family in understanding the disease process and maintaining hope for control of the fibrosis. It is important to prevent respiratory infections. Teach the client and family about the manifestations of infection and encourage them to avoid respiratory irritants, crowds, and those with known infections.

Home oxygen is needed by the time the client becomes symptomatic because significant fibrosis has already occurred. Instruct him or her about oxygen use as a continuous therapy. Fatigue is a major problem. Instruct the client and family about energy conservation measures (see Energy Conservation [Chronic Obstructive Pulmonary Disease] on p. 603). Activity limitations and rest help reduce the work of breathing and oxygen consumption (see Chart 39-9).

Support the client's need to be as independent as possible and encourage him or her to pace activities and accept assistance as needed. The disease is costly because the client is often unable to work and may need home care.

> **Meeting HEALTHY PEOPLE 2010 Objectives**
>
> **TOBACCO USE**
>
> *Objective 3.1: Reduce to 13%, the proportion of adults (18 and older) who use tobacco.*
>
> Teach the client who smokes cigarettes the following techniques to quit smoking:
>
> - Make a list of the reasons you want to stop smoking (e.g., your health and the health of those around you, saving money, social reasons).
> - Set a date to stop smoking and keep it. Decide whether you are going to begin to cut down on the amount you smoke or are going to stop "cold turkey." Whatever way you decide to do it, keep this important date!
> - Ask for help from those around you. Find someone who wants to quit smoking and "buddy up" for support. Look for assistance in your community, such as formal smoking cessation programs, counselors, and certified acupuncture specialists or hypnotists.
> - Consult your health care provider about nicotine replacement therapy (i.e., patch, gum, etc.).
> - Remove ashtrays and lighters from your view.
> - Talk to yourself! Remind yourself of all the reasons you want to quit.
> - Think of a way to reward yourself with the money you save from not smoking for a year.
> - Avoid places that might tempt you to smoke. If you are used to having a cigarette after meals, get up from the table as soon as you are finished eating. Think of new things to do at times when you used to smoke.
> - Find activities that keep your hands busy: needlework, painting, gardening, even holding a pencil.
> - Take five deep breaths of clean, fresh air through your nose and out your mouth if you feel the urge to smoke.
> - Keep plenty of healthy, low-calorie snacks, such as fruit and vegetables, on hand to nibble on. Try sugarless gum or mints as a substitute for tobacco.
> - Drink at least eight glasses of water each day.
> - Begin an exercise program with the approval of your health care provider. Be aware of the positive, healthy changes in your body since you stopped smoking.
> - List the many reasons why you are glad that you quit. Keep the list handy as a reminder of the positive things you are doing for yourself.
> - Think of each day without tobacco as a major accomplishment. It is!!

In the later stages of the disease, the focus is to reduce the sensation of dyspnea. This is often accomplished with the use of oral, parenteral, or nebulized morphine. Provide information about hospice, which supports and coordinates resources to meet the needs of the client and family when the prognosis for survival is less than 6 months.

OCCUPATIONAL PULMONARY DISEASE

PATHOPHYSIOLOGY

Exposure to occupational or environmental fumes, dust, vapors, gases, bacterial or fungal antigens, and allergens can result in a variety of respiratory disorders. Depending on the degree, frequency, and intensity of exposure, and on the specific disease, clients may have acute reversible effects or chronic lung disease. All occupational pulmonary diseases are made worse by cigarette smoking. Thus smoking cessation efforts are very important (see the Meeting Healthy People 2010 Objectives box above).

CHART 33-12

KEY FEATURES of
Common Occupational Pulmonary Diseases

Disease and Category	Causes and Manifestations
Occupational Asthmas	
Latency (allergic) asthma	Airway narrowing related only to workplace exposures Atopic allergic response to industrial irritants Develops after a period of exposure (from several weeks to several years) Characterized by airflow limitation Usually resolves when exposure ceases Obstructive disease
Irritant-induced asthma	Manifestations only in the workplace First onset usually within 24 hours of exposure Common irritants: chlorine, ammonia, and phosgene Characterized by sloughing of epithelium, thickening of the basement membranes, and mucosal inflammation Early manifestations: cough, wheeze, and dyspnea High exposures can lead to pulmonary edema, acute respiratory distress syndrome, and death Permanent tissue changes in most cases Obstructive and restrictive disease
Pneumoconiosis	
Silicosis	Chronic fibrosis from long-term inhalation of silica dust Found among people working in mines, stone quarries, foundries, and in the following industries: glass-making, pottery, sandblasting, tile and brick making, soap and polishes, and manufacture of filters Characterized by nodule formation between alveoli, leading to fibrosis Manifestations: dyspnea on exertion, fatigue, weight loss, reduced lung volume, and upper lobe fibrosis Restrictive disease
Coal miner's disease (black lung disease)	Massive deposits of coal dust in the lungs leading to diffuse fibrosis Develops earlier among miners who smoke Early manifestations are similar to bronchitis Emphysema is a late development Restrictive disease
Diffuse Interstitial Fibrosis	
Asbestosis	Occurs among people who work in asbestos mines, building construction/remodeling, and shipyards Characterized by diffuse pleural thickening and diaphragmatic calcification Restrictive disease
Talcosis	Occurs among people who work in industries that manufacture paint, ceramics, roofing materials, cosmetics, and rubber goods Restrictive disease
Berylliosis	Occurs among people who work in industries where metal is heated (steel mills, welding) or metal is machined, creating dust Has a genetic component for increased susceptibility to disease after beryllium exposure Restrictive disease
Extrinsic Allergic Alveolitis	
"Farmer's lung" "Bird fancier's lung" "Machine operator's lung"	Hypersensitivity pneumonitis as an immunologic response to inhaling dust or chemical that contains bacterial or fungal antigens Characterized by formation of granulomas with central necrosis in the alveoli and surrounding blood vessels Restrictive disease

Many occupational diseases have an onset of symptoms long after the initial exposure to the offending agent. The client's personal history can provide clues about the presence and cause of occupational pulmonary diseases. Common occupational pulmonary diseases include occupational asthma, pneumoconiosis, diffuse interstitial fibrosis, and extrinsic allergic alveolitis. Chart 33-12 lists the key features of these disorders.

COLLABORATIVE MANAGEMENT

Assessment

Consider an occupational cause for all clients with new-onset asthma or dyspnea. Obtain a thorough history of occupational exposure and onset of symptoms because there may or may not be a latency period between exposure and onset of symptoms. Determine whether the symptoms are acute or chronic. Ask the client about the use of inhalation protection and about cigarette smoking.

Interventions

Prevention is important to avoiding disability from occupationally related disease. Stress the importance of using special respirators and ensuring adequate ventilation when working in potentially harmful environments.

The client with occupational asthma with a latency period should be removed from the site of exposure, transferred to a job without exposure, and treated with medications for asthma. Nursing care is similar to the care for

TABLE 33-5 Features of the Major Types of Lung Cancer

Category and Type	Characteristics
Small cell lung cancer (SCLC)	20% of all lung cancers 99% association with cigarette smoking Fast growing Usually metastatic at time of diagnosis Paraneoplastic syndromes common Surgical resection not helpful Treatment regimen: combination chemotherapy
Non–small cell lung cancer (NSCLC)	Surgical resection helpful for stage I and II disease Combination chemotherapy helpful Targeted therapy helpful Radiation used for cure if disease is confined to the chest
Epidermoid carcinoma	30% of all lung cancers Strongly associated with cigarette smoking Slower growing, less invasive Found in bronchi and peripheral lung tissue
Adenocarcinoma	30%-35% of all lung cancers Incidence similar for smokers and nonsmokers Most common lung cancer in women Metastasis occurs early Found in peripheral lung tissue
Large cell	≈10% of all lung cancers Slow growing Found in peripheral lung tissue

asthma not caused by the workplace environment. Refer the client to a social worker, who provides information regarding compensation and pensions.

Nursing interventions for clients with occupational lung restrictive disease are the same as for those with emphysema. Hypoxemic clients require supplemental oxygen. In addition, respiratory therapies to promote sputum clearance are essential.

LUNG CANCER

PATHOPHYSIOLOGY

Lung cancer is a leading cause of cancer-related deaths worldwide. In the United States, more deaths from lung cancer occur each year than from prostate cancer, breast cancer, and colon cancer combined. The American Cancer Society estimates that more than 186,000 new cases of lung cancer are diagnosed each year and that more than 165,000 deaths occur each year from lung care. The overall 5-year survival rate for all clients with lung cancer is only 14%. This poor long-term survival rate is due to the fact that most lung cancers are diagnosed at a late stage, when metastasis is present. Only 15% of clients have small tumors and localized disease at the time of diagnosis (American Cancer Society, 2005).

Despite many advances in cancer treatment, the prognosis for lung cancer remains poor unless the tumor can be removed completely by surgery. Treatment of lung cancer is often aimed toward relieving symptoms **(palliation)** rather than cure, because of the presence of metastasis.

More than 90% of all primary lung cancers arise from the bronchial epithelium. These cancers are collectively called

TABLE 33-6 Endocrine Paraneoplastic Syndromes Associated with Lung Cancer

Ectopic Hormone	Manifestation
Adrenocorticotropic hormone (ACTH)	Cushing's syndrome
Antidiuretic hormone	Syndrome of inappropriate antidiuretic hormone (SIADH) ▪ Weight gain ▪ General edema ▪ Dilution of serum electrolytes
Follicle-stimulating hormone (FSH)	Gynecomastia
Parathyroid hormone	Hypercalcemia
Ectopic insulin	Hypoglycemia

bronchogenic carcinomas. Lung cancers can be classified according to their histologic cell type as small cell lung cancer (SCLC), epidermoid (squamous cell) cancer, adenocarcinoma, and large cell cancer (Table 33-5). The last three types are now referred to as non–small cell lung cancer (NSCLC) because of their similar responses to treatment. Chapter 27 discusses the general mechanisms and processes of cancer development.

Metastasis

Lung cancers **metastasize** (spread) by direct extension, through the blood and invading lymph glands and vessels. Tumors in the bronchial tubes can grow and obstruct the bronchus partially or completely. Tumors in other areas of lung tissue can grow so large that they can cause airway obstruction by compressing the airway. Tumors in the edges of the lungs spread and can compress the alveoli, nerves, blood vessels, and lymph vessels.

The patterns of metastasis depend on the type of tumor cell and the location of the tumor. Lung lymph nodes, as well as more distant lymph nodes, can be invaded.

Hematogenous (bloodborne) metastasis of lung cancer is due to invasion of blood vessels in the lungs. Tumor pieces **(emboli)** spread to distant body areas. These sites of metastasis include the bone, liver, brain, and adrenal glands.

Additional manifestations, known as **paraneoplastic syndromes,** complicate certain lung cancers. The paraneoplastic syndromes are caused by hormones secreted by tumor cells. Paraneoplastic syndrome commonly occurs with SCLC. Tables 33-6 and 33-7 list the endocrine and nonendocrine paraneoplastic syndromes, respectively, that may occur with lung cancer.

Staging

Lung cancer is staged at diagnosis to assess the size and extent of the disease. These factors are correlated to survival rate. The staging of lung cancer is based on the TNM system (T, primary *t*umor; N, regional lymph *n*odes; M, distant *m*etastasis). Table 33-8 shows the TNM system for lung cancer staging. Higher numbers represent later stages and less chance for cure or long-term survival.

Etiology and Genetic Risk

Lung cancers occur as a result of repeated exposure to inhaled substances that cause chronic tissue irritation or inflammation. Cigarette smoking is the major risk factor and

TABLE 33-7 Nonendocrine Paraneoplastic Syndromes Associated with Lung Cancer

Tissue/System	Manifestation
Connective tissue	Arthralgia Digital clubbing
Hematologic system	Anemia Leukocytosis Thrombocytopenia purpura Polycythemia Thrombocytosis
Neuromuscular system	Peripheral neuropathy Carcinomatous myopathy Cortical cerebellar degeneration Seizure Polymyositis Myasthenia-like syndrome
Integumentary system	Dermatomyositis Scleroderma Acanthosis nigricans
Vascular system	Thrombophlebitis Nonbacterial endocarditis
Renal system	Arterial thrombosis Nephrotic syndrome Proteinuria

is responsible for 85% of all lung cancer deaths (American Cancer Society, 2004). The risk for lung cancer is directly related to the total exposure to cigarette smoke as determined by the number of years of smoking and number of cigarettes smoked per day. Pipe and cigar smoking also increase risk. The incidence of lung cancer decreases when smoking stops, and after 15 years of smoking cessation, it approaches that of those who have never smoked. About 50,000 ex-smokers, however, develop lung cancer in the United States each year.

Nonsmokers exposed to "passive," or "secondhand," smoke also have a greater risk for lung cancer than do nonsmokers who are minimally exposed to cigarette smoke. Passive smoke has many of the carcinogens found in inhaled, or "mainstream," tobacco smoke.

Other risk factors for lung cancer include chronic exposure to asbestos, beryllium, chromium, coal distillates, cobalt, iron oxide, mustard gas, petroleum distillates, radiation, tar, nickel, and uranium. Air pollution that contains benzopyrenes and hydrocarbons also increase the risk for lung cancer.

Genetic Considerations

Variation is seen in lung cancer development among people with similar smoking histories, suggesting that genetic factors can influence susceptibility. Differences in two different genes are associated with differences in personal susceptibility to lung cancer. One of the P450 enzymes, CYP2D6, activates carcinogens present in tobacco. People who have a mutated CYP2D6 gene do not activate the tobacco carcinogen and are less susceptible to lung cancer even if they smoke. About 10% of the U.S. population has this "resistance to lung cancer" gene. Another enzyme, glutathione S transferase, detoxifies and clears carcinogens from the body. Women who are missing this active enzyme are less able to clear carcinogens and are thus at greater risk for lung cancer if they are exposed to tobacco smoke. Men missing this enzyme do not have a greater risk for lung cancer.

TABLE 33-8 TMN Stage Grouping for Lung Cancer

Stage	Tumors	Nodes	Distant Metastasis
Occult carcinoma	T_x	N_0	M_0
Stage 0	T_{IS}	Carcinoma in situ	
Stage I	T_1 T_2	N_0 N_0	M_0 M_0
Stage II	T_1 T_2	N_1 N_1	M_0 M_0
Stage IIIa	T_3 T_3 $T_{1\text{-}3}$	N_0 N_1 N_2	M_0 M_0 M_0
Stage IIIb	Any T T_4	N_3 Any N	M_0 M_0
Stage IV	Any T	Any N	M_1

From Mountain, C.F., Greenberg, M.D., & Fraire, A.E. (1991). Tumor stages in non–small cell carcinoma of the lung. *Chest, 99*(5), 1258-1260.

Incidence/Prevalence

Lung cancer is a major health problem throughout the world. It represents 13% of new cancers in both men and women.

HEALTH PROMOTION/ILLNESS PREVENTION

Primary prevention for lung cancer is directed at reducing tobacco smoking. Educational strategies start with elementary school children to discourage them from beginning to smoke. Nurses are actively involved in encouraging nonsmokers not to begin to smoke, in promoting smoking cessation programs, and in establishing a smoke-free environment. Such educational strategies have been successfully used in the United States (see the Meeting Healthy People 2010 Objectives box on p. 611). Encourage nonsmokers to avoid passive, or secondhand, smoke by avoiding environmental exposure.

Teach workers in industrial settings about safety precautions, such as wearing specialized masks and protective clothing, to reduce occupational hazards. Encourage people who are at high risk for lung cancer development to seek frequent health examinations.

Urge clients being treated for lung cancer to quit smoking. The actual diagnosis of the disease and its treatment time represent "teachable moments." Nearly 80% of lung cancer survivors (those who live 5 years or longer after diagnosis) who quit smoking remain nonsmokers. Many survivors also engage in other healthy lifestyle changes. (See the Evidence-Based Practice for Nursing box on p. 615.)

COLLABORATIVE MANAGEMENT

Assessment

HISTORY

Ask the client about risk factors, including smoking, hazards in the workplace, and warning signals (Table 33-9). Have the client describe how many packs of cigarettes per day have been smoked for how many years to determine the pack-year smoking history.

Ask about the presence of lung cancer manifestations, such as hoarseness, cough, sputum production, hemoptysis, shortness of breath, or change in endurance. Many mani-

EVIDENCE-BASED PRACTICE for Nursing

Lung cancer survivors participate in healthy behaviors

Evangelista, L., Sarna, L., Brecht, M., Padilla, G., & Chen, J. (2003). Health perceptions and risk behaviors of lung cancer survivors. *Heart & Lung, 32*(2), 131-139.

This study sought to determine to what degree lung cancer survivors maintain the healthy lifestyle changes started at the time of diagnosis. Survivorship was defined as a minimum of 5 disease-free years after the initial cancer treatment. One hundred and forty-two survivors of non–small cell lung cancer (NSCLC) were asked to complete a battery of questionnaires to determine their perceptions of their own health status, their maintenance of healthy lifestyle changes, and exposure to high-risk environments. The reported smoking status was confirmed by urinary cotinine biomarker. This test measures the presence of a nicotine metabolite in the urine. Ingestion of nicotine in any form results in the formation of cotinine as a metabolite.

Participants ranged from 5 to 21 years of survival after initial diagnosis with a mean survival of 10 years. The majority of participants (70%) perceived their overall health status to be in the good to excellent range. Most participants who used tobacco had quit at diagnosis and were able to maintain this important lifestyle change. Only 19 participants (13%) continued to use tobacco after diagnosis. More than one fourth of the participants reported continued exposure to secondhand smoke.

Level of Evidence: 3—Well-designed trial without randomization—cohort study.

Critique. The study was well designed and implemented for its purpose. Using multiple tools with established validity and reliability increase the credibility of the findings. Major strengths include the large sample size, use of a highly sensitive biomarker to confirm smoking status, and the direct collection of physical parameters to establish body mass index.

Implications for Nursing. The overall 5-year survival rate for clients with NSCLC is only 20%. About 2% of these clients develop a second primary lung cancer. Smoking cession is linked to longer survivorship after a lung cancer diagnosis and treatment. Lung cancer diagnosis represents a "teachable moment" when the benefits of smoking cessation are perceived as high. Even though it is gratifying to find that most of the participants who stopped smoking were able to maintain this lifestyle change, a substantial number continued to smoke. Even more disturbing was the number of participants who remain exposed to secondhand smoke. Nurses need to stress the benefits of smoking cessation and of avoiding secondhand smoke in this population.

festations are common and may have been present for years. Ask the client to describe any recent changes in symptoms or if position affects symptoms.

Assess for chest pain or discomfort, which can occur at any stage of tumor development. Chest pain may be localized or on just one side and can range from mild to severe. Ask about any sensation of fullness, tightness, or pressure in the chest, which may suggest obstruction. A piercing chest pain or pleuritic pain may occur on inspiration. Pain radiating to the arm results from tumor invasion of nerve plexuses in advanced disease.

PHYSICAL ASSESSMENT/CLINICAL MANIFESTATIONS—PULMONARY

OBSERVATION. Manifestations of lung cancer are often nonspecific and appear late in the disease process. Specific manifestations depend on the type and location of the tumor. Chills, fever, and cough may be related to pneumonitis or bronchitis that occur with obstruction. Assess sputum quantity and quality. Blood-tinged sputum may occur with bleeding from a tumor. Hemoptysis is a later finding in the course of the disease. If infection or necrosis is present, sputum may be purulent and copious.

TABLE 33-9 Warning Signals Associated with Lung Cancer

- Hoarseness
- Change in respiratory pattern
- Persistent cough or change in cough
- Blood-streaked sputum
- Rust-colored or purulent sputum
- Frank hemoptysis
- Chest pain or chest tightness
- Shoulder, arm, or chest wall pain
- Recurring episodes of pleural effusion, pneumonia, or bronchitis
- Dyspnea
- Fever associated with one or two other signs
- Wheezing
- Weight loss
- Clubbing of the fingers

Breathing patterns may be labored or painful. An obstructive breathing pattern may occur as prolonged exhalation alternating with periods of shallow breathing. Rapid, shallow breathing occurs with pleuritic chest pain and an elevated diaphragm. Inspiratory efforts are reduced in advanced disease. Look for abnormal retractions, the use of accessory muscles, flared nares, stridor, and asymmetric diaphragmatic movement on inspiration. Dyspnea and wheezing may be present with airway obstruction. Ask about the client's level of dyspnea at rest, with activity, and in the supine position (orthopnea).

PALPATION. You may find areas of tenderness or masses when palpating the chest wall. Increased vibrations felt on the chest wall **(fremitus)** indicate areas of the lung where airspaces are replaced with tumor or fluid. Fremitus is decreased or absent when the bronchus is obstructed. The trachea may be displaced from midline if a mass is present in the area.

PERCUSSION. Lung areas with masses sound dull or flat rather than hollow or resonant on chest percussion.

AUSCULTATION. Breath sounds may change with the presence of a tumor. Wheezes indicate partial obstruction of airflow in passages narrowed by tumors. Decreased or absent breath sounds indicate complete obstruction of an airway by a tumor or fluid. Increased loudness or sound intensity of the voice while listening to breath sounds indicates increased density of lung tissue from tumor compression. A pleural friction rub is heard when inflammation also is present.

PHYSICAL ASSESSMENT/CLINICAL MANIFESTATIONS—NONPULMONARY

Many other systems can be affected by lung cancer and have changes at the time of diagnosis. Heart sounds may be muffled by a tumor or fluid around the heart (cardiac tamponade). Dysrhythmias may occur as a result of hypoxemia or direct pressure of the tumor on the heart. Cyanosis of the lips and fingertips or clubbing of the fingers may be present (see Figure 33-10).

Bones become thin with tumor invasion and break easily. The client may have bone pain or pathologic fractures.

Late manifestations of lung cancer usually include fatigue, weight loss, anorexia, dysphagia, and nausea and vomiting. Superior vena cava syndrome may result from tumor pressure in or around the vena cava. This syndrome is an emergency (see Chapter 28). Lethargy and somnolence may develop, and the client may have confusion or personality changes as a result of brain metastasis. Bowel and bladder tone or function may be affected by tumor spread to the spine and spinal cord.

PSYCHOSOCIAL ASSESSMENT

The poor prognosis for lung cancer has made it a much-feared disease. Lung cancer manifestations, especially dyspnea, add to the client's fear and anxiety. The client with a history of cigarette smoking may feel guilt and shame. Convey acceptance and interact with the client in a nonjudgmental way.

Few clients with lung cancer are cured or live 5 years after diagnosis. Many are given limited palliative treatment for symptom relief. Fear of pain and death is common.

DIAGNOSTIC ASSESSMENT

The diagnosis of lung cancer is made by direct examination of cancer cells. Cytologic examination of early morning sputum specimens may identify tumor cells; however, cancer cells may not be present in the sputum. When pleural effusion is present, fluid can be obtained by thoracentesis for cytology.

Lung lesions may be first identified on chest x-rays. Computed tomography (CT) examinations are then used to identify the lesions more clearly. Usually, the entire chest is scanned at 5- to 10-mm slices and the suspicious areas are then scanned at 1- to 2-mm slices for the highest resolution.

Fiberoptic bronchoscopy provides direct visibility of the tracheobronchial tree. Specimens and bronchial brushings can be obtained with this technique, especially when lesions are located within or close to an airway. Needle biopsy during bronchoscopy also may be used to obtain cancer cells.

A thoracoscopy may be performed through a video-assisted thoracoscope entering the chest cavity via small incisions through the chest wall. This procedure allows direct visualization of the lung tissue. To identify metastasis in mediastinal lymph nodes, a mediastinoscopy may be performed through a small chest incision.

Other diagnostic studies may be needed to determine how widely the cancer has spread. Such tests include needle biopsy of lymph nodes, direct surgical biopsy, and thoracentesis with pleural biopsy. Magnetic resonance imaging (MRI) and radionuclide scans of the liver, spleen, brain, and bone help determine the location of metastatic tumors. Pulmonary function tests and arterial blood gas (ABG) analysis help determine the overall respiratory status. Positron emission tomography (PET) scanning is becoming the most thorough way to find metastases. Together, these tests help determine the extent of the cancer and the best methods to treat it.

Interventions for Cure

Interventions for the client with lung cancer can be aimed at curing the disease, increasing the client's survival time, and enhancing the client's quality of life through palliation. Both nonsurgical and surgical interventions are used to achieve these aims. Some clients with lung cancer may undergo interventions for all three aims at different stages in the disease process.

NONSURGICAL MANAGEMENT

Chemotherapy. Chemotherapy is often the treatment of choice for lung cancers, especially small cell lung cancer (SCLC). It may be used alone or as adjuvant therapy in combination with surgery for non–small cell lung cancer (NSCLC). Table 33-10 lists common agents used in combination for treatment of lung cancer. The exact combination of drugs used may vary depending on the response of the tumor and the overall health of the client.

TABLE 33-10 Common Chemotherapy Agents Used in the Treatment of Lung Cancer*

Generic Name	Trade Name
Carboplatin	Paraplatin
Cisplatin	Platinol
Docetaxel	Taxotere
Gemcitabine	Gemzar
Irinotecan	Camptosar
Paclitaxel	Taxol
Vinorelbine	Navelbine

*This listing is not comprehensive and only lists the most commonly used current agents. Regimens vary. Combinations usually include a platinum-based drug with an antimitotic. See Table 28-6 for more information on chemotherapeutic agents.

Side effects that occur with chemotherapy for lung cancer include **alopecia** (hair loss), nausea and vomiting, open sores on mucous membranes **(mucositis),** immunosuppression, anemia, and **thrombocytopenia** (decreased numbers of platelets).

Reassure clients that hair loss is temporary. Hair regrowth begins about 1 month after chemotherapy is completed. Hair loss can be disguised by the use of wigs, scarves, turbans, and caps.

The chemotherapy agents used for lung cancer treatment are **emetogenic** (inducing nausea and vomiting). Many effective antiemetic drugs are available. Usually one or more antiemetics are given before and after chemotherapy. Drugs used to control chemotherapy-induced nausea and vomiting are listed in Chart 28-5. Client response to antiemetic therapy varies, and the drug combinations are individualized for best effect.

Frequent mouth assessment and oral hygiene are key in managing mucositis. Stress the importance of good, frequent oral hygiene, including tooth cleaning and mouth rinsing. Instruct clients to use a soft-bristled toothbrush or disposable mouth sponges and to avoid using dental floss and water-pressure gum cleaners (such as a WaterPik).

Immunosuppression, which greatly increases the risk for infection, is the major dose-limiting side effect of chemotherapy for lung cancer. Immunosuppression can be managed by the use of biological response modifiers (BRMs) to stimulate bone marrow production of immune system cells. Teach the client and family about precautions to take to reduce the client's chances of developing an infection (see Chart 28-8). (See Chapter 28 for more information about chemotherapy and associated nursing care.)

Genetic Considerations

An experimental treatment for advanced NSCLC takes advantage of genetic differences in cancer cells. A "targeted therapy" is erlotinib (Tarceva). This once-a-day tablet inhibits the enzyme tyrosine kinase from activating the epidermal growth factor receptors on lung cancer cells. With the receptor inactivated, cancer cell growth is slowed significantly. Although this drug is too new to know whether its use will cure NSCLC, it is extending the life spans of some clients by as much as 2 years. Because this drug targets the cancer cell receptors, the side effects on normal cells are minimal.

Radiation Therapy. Radiation therapy can be an effective treatment for locally advanced lung cancers confined to the chest. Best results are seen when radiation is used in addition to surgery or chemotherapy. Radiation may be performed before surgery to shrink the tumor and make resection easier.

Usually radiation therapy for lung cancer is performed daily for a 5- to 6-week period. Only the areas thought to have cancer are in the radiation path. The immediate side effects of this treatment are skin irritation and peeling, fatigue, nausea, and taste changes. Some clients have esophagitis during therapy. Narrowing of the esophagus can occur as a late response to radiation therapy for lung cancer.

Skin care in the radiation-treated area can be difficult. If the area has been marked with a dye to outline the areas for radiation, instruct the client not to wash off the markings. The use of ink or dye markings is rare, with most cancer centers using small permanent tattoos to mark the area. Instruct clients not to use lotions or ointments on the skin of the chest unless the radiologist prescribes them. Because skin in the radiation path is more sensitive to sun damage, advise clients to avoid direct skin exposure to the sun during treatment and for at least 1 year after radiation is completed.

SURGICAL MANAGEMENT. Surgery is the main treatment for stage I and stage II NSCLC. Total removal of a non–small cell primary lung cancer is undertaken in hope of achieving a cure. If complete resection is not possible, the surgeon removes the bulk of the tumor. The specific surgery depends on the stage of the cancer and the client's overall health and functional status. The procedure may involve only a thoracotomy with tumor removal. More often, lung cancer surgery involves removal of a lung segment, lobe **(lobectomy),** or entire lung **(pneumonectomy).**

Preoperative Care. The goals of care before surgery are to relieve anxiety and promote the client's participation (see Chapter 20 for routine preoperative care). Encourage the client to express fears and concerns, reinforce the surgeon's explanation of the surgical procedure, and provide education related to what is expected after surgery. Teach about the probable location of the surgical incision, shoulder exercises, and about the chest tube and drainage system (except after pneumonectomy).

Operative Procedures. Three types of incisions can be made depending on the location of the cancer: posterolateral, anterolateral, and median sternotomy (Figure 33-13). The incisions are large and are held open with retractors during surgery, contributing to pain after surgery.

A segmental resection **(segmentectomy)** is a lung resection that includes the bronchus, pulmonary artery and vein, and tissue of the involved lung segment or segments, which are divisions of lobes. A **wedge resection** is removal of the peripheral portion of small, localized areas of disease. A **lobectomy** is the removal of an entire lung lobe. A **pneumonectomy** is the removal of an entire lung, including all blood vessels. The bronchus to that lung is severed and sutured.

Postoperative Care. General care of the client after thoracotomy is reviewed in the Plan of Care on pp. 618 to 622. Care after surgery for clients who have undergone thoracotomy (except for pneumonectomy) requires closed-chest drainage to drain air and blood that accumulate in the pleural space. A **chest tube,** a drain placed in the pleural space to restore intrapleural pressure, allows re-expansion of the lung (Figure 33-14). The chest tube also prevents air and fluid from returning to the chest. The drainage system consists of one or more chest tubes or drains, a collection container placed below the chest level, and a water seal to keep air from entering the chest. The drainage system may use actual bottles (Figure 33-15) or, more often, a disposable self-contained system (Figure 33-16). The basic principles of gravity and pressure are the same with both systems.

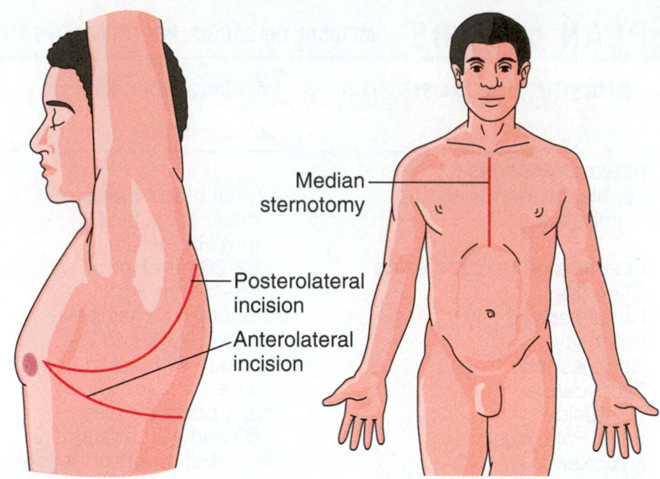

Figure 33-13 ■ Common incision locations for partial or total pneumonectomy.

Chest Tube Placement. The tip of the tube used to drain air is placed near the front lung apex (see Figure 33-14). The tube that drains liquid is placed on the side near the base of the lung. After lung surgery, two tubes, anterior and posterior, are used. The puncture wounds are covered with airtight dressings.

The chest tube is connected to about 6 feet of tubing that leads to a collection device or bottle placed several feet below the chest. The tubing allows the client to turn and move easily. Keeping the collection device below the chest allows gravity to drain the pleural space. When two chest tubes are inserted, they are joined by a Y-connector near the client's body; the 6 feet of tubing are attached to the Y-connector.

Drainage System. The chest drainage system uses a water seal mechanism that acts as a one-way valve to prevent air or liquid from moving back into the chest cavity. Earlier chest drainage consisted of one-, two-, and three-bottle systems. These bulky glass bottle systems have been replaced with one-piece disposable chest drainage devices. The Pleur-Evac system is a common device using a one-piece disposable plastic unit with three chambers. It duplicates the three-bottle system.

The three-bottle system (see Figure 33-15) is used to explain the principles and actions of water-seal chest drainage. The three bottles are connected to one another. The tube(s) from the client is(are) connected to the first bottle (or chamber) in the series of three. This bottle (chamber) is the collection container. The second bottle (chamber) in the series is the water seal to prevent air from moving back up the tubing system and into the chest. The third bottle (chamber), when suction is applied, is the suction regulator.

BOTTLE ONE. In setting up the system, bottle one (nearest to the client) does not at first have fluid in it. The tubing

Text continued on p. 623.

PLAN of CARE — MEDICAL DIAGNOSIS: POSTOPERATIVE THORACOTOMY

NURSING DIAGNOSIS NO. 1 ■ Impaired Gas Exchange

RELATED FACTORS

Ventilation-perfusion imbalance

DEFINING CHARACTERISTICS

Dyspnea
Nasal flaring
Irritability
Restlessness
Tachycardia
Confusion
Skin: Pale, dusky
Hypoxemia
Breathing: Abnormal rate; abnormal depth
Arterial blood gases: Abnormal

Expected Outcomes

Arterial blood gases remain: pO_2 80-100 mm Hg; $pHCO_3$ 22-26 mm Hg; pCO_2 35-45 mm Hg
Arterial pH remains between 7.35 and 7.45
Has skin with warm undertones
Has a pulse between 60 and 100 beats/min
No verbal report or observation of irritability
No verbal report or observation of restlessness
Has a respiratory rate that remains between 11 and 22 breaths/min
Has respirations that remain regular and deep

Nursing Interventions	Rationales
NIC Airway Management	
D Place the client in semi-Fowler's position, if possible.	Semi-Fowler's position ensures that abdominal contents do not press against the diaphragm and restrict chest expansion.
Encourage the client to cough frequently, or suction the client as necessary.	Coughing or suction will rid the airway of secretions.
D Encourage the client to take slow, deep breaths; to turn; and to cough.	Effective aeration and cough will help rid the body of secretions. Frequent position changes will prevent secretions from pooling in one area.
Assist the client with an incentive spirometer, as appropriate.	Incentive spirometry encourages the client to deep breathe.
Administer humidified air or oxygen, as appropriate.	Humidified air will soothe respiratory passages. Increased oxygen will elevate the amount of oxygen in the alveoli available for exchange.
Regulate fluid intake to optimize fluid balance.	Fluids will help keep lung secretions thin and easier to cough out of the airways.
NIC Respiratory Monitoring	
D Monitor rate, rhythm, depth, and effort of respirations.	Changes in respiratory rate, rhythm, depth, or effort may signal a descent into respiratory failure.
Note chest movement, watching for symmetry, use of accessory muscles, and supraclavicular and intercostal muscle retractions.	The use of accessory muscles indicates increased respiratory effort.
Note location of trachea.	A deviated trachea may indicate a tension pneumothorax.
Auscultate breath sounds, noting areas of decreased/absent ventilation and the presence of adventitious sounds.	Absent breath sounds or adventitious breath sounds indicate poor gas exchange or poor movement of air through the airways.
Monitor for increased restlessness, anxiety, and air hunger.	A change in the client's level of consciousness is the earliest sign of deterioration in effective oxygenation.
Note changes in SaO_2, SvO_2, end tidal CO_2, and ABG values, as appropriate.	These tests are indicators of the effectiveness of gas exchange or gas transport.
D Monitor for dyspnea and the events that improve and worsen it.	Events that improve dyspnea should be encouraged, and events that worsen dyspnea need to be avoided.
NIC Oxygen Therapy	
Maintain airway patency.	Oxygen requires free passage to the lungs.
Monitor the effectiveness of oxygen therapy, as appropriate.	Pulse oximetry and ABGs reflect oxygen concentrations in the blood or attached to red blood cells.

D Indicates tasks that can be delegated to unlicensed assistive nursing personnel at the discretion of the nurse.

PLAN of CARE MEDICAL DIAGNOSIS: POSTOPERATIVE THORACOTOMY—*cont'd*

NURSING DIAGNOSIS NO. 1 ■ Impaired Gas Exchange—*cont'd*

	Expected Outcomes	Nursing Interventions	Rationales
		Monitor the client's anxiety related to the need for oxygen therapy.	Oxygen deprivation causes the sympathetic nervous system to secrete stress hormones, which are interpreted subjectively as anxiety.
		Provide for oxygen when the client is transported.	Portable oxygen should be provided when transporting a client who requires supplemental oxygen.
		Other Interventions	
		Advise the client to limit caffeine intake.	Caffeine causes diuresis and increases the risk of dehydration.
		Check chest tubes hourly.	Tube connections must be checked to ensure sterility and patency.
		Tape tubing junctions.	Taping prevents accidental disconnections.
		Position the drainage tube to prevent kinks and large loops of tubing.	Kinks and large loops of tubing can block drainage and prevent lung re-expansion.
		Observe the type and amount of drainage hourly, and mark the fluid level and time on the drainage system.	Notify the physician if more than 100 mL/hr drains. Excessive drainage may indicate hemorrhage.
		Check the water seal chamber for unexpected bubbling.	Bubbling may indicate an air leak in the system.
		Administer antibiotics as prescribed.	Infection of the lung tissue causes inflammation and exudate, which interferes with oxygen diffusion into the vascular system.
		Encourage the client to have a pneumococcal vaccination and to be revaccinated if the original vaccination is 5 to 10 years old.	The vaccine will lower the severity of illness and reduce the risk of serious complications or death.

NURSING DIAGNOSIS NO. 2 ■ Acute Pain

	Expected Outcomes	Nursing Interventions	Rationales
RELATED FACTORS		NIC **Pain Management**	
Injury agents (biologic, chemical, physical, psychological)	Denies experiencing pain greater than a 5 on a 0 to 10 pain scale	Perform a comprehensive assessment of pain to include location, characteristics, onset/duration, frequency, quality, intensity or severity of pain, and precipitating factors.	A plan for pain management must be based on the client's unique responses to pain.
DEFINING CHARACTERISTICS	No verbal report or observation of guarding or protective gestures		
Verbal or coded report of pain	No verbal report or observation of alteration in sleep patterns		
Observed evidence of pain	No verbal report or observation of alteration in activity level		
Behavior: Guarding			
		Reduce or eliminate factors that precipitate or increase the pain experience.	Preventing a pain experience is preferred to trying to control or eliminate pain.
		Select and implement a variety of measures to facilitate pain relief, as appropriate.	Pharmacologic, nonpharmacologic, and interpersonal strategies may provide pain relief depending on the client's unique responses to the therapeutic interventions.

Continued

PLAN of CARE MEDICAL DIAGNOSIS: POSTOPERATIVE THORACOTOMY—*cont'd*

NURSING DIAGNOSIS NO. 2 ■ Acute Pain—*cont'd*

Expected Outcomes	Nursing Interventions	Rationales
	Use pain control measures before pain becomes severe.	Medicating the client in a timely manner prevents pain from reaching acutely unpleasant levels.
	Teach the use of nonpharmacologic techniques before, after and, if possible, during painful activities; before pain occurs or increases; and along with other pain relief measures.	Nonpharmacologic techniques help the client establish a sense of control over his or her pain experience.
	NIC **Analgesic Administration**	
	Monitor vital signs before and after administering narcotic analgesics with first-time dose or if unusual signs are noted.	Narcotic analgesics may depress respirations or cause other adverse effects.
	Choose the IV rather than the IM route for frequent pain medication injections, when possible.	The IV route avoids tissue trauma and unpredictable absorption of medication.
	Administer analgesics around-the-clock.	Administration around-the-clock prevents peaks and troughs of analgesia, especially with severe pain.
	D Evaluate the effectiveness of analgesics at regular frequent intervals after each administration, but especially after the initial dose; also observe for any manifestations of untoward effects.	Frequent evaluation of analgesic effectiveness permits the nurse to adjust the dose and timing interval to the client's need and provides an early warning of adverse responses.
	Implement actions to decrease the untoward effects of analgesics.	Actions taken to prevent predictable but unwanted effects of narcotic analgesics (e.g., constipation) increase client comfort.
	Instruct the client to request PRN pain medication before the pain is severe.	Pain may be managed with lower doses of analgesics and fewer untoward effects if PRN drugs are used before pain becomes severe.
	Teach about the use of analgesics, strategies to decrease side effects, and expectations for involvement in decisions about pain relief.	Information about analgesics and the expectation for client involvement increase the client's sense of control over his or her pain.
	NIC **Patient-Controlled Analgesia (PCA) Administration**	
	Validate that the client can use a PCA device.	To use a PCA device, the client must be able to communicate, comprehend explanations, and follow directions.
	Document the client's pain, amount and frequency of drug dosing, and response to pain treatment in a pain flow sheet.	Information on the pain flow sheet will assist the health care team to adjust the analgesic regimen to the client's needs.

D Indicates tasks that can be delegated to unlicensed assistive nursing personnel at the discretion of the nurse.

PLAN of CARE MEDICAL DIAGNOSIS: POSTOPERATIVE THORACOTOMY—*cont'd*

NURSING DIAGNOSIS NO. 2 ■ Acute Pain—*cont'd*

Expected Outcomes	Nursing Interventions	Rationales
	Teach the client and family how to use the PCA device.	The device will not be used if the client and/or family do not know how to use or are afraid of the device.
	Teach the client how to titrate doses up or down depending on respiratory rate, pain intensity, and pain quality.	The client may prevent severe pain and untoward effects by judicious use of the PCA.
	NIC **Environmental Management: Comfort**	
	Determine sources of discomfort, such as damp dressings, positioning of tubing, constrictive dressings, wrinkled bed linens, and environmental irritants.	Control of environmental discomforts may decrease the need for pharmacologic intervention.
	D Position the client to facilitate comfort.	The nurse may decrease sources of discomfort by using principles of body alignment, supporting with pillows, supporting joints during movement, splinting over incisions, and immobilizing painful body parts.
	Other Interventions	
	Refer the client to the Pain Advisory Committee.	The Pain Advisory Committee is a multidisciplinary committee with wide expertise in pain relief interventions.
	Consider the use of alternative therapies such as yoga, meditation, spirituality, and/or religion.	The experience of meditation and prayer and the reflection on meaning may help the patient to relax, thereby easing the muscle tension that contributes to pain sensation.
	Consider the use of alternative therapies such as imagery, aromatherapy, music, touch, and laughter/humor.	Cognitive and behavioral strategies may serve as adjuncts to or replacements for pharmacologic or surgical interventions for chronic pain. Each therapy has a differing mode of action that may or may not benefit the patient.
	Manage continuous cutaneous opioid analgesia, neuraxial analgesia, intraspinal analgesia, or transdermal analgesia, as needed.	Methods of delivering analgesia other than the traditional IV route may provide substantial pain relief in a form that the client may tolerate with fewer untoward effects.
	Continuing Care Considerations	
	Refer the client to an advanced practice nurse pain specialist, social worker, home care nurse, and/or psychologist, as appropriate.	Health care team members are able to provide continuing support for the client facing chronic pain.

Continued

PLAN of CARE MEDICAL DIAGNOSIS: POSTOPERATIVE THORACOTOMY—*cont'd*

NURSING DIAGNOSIS NO. 3 ■ Activity Intolerance

	Expected Outcomes	Nursing Interventions	Rationales
RELATED FACTORS Imbalance between oxygen supply/demand **DEFINING CHARACTERISTICS** Verbal report: Fatigue Abnormal heart rate or blood pressure response to activity Exertional discomfort Dyspnea	Denies discomfort with exertion No verbal report or observation of dyspnea with exertion Has no electrocardiographic evidence of dysrhythmias or ischemia Denies fatigue Denies weakness Has a heart rate that remains regular and strong with activity	NIC **Energy Management** Monitor the client for evidence of excess physical and emotional fatigue.	Extended periods of inactivity may place the client at risk for excessive fatigue when carrying out desired activities.
		Monitor cardiorespiratory response to activity.	Tachycardia, other dysrhythmias, dyspnea, diaphoresis, pallor, hemodynamic pressures, and respiratory rate increases may result from increased activity.
		Monitor nutritional intake.	Ensure that the client has adequate energy resources.
		D Reduce physical discomforts.	Physical discomforts could interfere with cognitive function and self-monitoring/regulation of activity.
		Arrange physical activities (e.g., avoid activity immediately after meals).	Such an arrangement reduces competition for oxygen supply to vital body functions.
		D Encourage alternate rest and activity periods.	This avoids extended periods of either activity or exercise.
		Plan activities for periods when the client has the most energy.	The client will be better able to manage activities during peak energy periods.
		D Assist the client to sit on the side of the bed ("dangle") if unable to transfer or walk.	Sitting on the edge of the bed helps the client avoid orthostatic hypotension during transfer.
		Instruct the client to recognize manifestations of exercise tolerance/intolerance during and after exercise sessions.	Light-headedness; shortness of breath; more than the usual muscle, skeletal, or joint pain; weakness; extreme fatigue; angina; profuse sweating; and palpitations indicate that the exercise program is more taxing than the client can undertake.
		Establish a follow-up schedule.	Follow-up schedules should assist in maintaining motivation, assist in problem solving, and monitor progress.
		Other Interventions Instruct the client/significant other to recognize manifestations of fatigue.	Symptoms of undue fatigue require a reduction in activity.
		Provide assistive devices, as appropriate.	Splints, special hand tools, or other devices may assist the client to carry out desired activities with less energy expenditure.
		Consider the use of complementary and alternative therapies.	Complementary and alternative therapies may be used to cope with chronic disease and disability, especially if chronic pain is a problem.
		Continuing Care Considerations Collaborate with the client/family and the rehabilitation team.	Effective interdisciplinary interventions facilitate the client's ability to manage his or her life.

D Indicates tasks that can be delegated to unlicensed assistive nursing personnel at the discretion of the nurse.

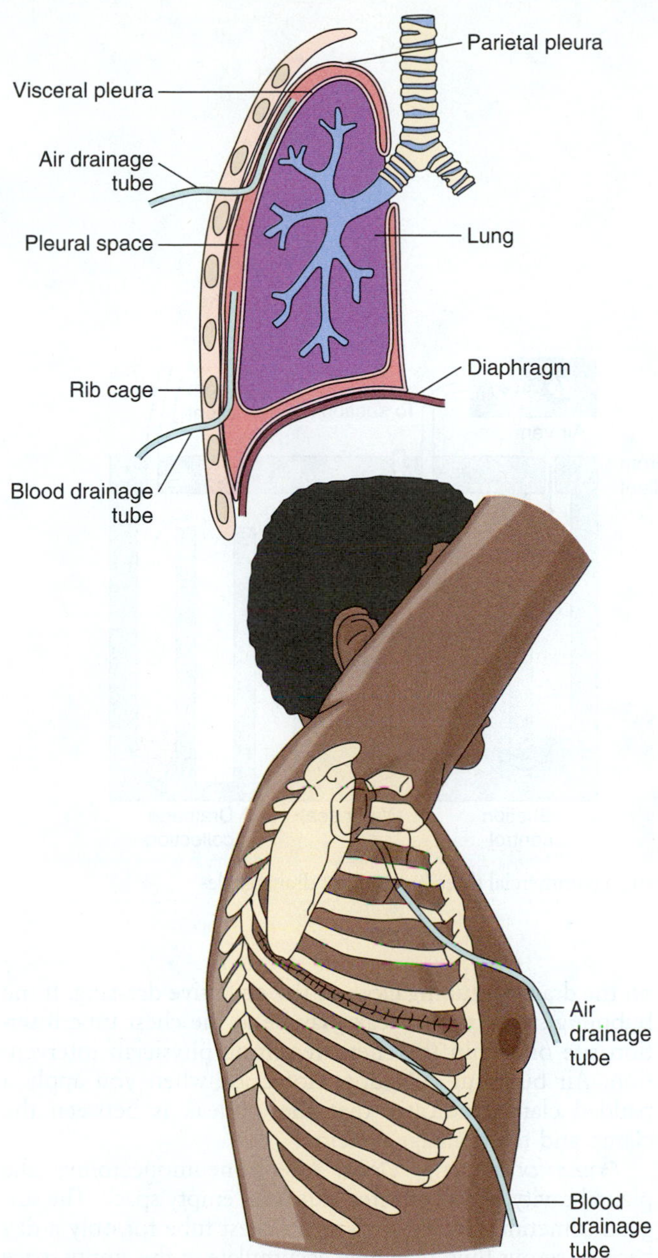

Figure 33-14 ■ Chest tube placement.

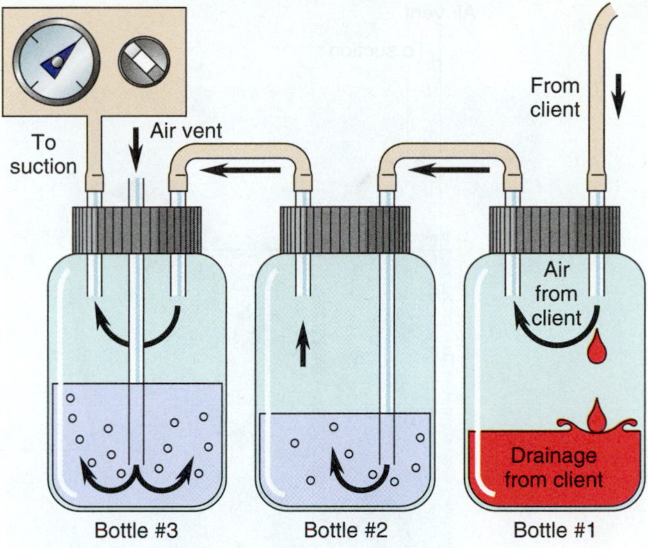

Figure 33-15 ■ Three-bottle chest drainage system.

from the client penetrates shallowly into the bottle, as does the tube connecting with bottle two. *It is critical that the stopper remain tightly connected to the bottle to maintain a closed system. If the stopper loosens and the chest tube is unclamped, the negative pressure in the pleural space will pull air into the space and cause a pneumothorax.*

Bottle (chamber) one collects the fluid draining from the client. This fluid is measured hourly during the first 24 hours. *The fluid must never come into direct contact with either the tube draining from the client or the tube connecting this bottle to bottle two.* If the tubing from the client enters the fluid, drainage stops.

BOTTLE TWO. Bottle two is the water seal that prevents air from entering the client's pleural space. Air from the pleural space also enters bottle one but moves immediately to bottle two through the connecting tube. This tube must always be under the water level in bottle two to prevent air from returning to the client. The bubbling of the water in bottle two indicates air drainage from the client. Bubbling is usually seen when intrathoracic pressure is greater than atmospheric pressure, such as when the client exhales, coughs, or sneezes. When the air in the pleural space has been removed, bubbling stops. A blocked or kinked chest tube also can cause bubbling to stop. Excessive bubbling in the second bottle may indicate an air leak. The water in the long tube of the second bottle rises and falls slightly with the client's respiratory cycle. A rise of 2 to 4 inches during inhalation and a fall during exhalation are normal. An absence of fluctuation may mean that the chest tube is obstructed, the expanded lung has blocked the eyelets of the chest tube, or no more air is leaking into the pleural space.

If the system consisted only of two bottles, drainage could occur only by gravity. Then, the second tube in the second bottle would be open to the air to prevent a buildup of pressure that could hinder air drainage.

BOTTLE THREE. The third bottle is the suction control bottle of the system. This stopper has three tubing connections: a short tube from the second bottle, a long open tube dipped into the water, and a short tube connecting to the suction unit. Suction enhances the pressure difference between the pleural space and the drainage system, causing the pressure to drop inside the system by 15 to 20 cm. Although the amount of suction generated by the suction unit can be increased, the amount of suction in the system is determined not by the suction unit but by the depth of the open tube in the water. While suction is applied, gentle bubbling is seen in the chamber.

COMMERCIAL CHEST DRAINAGE UNITS. Chest drainage units are self-contained units that work in exactly the same way that the three-bottle system does. From right to left, the system contains chambers for drainage, a water seal, and suction control (see Figure 33-16). The plastic devices reduce the risk of breakage or contamination of the drainage system and allow the client increased mobility.

Check hourly to ensure the sterility and patency of any chest drainage system. Tape tubing junctions to prevent ac-

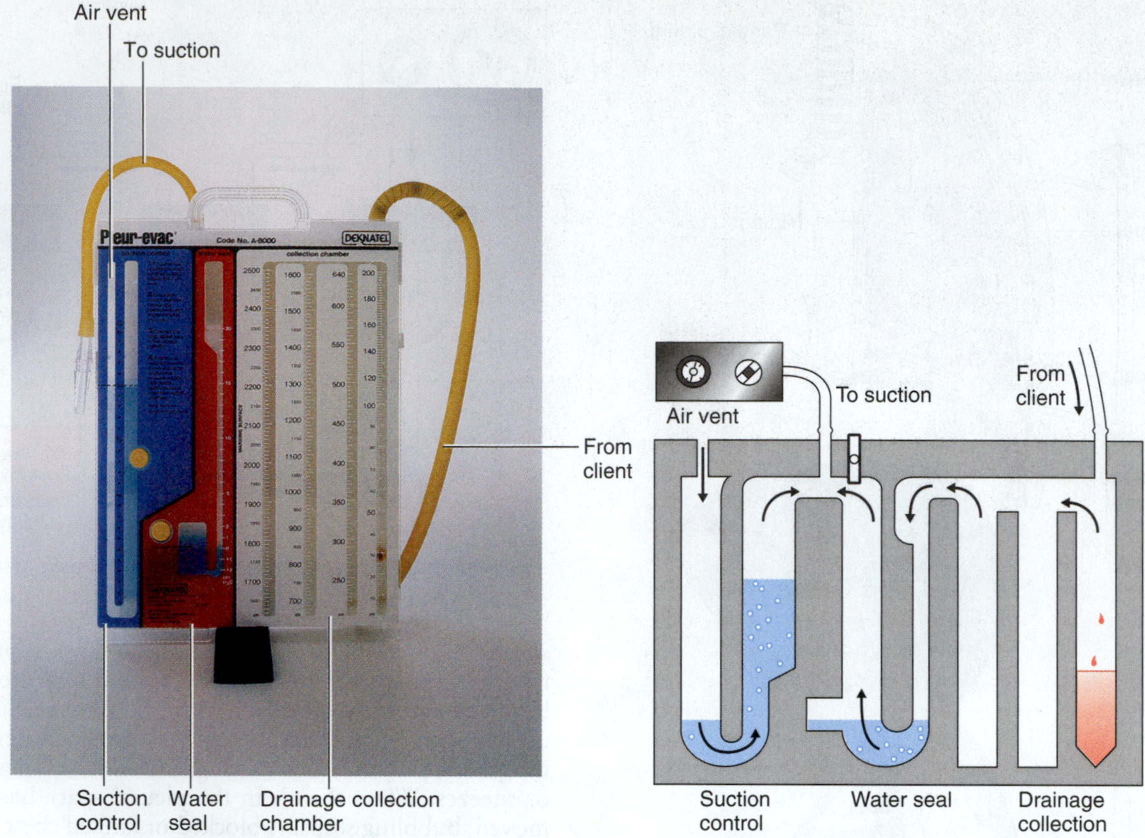

Figure 33-16 ■ *Left,* The Pleur-Evac drainage system, a commercial three-bottle chest drainage device. *Right,* Schematic of the drainage device.

cidental disconnections, and keep an occlusive dressing at the chest tube insertion site. Keep sterile gauze at the bedside to cover the insertion site immediately if the chest tube becomes dislodged. Also keep padded clamps at the bedside for use if the drainage system is interrupted. Position the drainage tubing to prevent kinks and large loops of tubing, which can block drainage and prevent lung re-expansion. Avoid vigorous stripping of the chest tube. Use gentle milking of the tube to move blood clots and prevent obstruction.

Assess the client's respiratory status and document the amount and type of drainage hourly. Usually the drainage in bottle one or chamber one is not emptied unless the container is so full that the fluid is in danger of coming into contact with the chest drainage tube. For the bottle system, place a tape marking for volume on the side of the bottle. When you check the volume, mark the fluid level and the time on the tape. The self-contained systems have calibrations on the collection chamber. Record the amount of hourly drainage. Notify the physician of drainage if more than 100 mL/hr occurs. After the first 24 hours, assess drainage at least every 8 hours.

Check the water seal chamber for unexpected bubbling created by an air leak in the system. Bubbling is normal during forceful expiration or coughing because air in the chest is being expelled. Continuous bubbling indicates an air leak that must be identified. Notify the physician if bubbling occurs continuously in the water seal bottle or chamber. On the physician's prescription, gently apply a padded clamp on the drainage tubing close to the occlusive dressing. If the bubbling stops, the air leak may be at the chest tube insertion site or within the chest, requiring physician intervention. Air bubbling that does not cease when you apply a padded clamp indicates that the air leak is between the clamp and the drainage system.

Pneumonectomy Care. After pneumonectomy, the pleural cavity on the affected side is an empty space. The surgeon sometimes inserts a clamped chest tube for only a day because serous fluid may then accumulate in the empty space and create adhesions, which reduce mediastinal shift toward the affected side. Closed-chest drainage is not usually used.

Complications of a pneumonectomy can include empyema and the development of a bronchopleural fistula. Positioning of the client after pneumonectomy varies according to surgeon preference and the client's comfort. Some surgeons want the client placed on the nonoperative side immediately after a pneumonectomy to reduce stress on the bronchial stump incision. Others prefer that the client be placed on the operative side to allow fluids to fill in the space formerly taken up by the lungs.

Interventions for Palliation

Oxygen Therapy. If the client is hypoxemic, supplemental oxygen is provided. Even if the client is not overtly hypoxemic, the physician may prescribe oxygen to relieve dyspnea and anxiety. Humidification is used with oxygen therapy for the client with lung cancer. (See Chapter 31 for issues related to home oxygen therapy.)

Drug Therapy. Bronchodilators and corticosteroids are prescribed for the client with bronchospasm to decrease bronchospasm, inflammation, and edema. Mucolytics may be of use to ease removal of thick mucus and sputum. Bacterial infections are treated with the appropriate antibiotic therapy.

Radiation Therapy. Radiation therapy can help relieve hemoptysis, obstruction of the bronchi and great veins (superior vena cava syndrome), **dysphagia** (difficulty swallowing) from esophageal compression, and pain resulting from bone metastasis. Usually radiation for palliation uses higher doses for shorter periods of time. Skin care issues and fatigue are the same as those occurring with radiation therapy for cure.

Laser Therapy. Lasers may be used to remove bronchial obstruction when tumors are accessible by bronchoscopy. The obstruction is debulked, and the airway is reopened. Laser therapy does not cause systemic or toxic effects and is usually well tolerated.

Thoracentesis and Pleurodesis. Pleural effusion can be a problem for the client with lung cancer. The excess fluid increases dyspnea, discomfort, and the risk for infection. The goal of treatment is to remove pleural fluid and prevent its formation. Fluid can be removed rapidly through suction after the placement of a large needle or catheter into the intrapleural space **(thoracentesis).** Fluid removal temporarily relieves hypoxia; however, the fluid can rapidly reform in the pleural space.

Another technique to relieve pleural effusion is to insert a chest tube to drain the fluid and to instill a **sclerosing** agent. The agent is an irritant that causes inflammation. The aim of thoracentesis and sclerosis is to create a **pleurodesis,** an inflammation that causes the pleura to stick to the chest wall and prevent formation of effusion fluid.

The procedure can be performed under local anesthesia at the bedside or in an operating room. Usually the client is also given an analgesic or sedative. Once the sclerosing agent is instilled, the chest tube is clamped to prevent drainage of the agent. Chart 33-13 reviews best practices for care of the client undergoing pleurodesis.

Dyspnea Management. The client with lung cancer tires easily and is often most comfortable resting in a semi-Fowler's position. Dyspnea is reduced with oxygen, use of a morphine drip, and positioning for comfort. The severely dyspneic client may be most comfortable sitting in a lounge chair or reclining chair.

Pain Management. The client with lung cancer may have chest pain and pain radiating to the arm. With bone metastasis, the client may also have bone pain. Perform a complete pain assessment with attention to onset, intensity, quality, duration, and the client's description of the pain. The goal of therapy is to help the client to be as pain free and as comfortable as possible.

Pharmacologic management with opioid drugs as oral, parenteral, or transdermal preparations is needed. Nonpharmacologic measures, such as positioning, hot or cold compresses, distractions, and guided imagery, may also be helpful. Prescribed analgesics are most effective when given around-the-clock. Additional PRN analgesics are used for breakthrough pain. Ongoing assessment and evaluation of the effectiveness of the pain control regimen is a primary nursing responsibility.

Hospice and End-of-Life Issues. For the client in the terminal phase of lung cancer, a referral to a hospice program can be beneficial. Hospice programs provide support to the terminally ill client and the family by meeting physical and psychosocial needs, adjusting the palliative care regimen as needed, making home visits, and providing volunteers for errands and respite care. (See Chapter 9 for a more complete discussion of end-of-life issues.) The American Cancer Society may also be able to provide assistance through support groups for clients and families or through the use of equipment, such as a hospital bed or bedside commode.

CHART 33-13

BEST PRACTICE for
The Client Undergoing Pleurodesis

- Reinforce explanation of the pleurodesis and inform the client that medication will be provided to promote comfort before the procedure. (The physician may administer IV analgesia/sedation immediately before the procedure.)
- Ensure that the chest tube is clamped after instillation of the sclerosing agent.
- Monitor vital signs and respiratory status at the completion of the procedure and then at least every 30 minutes until the effects of the IV medication have dissipated.
- Thereafter, monitor vital signs every 4 hours for 24 hours. (The client may experience a low-grade fever. Pleurodesis creates pleuritis between the visceral and parietal layers, thus preventing reaccumulation of fluid.)
- If a rotation schedule is ordered, assist the client to the correct position for appropriate time frames and provide reassurance.
- Unclamp the chest tube after completion of the rotation schedule or at the specified time ordered by the physician.
- Assess chest tube drainage and document the amount and character of the drainage.
- Perform a complete respiratory assessment every 2 hours and observe for manifestations of distress, including those of pneumothorax.
- Analgesics may be administered as needed to promote the client's comfort.
- When drainage has decreased (<150 mL in 12 to 24 hours), the physician may remove the chest tube. Maintain an occlusive dressing at the insertion site for a minimum of 48 hours.

GET READY for the NCLEX Examination!

KEY POINTS

Safe Effective Care Environment

- When using aerosolized drugs or other chemicals, close the door to the room where they are being used.
- Use gloves when obtaining a sputum specimen.
- Ensure there are no open flames or combustion hazards in rooms where oxygen is in use.

Health Promotion and Maintenance

- Teach clients who come into contact with inhalation irritants in their workplaces or for leisure time activities, to use a mask to avoid respiratory contact with these substances.
- Inform all clients who smoke that smoking increases the risk for development of many pulmonary problems.
- Assist clients interested in smoking cessation to find an appropriate smoking cessation program.
- Encourage older adults who are confined to bed for any reason or who are recovering from surgery to turn, cough, and deep breathe at least every 2 hours.

- Encourage all clients older than 50 years of age and anyone with a respiratory problem to receive a yearly influenza vaccination.
- Teach all clients who smoke the warning signs of lung cancer.

Psychosocial Integrity

- Assess the degree to which breathing problems interfere with the client's ability to perform activities of daily living.
- Pace your interview to match the learning needs and style of the individual client.
- Allow the client the opportunity to express fear or anxiety regarding the diagnosis of cancer or the treatment regimen.
- Allow clients to verbalize feelings about changes in appearance resulting from cancer therapy.
- Explain all diagnostic procedures, restrictions, and follow-up care to the client scheduled for tests.
- Help clients use strategies to improve their appearance when alopecia occurs.
- Refer clients and family members to local cancer resources and support groups.

Physiological Integrity

- Monitor the rate and depth of respiration at least every hour for any client with hypercarbia and CO_2 narcosis who is receiving oxygen by mask or nasal cannula.
- Document any known specific allergies that have respiratory manifestations.
- Assess the airway and breathing effectiveness for any client who experiences shortness of breath or any change in mental status.
- Assess the client's respiratory status every 15 minutes for at least the first 2 hours after undergoing an endoscopic test for respiratory disorders.
- Apply oxygen to anyone who is hypoxemic.
- Ensure that oxygen therapy delivered to the client is humidified (and warmed, when possible).
- Monitor arterial blood gases and oxygen saturation of all clients receiving oxygen therapy.
- Teach clients receiving radiation therapy how to care for the skin in the radiation path (see Chart 28-2).

ADDITIONAL STUDY RESOURCES

Go to your Student CD-ROM for Review Questions for the NCLEX Examination.

evolve Go to http://evolve.elsevier.com/Iggy/ for Integrated Management of Care Questions for the NCLEX Examination.

SELECTED BIBLIOGRAPHY

Asterisk indicates a classic or definitive work on this subject.

Aberle, M., & McLeskey, S. (2003). Biology of lung cancer with implications for new therapies. *Oncology Nursing Forum, 30*(2), 273-280.

Ackley, B., & Ladwig, G. (2002). *Nursing diagnosis handbook: A guide to planning care* (5th ed.). St. Louis: Mosby.

Adiutori, D. (2000). Primary pulmonary hypertension: A review for advanced practice nurses. *MEDSURG Nursing, 9*(5), 255-264.

American Cancer Society. (2005). *Cancer facts and figures-2005.* Report No. 01-300M-No. 5008.05. Atlanta: Author.

Asch-Goodkin, J. (2000). Eliminating disparities in asthma management. *Patient Care for the Nurse Practitioner, 3*(5), 68-83.

Ayes, D.M., & Lappin, J.S. (2004). Act fast when your patient has dyspnea. *Nursing 2004, 34*(7), 36-41.

Bernier, M., & Leonard, B. (2001). Pulmonary rehabilitation after acute COPD exacerbation. *Critical Care Clinics of North America, 13*(3), 375-387.

Boyle, A., & Locke, D. (2004). Update on chronic obstructive pulmonary disease. *MEDSURG Nursing, 13*(1), 42-48.

Brubacher, S., Gobel, B. (2003). Use of the Pleurx Pleural catheter for the management of malignant pleural effusions. *Clinical Journal of Oncology Nursing, 7*(1), 35-38.

*Centers for Disease Control and Prevention. (1998). Forecasted state-specific estimates of self-reported asthma prevalence-United States, 1998. *Morbidity and Mortality Weekly Report, 47*(47), 1022-1025.

Centers for Disease Control and Prevention. (2003). Asthma prevalence, health care use, and mortality, 2000-2001. National Center for Health Statistics. Available at http://www.cdc.gov/nchs/products/pubs/pubd/hestats/asthma/asthma.htm.

Chatila, W., et al. (2003). Respiratory failure after lung transplantation. *Chest, 123*(1), 165-173.

Cody, M. (2001). Is there help for a smoker? Understanding nicotine replacement therapy. *The American Journal for Nurse Practitioners, 5*(4), 32-41.

Cordes, M.E., & Brueggen, C. (2003). Diffuse malignant pleural mesothelioma: Part II. Symptom management. *Clinical Journal of Oncology Nursing, 7*(5), 545-552.

Dabbs, A., et al. (2003). Pattern and predictors of early rejection after lung transplantation. *American Journal of Critical Care, 12*(6), 497-507.

Dochterman, J., & Bulechek, G. (Eds.). (2004). *Nursing interventions classification (NIC)* (4th ed.). St. Louis: Mosby.

Dunn, N. (2001). Keeping COPD patients out of the ED. *RN, 64*(2), 33-37.

Duquette, S., LaLonde, L.C., & Traiger, G. (2000). Living-donor lobar lung transplantation: A case study. *Critical Care Nurse, 20*(1), 69-80.

Eells, P. (2004). Advances in prostacyclin therapy for pulmonary arterial hypertension. *Critical Care Nurse, 24*(2), 42-54.

Evangelista, L., et al. (2003). Health perceptions and risk behaviors of lung cancer survivors. *Heart & Lung, 32*(2), 131-139.

Facts and Comparisons. (2004). *Drug facts and comparisons* (58th ed.). St. Louis: Author.

Fehrenbach, C. (2002). Chronic obstructive pulmonary disease. *Nursing Standard, 17*(10), 45-52.

*Gazarian, P.K. (1997). Teaching your patient to use a metered-dose inhaler: The direct route for asthma therapy. *Nursing97, 27*(10), 52-54.

Gift, A., et al. (2004). Symptom clusters in elderly patients with lung cancer. *Oncology Nursing Forum, 31*(2), 203-210.

Goodfellow, L., & Jones, M. (2002). Bronchial hygiene therapy. *American Journal of Nursing, 102*(1), 37-43.

Goodwin, J., & Coleman, E. (2003). Exploring measures of functional dependence in the older adult with cancer. *MEDSURG Nursing, 12*(6), 359-366.

Green, F. (2002). Overview of pulmonary fibrosis. *Chest, 122*(6), 334S-339S.

Halpern, M., et al. (2003). Asthma: Resource use and costs for inhaled corticosteroid vs leukotriene modifier treatment–a meta-analysis. *Journal of Family Practice, 52*(5), 382-389.

Houfek, J., & Atwood, J. (2003). Genetic susceptibility to lung cancer: Implications for smoking cessation. *MEDSURG Nursing, 12*(1), 45-49.

Jablonski, R. (2000). Discovering asthma in the older adult. *Nurse Practitioner, 25*(3), 14, 24-25, 29-39.

Janson, S. (2000). Biologic markers of airway inflammation in asthma. *AACN Clinical Issues: Advanced Practice in Acute and Critical Care, 11*(2), 232-240.

Jones, A., & Rowe, B. (2000). Bronchopulmonary hygiene physical therapy and chronic obstructive pulmonary disease: A systematic review. *Heart and Lung, 29*(2), 125-135.

Judson, M. (2000). Clinical aspects of pulmonary sarcoidosis. *Journal of the South Carolina Medical Association, 96*(1), 9-17.

Kreamer, K. (2003). Getting the lowdown on lung cancer. *Nursing2003, 33*(11), 36-42.

Lanuza, D., Lefaiver, C., & Farcas, G. (2000). Research on the quality of life of lung transplant candidates and recipients: An integrative review. *Heart and Lung, 29*(3), 180-195.

Lindell, K., & Jacobs, S. (2003). Idiopathic pulmonary fibrosis, *American Journal of Nursing, 103*(4), 32-42.

Maliski, S., et al. (2003). The aftermath of lung cancer. *Cancer Nursing, 26*(3), 237-244.

McCance, K., & Huether, S. (2002). *Pathophysiology: The biologic basis for disease in adults and children* (4th ed.). St. Louis: Mosby.

McConnell, E. (2002). Teaching your patient to use a metered-dose inhaler. *Nursing2002, 32*(2), 73.

McHale, J., & Barth, M. (2000). Nursing care after pneumonectomy in patients with invasive pulmonary aspergillosis. *Critical Care Nurse, 20*(1), 37-44.

Meek, P. (2000). Influence of attention and judgment on perception of breathlessness in healthy individuals and patients with chronic obstructive pulmonary disease. *Nursing Research, 49*(1), 11-19.

Miracle, V. (2001). Taking the wind out of asthma. *Dimensions in Critical Care Nursing, 20*(1), 2-9.

Moorhead, S., Johnson, M., & Maas, M. (Eds.). (2004). *Nursing outcomes classification (NOC)* (3rd ed.). St. Louis: Mosby.

National Heart, Lung, and Blood Institute. (2003). *Global initiative for chronic obstructive pulmonary disease: Global strategy for the diagnosis, management, and prevention of chronic obstructive pulmonary disease.* NIH Publication No. 2701A. Rockville, MD. Author.

Nield, M. (2000). Dyspnea self-management in African-Americans with chronic lung disease. *Heart and Lung, 29*(1), 50-55.

Nussbaum, R., McInnes, R., & Willard, H. (2001). *Thompson & Thompson: Genetics in medicine* (6th ed.). Philadelphia: W.B. Saunders.

O'Neill, E. (2002). Illness representations and coping of women with chronic obstructive pulmonary disease: A pilot study. *Heart & Lung, 31*(4), 295-302.

Petty, M. (2003). Lung and lung-heart transplantation: Implications for nursing care when hospitalized outside the transplant center. *MEDSURG Nursing, 12*(4), 250-259.

Petty, T. (2003). Helping patients with COPD breathe easier. *Consultant, 43*(6), 687-688.

Phillip, M. (2000). Primary pulmonary hypertension. *MEDSURG Nursing, 9*(1), 17-20.

Pope, B. (2004). Chronic obstructive pulmonary disease. *Nursing2004, 34*(3), 56-57.

Puntillo, K., & Ley, J. (2004). Appropriately timed analgesics control pain due to chest tube removal. *American Journal of Critical Care, 13*(4), 292-301.

Reinke, L., & Hoffman, L. (2000). Asthma education: Creating a partnership. *Heart and Lung, 29*(3), 225-236.

Rogers, P., & Armstrong, I. (2002). Pulmonary hypertension. *Nursing Standard, 16*(24), 45-54.

Rosenberg, H., & Resnick, B. (2003). Exercise intervention in patients with chronic obstructive pulmonary disease. *Geriatric Nursing, 24*(2), 91-95.

Sabo, J., & Nord, P. (2000). Intravenous epoprostenol: A new therapy for primary pulmonary hypertension. *Critical Care Nurse, 20*(6), 31-40.

Sarna, L., et al. (2001). Barriers to tobacco cessation in clinical practice: Report from a national survey of oncology nurses. *Nursing Outlook, 49*(4), 166-172.

Silverman, E., et al. (2003). Current management of bronchiectasis: Review and 3 cases. *Heart & Lung, 32*(1), 59-64.

Simmons, P., & Simmons, M. (2004). Informed nursing practice: The administration of oxygen to patients with COPD. *MEDSURG Nursing, 13*(2), 82-85.

Smaha, D. (2001). Asthma emergency care: National guidelines summary. *Heart & Lung, 30*(6), 472-474.

Thomas, M. (2003). Epidermal growth factor receptor tyrosine kinase inhibitors: Application in non-small cell lung cancer. *Cancer Nursing, 26*(6S), 21S-25S.

Tishelman, C., Degner, L., & Mueller, B. (2000). Measuring symptom distress in patients with lung cancer. *Cancer Nursing, 23*(2), 82-90.

Togger, D., & Brenner, P. (2001). Metered dose inhalers. *American Journal of Nursing, 102*(10), 26-38.

Walker, A. (2003). Updates in small cell lung cancer treatment. *Clinical Journal of Oncology Nursing, 7*(5), 563-568.

Wong, D. (2001). COPD: Overview and update. *The American Journal for Nurse Practitioners, 5*(5), 9-25.

Wu, C., et al. (2001). Coping behaviors of individuals with chronic obstructive pulmonary disease. *MEDSURG Nursing, 10*(6), 315-320.

CHAPTER 34

Interventions for Clients with Infectious Problems of the Respiratory Tract

M. LINDA WORKMAN

LEARNING OUTCOMES

After studying this chapter, you should be able to:

1. Explain the consequences of an untreated streptococcal infection of the upper respiratory tract.
2. Identify adults at highest risk for contracting influenza.
3. Develop a teaching plan to prevent influenza in the older adult.
4. Identify clients at risk for developing community-acquired or hospital-acquired pneumonia.
5. Compare the manifestations of pneumonia in the younger adult with those exhibited by the older adult client with pneumonia.
6. Describe the mechanisms of action, side effects, and nursing implications of drug therapy for pneumonia.
7. Identify adults at risk for tuberculosis (TB).
8. Interpret correctly the TB test results for a person with normal immune function and a person with human immunodeficiency virus/acquired immunodeficiency syndrome (HIV/AIDS).
9. Describe the mechanisms of action, side effects, and nursing implications of drug therapy for TB.
10. Develop a community-based teaching plan for continuing care of the client with active TB.
11. Compare the early and late manifestations of inhalation anthrax with those of other lower respiratory infections.

Go to your Student CD-ROM for Review Questions for the NCLEX Examination keyed to these Learning Outcomes.

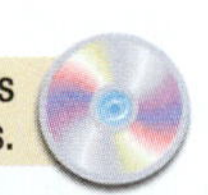

DISORDERS OF THE NOSE AND SINUSES

Rhinitis

PATHOPHYSIOLOGY

Rhinitis, an inflammation of the nasal mucosa, is the most common problem of nose and sinuses. Inflammation can be caused by infection (viral or bacterial) or contact with allergens. Often an allergic rhinitis will make the mucous membranes more susceptible to invasion, and an infection will accompany the allergy.

Allergic rhinitis, often called *hay fever* or *allergies,* is triggered by hypersensitivity reactions to airborne allergens, especially plant pollens or molds (see Chapter 26). Some episodes are "seasonal" in that they tend to recur at the same time each year and last only a few weeks. *Chronic rhinitis* occurs either intermittently with no seasonal pattern or continuously whenever the person is exposed to allergens such as dust, animal dander, wool, and foods (e.g., seafood). Other causes of rhinitis include a "rebound" nasal congestion from overuse of nose drops or sprays **(rhinitis medicamentosa)** and chronic nasal inhalation of cocaine.

Acute viral rhinitis (**coryza,** or the common cold) is caused by any one of at least 200 viruses. It spreads from person to person by droplets from sneezing or coughing. Colds are most contagious in the first 2 to 3 days after symptoms appear. Colds are self-limiting unless a bacterial infection occurs at the same time. Complications occur most often in immunosuppressed people and older adults, especially if they live or work in crowded conditions or in group settings (e.g., long-term care facility).

COLLABORATIVE MANAGEMENT

Assessment

In both acute and chronic allergic rhinitis, the presence of the **allergen** (offending substance) causes a release of natural chemicals, such as histamine, from white blood cells in the nasal mucosa. These chemicals bind to blood vessel receptor sites, causing local blood vessel dilation and capillary leak, leading to edema and swelling of the nasal mucosa. The resulting symptoms include headache, nasal irritation, sneezing, nasal congestion, **rhinorrhea** (watery drainage from the nose), and itchy, watery eyes.

Viral or bacterial invasion of the nasal passages causes the same local tissue responses as allergic rhinitis. Often the client also has systemic manifestations, including a sore, dry throat and a low-grade fever.

Interventions

Management of the client with any type of rhinitis focuses on symptom relief and client education. Instruct the client in the correct use of the drug therapy prescribed.

Drug Therapy. Drugs, including antihistamines and decongestants, are prescribed but must be used with caution in the older adult because of side effects such as vertigo, hypertension, urinary retention, and insomnia. Antihistamines block the chemicals released by white blood cells from binding to receptor sites on blood vessels and nasal tissues, preventing local edema and itching. Decongestants work by constricting blood vessels, thus decreasing edema. Antipyretics are given if fever is present. Antibiotics are prescribed only for bacterial rhinitis. Rhinitis caused by overuse of nose drops or sprays is treated by discontinuing the offending drug. Steroid nasal sprays may be used to decrease the rebound nasal congestion during the time immediately after discontinuing the drug.

Complementary and Alternative Therapies. Some people are able to decrease the severity of acute viral rhinitis with the use of complementary and alternative therapy early in the course of the problem. Agents often used are Echinacea, large doses of vitamin C, and zinc preparations such as COLD-EEZE or Zicam. It is not clear how these agents reduce symptom severity or duration of illness, but it is believed they may help increase nonspecific immune function.

Supportive Therapy. Instruct the client about the importance of rest (8 to 10 hours a day) and fluid intake of at least 2000 mL/day (about eight glasses) unless other health problems (e.g., heart failure, chronic renal failure) limit this amount. Humidifying the air helps to relieve congestion. Ways to increase humidity include using a room humidifier, inhaling steam from a pan of boiled water after removing it from the heat, or breathing steamy air in the bathroom after running hot shower water.

The client is most likely to spread the infection during the first 2 to 3 days after symptoms begin. Teach the client to reduce the risk of spreading the cold by thoroughly washing hands, especially after nose blowing or sneezing. Instruct the client to avoid close contact with people who are more susceptible to infection, such as older adults, infants, and anyone who has a chronic respiratory problem. An uncomplicated cold typically subsides within 7 to 10 days.

The client with recurrent allergic rhinitis can have allergy testing to determine the cause. The client may prevent further episodes by avoiding the allergen or using desensitization therapy (see Chapter 26).

Sinusitis

PATHOPHYSIOLOGY

Sinusitis is an inflammation of the mucous membranes of one or more of the sinuses. Swelling can obstruct the flow of secretions from the sinuses, which may then become infected. The disorder often follows rhinitis. Other conditions leading to sinusitis include deviated nasal septum, polyps, tumors, inhaled air pollutants or cocaine, facial trauma, nasal intubation, dental infection, or decreased immune function. In chronic sinusitis, the mucous membrane is permanently thickened from repeated inflammation.

The most common organisms causing sinus infection are *Streptococcus pneumoniae, Haemophilus influenzae, Diplococcus,* or *Bacteroides*. Sinusitis most often develops in the maxillary and frontal sinuses. Complications include cellulitis, abscess, and meningitis.

Diagnosis is made on the basis of the client's history and manifestations. Transillumination of the affected sinus is decreased. Other diagnostic tests for sinusitis include sinus x-rays, endoscopic examination, and computed tomography (CT).

COLLABORATIVE MANAGEMENT

Assessment

The manifestations of sinusitis include nasal swelling and congestion, headache, facial pressure, pain (usually worse when the head is in a dependent position), tenderness to touch over the involved area, low-grade fever, cough, and purulent or bloody nasal drainage.

Interventions

NONSURGICAL MANAGEMENT. Treatment includes the use of broad-spectrum antibiotics (e.g., amoxicillin), analgesics for pain and fever (e.g., acetaminophen [Tylenol, Atasol✱]), decongestants (e.g., phenylephrine [Neo-Synephrine]), steam humidification, hot and wet packs over the sinus area, and nasal saline irrigations. Instruct the client to increase fluid intake to more than 10 glasses of water or juice per day unless another medical problem requires fluid restriction. If this treatment plan is not successful, the client may need to be evaluated with sinus films and CT. Surgical intervention may be needed.

SURGICAL MANAGEMENT

Antral Irrigation. Antral irrigation, also known as *maxillary antral puncture* and *lavage,* is an outpatient procedure. With the client under local anesthesia, a large-gauge needle is inserted into the maxillary sinus on the affected side. Fluid or pus is drained from the sinus. The sinus is then irrigated with saline solution, an antibiotic solution, or both.

Other Surgical Procedures. If antral irrigation is not successful, other surgical procedures may be used to open the sinus cavities. In the Caldwell-Luc procedure, the surgeon makes an incision under the upper lip into the maxillary sinus. The infected mucosa is then removed. With the

CHART 34-1

BEST PRACTICE for
Postoperative Care for Clients with Sinus Surgery

- Place the client in the semi-Fowler's position to promote drainage and prevent swelling.
- Perform gentle oral hygiene to promote healing and prevent injury to the surgical incision.
- Use ice compresses as prescribed for 24 hours.
- Change the "mustache" dressing under the nose as needed, and record the type and amount of drainage.
- Instruct the client to eat soft foods and increase fluid intake.
- Instruct the client to limit the Valsalva maneuver (no coughing, blowing the nose, or straining at stool) for at least 2 weeks postoperatively to prevent bleeding and tissue damage.

nasal antral window procedure, the surgeon makes an opening in the front portion of the lower nasal bone to improve drainage through the nares. After either procedure, the client may have difficulty eating for a few days because of pain and swelling. Chart 34-1 describes the best practices for postoperative care for clients undergoing these procedures. When the ethmoid sinuses need to be opened, the surgeon uses an external incision along the side of the nose from the middle of the eyebrow (Weber-Ferguson incision).

Endoscopic Sinus Surgery. Endoscopic sinus surgery is a common method of diagnosing and treating sinus disorders. Direct inspection of the sinuses through a sinus endoscope is completed with the client under general anesthesia in an outpatient surgical center. The procedure takes only minutes, although the nasal mucosa may take from 4 to 6 weeks to heal. The client goes home the same day and can return to work in 4 to 5 days. Instruct the client to use saline nasal sprays frequently (every 2 to 4 hours) to prevent mucosal crusting and promote healing.

DISORDERS OF THE ORAL PHARYNX AND TONSILS

Pharyngitis

PATHOPHYSIOLOGY

Pharyngitis, or "sore throat," is a common inflammation of the mucous membranes of the pharynx. It accounts for more than 15 million office visits each year in the United States. This condition often occurs with acute rhinitis and sinusitis.

Acute pharyngitis has many causes (Table 34-1). The most common bacteria causing pharyngitis is group A beta-hemolytic *Streptococcus*, but most adult cases are caused by a virus. The incidence of infection is highest between late fall and spring, especially in colder climates.

TABLE 34-1 Causes of Pharyngitis

Bacterial Causes	Other Causes
Streptococcus	*Chlamydia*
Staphylococcus	*Mycoplasma pneumoniae*
Haemophilus influenzae	*Candida*
Pneumococcus	Physical and chemical causes
Corynebacterium diphtheriae	Alcohol
Neisseria gonorrhoeae	Tobacco
Viral Causes	Heat
Adenovirus	Irritants
Rhinovirus	Dehydration
Epstein-Barr virus	Trauma
Cytomegalovirus (CMV)	
Influenza virus	
Parainfluenza virus	
Herpesvirus	
Coxsackievirus A	
Echovirus	

COLLABORATIVE MANAGEMENT

Assessment

The client with pharyngitis has throat soreness and dryness, throat pain, pain on swallowing **(odynophagia),** difficulty in swallowing **(dysphagia),** and fever. Viral and bacterial pharyngitis are often difficult to distinguish on physical assessment. When inspecting a throat infected with either virus or bacteria, you may see mild to severe **hyperemia** (redness) with or without enlarged tonsils and with or without exudate. Ask the about nasal discharge, which can vary from thin and watery to thick and purulent. Lymph node enlargement in the neck occurs with both viral and bacterial pharyngitis. When a tonsillar abscess occurs with pharyngitis, the client may have a "hot potato" voice, a thickened voice of poor quality.

Bacterial infections are more often associated with enlarged red tonsils, exudate, purulent nasal discharge, and local lymph node enlargement. Chart 34-2 compares the manifestations of viral and bacterial pharyngitis. Viral pharyngitis is contagious for 2 to 3 days. Symptoms usually subside within 3 to 10 days after onset, and the disease is usually self-limiting.

Bacterial pharyngitis, such as group A streptococcal infection, can lead to serious medical complications (Table 34-2), including acute glomerulonephritis (Chapter 74) and rheumatic fever carditis. Acute glomerulonephritis may occur 7 to 10 days after the acute infection, and rheumatic fever may develop 3 to 5 weeks after the acute infection.

Throat cultures are important in distinguishing viral from a group A beta-hemolytic streptococcal infection; however, the results are not entirely accurate. False-negative cultures can occur, some of which are due to incorrect throat culture technique. The organisms are not uniformly distributed throughout the throat and can be missed during swabbing. To obtain a specimen, rub a cotton swab first over the right tonsillar area, moving across the right arch, the uvula, and then across the left arch to the left tonsillar area. The cotton swab is streaked on a blood agar plate, which is then incubated for 24 to 48 hours.

Many types of rapid tests and screens for group A beta-hemolytic streptococcal antigen are available. These tests vary in specificity and sensitivity and cost about the same as a culture and sensitivity, but the results are available more quickly than standard cultures. Two common tests are the GenProbe and the OIA (Optical Immunoassay).

A complete blood count (CBC) is performed when the client's condition is severe or does not improve. Clients who need a CBC are those who have high fevers, lethargy, or manifestations of complications. A CBC may indicate other causes of pharyngitis.

When taking a history, ask about the client's recent contacts (within the last 10 days) with people who have been ill. Specifically ask whether the client has been ill with symptoms of a cold or upper respiratory tract infection recently. Document any previous history of streptococcal infections,

CHART 34-2

KEY FEATURES of
Acute Viral and Bacterial Pharyngitis

Feature	Viral Pharyngitis	Bacterial Pharyngitis
Temperature	Low-grade or no fever	High temperature (>101° F [38° C], and usually 102°-104° F [38.5°-40° C])*
Ear manifestations	Retracted or dull tympanic membrane	Retracted or dull tympanic membrane
Throat manifestations	Scant or no tonsillar exudate Slight erythema of pharynx and tonsils	Severe hyperemia of pharyngeal mucosa, tonsils, and uvula Erythema of tonsils with yellow exudate
Neck manifestations	Possible lymphadenopathy	Anterior cervical lymphadenopathy and tenderness
Skin manifestations	No rash	Possible scarlatiniform rash Possible petechiae on chest or abdomen or both
Dysphagia, odynophagia	Present	Present
Other symptoms	No cough Rhinitis Mild hoarseness Headache	No cough Voice characterized by pain on voicing and slurred speech Headache Arthralgia Myalgia
Laboratory data	Complete blood count usually normal White blood cell count usually lower than 10,000/mm³ Negative throat culture results	Complete blood count abnormal White blood cell count usually >12,000/mm³* Throat culture results positive for beta-hemolytic streptococcus
Onset	Gradual	Abrupt

*May not be present in adults over 65 years of age.

TABLE 34-2 Complications of Group A Streptococcal Infection

- Rheumatic fever
- Acute glomerulonephritis
- Peritonsillar abscess
- Retropharyngeal abscess
- Otitis media
- Sinusitis
- Mastoiditis
- Bronchitis
- Pneumonia
- Scarlet fever

rheumatic fever, valvular heart disease, or penicillin allergy. Because diphtheria (*Corynebacterium diphtheriae*) can cause pharyngitis, ask about and document whether the client has had a diphtheria immunization.

Interventions

Most sore throats in adults are viral and do not require antibiotic therapy. Treatment includes rest, increased fluid intake, humidifying the air, analgesics for pain, warm saline gargles, and throat lozenges containing mild anesthetics.

The management of bacterial pharyngitis involves the use of antibiotics and the same supportive care provided for viral pharyngitis. For streptococcal infection, an oral penicillin or cephalosporin is prescribed. Drugs from the macrolide class (e.g., azithromycin or erythromycin) are recommended if the client is allergic to penicillin. *Stress the importance of completing the entire antibiotic prescription, even when symptoms improve or subside.* If the client cannot tolerate the drug, notify the physician so that the antibiotic can be changed. If adherence is a concern or if the client cannot swallow pills, long-acting penicillin can be given intramuscularly in a single dose.

The client should be re-evaluated if there is no improvement in 3 days or if manifestations are still present after completion of the antibiotic course. Persistent bacterial pharyngitis may occur with immunosuppression. Any client whose bacterial pharyngitis does not improve with antibiotics should consider HIV testing.

A rare complication of pharyngitis in adults is infection of the epiglottis and supraglottic structures **(epiglottitis).** The epiglottis is a flaplike structure that closes over the trachea during swallowing to prevent aspiration. An inflamed epiglottis can swell and obstruct the airway, causing a medical emergency. *Any client with pharyngitis who has stridor or indications of airway obstruction should be immediately evaluated by a health care provider in a setting in which intubation or tracheostomy can be performed quickly and safely.*

Teach the client how to take his or her oral temperature accurately every morning and evening until the infection resolves. The client is not contagious after 24 hours of antibiotic therapy. Family members or close contacts who also have a sore throat should be evaluated, and a throat culture may be indicated.

Tonsillitis

PATHOPHYSIOLOGY

Tonsillitis is an inflammation and infection of the tonsils and lymphatic tissues located on each side of the throat. The tonsils are lymphatic tissue shaped like a small almond. Each tonsil is covered by a mucous membrane and has small valleys **(crypts)** across the surface. Tonsils filter organisms and protect the respiratory tract from infection.

Tonsillitis is a contagious airborne infection. Acute or chronic tonsillitis can occur in any age group, but it is less common in adults. The infection is usually more severe when it occurs in adolescents or adults.

Acute tonsillitis usually lasts 7 to 10 days and is usually caused by bacteria. The most common organism is *Streptococcus.* Other bacterial causes include *Staphylococcus aureus, H. influenzae,* and *Pneumococcus.* Viruses also cause tonsillitis. Chronic tonsillitis may result from an unresolved acute infection or recurrent infections.

COLLABORATIVE MANAGEMENT

Assessment

Chart 34-3 lists the manifestations of acute tonsillitis. Diagnostic tests often used to rule out other causes of the sore throat and fever include a complete blood count (CBC), throat culture and sensitivity (C&S) studies, and Monospot test. If respiratory symptoms are present, chest x-rays may be needed. The white blood cell count is elevated in bacterial infections. Throat C&S studies identify the causative organism and direct the choice of drug therapy.

Interventions

The health care provider prescribes antibiotics (usually penicillin or azithromycin) for 7 to 10 days. Warm saline throat gargles, analgesics, antipyretics, and lozenges with topical anesthetic agents may provide symptom relief.

Surgical intervention for tonsillitis may be needed for recurrent acute infections (especially group A beta-hemolytic streptococcal infections), chronic infections that have not responded to antibiotic therapy, a peritonsillar abscess, and enlarged tonsils or adenoids that obstruct the airway.

Surgery is usually performed after the client has recovered from an acute tonsillitis and no infection is present (except with an acute peritonsillar abscess).

Surgery may involve complete tonsil removal (for chronic infection) or a partial tonsil removal for obstruction without infection. A common procedure to remove the tonsils is dissection and snare, although laser tonsillectomy, radiothermal ablation tonsillectomy, and tonsil "shaving" are being used increasingly. The adenoids may be removed at the same time. A tonsillectomy and adenoidectomy (T&A) is usually performed with the adult client under general anesthesia. After surgery, assess for airway clearance, provide pain relief, and monitor for excessive bleeding.

Peritonsillar Abscess

PATHOPHYSIOLOGY

Peritonsillar abscess (PTA), or *quinsy*, is a complication of acute tonsillitis. The infection spreads from the tonsil to the surrounding tissue, which forms an abscess. The most common cause of PTA is group A beta-hemolytic streptococcus.

CHART 34-3

KEY FEATURES of Acute Tonsillitis

- Sudden onset of a mild to severe sore throat
- Fever
- Muscle aches
- Chills
- Dysphagia, odynophagia (painful swallowing of food)
- Pain in the ears
- Headache
- Anorexia
- Malaise
- "Hot potato" voice (thickened voice of poor quality)
- Tonsils visually swollen and red with pus
- Tonsils may be covered with a white or yellow exudate
- Purulent drainage may be expressed by pressing a tonsil
- Uvula visually edematous or inflamed
- Cervical lymph nodes usually tender and enlarged

COLLABORATIVE MANAGEMENT

Signs of infection are pronounced on examination. Pus forms behind the tonsil and causes one-sided swelling with deviation of the uvula. The swelling may cause the client to drool, have severe throat pain radiating to the ear, have a voice change, and have difficulty swallowing. The client may also have a tonic contraction of the muscles of chewing **(trismus)** and have difficulty breathing.

Outpatient management with antibiotic therapy and percutaneous needle aspiration of the abscess is usually needed. The client usually improves in 36 hours. *Stress the importance of completing the antibiotic regimen and of coming to the emergency department quickly if symptoms of obstruction appear (drooling and stridor).* Instruct the client about comfort measures (e.g., warm saline gargles or irrigations, an ice collar, analgesics). Hospitalization is required when the client's airway is in jeopardy or when the infection does not respond to antibiotic therapy. Incision and drainage **(I&D)** of the abscess, plus additional antibiotic therapy, may be needed. A tonsillectomy may be performed to prevent recurrence.

DISORDERS OF THE LARYNX AND LUNGS

Laryngitis

PATHOPHYSIOLOGY

Laryngitis is an inflammation of the mucous membranes lining the larynx and may or may not include edema of the vocal cords. It can occur as a single problem or occur with upper respiratory infections. Laryngitis also can be a manifestation of a related disease process, such as throat or lung cancer. Common causes include exposure to irritating inhalants and pollutants (chemical agents, tobacco, alcohol, and smoke), overuse of the voice, inhalation of volatile gases (e.g., glue, paint thinner, butane), or intubation. An increasingly common cause of recurrent laryngitis is gastroesophageal reflux disease (GERD).

COLLABORATIVE MANAGEMENT

Assess the client for acute hoarseness, dry cough, and difficulty swallowing. Complete but temporary voice loss **(aphonia)** also may occur. A laryngeal mirror is used to examine the larynx visually and to identify inflammation, polyps, edema, or tumor. If suspicious lesions are present, an x-ray, computed tomography (CT), or fiberoptic laryngoscopic examination may be needed. Clients who may have a disorder other than acute laryngitis are referred to an ear, nose, and throat (ENT) specialist.

Nursing management is aimed toward symptom relief and prevention. Treatment consists of voice rest, steam inhalations, increased fluid intake, and throat lozenges. The health care provider may prescribe antibiotic therapy and bronchodilators when sinusitis, bronchitis, or a bacterial infection is also present. Inform the client and family about relief measures; infection prevention; and avoidance of alcohol, tobacco, and pollutants.

Preventive therapy is aimed toward increasing the client's and family's awareness of the hazards of tobacco and alcohol use. Emphasize the activities that place an added strain on the larynx, such as singing, cheering, public speaking, heavy lifting, and whispering. Speech therapy is used when vocal cord injury occurs with laryngitis and for any voice disorder. For recurrent bouts of laryngitis, further medical and voice evaluation is indicated.

Influenza

PATHOPHYSIOLOGY

Influenza, or "flu," is a highly contagious acute viral respiratory infection that can occur in adults of all ages. Epidemics are common and lead to complications of pneumonia or death, especially in older adults or debilitated or immunocompromised clients. Hospitalization may be required. Influenza may be caused by one of several viruses, usually referred to as A, B, and C.

The client with influenza usually has a severe headache, muscle aches, fever, chills, fatigue, weakness, and anorexia. Manifestations of sore throat, cough, and rhinorrhea (watery discharge from the nose) generally follow the initial symptoms for a week or longer. Most clients continue to feel fatigued for 1 to 2 weeks after the acute episode has resolved.

HEALTH PROMOTION/ILLNESS PREVENTION

Vaccinations for the prevention of influenza are widely available. The vaccine is changed every year on the basis of which specific viral strains are most likely to pose a problem during the influenza season (i.e., late fall and winter). Influenza vaccinations can be taken as an intramuscular injection (Fluviron, Fluzone) or as an intranasal spray (FluMist). People recommended to receive the vaccine each year include those older than 50 years of age, people with chronic illness or immune compromise, those living in institutions, and health care personnel providing direct care to clients (Centers for Disease Control and Prevention [CDC], 2000).

◆COLLABORATIVE MANAGEMENT

Viral infections do not respond to traditional antibiotic therapy. Antiviral agents may be effective for prevention and treatment of some types of influenza. Amantadine (Symmetrel) and rimantadine (Flumadine) have been effective in the prevention and treatment of influenza A. Ribavirin (Virazole) has been used for severe influenza B. Newer antivirals include zanamivir (Relenza), which is used as an oral inhalant, and oseltamivir (Tamiflu), which is an oral tablet. Both these antivirals prevent viral spread in the respiratory tract by inhibiting a viral enzyme (neuraminidase) that allows the virus to penetrate respiratory cells. These agents shorten the duration of influenzas A or B if taken within 24 to 48 hours after the onset of manifestations. Both agents also may be used for prevention.

Advise the client to stay in bed for several days and drink large amounts of fluids unless another medical problem requires fluid restriction (e.g., kidney disease or heart failure). Saline gargles may ease sore throat pain. Antihistamines may reduce the rhinorrhea. Other supportive and comfort measures are the same as those for acute rhinitis.

Pneumonia

PATHOPHYSIOLOGY

Pneumonia is an excess of fluid in the lungs resulting from an inflammatory process. The inflammation is triggered by many infectious organisms and by inhalation of irritating agents. Infectious pneumonias are categorized as community-acquired (CAP) or hospital-acquired **(nosocomial),** depending on where the client was exposed to the infectious agent. This distinction is important because nosocomial pneumonias are more likely to be resistant to antibiotics than are CAPs.

The inflammation occurs in the interstitial spaces, the alveoli, and often the bronchioles. The process begins when organisms penetrate the airway mucosa and multiply in the alveolar spaces. To do this, they must survive the lung's many defenses against microbial invasion, including the inflammatory response. White blood cells migrate to the area of infection, causing local capillary leak, edema, and exudate. These fluids collect in and around the alveoli, and the alveolar walls thicken. Both events reduce gas exchange and lead to hypoxemia. Red blood cells and fibrin also move into the alveoli. The capillary leak spreads the infection to other areas of the lung. If the organisms move into the bloodstream, sepsis results; if the infection extends into the pleural cavity, empyema results.

The fibrin and edema of inflammation stiffen the lung, reducing compliance and decreasing the vital capacity (VC). Alveolar collapse **(atelectasis)** further reduces the ability of the lungs to oxygenate the blood moving through it. As a result, arterial oxygen tension falls, causing **hypoxemia** (insufficient oxygen in the blood).

Pneumonia may occur as lobar pneumonia with **consolidation** (solidification, lack of air spaces) in a segment or an entire lobe of the lung or as bronchopneumonia with diffusely scattered patches around the bronchi. The extent of lung involvement after the organism invades depends on the host defenses. Bacteria multiply quickly in a person whose immune system is compromised. Tissue necrosis results when organisms form an abscess that perforates the bronchial wall.

Etiology

In general, people develop pneumonia when their immune systems are unable to combat the virulence of the invading organisms. Organisms from the environment, invasive devices, equipment and supplies, staff, or from other people can invade the body. Risk factors are listed in Table 34-3. Pneumonia can be caused by bacteria, viruses, mycoplasmas, fungi, rickettsiae, protozoa, and helminths (worms) (Table 34-4). Noninfectious causes of pneumonia include inhalation of toxic gases, chemicals, smoke, and aspiration of water, food, fluid, and vomitus.

Incidence/Prevalence

In the United States, two to four million cases of pneumonia occur each year, and it is the fifth leading cause of death (CDC, 2003b). The highest incidence among adults occurs in older adults, nursing home residents, hospitalized clients, and those being mechanically ventilated. Community-acquired pneumonia (CAP) is more common than nosocomial pneumonia and occurs in late fall and winter as a complication of

TABLE 34-3 Risk Factors Associated with Pneumonia

Community-Acquired Pneumonias
- Older adult
- No history of pneumococcal vaccination
- No history of having received the influenza vaccine in the previous year
- Chronic or other coexisting condition
- Recent history of or exposure to viral or influenza infections
- History of tobacco or alcohol use

Nosocomial Pneumonias
- Older adult
- Chronic lung disease
- Gram-negative colonization of the oropharynx and stomach
- Altered level of consciousness
- Aspiration
- Endotracheal, tracheostomy, or nasogastric tube
- Poor nutritional status
- Immunocompromised status (from disease, medications)
- Medications that increase gastric pH (histamine [H_2] blockers, antacids) or alkaline tube feedings
- Mechanical ventilation (ventilator acquired pneumonia [VAP])

TABLE 34-4 Common Organisms Causing Pneumonia*

Community-Acquired Pneumonias
- *Streptococcus pneumoniae* (Gram positive)
- *Staphylococcus aureus* (Gram positive)
- *Haemophilus influenzae* (Gram negative)
- *Legionella pneumophila* (Gram negative)
- *Mycoplasma pneumoniae* (smallest free-living organism)
- *Chlamydia pneumoniae* (parasite)

Nosocomial Pneumonias
- *Staphylococcus aureus* (Gram positive)
- *Pseudomonas aeruginosa* (Gram negative)
- *Enterobacter* organisms (Gram negative)
- *Klebsiella* organisms (Gram negative)
- *Haemophilus influenzae* organisms (Gram negative)
- *Acinetobacter* organisms (Gram negative)
- *Candida albicans* (fungus)

*Because of various factors that influence the incidence of the pathogenic causes of pneumonia, these organisms are listed loosely in order of incidence.

influenza. Hospital-acquired pneumonia is a common nosocomial infection. Nosocomial pneumonia has a 20% to 50% mortality; the highest incidence is in those clients infected with *Pseudomonas aeruginosa*, *Acinetobacter*, other "high-risk" organisms, or secondary bacteremia. Mortality also is higher in clients who have complications (Table 34-5).

CONSIDERATIONS FOR OLDER ADULTS

Pneumonia and influenza are the third leading cause of death for clients older than 85 years of age. The death rate for clients older than 64 years of age is steadily increasing (CDC, 2003b).

HEALTH PROMOTION/ILLNESS PREVENTION

Of the different types of pneumonia organisms, the most common are 6B, 23F, 14, 9V, 19A, and 19F. All these types are included in the pneumococcal vaccine. Client education is important in the prevention of pneumonia (Chart 34-4), as is making the vaccines readily available to those most at risk.

Other prevention techniques include strict handwashing to avoid the spread of organisms. Respiratory therapy equipment must be well maintained and decontaminated or changed as recommended. Use sterile water rather than tap water in gastrointestinal tubes, and institute aspiration precautions as indicated. Specific interventions to prevent aspiration are discussed in Chapter 31.

TABLE 34-5 Common Complications of Pneumonia

Complication	Definition
Hypoxemia	Arterial oxygen <80 mm Hg
Ventilatory failure	Lungs unable to move gas in and out of lungs mechanically, resulting in hypoxemia and hypercarbia
Atelectasis	Collapse of the affected alveoli and associated lobes of the lungs
Pleural effusion	Collection of fluid in the pleural space (usually sterile fluid that resolves)
Pleurisy	Pain caused by friction between layers of pleura

CHART 34-4

CLIENT EDUCATION GUIDE
Preventing Pneumonia

- Know whether you are at risk for pneumonia.
- Have the annual influenza vaccine after discussing appropriate timing of the vaccination with your primary health care provider.
- Discuss the pneumococcal vaccine with your primary health care provider, and have the vaccination as recommended.
- Avoid crowded public areas during flu and holiday seasons.
- Cough, turn, move about, and perform deep-breathing exercises as directed by your nurse or other health care professional.
- If you are using respiration equipment at home, clean the equipment as you have been taught.
- Avoid indoor pollutants, such as dust, secondhand (passive) smoke, and aerosols.
- If you do not smoke, do not start.
- If you smoke, seek professional help on how to stop (or at least decrease) your habit.
- Be sure to get enough rest and sleep on a daily basis.
- Eat a healthy, balanced diet and take in a sufficient amount of nonalcoholic fluids each day.

COLLABORATIVE MANAGEMENT

PHARM e REVIEW

The Concept Map on p. 635 addresses assessment and nursing care issues related to clients who have pneumonia.

Assessment

HISTORY

In taking the history from the client who may have pneumonia, consider the risk factors for infection (see Table 34-3). Obtain the information from a family member if the client is confused or too dyspneic. Document age; living, work, or school environment; diet, exercise, and sleep routines; swallowing problems; presence of a nasogastrointestinal tube; tobacco and alcohol use; past and current use of drugs; and his-

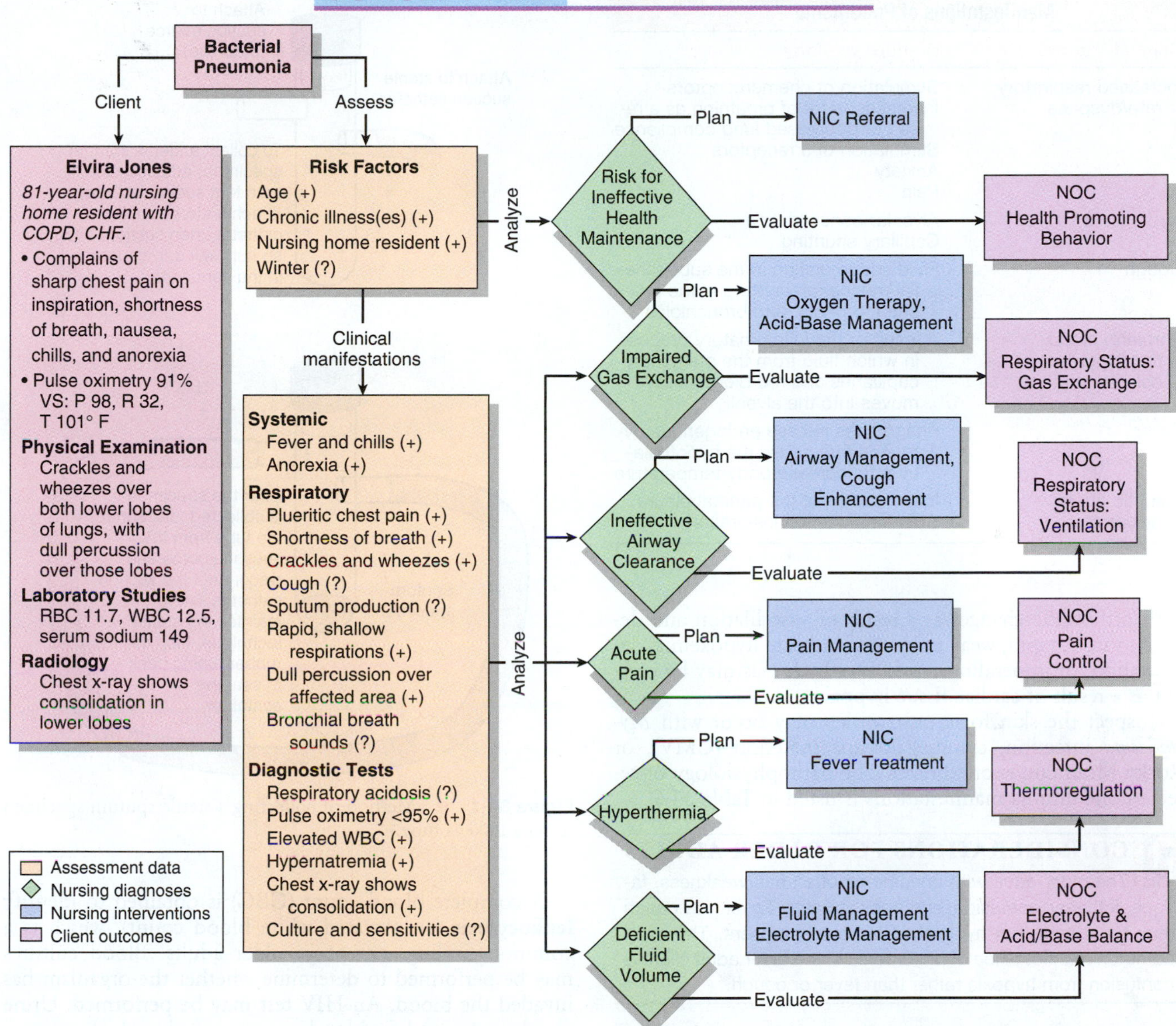

Concept Map by Elaine Bishop Kennedy, EdD, RN

tory of drug addiction or injection drug use. Ask the client about past respiratory illnesses and whether he or she has been exposed to influenza or pneumonia or has had a recent viral infection. Ask about recent skin rashes, insect bites, or exposure to animals.

If the client has chronic respiratory problems, ask whether respiratory equipment is used in the home. Assess whether the client's home cleaning level is adequate to prevent infection. Ask the client when the last influenza or pneumococcal vaccine was taken.

PHYSICAL ASSESSMENT/CLINICAL MANIFESTATIONS

First observe the client's general appearance. Many clients with pneumonia have flushed cheeks, bright eyes, and an anxious expression. The client may have chest or pleuritic pain or discomfort, myalgia, headache, chills, fever, cough, tachycardia, dyspnea, tachypnea, and sputum production. Severe chest muscle weakness also may be present from sustained coughing.

Observe the client's breathing pattern, position, and use of accessory muscles. The hypoxic client may be uncomfortable in a lying position and sit upright, balancing with the hands. Assess the client's cough and the amount, color, consistency, and odor of sputum produced.

Crackles are heard with auscultation when there is fluid in interstitial and alveolar areas. Wheezing may be heard as a result of inflammation and exudate in the airways. Bronchial breath sounds are heard over areas of density or consolidation. Tactile fremitus is increased over areas of pneumonia, and percussion is dulled in these areas. Chest expansion may be diminished or unequal on inspiration.

In evaluating vital signs, compare the results with baseline values. The client with pneumonia is likely to be hypotensive

TABLE 34-6 Pathophysiology of Selected Clinical Manifestations of Pneumonia

Clinical Manifestation	Pathophysiology
Increased respiratory rate/dyspnea	Stimulation of chemoreceptors Increased work of breathing as a result of decreased lung compliance Stimulation of J receptors Anxiety Pain
Hypoxemia	Alveolar consolidation Capillary shunting
Cough	Fluid accumulation in the subepithelial mechanoreceptors in the trachea, bronchi, and bronchioles
Purulent, blood-tinged, or rust-colored sputum	A result of the inflammatory process in which fluid from the pulmonary capillaries and red blood cells moves into the alveoli
Fever	Phagocytes release endogenous pyrogens that cause the hypothalamus to increase body temperature
Pleuritic chest discomfort	Inflammation of the parietal pleura causes pain on inspiration

with orthostatic changes as a result of vasodilation and dehydration. A rapid, weak pulse may indicate hypoxemia, dehydration, or impending shock. Dysrhythmias may be present as a result of cardiac tissue hypoxia.

Inspect the skin for a rash, which may occur with *Mycoplasma* infection, cytomegalovirus infection (CMV), or Rocky Mountain spotted fever. The pathophysiology of selected pneumonia manifestations is listed in Table 34-6.

CONSIDERATIONS FOR OLDER ADULTS

The older adult with pneumonia often has weakness, fatigue, lethargy, confusion, and poor appetite. Fever and cough may be absent, but hypoxemia is usually present. The most common manifestation of pneumonia in the older adult client is confusion from hypoxia rather than fever or cough.

PSYCHOSOCIAL ASSESSMENT

The client with pneumonia often has pain, fatigue, and dyspnea, all of which promote anxiety. Assess anxiety by looking at the client's facial expression and general tenseness of facial and shoulder muscles. Listen to the client carefully and use a calm, slow approach to assessment. Because of airway obstruction and muscle fatigue, the client with dyspnea speaks in broken sentences. Keep the interview short if the client has significant dyspnea or breathing discomfort.

LABORATORY ASSESSMENT

Sputum is obtained and examined by Gram stain, culture, and sensitivity testing; however, the responsible organism is not identified about 50% of the time. A sputum sample is easily obtained from the client who can cough into a specimen container. Extremely ill clients may need suctioning to obtain a sputum specimen. In these situations, a sputum specimen is obtained by sputum trap (Figure 34-1) during suctioning.

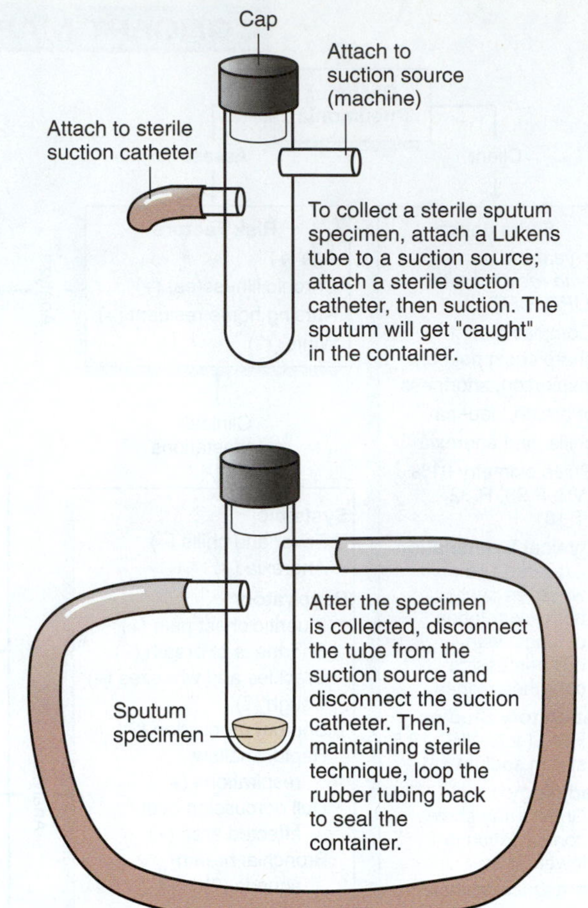

Figure 34-1 ■ Method of collecting a sterile sputum specimen using a Lukens tube.

A complete blood count (CBC) is obtained to identify **leukocytosis** (an elevated white blood count), which is a common finding, except in older adults. Blood cultures may be performed to determine whether the organism has invaded the blood. An HIV test may be performed. Urine may be examined for blood, pus, or protein, which may occur in the septic client with pneumonia.

Arterial blood gases (ABGs) determine baseline arterial oxygen and carbon dioxide levels and help identify a need for supplemental oxygen. Serum electrolyte, blood urea nitrogen (BUN), and creatinine levels also are assessed. A high BUN level may occur as a result of dehydration. Hypernatremia occurs with dehydration as a result of fever and decreased fluid intake.

RADIOGRAPHIC ASSESSMENT

Pneumonia usually appears on chest x-ray as an area of increased density. It may involve a lung segment, a lobe, one lung, or both lungs. In the older adult, the chest x-ray is essential for early diagnosis of pneumonia because symptoms are often vague.

OTHER DIAGNOSTIC ASSESSMENTS

Pulse oximetry is used to assess for hypoxemia. More invasive tests may be needed, such as transtracheal aspiration, bronchoscopy, or direct needle aspiration of the lung to obtain lower airway specimens. Thoracentesis is most often used in clients who have an accompanying pleural effusion.

Critical Thinking Challenge

When you bring the morning medications to your 86-year-old male client in the long-term care facility, he does not know who you are. This problem is a change from yesterday, when he told you all about the visit 4 days earlier from his daughter, who teaches kindergarten, and his three grandchildren. You note that he has not eaten or had anything to drink from his breakfast tray. Because he is diabetic, you hold the morning dose of his oral antidiabetic agent. Concerned, you check his vital signs, which are as follows: T 99.0, P 110 and thready, R 34, BP 96/60. All these values are different from his usual morning vital sign values. You are concerned that he may either have pneumonia or urosepsis.

1. What additional assessment data should you obtain?
2. What risk factors does he have for urosepsis?
3. What risk factors does he have for pneumonia?
4. Should you notify his physician or nurse practitioner?
5. What should you do about his oral antidiabetic medication and other morning medications (Lasix, multivitamin, captopril)?
6. Should you apply oxygen? If so, how?

evolve For suggested answer guidelines, go to http://evolve.elsevier.com/Iggy/.

Analysis

COMMON NURSING DIAGNOSES AND COLLABORATIVE PROBLEMS

The following are priority nursing diagnoses for clients with pneumonia:

1. Impaired Gas Exchange related to effects of alveolar-capillary membrane changes
2. Ineffective Airway Clearance related to effects of infection, excessive tracheobronchial secretions, fatigue and decreased energy, chest discomfort, and muscle weakness

A primary collaborative problem for the client with pneumonia is Potential for Sepsis.

ADDITIONAL NURSING DIAGNOSES AND COLLABORATIVE PROBLEMS

In addition to the common nursing diagnoses and collaborative problems, clients with pneumonia may have one or more of the following:

- Acute Pain related to effects of inflammation of parietal pleura, coughing
- Deficient Fluid Volume related to increased respiratory rate.
- Deficient Fluid Volume related to fever, infection, and increased metabolic rate
- Disturbed Sleep Pattern related to pain, dyspnea, unfamiliar environment (hospitalization)
- Potential for Pleural Effusion

Planning and Implementation

IMPAIRED GAS EXCHANGE

NOC **PLANNING: EXPECTED OUTCOMES.** The client with pneumonia is expected to have adequate gas exchange. The following are indicators of adequate gas exchange:

- Maintenance of SaO_2 of at least 95%
- Absence of cyanosis
- Maintenance of cognitive orientation

INTERVENTIONS. NIC interventions for the client with pneumonia are listed in Chart 34-5. Interventions to treat and manage impaired gas exchange are similar to those for the client with chronic airflow limitation (CAL) (see Chapter 33). In pneumonia, oxygen is the gas exchange affected most; therefore, hypoxemia is the primary problem. Carbon dioxide retention is not common in pneumonia.

Incentive spirometry, also referred to as **sustained maximal inspiration,** is a type of bronchial hygiene used in pneumonia. The objective is to improve inspiratory muscle performance and to prevent or reverse **atelectasis** (alveolar collapse). Instruct the client to exhale fully; then place the mouthpiece in his or her mouth; and take a long, slow, deep breath for 3 to 5 seconds. Evaluate technique, and record the volume of air inspired. Instruct the client to perform 5 to 10 breaths per session every hour while awake.

INEFFECTIVE AIRWAY CLEARANCE

NOC **PLANNING: EXPECTED OUTCOMES.** The client with pneumonia is expected to maintain a patent airway. Indicators are the following:

- Effective cough
- Absence of pallor or cyanosis
- Absence of crackles and wheezes on auscultation
- Decreased tactile fremitus

INTERVENTIONS. For the client with pneumonia, interventions for ineffective airway clearance are similar to those for COPD or asthma. Because of fatigue, muscle weakness, chest discomfort, and excessive secretions, the client with pneumonia often has difficulty clearing secretions. Help the client to cough and deep breathe at least every 2 hours. The alert client may use an incentive spirometer to facilitate deep breathing and stimulate coughing. Chest physiotherapy (CPT or chest PT) is no longer recommended for uncomplicated pneumonia. Dehydration should be avoided, but there is no evidence that hydration helps to clear secretions. Adequate hydration may help to thin secretions and make them easier to remove. Monitor intake and output to ensure adequate hydration when fever and tachypnea are present.

The health care provider prescribes bronchodilators, especially beta-2 agonists (see Chart 33-5), when bronchospasm is part of the disease process. They are initially given by aerosol nebulizer and then by metered-dose inhaler (see Chart 33-5). Inhaled steroids are rarely used with acute pneumonia except when the client also has bronchial asthma or respiratory failure.

POTENTIAL FOR SEPSIS

NOC **PLANNING: EXPECTED OUTCOMES.** The client with pneumonia is expected to be free of the invading organism and to return to a pre-pneumonia health status. Indicators are the following:

- Absence of fever
- Absence of pathogens in blood and sputum cultures
- White blood cell count and differential within normal limits

INTERVENTIONS. The key to effective treatment of pneumonia is eradication of the organism causing the infection. Anti-infectives are given for all types of pneumonias

CHART 34-5

NIC **INTERVENTION ACTIVITIES for**
The Client with Pneumonia

Cough Enhancement: *Promotion of deep inhalation by the client with subsequent generation of high intrathoracic pressures and compression of the underlying lung parenchyma for the forceful expulsion of air*

- Assist client to a sitting position with neck slightly flexed, shoulders relaxed, and knees flexed.
- Encourage client to take several deep breaths.
- Encourage client to take a deep breath, hold it for 2 seconds, and cough two or three times in succession.
- Instruct client to inhale deeply, bend forward slightly, and perform three or four huffs (against an open glottis).
- Instruct client to inhale deeply several times, to exhale slowly, and to cough at the end of exhalation.
- Initiate lateral chest wall rib spring techniques during the expiration phase of the cough maneuver, as appropriate.
- Instruct client to follow coughing with several maximal inhalation breaths.
- Encourage use of incentive spirometry, as appropriate.
- Promote systemic fluid hydration, as appropriate.

Oxygen Therapy: *Administration of oxygen and monitoring of its effectiveness*

- Clear oral, nasal, and tracheal secretions, as appropriate.
- Restrict smoking.
- Maintain airway patency.
- Set up oxygen equipment and administer through a heated, humidified system.
- Administer supplemental oxygen as ordered.
- Monitor the oxygen liter flow.
- Monitor position of oxygen delivery device.
- Instruct client about importance of leaving oxygen delivery device on.
- Periodically check oxygen delivery device to ensure that the prescribed concentration is being delivered.
- Monitor the effectiveness of oxygen therapy (e.g., pulse oximetry, ABGs), as appropriate.
- Ensure replacement of oxygen mask/cannula whenever the device is removed.
- Monitor client's ability to tolerate removal of oxygen while eating.
- Change oxygen delivery device from mask to nasal prongs during meals, as tolerated.
- Observe for signs of oxygen-induced hypoventilation.
- Monitor for signs of oxygen toxicity and absorption atelectasis.
- Monitor client's anxiety related to need for oxygen therapy.
- Monitor for skin breakdown from friction of oxygen device.
- Provide for oxygen when client is transported.

Respiratory Monitoring: *Collection and analysis of client data to ensure airway patency and adequate gas exchange*

- Monitor rate, rhythm, depth, and effort of respirations.
- Note chest movement, watching for symmetry, use of accessory muscles, and supraclavicular and intercostal muscle retractions.
- Monitor breathing patterns: bradypnea, tachypnea, hyperventilation, Kussmaul respirations, Cheyne-Stokes respirations, apneustic Biot's respiration, and ataxic patterns.
- Palpate for equal lung expansion.
- Monitor for diaphragmatic muscle fatigue (paradoxical motion).
- Auscultate breath sounds, noting areas of decreased/absent ventilation and presence of adventitious sounds.
- Determine the need for suctioning by auscultating for crackles and rhonchi over major airways.
- Auscultate lung sounds after treatments to note results.
- Monitor for increased restlessness, anxiety, and air hunger.
- Note changes in Sao_2, Svo_2, end tidal CO_2, and ABG values, as appropriate.
- Monitor client's ability to cough effectively.
- Note onset, characteristics, and duration of cough.
- Monitor client's respiratory secretions.
- Monitor for dyspnea and events that decrease and worsen it.
- Monitor chest x-ray reports.
- Place the client on side, as indicated, to prevent aspiration; log roll if cervical aspiration is suspected.
- Institute respiratory treatments (e.g., nebulizer), as needed.

NIC intervention activities selected from Dochterman, J.M., & Bulechek, G.M. (Eds.). (2004). *Nursing interventions classification (NIC)* (4th ed.). St. Louis: Mosby.
ABG, Arterial blood gas; Sao_2, arterial oxygen saturation; Svo_2, venous oxygen saturation; CO_2, carbon dioxide.

except those caused by viruses. The health care provider prescribes anti-infective therapy. The exact drug or drugs are determined by the organism suspected or identified, whether the pneumonia is community-acquired (CAP) or hospital-acquired, and whether the client has other conditions or factors that increase the risk for complication (Table 34-7). Initial treatment is based on the manifestations, prior experience, and the most common organisms causing pneumonia in that geographic region. The initial therapy may be continued if the specific organism is not identified.

The client may be able to be switched from intravenous (IV) to oral therapy in 2 or 3 days, depending on the response (e.g., stable clinical condition, afebrile). The course of anti-infective therapy varies with the drug used and the organism(s) involved. Usually anti-infectives are used for 7 to 10 days for a client with uncomplicated CAP and up to 21 days for an immunocompromised client.

Drug resistance is becoming increasingly common, especially for infections with *Streptococcus pneumoniae*. This problem is known as drug-resistant *S. pneumoniae,* or DRSP. DRSP is most common among people over 65 years of age and among those who became infected as a result of exposure to young children from a day-care environment.

For pneumonia resulting from aspiration of food or stomach contents, interventions focus on prevention of lung damage and treating the infection. Aspiration of acidic substances (e.g., vomitus or stomach contents) can cause widespread inflammation, leading to acute respiratory distress syndrome (ARDS) and permanent lung damage. In these conditions, steroids and nonsteroidal anti-inflammatory agents are used with antibiotics to reduce the inflammatory response.

Community-Based Care

The client needs to continue the anti-infective drugs as prescribed. An important nursing role is to reinforce, clarify, and provide information to the client and family as indicated.

HOME CARE MANAGEMENT

No special changes are needed in the home. If the home consists of more than one story, the client may prefer to stay on one floor for a few weeks because stair climbing may increase fatigue and dyspnea. Bath and hygiene needs may be met by using a bedside commode if a bathroom is not located on the level the client is using. Home care needs will depend on the client's level of fatigue, dyspnea, and family and social support.

TABLE 34-7 Recommended Drug Categories for the Treatment of Pneumonia

Pneumonia Type	Recommended Drug Categories with Alternatives
Community-Acquired Pneumonias	
Age <60 yr with no comorbidity	Cefuroxime (add erythromycin if concern for *Mycoplasma, Chlamydia*, or *Legionella* is high) Azithromycin (alternative if client is allergic to penicillin/cephalosporin or is erythromycin intolerant) Levofloxacin (if client is macrolide* intolerant or pneumonia fails to resolve)
Age >60 or <60 yr with comorbidity	Ceftriaxone and azithromycin (or erythromycin) Levofloxacin (alternative if macrolide intolerant or pneumonia fails to resolve) Trovafloxacin
Aspiration pneumonia	Ampicillin/sulbactam and clindamycin Trovafloxacin (alternative if penicillin/cephalosporin allergy) Ceftriaxone and clindamycin
Hospital-Acquired (Nosocomial) Pneumonias	
Gram-positive infections	Ticarcillin/clavulanate Vancomycin Imipenem/cilastatin Piperacillin/tazobactam Cefepime and metronidazole
Gram-negative infections	Ciprofloxacin Aminoglycoside (amikacin, gentamicin) if renal function is stable Ceftazidime Aztreonam Ticarcillin

*Macrolides include erythromycin, azithromycin, clarithromycin, and dirithromycin.

CHART 34-6

FOCUSED ASSESSMENT of
The Client Recovering from Pneumonia

Ascertain whether the client has had any of the following:
- Chills
- Fever
- Persistent cough
- Dyspnea
- Wheezing
- Hemoptysis
- Increased sputum production
- Chest discomfort
- Increasing fatigue
- Any other symptoms that have failed to resolve

Assess the client for the following:
- Fever
- Diaphoresis
- Cyanosis, especially around the mouth or conjunctiva
- Dyspnea, tachypnea, or tachycardia
- Adventitious or abnormal breath sounds
- Weakness

The long recovery phase of pneumonia, especially in the older client, can be frustrating and perhaps depressing. Fatigue, weakness, and a residual cough can last for weeks. Some clients fear they will never return to a "normal" level of functioning. It is important to prepare the client for the course of the disease and to offer reassurance that complete recovery will occur. Early after discharge, a home health nursing assessment may be helpful (Chart 34-6).

HEALTH TEACHING

Review all drugs with the client and family and emphasize completing anti-infective therapy. Instruct the client to notify the health care provider if chills, fever, persistent cough, dyspnea, wheezing, hemoptysis, increased sputum production, chest discomfort, or increasing fatigue recurs or if symptoms fail to resolve. Emphasize the importance of getting plenty of rest and gradually increasing exercise.

An important aspect of education for the client and family is the avoidance of upper respiratory tract infections and viruses. Instruct the client to avoid crowds (especially in the fall and winter when viruses are prevalent), people who have a cold or flu, and exposure to irritants such as smoke. An annual influenza vaccine is recommended, and the pneumococcal vaccine is currently recommended once every 5 years (possibly more often for clients at high-risk). A balanced diet and adequate fluid intake are essential.

HEALTH CARE RESOURCES

Inform clients who smoke that smoking is a risk factor for pneumonia. Provide them with information on smoking-cessation classes through the American Lung Association (ALA) and American Cancer Society. The health care provider may prescribe nicotine patches. *Warn the client of the danger of myocardial infarction if smoking is continued while using the patches.* Urge the client to enroll in a smoking-cessation program to assist in the nicotine withdrawal process in conjunction with nicotine patches. Give him or her information booklets on pneumonia provided by the ALA. Urge the client who has not already been vaccinated against influenza or pneumonia to take this preventive measure when the pneumonia has resolved.

Evaluation: Outcomes

Evaluate the care of the client with pneumonia on the basis of the identified nursing diagnoses and collaborative problems. The expected outcomes are that the client:
- Attains or maintains adequate gas exchange
- Maintains patent airways
- Is free of the invading organism
- Returns to his or her pre-pneumonia health status

Specific indicators for these outcomes are listed for each nursing diagnosis and collaborative problem under the Planning and Implementation section (see earlier).

Severe Acute Respiratory Syndrome (SARS)

A new respiratory infection was first identified in China early in November 2002. At first appearing as an atypical pneumonia, the infection has been termed **severe acute respiratory syndrome,** or **SARS.** As of July 2003, more than 8400 cases of SARS had been reported to the World Health Organization, 325 cases in North America. In more affluent countries, the mortality rate is 8%. This rate is higher in less affluent countries.

PATHOPHYSIOLOGY

The cause of SARS is a new virus from a family of virus types known as *coronaviruses.* These viruses have ribonucleic acid (RNA) as their genetic material and have many projections that look like a halo or "corona" when examined by electron microscopes. This family of viruses causes many forms of the common cold. The new virus is a mutated form of the coronavirus and is more virulent than most members of this virus family. The virus infects cells of the respiratory tract, triggering an inflammatory response. It stays in the respiratory passageways rather than spreading into the blood because it grows best at temperatures slightly lower than the normal core body temperature.

The virus is easily spread by airborne droplets from infected people through sneezing, coughing, and talking. It can contaminate surfaces and objects, although it does not survive on nonliving surfaces for long periods. People at greatest risk for SARS are those in close direct contact with an infected person. The portals of entry for infection with the virus are the mucous membranes of the eyes, nose, and mouth.

◆COLLABORATIVE MANAGEMENT

◆Assessment

The manifestations of SARS are the same as those of any respiratory infection. Usually, the client has a fever higher than 100.4° F (38.0° C), a headache, and general body aches. Mild cold symptoms of a runny nose, sore throat, and watery eyes may also be present. Within 2 to 7 days, the client develops a dry cough and has difficulty breathing. Hypoxia, with cyanosis, low oxygen saturation, and a feeling of breathlessness, indicates more severe illness. Chest x-rays show a pattern similar to pneumonia or other respiratory distress syndromes.

Diagnosis is made by the manifestations and by ruling out other causes of the symptoms. No rapid test specific for this disorder exists at this time. About 28 days after the infection starts, a blood test for antibodies to the virus or pieces of the RNA from the virus can confirm the diagnosis (usually the client is well by this time).

◆Interventions

No known effective treatment for this infection exists at this time. Standard antibiotic agents and antiviral drugs are not able to kill the virus or prevent its replication. Interventions are supportive to allow the client's own immune system to fight the infection. Oxygen is given when hypoxia or breathlessness is present. Respiratory treatments to dilate the bronchioles and move respiratory secretions are used. If gas exchange is not improved with oxygen therapy alone, intubation and mechanical ventilation may be needed. Antibiotics are used to treat a bacterial pneumonia that may occur with SARS.

PREVENTION OF INFECTION SPREAD

A major nursing responsibility is the prevention infection spread. Handwashing is a key prevention intervention. Gloves may be used but are not a replacement for good handwashing. Use airborne and contact precautions with clients who are suspected to have SARS. Use gowns and eye protection when coming into direct contact with the client. Airborne isolation is recommended. When the client is out of the isolation environment, he or she must wear a mask. If for some reason the client cannot wear a mask, all other people in the environment should wear a mask.

When performing procedures that normally induce coughing or promote aerosolization of particles (e.g., suctioning, using a positive-pressure face mask, obtaining a sputum culture, or giving aerosolized treatments), be sure to protect yourself and other health care workers. Wear a disposable particulate mask respirator (e.g., N-95, N-99, or N-100) and protective eyewear during such procedures. Keep the door to the client's room closed. Avoid touching your face with contaminated gloves. Wash your hands after you remove the gown, gloves, eyewear, and face shield and whenever you leave the client's room. Wear clean gloves when disinfecting contaminated surfaces or equipment.

Pulmonary Tuberculosis

PATHOPHYSIOLOGY

Tuberculosis (TB) is a highly communicable disease caused by *Mycobacterium tuberculosis.* It is the most common bacterial infection worldwide. The organism is transmitted via **aerosolization** (i.e., an airborne route). When a person with active TB coughs, laughs, sneezes, whistles, or sings, droplets become airborne and may be inhaled by others. Far more people are infected with the bacillus than actually develop active TB.

The bacillus multiplies freely when it reaches a susceptible site (bronchi or alveoli). An exudative response occurs, causing a nonspecific pneumonitis. With the development of acquired immunity, further growth of bacilli is controlled in most initial lesions. These lesions usually resolve and leave little or no residual bacilli. Only a small percentage of people initially infected will develop active TB (5% to 15%). The greatest risk for active TB among people who are HIV negative is during the first 2 years after infection.

Cell-mediated immunity develops 2 to 10 weeks after infection and is manifested by a positive reaction to a tuberculin test. The primary infection may be so small that it does not appear on a chest x-ray. The process of infection occurs in the following order:

1. The granulomatous inflammation created by the tubercle bacillus in the lung becomes surrounded by collagen, fibroblasts, and lymphocytes.
2. **Caseation necrosis** (necrotic tissue being turned into a granular mass) occurs in the center of the lesion. If this area shows on x-ray, it is called **Ghon tubercle,** or the primary lesion.

Areas of caseation then undergo resorption, degeneration, and fibrosis. These necrotic areas may calcify **(calcification)** or liquefy **(liquefaction).** If liquefaction occurs, the liquid

TABLE 34-8 American Lung Association Classification of Tuberculosis

Class	Criteria
0	No TB exposure, not infected
1	TB exposure, no evidence of infection
2	TB infection, no disease
3	TB clinically active (clients with completed diagnostic evidence of TB—both a significant reaction to TB skin test and clinical or x-ray evidence of TB)
4	TB: not clinically active (clients with history of TB or abnormal chest x-ray film but no significant TB skin test reaction or clinical evidence)
5	TB: suspect (diagnosis pending); used during diagnostic testing of suspect clients for no longer than 3 mo

material then empties into a bronchus, and the evacuated area becomes a cavity **(cavitation).** Bacilli continue to grow in the necrotic cavity wall and spread via lymph channels into new areas of the lung.

A lesion also may progress by direct extension if bacilli multiply rapidly during inflammation. The lesions may extend through the pleura, resulting in pleural or pericardial effusion. **Miliary** or **hematogenous TB** is the spread of TB throughout the body when a large number of organisms enter the blood. Many tiny, discrete nodules scattered throughout the lung are seen on chest x-ray. The brain, meninges, liver, kidney, or bone marrow can become infected as a result of spread through the blood.

Initial infection is seen more often in the middle or lower lobes of the lung. The local lymph nodes are infected and enlarged. An asymptomatic period usually follows the primary infection and can last for years or decades before clinical symptoms develop. *An infected individual is not infectious to others until manifestations of disease occur.*

Secondary TB is a reactivation of the disease in a previously infected person. Reactivation is more likely when defenses are lowered, which may be part of the reason older adults and people with HIV disease are at greater risk for TB. The upper lobes are the most common site of reactivation and are referred to as **Simon's foci.** The ALA's TB classification is shown in Table 34-8.

Etiology

Mycobacterium tuberculosis is a nonmoving, slow-growing, acid-fast rod transmitted via the airborne route. People who are most often infected are those having repeated close contact with an infectious person who has not yet been diagnosed with TB. The risk of transmission is reduced after the infectious person has received proper medication for 2 to 3 weeks, clinical improvement occurs, and acid-fast bacilli [AFB] in the sputum are reduced.

Incidence/Prevalence

The incidence of TB has been steadily increasing in the United States and worldwide for two decades. The increase is related to the onset of HIV infection. In the United States, the following people are at greatest risk for development of TB:

- Those in constant, frequent contact with an untreated individual
- Those who have immune dysfunction or HIV
- Individuals who live in crowded areas such as long-term care facilities, prisons, and mental health facilities
- Older and homeless people
- Abusers of injection drugs or alcohol
- Lower socioeconomic groups
- Foreign immigrants (especially from Mexico, the Philippines, and Vietnam)

COLLABORATIVE MANAGEMENT

Assessment

Early detection of tuberculosis (TB) depends on subjective findings rather than on observable symptoms. TB has a slow onset, and many clients are not aware of symptoms until the disease is advanced. *A diagnosis of TB should be considered for any client with a persistent cough or other symptoms compatible with TB, such as weight loss, anorexia, night sweats, hemoptysis, shortness of breath, fever, or chills.*

HISTORY

Assess the client's past exposure to TB. Ask about the client's country of origin and travel to foreign countries where there is a high incidence of TB. It is important to ask about the results of any previous tests for TB. Also ask whether the client has had bacillus Calmette-Guérin (BCG) vaccine. The BCG vaccine contains attenuated tubercle bacilli and is used in many countries to produce increased resistance to TB. *Anyone who has received BCG vaccine within the previous 10 years will have a positive skin test that can complicate interpretation.* Usually the size of the skin response decreases each year after BCG vaccination. These clients should be evaluated for TB with a chest x-ray. The effectiveness of BCG vaccine in preventing TB is controversial, and it is not used for this purpose in the United States.

PHYSICAL ASSESSMENT/CLINICAL MANIFESTATIONS

The client with TB has progressive fatigue, lethargy, nausea, anorexia, weight loss, irregular menses, and a low-grade fever. Manifestations may have been present for weeks or months. Night sweats may occur with the fever. The client has a cough and mucopurulent sputum, which may be streaked with blood. Chest tightness and a dull, aching chest pain occur with the cough.

Physical examination of the chest does not provide conclusive evidence of TB. You may hear dullness with percussion over involved the lung fields, bronchial breath sounds, crackles, and increased transmission of spoken or whispered sounds. Partial obstruction of a bronchus from endobronchial disease or compression by lymph nodes may produce localized wheezing.

DIAGNOSTIC ASSESSMENT

A diagnosis of TB is suggested by the manifestations and a positive smear for acid-fast bacillus. Sputum is obtained, smeared on a slide, and stained with a red dye. After the slide has dried, it is treated with an acid alcohol to remove the stain. TB does not destain with this procedure and remains red. The acid-fast bacillus test is not specific for TB (other organisms are also acid-fast), but it is used as a quick method to determine whether TB treatment and precautions should be started until more definitive testing can be completed.

Sputum culture of *M. tuberculosis* confirms the diagnosis. Traditional cultures are slow growing, requiring weeks to determine a positive or negative result. Newer techniques (BACTEC) enhance culture growth and allow identification 1 to 3 weeks instead of 4 to 6 weeks. After drugs are started, sputum samples are obtained again to determine therapy effectiveness. Cultures are usually negative after 3 months of treatment.

The polymerase chain reaction (PCR) assay is used for rapid identification of mycobacteria in selected situations. This test amplifies the organism's genetic material (DNA) and identifies the organism within hours instead of weeks. Although highly accurate, its high cost and limited availability limit the widespread use of this test as a TB screening or diagnostic tool.

The tuberculin test (Mantoux test) result is the most commonly used reliable test of TB infection. A small amount (0.1 mL) of purified protein derivative (PPD) is given intradermally in the forearm. An area of induration (not just redness) measuring 10 mm or greater in diameter 48 to 72 hours after injection indicates exposure to and infection with TB. Recent studies indicate that a reading after 72 hours rather than after just 48 hours is more accurate. The incidence of false-negative readings is greater at 48 hours. (See the Evidence-Based Practice for Nursing box at right). *A positive reaction does not mean that active disease is present but indicates exposure to TB or the presence of inactive (dormant) disease.* A reaction of 5 mm or greater is considered positive in people with HIV infection. A reduced skin reaction or a negative skin test does not rule out TB disease or infection of the very old or anyone who is severely immunocompromised. This condition is called **anergy.**

Screening is performed yearly for anyone at high risk for coming into contact with people infected with TB. Screening is particularly important for foreign-born people and migrant workers. Participation in screening programs is enhanced when programs are delivered in a culturally sensitive and nonthreatening manner.

Once a person's skin test is positive for TB, a chest x-ray is needed to detect clinically active TB or old, healed lesions. Caseation and inflammation may be seen on the x-ray if the disease is active. Clients are instructed to seek medical attention if they have manifestations of TB.

The chest x-rays of HIV-infected clients may be normal or may show infiltrates in any lung zone along with hilar lymph node enlargement.

Common Nursing Diagnoses and Collaborative Problems

Nursing diagnoses and collaborative problems that may apply to clients with TB include the following:

- Impaired Gas Exchange related to disease progression
- Ineffective Airway Clearance related to increased secretions or fatigue
- Deficient Knowledge (Infection Control, Therapeutic Regimen, Nutrition) related to lack of exposure or information misinterpretation
- Fatigue related to poor tissue oxygenation and increased metabolism
- Imbalanced Nutrition: Less Than Body Requirements related to increased metabolism, poor appetite, drug regimen, or fatigue
- Social Isolation related to altered state of wellness or changed appearance

EVIDENCE-BASED PRACTICE for Nursing

Time makes a difference

Singh, D., Sutton, C., & Woodcock, A. (2002). Tuberculin test measurement: Variability due to the time of reading. *Chest, 122*(4), 1299-1301.

This study sought to compare the 48-hour results of the Mantoux purified protein derivative (PPD) testing for tuberculosis (TB) with those obtained at 72 hours after intradermal injection. The Mantoux test is the most frequently used method to identify latent TB infection worldwide. Historically, test results are recommended to be read at either 48 hours or 72 hours after the initial intradermal injection; however, it is not known whether the timing of these two readings are truly comparable.

A total of 116 healthy adult volunteers were injected with 10 units of the PPD, and the skin test results were read at both 48 hours and 72 hours for all subjects. None of the subjects had a history of tuberculosis, HIV disease, IV drug use, or recent exposure to tuberculosis. Among the 116 subjects, 106 had a history of vaccination with bacillus Calmette-Guérin (BCG) and would be expected to have a positive PPD test result, defined as an area of induration greater than 15 mm. Areas of induration were significantly greater at the 72-hour reading than at the 48-hour reading. The number of subjects considered to have a positive PPD test at 48 hours was 28 and the number of subjects considered to have a positive PPD test at 72 hours was 36. Thus, the 48 hour reading yielded a false negative result in 8 subjects (22%).

Level of Evidence: 3—Well-designed trial without randomization; time series.

Critique. The major problem with this study was a failure to control inter-rater reliability among the observers/readers of the PPD test.

Implications for Nursing. Nurses are often responsible for conducting mass TB screening programs in schools, student health services, inpatient and outpatient settings, health fairs, and places of employment. With an option of evaluating the test at either 48 or 72 hours, the scheduling of tested persons to return for evaluation in 48 hours may result in a significant number of false-negative results. Such people would not be further evaluated and would pose a public health risk. Thus, when planning TB screenings, nurses should either schedule test readings at 72 hours or, if readings show any induration at 48 hours, the person should return for a second evaluation at 72 hours.

Critical Thinking Challenge

You are the outpatient nurse in the infectious disease clinic. The client is a 62-year-old registered nurse who works at a prison clinic/hospital. She has type 2 diabetes, hypertension, and gastroesophageal reflux disease (GERD), and she had a mastectomy 7 years ago for breast cancer. She has smoked since she was 17 years of age (two packs per day). Her prescribed drugs include lisinopril (Zestril), tamoxifen (Nolvadex, Tamofen✱), omeprazole (Prilosec, Losec✱), and metformin (Glucophage). On screening last week, her PPD had an indurated area of 5 mm 48 hours after the injection and 20 mm 72 hours after the injection.

1. Does this woman have active TB?
2. What are her risk factors for TB?
3. Calculate her smoking history in pack years.
4. What assessment data should you obtain?

evolve For suggested answer guidelines, go to http://evolve.elsevier.com/Iggy/.

Interventions

Combination drug therapy is the most effective method of treating TB and preventing transmission. Increasing the

CHART 34-7

DRUG THERAPY for Tuberculosis*

Drug	Usual Dosage	Nursing Interventions	Drug Action/Rationale for Use
Isoniazid (INH)	5 mg/kg PO, IM (maximum 300 mg) daily; 15 mg/kg (maximum 900 mg) biweekly	Observe for drug interactions, which may inhibit drug metabolism of phenytoin, carbamazepine, primidone, and warfarin. Instruct the client to take on empty stomach and avoid antacids. Monitor for signs of hepatitis and neurotoxicity effects.	Isoniazid inhibits the synthesis of mycolic acids and acts to kill actively growing organisms in the extracellular environment and inhibits the growth of dormant organisms in the macrophages and caseating granulomas.
Rifampin (RIF)	10 mg/kg PO (maximum 600 mg) daily or biweekly	Instruct the client that secretions, including urine, will be orange colored and that the drug will permanently discolor soft contact lenses. Observe for drug interactions, which may enhance elimination of theophylline, steroids, opioids, oral hypoglycemics, warfarin, and occasionally vitamin D. Observe for hepatotoxic effects. RIF decreases effectiveness of oral contraceptives.	RIF has the unique ability to kill slower growing organisms that reside in the caseating granuloma and macrophage.
Pyrazinamide (PZA)	15-30 mg/kg PO (maximum 2000 mg) daily; 50 mg/kg biweekly	Observe for hepatotoxic effects.	Pyrazinamide is the most active drug at killing mycobacteria present in macrophages. The acidic environment in the macrophage inhibits most agents.
Ethambutol (EMB)	15 mg/kg daily PO; 50 mg/kg biweekly	Obtain baseline visual acuity and color discrimination, especially to the color green. Repeat testing every 1-2 mo.	Ethambutol inhibits bacterial ribonucleic acid (RNA) synthesis. It is slow acting and must be used in combination with other bactericidal agents.
Streptomycin (SM)	1000 mg IM, IV over 1 hr, daily for 2 mo followed by biweekly injections until treatment is completed	Obtain baseline audiometric test every 1-2 mo. It can impair the eighth cranial nerve. Older clients are especially susceptible.	Streptomycin is an aminoglycoside antibiotic that is active against extracellular organisms only.
Amikacin	15 mg/kg daily IM, IV (usual dose 1 g)	Ensure adequate hydration, monitor renal function and hearing. Amikacin can lead to renal toxicity and ototoxicity.	Amikacin is an aminoglycoside antibiotic that can be used if streptomycin is not available.
Rifapentine (Priftin)	600 mg twice weekly	Doses must be separated by at least 72 hr. Instruct the client that metabolism of other drugs may be faster, causing lower blood concentrations and a need for higher doses (especially for antidiabetic drugs, barbiturates, and antibiotics). Instruct female clients to use additional forms of birth control, because this drug decreases the effectiveness of oral contraceptives. Observe for hepatotoxic effects.	Rifapentine has high bacteriostatic and bactericidal action against slow-growing intracellular bacteria.

*Newer drugs contain combinations of rifampin and isoniazid (Rifamate) or of rifampin, isoniazid, and pyrazinamide (Rifater).

number of clients with TB who complete curative therapy is a major focus for Healthy People 2010 (see the Meeting Healthy People 2010 Objectives box on p. 644). Active TB is treated with a combination of drugs to which the organism is sensitive. Therapy continues until the disease is under control. The use of multiple-drug regimens destroys organisms as quickly as possible and reduces the emergence of drug-resistant organisms. Current therapy uses isoniazid (INH) and rifampin throughout the therapy; pyrazinamide is added for the first 2 months (Chart 34-7). This protocol shortens the therapy from 6 to 12 months to 6 months. Ethambutol or streptomycin may be added to the regimen as the fourth drug.

Strict adherence to the prescribed drug regimen is crucial for suppressing the disease. Thus your major role is teaching the client about drug therapy. Accurate information provided

Meeting HEALTHY PEOPLE 2010 Objectives

TUBERCULOSIS

Objective 22.25: Increase to at least 90% the proportion of all tuberculosis patients who complete curative therapy within 12 months.

- Teach all clients to have yearly TB skin tests.
- Assist clients who have a positive TB skin test to have follow-up screening for a definitive diagnosis.
- Develop culturally appropriate education materials.
- Ensure that education materials are written or presented at no greater than a fourth-grade literacy level.
- Educate those clients who are diagnosed with TB to:
  - Take all medication as prescribed
  - Keep all follow-up appointments
  - Identify contacts
- Implement a direction observation therapy (DOT) program for those clients who have not consistently taken medication as prescribed.
- Refer clients who do not have money for medications to the appropriate resource for obtaining low-cost or no-cost TB drugs.

in multiple formats (e.g., pamphlets, videos, drug-schedule worksheets) can be of value in client education. An anxious client may not absorb information well. You may need to repeat the information and obtain the help of family members. To determine whether the client understands how to take the drugs, ask him or her to describe the treatment regimen, major side effects, and when to call the health care agency and physician.

TB is often treated outside the acute care setting, with the client convalescing in the home setting. Airborne precautions are not necessary in this setting because family members have already been exposed; however, all members of the household need to undergo TB testing. Instruct the client to cover the mouth and nose when coughing or sneezing, to place used tissues in plastic bags, and to wear a mask when in contact with crowds until the drugs suppress infection.

Tell the client sputum specimens are needed every 2 to 4 weeks once drug therapy is initiated. When the results of three sputum cultures are negative, the client is no longer infectious and may return to former employment. Remind him or her to avoid exposure to any inhalation irritants because they can cause further lung damage.

The hospitalized client with active TB is placed under Airborne Precautions (see Chapter 29) in a well-ventilated room. The room should have at least six exchanges of fresh air per minute and should be ventilated to the outside if possible. All health care workers must wear a N95 or high-efficiency particulate air (HEPA) respirator when caring for the client (Figure 34-2). When there is risk of hand and clothing contamination, implement standard precautions by using appropriate barrier protection (i.e., gowns and gloves). Perform thorough handwashing before and after client care. Precautions are discontinued when the client is no longer considered infectious.

The TB drugs may cause the client to have nausea. Teach him or her to prevent nausea by taking the daily dose at bedtime. Antiemetics may also prevent this problem. Instruct the client about the need for a well-balanced diet to promote healing. An increased intake of foods that are rich in iron, protein, and vitamin C is recommended for the client with TB. Consult with the nutritionist for specialized needs.

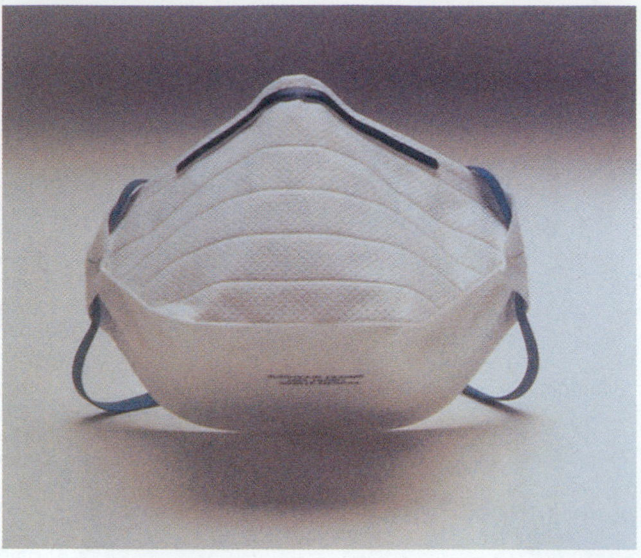

Figure 34-2 ■ A high-efficiency particulate air (HEPA) respirator used in the care of clients with active or "rule-out" tuberculosis. (Courtesy of Uvex Safety, Smithfield, RI.)

The client with TB may have changes in physical stamina and also faces concerns about the prognosis of the disease. Be realistic in offering a positive outlook for the client who adheres to the drug regimen. Tell him or her that fatigue will diminish as the treatment progresses. With current resistant strains of TB, however, you must emphasize that not taking the drugs as prescribed could lead to an infection that is difficult to treat or has total drug resistance.

Community-Based Care

HOME CARE MANAGEMENT

Most clients with TB are managed outside the hospital; however, clients may be diagnosed with TB while in the hospital if pneumonia is suspected or other complications exist. Discharge may be delayed if the living situation is high risk or if nonadherence is likely. Consult with the social service worker in the hospital or the community health nursing agency to ensure that the client is discharged to the appropriate environment with continued supervision.

HEALTH TEACHING

Instruct the client to follow the drug regimen exactly as prescribed and always to have a supply on hand. Teach about side effects and ways of reducing them to ensure adherence. Remind the client that the disease is usually no longer contagious after drugs have been taken for 2 to 3 consecutive weeks and clinical improvement is seen; however, he or she must continue with the prescribed drugs for 6 months or longer as prescribed. Directly observed therapy (DOT), in which the nurse or other health care provider watches the client swallow the drugs, may be indicated in some situations. This practice contributes to more treatment successes, fewer relapses, and less drug resistance.

The client who has weight loss and severe lethargy should gradually resume his or her usual activities. Proper nutrition must be maintained to prevent recurrence of infection.

To help with concerns about the contagious aspect of the infection, provide the client with information about TB. A key to preventing transmission is identifying those in close contact with the infected person so that they can be tested and treated if needed. Health care professionals have an important role in this aspect of care. Identified contacts are assessed with a TB test and possibly a chest x-ray to determine TB infection status. Multidrug therapy may be indicated. In addition, certain high-risk contacts receive prophylactic therapy, usually with INH.

HEALTH CARE RESOURCES

Instruct the client to receive follow-up care by a health care provider for at least 1 year during active treatment. The American Lung Association (ALA) can provide free information to the client about the disease and its treatment. In addition, Alcoholics Anonymous and other health care resources for clients with alcoholism are available if needed. Assist the client who uses illicit drugs to locate a drug treatment program. Urge smokers to quit, and assist them in finding an appropriate smoking-cessation program.

Critical Thinking Challenge

The client (a 62-year-old registered nurse) is confirmed to have active TB. She lives at home with her husband, who is 70 years old and has moderate heart failure. She is the sole support of the family and is concerned about when she can go back to work. Her prescribed drug regimen for the first 2 months includes the following:

- Isoniazid (INH) 250 mg taken orally (PO) daily
- Rifampin (RIF) 500 mg PO daily
- Pyrazinamide (PZA) 750 mg PO daily
- Ethambutol (EMB) 750 mg PO daily

If her cultures indicate that the organism causing her infection is not drug resistant and if the sputum culture at 2 months is negative, the PZA and EMB will be discontinued and she will continue to take the INH and RIF daily for an additional 4 months.

1. When can this client go back to work?
2. Should this client's husband be tested? Why or why not?
3. Are there any issues or special considerations for the prescribed TB drug therapy and the client's other drug regimen?
4. Is this client a candidate for DOT? Why or why not?
5. What specific precautions or actions will you recommend that this client make in her home care?

evolve For suggested answer guidelines, go to http://evolve.elsevier.com/Iggy/.

Lung Abscess

PATHOPHYSIOLOGY

A lung abscess is a localized area of lung destruction caused by liquefaction necrosis, which is usually related to pyogenic bacteria. Clients with this problem often have a history of pneumonia, aspiration of oropharyngeal contents, or obstruction as a result of a tumor or foreign body. Other causes of aspiration leading to lung abscess formation include any condition that alters the ability to swallow, such as alcoholic blackouts, seizure disorders, other neurologic deficits, and swallowing disorders. Bronchial obstruction may cause a necrotizing process in the lung that eventually becomes an abscess.

Multiple abscesses and cavities form in clients with tuberculosis (TB) or fungal infections of the lung. Immunosuppressed clients, such as those receiving chemotherapy or those with a disease such as leukemia or AIDS, are at high risk for fungal infections. Most common organisms are anaerobic bacteria, *Staphylococcus* or other gram-positive organisms, or gram-negative or opportunistic infections such as fungi.

COLLABORATIVE MANAGEMENT

Assessment

Ask the client about any recent history of influenza, pneumonia, febrile illness, cough, and foul-smelling sputum production. Ask about the sputum color and odor and about any **pleuritic chest pain** (a stabbing pain on taking a deep breath). Often the client is febrile, pale, fatigued, and cachectic. Auscultation may reveal decreased breath sounds, and there is dullness on percussion in the involved area. Bronchial breath sounds and crackles are often heard over the site of the lesion. A chest x-ray and sputum samples are needed for the diagnosis.

Interventions

Nursing diagnoses and interventions for the client with pneumonia also apply to the client with a lung abscess. Treatment involves antibiotics and drainage of the abscess. More than one antibiotic may be prescribed. Provide frequent mouth care and observe for oral overgrowth of *Candida albicans.*

Inhalation Anthrax

PATHOPHYSIOLOGY

Inhalation anthrax (also known as respiratory anthrax) is a bacterial infection caused by the gram-positive, rod-shaped organism *Bacillus anthracis,* which lives as a spore in contaminated soil. Infection with this organism can occur through the skin, the intestinal tract, or the lungs. Inhalation anthrax is a rare natural occurrence in the United States, but it has a fatality rate of nearly 100% without treatment. It is not spread by person-to-person contact. Because the inhalation form of the disease is so rare, any occurrence is considered unnatural or an intentional act of bioterrorism.

This organism first forms a **spore,** an encapsulated organism that is inactive. When many spores are inhaled into the deep parts of the lungs, macrophages engulf them. Once inside the macrophage, the organism leaves its capsule and replicates. The active bacteria produce several toxins that they release into the infected tissues and the blood. These toxins increase the virulence of the organism by creating massive edema in infected tissues, suppressing neutrophil action, causing hemorrhage, and destroying both lung cells and white blood cells. The infected macrophages carry the organisms to the hilar and mediastinal lymph nodes. From these nodes, the organisms can enter the blood and spread rapidly, causing sepsis and meningitis.

COLLABORATIVE MANAGEMENT

Assessment

Inhalation anthrax is a two-stage illness, and manifestations may not begin until as long as 8 weeks after exposure to the organism. Manifestations are listed in Chart 34-8.

CHART 34-8

KEY FEATURES of
Inhalation Anthrax

Prodromal Stage (Early)	Fulminant Stage (Late)
Fever Fatigue Mild chest pain Dry cough No manifestations of upper respiratory infection Mediastinal "widening" on chest x-ray	Sudden onset of breathlessness Dyspnea Diaphoresis Stridor on inhalation and exhalation Hypoxia High fever Mediastinitis Pleural effusion Hypotension Septic shock

PRODROMAL STAGE

The first stage, the "prodromal" stage, is difficult to differentiate from influenza or pneumonia. Manifestations are nonspecific. In this stage, clients have a fever, some fatigue, mild chest pain, and a dry, harsh cough. *A special feature of inhalation anthrax is that it is **not** accompanied by upper respiratory manifestations of rhinitis, headache, watery eyes, or sore throat.* Usually, the client starts to feel better, and symptoms improve in 2 to 4 days.

Although diagnosis is difficult at this stage, if the client begins appropriate antibiotic therapy, the likelihood of survival is high. Diagnostic tests may show a slightly elevated white blood cell count with increasing numbers of band neutrophils. Other indicators of inhalation anthrax that may be detectable at this time are positive Gram stain of the serum and a mediastinal "widening" on chest x-ray as the lymph nodes in the area greatly enlarge. After several days, blood cultures may be positive for the organism and the genetic material of the bacteria may be detected through the amplification process of the polymerase chain reaction (PCR). These more definitive diagnostic tests may not be evident, however, until the disease has progressed to the fulminant stage.

FULMINANT STAGE

The second or "fulminant" stage begins after the client feels a little better. Usually there is a sudden onset of a feeling of breathlessness. This sensation rapidly progresses to severe respiratory distress, dyspnea, diaphoresis, stridor on inhalation and exhalation, and cyanosis. The client has a high fever. Mediastinitis and pleural effusions develop. As the disease spreads through the blood, causing septic shock and meningitis, death often occurs within 24 to 36 hours after the onset of breathlessness even if antibiotics are started in this stage.

Interventions

The naturally occurring organism has a cell wall and is sensitive to many antibiotics, including the penicillins and the cephalosporins; however, it is thought that organisms grown for bioterrorism may have been altered to be resistant to these antibiotics. Therefore the antibiotics used for suspected or diagnosed inhalation anthrax include combination therapy with ciprofloxacin, doxycycline, and amoxicillin (Chart 34-9). The same drugs are used individually in oral form for prophylaxis when people have been exposed to inhalation anthrax.

CHART 34-9

DRUG THERAPY for
Prophylaxis and Treatment of Inhalation Anthrax

Prophylaxis	Treatment
Ciprofloxacin (Cipro) 500 mg PO twice daily *Or* Doxycycline (Vibramycin) 100 mg PO twice daily *Or* *(if organism is proven susceptible to penicillin)* Amoxicillin (Amoxil, Trimox) 500 mg q8h	Ciprofloxacin (Cipro I.V.) 400 mg IV q12h *Or* Doxycycline (Doxy 100) 100 mg IV q12h *Plus one or two of the following secondary agents (parenteral form; dosage based on client's weight and age)* Rifampin (RIF) Clindamycin (Cleocin) Vancomycin (Vancocin, Vancoled)
Prophylaxis must continue for 60 days (or longer if exposure was heavy)	**Treatment with intravenous drugs continues for at least 7 days. When the response is good and the client improves, IV drugs are changed to oral agents and are continued for at least 60 days.**

Teach clients with any type of lower respiratory infection to be especially vigilant for changes after they think they are getting well. They need to seek medical attention immediately on having a setback that starts with breathlessness.

Pulmonary Empyema

PATHOPHYSIOLOGY

Empyema is a collection of pus in the pleural space. The most common cause of empyema is pulmonary infection, lung abscess, or infected pleural effusion. Pneumonia or lung abscess can spread across the pleura. Lymph node obstruction can cause a **retrograde** (backward) flood of infected lymph into the pleural space. In addition, a liver abscess or abdominal abscess can spread through the lymphatic system into the lung area. Thoracic surgery and chest trauma can introduce bacteria directly into the pleural space, leading to empyema. Blood from trauma may collect in the pleural space. Poor drainage of this blood promotes infection.

COLLABORATIVE MANAGEMENT

Assessment

Important history findings include recent febrile illness (including pneumonia), chest pain, dyspnea, cough, and trauma. Observe and document the character of the sputum. Chest wall motion may be reduced on physical examination. If a pleural effusion is present, fremitus may be decreased or absent on palpation, percussion may sound flat, and breath sounds are decreased on auscultation. With compression of lung tissue near the effusion, abnormal breath sounds include bronchial breath sounds, egophony, and whispered pectoriloquy (see Chapter 30).

Some clients have fever, chills, night sweats, and weight loss. If there is cardiac compromise, the client may be hypotensive because of a mediastinal deviation. The PMI (point of maximal impulse) may be displaced on cardiac palpation.

A chest x-ray is ordered, and a sample of the pleural fluid is obtained via thoracentesis for help in making the diagnosis (see Chapter 30). Empyema fluid is thick, opaque, exudative, and foul smelling. The pleural fluid is sent to the laboratory and is analyzed for color, red blood cell count, white blood cell count and differential, glucose and protein levels, lactate dehydrogenase (LDH), and pH. Gram stains, acid-fast stains, and cytology studies are also performed. A protein level higher than 3 g/100 mL indicates an exudative process.

Interventions

Therapy for empyema is focused on emptying the empyema cavity, re-expanding the lung, and controlling the infection. Antibiotics appropriate for the identified organism are prescribed. Closed-chest drainage (see Chapter 33) is used to promote lung expansion. The health care provider places one or more chest tubes in the lower parts of the empyema sac. Underwater seal drainage is used without suction initially, but suction may be added if the lung fails to expand with gravity drainage alone. The tube is removed when the lung is fully expanded and the infection is under control. Open thoracotomy and removal of a portion of the pleura may be needed for thick pus or marked pleural thickening. Nursing considerations are the same as those for clients with a pleural effusion, pneumothorax, or infection.

GET READY for the NCLEX Examination!

KEY POINTS

Safe Effective Care Environment

- Teach clients with respiratory infections to limit infection spread by washing hands after blowing the nose or using a tissue.
- Instruct clients that colds are most easily spread to others during the first 2 to 3 days after symptoms begin.
- Ask clients from other countries whether or not they have had BCG as a vaccination against TB. Clients who have had BCG usually have a large, positive reaction to a PPD skin test, making the test less reliable as an indicator of active TB disease.
- Use airborne precautions for any client who has TB or SARS manifestations until proven otherwise.
- Keep the door to the room of any client with a respiratory infection closed until the cause of the infection is identified.

Health Promotion and Maintenance

- Receive a yearly influenza vaccination because you come into contact more frequently with infected people and also because you can have a mild or subclinical case of influenza and spread it to people who are immunocompromised.
- Urge all adults over 50 years of age, anyone who has a chronic respiratory problem, and anyone who is immunocompromised to any degree to receive yearly influenza vaccinations.
- Urge all adults over 50 years of age, anyone who has a chronic respiratory problem, and anyone who is immunocompromised to any degree to receive the pneumonia vaccination.
- Stress to clients that they should complete the medication regimen for any respiratory infection for which anti-infective therapy has been prescribed.
- Urge all people to quit smoking or using tobacco in any form.
- Encourage family members of clients with TB who live at home to ensure good ventilation of the home with open windows whenever possible.

Psychosocial Integrity

- Assess any older client who has acute confusion for pneumonia (remembering that they may not have a cough or fever).
- Assure the family of an older adult client with pneumonia who is confused that the new-onset confusion is temporary.
- Reassure the client who feels depressed by the degree of fatigue felt and the activity intolerance experienced that the recovery times for influenza and pneumonia are long (weeks to months), especially for the older adult.
- Inform clients who may be afraid of contracting inhalational anthrax that this disease is not transmitted by person-to-person contact.
- Inform clients who have a positive TB test that far more people are infected with the bacillus than have active TB disease.
- Assess the likelihood of adherence to the drug regimen for clients with TB.
- Identify clients who may require a directly observed therapy (DOT) program in which they must be directly observed by a health care professional while swallowing the drug.
- Assess the degree of social interaction for clients receiving drug therapy for active TB on an outpatient basis.

Physiological Integrity

- Teach all clients with a respiratory infection of bacterial origin to complete all anti-infective therapy as prescribed.
- Urge clients to limit the use of decongestant nasal sprays to no more than 4 days.
- Teach clients with allergic rhinitis to avoid contact with the offending allergen(s).
- Caution older adults using antihistamines that these drugs may make hypertension worse.
- Treat epiglottitis in an adult as an emergency because it can lead to complete respiratory obstruction.
- Assess the client receiving rifampin or rifapentine as drug therapy for TB for any manifestation of liver impairment (dark urine, clay-colored stools, anorexia, jaundiced sclera or hard palate).
- Inform women taking rifampin or rifapentine as drug therapy for TB that these drugs reduce the effectiveness of oral contraceptives and that another form of birth control should be considered while on this therapy.

ADDITIONAL STUDY RESOURCES

Go to your Student CD-ROM for Review Questions for the NCLEX Examination.

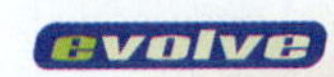

Go to http://evolve.elsevier.com/Iggy/ for Integrated Management of Care Questions for the NCLEX Examination.

SELECTED BIBLIOGRAPHY

Asterisk indicates a classic or definitive work on this subject.

Ackley, B., & Ladwig, G. (2002). *Nursing diagnosis handbook: A guide to planning care* (5th ed). St. Louis: Mosby.

Baek, C., et al. (2000). Polymerase chain reaction detection of *Mycobacterium tuberculosis* from fine-needle aspirate for the diagnosis of cervical tuberculosis lymphadenitis. *Laryngoscope, 110*(1), 30-34.

Bhattacharyya, N., Kepnes, L., & Shapiro, J. (2001). Efficacy and quality of life impact on adult tonsillectomy. *Archives of Otolaryngology & Head and Neck Surgery, 127*(11), 1347-1350.

Bridges, C., et al. (2002). Prevention and control of influenza: Recommendations of the Advisory Committee on Immunization Practices (ACIP). *Morbidity & Mortality Weekly Report, 51*(RR03), 1-31.

Brooks, J. (2001). Postoperative nosocomial pneumonia: Nurse sensitive interventions. *AACN Clinical Issues for Advanced Practice in Acute and Critical Care, 12*(2), 305-323.

*Centers for Disease Control and Prevention. (1999). Progress toward the elimination of tuberculosis–United States, 1998. *Morbidity and Mortality Weekly Report, 48*(33), 732-736.

Centers for Disease Control and Prevention. (2001). Notice to readers: Considerations for distinguishing influenza-like illness from inhalational anthrax. *Morbidity and Mortality Weekly Report, 50*(44), 984-986.

Centers for Disease Control and Prevention. (2003a). *Guidelines and recommendations: Interim domestic infection control precautions for aerosol-generating procedures on patients with severe acute respiratory syndrome (SARS).* Department of Health and Human Services, May 20, 2003.

Centers for Disease Control and Prevention. (2003b). *Health, United States, 2003.* Department of Health and Human Services, March 11, 2004.

Centers for Disease Control and Prevention. (2003c). Update: Influenza activity–United States, 2002-03 season. *Morbidity and Mortality Weekly Report, 52*(02),26-28.

Centers for Disease Control and Prevention. (2003d) *Updated interim U.S. case definition for severe acute respiratory syndrome (SARS).* Department of Health and Human Services, July 11, 2003.

Connally, M. (2001). Black, white, and shades of gray: Common abnormalities in chest radiographs. *AACN Clinical Issues for Advanced Practice in Acute and Critical Care, 12*(2), 259-269.

Dochterman, J., & Bulechek, G. (Eds) (2004). *Nursing interventions classification (NIC)* (4th ed). St. Louis: Mosby.

Dreher, M., et al. (2004). What you need to know about SARS now! *Nursing 2004, 34*(1), 58-63.

Ebersole, P., Hess, P., & Luggen, A. (2004). *Toward healthy aging: Human needs and nursing response* (6th ed). St. Louis: Mosby.

Eckler, J. (2002). Keeping pulmonary tuberculosis at bay. *Nursing 2002, 32*(12), 70.

Facts and Comparisons. (2004). *Drug facts and comparisons* (58th ed). St. Louis: Author.

Frakes, M. & Evans, T. (2004). TB: Your vigilance is vital. *RN, 67* (11), 30-35.

Goldrick, B. (2003). Adult respiratory infections. *American Journal of Nursing, 103*(10), 65.

Goldrick, B. (2004a). Is SARS reemerging? *American Journal of Nursing, 104*(7), 28-29.

Goldrick, B. (2004b). 21st-century emerging and reemerging infections: Where do we go from here? *American Journal of Nursing, 104*(1), 67-70.

Goolsby, M. (2001). Viral upper respiratory infections. *Journal of the American Academy of Nurse Practitioners, 13*(2), 50-54.

Harris, J., & Miller, T. (2000). Preventing nosocomial pneumonia: Evidenced-based practice. *Critical Care Nurse, 20*(1), 51-67.

Harris, J., et al. (2000). Risk factors for nosocomial pneumonia in critically ill trauma patients. *AACN Clinical Issues, 11*(2), 198-231.

Havas, T. (2002). Obstructive adenoid tissue: An indication for power-shaver adenoidectomy. *Archives of Otolaryngology & Head and Neck Surgery, 128*(7), 789-791.

Hodnicki, D. (2001). Anthrax. *The American Journal for Nurse Practitioners, 5*(10), 21-24.

Johnson, J., & Force, R. (2000). Oseltamivir for flu prevention. *Journal of Family Practice, 49*(2), 183-184.

Kearney, K. (2001). Epiglottitis. *American Journal of Nursing, 101*(8), 37-38.

*Krouse, J. (1999). Introduction to sinus disease: I, Anatomy and physiology. *ORL–Head and Neck Nursing, 17*(2), 7-12.

*Krouse, J., & Krouse, H. (1999). Introduction to sinus disease: II, diagnosis and treatment. *ORL–Head and Neck Nursing, 17*(3), 6-17.

Leiner, S. (2000). Acute pharyngitis with lifelong implications. *The Nurse Practitioner, 25*(4), 119-122.

McCance, K., & Huether, S. (2002). Pathophysiology: *The biologic basis for disease in adults and children* (4th ed), St. Louis: Mosby.

Meredith, P. (2001). Community acquired pneumonia. *The American Journal for Nurse Practitioners, 5*(6), 9-17.

Moorhead, S., Johnson, M., & Maas, M. (Eds.). (2004). *Nursing outcomes classification (NOC)* (3rd ed). St. Louis: Mosby.

Orgill. R., Krempl, G., & Medina, J. (2002). Acute pain management following laryngectomy. *Archives of Otolaryngology & Head and Neck Surgery, 128*(7), 829-832.

Patel, N., & Criner, G. (2003). Community-acquired pneumonia in the elderly: Update on treatment strategies. *Consultant, 43*(6), 689-701.

Schultz, R. (2002). Straight talk about community-acquired pneumonia. *Nursing 2002, 32*(1), 46-49.

Singh, D., Sutton, C., & Woodcock, A. (2002). Tuberculin test measurement: Variability due to the time of reading. *Chest, 122*(4), 1299-1301.

Spencer, D., Whitman, K., & Morton, P. (2001). Inhalational anthrax. *MEDSURG Nursing, 10*(6), 308-312.

Spiegel, J., et al. (2000). Acute laryngitis. *Ear, Nose, and Throat Journal, 79*(7), 488.

Tasota, F., Henker, R., & Hoffman, L. (2002). Anthrax as a biological weapon: An old disease that poses new threats. *Critical Care Nurse, 22*(5), 21-34.

Thaler, E. (2002). Postoperative care after endoscopic sinus surgery. *Archives of Otolaryngology & Head and Neck Surgery, 128*(10), 1204-1208.

U.S. Department of Health and Human Services (2001). Update: Investigation of bioterrorism-related anthrax and adverse events from antimicrobial prophylaxis. *Morbidity and Mortality Weekly Report, 50*(44), 973-976.

Vergis, E., et al. (2000). Azithromycin vs cefuroxime plus erythromycin for empirical treatment of community-acquired pneumonia in hospitalized patients. *Archives of Internal Medicine, 160*(9), 1294-1300.

Wan, G.W., Lu, S., & Tsai, Y. (2004). Polymerase chain reaction used for the detection of airborne *Mycobacterium tuberculosis* in health care settings. *American Journal of Infection Control, 32*(1), 17-22.

West, J. (2002). Acute upper airway infections. *British Medical Journal, 61*(1), 215-230.

Woods, A. (2002). Anthrax: New threat from an ancient microbe. *Nursing 2002, 32*(1), 44-45.

Workman, M.L. (2003). The cellular basis of bacterial infection. *Critical Care Clinics of North America, 15*(1), 1-11.

World Health Organization (WHO). Epidemic surveys–Severe acute respiratory syndrome (SARS). July 10, 2003.

CHAPTER 35

Interventions for Critically Ill Clients with Respiratory Problems

JOHN M. CLOCHESY

LEARNING OUTCOMES

After studying this chapter, you should be able to:

1. Identify clients at risk for development of pulmonary embolism.
2. Describe the clinical manifestations of pulmonary embolism.
3. Use laboratory data and clinical manifestations to determine the presence of acidosis.
4. Describe the precautions to use for clients receiving heparin or warfarin.
5. Develop a community-based teaching plan for the client who has had a pulmonary embolism.
6. Compare the features of respiratory failure of ventilatory origin with those of respiratory failure of oxygenation origin.
7. Use laboratory data and clinical manifestations to determine the adequacy of ventilatory interventions.
8. Describe the indications for intubation.
9. Prioritize nursing care for the conscious client being mechanically ventilated.
10. Develop interventions to communicate effectively with a client who is unable to talk as a result of intubation.
11. Identify clients at risk for development of pneumothorax.

Go to your Student CD-ROM for Review Questions for the NCLEX Examination keyed to these Learning Outcomes.

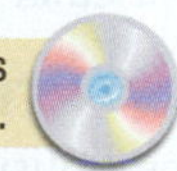

Acute or chronic respiratory problems can progress to a life-threatening emergency and death, even with prompt treatment. Anyone can have an acute injury or problem that results in severe respiratory impairment. Older adults, however, are more at risk for developing critical respiratory problems or complications. The client who is short of breath is also anxious and fearful. You must therefore be prepared to manage both the physical and emotional needs of the client during any respiratory emergency.

PULMONARY EMBOLISM

PATHOPHYSIOLOGY

A **pulmonary embolism (PE)** is a collection of particulate matter (solids, liquids, or gaseous substances) that enters venous circulation and lodges in the pulmonary vessels. Large emboli obstruct pulmonary blood flow, leading to decreased systemic oxygenation, pulmonary tissue hypoxia, and potential death. Any substance can cause an embolism, but a blood clot is the most common.

Pulmonary embolism is the most common acute pulmonary disease (90%) among hospitalized clients. In most people with PE, a blood clot from a deep vein thrombosis (DVT) breaks loose from one of the veins in the legs or the pelvis. The thrombus breaks off, travels through the vena cava and right side of the heart, and then lodges in a smaller blood vessel in the lung. Platelets collect with the embolus, triggering the release of substances that cause blood vessel constriction. Widespread pulmonary vessel constriction and pulmonary hypertension impair gas exchange. Deoxygenated blood shunts into the arterial circulation, causing hypoxemia. About 12% of clients with PE do *not* have hypoxemia.

Etiology

The following are major risk factors for DVT leading to PE:

- Prolonged immobilization
- Central venous catheters
- Surgery
- Obesity
- Advancing age
- Hypercoagulability
- History of thromboembolism
- Cancer diagnosis

In addition, smoking, pregnancy, estrogen therapy, heart failure, stroke, cancer (particularly lung or prostate), Trousseau's syndrome, and trauma increase the risk for DVT and PE.

Fat, oil, air, tumor cells, amniotic fluid, foreign objects (e.g., broken intravenous [IV] catheters), injected particles, and infected fibrin clots or pus can enter the venous system and cause PE. Fat emboli from fracture of a long bone and oil emboli from diagnostic procedures do not impede blood flow; instead, they cause blood vessel injury and acute respiratory distress syndrome (ARDS). Amniotic fluid embolus has a mortality rate of 80% to 90% and occurs as a rare complication childbirth, abortion, or amniocentesis. Septic emboli often arise from a pelvic abscess, an infected IV catheter, and nonsterile injections of illegal drugs. The problem with septic emboli lies in the toxic effects of the infection more than in the vascular occlusion.

Incidence/Prevalence

Pulmonary embolism affects at least 500,000 people a year in the United States, about 10% of whom die. Many die within 1 hour of the onset of symptoms or before the diagnosis has even been suspected.

HEALTH PROMOTION/ILLNESS PREVENTION

Although pulmonary embolism (PE) can occur in healthy people and may give no warning, it occurs more often in some situations. Thus prevention of conditions contributing to PE is a major nursing concern. Preventive actions for PE are those that also prevent venous stasis and DVT. Best practices for PE prevention are outlined in Chart 35-1.

Lifestyle changes can help reduce the risk for PE. Urge clients to stop smoking cigarettes, especially women who take oral contraceptives. Reducing weight and becoming more physically active, such as walking one or more miles each day, can dramatically reduce risk for PE. Teach clients who are traveling for long periods to drink plenty of water, change positions often, avoid crossing the legs, and get up from the sitting position at least 5 minutes out of every hour. Actions to prevent DVT and PE during the perioperative period are described in Chapters 20, 21, and 22.

For clients with a known risk for PE, small doses of prophylactic subcutaneous heparin may be prescribed every 8 to 12 hours. Heparin prevents excessive coagulation in clients immobilized for a prolonged period, after trauma or surgery, or when restricted to bedrest. Occasionally, a drug to reduce platelet aggregation, such as clopidogrel (Plavix), is used in place of heparin.

CHART 35-1

BEST PRACTICE for
Prevention of Pulmonary Embolism

- Initiate passive and active range-of-motion exercises for the extremities of immobilized and postoperative clients.
- Ambulate postoperative clients soon after surgery.
- Use antiembolism and pneumatic compression stockings and devices postoperatively.
- Avoid the use of tight garters, girdles, and constricting clothing.
- Prevent pressure under the popliteal space (such as with a pillow).
- Perform a comprehensive appraisal of peripheral circulation.
- Elevate the affected limb 20 degrees or greater, above the level of the heart, to improve venous return, as appropriate.
- Change client position every 2 hours or ambulate as tolerated.
- Prevent injury to the vessel lumen by preventing local pressure, trauma, infection, or sepsis.
- Refrain from massaging or compressing leg muscles.
- Instruct client not to cross legs.
- Administer prophylactic low-dose anticoagulant and antiplatelet medication.
- Instruct the client to avoid activities that result in the Valsalva maneuver.
- Administer medications that will prevent episodes of the Valsalva maneuver as appropriate.
- Instruct the client and family on appropriate precautions.
- Encourage smoking cessation.

COLLABORATIVE MANAGEMENT

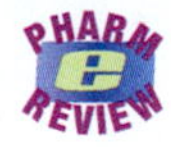

Assessment

HISTORY

Ask any client with sudden onset of breathing difficulty about the risk factors for PE, especially a history of DVT, recent surgery, or prolonged immobilization.

PHYSICAL ASSESSMENT/CLINICAL MANIFESTATIONS

RESPIRATORY MANIFESTATIONS. Chart 35-2 outlines the key features of PE. Assess the client for dyspnea occurring with tachypnea, tachycardia, and pleuritic chest pain (sharp, stabbing-type pain on inspiration). These symptoms are found in 80% of clients who have PE. Other symptoms vary depending on the severity and the type of embolism. Breath sounds may be normal, but crackles occur in 50% of clients with PE. Often a dry cough is present. **Hemoptysis** (blood sputum) may result from pulmonary infarction.

CARDIAC MANIFESTATIONS. Assess for distended neck veins, **syncope** (fainting or loss of consciousness), cyanosis, and hypotension. Hypotension associated with massive emboli results from acute pulmonary hypertension and impeded forward blood flow. Often abnormal heart sounds, such as an S_3 or S_4 sound occur. Electrocardiogram findings are abnormal, nonspecific, and transient. T-wave changes and

CHART 35-2

KEY FEATURES of
Pulmonary Embolism

Symptoms
- Dyspnea, sudden onset
- Pleuritic chest pain
- Apprehension, restlessness
- Feeling of impending doom
- Cough
- Hemoptysis

Signs
- Tachypnea
- Crackles
- Pleural friction rub
- Tachycardia
- S_3 or S_4 heart sound
- Diaphoresis
- Fever, low-grade
- Petechiae over chest and axillae
- Decreased arterial oxygen saturation (Sao_2)

ST-segment abnormalities develop in 50% of clients, but left- and right-axis deviations occur with equal frequency.

MISCELLANEOUS MANIFESTATIONS. A low-grade fever may be present. Petechiae may be present on the skin over the chest and in the axillae. Some clients have more vague symptoms resembling the flu, such as nausea, vomiting, and general malaise.

LABORATORY ASSESSMENT

The hyperventilation triggered by hypoxia and pain first leads to respiratory alkalosis, indicated by low partial pressure of arterial carbon dioxide ($Paco_2$) values on arterial blood gas (ABG) analysis. The alveolar-arterial (A-a) gradient is increased. The "friendlier" Pao_2-Fio_2 (fraction of inspired oxygen) ratio is commonly used to assess shunt because it does not require use of the complex A-a gradient formula. As blood is shunted without picking up oxygen from the lungs, the $Paco_2$ level starts to rise, indicating respiratory acidosis. Later metabolic acidosis results from accumulation of lactic acid due to tissue hypoxia.

Even if ABG studies and pulse oximetry show hypoxemia, these results alone are not sufficient for the diagnosis of PE. A client with a small embolus may not be hypoxemic, and PE is not the only cause of hypoxemia.

RADIOGRAPHIC ASSESSMENT

A chest x-ray may show evidence of a PE if it is large. Some lung infiltration may be present around the embolism site. However, the chest x-ray may not show any acute changes. Spiral computed tomography (CT) scans are often used to diagnose PE.

In a few clients the physician performs a transesophageal echocardiography (TEE) (see Chapter 36) for help in detecting PE. Doppler ultrasound studies or impedance plethysmography (IPG) may be used to document the presence of DVT and to support a diagnosis of PE.

PSYCHOSOCIAL ASSESSMENT

The onset of symptoms is usually abrupt, making the client with PE anxious and fearful. Hypoxemia may cause the client to have a sense of impending doom and increased restlessness. The emergency nature of the disorder and admission to an intensive care unit (ICU) increase the client's anxiety and fear of death.

Critical Thinking Challenge

The client is a 36-year-old woman who had a laminectomy yesterday for a ruptured lumbar disk. She has had pain for several months and has been unable to participate in her usual exercise program. She smokes one pack of cigarettes per day and drinks about two glasses of wine per week. Her other medications include oral contraceptives, ibuprofen PRN for joint and muscle pain, and sumatriptan (Imitrex) several times a month for migraine headaches. When you go to assess her this morning, she tells you that she is nauseated and having some chest pain.

1. What risk factors does she have for a pulmonary embolism?
2. For what other clinical manifestations should you assess?
3. Is oxygen by mask appropriate for this client? Why or Why not?
4. What other actions should you initiate?

evolve For suggested answer guidelines, go to http://evolve.elsevier.com/Iggy/.

Analysis

COMMON NURSING DIAGNOSES AND COLLABORATIVE PROBLEMS

The primary collaborative problem for clients with PE is Hypoxemia. The following are priority nursing diagnoses for clients with PE:

1. Decreased Cardiac Output related to acute pulmonary hypertension
2. Anxiety related to hypoxemia and life-threatening illness
3. Risk for Injury (Bleeding) related to anticoagulation or fibrinolytic therapy

ADDITIONAL NURSING DIAGNOSES AND COLLABORATIVE PROBLEMS

In addition to the common nursing diagnoses and collaborative problems, clients with PE may have one or more of the following:

- Impaired Gas Exchange related to disrupted pulmonary perfusion and increased dead space
- Fatigue related to hypoxemia
- Impaired Oral Mucous Membrane related to oxygen therapy
- Acute Confusion related to hypoxemia
- Disturbed Sleep Pattern related to the ICU environment

Planning and Implementation

HYPOXEMIA

When a client has a sudden onset of dyspnea and pleuritic chest pain, notify the physician. Reassure the client and assist him or her to a position of comfort with the head of the bed elevated. Prepare for oxygen therapy and blood gas analysis while continuing to monitor and assess for other manifestations.

NOC **PLANNING: EXPECTED OUTCOMES.** The client with PE is expected to have adequate tissue perfusion in all major organs. The following are indicators of adequate perfusion:

- ABGs within normal limits
- Pulse oximetry above 95%
- Cognitive status not compromised
- Absence of pallor or cyanosis

INTERVENTIONS. Nonsurgical management of PE is most common. In some cases, surgery may be needed in addition to drug therapy. NIC intervention activities for the client with PE are listed in Chart 35-3.

NONSURGICAL MANAGEMENT. Goals of management for PE are to increase alveolar gas exchange, improve pulmonary perfusion, minimize risk for further thromboembolism, and prevent complications. Interventions include oxygen therapy, monitoring, and anticoagulation or fibrinolytic therapy.

Oxygen Therapy. Oxygen therapy is important for the client with PE (see Chapter 31). The severely hypoxemic client may need mechanical ventilation and close monitoring with arterial blood gas (ABG) studies. In less severe cases, oxygen may be applied by nasal cannula or mask. Use pulse oximetry to monitor oxygen saturation and determine the degree of hypoxemia.

Monitoring. Assess the client continually for any changes in status. Check vital signs, lung sounds, and cardiac and respiratory status at least every 1 to 2 hours. Document increasing dyspnea, dysrhythmias, distended neck veins, and pedal or sacral edema. Assess for crackles and other abnormal sounds on auscultation of the lungs along with cyanosis of the lips, conjunctiva, oral mucosa, and nail beds.

Anticoagulation/Fibrinolytic Therapy. The health care provider may prescribe anticoagulation to keep the embolus from enlarging and to prevent the formation of new clots. Active bleeding, stroke, and recent trauma are relative contraindications for this therapy. Before proceeding, each client is evaluated to determine the risk versus the benefit of therapy.

Heparin is usually used unless the PE is massive or is accompanied by hemodynamic instability. A fibrinolytic drug may then be used to break up the existing clot. Review the client's partial thromboplastin time (PTT)–also called activated partial thromboplastin time (aPTT)–before therapy is started, every 4 hours when therapy begins, and daily thereafter. Therapeutic PTT values usually range between 1.5 and 2.5 times the control value.

Some fibrinolytic drugs, such as alteplase (Activase, tPA) and urokinase (Abbokinase), are approved for use in treatment of PE. Specific criteria for use of these drugs are massive PE (those that obstruct blood flow to a lobe or multiple segments) and emboli that induce hemodynamic instability that includes failure to maintain blood pressure without supportive measures. *In addition to greatly increased risk for bleeding with the use of fibrinolytic drugs, urokinase use can induce allergic responses and anaphylaxis. Such reactions usually occur within the first hour of starting the urokinase infusion. If a reaction occurs, stop the infusion and prepare to give IV antihistamine, corticosteroids, or adrenergic agonists.*

Heparin therapy usually continues for 5 to 10 days. Most clients are started on a regimen of oral anticoagulants, such as warfarin (Coumadin, Warfilone✱), on the third day of heparin use. Therapy with both heparin and warfarin continues until the client has an International Normalized Ratio (INR) of 2.0 to 3.0. To facilitate early discharge, a low-molecular-weight heparin (e.g., dalteparin or enoxaparin) is often used along with the warfarin. Monitor the INR daily. Warfarin use continues for 3 to 6 weeks, but some clients at high risk may take warfarin indefinitely. Charts 35-4 and 35-5 list drugs used and laboratory tests monitored. Anticoagulants and associated nursing care are also discussed in Chapters 39, 41, and 42.

CHART 35-3

NIC INTERVENTION ACTIVITIES for The Client with Pulmonary Embolism

Embolus Care: Pulmonary: *Limitation of complications for a client experiencing, or at risk for, occlusion of pulmonary circulation*

- Evaluate chest pain (e.g., intensity, location, radiation, duration, and precipitating and alleviating factors).
- Auscultate lung sounds for crackles or other adventitious sounds.
- Monitor respiratory pattern for symptoms of respiratory difficulty (e.g., dyspnea, tachypnea, and shortness of breath).
- Monitor determinants of tissue oxygen delivery (e.g., Pao_2, Sao_2, and hemoglobin levels and cardiac output), if available.
- Monitor for symptoms of inadequate tissue oxygenation (e.g., pallor, cyanosis, and sluggish capillary refill).
- Monitor for symptoms of respiratory failure (e.g., low Pao_2 and elevated $Paco_2$ levels and respiratory muscle fatigue).
- Encourage good ventilation (e.g., incentive spirometry and cough and deep breathe every 2 hours).
- Monitor lab values for changes in oxygenation or acid-base balance, as appropriate.
- Instruct the client and/or family regarding diagnostic procedures (e.g., V/Q scan), as appropriate.
- Encourage the client to relax.
- Monitor side effects of anticoagulant medications, if appropriate.

NIC intervention activities selected from Dochterman, J.M., & Bulechek, G.M. (Eds.). (2004). *Nursing interventions classification (NIC)* (4th ed.). St. Louis: Mosby.

Pao_2, partial pressure of arterial oxygen; *Sao_2*, arterial oxygen saturation; *$Paco_2$*, partial pressure of arterial carbon dioxide.

SURGICAL MANAGEMENT. Two surgical procedures for the management of PE are embolectomy and inferior vena cava interruption.

Embolectomy. When fibrinolytic therapy is contraindicated in a client with massive or multiple large pulmonary emboli with shock, surgical embolectomy may be needed. **Embolectomy** is the removal of the embolus or emboli from the pulmonary blood vessels.

Inferior Vena Cava Interruption. The physician considers placing a vena cava filter as a lifesaving measure by preventing further embolus formation for some clients. Candidates for this procedure include clients with an absolute contraindication to anticoagulation, recurrent or major bleeding while receiving anticoagulants, septic PE, and those undergoing pulmonary embolectomy. Placement of a vena cava filter is detailed in Chapter 38.

DECREASED CARDIAC OUTPUT

NOC **PLANNING: EXPECTED OUTCOMES.** The client with PE is expected to have adequate circulation. The following are indicators of adequate circulation:

- Maintenance of pulse rate and blood pressure within the normal ranges
- Maintenance of a urine output of at least 30 mL/hr
- Absence of cyanosis

INTERVENTIONS. In addition to the interventions used for hypoxemia, IV fluid therapy and drug therapy are used to increase cardiac output.

Intravenous Fluid Therapy. Place and maintain IV access for fluid and drug therapy. Fluid therapy involves giving crystalloid solutions to restore plasma volume and prevent shock (see Chapter 40). Continuously monitor the electrocardiogram (ECG), pulmonary artery,

CHART 35-4

DRUG THERAPY for Pulmonary Embolism

Drug	Usual Dosage	Nursing Interventions	Rationales
Heparin sodium (Hepalean✱)	5000-10,000 units IVP initially; then dose adjustment is based on PTT, 1300 units/hr on continuous drip or, less preferably, intermittent infusion	Monitor PTT. Know expected therapeutic PTT range for each client. Report PTT results. Monitor client for bleeding or bruising. Rebolus every time infusion is increased.	Ongoing assessment helps detect side effects and prevent complications. Reporting enables the physician to begin early treatment of a prolonged PTT.
		Do not use with salicylates.	An increased anticoagulation effect can occur with salicylates.
		Monitor platelets daily for thrombocytopenia.	Heparin-induced thrombocytopenia (HIT) a type of arterial thrombosis, can occur.
		Have the antidote, protamine sulfate, available.	Being prepared for an emergency helps prevent further complications.
		Avoid puncture sites and apply pressure to venipuncture and IM injection sites.	Pressure at puncture sites helps promote clotting.
		Avoid use of firm toothbrushes, straight razors, and rectal thermometers.	Safety measures help prevent bleeding.
Enoxaparin (Lovenox)	1 mg/kg SC q12h	Same as with unfractionated heparin.	Same as with unfractionated heparin.
Warfarin sodium (Coumadin, Warfilone sodium✱)	10-15 mg PO for 3 days initially; then dose adjustment is based on INR, usually 5-10 mg PO daily	Monitor INR. Know expected therapeutic INR range for each client. Report INR results. Monitor the client for bleeding or bruising.	Ongoing assessment helps detect side effects and prevent complications. Reporting enables the physician to begin early treatment of a prolonged INR.
		Monitor for fever and skin rash.	Adverse drug reaction can occur.
		Consult the pharmacist about potential drug interactions.	There are many drug interactions with warfarin.
		Have the antidote, vitamin K, available.	Being prepared for an emergency helps prevent further complications.
		Apply pressure to venipuncture and IM injection sites.	Pressure at puncture sites helps promote clotting.
		Avoid use of firm toothbrushes, straight razors, and rectal thermometers.	Safety measures help prevent bleeding.
		Teach the client which foods are high in vitamin K.	Food sources of vitamin K will alter INR.
Alteplase (tissue plasminogen activator, recombinant; tPA; Activase)	100 mg IV infusion over 2 hr	Assess for internal and external bleeding.	Bleeding is the most common adverse effect.
		Reconstitute with sterile water without preservative immediately before use.	Recommended preparation ensures drug stability.
Med Error Alert! *Enoxaparin can be given only subcutaneously, NOT intravenously or intramuscularly.*		Administer with caution to clients who have been receiving aspirin, dipyridamole, heparin, or other anticoagulants.	Other drugs with anticoagulation effects increase the risk of bleeding.

IVP, Intravenous push, or bolus; *PTT*, partial thromboplastin time; *INR*, International Normalized Ratio; *SC*, subcutaneously.

and central venous/right atrial pressures of the client receiving IV fluids because increased fluids can worsen pulmonary hypertension and contribute to right-sided heart failure.

Drug Therapy. When IV therapy alone is not effective in improving cardiac output, drug therapy with agents that increase myocardial contractility **(positive inotropic agents)** may be prescribed. Such agents include milrinone (Primacor) and dobutamine (Dobutrex). Assess the client's cardiac status hourly during therapy with inotropic agents. Vasodilators, such as nitroprusside (Nipride, Nitropress), may be used to decrease pulmonary artery pressure if it is impeding cardiac contractility.

ANXIETY

NOC PLANNING: EXPECTED OUTCOMES. The client with PE is expected to have a reduction in the level of anxiety. Indicators include that the client consistently demonstrates the following behaviors:

- Verbalization of reduced anxiety

CHART 35-5

LABORATORY PROFILE

Blood Tests Used to Monitor Anticoagulation Therapy

Test	Normal Range	Significance of Abnormal Findings
Partial thromboplastin time (PTT, aPTT [APTT])	Normal values for each local laboratory may vary. When activator reagents are used by the laboratory, the normal clotting time is shortened. Common normal ranges are 20-30 sec in some laboratories and 30-40 sec in others. Therapeutic range for PE is 1.5-2.5 times the normal value (e.g., if normal is 20-30 sec, then therapeutic range is 40-75 sec).	*Subtherapeutic times* may signify that the client is not receiving enough heparin to prevent extension of the blood clot. An increase in the dosage or rate of infusion is usually indicated. *Therapeutic times* mean that the clotting time is increased from normal, but this increase is indicated in the case of PE. *Prolonged times* in clients with PE (i.e., >75 sec) indicate that the client is at risk of serious spontaneous bleeding. Heparin is usually held or decreased unit the PTT drops back into the therapeutic range.
Prothrombin time (protime, PT)	11-12.5 sec Therapeutic range for anticoagulant therapy in PE is 1.5-2 times the normal or control value in seconds. Control values can vary day to day because reagents used may vary. If INR values are reported with the PT, therapeutic range for PE is 2.5-3.0, or, 3.0-4.5 for recurrent PE.	*Subtherapeutic values* may signify that the client is not receiving enough warfarin. An increase in the dosage is usually indicated. *Therapeutic values* mean that the protime is increased from normal, but this increase is indicated in the case of PE. *Prolonged values* in the treatment of PE indicate that the client is at risk for bleeding. The warfarin dose is usually decreased or held, the client is instructed to eat foods high in vitamin K, or an injection of vitamin K may be given.

PE, Pulmonary embolism; *INR*, International Normalized Ratio; *aPTT* or *APTT*, activated partial thromboplastin time.

- Absence of distress, irritability, and facial tension
- Effective use of coping strategies

INTERVENTIONS. The client with PE is anxious and fearful for many reasons. Interventions for reducing anxiety in clients with PE include oxygen therapy (see the interventions for hypoxemia, p. 652), communication, and drug therapy.

Communication. Acknowledge the anxiety and the client's perception of a life-threatening situation. Speaking calmly and clearly, assure him or her that appropriate measures are being taken. When giving drugs, changing position, taking vital signs, or assessing the client, explain the rationale and share information.

Drug Therapy. If the client's anxiety increases or prevents adequate rest, an antianxiety drug may be prescribed. Unless the client is intubated and mechanically ventilated, agents that have a sedating effect are avoided.

RISK FOR INJURY (BLEEDING)

NOC **PLANNING: EXPECTED OUTCOMES.** The client with PE is expected to remain free from bleeding. Indicators are the following:

- Absence of bruising or petechiae
- Maintenance of hematocrit and hemoglobin within the normal range

INTERVENTIONS. As a result of anticoagulation or fibrinolytic therapy, the client's ability to start and continue the blood-clotting cascade when injured is seriously impaired, and the risk for bleeding is high. Your major objectives are to protect the client from situations that could lead to bleeding and to monitor closely the amount of bleeding that is occurring.

Assess often for evidence of bleeding in the form of oozing, confluent ecchymoses, petechiae, or purpura. Examine all stools, urine, nasogastric drainage, and vomitus visually for the appearance of blood, and test for occult blood. Measure any blood loss as accurately as possible. Measure the client's abdominal girth every 8 hours. Increases in abdominal girth can indicate internal hemorrhage. Best practices to prevent bleeding are outlined in Chart 35-6.

Monitor laboratory values daily. Review the complete blood count (CBC) results to determine the client's risk for bleeding and whether actual blood loss has occurred. If the client has severe blood loss, packed red blood cells may be prescribed (see the discussion of transfusion therapy in Chapter 43). Monitor the platelet count. A decreasing count may indicate ongoing clotting or development of heparin-induced thrombocytopenia (HIT) caused by the formation of anti-heparin antibodies.

Community-Based Care

The client with PE is discharged after the hemodynamic consequences of embolism have been resolved. Anticoagulation therapy usually continues after discharge.

HOME CARE MANAGEMENT

Some clients are discharged to home with minimal risk for recurrence and no permanent physiologic changes. Others may have extensive lung damage and need home and lifestyle modifications.

Clients with extensive lung damage may have activity intolerance and become fatigued easily. The living arrangements may need to be modified so that clients can spend all or most of the time on one floor and avoid stair climbing. Depending on the degree of impairment, clients may require some or much assistance with activities of daily living.

HEALTH TEACHING

The client with PE may continue anticoagulation therapy for weeks, months, or years after discharge, depending on

CHART 35-6

BEST PRACTICE for
Bleeding Precautions

- Handle the client gently.
- Use a lift sheet when moving or positioning the client in bed.
- Avoid IM injections and venipunctures.
- When injections are necessary, use the smallest gauge needle appropriate for the task.
- Apply firm pressure to the needle stick site for 10 minutes or until the site no longer oozes blood.
- Apply ice to areas of trauma.
- Test all urine and stool for the presence of occult blood.
- Check IV sites every 2 hours for bleeding.
- Avoid trauma to rectal tissue:
  - Do not take temperatures rectally.
  - Do not give enemas.
  - Administer well-lubricated suppositories with caution.
- Measure abdominal girth daily.
- If the client is to be shaved, use an electric shaver.
- Use a soft-bristled toothbrush or tooth sponge for oral care.
- Inspect the mouth and gums for bleeding every 4 hours.
- Pad the side rails of the bed.
- Encourage the client not to blow the nose or insert objects into the nose.
- If the client is to ambulate, ensure that the footwear has a firm sole.

the risks for PE. Teach the client and family about bleeding precautions, activities to reduce the risk for deep vein thrombosis (DVT) and recurrence of PE, complications, and the need for follow-up care (Chart 35-7).

HEALTH CARE RESOURCES

For clients continuing with anticoagulation therapy, a home care nurse usually visits at least once per week to draw blood and perform an assessment (see Chart 35-8 for a focused assessment guide). Clients with severe dyspnea may need home oxygen therapy. Respiratory therapy treatments can be performed in the home. The nurse or case manager coordinates arrangements for oxygen and other respiratory therapy to be available if needed at home.

Critical Thinking Challenge

The client described earlier with a PE is going home. She will continue warfarin therapy for at least 1 month.

1. What will you tell this client about warfarin therapy?
2. Is this client still at risk for a PE? Why or why not?
3. How can this client reduce her risk for PE?

evolve For suggested answer guidelines, go to http://evolve.elsevier.com/Iggy/.

Evaluation: Outcomes

Evaluate the care of the client with PE on the basis of the identified nursing diagnoses and collaborative problems. The expected outcomes are that the client:

- Attains and maintains adequate gas exchange and oxygenation
- Does not experience hypovolemia and shock
- Remains free from bleeding episodes
- States that levels of anxiety are reduced
- Uses effective coping strategies

Specific indicators for these outcomes are listed for each nursing diagnosis and collaborative problem under the Planning and Implementation section (see earlier).

CHART 35-7

CLIENT EDUCATION GUIDE
The Client After Pulmonary Embolism

- Use an electric shaver.
- Use a soft-bristled toothbrush, and do not floss.
- Do not have dental work done without consulting your health care provider.
- Do not take aspirin or aspirin-containing products. Read the labels of all over-the-counter medications to be sure that the product does not contain aspirin or salicylates.
- Do not participate in contact sports or in any activity in which you might be bumped, scraped, or scratched.
- Apply ice immediately to any site of injury.
- Avoid anal intercourse.
- Take a stool softener to prevent straining during a bowel movement.
- Do not use enemas or rectal suppositories.
- Do not wear clothing that is tight or rubs.
- Avoid bending over at the waist.
- Avoid positions in which your knees are bent for any length of time.
- Wear elastic stockings as prescribed.
- Avoid prolonged sitting or standing.
- Avoid blowing your nose or placing objects in your nose. If you must blow your nose, do so gently without blocking either nasal passage.
- Take the prescribed dosage of medication at the precise time it was prescribed to be taken.
- Do not stop taking the medication abruptly or without a physician's prescription.
- Notify your doctor if you:
  - Have an injury and persistent bleeding results.
  - Have excessive menstrual bleeding.
  - See blood in your urine or bowel movement.
  - Notice large bruises or areas of small red or purple marks over the skin.

ACUTE RESPIRATORY FAILURE

PATHOPHYSIOLOGY

Acute respiratory failure is classified by blood gas abnormalities. The critical values are partial pressure of arterial oxygen (PaO_2) less than 60 mm Hg, arterial oxygen saturation (SaO_2) less than 90%, or partial pressure of arterial carbon dioxide ($PaCO_2$) greater than 50 mm Hg occurring with acidemia (pH <7.30). Acute respiratory failure is further defined as *ventilatory failure, oxygenation failure,* or a *combination of both ventilatory and oxygenation failure.* Whatever the underlying problem, the client in acute respiratory failure is always hypoxemic.

Ventilatory Failure

Ventilatory failure is the type of ventilation-perfusion ($\dot{V}/\dot{Q}$) mismatch in which perfusion is normal but ventilation is inadequate. Ventilatory failure occurs when the thoracic pressure does not change sufficiently to permit air movement into and out from the lungs. As a result, too little oxygen reaches the alveoli and carbon dioxide is retained. Both problems lead to hypoxemia.

Ventilatory failure is often the result of any of the following three problems: a mechanical abnormality of the lungs or chest wall, a defect in the respiratory control center in the brain, or impaired ventilatory muscle function, especially the diaphragm. Ventilatory failure is defined by a $PaCO_2$ level above 45 mm Hg in clients who have otherwise healthy lungs.

CHART 35-8

HOME CARE ASSESSMENT of The Client After Pulmonary Embolism

Assess respiratory status.
- Observe rate and depth of ventilation.
- Auscultate lungs.
- Examine nail beds and mucous membranes for evidence of cyanosis.
- Take a pulse oximetry reading.
- Ask the client if chest pain or shortness of breath is experienced in any position.
- Ask the client about the presence of sputum and its color and character.

Assess cardiovascular status.
- Take vital signs, including apical pulse, pulse pressure; assess for presence or absence of orthostatic hypotension and quality and rhythm of peripheral pulses.
- Take blood pressure in both arms.
- Note presence or absence of peripheral edema.
- Examine hand vein filling in the dependent position.
- Examine neck vein filling in the recumbent and sitting positions.

Assess lower extremities for deep vein thrombosis.
- Examine lower legs and compare with each other for the following:
  - General edema
  - Calf swelling
  - Surface temperature
  - Presence of red streaks or cordlike palpable structure
- Measure calf circumference.
- Ask the client to dorsiflex and plantarflex each foot. Note the ease with which the client can do this, and ask whether pain is experienced in either position.
- Gently squeeze the calf of each leg laterally and from front to back. Ask the client whether pain or tenderness is experienced with either maneuver.

Assess for evidence of bleeding.
- Examine the mouth and gums for oozing or frank bleeding.
- Examine all skin areas for bruising or petechiae.
- If the client voids during the visit, test the urine for occult blood.

Assess cognition and mental status.
- Level of consciousness
- Orientation to time, place, and person
- Can the client accurately read a seven-word sentence containing no words greater than three syllables?

Assess the client's understanding of illness and compliance with treatment.
- Manifestations to report to health care provider
- Medication plan (correct timing and dose)
- Bleeding precautions
- Prevention of deep vein thrombosis

Oxygenation Failure

In oxygenation failure, thoracic pressure changes are normal, and air moves in and out without difficulty but does not oxygenate the pulmonary blood sufficiently. Oxygenation failure occurs in the type of $\dot{V}/\dot{Q}$ mismatch in which air movement *(ventilation)* is normal but lung perfusion is decreased.

Combined Ventilatory and Oxygenation Failure

Combined ventilatory and oxygenation failure involves poor respiratory movements **(hypoventilation).** Gas exchange at the alveolar-capillary membrane is inadequate so that too little oxygen reaches the blood and carbon dioxide is retained. The condition may or may not include poor lung perfusion. When lung perfusion is not adequate, $\dot{V}/\dot{Q}$ mismatch occurs and both ventilation and perfusion are inadequate. This type of respiratory failure leads to a more profound hypoxemia than either ventilatory failure or oxygenation failure alone.

TABLE 35-1 Common Causes of Ventilatory Failure

Extrapulmonary Causes

Neuromuscular disorders
- Multiple sclerosis
- Myasthenia gravis
- Guillain-Barré syndrome
- Poliomyelitis

Spinal cord injuries affecting nerves to intercostal muscles

Central nervous system dysfunction
- Stroke
- Cerebral edema
- Increased intracranial pressure
- Meningitis

Chemical depression
- Opioid analgesics
- Sedatives
- Anesthetic agents

Kyphoscoliosis

Massive obesity

Sleep apnea

External obstruction/constriction

Intrapulmonary Causes

Airway disease
- Chronic obstructive pulmonary disease
- Asthma

Ventilation-perfusion ($\dot{V}/\dot{Q}$) mismatch
- Pulmonary embolism
- Pneumothorax
- Acute respiratory distress syndrome (ARDS)
- Amyloidosis
- Pulmonary edema
- Interstitial fibrosis

Etiology

VENTILATORY FAILURE

Many diseases and conditions can result in ventilatory failure. Causes of ventilatory failure are categorized as either **extrapulmonary** (involving nonpulmonary tissues but affecting respiratory function) or **intrapulmonary** (disorders of the respiratory tract). Table 35-1 lists common causes of ventilatory failure.

OXYGENATION FAILURE

Many lung diseases and problems can cause oxygenation failure. Problems include impaired diffusion of oxygen at the alveolar level, right-to-left shunting of blood in the pulmonary vessels, $\dot{V}/\dot{Q}$ mismatch, breathing air with a low partial pressure of oxygen (a rare problem), and abnormal hemoglobin that fails to bind oxygen. In one type of $\dot{V}/\dot{Q}$ mismatch, areas of the lungs are still being perfused, but gas exchange is unable to occur, which leads to hypoxemia. An extreme example of $\dot{V}/\dot{Q}$ mismatch is a right-to-left shunt. A normal shunt is less than 5% of cardiac output. With a right-to-left shunt, even more venous blood is not oxygenated, and applying 100% oxygen does not correct the

TABLE 35-2 Common Causes of Oxygenation Failure

- Low atmospheric oxygen concentration
  - High altitudes
  - Smoke inhalation
  - Carbon monoxide poisoning
- Pneumonia
- Congestive heart failure with pulmonary edema
- Pulmonary embolism (PE)
- Acute respiratory distress syndrome (ARDS)
- Interstitial pneumonitis-fibrosis
- Abnormal hemoglobin
- Hypovolemic shock
- Hypoventilation
- Complications of nitroprusside therapy
  - Thiocyanate toxicity
  - Methemoglobinemia

problem. A classic cause of such a $\dot{V}/\dot{Q}$ mismatch is acute respiratory distress syndrome (ARDS). Table 35-2 lists specific causes of oxygenation failure.

COMBINED VENTILATORY AND OXYGENATION FAILURE

A combination of ventilatory failure and oxygenation failure occurs in clients who have abnormal lungs, such as those who have any form of **chronic airflow limitation (CAL),** such as chronic bronchitis, emphysema, or asthma. The bronchioles and alveoli are diseased (causing oxygenation failure), and the work of breathing increases until the respiratory muscles are unable to function effectively (causing ventilatory failure). Acute respiratory failure results. This process can also occur in clients who have cardiac failure along with respiratory failure. This problem is serious because the cardiac system cannot compensate for the hypoxia by increasing the cardiac output.

COLLABORATIVE MANAGEMENT

Assessment

Assess for **dyspnea** (perceived difficulty breathing), the hallmark of respiratory failure. Evaluate dyspnea with the use of a dyspnea assessment guide (Figure 35-1). Depending on the process, nature, and course of the underlying problem, the client may or may not be aware of changes in the work of breathing. In addition, the client needs to be alert enough to perceive the sensation of breathlessness.

Dyspnea is more intense when it develops rapidly. Slowly progressive respiratory failure may first be noticed as dyspnea on exertion (DOE) or when lying down. The client may have **orthopnea,** finding it is easier to breathe in an upright position. In the client with chronic respiratory problems, a minor increase in dyspnea from baseline may represent severe gas exchange problems.

Assess for a change in the client's respiratory rate or pattern, a change in lung sounds, and manifestations of hypoxemia and hypercarbia. Pulse oximetry may show decreased oxygen saturation, but an arterial blood gas (ABG) analysis is needed for the most accurate assessment of oxygenation. The health care provider reviews the ABG studies to identify the degree of hypercarbia and hypoxemia.

Interventions

Oxygen therapy is prescribed in acute respiratory failure to keep the partial pressure of arterial oxygen (PaO_2) level

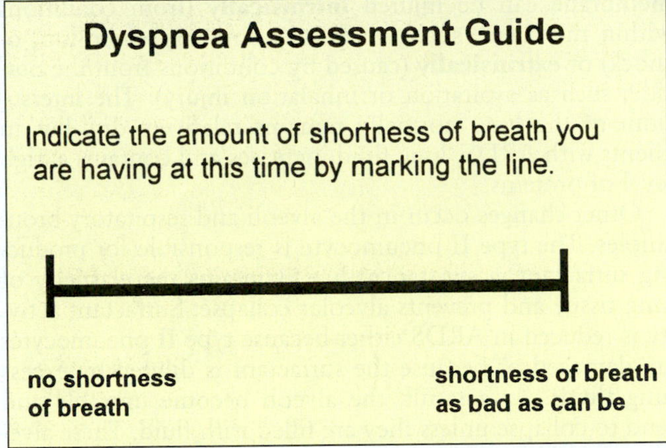

Figure 35-1 ■ A dyspnea assessment tool. (Modified from Gift, A. [1989]. A dyspnea assessment guide. *Critical Care Nurse, 9*[8], 79. Used with permission.)

above 60 mm Hg while treating the underlying cause of the respiratory failure. Oxygen therapy is discussed in detail in Chapter 31. If supplemental oxygen does not maintain acceptable PaO_2 levels, mechanical ventilation may be needed.

Help the client find a position of comfort that allows easier breathing. To decrease the anxiety occurring with dyspnea, assist the client in using relaxation, diversion, and guided imagery. Start energy-conserving measures, such as minimal self-care and no unnecessary procedures. Pulmonary drugs given systemically or by metered dose inhaler (MDI) may be prescribed to widen the bronchioles and decrease inflammation to promote gas exchange. Teach the client how to use the inhaler and about the drugs. Encourage deep breathing and other breathing exercises.

ACUTE RESPIRATORY DISTRESS SYNDROME

PATHOPHYSIOLOGY

Acute respiratory distress syndrome (ARDS) is acute respiratory failure with the following indicators:

- Hypoxemia that persists even when 100% oxygen is given
- Decreased pulmonary compliance
- Dyspnea
- Noncardiac-associated bilateral pulmonary edema
- Dense pulmonary infiltrates on x-ray (ground-glass appearance)

Often ARDS occurs after an acute traumatic event in people with no previous pulmonary disease. The mortality rate is 50% to 60% even when intensive interventions are used. Other terms for ARDS include **noncardiogenic pulmonary edema, adult respiratory distress syndrome**, and the former term **shock lung.**

Despite different causes of lung injury in ARDS, a systemic inflammatory response is the common pathway in its development. Thus the manifestations of ARDS are similar regardless of the cause. The major site of injury in the lung is the alveolar-capillary membrane, which is normally permeable to only small molecules. The alveolar-capillary membrane can be injured **intrinsically** (from conditions within the client, such as sepsis, pulmonary embolism, or shock) or **extrinsically** (caused by conditions from the outside, such as aspiration or inhalation injury). The interstitium of the lung normally remains relatively dry, but in clients with ARDS, lung fluid increases and contains a high level of proteins.

Other changes occur in the alveoli and respiratory bronchioles. The type II pneumocyte is responsible for producing surfactant, a substance that maintains the elasticity of lung tissue and prevents alveolar collapse. Surfactant activity is reduced in ARDS either because type II pneumocytes are damaged or because the surfactant is diluted by excess lung fluids. As a result, the alveoli become unstable and tend to collapse unless they are filled with fluid. These alveoli can no longer participate in gas exchange. As a result, edema forms around terminal airways, which are compressed, closed, and can be destroyed. Lung volume is further reduced, and there is even less **compliance** (elasticity). As fluid continues to leak in more lung areas, fluid, protein, and blood cells collect in the alveoli and the interstitial space between the alveoli. Lymph channels are compressed and ineffective. Poorly ventilated alveoli receive blood but cannot oxygenate it, increasing the shunt. Hypoxemia and ventilation-perfusion (V/Q) mismatch result.

Etiology

Acute respiratory distress syndrome (ARDS) has many causes (Table 35-3). Some causes involve direct injury to lung tissue; others do not directly involve the respiratory system. Serious nervous system injury, such as head or spinal trauma, strokes, tumors, and sudden increases in cerebrospinal fluid pressure, may cause massive sympathetic discharge. Systemic blood vessel constriction results, with movement of large volumes of blood into lung circulation. Lung hydrostatic pressure increases and probably causes lung injury. Any problems that cause cerebral hypoxia can lead to the same type of lung injury.

Some factors produce ARDS by direct injury to the lung. For example, aspiration of gastric contents may obstruct or burn the airway when the gastric contents are highly acidic (pH less than 2.5). In such a direct injury, type I pneumocytes are destroyed. Injured capillaries allow protein and cells to escape from the blood vessels into lung tissues. Radiation, near-drowning, and inhalation of toxic gases all injure the alveolar and capillary tissue layers. Trauma, sepsis, drowning, and burns also cause the release of thromboplastins, which form fibrin clots in the peripheral blood. The clots, together with platelets and leukocytes, are filtered out in the lung. In many cases of ARDS, especially after trauma, clot production is increased and clot breakdown **(fibrinolysis)** is reduced. As a result, small emboli remain in the lung. Disseminated intravascular coagulation (DIC) plays a role in some clients.

TABLE 35-3 Common Causes of Acute Respiratory Distress Syndrome

- Shock
- Trauma
- Serious nervous system injury
- Pancreatitis
- Fat and amniotic fluid emboli
- Pulmonary infections
- Sepsis
- Inhalation of toxic gases (smoke, oxygen)
- Pulmonary aspiration
- Drug ingestion (e.g., heroin, opioids, aspirin)
- Hemolytic disorders
- Multiple blood transfusions
- Cardiopulmonary bypass
- Near-drowning (especially in fresh water)

Incidence/Prevalence

The actual incidence of ARDS is unknown, although a 2003 estimate suggested that 150,000 cases of ARDS occur yearly in the United States.

HEALTH PROMOTION/ILLNESS PREVENTION

A major goal in the prevention of ARDS is early recognition of clients at high risk for the syndrome. Because clients who aspirate gastric contents are at great risk, you must closely assess and monitor clients receiving tube feeding and those with neurologic problems that impair swallowing and gag reflexes. Follow meticulous infection control guidelines, including handwashing, invasive catheter and wound care, and body substance precautions. In addition, carefully observe clients who are being treated for any health problem associated with ARDS.

◆COLLABORATIVE MANAGEMENT

◆Assessment

PHYSICAL ASSESSMENT/CLINICAL MANIFESTATIONS

Assess the client's breathing and determine whether increased work of breathing is evident, as indicated by hyperpnea, grunting respiration, cyanosis, pallor, and retraction **intercostally** (between the ribs) or **substernally** (below the ribs). Document sweating and any change in mental status. No abnormal lung sounds are present on auscultation because the edema of ARDS occurs first in the interstitial spaces and not in the airways. Monitor vital signs at least hourly to assess for hypotension, tachycardia, and dysrhythmias.

DIAGNOSTIC ASSESSMENT

The diagnosis of ARDS is established by a lowered partial pressure of arterial oxygen (PaO_2) value, determined by arterial blood gas (ABG) measurements. Because a widening alveolar oxygen gradient (increased fraction of inspired oxygen [FIO_2] does not yield corresponding increased PaO_2 levels) develops with increased shunting of blood, the client has a progressive need for higher concentrations of oxygen. The client with ARDS is poorly responsive to high concentrations of oxygen **(refractory hypoxemia),** however, and often needs intubation and mechanical ventilation. A large difference between the predicted and actual alveolar oxygen tension indicates shunting. Sputum cultures obtained through bronchoscopy with protective brushings and by transtracheal aspiration are performed to determine if a lung infection also is present.

The chest x-ray usually shows diffuse haziness or a "whited-out" (ground-glass) appearance of the lung. An electrocardiogram (ECG) rules out cardiac problems and usually reveals no specific changes. Pulmonary artery (Swan-Ganz) catheter placement and hemodynamic monitoring is a diagnostic tool. In the client with ARDS, the pulmonary capillary wedge pressure (PCWP) is usually low to normal. This pressure differs from that in the client with cardiac-induced pulmonary edema, where the PCWP is above 18 mm Hg.

Common Nursing Diagnoses and Collaborative Problems

Nursing diagnoses and collaborative problems that may apply to clients with ARDS include the following:

- Anxiety related to hypoxemia, life-threatening illness, and loss of control
- Impaired Gas Exchange related to disrupted pulmonary ventilation and perfusion
- Fatigue related to hypoxemia and systemic inflammation
- Disturbed Sleep Pattern related to the intensive care unit (ICU) environment
- Imbalanced Nutrition: Less than Body Requirements related to presence of endotracheal tube, chemical paralysis, increased metabolic rate
- Risk for Injury related to elevated FIO_2 or barotrauma
- Potential for Ventilator-Associated Pneumonia (VAP)

Interventions

The client with ARDS often needs endotracheal intubation and mechanical ventilation with positive end-expiratory pressure (PEEP) or continuous positive airway pressure (CPAP). Sedation and paralysis may be needed for adequate ventilation and for reducing oxygen requirements. Because one of the side effects of PEEP is tension pneumothorax, you must assess lung sounds hourly and suction as needed to maintain a patent airway. Positioning may be important in promoting gas exchange.

Drug and Fluid Therapy. Corticosteroids may be used in the treatment of ARDS because they decrease white blood cell movement and stabilize the capillary membrane. Their effectiveness, however, has not been determined. It is thought that they may help minimize the fibrosis that occurs in late ARDS. Antibiotics are used to treat infections when organisms are identified.

Many interventions are under investigation, but none has been effective in decreasing mortality. Some of these interventions include agents that modify the inflammatory responses and oxidative stress (vitamins C and E, *N*-acetylcysteine), nitric oxide, surfactant replacement, and prone positioning.

The optimal fluid therapy for the client with ARDS remains unknown. Red blood cell transfusion may expand vascular volume. Fluid volume is titrated to maintain adequate cardiac output and tissue perfusion. Diuretics may help to decrease lung edema, but care should be taken to prevent dehydration and hypotension.

Nutrition Therapy. The client with ARDS is at risk for malnutrition, which further compromises the respiratory system and the immune response. Diaphragm function is also reduced. Therefore enteral nutrition (tube feeding) or parenteral nutrition (hyperalimentation) is started as soon as possible.

Case Management. Case management of the client with ARDS focuses on the phases of ARDS rather than day-to-day care. The course of ARDS and its management are divided into four phases:

Phase 1. This phase includes early changes with the client having dyspnea and tachypnea. Early interventions focus on supporting the client and providing oxygen.

Phase 2. Patchy infiltrates form from increasing pulmonary edema. Interventions include mechanical ventilation and prevention of complications.

Phase 3. This phase occurs over days 2 to 10, and the client has progressive hypoxemia that responds poorly to high levels of oxygen. Interventions focus on maintaining adequate oxygen transport, preventing complications, and supporting the failing lung until it has had time to heal.

Phase 4. Pulmonary fibrosis with progression occurs after 10 days. This phase is irreversible and is often called "late" or "chronic" ARDS. Clients who survive this stage will have some permanent lung changes. Interventions focus on preventing sepsis, pneumonia, and multiple organ dysfunction syndrome (MODS) as well as weaning the client from the ventilator. The client in this phase may be ventilator dependent for weeks to months. Care may occur in specialized units or facilities that focus on rehabilitation and long-term weaning. Some clients may not be weanable and may go home or to long-term care dependent on mechanical ventilation.

THE CLIENT REQUIRING INTUBATION AND VENTILATION

PATHOPHYSIOLOGY

With mechanical ventilation, the client who has severe problems of gas exchange may be supported until the underlying problem resolves or improves. Usually mechanical ventilation is a temporary life-support technique. The need for this support may be lifelong, especially for clients with chronic, progressive neuromuscular diseases that reduce effective ventilation.

Mechanical ventilation is most often used for clients with hypoxemia and progressive alveolar hypoventilation with respiratory acidosis. The hypoxemia is usually due to pulmonary shunting of blood when other methods of oxygen delivery do not provide a sufficiently high fraction of inspired oxygen (FIO_2). Mechanical ventilation may be used for clients who need respiratory support after surgery, who are barely maintaining adequate gas exchange at the cost of expending energy with the high work of breathing, or who require general anesthesia or heavy sedation to allow diagnostic or therapeutic interventions.

COLLABORATIVE MANAGEMENT

Assessment

Assess the client about to be intubated in the same way as for other breathing problems. Once mechanical ventilation has been started, assess the respiratory system on an ongoing basis. Monitor and assess for complications related to the artificial airway or ventilator as well as for those related to mechanical ventilation.

Common Nursing Diagnoses and Collaborative Problems

Nursing diagnoses and collaborative problems that may apply to clients requiring mechanical ventilation include the following:

- Impaired Verbal Communication related to physical barrier.

- Disturbed Sleep Pattern related to interruptions for monitoring, noisy environment.
- Death Anxiety related to loss of independent breathing ability.
- Impaired Oral Mucous Membrane related to presence of endotracheal tube.
- Potential for Ventilator-Associated Pneumonia

Interventions

Endotracheal Intubation. The client who needs mechanical ventilation must have an artificial airway. The most common type of artificial airway for a short-term basis is the endotracheal (ET) tube. A tracheostomy is usually considered if the client requires an artificial airway for longer than 10 to 14 days, (see Chapter 31) to reduce tracheal and vocal cord damage.

The goals of intubation are to maintain a patent airway, provide a means to remove secretions, and provide ventilation and oxygen. Indications for intubation are listed in Table 35-4.

Endotracheal Tube. An ET tube is a long polyvinyl chloride tube that is passed through the mouth or nose and into the trachea (Figure 35-2). When properly positioned, the tip of the ET tube rests about 0.8 to 1.2 inches (2 to 3 cm) above the **carina** (the point at which the trachea divides into the right and left mainstem bronchi). Oral intubation is the easiest and quickest method of establishing an airway and is often performed as an emergency procedure. Because of increased problems with sinusitis, the nasal route is reserved for facial or oral traumas and surgeries and when oral intubation is not possible. The nasal route is not used if the client has a blood dyscrasia. An anesthesiologist, nurse anesthetist, or pulmonologist usually performs the intubation.

An ET tube has several parts (see Figure 35-2). The shaft of the tube has a radiopaque line running the length of the tube. This line shows on x-ray and is used to determine correct tube placement. Short horizontal lines (depth markings) are used to place the tube correctly at the nares or mouth (at the incisor tooth) and to identify how far the tube has been inserted.

The cuff at the distal end of the tube is inflated after placement and can create a seal between the trachea and the cuff. The seal ensures delivery of a set tidal volume when mechanical ventilation is used. When the cuff is inflated to an adequate sealing volume, no air can pass around the cuff to the vocal cords, nose, or mouth. Thus the client is not able to talk when the cuff is inflated. The cuff should be inflated using minimal-leak or no-leak techniques.

The pilot balloon with a one-way valve permits air to be inserted into the cuff and prevents air from escaping. This balloon is a guide for determining whether air is present in the cuff, but it does not show how much or how little air is present.

The universal adaptor connects the ET tube to ventilator tubing or to other types of oxygen delivery systems. The endotracheal tube size is listed on the shaft of the tube. Adult tube sizes range from 7 to 9 mm. Tube size selected is based on the size of the client.

Preparing for Intubation. You must know the proper procedure for summoning intubation personnel in your facility to the bedside in an emergency situation. Explain the procedure to the client as clearly as possible. Basic life support measures, such as the establishment of a patent airway and the delivery of 100% oxygen by a manual resuscitation bag with a face mask, are crucial to the client's survival until help arrives.

In an emergency, bring the code (or "crash") cart, airway equipment box, and suction equipment (often already on the code cart) to the bedside. Maintain a patent airway through positioning and the insertion of an oral or nasopharyngeal airway until the client is intubated. During intubation, continuously monitor for changes in vital signs, signs of hypoxia or hypoxemia, dysrhythmias, and aspiration. Ensure that each intubation attempt lasts no longer than 30 seconds, preferably less than 15 seconds. After 30 seconds, provide oxygen by means of a mask and manual resuscitation bag to prevent hypoxia and cardiac arrest. Suction as necessary.

Verifying Tube Placement. Immediately after an ET tube is inserted, placement must be verified. The most accurate way to verify placement is by checking end-tidal carbon

TABLE 35-4 Major Indications for Intubation

- Airway protection when the client loses reflexes because of anesthesia, medications, disease, or decreased level of consciousness
- To provide positive pressure or high oxygen concentration
- To bypass airway obstruction
- Facilitating pulmonary hygiene and suctioning of secretions when the client cannot handle secretions (as in diseases of chronic airflow limitation)

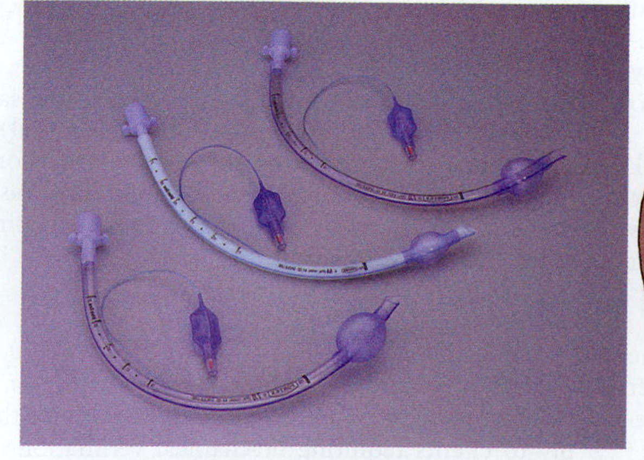

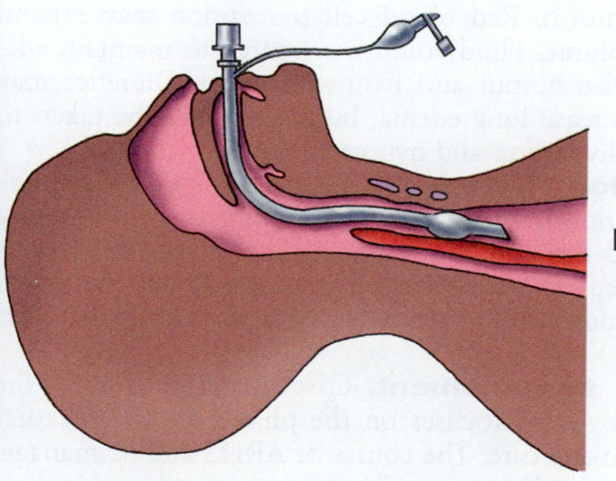

Figure 35-2 ■ **A,** Endotracheal tubes. (Courtesy of Sims Porter, Inc.) **B,** Correct placement of an oral endotracheal tube.

dioxide level. Assess for breath sounds bilaterally, symmetrical chest movement, and air emerging from the ET tube. If breath sounds and chest wall movement are absent on the left side, the tube may be in the right mainstem bronchus. The person intubating the client should be able to reposition the tube without repeating the entire intubation procedure.

Auscultate over the stomach to rule out esophageal intubation. If the tube is in the stomach, louder breath sounds are heard over the stomach than over the chest, and the abdomen may be distended. Continuously monitor chest wall movement and breath sounds until tube placement is verified by chest x-ray.

Stabilizing the Tube. The nurse, respiratory therapist, or anesthesia personnel stabilize the ET tube at the mouth or nose. The tube is marked at the level where it touches the incisor tooth or naris. Two people working together use a head halter technique to secure the tube. Chart 35-9 outlines best practices for securing an oral or nasal ET tube.

An oral airway may be inserted to keep the client from biting an oral tube. One person stabilizes the tube at the correct position and prevents head movement while a second person applies the tape. After the procedure is completed, verify and document the presence of bilateral and equal breath sounds and the level of the tube.

Nursing Care. Assess tube placement, minimal cuff leak, breath sounds, and chest wall movement regularly. Prevent pulling or tugging on the tube by the client to prevent dislodgment or "slipping" of the tube, and check the pilot balloon to ensure that the cuff is inflated. Suctioning, coughing, and speaking attempts can cause dislodgment. Neck flexion moves the tube away from the carina; neck extension moves the tube closer to the carina. Rotation of the head also causes the tube to move. Mouth secretions and tongue movement can loosen the tape and malposition the tube. When other measures fail, apply soft wrist restraints, as prescribed, for the client who is pulling on the tube. *Restraints are used as a last resort to prevent accidental extubation.* Adequate sedation (chemical restraint) may be needed to decrease agitation or prevent extubation. Obtain permission for restraints from the client or family. More information on airway management is found in Chapter 31.

Complications of an ET or nasotracheal tube can occur during placement, while in place, during extubation, or after extubation (either early or late). Trauma and complications can occur to the face; eye; nasal and paranasal areas; oral, pharyngeal, bronchial, tracheal, and pulmonary areas; esophageal and gastric areas; and cardiovascular, musculoskeletal, and neurologic systems.

Mechanical Ventilation. Mechanical ventilation to support and maintain respiratory function is widely used on medical-surgical units, in nursing homes, and in the home setting as well as in critical care units. The nurse plays a pivotal role in the coordination of care and the prevention of complications. Chart 35-10 reviews best practices for care of the client during mechanical ventilation.

The goals of mechanical ventilation are to improve oxygenation and ventilation and to decrease the work needed for an effective breathing pattern. Mechanical ventilation is used to support the client until lung function is adequate or until the acute episode has passed. *A ventilator does not cure diseased lungs; it provides ventilation until the client is able to resume the process of breathing.* It is important to remember why the client is using the ventilator so that management efforts also focus on correcting the causes of the respiratory failure. If normal oxygenation, ventilation, and respiratory muscle strength are achieved, mechanical ventilation can be discontinued.

Types of Ventilators. A wide variety of ventilators are available. The ventilator selected depends on the severity of the disease process and the length of time ventilator support is needed. Two major types of ventilators are negative-pressure and positive-pressure ventilators.

Negative-Pressure Ventilators. The negative-pressure ventilator is noninvasive and works by changing pressures in the chest cavity rather than by forcing air directly into the lungs (Figure 35-3). The iron lung, widely used during the poliomyelitis epidemic in the 1940s, is the classic negative-pressure ventilator. The client is placed in an airtight tube that surrounds either the chest area or the entire body and leaves the head exposed. During inspiration, with the expansion of the chest wall, negative pressure is generated in the chest cavity. Because of the pressure gradient, air moves from the atmosphere *(higher pressure)* into the thoracic cavity *(lower pressure).* At a preset time, negative pressure ceases and expiration occurs. Thus negative-pressure ventilators create pressure gradients that mimic normal ventilation.

Newer negative-pressure ventilators include the cuirass, poncho, and body wrap. These ventilators, which encase only the body trunk, are used for clients with neuromuscular disease, central nervous system problems, spinal cord injuries, and chronic obstructive pulmonary disease (COPD). Clients may use negative-pressure ventilation for home nighttime breathing support so that their muscles can rest. An artificial airway is not required. Newer models are lightweight and easy to use. The enclosing ventilator makes some direct nursing care more difficult. The client must be able to clear oral secretions and must have compliant (elastic) lungs to benefit from this mode of ventilation.

Positive-Pressure Ventilators. The positive-pressure ventilator is widely used in the acute care setting. During inspiration, pressure is generated that pushes air into the lungs and expands the chest. In most instances, an endotracheal (ET) tube or tracheostomy is needed. Positive-pressure ventilators are classified by the mechanism that ends inspiration and starts expiration. Inspiration is terminated or cycled in three major ways: pressure cycled, time cycled, or volume cycled.

PRESSURE-CYCLED VENTILATORS. Pressure-cycled ventilators (now rarely used) push air into the lungs until a preset airway pressure is reached. Tidal volumes and inspiratory time vary. Pressure-cycled ventilators are used for short periods, such as just after surgery and for respiratory therapy.

TIME-CYCLED VENTILATORS. Time-cycled ventilators push air into the lungs until a preset time has elapsed. Tidal volume and pressure vary, depending on the needs of the client and the type of ventilator.

VOLUME-CYCLED VENTILATORS. Volume-cycled ventilators push air into the lungs until a preset volume is delivered. A constant tidal volume is delivered regardless of the pressure needed to deliver the tidal volume. A set pressure limit, however, prevents excessive pressure from being exerted on the lungs. The advantage of this type of ventilator is that a constant tidal volume is delivered regardless of the

CHART 35-9

BEST PRACTICE for Securing an Oral and Nasal Endotracheal Tube

Little evidence is available to provide clinical direction on the best method to secure endotracheal (ET) and nasotracheal tubes; however, adhesive tape is the easiest, cheapest, and most frequently used.

Adhesive tape may be irritating to the skin, and frequent tape changes may disrupt the skin integrity. An additional reported complication is nosocomial cutaneous mucomycosis occurring around the surgical tape securing the ET tube. Protecting the skin, especially on the face, is a high priority for clients and nurses. This must be balanced against making sure the ET tube is not dislodged. A simple yet effective method of securing the oral and nasotracheal tube is demonstrated here:

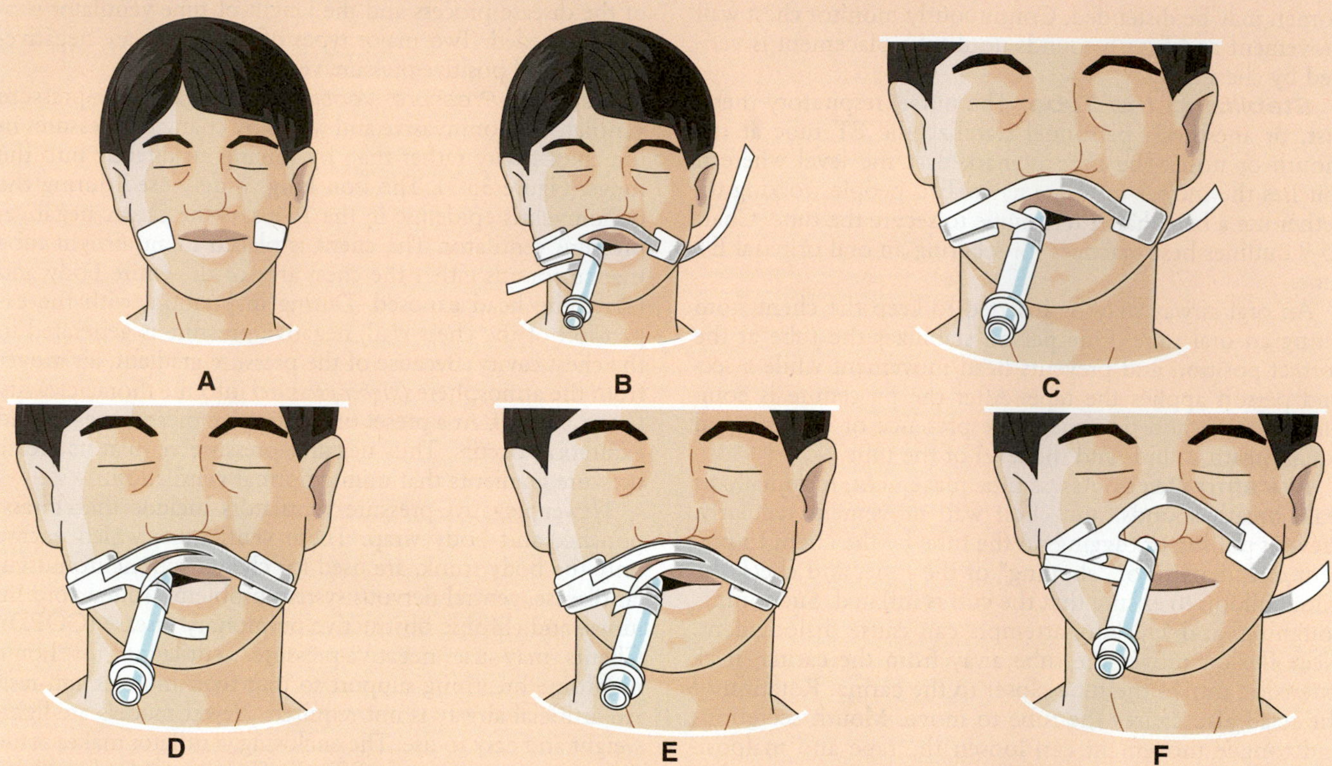

1. Prepare the skin by shaving the cheeks and upper lip, if possible.
2. Protect the skin by applying tincture of benzoin to the skin and ET tube and allow to dry (Mastisol may also be used, but Detachol must be used before removing the tape); then apply a 1 × 3-inch piece of thin DuoDerm or other protective or hydrocolloid membrane to the skin on the cheeks *(A)*.
3. Take a 30-inch (about 2½-foot) piece of adhesive tape and lay it on a flat surface, sticky side up. Take another piece of tape (about 10 inches), and cover the middle portion of the tape (sticky side to sticky side) to protect the back of the client's neck. A tongue blade on each end folded over can keep it from getting tangled or sticking prematurely.
4. Place the tape behind the client's neck. Remove the tongue blades, and place the tape on the protective membrane up to the end of the mouth on each side. Trim the tape as needed and split each end of the tape.
5. Take the upper part of one end of the tape, and place it on the upper lip. Take the lower part of the tape and wrap it securely around the tube *(B, C)*. Take the upper part of the other end of the tape, place it on the upper lip, and wrap the lower part securely around the tube *(D, E)*. Do not have the tube too far to either side of the mouth, or it can cause skin breakdown in the corner of the mouth or lips.
6. The same method can be used for nasal tubes, but do not tape the tube too tightly to the nose or skin breakdown will occur on the nares *(F)*.
7. Always tape the tube to the upper lip; never the lower. The lower jaw moves too much with attempts to speak or oral care, which will move the tube and cause irritation and discomfort for the client. The tape should be inspected at least every shift for signs of loosening or skin irritation or breakdown, especially with increased oral secretions. Tightness of the tape should also be checked each shift if swelling in the face and neck occurs or if there is an increase in fluid retention (as in anasarca, sepsis, or acute respiratory distress syndrome).

An additional technique for securing tubing that can decrease ET tube movement and provide a fulcrum for pulling on ventilator tubing is to attach a 6-inch (50-mL) piece of flexible ventilator tubing between the ET tube adaptor and the Y-connector of the ventilator tubing. The procedure for this technique is as follows:

1. Shave the chest or clean with alcohol a portion of the chest at right angles to the angle of Louis. Apply tincture of benzoin and allow to dry.
2. Prepare Montgomery straps by taking two 6-inch pieces of 2-inch wide adhesive tape. Double-back one end of each piece of tape, and cut a small hole in the ends that are doubled over.
3. Apply the tape to the prepared chest with the ends with the hole over each other. Take a 12-inch piece of twill (trach) tape, and thread through both holes. Position the tubing with the Y-connector over the holes and tie into place. This procedure allows all pulling on the tubing to place strain on the tape (straps) and not on the face or the tube. Caution should be taken if clients have increased partial pressure of arterial carbon dioxide retention, and end-tidal carbon dioxide monitoring may be useful when weaning.

CHART 35-10

BEST PRACTICE for
Care of the Client Receiving Mechanical Ventilation

- At least once every shift check to be sure the ventilator settings are set as prescribed.
- Check to be sure alarms are set (especially low-pressure and low-exhaled volume).
- Observe the exhaled volume digital display to be sure the client is receiving the prescribed tidal volume.
- Empty ventilator tubings when moisture collects. Never empty fluid in the tubing back into the cascade.
- Ensure adequate humidity by keeping delivered air temperature maintained at body temperature.
- If the client is on PEEP, observe the peak airway pressure dial to determine the proper level of PEEP.
- Assess the client's respiratory status each shift and as needed:
  - Observe the client's color (especially lips and nail beds).
  - Observe the client's chest for bilateral expansion.
  - Auscultate the lungs for crackles, rhonchi, wheezes, equal breath sounds, and decreased or absent breath sounds.
  - Obtain pulse oximetry reading.
  - Evaluate ABGs as indicated.
- Take vital signs at least every 4 hours.
- Be sure the tracheostomy cuff (or the endotracheal cuff) is adequately inflated to ensure tidal volume.
- Administer mouth care every 2 to 4 hours.
- Observe the client's need for tracheal/oral/nasal suctioning every 2 hours. Provide adequate suctioning as needed.
- Provide tracheostomy care every shift.
- Change tracheostomy tape or endotracheal tube tape as needed. Observe the client's mouth around the endotracheal tube for pressure sores.
- Move the oral endotracheal tube to the opposite side of the mouth once every 24 hours to prevent ulcers.
- Maintain accurate intake and output records to monitor fluid balance.
- Turn the client at least every 2 hours, and get the client out of bed as prescribed to promote pulmonary hygiene and prevent complications of immobility.
- Schedule treatments and nursing care at intervals to provide rest.
- Explain all procedures and treatments; provide access to a call bell; visit the client frequently.
- Include the client and his or her family in care whenever possible (especially suctioning and tracheostomy care).
- Provide a letter board or pencil and paper for communication. Request consultation with a speech therapist for assistance, if necessary.
- Observe ventilated clients for gastrointestinal distress (diarrhea, constipation, tarry stools).
- Document pertinent observations in the client's medical record (chart).
- Administer muscle-paralyzing agents, sedatives, and narcotic analgesics, as appropriate.
- Monitor the effectiveness of mechanical ventilation in terms of the client's physiologic and psychological status.
- Initiate relaxation techniques as appropriate.
- Monitor the client's progress on current ventilator settings and make appropriate changes as indicated.
- Monitor for adverse effects of mechanical ventilation: infection, barotrauma, reduced cardiac output.
- Position to facilitate ventilation/perfusion matching ("good lung down"), as appropriate.
- Monitor the effects of ventilator changes on oxygenation and the client's subjective response.
- Monitor readiness to wean.

Courtesy Our Lady of Lourdes Medical Center, Camden, NJ.
PEEP, Positive end-expiratory pressure; *ABGs*, arterial blood gases.

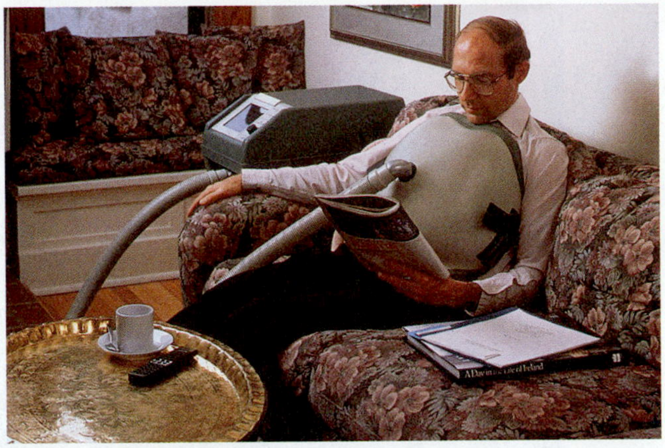

Figure 35-3 ■ A negative-pressure ventilator. Lifecare Chest Shell. (From Hill, N. [1986]. Clinical application of body ventilators. *Chest*, 90[6], 900. Used with permission.)

changing compliance of the lungs and chest wall or the airway resistance.

MICROPROCESSOR VENTILATORS. Microprocessor ventilators are computer-managed, positive-pressure ventilators. A microprocessor is built into the ventilator to allow ongoing monitoring of ventilatory functions, alarms, and client conditions. It often has components of volume-, time-, and pressure-cycled ventilators. The microprocessor ventilator is more responsive to clients who have severe lung disease and those who need prolonged weaning trials. Examples include the Draeger Evita XL and Puritan-Bennett 840.

Modes of Ventilation. The mode of ventilation is the way in which the client receives breaths from the ventilator.

Assist-Control Ventilation. Assist-control (AC) ventilation is the mode used most often and is mainly a resting mode. The ventilator takes over the work of breathing for the client. The tidal volume and ventilatory rate are preset. If the client does not trigger spontaneous breaths, a minimal ventilatory pattern is established. The ventilator is programmed to respond to the client's inspiratory effort if he or she does initiate a breath. In this case, the ventilator delivers the preset tidal volume while allowing the client to control the rate of breathing.

A disadvantage of the AC mode is that if the client's spontaneous ventilatory rate increases, the ventilator continues to deliver a preset tidal volume with each breath. The client may then hyperventilate, and respiratory alkalosis occurs. Causes of hyperventilation, such as pain, anxiety, or acid-base imbalances, must be corrected.

Synchronized Intermittent Mandatory Ventilation. Synchronized intermittent mandatory ventilation (SIMV) is similar to AC ventilation in that tidal volume and ventilatory rate are preset. If the client does not breathe, a minimal ventilatory pattern is established. Unlike the AC mode, SIMV allows spontaneous breathing at the client's own rate and tidal volume between the ventilator breaths. SIMV can be used as a main ventilatory mode or as a weaning mode. When used for weaning, the number of mechanical breaths (SIMV breaths) is gradually decreased (e.g., from 12 to 2), and the client gradually resumes spontaneous breathing.

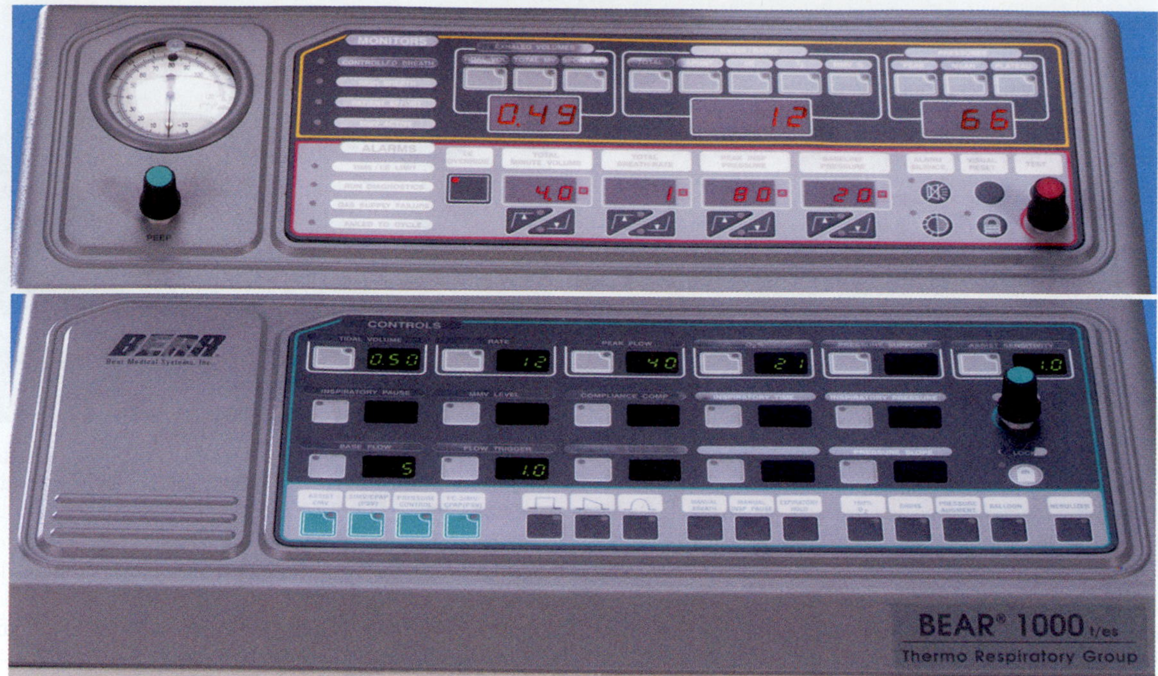

Figure 35-4 ■ Display signals and alarms *(top)* and control panel *(bottom)* of a typical volume-cycled ventilator. (Bear 1000t/es Adult Volume Ventilator. Courtesy Bear Medical Systems, Thermo Respiratory Group, Palm Springs, CA.)

The mandatory ventilator breaths are delivered when the client is ready to inspire. This action promotes synchrony between the ventilator and the client.

Bi-level Positive Airway Pressure. Bi-level positive airway pressure (BiPAP) provides noninvasive pressure support ventilation by nasal or face mask. Whereas BiPAP is most often used for clients with sleep apnea, it may be used for clients with ventilatory muscle fatigue to avoid the more invasive endotracheal intubation or tracheostomy.

Other Modes of Ventilation. Newer modes of ventilation, such as pressure support and continuous flow (flow-by), are part of most microprocessor ventilators. Both types decrease the work of breathing and are often used for weaning clients from mechanical ventilation. Other modes are maximum mandatory ventilation (MMV), inverse inspiration-expiration (I/E) ratio, permissive hypercarbia, airway pressure–release ventilation, proportional assist ventilation, high-frequency ventilation, and high-frequency oscillation. Many of these modes use special ventilators, tubing, or airways.

Ventilator Controls and Settings. The volume-cycled ventilator is the most widely used ventilator in the acute care setting. Regardless of the type of volume-cycled ventilator used, the controls and types of settings are universal (Figure 35-4). The physician prescribes the ventilator settings, and usually the ventilator is readied or set up by the respiratory department. The nurse assists in connecting the client to the ventilator and monitors the ventilator settings.

Tidal Volume. Tidal volume (V_T) is the volume of air the client receives with each breath. It can be measured on either inspiration or expiration. The average prescribed V_T ranges between 7 and 10 mL/kg of body weight (see the Evidence-Based Practice for Nursing box at right). Adding a zero to the weight of clients in kilograms gives an estimate of tidal volume.

EVIDENCE-BASED PRACTICE for Nursing

Less is better for tidal volumes

The Acute Respiratory Distress Syndrome Network. (2000). Ventilation with lower tidal volumes as compared with traditional tidal volumes for acute lung injury. *The New England Journal of Medicine, 342*(18), 1301-1308.

Traditionally, tidal volumes from 10 to 15 mg/kg body weight are used in mechanical ventilation; however, these volumes may cause stretch-induced lung injury in clients with acute lung injury and acute respiratory distress syndrome (ARDS; so-called volu-trauma). The purpose of this study was to compare these volumes with a lower tidal volume and evaluate clinical outcomes.

Clients were enrolled in a multicenter, randomized clinical trial. The trial compared traditional treatment (tidal volume of 12 mL/kg and plateau pressure of ≤50 cm water) with the treatment group (tidal volume of 6 mL/kg and plateau pressure of ≤30 cm of water or less). The outcomes were death before discharge or breathing without assistance and number of days without ventilator use from day 1 to day 28. The trial was stopped prematurely because mortality was lower in the treatment group as well as because of the greater number of days without ventilator use during the first 28 days.

Level of Evidence: 2—At least one properly designed randomized control trial of appropriate size (multisite).

Critique. This study has major implications for decreasing complications related to use of mechanical ventilation. Lessening the effect of volu-trauma can impact costs and length of stay as well functional status post-hospitalization. The study has limitations however, in that volume-assist control mode was used until the client was weaned. This is not consistently used in clinical practice; synchronized intermittent mandatory ventilation (SIMV) is more commonly used.

Implications for Nursing. Decreasing complications is a major role for nurses in critical care. Clients on mechanical ventilation are vulnerable to numerous insults and diligent care is required to assess and intervene when an untoward event occurs. This treatment change is simple yet may impact the survival of clients with acute lung injury and ARDS.

Rate, or Breaths per Minute. Rate, or breaths/min, is the number of ventilator breaths delivered per minute. The rate is usually set between 10 and 14 breaths/min.

Fraction of Inspired Oxygen. The **fraction of inspired oxygen** (FIO_2) is the oxygen level delivered to the client. The prescribed FIO_2 is determined by the arterial blood gas (ABG) value and the client's condition. Ventilators can provide 21% to 100% oxygen, depending on need.

The oxygen delivered to the client is warmed to body temperature (98.6° F [37° C]) and humidified to 100%. Humidification and warming are needed because upper air passages of the respiratory tree, which normally warm, humidify, and filter air, are bypassed. Humidification and warming prevent mucosal damage and ease clearance of secretions.

Sighs. **Sighs** are volumes of air that are 1.5 to 2 times the set tidal volume, delivered 6 to 10 times/hr. These may be used to prevent atelectasis in special circumstances. Sighs are rarely used, however, because they can cause **barotrauma** (lung damage from excessive pressure) and have not been shown to be useful.

Peak Airway (Inspiratory) Pressure. Peak airway (inspiratory) pressure (PIP) indicates the pressure needed by the ventilator to deliver a set tidal volume at a given dynamic compliance. The PIP value appears on the display on the front or top of the ventilator. Peak pressure is the highest pressure reached during inspiration. Monitoring trends in PIP reflect changes in resistance of the lungs and resistance in the ventilator. An increased PIP reading means increased airway resistance in the client or the ventilator tubing (bronchospasm, or pinched tubing), increased amount of secretions, pulmonary edema, or decreased pulmonary compliance (the lungs or chest wall are "stiffer" or harder to inflate). An upper pressure limit is set on the ventilator to prevent barotrauma. When the limit is reached, the high-pressure alarm sounds, and the remaining volume is not given.

Continuous Positive Airway Pressure. Continuous positive airway pressure (CPAP) applies positive airway pressure throughout the entire respiratory cycle for spontaneously breathing clients. Sedating drugs are given cautiously or not at all when the client is receiving CPAP so that respiratory effort is not suppressed. CPAP keeps the alveoli open during inspiration and prevents alveolar collapse during expiration. This process increases functional residual capacity (FRC), improves gas exchange, and improves oxygenation.

The most common use of CPAP is to help in the weaning process. During CPAP, no ventilator breaths are delivered. The ventilator just delivers oxygen and provides monitoring and an alarm system. The respiratory pattern is determined by the client's efforts. Normal levels of CPAP are 5 to 15 cm H_2O, adjusted to promote adequate oxygenation. If no pressure is set on the ventilator, the client receives no positive pressure. Thus, the client is then using the ventilator as a T-piece with alarms.

Modifications of CPAP include nasal CPAP and bi-level positive airway pressure (BiPAP). These modifications are used for select problems.

Positive End-Expiratory Pressure. Positive end-expiratory pressure (PEEP) is positive pressure exerted during the expiratory phase of ventilation. PEEP improves oxygenation by enhancing gas exchange and preventing atelectasis. It is used to treat persistent hypoxemia that does not improve with an acceptable oxygen delivery level. PEEP is often added when the partial pressure of arterial oxygen (PaO_2) remains low with an FIO_2 of 50% to 70% or greater.

The need for PEEP indicates a severe gas-exchange problem. It is important to lower the FIO_2 delivered whenever possible. Prolonged use of a high FIO_2 can damage lungs from the toxic effects of oxygen. PEEP prevents alveoli from collapsing because the lungs are kept partially inflated so that alveolar-capillary gas exchange is promoted throughout the ventilatory cycle. The effect should be an increase in arterial blood oxygenation so that the FIO_2 can be decreased.

Positive end-expiratory pressure (PEEP) is "dialed in" with the PEEP dial on the control panel. The amount of PEEP is usually 5 to 15 cm H_2O and is read (monitored) on the peak airway pressure dial, the same dial used to read the PIP. When PEEP is added, the dial does not return to zero at the end of exhalation; rather, it returns to a baseline that has been increased from zero by the amount of PEEP applied.

Flow. **Flow** is how fast the ventilator delivers each breath. It is usually set at 40 L/min. *If a client is agitated, is restless, has a widely fluctuating pressure reading on inspiration, or has other signs of air hunger, the flow may be set too low. Increasing the flow should be tried before using chemical restraints.*

Other Settings. Other settings may be used, depending on the type of ventilator and mode of ventilation. Examples include inspiratory and expiratory cycle, waveform, expiratory resistance, and plateau.

Nursing Management. The use of mechanical ventilation involves a complex decision-making process for both the client/family and the interdisciplinary health care team. The physical and psychological concerns of the client and family must be addressed because the mechanical ventilator often causes them anxiety. You must carefully explain the purpose of the ventilator and acknowledge that the client might feel some different sensations. Encourage the client and family to express their concerns. Act as the coach to help and support the client and family through this experience. In an emergency, explanations may not occur until the emergency has been controlled. Clients undergoing mechanical ventilation in intensive care units (ICUs) often experience delirium, or "ICU psychosis." These clients need frequent, repeated explanations and reassurance.

When caring for a ventilated client, you must be concerned with the client first and the ventilator second. It is vital that you understand why mechanical ventilation is needed. Causes such as excessive amounts of secretions, sepsis, and trauma require different interventions to allow ventilator independence. In addition, you must understand the client's chronic health problems, especially chronic obstructive pulmonary disease (COPD), left-sided heart failure, anemia, and malnutrition. These problems may slow weaning from mechanical ventilation and warrant close monitoring and intervention.

Three nursing goals in caring for the client with mechanical ventilation are to monitor and evaluate the response to the ventilator, manage the ventilator system safely, and prevent complications.

Monitoring the Client's Response. A major nursing responsibility is to monitor and evaluate the client's response to the ventilator. Assess vital signs and listen to breath sounds every 30 to 60 minutes at first. Monitor respiratory parameters (e.g., capnography and pulse oximetry), and check arterial blood gas (ABG) values. Vital signs change during hypercarbia and hypoxemia.

Assess the breathing pattern in relation to the ventilatory cycle to determine whether the client is tolerating or fighting the ventilator. Assess and record breath sounds, including bilateral equal breath sounds to ensure proper endotracheal (ET) tube placement. To determine the need for suctioning, observe secretions for type, color, and amount.

Assess the area around the ET tube or tracheostomy site at least every 4 hours for color, tenderness, skin irritation, and drainage. This monitoring provides information to guide the client's activities, such as weaning, physical or occupational therapy, and self-care. Pace activities so that oxygenation and ventilation are adequate. Interpret ABG values to evaluate ventilation and suggest ventilator settings that help the client.

Because you as the nurse spend the most time with the client, you are most likely to be the first person to recognize slight changes in vital signs or ABG values, fatigue, or distress. Promptly confer with the physician and implement the appropriate interventions.

While monitoring and evaluating the client's clinical status, also serve as a resource for the psychological needs of the client and family. Anxiety can reduce the tolerance of mechanical ventilation. Skilled and sensitive nursing care promotes psychological well-being and promotes synchrony with the ventilator. Because the client cannot speak, communication can be frustrating and anxiety producing. The client and family may panic because they believe that the voice has been lost. Reassure them that the ET tube prevents speech temporarily.

Plan methods of communication to meet the client's needs. Magic Slates, writing paper, computers, and tracheostomy tubes that permit talking are ways to facilitate communication. Finding a successful means for communication is important because the client often feels isolated as a result of the inability to speak. Try to anticipate the client's needs and provide easy access to frequently used belongings. Visits from family, friends, and pets and keeping a call light within reach are some ways of giving clients a sense of control over the environment. Urge the client to participate in self-care.

Managing the Ventilator System. Ventilator settings are prescribed by the physician. These settings include tidal volume, respiratory rate, fraction of inspired oxygen (FIO_2), mode of ventilation (assist-control [AC] ventilation, synchronized intermittent mandatory ventilation [SIMV]), and adjunctive modes, such as positive end-expiratory pressure (PEEP), pressure support, or continuous flow.

Perform and document ventilator checks according to the standards of the unit or facility. Respond promptly to alarms. During a ventilator check, compare the prescribed ventilator settings with the actual settings. Check the level of water in the humidifier and the temperature of the humidifying system to ensure that they are not too high. Temperature extremes damage the airway mucosa. Remove any condensation in the ventilator tubing by draining water into drainage collection receptacles, and empty them every shift. To prevent bacterial contamination, do not allow tubing moisture and water to enter the humidifier.

Mechanical ventilators have alarm systems that warn of a problem with either the client or the ventilator. *Alarm systems must be activated and functional at all times.* If the cause of the alarm cannot be determined, ventilate the client manually with a resuscitation bag until the problem is corrected by another health care professional. The two major alarms on a ventilator indicate either a high pressure or a low exhaled volume. Table 35-5 lists nursing interventions for various causes of ventilator alarms.

Provide proper care of the ET or tracheostomy tube. Maintain a patent airway by suctioning as needed. The following are indications for suctioning in the ventilated client:

- Presence of secretions
- Increased peak airway (inspiratory) pressure (PIP)
- Presence of rhonchi (wheezes)
- Decreased breath sounds

Careful maintenance of the ET or tracheostomy tube also ensures a patent airway. Assess the tube's position at least every 2 hours, especially for the client whose airway is attached to heavy ventilator tubing that may pull on the tracheostomy or ET tube. Position the ventilator tubing in such a way that the client can move without pulling on the ET or tracheostomy tube. The ET tube can move and slip into the right mainstem bronchus. To detect changes in the tube's position, mark the level at which the tube touches the client's teeth or nose. Give mouth care at least every shift for oral hygiene and to prevent loosening of the tape that holds the tube.

Preventing Complications. Most complications are due to the positive pressure from the ventilator. Nearly every body system is affected.

CARDIAC COMPLICATIONS. Cardiac problems from mechanical ventilation include hypotension and fluid retention. Hypotension is caused by positive pressure that increases thoracic pressure and inhibits blood return to the heart. The decreased venous return decreases cardiac output, reflected as hypotension. Hypotension is most often seen in clients who are dehydrated or need high PIP for ventilation. Teach the client to avoid a **Valsalva maneuver** (bearing down while holding the breath) and to prevent constipation, which could result in a Valsalva maneuver.

Fluid is retained because of decreased cardiac output. The kidneys receive less blood flow, which then stimulates the renin-angiotensin-aldosterone system to retain fluid. Also, humidified air in the ventilator system contributes to fluid retention. If humidification is not adequate, the airways become dehydrated and the secretions solidify. Monitor the client's fluid intake and output, weight, hydration, and signs of hypovolemia.

LUNG COMPLICATIONS. The lungs can experience **barotrauma** (damage to the lungs by positive pressure), **volutrauma** (damage to the lung by excess volume delivered to one lung over the other), and acid-base imbalance. Barotrauma includes pneumothorax, subcutaneous emphysema, and pneumomediastinum. Clients at highest risk for barotrauma have chronic airflow limitation (CAL), have blebs, are on PEEP, have dynamic hyperinflation, or require high pressures to ventilate the lungs (because of decreased compliance or "stiff" lungs, as seen in acute respiratory distress syndrome [ARDS]). Blood gas abnormalities can be corrected by ventilator changes and adjustment of fluid and electrolyte imbalances.

GASTROINTESTINAL AND NUTRITIONAL COMPLICATIONS. Gastrointestinal (GI) alterations result from the stress of mechanical ventilation. Stress ulcers occur in about

TABLE 35-5 Nursing Interventions for Various Causes of Ventilator Alarms

Cause	Nursing Interventions
High-Pressure Alarm (sounds when peak inspiratory pressure reaches the set alarm limit [usually set 10-20 mm Hg above the client's baseline PIP])	
There is an increased amount of secretions in the airways or a mucous plug.	Suction as needed.
The client coughs, gags, or bites on the oral ET tube.	Insert oral airway to prevent biting on the ET tube.
The client is anxious or fights the ventilator.	Provide emotional support to decrease anxiety. Increase the flow rate. Explain all procedures to the client. Provide sedation or paralyzing agent per the physician's prescription.
Airway size decreases related to wheezing or bronchospasm.	Auscultate breath sounds. Consult with the physician for management of bronchospasm.
Pneumothorax occurs.	Auscultate breath sounds. Consult with the physician about a new onset of decreased breath sounds or unequal chest excursion, which may be due to pneumothorax.
The artificial airway is displaced; the ET tube may have slipped into the right mainstem bronchus.	Assess the chest for unequal breath sounds and chest excursion. Obtain a chest x-ray as ordered to evaluate the position of the ET tube. After the proper position is verified, tape the tube securely in place.
Obstruction in tubing occurs because the client is lying on the tubing or there is water or a kink in the tubing.	Assess the system, moving from the artificial airway toward the ventilator. Empty water from the ventilator tubing, and remove any kinks.
There is increased PIP associated with deliverance of a sigh.	Consult with respiratory therapist or physician to adjust the pressure alarm.
Decreased compliance of the lung is noted; a trend of gradually increasing PIP is noted over several hours or a day.	Evaluate the reasons for the decreased compliance of the lungs. Increased PIP occurs in ARDS, pneumonia, or any worsening of pulmonary disease.
Low Exhaled Volume (or Low-Pressure) Alarm (sounds when there is a disconnection or leak in the ventilator circuit or a leak in the client's artificial airway cuff)	
A leak in the ventilator circuit prevents breath from being delivered.	Assess all connections and all ventilator tubings for disconnection.
The client stops spontaneous breathing in the SIMV or CPAP mode or on pressure support ventilation.	Evaluate the client's tolerance of the mode.
A cuff leak occurs in the ET or tracheostomy tube.	Evaluate the client for a cuff leak. A cuff leak is suspected when the client is able to talk (air escapes from the mouth) or when the pilot balloon on the artificial airway is flat (see section on tracheostomy tubes in Chapter 31).

ARDS, Acute respiratory distress syndrome; *CPAP*, continuous positive airway pressure; *ET*, endotracheal; *PIP*, Peak inspiratory pressure; *SIMV*, synchronized intermittent mandatory ventilation.

25% of clients receiving mechanical ventilation. Antacids, sucralfate (Carafate, Sulcrate✱), and histamine blockers such as ranitidine (Zantac) or proton-pump inhibitors such as esomeprazole (Nexium) are often prescribed as soon as the client is intubated. Changes in thoracic and abdominal cavity pressure can lead to a paralytic ileus. This problem affects absorption of nutrients through the GI system, requiring short-term parenteral nutritional support.

Malnutrition is a common problem in clients receiving mechanical ventilation. Because many other acute or life-threatening events occur at the same time, nutrition is often neglected. Malnutrition is an extreme problem for these clients and is a major reason why they cannot be weaned from the ventilator. In malnourished clients the respiratory muscles lose mass and strength. The diaphragm, the major muscle of inspiration, is affected early in this process. When the diaphragm and other respiratory muscles are weakened, ineffective breathing results, fatigue occurs, and the client cannot be weaned from the ventilator.

A balanced diet is essential whenever a ventilator is used. Furthermore, nutrition for the client with chronic obstructive pulmonary disease (COPD) requires that special attention be given to the percentage of carbohydrates in the diet. During metabolism, carbohydrates are broken down to glucose, which then produces energy, carbon dioxide, and water. Excessive carbohydrate loads increase carbon dioxide production, which the client with COPD may be unable to exhale. Hypercarbic respiratory failure results. Nutritional formulas with a higher fat content (e.g., Pulmocare, Nutri-Vent, intralipids) are calorie sources to combat this problem.

Electrolyte replacement is also important. Electrolytes have a major impact on ventilatory muscle function. Closely monitor potassium, calcium, magnesium, and phosphate levels, and replenish deficits as prescribed.

INFECTION. Infections are always a potential threat for the client using a ventilator. The ET or tracheostomy tube bypasses the body's normal process of filtering air and provides a direct access for bacteria to the lower parts of the respiratory system. Often within 48 hours the artificial airway is colonized with bacteria, which promotes pneumonia development. Aspiration of colonized fluid from the mouth or the stomach can be a source of infection. Pneumonia pro-

RESOURCE MANAGEMENT

THE CLIENT BEING MECHANICALLY VENTILATED

Cost of Care

Long-term mechanical ventilation is associated with 47% in-hospital mortality, with only 35% of clients surviving at 1 year. Many of the survivors of long-term mechanical ventilation have a need for continued care in an extended care facility. Many report a poor quality of life.

Caregivers of those who have required long-term mechanical ventilation report poor physical health and depression with those whose family member require extended institutional care reporting greater depression than those living at home.

Implications for Nursing

The likelihood of the need for continued care in an extended care facility and the risk of death during the first year following hospital discharge are common features of the population requiring prolonged mechanical ventilation. These factors need to be included in discussions of treatment options that the nurse and other members of the health care team have with clients and their families.

Data from Douglas, S.L., et al. (2002). Survival and quality of life: Short-term versus long-term ventilator patients. *Critical Care Medicine, 30*(12), 2655-2662; and Douglas, S.L., & Daly, B.J. (2003). Caregivers of long-term ventilator patients: Physical and psychological outcomes. *Chest, 123*(4), 1073-1081.

longs hospital stay and increases morbidity. *Infection prevention through strict adherence to infection control, especially handwashing, during suctioning and care of the tracheostomy or ET tube is essential.* To prevent pneumonia, implement ongoing oral care and pulmonary hygiene, including chest physiotherapy, postural drainage, and turning and positioning. More information on pneumonia can be found in Chapter 34.

MUSCULAR COMPLICATIONS. Muscle deconditioning can occur because of immobility. Having the client get out of bed, ambulate with assistance, and perform exercises not only improve muscle strength but also boost morale, facilitate gas exchange, and promote oxygen delivery to all muscles.

VENTILATOR DEPENDENCE. Another complication of mechanical ventilation is ventilator dependence, or inability to wean. Ventilator dependence can be psychological or physiologic, but more often it has a physiologic basis. The longer a client uses a ventilator, the more difficult is the weaning process because the ventilatory muscles fatigue and cannot assume breathing. The cost of maintaining a client with long-term ventilation is great in terms of both actual direct costs and the personal cost of caregivers (see the Resource Management box above). The health care team uses every method of weaning before a client is declared unweanable.

Along with the physician, social worker or psychologist, and a member of the clergy, discuss with the family and the client, as able, the client's quality of life, goals, and values. In accordance with this discussion, make arrangements for home ventilation, nursing home placement, or withdrawal of life support (in terminal cases). Family members who are responsible for providing care to clients receiving long-term mechanical ventilation are at risk for decline in physical health and for depression. These problems occur among caregivers of clients who are placed in care facilities as well as those who are cared for in the home (see the Evidence-Based Practice for Nursing box at right). Special units and facilities are available to maximize the rehabilitation and weaning of ventilator-dependent clients.

EVIDENCE-BASED PRACTICE for Nursing

Caregivers do not care for themselves

Douglas, S., & Daly, B. (2003). Caregivers of long-term ventilator patients: Physical and psychological outcomes. *Chest, 123*(4), 1073-1081.

This prospective, longitudinal, descriptive study examined the physical and psychosocial responses of caregivers of clients requiring long-term ventilation (LTV) either in the home or in a nonacute institutional setting. The purpose of the study was to describe the effects of caring for a client receiving LTV on depression, burden, role overload, and the physical health of caregivers at the time of hospital discharge and 6 months after discharge. This study was part of a larger study to examine the outcomes of clients receiving continuous mechanical ventilation after hospital discharge.

Study participants were caregivers of 135 clients who required LTV after discharge from an acute care setting. *Caregiver* was defined as the adult person who gives the majority of needed care to the client receiving LTV. Caregivers were either self-identified or identified by the client receiving LTV. Caregivers were interviewed both at the time of the client's discharge from the hospital and again 6 months later. Of the clients in the study, 77 had the same caregiver at 6 months as they did at discharge. Interview and data collection instruments used in the study were well-established and had acceptable levels of reliability and validity. Interviewers were trained to use the instruments appropriately, and interrater reliabilities remained at 90% or higher throughout the study period.

The results of the study showed that caregivers overall, experienced a decline in physical health, an increase in depression, and an increase in perceived role overload. About 15% of the subjects had manifestations of severe depression. Interestingly, subjects who were caregivers of clients in institutions had greater depression than did the caregivers of clients residing at home. The results of this study were consistent with those of studies examining caregiver responses for other populations, although the subjects in this study had higher depression scores than those reported among other caregiver groups.

Level of Evidence: 3—Well-designed study without randomization.

Critique. The study was well-designed and well-implemented. The methods and instruments used were appropriate for the questions posed by the study. Study limitations include self-identification and varied definition of the term *caregiver,* the high rate of "false-negative" results of one instrument in assessing depression compared with clinical manifestations, and a limited sample size.

Implications for Nursing. The ongoing care needs of a client requiring LTV place stress and burden on family member caregivers. This burden is still present even when the client is cared for in a long-term care facility. Nurses need to urge caregivers to care for themselves physically and emotionally. Assisting caregivers to find and use respite resources, to share the burden of care with others, and to participate in support groups are all actions that nurses can use to reduce the caregiver's stress and burden. An important intervention for nursing is to assess the caregiver on an ongoing basis for manifestations of depression and to identify caregivers who are at risk for severe depression.

Weaning. *Weaning* is the process of going from ventilatory dependence to spontaneous breathing. The weaning process is prolonged if complications develop. Many complications can be avoided through skillful nursing care. For example, turning and positioning the client not only promote comfort and prevent skin breakdown but also improve gas exchange and prevent pneumonia and atelectasis. Table 35-6 lists various weaning techniques.

TABLE 35-6 Weaning Methods

Synchronous Intermittent Mandatory Ventilation
- The client breathes between the machine's preset breaths/min rate.
- The machine is initially set on an SIMV rate of 12, meaning the client receives a minimum of 12 breaths/min by the ventilator.
- The client's respiratory rate will be a combination of ventilator breaths and spontaneous breaths.
- As the weaning process ensues, the physician prescribes gradual decreases in the SIMV rate, usually at a decrease of 1 to 2 breaths/min.

T-Piece Technique
- The client is taken off the ventilator for short periods (initially 5 to 10 minutes) and allowed to breathe spontaneously.
- The ventilator is replaced with a T-piece (see Chapter 31) or CPAP, which delivers humidified oxygen.
- The prescribed FIO_2 may be higher for the client on the T-piece than on the ventilator.
- Weaning progresses as the client is able to tolerate progressively longer periods off the ventilator.
- Nighttime weaning is not usually attempted until the client is able to maintain spontaneous respirations most of the day.

Pressure Support Ventilation
- PSV allows the client's respiratory effort to be augmented by a predetermined pressure assist from the ventilator.
- As the weaning process ensues, the amount of pressure applied to inspiration is gradually decreased.
- Another method of weaning with PSV is to maintain the pressure but gradually decrease the ventilator's preset breaths/min rate.

CPAP, Continuous positive airway pressure; *FIO_2*, fraction of inspired oxygen; *PSV*, pressure support ventilation; *SIMV*, synchronized intermittent mandatory ventilation.

CONSIDERATIONS FOR OLDER ADULTS

The older client, especially one who has smoked or who has a chronic lung problem such as COPD, is at risk for ventilator dependence and failure to wean. Age-related changes, such as increased chest wall stiffness, reduced ventilatory muscle strength, and decreased lung elasticity, reduce the likelihood of weaning. The usual manifestations of ventilatory failure—hypoxemia and hypercarbia—may be less obvious in the older adult, and other clinical measures of oxygenation, such as a change in mental status, must be used.

Extubation. **Extubation** is the removal of the endotracheal (ET) tube. The tube is removed when the need for intubation has been resolved. Before removal, explain the procedure. Set up the prescribed oxygen delivery system at the bedside, and bring in the equipment for emergency reintubation. Hyperoxygenate the client and thoroughly suction both the ET tube and the oral cavity. Then rapidly deflate the cuff of the ET tube and remove the tube at peak inspiration. Immediately instruct the client to cough. It is normal for large amounts of oral secretions to collect. Give oxygen by face mask or nasal cannula. The fraction of inspired oxygen (FIO_2) is usually prescribed at 10% higher than the level used while the ET tube was in place.

Monitoring after extubation is essential. Monitor the vital signs every hour initially, assessing the ventilatory pattern and for manifestations of respiratory distress. It is common for clients to be hoarse and have a sore throat for a few days after extubation. Instruct the client to sit in a semi-Fowler's position, take deep breaths every half-hour, use an incentive spirometer every 2 hours, and limit speaking in the immediate period after extubation. These measures help gas exchange, decrease laryngeal edema, and reduce vocal cord irritation. Observe closely for respirator fatigue and airway obstruction (see Chapter 31).

Early manifestations of obstruction are mild dyspnea, coughing, and the inability to expectorate secretions. Notify the physician at the onset of these problems. The physician then evaluates the need for reintubation. ***Stridor*** *is a high-pitched, crowing noise during inspiration caused by laryngospasm or edema above or below the glottis. This sound is a late manifestation of a narrowed airway and requires prompt attention.* Racemic epinephrine, a topical aerosol vasoconstrictor, is given, and reintubation may be needed.

CHEST TRAUMA

Chest injuries are responsible for about 25% of all civilian traumatic deaths. More than 50% of the injured die before arriving at health care facilities. Only 5% to 15% of all chest injuries require thoracotomy. The remainder can be treated with basic resuscitation, intubation, or chest tube placement. The initial emergency approach to all chest injuries is ABC (*a*irway, *b*reathing, *c*irculation) followed by rapid assessment and treatment of life-threatening conditions.

Pulmonary Contusion

PATHOPHYSIOLOGY

Pulmonary contusion, a potentially lethal injury, is the most common chest injury seen in the United States. After a contusion, respiratory failure develops over time rather than immediately. This condition most often follows injuries caused by rapid deceleration during vehicular accidents. Hemorrhage occurs in and between the alveoli. The resulting edema decreases pulmonary compliance and reduces the area for gas exchange. The client becomes hypoxemic and dyspneic. The bronchial mucosa is irritated and secretions increase.

◆COLLABORATIVE MANAGEMENT

◆Assessment

Clients with pulmonary contusion may be asymptomatic at first and can later develop respiratory failure. These clients present with hemoptysis, decreased breath sounds, crackles, and wheezes. Initially, the chest x-ray may show no abnormalities. A hazy opacity in the lobes or parenchyma may develop over several days. If there is no disruption of the parenchyma, resorption of the lesion often occurs without treatment.

◆Interventions

Treatment includes maintenance of ventilation and oxygenation. Central venous pressure (CVP) is monitored closely, and fluid intake is restricted as needed. The client in obvious respiratory distress may need mechanical ventilation with positive end-expiratory pressure (PEEP) to inflate the lungs.

A vicious cycle occurs in which more muscle effort is needed for ventilating a lung with a contusion and the client becomes progressively hypoxemic. This situation causes the client to tire easily, have reduced gas exchange, and become more fatigued and hypoxemic. Flail chest may also occur when pulmonary contusion occurs with parenchymal damage.

This condition often leads to acute respiratory distress syndrome (ARDS).

Rib Fracture

PATHOPHYSIOLOGY

After chest-wall contusion, rib fractures are the next most common injury to the chest wall. Rib fractures most often result from direct blunt trauma to the chest. Direct force applied to the ribs fractures them and drives the bone ends into the thorax. Thus there is a risk for intrathoracic injury, such as pulmonary contusion or pneumothorax, which occurs most often if ribs one through four are fractured.

COLLABORATIVE MANAGEMENT

The client has pain on movement and splints the chest defensively. Splinting reduces breathing depth and leads to inadequate clearance of pulmonary secretions. If the client has pre-existing pulmonary disease, the risk for atelectasis and pneumonia increases. Clients with injuries to the first or second ribs, flail chest, seven or more fractured ribs, or expired volumes of less than 15 mL/kg often have an intrathoracic injury and a poor prognosis.

Treatment for uncomplicated rib fractures is nonspecific because the fractured ribs reunite spontaneously. The chest is usually not splinted by tape or other materials. The main focus is to decrease pain so that adequate ventilation is maintained. An intercostal nerve block may be used if pain is severe. Potent analgesics that cause respiratory depression are avoided.

Flail Chest

PATHOPHYSIOLOGY

Flail chest is the inward movement of the thorax during inspiration, with outward movement during expiration. It usually involves one side of the chest and results from multiple rib fractures caused by blunt chest trauma leaving a segment of the chest wall loose. Flail chest often occurs in high-speed vehicular crashes. It is more common in older clients and has a high mortality rate (40%).

The movement of this loose segment becomes paradoxic to the expansion and contraction of the rest of the chest wall. Flail chest can also occur from bilateral separations of the ribs from their cartilage connections to each other anteriorly, without an actual rib fracture. This condition can occur during cardiopulmonary resuscitation on an older adult. Other injuries to the lung tissue under the flail segment may be present. Gas exchange is impaired, as is the ability to cough and clear secretions. Defensive splinting further reduces the client's ability to exert the extra effort required for breathing and may contribute later to failure to wean.

COLLABORATIVE MANAGEMENT

Assessment

Assess the client with a flail chest for paradoxic chest movement, dyspnea, cyanosis, tachycardia, and hypotension. **Paradoxic chest movement** is the "sucking inward" of the loose chest area during inspiration and a "puffing out" of the same area during expiration. The client is often anxious, short of breath, and in pain.

Interventions

Interventions include humidified oxygen, pain management, promotion of lung expansion through deep breathing and positioning, and secretion clearance by coughing and tracheal aspiration.

The client with a flail chest may be treated conservatively with vigilant respiratory care. Mechanical ventilation may be needed if respiratory failure or shock occurs. Monitor arterial blood gas (ABG) values closely, along with vital capacity. With severe hypoxemia and hypercarbia, the client is intubated and mechanically ventilated with PEEP. With pulmonary contusion or an underlying pulmonary disease, the risk for respiratory failure increases. Flail chest is best stabilized by positive-pressure ventilation rather than surgical intervention. Surgical stabilization is used only in extreme cases of flail chest.

Monitor the client's vital signs and fluid and electrolyte balance closely so that hypovolemia or shock can be treated immediately. If the client has a pulmonary contusion, monitor central venous pressure (CVP) and give IV fluids as prescribed. Assess for pain and intervene to relieve the pain. Analgesic drugs by IV, epidural, or nerve block route may be prescribed.

Give psychosocial support to the extremely anxious client by explaining all procedures, talking slowly, and allowing time to verbalize feelings and concerns.

Pneumothorax

PATHOPHYSIOLOGY

Any chest injury that allows air to enter the pleural space results in a rise in intrathoracic pressure and a reduction in vital capacity. Severity depends on the amount of pulmonary collapse produced. Pneumothorax is often caused by blunt chest trauma and may occur with some degree of hemothorax. The pneumothorax can be open (pleural cavity is exposed to outside air, as through an open wound in the chest wall) or closed.

COLLABORATIVE MANAGEMENT

Assessment findings commonly include the following:

- Reduced breath sounds on auscultation
- Hyperresonance on percussion
- Prominence of the involved side of the chest, which moves poorly with respirations
- Deviation of the trachea away from (closed) or toward (open) the affected side

In addition, the client may have pleuritic pain, tachypnea, and **subcutaneous emphysema** (air under the skin in the subcutaneous tissues).

A chest x-ray is used for diagnosis. Chest tubes may be needed to allow the air to escape and the lung to reinflate.

Tension Pneumothorax

PATHOPHYSIOLOGY

Tension pneumothorax, a rapidly developing and life-threatening complication of blunt chest trauma, results from an air leak in the lung or chest wall. Air forced into the chest cavity causes complete collapse of the affected lung. Air that enters the pleural space during inspiration does not exit during expiration. As a result, air continues to accumulate under pressure, compressing blood vessels, and limiting venous return. Because this process leads to decreased filling of the heart, cardiac output is reduced. If not promptly detected and treated, tension pneumothorax is quickly fatal. Causes of tension pneumothorax are blunt chest trauma, mechanical ventilation with positive end-expiratory pressure (PEEP), closed-chest drainage (chest tubes), and insertion of central venous access catheters.

COLLABORATIVE MANAGEMENT

Assessment

Assessment findings with tension pneumothorax include the following:

- Asymmetry of the thorax
- Tracheal deviation to the unaffected side
- Respiratory distress
- Absence of breath sounds on one side
- Distended neck veins
- Cyanosis
- Hypertympanic sound on percussion over the affected side

Pneumothorax is detectable on a chest x-ray. ABG assays show hypoxia and respiratory alkalosis.

Interventions

A large-bore needle is inserted into the second intercostal space in the midclavicular line of the affected side as initial treatment for tension pneumothorax. After this measure is completed, a chest tube is placed into the fourth intercostal space, and the other end is attached to a water seal drainage system until the lung reinflates.

Hemothorax

PATHOPHYSIOLOGY

Hemothorax is a common problem occurring after blunt chest trauma or penetrating injuries. A *simple* hemothorax is a blood loss of less than 1500 mL into the chest cavity; a *massive* hemothorax is a blood loss of more than 1500 mL.

Bleeding is caused by injury to the lung tissue, such as pulmonary contusions or lacerations, that can occur with rib and sternal fractures. Massive intrathoracic bleeding in blunt chest trauma may stem from the heart, great vessels, or the intercostal arteries.

COLLABORATIVE MANAGEMENT

Assessment

Physical assessment findings vary with the size of the hemothorax. If the hemothorax is small, the client may be asymptomatic. If the hemothorax is larger, the client may have respiratory distress. In addition, breath sounds are reduced on auscultation. Percussion on the involved side results in a dull sound. Blood in the pleural space is visible on a chest x-ray and confirmed by diagnostic thoracentesis.

Interventions

Interventions are aimed at removing the blood in the pleural space to normalize pulmonary function and to prevent infection. Anterior and posterolateral chest tubes are inserted to evacuate the pleural space. Carefully monitor the chest tube drainage. The physician evaluates chest x-rays serially to determine treatment effectiveness.

An open thoracotomy may be needed when there is initial evacuation of 1500 to 2000 mL of blood or persistent bleeding at the rate of 200 mL/hr over 3 hours. Monitor the vital signs, blood loss, and overall intake and output. Assess the client's response to the chest tubes, and infuse IV fluids and blood as prescribed. Autotransfusion of the blood lost through chest drainage may be considered.

Tracheobronchial Trauma

PATHOPHYSIOLOGY

Most tears of the tracheobronchial tree result from severe blunt trauma or rapid deceleration. The tears often involve the mainstem bronchi. Injuries to the trachea usually occur at the junction of the trachea and cricoid cartilage. These injuries are often caused by striking the neck against the dashboard or steering wheel during a motor-vehicle crash. Clients with lacerations of the trachea develop massive air leaks, which cause air to enter the mediastinum and extensive subcutaneous emphysema. Upper-airway obstruction may also occur, causing severe respiratory distress and inspiratory stridor. Large tracheal tears are managed by cricothyroidotomy or tracheotomy below the level of injury. A client with a torn mainstem bronchus may develop a tension pneumothorax rapidly once he or she is intubated and ventilated with positive pressure.

COLLABORATIVE MANAGEMENT

Assess the client for hypoxemia by ABG assays. Apply oxygen as needed. Depending on the degree of injury, the client may need mechanical ventilation or surgical repair. Assess vital signs every 15 minutes because the client is likely to be hypotensive and in shock. Continue to assess for subcutaneous emphysema and auscultate the lungs every 1 to 2 hours. Decreased breath sounds or wheezing may indicate further obstruction, atelectasis, or pneumothorax. Care of the client with a tracheostomy is discussed in Chapter 31.

GET READY for the NCLEX Examination!

KEY POINTS

Safe Effective Care Environment

- Use aseptic technique when caring for a client requiring pulmonary suctioning.
- Identify clients in your setting who are at risk for developing a pulmonary embolism.
- Use bleeding precautions for any client receiving anticoagulant or fibrinolytic therapy (see Chart 35-6).
- Keep antidotes available when clients are receiving heparin (antidote is protamine) or warfarin (antidote is vitamin K).
- Inspect the oral mucous membranes each shift for anyone who has an endotracheal tube.
- Ensure that alarm systems on mechanical ventilators are activated and functional at all times.

Health Promotion and Maintenance

- Teach clients ways to promote venous return and avoid deep vein thrombosis (DVT), especially when traveling long distances (see Chart 35-1).
- Use aspiration precautions for any client with an altered level of consciousness, poor gag reflex, neurologic impairment, or who has an endotracheal tube.
- Check the client with ARDS hourly for oxygen saturation, vital sign changes, or any indication of increased work of breathing such as cyanosis, pallor, and retractions.
- Assess all clients with blunt chest trauma for position of the trachea and bilateral breath sounds.
- Encourage all people to use proper safety restraints when driving or riding in motor vehicles.

Psychosocial Integrity

- Allow the client and family members the opportunity to express fear or anxiety regarding a change in breathing status or the possibility of intubation and mechanical ventilation.
- Explain all diagnostic procedures, restrictions, and follow-up care to the client scheduled for tests.
- Teach family members ways to communicate with a client who is intubated or being mechanically ventilated.
- Reassure intubated clients that speech loss is temporary.
- Remember that clients who are receiving mechanical ventilation and are being chemically paralyzed may have sensations of all types (can hear and can feel pain).

Physiological Integrity

- Notify the physician immediately for any client who develops sudden-onset respiratory difficulty.
- Check oxygen saturation by pulse oximetry for any client who has respiratory difficulty or who develops acute confusion.
- Evaluate arterial blood gas values to determine the severity of hypoxia and the client's response to therapy.
- Apply oxygen to anyone who is hypoxemic.
- Ensure that oxygen therapy delivered to the client is humidified (and warmed, when possible).
- Assess lung sounds bilaterally each hour for clients who are receiving PEEP.
- Check all ventilator settings against the prescription at least once per shift.
- Administer pain medications to clients who have rib fractures and encourage deep breaths.
- Maintain a patent airway on all clients who experience trauma.

ADDITIONAL STUDY RESOURCES

Go to your Student CD-ROM for Review Questions for the NCLEX Examination.

evolve Go to http://evolve.elsevier.com/Iggy/ for Integrated Management of Care Questions for the NCLEX Examination.

SELECTED BIBLIOGRAPHY

Asterisk indicates a classic or definitive work on this subject.

The Acute Respiratory Distress Syndrome Network. (2000). Ventilation with lower tidal volumes as compared with traditional tidal volumes for acute lung injury. *New England Journal of Medicine, 352*(18), 1301-1308.

Andrews, C. (2002). Emergency: Preventing air embolism. *American Journal of Nursing, 102*(1), 35-36.

Austan, F. (2002). Management of respiratory failure with noninvasive positive pressure ventilation and heliox adjunct. *Heart & Lung, 31*(3), 214-218.

Ayers, D., & Lappin, J. (2004). Act fast when your patient has dyspnea. *Nursing 2004, 34*(7), 36-41.

Balas, M. (2000). Prone positioning of patients with acute respiratory distress syndrome: Applying research to practice. *Critical Care Nurse, 20*(1), 24-36.

*Baldwin-Myers, A., et al. (1994). *Standards of care for the ventilator-assisted individual: A comprehensive management plan from hospital to home.* Loma Linda, CA: Loma Linda University/Respiratory Nursing Society.

Behnia, M., & Garrett, K. (2004). Association of tension pneumothorax with use of small-bore chest tubes in patients receiving mechanical ventilation. *Critical Care Nurse, 24*(1), 64-66.

*Burns, S. (1998). Making weaning easier: Pathways and protocols that work. *Critical Care Nursing Clinics of North America, 11*(4), 465-479.

*Burns, S. (1999). The long-term mechanically ventilated patient: An outcomes management approach. *Critical Care Nursing Clinics of North America, 10*(1), 87-97.

*Burns, S.M. (1999). Weaning from long-term mechanical ventilation. In C.M. Chulay & S.M. Burns (Eds.), *Care of the mechanically ventilated patient series.* Aliso Viejo, CA: American Association of Critical Care Nurses.

Carroll, P. (2002). Procedural sedation: Capnography's heightened role. *RN, 65*(10), 54-63.

*Clochesy, J., Daly, B., & Montenegro, H. (1995). Weaning chronically critically ill adults from mechanical ventilatory support: A descriptive study. *American Journal of Critical Care, 4*(2), 93-99.

Connelly, B., Gunzerath, L., & Knebel, A. (2000). A pilot study exploring mood state and dyspnea in mechanically ventilated patients. *Heart & Lung, 29*(3), 173-179.

Davies, P. (2002). Guarding your patient against ARDS. *Nursing 2002, 32*(3), 36-42.

Dochterman, J., & Bulechek, G. (eds). (2004). *Nursing interventions classification (NIC)* (4th ed). St. Louis: Mosby.

Douglas, S., & Daly, B. (2003). Caregivers of long-term ventilator patients: Physical and psychological outcomes. *Chest, 123*(4), 1073-1081.

Douglas, S., et al. (2002). Survival and quality of life: Short-term versus long-term ventilator patients. *Critical Care Medicine, 30*(12), 2655-2662.

Ebersole, P., Hess, P., & Luggen, A. (2004). *Toward healthy aging: Human needs and nursing response* (6th ed). St. Louis: Mosby.

Ellstrom, K. (2000). Relationship of psychoneurological, physiological, and environmental constructs to risk of unplanned extubation and outcomes in medical ICU patients. Doctoral Disseration, University of California Los Angeles.

El-Masri, M., Williamson, K., & Fox-Wasylyshyn, S. (2004). Severe acute respiratory syndrome: Another challenge for critical care nurses. *AACN Clinical Issues: Advanced Practice in Acute and Critical Care, 15*(1), 150-159.

Facts and Comparisons. (2004). *Drug facts and comparisons* (58th ed). St. Louis: Author.

Frawley, P., & Habashi, N. (2001). Airway pressure release ventilation: Theory and practice. *AACN Clinical Issues: Advanced Practice in Acute and Critical Care, 12*(2), 235-246.

Giuliano, K., & Higgins, T. (2005). New generation pulse oximetry in the care of critically ill patients. *American Journal of Critical Care, 14*(1), 26-37.

Greifzu, S. (2002). Caring for the chronically critically ill. *RN, 65*(7), 42-44, 46, 48-49.

Hanneman, S. (2004). Weaning from short-term mechanical ventilation. *Critical Care Nurse, 24*(1), 70-73.

Happ, M.B. (2000). Preventing treatment interference: The nurse's role in maintaining technological devices. *Heart and Lung,* 29(1), 60-69.

Happ, M.B. (2001). Communicating with mechanically ventilated patients: State of the science. *AACN Clinical Issues: Advanced Practice in Acute and Critical Care, 12*(2), 247-258.

Howard, A., et al. (2004). Comparison of 3 methods of detecting acute respiratory distress syndrome: Clinical screening, chart review, and diagnostic coding. *American Journal of Critical Care, 13*(1), 59-64.

Kleinpell, R. (2003). The role of the critical care nurse in the assessment and management of the patient with severe sepsis. *Critical Care Clinics of North America, 15*(1), 27-34.

Marion, B. (2001). A turn for the better: "Prone positioning" of patients with ARDS. *American Journal of Nursing, 101*(5), 26-34.

Marini, J.J.,, & Gattinoni, L. (2004). Ventilatory management of acute respiratory syndrome: A consensus of two. *Critical Care Medicine, 32*(1), 250-255.

McCance, K., & Huether, S. (2002). *Pathophysiology: The biologic basis for disease in adults and children* (4th ed). St. Louis: Mosby.

Mitchell, D. (2004). Vent injury: How to avoid it. *RN, 67*(7), 54-59.

Moorhead, S., Johnson, M., & Maas, M. (Eds.). (2004). *Nursing outcomes classification (NOC)* (3rd ed). St. Louis: Mosby.

O'Bryan, L., Von Rueden, K., & Malila, F. (2002). Evaluating ventilator weaning best practice: A long-term acute care hospital systemwide quality initiative. *AACN Clinical Issues, 13*(4), 567-576.

O'Keefe, G. et al. (2001). Indicators of fatigue and of prolonged weaning from mechanical ventilation in surgical patients. *World Journal of Surgery, 25*(1), 98-103.

Pfeifer, L., et al. (2001). Preventing ventilator-associated pneumonia. *American Journal of Nursing, 101*(8), 24AA-24GG.

Phelan, B., Cooper, D., & Sangkachand, P. (2002). Prolonged mechanical ventilation and tracheostomy in the elderly. *AACN Clinical Issues, 13*(1), 84-93.

Pierce, L. (2000). Traditional and nontraditional modes of mechanical ventilation. *Critical Care Nurse, 20*(1), 81-84.

Pruitt, W. (2004). Manual ventilation by one or two rescuers. *Nursing 2004, 34*(11), 43-45.

Richmond, A., Jarog, D., & Hanson, V. (2004). Unplanned extubation in adult critical care: Quality improvement and education payoff. *Critical Care Nurse, 24*(1), 32-37.

Seay, S., Gay, S., & Strauss, M. (2002). Emergency: Managing tracheostomy decannulation and displacement. *American Journal of Nursing, 102*(3), 59,61-63.

Spritzer, C. (2003). Unraveling the mysteries of mechanical ventilation: A helpful step-by-step guide. *Journal of Emergency Nursing, 29*(1), 29-36.

St. John, R. (2004). Airway management. *Critical Care Nurse, 24*(2), 93-96.

Veronesi, J. (2004). Blunt chest injuries. *RN, 67*(3), 48-54.

Winkelman, C. (2004). Inactivity and inflammation: Selected cytokines as biologic mediators in muscle dysfunction during critical illness. *AACN Clinical Issues: Advanced Practice in Acute and Critical Care, 15*(1), 74-82.

Woodruff, D. (2003). Protect your patient while he's receiving mechanical ventilation. *Nursing 2003, 33*(7), 32hn1-32hn4.

Yagan, M., White, D., & Staab, J. (2000). Sedation of the mechanically ventilated patient. *Critical Care Nursing Quarterly, 22*(4), 90-100.

Yantis, M.A. (2003). Assisting patients using positive airway pressure therapy. *Home Healthcare Nurse, 21*(3), 160-165.

Yosefy, C., et al. (2003). BiPAP ventilation as assistance for patients presenting with respiratory distress in the department of emergency medicine. *American Journal of Respiratory Medicine, 2*(4), 343-347.

UNIT EIGHT

PROBLEMS of CARDIAC OUTPUT and TISSUE PERFUSION

Management of Clients with Problems of the Cardiovascular System

CHAPTER

36 Assessment of the Cardiovascular System

DEANNE A. BLACH

LEARNING OUTCOMES

After studying this chapter, you should be able to:

1. Review the anatomy and physiology of the cardiovascular system.
2. Describe cardiovascular changes associated with aging.
3. Identify factors that place clients at risk for cardiovascular problems.
4. Perform appropriate physical assessment for clients with cardiovascular problems.
5. Interpret laboratory test findings for clients with suspected or actual cardiovascular disease.
6. Explain and pre- and post-test care associated with diagnostic cardiovascular testing.
7. Explain the purpose of hemodynamic monitoring.

Go to your Student CD-ROM for Review Questions for the NCLEX Examination keyed to these Learning Outcomes.

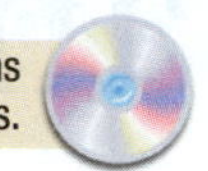

In every year since 1900 (except 1918), cardiovascular disease (CVD) has been the number one cause of death in the United States. It remains the major cause of mortality in the twenty-first century, resulting in 42% of all deaths, or nearly one million deaths, each year in the United States. CVD kills more people than the next five causes of death combined, including cancer, chronic lower respiratory diseases, accidents, diabetes, influenza, and pneumonia. It is the leading cause of death for women. In addition, the American Heart Association (AHA) estimates that about one in five people has experienced, and is living with some form of CVD (AHA, 2002).

ANATOMY AND PHYSIOLOGY REVIEW

Heart

Structure

The human heart is a cone-shaped, hollow, muscular organ located in the mediastinum between the lungs (Figure 36-1). It is about the size of an adult fist. The heart rests on the diaphragm, tilting forward and to the left in the client's chest. Each beat of the heart pumps about 60 mL of blood, or 5 L/min. During strenuous physical activity, the heart can double the amount of blood pumped to meet the increased oxygen needs of the peripheral tissues.

The heart is encapsulated by a protective covering called the *pericardium* (see Figure 36-2). Cardiac muscle tissue is composed of three layers: epicardium, myocardium, and endocardium. The *epicardium,* the outer surface, is a thin, transparent tissue. The *myocardium,* the middle layer, is composed of striated muscle fibers interlaced into bundles. This layer is responsible for the contractile force of the heart. The innermost layer, the *endocardium,* is composed of endothelial tissue. This tissue lines the inside of the chambers of the heart and covers the four heart valves.

CHAMBERS OF THE HEART

A muscular wall (septum) separates the heart into two halves: right and left. Each half has an upper chamber (atrium) and a lower chamber (ventricle) (see Figure 36-2).

RIGHT SIDE. The right atrium (RA) is a thin-walled structure that receives deoxygenated venous blood (venous return) from all peripheral tissues by way of the superior and inferior venae cavae and from the heart muscle by way of the coronary sinus. Most of this venous return flows passively from the RA, through the opened tricuspid valve, and to the right ventricle during ventricular diastole, or filling. The remaining venous return is actively propelled by the RA into the right ventricle during atrial systole, or contraction.

The right ventricle is a flat muscular pump located behind the sternum. The right ventricle generates enough pressure (about 25 mm Hg) to close the tricuspid valve, open the pulmonic valve, and propel blood into the pulmonary artery and the lungs. The workload of the right ventricle is light compared with that of the left ventricle because the pulmonary system is normally a low-pressure system, which imposes less resistance to flow.

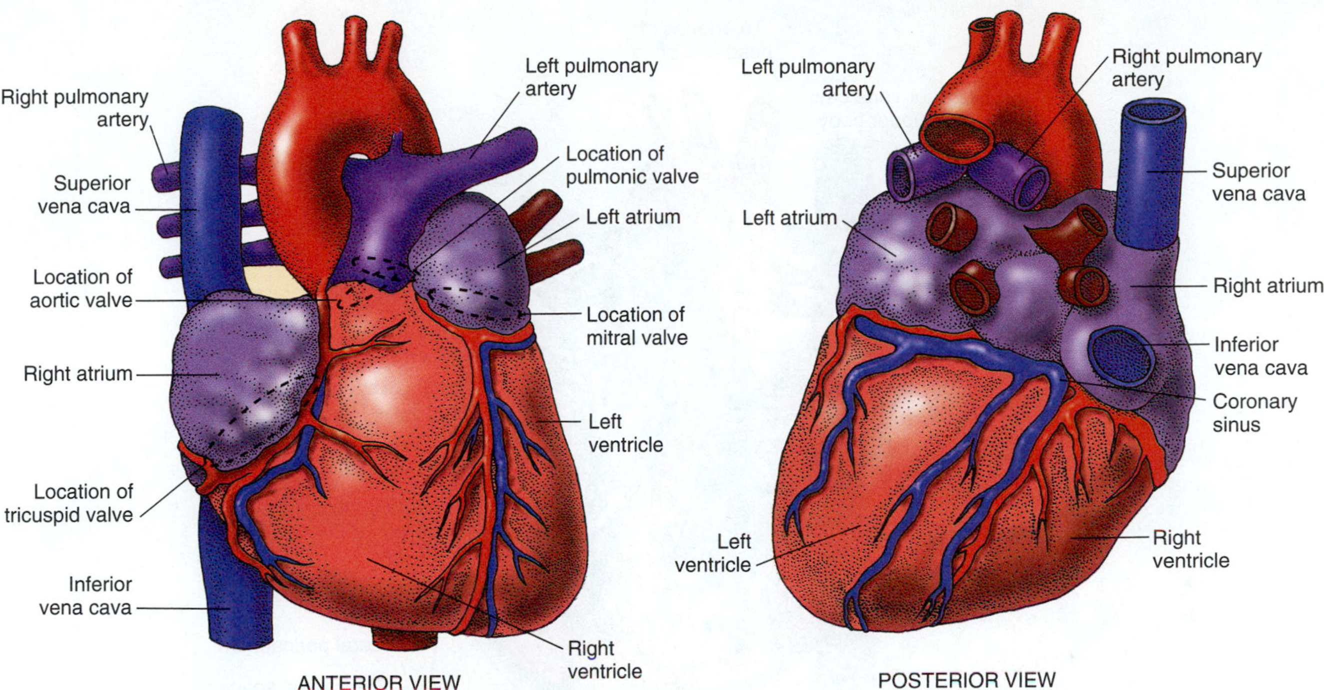

Figure 36-1 ■ Surface anatomy of the heart.

LEFT SIDE. After blood is reoxygenated in the lungs, it flows freely from the four pulmonary veins into the left atrium. Blood then flows through an opened mitral valve into the left ventricle during ventricular diastole. When the left ventricle is almost full, the left atrium contracts, pumping the remaining blood volume into the left ventricle. With systolic contraction, the left ventricle generates enough pressure (approximately 120 mm Hg) to close the mitral valve and open the aortic valve. Blood is propelled into the aorta and into the systemic arterial circulation. Blood flow through the heart is shown in Figure 36-2.

The left ventricle is ellipsoid in shape and is the largest and most muscular chamber of the heart. Its wall is two to three times the thickness of the right ventricular wall. The left ventricle must generate a higher pressure than the right ventricle because it must contract against a high-pressure systemic circulation, which imposes a greater resistance to blood flow.

Blood is propelled from the aorta throughout the systemic circulation to the various tissues of the body; blood returns to the RA because of pressure differences. The pressure of blood in the aorta of a young adult averages about 100 to 120 mm Hg, whereas the pressure of blood in the RA averages about 0 to 5 mm Hg. These differences in pressure produce a pressure gradient, with blood flowing from an area of higher pressure to an area of lower pressure. The heart and vascular structures are responsible for maintaining these pressures.

HEART VALVES

The four cardiac valves are responsible for maintaining the forward flow of blood through the chambers of the heart (see Figure 36-2). These valves open and close passively in response to pressure and volume changes within the cardiac chambers. The cardiac valves are classified into two types: atrioventricular (AV) valves and semilunar valves. Both AV valves are supported by chordae tendineae, which keep them from everting into the atria during systole.

ATRIOVENTRICULAR VALVES. The AV valves separate the atria from the ventricles. The tricuspid valve is composed of three leaflets and separates the RA from the right ventricle. The mitral (bicuspid) valve is composed of two leaflets and separates the left atrium from the left ventricle.

During ventricular diastole, the valves act as funnels and facilitate the flow of blood from the atria to the ventricles. During systole, the valves close to prevent the backflow (regurgitation) of blood into the atria.

SEMILUNAR VALVES. The two semilunar valves are the pulmonic valve and the aortic valve. The pulmonic valve separates the right ventricle from the pulmonary artery. The aortic valve separates the left ventricle from the aorta. Each semilunar valve consists of three cuplike cusps, or pockets, around the inside wall of the artery. These cusps prevent blood from flowing back into the ventricles during ventricular diastole. During ventricular systole, these valves are open to permit blood flow into the pulmonary artery and the aorta.

CORONARY ARTERIES

The heart muscle receives blood to meet its metabolic needs through the coronary arterial system (Figure 36-3). The coronary arteries originate from an area on the aorta just beyond the aortic valve. The two main coronary arteries are the left coronary artery (LCA) and the right coronary artery (RCA).

Coronary artery blood flow to the myocardium occurs primarily during diastole, when coronary vascular resistance is minimized. To maintain adequate blood flow through the coronary arteries, **mean arterial pressure (MAP)** must be at least 60 mm Hg. A MAP of between 60 and 70 mm Hg is necessary to maintain perfusion of major body organs, such as the kidneys and brain.

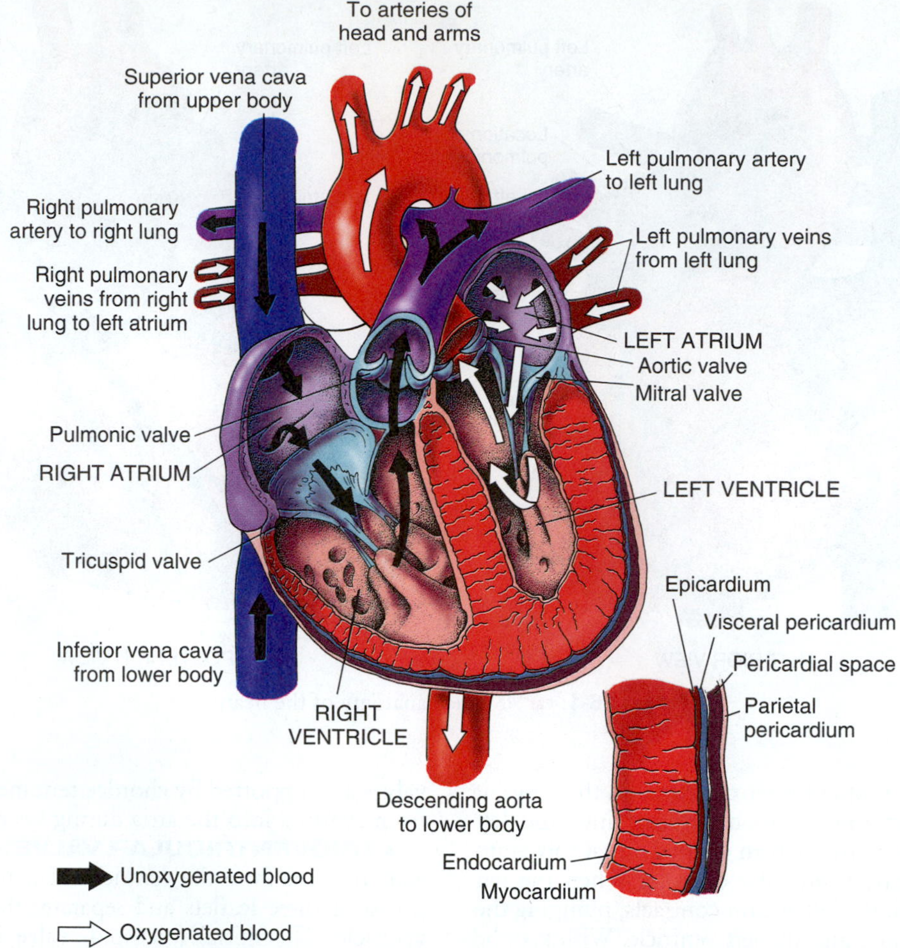

Figure 36-2 ■ Blood flow through the heart.

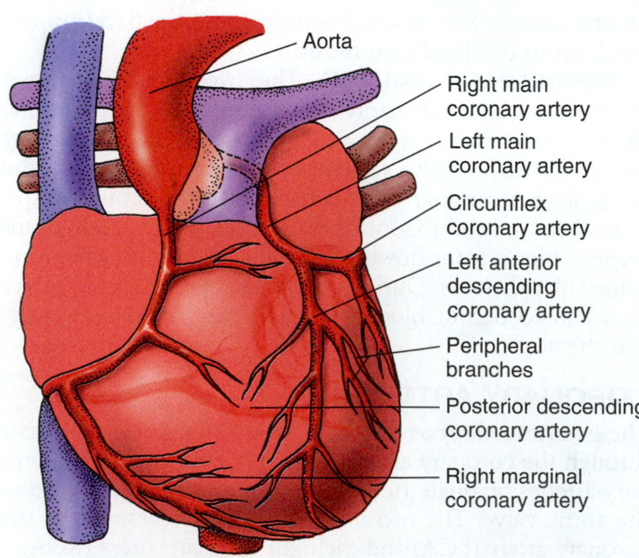

Figure 36-3 ■ Coronary arterial system.

LEFT MAIN ARTERY. The left main artery divides into two branches: the left anterior descending (LAD) and the circumflex coronary artery (LCX). The LAD branch descends toward the anterior wall and the apex of the left ventricle. It supplies blood to portions of the left ventricle, ventricular septum, chordae tendineae, papillary muscle, and, to a lesser extent, the right ventricle.

The LCX descends toward the lateral wall of the left ventricle and apex. It supplies blood to the left atrium, the lateral and posterior surfaces of the left ventricle, and sometimes portions of the interventricular septum. In 45% of people, the LCX supplies the sinoatrial (SA) node, and in 10% of people it supplies the AV node. Peripheral branches (diagonal and obtuse marginal) arise from the LAD and LCX and form an abundant network of vessels throughout the entire myocardium.

RIGHT CORONARY ARTERY. The RCA originates from the right sinus of Valsalva, encircles the heart, and descends toward the apex of the right ventricle. The RCA supplies the RA, right ventricle, and inferior portion of the left ventricle. The branching pattern of the coronary arteries varies considerably among individuals.

Function

ELECTROPHYSIOLOGIC PROPERTIES OF THE HEART

The electrophysiologic properties of heart muscle are responsible for regulating heart rate (HR) and rhythm. Cardiac muscle cells possess the characteristics of automaticity, excitability, conductivity, contractility, and refractoriness.

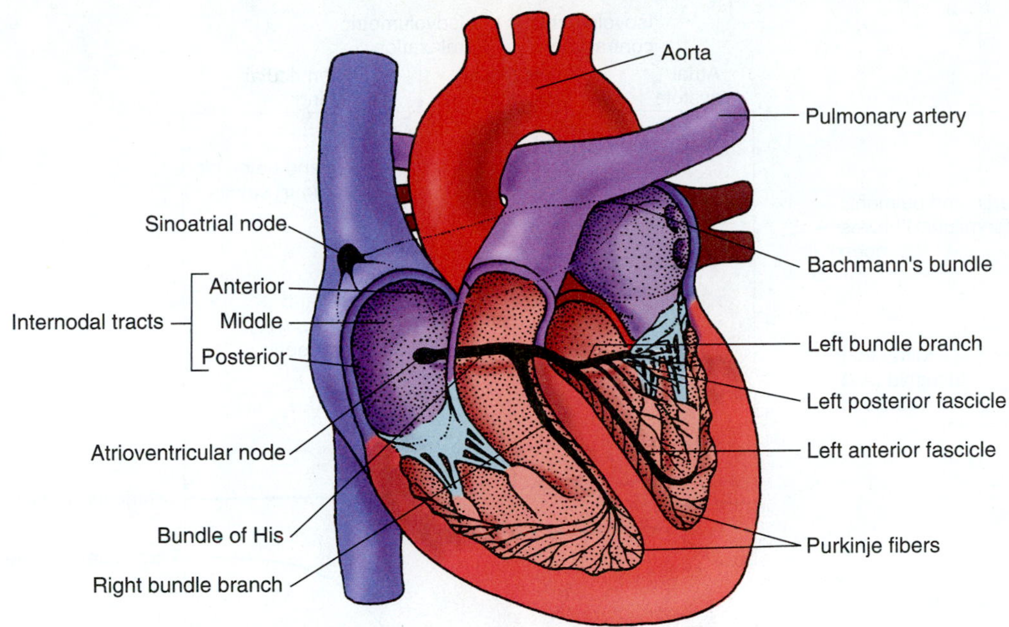

Figure 36-4 ■ Conduction system of the heart.

Automaticity refers to the ability of all cardiac cells to initiate an impulse spontaneously and repetitively. **Excitability** is the ability of the cells to respond to a stimulus by initiating an impulse **(depolarization). Conductivity** means that cardiac cells transmit the electrical impulses they receive. Because the cells possess the property of **contractility,** they also contract in response to an impulse. **Refractoriness** means that cardiac cells are unable to respond to a stimulus until they have recovered (repolarized) from the previous stimulus. These properties are described more completely in Chapter 37.

CONDUCTION SYSTEM OF THE HEART

The cardiac conduction system is composed of specialized tissue capable of rhythmic electrical impulse formation (Figure 36-4). It can conduct impulses much more rapidly than other cells located in the myocardium. The SA node, located at the junction of the RA and the superior vena cava, is considered the main regulator of HR. The SA node is composed of pacemaker cells, which spontaneously initiate impulses at a rate of 60 to 100 times/min, and myocardial working cells, which transmit the impulses to the surrounding atrial muscle.

An impulse from the SA node initiates the process of depolarization and hence the activation of all myocardial cells. The impulse travels through both atria to the atrioventricular (AV) node located in the junctional area. After the impulse reaches the AV node, conduction of the impulse is delayed briefly. This delay allows the atria to contract completely before the ventricles are stimulated to contract. The intrinsic rate of the AV node is 40 to 60 beats/min.

The bundle of His is a continuation of the AV node and is located in the interventricular septum. It divides into the right and left bundle branches. The bundle branches extend downward through the ventricular septum and fuse with the Purkinje fiber system. The Purkinje fibers are the terminal branches of the conduction system and are responsible for carrying the wave of depolarization to both ventricular walls. Purkinje fibers can act as an intrinsic pacemaker, but their discharge rate is only 20 to 40 beats/min.

Animation: Cardiac Cycle

SEQUENCE OF EVENTS DURING THE CARDIAC CYCLE

The phases of the cardiac cycle are generally described in relation to changes in pressure and volume in the left ventricle during filling (diastole) and ventricular contraction (systole) (Figure 36-5). **Diastole,** normally about two thirds of the cardiac cycle, consists of relaxation and filling of the atria and ventricles, whereas **systole** consists of the contraction and emptying of the atria and ventricles.

Cardiac-muscle contraction results from the release of large numbers of calcium ions from the sarcoplasmic reticulum. These ions diffuse into the **myofibril sarcomere** (the basic contractile unit of the myocardial cell). Calcium ions promote the interaction of actin and myosin protein filaments, causing these filaments to link and overlap. Cross-bridges, or linkages, are formed as the protein filaments slide over or overlap each other. These cross-bridges act as force-generating sites. The sliding of these protein filaments of multiple myofibril sarcomeres shortens the sarcomeres, producing myocardial contraction.

Cardiac muscle relaxes when calcium ions are pumped back into the sarcoplasmic reticulum, causing a decrease in the number of calcium ions around the myofibrils. This reduced number of ions causes the protein filaments to disengage or dissociate, the sarcomere to lengthen, and the muscle to relax.

MECHANICAL PROPERTIES OF THE HEART

The electrical and mechanical properties of cardiac muscle determine the function of the cardiovascular system. The heart is able to adapt to various pathophysiologic conditions (e.g., stress, infections, hemorrhage) to maintain adequate blood flow to the various body tissues. Blood flow from the heart into the systemic arterial circulation is measured clinically as cardiac output (CO), the amount of blood pumped from the

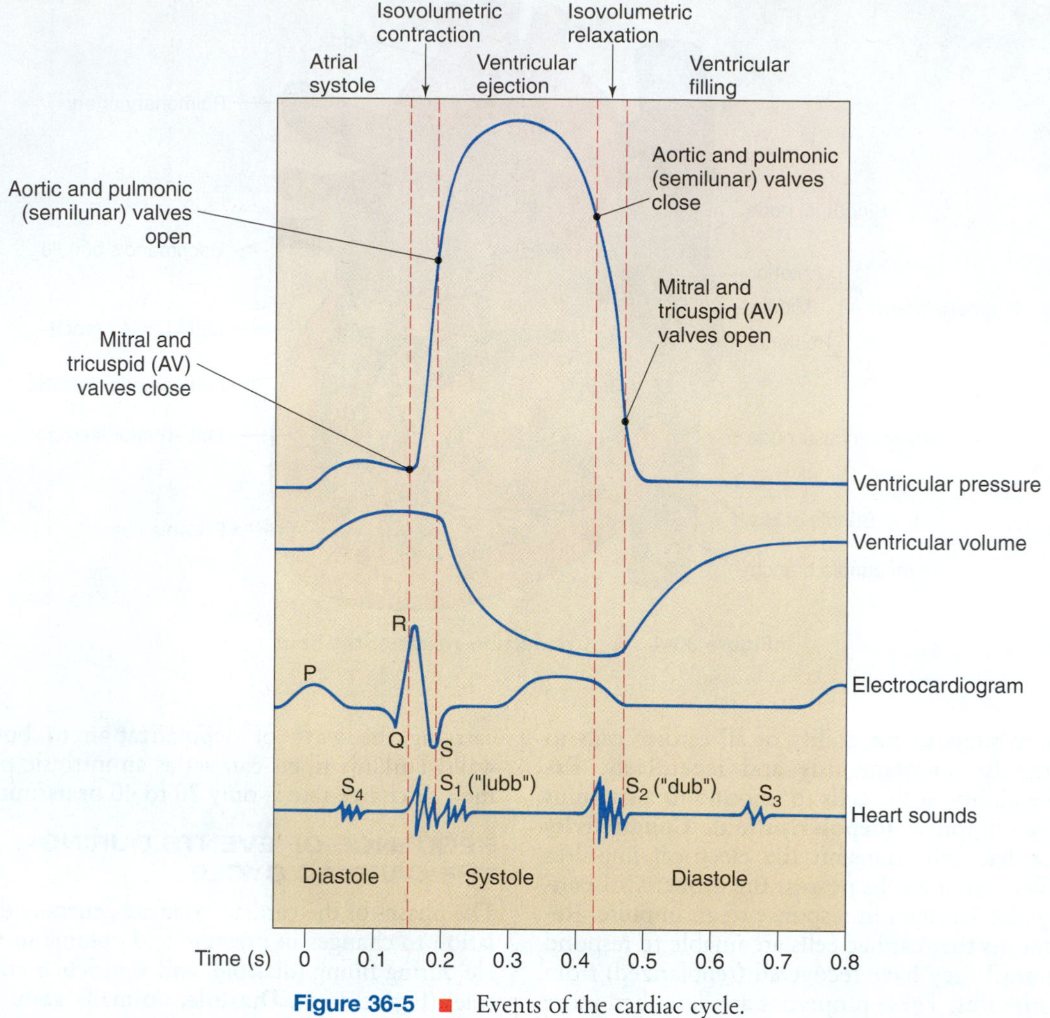

Figure 36-5 ■ Events of the cardiac cycle.

left ventricle each minute. CO depends on the relationship between heart rate (HR) and stroke volume (SV); it is the product of these two variables:

Cardiac output = Heart rate × Stroke volume

CARDIAC OUTPUT AND CARDIAC INDEX. **Cardiac output (CO)** is the volume of blood (in liters) ejected by the heart each minute. In adults the CO ranges from 4 to 7 L/min. Because cardiac output requirements vary according to body size, the cardiac index is calculated to adjust for differences in body size. The **cardiac index** can be determined by dividing the CO by the body surface area. The normal range is 2.7 to 3.2 L/min/m² of body surface area.

HEART RATE. Heart rate (HR) refers to the number of times the ventricles contract each minute. The normal resting HR for an adult is between 60 and 100 beats/min. Increases in HR increase myocardial oxygen demand. The HR is extrinsically controlled by the autonomic nervous system (ANS), which adjusts rapidly when necessary to regulate cardiac output. The parasympathetic (vagus nerve) system slows the HR, whereas sympathetic stimulation has an excitatory effect. An increase in circulating endogenous catecholamines (e.g., epinephrine and norepinephrine) usually causes an increase in HR and vice versa. Many cardiovascular drugs, including beta blockers and calcium channel blockers, mimic this pattern by decreasing the HR.

Other factors, such as the central nervous system (CNS) and baroreceptor (pressoreceptor) reflexes, influence the effects of the ANS on HR. Pain, fear, and anxiety can increase the HR. The baroreceptor reflex acts as a negative-feedback system. If a client experiences hypotension, the baroreceptors in the aortic arch sense a lowered pressure in the blood vessels. A signal is then relayed to the parasympathetic system to have less of an inhibitory effect on the sinoatrial (SA) node; this results in a reflex increase in HR.

STROKE VOLUME. **Stroke volume** (SV) is the amount of blood ejected by the left ventricle during each systole. Several variables influence stroke volume and, ultimately, CO. These variables include HR, preload, afterload, and contractility.

PRELOAD. **Preload** refers to the degree of myocardial fiber stretch at the end of diastole and just before contraction. The stretch imposed on the muscle fibers results from the volume contained within the ventricle at the end of diastole. Preload is determined by the amount of blood returning to the heart from both the venous system (right heart) and the pulmonary system (left heart) (left ventricular end-diastolic volume (LVED).

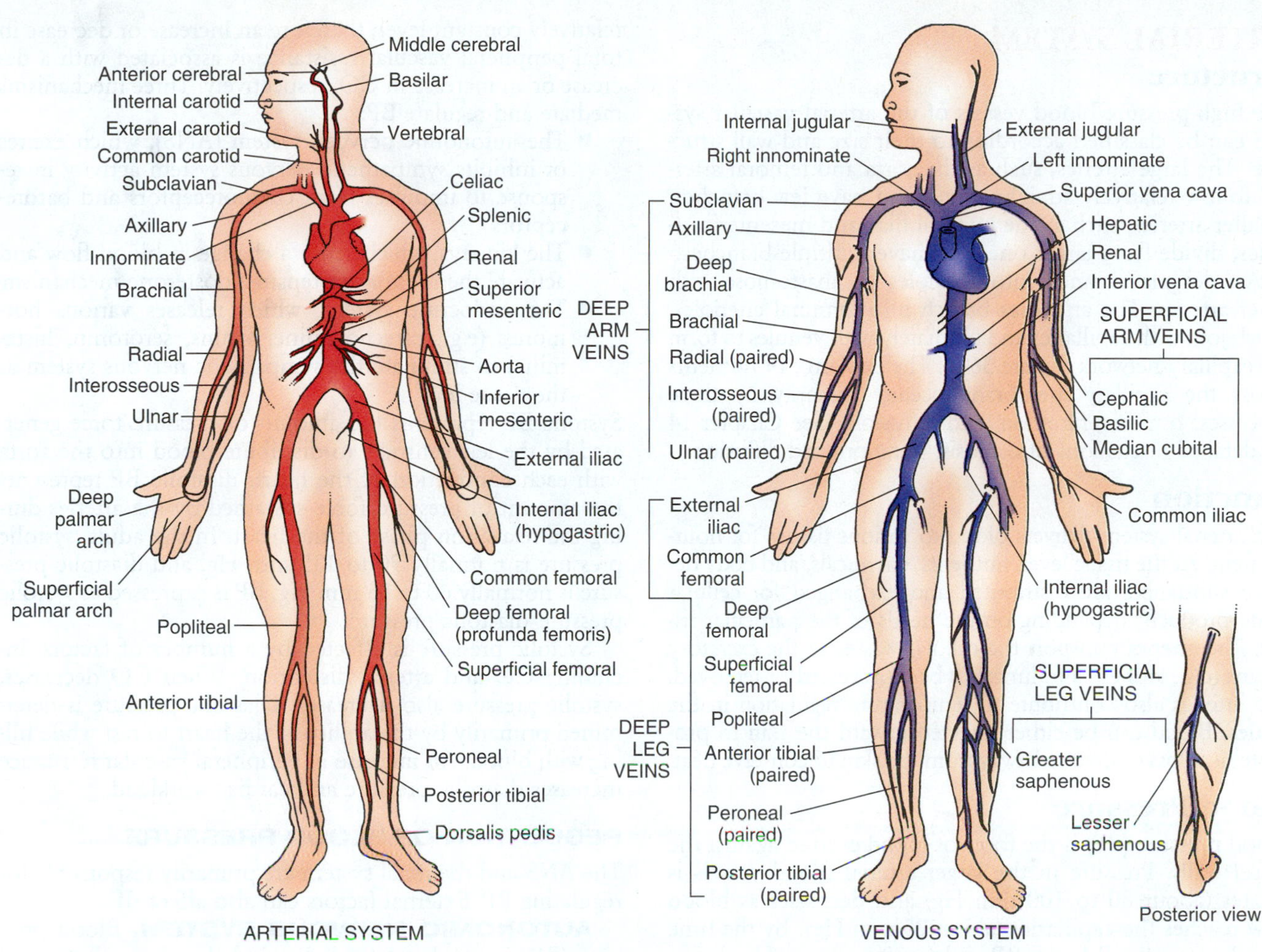

Figure 36-6 ■ Anatomy of the arterial and venous systems.

An increase in ventricular volume increases muscle-fiber length and tension, thereby enhancing contraction and improving stroke volume. This statement is derived from Starling's law of the heart: The more the heart is filled during diastole (within limits), the more forcefully it contracts. Excessive filling of the ventricles results in excessive LVED volume and pressure, however, and may result in decreased cardiac output.

AFTERLOAD. Another determinant of stroke volume, **afterload,** is the pressure or resistance that the ventricles must overcome to eject blood through the semilunar valves and into the peripheral blood vessels. The amount of resistance is directly related to arterial blood pressure and the diameter of the blood vessels.

Impedance, the peripheral component of afterload, is the pressure that the heart must overcome to open the aortic valve. The amount of impedance depends on aortic compliance and total systemic vascular resistance, a combination of blood viscosity and arteriolar constriction. A decrease in stroke volume can result from an increase in afterload without the benefit of compensatory mechanisms.

CONTRACTILITY. Contractility also affects stroke volume and CO. Myocardial contractility is the force of cardiac contraction independent of preload. Contractility is increased by factors such as sympathetic stimulation, calcium release, and positive inotropic drugs. Factors such as hypoxia and acidemia decrease contractility.

Animation: Blood Flow

Vascular System

The vascular system serves several purposes:

- To provide conduits for blood to travel from the heart to nourish the various tissues of the body
- To carry cellular wastes to the excretory organs
- To allow lymphatic flow to drain tissue fluid back into the circulation
- To return blood to the heart for recirculation

This system of conduits depends on an efficient heart and patent blood vessels to regulate and maintain systemic and regional blood flow and temperature.

The vascular system is divided into the arterial system and the venous system (Figure 36-6). In the arterial system, blood moves from the larger conduits to a network of smaller blood vessels, called arterioles, that meet the capillary bed. In the venous system, blood travels from the capillaries to the venules and to the larger system of veins, eventually returning in the venae cavae to the heart for recirculation.

ARTERIAL SYSTEM

Structure

The high-pressure blood vessels of the arterial vascular system can be classified according to their size and wall structure. The large arteries, such as the aorta and femoral arteries, follow relatively straight routes and have few branches. Smaller arteries, such as the internal iliac and mesenteric arteries, divide from larger ones and have multiple branches.

Arteries may branch into arterioles or anastomose with other arteries. The arterioles branch into terminal arterioles, which join with capillaries and ultimately with venules to form the capillary network (Figure 36-7). The exchange of nutrients across the capillary membrane occurs primarily by three processes: osmosis, filtration, and diffusion. (See Chapter 14 for detailed discussions of osmosis, filtration, and diffusion.)

Function

The arterial system delivers blood to various tissues for nourishment. At the tissue level, nutrients, chemicals, and body defense substances are distributed and exchanged for cellular waste products, depending on the needs of the particular tissue. The arteries transport the cellular wastes to the excretory organs (e.g., kidneys and lungs) to be reprocessed or removed. The arteries also contribute to temperature regulation in the tissues. Blood can be either directed toward the skin to promote heat loss or diverted away from the skin to conserve heat.

Blood Pressure

Blood pressure (BP) is the force of blood exerted against the vessel walls. Pressure in the larger arterial blood vessels is greater (about 80 to 100 mm Hg) and decreases as blood flow reaches the capillaries (about 25 mm Hg). By the time blood enters the RA, the BP is about 0 to 5 mm Hg.

INDIRECT MEASUREMENT OF BLOOD PRESSURE

The BP in the arterial system is determined primarily by the quantity of blood flow or cardiac output (CO) as well as by the resistance in the arterioles:

Blood pressure = Cardiac output × Peripheral vascular resistance

Any factor that increases CO or total peripheral vascular resistance increases the BP. In general, BP is maintained at a relatively constant level; therefore an increase or decrease in total peripheral vascular resistance is associated with a decrease or an increase in CO, respectively. Three mechanisms mediate and regulate BP:

- The autonomic nervous system (ANS), which excites or inhibits sympathetic nervous system activity in response to impulses from chemoreceptors and baroreceptors
- The kidneys, which sense a change in blood flow and activate the renin-angiotensin-aldosterone mechanism
- The endocrine system, which releases various hormones (e.g., catecholamine, kinins, serotonin, histamine) to stimulate the sympathetic nervous system at the tissue level

Systolic BP represents the amount of pressure/force generated by the left ventricle to distribute blood into the aorta with each contraction of the heart; diastolic BP represents the amount of pressure/force sustained by the arteries during the relaxation phase of the heart. In the adult, systolic pressure is normally 90 to 135 mm Hg, and diastolic pressure is normally 60 to 85 mm Hg. BP is expressed as systolic pressure/diastolic pressure.

Systolic pressure is affected by a number of factors, including CO and arterial distention. When CO decreases, systolic pressure also decreases. Diastolic pressure is determined primarily by the ability of the heart to rest while filling with blood. An increase in peripheral vascular resistance increases diastolic pressure and cardiac workload.

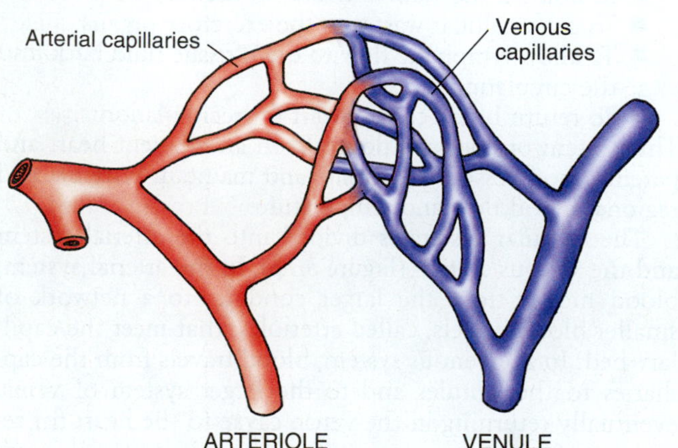

Figure 36-7 ■ Structure of the capillary bed.

REGULATION OF BLOOD PRESSURE

The ANS and the renal system are primarily responsible for regulating BP. External factors can also affect BP.

AUTONOMIC NERVOUS SYSTEM. Blood pressure (BP) is regulated by balancing the sympathetic and parasympathetic nervous systems of the ANS. Changes in sympathetic and parasympathetic activity are responses to messages sent by the sensory receptors in the various tissues of the body. These receptors, including the baroreceptors, chemoreceptors, and stretch receptors, respond differently to the biochemical and physiologic changes of the body.

Baroreceptors in the arch of the aorta and at the origin of the internal carotid arteries are stimulated when the arterial walls are stretched by an increased BP. Impulses from these baroreceptors inhibit the vasomotor center, which is located in the pons and the medulla. Inhibition of this center results in a drop in BP.

Several 1- to 2-mm collections of tissue have been identified in the bifurcations of the carotid arteries and along the aortic arch. These carotid and aortic bodies contain specialized **chemoreceptors** that are sensitive primarily to hypoxemia (a decrease in the partial pressure of arterial oxygen [PaO_2]). When stimulated, the carotid chemoreceptors send impulses along Hering's nerves, and the aortic chemoreceptors send impulses along the vagus nerves to activate a vasoconstrictor response.

The chemoreceptors are also stimulated by hypercapnia (an increase in partial pressure of arterial carbon dioxide [$PaCO_2$]) and acidosis. The direct effect of carbon dioxide on the CNS, however, is 10 times stronger than the effect it produces by stimulating the chemoreceptors.

Stretch receptors found in the venae cavae and the right atrium (RA) are sensitive to pressure or volume changes.

When a client is hypovolemic, the stretch receptors in the blood vessels sense a reduced volume or pressure and send fewer impulses to the CNS. This reaction stimulates the sympathetic nervous system to increase the heart rate (HR) and constrict the peripheral blood vessels.

RENAL SYSTEM. The renal system also helps to regulate cardiovascular activity. When renal blood flow or pressure decreases, the kidneys retain sodium and water. BP tends to rise because of fluid retention and activation of the renin-angiotensin-aldosterone mechanism. This mechanism results in vasoconstriction and sodium retention (and thus fluid retention). Vascular volume is also regulated by the release of antidiuretic hormone (vasopressin) from the posterior pituitary gland (see Chapter 14).

EXTERNAL FACTORS. Other factors can influence the activity of the cardiovascular system. Emotional behaviors (e.g., excitement, pain, anger) stimulate the sympathetic nervous system to increase BP and HR. Increased physical activity such as exercise increases BP and pulse rate. Body temperature can affect the metabolic needs of the tissues, thereby influencing the delivery of blood. In hypothermia, tissues require fewer nutrients and blood pressure falls. In hyperthermia, the metabolic requirement of the tissues is greater, and BP and pulse rate rise.

VENOUS SYSTEM

Structure

The venous system is composed of a series of veins that are located adjacent to the arterial system (see Figure 36-6). A second superficial venous circulation runs parallel to the subcutaneous tissue of the extremity. These two venous systems are connected by communicating veins that provide a means for blood to travel from the superficial veins to the deep veins. Blood flow is directed toward the deep venous circulation.

The venules collect blood from the capillaries and the terminal arterioles. White blood cells also enter and exit the body tissues at the venules. Venules branch into veins, which are low-pressure blood vessels. Veins have the ability to accommodate large shifts in volume with minimal changes in venous pressure. This flexibility allows the venous system to accommodate the administration of intravenous (IV) fluids and blood transfusions, blood loss, and dehydration. All veins in the superficial and deep venous systems in the legs (except the smallest and the largest veins) have valves that direct blood flow back to the heart; this prevents retrograde flow (backflow). The force that propels the blood forward in the veins is skeletal muscle in the extremities.

Function

The primary function of the venous system is to complete the circulation of blood by returning blood from the capillaries to the right side of the heart. The venous system also acts as a reservoir for a large portion of the blood volume. In contrast to the arterial system, which consists of a high-pressure, continuous flow system through relatively rigid conduits, the venous system consists of a low-pressure, intermittent flow system through collapsible tubes that work against the effects of gravity.

Gravity exerts an increase in hydrostatic pressure (capillary blood pressure) when the client is in an upright position, which delays venous return. Hydrostatic pressure is lessened when the client is lying down, and thus there is less hindrance of venous return to the heart.

Cardiovascular Changes Associated with Aging

A number of physiologic changes in the cardiovascular system occur with advancing age (Chart 36-1). Many of these changes result in a loss of cardiac reserve. Thus these changes are usually not evident when the older adult is resting. They become apparent only when the person is physically or emotionally stressed and the heart cannot meet the increased metabolic demands of the body.

ASSESSMENT TECHNIQUES

History

A thorough history must be obtained, including demographic data, personal and family history, diet, socioeconomic status, and a functional assessment. The focus of the history is on obtaining information relative to client's risk factors and symptoms of cardiovascular disease (Chart 36-2).

DEMOGRAPHIC DATA

Demographic data include the client's age, gender, and ethnic origin. The incidence of conditions such as coronary artery disease (CAD) and valvular disease increases with age (AHA, 2002). The incidence of CAD also varies with the client's gender. Men have a higher baseline risk for CAD than women of all ages, except in the oldest age group of 80 years and older (National Cholesterol Education Program [NCEP], 2002). Postmenopausal women are two to three times more likely than premenopausal women to have CAD. The incidence for CAD in women is about 10 years later than for men and 20 years later for myocardial infarction (MI) and death to occur (AHA, 2002). After an acute MI, women tend to die more frequently and have survival disadvantages compared with men.

White women with abdominal obesity (greater waist circumference than hip circumference) are more likely to experience cardiovascular disease (CVD) than are white women with fat distributed in their buttocks, hips, and thighs (greater hip circumference than waist circumference). Clients with an early onset of obesity (during adolescence) and an elevated waist-hip ratio appear to be at especially high risk for cardiovascular disease. Diabetes mellitus is also a major risk factor, especially in women.

Age, gender, ethnic background, and family history of CVD are considered nonmodifiable or uncontrollable risk factors for CVD. Modifiable risk factors (e.g., high blood pressure, smoking, excessive blood cholesterol), if controlled, can reduce the risk of heart disease. These factors are discussed under Modifiable Risk Factors beginning on p. 685.

FAMILY HISTORY AND GENETIC RISK

Review the family history, and obtain information about the age, health status, and cause of death of immediate family members. A positive family history for CAD in a first-degree relative (parent, sibling, or child) is a major risk factor. This risk factor is more significant than other risk factors such as hy-

CHART 36-1

NURSING FOCUS on the OLDER ADULT

Changes in the Cardiovascular System Related to Aging

Change	Nursing Interventions	Rationales
Cardiac Valves		
Calcification and mucoid degeneration occur, especially in mitral and aortic valves.	Assess heart rate and rhythm and heart sounds for murmurs. Question clients about dyspnea.	Murmurs may be detected before other symptoms. Valvular abnormalities may result in rhythm changes.
Conduction System		
Pacemaker cells decrease in number. Fibrous tissue and fat in the sinoatrial node increase. Few muscle fibers remain in the atrial myocardium and bundle of His. Conduction time increases.	Assess the electrocardiogram (ECG) and heart rhythm for dysrhythmias or a heart rate less than 60 beats/min.	The sinoatrial (SA) node may lose its inherent rhythm. Atrial dysrhythmias occur in 50%-90% of older adults; 80% of older adults experience premature ventricular contractions (PVCs).
Left Ventricle		
The size of the left ventricle increases. The left ventricle becomes stiff and less distensible. Fibrotic changes in the left ventricle decrease the speed of early diastolic filling by about 50%.	Assess the ECG for a widening QRS complex and a longer QT interval. Assess the heart rate at rest and with activity. Assess for activity intolerance.	Ventricular changes result in decreased stroke volume, ejection fraction, and cardiac output during exercise; the heart is less able to meet increased oxygen demands. Maximum heart rate with exercise is decreased. The heart is less able to meet increased oxygen demands.
Aorta and Other Large Arteries		
The aorta and other large arteries thicken and become stiffer and less distensible. Systolic blood pressure increases to compensate for the stiff arteries. Systemic vascular resistance increases as a result of less distensible arteries; therefore the left ventricle pumps against greater resistance, contributing to left ventricular hypertrophy.	Assess blood pressure. Note increases in systolic, diastolic, and pulse pressures. Assess for activity intolerance and shortness of breath. Assess the peripheral pulses.	Hypertension may occur and must be treated to avoid target organ damage.
Baroreceptors		
Baroreceptors become less sensitive.	Assess the client's blood pressure with the client lying and then sitting or standing. Assess for dizziness when the client changes from a lying to a sitting or standing position. Teach the client to change positions slowly.	Orthostatic (postural) and postprandial changes occur because of ineffective baroreceptors. Changes may include blood pressure decreases of 10 mm Hg or more, dizziness, and fainting.

pertension, obesity, diabetes, or sudden cardiac death. The younger the age of onset and the more first-degree relatives are affected, the greater the risk for CAD (NCEP, 2002).

Heart disease has many contributory factors, including a genetic tendency. Researchers have found a gene mutation called *R1141X,* which appears in a gene called *ABCCG.* The mutation causes pseudoxanthoma elasticum (PXE), a rare connective tissue disorder that causes the cardiac muscle fibers to calcify in the coronary arteries and contributes to high BP. People with CAD are four times more likely to have the mutation (Trip et al., 2001). Genetic screening for PXE and aggressive strategies to reduce modifiable risk factors may help reduce the incidence of heart disease.

PERSONAL HISTORY

Review the client's history, noting any major illnesses such as diabetes mellitus, renal disease, anemia, high BP, stroke, bleeding disorders, connective tissue diseases, chronic pulmonary diseases, heart disease, and thrombophlebitis. These conditions can influence the client's cardiovascular status.

Ask about previous treatment for CVD, identify previous diagnostic procedures (e.g., electrocardiography, cardiac catheterization), and request information about any medical or invasive treatment of CVD. It is important to ask specifically about recurrent tonsillitis, streptococcal infections, and rheumatic fever because these conditions may lead to valvular abnormalities of the heart. In addition, inquire about any known congenital heart defects. Many clients with congenital heart problems are living into adulthood because of improved treatment and surgical modalities.

Clients are asked in detail about their medication history, beginning with any current or recent use of prescription or over-the-counter (OTC) medications or herbal/natural products (e.g., ginseng). Inquire about known sensitivities to any drug and the nature of the reaction (e.g., nausea, rash). Clients should be asked whether they have recently used cocaine or any IV "street" drugs because these substances may be associated with chest pain or endocarditis.

Ask female clients whether they are taking oral contraceptives or an estrogen replacement. There is an increased

CHART 36-2

Cardiovascular Assessment
USING GORDON'S FUNCTIONAL HEALTH PATTERNS

Health Perception-Health Management
- What advice has your health care provider offered you about exercise, diet, or smoking?
- Are you able to follow that advice?
- What medications (both over-the-counter and prescription) are you supposed to be taking?
- Are you taking them as suggested or prescribed?
- What problems have you had with the medications?

Nutrition-Metabolic
- What is your usual daily diet? (Analyze the diet for saturated fat, cholesterol, total calorie, and sodium content.)
- How much fluid do you drink daily? Are you thirsty?
- What do you weigh? When did you last weigh yourself?
- How often do you weigh yourself?
- What is your height?
- Do you know your cholesterol level? What is it?
- How often do you feel nauseated or not interested in eating?
- Do your feet/ankles swell during the day? At night, too?

Elimination
- How often do you urinate in the daytime?
- How often do you wake up at night to urinate?

Activity/Exercise
- What is the most strenuous exercise you did last week?
- How active are you compared with 6 months ago? 1 year ago?
- How often do you feel fatigued or tired?
- Can you climb a flight of stairs and walk a block without feeling short of breath or experiencing chest pain?
- Do you experience leg cramps when you walk or climb stairs?

Sleep/Rest
- Where do you sleep? (In bed? In a lounge chair?)
- How many pillows do you sleep on?
- Do you ever wake up at night short of breath?
- What happens when you wake up short of breath?
- Do you ever wake up at night with pain or cramps in your legs? How do you relieve that sensation?

Cognitive/Perceptual
- How is your memory? What does your family say about your memory?
- How often do you feel dizzy, disoriented, or faint?
- Do you ever have chest discomfort? How often? What precipitates it? What is it like? How do you relieve it? What is its level on a scale of 0 to 10?
- Do you ever have leg or buttock pain? What are its characteristics?
- How do you learn best?

Role/Relationship
- What is your job?
- What does a day's work entail?
- What are your family responsibilities?
- With whom do you live?
- Who is available to help you?

Sexuality/Reproductive
- Has your ability to engage in sexual activity changed in the past year?
- If so, how?
- Do you take any medications that affect your sexual response? If so, what?

Coping/Stress Tolerance
- What do you think has been happening to you?
- How do you respond to being caught in a traffic jam or meeting a deadline?
- What do you do to relax?
- What do you do when you feel stressed?

Based on Gordon, M. (2002). *Manual of nursing diagnosis* (10th ed.). St. Louis: Mosby.

incidence of myocardial infarction (MI) and stroke in women over the age of 35 who take oral contraceptives, but only if they smoke, have diabetes, or have hypertension.

DIET HISTORY

A diet history includes the client's recall of food and fluid intake during a 24-hour period, self-imposed or medically prescribed dietary restrictions or supplementations, and the amount and type of alcohol consumption. The dietitian reviews the type of foods selected by the client for the amount of sodium, sugar, cholesterol, fiber, and fat. Working with the dietitian, explore the client's attitude toward food, knowledge level of essential and nonessential dietary elements, and willingness to make changes in the diet. Cultural beliefs and economic status can influence the choice of food items and therefore must be reviewed. Family members or significant others who are responsible for shopping and cooking are included in this discussion.

SOCIOECONOMIC STATUS

The social history includes information about the client's domestic situation, such as marital status, number of children, household members, living environment, and occupation. Identification of support systems is especially important in exploring the possibility that the client might have difficulty paying for medications or treatment.

Ask about the client's occupation, including the type of work performed and the requirements of the specific job. For instance, does the job involve lifting of heavy objects? Is the job emotionally stressful? What does a day's work entail? Does the client's job require him or her to be outside in extreme weather conditions?

MODIFIABLE RISK FACTORS

Personal habits that are risk factors for heart disease include cigarette smoking, physical inactivity, obesity, psychological variables, and certain chronic diseases. These factors are considered modifiable or controllable risk factors. Inquire about each of the following modifiable risk factors.

Cigarette Smoking

Cigarette smoking is a major risk factor for cardiovascular disease (CVD), specifically coronary artery disease (CAD) and peripheral vascular disease (PVD) (AHA, 2002). According to the U.S. Department of Health and Human Services (DHHS), cigarette smoking is directly responsible for 21% of all deaths from CAD. Three compounds in cigarette smoke have been implicated in the development of CAD: tar, nicotine, and carbon monoxide. Smoking costs

Americans more than $157 billion each year in medical care (AHA, 2002).

The risks to the cardiovascular system from cigarette smoking appear to be dose related, noncumulative, and transient. The smoking history should include the number of cigarettes smoked daily, the duration of the smoking habit, and the age of the client when smoking started. A person who smokes fewer than four cigarettes per day has twice the risk of CVD disease of a person who does not smoke; a person who smokes more than 20 cigarettes per day has four times the risk. Typically the smoking history is recorded in **pack-years,** which is the number of packs per day multiplied by the number of years the client has smoked.

Inquire about the client's desire to quit, past attempts to quit, and the methods used. Ascertain nicotine dependence by asking questions such as the following:

- How soon after you wake up in the morning do you smoke?
- Do you find it difficult not to smoke in places where smoking is prohibited?
- Do you smoke when you are ill?

Clients should be directed to smoking-cessation programs through the support of group meetings and new behavioral and pharmacologic approaches (including nicotine replacement patches and bupropion). Few physicians are trained to implement these programs. Identifying experienced health care providers who can implement smoking cessation programs for clients is a priority. A structured program is essential to provide the support necessary to quite smoking.

Three to four years after a client has stopped smoking, his or her cardiovascular risk appears to be similar to that of a person who has never smoked. Be sure to ask clients who do not currently smoke whether they have ever smoked and when they quit. Passive smoke significantly reduces the blood flow velocity in health young adults' coronary arteries (JAMA, 2001), and the risk of dying increases by 30% among those who are exposed to secondhand smoke (AHA, 2002).

Physical Inactivity

A sedentary lifestyle is also considered a significant risk factor in the development of heart disease. Regular physical activity promotes cardiovascular fitness and produces beneficial changes in blood pressure and levels of blood lipids and clotting factors. Unfortunately few people in the United States engage in the recommended exercise guidelines: 30 minutes daily of light to moderate exercise, which is equivalent to a 30-minute brisk walk. According to the American Heart Association (AHA), only 22% of Americans engage in this much exercise five times a week, and only 15% engage in vigorous physical activity (enough to promote cardiopulmonary fitness) three times a week (AHA, 2002). Increased physical exercise should be encouraged in accordance with a person's overall health status as part of a lifestyle change to reduce the risk for CAD (NCEP, 2002). Ask clients about the type of exercise they perform, how long a period they have participated in the exercise, and the frequency and intensity of the exercise.

Obesity

About 64% of American adults are **overweight** when defined as a body mass index (BMI) of 25 to 30 compared with 56% in 1994. **Obesity,** defined as a BMI greater than 30, increased from 23% in 1994 to 31% in 2002 (JAMA, 2002). It is particularly a problem for African-American women, Mexican Americans, and native Hawaiians (AHA, 2002). The Framingham Heart Study confirmed that obesity is a strong indicator of cardiovascular disease (CVD), especially when abdominal obesity is present (D'Agostino et al., 2001). It is also associated with hypertension, hyperlipidemia, and diabetes; all are known contributors to CVD.

Psychological Factors

A variety of psychological factors are more vulnerable to the development of heart disease. People who are highly competitive, overly concerned about meeting deadlines, and often hostile or angry are at higher risk for heart disease. Psychological stress, anger, depression, and hostility are all closely associated with risk of developing heart disease.

You might ask the client, "Have you ever experienced road rage?" or "How do you respond when you have to wait for an appointment?" Chronic anger and hostility appear to be closely associated with CVD. The constant arousal of the sympathetic nervous system (ANS) as a result of anger may influence blood pressure, serum fatty acids and lipids, and clotting mechanisms. Observe the client and determine his or her response to stressful situations.

Critical Thinking Challenge

Your client is a middle-aged African-American man, an accountant with a 20-year history of hypertension treated with a beta blocker and diuretic. He works long hours, his eating habits are poor, and he is 35 pounds overweight. He smoked a pack of cigarettes every day for 23 years but recently quit. His father died at age 55 of a myocardial infarction (MI). The client's total cholesterol is 242 mg/dL, his low-density lipoprotein (LDL) is 150 mg/dL, and his high-density lipoprotein (HDL) is 30 mg/dL. He was recently told at work that layoffs are likely; he is supporting two children in college and has one child with an addiction problem living at home. His mother has been living with the family since the loss of her husband 2 years ago.

1. How could this client modify his lifestyle further to help decrease his risk of cardiac disease?
2. What is the significance of his nonmodifiable risk factors?
3. What cultural and age-related variables should be considered in health teaching for this client?
4. What psychosocial issues need to be addressed?

evolve For suggested answer guidelines, go to http://evolve.elsevier.com/Iggy/.

CURRENT HEALTH PROBLEMS

Inquiring about major concerns helps to establish priorities in nursing care and management. The client is asked to describe his or her health concerns. Expand on the description of these concerns by obtaining information about their onset, duration, chronology, frequency, location, quality, intensity, associated symptoms, and precipitating, aggravating, and relieving factors. Major symptoms identified by clients with CVD include chest pain or discomfort, dyspnea, fatigue, palpitations, weight gain, syncope, and extremity pain.

Chronic Disease

Clients who have diabetes mellitus, hyperlipidemia, or hypertension are also at risk for cardiovascular problems. Those who are not diagnosed or are not compliant with the treatment plan have a much higher risk than those who are following the direction of a health care provider. These chronic illnesses are discussed elsewhere in this text.

Pain or Discomfort

Pain or discomfort, a common symptom of heart disease, can result from ischemic heart disease, pericarditis, and aortic dissection. Chest pain can also be due to noncardiac conditions such as pleurisy, pulmonary embolus, hiatal hernia, and anxiety. Thoroughly evaluate the nature and characteristics of the chest pain. Because pain resulting from myocardial ischemia is life threatening and can lead to serious complications, its cause should be considered ischemic (reduced or obstructed blood flow to the myocardium) until proven otherwise.

When assessing for pain, use alternative terms such as "discomfort," "heaviness," "pressure," and "indigestion." Some clients, especially women, do not experience pain in the chest but instead feel discomfort or indigestion. The client may also describe the sensation as aching, choking, strangling, tingling, squeezing, constricting, or viselike.

WOMEN'S HEALTH CONSIDERATIONS

Women respond uniquely to heart disease, often differing from the classic symptoms presented by men. Men typically have substernal pain occurring with activity or stress; the pain is often relieved by rest. Subtle symptoms and atypical chest pain are more common in women, who may not respond to rest or medication. Women report more back pain, indigestion, nausea, vomiting, and anorexia. Therefore, antacids, rather than nitroglycerin, may relieve their pain (DeVon & Zerwic, 2003).

Ask the client to identify when the pain was first noticed (onset):

- Did the pain begin suddenly or develop gradually (manner of onset)?
- How long did it last (duration)?

If the client has repeated painful episodes, assess how often the pain occurs (frequency). Ask whether this pain is different from any other episodes of pain. Ask the client to describe what activities he or she was doing when it first occurred, such as sleeping, arguing, or running (precipitating factors). The client can be asked to point to the area where the chest pain occurred (location) and to describe how the pain spread (radiation).

In addition, the client describes how the pain feels and whether it is sharp or dull (quality). To understand the severity of the pain, ask the client to grade it from 0 to 10, with 0 indicating an absence of pain and 10 indicating severe pain (intensity). The client may also report other signs and symptoms that occur at the same time (associated symptoms), such as dyspnea, diaphoresis, nausea, and vomiting. Other factors that need to be addressed are those that may have made the chest pain worse (aggravating factors) or less intense (relieving factors). Chest pain can arise from a variety of sources (Table 36-1). By obtaining the appropriate information, you may assist in identifying the source of the chest discomfort.

Dyspnea

Dyspnea can occur as a result of both cardiac and pulmonary disease. Dyspnea is described as difficult or labored breathing and is experienced as uncomfortable breathing or shortness of breath. When obtaining the client's history, as-

TABLE 36-1 Assessment of Chest Discomfort: How Various Types of Chest Pain Differ

Onset	Quality and Severity	Location and Radiation	Duration and Relieving Factors
Angina Sudden, usually in response to exertion, emotion, or extremes, in temperature	Squeezing, vise-like pain	Substernal; may spread across the chest and the back and/or down the arms	Usually lasts less than 15 min; relieved with rest, nitrate administration, or oxygen therapy
Myocardial Infarction Sudden, without precipitating factors, often in early morning	Intense stabbing, viselike pain or pressure, severe	Substernal; may spread throughout the anterior chest and to the arms, jaw, back, or neck	Usually last 30 min or longer or is relieved with opioids
Pericarditis Sudden	Sharp, stabbing, moderate to severe	Substernal; usually spreads to the left side or the back	Intermittent; relieved with sitting upright, analgesia, or administration of anti-inflammatory agents
Pleuropulmonary Variable	Moderate ache, worse on inspiration	Lung fields	Continuous until the underlying condition is treated or the client has rested
Esophageal-Gastric Variable	Squeezing, heartburn, variable severity	Substernal; may spread to the shoulders or the abdomen	Variable; may be relieved with antacid administration, food intake, or taking a sitting position
Anxiety Variable, may be in response to stress or fatigue	Dull ache to sharp stabbing; may be associated with numbness in fingers	Usually the left side of chest without radiation	Usually lasts a few minutes

certain what factors precipitate and relieve dyspnea, what level of activity produces dyspnea, and the client's body position when dyspnea occurred.

There are several types of dyspnea. Dyspnea that is associated with activity, such as climbing stairs, is referred to as dyspnea on exertion (DOE). This is usually an early symptom of heart failure and may be the only symptom experienced by women.

The client with advanced heart disease may experience orthopnea, or dyspnea that appears when he or she lies flat. The client may use several pillows at night to elevate the head and chest or may sleep in a recliner to prevent nighttime breathlessness. The severity of orthopnea is measured by the number of pillows or the amount of head elevation needed to provide restful sleep. Orthopnea is usually relieved within a matter of minutes by sitting up or standing.

Paroxysmal nocturnal dyspnea (PND) develops after the client has been lying down for several hours. In this position, blood from the lower extremities is redistributed to the venous system, which increases venous return to the heart. A diseased heart is unable to compensate for the increased volume and is ineffective in pumping the additional fluid into the circulatory system. Pulmonary congestion results. The client awakens abruptly, often with a feeling of suffocation and panic. The client usually sits upright with the legs dangled over the bedside to relieve the dyspnea. This sensation may last for 20 minutes before disappearing.

Fatigue

Fatigue may be described as a feeling of tiredness or weariness resulting from activity. The client may complain that a certain activity takes longer to complete or that he or she tires easily after activity. Although fatigue in itself is not diagnostic of heart disease, many people with heart failure are limited by leg fatigue during exercise. Fatigue that occurs after mild activity and exertion usually indicates inadequate cardiac output (due to low stroke volume) and anaerobic metabolism in skeletal muscle. It can also accompany other symptoms or may be an early indication of heart disease in women.

Question the client to determine the time of day he or she experiences fatigue as well as the activities that he or she can perform. Fatigue resulting from decreased cardiac output is often worse in the evening. Ask whether the client can perform the same activities as he or she could perform a year ago or the same activities as others of the same age. Often the client limits activities in response to fatigue and unless questioned is unaware how much less active he or she has become.

Palpitations

A feeling of fluttering in the chest, an unpleasant awareness of the heartbeat, and an irregular heartbeat are referred to as **palpitations.** Palpitations may result from a change in heart rate or rhythm or from an increase in the force of heart contractions. Rhythm disturbances that may cause palpitations include paroxysmal supraventricular tachycardia, premature contractions, and sinus tachycardia. Those that occur during or after strenuous physical activity, such as running and swimming, may indicate overexertion or possibly heart disease. Noncardiac factors that may precipitate palpitations include anxiety, stress, fatigue, insomnia, hyperthyroidism, and the ingestion of caffeine, nicotine, or alcohol. Ask the client about specific factors that that precipitate the client's palpitations.

Weight Gain

A sudden weight increase of 2.2 pounds (1 kg) can result from an accumulation of excessive fluid (1 L) in the interstitial spaces. Weight gain is the best indicator of fluid retention. This condition is commonly known as **edema.** It is possible for weight gains of up to 10 to 15 pounds (4.5 to 6.8 kg, or 4 to 7 L of fluid) to occur before edema is apparent. Inquire whether the client has noticed a tightness of shoes, indentations from socks, or tightness of rings.

Syncope

Syncope refers to a transient loss of consciousness. The most common cause is decreased perfusion to the brain. Any condition that suddenly reduces cardiac output, resulting in decreased cerebral blood flow, can potentiate a syncopal episode. Conditions such as cardiac rhythm disturbances, especially ventricular dysrhythmias, and valvular disorders, such as aortic stenosis, may potentiate this symptom.

Near-syncope refers to dizziness with an inability to remain in an upright position. Explore the circumstances that lead to dizziness or syncope.

CONSIDERATIONS FOR OLDER ADULTS

Syncope in the aging individual may result from hypersensitivity of the carotid sinus bodies in the carotid arteries. Pressure applied to these arteries while turning the head, shrugging shoulders, or other performing a Valsalva maneuver (bearing down during defecation) may stimulate a vagal response. A decrease in blood pressure and heart rate can result, which can produce syncope. This type of syncopal episodes may also result from postural (orthostatic) or postprandial (after eating) hypotension as a result of this response.

Extremity Pain

Extremity pain may be caused by two conditions: ischemia from atherosclerosis and venous insufficiency of the peripheral blood vessels. Clients who report a moderate to severe cramping sensation in their legs or buttocks associated with an activity such as walking have intermittent claudication related to reduced arterial tissue perfusion. Claudication pain is usually relieved by resting or lowering the affected extremity to decrease tissue demands or to enhance arterial blood flow. Leg pain that results from prolonged standing or sitting is related to venous insufficiency from either incompetent valves or venous obstruction. This pain may be relieved by elevating the extremity.

FUNCTIONAL HISTORY

After the history of the client's cardiovascular status is obtained, he or she may be classified according to the New York Heart Association's Functional Classification (Table 36-2). The four classifications (I, II, III, and IV) depend on the degree to which ordinary physical activities (routine activities of daily living [ADLs]) are affected by heart disease. The Killip Classification provides a more objective description of the hemodynamics of heart failure and is described in Chapter 41.

Physical Assessment

A thorough physical assessment is the foundation for the nursing database and the formation of nursing diagnoses and collaborative problems. Any changes noted during the course of illness can be compared with this initial database. Evaluate the client's vital signs on admission to the hospital or during the initial visit to the clinic or health care provider's office.

GENERAL APPEARANCE

Physical assessment begins with the client's general appearance. Assess the following areas: general build and appearance, skin color, distress level, level of consciousness, shortness of breath, position, and verbal responses.

Clients can have left- or right-sided heart failure, or both. As a result, poor cardiac output and decreased cerebral perfusion may cause confusion, memory loss, and slowed verbal responses. Clients with chronic heart failure may also appear malnourished, thin, and cachectic. Late signs of severe right-sided heart failure are ascites, jaundice, and anasarca (generalized edema) as a result of prolonged congestion of the liver. Heart failure may also cause fluid retention and may be manifested by obvious generalized dependent edema. Chapter 38 differentiates right and left failure in detail.

INTEGUMENTARY SYSTEM

Assessment and evaluation of the integumentary system are determined primarily by the color and temperature of the skin. The best areas in which to assess circulation include the nail beds, mucous membranes, and conjunctival mucosa because small blood vessels are located near the surface of the skin.

TABLE 36-2 New York Heart Association Functional Classification of Cardiovascular Disability

Class I
- Clients with cardiac disease but without resulting limitations of physical activity
- Ordinary physical activity does not cause undue fatigue, palpitation, dyspnea, or anginal pain

Class II
- Clients with cardiac disease resulting in slight limitation of physical activity
- They are comfortable at rest
- Ordinary physical activity results in fatigue, palpitation, dyspnea, or anginal pain

Class III
- Clients with cardiac disease resulting in marked limitation of physical activity
- They are comfortable at rest
- Less than ordinary physical activity causes fatigue, palpitation, dyspnea, or anginal pain

Class IV
- Clients with cardiac disease resulting in inability to carry on any physical activity without discomfort
- Symptoms of cardiac insufficiency or of the anginal syndrome may be present, even at rest
- If any physical activity is undertaken, discomfort is increased

Excerpted from *Diseases of the heart and blood vessels—nomenclature and criteria for diagnosis* (6th ed.). Boston: Little, Brown; copyright 1964 by the New York Heart Association.

Skin Color

If there is normal blood flow or adequate perfusion to a given area in light-colored skin, it appears pink, perhaps rosy in color, and it is warm to the touch. Decreased perfusion is depicted as cool, pale, and moist skin. Pallor is characteristic of anemia and can be seen in areas such as the nail beds, palms, and conjunctival mucous membranes.

A bluish or darkened discoloration of the skin and mucous membranes in light-skinned individuals is referred to as **cyanosis.** This condition results from an increased amount of deoxygenated hemoglobin. It is not an early sign of decreased perfusion but occurs later with other symptoms. Dark-skinned individuals may experience cyanosis as a graying of the same tissues.

Central cyanosis involves decreased oxygenation of the arterial blood in the lungs and appears as a bluish tinge of the conjunctivae and the mucous membranes of the mouth and tongue. Central cyanosis may indicate impaired lung function or a right-to-left shunt found in congenital heart conditions. Because of impaired circulation, there is marked desaturation of hemoglobin in the peripheral tissues, which produces a bluish or darkened discoloration of the nail beds, earlobes, lips, and toes.

Peripheral cyanosis occurs when blood flow to the peripheral vessels is decreased by peripheral vasoconstriction. The clamping down of the peripheral blood vessels results from a low cardiac output or an increased extraction of oxygen from the peripheral tissues. Peripheral cyanosis localized in an extremity is usually a result of arterial or venous insufficiency. **Rubor** (dusky redness) that replaces pallor is a dependent foot suggests arterial insufficiency.

Skin Temperature

Skin temperature can be assessed for symmetry by touching different areas of the client's body (e.g., arms, hands, legs, feet) with the dorsal surface of the hand or fingers. Decreased blood flow results in decreased skin temperature. Skin temperature is lowered in several clinical conditions, including heart failure, peripheral vascular disease, and shock.

EXTREMITIES

Assess the client's hands, arms, feet, and legs for skin changes, vascular changes, clubbing, and edema. Skin mobility and turgor are affected by fluid status. Dehydration and aging reduce skin turgor, and edema decreases skin mobility. Vascular changes in an affected extremity may include paresthesia, muscle fatigue and discomfort, numbness, pain, coolness, and loss of hair distribution from a reduced blood supply.

Clubbing of the fingers and toes results from chronic oxygen deprivation in these tissue beds. Clubbing is characteristic in clients with advanced chronic pulmonary disease, congenital heart defects, and cor pulmonale. Clubbing can be identified by assessing the angle of the nail bed. The angle of the normal nail bed is 160 degrees. With **clubbing,** the nail straightens out to an angle of 180 degrees, and the base of the nail becomes spongy. Figure 36-8 describes assessment of clubbing using the Schamroth method.

Peripheral edema is a common finding in clients with cardiovascular problems. The location of edema helps to determine its potential cause. Bilateral edema of the legs may be

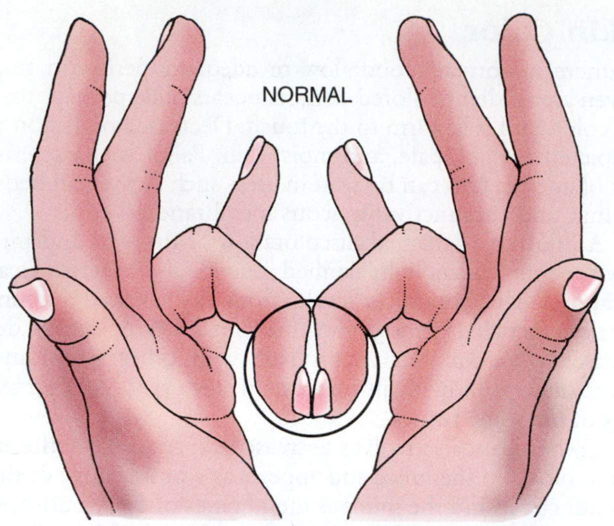

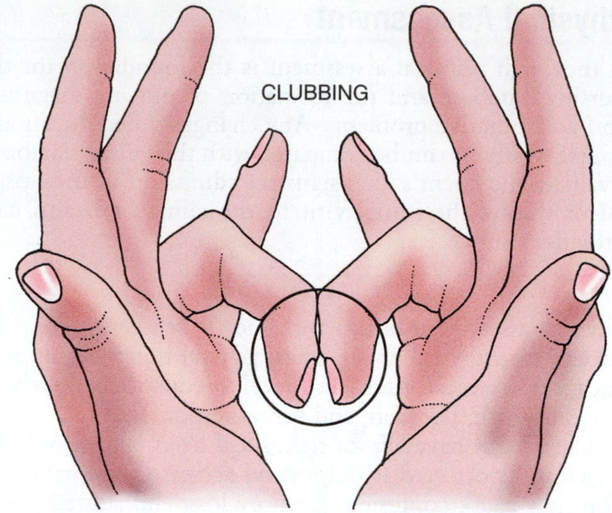

Figure 36-8 ■ Assessment of clubbing by the Schamroth method. The client places the fingernails of the ring fingers together and holds them up to a light. If the examiner can see a diamond shape between the nails, there is no clubbing. Clubbing is identified by the absence of the diamond shape.

seen in clients with heart failure or chronic venous insufficiency. Abdominal and leg edema can be seen in clients with heart disease and cirrhosis of the liver. Localized edema in one extremity may be the result of venous obstruction (thrombosis) or lymphatic blockage of the extremity (lymphedema). Edema may also be noted in dependent areas, such as the sacrum, when a client is confined to bed. In other clients, edema results from third spacing, such as when plasma proteins decrease.

Document the location of edema as precisely as possible (e.g., midtibial or sacral) and the number of centimeters from an anatomic landmark. The extent of edema can be characterized as mild, moderate, and severe (or 1, 2, 3, or 4). However, these values are not precise and are subjective. Determine whether the edema is pitting (the skin can be indented) or nonpitting.

Blood Pressure

Arterial blood pressure is measured indirectly by sphygmomanometry (Chart 36-3). This technique of measurement is described in greater detail in nursing skills textbooks.

The National High Blood Pressure Education Program Joint National Committee on Prevention, Detection, Evaluation, and Treatment of High Blood Pressure (2002) has recommended a new system of categorizing levels of blood pressure. High normal blood pressure is considered a systolic reading of 130 to 139 mm Hg or a diastolic pressure of 85 to 89. A blood pressure that exceeds 135/85 mm Hg increases the workload of the left ventricle and oxygen consumption of the myocardium. Approximately 50 million Americans (one out every five Americans) have **hypertension,** which is defined as a blood pressure greater than 140/90 mm Hg.

A new category has been designated **prehypertension.** This classification includes blood pressure (BP) readings of 120 to 139 mm Hg systolic or 80 to 89 mm Hg diastolic. Prehypertensive clients are at a higher risk to develop hypertension. Normal BP is classified as systolic pressure less than 120 mm Hg and diastolic blood pressure less than 80 mm Hg. Although the cause of hypertension is not known in 90% of people, it can be effectively controlled with lifestyle modification or medication. Hypertension is a cause of approximately five million deaths each year on its

CHART 36-3

BEST PRACTICE for
Accurate Blood Pressure Measurement

Select the proper cuff size.
- Adult cuff size is 12 to 14 cm wide and 30 cm long.
- Pediatric cuffs vary in width and length.
- Larger adult cuff size is 18 to 20 cm in width.

Ensure that equipment is properly assembled and calibrated.
- The cuff bladder should be intact inside the cuff.
- The sphygmomanometer should be calibrated to 0 mm Hg every few months to ensure reliability.

The cuff must be placed above the area to be auscultated (e.g., if the right arm is used, the cuff is placed above the brachial artery).

Follow these steps to ensure correct blood pressure measurement and recording:
- After palpating the brachial or radial pulse, inflate the cuff 30 mm Hg above the level at which those pulses disappear. Release the cuff slowly to palpate the systolic pressure. Reinflate the cuff, and auscultate the systolic and diastolic pressures. The auscultated pulses are referred to as the *Korotkoff sounds.*
- Record measurements on both arms to rule out dissecting aortic aneurysm, coarctation of the aorta, vascular obstruction, and possibly errors in measurement. Perform subsequent readings on the extremity with the highest pressure.
- If the client's arms are inaccessible (after amputation or mastectomy), you can obtain readings using the client's thigh or calf. Auscultate the popliteal artery or the posterior tibial artery, respectively.
- Obtain and record the client's blood pressure with the client in different positions, including supine, sitting, and standing positions.
- Record the position of the client and the site used to obtain the blood pressure.

own and is a major contributor to the development of CAD and heart failure.

A BP less than 90/60 mm Hg may be inadequate for providing proper and sufficient nutrition to body cells. In certain circumstances, such as shock and hypotension, the Korotkoff sounds are less audible or are absent. In these cases palpate the BP, use an ultrasonic device (Doppler device), or obtain a direct measurement by arterial catheter. When BP is palpated, the diastolic pressure is usually not obtainable. More information on direct measurement of arterial pressure is available under Hemodynamic Monitoring on p. 703.

POSTURAL BLOOD PRESSURE

Clients may report dizziness or light-headedness when they move from a flat, supine position to a sitting or a standing position at the edge of the bed. Normally these symptoms are transient and pass quickly; pronounced symptoms may be due to postural hypotension. **Postural (orthostatic) hypotension** occurs when the BP is not adequately maintained while moving from a lying to a sitting or standing position. It is defined as a decrease of more than 20 mm Hg of the systolic pressure or more than 10 mm Hg of the diastolic pressure as well as a 10% to 20% increase in heart rate. The causes of postural hypotension include medications, depletion of blood volume, prolonged bedrest, and age-related changes or disorders of the ANS.

To detect orthostatic changes in BP, first measure the BP when the client is supine. After remaining supine for at least 3 minutes, the client changes position to sitting or standing. Normally systolic pressure drops slightly or remains unchanged as the client rises, whereas diastolic pressure rises slightly. After the position change, a time delay of 1 to 5 minutes should be permitted before auscultating BP and palpating and counting the radial pulse. The cuff should remain in the proper position on the client's arm. Observe and record any signs or symptoms of distress. If the client is unable to tolerate the position change, he or she is returned to the previous position of comfort.

PARADOXICAL BLOOD PRESSURE

Paradoxical blood pressure is defined as an exaggerated decrease in systolic pressure by more than 10 mm Hg during the inspiratory phase of the respiratory cycle (normal is 3 to 10 mm Hg). Certain clinical conditions that potentially alter the filling pressures in the right and left ventricles may produce a paradoxical BP. Such conditions include pericardial tamponade, constrictive pericarditis, and pulmonary hypertension. During inspiration the filling pressures normally decrease slightly; however, the decreased fluid volume in the ventricles resulting from these pathologic conditions produces an exaggerated or marked reduction in cardiac output. The procedure for assessing a paradoxical BP is found in Chapter 39, Chart 39-12.

PULSE PRESSURE

The difference between the systolic and diastolic values is referred to as pulse pressure. A normal pulse pressure for an adult is 30 to 40 mm Hg. This value can be used as an indirect measure of cardiac output.

Narrowed pulse pressure is rarely normal and results from increased peripheral vascular resistance or decreased stroke volume in clients with heart failure, hypovolemia, or shock. Narrowed pulse pressure can also be seen in clients who have mitral stenosis or regurgitation. An increased pulse pressure may be seen in clients with slow heart rates, aortic regurgitation, atherosclerosis, hypertension, and aging.

Ankle Brachial Index

The **ankle brachial index (ABI)** can be used to assess the vascular status of the lower extremities. A BP cuff is applied to the lower extremities just above the malleoli. The systolic pressure is measured by Doppler ultrasound at both the dorsalis pedis and posterior tibial pulses. The higher of these two pressures is then divided by the higher of the two brachial pulses to obtain the ABI.

Normal values for ABI are 1 or higher because BP in the legs is usually higher than BP in the arms. ABI values less than 0.80 usually indicate moderate vascular disease, whereas values less than 0.50 indicate severe vascular compromise.

A **toe brachial pressure index (TBPI)** may be performed instead of or in addition to the ABI to determine arterial perfusion in the feet and toes. It is defined as toe systolic pressure divided by brachial (arm) systolic pressure (Bonham, 2003).

VENOUS AND ARTERIAL PULSES

Venous Pulses

Observe the venous pulsations in the neck to assess the adequacy of blood volume and central venous pressure (CVP). Specially trained or critical care nurses can assess **jugular venous pressure (JVP)** to estimate the filling volume and pressure on the right side of the heart. An increase in JVP causes **jugular venous distention (JVD).**

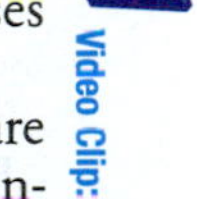

Video Clip: Pulses, Lower Extremities

Normally the JVP is 3 to 10 cm H_2O. Increases in JVP are usually caused by right ventricular failure. Other causes include tricuspid regurgitation or stenosis, pulmonary hypertension, cardiac tamponade, constrictive pericarditis, hypervolemia, and superior vena cava obstruction.

Arterial Pulses

Assessment of arterial pulses provides information about vascular integrity and circulation. For clients with suspected or actual vascular disease, all major peripheral pulses, including the temporal, carotid, brachial, radial, ulnar, femoral, popliteal, posterior tibial, and dorsalis pedis pulses, need to be assessed for presence or absence, amplitude, contour, rhythm, rate, and equality. Examine the peripheral arteries in a head-to-toe approach with a side-to-side comparison (Figure 36-9).

Animation: Pulse Variations

A hypokinetic pulse is a weak pulse indicative of a narrow pulse pressure. It is seen in clients with hypovolemia, aortic stenosis, and decreased cardiac output. A hyperkinetic pulse is a large, "bounding" pulse caused by an increased ejection of blood. It is seen in clients with a high cardiac output (with exercise or thyrotoxicosis) and in those with increased sympathetic system activity (with pain, fever, or anxiety).

In **pulsus alternans,** a weak pulse alternates with a strong pulse despite a regular heart rhythm. It is seen in clients with severely depressed cardiac function. Clients may be asked to hold their breath to exclude any false readings. You can palpate the brachial or radial arteries to assess this condition, but it is more accurately assessed by auscultation of blood pressure.

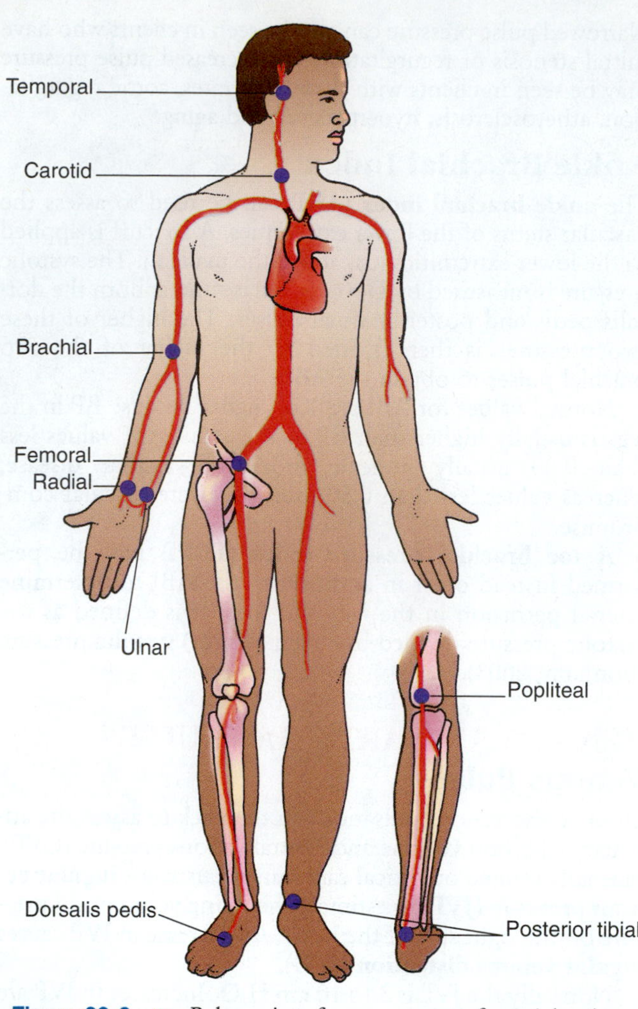

Figure 36-9 ■ Pulse points for assessment of arterial pulses.

▶ Video Clip: Carotid Artery

Auscultation of the major arteries (e.g., carotid and aorta) is necessary to assess for bruits. **Bruits** are swishing sounds that may develop in narrowed arteries and are usually associated with atherosclerotic disease. Assess for the absence or presence of bruits by placing the bell of the stethoscope over the skin of the carotid artery while the client holds his or her breath. Normally there are no sounds if the artery has uninterrupted blood flow. A bruit may develop when the internal diameter of the vessel is narrowed by 50% or more, but this does not indicate the severity of disease in the arteries.

PRECORDIUM

Assessment of the precordium (the area over the heart) involves inspection, palpation, percussion, and auscultation. In most settings the medical-surgical nurse seldom performs precordial palpation and percussion; however, the critical care nurse should perform a complete assessment. Place the client in a supine position, with the head of the bed slightly elevated for comfort. Some clients may require elevation of the head of the bed to 45 degrees for ease and comfort in breathing.

▶ Video Clip: Anterior Chest

Inspection

A cardiac examination is usually performed in a systematic order, beginning with inspection. Inspect the chest from the side, at a right angle, and downward over areas of the precordium where vibrations are visible. Cardiac motion is of low amplitude, and sometimes the inward movements are more easily detected by the naked eye.

Examine the entire precordium, focusing on the precordial areas (Figure 36-10) and noting any prominent precordial pulses. Movement over the aortic, pulmonic, and tricuspid areas is abnormal. Pulses in the mitral area (the apex of the heart) are considered normal and are referred to as the **apical impulse,** or the **point of maximal impulse (PMI).** The apical impulse should be located at the left fifth intercostal space (ICS) in the midclavicular line. If the apical impulse appears in more than one ICS and has shifted lateral to the midclavicular line, it may indicate left ventricular hypertrophy.

Video Clip: Auscultatory Landmarks ◀

Palpation

Palpate with the fingers and the most sensitive part of the palm of the hand to detect precordial motion and thrills, respectively. Continue to palpate by inching your hand in a Z pattern along the chest, starting with the aortic area and passing through all seven areas. Turning the client on his or her left side brings the heart closer to the surface of the chest. This may be helpful in achieving maximum tactile sensitivity during the assessment.

An abnormal forceful thrust accompanied by a sustaining outward movement over the left anterior side of the chest usually indicates left ventricular enlargement. An outward systolic lift along the left sternal border that extends from the fourth to the fifth ICS represents right ventricular enlargement.

Heaves and **lifts** are terms used to describe pulsations associated with valvular diseases or pulmonary hypertension. **Thrills** are vibrations associated with turbulent blood flow caused by abnormal heart valve function (mitral regurgitation, tricuspid regurgitation, and pulmonic stenosis). Specially trained nurses or primary care practitioners usually assess for these abnormalities.

Animation: Auscultation of Heart Valves ◀

Percussion

Cardiac size is determined most accurately by chest x-ray; percussion is now rarely used to determine the size of the heart. The size of the left ventricle, however, can be estimated by locating the apical impulse by inspection and palpation.

Auscultation

Auscultation evaluates heart rate and rhythm, cardiac cycle (systole and diastole), and valvular function. The technique of auscultation requires a good-quality stethoscope and extensive clinical practice. As a medical-surgical nurse, it is important to be familiar with normal heart sounds. Identifying common abnormal heart sounds becomes important when in critical care, telemetry, and advanced practice areas.

Evaluate heart sounds in a systematic order. Examination usually begins at the aortic outflow tract area and progresses slowly to the apex of the heart. The diaphragm of the stethoscope is pressed tightly against the chest to listen for high-frequency sounds and is useful in listening to the first and second heart sounds and high-frequency murmurs. Repeat the progression from the base to the apex of the heart using the bell of the stethoscope, which is held lightly against the chest. The bell is able to screen out high-frequency sounds and is useful in listening for low-frequency gallops (diastolic filling sounds) and murmurs.

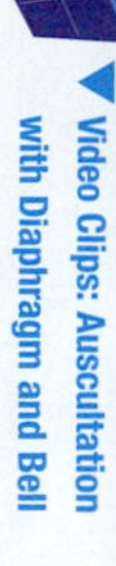

◀ Video Clips: Auscultation with Diaphragm and Bell

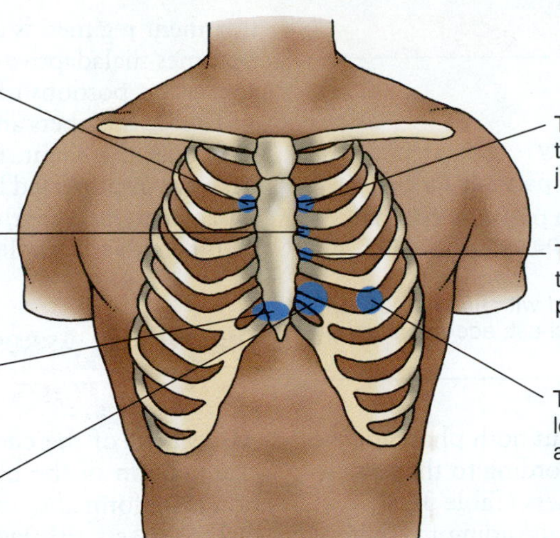

Figure 36-10 ■ Areas for myocardial inspection, palpation, and auscultation.

Attention is given to the areas in Figure 36-10 (except the epigastric area). Auscultation checks for heart rate and rhythm, murmurs, extrasystolic sounds, and rubs in the presence of a current or suspected cardiac problem.

NORMAL HEART SOUNDS

The first heart sound (S_1) is created by the closure of the mitral and tricuspid valves (atrioventricular valves) (see Figure 36-5). When auscultated, the first heart sound is softer and longer; it is of a low pitch and is best heard at the lower left sternal border or the apex of the heart. It may be identified by palpating the carotid pulse while listening. S_1 marks the beginning of ventricular systole and occurs right after the QRS complex on the electrocardiogram (ECG).

The first heart sound can be accentuated or intensified in conditions such as exercise, hyperthyroidism, and mitral stenosis. A decrease in sound intensity occurs in clients with mitral regurgitation and heart failure.

The second heart sound (S_2) is caused mainly by the closing of the aortic and pulmonic valves (semilunar valves) (see Figure 36-5). S_2 is characteristically shorter. It is higher pitched and is heard best at the base of the heart at the end of ventricular systole.

The splitting of heart sounds is often difficult to differentiate from diastolic filling sounds (gallops). A splitting of S_1 (closure of the mitral valve followed by closure of the tricuspid valve) occurs physiologically because left ventricular contraction occurs slightly before right ventricular contraction. Closure of the mitral valve is louder than closure of the tricuspid valve, however, so splitting is often not heard. Normal splitting of S_2 occurs because of the longer systolic phase of the right ventricle. Splitting of S_1 and S_2 can be accentuated by inspiration (increased venous return), and it narrows during expiration.

ABNORMAL HEART SOUNDS

PARADOXICAL SPLITTING. Abnormal splitting of S_2 is referred to as *paradoxical splitting* and is characteristic of a wider split heard on expiration. Paradoxical splitting of S_2 is heard in clients with severe myocardial depression that causes early closure of the pulmonic valve or a delay in aortic valve closure. Such conditions include myocardial infarction (MI), left bundle-branch block, aortic stenosis, aortic regurgitation, and right ventricular pacing.

GALLOPS AND MURMURS. Gallops and murmurs are common abnormal heart sounds that may occur with heart disease, but they can occur in some healthy individuals.

GALLOPS. Diastolic filling sounds (S_3) and (S_4) are produced when blood enters a noncompliant chamber during rapid ventricular filling. The third heart sound (S_3) is produced during the rapid passive filling phase of ventricular diastole when blood flows from the atrium to a noncompliant ventricle. The sound arises from vibrations of the valves and supporting structures. The fourth heart sound (S_4) occurs as blood enters the ventricles during the active filling phase at the end of ventricular diastole.

S_3 is termed **ventricular gallop,** and S_4 is referred to as **atrial gallop.** These sounds can be caused by decreased compliance of either or both ventricles. You can best hear left ventricular diastolic filling sounds with the client on his or her left side. The bell of the stethoscope is placed at the apex and at the left lower sternal border during expiration.

An S_3 heart sound is most likely to be a normal finding in children or young adults up to 30 years of age. An S_3 gallop in clients older than 35 years of age is considered abnormal and represents a decrease in left ventricular compliance. S_3 can be detected as an early sign of heart failure or as a ventricular septal defect.

An atrial gallop (S_4) may be heard in clients with hypertension, anemia, ventricular hypertrophy, MI, aortic or pulmonic stenosis, and pulmonary emboli. It may also be heard with advancing age because of a stiffened ventricle.

The auscultation of both S_3 and S_4, called a *summation* or a *quadruple gallop,* is an indication of severe heart failure. If the quadruple rhythm is present and the client has tachycardia (a shortened diastole), the two sounds may actually fuse to produce a rhythm that sounds like a horse galloping.

MURMURS. Murmurs reflect turbulent blood flow through normal or abnormal valves. They are classified according to their timing in the cardiac cycle: systolic murmurs (e.g., aortic stenosis and mitral regurgitation) occur between S_1 and S_2, whereas diastolic murmurs (e.g., mitral stenosis and aortic regurgitation) occur between S_2 and S_1. Murmurs can occur during presystole, midsystole, or late

TABLE 36-3 Grading of Heart Murmurs

Grade I	Very faint
Grade II	Faint but recognizable
Grade III	Loud but moderate in intensity
Grade IV	Loud and accompanied by a palpable thrill
Grade V	Very loud, accompanied by a palpable thrill, and audible with the stethoscope partially off the client's chest
Grade VI	Extremely loud, may be heard with the stethoscope slightly above the client's chest, accompanied by a palpable thrill

systole or diastole or can last throughout both phases of the cardiac cycle. They are also graded according to their intensity, depending on their level of loudness (Table 36-3).

Describe the location of a murmur according to where it is best heard on auscultation. Some murmurs transmit or radiate from their loudest point to other areas, including the neck, the back, and the axilla. The configuration is described as crescendo (increases in intensity) or decrescendo (decreases in intensity). The quality of murmurs can be further characterized as harsh, blowing, whistling, rumbling, or squeaking. They are also described by pitch, usually high or low.

PERICARDIAL FRICTION RUB. A **pericardial friction rub** originates from the pericardial sac and occurs with the movements of the heart during the cardiac cycle. Rubs are usually transient and are a sign of inflammation, infection, or infiltration. Pericardial friction rubs may be heard in clients with pericarditis resulting from MI, cardiac tamponade, or post-thoracotomy.

Psychosocial Assessment

To most people, the heart is a symbol of their ability to exist, survive, and love. A client with a heart-related illness, whether acute or chronic, usually perceives it as a major life crisis. The client, families, and significant others confront not only the possibility of death but also fears about pain, disability, lack of self-esteem, physical dependence, and changes in family dynamics. You may assess the meaning of the illness to the client and family members by asking, "What do you understand about what happened to you (or the client)?" and "What does that mean to you?" When the client or family members perceive the stressor as overwhelming, formerly adequate support systems may no longer be effective. In these circumstances, the client and family members attempt to cope to regain a sense or feeling of control.

Coping behaviors vary among clients. Those who feel helpless to meet the demands of the situation may exhibit behaviors such as disorganization, fear, and anxiety. You may ask the client or family members, "Have you ever encountered such a situation before?" "How did you manage that situation?" and "To whom can you turn for help?" The answers to these questions often reassure the client that he or she has encountered difficult situations in the past and has the ability and resources to cope with them.

A common and normal response is *denial,* which is a defense mechanism that enables the client to cope with threatening circumstances. The client may deny that he or she has the current cardiovascular condition, may state that it was present but is now absent, or may be excessively cheerful. Denying the seriousness of the illness while following the treatment regimen is a protective response; however, denial becomes maladaptive when the client is noncompliant with significant portions of medical and nursing care.

Family members and significant others may be more anxious than the client. Often they recall all events of the illness, are unprotected by denial, and are afraid of recurrence. Disagreements often occur between the client and family members over compliance with appropriate follow-up care.

Diagnostic Assessment

LABORATORY TESTS

Assessment of the client with cardiac dysfunction includes examination of the blood for abnormalities. The examination is performed to establish a diagnosis, detect concurrent disease, assess risk factors, and monitor response to treatment. Normal values for serum cardiac enzymes and serum lipids are listed in Chart 36-4.

Serum Markers of Myocardial Damage

Events leading to cellular injury cause a release of enzymes from intracellular storage, and circulating levels of these enzymes are dramatically elevated. Acute myocardial infarction (MI), also known as acute coronary syndrome, can be confirmed by abnormally high levels of enzymes or isoenzymes. These serum studies are commonly referred to as *cardiac markers.*

TROPONIN

Troponin is a myocardial muscle protein released into the bloodstream with injury to myocardial muscle. Troponin T and I are not found in healthy clients, so any rise in values indicates cardiac necrosis or acute MI. Specific markers of myocardial injury, troponin T and I have a wide diagnostic time frame, making them useful for clients who present several hours after the onset of chest pain. Even low levels of troponin T should be treated vigorously because of increased risk of death from cardiovascular disease (CVD). Obtaining cardiac markers at the bedside in the emergency department can be done as "point of care" (POC) testing for clients experiencing or at risk for acute MI with results available within 15 to 20 minutes. These markers are evaluated in addition to clinical signs and symptoms and ECG changes when identifying at-risk clients.

CREATINE KINASE (CK)-MB

Creatine kinase (CK) is an enzyme specific to cells of the brain, myocardium, and skeletal muscle. The appearance of CK in the blood indicates tissue necrosis or injury, with CK levels following a predictable rise and fall during a specified period. Cardiac specificity must be determined by measuring isoenzyme activity. There are three isoenzymes of CK: CK-MM is the predominant isoenzyme of skeletal muscle; CK-MB is found in myocardial muscle; and CK-BB occurs in the brain. CK-MB activity is most specific for MI and shows a predictable rise and fall during 3 days; a peak level occurs approximately 24 hours after the onset of chest pain.

Treatment modalities for early intervention after acute MI and acute ischemia require more rapid diagnosis of MI. An assay using monoclonal anti–CK-MB antibodies (stat CK) can detect myocardial necrosis accurately 3 hours after

CHART 36-4

LABORATORY PROFILE
Cardiovascular Assessment

Normal Range	Significance of Abnormal Findings
Serum Cardiac Enzymes	
Creatine kinase (CK) *Females*: 30-135 units/L *Males*: 55-170 units/L Values higher after exercise	Elevations indicate possible brain myocardial, and skeletal muscle necrosis or injury.
CK-MM (CK_3) 100% of total CK	Elevations occur with muscle injury.
CK-MB (CK_2) 0% of total CK	Elevations occur with myocardial injury or after percutaneous transluminal angioplasty and intracoronary streptokinase infusion.
CK-BB (CK_1) 0%	Elevations occur with brain tissue injury.
Serum Lipids	
Total lipids 400-1000 mg/dL	Elevation indicates increased risk of coronary artery disease (CAD).
Cholesterol 122-200 mg/dL, or 3.16-6.5 mmol/L *Older adult (>70 yr)*: 144-280 mg/dL	Elevation indicates increased risk of CAD.
Triglycerides *Females*: 35-135 mg/dL *Males*: 40-160 mg/dL *Older adult (>65 yr)*: 55-260 mg/dL	Elevation indicates increased risk of CAD.
Plasma high-density lipoproteins (HDLs) *Females*: mean 55-60 mg/dL *Males*: mean, 45-50 mg/dL Older adult range increases with age	Elevations protect against CAD.
Plasma low-density lipoproteins (LDLs) 60-180 mg/dL *Older adult (>65 yr)*: 92-221 mg/dL	Elevation indicates increased risk of CAD.
HDL: LDL ratio 3:1	Elevated ratios may protect against CAD.
VLDL 25%-50%	Elevated level indicates risk of CAD.
C-reactive protein (CRP) <1.0 mg/dL	Elevation may indicate tissue infarction or damage.
Serum Markers	
Troponins Cardiac troponin T <0.2 ng/mL Cardiac troponin I <0.03 ng/mL	Elevations indicate myocardial injury or infarction.
Myoglobin <90 mcg/L	Elevation indicates myocardial infarction.

VLDL, Very-low-density lipoproteins.

emergency department admission when examined with an electrocardiogram (ECG). Two subforms of CK-MB ($CK\text{-}MB_1$ and $CK\text{-}MB_2$) have also been identified. Abnormal elevations of these CK subforms may occur as early as 2 hours after MI. These subforms remain elevated for up to 12 hours after MI and appear to be very sensitive and specific early diagnostic markers of MI.

MYOGLOBIN

Another early marker of an MI is myoglobin. **Myoglobin**, a low-molecular-weight heme protein found in cardiac and skeletal muscle, is the earliest marker detected–as early as 2 hours after an MI with rapid decline after 7 hours. Because myoglobin is not cardiac specific, is found in skeletal and cardiac muscle, and is detected very early in the bloodstream makes its clinical usefulness more limited than troponin.

Serum Lipids

Elevated lipid levels are considered a risk factor for coronary artery disease (CAD). Cholesterol, triglycerides, and the protein components of high-density lipoproteins (HDL) and low-density lipoproteins (LDL) are evaluated to assess a client's degree of risk for CAD. The risk for CAD is three times greater in clients with a serum cholesterol level greater than 260 mg/dL than in clients with a serum level less than 200 mg/dL.

Each of the lipoproteins contains varying proportions of cholesterol, triglyceride, protein, and phospholipid. HDL contains mainly protein and 20% cholesterol, whereas LDL is predominantly cholesterol. Elevated LDL levels are positively correlated with CAD, whereas elevated HDL levels are negatively correlated and appear to be a protective factor.

A nonfasting blood sample for the measurement of serum cholesterol levels is acceptable. If triglycerides are to be evaluated with cholesterol, the health care provider requests the specimen after a 12-hour fast.

Homocysteine

Homocysteine is an amino acid that is produced when proteins breaks down. A certain amount of homocysteine is present in the blood, but elevated values may be an independent risk factor for the development of CVD. Although the relationship between homocysteine and CVD remains controversial, some studies suggest that elevated levels of homocysteine increase the risk of CVD as much as smoking and hyperlipemia, especially in women. A scientific advisory from the American Heart Association to reduce total homocysteine recommends screening for total homocysteine in high-risk clients who have a personal or family history of premature heart disease. Clients usually fast for 10 to 12 hours before the test, and the blood must be separated and frozen within 1 hour of collection. A level less than 12 mmol/dL is considered optimal.

Client education should emphasize the nutritional aspect in decreasing homocysteine levels. By eating foods rich in B complex vitamins, especially folic acid, homocysteine levels can be reduced and may decrease the risk for CVD. Some health care providers prescribe supplemental folic acid to clients with high homocysteine levels. Encourage the client to consume a diet high in folate, vitamin B_6, and vitamin B_{12}, such as in vegetables, fruits, legumes, meats, fish, and fortified grains and cereals.

C-Reactive Protein

Recent studies have shown that inflammation is a common and critical component to the development of atherothrombosis. **Highly sensitive C-reactive protein (hsCRP)** has been the most studied marker of inflammation. Any inflammatory process can produce CRP in the blood. Elevations are also seen with hypertension, infection, and smoking. A level less than 1 mg/dL is considered low risk; a level over 3 mg/dL places the client at high risk for heart disease. The most useful time to measure CRP appears to be for risk assessment in middle-aged or older persons. Cholesterol-lowering drugs known as *statins* are promoted because they may modify the anti-inflammatory process. Clients may reduce their CRP level with a low-fat, low-cholesterol diet; smoking cessation; exercise; statins; and aspirin.

Blood Coagulation Tests

Blood coagulation tests evaluate the ability of the blood to clot and are important in clients with a greater tendency to form thrombi (e.g., clients with atrial fibrillation, prosthetic valves, or infective endocarditis). They are also important for clients receiving anticoagulant therapy (e.g., during cardiac surgery, after thrombolytic therapy, and during treatment of an established thrombus).

PROTHROMBIN TIME AND INTERNATIONAL NORMALIZED RATIO

Prothrombin time (PT) and International Normalized Ratio (INR) are used when initiating and maintaining therapy with oral anticoagulants, such as sodium warfarin (Coumadin, Warfilone✱). They measure the activity of prothrombin, fibrinogen, and factors V, VII, and X. INR is the most reliable way to monitor anticoagulant status in warfarin therapy. The therapeutic ranges vary significantly based on the reason for the anticoagulation and the client's history.

PARTIAL THROMBOPLASTIN TIME

Partial thromboplastin time (PTT) is assessed in clients who are receiving heparin (Hepalean✱). It measures deficiencies in all coagulation factors except VII and XIII.

Arterial Blood Gases

Arterial blood gas (ABG) determinations are often obtained in clients with CVD. Determination of tissue oxygenation, carbon dioxide removal, and acid-base status is essential to appropriate intervention and treatment. (See Chapter 18 for a complete discussion of ABGs.)

Serum Electrolytes

Fluid and electrolyte balance is essential for normal cardiovascular performance. Cardiac manifestations often occur when there is an imbalance in either fluids or electrolytes in the body. For example, the cardiac effects of hypokalemia (low serum potassium level) include increased electrical instability, ventricular dysrhythmias, and an increased risk of digitalis toxicity. The effects of hyperkalemia on the myocardium include slowed ventricular conduction, peaked T waves on the ECG, and contraction followed by asystole (cardiac standstill).

Cardiac manifestations of hypocalcemia are ventricular dysrhythmias, a prolonged QT interval, and cardiac arrest. Hypercalcemia shortens the QT interval and causes AV block, digitalis hypersensitivity, and cardiac arrest.

Serum sodium values reflect fluid balance and may be decreased, indicating a fluid excess in clients with heart failure (dilutional hyponatremia).

Because magnesium regulates some aspects of myocardial electrical activity, hypomagnesemia has been implicated in some forms of rapid ventricular dysrhythmias. Another manifestation of hypomagnesemia is hypokalemia that is unresponsive to potassium replacement.

Complete Blood Count

The erythrocyte (red blood cell) count is usually decreased in rheumatic fever and infective endocarditis. It is increased in heart diseases characterized by inadequate tissue oxygenation.

Decreased hematocrit and hemoglobin levels (e.g., caused by hemorrhage or hemolysis from prosthetic valves) indicate anemia and can lead to angina or aggravate heart failure. Vascular volume depletion with hemoconcentration (e.g., hypovolemic shock and excessive diuresis) results in an elevated hematocrit.

The leukocyte (white blood cell) count is typically elevated after an MI and in various infectious and inflammatory diseases of the heart (e.g., infective endocarditis and pericarditis).

Critical Thinking Challenge

A middle-aged man, an accountant, with multiple cardiovascular risk factors comes to the emergency department with complaints of a dull, aching feeling in his shoulder and arm. His admission laboratory results include creatinine kinase of 190 units/L, troponin level of greater than 2.0 ng/mL, and C-reactive protein of 1.0 mg/dL.

1. What additional assessment should you perform for this client?
2. What is the significance of each of these test results?
3. How might the client's cardiac markers differ from hospital admission to discharge?

evolve For suggested answer guidelines, go to http://evolve.elsevier.com/Iggy/.

RADIOGRAPHIC EXAMINATIONS

Chest Radiography

Posteroanterior and left lateral x-ray views of the chest are routinely obtained to determine the size, silhouette, and position of the heart. In acutely ill clients, a simple anteroposterior (AP) view is obtained at the bedside. Cardiac enlargement, pulmonary congestion, cardiac calcifications, and placement of central venous catheters, endotracheal tubes, and hemodynamic monitoring devices are assessed by x-ray.

Angiography

Angiography of the arterial vessels, or **arteriography,** is an invasive diagnostic procedure that involves fluoroscopy and the use of contrast media. This procedure is performed when an arterial obstruction, narrowing, or aneurysm is suspected. The radiologist performs selective arteriography to evaluate specific areas of the arterial system. For example, a coronary arteriography, which is performed during left-sided cardiac catheterization, assesses arterial circulation within the heart. Angiography can also be performed on arteries in the extremities, mesentery, and cerebrum. Angiography is discussed under the appropriate associated diseases elsewhere in this text.

TABLE 36-4 Indications for Cardiac Catheterization

- To confirm suspected heart disease, including coronary artery disease, myocardial disease, valvular disease, and valvular dysfunction
- To determine the location and extent of the disease process
- To assess the following:
  - Stable, severe angina unresponsive to medical management
  - Unstable angina pectoris
  - Uncontrolled heart failure, ventricular dysrhythmias, or cardiogenic shock associated with acute myocardial infarction, papillary muscle dysfunction, ventricular aneurysm, or septal perforation
- To determine best therapeutic option (percutaneous transluminal coronary angioplasty, stents, coronary artery bypass graft, valvulotomy versus valve replacement)
- To evaluate effects of medical or invasive treatment on cardiovascular function, percutaneous transluminal coronary angioplasty, or coronary artery bypass graft patency

TABLE 36-5 Complications of Cardiac Catheterization

Right-Sided Heart Catheterization
- Thrombophlebitis
- Pulmonary embolism
- Vagal response

Left-Sided Heart Catheterization and Coronary Arteriography
- Myocardial infarction
- Stroke
- Arterial bleeding or thromboembolism
- Dysrhythmias

Right-Sided or Left-Sided Heart Catheterization*
- Cardiac tamponade
- Hypovolemia
- Pulmonary edema
- Hematoma or blood loss at insertion site
- Reaction to contrast medium

*In addition to those cited for each procedure.

Cardiac Catheterization

The most definitive, but most invasive, test in the diagnosis of heart disease is cardiac catheterization. **Cardiac catheterization** may include studies of the right or left side of the heart and the coronary arteries. Some of the most common indications for cardiac catheterization are listed in Table 36-4.

CLIENT PREPARATION. Assessment of the client's physical and psychosocial readiness and knowledge level is an important aspect of client preparation because many clients have anxiety and fear about cardiac catheterization. Most individuals are very anxious and fearful about the procedure.

Review the purpose of the procedure, inform the client about the length of the procedure, state who will be present, and describe the appearance of the catheterization laboratory. The client is also informed about the sensations that may be experienced during the procedure, such as palpitations (as the catheter is passed up to the left ventricle), a feeling of heat or a hot flash (as the medium is injected into either side of the heart), and a desire to cough (as the medium is injected into the right side of the heart). Written or illustrated materials or videotapes may be used, if available, to assist in the client's understanding.

The risks of cardiac catheterization are usually explained by the interventional cardiologist. The risks vary with the procedures to be performed and the client's physical status (Table 36-5). Several complications may follow coronary arteriography, such as the following:

- Myocardial infarction (MI)
- Stroke
- Arterial bleeding
- Thromboembolism
- Lethal dysrhythmias
- Death

The cardiologist or radiologist obtains a written informed consent from the client or responsible party prior to the procedure.

The client may be admitted to the hospital on the day of the catheterization procedure. Standard preoperative tests are performed, which usually include a chest x-ray, complete blood count, coagulation studies, and 12-lead ECG. The client receives nothing by mouth after midnight or has only a liquid breakfast if the catheterization is to take place in the afternoon. The catheterization site is shaved and antiseptically prepared according to the institution's policy.

Nursing assessment before the procedure includes measuring the client's vital signs, auscultating the heart and the lungs, and evaluating the peripheral pulses. Question the client about any history of allergy to iodine-based contrast agents. An antihistamine or steroid may be given to a client with a positive history or to prevent a reaction. A mild sedative is usually administered before the procedure. If the client normally takes a digitalis preparation or diuretic, it is usually withheld before the catheterization.

PROCEDURE. The client is taken to the cardiac catheterization laboratory (sometimes referred to as the "cath lab"), placed in the supine position on the x-ray table, and securely strapped to the table. Inform the client that this precaution is necessary because the table turns like a cradle during the procedure. The physician injects a local anesthetic at the insertion site. During the procedure, the client is instructed to report any chest pain, pressure, or other symptoms to the staff.

RIGHT-SIDED HEART CATHETERIZATION. The right side of the heart is catheterized first and may be the only side examined. The cardiologist inserts a catheter through the femoral vein to the inferior vena cava or through the basilic vein to the superior vena cava. The catheter is advanced through either the inferior or the superior vena cava and, guided by fluoroscopy, is advanced through the right atrium (RA), through the right ventricle and, at times, into the pulmonary artery (Figure 36-11). Intracardiac pressures (right atrial, right ventricular, pulmonary artery, and pulmonary artery wedge pressures) and blood samples are obtained. A contrast medium is usually injected to detect any cardiac shunts or regurgitation from the pulmonic or tricuspid valves.

LEFT-SIDED HEART CATHETERIZATION. In a left-sided heart catheterization, the cardiologist advances the catheter against the blood flow from the femoral or brachial artery up the aorta, across the aortic valve, and into the left ventricle. Alternatively the cardiologist may pass the catheter from the right side of the heart through the atrial septum, using a special needle to puncture the septum. Intracardiac pressures and blood samples are obtained. The pressures of the left atrium, left ventricle, and aorta, as well as mitral and aortic valve status, are evaluated. The cardiologist injects contrast dye into the ventricle; cineangiograms

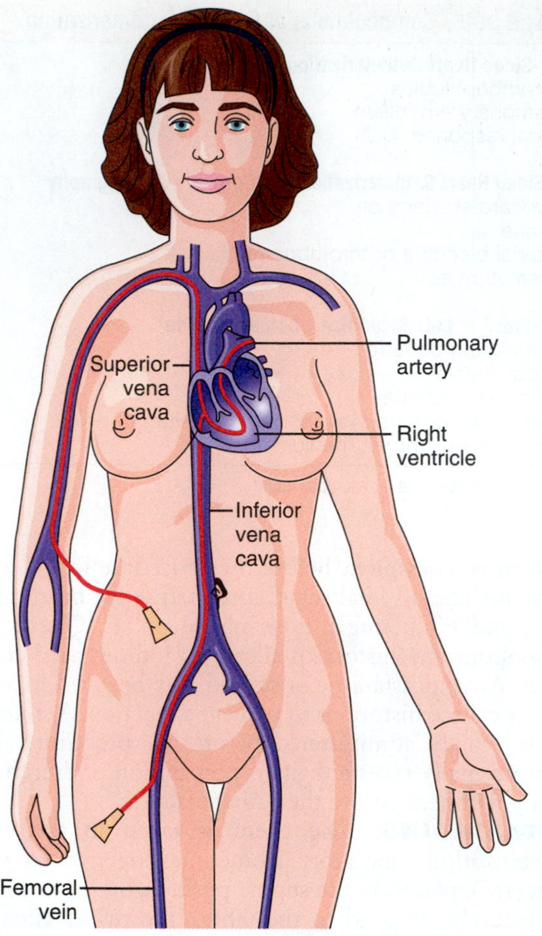

Figure 36-11 ■ Right-sided heart catheterization. The catheter is inserted into the femoral vein and advanced through the inferior vena cava (or, if into an antecubital or basilic vein, through the superior vena cava), right atrium, and right ventricle and into the pulmonary artery.

(rapidly changing films) evaluate left ventricular motion. Calculations are made regarding end-systolic volume, end-diastolic volume, stroke volume, and ejection fraction.

CORONARY ARTERIOGRAPHY. The technique for coronary arteriography is the same as for left-sided heart catheterization. The catheter is advanced into the aortic arch and positioned selectively in the right or left coronary artery. Injection of a contrast medium permits visualization of the coronary arteries. By assessing the flow of the medium through the coronary arteries, information about the site and severity of coronary lesions is obtained.

INTRAVASCULAR ULTRASONOGRAPHY. An alternative to injecting a medium into the coronary arteries is **intravascular ultrasonography (IVUS),** which introduces a flexible catheter with a miniature transducer at the distal tip to visualize the coronary arteries. The transducer emits sound waves, which reflect off the plaque and the arterial wall, creating an image of the blood vessel. IVUS is more reliable than angiography in indicating plaque distribution and composition, arterial dissection, and degree of stenosis of the occluded artery.

FOLLOW-UP CARE. After cardiac catheterization, the client is typically restricted to bedrest, and the insertion site extremity is kept straight. A soft knee brace can be applied to prevent bending of the affected extremity. Some cardiologists allow the head of the bed to be elevated up to 30 or 45 degrees during the period of bedrest, whereas other cardiologists prefer that the client remain supine. Current practice is for clients to remain in bed for 4 to 6 hours unless a special closure is used. Several arterial closure devices are available during the procedure to eliminate the need for manual compression or sandbags after the catheterization. Examples include arteriotomy sutures and collagen plugs to seal the insertion site.

There are many post-catheterization nursing responsibilities. Monitor vital signs every 15 minutes for 1 hour, then every 30 minutes for 2 hours or until vital signs are stable, and then every 4 hours or according to hospital policy. Assess the insertion site for bloody drainage or hematoma formation. Peripheral pulses in the affected extremity, as well as skin temperature and color, are monitored with every vital sign check.

Observe for complications of cardiac catheterization (see Table 36-5). Complaints of pain and discomfort at the insertion site, chest pain, nausea, or feelings of light-headedness should be reported. The client is recovered in the postanesthesia care unit or other specialty area where monitored beds are located. Because the contrast medium acts as an osmotic diuretic, monitor urine output and ensure that the client receives sufficient oral and IV fluids for adequate excretion of the medium. Pain medication for insertion site or back discomfort may be given as prescribed.

If the client experiences chest pain, dysrhythmias, bleeding, hematoma formation, or a dramatic change in peripheral pulses in the affected extremity, contact the physician immediately and provide prompt intervention. Neurologic changes, such as visual disturbances, slurred speech, swallowing difficulties, and extremity weakness, should also be reported.

OTHER DIAGNOSTIC TESTS

Electrocardiography

The **electrocardiogram (ECG)** is a routine part of every cardiovascular evaluation and is one of the most valuable diagnostic tests. Various forms are available: resting ECG, continuous ambulatory ECG (Holter monitoring), exercise ECG (stress test), and signal-averaged ECG. The resting ECG provides information about cardiac dysrhythmias, myocardial ischemia, the site and extent of MI, cardiac hypertrophy, electrolyte imbalances, and the effectiveness of cardiac drugs. The normal ECG pattern of one cardiac cycle is illustrated in Figure 36-12. Further discussion of the interpretation and evaluation of normal and abnormal patterns is found in Chapter 37.

RESTING ELECTROCARDIOGRAPHY

The ECG graphically records the electrical current generated by the heart. This current is measured by electrodes that are placed on the skin and connected to an amplifier and strip chart recorder (Figure 36-13). In the standard 12-lead ECG, five electrodes attached to the arms, legs, and chest measure current from 12 different views or leads: three bipolar limb leads (Figure 36-14), three unipolar augmented leads (Figure 36-15), and six unipolar precordial leads (Figure 36-16). Placement of the leads allows the health care provider to view myocardial electrical conduction from different axes or positions, identifying sections of the heart in which electrical conduction is abnormal.

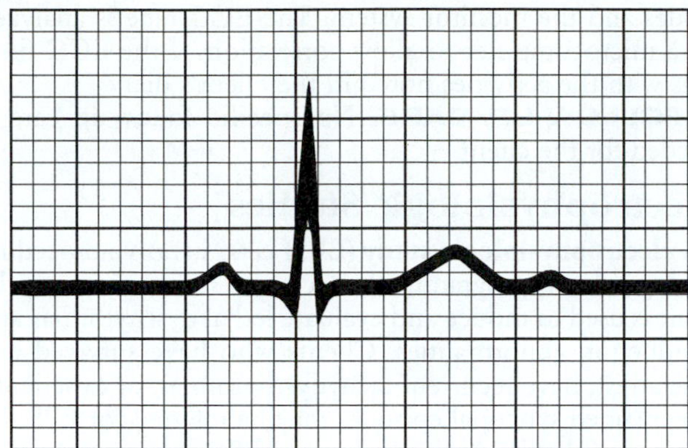

Figure 36-12 ■ A normal ECG pattern in lead II.

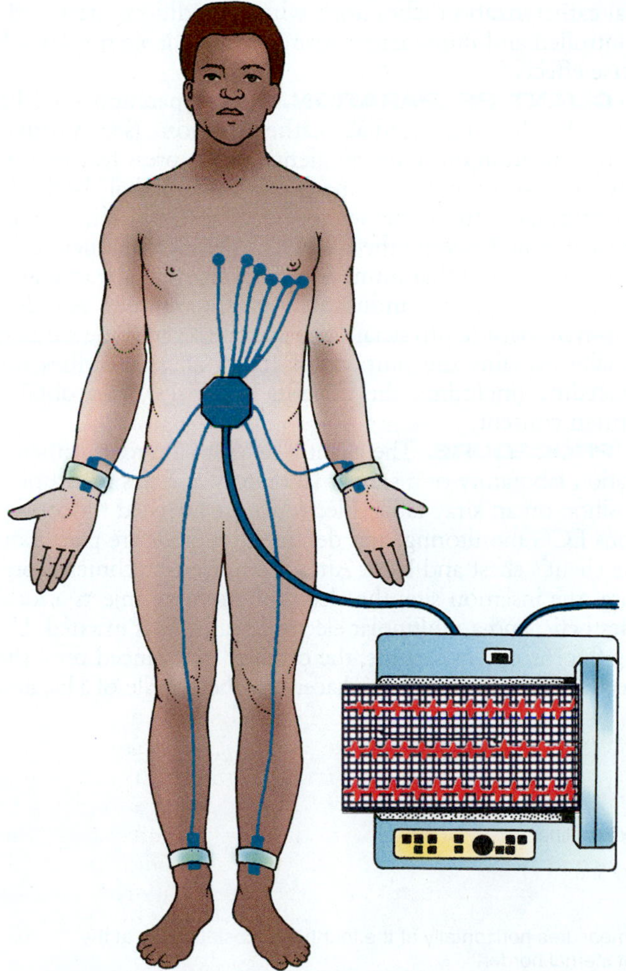

Figure 36-13 ■ Electrode placement for a 12-lead ECG.

CLIENT PREPARATION. Explain the purpose and procedure of the resting ECG, inform the client that the test is safe and painless, and remind him or her to lie as still as possible during the test.

PROCEDURE. The ECG is performed with the client in a supine position with the chest exposed. Before applying the electrodes, the nurse or the technician washes the skin to reduce skin oils and improve electrode contact. To ensure good contact between the skin and the electrodes for the limb leads, the electrodes should be placed on a flat surface above the wrists and the ankles. A total of 10 electrodes are used for a standard ECG and are attached to lead wires that connect to the ECG machine. The 12-lead ECG reading is obtained by selecting the indicators on the machine.

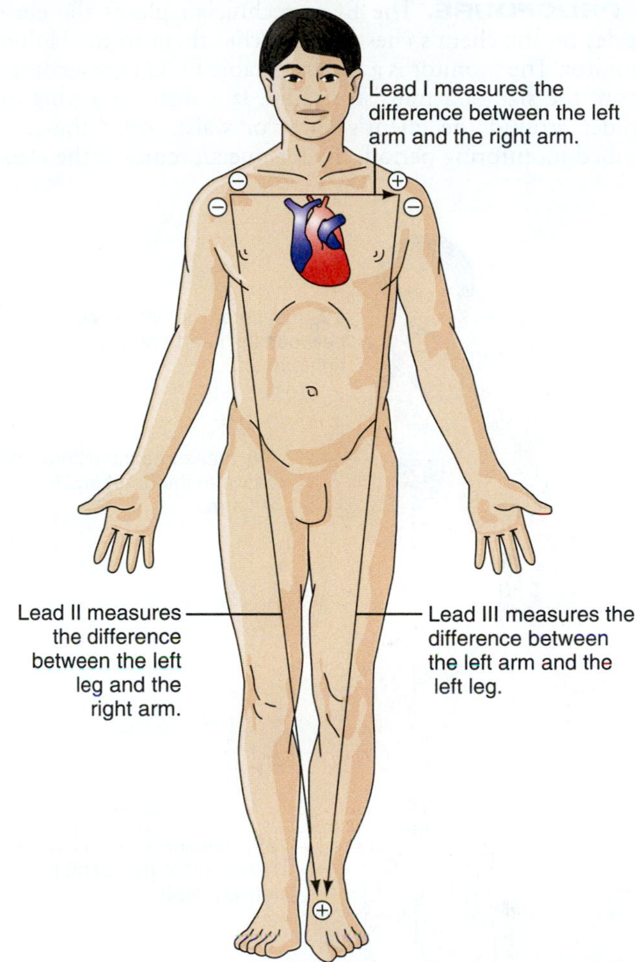

Figure 36-14 ■ Standard ECG limb leads.

FOLLOW-UP CARE. No specific follow-up care is warranted.

AMBULATORY ELECTROCARDIOGRAPHY

Ambulatory ECG (also called *Holter monitoring*) allows continuous recording of cardiac activity during an extended period (usually 24 hours) while the client is performing his or her usual activities of daily living (ADLs). The ambulatory ECG allows the assessment and correlation of dyspnea, chest pain, CNS symptoms (e.g., light-headedness and syncope), and palpitations with actual cardiac events and the client's activities.

CLIENT PREPARATION. Encourage the client to maintain a normal day's schedule. He or she is instructed to keep a diary, or log, in which to note the time of activities (e.g., eating, sleeping, walking, working) and to record any symptoms such as chest pain, light-headedness, fainting, and palpitations. Instruct the client to avoid operating heavy machinery, using electric shavers and hair dryers, and bathing or showering because these activities may interfere with the ECG recorder. If the client is hospitalized, the nurse may need to make the diary entries.

PROCEDURE. The ECG technician places the electrodes on the client's chest and attaches them to the Holter monitor. The monitor is a small portable ECG tape recorder about the size of a transistor radio. It is worn in a sling or holder around the client's chest or waist. After the prescribed monitoring period, the technician removes the electrodes and the monitor system. The ECG tape is analyzed by a microcomputer to allow correlation of the ECG findings with the activities noted in the client's diary.

FOLLOW-UP CARE. No specific follow-up care is needed for the client.

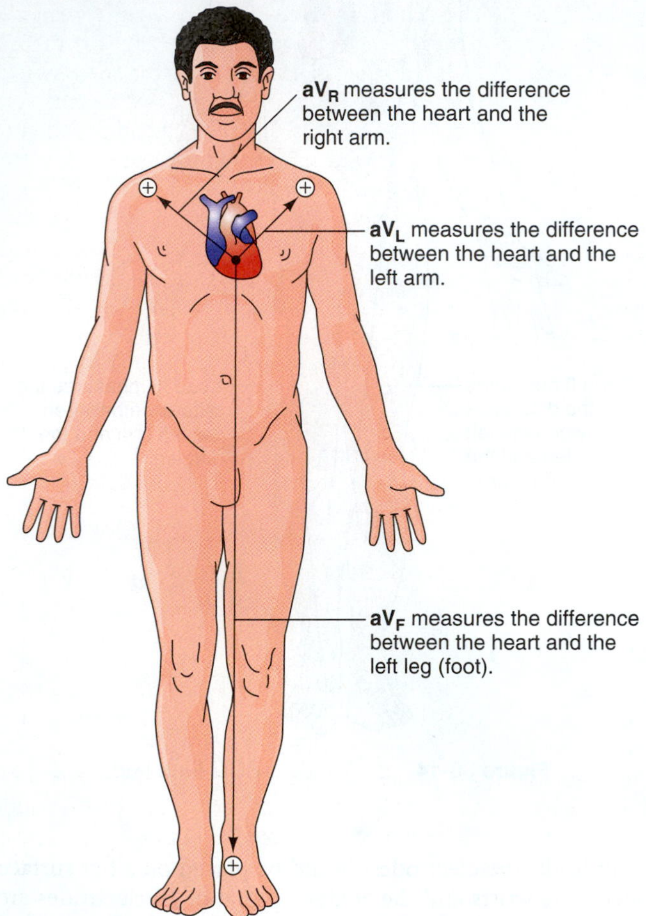

Figure 36-15 ■ Unipolar augmented ECG leads.

Electrophysiologic Studies

An **electrophysiologic study (EPS)** is an invasive procedure during which programmed electrical stimulation of the heart is used to induce and evaluate lethal dysrhythmias and conduction abnormalities. Clients who have survived cardiac arrest, have recurrent tachydysrhythmias, or experience unexplained syncopal episodes may be referred for EPS. Induction of the dysrhythmia during EPS permits accurate diagnosis of the dysrhythmia and aids in the search for an effective treatment. These procedures have risks similar to those for cardiac catheterization and are performed in a special catheterization laboratory, where conditions are strictly controlled and immediate treatment is available for any adverse effects.

CLIENT PREPARATION. The preparation for EPS parallels that for cardiac catheterization (see Cardiac Catheterization on p. 697). Clients may express fear or anxiety because attempts are made to induce lethal dysrhythmias similar to those that led to the initial hospitalization or resuscitation. Reassure the client that EPS is a planned, controlled event and that immediate treatment will be available for any dysrhythmia induced during the studies. An electrophysiologist (a physician who specializes in these studies) usually explains the purpose of the studies, describes the procedure (including the benefits and risks), and obtains written consent.

PROCEDURE. The client is taken to a cardiac catheterization laboratory or a similar laboratory and lies in a supine position on an x-ray table. Electrodes are attached for continuous ECG monitoring, and defibrillation pads are placed on the client's chest and back. After the nurse or technician prepares the insertion site, the electrophysiologist injects a local anesthetic, and a multipolar electrode catheter is inserted. Using fluoroscopy as a guide, the catheter is advanced until the electrodes rest in the RA, adjacent to the bundle of His, and

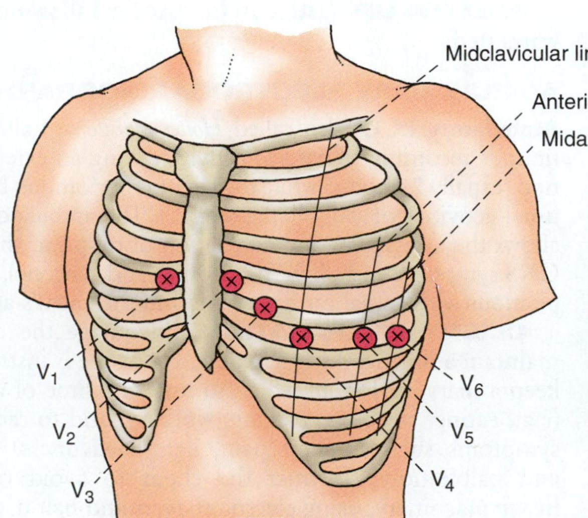

Figure 36-16 ■ Unipolar precordial ECG leads.

in the right ventricle. Additional electrodes may be placed for endocardial mapping.

During EPS, baseline conduction times can be measured: the AH interval (conduction time from the RA through the His bundle) and the HV interval (conduction time from the proximal His bundle to the ventricular myocardium). The catheter may be programmed to pace at varying rates to determine the function of the SA and AV node, or it may be programmed to deliver premature paced stimuli in an effort to initiate and evaluate tachydysrhythmia.

If the dysrhythmia is induced, it may terminate spontaneously or be treated by the physician. The physician might elect to use properly timed stimuli, rapid pacing, medications, or countershock to terminate the dysrhythmia.

The client is advised to inform the staff about any symptoms that he or she experiences. During rapid pacing, the client may be aware of the rapid heartbeat and state that he or she is experiencing palpitations. The client may also experience chest pain or loss of consciousness if he or she becomes hypotensive. The client often experiences back discomfort during the procedure because he or she must remain supine for 2 to 6 hours. Pain may develop at the insertion site as the anesthetic wears off.

FOLLOW-UP CARE. Follow-up care for EPS is the same as for cardiac catheterization. Comfort measures may be provided to alleviate back discomfort, including massage and position changes. If the client lost consciousness during the procedure and received electrical cardioversion or defibrillation, he or she may complain of chest discomfort over the area where the electrical current was applied. Assess the skin for any signs of redness, swelling, or burns. In addition, there may be memory loss for the events during the procedure; if so, provide reassurance and calmly explain the events of the procedure.

Exercise Electrocardiography (Stress Test)

The **exercise electrocardiography** test (also known as exercise tolerance, or **stress test**) assesses cardiovascular response to an increased workload. The stress test helps to determine the functional capacity of the heart and screens for asymptomatic coronary artery disease. Dysrhythmias that develop during exercise may be identified, and the effectiveness of antidysrhythmic drugs can be evaluated.

CLIENT PREPARATION. Because there are risks associated with exercising, the client must be adequately informed about the purpose of the test, the procedure, and the risks involved. Written consent must be obtained. Anxiety and fear are common before stress testing. Therefore assure the client that the procedure is performed in a controlled environment where prompt nursing and medical attention is available.

The client is instructed to get plenty of rest the night before the procedure. He or she may have a light meal 2 hours before the test but should avoid smoking or drinking alcohol or caffeine-containing beverages on the day of the test. The cardiologist decides whether the client should stop taking any cardiac medications. He or she is advised to wear comfortable, loose clothing and rubber-soled, supportive shoes. Instruct the client to tell the physician if symptoms such as chest pain, dizziness, shortness of breath, and an irregular heartbeat are experienced during the test.

Before the stress test, a resting 12-lead ECG, cardiovascular history, and physical examination are performed to check for any ECG abnormalities or medical factors that might interfere with the test.

Emergency supplies such as cardiac drugs, a defibrillator, and other necessary resuscitation equipment are available in the room in which the stress test is performed. It is important to be proficient in the use of resuscitation equipment when assisting the physician because chest pain, dysrhythmias, and other ECG changes may occur during this test.

PROCEDURE. The technician places electrodes on the client's chest and attaches them to a multilead monitoring system. Note baseline blood pressure (BP), heart rate (HR), and respiratory rate. The two major modes of exercise available for stress testing are pedaling a bicycle ergometer and walking on a treadmill. A bicycle ergometer has a wheel operated by pedals that can be adjusted to increase the resistance to pedaling. The treadmill is a motorized device with an adjustable conveyor belt; it can reach speeds of 1 to 10 miles/hr and can also be adjusted from a flat position to a 22-degree gradient.

After the client is shown how to use the bicycle or to walk on the treadmill, he or she begins to exercise. During the test, the BP and electrocardiogram (ECG) are closely monitored as the resistance to cycling or the speed and incline of the treadmill are increased. The client exercises until one of the following occurs:

- A predetermined HR is reached and maintained.
- Signs and symptoms such as chest pain, fatigue, extreme dyspnea, vertigo, hypotension, and ventricular dysrhythmias appear.
- Significant ST-segment depression occurs.

FOLLOW-UP CARE. After the test, the nurse continues to monitor the ECG and BP until the client has completely recovered. After the client has recovered, he or she can return home if the test was performed on an ambulatory basis. Advise the client to avoid a hot shower for 1 to 2 hours after the test because this may precipitate hypotension. If the client does not recover but continues to have pain or ventricular dysrhythmias or appears medically unstable, he or she is admitted to a telemetry unit for observation.

For clients who are unable to exercise because of conditions such as peripheral vascular disease or arthritis, pharmacologic stress testing with agents such as dobutamine may be indicated. The nursing considerations are similar to those for the client who has undergone an exercise electrocardiography.

Echocardiography

As a noninvasive, risk-free test, echocardiography is easily performed at the bedside or on an ambulatory care basis. **Echocardiography** uses ultrasound waves to assess cardiac structure and mobility, particularly of the valves. ECGs help to assess and diagnose cardiomyopathy, valvular disorders, pericardial effusion, left ventricular function, ventricular aneurysms, and cardiac tumors.

CLIENT PREPARATION. There is no special preparation for echocardiography. Inform the client that the test is painless and takes 30 to 60 minutes to complete. The client is instructed to lie quietly during the test and on his or her left side with the head elevated 15 to 20 degrees.

PROCEDURE. During an echocardiogram, a small transducer lubricated with gel to facilitate movement and conduction is placed on the client's chest at the level of the third or fourth intercostal space near the left sternal border. The transducer transmits high-frequency sound waves and receives them as they are reflected from different structures. These echoes are usually videotaped simultaneously with the echocardiogram and can be recorded on graph paper for a permanent record.

After the images are taped, cardiac measurements that require several images can be obtained. Routine measurements include chamber size, ejection fraction, and flow gradient across the valves.

FOLLOW-UP CARE. There is no specific follow-up care for a client who has undergone an echocardiogram.

Pharmacologic Stress Echocardiogram

A slightly more aggressive form of echocardiogram is a **pharmacologic stress echocardiogram** using either dobutamine or adenosine. This test is usually used when clients cannot tolerate exercise. Dobutamine (Dobutrex) increases the heart's contractility; adenosine (Adenocard) is a coronary artery dilator. Clients are required to have nothing by mouth (NPO status) for 3 to 6 hours before the test, except for sips of water with medications. The technician ensures that IV access is present before the procedure and monitors BP and pulse continuously throughout the procedure. After the procedure, vital signs are monitored until BP returns to baseline and the pulse rate slows to less than 100 beats/min.

Transesophageal Echocardiography

Echocardiograms may also be performed transesophageally (through the esophagus). **Transesophageal echocardiography (TEE)** examines cardiac structure and function with an ultrasound transducer placed immediately behind the heart in the esophagus or stomach. The transducer provides especially detailed views of posterior cardiac structures such as the left atrium, mitral valve, and aortic arch. Preparation and follow-up are similar to that for an upper gastrointestinal endoscopic examination (see Chapter 56).

Myocardial Nuclear Perfusion Imaging

The use of radionuclide techniques in cardiovascular assessment is called **myocardial nuclear perfusion imaging (MNPI).** Cardiovascular abnormalities can be viewed, recorded, and evaluated using radioactive tracer substances. These studies are useful for detecting myocardial infarction (MI) and decreased myocardial blood flow and for evaluating left ventricular ejection. Conducting myocardial nuclear imaging tests, in conjunction with exercise or the administration of vasodilating agents such as dipyridamole and adenosine, allow clearer identification of how the heart responds to stress.

CLIENT PREPARATION. Inform the client that the tests are relatively noninvasive. Because the amount of radioisotope is small, radiation exposure risks are minimal. If a dilating agent is to be used, the client is advised to abstain from cigarettes and caffeinated food or drinks for 4 hours before administration of the vasodilator.

PROCEDURE. Common tests in nuclear cardiology include technetium (^{99m}Tc) pyrophosphate scanning, thallium imaging, and multigated cardiac blood pool imaging.

TECHNETIUM PYROPHOSPHATE SCANNING. For this scan, a small dose of ^{99m}Tc pyrophosphate is injected into the antecubital vein. The client waits at least 2 hours while the renal system clears the unbound technetium. A gamma-scintillation camera scans the heart to identify the areas of increased uptake of the radioisotope. The radioisotope accumulates in damaged myocardial tissue and is referred to as a "hot spot." This test helps to detect an acute MI and define its location and size, but it does not show an old infarction.

THALLIUM IMAGING. For thallium imaging, a small dose of thallium-201 (^{201}Tl) is injected into the client's antecubital vein. A nuclear camera takes images of the heart 10 minutes later to detect areas of normal blood flow and intact cells, which rapidly take up the thallium. Necrotic or ischemic tissue does not take up the radioisotope and appears as "cold spots" on the scan. Scanning is repeated in 2 to 4 hours to evaluate thallium clearance.

Thallium imaging may be performed with the client at rest or during an exercise test. Dipyridamole (Persantine, Apo-Dipyridamole✱) is administered before the Persantine thallium test. Dobutamine hydrochloride (Dobutrex) or adenosine (Adenocard) may be given instead. By causing vasodilation, these drugs simulate the effects of exercise and are used for clients who are unable to exercise on a bike or treadmill. These medications may cause flushing, headache, dyspnea, and chest tightness for a few moments after injection.

Thallium imaging performed during an exercise test may demonstrate perfusion deficits not apparent at rest. First, the stress test procedure is performed (see Exercise Electrocardiography [Stress Test], p. 701). After the client reaches maximum activity level, a small dose of ^{201}Tl is injected intravenously. The client continues to exercise for approximately 1 to 2 minutes, after which the scanning is performed. Nuclear cardiologists often compare the resting and stress images to differentiate between fixed and reversible defects in the myocardium.

Thallium imaging is used to assess myocardial scarring and perfusion, to detect the location and extent of an acute or chronic MI, evaluate graft patency after coronary bypass surgery, and evaluate antianginal therapy, thrombolytic therapy, or balloon angioplasty.

CARDIAC BLOOD POOL IMAGING. Cardiac blood pool imaging is a noninvasive test for evaluating cardiac motion and calculating ejection fraction. It uses a computer to synchronize the client's electrocardiogram (ECG) with pictures taken by a gamma-scintillation camera. The technician attaches the client to an ECG and injects a small amount of ^{99m}Tc intravenously. The radioisotope is not taken up by tissue but remains "tagged" to red blood cells in the circulation. The camera may take pictures of the radioactive material as it makes its first pass through the heart.

During **multigated blood pool scanning,** the computer breaks the time between R waves on the ECG into fractions of a second, called "gates." The camera records blood flow through the heart during each of these gates. By analyzing the information from multiple gates, the computer can evaluate the ventricular wall motion and calculate ejection fraction (percentage of the left ventricular volume that is ejected with each contraction) and ejection velocity. Areas of decreased, absent, or paradoxical movement of the left ventricle may also be identified.

POSITRON EMISSION TOMOGRAPHY. Positron emission tomography (PED) scans are used to compare cardiac perfusion and metabolic function and differentiate normal from diseased myocardium. The technician administers the first radioisotope (nitrogen-13-ammonia) and then begins a 20-minute scan to detect myocardial perfusion. Next the technician administers a second radioisotope (fluoro-18-deoxyglucose). After a pause, a second scan is performed to detect the metabolically active myocardium, which is using glucose.

The two scans are compared. In a normal heart, performance and metabolic function will match. In an ischemic heart, there will be a mismatch: a reduction in perfusion and increased glucose uptake by the ischemic myocardium. The scanning procedure takes 2 to 3 hours, and the client may be asked to use a treadmill or exercise bicycle in conjunction with the scan.

FOLLOW-UP CARE. Depending on which test is performed, the client may complain of fatigue or discomfort at the antecubital injection site. If a stress test was paired with the study, the client will need follow-up care for the stress test.

Magnetic Resonance Imaging

Magnetic resonance imaging (MRI) is a noninvasive diagnostic option. An image of the heart or great vessels is produced through the interaction of magnetic fields, radio waves, and atomic nuclei showing hydrogen density. Simply put, the radio waves "bounce off" the body tissue being examined. Because each tissue has its own density, the computer image clearly differentiates between different types of tissues. MRI permits determination of cardiac wall thickness, chamber dilation, valve and ventricular function, and blood movement in the great vessels. Improved MRI techniques allow coronary artery blood flow to be mapped with nearly the accuracy of a cardiac catheterization.

Before an MRI, ensure that the client has removed all metallic objects, including watches, jewelry, clothing with metal fasteners, and hair clips. Clients with pacemakers should not undergo an MRI because the magnetic fields can deactivate the pacemaker. Approximately 5% of clients experience claustrophobia during the 15 to 60 minutes required to complete the scan.

Electronic-Beam Computed Tomography Scan

Electronic-beam computed tomography (EBCT) is a valuable tool in cardiovascular diagnostics. This test helps to determine whether calcifications are present in the arteries; calcifications are a common component of arterial plaque.

Hemodynamic Monitoring

Hemodynamic monitoring is an invasive system used in critical care areas to provide quantitative information about vascular capacity, blood volume, pump effectiveness, and tissue perfusion. Hemodynamic monitoring directly measures pressures in the heart and great vessels. These procedures are usually performed for more seriously ill clients and can provide more accurate measurements of blood pressure, heart function, and volume status.

Hemodynamic monitoring does involve significant risks, although complications are uncommon. Therefore informed consent is required. After obtaining consent, the nurse prepares a pressure-monitoring system. The components of this system are a catheter with an infusion system, a transducer, and a monitor. The catheter receives the pressure waves (mechanical energy) from the heart or the great vessels. The transducer converts the mechanical energy into electrical energy, which is displayed as waveforms or numbers on the monitor. Patency of the catheter is maintained with a slow continuous flush of normal saline, usually infused at 3 to 4 mL/hr under pressure to prevent the back up of blood and occlusion of the catheter.

To prepare the transducer, balance and calibrate it according to hospital policy and the manufacturer's specifications. Finally, identify the phlebostatic axis (Chart 36-5) and level the transducer to it. When the monitoring system is prepared, the physician inserts the catheter.

CHART 36-5

BEST PRACTICE for
Identification of the Phlebostatic Axis

1. Position the client supine.
2. Palpate the fourth intercostal space at the sternum.

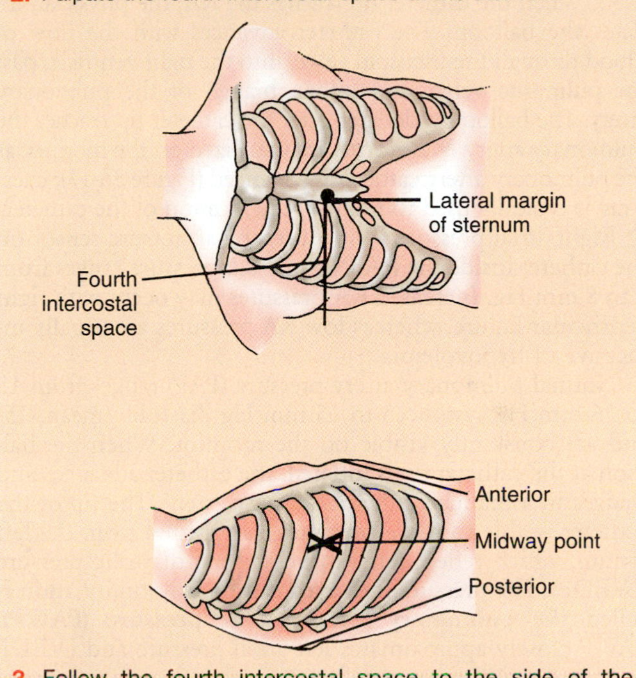

3. Follow the fourth intercostal space to the side of the client's chest.
4. Determine the midway point between anterior and posterior.
5. Find the intersection between the midway point and the line from the fourth intercostal space, and mark it with an X in indelible ink. This is the phlebostatic axis.

RIGHT ATRIAL, PULMONARY ARTERY, AND PULMONARY WEDGE PRESSURES

A pulmonary artery catheter is a multi-lumen catheter with the capacity to measure right atrial and indirect left atrial pressures or pulmonary artery wedge pressure (PAWP), also known as the **pulmonary artery occlusive pressure (PAOP).** A cardiac output measurement may also be obtained, as well as cardiac index and systemic and pulmonary vascular resistance.

CLIENT PREPARATION. The physician explains the procedure and advises the client and family members or significant others of the risks. The physician then obtains written consent for the procedure. The client and family should understand that the hemodynamic monitoring system represents an assessment tool. Although it is used to guide therapy, it is not itself a treatment. Ask the client to remain still and in the supine or Trendelenburg position for insertion of the catheter.

PROCEDURE. The physician inserts a balloon-tipped catheter percutaneously through a large vein, usually the internal jugular or subclavian, and directs it to the right atrium (RA). When the catheter tip reaches the RA, the physician inflates the balloon. The catheter advances with the flow of blood through the tricuspid valve, into the right ventricle, past the pulmonic valve, and into a branch of the pulmonary artery. The balloon is deflated after the catheter tip reaches the pulmonary artery. Waveforms are visualized on the monitor as the pulmonary artery catheter is advanced (Figure 36-17); chest x-ray is typically used to monitor the location of the catheter.

Right atrial pressure is measured by a pressure sensor on the catheter inside the RA. Normal RA pressure ranges from 1 to 8 mm Hg. Increased RA pressures may occur with right ventricular failure, whereas low RA pressures are usually indicative of hypovolemia.

Normal pulmonary artery pressure (PAP) ranges from 15 to 26 mm Hg systolic/5 to 15 mm Hg diastolic (mean, 15) and are constantly visible on the monitor. When the balloon at the catheter tip is inflated, the catheter advances and wedges in a branch of the pulmonary artery. The tip of the catheter is able to sense pressures transmitted from the left atrium, which reflect left ventricular end-diastolic pressure (LVEDP). The pressure measured during balloon inflation is called the **pulmonary artery wedge pressure (PAWP).** PAWP closely approximates left atrial pressure and LVEDP in clients with normal left ventricular function, normal heart rates, and no mitral valve disease. The PAWP is a mean pressure and normally ranges between 4 and 12 mm Hg.

Elevated PAWP measurements may indicate left ventricular failure, hypervolemia, mitral regurgitation, or intracardiac shunt. A decreased PAWP is seen with hypovolemia or afterload reduction. Individual values may be less important than the trend in values.

FOLLOW-UP CARE. The critical care nurse obtains and records RA pressure, PAP, and PAWP at appropriate intervals (usually every 1 to 4 hours). The trend of these pressures helps to guide medical therapy. During pressure recording, it is important that the transducer be at the level of the phlebostatic axis and that the client's position be appropriate. The client is usually supine with the head elevated up to 45 degrees during hemodynamic readings, although the client's position may not affect results (see the Evidence-Based Practice for Nursing box on p. 705). If the balloon remains in the wedge position after PAWP measurement, try to change the catheter's position by asking the client to cough or by changing the client's position. If these methods are not successful, notify the physician immediately.

Change the occlusive dressing over the catheter aseptically according to hospital policy. Inspect the insertion site for redness, induration, swelling, drainage, and intactness of the sutures. Detailed discussion of the management and care of clients with pulmonary artery catheters can be found in textbooks on critical care nursing.

Be sure to assess for a number of complications associated with pulmonary artery catheters. For example, pulmonary infarction or pulmonary rupture may occur if the catheter remains in the wedge position. Air embolism is possible if the balloon has ruptured and repeated attempts are made to inflate it. Ventricular dysrhythmias may occur during insertion or if the catheter tip slips back into the right ventricle and irritates the myocardium. Thrombus and embolus formation may occur at the catheter site. Infection may result, and bleeding may be pronounced if the infusion system becomes disconnected.

CARDIAC OUTPUT

Cardiac output can be measured using the thermodilution method when the client has a pulmonary artery catheter with a thermistor. A specified amount (5 or 10 mL) of iced

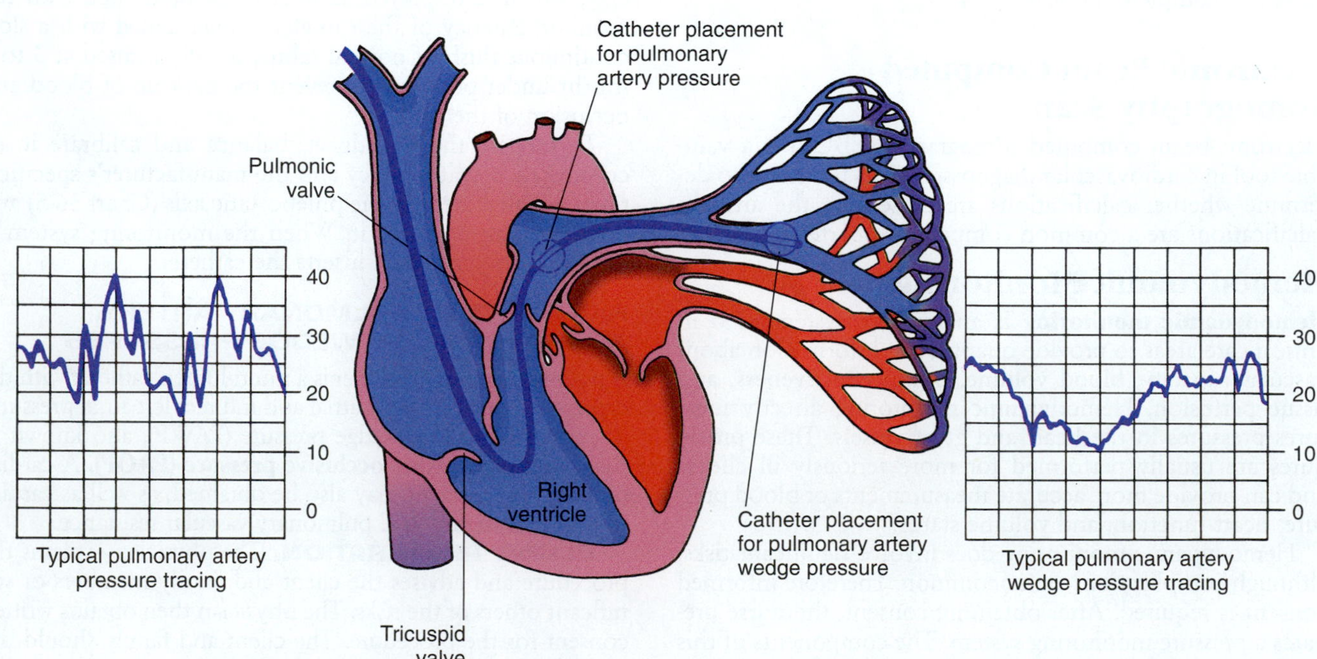

Figure 36-17 ■ Cardiac pressure waveforms can be visualized on the monitor.

or room-temperature IV solution (normal saline or dextrose in water) is injected into the proximal port of the catheter. The solution mixes with the blood in the RA and travels with the flow of blood through the heart. A temperature-sensitive device located on the tip of the catheter in the pulmonary artery registers and senses the change in blood temperature. This information is transmitted to a cardiac output computer, which displays a digital value. Nursing research continues to confirm that client positioning may not affect cardiac output readings (see the Evidence-Based Practice for Nursing box below).

MIXED VENOUS OXYGEN SATURATION MONITORING

Mixed venous oxygen saturation (SvO_2) reflects the balance between the client's oxygen supply and demand. SvO_2 may be measured with a pulmonary artery catheter with fiberoptics. Light travels down one optical fiber, is reflected by the red blood cells according to the oxygen saturation of the hemoglobin, and returns to an optical module for interpretation and continuous display. The normal range for SvO_2 is 60% to 80%. Using SvO_2 monitoring individualizes the plan of care so that the SvO_2 remains in the normal range and the client's oxygen supply and demand are in balance.

EVIDENCE-BASED PRACTICE for Nursing

What is the effect of the different positions on the accuracy of cardiac output readings?

Giuliano, K.K., et al. (2003). Backrest angle and cardiac output measurements in critically ill patients. *Nursing Research*, 52(4), 242-248.

The purpose of this study was to determine whether different position changes affect continuous cardiac output (CO) measurements in critical care clients with head elevation angles of 0 degrees, 30 degrees, and 45 degrees, at time intervals of 0 minutes, 5 minutes, and 10 minutes after changing positions.

The 26 adult critical care clients were recruited in an adult intensive care unit (ICU), and all had a cardiac output catheter in place for continuous CO measurements. Four repeated measures of analysis of variance (ANOVA) were done, one for each dependent variable: continuous cardiac index, stroke value, heart rate, and mean arterial pressure. No significant differences were found across the nine different measurement conditions. The lack of CO change in different positions was determined not to be due to compensatory changes within the CO determinants of stroke volume and heart rate.

Level of Evidence: 6—This study was small but was well-controlled research.

Critique. This study was conducted by a qualified nurse researcher and expert critical care nurses with critical care registered nurse (CCRN) status. The research question was answered using single-group, repeated-measures ANOVA with two participant factors: time and backrest angle. A repeated-measures ANOVA was used for this study because repeated measurements of cardiac index were done on each individual in the study. This allowed each person to serve as his or her own control. It also permitted a descriptive comparison to other studies, which used repeated measure ANOVA; however, the sample is small, and only one unit was used.

Implications for Nursing. These findings add to the growing body of evidence about positioning in current practice and support earlier research indicating that critically ill clients need not to be repositioned unnecessarily solely for the purpose of obtaining a cardiac output. It adds to other empirical data in demonstrating that CO measurements can be taken in different positions without significantly affecting the results.

SYSTEMIC INTRA-ARTERIAL MONITORING

Direct measurement of arterial BP is by invasive arterial catheter in critically ill clients. The physician or specially trained nurse inserts an intra-arterial catheter into the radial or femoral artery. After the physician has inserted the catheter, it is attached to pressure tubing. A normal saline flush solution is infused constantly under pressure to maintain the integrity of the system. A transducer attached to the tubing allows continuous direct monitoring of the arterial BP. Direct measurements of BP are usually 10 to 15 mm Hg greater than indirect (cuff) measurements. The arterial catheter may also be used to obtain blood samples for arterial blood gas values and other blood tests.

Because the arterial vasculature is a high-pressure system, frequent assessment of the arterial site and infusion system is essential. Note any bleeding around the intra-arterial catheter or any loose connections and correct the situation immediately. Collateral circulation must be assessed by Doppler or Allen's tests before and while the arterial catheter is in place. Color, pulse, and temperature distal to the insertion site should be scrupulously monitored for any early signs of circulatory compromise. Complications of systemic intra-arterial monitoring may include pain, infection, arteriospasm, or obstruction at the site with the potential for distal infarction, air embolism, and hemorrhage.

Impedance Cardiography

Unlike conventional hemodynamic monitoring, **impedance cardiography (ICG)** is a flexible and fast–acting noninvasive monitoring system that consists of four ICG electrodes, four electrocardiogram (ECG) electrodes, and a portable ICG monitor. Simply stated, it measures the total impedance (resistance) to the flow of electricity in the heart. ICG can be used in any setting: intensive care unit (ICU), emergency department (ED), and in the home. ICG is used to assess, plan, and individualize the treatment plan for clients with heart failure, severe trauma, or fluid management. It provides measures of thoracic fluid, left ventricular function (cardiac output and cardiac index), preload, afterload, and contractility of the heart.

GET READY for the NCLEX Examination!

KEY POINTS

Safe Effective Care Environment

- Assess the older adult for cardiovascular changes associated with aging as described in Chart 36-1.
- Assess clients for allergy to iodine-based contrast media before having diagnostic tests requiring a contrast agent.
- Following invasive cardiovascular diagnostic testing, such as angiography and cardiac catheterization, monitor the insertion site for bleeding and hematoma formation.
- Assess vital signs carefully in clients having invasive cardiovascular testing; report new dysrhythmias following testing.

Health Promotion and Maintenance

- Identify clients at risk for cardiovascular disease, especially those with hyperlipidemia, hypertension, excess weight, physical inactivity, smoking, psychological stress, a positive family history, and diabetes.

- Teach clients how to reduce the risk of heart disease through exercise, diet modification, smoking cessation, and medications, as needed.
- Inform clients that genetics and other nonmodifiable risk factors, such as family history and gender, contribute to the development of CAD.

Psychosocial Integrity

- Discuss with the client any feelings or concerns he or she might have about the stress of cardiac illness, diagnostic testing, or other issues and use therapeutic measures to decrease anxiety.
- Recognize that denial is a common and normal response to help clients cope with threatening circumstances.
- Be aware that coping behaviors of clients who have cardiovascular problems vary from client to client.
- Allow the client to express feelings about an actual or perceived loss of health or social status related to cardiovascular disease.

Physiological Integrity

- Assess the client's complaint of pain to differentiate between the pain of angina and myocardial infarction (MI) from other noncardiac causes; discomfort, indigestion, squeezing, heaviness, and "viselike" are common terms used to describe chest pain of cardiac origin.
- Recall that syncope is a transient loss of consciousness and is common in older adults.
- Use jugular venous pressure to assess the filling volume and pressure on the right side of the heart.
- Assess for bruits, which are swishing sounds that develop in narrowed arteries.
- Auscultate the heart for normal first and second sounds, as well as for abnormalities such as an S_3, S_4, murmur, or gallop.
- Monitor serum markers of myocardial damage and other cardiac related laboratory tests as listed in Chart 36-4.
- Assess clients having cardiac catheterizations for potential complications as listed in Table 36-5.
- Directly assess cardiac pressures and cardiac output when clients have invasive hemodynamic monitoring systems.

ADDITIONAL STUDY RESOURCES

Go to your Student CD-ROM for Review Questions for the NCLEX Examination.

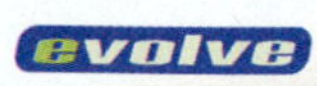

Go to http://evolve.elsevier.com/Iggy/ for Integrated Management of Care Questions for the NCLEX Examination.

SELECTED BIBLIOGRAPHY

Asterisk indicates a classic or definitive work on this subject.

American Heart Association. (2002). *Heart disease and stroke statistics–2003 update.* Dallas: Author.

Beyerle, K. (2002). Point of care testing of cardiac markers aids patient experiencing or at risk for acute myocardial infarction. *Nursing Management, 33*(9), 37-39.

Bonham, P.A. (2003). Determining the toe brachial pressure index. *Nursing 2003, 33*(9), 54-55.

Bridges, E.J., et al. (2000). Effect of the 30° lateral recumbent position in pulmonary artery and pulmonary artery wedge pressures in critically ill adult cardiac surgery patients. *American Journal of Critical Care, 9*(4), 262-275.

Burke, A.P., et al. (2002). Traditional risk factors and the incidence of sudden coronary death with and without coronary thrombosis in blacks. *Circulation, 105*(4), 419-424.

Cheek, D., & Cesan, A. (2003). What's different about heart disease in women? *Nursing 2003, 33*(8), 36-43.

Coffey, M., Crowder, G.K. & Cheek, D.J. (2003). Reducing coronary artery disease by decreasing homocysteine levels. *Critical Care Nurse, 23*(1), 25-30.

Critchley, J.A., & Capewell, S. (2003). Mortality risk reduction associated with smoking cessation in patients with coronary heart disease. *Journal of the American Medical Association, 290*(1), 86-97.

Crook, J., & Woody, F. (2003). Rapidly identify CHF with POC advances. *Nursing Management, 34*(1), 48-49.

D'Agostino, R.B., et al., for the CHS Risk Prediction Group (2001). Validation of the Framingham coronary heart disease prediction scores. *Journal of the American Medical Association, 286*(2), 180-187.

DeVon, H.A., & Zerwic, J.J. (2003). The symptoms of unstable angina: Do women and men differ? *Nursing Research, 52*(2), 108-118.

Fletcher, S.W., & Colditz, G.A. (2002). Failure of estrogen plus progestin therapy for prevention. *Journal of the American Medical Association, 288*(3), 366-368.

Funk, M., et al. (2002). Racial differences in the use of cardiac procedures in patients with acute myocardial infarction. *Nursing Research, 51*(3), 148-157.

Futterman, L., & Lemberg, L. (2002). High sensitivity C-reactive protein is the most effective prognostic measurement of acute coronary events. *American Journal of Critical Care, 11*(5), 482-486.

Gibbons, R.J., et al. (2002). *ACC/AHA 2002 guideline update for the management of patients with chronic stable angina: a report of the American College of Cardiology/American Heart Association Task Force on Practice Guidelines* (Committee to Update the 1999 Guidelines for the Management of Patient with Chronic Stable Angina). Accessed July 25, 2003, from http://www.acc.org/clinical/guidelines/stable/stable.pdf.

Giuliano, K.K, et al. (2003). Backrest angle and cardiac output measurement in critically ill patients. *Nursing Research, 52*(4), 242-248.

Groeneveld, P.W., Heidenreich, P.A., & Garber, A.M. (2003). Racial disparity in cardiac procedures and mortality among long-term survivors of cardiac arrest. *Circulation, 108*(3), 286-291.

Jarvis, C. (2004). *Physical examination and health assessment.* 4th ed. St. Louis: Elsevier Science.

Khattar, R.S., et al. (2001). Effect of aging on the prognostic significance of ambulatory systolic, diastolic, and pulse pressure in essential hypertension. *Circulation, 104*(7), 783-790.

Maas, M.L., et al. (2001). *Nursing care of older adults: Diagnoses, outcomes, and interventions.* St. Louis: Mosby.

Mehta, M. (2003). Assessing cardiovascular status. *Nursing 2003, 33*(1), 56-57.

Natarajan, et al. (2003). Sex differences in risk for coronary heart disease mortality associated with diabetes and established coronary heart disease. *Archives of Internal Medicine, 163*(14), 1735-1740.

National Cholesterol Education Program (2002). *Third report of the Expert Panel on Detection, Evaluation, and Treatment of High Blood Cholesterol in Adults (Adult Treatment Panel III).* Bethesda: National Heart, Lung, and Blood Institute, NIH Publication No. 02-5215.

National Heart, Lung, and Blood Institute (2002). *Postmenopausal hormone therapy: facts about postmenopausal hormone therapy.* Bethesda: NIH Publication No. 02-5200. Accessed August 8, 2003, from http://www.nhlbi.nih.gov/health/women/pht_facts.

National High Blood Pressure Education Program (2002). *Primary prevention of hypertension: clinical and public health advisory.* Bethesda: National Heart, Lung, and Blood Institute, NIH Publication No. 02-5076.

National High Blood Pressure Education Program (2003). *The seventh report of the Joint National Committee on Prevention, Detection, Evalua-*

tion, and Treatment of High Blood Pressure. Bethesda: National Heart, Lung, and Blood Institute, NIH Publication No. 03-5233.

*New York Heart Association Criteria Committee. (1964). *Diseases of the heart and blood vessels: Nomenclature and criteria for diagnosis* (6th ed.). Boston: Little, Brown.

Oliver-McNeil, S., & Artinian, N.T. (2003). Women's perceptions of personal cardiovascular risk and their risk-reducing behaviors. *American Journal of Critical Care, 11*(3), 221-227.

Otsuka, R., et al. (2001). Acute effects of passive smoking on the coronary circulation in healthy young adults. *Journal of the American Medical Association, 286,* 436-441.

Pagana, K.D., & Pagana, T.J. (2002). *Manual of diagnostic and laboratory tests* (2nd ed.). St. Louis: Mosby.

Paternak, R.C., et al. (2002). ACC/AHA/ NHLBI advisory on the use and safety of statins. *Journal of American College of Cardiology, 40,* 567-572.

Rauscher, F.M., et al. (2003). Aging, progenitor cell exhaustion, and atherosclerosis. *Circulation, 108*(4), 457-462.

Samara, J.N., & Popkin, B.M. (2003). Patterns and trends in food portion sizes, 1977-1998. *Journal of the American Medical Association, 290,* 450-453.

Sever, P.S., et al. (2003). Prevention of coronary and stroke events with atorvastatin in hypertensive patients who have average or lower than average cholesterol concentrations, in the Anglo-Scandinavian cardiac outcomes trial-lipid lowering arm (ASCOT-LLA): a multicentre randomized controlled trial. *The Lancet, 361,* 1149-1158.

Siomko, A.J. (2000). Demystifying cardiac markers. *American Journal of Nursing, 100*(1), 36-41.

*A Statement for Healthcare Professionals from the AHA Task Force on Risk Reduction. Primary Prevention of Coronary Heart Disease: Guidance from Framingham. (1998). AHA Scientific Statement. *Circulation, 97*(18), 1876-1887.

Turner, M.A. (2000). Monitoring hemodynamics noninvasively. *Nursing2000, 30*(5), 32cc1-32cc8.

Vakili, B.A., Kaplan, R.C., & Brown, D.L. (2001). Sex-based differences in early mortality of patients undergoing primary angioplasty for first acute myocardial infarction. *Circulation, 104*(25), 3034-3039.

Valli, G., & Giardina, E.G. (2002). Benefits, adverse effects and drug interactions of herbal therapies with cardiovascular effects. *Journal of American College of Cardiology, 39,* 1083-1095.

Writing Group for the Women's Health Initiative Investigators (2002). Risks and benefits of estrogen plus progestin in healthy postmenopausal women. *Journal of the American Medical Association-Express, 288,* 321-333.

Yeh, E.T.H., et al. (2001). C-reactive protein: Linking inflammation to cardiovascular complications. *Circulation, 104*(9), 974-979.

CHAPTER 37

Interventions for Clients with Dysrhythmias

PAMELA C. ZICKAFOOSE

LEARNING OUTCOMES

After studying this chapter, you should be able to:

1. Correlate the components of the electrocardiogram (ECG) with the cardiac conduction system.
2. Analyze a rhythm strip or ECG tracing to identify common cardiac dysrhythmias.
3. Identify typical physical assessment findings associated with common dysrhythmias.
4. Prioritize nursing diagnoses for clients experiencing dysrhythmias.
5. Plan care for clients experiencing common dysrhythmias.
6. Implement appropriate treatment modalities, including antidysrhythmic drugs, for common and lethal dysrhythmias.
7. Develop a teaching plan for clients experiencing common dysrhythmias.
8. Explain the purpose and types of pacing used as interventions for clients with dysrhythmias.
9. Differentiate between defibrillation and cardioversion, identifying the indications for the use of each.
10. Plan community-based care for a client after pacemaker or implantable cardioverter/defibrillator insertion.

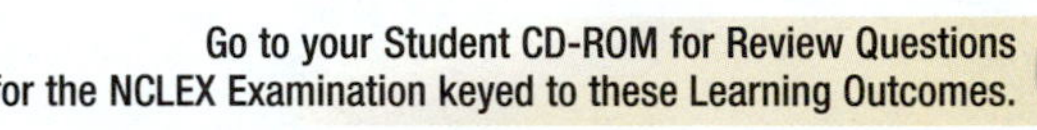

Cardiac dysrhythmias are abnormal rhythms of the heart's electrical system. Some dysrhythmias are life threatening, and others are benign. They are the result of disturbances of cardiac electrical impulse formation, conduction, or both. Many diseases (coronary artery disease [CAD] leading to ischemia and myocardial infarction [MI] are most common) as well as electrolyte imbalance, changes in oxygenation, and drug toxicity can affect the electrical activity of the heart, causing dysrhythmias. A dysrhythmia can markedly change the cardiac output and cause deterioration in vital signs. Although more common in older adults, dysrhythmias can occur in people of any age. To interpret and treat dysrhythmias correctly, an understanding of cardiac electrophysiology, the conduction system of the heart, and the principles of electrocardiography are needed.

REVIEW OF CARDIAC ELECTROPHYSIOLOGY

Electrophysiologic Properties

The electrophysiologic properties of cardiac cells regulate heart rate and rhythm. Specialized cardiac muscle cells possess unique properties: automaticity, excitability, conductivity, and contractility.

AUTOMATICITY

Automaticity (pacing function) is the ability of cardiac cells to generate an electrical impulse spontaneously and repetitively. Normally only primary pacemaker cells (SA node, AV junction) possess the ability to generate an electrical impulse. Under certain conditions, such as myocardial ischemia (decreased blood flow), electrolyte imbalance, hypoxia, drug toxicity, an abnormally configured electrical system, and infarction (cell death), any cardiac cell may generate electrical impulses independently and create dysrhythmias. Disturbances in automaticity may involve either an increase or a decrease in pacing function.

EXCITABILITY

Excitability is the ability of nonpacemaker myocardial cells to respond to an electrical impulse generated from pacemaker cells and to depolarize. Depolarization occurs when the normally negatively charged cells develop a positive charge.

CONDUCTIVITY

Conductivity is the ability to transmit an electrical stimulus from cell membrane to cell membrane. Consequently, excitable cells depolarize in rapid succession from cell to cell until all cells have depolarized. The wave of depolarization gives rise to the deflections of the electrocardiogram (ECG) waveforms that are recognized as the P wave and the QRS complex. Disturbances in conduction result when conduction is too rapid or too slow, when there is a total blockage of the pathway, or when there is an abnormal pathway that the electrical impulse travels. Re-entry is a situation in which a misdirected electrical impulse re-excites a conduction pathway through which it has already passed. Re-entry results in tachycardia.

CONTRACTILITY

Contractility is the ability of atrial and ventricular muscle cells to shorten their fiber length in response to electrical stimulation, generating sufficient pressure to propel blood forward. Contractility is the mechanical activity of the heart.

Action Potential

The cardiac cell membrane (sarcolemma) exhibits selective permeability to ions. An ion is an electrically charged particle. The selective permeability creates an electrical imbalance, known as an **action potential,** across the cell membrane. The cardiac cell at rest has an internal negative charge, whereas the charge outside the cell is positive. The state of electrical imbalance of the resting cell is called **resting membrane potential**.

Cardiac Conduction System

The cardiac conduction system consists of specialized cells (Figure 37-1). The conduction system is responsible for the generation and conduction of electrical impulses that cause atrial and ventricular depolarization. The conduction system consists of the sinoatrial node, atrioventricular junctional area, and bundle branch system.

SINOATRIAL NODE

The conduction system begins with the **sinoatrial (SA) node** (also called the sinus node), located close to the epicardial surface of the right atrium near its junction with the superior vena cava. The SA node is the heart's primary pacemaker. It can spontaneously and rhythmically generate electrical impulses at a rate of 60 to 100 beats/min, possessing the greatest degree of automaticity.

The SA node is richly supplied by the sympathetic and parasympathetic nervous systems, which accelerate and decelerate the rate of discharge of the sinus node, respectively. This process results in changes in the heart rate.

Impulses from the sinus node move directly through atrial muscle and lead to atrial depolarization, which is reflected in a P wave on the ECG. Atrial muscle contraction should follow. Within the atrial muscle are slow and fast conduction pathways leading to the atrioventricular (AV) node.

ATRIOVENTRICULAR JUNCTIONAL AREA

The **atrioventricular (AV) junctional** area consists of a transitional cell zone, the AV node itself, and the bundle of His. The AV node lies just beneath the right atrial endocardium, between the tricuspid valve and the ostium of the coronary sinus. Here T-cells (transitional cells) cause impulses to slow down or to be delayed in the AV node before proceeding to the ventricles. This delay is reflected in the PR segment on the ECG. This slow conduction provides a short delay, allowing the atria to contract and the ventricles to fill. The contraction is known as "atrial kick" and contributes additional blood volume for a greater cardiac output. The AV node is also controlled by both the sympathetic and the parasympathetic nervous systems. The bundle of His connects with the distal portion of the AV node and continues to perforate the interventricular septum.

BUNDLE BRANCH SYSTEM

The bundle of His extends as a right bundle branch down the right side of the interventricular septum to the apex of the right ventricle. On the left side it extends as a left bundle branch, which further divides into two fascicles.

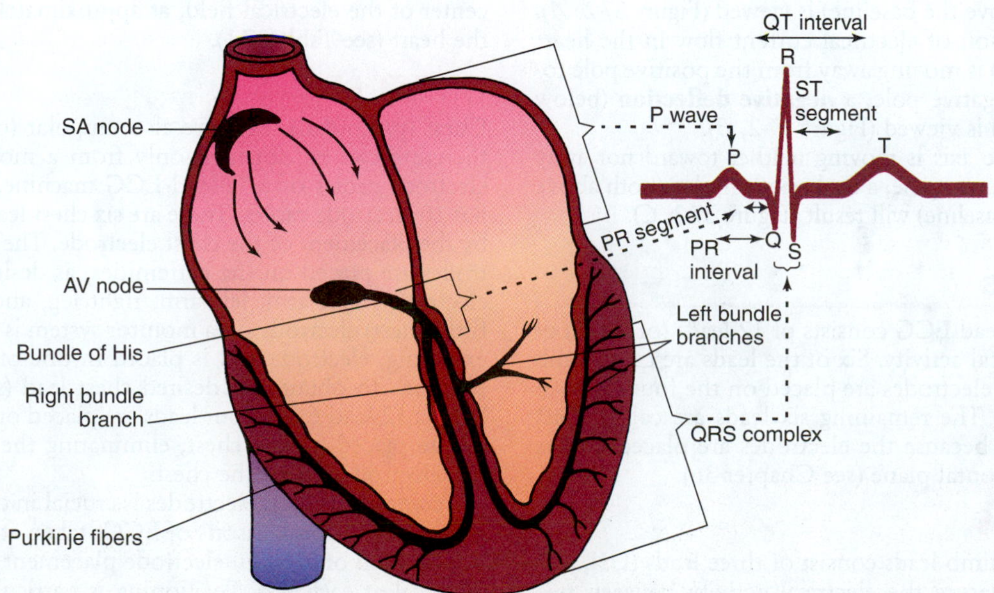

Figure 37-1 ■ The cardiac conduction system.

At the ends of both the right and left bundle branch systems are the Purkinje fibers. These fibers are an interweaving network located on the endocardial surface of both ventricles, from apex to base. The fibers then partially penetrate into the myocardium. **Purkinje cells** make up the bundle of His, bundle branches, and terminal Purkinje fibers. These cells are responsible for the rapid conduction of electrical impulses throughout the ventricles, leading to ventricular depolarization and the subsequent ventricular muscle contraction. A few nodal cells in the ventricles also occasionally demonstrate automaticity, giving rise to ventricular beats or rhythms.

ELECTROCARDIOGRAPHY

The **electrocardiogram (ECG)** provides a graphic representation, or picture, of cardiac electrical activity. The weak cardiac electrical currents are transmitted to the body surface. Electrodes, consisting of a conductive gel on an adhesive pad, are placed on specific sites on the body and attached to cables connected to an ECG machine or to a monitor. The cardiac electrical current is transmitted via the electrodes and through the lead wires to the machine or monitor, which displays the cardiac electrical activity.

A **lead** provides one view of the heart's electrical activity. Multiple leads, or views, can be obtained. Electrode placement is the same for male and female clients.

Lead systems are made up of a positive pole and a negative pole. An imaginary line joining these two poles is called the **lead axis**. The direction of electrical current flow in the heart is the **cardiac axis**. The relationship between the cardiac axis and the lead axis is responsible for the deflections seen on the ECG pattern:

- The baseline is the isoelectric line. It occurs when there is no current flow in the heart after complete depolarization and also after complete repolarization. Positive deflections occur above this line, and negative deflections occur below it. Deflections represent depolarization and repolarization of cells.
- If the direction of electrical current flow in the heart (cardiac axis) is toward the positive pole, a **positive deflection** (above the baseline) is viewed (Figure 37-2, *A*).
- If the direction of electrical current flow in the heart (cardiac axis) is moving away from the positive pole toward the negative pole, a **negative deflection** (below the baseline) is viewed (Figure 37-2, *B*).
- If the cardiac axis is moving neither toward nor away from the positive pole, a biphasic complex (both above and below baseline) will result (Figure 37-2, *C*).

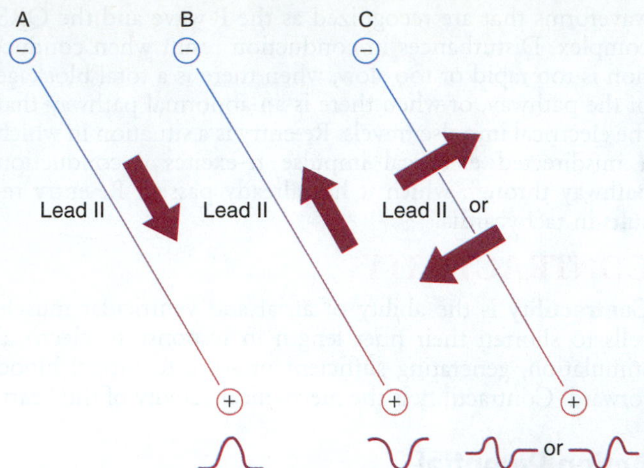

Figure 37-2 ■ **A,** The cardiac axis (bold arrow) is parallel to the lead axis (the line between the negative and the positive electrodes), going toward the positive electrode; a positive deflection is inscribed. **B,** The cardiac axis is parallel to the lead axis, going toward the negative electrode; a negative deflection is inscribed. **C,** The cardiac axis is perpendicular to the lead axis, going neither toward the positive electrode nor toward the negative electrode; a biphasic deflection is inscribed.

Lead Systems

The standard 12-lead ECG consists of 12 leads (or views) of the heart's electrical activity. Six of the leads are called limb leads because the electrodes are placed on the four limbs in the frontal plane. The remaining six leads are called chest (precordial) leads because the electrodes are placed on the chest in the horizontal plane (see Chapter 36).

LIMB LEADS

Standard bipolar limb leads consist of three leads (I, II, and III) that each measure the electrical activity between two points and a fourth lead (right leg) that acts solely as a ground electrode (Table 37-1; see also Chapter 36). Of the three measuring leads, the right arm is always negative, the left leg is always positive, and the left arm can be either positive or negative. Bipolar leads can be obtained by using a monitor with either three or five electrode cables or a 12-lead ECG machine.

Unipolar limb leads consist of a positive electrode only. These leads can be obtained only by using a monitor with four or five electrode cables or a 12-lead ECG machine. The unipolar limb leads are aVR, aVL, and aVF, with *a* meaning augmented. *V* is a designation for a unipolar lead. The third letter denotes the positive electrode placement: *R* for right arm, *L* for left arm, and *F* for foot (left leg). The positive electrode is at one end of the lead axis. The other end is the center of the electrical field, at approximately the center of the heart (see Table 37-1).

CHEST LEADS

Chest (precordial) leads are also unipolar (or V) leads and therefore can be obtained only from a monitor with five electrode cables or a 12-lead ECG machine, which usually has 10 electrode cables. There are six chest leads, determined by the placement of the chest electrode. The four limb electrodes are placed on the extremities, as designated on each electrode (right arm, left arm, right leg, and left leg). The fifth (chest) electrode on a monitor system is the positive, or exploring, electrode and is placed in one of six designated positions to obtain the desired chest lead (see Table 37-1). With a 12-lead ECG, four leads are placed on the limbs and six are placed on the chest, eliminating the need to move any electrodes about the chest.

Positioning of the electrodes is crucial in obtaining an accurate ECG. Comparisons of ECGs taken at different times will be valid only when electrode placement is accurate and identical at each test. Positioning is particularly important when serving clients with chest deformities or large breasts.

TABLE 37-1 Electrode Placement for 12 Leads

Lead	Negative Electrode	Positive Electrode	Ground Electrode
I	Right arm or under the right clavicle	Left arm or under the left clavicle	Right leg or lowest rib, left midclavicular line
II	Right arm or under the right clavicle	Left leg or lowest rib, left midclavicular line	Right leg or under the left clavicle
III	Left arm or under the left clavicle	Left leg or lowest rib, left midclavicular line	Right leg or under the right clavicle
aVR	Average potential of left arm (or under the left clavicle) and left leg (or lowest rib, left midclavicular line)	Right arm or under the right clavicle	Right leg or lowest rib, right midclavicular line
aVL	Average potential of right arm (or under the right clavicle) and left leg (or lowest rib, left midclavicular line)	Left arm or under the left clavicle	Same as for aVR
aVF	Average potential of right arm (or under the right clavicle) and left arm (or under the left clavicle)	Left leg or lowest rib, left midclavicular line	Same as for aVR
V_1	Average potential of right arm, left arm, and left leg	Fourth intercostal space (ICS), right sternal border	Same as for aVR
V_2	Same as for V_1	Fourth ICS, left sternal border	Same as for aVR
V_3	Same as for V_1	Midway between V_2 and V_4	Same as for aVR
V_4	Same as for V_1	Fifth ICS, left midclavicular line	Same as for aVR
V_5	Same as for V_1	Horizontal to V_4, left anterior axillary line	Same as for aVR
V_6	Same as for V_1	Horizontal to V_4, left midaxillary line	Same as for aVR

Clients may be asked to displace the breast to ensure proper electrode placement.

While obtaining a 12-lead ECG, the client should be as still as possible in a semi-reclined position, breathing normally. Any repetitive movement will cause artifact and could lead to inaccurate interpretation of the ECG.

Often nurses are responsible for obtaining 12-lead ECGs, but more commonly technicians are trained to take 12-lead ECGs in various health care settings. It is imperative that the technician notify the nurse or physician of any suspected abnormality. A nurse may direct a technician to take a 12-lead ECG on a client experiencing chest pain to observe for diagnostic changes, but it is ultimately the physician's responsibility to interpret the ECG.

Continuous Electrocardiographic Monitoring

PROCEDURE

For continuous electrocardiographic (ECG) monitoring, the electrodes are not placed on the limbs because movement of the extremities causes "noise," or motion artifact, on the ECG signal. Place the electrodes on the trunk, a more stable area, to minimize such artifacts and to obtain a clearer signal. If the monitoring system provides five electrode cables, place the electrodes as follows:

- Right arm electrode just below the right clavicle
- Left arm electrode just below the left clavicle
- Right leg electrode on the lowest palpable rib, on the right midclavicular line
- Left leg electrode on the lowest palpable rib, on the left midclavicular line
- Fifth electrode placed to obtain one of the six chest leads

With this placement, the monitor lead select control may be changed to provide lead I, II, III, aVR, aVL, or aVF or one chest lead. The monitor automatically alters the polarity of the electrodes to provide the lead selected.

If the monitoring system provides only three electrode cables, place the right arm, the left arm, and the left leg electrodes as described. In this case, the lead selected provides only lead I, II, or III.

The popular MCL_1 lead is a modified *(M)* bipolar chest *(C)* lead. It approximates the V_1 lead without requiring a five-electrode cable monitoring system because it is a bipolar lead system. To obtain MCL_1, place the negative electrode just below the left *(L)* midclavicle and the positive electrode in the V_1 position. The ground electrode can be placed anywhere but is usually placed under the right clavicle. Use this lead for bedside or telemetry monitoring to differentiate left from right electrical activity, such as left from right bundle branch block or left from right premature ventricular complexes, and to differentiate certain supraventricular beats from ventricular ectopic beats. Another bipolar lead, MCL_6, is frequently used. It can be achieved by placing the negative and ground electrodes as for MCL_1 and moving the positive electrode to the V_6 position. This approximates the V_6 lead. It is used for the same reasons as is the MCL_1.

The clarity of continuous ECG monitor recordings is affected by skin preparation and electrode quality. To ensure the best signal transmission and to decrease skin impedance, clean the skin and shave the area if needed. Make sure the area for electrode placement is dry. The gel on each electrode must be moist and fresh. Attach the electrode to the lead cable and then to the contact site. The contact site should be free of any lotion, tincture, or other substance that increases skin impedance. Electrodes cannot be placed on irritated skin or over scar tissue. The application of electrodes may be done by assistive nursing personnel, but the nurse must determine which lead to select and check for correct electrode placement. Assess the quality of the ECG rhythm transmission to the monitoring system, and assess and manage the client.

TELEMETRY

The ECG cables can be attached directly to a wall-mounted monitor (a hard-wired system) if the client's activity is restricted to bedrest and sitting in a chair, as in a critical care unit. For an ambulatory client, the ECG cable is attached to a battery-operated transmitter (a **telemetry** system) held in a pouch worn by the client. The ECG is transmitted via antennae located in strategic places, usually in the ceiling, to a remote monitor. Telemetry allows freedom of movement within a certain radius without losing transmission of the ECG.

Some acute care facilities employ monitor technicians who are educated in ECG rhythm interpretation and are responsible for the following:

- Watching a bank of monitors on a unit
- Printing ECG rhythm strips routinely and as needed
- Interpreting rhythms
- Communicating with the nurse to report the client's rhythm and significant changes

The technical support is particularly helpful on a telemetry unit that does not have monitors at the bedside. The nurse is reasonably assured that the ECG rhythm is being monitored "continuously," although some rhythms will not be observed by technicians. The nurse remains ultimately responsible for accurate ECG rhythm interpretation as well as for client assessment and management.

Some units have full-disclosure monitors, which continuously store ECG rhythms in memory up to a maximum amount of time, allowing nurses and physicians to access and print them for more thorough assessment and management of clients with dysrhythmias. Routine strips, as well as any changes in rhythm, are printed and documented in the client's record.

The physician is responsible for determining when monitoring can be suspended, such as when the client is showering. The health care provider also determines whether monitoring is needed during off-unit testing procedures and for transportation to other facilities. Collaborate with the physician in making these determinations.

Prehospital personnel, such as paramedics and emergency medical technicians (EMTs) with advanced training, frequently monitor a client's ECG rhythm at the scene and en route to a health care facility. They function under medical direction and protocols but may also be in communication with a nurse in the emergency department.

Electrocardiographic Paper

The electrocardiogram (ECG) strip is printed on graph paper (Figure 37-3), with each small block measuring 1 mm in height and width. ECG recorders and monitors are standardized at a speed of 25 mm/sec. Time is measured on the horizontal axis. At this speed, each small block represents 0.04 second. Five small blocks make up one large block, defined by darker bold lines and representing 0.20 second. Five large blocks represent 1 second, and 30 large blocks represent 6 seconds. Vertical lines in the top margin of the graph paper are usually 15 large blocks apart, representing 3-second segments.

Electrocardiographic Complexes, Segments, and Intervals

Complexes that make up a normal ECG consist of a P wave, a QRS complex, a T wave, and possibly a U wave. Segments include the PR segment, the ST segment, and the TP segment. Intervals include the PR interval, the QRS duration, and the QT interval (Figure 37-4).

P WAVE

The **P wave** is a deflection representing atrial depolarization. The shape of the P wave may be a positive, negative, or biphasic deflection, depending on the lead selected. When the electrical impulse is consistently generated from the sinoatrial (SA) node, the P waves have a consistent shape in a given lead. If an impulse is then generated from a different (ectopic) focus, such as atrial tissue, the shape of the P wave changes in that lead, indicating that an ectopic focus has fired.

PR SEGMENT

The **PR segment** is the isoelectric line from the end of the P wave to the beginning of the QRS complex, when the electrical impulse is traveling through the atrioventricular (AV) node, where it is delayed. It then travels through the ventricular conduction system to the Purkinje fibers.

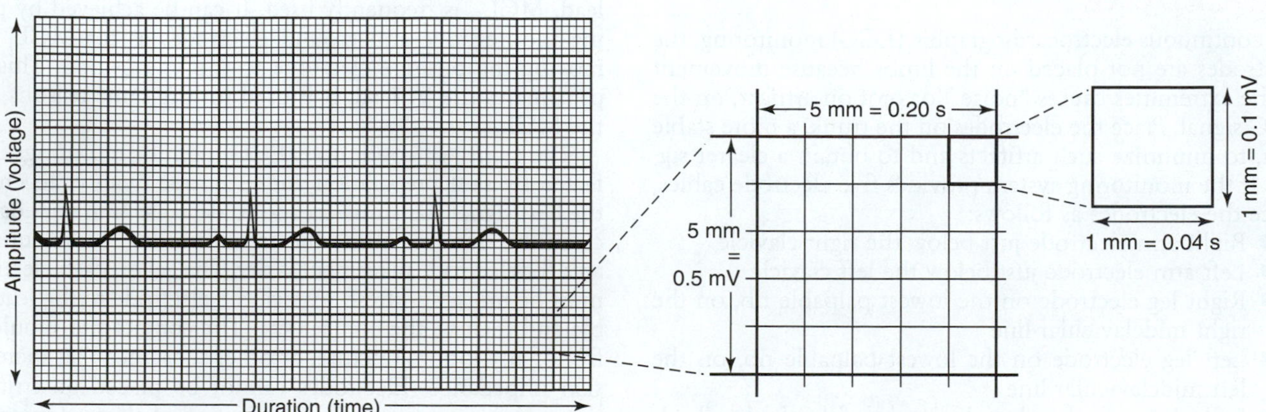

Figure 37-3 ■ Electrocardiographic waveforms are measured in amplitude (voltage) and duration (time).

PR INTERVAL

The **PR interval** is measured from the beginning of the P wave to the end of the PR segment. It represents the time required for atrial depolarization as well as the impulse delay in the AV node and the travel time to the Purkinje fibers. It normally measures from 0.12 to 0.20 second (five small blocks).

QRS COMPLEX

The **QRS complex** represents ventricular depolarization. The shape of the QRS complex depends on the lead selected. The Q wave is the first negative deflection and is not present in all leads. When present, it is small and represents initial ventricular septal depolarization. When the Q wave is abnormally present in a lead, it represents myocardial

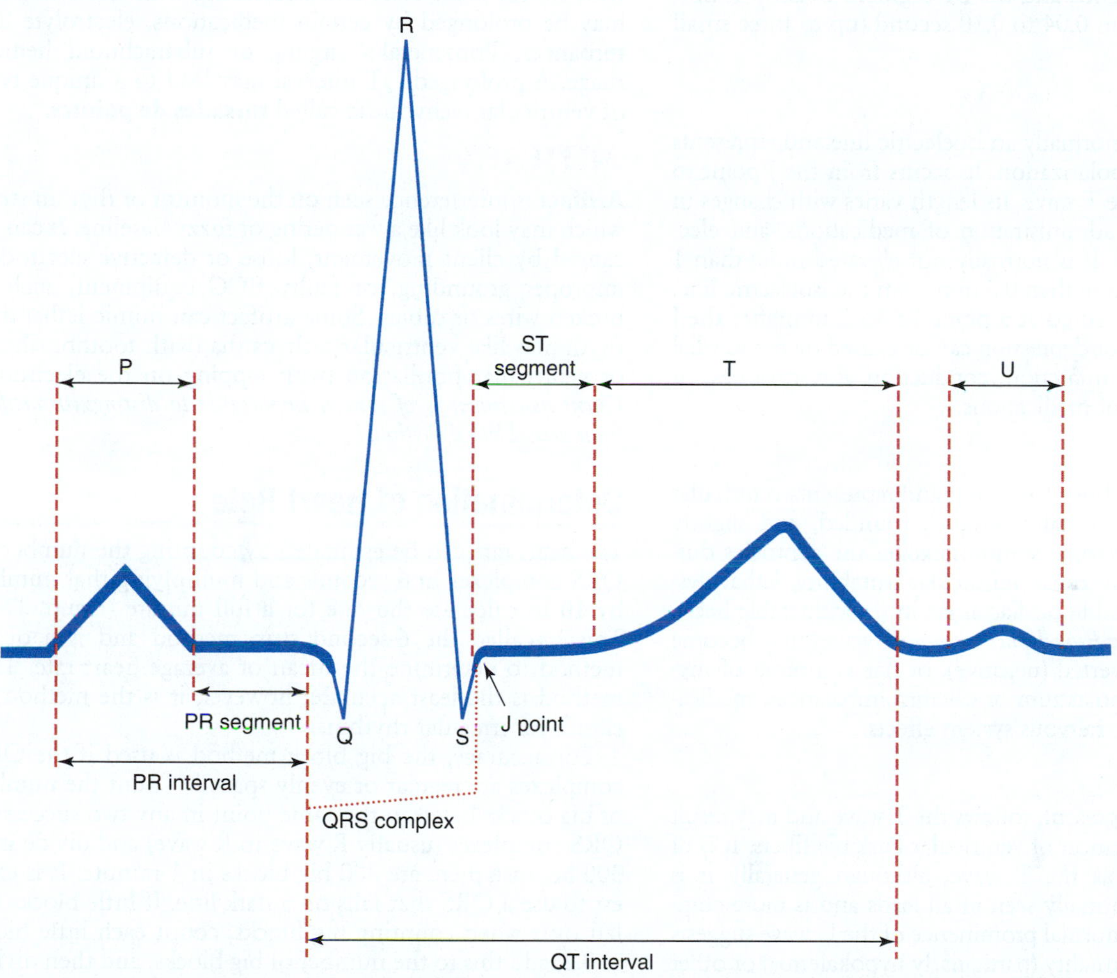

P wave:	Represents atrial depolarization.
PR segment:	Represents the time required for the impulse to travel through the AV node, where it is delayed, and through the bundle of His, bundle branches, and Purkinje fiber network, just before ventricular depolarization.
PR interval:	Represents the time required for atrial depolarization as well as impulse travel through the conduction system and Purkinje fiber network, inclusive of the P wave and PR segment. It is measured from the beginning of the P wave to the end of the PR segment.
QRS complex:	Represents ventricular depolarization and is measured from the beginning of the Q (or R) wave to the end of the S wave.
J point:	Represents the junction where the QRS complex ends and the ST segment begins.
ST segment:	Represents early ventricular repolarization.
T wave:	Represents ventricular repolarization.
U wave:	Represents late ventricular repolarization.
QT interval:	Represents the total time required for ventricular depolarization and repolarization and is measured from the beginning of the QRS complex to the end of the T wave.

Figure 37-4 ■ The components of a normal electrocardiogram.

necrosis (cell death). The R wave is the first positive deflection. It may be small, large, or absent, depending on the lead. The S wave is a negative deflection following the R wave and is not present in all leads.

QRS DURATION

The **QRS duration** represents the time required for depolarization of both ventricles. It is measured from the beginning of the QRS complex to the J point (the junction where the QRS complex ends and the ST segment begins). It normally measures from 0.04 to 0.10 second (up to three small blocks).

ST SEGMENT

The **ST segment** is normally an isoelectric line and represents early ventricular repolarization. It occurs from the J point to the beginning of the T wave. Its length varies with changes in the heart rate, the administration of medications, and electrolyte disturbances. It is normally not elevated more than 1 mm or depressed more than 0.5 mm from the isoelectric line. Its amplitude is measured at a point 1.5 to 2 mm after the J point. ST elevation or depression can be caused by myocardial injury, ischemia or infarction, conduction abnormalities, or the administration of medications.

T WAVE

The **T wave** follows the ST segment and represents ventricular repolarization. It is usually positive, rounded, and slightly asymmetric. If an ectopic stimulus excites the ventricles during this time, it may cause ventricular irritability, lethal dysrhythmias, and possible cardiac arrest in the vulnerable heart. This is known as the *R-on-T phenomenon.* T waves may become tall and peaked, inverted (negative), or flat as a result of myocardial ischemia, potassium or calcium imbalances, medications, or autonomic nervous system effects.

U WAVE

The **U wave,** when present, follows the T wave and may result from slow repolarization of ventricular Purkinje fibers. It is of the same polarity as the T wave, although generally it is smaller. It is not normally seen in all leads and is more common in lead V_3. Abnormal prominence of the U wave suggests an electrolyte abnormality (particularly hypokalemia) or other disturbance. Correct identification is important so that it is not mistaken for a P wave. If in doubt, notify the health care provider and request that a potassium level be obtained.

QT INTERVAL

The **QT interval** represents the total time required for ventricular depolarization and repolarization. The QT interval is measured from the beginning of the QRS complex to the end of the T wave. This interval varies with the client's age and gender and changes with the heart rate, lengthening with slower heart rates and shortening with faster rates. It may be prolonged by certain medications, electrolyte disturbances, Prinzmetal's angina, or subarachnoid hemorrhage. A prolonged QT interval may lead to a unique type of ventricular tachycardia called **torsades de pointes.**

ARTIFACT

Artifact is interference seen on the monitor or rhythm strip, which may look like a wandering or fuzzy baseline. It can be caused by client movement, loose or defective electrodes, improper grounding, or faulty ECG equipment, such as broken wires or cables. Some artifact can mimic lethal dysrhythmias like ventricular tachycardia (with toothbrushing) or ventricular fibrillation (with tapping on the electrode). *Client assessment is of utmost importance to distinguish artifact from actual lethal rhythms!*

Determination of Heart Rate

The heart rate can be estimated by counting the number of QRS complexes in 6 seconds and multiplying that number by 10 to calculate the rate for a full minute (Figure 37-5). This is called the 6-second strip method and is a quick method to determine the mean or average heart rate. This method is the least accurate; however, it is the method of choice for irregular rhythms.

For accuracy, the big block method is used if the QRS complexes are regular or evenly spaced. Count the number of big blocks between the same point in any two successive QRS complexes (usually R wave to R wave) and divide into 300 because there are 300 big blocks in 1 minute. It is easiest to use a QRS that falls on a dark line. If little blocks are left over when counting big blocks, count each little block as 0.2, add this to the number of big blocks, and then divide by 300 (Figure 37-6).

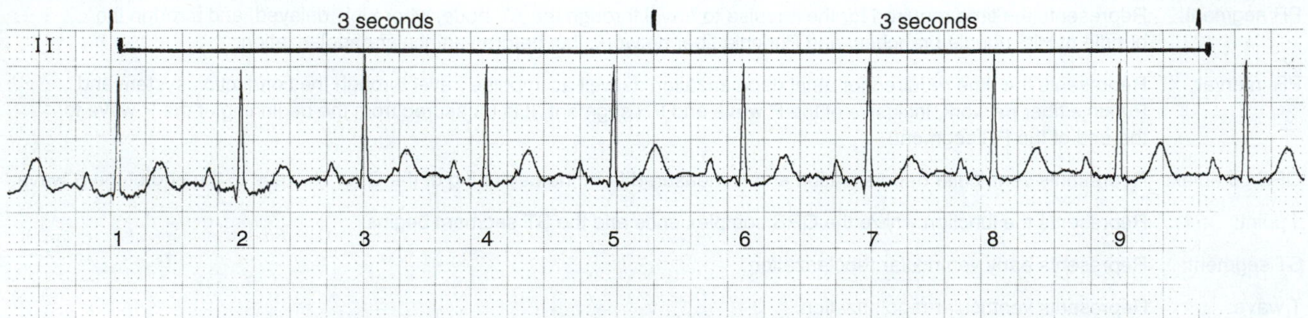

Figure 37-5 ■ Each segment between the dark lines (above the monitor strip) represents 3 seconds when the monitor is set at a speed of 25 mm/sec. To estimate the ventricular rate, count the QRS complexes in a 6-second strip and then multiply that number by 10 to estimate the rate for 1 minute. In this example, there are 9 QRS complexes in 6 seconds. Therefore the heart rate can be estimated to be 90 beats/min.

Count the number of large blocks in an interval and divide into 300 (the number of large blocks in 1 minute). For example, three large blocks equals a heart rate of 100 beats/min (300/3 = 100).

Another method (called the memory method) relies on memorization of the following sequence: 300, 150, 100, 75, 60, 50, 43, 37, 33, 30. This is the big block method with the math already done. Find a QRS complex that falls on the dark line representing 0.2 second or a big block, and count backwards to the next QRS complex. Each dark line is a memorized number. This is the method most widely used in hospitals for calculating heart rates for regular rhythms.

Commercially prepared electrocardiogram (ECG) rate rulers are based on these calculations and may be used for regular rhythms. Current monitoring systems will display a continuous heart rate and print the heart rate on the ECG strip. Use caution and confirm that the rate is correct by assessing the client's heart rate directly. Many factors can incorrectly alter the rate displayed by the monitor.

Electrocardiographic Rhythm Analysis

Analysis of an ECG rhythm strip requires a systematic approach using a five-step method facilitated by use of a measurement tool called an **ECG caliper** (Chart 37-1):

1. ***Determine the heart rate.*** If the atrial and ventricular rhythms are regular, the nurse may use any of the methods previously described to calculate the heart rate. If the rhythms are irregular, the nurse must use the 6-second strip method for accuracy. Normal heart rates fall between 60 and 100 beats/min. If the rate is less than 60 beats/min, this is **bradycardia.** If the rate is greater than 100 beats/min, this is **tachycardia.**
2. ***Determine the heart rhythm.*** Heart rhythms can be either regular or irregular. Irregular rhythms can be regularly irregular, occasionally irregular, or irregularly irregular. Check the regularity of the atrial rhythm by assessing the P-P intervals, placing one caliper point on a P wave, and placing the other point on the precise spot on the next P wave. Then move the caliper from P wave to P wave along the entire strip ("walking out" the P waves) to determine the regularity of the rhythm. P waves of a different shape (ectopic waves), if present, create an irregularity and do not walk out with the other P waves. A slight irregularity in the P-P intervals, varying no more than three small blocks, is considered essentially regular if the P waves are all of the same shape. This alteration is caused by changes in intrathoracic pressure during the respiratory cycle.

   Check the regularity of the ventricular rhythm by assessing the R-R intervals, placing one caliper point on a portion of the QRS complex (usually the most prominent portion of the deflection) and the other point on the precise spot of the next QRS complex. Move the caliper from QRS complex to QRS complex along the entire strip (walking out the QRS complexes) to determine the regularity of the rhythm. QRS complexes of a different shape (ectopic QRS complexes), if present, create an irregularity and do not "walk out" with the other QRS complexes. A slight irregularity of no more than three small blocks between intervals is considered essentially regular if the QRS complexes are all of the same shape.
3. ***Analyze the P waves.*** Check that the P-wave shape is consistent throughout the strip, indicating that atrial depolarization is occurring from impulses originating from one focus, normally the SA node. Determine whether there is one P wave occurring before each QRS complex, establishing that a relationship exists between the P wave and the QRS complex. This relationship indicates that

CHART 37-1

BEST PRACTICE for
Electrocardiographic Rhythm Analysis

1. Determine the heart rate.
2. Determine the heart rhythm.
3. Analyze the P waves.
4. Measure the P-R interval.
5. Measure the QRS duration.
6. Interpret the rhythm.

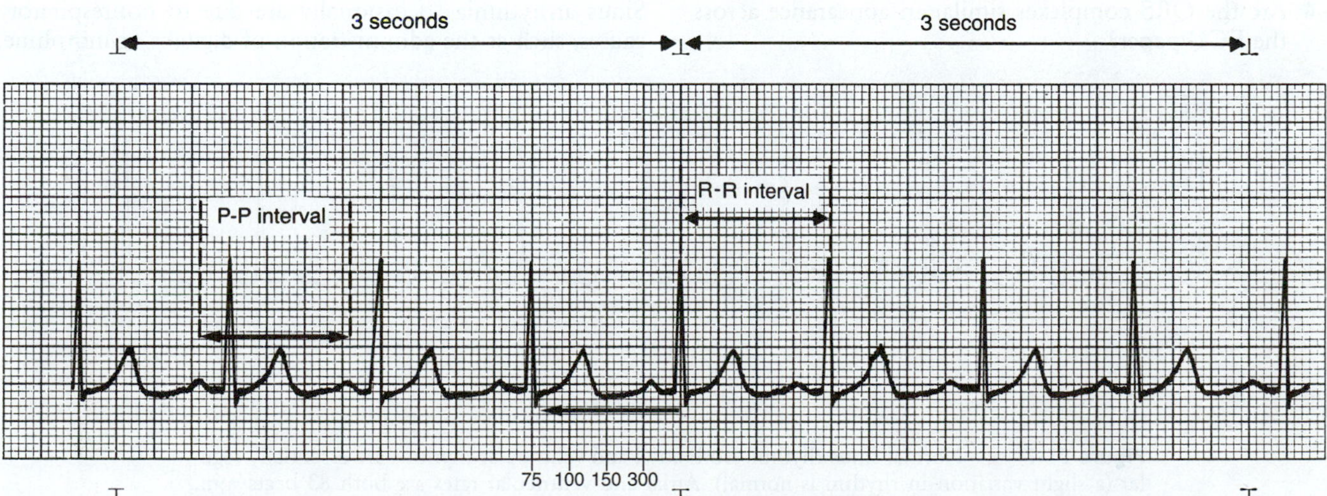

Figure 37-6 ■ In this example, the heart rate using the big block method is 300 ÷ 4 big blocks (between QRS complexes), or 75 beats/min. The memory method is also demonstrated with a heart rate of 75 beats/min.

an impulse from one focus is responsible for both atrial and ventricular depolarization. The nurse may observe more than one P wave shape, more P waves than QRS complexes, absent P waves, or P waves coming after the QRS, each indicating that a dysrhythmia exists. Ask these five questions when analyzing P waves:

- Are P waves present?
- Are the P waves occurring regularly?
- Is there one P wave for each QRS complex?
- Are the P waves smooth, rounded and upright in appearance, or are they inverted?
- Do all the P waves look similar?

4. *Measure the PR interval.* Place one caliper point at the beginning of the P wave and the other point at the end of the PR segment. The PR interval normally measures between 0.12 and 0.20 second. The measurement should be constant throughout the strip. The PR interval is unable to be determined if there are no P waves or if P waves occur after the QRS complex. Ask these three questions about the PR interval:
   - Are PR intervals greater than 0.20 second?
   - Are PR intervals less than 0.12 second?
   - Are PR intervals constant across the ECG strip?
5. *Measure the QRS duration.* Place one caliper point at the beginning of the QRS complex and the other at the J point, where the QRS complex ends and the ST segment begins. The QRS duration normally measures between 0.04 and 0.10 second. The measurement should be constant throughout the entire strip. Check that the QRS complexes are consistent throughout the strip. When the QRS is narrow (0.10 second or less), this indicates that the impulse was not formed in the ventricles and is referred to as supraventricular or "above the ventricles." When the QRS complex is wide (greater than 0.10 second), this indicates that the impulse is either of ventricular origin or of supraventricular origin with aberrant conduction, meaning deviating from the normal course or pattern. More than one QRS complex pattern or occasionally missing QRS complexes may be observed, indicating a dysrhythmia. Ask these questions to evaluate QRS intervals:
   - Are QRS intervals less than or greater than 0.12 second?
   - Are the QRS complexes similar in appearance across the ECG paper?
6. *Interpret the rhythm.* Using these rules, you can interpret the cardiac rhythm and differentiate normal and abnormal cardiac rhythms.

NORMAL RHYTHMS

Normal Sinus Rhythm

Normal sinus rhythm (NSR) is the rhythm originating from the sinoatrial (SA) node (dominant pacemaker) that meets the following electrocardiographic (ECG) criteria (Figure 37-7):

- *Rate:* Atrial and ventricular rates of 60 to 100 beats/min
- *Rhythm:* Atrial and ventricular rhythms regular
- *P waves:* Present, consistent configuration, one P wave before each QRS complex
- *PR interval:* 0.12 to 0.20 second and constant
- *QRS duration:* 0.04 to 0.10 second and constant

Sinus Arrhythmia

Sinus arrhythmia is a variant of NSR. It results from changes in intrathoracic pressure during breathing. In this context the term *arrhythmia* does not denote an absence of rhythm, as the term suggests. Instead, the heart rate increases slightly during inspiration and decreases slightly during exhalation. This irregular rhythm is frequently observed in healthy children as well as adults.

Sinus arrhythmia has all the characteristics of NSR except for its irregularity. The P-P and R-R intervals vary, with the difference between the shortest and the longest intervals being greater than 0.12 second (three small blocks):

- *Rate:* Atrial and ventricular rates are between 60 and 100 beats/min.
- *Rhythm:* Atrial and ventricular rhythms are irregular, with the shortest P-P or R-R interval varying at least 0.12 second from the longest P-P or R-R interval.
- *P waves:* One P wave before each QRS complex; consistent configuration.
- *PR interval:* Normal, constant.
- *QRS duration:* Normal, constant.

Sinus arrhythmias occasionally are due to nonrespiratory causes, such as the administration of digitalis or morphine.

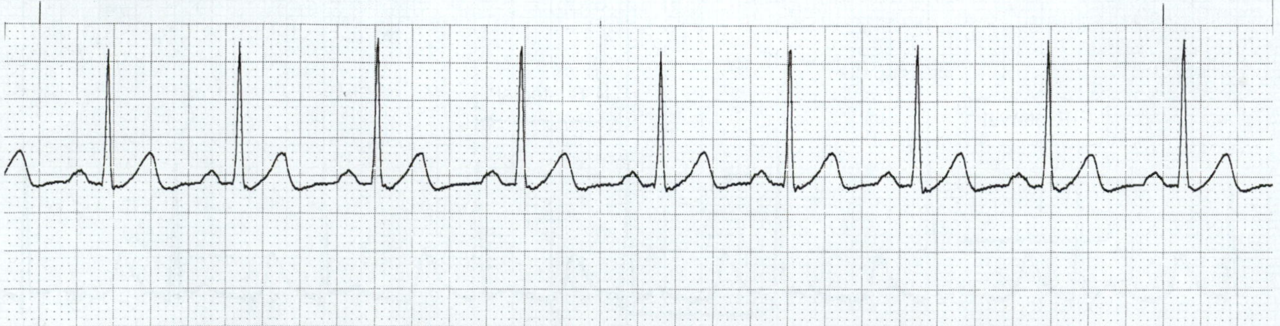

Figure 37-7 ■ Normal sinus rhythm. Both atrial and ventricular rhythms are essentially regular (a slight variation in rhythm is normal). Atrial and ventricular rates are both 83 beats/min. There is one P wave before each QRS complex, and all the P waves are of a consistent morphology, or shape. The PR interval measures 0.18 second and is constant; the QRS complex measures 0.06 second and is constant.

These drugs enhance vagal tone and cause decreased heart rate and irregularity unrelated to the respiratory cycle.

DYSRHYTHMIAS

OVERVIEW

Any disorder of the heartbeat uses the term *dysrhythmia.* Historically, the term **arrhythmia** has been used in the literature; however, it means an absence of cardiac rhythm. Although the terms are often used interchangeably, **dysrhythmia,** which means a disturbance in cardiac rhythm, is more accurate.

Dysrhythmias result from the following:

- A disturbance in the relationship between electrical conductivity and the mechanical response of the myocardium
- A disturbance in impulse formation (either from an abnormal rate or from an ectopic focus)
- A disturbance in impulse conduction (delays and blocks)
- The combination of several mechanisms

Although many dysrhythmias have no clinical manifestations, many others have serious consequences. A summary of key features is provided in Chart 37-2.

Dysrhythmia Terminology

TACHYDYSRHYTHMIAS

Tachydysrhythmias are heart rates greater than 100 beats/min. These rhythms may have serious hemodynamic consequences in the adult client with coronary artery disease (CAD). Coronary artery blood flow occurs predominantly during diastole, when the aortic valve is closed, and is determined by diastolic time and blood pressure in the root of the aorta. The following three points are important to understanding and appreciating the seriousness of tachydysrhythmias:

- Tachydysrhythmias shorten the diastolic time and therefore the coronary perfusion time (the amount of time available for blood to flow through the coronary arteries to the myocardium).
- Tachydysrhythmias initially increase cardiac output and blood pressure. However, a continued rise in heart rate decreases the ventricular filling time because of a shortened diastole, decreasing the stroke volume. Consequently, cardiac output and blood pressure will begin to decrease, reducing aortic pressure and therefore coronary perfusion pressure.
- Tachydysrhythmias increase the work of the heart, increasing myocardial oxygen demand.

The client with a tachydysrhythmia may have palpitations; chest discomfort; pressure or pain from myocardial ischemia or infarction; restlessness; anxiety; pale, cool skin; and syncope from hypotension. Tachydysrhythmias may also lead to heart failure. Presenting symptoms of heart failure may include dyspnea, orthopnea, pulmonary crackles, distended neck veins, fatigue, and weakness (see Chapter 38).

CHART 37-2

KEY FEATURES of
Sustained Tachydysrhythmias and Bradydysrhythmias

- Chest discomfort, pressure, or pain, which may radiate to the jaw, the back, or the arm
- Restlessness, anxiety, nervousness, confusion
- Dizziness, syncope
- Palpitations (in tachydysrhythmias)
- Change in pulse strength, rate, and rhythm
- Pulse deficit
- Shortness of breath, dyspnea
- Tachypnea
- Pulmonary crackles
- Orthopnea
- S_3 or S_4 heart sounds
- Jugular venous distention
- Weakness, fatigue
- Pale, cool, skin; diaphoresis
- Nausea, vomiting
- Decreased urine output
- Delayed capillary refill
- Hypotension

BRADYDYSRHYTHMIAS

Bradydysrhythmias are characterized by a heart rate less than 60 beats/min. These rhythms can also have serious hemodynamic consequences. Consider the following three points:

- Myocardial oxygen demand is reduced from the slow heart rate, which is beneficial.
- Coronary perfusion time may be adequate because of a prolonged diastole, which is desirable.
- Coronary perfusion pressure may decrease if the heart rate is too slow to provide adequate cardiac output and blood pressure; this is a serious consequence.

Therefore the client may tolerate the bradydysrhythmia well if the blood pressure is adequate. If the blood pressure is not adequate, symptomatic bradydysrhythmias may lead to myocardial ischemia or infarction, dysrhythmias, hypotension, and heart failure.

PREMATURE COMPLEXES

Premature complexes are early complexes. They occur when a cardiac cell or cell group, other than the sinoatrial (SA) node, becomes irritable and fires an impulse before the next sinus impulse is generated. The abnormal focus is called an *ectopic focus* and may be generated by atrial, junctional, or ventricular tissue. Following the premature complex, there is a pause before the next normal complex, creating an irregularity in the rhythm. The client with premature complexes may be unaware of them or may feel palpitations or a "skipping" of the heartbeat. If premature complexes, especially those that are ventricular, become more frequent, the client may experience symptoms of decreased cardiac output.

REPETITIVE RHYTHMS

Premature complexes may occur repetitively in a rhythmic fashion:

- **Bigeminy** exists when normal complexes and premature complexes occur alternately in a repetitive two-beat pattern, with a pause occurring after each premature complex so that complexes occur in pairs.
- **Trigeminy** is a repetitive three-beat pattern, usually occurring as two sequential normal complexes followed by a premature complex and a pause, with the same pattern repeating itself in triplets.

- **Quadrigeminy** is a repetitive four-beat pattern, usually occurring as three sequential normal complexes followed by a premature complex and a pause, with the same pattern repeating itself in a four-beat pattern.

Such patterns may occur with atrial, junctional, or ventricular premature complexes. Clients may be unaware of the premature beats, or they may feel palpitations.

ESCAPE COMPLEXES AND RHYTHMS

Escape complexes or escape rhythms may occur when the SA node fails to discharge or is blocked or when a sinus impulse fails to depolarize the ventricles because of an atrioventricular (AV) nodal block. Escape complexes or rhythms serve as a secondary or escape pacemaker and are seen after a pause. Such impulses may originate from AV junctional or ventricular tissue. They cease when the SA node or the AV node regains the ability to function normally. If there are pauses followed by escape beats or rhythms, clients may feel light-headed, dizzy, or faint during the pause.

Classification of Dysrhythmias

Dysrhythmias are classified according to their site of origin. The sites include the SA node, atrial tissue, AV node, junctional tissue, and ventricular tissue. Dysrhythmias may be caused by a disturbance in impulse formation or by conduction delays or blocks. The incidence and the prevalence of dysrhythmias are not precisely known because they usually result from an underlying condition, such as heart disease. The incidence of dysrhythmias increases with age. A summary of the common dysrhythmias and their treatment is provided in Table 37-2.

SINUS DYSRHYTHMIAS

The sinus node is the **pacemaker** in all sinus dysrhythmias. Innervation from sympathetic and parasympathetic nerve fibers is normally in balance to ensure a normal sinus rhythm (NSR). An imbalance increases or decreases the rate of SA node discharge either as a normal response to activity or physiologic changes or as a pathologic response to disease.

SINUS TACHYCARDIA

PATHOPHYSIOLOGY. Dominant sympathetic nervous system stimulation of the heart or vagal inhibition results in an increased rate of SA node discharge, which increases the heart rate.

When the rate of SA node discharge exceeds 100 beats/min, the rhythm is called **sinus tachycardia** (Figure 37-8, *A*). Sinus tachycardia, with heart rates of 200 to 220 beats/min, is normal in infants and children. The rate gradually decreases until age 10 years. From age 10 years to adulthood, the heart rate normally does not exceed 100 beats/min except in response to activity and then usually does not exceed 160 beats/min. Rarely the heart rate reaches 180 beats/min. Sinus tachycardia initially enhances cardiac output and blood pressure. However, sustained increases in heart rate decrease coronary perfusion time, diastolic filling time, and coronary perfusion pressure while increasing myocardial oxygen demand.

Increased sympathetic stimulation is a normal response to physical activity but may also be caused by anxiety, pain,

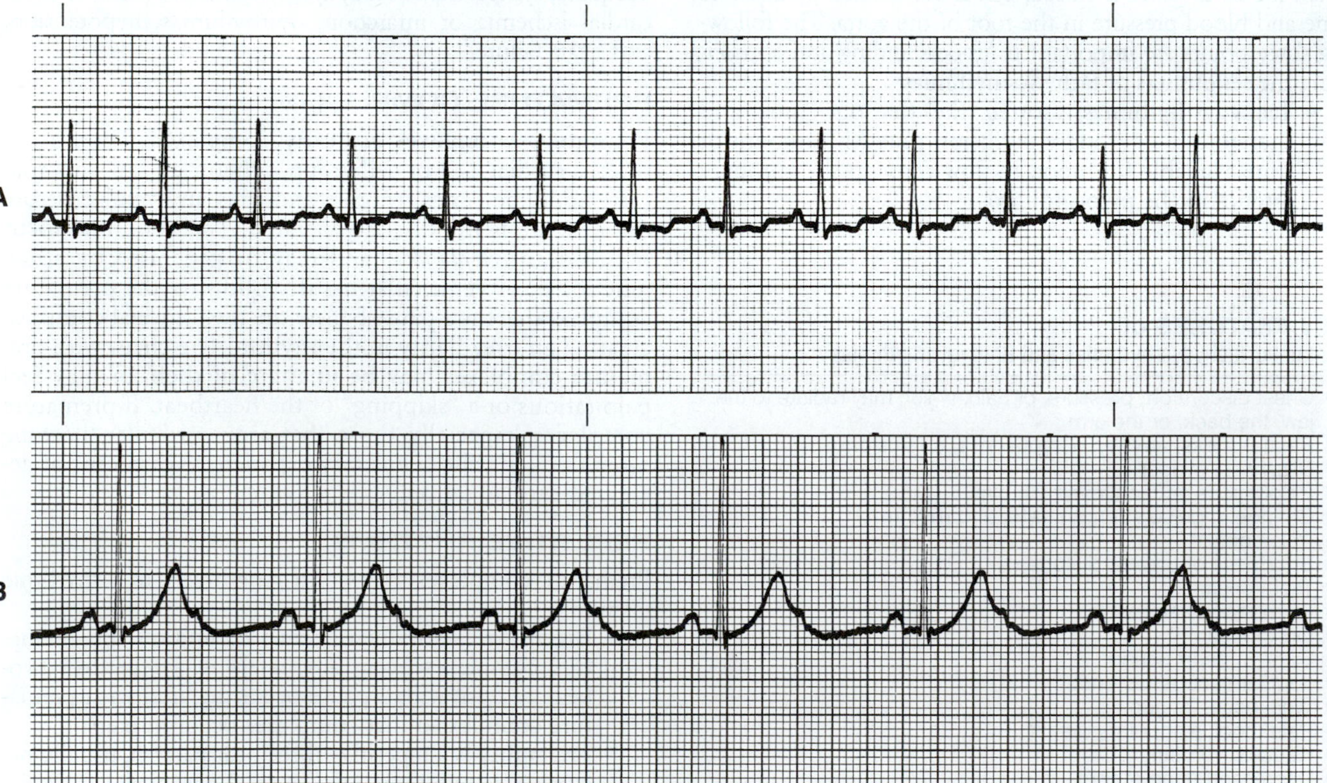

Figure 37-8 ■ Sinus rhythms. **A,** Sinus tachycardia (heart rate, 110 beats/min; PR interval, 0.12 second; QRS complex, 0.08 second). **B,** Sinus bradycardia (heart rate, 52 beats/min; PR interval, 0.18 second; QRS complex, 0.08 second).

TABLE 37-2 Common Dysrhythmias and Their Treatment

Dysrhythmia	Treatment
Sinus tachycardia	Correction of the underlying problem (e.g., fever, hypovolemia, pain, anxiety, or CHF) Beta-adrenergic blockade if increased catecholamine secretion is the underlying problem
Sinus bradycardia	Treatment is necessary only if the client is symptomatic (has hypotension, diaphoresis, chest discomfort or pain, pulmonary congestion, or altered level of consciousness) ▪ Atropine ▪ Pacemaker ▪ Avoidance of parasympathetic stimulation, such as prolonged suctioning or stimulation of the gag reflex
Premature Beats and Ectopic Rhythms	
Supraventricular beats (PACs, PJCs)	Correction of any underlying problem (e.g., anxiety, stress, caffeine or nicotine intake, CHF, effects of drugs, COPD, or asthma) Medication administration ▪ Propranolol ▪ Sedatives
Supraventricular rhythms	Correction of any underlying problem (e.g., CHF, COPD, asthma, stress, or drugs) Medication administration ▪ Diltiazem ▪ Adenosine ▪ Digitalis ▪ Propranolol ▪ Esmolol ▪ Amiodarone Vagal stimulation with carotid massage Valsalva maneuvers Overdrive atrial pacing Synchronized cardioversion if the above measures are unsuccessful
Premature ventricular complexes and ventricular tachycardia (not sustained)	Correction of any underlying problem (e.g., infection, electrolyte imbalance, effects of drugs, myocardial infarction, hypoxia CHF, stress, fatigue, or nicotine) Medication administration ▪ Lidocaine bolus and infusion ▪ Procainamide bolus and infusion ▪ Magnesium sulfate infusion ▪ Class I and II antidysrhythmics ▪ Amiodarone Restoration of electrolyte balance
Atrial flutter	Medication administration ▪ Diltiazem ▪ Amiodarone ▪ Propranolol ▪ Esmolol ▪ Ibutilide ▪ Digitalis Atrial overdrive pacing Cardioversion Catheter or surgical ablation
Atrial fibrillation	Medication administration ▪ Amiodarone ▪ Diltiazem ▪ Ibutilide ▪ Verapamil Anticoagulation Atrial overdrive pacing Cardioversion Surgery
Escape beats and rhythms	Correction of the underlying cause if the client is symptomatic Atropine administration Pacemaker Isoproterenol administration if pacemaker unavailable
Conduction Delays	
First-degree AV block	Treatment necessary only if the client is symptomatic Withhold digitalis (if the cause) Atropine administration if block is associated with symptomatic bradycardia
Second-degree AV block type I	Same as for first-degree AV block
Second-degree AV block type II	Pacemaker Isoproterenol administration if pacemaker unavailable
Third-degree AV block	Pacemaker Isoproterenol administration if pacemaker unavailable
Life-Threatening Dysrhythmias	
Sustained ventricular tachycardia	Medication administration ▪ Lidocaine bolus and infusion ▪ Procainamide bolus and infusion ▪ Amiodarone ▪ Magnesium sulfate infusion If unstable: synchronized cardioversion If pulseless: defibrillation, CPR
Ventricular fibrillation	Defibrillation CPR Medication administration ▪ Vasopressin ▪ Epinephrine ▪ Amiodarone ▪ Magnesium sulfate
Ventricular asystole	CPR Medication administration ▪ Epinephrine ▪ Atropine ▪ Pacemaker

AV, atrioventricular; *CHF*, congestive heart failure; *COPD*, chronic obstructive pulmonary disease; *CPR*, cardiopulmonary resuscitation; *PACs*, premature atrial complexes; *PJCs*, premature junctional complexes.

stress, fear, fever, anemia, hypoxemia, hyperthyroidism, and pulmonary embolism. Drugs such as catecholamines, atropine, caffeine, alcohol, nicotine, aminophylline, and thyroid medications may also increase the heart rate. In some cases, sinus tachycardia is a compensatory response to decreased cardiac output or blood pressure, as occurs in hypovolemia, shock, myocardial infarction (MI), and heart failure.

PHYSICAL ASSESSMENT/CLINICAL MANIFESTATIONS. The client may be asymptomatic except for the increased pulse rate. However, if the rhythm is not well tolerated, he or she may become symptomatic. Assess for fatigue, weakness, shortness of breath, orthopnea, neck vein distention, decreased oxygen saturation, and decreased blood pressure. Also assess for restlessness and anxiety from decreased cerebral perfusion and for decreased urine output from decreased renal perfusion. The adult client may also experience anginal pain and palpitations. The electrocardiographic (ECG) pattern may show T-wave inversion or ST-segment elevation or depression in response to myocardial ischemia.

INTERVENTIONS. Collaborate with the health care provider to identify the cause of sinus tachycardia and select the appropriate treatment. The goal is to decrease the heart rate to normal levels by treating the underlying cause. For example, if the client has angina, administer oxygen, help the client to rest, and administer nitroglycerin or morphine as prescribed. Diuretics and inotropic agents may be given for heart failure. Initiate intravascular volume replacement for hypovolemia, administer antipyretics and antibiotics to the client with fever and infection, or provide comfort measures and administer analgesics or opioids to the client with noncardiac pain, as prescribed. Maintain the client on bedrest if the tachycardia is causing hypotension or weakness.

Collaborate with the respiratory therapist, when indicated, to oxygenate and suction the client with hypoxemia from excessive airway secretions. Beta-adrenergic blocking agents may also be prescribed for the client with inappropriate sympathetic nervous system stimulation. Emotional support and relevant teaching are important for the client and family.

SINUS BRADYCARDIA

PATHOPHYSIOLOGY. Dominance of the parasympathetic nervous system, with excessive vagal stimulation to the heart, causes a decreased rate of sinus node discharge. This slows the heart rate and decreases the speed of conduction through the AV node and conduction system. When the rate of sinus node discharge is less than 60 beats/min in adults or lower, the normal range in infants and children, the rhythm is called **sinus bradycardia** (Figure 37-8, *B*). Sinus bradycardia increases coronary perfusion time, but it may decrease coronary perfusion pressure. However, myocardial oxygen demand is decreased.

Increased parasympathetic stimulation of the heart by the vagus nerve is a normal response to decreased physical activity. It also often occurs in well-conditioned athletes because the strong heart muscle is extremely efficient in providing an adequate stroke volume while not requiring a higher heart rate for a normal cardiac output. Excessive vagal stimulation may result from carotid sinus massage, vomiting, suctioning, Valsalva maneuvers (e.g., bearing down for a bowel movement or gagging), ocular pressure, or pain. Sinus bradycardia may also result from hypoxia, inferior wall MI, and the administration of drugs such as beta-adrenergic blocking agents, calcium channel blockers, and digitalis.

PHYSICAL ASSESSMENT/CLINICAL MANIFESTATIONS. The client may be asymptomatic except for the decreased pulse rate. At times, however, the rhythm may not be well tolerated. Assess the client for dizziness, weakness, syncope, confusion, hypotension, diaphoresis (excessive sweating), shortness of breath, ventricular ectopy (superficial beats), and anginal pain. T-wave inversion or ST-segment elevation or depression may occur in response to myocardial ischemia.

INTERVENTIONS. If the client is symptomatic and the underlying cause cannot be determined, the treatment of choice is atropine administration, given as prescribed to increase the heart rate to about 60 beats/min. Oxygen should be applied. If the heart rate does not increase sufficiently, an external pacemaker may be applied to increase the heart rate. However, if atropine administration succeeds in achieving an adequate heart rate but the client remains hypotensive, initiate intravascular volume replacement as prescribed rather than administering another dose of atropine. Excessive atropine may induce tachycardia and myocardial ischemia. If a medication is suspected to be the cause, withhold the drug and notify the physician.

Critical Thinking Challenge

During physical assessment class you find your female nursing student partner, who is on the track team, has an apical pulse of 44 beats/min with a regular heart rhythm. She states she sometimes has chest pain and shortness of breath after running.

1. What other assessment data are needed?
2. What cardiac dysrhythmia is expected on the ECG recording?
3. Does this dysrhythmia need treatment? Why or why not?

evolve For suggested answer guidelines, go to http://evolve.elsevier.com/Iggy/.

ATRIAL DYSRHYTHMIAS

With atrial dysrhythmias, the focus of impulse generation shifts away from the sinus node to the atrial tissue, which acts as an ectopic pacemaker for one or more beats. The shift changes the axis (direction) of atrial depolarization, resulting in a P-wave shape that differs from that of P waves with a sinus node origin. The most common atrial dysrhythmias are premature atrial complexes, supraventricular tachycardia, atrial flutter, and atrial fibrillation.

PREMATURE ATRIAL COMPLEXES

PATHOPHYSIOLOGY. A **premature atrial complex (PAC)** occurs when atrial tissue becomes irritable. This ectopic focus fires an impulse before the next sinus impulse is due, thus usurping the sinus pacemaker (Figure 37-9). The premature P wave from the atrial focus is early and has a shape different from that of the P wave generated from the sinus node. The premature P wave may not always be clearly visible because it can be hidden in the preceding T wave. The T wave must be closely examined for any change in shape and compared with other T waves to reveal a hidden P wave. A PAC is usually followed by a pause.

The causes of atrial irritability include stress; fatigue; anxiety; inflammation; infection; intake of caffeine, nicotine, or alcohol; and the administration of drugs such as cate-

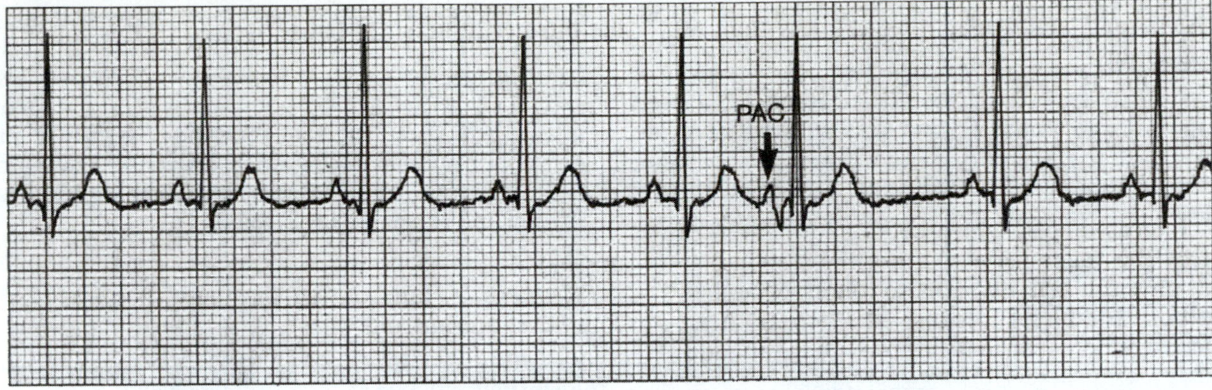

Figure 37-9 ■ Normal sinus rhythm with a premature atrial complex (PAC) at arrow.

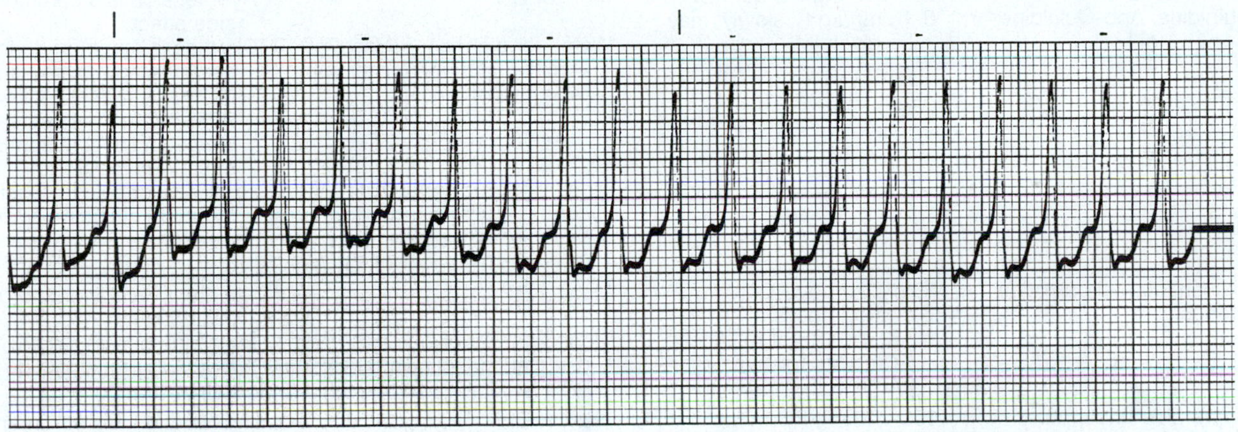

Figure 37-10 ■ Sustained supraventricular tachycardia in a client with Wolff-Parkinson-White syndrome. Heart rate is 200 beats/min.

cholamines, sympathomimetics, amphetamines, digitalis, or anesthetic agents. PACs may also result from myocardial ischemia, hypermetabolic states, electrolyte imbalance, or atrial stretch, as may occur with congestive heart failure, valvular disease, and pulmonary hypertension with cor pulmonale.

PHYSICAL ASSESSMENT/CLINICAL MANIFESTATIONS. The client is usually asymptomatic except for possible heart palpitations because PACs usually have no hemodynamic consequences.

INTERVENTIONS. No intervention is usually needed except to treat the cause, such as heart failure or valvular disease. If PACs occur frequently, they may signal the onset of more serious atrial tachydysrhythmias and therefore may warrant treatment. Administration of prescribed type IA antidysrhythmics or other drugs may be warranted. Teach the client measures to manage stress and substances to avoid that are known to increase atrial irritability.

SUPRAVENTRICULAR TACHYCARDIA

PATHOPHYSIOLOGY. Supraventricular tachycardia (SVT) involves the rapid stimulation of atrial tissue at a rate of 100 to 280 beats/min, with a mean of 170 beats/min in adults (Figure 37-10) and 200 to 300 beats/min in children. SVT is most often due to a re-entry mechanism in which one impulse circulates repeatedly throughout the atrial pathway, restimulating the atrial tissue at a rapid rate. The term **paroxysmal supraventricular tachycardia (PSVT)** is used when the rhythm is intermittent, initiated suddenly by a premature complex such as a PAC, and terminated suddenly with or without intervention.

During SVT the P waves have a shape different from that of sinus P waves. The P waves may not be visible, especially if there is a 1:1 conduction with rapid rates because the P waves are embedded in the preceding T wave.

The causes of SVT are the same as those for PACs. SVT may occur in healthy young people without evidence of heart disease, especially women under 40 years of age. The condition commonly occurs in clients with a pre-excitation syndrome, such as **Wolff-Parkinson-White (WPW) syndrome.**

PHYSICAL ASSESSMENT/CLINICAL MANIFESTATIONS. The clinical manifestations depend on the duration of the SVT and the rate of the ventricular response. In clients with a sustained rapid ventricular response, assess for palpitations, weakness, fatigue, shortness of breath, nervousness, anxiety, hypotension, and syncope. Hemodynamic deterioration may occur if the rate does not sustain adequate blood pressure. In that case SVT can result in angina, heart failure, and shock. With a nonsustained or slower ventricular response, the client may be asymptomatic except for transient palpitations.

INTERVENTIONS. If SVT occurs in a healthy person and terminates spontaneously, no intervention is necessary other than eliminating identified causative factors. If it is recurrent, the client should be studied in the electrophysiology laboratory. The preferred treatment for recurrent SVT is radiofrequency catheter ablation. In sustained SVT with a rapid ventricular response, the goals of treatment are to decrease the ventricular response, convert the dysrhythmia to a sinus rhythm, and treat the cause. Vagal stimulation (e.g., carotid massage) may be successful, but often only transiently, and must be performed only by a physician.

Administer oxygen and prescribed antidysrhythmic drugs, such as diltiazem (Cardizem), which slow the ventricular rate by increasing the AV block (Chart 37-3). Some may also succeed in converting the dysrhythmia. In the severely compromised client, the nurse may assist the physician in attempting atrial overdrive pacing or in delivering a synchronized electrical shock (cardioversion) to re-establish an organized rhythm and regain cardiac stability.

CHART 37-3

DRUG THERAPY for Dysrhythmias

Drug	Usual Dosage	Nursing Interventions	Rationales
Class I Drugs			
Type IA			
Quinidine sulfate (quinidine, Apo-Quinidine✱)	300-600 mg PO q8-12h 6-10 mg/kg IV slowly; may be given IM	Monitor BP.	Hypotension is a common side effect.
		Watch for diarrhea, nausea, or vomiting and administer with food if these occur.	Diarrhea is common during early therapy. Diarrhea and other gastrointestinal symptoms often decrease when quinidine is administered with food.
		Monitor for widening QRS complex, prolonged QT interval, heart block, onset or increase in number of PVCs.	Toxic side effects necessitate stopping quinidine administration.
Procainamide hydrochloride (Pronestyl)	50 mg/kg/day PO in 4 divided doses 20-30 mg IV, not to exceed 17 mg/kg, followed by infusion of 1-4 mg/min	Monitor BP.	Hypotension warrants drug discontinuation.
		Monitor for widening QRS complex, prolonged QT or PR interval, or heart block.	Toxic side effects necessitate stopping procainamide administration.
Disopyramide phosphate (Norpace)	100-200 mg PO q6h	Monitor BP.	Hypotension is a common side effect.
		Watch for shortness of breath and weight gain.	Disopyramide can cause heart failure in a client with CAD.
		Monitor for widening QRS complex, prolonged QT or PR interval, or heart block.	Toxic side effects necessitate stopping disopyramide administration.
Type IB			
Lidocaine (Xylocaine)	1-1.5 mg/kg IV bolus, then 0.5-0.75 mg/kg IV boluses q5-10min to a loading dose of 3 mg/kg, followed by 2-4 mg/min infusion. For VF or pulseless VT: 1-1.5 mg/kg IV bolus q3-5min to a loading dose of 3 mg/kg, followed by 2-4 mg/min infusion	Watch for confusion, paresthesias, slurring of speech, drowsiness, or seizure activity.	CNS adverse effects predominate; they may require a decrease in dosage or discontinuation of the infusion.
Mexiletine hydrochloride (Mexitil)	200-300 mg PO q8h with food 125-250 mg IV bolus for 5-10 min 0.5-1.5 mg/min infusion	Monitor BP and heart rate.	Hypotension and bradycardia may occur.
		Assess for tremors, blurred vision, dizziness, ataxia, or confusion.	CNS adverse reactions predominate.
Tocainide hydrochloride (Tonocard)	400 mg PO q8h initially 400-800 mg PO q8h Maximum of 2.4 g daily Take with food	Watch for tremors.	Tremors indicate that the maximum dose is being approached.
		Monitor heart rate and BP.	Bradycardia and hypotension may occur.
		Teach client to report shortness of breath, wheezing, chest pain, or cough as well as dyspnea and distended neck veins or swelling of the extremities.	Pulmonary fibrosis is a serious side effect, which necessitates discontinuation of the drug; the drug may also cause CHF.

AV, Atrioventricular; *BP*, blood pressure; *CAD*, coronary artery disease; *CHF*, congestive heart failure; *CNS*, central nervous system; D_5W, 5% dextrose in water; *EMD*, electromechanical dissociation; *PEA*, pulseless electrical activity; *PSVT*, premature supraventricular tachycardia; *PVC*, premature ventricular complex; *SVT*, supraventricular tachycardia; *VF*, ventricular fibrillation; *VT*, ventricular tachycardia.

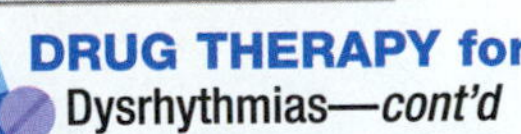

DRUG THERAPY for Dysrhythmias—*cont'd*

Drug	Usual Dosage	Nursing Interventions	Rationales
Class I Drugs—*cont'd*			
Type IC			
Flecainide acetate (Tambocor)	100 mg PO twice daily Maximum dose of 400 mg daily	Monitor for an increase in frequency and severity of dysrhythmias.	Flecainide can induce dysrhythmias.
		Monitor heart rate and BP.	Bradycardia and hypotension may occur.
		Monitor for CHF dizziness, visual disturbances, paresthesias, and tremors.	Side effects may require a decrease in dosage or discontinuation of the drug.
Propafenone hydrochloride (Rythmol)	150-300 mg PO q8h	Monitor for an increase in dysrhythmias.	Propafenone can induce dysrhythmias.
		Monitor heart rate and BP.	Bradycardia and hypotension may occur.
		Monitor for CNS effects, dizziness, anxiety, ataxia, insomnia, confusion, and seizures, as well as CHF and gastrointestinal distress.	Side effects may require a decrease in dosage or discontinuation of the drug.
Class II Drugs			
Propranolol hydrochloride (Inderal, Apo-Propranolol✱)	10-80 mg PO four times daily before meals 0.1 mg/kg slow IV bolus divided into 3 equal doses given at intervals of 2-3 min at rate of 1 mg/min	Monitor heart rate and BP.	Bradycardia and decreased BP are expected effects.
		Assess for shortness of breath or wheezing.	$Beta_2$-blocking effects on the lungs can cause bronchospasm.
		Assess for insomnia, fatigue, and dizziness.	Side effects may require decrease in dosage or discontinuation of the drug.
Acebutolol hydrochloride (Sectral)	600-1200 mg PO daily	Monitor heart rate and BP.	Bradycardia and decreased BP are expected effects.
		Assess for shortness of breath or wheezing.	$Beta_2$-blocking effects on the lungs can cause bronchospasm.
		Assess for insomnia, fatigue, and dizziness.	Side effects may require a decrease in dosage or discontinuation of the drug.
Esmolol hydrochloride (Brevibloc)	Initially, 500 mcg/kg/min for 1 min, then 50 mcg/kg/min for 4 min IV Titrate up if necessary	Monitor heart rate and BP.	Bradycardia and decreased BP are expected effects.
		Assess for shortness of breath or wheezing.	$Beta_2$-blocking effects on the lungs can cause bronchospasm.
		Assess for insomnia, fatigue, and seizures.	Side effects may require a decrease in dosage or discontinuation of the drug.
Sotalol hydrochloride (Betapace)	Initial dose of 80 mg PO twice daily Dosage may be increased every 2-3 days, if necessary, to 240-320 mg daily in 2-3 divided doses	Assess ECG rhythm for torsades de pointes and other serious new ventricular dysrhythmias.	Sotalol may have proarrhythmic effects.
		Assess for fatigue, bradycardia, dyspnea, CHF, chest pain, hypotension, dizziness, hypoglycemia, nausea, and vomiting.	Adverse reactions may warrant drug discontinuation.
		Sotalol should not be administered to clients with hypokalemia or hypomagnesemia before correction of these imbalances.	Hypokalemia or hypomagnesemia may prolong the QT interval and cause torsades de pointes.
		Sotalol is contraindicated in clients with bronchial asthma, sinus bradycardia, or second- and third-degree AV block (unless a functioning pacemaker is present), prolonged QT syndrome, cardiogenic shock, or CHF.	Sotalol has beta-blocking (class II) effects and class III effects.

Continued

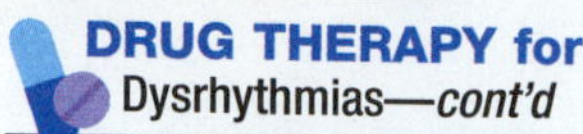

DRUG THERAPY for
Dysrhythmias—*cont'd*

Drug	Usual Dosage	Nursing Interventions	Rationales
Class III Drugs Amiodarone hydrochloride (Cordarone)	800-1600 mg PO daily in divided doses for 1-3 wk, then 600-800 mg daily for 1 mo, then 200-600 mg daily (average of 400 mg daily) Rapid loading dose: 150 mg IV over first 10 min (15 mg/min); slow loading dose: 360 mg IV over next 6 hr (1 mg/min); maintenance infusion: 540 mg IV over next 18 hr (0.5 mg/min), then 720 mg/24 hr (0.5 mg/min)	Use volumetric infusion pump and PVC tubing with in-line filter and infuse via central line.	Drug is irritating to peripheral vasculature; drug is more stable in glass bottle.
		Rapid-loading IV dose must not be administered faster than 10 min. Must stay with client and monitor heart rate and BP.	Hypotension may occur. It should be treated by slowing the infusion and other standard therapy. Cordarone should not be discontinued unless necessary.
		Continually monitor ECG rhythm during IV infusion; measure QT and QT_c.	Bradycardia and AV block may occur and are treated by slowing the infusion rate and providing pacemaker therapy, if necessary. May cause a worsening of ventricular dysrhythmias.
		Assess the client's knowledge of the treatment regimen and side effects.	Drug has major side effects, which make noncompliance a problem; clients may take the drug for 1½-3 mo before full clinical effects are apparent.
		Monitor heart rate, BP, and cardiac rhythm when initiating therapy.	Bradycardia, hypotension, and worsening dysrhythmia can occur.
		Teach clients to report any muscle weakness, tremors, or difficulty with ambulation.	Muscle-related side effects usually develop during the first week of treatment.
		Teach clients to report shortness of breath, cough, pleuritic pain, or fever.	Pulmonary side effects may indicate drug-induced pulmonary toxicity.
		Teach clients to report any visual disturbances and to wear sunglasses outdoors in the daytime if they have photophobia.	Corneal pigmentation occurs in most clients but generally does not interfere with vision; if it does, the dosage is decreased.
		Teach clients to use barrier sunscreens.	Photosensitivity reactions may occur.
		Teach clients to report any signs of thyroid problems or hepatotoxicity.	Thyroid problems or hepatotoxicity may occur, necessitating a decrease in dosage or discontinuation of the drug.
Ibutilide fumarate (Corvert)	1 mg IV over 10 min for clients >60 kg; 0.01 mg/kg over 10 min for clients <60 kg May repeat dose 10 min after completion of first infusion if necessary	Stop infusion as soon as dysrhythmia is terminated, or in event of sustained or nonsustained VT, or marked prolongation of QT or QT_c.	Drug may cause potentially fatal dysrhythmias.
		Observe clients with continuous ECG monitoring and measure QT or QT_c for at least 4 hr following infusion or until QT_c has returned to baseline.	Acute ventricular dysrhythmias must be promptly identified and treated. Client may develop heart blocks.
		Clients with atrial fibrillation of >2-3 days' duration must be adequately anticoagulated for at least 2 wk.	Atrial fibrillation is associated with formation of thrombi in atrial chambers.
		Hypokalemia and hypomagnesemia must be corrected before Covert infusion.	This is important to reduce potential for proarrhythmia effects.

AF, Atrioventricular; *BP,* blood pressure; *CAD,* coronary artery disease; *CHF,* congestive heart failure; *CNS,* central nervous system; *D_5W,* 5% dextrose in water; *EMD,* electromechanical dissociation; *PEA,* pulseless electrical activity; *PSVT,* premature supraventricular tachycardia; *PVC,* premature ventricular complex; *SVT,* supraventricular tachycardia; *VF,* ventricular fibrillation; *VT,* ventricular tachycardia.

CHART 37-3

DRUG THERAPY for
Dysrhythmias—*cont'd*

Drug	Usual Dosage	Nursing Interventions	Rationales
Class III Drugs—cont'd			
Dofetilide (Tikosyn)	125-500 mcg PO twice daily	Teach clients to change positions slowly.	Orthostatic hypotension is a common side affect of the drug.
		Inform clients that dosages will be adjusted, depending on the client's creatinine clearance level.	The client must have adequate creatinine clearance to prevent drug toxicity.
		Monitor clients on telemetry for several days; observe for and report bradycardia and hypotension.	Bradycardia and hypotension are common side effects.
Class IV Drugs			
Verapamil hydrochloride (Calan, Isoptin✱)	2.5-5 mg IV for 1-2 min for narrow-complex SVT or PSVT, after 15-30 min may give 5-10 mg IV for 1-2 min, if necessary, and repeat to a maximum of 20 mg 80-120 mg PO q6-8h	Monitor heart rate and BP.	Bradycardia and hypotension are common side effects.
		Teach clients to remain recumbent for at least 1 hr after IV administration.	Hypotension may occur; may be reversed with calcium chloride ($CaCl_2$), 0.5-1 g slow IV.
		Teach clients to change positions slowly when receiving oral therapy.	Dizziness and orthostatic hypotension often occur until tolerance develops.
		Teach clients to report dyspnea, orthopnea, distended neck veins, or swelling of the extremities.	Heart failure may occur, necessitating a decrease in dosage or discontinuation of the drug.
Diltiazem hydrochloride (Cardizem)	0.25 mg/kg IV for 2 min After 15 min, give 0.35 mg/kg IV for 2 min 5-15 mg/hr IV infusion	Monitor heart rate and BP.	Bradycardia and hypotension are common side effects.
		Teach clients to remain recumbent for at least 1 hr after IV administration.	Hypotension may occur.
		Teach clients to report dyspnea, orthopnea, distended neck veins, or swelling of the extremities.	Heart failure may occur, necessitating a decrease in dosage or discontinuation of the drug.
Other Drugs			
Digoxin (Lanoxin, Novodigoxin✱)	Rapid digitalization: 0.5-1 mg PO or IV initially; 0.125-0.5 mg PO q6h or IV until a total of 1-1.5 mg is reached Maintenance: 0.125-0.25 mg PO or IV daily or every other day (may be less for older adults)	Assess apical heart rate for 1 min before each dose.	Decreased heart rate is an expected response, but bradycardia may indicate toxicity.
		Assess for sudden increase in heart rate and change of rhythm from regular to irregular, or irregular to regular.	Changes in heart rate or rhythm may indicate toxicity.
		Teach clients to report anorexia, nausea, vomiting, diarrhea, paresthesias, confusion, or visual disturbances.	Side effect can indicate toxicity.
		Monitor serum potassium levels.	Hypokalemia increases the risk of toxicity and ventricular dysrhythmias.
		Monitor serum creatinine levels.	Impaired renal function can cause toxicity; the dosage is altered if this occurs.
Atropine sulfate	0.5-1 mg IV bolus may be repeated q3-5min, if necessary, to a maximum of 0.04 mg/kg For asystole, PEA, or EMD: 1 mg IV bolus q3-5min, if necessary, to a total of 0.04 mg/kg	Monitor heart rate and rhythm after administration.	Increased heart rate is expected.
		Assess for chest pain after administration.	Increased heart rate may cause ischemia in clients with CAD.
		Assess for urinary retention and dry mouth after administration.	Atropine is an anticholinergic agent.
		Avoid using in clients with angle-closure glaucoma.	Atropine increases intraocular pressure.

Continued

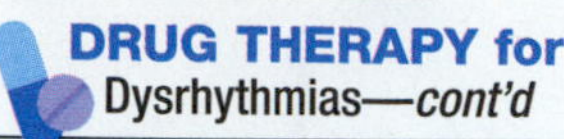

CHART 37-3

DRUG THERAPY for Dysrhythmias—*cont'd*

Drug	Usual Dosage	Nursing Interventions	Rationales
Other Drugs—*cont'd*			
Adenosine (Adenocard)	6 mg IV for 1-3 sec followed by 20-mL saline flush; may repeat in 1-2 min, if necessary, at 12 mg IV for 1-3 sec with 20-mL flush; may repeat 12 mg IV after 1-2 min if necessary	Monitor heart rate and rhythm after administration.	A short period of asystole is common after administration; bradycardia and hypotension may occur.
		Assess clients for facial flushing, shortness of breath, dyspnea, and chest pain.	These side effects commonly occur.
		Assess clients for recurrence of PSVT or ventricular ectopy.	Recurrence of PSVT is common; PVCs may occur.
Magnesium sulfate	1-2 g diluted in 100 mL of D_5W administered for 1-2 min for VF or VT	Assess ECG rhythm for conversion to sinus rhythm.	Hypomagnesemia may precipitate refractory VF.
	1-2 g in 50-100 mL of D_5W for 5-60 min for loading dose; 0.5-1 g/hr for 24 hr for supplementation	Assess clients for facial flushing, hypotension, and respiratory and CNS depression.	Magnesium sulfate causes vasodilation and respiratory and CNS depression.

AF, Atrioventricular; *BP,* blood pressure; *CAD,* coronary artery disease; *CHF,* congestive heart failure; *CNS,* central nervous system; *D_5W,* 5% dextrose in water; *EMD,* electromechanical dissociation; *PEA,* pulseless electrical activity; *PSVT,* premature supraventricular tachycardia; *PVC,* premature ventricular complex; *SVT,* supraventricular tachycardia; *VF,* ventricular fibrillation; *VT,* ventricular tachycardia.

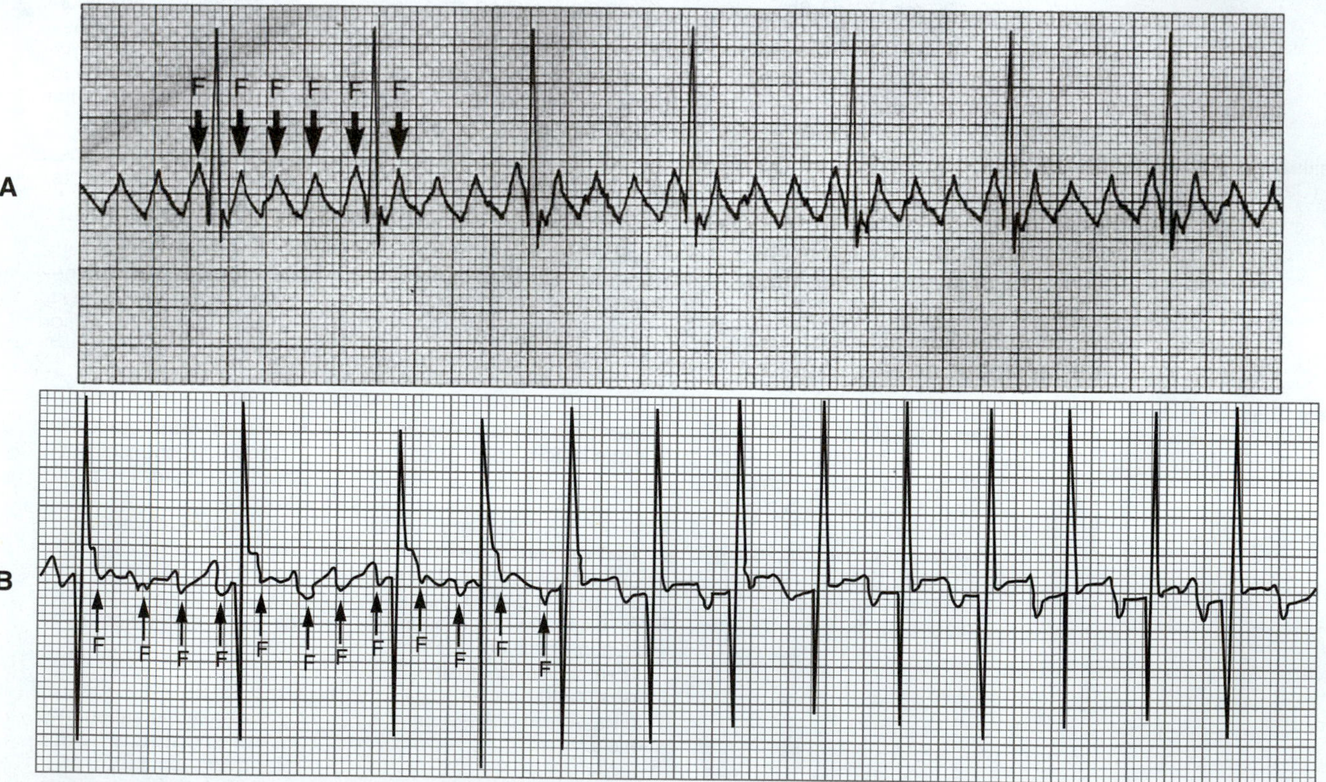

Figure 37-11 ■ Atrial dysrhythmias. **A,** Atrial flutter (F) with 4:1 block. The atrial rate is 280 beats/min; the ventricular rate is 70 beats/min. **B,** Atrial flutter with 4:1 conduction and then an 11-beat run with 2:1 conduction.

ATRIAL FLUTTER

PATHOPHYSIOLOGY. Atrial flutter is rapid atrial depolarization occurring at a rate of 250 to 350 times per minute. The most common rate is about 300 times per minute. An atrioventricular (AV) node blocks the number of impulses that reach the ventricles as a protective mechanism (Figure 37-11, *A*). When untreated, atrial flutter results in a 2:1 block (Figure 37-11, *B*). In general, when the ventricular rate is 150 beats/min, suspect atrial flutter with 2:1 block and carefully scrutinize the electrocardiographic (ECG) baseline for evidence of atrial flutter waves.

Atrial flutter may be caused by rheumatic or ischemic heart disease, heart failure (CHF), AV valve disease, pre-excitation syndromes, septal defects, pulmonary emboli, thyrotoxicosis, alcoholism, or pericarditis.

PHYSICAL ASSESSMENT/CLINICAL MANIFESTATIONS. The clinical manifestations depend on the rate of ventricular response. Assess the client for palpitations,

EVIDENCE-BASED PRACTICE for Nursing

Drug-induced QT prolongation in women during the menstrual cycle

Rodriquez, I., et al. (2001). Drug-induced QT prolongation in women during the menstrual cycle. *Journal of the American Medical Association, 285*(10), 1322-1326.

Ibutilide is an antiarrhythmic agent used for termination of atrial fibrillation and flutter. The purpose of this quantitative research study was to determine whether the degree of QT prolongation in response to ibutilide varies with the menstrual cycle phase and to compare QT prolongation between women and men.

Results indicated that the mean QT interval corrected for heart rate (QTc) after ibutilide infusion was greater for women during menses and the ovulatory phase compared with women during the luteal phase and compared with men. Menstrual cycle and gender differences exist in QTc responses to ibutilide, with the greatest increase in QTc corresponding to the first half of the menstrual cycle. Women are more likely than men to develop ibutilide-induced torsades de pointes.

Level of Evidence: 6—The study used a small sample, but it controlled for selected variables.

Critique. A sample of 38 men and 20 women were given a low dose of ibutilide. This dose was one third lower than normally given for rhythm conversion. Therefore the findings might be even greater when normal dosages are used in practice. Sample size was calculated to allow detection of a 30% difference in QTc prolongation between menstrual cycle phases and each gender, with an alpha of 0.05 and power of 0.80. One limitation is that this is the first study to compare QT-prolonging effects during the phases of the menstrual cycle. Differences in gender were the only statistically significant finding for QTc prolongation, although differences were noted among women in various life stages.

Implications for Nursing. Nurses are responsible for administering, monitoring, and reporting the results of ibutilide infusions. Prolonged QT intervals can lead to the development of serious ventricular dysrhythmias, such as ventricular tachycardia, ventricular fibrillation, and torsades de pointes. Dosages of antiarrhythmic medications may be adjusted or medications discontinued based on QT interval calculations. Nurses must know how to calculate the QTc accurately for client safety. It is generally accepted that a normal QTc is between 0.35 and 0.45 seconds. It is important to assess menstrual history as well as kidney function before the administration of antidysrhythmics that prolong the QT interval in women.

weakness, fatigue, shortness of breath, nervousness, anxiety, syncope (loss of consciousness), angina, and evidence of heart failure and shock. Carotid sinus massage transiently decreases the ventricular rate to facilitate rhythm interpretation, but it can be performed only by the physician. The client with a normal ventricular rate is usually asymptomatic. If the ventricular rate is below 100 beats/min, the term **controlled ventricular response** is used; above 100 bpm is called **rapid ventricular response.**

INTERVENTIONS. The treatment goals are the same as those for supraventricular tachycardia (SVT). Administer oxygen and prescribed drugs, such as ibutilide (Corvert), amiodarone (Cordarone), and diltiazem (Cardizem), to slow the rapid ventricular response. Studies on the effects of some of these drugs in women compared with men have been conducted to ensure their effectiveness and safety (see Evidence-Based Practice for Nursing box above).

If the client is hemodynamically compromised, cardioversion is the treatment of choice. Rapid atrial overdrive pacing may be attempted or radiofrequency catheter ablation may be necessary if the client does not respond to these therapies. These therapies are discussed later in this chapter.

RESOURCE MANAGEMENT

ATRIAL FIBRILLATION

Cost of Care

- The costs associated with the treatment of atrial fibrillation (AF) are enormous. Clients with AF make up the largest group of those hospitalized with *any* dysrhythmia, including all the life-threatening ventricular dysrhythmias combined.
- Hospital stays for AF are the longest of any hospitalizations wherein the principal diagnosis is a dysrhythmia.
- Economists estimate the annual cost of treating AF at a staggering one billion dollars.
- More than two million people in the United States have AF, requiring more than 365,000 hospitalizations each year.
- The estimated cost for each 4-day hospital stay is over $7,000 but may cost as much as $20,000.

Implications for Nursing

- Early detection and appropriate management of AF must be a priority; health promotion, especially for the older adult, is essential, and health teaching must target the components of treatment in a clear, concise manner that is individualized to the client.
- Evaluations of any older adult should include assessment for AF.
- Once AF is identified, restoration of normal sinus rhythm is crucial to prevent strokes and improve quality of life.

Data from Yee, C.A., & Rozewicz, B. (2003). Getting to the heart of atrial fibrillation. *Nursing Management, 34*(9), 21-27.

ATRIAL FIBRILLATION

PATHOPHYSIOLOGY. Atrial fibrillation (AF) is the most common dysrhythmia found in clinical practice. About 2.2 million Americans are affected with AF, and sustained AF increases with age. Ten percent of persons over the age of 80 years develop AF. Men are more likely to develop AF and women are more likely to die of AF (Josephson & McMullen, 2003). It is estimated that by the year 2050, the incidence of AF will increase to 5.6 million people, half of them females (Benson & Powless, 2003). With millions of cases of intermittent or sustained AF occurring each year in the United States, health care costs are soaring (see the Resource Management box above).

Multiple rapid impulses from many atrial foci, at a rate of 350 to 600 times per minute, depolarize the atria in a totally disorganized manner. The result is chaos, with no P waves, no atrial contractions, loss of the atrial kick, and an irregular ventricular response (Figure 37-12). The atria merely quiver in fibrillation (commonly called "A fib"). Recurrent episodes of AF eventually lead to sustained AF. Dilation and blood stagnation in the atria can lead to thrombus formation, and this increases the risk of stroke or other embolic events (Josephson & McMullen, 2003). In addition, AF causes a decrease in cardiac output, further compromising the heart's perfusion ability.

Atrial fibrillation occurs most commonly in clients with underlying cardiac disease. Cardiac damage may precede or cause AF. Of all acute myocardial infarctions (MIs), 10% to 15% are complicated by new onset of AF (Josephson & McMullen, 2003). It may also occur in clients with the following conditions:

- MI
- Rheumatic heart disease with mitral stenosis
- Atrial septal defect
- Heart failure
- Cardiomyopathy

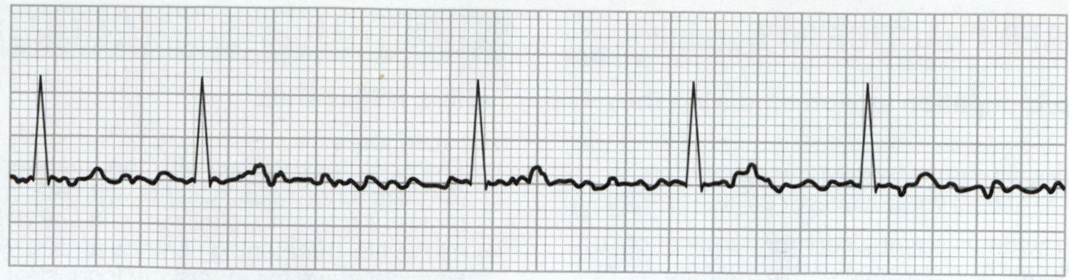

Figure 37-12 ■ Atrial dysrhythmias. Atrial fibrillation. (From Huszar, R.J. [2002]. *Pocket guide to basic dysrhythmias* [3rd ed.]. St. Louis: Mosby.)

- Hyperthyroidism
- Pulmonary emboli
- Wolff-Parkinson-White (WPW) syndrome
- Congenital heart disease
- Chronic constrictive pericarditis

Atrial fibrillation commonly occurs following cardiac surgery, in which case it is most often transient and usually responds well to treatment.

PHYSICAL ASSESSMENT/CLINICAL MANIFESTATIONS. Atrial fibrillation may be intermittent or chronic. Symptoms depend on the ventricular rate. If the ventricular rate is rapid, the presenting symptoms may be as described for supraventricular tachycardia (SVT). Because of loss of the atrial kick, however, the client in uncontrolled AF is at greater risk for an inadequate cardiac output. Assess the client for the presence of a pulse deficit, fatigue, weakness, shortness of breath, distended neck veins, dizziness, decreased exercise tolerance, anxiety, syncope, palpitations, chest discomfort or pain, and hypotension.

The client is also at risk for pulmonary embolism. Thrombi may accumulate within the right atrium and transported through the right ventricle to the lungs. Assess for shortness of breath, chest pain, hemoptysis, and a feeling of impending doom.

In addition, the client is at risk for systemic emboli, particularly an embolic stroke, which may cause severe neurologic impairment or death. Because about one third of clients with AF have thromboemboli, be sure to assess the client for evidence of embolic events. Changes in mentation, speech, sensory function, and motor function are particularly noted. Assess pulses, urine output, back pain, and complaints of gastrointestinal (GI) disturbances. Report any of these symptoms to the health care provider immediately. Clients with AF who have valvular disease are particularly at risk for thromboemboli.

INTERVENTIONS. Treatment is the same as for atrial flutter. In addition, the nurse may administer anticoagulants, such as heparin, enoxaparin (Lovenox), and sodium warfarin, as prescribed by the physician for clients considered at high risk for emboli. Before elective cardioversion, the health care provider prescribes anticoagulation therapy for about 6 weeks to prevent a thromboembolic event if the rhythm is successfully converted. To assess for the presence of atrial clots, a contraindication for cardioversion, the physician may order a transesophageal echocardiogram (TEE) before attempting emergency cardioversion (see Chapter 36). AF of greater than 12 months' duration is not likely to respond to attempts at conversion to sinus rhythm by drug therapies and may fail to respond to cardioversion. Cardioversion is discussed later in this chapter.

Clients with recurring, symptomatic AF resistant to medical therapies may be treated with radiofrequency catheter ablation to the bundle of His to interrupt all conduction between the atria and the ventricles. However, this treatment requires implantation of a permanent ventricular pacemaker and does not stop the atria from fibrillating. The atrial kick is not restored, and clients remain at risk for embolic events.

Clients in AF with decompensation may benefit from the **maze procedure,** an open chest surgical technique often performed with coronary artery bypass grafting (CABG). For the procedure, electrophysiologic mapping studies are done to confirm the diagnosis of AF. The surgeon places a maze of sutures in strategic places in the atrial myocardium, pulmonary artery, and possibly the superior vena cava to prevent electrical circuits from developing and perpetuating AF. Sinus impulses can then depolarize the atria before reaching the AV node and preserve the atrial kick. Postoperative care is similar to that after other open-heart surgical procedures (see Chapter 41).

JUNCTIONAL DYSRHYTHMIAS

Nodal cells in the atrioventricular (AV) junctional area can generate electrical impulses and are therefore secondary or latent pacemaker cells. They have a slower rate of discharge, usually 40 to 60 beats/min, and are usually suppressed. Occasionally these cells do generate impulses as an escape pacemaker when the sinus node is excessively slow, or the cells may do so inappropriately as irritable rhythms. These rhythms are most commonly transient, and clients usually remain hemodynamically stable.

VENTRICULAR DYSRHYTHMIAS

The ventricles have the fewest nodal cells and are the slowest pacemaker, generally being overcome by faster, higher pacemakers. However, irritable ventricular cells may generate electrical impulses and fire prematurely. Because the impulse originates in and depolarizes one ventricle first, then spreads to depolarize the other, the resultant QRS complex is wide, usually measuring greater than 0.12 second. The QRS complex is bizarre or oddly shaped, looking different from the normal QRS complexes. The repolarization sequence is also different so that the T wave is large and usually occurs in a direction opposite to the largest deflection of the QRS complex. The impulse most commonly is blocked in the AV node and cannot proceed further with retrograde conduction so that the atria and the sinoatrial (SA) node are usually not affected by the ventricular impulse. The atrial rhythm typically remains regular unless the underlying rhythm is sinus arrhythmia.

IDIOVENTRICULAR RHYTHM (VENTRICULAR ESCAPE RHYTHM)

PATHOPHYSIOLOGY. During an **idioventricular rhythm** (ventricular escape rhythm), the ventricular nodal cells pace the ventricles. Because their inherent rate of firing is slow, the rate is usually less than 40 beats/min. If P waves are seen, they are independent of the QRS complexes and are not related (AV dissociation).

Idioventricular rhythm is seen as a rhythm in the dying heart, where downward displacement of the pacemaker has occurred. Pulseless electrical activity (PEA) is characterized by no palpable pulse and therefore no perfusion, although electrical activity is displayed on the monitor. Common causes of PEA are hypovolemia, hypoxia, acidosis, hyperkalemia or hypokalemia, hypothermia, drug overdose, tension pneumothorax, coronary or pulmonary thrombosis, and cardiac tamponade.

PHYSICAL ASSESSMENT/CLINICAL MANIFESTATIONS. Because idioventricular pacemakers are unstable, unreliable, and slow, the client is hypotensive and in shock or, most typically, pulseless and therefore in cardiac arrest. Assess the client's airway, breathing, circulation, level of consciousness, and oxygenation.

EMERGENCY CARE: IDIOVENTRICULAR RHYTHMS. Usually idioventricular rhythms require immediate resuscitation measures, unless there is a do-not-resuscitate (DNR) order. Initiate cardiopulmonary resuscitation (CPR) and summon assistance. The team may initiate advanced cardiac life support (ACLS) measures, including epinephrine administration, intravascular volume replacement, and other measures. The physician may attempt pacemaker therapy or discontinue resuscitation efforts.

PREMATURE VENTRICULAR COMPLEXES

PATHOPHYSIOLOGY. Premature ventricular complexes (PVCs) result from increased irritability of ventricular cells. PVCs are early ventricular complexes followed by a pause. When multiple PVCs are present, the QRS complexes may be unifocal or uniform, meaning that they are of the same shape (Figure 37-13, *A*) or multifocal or multiform, meaning that they are of different shapes (Figure 37-13, *B*). PVCs frequently occur in repetitive rhythms, such as bigeminy, trigeminy, and quadrigeminy. Two sequential PVCs are a pair, or couplet. Three or more successive PVCs are usually called nonsustained ventricular tachycardia (NSVT) (Figure 37-13, *C*).

Premature ventricular contractions are common, and their frequency increases with age. PVCs may be insignificant or may occur with myocardial ischemia or MI, CHF, chronic hypoxemia, chronic airway limitation (CAL), anemia, hypokalemia, or hypomagnesemia. The administration of catecholamines, sympathomimetic drugs, and digitalis, as well as acidosis, anesthesia, stress, nicotine intake, ingestion of caffeine and alcohol, infection, trauma, or surgery, can also cause PVCs. Postmenopausal women often find that caffeine causes palpitations and PVCs.

PHYSICAL ASSESSMENT/CLINICAL MANIFESTATIONS. The client may be asymptomatic or may experience palpitations or chest discomfort caused by increased stroke volume of the normal beat after the pause. Peripheral pulses may be diminished or absent with the PVCs themselves because the decreased stroke volume of the premature beats may decrease peripheral perfusion. Because other rhythms also cause widened QRS complexes, it is essential that the nurse assess whether the premature complexes perfuse to the extremities. This is done by palpating the carotid, brachial, or femoral arteries while observing the monitor for widened complexes or auscultating for the apical heart sounds. With acute MI, PVCs may be considered warning dysrhythmias, possibly heralding the onset of ventricular tachycardia (VT) or ventricular fibrillation (VF). For a client with chest discomfort or pain, the nurse reports to the physician whether PVCs increase in frequency, are multiform, are R-on-T phenomena, or occur in runs of VT.

INTERVENTIONS. If there is no underlying heart disease, PVCs are not usually treated other than by eliminating any contributing cause (e.g., caffeine, stress). With acute myocardial ischemia or MI, the nurse treats significant PVCs by administering oxygen and amiodarone (Cordarone) as prescribed. If an MI occurs, administer other drugs as prescribed, including procainamide (Pronestyl), magnesium sulfate, and quinidine (see Chart 37-3). Potassium is administered as prescribed for replacement therapy if hypokalemia is the cause.

VENTRICULAR TACHYCARDIA

PATHOPHYSIOLOGY. Ventricular tachycardia (VT), sometimes referred to as "V tach," occurs with repetitive firing of an irritable ventricular ectopic focus, usually at a rate of 140 to 180 beats/min or more (Figure 37-14). VT may result from increased automaticity or a re-entry mechanism. It may be intermittent, as in three or more self-limiting beats (nonsustained VT), or sustained, lasting longer than 15 to 30 seconds. The sinus node may continue to discharge independently, depolarizing the atria but not the ventricles (atrioventricular [AV] dissociation), although P waves are seldom seen in sustained VT.

Ventricular tachycardia may occur in clients with ischemic heart disease, MI, cardiomyopathy, hypokalemia, hypomagnesemia, valvular heart disease, heart failure, drug toxicity, hypotension, or ventricular aneurysm. In clients who go into cardiac arrest, VT is commonly the initial rhythm before deterioration into ventricular fibrillation (VF) as the terminal rhythm. VT is not common in infants and children unless they have cardiac disease.

PHYSICAL ASSESSMENT/CLINICAL MANIFESTATIONS. Clinical manifestations of sustained VT partially depend on the ventricular rate. Slower rates are better tolerated. Clients may be hemodynamically compromised if the cardiac output decreases because of the shortened ventricular filling time and loss of the atrial kick. In some clients, VT causes cardiac arrest. Assess the client's airway, breathing, circulation, level of consciousness, and oxygenation.

INTERVENTIONS. For the *stable* client with sustained VT, administer oxygen, and confirm the rhythm via a 12-lead electrocardiogram (ECG). Amiodarone, lidocaine, or magnesium sulfate may be given. Current advanced cardiac life support (ACLS) guidelines state that elective cardioversion is highly recommended for stable VT. The physician may prescribe an oral antidysrhythmic agent, such as mexiletine (Mexitil) or sotalol (Betapace, Sotacor✱).

EMERGENCY CARE: VENTRICULAR TACHYCARDIA. For the client with unstable VT with a pulse, the physician or ACLS-qualified nurse administers emergency cardioversion followed by oxygen and antidysrhythmic therapy (Chart 37-4). Rapid atrial or ventricular overdrive pacing can be used if the VT is related to a significant bradydysrhythmia.

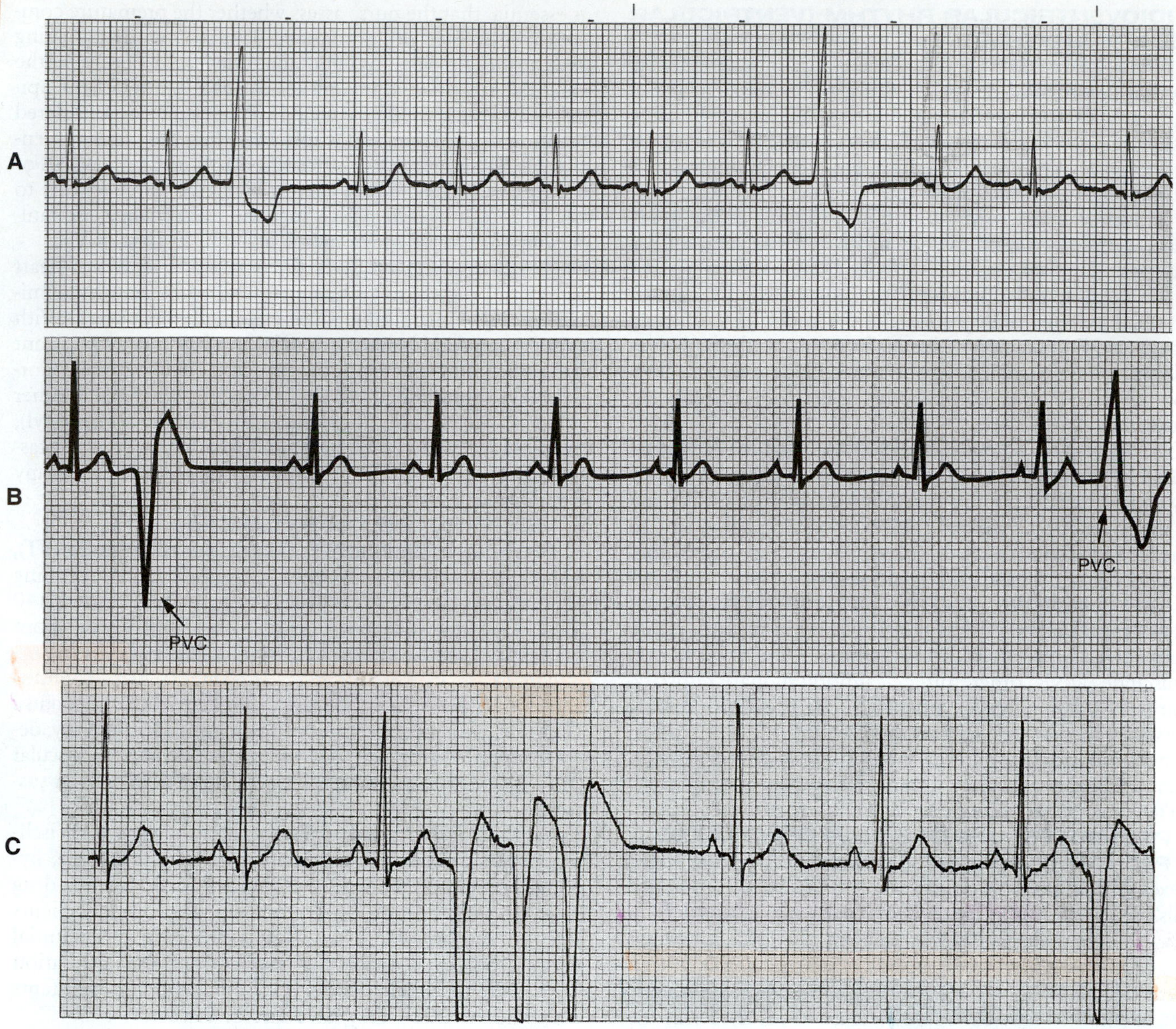

Figure 37-13 ■ Ventricular dysrhythmias. **A,** Normal sinus rhythm with unifocal premature ventricular complexes (PVCs). **B,** Normal sinus rhythm with multifocal PVCs (one negative and the other positive). **C,** Normal sinus rhythm with three consecutive PVCs (nonsustained ventricular tachycardia) and another unifocal PVC.

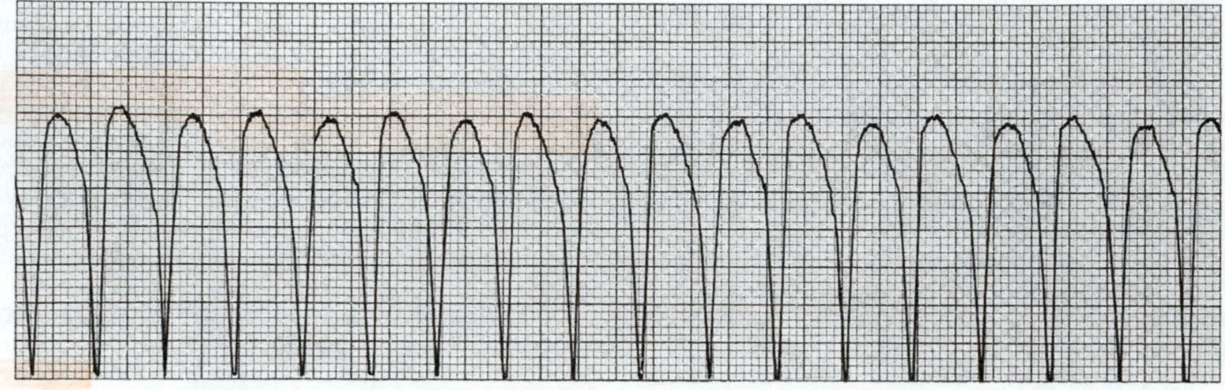

Figure 37-14 ■ Ventricular dysrhythmias. Sustained ventricular tachycardia at a rate of 166 beats/min.

CHART 37-4

BEST PRACTICE for
Emergency Care of Unstable Ventricular Tachycardia

EMERGENCY CARE

- Assist the physician with cardioversion.
- Provide oxygen and antidysrhythmic drugs as prescribed.
- Teach the client how to perform cough cardiopulmonary resuscitation (CPR), if ordered.
- Assist with or provide defibrillation (if you are certified in advanced cardiac life support [ACLS]).
- Initiate CPR if the client does not respond to the preceding measures.
- Maintain a patent airway at all times. Administer oxygen.
- Monitor airway, breathing, and circulation.
- Monitor the client for premature ventricular complexes (PVCs) and the recurrence of ventricular tachycardia (VT).
- Assess for manifestations of myocardial infarction, hypokalemia, or hypomagnesemia.

With pulseless VT, the physician or ACLS-qualified nurse or other health care provider must *immediately* defibrillate the client or initiate CPR and defibrillate as soon as possible. If the client remains pulseless, the nurse or other health care provider must resume CPR and full resuscitative measures following defibrillation. This includes airway management and administration of oxygen, epinephrine, vasopressin, and antidysrhythmic therapy with amiodarone (Cordarone), magnesium sulfate, and procainamide (Pronestyl).

If the rhythm has been successfully converted, attention is given to treating reversible causes of VT, such as myocardial ischemia, acidosis, hypokalemia, and hypomagnesemia. Ensure that oxygen therapy and antidysrhythmic agent administration are continued, and monitor the client closely for premature ventricular complexes (PVCs) and the recurrence of VT. The client with recurrent, medically refractory VT should be studied in the electrophysiology laboratory and may benefit from radiofrequency catheter ablation. Implantation of a cardioverter/defibrillator is often performed in clients who have experienced recurrent VT (see later).

VENTRICULAR FIBRILLATION

PATHOPHYSIOLOGY. Ventricular fibrillation (VF), sometimes called "V fib," is the result of electrical chaos in the ventricles. Impulses from many irritable foci fire in a totally disorganized manner so that ventricular contraction cannot occur. There are no recognizable deflections. Instead, there are irregular undulations of varying amplitudes, from coarse to fine (Figure 37-15, *A*). The ventricles merely quiver, consuming a tremendous amount of oxygen. There is no cardiac output or pulse and therefore no cerebral, myocardial, or systemic perfusion. This rhythm is *rapidly fatal* if not successfully terminated within 3 to 5 minutes.

Ventricular fibrillation may be the first manifestation of coronary artery disease (CAD). Clients with myocardial infarction (MI) are at great risk for VF, which may also occur in clients with myocardial ischemia, hypokalemia, hypomagnesemia, hemorrhage, antidysrhythmic therapy, rapid supraventricular tachydysrhythmias (SVTs), shock, asynchronous pacing with competition, or severe metabolic disease. VF also occurs following surgery or trauma.

PHYSICAL ASSESSMENT/CLINICAL MANIFESTATIONS. On initiation of VF, the client becomes faint, immediately loses consciousness, and becomes pulseless and apneic. There is no blood pressure, and heart sounds are absent. Respiratory and metabolic acidosis develop. Seizures

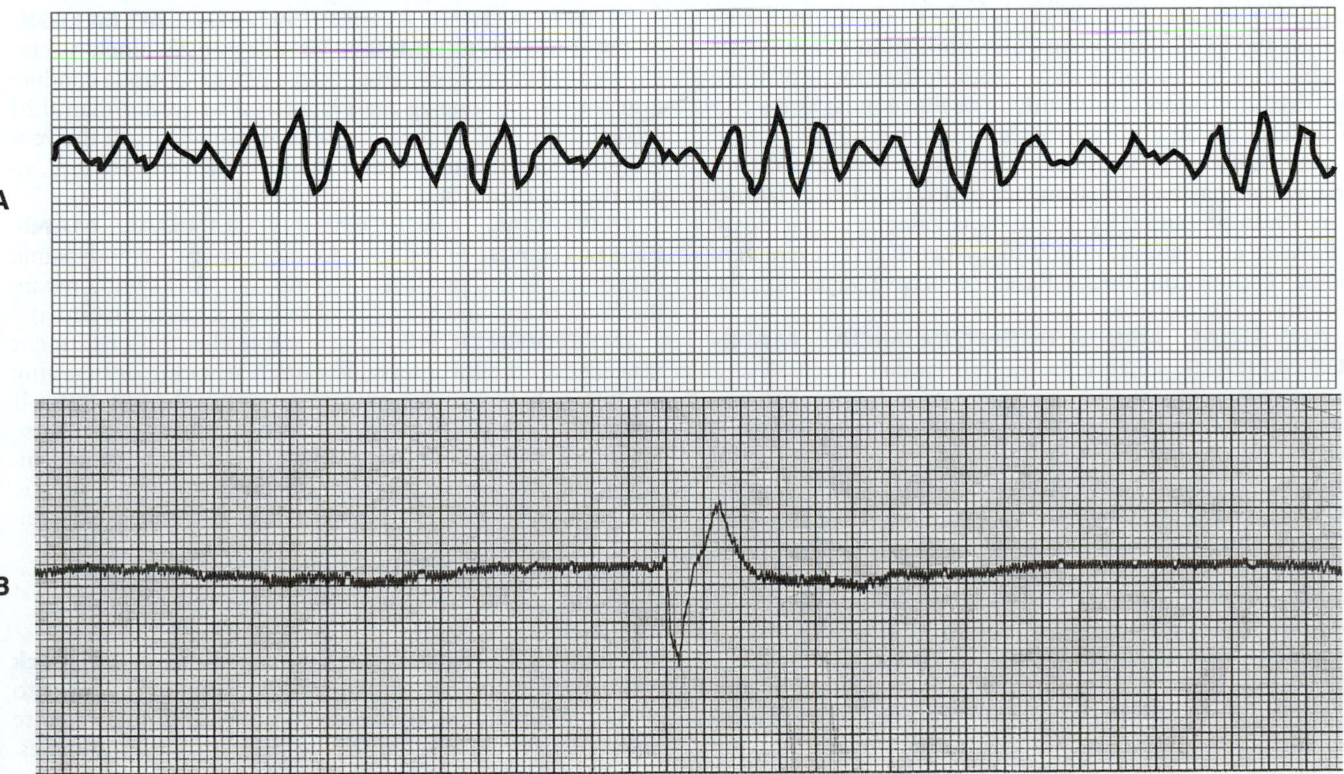

Figure 37-15 ■ Ventricular dysrhythmias. **A,** Coarse ventricular fibrillation. **B,** Ventricular asystole with one idioventricular complex.

may occur. Within minutes, the pupils become fixed and dilated, and the skin becomes cold and mottled. Death ensues without prompt restoration of an organized rhythm and cardiac output.

EMERGENCY CARE: VENTRICULAR FIBRILLATION. The goals of treatment are to terminate VF promptly and convert it to an organized rhythm. Therefore the priority is to defibrillate the client *immediately* according to ACLS protocol. If a defibrillator is not readily available, CPR must be continued until the defibrillator arrives.

If the VF does not terminate after three rapid successive shocks of increasing energy, the nurse and resuscitation team resume CPR and provide airway management. They also administer oxygen and antidysrhythmic therapy with vasopressin, epinephrine, amiodarone, procainamide (Pronestyl), lidocaine, and magnesium sulfate, along with attempting defibrillation frequently. If VF is successfully converted to an organized rhythm, the nurse continues supportive therapy and assists the physician in treating potential causes of VF and preventing its recurrence.

VENTRICULAR ASYSTOLE

PATHOPHYSIOLOGY. Ventricular asystole, sometimes called *ventricular standstill,* is the complete absence of any ventricular rhythm (Figure 37-15, *B*). There are no electrical impulses in the ventricles and therefore *no* ventricular depolarization, no QRS complex, no contraction, no cardiac output, and no pulse, respirations, or blood pressure. The client is in full cardiac arrest. The sinoatrial (SA) node, in some cases, may continue to fire and depolarize the atria, with only P waves seen on the electrocardiogram (ECG). The sinus impulses, however, do not conduct to the ventricles, and QRS complexes remain absent. In most cases, the entire conduction system is electrically silent, with no P waves seen on the ECG. There is only a mildly undulating line on the ECG. Fine ventricular fibrillation (VF) may resemble asystole in some leads. Because treatment of these two rhythms differs significantly, the nurse must assess two ECG leads for an accurate rhythm interpretation.

Ventricular asystole usually results from myocardial hypoxia, which may be a consequence of advanced heart failure. It may also be caused by severe hyperkalemia and acidosis. If P waves are seen, asystole is likely because of severe ventricular conduction blocks. Rarely, excessive vagal stimulation may cause asystole.

PHYSICAL ASSESSMENT/CLINICAL MANIFESTATIONS. Clients are in full cardiac arrest with a loss of consciousness and an absence of pulse, respirations, and blood pressure. Ventricular asystole is often unresponsive to resuscitation measures and fatal.

EMERGENCY CARE: VENTRICULAR ASYSTOLE. The goal of treatment is to restore cardiac electrical activity. The nurse or other health care provider initiates CPR immediately (unless there is a DNR order) and summons assistance. Another ECG lead is assessed to ensure that the rhythm is asystole and not fine VF, which warrants immediate defibrillation. Do NOT shock asystole. The nurse and resuscitation team manage the airway and administer oxygen, epinephrine, and atropine. The nurse assists the physician with the initiation of noninvasive pacing or invasive transvenous or epicardial pacing, although pacemaker therapy is generally not effective. The prognosis for clients with asystole is poor. Health care providers should consider termination of resuscitation efforts if there is no response after successful initiation of standard interventions when cessation is approved by an authorized physician. Nurses should know the criteria for termination of CPR and ACLS based on current facility and state legal policies.

An emerging clinical practice is allowing or encouraging family presence at resuscitation attempts. Interviews conducted with family members and significant others revealed this to be a positive experience. It allowed closure after the death of a loved one. Although there may be staff resistance and some limits to family presence, research shows a strong therapeutic effect from this practice (Eichhorn et al., 2001).

ATRIOVENTRICULAR BLOCKS

Atrioventricular (AV) blocks exist when supraventricular impulses are excessively delayed or totally blocked in the AV node or intraventricular conduction system. Conduction may be transiently or permanently abnormal for a number of reasons. The SA node continues to function normally, and atrial depolarizations and P waves occur regularly. Because of the conduction dysfunction, ventricular depolarizations and QRS complexes are either delayed or blocked.

The following are the different degrees of heart blocks:

- In *first-degree* AV block, all sinus impulses eventually reach the ventricles.
- In *second-degree* heart block, some sinus impulses reach the ventricles, but others do not because they are blocked.
- In *third-degree* heart block (complete heart block), none of the sinus impulses reaches the ventricles. The ventricles are therefore depolarized by a second, independent pacemaker.

AV blocks are differentiated by their PR intervals.

FIRST-DEGREE ATRIOVENTRICULAR BLOCK

PATHOPHYSIOLOGY. First-degree AV block is actually a conduction delay rather than a block. AV node conduction is slow, prolonging the PR interval to greater than 0.20 second. However, all sinus impulses eventually reach the ventricles. The underlying rhythm must still be identified (e.g., sinus rhythm with first-degree AV block (Figure 37-16, *A*).

PHYSICAL ASSESSMENT/CLINICAL MANIFESTATIONS. First-degree AV block has no hemodynamic consequences and produces no symptoms. Any symptoms are the result of the underlying rhythm (e.g., sinus bradycardia).

INTERVENTIONS. In the stable client, no treatment is needed. If the PR interval is particularly long or is getting progressively longer, the nurse must notify the physician. If the first-degree AV block is due to drug therapy, the nurse must withhold the offending drug and notify the physician. When first-degree AV block is associated with symptomatic bradycardia, oxygen is administered as prescribed to accelerate AV conduction.

SECOND-DEGREE ATRIOVENTRICULAR BLOCK TYPE I (WENCKEBACH OR MOBITZ TYPE I)

PATHOPHYSIOLOGY. In **second-degree AV block type I,** each successive sinus impulse takes a little longer to conduct through the impaired AV node, until one impulse is completely blocked and fails to depolarize the ventricles. This block results in a nonconducted or dropped beat (missing QRS complex). There is progressive prolongation of the PR interval, followed by a dropped beat and a pause (a char-

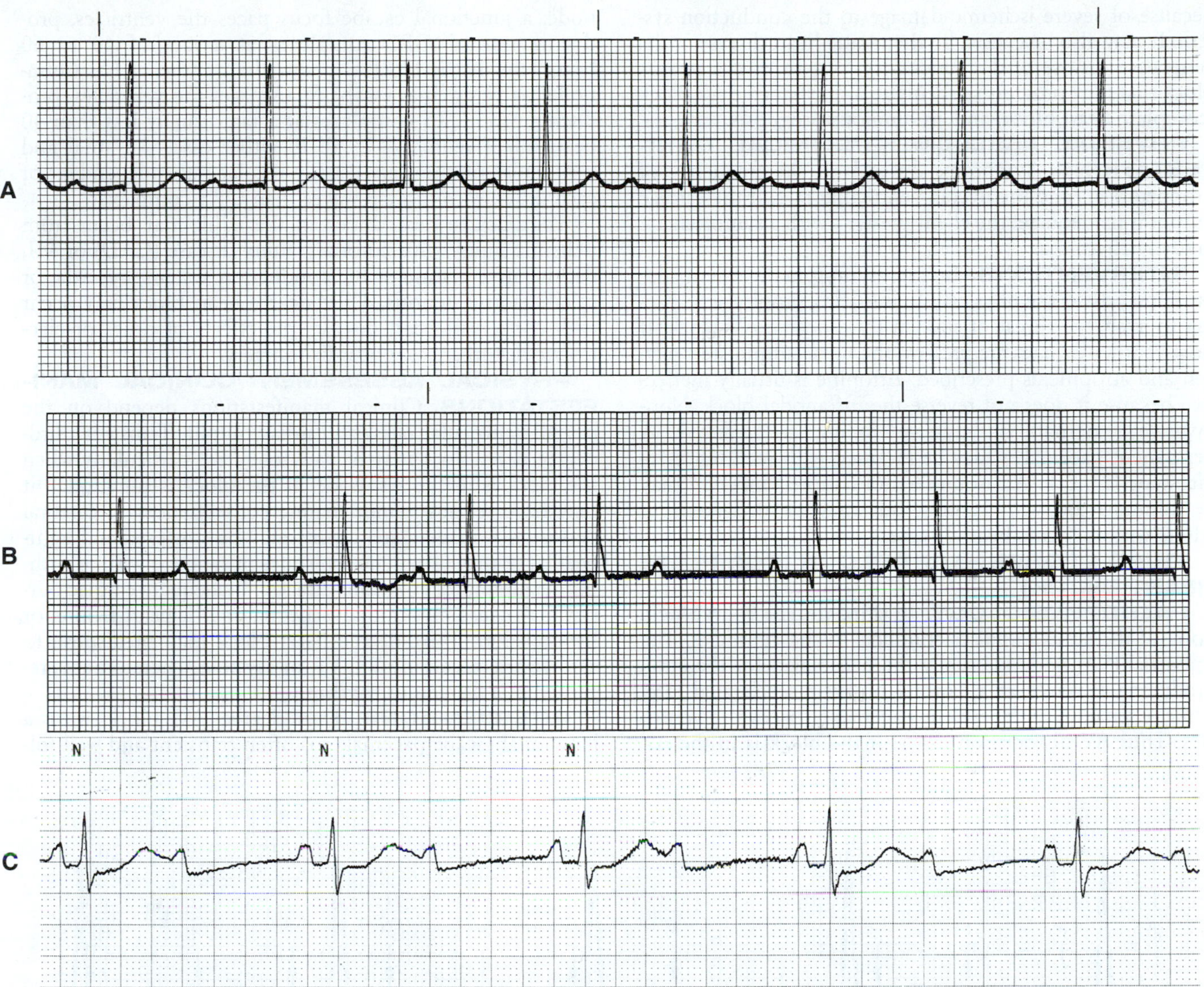

Figure 37-16 ■ Atrioventricular (AV) blocks. **A,** Normal sinus rhythm with first-degree AV block (PR interval, 0.36 second). **B,** Second-degree AV block type I (Wenckebach AV) with an irregular rhythm, grouped beating, and progressive prolongation of the PR interval until a P wave is completely blocked and not followed by a QRS complex. **C,** Second-degree AV block type II (Mobitz II) with 2:1 conduction, a constant PR interval, and wide QRS complex.

acteristic feature of this rhythm). Because of the dropped QRS complex, each group normally has one more P wave than QRS complexes (Figure 37-16, *B*).

PHYSICAL ASSESSMENT/CLINICAL MANIFESTATIONS. The client is usually asymptomatic if the frequency of dropped beats and the overall ventricular rate do not decrease the cardiac output. If the ventricular rate is too slow, decreasing the cardiac output, the client will have symptoms of a symptomatic bradydysrhythmia. This rhythm is usually transient and terminates spontaneously.

INTERVENTIONS. No intervention is required in the stable client because this rhythm rarely progresses to a more severe block. In the symptomatic client, administer oxygen and atropine as prescribed. If atropine is not successful in speeding AV nodal conduction time and increasing the heart rate, initiate pacemaker therapy as ordered and notify the physician.

SECOND-DEGREE HEART BLOCK TYPE II (MOBITZ TYPE II)

PATHOPHYSIOLOGY. In Mobitz type II block, the block is actually infranodal, occurring below the bundle of His. It involves a constant block in one of the bundle branches, resulting in a wide QRS complex in conducted beats and an intermittent block in the other bundle branch, resulting in dropped beats because both bundles are blocked (P waves are not followed by a QRS complex). Because the block is not in the AV node, sinus impulses that conduct to the ventricles always do so with a constant PR interval. Impulses may be blocked randomly, making the ventricular rhythm irregular. Alternatively, the impulses may be blocked at regular intervals, such as in 2:1 block, in which case the ventricular rhythm is regular (Figure 37-16, *C*).

Second-degree AV block type II is less common than type I. It may occur in the adult with an anterior wall MI because of severe ischemic damage to the conduction system. It may also be caused by rheumatic heart disease or degenerative disease of the conduction system. It is a serious block that may progress suddenly to a third-degree AV block (complete heart block) and an ominous prognosis.

PHYSICAL ASSESSMENT/CLINICAL MANIFESTATIONS. Symptoms depend on the frequency of dropped beats and the overall ventricular rate. If the cardiac output is inadequate, the client presents with a symptomatic bradydysrhythmia.

INTERVENTIONS. In the asymptomatic client, the nurse may assist the physician in initiating prophylactic pacing to avert the threat of sudden third-degree AV block. If slow ventricular rates are present, the nurse administers oxygen and atropine as prescribed. Atropine is usually ineffective because it does not reverse the infranodal block. Noninvasive (external) or invasive pacing is preferred. A permanent pacemaker may be required with recurrent Mobitz type II block. An isoproterenol (Isuprel) infusion may be administered with caution but may be dangerous in adults with ischemic heart disease.

THIRD-DEGREE HEART BLOCK (COMPLETE HEART BLOCK)

PATHOPHYSIOLOGY. In **third-degree heart block,** none of the sinus impulses conducts to the ventricles. The sinoatrial (SA) node is usually the pacemaker for the atria, producing P waves at a normal or even accelerated rate, while a separate, independent pacemaker paces the ventricles. Thus AV dissociation exists. If the block is in the AV node, a junctional escape focus paces the ventricles, producing normal QRS complexes at a rate of 40 to 60 beats/min. If the block is below the bundle of His (infranodal), a ventricular escape focus paces the ventricles, producing wide QRS complexes at a rate usually less than 40 beats/min (Figure 37-17, *A*). In either case, the atrial and ventricular rhythms are usually regular but independent of each other, with more P waves than QRS complexes.

Third-degree heart block in the adult may occur from ischemic injury with coronary artery disease (CAD) or MI, degenerative disease of the conduction system, hypoxia, or calcific aortic stenosis. Third-degree heart block may occur with congenital heart disease, the effects of drugs or electrolyte disturbances, or cardiac surgery.

PHYSICAL ASSESSMENT/CLINICAL MANIFESTATIONS. Clinical manifestations depend on the overall ventricular rate and cardiac output. Transient third-degree heart block may be well tolerated, particularly when the block is in the AV node. If the block is infranodal, it may have serious hemodynamic consequences. If cerebral perfusion is inadequate, clients may be confused and lightheaded or may experience episodes of syncope with or without seizures (Stokes-Adams attacks). Inadequate cardiac output may cause myocardial ischemia or MI, heart failure, or hypotension. Third-degree heart block may predispose to cardiac arrest, causing VT, VF, or asystole. Therefore it is regarded as a dangerous rhythm.

INTERVENTIONS. Third-degree AV block with a junctional escape pacemaker is often transient and well tol-

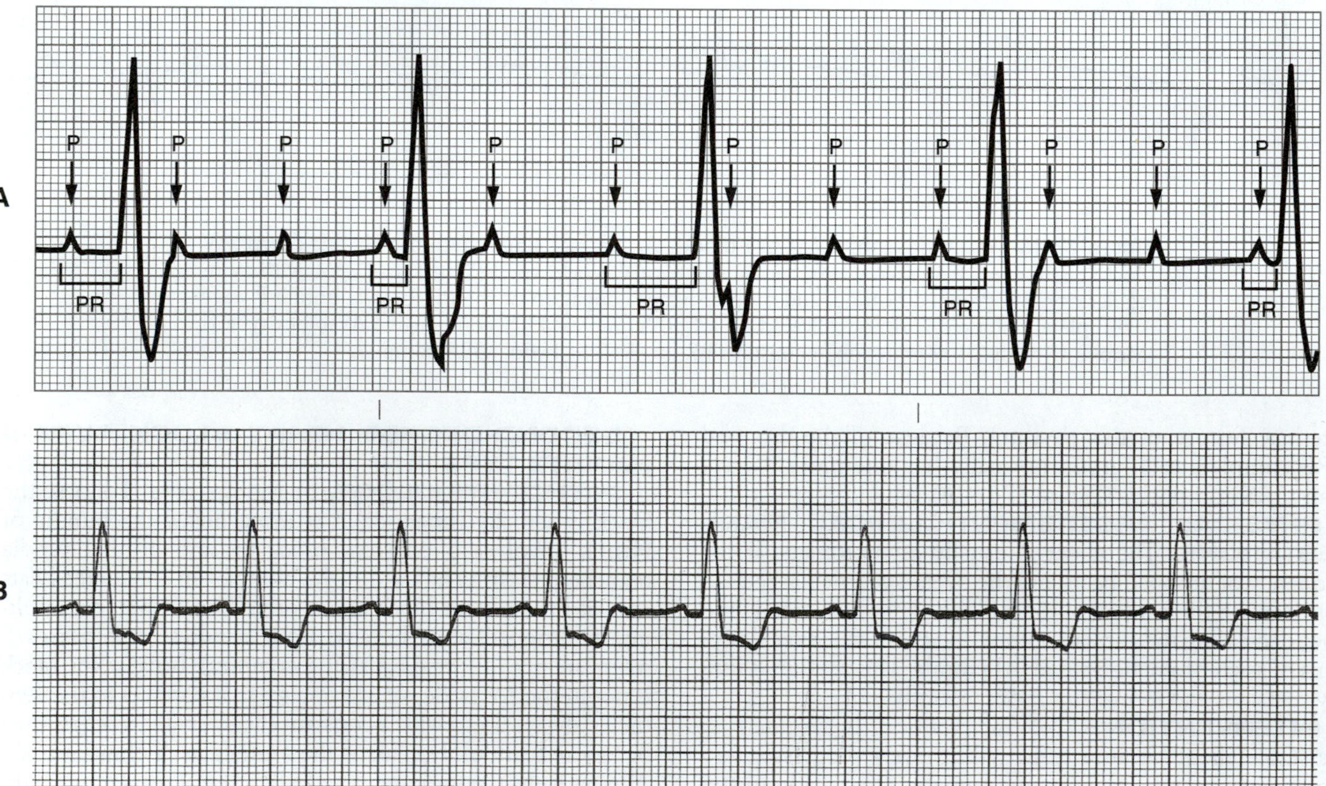

Figure 37-17 ■ Atrioventricular (AV) blocks. **A,** Third-degree AV block with regular atrial and ventricular rhythms, inconstant PR intervals (AV dissociation), and a ventricular escape focus pacing the ventricles at a rate of 38 beats/min, with wide QRS complexes. **B,** Normal sinus rhythm with bundle branch block (wide QRS complexes measuring 0.12 second).

erated. If the client is symptomatic, administer oxygen and atropine as prescribed. Clients with third-degree heart block with a ventricular escape pacemaker are frequently symptomatic. Administer oxygen and assist the physician in initiating pacing to avert the threat of cardiac arrest. Atropine is usually not successful in infranodal blocks with wide QRS complexes. Cautious use of isoproterenol (Isuprel) infusions may be necessary as a temporary measure while awaiting pacemaker therapy but is dangerous in clients with acute myocardial infarction. Implantation of a permanent pacemaker may be required for clients with recurrent third-degree infranodal block.

BUNDLE BRANCH BLOCKS

PATHOPHYSIOLOGY. Bundle branch block is a conduction delay or block within one of the two main bundle branches below the bifurcation of the bundle of His. When one bundle branch is blocked, the supraventricular impulse is able to descend only down the unblocked bundle branch and to depolarize that ventricle. The other ventricle is depolarized afterward as the wave of depolarization from the first ventricle proceeds from cell to cell to the other ventricle. Such slow depolarization prolongs the QRS duration to 0.12 second or longer. The underlying rhythm is usually sinus in origin (e.g., sinus rhythm with bundle branch block) (Figure 37-17, *B*).

Bundle branch block may be a temporary or a permanent conduction disorder. Right or left bundle branch blocks are occasionally seen in clients with normal hearts. More commonly they are seen in clients with cardiovascular disease, such as congenital heart disease, rheumatic heart disease, ventricular hypertrophy, cardiomyopathy, severe aortic stenosis, chronic degenerative disease of the conduction system, or fibrotic scarring of the conduction system. Transient bundle branch block may be seen with acute conditions such as coronary insufficiency, MI, or heart failure; during right-sided heart catheterization; or with rapid supraventricular rates.

PHYSICAL ASSESSMENT/CLINICAL MANIFESTATIONS. No clinical manifestations are specifically related to bundle branch block. Notify the physician when a new bundle branch block develops, especially in the client with an acute MI. The conduction disorder may deteriorate to a more significant block requiring pacemaker therapy.

INTERVENTIONS. No interventions are specifically related to bundle branch block. Assess the client during alterations in heart rate for symptoms of hemodynamic compromise, which are reported to the physician. Ensure that the client is resting and has adequate ventilation and oxygenation.

COLLABORATIVE MANAGEMENT

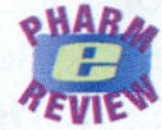

Analysis

COMMON NURSING DIAGNOSES AND COLLABORATIVE PROBLEMS

The following are priority nursing diagnoses for all clients with dysrhythmias:

1. Decreased Cardiac Output related to altered heart rate/rhythm
2. Ineffective Tissue Perfusion related to reduction of arterial blood flow

ADDITIONAL NURSING DIAGNOSES AND COLLABORATIVE PROBLEMS

In addition to the common nursing diagnoses, clients with dysrhythmias may have one or more of the following:

- Impaired Gas Exchange related to ventilation-perfusion imbalance
- Ineffective Coping related to uncertainty and situational crisis
- Activity Intolerance related to imbalance between oxygen supply/demand
- Deficient Knowledge related to cause and treatment of dysrhythmia

An additional collaborative problem is Potential for Pulmonary Edema.

Planning and Implementation

DECREASED CARDIAC OUTPUT AND INEFFECTIVE TISSUE PERFUSION

NOC **PLANNING: EXPECTED OUTCOMES.** The client with dysrhythmias is expected to have adequacy of blood flow ejected from the left ventricle to support systemic perfusion pressure. Indicators include that the following will not be compromised in the client:

- Apical heart rate
- Systolic and diastolic blood pressure
- Activity tolerance
- Cognitive status
- Skin color
- Peripheral pulses
- Ejection fraction

Additional indicators include that the client will not have any of the following:

- Dysrhythmias
- Abnormal heart sounds
- Angina
- Dyspnea
- Fatigue
- Pulmonary edema

INTERVENTIONS. The nurse's major role is to assess for complications and monitor the client for response to treatment (Chart 37-5). Interventions are specific to the type of dysrhythmia, the cause, the effect it has on cardiac output, and the risk it presents to the client. Interventions for specific dysrhythmias are summarized in Table 37-2.

NIC **CARDIAC CARE.** Monitor or direct assistive nursing personnel to monitor the client's electrocardiographic (ECG) rhythm or assess the client for manifestations associated with dysrhythmias, such as abnormal pulse rate and rhythm, palpitations, chest pain, syncope, decreased blood pressure, and dyspnea.

Assess the client's apical and radial pulses for a full minute for any irregularity, which may occur with premature beats, escape beats, atrial fibrillation (AF), or second-degree heart blocks. If the apical pulse rate differs from the radial pulse rate, a pulse deficit exists and suggests that not all beats are perfusing. Clinical manifestations of sustained tachydysrhythmias and bradydysrhythmias are summarized in Chart 37-2.

In a critical care setting, if the client has a pulmonary artery catheter and an arterial line, his or her hemodynamic profile is reviewed to determine the physiologic effects of

CHART 37-5

NIC INTERVENTION ACTIVITIES for The Client with Dysrhythmias

Cardiac Care: *Limitation of complications resulting from an imbalance between myocardial oxygen supply and demand for a client with symptoms of impaired cardiac function*

- Evaluate chest pain (e.g., intensity, location, radiation, duration, and precipitating and alleviating factors).
- Perform a comprehensive appraisal of peripheral circulation (e.g., check peripheral pulses, edema, capillary refill, color, and temperature of extremity).
- Monitor cardiovascular status.
- Document cardiac dysrhythmias.
- Monitor vital signs frequently.
- Evaluate the client's response to ectopy or dysrhythmias.
- Monitor appropriate laboratory values (e.g., cardiac enzymes, electrolyte levels).
- Provide antiarrhythmic therapy according to unit policy (e.g., antiarrhythmic medication, cardioversion, or defibrillation), as appropriate.
- Monitor client's response to antiarrhythmic medications.
- Arrange exercise and rest periods to avoid fatigue.
- Monitor the client's activity tolerance.
- Monitor for dyspnea, fatigue, tachypnea, and orthopnea.
- Promote stress reduction.
- Instruct the client on the importance of immediately reporting any chest discomfort.
- Offer spiritual support to the client and/or family (e.g., contact clergy), as appropriate.

NIC intervention activities selected from Dochterman, J.M., & Bulechek, G.M. (Eds.) (2004). *Nursing interventions classification (NIC)* (4th ed.). St. Louis: Mosby. No part of this work is to be altered without prior written permission from the Publisher.

the dysrhythmia. Also assess the psychosocial impact of dysrhythmias on clients and families and the effectiveness of their coping mechanisms.

Assessment of the client's past and current history is essential because dysrhythmias are associated with both acute and chronic disorders as well as with medical and surgical therapies. Review the interpretation of the client's 12-lead ECG and other ECG diagnostic tests, such as the Holter monitor, event monitor, or signal-averaged ECG.

NONSURGICAL MANAGEMENT. Nonsurgical management of dysrhythmias includes drug therapy, vagal maneuvers, temporary pacing, cardioversion, cardiopulmonary resuscitation (CPR), defibrillation, and catheter ablation.

Drug Therapy. Pharmacologic therapy administered for the control of dysrhythmias often includes drugs from one or more classes of antidysrhythmic agents (see Chart 37-3). The Vaughn-Williams classification is commonly used to classify drugs according to their effects on the action potential of cardiac cells. Other drugs also have antidysrhythmic effects but do not fit the Vaughn-Williams classification.

Vaughn-Williams Classification. Class I antidysrhythmics are membrane-stabilizing agents, stabilizing phase 4 to decrease automaticity. The three subclassifications in this group include type IA drugs, which moderately slow conduction and prolong repolarization, prolonging the QT interval. These drugs are used to treat or to prevent supraventricular and ventricular premature beats and tachydysrhythmias, but they are not as commonly used as other drugs. Examples include quinidine sulfate and procainamide hydrochloride (Pronestyl). Type IB drugs shorten repolarization. These drugs are used to treat or prevent ventricular premature beats, ventricular tachycardia (VT), and ventricular fibrillation (VF). Examples include lidocaine and mexiletine hydrochloride (Mexitil). Type IC drugs markedly slow conduction and widen the QRS complex. These drugs are used primarily to treat or to prevent recurrent, life-threatening ventricular premature beats, VT, and VF. Examples include flecainide acetate (Tambocor) and propafenone hydrochloride (Rythmol).

Class II antidysrhythmics control dysrhythmias associated with excessive beta-adrenergic stimulation by competing for receptor sites and thereby decreasing heart rate and conduction velocity. Beta-adrenergic blocking agents, such as propranolol (Lopressor) and esmolol hydrochloride (Brevibloc), are class II drugs. They are used to treat or to prevent supraventricular and ventricular premature beats and tachydysrhythmias. Sotalol hydrochloride (Betapace, Sotacor✱) is an antidysrhythmic agent with both noncardioselective beta-adrenergic blocking effects (class II) and action potential duration prolongation properties (class III). It is an oral agent recommended for the treatment of documented ventricular dysrhythmias, such as VT, that are life threatening.

Class III antidysrhythmics lengthen the absolute refractory period and prolong repolarization and the action potential duration of ischemic cells. Class III drugs include amiodarone (Cordarone) and ibutilide (Covert) and are used to treat or prevent ventricular premature beats, VT, and VF.

Class IV antidysrhythmics impede the flow of calcium into the cell during depolarization, thereby depressing the automaticity of the sinoatrial (SA) and atrioventricular (AV) nodes, decreasing the heart rate, and prolonging the AV nodal refractory period and conduction. Calcium channel blockers, such as verapamil hydrochloride (Calan, Isoptin✱) and diltiazem hydrochloride (Cardizem), are class IV drugs. They are used to treat supraventricular tachycardia (SVT), atrial flutter, and atrial fibrillation (AF) to slow down the ventricular response.

Other Antidysrhythmic Drugs. Other drugs, such as digoxin, atropine, adenosine, and magnesium sulfate, are frequently used to treat dysrhythmias. Digoxin (Lanoxin, Novodigoxin✱) increases vagal tone, slowing AV nodal conduction. It is useful in treating supraventricular tachydysrhythmias, particularly chronic AF, by controlling the rate of ventricular response. However, digoxin does not convert AF to sinus rhythm. Atropine is a parasympatholytic or vagolytic agent. It is used to treat vagally induced symptomatic bradydysrhythmias. Adenosine is an endogenous nucleoside that slows AV nodal conduction to interrupt re-entry pathways. It is effective in terminating paroxysmal SVT, a re-entrant tachydysrhythmia. Magnesium sulfate is an electrolyte administered to treat refractory VT or VF because these clients may be hypomagnesemic, with increased ventricular irritability.

Emergency Cardiac Drugs. In addition to antidysrhythmics, several other drugs are used during cardiac arrest (Chart 37-6). Epinephrine (Adrenalin) is a first-line agent in all cardiac arrests. It is given predominantly for its alpha-adrenergic effects to increase vasomotor tone for myocardial and cerebral perfusion. Its beta-adrenergic effects may stimulate the heart and increase myocardial contractility to improve cardiac output. Vasopressin has potent vasoconstricting effects and has been shown to be equivalent to epinephrine in VF and pulseless VT. It has a long half-life and is given one

CHART 37-6

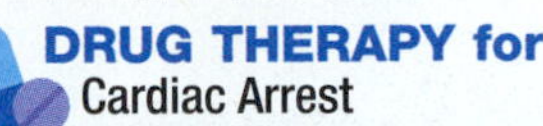

DRUG THERAPY for Cardiac Arrest

Drug	Usual Dosage	Nursing Interventions	Rationales
Epinephrine (Adrenalin)	1-mg IV bolus followed by 20-mL saline flush q3-5min If this fails, consider 2-5 mg IV bolus q3-5min; 1-mg, 3-mg, and 5-mg IV boluses (3 min apart); or 0.1 mg/kg IV bolus q3-5 min If necessary give endotracheally with dose at least 2-2½ times the IV dose	Monitor for return of rhythm and pulse when used for asystole or VF.	Return of rhythm and pulse is the expected response.
		Assess for tachycardia, dysrhythmias, or hypertension.	Adverse reactions can occur with a dramatic response.
		Assess for the development of coarse VF when given during the VF.	This may improve the response to defibrillation.
Amiodarone hydrochloride (Cordarone)	300 mg IV push for cardiac arrest in VF/pulseless VT 150 mg IVP over 10 min (15 mg/min), followed by 360 mg IV over next 6 hr (1 mg/min), followed by 540 mg IV over next 18 hr (0.5 mg/min) After first 24 hr, continue maintenance infusion of 720 mg/24 hr (0.5 mg/min)	Monitor for return of rhythm and pulse when used for recurrent unstable VT or VF.	Return of rhythm and pulse is the expected response.
		Use with extreme caution in clients receiving other antidysrhythmics.	Amiodarone reduces the hepatic and renal clearance of certain antiarrhythmics, specifically procainamide, quinidine, and flecainide.
		Use caution in clients with pulmonary, hepatic, or thyroid disease.	Amiodarone can cause fatal toxicity, especially in clients receiving more than 600 mg daily.
		Perform continuous cardiac monitoring while the client is receiving the loading dose.	There is a slow onset of antiarrhythmic effect and a high risk of life-threatening arrhythmias.
Dopamine hydrochloride (Intropin)	2.5-5 mcg/kg/min IV infusion; titrate to desired clinical response 1-2 mcg/kg/min for renal and mesenteric vasodilation 2-10 mcg/kg/min for beta-adrenergic effects 10-20 mcg/kg/min for alpha-adrenergic effects	Assess clients for increased BP.	Increased BP is the expected response.
		Monitor for tachycardia, dysrhythmias, or hypertension.	Adverse reactions may occur.
		Monitor IV site for infiltration.	Extravasation of drug can occur, causing necrosis.
		Assess for urine output <30 mL/hr, pallor, cyanosis, pain, or numbness in the extremities.	Dosages >10 mcg/kg/min cause vasoconstriction of renal and peripheral blood vessels; dosages of 2-5 mcg/kg/min may improve urine output by causing renal vasodilation and improving renal blood flow.
Dobutamine hydrochloride (Dobutrex)	2-20 mcg/kg/min IV infusion	Assess for increased BP.	Increased BP is the expected response.
		Assess for hypertension and dysrhythmias.	Adverse reactions may occur.
Norepinephrine (Levophed)	0.5-1 mcg/min IV infusion, titrate to desired effect, up to 8-30 mcg/min	Assess for increased BP.	Increased BP is the expected response.
		Monitor for bradycardia.	Reflex bradycardia may occur with a rise in BP.
		Monitor for hypertension and dysrhythmias.	Adverse reactions may occur with a dramatic response.
		Administer drug through central IV line.	Extravasation can occur.
		Assess for urine output <30 mL/hr, pallor, cyanosis, pain, or numbness in the extremities.	Norepinephrine is a powerful vasoconstrictor.
		Assess for chest pain after resuscitation.	Norepinephrine increases myocardial oxygen demand.

VF, Ventricular fibrillation; *VT*, ventricular tachycardia.

Continued

CHART 37-6

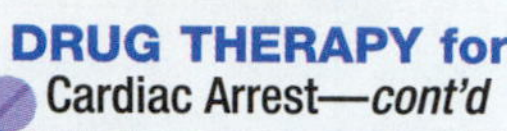

DRUG THERAPY for Cardiac Arrest—*cont'd*

Drug	Usual Dosage	Nursing Interventions	Rationales
Sodium bicarbonate	1 mEq/kg IV bolus given after the first 10 min of cardiac arrest if necessary 0.5 mEq/kg IV bolus q10min thereafter if necessary	Assess arterial blood gas values for metabolic acidosis.	Administration without evidence of metabolic acidosis can result in alkalosis, which can hinder resuscitation efforts.
Isoproterenol (Isuprel)	2-10 mcg/min IV infusion; titrate to desired clinical response	Assess for increased heart rate. Assess for tachycardia, hypotension, or hypertension. Assess for chest pain after resuscitation. Monitor for ventricular dysrhythmias.	Increased heart rate is the expected response. Adverse reactions may occur with a dramatic response. Isoproterenol increases myocardial oxygen demand. Isoproterenol increases ventricular irritability, especially in clients who are hypokalemic or who are receiving digitalis.
Calcium chloride ($CaCl_2$)	2-4 mg/kg IV slowly; may repeat q10min if necessary	Calcium chloride is indicated only for cardiac arrest associated with hyperkalemia, hypocalcemia, or calcium channel blocker toxicity.	Calcium chloride may cause cellular damage and cerebrovascular spasm.
Vasopressin	40 units IV bolus, one time	Monitor for return of rhythm and pulse when used for VF or pulseless VT.	Return of rhythm and pulse is the expected response.

VF, Ventricular fibrillation; *VT*, ventricular tachycardia.

time as an intravenous (IV) bolus of 40 units. Dopamine hydrochloride (Intropin) is generally used for its beta-adrenergic effects after cardiac arrest but may be used for its alpha-adrenergic effects during resuscitation. Dobutamine hydrochloride (Dobutrex) is a beta-adrenergic agent used to improve myocardial contractility and increase cardiac output.

Norepinephrine (Levophed) or phenylephrine hydrochloride (Neo-Synephrine) may be used for their alpha-adrenergic effects to increase vasomotor tone and increase perfusion pressure. Sodium bicarbonate, along with regular insulin and calcium chloride, is administered during cardiac arrest for clients who are hyperkalemic. It may also be used, if necessary, to treat a documented bicarbonate metabolic acidosis, as occurs in diabetic ketoacidosis or tricyclic antidepressant overdose. In addition to hyperkalemia, calcium chloride is given for hypocalcemia or calcium channel blocker toxicity because it may cause cell damage and cerebrovascular vasospasm. Isoproterenol (Isuprel) is indicated to increase the heart rate in heart transplant clients, but pacing is preferred.

Vagal Maneuvers. Vagal maneuvers induce vagal stimulation of the cardiac conduction system, specifically the SA and AV nodes. Vagal maneuvers may be attempted to terminate supraventricular tachydysrhythmias and include **carotid sinus massage** and **Valsalva maneuvers.** The results of these interventions, however, are often temporary and further therapy must be initiated.

Carotid Sinus Massage. The physician massages over one carotid artery for a few seconds, observing for a change in cardiac rhythm. Massaging the carotid sinus causes vagal stimulation, slowing SA and AV nodal conduction. Prepare the client for the procedure, instruct him or her to turn the head slightly away from the side to be massaged, and observe the cardiac monitor for a change in rhythm. An electrocardiographic (ECG) rhythm strip is recorded before, during, and after the procedure. After the procedure, assess vital signs and the level of consciousness. Complications include bradydysrhythmias, asystole, VF, and cerebral damage. Because of these risks, carotid massage is *not* commonly performed. A defibrillator and resuscitative equipment must be immediately available during the procedure.

Valsalva Maneuvers. To stimulate a vagal reflex, the health care provider instructs the client to bear down as if straining to have a bowel movement. Prepare the client for the procedure, assess the heart rate, heart rhythm, and blood pressure; observe the cardiac monitor; and record an ECG rhythm strip before, during, and after the procedure to determine the effect of therapy.

Unintended vagal stimulation sometimes occurs, and the nurse must be cautious when performing procedures that may inadvertently cause vagal stimulation. For example, tracheal suctioning, enema administration, and rectal temperature checks can stimulate the vagus nerve and decrease the heart rate inappropriately. Instruct the client not to strain during bowel movements and to avoid constipation through proper diet and exercise. Stool softeners may be prescribed. Instruct the client to avoid inducing gagging during oral hygiene, which triggers a vagal response. Monitor the heart rate and rhythm of a client who is vomiting because a vagal reflex can result. Some clients experience a vagal response when raising their arms above their head and must be instructed to avoid this movement.

Temporary Pacing. Temporary pacing is a nonsurgical intervention that provides a timed electrical stimulus to the heart when either the impulse initiation or the intrinsic conduction system of the heart is defective. The electrical stimulus then spreads throughout the heart to depo-

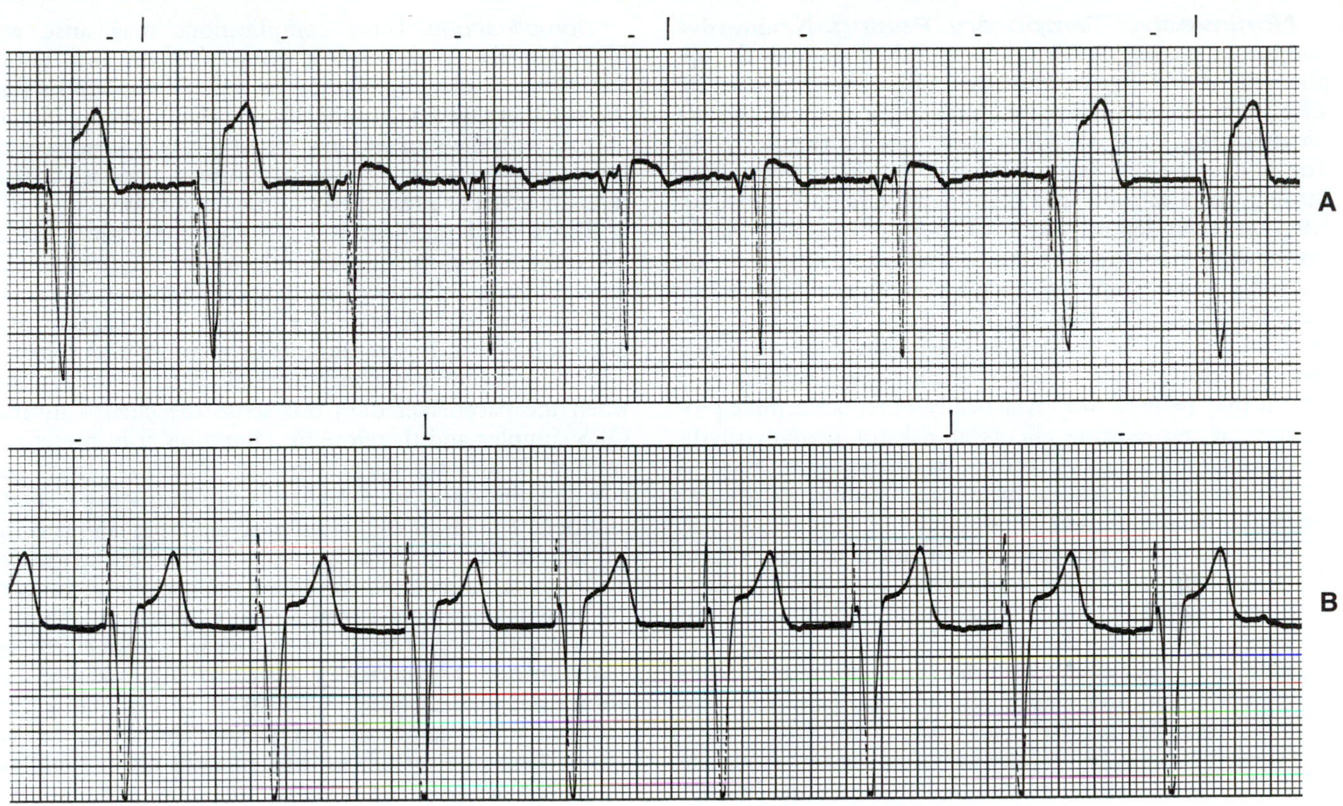

Figure 37-18 ■ Modes of pacing. **A,** Synchronous (demand) ventricular pacing. **B,** Asynchronous (fixed-rate) ventricular pacing at a rate of 70 beats/min.

larize the cells, which should be followed by contraction and cardiac output. Electrical stimuli may be delivered to the right atrium or right ventricle (single-chamber pacemakers) or to both (dual-chamber pacemakers).

When a pacing stimulus is delivered to the heart, a spike (or pacemaker artifact) is seen on the monitor or ECG strip. The spike should be followed by evidence of depolarization (i.e., a P wave, indicating atrial depolarization, or a QRS complex, indicating ventricular depolarization). This pattern is referred to as *capture,* indicating that the pacemaker has successfully depolarized, or captured, the chamber.

Temporary pacing is generally initiated in clients with symptomatic, atropine-refractory bradydysrhythmias, particularly second-degree heart block type II and third-degree heart block, or in clients with asystole. Temporary pacing may also be initiated prophylactically in hemodynamically stable clients with left bundle branch block in certain situations, such as insertion of a pulmonary artery catheter.

A different type of pacing may be used to terminate symptomatic tachydysrhythmias. Occasionally **atrial overdrive pacing** is attempted to terminate atrial tachydysrhythmias, such as atrial flutter or atrial fibrillation (AF). Overdrive pacing is accomplished by rapidly pacing the atrium to capture the heart and control depolarization, followed by no pacing, in the hope that the sinus node will regain control of the heart. Ventricular overdrive pacing may be done to terminate ventricular tachydysrhythmias in much the same way. Overdrive pacing is usually performed by the physician or advanced practice nurse who is specially trained. Have emergency equipment available in case the client becomes more unstable or goes into cardiac arrest.

Modes of Pacing. The two basic modes of pacing are synchronous (demand) pacing and asynchronous (fixed-rate) pacing.

Synchronous Pacing. Temporary pacing is most commonly done in the **synchronous (demand) mode.** The pacemaker's sensitivity is set to sense the client's own beats. When the client's intrinsic rate is above the rate set on the pulse generator, the pacemaker is inhibited from firing. When the client's rate is below that set on the generator, the pacemaker fires electrical impulses to stimulate depolarization (Figure 37-18, *A*).

Asynchronous Pacing. The **asynchronous (fixed-rate) mode** is used when the client is asystolic or profoundly bradycardic, as may occur after open-heart surgery. When the pulse generator is set in an asynchronous mode, it does not sense any intrinsic beats of the client. The pacemaker continues to fire at a fixed rate as set on the generator, regardless of the intrinsic rhythm. This continued firing is not a problem as long as the client remains asystolic or has a rate slower than the pacemaker rate because all beats come from the pacemaker and there is no competition from the client's beats (Figure 37-18, *B*). If the client's rate increases and equals or exceeds the pacemaker rate, however, competition (undersensing) is noted. The danger is that a pacemaker stimulus may reach the heart during the vulnerable period of repolarization (R-on-T phenomenon, with the pacer spike falling on the T wave) and possibly induce ventricular fibrillation (VF). Observe for pacemaker competition, and set the pacemaker to a synchronous mode to avert potential problems.

The two basic types of temporary pacing are noninvasive (external) temporary pacing and invasive temporary pacing.

Noninvasive Temporary Pacing. **Noninvasive temporary pacing (NTP)** is accomplished through the application of two large external electrodes. The electrodes are attached to an external pulse generator, which can operate on alternating current (AC) or battery power (Figure 37-19). The generator emits electrical pulses, which are transmitted through the electrodes and then transcutaneously to stimulate ventricular depolarization when the client's heart rate is slower than the rate set on the pacemaker.

Noninvasive temporary pacing is used as an emergency measure to provide demand ventricular pacing in a profoundly bradycardic or asystolic client until invasive pacing can be instituted or the client's intrinsic rate returns to normal. It may be used prophylactically when performing procedures or transporting clients at risk for bradydysrhythmias. However, it is used only as a temporary measure to maintain heart rate and perfusion until a more permanent method of pacing is used.

Procedure. In a nonemergent situation, explain NTP to the client and prepare the equipment. Wash the skin with soap and water. To prevent skin abrasion, the skin must not be shaved. Do not rub the skin or apply alcohol or tinctures on the skin because electrical current flows from the patches through the skin and causes discomfort. Apply the large posterior electrode on the client's back, between the spine and the left scapula, behind the heart (see Figure 37-19). The electrode should not be placed higher over bone because bone is a poor conductor of electrical current. The anterior electrode is then applied on the chest, between the V_2 and the V_5 positions, over the heart. The electrode cannot be placed over female breast tissue. Displace the breast tissue to position the electrode underneath the breast.

Set the pacing rate as ordered, and establish the stimulation threshold, the lowest current that achieves capture with each pacing spike followed by a QRS complex. The QRS complex is wide because one ventricle depolarizes first, followed by the other. The electrical current is then set 10% above threshold levels.

Palpate the right radial or carotid pulse, and assess the blood pressure using the client's right arm, ensuring that each paced beat is perfused. Vital signs are not taken on the left side of the body because they may not be accurate, particularly if a high milliamperage is used.

Complications. Three complications may arise with NTP. The first is discomfort from cutaneous and muscle stimulation and skin irritation as well as diaphoresis from the patch electrodes. Ensure that the electrodes are in good contact with the skin and in the best location to achieve the lowest threshold for consistent capture. Analgesics or sedatives are given as prescribed to provide comfort.

The second problem is loss of capture, which occurs when the pacing spike is not followed by a QRS complex. Ensure that the electrodes are in good contact with the skin and, if necessary, increase the current until capture is regained; however, higher currents cause more discomfort.

The third problem is inappropriate pacing, which occurs when the pacemaker does not sense the client's intrinsic QRS complex and therefore fires impulses at its preset rate, competing with the client's rhythm. Assess electrode contact and the effect of the client's position on pacemaker function. The client may need to avoid lying on his or her left side. If diaphoresis has caused poor contact and the electrodes must be replaced, first turn the pacemaker function off to avoid receiving electrical shocks when touching the gel side of the electrodes. Then replace with fresh electrodes.

Invasive Temporary Pacing. An **invasive temporary pacemaker** system consists of an external battery-operated pulse generator and pacing electrodes, or lead wires. These wires attach to the generator on one end and are in contact with the heart on the other end. Electrical pulses, or stimuli, are emitted from the negative terminal of the generator, flow through a lead wire, and stimulate the cardiac cells to depolarize. The current seeks ground by returning through the other lead wire to the positive terminal of the generator, thus completing a circuitous route. The intensity of electrical current is set by selecting the appropriate current output, measured in milliamperes.

The client does not usually feel invasive pacemaker stimuli; however, clients occasionally feel an uncomfortable sensation from the stimuli if strong electrical currents (high milliamperage) are delivered by the pacemaker. The discomfort may be alleviated by decreasing the current if possible.

Complications. Complications of invasive temporary pacing may be serious and include the following:

- Infection or hematoma at the pacemaker wire insertion site

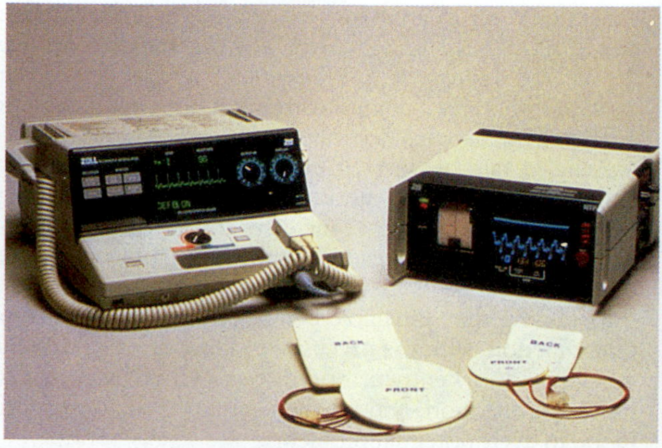

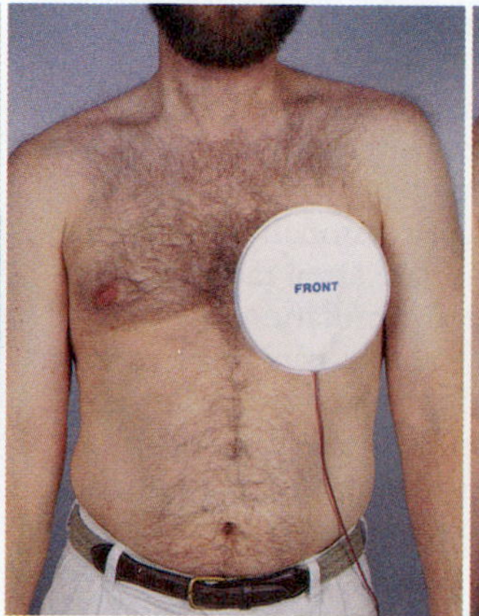

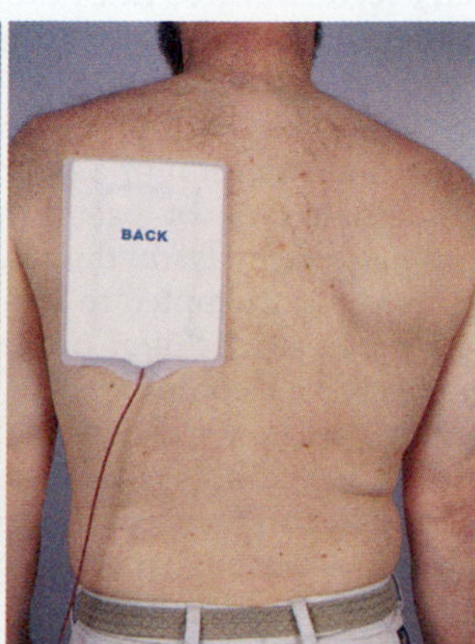

Figure 37-19 ■ Equipment and electrode placement for transcutaneous external pacing. (Courtesy Zoll Medical Corporation, Burlington, MA.)

- Ectopic complexes (usually premature ventricular complexes [PVCs]) caused by irritability from the pacing wire in the ventricle, use of high current, or undersensing with pacemaker competition
- Loss of capture, noted by the presence of a pacing stimulus or spike but no QRS complex
- Undersensing or pacemaker competition, noted when pacing stimuli occur at a fixed rate in the presence of an adequate intrinsic rhythm
- Oversensing, noted when the pacemaker fails to fire in the presence of an inadequate intrinsic rhythm
- Electromagnetic interference, noted by altered generator variables
- Stimulation of the chest wall or diaphragm, noted by rhythmic contraction of the chest-wall muscles or hiccups with the use of high current or from lead wire perforation, which could cause cardiac tamponade

Prevention of Microshock. When the metal external ends of lead wires are not attached to a pulse generator, insulate the wire ends to prevent microshock. The fingertips of rubber gloves work well for this purpose, and the wire ends may then be looped and covered with nonconductive tape. All electrical equipment in the room must be properly grounded using a three-pronged plug. Report faulty electrical equipment, such as frayed or broken electrical wires, to the biomedical engineering department. Neither the client nor the bed should be in contact with such equipment. The risk is that ungrounded electrical current may conduct through the lead wire, stimulate the heart, and induce ventricular fibrillation (VF). Remember to wear rubber gloves when touching any of the wires. Static electricity may be conducted from your hands to the client, causing dysrhythmias if gloves are not worn.

Cardiopulmonary Resuscitation. Management of the client in cardiac arrest depends on prompt recognition and therapeutic interventions for successful reversal of a potentially fatal event.

When cardiac arrest occurs, cardiac output ceases. The underlying rhythm is usually ventricular tachycardia (VT), ventricular fibrillation (VF), or asystole. In rare instances, cardiac arrest occurs in the presence of an organized electrocardiographic (ECG) rhythm but with no effectual mechanical response, a condition referred to as pulseless electrical activity (PEA). Without cardiac output, the client is pulseless and becomes unconscious because of inadequate cerebral perfusion. Shortly after cardiac arrest, respiratory arrest occurs.

Cardiopulmonary resuscitation (CPR) must be initiated immediately to help prevent brain damage and death. When finding an unresponsive client, confirm unresponsiveness and call 911 or the emergency response team before initiating CPR. The initial priorities are as follows:

- Maintenance of a patent airway
- Ventilation with a mouth-to-mask device
- Chest compressions

As soon as help arrives, a board is placed under the client who is not on a firm surface. To make room for the resuscitation team and the crash cart, the nurse commands that the area be cleared of movable items and unnecessary personnel.

Complications of CPR include rib fractures, fracture of the sternum, costochondral separation, lacerations of the liver and spleen, pneumothorax, hemothorax, cardiac tamponade, lung contusions, and fat emboli. The goal of resuscitation is the rapid return of a pulse, blood pressure, and consciousness. This is rarely achieved by CPR and basic measures alone. More definitive therapy must be initiated as soon as possible with advanced cardiac life support (ACLS) measures, including defibrillation, if warranted.

The goal is to be able to give a defibrillatory shock within 5 minutes of collapse outside of a hospital and within 3 minutes in a hospital. To help meet this goal, automated external defibrillators (AEDs) should be placed where there is a probability of at least one sudden cardiac arrest every 5 years, such as on airplanes.

Advanced Cardiac Life Support. When the crash cart arrives, apply ECG electrodes to the client's chest and turn on the monitor. Direct the team to continue CPR and continue to coordinate the personnel who respond to the emergency. If the client is found to be in VF or pulseless VT, the immediate priority is to defibrillate. Following defibrillation, CPR is resumed. An oropharyngeal airway is inserted to facilitate proper ventilation. A manual resuscitation bag (MRB) with mask is attached to an oxygen flowmeter set at 10 to 15 L/min. Direct the person managing the airway to ventilate the lungs with the MRB, maintaining the proper head-tilt, chin-lift position of the client. Initiate two large-bore IV lines if the client does not have any, infusing normal saline. These lines provide access for emergency drug administration. Suction equipment is also set up, with a tonsillar suction tube for suctioning vomitus and a suction catheter for endotracheal suctioning. Carotid or femoral pulse checks with or without chest compressions, blood pressure measurements, and pupil assessments are done at frequent intervals. Document all assessments and findings, therapeutic measures, and the client's responses throughout the resuscitation.

Additional measures include endotracheal intubation with ventilation and oxygenation, IV administration of emergency cardiac drugs, and occasionally external pacing. Chest compressions are continued as long as the client remains pulseless or until a physician decides to terminate resuscitation attempts.

Cardioversion. **Cardioversion** is a synchronized countershock that may be performed in emergencies for hemodynamically unstable ventricular or supraventricular tachydysrhythmias or electively for stable tachydysrhythmias that are resistant to medical therapies. If the client has been taking digitalis, the drug is withheld for up to 48 hours preceding an elective cardioversion, as prescribed. Digitalis increases ventricular irritability and puts the client at risk for VF after the countershock. For elective cardioversion for atrial flutter or fibrillation, the client must take anticoagulants for 4 to 6 weeks before the procedure to prevent embolization of clots from the heart to the brain or lungs.

The shock depolarizes a critical mass of myocardium simultaneously during intrinsic depolarization. It is intended to stop the re-entry circuit and allow the sinus node to regain control of the heart. Emergency equipment must be available during the procedure. The physician, advance practice nurse (e.g., nurse practitioner), or other qualified nurse explains the procedure to the client and assists him or her in signing a consent form unless the procedure is an emergency for a life-threatening dysrhythmia. Because the client is usually conscious, an anesthesiologist may administer a short-acting anesthetic agent as IV sedation.

The defibrillator should be set in the synchronized mode. This avoids discharging the shock during the vulnerable period (T wave), which may increase ventricular irritability, causing ventricular fibrillation (VF). Charge the defibrillator to the energy level requested, usually starting at a low rate. Ensure that the oxygen delivery device has been removed and turned away from the client. Oxygen supports combustion, and a fire may result if there is arcing from the paddles. One paddle is placed to the left of the precordium, and the other is placed on the right next to the sternum and just below the clavicle. Arcing is usually due to improper paddle contact on the chest. At least 25 pounds of pressure should be applied to each paddle to prevent arcing.

The health care provider loudly and clearly commands all personnel to clear contact with the client and the bed, as required for electrical safety. Ensure compliance of all personnel before delivering the shock. The buttons on the paddles are held down until a shock is delivered. There may be a short period before the energy is delivered while the defibrillator is synchronizing with the client's cardiac rhythm.

Another method of delivering synchronized cardioversion is known as the "hands off" method. Special patches are placed on the front and back of the client's thorax or upper right sternal area to deliver the shock. This procedure provides additional safety for the client as well as for the health care personnel.

After cardioversion, assess the client's response and heart rhythm. Therapy is repeated as ordered, if necessary, until the desired result is obtained or alternative therapies are considered. If the client's condition deteriorates into VF after cardioversion, ensure that the synchronizer is turned off so that immediate defibrillation can be administered. Most defibrillators have a dial to turn between synchronous and asynchronous modes.

Nursing care after cardioversion includes the following:

- Maintaining a patent airway
- Administering oxygen
- Assessing vital signs and the level of consciousness
- Administering antidysrhythmic drug therapy
- Monitoring for dysrhythmias
- Assessing for chest burns from paddle edges that may not have been on the conductive pad
- Providing emotional support
- Documenting the results of cardioversion

Defibrillation. **Defibrillation,** an asynchronous countershock, depolarizes a critical mass of myocardium simultaneously to stop the re-entry circuit, allowing the sinus node to regain control of the heart. Early defibrillation is critical in terminating pulseless VT or VF. It must not be delayed for any reason after the equipment and skilled personnel are present. The earlier defibrillation is performed, the greater the chance of survival.

If a defibrillator is not immediately available, an ACLS-qualified nurse may deliver a precordial thump to a pulseless client in VF. There is a slight chance that it may succeed in terminating the VF. A **precordial thump** is performed by striking the lower half of the sternum with a closed fist from a height of 8 to 12 inches (12 to 30 cm) above the sternum. If the client remains in VF, CPR is resumed and the nurse prepares for defibrillation. The defibrillator is charged to 200 Joules, 300 Joules, and 360 Joules for three successive countershocks on a monophasic defibrillator. More effective biphasic defibrillators that allow a lower DC shock and cause less damage to the myocardium are available in some facilities. Before defibrillation, loudly and clearly command all personnel to clear contact with the client and the bed, and ensure their compliance before delivering the shock. Depress the shock buttons on the defibrillator, and the energy is immediately released (see Figure 37-19). Repeat up to three times as needed for VF or pulseless VT. Then continue with the ACLS protocol. Nursing care for defibrillation is the same as for cardioversion.

Automatic External Defibrillation. The American Heart Association promotes the use of automatic external defibrillators (AEDs) for use by laypersons and health care providers responding to cardiac arrest emergencies. These devices are now found in public places such as malls and commercial jets. The client in cardiac arrest must be on a firm, dry surface. The rescuer places two large adhesive-patch electrodes on the client's chest in the same positions as for defibrillator paddles. The rescuer stops CPR and commands anyone present to move away, ensuring that no one is touching the client. This measure eliminates motion artifact when the machine analyzes the rhythm. The rescuer presses the "analyze" button on the machine. After rhythm analysis, which may take up to 30 seconds, the machine either advises that a shock is necessary or advises that a shock is not indicated. Shocks are recommended for VF or pulseless VT only.

After issuing a command to clear all contact with the client, the rescuer charges the defibrillator and presses both discharge buttons on the machine simultaneously, delivering the first shock at 200 Joules. The shock is delivered through the patches, so it is hands-off defibrillation, which is safer for the rescuer. The rescuer then presses the analyze button again, repeating the sequence. With sustained VF or VT, two more shocks may be delivered, with the third at 360 Joules. If the client remains in cardiac arrest, CPR is performed for 1 minute, and then another series of three shocks may be delivered, each at 360 Joules. It is imperative that ACLS be provided as soon as possible. Use of automatic external defibrillators (AEDs) results in earlier defibrillation of clients and therefore a greater chance of successful rhythm conversion and survival.

Critical Thinking Challenge

On the medical-surgical unit, there is a loud crash in the visitors lounge. You find a middle-aged visitor who is pulseless and without respiration on the floor.

1. What should you do first?
2. What actions will the cardiac arrest team take?
3. What cardiac rhythms could be present when the monitor is attached?
4. What treatment modalities should be anticipated for each possible rhythm?

evolve For suggested answer guidelines, go to http://evolve.elsevier.com/Iggy/.

Radiofrequency Catheter Ablation. **Radiofrequency catheter ablation** is an invasive procedure that may be used to abolish an irritable focus causing a supraventricular or ventricular tachydysrhythmia. The client must first undergo electrophysiologic studies and mapping procedures to locate the focus. Then radiofrequency waves are delivered to abolish the irritable focus. When ablation is performed in the AV nodal or His bundle area, damage may also occur to the normal conduction system, causing heart blocks and requiring implantation of a permanent pacemaker.

SURGICAL MANAGEMENT. Clients who experience life-threatening dysrhythmias may require surgical treatment for long-term management. The type of treatment depends on the nature of the dysrhythmia. Procedures include permanent pacing, coronary artery bypass grafting (CABG), aneurysmectomy, insertion of an implantable cardioverter/defibrillator, and open-chest cardiac massage.

Permanent Pacing. Permanent pacemaker insertion is performed for the resolution of conduction disorders that are not temporary, including complete heart block and sick sinus syndrome. Permanent pacemakers are usually powered by a lithium battery and have an average life span of 10 years. After the battery power is depleted, the generator must be replaced, a procedure done with the client under local anesthesia. Some pacemakers are nuclear powered and have a life span of 20 years or longer. Other pacemakers can be recharged externally.

A new type of pacemaker may be utilized to coordinate contractions between the right and left ventricles. In addition to pacing used in the right side of the heart, an additional lead is placed in the left lateral wall of the left ventricle through the coronary sinus. This procedure allows synchronized depolarization of the ventricles and is used in clients with moderate to severe heart failure to improve functional ability.

Surgical Procedures. The surgeon most commonly implants the pulse generator in a surgically made subcutaneous pocket at the shoulder in the right or left subclavicular area. The leads are introduced transvenously via the cephalic or the subclavian vein to the endocardium on the right side of the heart. After the procedure, the nurse monitors the client's electrocardiographic (ECG) rhythm to ensure that the pacemaker is functioning correctly. The implantation site is assessed for evidence of bleeding, swelling, redness, tenderness, or infection. The dressing over the site should remain clean and dry, and the client should be afebrile and have stable vital signs. The physician orders activity restrictions to enhance lead fixation. After 24 hours, activity is gradually increased. Complications of permanent pacemakers are similar to those for temporary invasive pacing.

Pacemaker checks are done on an ambulatory care basis at regular intervals. Reprogramming may be warranted if pacemaker problems develop. The pulse generator is interrogated using an electronic device to determine the pacemaker settings and battery life.

For clients who live far from the pacemaker clinic or physician's office, pacemaker information can be sent via transtelephonic transmission of data. The client attaches ECG electrodes to the wrists and places the telephone receiver in a transmitting unit. The sound signals are relayed via telephone lines to the clinic or office, where they are converted and recorded as the client's ECG rhythm strip and information about the pacemaker variables. The nurse stresses the need to keep clinic appointments for more detailed pacemaker checks and reprogramming, if necessary, as well as assessment.

Critical Thinking Challenge

Your client recently admitted from the ED with chest pain complains of nausea and suddenly develops third-degree heart block. The physician orders external cardiac pacing.

1. How should you prepare the client for this procedure?
2. How should the external pacer pads be applied?

External pacemaking fails, and the physician tells you to prepare for insertion of a temporary pacemaker.

3. What is the difference between a temporary pacemaker and external cardiac pacing?
4. What health teaching should you do in preparation for this treatment modality?

evolve For suggested answer guidelines, go to http://evolve.elsevier.com/Iggy/.

Coronary Artery Bypass Grafting. Coronary artery bypass grafting (CABG) is performed if the cause of the dysrhythmia is coronary artery insufficiency that is unresponsive to medical therapy. This procedure is described in Chapter 41.

Aneurysmectomy. Ventricular aneurysms are a complication of myocardial infarction (MI) and may be the source of intractable ventricular tachydysrhythmias. The surgeon resects the aneurysm, a dyskinetic or ballooning portion of the ventricular wall. Resection of the area eliminates the dangerous irritable focus and thus the cause of the dysrhythmias. Care of the client is similar to that for CABG, described in Chapter 41.

Insertion of Implantable Cardioverter/Defibrillator. The implantable cardioverter/defibrillator (ICD) is indicated for clients who have experienced one or more episodes of spontaneous sustained ventricular tachycardia (VT) or ventricular fibrillation (VF) unrelated to a MI or other causes amenable to correction.

Clients undergo electrophysiologic studies to assess the inducibility of VTs and their response to medication. If the dysrhythmias can be induced despite medical therapy, the client is considered a candidate for ICD implantation. Collaborate with the physician and the electrophysiology nurse to prepare the client for an ICD. A psychological profile is done to determine whether the client will be able to cope with the discomfort and fear associated with internal defibrillation from the ICD.

The leads are introduced percutaneously, and the generator is implanted in the left pectoral area, similar to a permanent pacemaker insertion procedure. This procedure is performed in the electrophysiology laboratory.

If the ICD therapies are not successful and the client remains in VF or pulseless VT, the qualified nurse or health care provider must promptly externally defibrillate the client.

The generator may be activated or deactivated by the physician's placing a magnet over the implantation site for a few moments. The client requires close monitoring in the postimplantation period for the occurrence of dysrhythmias and complications such as bleeding and cardiac tamponade. The nurse must know whether the ICD is activated or deactivated. Care of the client is similar to that following implantation of a permanent pacemaker.

Open-Chest Cardiac Massage. When external chest compressions and advanced cardiac life support measures are unsuccessful in resuscitating a client in cardiac arrest, the physician may decide whether to perform open-chest cardiac massage through a thoracotomy approach or through the median sternotomy incision in post–cardiac surgery clients. Internal defibrillation may also be performed. Open-chest cardiac massage is usually reserved for the client who goes into cardiac arrest during cardiac surgery, often because of cardiac tamponade. It may also be beneficial but is rarely indicated for hypothermia, crushing or penetrating chest injuries, penetrating abdominal trauma, or chest deformities prohibiting external chest compressions. This procedure is a drastic measure that frequently results in devastating consequences for the client.

Critical Thinking Challenge

The physician is performing an elective cardioversion on a client with symptomatic atrial flutter. Suddenly you note the cardiac rhythm on the monitor changes to ventricular fibrillation.

1. What electrical procedure should be used for ventricular fibrillation?
2. What is the difference between defibrillation and synchronized cardioversion?
3. What is the procedure for cardioversion/defibrillation, and what safety precautions should be used?

evolve For suggested answer guidelines, go to http://evolve.elsevier.com/Iggy/.

Community-Based Care

For many clients, dysrhythmias are a chronic disorder resulting from chronic cardiac and pulmonary diseases. Clients may be cared for in a variety of settings, including the acute care hospital, subacute unit, traditional nursing home, or their own home. They are admitted to the hospital when they experience life-threatening or potentially life-threatening dysrhythmias, often associated with an acute disorder. Others can be managed with office or clinic visits or in other settings.

HOME CARE MANAGEMENT

Clients discharged from the hospital may have considerable needs, often more related to their underlying chronic diseases than to their dysrhythmias, which should be essentially controlled by drug or device therapy. A case manager or care coordinator can assess the need for health care resources and coordinate access to services.

The focus of the home care nurse's interventions is assessment and health teaching. Clients and families often fear recurrence of a life-threatening dysrhythmia. Clients with an ICD may dread or fear the activation of the ICD. The community-based nurse provides the client and family members with an opportunity to verbalize their concerns and fears. Provide emotional support as well as information about support groups in the community, and make appropriate referrals. Assess the client for possible side effects of antidysrhythmic agents or complications from a pacemaker or ICD.

HEALTH TEACHING

PREVENTION OF RECURRENCE. Clients who have experienced a dysrhythmia associated with an acute disorder, such as electrolyte imbalance or ischemia related to an MI, are instructed in the prevention, early recognition, and management of that disorder. Teach the client and family about lifestyle modifications designed to prevent, decrease, or control the occurrence of dysrhythmias, as outlined in Chart 37-7. This teaching may be provided in the acute care setting, physician's office, health care clinic, or home setting.

CHART 37-7

CLIENT EDUCATION GUIDE
How to Prevent or Decrease Dysrhythmias

For Clients at Risk for Vasovagal Attacks Causing Bradydysrhythmias

- Avoid doing things that stimulate the vagus nerve, such as raising your arms above your head, applying pressure over your carotid artery, applying pressure on your eyes, bearing down or straining during a bowel movement, and stimulating a gag reflex when brushing your teeth or putting objects in your mouth.

For Clients with Premature Beats and Ectopic Rhythms

- Take the medications that have been prescribed for you, and report any adverse effects to your physician.
- Stop smoking, avoid caffeinated beverages as much as possible, and drink alcohol only in moderation.
- Learn ways to manage stress and avoid getting too tired.

For Clients with Ischemic Heart Disease

- If you have an angina attack, treat it promptly with rest and nitroglycerin administration as prescribed by your physician. This decreases your chances of experiencing a dysrhythmia.
- If chest pain is not relieved after taking the amount of nitroglycerin that has been prescribed for you, seek medical attention promptly. Also, seek prompt medical attention if the pain becomes more severe or you experience other symptoms, such as sweating, nausea, weakness, and palpitations.

For Clients at Risk for Potassium Imbalance

- Know the symptoms of decreased potassium levels, such as muscle weakness and cardiac irregularity.
- Eat foods high in potassium, such as tomatoes, beans, prunes, avocados, bananas, strawberries, and lettuce.
- Take the potassium supplements that have been prescribed for you.

DRUG THERAPY. Clients and designated caregivers must have a thorough understanding of the prescribed medications, including antidysrhythmic agents. Pharmacies provide written instructions with filled prescriptions. Teach clients and families the generic and trade names of their drugs as well as the drugs' purposes, using basic terms that are easily understood. Clear instructions regarding dosage schedules and common side effects are important (see Chart 37-3). Emphasize the importance of reporting these side effects and any dizziness, nausea, vomiting, chest discomfort, or shortness of breath to the health care provider. Chart 37-8 highlights special considerations for older adults receiving antidysrhythmic therapy.

PULSE CHECK. Teach all clients and their significant others or family members how to take a pulse. Instruct them to report any signs of a change in heart rhythm, such as a significant decrease in pulse rate, a rate greater than 100 beats/min, or increased rhythm irregularity.

PACEMAKER. Clients who have a permanent pacemaker are given written and verbal information about the type and settings of their pacemaker. They are taught to report any pulse rate lower than that set on the pacemaker. Review the proper care of the pacemaker insertion site and the importance of reporting any fever or any redness, swelling, or drainage at the pacemaker insertion site. If the surgical incision is near either shoulder, teach and demonstrate range-

CHART 37-8

NURSING FOCUS on the OLDER ADULT

Dysrhythmias

Older adults are at increased risk for dysrhythmias because of changes in their cardiac conduction system. The sinoatrial node has fewer pacemaker cells. There is a loss of fibers in the bundle branch system. Therefore older adults are at risk for sinus node dysfunction and may require pacemaker therapy. The most common dysrhythmias are premature atrial contractions, premature ventricular contractions, and atrial fibrillation. Dysrhythmias tend to be more serious in older clients because of underlying heart disease, causing cardiac decompensation. Consequently, blood flow to organs, which may already be decreased because of the aging process, is further compromised, leading to multisystem organ dysfunction. The following are special nursing considerations for the older client with dysrhythmias:

- Evaluate the client with dysrhythmias immediately for the presence of a life-threatening dysrhythmia or hemodynamic deterioration.
- Assess the client with a dysrhythmia for angina, hypotension, heart failure, and decreased cerebral and renal perfusion.
- Consider the following causes of dysrhythmias when taking the client's history: hypoxia, drug toxicity, electrolyte imbalances, heart failure, and myocardial ischemia or infarction.
- Assess the client's level of education, hearing, learning style, and ability to understand and recall instructions to determine the best approaches for teaching.
- Assess the client's ability to read written instructions.
- Teach the client the generic and trade names of prescribed antidysrhythmic drugs as well as their purposes, dosage, side effects, and special instructions for their use.
- Provide clear written instructions in basic language and easy-to-read print.
- Provide a written drug dosage schedule for the client, taking into account all the medications the client is taking and possible drug interactions.
- Assess the client for possible side effects or adverse reactions to drugs considering the client's age and health status.
- Teach the client to take his or her pulse and to report significant changes in heart rate or rhythm to the physician.
- Inform the client of available resources for blood pressure and pulse checks, such as blood pressure clinics, home health agencies, and cardiac rehabilitation programs.
- Instruct the client on the importance of keeping follow-up appointments with the physician and reporting symptoms promptly.
- Include the client's family members or significant other in all teaching whenever possible.
- Instruct the client to avoid drinking caffeinated beverages, to stop smoking, to drink alcohol only in moderation, and to follow his or her prescribed diet.

of-motion exercises to perform to prevent shoulder stiffness.

Clients with pacemakers are also instructed to keep hand-held cellular phones at least 6 inches away from the generator, with the handset on the ear opposite the side of the generator. Teach them to avoid sources of strong electromagnetic fields, such as magnets and telecommunications transmitters. These may cause interference and could change the pacemaker settings, causing a malfunction. Magnetic resonance imaging (MRI) is contraindicated. Instruct clients to carry a pacemaker identification card and to wear a medical alert bracelet. Chart 37-9 outlines the major points for client and family teaching after the insertion of a permanent pacemaker.

IMPLANTABLE CARDIOVERTER/DEFIBRILLATOR. Clients with an implantable cardioverter/defibrillator (ICD) usually continue to receive antidysrhythmic drugs after discharge from the hospital. Provide clear instructions

CHART 37-9

CLIENT EDUCATION GUIDE

Permanent Pacemakers

- Follow the instructions for pacemaker site skin care that have been specifically prepared for you. Report any fever or redness, swelling, or drainage from the incision site to your physician.
- Keep your pacemaker identification card in your wallet, and wear a medical alert bracelet.
- Take your pulse for 1 full minute at the same time each day, and record the rate in your pacemaker diary. Take your pulse any time you feel symptoms of a possible pacemaker failure, and report your heart rate and symptoms to your physician.
- Know the rate at which your pacemaker is set and the basic functioning of your pacemaker. Know what rate changes to report to your physician.
- Do not apply pressure over your generator. Avoid tight clothing or belts.
- You may take baths or showers without concern for your pacemaker.
- Inform other physicians and dentists that you have a pacemaker. Certain tests they may wish to perform (such as magnetic resonance imaging) could affect or damage your pacemaker.
- Know the indications of battery failure for your pacemaker as you were instructed, and report these findings to your physician if they occur.
- Do not operate electrical appliances directly over your pacemaker site because this may cause your pacemaker to malfunction.
- Do not lean over electrical or gasoline engines or motors. Be sure that electrical appliances or motors are properly grounded.
- Avoid all transmitter towers for radio, television, and radar. Radio, television, other home appliances, and antennas do not pose a hazard.
- Be aware that antitheft devices in stores may cause temporary pacemaker malfunction. If symptoms develop, move away from the device.
- Inform airport personnel of your pacemaker before passing through a metal detector, and show them your pacemaker identification card. The metal in your pacemaker will trigger the alarm in the metal detector device.
- Stay away from any arc welding equipment.
- Be aware that it is safe to operate a microwave oven unless it does not have proper shielding (old microwave ovens) or is defective.
- Report any of the following symptoms to your physician if you experience them: difficulty breathing, dizziness, fainting, chest pain, weight gain, and prolonged hiccupping. If you have any of these symptoms, check your pulse rate and call your physician.
- If you feel symptoms when near any device, move 5 to 10 feet away from it and then check your pulse. Your pulse rate should return to normal.
- Keep all of your physician and pacemaker clinic appointments.
- Take all medications prescribed for you as instructed.
- Follow your prescribed diet.
- Follow instructions on restrictions on physical activity, such as no sudden, jerky movement for 8 weeks to allow the pacemaker to settle in place.

about the purposes of the medications, the dosage schedules, special instructions for taking the medications, and side effects that need to be reported. If clients experience an internal defibrillator shock, they must sit or lie down immediately and notify the physician. Some clients describe the experience of a shock as a quick thud or kick in the chest, whereas others relate severe pain similar to that of external defibrillation. Inform family members that they may feel an electrical shock if

CHART 37-10

CLIENT EDUCATION GUIDE
Implantable Cardioverter/Defibrillator

- Follow the instructions for implantable cardioverter defibrillator (ICD) site skin care that have been specifically prepared for you.
- Report to your physician any fever or redness, swelling, soreness, or drainage from your incision site.
- Do not wear tight clothing or belts that could cause irritation over the ICD generator.
- Avoid activities that involve rough contact with the ICD implantation site.
- Keep your ICD identification card in your wallet and consider wearing a medical alert bracelet.
- Know the basic functioning of your ICD device and its rate cutoff as well as the number of consecutive shocks it can deliver.
- Avoid magnets directly over your ICD because they can inactivate the device. If beeping tones are coming from the ICD, move away from the electromagnetic field immediately (within 30 seconds) before the inactivation sequence is completed, and notify your physician.
- Inform all physicians and dentists caring for you that you have an ICD implanted because certain diagnostic tests and procedures must be avoided to prevent ICD malfunction. These include diathermy, electrocautery, and nuclear magnetic resonance tests.
- Avoid other sources of electromagnetic interference, such as devices emitting microwaves (not microwave ovens); transformers; radio, television, and radar transmitters; large electrical generators; metal detectors, including handheld security devices at airports; antitheft devices; arc welding equipment; and sources of 60-cycle (Hz) interference. Also avoid leaning directly over the alternator of a running motor of a car or boat.
- Report to your physician symptoms such as fainting, nausea, weakness, blackout, and rapid pulse rates.
- Take all medications prescribed for you as instructed.
- Follow instructions on restrictions on physical activity, such as not swimming, driving motor vehicles, or operating dangerous equipment.
- Follow your prescribed diet.
- Keep all physician and ICD clinic appointments.
- Sit or lie down immediately if you feel dizzy or faint to avoid falling if the ICD discharges.
- Postemergency telephone numbers.
- Know how to contact the local emergency medical services (EMS) systems in your community. Inform them in advance that you have an ICD so that they can be prepared if they need to respond to an emergency call for you.
- Know how to perform cough cardiopulmonary resuscitation (CPR) as instructed.
- Encourage family members to learn how to perform CPR. Family members should know that if they are touching you when the device discharges, they may feel a slight shock but that this is not harmful to them.
- Follow instructions on what to do if the ICD successfully discharges, after which you feel well. This may include maintaining a diary of the date, the time, activity preceding the shock, symptoms, the number of shocks delivered, and how you feel after the shock. The physician may wish to be notified each time the device discharges.
- Avoid strenuous activities that may cause your heart rate to meet or exceed the rate cutoff of your ICD because this causes the device to discharge inappropriately.
- Notify your physician if you are leaving town or are relocating for information regarding access to health care.

they are touching the client during delivery of the shock but that it is not harmful. Provide information about how to access the emergency medical services (EMS) system in the community. Recommend resources for the family to learn how to perform cardiopulmonary resuscitation (CPR).

Clients with an ICD are taught to avoid sources of strong electromagnetic fields, such as large electrical generators and radio or television transmitters. These may inhibit tachydysrhythmia detection and therapy or may cause inadvertent antitachycardial pacing or shocks. MRI is contraindicated for clients with ICDs. Handheld cellular phones must be at least 6 inches away from the generator, with the handset held to the ear opposite the side of the ICD. If the pulse generator emits a beeping sound or provides some other indicator, the client must move away from the area as quickly as possible to prevent deactivation of the device. The client with an ICD should carry an ICD identification card and wear a medical alert bracelet. Chart 37-10 highlights the important points for teaching clients and family members and significant others.

HEALTH CARE RESOURCES

The cardiac rehabilitation nurse typically provides written and oral information about dysrhythmias, antidysrhythmic drugs, pacemakers, and ICDs as well as information about cardiac exercise programs, educational programs, and support groups. The office or clinic nurse may also provide information about resources. Instruct the client on how to contact the local affiliate of the American Heart Association or the provincial affiliate of the Heart and Stroke Foundation in Canada for information about dysrhythmias, pacemakers, and CPR training.

Manufacturers of pacemakers and ICDs provide helpful booklets and videotapes to give clients and their families a better understanding of these therapies. Teach clients how to use transtelephonic systems for transmission of their rhythms to a clinic or health care provider's office. Stress the importance of keeping scheduled appointments for office visits with the cardiologist and pacemaker or ICD clinic. Instruct clients with an ICD to contact the local ambulance or paramedic services and emergency facilities to inform them that they have these devices implanted. The client and family are encouraged to attend pacemaker or ICD support groups.

Evaluation: Outcomes

Evaluate the care of the client with dysrhythmias on the basis of the identified nursing diagnoses and collaborative problems. The primary expected outcome is that the client will have adequacy of blood flow from the left ventricle to support systemic blood pressure. Specific indicators for these outcomes are listed for each nursing diagnosis under the Planning and Implementation section (see earlier).

GET READY for the NCLEX Examination!

KEY POINTS

Safe Effective Care Environment

- In collaboration with the health care team, assess clients at risk for dysrhythmias.
- Consult with other health care providers regarding a change in client status.
- Evaluate the effectiveness of medication administration and treatment modalities for clients with dysrhythmias.

- Utilize the correct procedure for electrical and client safety during use of a defibrillator for cardioversion/defibrillation.
- Use infection control precautions during resuscitation efforts for a client with a lethal dysrhythmia.

Health Promotion and Maintenance

- Teach clients with dysrhythmias the correct drug, dose, route, time, and side effects of prescribed medications, and to notify their physicians if adverse effects occur.
- Teach clients of all ages the importance of a balanced diet, regular exercise, caffeine limitation, and tobacco and alcohol cessation to prevent dysrhythmias.
- Teach family members cardiopulmonary resuscitation techniques to decrease their anxiety while living with a client with dysrhythmias.
- Teach clients the importance of adhering to their prescribed cardiac regimen, such as checking their pulse to ascertain pacemaker function.

Psychosocial Integrity

- Because dysrhythmias can be life threatening, assess clients' and family members' reactions to the diagnoses and their resources for coping.
- Allow the client opportunities to express feelings of anxiety and fear.
- Evaluate the effectiveness of clients/family members coping mechanisms with lifestyle changes associated with dysrhythmias.
- Provide age-appropriate care for clients with dysrhythmias.
- Explain emergency interventions to the client and family before performing them, if appropriate.
- Allow family members to be present during resuscitation efforts, if desired and allowed.

Physiological Integrity

- Assess clients with dysrhythmias for a decrease in cardiac output.
- Administer medications and evaluate/document their effectiveness.
- Monitor clients with dysrhythmias, including conducting a physical assessment and health history, as well as interpreting ECG rhythm strips. Report significant changes to the health care provider.
- Use Table 37-2 to provide appropriate interventions for clients with dysrhythmias.
- Identify and intervene in life-threatening situations by providing cardiopulmonary resuscitation, electrical therapy, or medication administration. Specifically, know the lethal rhythms of ventricular fibrillation, ventricular tachycardia without a pulse, and asystole.
- Use Charts 37-9 and 37-10 to educate clients with permanent pacemakers or ICDs.
- Evaluate the client's response to emergency interventions and recommend changes in treatment based on evaluation of his or her response.

ADDITIONAL STUDY RESOURCES

Go to your Student CD-ROM for Review Questions for the NCLEX Examination.

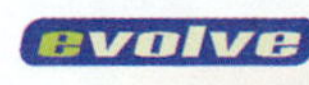

Go to http://evolve.elsevier.com/Iggy/ for Integrated Management of Care Questions for the NCLEX Examination.

SELECTED BIBLIOGRAPHY

Ackley, B.J., & Ladwig, G.B. (2004). *Nursing diagnosis handbook. A guide to planning care* (6th ed.). St. Louis: Mosby.

Adams-Hamoda, M.G., et al. (2003). Factors to consider when analyzing 12-lead electrocardiograms for evidence of acute myocardial ischemia. *American Journal of Critical Care, 12*(1), 9-18.

American Heart Association. (2000). *2000 handbook of emergency cardiovascular care for healthcare providers.* Dallas, TX: American Heart Association.

American Heart Association. (2000). Guidelines 2000 for cardiopulmonary resuscitation and emergency cardiovascular care. *Circulation, 102*(8), 112-124.

American Heart Association. (2001). *ACLS provider manual.* Dallas, TX: American Heart Association.

American Heart Association. (2001). *Heart and stroke statistical update.* Dallas, TX: American Heart Association.

Beasley, B.M. (2003). *Understanding EKGs–a practical approach* (2nd ed.). Upper Saddle River, NJ: Prentice Hall.

Benson, L.M., & Powless, D. (2003). Dofetilide and atrial fibrillation. *American Journal of Nursing, 103*(2), 64AA-GG.

Bosen, D.M. (2002). Atrio-ventricular nodal reentry tachycardia. *Dimensions of Critical Care Nursing, 21*(4), 134-140.

Conover, M.B. (2003). *Understanding electrocardiography* (8th ed.). St. Louis: Mosby.

Doherty, J.U., Fuchs, S., & Tecce, M.A. (2000). Ventricular arrhythmias. *Geriatrics, 55*(8), 26-33.

Ehrat, K.S. (2002). *The art of EKG interpretation.* Dubuque, IA: Kendall/Hunt.

Eichhorn, D., et al. (2001). Family presence during invasive procedures and resuscitation: hearing the voice of the patient. *American Journal of Nursing, 101*(5), 48-55.

Ellis, K.M. (2002). *EKG plain and simple-from rhythm strips to 12-leads.* Upper Saddle River, NJ: Prentice Hall.

Futterman, L.G., & Lemberg, L. (2002). Ambulatory electrocardiographic monitoring: Use of the implantable loop recorder in the evaluation of syncope. *Journal of Cardiovascular Nursing, 16*(3), 24-33.

Geiter, H.B., Jr. (2004). Getting back to basics with permanent pacemakers, Part I. *Nursing 2004, 34*(10), 32cc1-32cc4.

Goodman, D. (2001). Automatic external defibrillation. *Medsurg Nursing, 10*(5), 251-255.

Gulanick, M., et al. (2003). *Nursing care plans: Nursing diagnosis and intervention* (5th ed.). St. Louis: Mosby.

Harris, J. (2002). Biphase defibrillation. *Emergency Nurse, 10*(7), 33-38.

Harvard Medical School. (2002). Delivering the shock of a lifetime. *Harvard Health Letter, 27*(11), 4.

Hebbar, A.K, & Hueston, W.J. (2002). Management of common arrhythmias: Part I. Supraventricular arrhythmias. *American Family Physician, 65*(12), 2479-2487.

Hebbar, A.K, & Hueston, W.J. (2002). Management of common arrhythmias: Part II. Ventricular arrhythmias and arrhythmias in special populations . *American Family Physician, 65*(12), 2491-2497.

Householder-Hughes, S.D. (2002). Advanced cardiac life support for the new millennium. *Journal of Cardiovascular Nursing, 16*(3), 9-23.

Josephson, L., & McMullen, M. (2003). Atrial fibrillation. Beyond irregularly irregular: Learn to recognize and manage atrial fibrillation in its various forms. *Critical Care Choices, Nursing 2003 (suppl), 33*(5), 4-10.

Madrid, P., & Sendelbach, S. (2001). Heart-smarter drugs for resuscitation. *American Journal of Nursing, May 2001 Suppl,* 42-44.

McCloskey, J.C., & Bulechek, G.M. (2000). *Nursing interventions classification (NIC)* (3rd ed.). St. Louis: Mosby.

McComb, J.M., & Camm, A.J. (2002). Primary prevention of sudden cardiac death using implantable cardioverter defibrillators. *British Medical Journal, 325*(7372), 1050-1051.

McConnell, E.A. (2002). Using an automated external defibrillator. *Nursing 2002, 32*(10), 18.

Myerburg, R.J., & Castellanos, A. (2002). Electrode positioning for cardioversion of atrial fibrillation. *The Lancet, 360,* 1263-1264.

Nacrelli, G., et al. (2000). Amiodarone: what have we learned from clinical trials? *Clinical Cardiology, 23,*73-82.

Newton, J.L. (2000). Action stat: Amiodarone overdose. *Nursing 2000, 30*(2), 33.

Pagana, K.D., & Pagana, T.J. (2003). *Mosby's diagnostic and laboratory test reference* (6th ed.). St. Louis: Mosby.

Paulus, K., et al. (2002). Anterior-posterior versus anterior-lateral electrode positions for cardioversion of atrial fibrillation: A randomised (sic) trial. *The Lancet, 360,* 1275-1279.

Rodriquez, I., et al. (2001). Drug-induced QT prolongation in women during the menstrual cycle. *Journal of the American Medical Association, 285*(10), 1322-1326.

Schott, R. (2002). Wearable defibrillator. *Journal of Cardiovascular Nursing, 16*(3), 44-52.

Schwertz, D.W. (2003). Forward. *Journal of Cardiovascular Nursing, 18*(1), 6-10.

Skidmore-Roth, L. (2003). *Mosby's nursing drug reference.* St. Louis: Mosby.

Squires, A. (2000). Critical care: Teaching patients about telemetry. *Nursing 2000, 30*(7), 32cc1-32cc4.

Stahl, M.A., & Richards, N.M. (2002). Ventricular assist devices: Developing and maintaining a training and competency program. *Journal of Cardiovascular Nursing, 16*(3), 34-43.

Swearingen, P.L. (2003). *Manual of medical-surgical nursing care. Nursing interventions and collaborative management* (5th ed.). St. Louis: Mosby.

Swearingen, P.L., & Keen, J.H. (2001). *Manual of critical care nursing. Nursing interventions and collaborative management* (4th ed.). St. Louis: Mosby.

Thaler, M.S. (2002). *The only EKG book you'll ever need* (4th ed.). Philadelphia: Lippincott, Williams & Wilkins.

Urden, L.D., Stacy, K.M., & Lough, M.E. (2002). *Thelan's critical care nursing: Diagnosis and management* (4th ed.). St. Louis: Mosby.

Urden, L.D., Stacy, K.M., & Lough, M.E. (2003). *Priorities in critical care nursing* (4th ed.). St. Louis: Mosby.

White, E. (2000). Patients with implantable cardioverter defibrillators: Transition to home. *Journal of Cardiovascular Nursing, 14*(3), 42-52.

White, M.M. (2002). Psychosocial impact of the implantable cardioverter defibrillator: Nursing implications. *Journal of Cardiovascular Nursing, 16*(3), 53-61.

Woods, A. (2001). Calling all pacemakers. *Nursing 2001, 31*(1), 46-47.

Wooten, J.M. (2002). Drug-induced arrhythmias. *RN, 65*(1), 37-44.

Yee, C.A., & Rozewicz, B. (2003). Getting to the heart of atrial fibrillation. *Nursing Management, 34*(9), 21-27.

CHAPTER 38

Interventions for Clients with Cardiac Problems

ELAINE BISHOP KENNEDY • DONNA D. IGNATAVICIUS

LEARNING OUTCOMES

After studying this chapter, you should be able to:

1. Explain the pathophysiology of heart failure.
2. Compare and contrast left-sided and right-sided heart failure.
3. Perform a comprehensive assessment of clients experiencing heart failure.
4. Identify common nursing diagnoses and collaborative problems for clients with heart failure.
5. Evaluate the effects of interventions for reducing preload and afterload.
6. Identify common drug therapies to improve cardiac output.
7. Describe special considerations for older adults with heart failure.
8. Discuss the prevention of complications for clients with heart failure.
9. Prioritize nursing care for clients experiencing heart failure.
10. Identify essential focused assessments used by the home care nurse for clients with heart failure.
11. Compare and contrast common valvular disorders.
12. Discuss surgical management for clients with valvular disease.
13. Develop a teaching/learning plan for clients with valvular disease.
14. Differentiate between common cardiac inflammations and infections–endocarditis, pericarditis, and rheumatic carditis.
15. Discuss the legal/ethical aspects related to heart transplantation, including resource management.

Go to your Student CD-ROM for Review Questions for the NCLEX Examination keyed to these Learning Outcomes.

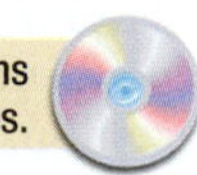

Although most Americans do not consider heart disease an incurable illness, more people die of heart disease than from the next seven leading causes of death combined. ". . . About 250,000 people a year die of coronary heart disease (CHD) without being hospitalized. That's about half of all deaths from CHD–more than 680 Americans each day" (American Heart Association [AHA], 2003). These deaths are usually the result of heart failure. One in five clients who develop heart failure die within one year. Women have a poorer survival rate than men, with fewer than 15% of women surviving longer than 8 to 12 years.

Long-term survival of clients with heart disease depends on client compliance with therapy and a coordinated interdisciplinary approach to ensure the best management of the illness and the highest possible quality of life. Therefore, as described in Chapter 3, high-risk clients are often targeted for case management to coordinate their care through the health care continuum.

HEART FAILURE

Heart failure, sometimes referred to as **pump failure,** is a general term for the inadequacy of the heart to pump blood throughout the body. This deficit causes insufficient perfusion of body tissues with vital nutrients and oxygen. Heart failure results from a number of acute and chronic cardiovascular problems that are discussed elsewhere in this text.

PATHOPHYSIOLOGY

Types of Heart Failure

The following are the major types of heart failure:

- Left-sided heart failure
- Right-sided heart failure
- High-output failure

LEFT-SIDED HEART FAILURE

Because the two ventricles of the heart represent two separate pumping systems, it is possible for one to fail by itself for a short period. Most heart failure begins with failure of the left ventricle and progresses to failure of both ventricles. Typical causes of **left-sided heart (ventricular) failure** include hypertensive, coronary artery, and valvular disease involving the mitral or aortic valve. Decreased tissue perfusion from poor cardiac output and pulmonary congestion from increased pressure in the pulmonary vessels indicate left ventricular failure.

Left-sided heart failure was formerly referred to as **congestive heart failure (CHF);** it may be acute or chronic and mild to severe. CHF can be further divided into two subtypes: systolic heart failure and diastolic heart failure.

SYSTOLIC HEART FAILURE. **Systolic heart failure (systolic ventricular dysfunction)** results when the heart is unable to contract forcefully enough during systole to eject adequate amounts of blood into the circulation. Preload increases with decreased contractility, and afterload increases as a result of increased peripheral resistance (e.g., hypertension) (McCance & Huether, 2002). The **ejection fraction** (the percentage of blood ejected from the heart during systole) drops from a normal of 50% to 70% to below 40%. As the ejection fraction decreases, tissue perfusion diminishes and blood accumulates in the pulmonary vessels. Manifestations of systolic dysfunction may include symptoms of inadequate tissue perfusion or pulmonary and systemic congestion.

DIASTOLIC HEART FAILURE. In contrast, **diastolic heart failure (diastolic ventricular function)** occurs when the left ventricle is unable to relax adequately during diastole. Inadequate relaxation or "stiffening" prevents the ventricle from filling with sufficient blood to ensure an adequate cardiac output; however, the ejection fraction may remain near normal (Martin, 2003). Diastolic failure represents about 20% to 40% of all heart failure, primarily in older adults and in women following a myocardial infarction. Symptoms of diastolic failure are similar to those of systolic dysfunction.

RIGHT-SIDED HEART FAILURE

Right-sided heart (ventricular) failure may be caused by left ventricular failure, right ventricular myocardial infarction, or pulmonary hypertension. In right-sided heart failure, the right ventricle is unable to empty completely. Increased volume and pressure develop in the systemic veins, and systemic venous congestion develops with peripheral edema.

HIGH-OUTPUT FAILURE

High-output failure can occur when cardiac output remains normal or above normal, unlike left- and right-sided heart failure, which are typically low-output states. High-output failure is caused by increased metabolic needs or hyperkinetic conditions, such as septicemia (fever), anemia, and hyperthyroidism. This type of heart failure is not as common as other types.

Classifications of Heart Failure

Heart failure (HF) can be classified using two approaches: staging of the disease or functional classification.

DISEASE STAGING

Staging of the disease is centered on its risk, evolution, and progression in four stages. Stage A indicates a high risk for HF without any structural heart changes or disorders. In stage B, the client has a structural disorder but has not developed any symptoms of the disease. The client in stage C has a current or past history of HF with a structural disorder, and stage D indicates end-stage disease. The client with stage D illness requires ongoing, chronic support and treatments, including possible hospice care or heart transplantation (Artinian, 2003).

A more popular method for staging HF is the Killip Classification System, which is based on the heart's hemodynamic ability. Table 41-3 in Chapter 41 outlines this system.

FUNCTIONAL CLASSIFICATION

HF may also be categorized by its effect on the client's functional status. The client is categorized according to the relationship between symptoms and activity level. Class I and II are less severe. Class III and IV indicate severe limitations in activity level and functional ability. Table 36-2 in Chapter 36 summarizes the New York Heart Association (NYHA) categories.

Compensatory Mechanisms

When cardiac output is insufficient to meet the demands of the body, compensatory mechanisms operate to improve cardiac output (Figure 38-1). Although these mechanisms may initially increase cardiac output, they eventually have a damaging effect on pump function. Compensatory mechanisms include the following:

- Sympathetic nervous system stimulation
- Renin-angiotensin system (RAS) activation
- Other neurohumoral responses
- Myocardial hypertrophy

SYMPATHETIC NERVOUS SYSTEM STIMULATION

In heart failure (HF), stimulation of the sympathetic nervous system (i.e., increasing catecholamines) as a result of tissue hypoxia represents the most immediate compensatory mechanism. Stimulation of the adrenergic receptors causes an increase in heart rate (beta adrenergic) and blood pressure from vasoconstriction (alpha adrenergic).

Because cardiac output (CO) is the product of heart rate (HR) and stroke volume (SV)–CO = HR × SV)–an increase in HR results in an immediate *increase in cardiac output.* An increase in HR is limited in its ability to compensate for decreased CO. If HR becomes too rapid, diastolic filling time is limited and CO may start to decline. An increase in HR also significantly increases oxygen demand by the myocardium. If the heart is poorly perfused because of arteriosclerosis, HF may worsen.

Stroke volume (SV) is also *improved* by sympathetic stimulation. Sympathetic stimulation increases venous return to the

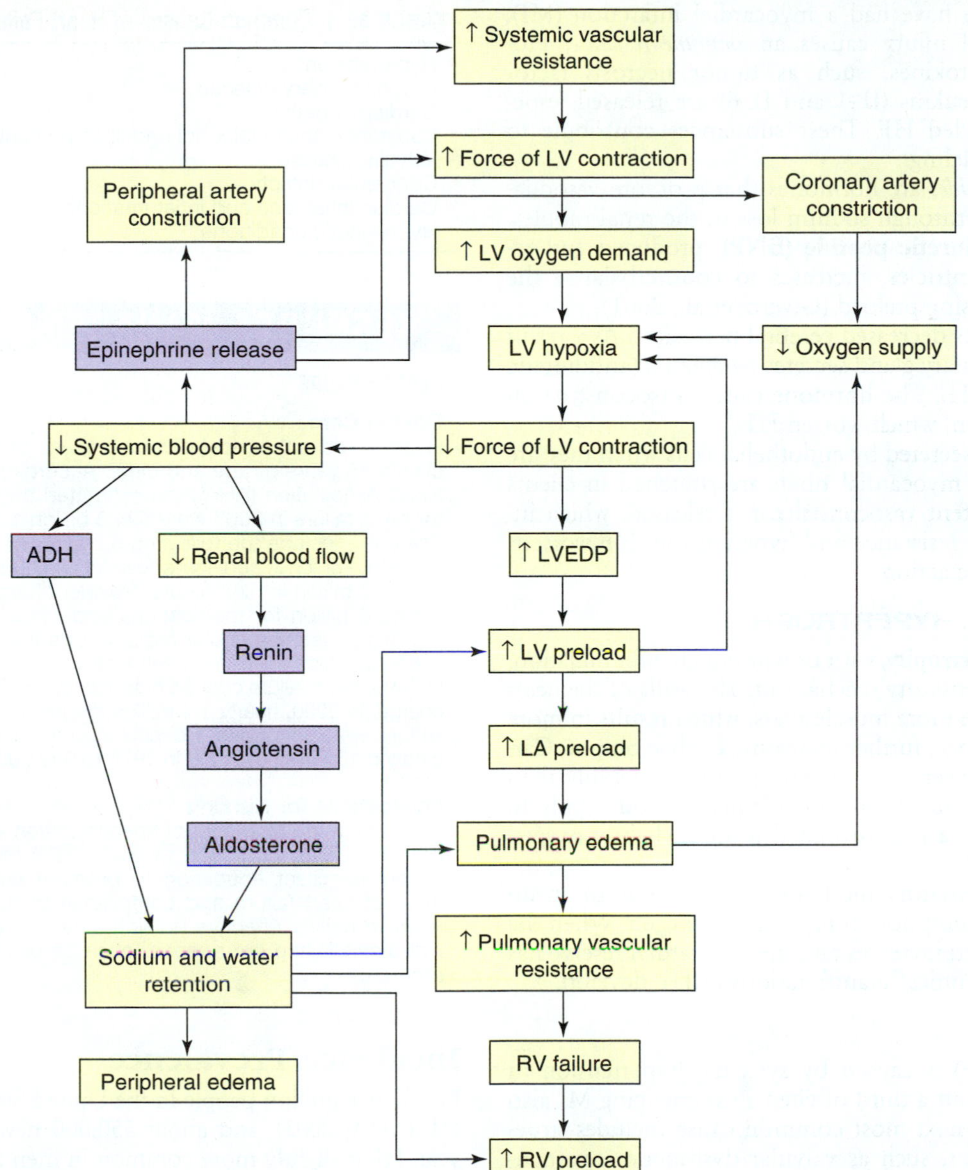

Figure 38-1 ■ Left-sided heart failure (congestive heart failure) from elevated systemic vascular resistance. Left heart failure leads to right heart failure. Systemic vascular resistance and preload are exacerbated by renal and adrenal mechanisms. *LV,* Left ventricular; *LVEDP,* left ventricular end-diastolic pressure; *LA,* left atrial; *ADH,* antidiuretic hormone; *RV,* right ventricular.

heart, which further stretches the myocardial fibers, causing dilation. In accordance with Starling's law of the heart, increased myocardial stretch results in more forceful contraction. More forceful contractions increase SV and CO. After a critical point is reached within the cardiac muscle, further volume and stretch will reduce the force of contraction and CO.

Sympathetic stimulation also results in *arterial vasoconstriction.* Constriction of the arteries has the benefit of maintaining blood pressure and improving tissue perfusion in low-output states; however, constriction of the arteries increases **afterload,** the resistance against which the heart must pump. Afterload is the major determinant of myocardial oxygen requirements. As afterload increases, the left ventricle requires more energy to eject its contents, and SV may decline.

RENIN-ANGIOTENSIN SYSTEM ACTIVATION

Reduced blood flow to the kidneys, a common occurrence in low-output states, results in activation of the renin-angiotensin system (RAS). Vasoconstriction becomes more pronounced in response to angiotensin II, and aldosterone secretion causes sodium and water retention. Preload and afterload increase; angiotensin II contributes to **ventricular remodeling,** resulting in progressive myocyte (myocardial cell) contractile dysfunction over time (McCance & Huether, 2002).

OTHER NEUROHUMORAL RESPONSES

In addition to the sympathetic nervous system and RAS responses, other mechanisms are activated when a client experiences heart failure (HF). Most of these actions contribute to worsening of the condition.

In clients who have had a myocardial infarction (MI), heart muscle cell injury causes an *immune response.* Proinflammatory cytokines, such as tumor necrosis factor (TNF) and interleukins (IL-1 and IL-6) are released, especially with left-sided HF. These substances contribute to ventricular remodeling.

Natriuretic peptides are hormones that promote vasodilation and diuresis through sodium loss in the renal tubules. The **B-type natriuretic peptide (BNP)**, produced and released by the ventricles, increases to counterbalance the RAS, thus decreasing preload (Givertz et al., 2001).

Low CO causes decreased cerebral perfusion. As a result the posterior pituitary gland secretes *vasopressin* (antidiuretic hormone, or ADH). The hormone causes vasoconstriction and fluid retention, which worsen HF.

Endothelin is secreted by endothelial cells when they are stretched. As the myocardial fibers are stretched in clients with HF, this potent vasoconstrictor is released, which increases peripheral resistance and hypertension. HF worsens as a result of these actions.

MYOCARDIAL HYPERTROPHY

Myocardial hypertrophy, with or without chamber dilation, is the final compensatory mechanism. The walls of the heart thicken to provide more muscle mass, which results in more forceful contractions, further increasing cardiac output. Cardiac muscle, however, may hypertrophy more rapidly than collateral circulation can provide adequate blood supply to the muscle. Often a hypertrophied heart is slightly oxygen deprived.

All the compensatory mechanisms contribute to an increase in the consumption of myocardial oxygen. When the demand for oxygen increases and the myocardial reserve has been exhausted, clinical manifestations of HF develop.

Etiology

Heart failure (HF) is caused by systemic hypertension in 75% of cases. About a third of clients experiencing MI also develop HF. The next most common cause includes structural heart changes, such as valvular dysfunction, particularly pulmonic or aortic stenosis, which cause pressure or volume overload on the heart. Common direct causes of HF are listed in Table 38-1.

CONSIDERATIONS FOR OLDER ADULTS

The use of certain drugs can also lead to heart failure (HF), especially in older adults. Long-term nonsteroidal anti-inflammatory drugs (NSAIDs), such as ibuprofen (Motrin), cause fluid and sodium retention. Many older adults take these drugs for arthritic pain and inflammation. Thiazolidinediones (TZDs) used for diabetics, such as pioglitazone (Actos) and rosiglitazone (Avandia), also cause fluid and sodium retention (Martin, 2003). These medications should be used with caution in the older adult population. These clients should be monitored closely by their health care provider.

Right-sided HF in the absence of left-sided HF is most often the result of pulmonary problems, such as chronic obstructive pulmonary disease (COPD) or cystic fibrosis. Acute respiratory distress syndrome (ARDS) may also cause right-sided HF.

TABLE 38-1 Common Causes of Heart Failure

- Hypertension
- Coronary artery disease
- Cardiomyopathy
- Substance abuse (alcohol and illicit/prescribed drugs)
- Valvular disease
- Congenital defects
- Cardiac infections and inflammations
- Hyperkinetic conditions

RESOURCE MANAGEMENT

HEART FAILURE

Cost of Care

Heart failure is the most common cause of hospitalization for clients 65 years of age and older. According to the American Heart Association (AHA), the estimated annual costs of care for heart failure in 2003 were $24.3 billion dollars (AHA, 2003). The costs include the following:

- $16.4 billion in additional hospital and nursing home charges
- $1.7 billion in health care provider charges
- $2.3 billion for medications and other medical durables (e.g., a left ventricular assist device [LVAD])
- $2.2 billion for home health care

In 1998, heart failure cost $3.6 million, or $5471 per hospital discharge. In 2000, nearly 1.4 million diagnostic cardiac catheterizations were performed. Hospital discharges for heart failure increased 165 from 377,000 in 1979 to 999,000 in 2000.

Implications for Nursing

Because of the high cost of hospitalization and nursing home care for clients with heart failure, nurses must be attuned to enhancing client education to promote client self-management of heart failure and compliance with therapy. Creative ways to deliver effective nursing care in the home to clients with heart failure are needed, such as disease management programs.

Incidence/Prevalence

Nearly five million people in the United States are living with HF (AHA, 2003), and about 550,000 new cases occur each year. HF is slightly more common in men than in women.

CONSIDERATIONS FOR OLDER ADULTS

The prevalence of heart failure (HF) steadily increases with aging. As many as 10% of people over 70 years of age have HF. About 80% of all hospital admissions for HF are clients older than 65 years of age (AHA, 2003). The cost of providing care for this number of people with HF is detailed in the Resource Management box above.

One of the Healthy People 2010 objectives for the United States is to reduce by 50% the number of hospitalizations of older adults with HF as the principal diagnosis. Interventions aimed at client and family education can help meet this objective (see the Meeting Healthy People 2010 Objectives box on p. 753).

COLLABORATIVE MANAGEMENT

PHARM e REVIEW

Assessment

Manifestations of HF depend on the type of failure, the ventricle involved, and the underlying cause. Impaired tissue perfusion, pulmonary congestion, and edema dominate

Meeting HEALTHY PEOPLE 2010 Objectives

CARDIAC DISEASE

Objective 12.6: To reduce hospitalizations of older adults with heart failure as the principal diagnosis.

- For clients hospitalized for heart failure, collaborate with the case manager for discharge planning, including adequate support in the community.
- Provide a continuing plan of care for clients and their families or other caregivers when the client is discharged from the hospital.
- If the client is discharged to home, call the client to check that he or she has no impending signs and symptoms of heart failure (the case manager may make calls).
- Teach the client and family or other caregiver about when to call the health care provider for health changes so the client can be treated at home.
- Ensure that the interdisciplinary team provides the client with follow-up care in the home or nursing home.

CHART 38-1

KEY FEATURES of
Left-Sided Heart Failure

Decreased Cardiac Output
- Fatigue
- Weakness
- Oliguria during the day
- Angina
- Confusion, restlessness
- Dizziness
- Tachycardia, palpitations
- Pallor
- Weak peripheral pulses
- Cool extremities

Pulmonary Congestion
- Hacking cough, worse at night
- Dyspnea/breathlessness
- Crackles or wheezes in lungs
- Frothy, pink-tinged sputum
- Tachypnea
- S_3/S_4 summation gallop

CHART 38-2

KEY FEATURES of
Right-Sided Heart Failure

Systemic Congestion
- Jugular (neck vein) distention
- Enlarged liver and spleen
- Anorexia and nausea
- Dependent edema (legs and sacrum)
- Distended abdomen
- Swollen hands and fingers
- Polyuria at right
- Weight gain
- Increased blood pressure (from excess volume) or decreased blood pressure (from failure)

the picture of left ventricular failure (Chart 38-1). Conversely, systemic venous congestion and peripheral edema are associated with right ventricular failure (Chart 38-2).

HISTORY

When obtaining a history, keep in mind the many conditions that can lead to HF. Carefully question the client about his or her medical history, including high blood pressure, angina, MI, rheumatic heart disease, valvular disorders, endocarditis, and pericarditis. Ask about the client's perception of his or her activity tolerance, breathing pattern, urinary pattern, and fluid volume status as well as his or her knowledge about HF

LEFT-SIDED HEART FAILURE. With left ventricular systolic dysfunction, cardiac output (CO) is diminished, leading to impaired tissue perfusion, anaerobic metabolism, and unusual fatigue. Assess activity tolerance by asking whether the client can perform normal activities of daily living (ADLs) or climb flights of stairs without fatigue or dyspnea. Many clients with HF experience weakness or fatigue with activity or have a feeling of heaviness in their arms or legs. Ask about their ability to perform simultaneous arm and leg work (e.g., walking while carrying a bag of groceries). Such activity may place an unacceptable demand on the failing heart. Question the client to identify their most strenuous activity in the past week. Many clients unconsciously limit their activities in response to fatigue or dyspnea and may not realize how limited they have become.

Perfusion to the myocardium is often impaired with left ventricular failure, and especially with cardiac hypertrophy. The client may report chest discomfort or may describe palpitations, skipped beats, or a fast heartbeat.

As the amount of blood ejected from the left ventricle diminishes, hydrostatic pressure builds in the pulmonary venous system and results in fluid-filled alveoli and pulmonary congestion. Thus cough is often an early manifestation of HF. The client in early HF describes the cough as irritating, nocturnal (at night), and usually nonproductive. As HF becomes very severe, the client may begin expectorating frothy, pink-tinged sputum–a sign of pulmonary edema.

Dyspnea also results from rising pulmonary venous pressure and pulmonary congestion. Carefully question the client about the presence of dyspnea and when and how it developed. The client may refer to dyspnea as "trouble in catching my breath," "breathlessness," or "difficulty in breathing."

As **exertional dyspnea** develops (also called dyspnea upon exertion [DUE]), the client often discontinues previously tolerated levels of activity because of shortness of breath. Dyspnea at rest in the recumbent (lying flat) position is known as **orthopnea.** Ask the client how many pillows he or she usually uses to sleep or whether he or she sleeps in an upright position in a bed or a chair.

Clients who describe sudden awakening with a feeling of breathlessness 2 to 5 hours after falling asleep have **paroxysmal nocturnal dyspnea (PND).** Sitting upright, dangling the feet, or walking usually relieves this condition.

RIGHT-SIDED HEART FAILURE. Signs of systemic congestion occur as the right ventricle fails, fluid is retained, and pressure builds in the venous system. Edema develops in the lower legs and ascends to the thighs and abdominal wall. Clients may note that their shoes fit more tightly, or their shoes or socks may leave indentations on their swollen feet. They have removed their rings because of swelling in their fingers and hands. Ask about weight gain. An adult may retain 4 to 7 L of fluid (10 to 15 pounds [4.5 to 6.8 kg]) before pitting edema occurs.

Gastrointestinal complaints of nausea and anorexia may be a direct consequence of liver engorgement resulting from fluid retention. In advanced HF, ascites and an increased abdominal girth may develop from the pronounced liver congestion. Another finding related to fluid retention is diuresis at rest. At rest, fluid in the peripheral tissue is mobilized and excreted, and the client describes frequent awakening at night to urinate.

Obtain a careful nutritional history, questioning the client about the use of salt and the types of food consumed. Ask about daily fluid intake. Clients with HF may experience increased thirst and take in excessive fluid (4000 to 5000 mL) because of sodium retention.

PHYSICAL ASSESSMENT/CLINICAL MANIFESTATIONS

The signs and symptoms of HF can be considered in the context of these components of the syndrome:

- Failure of the left ventricle as a pump with decreased tissue perfusion and pulmonary venous congestion
- Failure of the right ventricle as a pump with systemic venous congestion

LEFT-SIDED HEART FAILURE. Left ventricular failure is associated with decreased cardiac output and elevated pulmonary venous pressure. Left ventricular failure may appear clinically as weakness, fatigue, dizziness, confusion, pulmonary congestion, breathlessness, oliguria (scant urine output), or death (see Chart 38-1). Decreased blood flow to the major body organs can cause organ failure, especially renal failure.

Obtain the client's vital signs. When obtaining blood pressure (BP), note the presence or absence of an auscultatory gap or orthostatic (postural) hypotension. The **proportional pulse pressure** is calculated as follows:

$$\frac{\text{Systolic BP} - \text{Diastolic BP}}{\text{Systolic BP}}$$

A proportional pulse pressure less than 25% indicates severely compromised cardiac output (CO). The pulse may be tachycardiac, or it may alternate in strength **(pulsus alternans).** Take the apical pulse for a full minute, noting any irregularity in heart rhythm. An irregular heart rhythm resulting from premature atrial contractions (PACs), premature ventricular contractions (PVCs), or atrial fibrillation (AF) is common in HF. The sudden development of an irregular rhythm may further compromise CO. Carefully monitor the client's respiratory rate, rhythm, and character as well as oxygen saturation. The respiratory rate typically exceeds 20 breaths/min.

Determine whether the client is oriented to person, place, and time. A short mental status examination may be used if there are concerns about orientation. Objective data are important because in daily conversation many people are skillful at covering up memory losses.

Palpate the precordium. Increased heart size is common, with a displacement of the apical impulse to the left. A third heart sound, **(S_3) gallop,** an early diastolic filling sound indicating an increase in left ventricular pressure, may be heard on auscultation. A fourth heart sound (S_4) can also occur; it is not a sign of failure but is a reflection of decreased ventricular compliance.

Crackles and wheezes may be present on auscultation of the lungs. Late inspiratory crackles and fine profuse crackles that repeat themselves from breath to breath and do not diminish with coughing indicate HF. Crackles are produced by intra-alveolar fluid and are often noted first in the dependent areas of the lungs. Crackles usually develop in the bases and spread upward as the condition worsens. Identify the precise location of the crackles. Wheezes indicate a narrowing of the bronchial lumen caused by engorged pulmonary vessels.

RIGHT-SIDED HEART FAILURE. Right ventricular failure is associated with increased systemic venous pressures and congestion. Signs and symptoms are listed in Chart 38-2.

On inspection, assess the neck veins for distention and measure abdominal girth (see Chapter 36). Hepatomegaly (liver engorgement), hepatojugular reflux, and ascites may also be assessed. Abdominal fluid can reach volumes of more than 10 L.

Examine the client for dependent edema. In ambulatory clients, edema is normally located in the ankles and legs. When the client is restricted to bedrest, the sacrum is dependent and edema accumulates there. Edema is an extremely unreliable sign of HF, and therefore accurate daily weights are needed to document fluid retention. *Weight is the most reliable indicator of fluid gain or loss.*

PSYCHOSOCIAL ASSESSMENT

HF is usually a chronic, debilitating disease. A number of studies have found that anxiety is common in clients with HF (Artinian, 2003). These clients are usually frustrated about dealing with a chronic illness. Symptoms such as dyspnea increase their anxiety level.

Clients with advanced HF, especially those with New York Heart Association (NYHA) class III or IV HF, are at high risk for depression. It is not certain whether the functional impairments contribute to the depression or depression affects functional ability (Artinian, 2003). Hospitalized clients may be depressed, particularly those who have been rehospitalized for an acute episode of HF. Some individuals, however, do not manifest depression until they are in the community. Lifestyle changes and quality of life issues can precipitate depression many months after the initial diagnosis of HF.

Assess clients and their families for anxiety and depression. Ask them about their usual methods of coping as well as any history of depression. If anxiety is present, notify the health care provider for further assessment using an anxiety assessment tool, such as the Beck Anxiety Inventory or the Hospital Anxiety and Depression Scale. If depression is suspected, perform a thorough assessment using a tool such as the Geriatric Depression Scale or the Zung Self-Rating Depression Scale. In many hospitals, social workers or psychologists administer these tools.

If anxiety or depression occurs, the client may require treatment with medications and nonpharmacologic modalities, such as cognitive behavior therapy, biofeedback, or relaxation training.

Hope is a major determinant of well-being for clients in HF. Clients who are hopeful tend to feel better and are more socially involved. Asking clients about their activities and the significant people in their life and how often they are able to interact with them will provide information about client and family coping.

LABORATORY ASSESSMENT

Electrolyte imbalance may occur from complications of HF or as side effects of drug therapy, especially diuretic therapy. Regular evaluations of a client's serum electrolytes, including sodium, potassium, magnesium, calcium, and chloride, are essential. Any impairment of renal function resulting from inadequate perfusion causes elevated blood urea nitrogen, serum creatinine, and creatinine clearance levels. Urinalysis may reveal proteinuria and high specific gravity. Hemoglobin and hematocrit tests should be performed to identify HF resulting from anemia. If the client has fluid volume excess, the hematocrit levels may appear low as a result of hemodilution.

A new laboratory test for B-type natriuretic peptide (BNP) is used for diagnosing HF in clients with acute dyspnea. As discussed earlier, BNP is part of the neurohormonal response to decreased CO from either left or right ventricular dysfunction. An increase in BNP best differentiates between the dyspnea of HF and that associated with lung dysfunction.

Arterial blood gas values often reveal hypoxia (low oxygen level) because oxygen does not diffuse easily through fluid-filled alveoli. Respiratory alkalosis may occur because of hyperventilation; respiratory acidosis may occur because of carbon dioxide retention. Metabolic acidosis may indicate an accumulation of lactic acid.

CONSIDERATIONS FOR OLDER ADULTS

Thyroxine (T_4) and thyroid-stimulating hormone (TSH) levels should be determined in clients who are over 65 years of age, have atrial fibrillation, or have evidence of thyroid disease. Heart failure (HF) may be caused or aggravated by hypothyroidism or hyperthyroidism.

RADIOGRAPHIC ASSESSMENT

Chest x-rays can be helpful in diagnosing left ventricular failure. Typically the heart is enlarged (cardiomegaly), representing hypertrophy or dilation. Pleural effusions develop less often and generally reflect biventricular failure.

OTHER DIAGNOSTIC ASSESSMENTS

An electrocardiogram (ECG) is also performed. The ECG may demonstrate ventricular hypertrophy, dysrhythmias, and any degree of myocardial ischemia, injury, or infarction. It is not helpful in determining the presence or extent of HF.

Echocardiography is useful in diagnosing cardiac valvular changes, pericardial effusion, chamber enlargement, and ventricular hypertrophy. It can also be used to determine ejection fraction. Radionuclide studies (thallium imaging or technetium pyrophosphate scanning) can also indicate the presence and cause of HF. Multigated angiographic (MUGA) scans provide information about left ventricular ejection fraction and velocity, which are typically low in clients with HF.

Pulmonary artery catheters allow the assessment of cardiac function and volume status in acutely ill clients. These measurements can confirm the diagnosis and guide the management of HF. Right atrial pressure may be normal or elevated in left ventricular failure and is elevated in right ventricular failure. Pulmonary artery pressure (PAP) and pulmonary artery wedge pressure (PAWP) are elevated in left-sided HF because volumes and pressures are increased in the left ventricle. (See Chapter 36 for a more detailed description of these diagnostic assessments.)

Analysis

COMMON NURSING DIAGNOSES AND COLLABORATIVE PROBLEMS

The following are priority nursing diagnoses for clients with HF:

1. Impaired Gas Exchange related to ventilation perfusion imbalance
2. Decreased Cardiac Output related to altered contractility, preload, and afterload
3. Activity Intolerance related to an imbalance between oxygen supply and demand

The primary collaborative problem is Potential for Pulmonary Edema.

ADDITIONAL NURSING DIAGNOSES AND COLLABORATIVE PROBLEMS

In addition to the common nursing diagnoses and collaborative problems, clients with HF may have one or more of the following:

- Excess Fluid Volume related to compromised regulatory mechanism
- Acute Confusion related to delirium
- Ineffective Therapeutic Regimen Management related to social support deficits, complexity of therapeutic regimen, or knowledge deficit
- Anxiety related to stress, change in health status and role function, or threat of death
- Ineffective Tissue Perfusion: Cerebral related to mechanical reduction of arterial blood flow
- Impaired Physical Mobility related to limited cardiovascular endurance
- Risk for Ineffective Tissue Perfusion: Renal related to hypovolemia

Some clients are also at risk for the following collaborative problems:

- Potential for Pneumonia
- Potential for Dysrhythmias

Planning and Implementation

IMPAIRED GAS EXCHANGE

NOC **PLANNING: EXPECTED OUTCOMES.** The client with HF is expected to have adequate pulmonary tissue perfusion. Indicators include noncompromised status of the following:

- Pulmonary artery pressure (PAP)
- Respiratory function
- Respiratory rate
- Arterial blood gases and pH
- Oxygen saturation

INTERVENTIONS. The purpose of care is to promote an optimal spontaneous breathing pattern that maximizes oxygenation and maintains a normal carbon dioxide level in the blood (Chart 38-3).

NIC **Ventilation Assistance.** Monitor, or have assistive personnel monitor, the client's respiratory rate, rhythm, and quality every 1 to 4 hours and auscultate breath sounds. The oxygen content of the blood is often markedly reduced in clients who are experiencing pulmonary congestion. The nurse may titrate the amount of supplemental oxygen delivered to the client within a range prescribed by the health care provider to maintain oxygen saturation at 92% or greater.

If the client is experiencing respiratory difficulty, place him or her in a high Fowler's position with pillows under each arm to maximize chest expansion and improve oxygenation. Repositioning and performing coughing and deep breathing exercises every 2 hours help to improve oxygenation and prevent atelectasis.

CHART 38-3

NIC INTERVENTION ACTIVITIES for The Client with Heart Failure

Ventilation Assistance: *Promotion of an optimal spontaneous breathing pattern that maximizes oxygen and carbon dioxide exchange in the lungs*

- Monitor respiratory and oxygenation status.
- Initiate and maintain supplemental oxygen, as prescribed.
- Position to alleviate dyspnea.
- Auscultate breath sounds, noting areas of decreased or absent ventilation and presence of adventitious sounds.
- Position to minimize respiratory efforts (e.g., elevate the head of the bed and provide overbed table for client to lean on).
- Monitor the effects of position change on oxygenation: ABG, Sao_2, Svo_2, end tidal CO_2, Q_{sp}/Q_t, A-aDO_2 levels.

Hemodynamic Regulation: *Optimization of heart rate, preload, afterload, and contractility*

- Monitor and document heart rate, rhythm, and pulses.
- Monitor peripheral pulses, capillary refill, and temperature and color of extremities.
- Monitor pulmonary capillary/pulmonary artery wedge pressure and central venous/right atrial pressure, if appropriate.
- Administer vasodilator and/or vasoconstrictor medication, as appropriate.
- Administer positive inotropic/contractility medications.
- Maintain fluid balance by administering IV fluids or diuretics, as appropriate.
- Monitor intake/output, urine output, and client weight, as appropriate.
- Monitor electrolyte levels.
- Auscultate heart sounds.

Energy Management: *Regulating energy use to treat or prevent fatigue and optimize function*

- Monitor cardiorespiratory response to activity (e.g., tachycardia, other dysrhythmias, dyspnea, diaphoresis, pallor, hemodynamic pressures, and respiratory rate).
- Determine client's physical limitations.
- Encourage alternate rest and activity periods.
- Arrange physical activities to reduce competition for oxygen supply to vital body functions (e.g., avoid activity immediately after meals).
- Encourage physical activity (e.g., ambulation or performance of activities of daily living, consistent with client's energy resources).
- Monitor client's oxygen response (e.g., pulse rate, cardiac rhythm, and respiratory rate) to self-care or nursing activities.
- Teach client and significant other techniques of self-care that will minimize oxygen consumption (e.g., self-monitoring and pacing techniques for performance of activities of daily living).

NIC intervention activities selected from Dochterman, J.M., & Bulechek, G.M. (Eds.) (2004). *Nursing interventions classification (NIC)* (4th ed.). St. Louis: Mosby. No part of this work is to be altered without prior written permission from the Publisher.

ABG, Arterial blood gas, *CO_2,* carbon dioxide, *Sao_2,* saturation of arterial oxygen, *Svo_2,* saturation of venous oxygen, Q_{sp}/Q_t, physiologic blood flow per minute/cardiac output per minute; *A-aDO_2,* alveolar-arterial oxygen pressure difference.

DECREASED CARDIAC OUTPUT

NOC **PLANNING: EXPECTED OUTCOMES.** The client with HF is expected to have increased cardiac pump effectiveness. Indicators include noncompromised or mildly compromised:

- Systolic and diastolic blood pressure
- Apical pulse rate
- Ejection fraction
- Peripheral pulses
- Skin color

TABLE 38-2 Commonly Used Drug Classifications for Clients with Heart Failure

Angiotensin-converting enzyme (ACE) inhibitors
Diuretics
- High-ceiling
- Potassium-sparing

Human B-type natriuretic peptides
Nitrates
Inotropics
- Beta-adrenergic agonists
- Phosphodiesterase inhibitors
- Calcium sensitizers
- Digitalis

Beta-adrenergic blockers

- Urine output
- Cognitive status

INTERVENTIONS. Interventions are directed at optimizing the two major components of cardiac output (CO): stroke volume (SV) (determined by preload, afterload, and contractility) and heart rate (HR).

NONSURGICAL MANAGEMENT. Nonsurgical management relies primarily on a variety of medications (Table 38-2). If drug therapy is ineffective, other nonsurgical options are available.

NIC **Hemodynamic Regulation.** Interventions to improve stroke volume include reducing afterload, reducing preload, and improving cardiac muscle contractility. A major role of the nurse is to administer medications as prescribed, monitor for their therapeutic and adverse effects, and teach the client and family about drug therapy (see Chart 38-3).

Drugs That Reduce Afterload. By relaxing the arterioles, arterial vasodilators can reduce the resistance to left ventricular ejection (afterload) and improve CO. These drugs do not cause excessive vasodilation but reverse some of the inappropriate or excessive vasoconstriction common in HF.

Angiotensin-Converting Enzyme (ACE) Inhibitors. Clients with even mild heart failure (HF) resulting from left ventricular dysfunction should be given a trial of angiotensin-converting enzyme (ACE) inhibitors. ACE inhibitors are a group of arterial vasodilators such as enalapril (Vasotec), fosinopril (Monopril), and captopril (Capoten). In general, these drugs prolong and improve the quality of life for clients with HF. They enhance functional status, with 40% to 80% of clients showing an improvement in the NYHA class.

The ACE inhibitors suppress the renin-angiotensin system (RAS), which is activated in response to decreased renal blood flow. They prevent conversion of angiotensin I to angiotensin II, resulting in arterial resistance, arterial dilation, and increased SV. In addition, these drugs block aldosterone, which prevents sodium and water retention, thus decreasing fluid overload.

The health care provider usually starts doses of ACE inhibitors slowly and cautiously. The first dose of an ACE inhibitor is sometimes associated with a rapid drop in blood pressure (BP). Clients at risk for hypotension following ACE inhibitor administration have initial systolic BP less than 100 mm Hg, are older than 75 years of age, have a serum sodium level less than 137 mEq/L, or are volume depleted. Monitor BP for several hours after the initial dose and each time the dose is increased.

Clarify with the health care provider the guidelines for administering the vasodilator. For example, many clinicians maintain clients with HF at systolic BP ranging from 90 to 110 mm Hg. When such a BP is the maintenance level, assess the client for orthostatic hypotension, confusion, poor peripheral perfusion, and reduced urine output. Monitor serum potassium levels for hyperkalemia, serum creatinine for renal dysfunction, and the client for development of a cough while the client is receiving ACE inhibitors.

For clients with *acute* heart failure (HF), the health care provider may prescribe an intravenous (IV) push ACE inhibitor, such as Vasotec IV. Nursing implications for selected ACE inhibitors are described in Chapter 39 under Drug Therapy (Hypertension) and in Chart 39-3.

Human B-Type Natriuretic Peptides. Human B-type natriuretic peptides (hBNP) are one of the newest classes of drugs to treat *acute* HF. Endogenous BNP is released in response to decreased CO and causes *natriuresis,* or loss of sodium in the renal tubules, as well as vasodilation. Nesiritide (Natrecor) lowers PCWP and improves renal glomerular filtration. It is given as an IV bolus over 60 seconds, followed with a continuous infusion for up to 48 hours. When administering this drug, monitor BP and pulse carefully because it may cause dysrhythmias. Give Natrecor through a separate infusion line it because it is incompatible with heparin and most other parenteral medications.

Interventions That Reduce Preload. Ventricular fibers contract less forcefully when they are overstretched, such as in a failing heart. Interventions aimed at reducing preload attempt to decrease volume and pressure in the left ventricle, optimizing ventricular muscle stretch and contraction. Preload reduction is appropriate for HF accompanied by congestion with total body sodium and water overload.

Diet Therapy. In HF, diet therapy is aimed at reducing sodium and water retention.

In collaboration with the dietitian, the health care provider may restrict sodium intake in an attempt to decrease fluid retention. Many clients with HF need to omit only table salt (ingest no added salt) from their diet, thus reducing sodium intake to about 3 g daily.

If salt intake must be reduced further, the client may need to eliminate all salt in cooking as well as high-sodium foods, thus reducing sodium intake to 2 g daily. A dietitian is essential in helping to select foods that meet such a restricted therapeutic diet. About 25% of hospital admissions for clients with HF are due to excessive sodium intake. Therefore all clients must be advised to maintain an appropriate sodium restriction and avoid bingeing on high sodium foods (e.g., ham, bacon, pickles). Table 14-6 lists the sodium contents of some common foods.

Few clients are placed on severe fluid restrictions; however, clients with excessive aldosterone secretion may experience thirst and drink 3 to 5 L of fluid each day. As a result, their fluid intake may be limited to a more normal 2 L daily. Compliance with these simple strategies varies. When a fluid restriction is imposed on the hospitalized client, the nurse adjusts oral and IV therapy accordingly.

Weigh the client daily (1 kg of weight gain or loss equals 1 L of retained or lost fluid, respectively), and keep accurate records of fluid intake and output. The same scale should be used every morning before breakfast for the most accurate assessment of weight. The client's weight should decrease as excess fluid is excreted from the body.

Drug Therapy. Common drugs prescribed to reduce preload are diuretics and venous vasodilators. Chart 39-3 contains additional information about these medications.

Diuretics. The health care provider adds diuretics to the regimen when diet and fluid restriction have not been effective in managing the symptoms of systemic or pulmonary congestion associated with HF. Diuretics enhance the renal excretion of sodium and water by reducing circulating blood volume, decreasing preload, and reducing systemic and pulmonary congestion.

The type and dosage of diuretic prescribed depend on the degree of HF and renal function. High-ceiling (loop) diuretics, such as furosemide (Lasix, Furoside✱, Novosemide✱), torsemide (Demadex), and bumetanide (Bumex), are most effective for treating fluid volume overload. The practitioner may initially use a thiazide diuretic, such as hydrochlorothiazide (HydroDIURIL, Urozide✱) and metolazone (Zaroxolyn), for older clients with mild volume overload. Zaroxolyn is a long-acting agent and is therefore often given every second, third, or fourth day, depending on client need and tolerance.

The action of thiazide diuretics is self-limiting (i.e., diuresis decreases after edema fluid is lost); thus the excessive diuresis and dehydration that may occur with loop diuretics are uncommon occurrences with thiazide diuretics. Clients often prefer thiazide diuretics because of the gradual onset of diuresis.

Loop diuretics, nonetheless, are needed to ensure effective diuresis for many clients in HF. For clients with *acute* HF, Lasix or Bumex can be given by IV push (IVP). Lasix can be given in doses of 20 to 40 mg I, and increased by 20 mg every 2 hours until the desired response is obtained. The usual IV initial dose for Bumex is 1 to 2 mg once or twice daily, but it is more often given in a continuous infusion of 10 mg over 24 hours.

As HF progresses, many clients develop diuretic resistance with refractory edema. The health care provider may choose to treat this problem by administering two types of diuretics, most commonly a loop diuretic and a thiazide diuretic such as metolazone.

Monitor for and prevent potassium deficiency (hypokalemia) from diuretic therapy. The signs of hypokalemia are nonspecific neurologic and muscular complaints, such as generalized weakness, depressed reflexes, and irregular heart rate. Therefore the physician, nurse, and dietitian monitor serum potassium levels to accurately identify hypokalemia.

If the client's serum potassium level is less than 4.0 mEq/L, the health care provider has several alternatives:

- Add a potassium-sparing diuretic to the regimen (such as spironolactone [Aldactone])
- Request that clients further increase their dietary intake of potassium-rich foods
- Prescribe a potassium supplement

CONSIDERATIONS FOR OLDER ADULTS

Older clients receiving loop diuretics are particularly prone to dehydration, especially if they have type 2 diabetes mellitus. The nurse checks orthostatic blood pressures in the client receiving loop diuretics to detect volume depletion. The client is

Continued

weighed daily to detect the development of a slow, progressive weight loss despite an adequate diet. The nurse also looks for flat neck veins when the client is supine and for a loss of skin turgor. All these signs, plus disorientation in a very old client, may indicate excessive diuresis and volume depletion (Chart 38-4).

Clients being treated simultaneously with ACE inhibitors and diuretics may not experience hypokalemia. If their kidneys are not functioning well, they may develop hyperkalemia (elevated serum potassium level). Review the client's serum creatinine level. If the creatinine is greater than 1.8, notify the health care provider before administering supplemental potassium.

Venous Vasodilators. The health care provider may prescribe venous vasodilators (e.g., nitrates) for the client with HF with persistent dyspnea. Significant constriction of venous and arterial blood vessels occurs to compensate for reduced CO. Constriction reduces the volume of fluid that the vascular bed can hold and increases preload. Venous vasodilators may benefit from the following steps:

- Returning venous vasculature to a more normal capacity
- Decreasing the volume of blood returning to the heart
- Improving left ventricular function

Nitrates may be administered intravenously, orally, or topically. IV nitrates are used most often for *acute* HF. These drugs cause primarily venous vasodilation but also a significant amount of arteriolar vasodilation. It is essential to monitor the client's blood pressure when initiating nitrate therapy or increasing the dosage. Clients may initially report headache, but assure them that they will develop a tolerance to this effect and that the headache will cease or diminish. Acetaminophen (Tylenol, Exdol✦) can be given to help relieve discomfort.

Unfortunately, tolerance to the vasodilating effects develops when nitrates are uniformly administered during 24 hours. To prevent such tolerance, the health care provider may prescribe at least one 12-hour nitrate-free period out of every 24 hours (usually overnight). Nitrates, such as isosorbide (Imdur, Ismo) are prescribed to provide nitrate-free periods and reduce the problem of tolerance. Chapter 41 discusses nitrates in more detail.

Drugs That Enhance Contractility. Contractility of the heart can also be enhanced with drug therapy. Positive inotropic drugs are most commonly used, but vasodilators and beta adrenergic blockers may also be administered. For chronic HF, low-dose beta blockers are most commonly used. Digoxin (Lanoxin) may be prescribed to improve that client's symptoms, thereby decreasing dyspnea and improving activity. This older drug is very inexpensive. In some settings, nesiritide (Natrecor) may be administered for end-stage HF, although this medication is very expensive (see earlier discussion of Natrecor for acute HF).

CHART 38-4

NURSING FOCUS on the OLDER ADULT
Heart Failure

- Assess older clients with confusion for indications of heart failure. People older than 80 years of age often experience restlessness or confusion as the initial manifestation of heart failure.
- Auscultate the lungs carefully, recognizing that dependent crackles may not be an indication of heart failure in the older adult.
- Do not expect crackles to clear rapidly after treatment. Crackles may persist in the lung bases of older adults for an extended period after pulmonary congestion has decreased.
- Be especially alert for the signs of digitalis toxicity in the older client because it is common.
- If loop diuretics are used for diuresis, monitor the client closely for signs of excessive diuresis, dehydration, and hypokalemia.
- In older clients receiving drug therapy for heart failure, monitor for orthostatic hypotension. Cardiovascular changes associated with aging make this likely to develop.

Digitalis. Digoxin (Lanoxin, Novodigoxin✦), a cardiac glycoside, has been demonstrated to provide benefits for clients in heart failure (HF) with sinus rhythm and atrial fibrillation. "Dig" therapy reduces exacerbations of HF and hospitalizations when added to a regimen of angiotensin-converting enzyme (ACE) inhibitors, beta blockers, and diuretics. Digoxin increases functional capacity and improves hemodynamic parameters in clients with New York Heart Association (NYHA) class III and IV HF resulting from left systolic dysfunction. It may increase mortality, however, especially in older adults (McCance & Huether, 2002).

The potential benefits of digitalis derivatives include an increase in contractility, a reduction in heart rate (HR), a slowing of conduction through the atrioventricular node, and an inhibition of sympathetic activity while enhancing parasympathetic activity. Digitalis also may have a mild diuretic effect. Increased automaticity occurs with toxic digitalis levels or in the presence of hypokalemia (which increases sensitivity to digitalis), resulting in ectopic beats (premature ventricular contractions [PVCs]) may result.

Digoxin is erratically absorbed from the gastrointestinal tract. Many medications, especially antacids, interfere with its absorption. It is eliminated primarily by renal excretion.

The presentation of **digitalis toxicity** is often vague and nonspecific and includes anorexia, fatigue, and changes in mental status. Toxicity may cause nearly any dysrhythmia, but PVCs are most commonly noted. Carefully monitor the apical pulse rate and heart rhythm of clients receiving digoxin. The physician determines the desirable HR to achieve; many cardiologists prefer a rate less than 60 beats/min. Report the development of either an irregular rhythm in a client with a previously regular rhythm or a regular rhythm in a client with a previously irregular one. Monitor serum digoxin and potassium levels (hypokalemia potentiates digitalis toxicity) to identify toxicity.

Any medication that increases the workload of the failing heart also increases its oxygen requirement. Be alert for the possibility that the client may experience angina (chest pain) in response to digoxin.

CONSIDERATIONS FOR OLDER ADULTS

The half-life of digoxin in middle-aged adults is 36 hours; in older adults, who typically have diminished renal function, the half-life may be 48 hours or longer. Thus older clients are particularly susceptible to digoxin toxicity. Toxicity occurs in 10% to 20% of all clients taking digoxin, more commonly in older clients and clients with hypokalemia. Toxicity in older hypokalemic clients may be fatal, and therefore health teaching is essential.

Other Inotropic Drugs. Clients experiencing *acute* heart failure (HF) are candidates for IV medications that increase contractility, and these agents are often prescribed. For example, *beta-adrenergic agonists*, such as dobutamine (Dobutrex), are used for short-term treatment of acute episodes of HF. Dobutamine improves cardiac contractility and thus cardiac output and myocardial-systemic perfusion.

A more potent drug used for *acute* HF, milrinone (Primacor), functions as a vasodilator/inotropic medication with phosphodiesterase activity. Also known as a *phosphodiesterase inhibitor,* this drug increases cyclic adenosine monophosphate (cAMP), which enhances the entry of calcium into myocardial cells to increase contractile function. Like the beta-adrenergic drugs, Primacor is given intravenously.

Levosimendan (Simdax) is a calcium-sensitizing medication and a positive inotropic drug. It appears to bind to Troponin C in the heart muscle and therefore increases the contraction of the heart. Simdax is used most often in clients who have had or are at high risk for myocardial infarction. Chapter 41 discusses inotropic drugs in more detail.

Beta-Adrenergic Blockers. Beta blockers improve the condition of some clients in HF. It appears that prolonged exposure to increased levels of sympathetic stimulation and catecholamines worsens cardiac function. Beta-adrenergic blockade reverses this effect, improving morbidity, mortality, and quality of life for clients in HF.

Beta blockers must be started slowly for HF. In most cases, clients in HF should not be started on a beta blocker until their ACE inhibitor and diuretic doses have been stabilized for 2 weeks. Carvedilol (Coreg), metoprolol (Lopressor, Betaloc✱), and bisoprolol (Zebeta) are approved for treatment of HF. The first dose is extremely low, and the client is monitored either in the hospital or in the health care provider's office to detect bradycardia or hypotension.

Instruct the client to weigh daily while taking the beta blocker and to report any signs of worsening HF immediately. The health care provider gradually titrates the drug dose upward, and the client is evaluated at least weekly for changes in BP, pulse, activity tolerance, and orthopnea. A modest drop in BP is acceptable if the client remains asymptomatic and can stand without experiencing dizziness or a further drop in BP. The resting HR should remain between 55 and 60 and increase slightly with exercise. Activity tolerance improves, and less orthopnea is experienced. Most clients with mild and moderate HF demonstrate improved ejection fraction, decreased hospital admissions, and improvement in symptoms when beta blockers are added to their treatment regimens. The benefits of beta-blocker therapy accrue over a long period, not immediately.

For clients with *diastolic* HF, drug therapy has not been as effective. Calcium channel blockers, ACE inhibitors, and beta blockers have been used with various degrees of success.

Critical Thinking Challenge

You are a home care nurse visiting a 75-year-old widow with a long history of HF, myocardial infarction, pulmonary emphysema, hypertension, and type 2 diabetes mellitus. She is taking the following medications: Lasix, enalapril (Vasotec), digoxin, KCl, theophylline (Theo-Dur), and rosiglitazone (Avandia). She occasionally uses oxygen at night and sleeps sitting up in a lounge chair.

Today she complains that she "just doesn't feel right." Her pulse is 110, weak, and irregular, and her skin is pale and feels cooler than usual. She is dyspneic, has a respiratory rate of 34, and has crackles in her lung bases.

1. What additional information do you need to obtain?
2. What is the purpose of each of her medications?
3. What laboratory data would help diagnose her acute health problem?
4. What actions should you take at this time and why?

evolve For suggested answer guidelines, go to http://evolve.elsevier.com/Iggy/.

Other Nonsurgical Options. In addition to drug therapy, nonsurgical options, both noninvasive and invasive, may be used, including the following:

- Continuous positive airway pressure (CPAP)
- Cardiac resynchronization therapy (CRT)
- Investigative gene therapy

Continuous Positive Airway Pressure. **Continuous positive airway pressure (CPAP)** is a respiratory treatment that improves sleep apnea in clients with HF. It also improves cardiac output (CO) and ejection fraction (EF) by decreasing afterload and preload, blood pressure (BP), and dysrhythmias. Sleep apnea is directly correlated with coronary artery disease as a result of diminished oxygen supply to the heart during apneic episodes.

Cardiac Resynchronization Therapy. **Cardiac resynchronization therapy (CRT)** uses a permanent pacemaker alone or is combined with an implantable cardioverter-defibrillator to provide biventricular pacing. Electrical stimulation causes more synchronous ventricular contractions to improve EF, CO, and mean arterial pressure. This modality is indicated for clients with class III or IV HF and an EF of less than 35%. CRT improves the client's ability to perform activities of daily living (ADLs). Chapter 37 discusses pacing in more detail.

Gene Therapy. **Gene therapy** may be indicated for clients in end-stage HF who are not candidates for heart transplantation. This therapy replaces damaged genes with normal or modified genes by a series of injections of growth factor into the left ventricle. Although still investigative, this therapy has resulted in improved exercise tolerance and regrowth of cardiac cells (Bosen, 2003).

SURGICAL MANAGEMENT. Heart transplantation is still the ultimate choice for end-stage HF (see later). Several surgical procedures are available to improve CO in clients who are not candidates for a transplant or are awaiting transplant.

Ventricular Assist Devices. **Left ventricular assist devices (LVAD)** have been used for a number of years with varying success for clients awaiting heart transplantation. Recent studies have indicated that clients with end-stage HF who are ineligible for transplantation have shown improved survival rates with an LVAD compared with medical support alone (Bond et. al., 2003). Implantable, self-contained LVAD devices are now approved for long-term therapy. **Right ventricle assist devices (RVAD)** can be inserted for right ventricular failure as a result of pulmonary hypertension. Other clients require a bi-VAD as a "bridge to transplant" device. About 75% survive until a transplant is available (Bosen, 2003).

Newer Surgical Therapies. Several new therapies have been used to reshape the left ventricle in clients with heart failure (HF). Perioperative care is similar to the client experiencing a coronary artery bypass graft (CABG) (see Chapter 41). The procedures include the following:

- Partial left ventriculectomy (PLV)
- Endoventricular circular patch

- Acorn cardiac support device
- Myosplint

Also known as **heart reduction surgery,** PLV involves removing a triangle-shaped section of the weakened heart in the left lateral ventricle to reduce the ventricle's diameter and decrease wall tension. In **endoventricular circular patch** cardioplasty, the surgeon removes portions of the cardiac septum and left ventricular wall and grafts a circular patch (synthetic or autologous) into the opening. This procedure provides a more normal shape to the left ventricle to improve hemodynamics.

The **acorn cardiac support device** is a polyester mesh jacket that is placed over the ventricles to provide support and to avoid overstretching the myocardial muscle. The material for the jacket has been used for other procedures, such as vascular grafts. The mesh jacket appears to reduce hypertrophy of the heart muscle and assists with improvement of the EF.

The **Myosplint** is under investigation in Europe and the United States. Electrical stimulation of tension splints in the heart helps the ventricle change to a more normal shape.

ACTIVITY INTOLERANCE

NOC **PLANNING: EXPECTED OUTCOMES.** The client with HF is expected to take actions to manage energy for initiating and sustaining activity. Indicators include that the client consistently do the following:

- Balance activity and rest
- Use naps to restore energy
- Recognize energy limitations
- Organize activities to conserve energy
- Adapt lifestyle to energy level
- Report adequate endurance for activity

INTERVENTIONS. The purpose of interdisciplinary interventions is to regulate energy to prevent fatigue and optimize function (see Chart 38-3).

NIC **Energy Management.** The client in severe HF initially requires physical and emotional rest. On the first day of hospitalization, he or she may sit up in a chair for meals and perform basic leg exercises while out of bed. Nursing care should be organized to allow periods of rest. The interdisciplinary team observes and documents the client's physiologic response to activity.

As the client's condition improves, the physical therapist (PT) initiates ambulation, usually on hospital day 2. Check the blood pressure (BP), pulse, and oxygen saturation before and after the activity. A BP change of more than 20 mm Hg or a pulse increase of more than 20 beats/min may indicate that the activity is too stressful. Other indications of activity intolerance include dyspnea, fatigue, and chest pain. Ask a client displaying any of these symptoms to rate how hard he or she has been working on a scale of 1 to 20, with 20 being the maximum perceived exertion. If the client rates the exertion higher than 12, counsel him or her to slow down. If activity is tolerated, the PT steadily increases the activity level until the client is ambulating 200 to 400 feet several times per day.

If the client is able, the PT (or assistive nursing or PT personnel) might time him or her for 6 minutes while walking at a comfortable pace. The distance the client can walk can be used to determine his or her functional level and activity plan.

POTENTIAL FOR PULMONARY EDEMA

PLANNING: EXPECTED OUTCOMES. The client with HF is expected to be free of pulmonary edema. Indicators include that the client will have the following:

- No adventitious breath sounds
- Vital signs within normal limits
- Arterial blood gas values within normal limits

INTERVENTIONS. Monitor for manifestations of acute pulmonary edema, a life-threatening event that can result from severe HF. In pulmonary edema, the left ventricle fails to eject sufficient blood, and pressure increases in the lungs because of the accumulated blood. The increased pressure causes fluid to leak across the pulmonary capillaries and into the pulmonary interstitium.

Assess for early manifestations, such as crackles in the lung bases, dyspnea at rest, disorientation, and confusion, especially in older clients. Documentation of the precise location of the crackles is crucial because the level of the fluid ascends as the pulmonary edema worsens. The client in acute pulmonary edema is also extremely anxious, tachycardiac, and struggling for air. As pulmonary edema becomes more severe, he or she may have a moist cough productive of frothy, blood-tinged sputum, and his or her skin may be cold, clammy, or cyanotic.

The client diagnosed with pulmonary edema is admitted to the acute care hospital. The physician prescribes rapid-acting diuretics, such as Lasix or Bumex. Lasix is given intravenously over 1 to 2 minutes, usually at a starting dose of 40 mg, with another 40 mg repeated if needed in 30 minutes. Each increment of 40 mg of Lasix should be administered over 1 to 2 minutes to avoid ototoxicity. Bumex may be administered 1 to 2 mg IVP or as a continuous infusion to provide consistent fluid removal over 24 hours.

Oxygen is always used, and the client is placed in a high Fowler's position. IV morphine sulfate may be prescribed, 1 to 2 mg at a time, to reduce venous return (preload), decrease anxiety, and reduce the work of breathing. Monitor respiratory rate and BP closely. Nitroglycerin may be administered as a slow infusion to decrease preload and ease the oxygen demand on the heart. Monitor the client's BP closely while this medication is being given.

Insert a Foley catheter, if prescribed, to assess urine output after diuretic administration and to minimize exertion related to voiding. Diuresis normally begins within 5 minutes of the administration of IV Lasix and peaks at 30 minutes. Chart 38-5 summarizes the priority care for the client with acute pulmonary edema.

Clients often respond dramatically and quickly to these interventions, but their condition can also deteriorate rapidly because of pulmonary congestion and severe hypoxemia. Clients occasionally require bilateral positive airway pressure (biPAP) or intubation and ventilation to survive the acute episode (see Chapter 35 for a description of these modalities). A skilled nurse is needed to assist with intubation. If a client does not respond to other methods, vasodilators such as nitroglycerin or sodium nitroprusside may be administered intravenously, or inotropic support may be required. The client should be in an emergency department or intensive care unit (ICU), where the medications are carefully titrated via continuous infusion pumps and the client is closely assessed. Management of the client who is critically ill with HF is detailed in Chapter 41.

CHART 38-5

BEST PRACTICE for
Care of the Client with Pulmonary Edema

Emergency Care
- Identify the client's chief complaint.
- If the client's blood pressure is adequate, place the client in a high Fowler's position.
- Auscultate the client's lungs (posterior assessment).
- Ensure that vascular access is present, and check for patency.
- Provide oxygen as ordered.
- Provide an IV diuretic (usually furosemide) as prescribed.
- Anticipate urine output 5 to 15 minutes after diuretic administration; catheterize if ordered.

Continuing Care
- Monitor blood pressure, respiratory rate, pulse oximetry, pulse, cardiac rhythm, and the client's subjective report of ability to breathe.
- Provide additional medications as prescribed (usually morphine sulfate or nitroglycerin).
- Provide comfort measures and reassurance.
- Notify the health care provider if the client does not experience a rapid improvement and diuresis.

Community-Based Care

Clients who have not been adequately prepared for discharge or who do not have good community support and follow-up are at high risk for recurrent hospital admissions for heart failure (HF). In a case management system, the case manager or care coordinator assesses the client's needs for health care resources and facilitates appropriate placement. It is imperative that the case manager assess the available social supports. An inability to obtain help in activities such as food shopping and obtaining medications is a major contributor to hospital readmission. If home support is available, the client may be discharged home in the care of a family member or other caregiver. Home care nurses may direct the care, and aides may provide assistance with activities of daily living (ADLs).

Gorski and Johnson (2003) describe a collaborative approach between a case management and home health agency to manage clients with HF. The purpose of this disease management program was to improve clinical outcomes and decrease the cost of care through improved client education, evidence-based practice, and ongoing support. Results indicated that hospitalizations were reduced and clients were satisfied with their care.

If the client has multiple health problems or has been severely compromised by heart disease, he or she may require admission to a subacute unit or traditional nursing home for either transitional or long-term care. A variety of nontraditional approaches to the ambulatory care of clients with HF have been demonstrated to decrease rehospitalization rates. Costs involved in caring for the client with HF include a drug regimen that may be extensive. In one study, the overall mean monthly cost of medications for chronic HF was $440. Clients with class II and class III chronic HF had the highest costs of over $500 per month (Hussey et al., 2002).

HOME CARE MANAGEMENT

The focus of the home care nurse's interventions is assessment and health teaching, which is reimbursable by Medicare and other third-party payers. Chart 38-6 lists the major areas of assessment.

CHART 38-6

HOME CARE ASSESSMENT of
The Client with Heart Failure

Assess for signs of heart failure, including the following:
- Changes in vital signs (heart rate >100 beats/min at rest, new atrial fibrillation, blood pressure <90 or >150 systolic)
- Indications of poor tissue perfusion
  - Fatigue
  - Angina
  - Activity intolerance
  - Changes in mental status
  - Pallor or cyanosis
  - Cool extremities
- Indications of congestion
  - Presence of cough or dyspnea
  - Weight gain
  - Jugular venous distention and peripheral edema

Assess functional ability, including the following:
- Performance of activities of daily living
- Mobility and ambulation (review frequency and duration of walking, development of symptoms, and pulse rate)
- Cognitive ability

Assess nutritional status, including the following:
- Food and fluid intake
- Intake of sodium-rich foods
- Alcohol consumption
- Skin turgor

Assess home environment, including the following:
- Safety hazards, especially related to oxygen therapy
- Structural barriers affecting functional ability
- Social support (family, home health services)

Assess the client's compliance and understanding of illness and its treatment, including the following:
- Signs and symptoms to report to health care provider
- Dosages, effects, and side or toxic effects of medications
- When to report for laboratory and health care provider visits
- Ability to accurately weigh self on scale
- Presence of advanced directive
- Use of home oxygen, if appropriate

Assess client and caregiver coping skills

Clients with chronic HF must make many adjustments in their lifestyles. They must adhere to a medical regimen that includes dietary restrictions, activity prescriptions, and drug therapy. They need careful, concise explanations of the treatment plan. The community-based nurse in any setting encourages the client to verbalize fears and concerns about his or her illness and assists in exploring the appropriate coping skills. Client participation in treatment can help alleviate and control symptoms.

HEALTH TEACHING

Clients in HF and their nurses may have different priorities for health teaching. The Evidence-Based Practice for Nursing box on p. 762 describes a study that examined the perceived benefits of a home walking exercise program for clients with HF.

ACTIVITY SCHEDULE. For clients who qualify, Medicare usually provides reimbursement for assessment and teaching so that a home care nurse can continue teaching and assessment when the client returns home. Encourage clients with HF to stay as active as possible and to develop a regular exercise regimen. Those who are more active appear to have better outcomes. The primary outcome is development of a regular exercise routine (probably a home walking program) several times a week. Medicare and third-party payers typically

EVIDENCE-BASED PRACTICE for Nursing

Can a walk exercise program improve perceptions of well-being in clients with heart failure?

Corvera-Tindel, T., et al. (2002). Nurse-managed home walking program improves exercise duration and reduces symptoms in heart failure. VA HSR&D Annual Meeting, Washington, DC.

The purpose of this qualitative and quantitative research study was to compare the effects of a nurse-managed home walking exercise program on the functional status and quality of life in a group of advanced heart failure clients with a control group who carried out usual activities.

The progressive home walk exercise program was conducted over 12 weeks. The exercise periods progressed from once-a-day, 5 days a week, 10-minute periods to 60-minute periods five times a week with increasing exercise intensity. Clients were rated using a 6 Minute Walk Test (6MWT), Cardiac Quality of Life Index (C-QOL), Dyspnea-Fatigue Index (DFI), heart rate variability (HRV), as well as global ratings of symptoms and peak VO_2 and ventilatory threshold (CPX).

The sample (79 clients, all men, mean age 62.6) had a 79% (63) completion rate and a mean compliance rate of 74%. The 6MWT and the CPX showed that exercisers walked farther (p = 0.001) and longer (p = 0.02) than did the control group. Exercisers also reported improvement in dyspnea and fatigue scores (t = 2.42, p = 0.02) compared with the usual exercise group. The test measures were both objective and subjective and covered a range of issue associated with exercise and heart failure.

Level of Evidence: 5—The study used a randomized control sample of 79 clients.

Critique. The study used a randomized control sampling; however, all the subjects were men. One limitation, then, was that the study did not address women's response to a home walking exercise program. Another limitation was that racial or ethnic origins of the sample were not reported. The assumption is that all the subjects were white.

Implications for Nursing. Other studies have demonstrated that home exercise programs using stationary bicycles are effective in improving exercise tolerance. Such equipment may be expensive and thus pose a barrier to compliance. A home walking exercise program is a safe, low-cost alternative that appears to produce increases in exercise tolerance and decreases in dyspnea and fatigue.

do not reimburse for cardiac rehabilitation for HF, and paying for a cardiac rehabilitation program out of pocket is expensive.

Although most clients with HF appear to benefit from exercise programs, those with persistent crackles and uncontrolled edema despite medical therapy are not encouraged to exercise until their HF is stabilized. When exercise is indicated, teach the client to begin walking 200 to 400 feet per day. At home the client should try to walk at least three times a week and should slowly increase the amount of time walked (perhaps 10 minutes a week) over several months. If he or she experiences chest pain or pronounced dyspnea while exercising or experiences fatigue the next day, he or she is probably advancing the activity too quickly and should slow down. Encourage the client to keep an exercise diary that documents the time and duration of each exercise session as well as HR and any symptoms that occur with exercise.

INDICATIONS OF WORSENING HEART FAILURE. Many clients who are readmitted to hospitals for treatment of HF fail to seek medical attention promptly when symptoms recur. Instruct the client and caregiver to immediately report to the health care provider the occurrence of any of the following symptoms of worsening HF:

- Rapid weight gain (3 pounds in a week or 1 to 2 pounds overnight)
- Decrease in exercise tolerance lasting 2 to 3 days
- Cold symptoms (cough) lasting more than 3 to 5 days
- Excessive awakening at night to urinate
- Development of dyspnea or angina at rest or worsening angina
- Increased swelling in the feet, ankles, or hands

DRUG THERAPY. The health care provider or nurse provides oral and written instructions about the medication regimen. If digoxin is prescribed, teach the caregiver and client how to count a pulse rate. Assess their ability to accurately take and record the pulse rate. Chart 38-7 lists instructions for the client taking digoxin at home.

CHART 38-7

CLIENT EDUCATION GUIDE
Digoxin Therapy

- Establish one time of day to take this medication everyday.
- Continue taking this medication unless your health care provider tells you to stop.
- Do not take digoxin at the same time as antacids or cathartics (laxatives).
- Take your pulse rate before taking each dose of digoxin. Notify your health care provider of a change in pulse rate (60 to 100 beats/min is normal) or rhythm as well as increasing fatigue, muscle weakness, confusion, or loss of appetite (signs of digitalis toxicity).
- If you forget to take a dose, it may be delayed a few hours; however, if you do not remember it until the next day, you should take only your usual daily dose.
- Report for scheduled laboratory tests (such as potassium and digoxin levels).
- If potassium supplements are prescribed, continue the dose until told to stop by your health care provider.

Advise clients taking diuretics to take them in the morning to avoid waking during the night for voiding. After determining whether the client has a weight scale and can use it, emphasize the importance of weighing each morning. Although this simple intervention can greatly assist in managing HF, most clients do not weigh themselves regularly. Emphasize the relationship between weight gain, fluid retention, and HF. Daily weights indicate whether the client is losing or retaining fluid. Some motivated individuals are taught to use a sliding scale to adjust their daily diuretic dose depending on their daily weight, similar to the way a diabetic client adjusts an insulin dose based on the capillary glucose level. The home care nurse may reliably assess volume status by checking the pattern of daily weights.

Teach clients receiving angiotensin-converting enzyme (ACE) inhibitors to move slowly when changing positions, especially from a lying to a sitting position. Dizziness, lightheadedness, and cough need to be reported to the health care provider.

Clients taking diuretics and ACE inhibitors require that their serum potassium level and renal function be monitored at least every few months. Diuretics, especially loop diuretics such as Lasix and Bumex, deplete potassium and often cause hypokalemia. Conversely, ACE inhibitors may result in potassium retention. If potassium levels drop below 4.0 mEq/L, the primary care physician may prescribe potassium supplementation or add potassium-sparing diuretics such as spironolactone (Aldactone). Depending on the client's third-party payer, a dietitian may be consulted to provide information about potassium-rich foods to include in the diet.

DIET THERAPY. Clients with chronic HF are advised to restrict their dietary sodium. The home care nurse or dietitian provides written instructions on low- or restricted-sodium diets. A 3-g sodium diet is recommended for mild or moderate failure. Remind the client to avoid salty foods and table salt. Clients usually find this diet palatable and fairly easy to follow.

A 2-g sodium diet may be attempted for clients with severe HF. These clients are told not to add salt during or after meal preparation, to avoid milk and milk products, to use few canned or prepared foods, and to read food labels to determine sodium content. This diet is unpalatable, and for many clients the cost of low-sodium foods is a financial burden. Therefore the home care nurse or dietitian should assess the client for compliance.

Clients are instructed to confer with their health care provider if they want to use commercial salt substitutes. Most salt substitutes contain potassium, and the client's renal status and serum potassium level need to be considered before these products can be recommended. Clients may use lemon, garlic, and herbs to enhance the flavor of low-salt foods.

ADVANCE DIRECTIVES. About 50% of deaths from HF are sudden—many without any warning or worsening of symptoms. Because most of these deaths occur at home, it is important for the health care provider or home care nurse to discuss advance directives with the client and family. The family should be prepared to act in accordance with the client's wishes in the event of cardiac arrest. If resuscitation is desired, the family should know how to activate the Emergency Medical System (EMS) and how to provide cardiopulmonary resuscitation (CPR) until an ambulance arrives. If CPR is not desired, the client, family, and nurse should plan how the family will respond.

HEALTH CARE RESOURCES

A home care nurse may be needed to assess the client's adherence to medication and diet therapy and to monitor for worsening heart failure (HF). Clients with activity limitations benefit from the services of a home care aide. A dietitian might be consulted to assist with menu planning and teaching. Although participation in structured cardiac rehabilitation programs has been shown to be beneficial, referrals to such programs are not widespread because coverage is usually not provided by third-party payers.

In addition to home care support, other resources are available for client education and family support. The American Heart Association is an excellent community resource for pamphlets, books, cookbooks, and videotapes related to HF and heart disease. The organization also provides referrals to various local support groups for clients and their caregivers.

For equipment needs (e.g., home oxygen therapy, hospital bed), medical supply companies provide setup and maintenance services. Chapter 31 provides a detailed description of home oxygen therapy.

Evaluation: Outcomes

Evaluate the care of the client with HF on the basis of the identified nursing diagnoses and collaborative problems. The expected outcomes include that the client will:

- Have adequate pulmonary tissue perfusion
- Have increased cardiac pump effectiveness
- Take actions to manage energy
- Be free of pulmonary edema

Specific indicators for these outcomes are listed for each nursing diagnosis and collaborative problem under the Planning and Implementation section (see earlier).

Critical Thinking Challenge

Your 75-year-old home care client is admitted to the hospital with pulmonary edema. She is upset because her daughter and son-in-law are out of town and she does not know how to contact them to inform them of her hospital admission. Her best friend lives next door, but the friend does not drive.

1. What could you do to alleviate this client's anxiety?
2. What treatment do you anticipate for this client when she is hospitalized?
3. What options for follow-up care after discharge does she have?
4. What health teaching will she require?

evolve For suggested answer guidelines, go to http://evolve.elsevier.com/Iggy/.

VALVULAR HEART DISEASE

PATHOPHYSIOLOGY

Acquired valvular dysfunctions, in decreasing order of occurrence, are mitral stenosis, mitral regurgitation, mitral valve prolapse, aortic stenosis, and aortic regurgitation (Chart 38-8). The tricuspid valve is affected infrequently, primarily following endocarditis in IV drug abusers.

Mitral Stenosis

Mitral stenosis usually results from rheumatic carditis, which can cause valve thickening by fibrosis and calcification. Rheumatic fever is the most common cause of mitral stenosis. Nonrheumatic causes include atrial myxoma (tumor), calcium accumulation, and thrombus formation.

WOMEN'S HEALTH CONSIDERATIONS

Two thirds to three fourths of all clients with mitral stenosis are women. About two thirds of women with rheumatic mitral stenosis are younger than 45 years of age.

In mitral stenosis, the valve leaflets fuse and become stiff, and the chordae tendineae contract and shorten. The valve opening narrows, preventing normal blood flow from the left atrium to the left ventricle. As a result of these changes, left atrial pressure rises, the left atrium dilates, pulmonary artery pressures increase, and the right ventricle hypertrophies.

Pulmonary congestion and right-sided HF occur initially. Later, when the left ventricle receives insufficient blood volume, preload is decreased and cardiac output (CO) falls.

Clients with mild mitral stenosis are usually asymptomatic. As the valvular orifice narrows and pressure in the lungs increases, the client experiences dyspnea on exertion, orthopnea, paroxysmal nocturnal dyspnea (sudden dyspnea at night), and dry cough. Hemoptysis and pulmonary edema appear as pulmonary hypertension and congestion progress. Right-sided HF can cause hepatomegaly, neck vein distention, and pitting edema late in the disorder.

CHART 38-8

KEY FEATURES of Valvular Heart Disease

Mitral Stenosis	Mitral Insufficiency	Mitral Valve Prolapse	Aortic Stenosis	Aortic Insufficiency
Fatigue Dyspnea on exertion Orthopnea Paroxysmal nocturnal dyspnea Hemoptysis Hepatomegaly Neck vein distention Pitting edema Atrial fibrillation Rumbling, apical diastolic murmur	Fatigue Dyspnea on exertion Orthopnea Palpitations Atrial fibrillation Neck vein distention Pitting edema High-pitched holosystolic murmur	Atypical chest pain Dizziness, syncope Palpitations Atrial tachycardia Ventricular tachycardia Systolic click	Dyspnea on exertion Angina Syncope on exertion Fatigue Orthopnea Paroxysmal nocturnal dyspnea Harsh, systolic crescendo-decrescendo murmur	Palpitations Dyspnea Orthopnea Paroxysmal nocturnal dyspnea Fatigue Angina Sinus tachycardia Blowing, decrescendo diastolic murmur
S_1 S_2 S_1 S_2 S_1	S_1 S_2S_3 S_1 S_2S_3	click click S_1 S_2 S_1 S_2	S_1 S_2 S_1 S_2	S_1 S_2 S_1 S_2 S_1

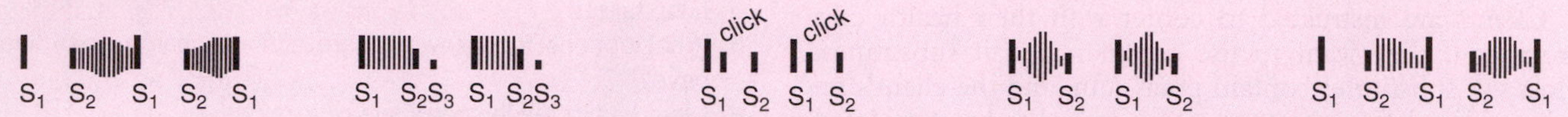

On palpation, the pulse may be normal, tachycardiac, or irregularly irregular (as in atrial fibrillation). Because the development of atrial fibrillation indicates that the client may decompensate, the physician should be notified immediately of the development of an irregularly irregular rhythm. A rumbling, apical diastolic murmur is noted on auscultation.

Mitral Regurgitation (Insufficiency)

The fibrotic and calcific changes occurring in **mitral regurgitation** (insufficiency) prevent the mitral valve from closing completely during *systole.* Incomplete closure of the valve allows the backflow of blood into the left atrium when the left ventricle contracts. During *diastole,* regurgitant output again flows from the left atrium to the left ventricle along with the normal blood flow. The increased volume must be ejected during the next systole. To compensate for the increased volume and pressure, the left atrium and ventricle dilate and hypertrophy.

Rheumatic heart disease is the predominant cause of mitral insufficiency. When it results from rheumatic heart disease, it usually coexists with some degree of mitral stenosis; it affects women more often than men. Nonrheumatic causes, more common in men, include papillary muscle dysfunction or rupture resulting from ischemic heart disease, infective endocarditis, and a congenital anomaly.

Mitral insufficiency usually progresses slowly; clients may remain symptom free for decades. Symptoms begin to occur when the left ventricle fails in response to increased blood volumes and include fatigue and chronic weakness as a result of reduced cardiac output (CO). Dyspnea on exertion and orthopnea develop later. A significant number of clients complain of anxiety, atypical chest pains, and palpitations. Assessment may reveal normal BP, atrial fibrillation (an irregularly irregular rhythm occurring in 75% of clients), or changes in respirations characteristic of left ventricular failure.

When right-sided HF develops, the neck veins become distended, the liver enlarges (hepatomegaly), and pitting edema is noted. A high-pitched systolic murmur at the apex, with radiation to the left axilla, is heard on auscultation. Severe regurgitation often exhibits a third heart sound (S_3).

Mitral Valve Prolapse

Mitral valve prolapse (MVP) occurs because the valvular leaflets enlarge and prolapse into the left atrium during systole. This abnormality is usually benign but may progress to pronounced mitral regurgitation.

Most clients with MVP are asymptomatic; however, they may report chest pain, palpitations, or exercise intolerance. Chest pain is usually atypical, with clients describing a sharp pain localized to the left side of the chest. Dizziness, **syncope** ("blackouts"), and palpitations may be associated with atrial or ventricular dysrhythmias.

A normal HR and BP is usually found on physical examination. A midsystolic click and a late systolic murmur may be audible at the apex. The intensity of the murmur is not related to the severity of the prolapse.

The etiology of MVP is variable and has been associated with conditions such as Marfan syndrome and other congenital cardiac defects (see Chapter 24 for a discussion on Marfan syndrome). Most often, however, no other cardiac abnormality is found. A familial occurrence is well established.

Mitral valve prolapse affects 5% to 10% of people. Although it is present in all age-groups, it is most common in women between 20 and 54 years of age.

Aortic Stenosis

In **aortic stenosis,** the aortic valve orifice narrows and obstructs left ventricular outflow during systole. This increased resistance to ejection or afterload results in ventricular hypertrophy. As stenosis progresses, cardiac output becomes fixed and unable to increase to meet the demands of the body during exertion, and symptoms develop. Eventually the left ventricle fails, volume backs up in the left atrium, and the pulmonary system becomes congested. Right-sided HF can occur late in the disease. *When the surface area of the valve becomes less than or equal to 1 cm, surgery is indicated on an urgent basis!*

The classic symptoms of aortic stenosis result from the fixed cardiac output: dyspnea, angina, and syncope occurring on exertion. When cardiac output falls in the late stages of the disease, the client experiences marked fatigue, debilitation, and peripheral cyanosis. A narrow pulse pressure is noted when the BP is examined. A diamond-shaped, systolic crescendo-decrescendo murmur is usually noted on auscultation.

Congenital valvular disease or malformation is the predominant etiologic factor in aortic stenosis. Bicuspid or unicuspid aortic valves are the primary reason for aortic stenosis in clients younger than 30 years and account for about 50% of the disease in clients 30 to 70 years of age. Rheumatic aortic stenosis is always concomitant with rheumatic disease of the mitral valve and develops in clients between 30 and 70 years of age. Atherosclerosis and degenerative calcification of the aortic valve are the predominant factors in people older than 70 years of age. Aortic stenosis has become the most common valvular disorder in countries with aging populations. Of clients with aortic stenosis, 80% are men.

Aortic Regurgitation (Insufficiency)

In clients with **aortic regurgitation,** the aortic valve leaflets do not close properly during diastole, and the *annulus* (the valve ring that attaches to the leaflets) may be dilated, loose, or deformed. This allows regurgitation of blood from the aorta back into the left ventricle during diastole. The left ventricle, in compensation, dilates to accommodate the greater blood volume and eventually hypertrophies.

Clients with aortic regurgitation remain asymptomatic for many years because of the compensatory mechanisms of the left ventricle. As the disease progresses and left ventricular failure occurs, the principal concerns are exertional dyspnea, orthopnea, and paroxysmal nocturnal dyspnea. Palpitations may be noted with severe disease, especially when the client lies on the left side. Nocturnal angina with diaphoresis often occurs.

On palpation, the nurse notes a "bounding" arterial pulse. The pulse pressure is usually widened, with an elevated systolic pressure and diminished diastolic pressure. The classic auscultatory finding is a high-pitched, blowing, decrescendo diastolic murmur.

Aortic insufficiency usually results from nonrheumatic conditions such as infective endocarditis, congenital anatomic aortic valvular abnormalities, hypertension, and Marfan syndrome (a rare, generalized, systemic disease of connective tissue). About 75% of clients with aortic regurgitation are men.

COLLABORATIVE MANAGEMENT

Assessment

A client with valvular disease may suddenly become ill or may slowly develop symptoms over many years. Information is collected about the client's family health history, including valvular or other forms of heart disease to which he or she may be genetically predisposed. Question the client about attacks of rheumatic fever and infective endocarditis, the specific dates when these occurred, and the use of antibiotic prophylaxis against the recurrence of rheumatic fever. Also question the client about a history of IV drug abuse. Discuss the client's fatigue level and tolerated activity level, the presence of angina or dyspnea, and the occurrence of palpitations, if present.

As part of the physical assessment, obtain the client's vital signs, inspect for signs of edema, palpate and auscultate the heart and lungs, and palpate the peripheral pulses. Findings consistent with valvular malformation are summarized in Chart 38-8.

In clients with mitral stenosis, the chest x-ray shows left atrial enlargement, prominent pulmonary arteries, and an enlarged right ventricle. In those with mitral regurgitation (insufficiency), the chest x-ray reveals an increased cardiac shadow, indicating left ventricular and left atrial enlargement.

In the later stages of aortic stenosis, the chest x-ray may show left ventricular enlargement and pulmonary congestion. Left atrial and left ventricular dilation appear on the chest x-ray of clients with aortic regurgitation (insufficiency). If HF is present, pulmonary venous congestion is also evident.

For valvular heart disease, echocardiography is the diagnostic procedure of choice because it is an excellent noninvasive tool for defining cardiac structure, movement of the valve leaflets, and size and function of the cardiac chambers. Exercise tolerance testing (ETT) and stress echocardiography are sometimes performed to evaluate symptomatic response, assess functional capacity, and enhance auscultatory findings. With either mitral or aortic stenosis, cardiac catheterization is often indicated to assess the severity of the stenosis and its other effects on the heart.

The health care provider also orders an electrocardiogram (ECG) to assess abnormalities such as left ventricular hypertrophy, as seen with mitral regurgitation and aortic regurgitation, or right ventricular hypertrophy, as seen in severe mitral stenosis. Atrial fibrillation is a common finding in both mitral stenosis and mitral regurgitation and may develop in aortic stenosis because of left atrial dilation.

Common Nursing Diagnoses and Collaborative Problems

Nursing diagnoses that may apply to clients with valvular heart disease include the following:

- Decreased Cardiac Output related to altered stroke volume
- Impaired Gas Exchange related to ventilation perfusion imbalance
- Activity Intolerance related to inability of the heart to meet metabolic demands during activity
- Acute Pain related to physiologic injury agent (hypoxia)

Interventions

Management of valvular heart disease depends on which valve is affected and the degree of valve impairment. Some clients can be managed with yearly monitoring and medications, whereas other clients require invasive procedures or heart surgery.

NONSURGICAL MANAGEMENT. Nonsurgical management focuses on drug therapy and rest. During the course of valvular disease, left ventricular failure with pulmonary or systemic congestion may develop. Diuretics, beta blockers, digoxin, and oxygen are often administered to improve the symptoms of heart failure (HF). Nitrates are administered cautiously to clients with aortic stenosis because of the potential for syncope associated with a reduction in left ventricular volume (preload). Vasodilators such as calcium channel blockers may be used to reduce the regurgitant flow for clients with aortic or mitral stenosis.

Prophylactic antibiotic therapy is required for all clients with valve disease before any invasive procedure. Procedures that require antibiotic coverage include bronchoscopy, endoscopy, sigmoidoscopy, colonoscopy, genitourinary instrumentation, surgery, and dental procedures of any type.

A major concern in valvular heart disease is maintaining cardiac output if atrial fibrillation develops. With mitral valvular disease, left ventricular filling is especially dependent on atrial contraction. When atrial fibrillation develops, there is no longer a single coordinated atrial contraction. Cardiac output can decrease by 25% to 30%, and HF may occur. Ineffective atrial contraction may also lead to the stasis of blood and thrombi in the left atrium. Monitor the client for the development of an irregular rhythm and notify the primary care provider if it develops. (See Chapter 37 for a detailed explanation of atrial fibrillation.)

The primary care provider usually institutes therapy to restore normal sinus rhythm or, if that is unsuccessful, to slow ventricular rate. The physician might elect to convert a client from atrial fibrillation to sinus rhythm using IV diltiazem (Cardizem, Apo-Diltiazem✱) or amiodarone (Cordarone, Pacerone). The client should be on a monitored unit where both cardiac rhythm and BP can be closely watched. Synchronized countershock (cardioversion) may be attempted if atrial fibrillation is rapid, the client decompensates, and the rhythm is unresponsive to medical treatment (see Chapter 37).

If the client remains in atrial fibrillation, low-dose amiodarone (Cordarone) or flecainide (Tambocor) is often prescribed to slow ventricular rate. Procainamide hydrochloride (Pronestyl hydrochloride, Procanbid) may be added to the regimen. A beta-blocking agent may also be considered to slow the ventricular response.

For valvular heart disease and chronic atrial fibrillation, anticoagulation with sodium warfarin (Coumadin, Warfilone✱) is usually a part of the medical treatment plan to prevent thrombus formation. A thrombus that forms on the wall of the heart is called a **mural thrombosis.** Thrombi may form in the atria or on defective valve segments, resulting in systemic emboli. If a portion breaks off and travels to the brain, one or more strokes may occur. Assess the client's baseline neurologic status and regularly reassess for neurologic changes.

Rest is often an important part of treatment. Activity may be limited because cardiac output (CO) cannot meet increased metabolic demands, and angina or HF can result. A balance of rest and exercise is needed to prevent muscle atrophy.

SURGICAL MANAGEMENT. Surgical repair or replacement of heart valves has a major effect on the prognosis of valvular heart disease. Correct timing is crucial. Repair or replacement of the valve is usually performed after symptoms of left ventricular failure have developed but before irreversible dysfunction occurs. Surgical therapy is the only definitive treatment of aortic stenosis and is recommended when angina, syncope, or dyspnea on exertion develops.

Reparative Procedures. Reparative procedures are gaining in popularity because of continuing problems with thrombi, endocarditis, and left ventricular dysfunction after valvular replacement. Reparative procedures do not result in a normal valve, but they usually "turn back the clock," resulting in a more functional valve and an improvement in cardiac output. Turbulent blood flow through the valve may persist, and degeneration of the repaired valve is possible.

Balloon Valvuloplasty. Balloon valvuloplasty, an invasive nonsurgical procedure, is possible for stenotic mitral and aortic valves; however, careful selection of clients is necessary. Valvuloplasty may be the initial treatment of choice for people with noncalcified, mobile mitral valves. Clients selected for aortic valvuloplasty are usually older and are at high risk for surgical complications or have refused operative treatment. The benefits of aortic valvuloplasty for aortic stenosis tend to be short lived, rarely lasting longer than 6 months.

When performing mitral valvuloplasty, the physician passes a balloon catheter from the femoral vein, through the atrial septum, and to the mitral valve. The balloon is inflated to enlarge the mitral orifice. For aortic valvuloplasty, the physician inserts the catheter through the femoral artery and advances it to the aortic valve, where it is inflated to enlarge the orifice. Valvuloplasty usually offers immediate relief of symptoms because the balloon has dilated the orifice and improved leaflet mobility. The results are comparable with those of surgical commissurotomy for appropriately selected clients.

After the procedure, observe the client closely for bleeding from the catheter insertion site and institute postangiogram precautions. Bleeding is likely after valvuloplasty because of the large size of the catheter. Also observe for signs of a regurgitant valve by closely monitoring heart sounds, CO, and heart rhythm. Because vegetations (thrombi) may have been dislodged from the valve, observe for any indication of systemic emboli (see Infective Endocarditis, p. 768).

Direct, or Open, Commissurotomy. Direct commissurotomy is accomplished with cardiopulmonary bypass during open heart surgery. The surgeon visualizes the valve, removes thrombi from the atria, incises the fused commissures (leaflets), and debrides calcium from the leaflets, widening the orifice.

Mitral Valve Annuloplasty. Mitral valve annuloplasty (reconstruction) is the reparative procedure of choice for most clients with acquired mitral insufficiency. To make the annulus (the valve ring that attaches to and supports the leaflets) smaller, the physician may suture the leaflets to an annuloplasty ring or take tucks in the client's annulus. Leaflet repair is often performed at the same time. Elongated leaflets may be shortened, and shortened leaflets may be repaired by lengthening the chordae that bind them in place. Perforated leaflets may be patched with synthetic grafts.

Annuloplasty and leaflet repair result in an annulus of the appropriate size and in leaflets that can close completely. Thus regurgitation is eliminated or markedly reduced.

Replacement Procedures. The development of *prosthetic* (synthetic) and *biologic* (tissue) valves has improved the surgical therapy and prognosis of valvular heart disease. Prosthetic valves come in a wide variety. Although prosthetic valves are durable, all clients must receive oral anticoagulation because of the possibility of clot formation.

Biologic valves may be **xenograft** (from other species), such as a porcine valve (from a pig) (Figure 38-2) or a bovine valve (from a cow). Because tissue valves are associated with little risk of clot formation, long-term anticoagulation is not indicated; however, xenografts are not as durable as prosthetic valves and usually must be replaced every 7 to 10 years. The durability of a xenograft is related to the age of the recipient. Calcium in the blood, which is present in larger quantities in younger clients, breaks down the valves.

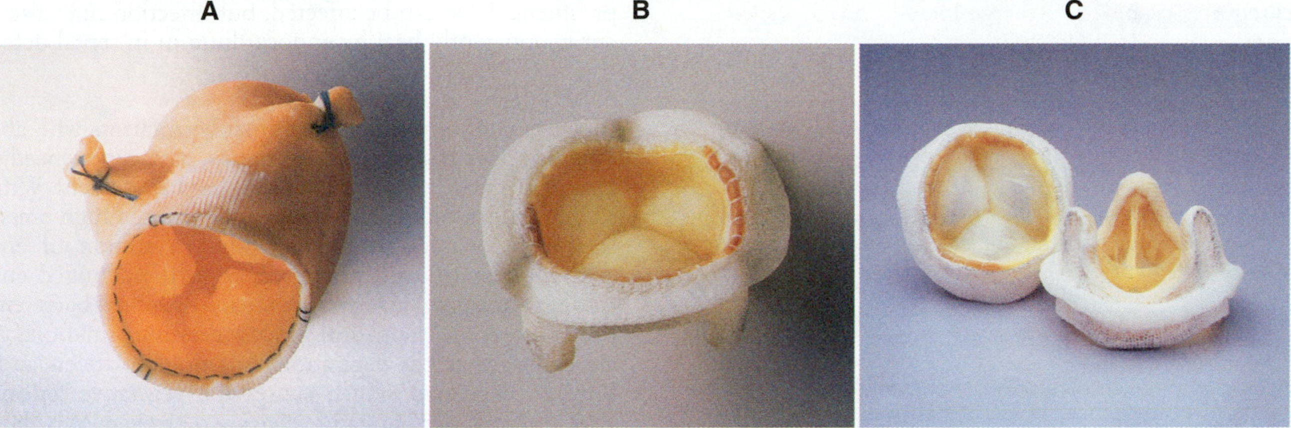

Figure 38-2 ■ Examples of biologic (tissue) heart valves. **A,** Freestyle, a stentless pig valve with no frame. **B,** Hancock II, a stented pig valve. **C,** Carpentier-Edwards pericardial bioprosthesis. (**A** and **B** courtesy of Medtronic, Inc., Minneapolis, MN; **C** courtesy of Baxter Healthcare Corporation, Edwards CVS Division, Santa Ana, CA.)

The older the client, the longer the xenograft will last. Valves donated from human cadavers and **pulmonary autographs** (relocation of the client's own pulmonary valve to the aortic position [Ross procedure]) are also being used for valve replacement.

An aortic valve is replaced with a mechanical valve for most symptomatic adults with aortic stenosis and aortic insufficiency. A tissue valve cannot be used because of the high pressure within the aorta.

Preoperative Care. Clients undergoing valve surgery have open heart surgery similar to the procedure for a coronary artery bypass graft (CABG) (see Chapter 41). Ideally, surgery is an elective and planned procedure. Instruct the client and family members or a significant other about the management of postoperative pain, incision care, and strategies to prevent respiratory complications (see Chapters 20 and 22). Teach clients receiving oral anticoagulants to stop taking them before surgery as the physician indicates, usually at least 72 hours before the procedure. Clients also need to have a preoperative dental examination. If dental caries or periodontal disease is present, these problems must be resolved before valve replacement.

Postoperative Care. Nursing interventions for open heart surgery for valve disorders are similar to those for a CABG (see Chapter 41); however, a few significant differences depend in part on the type of valvular surgery. Clients with mitral stenosis often have pulmonary hypertension and stiff lungs. Monitor respiratory status closely during weaning from the ventilator. Be especially vigilant for indications of bleeding in clients with aortic valve replacements because of a higher risk for postoperative hemorrhage.

Clients with valve replacements are also more likely to experience significant reductions in CO after surgery, especially those with aortic stenosis or left ventricular failure from mitral valve disease. Carefully monitor the client's CO and identifying any indications of pump failure. High filling pressures–pulmonary artery wedge pressure (PAWP) greater than 18 mm Hg–may be required to maintain an acceptable CO in the immediate postoperative period. Clients who have had valve replacements with prosthetic valves require lifetime prophylactic anticoagulation therapy to prevent thrombus formation.

Community-Based Care

The client with valvular heart disease may be discharged home on medical therapy or postoperatively after valve repair or replacement. Because fatigue is a common problem for clients, ensure that the home environment is conducive to providing rest while moving the client toward increased activity levels. Older clients with aortic stenosis may reside in long-term care.

HOME CARE MANAGEMENT

A home care nurse may be needed to help the client adhere to medication and activity schedules and to detect any problems, particularly with anticoagulant therapy. Clients who have undergone surgery may require a nurse for assistance with incision care. A home care aide may assist with activities of daily living if the client lives alone.

HEALTH TEACHING

The teaching plan for the client with valvular heart disease includes the following:

- The disease process
- Medications, including diuretics, vasodilators, beta blockers, calcium channel blockers, antibiotics, and anticoagulants
- The prophylactic use of antibiotics
- A plan of work, activity, and rest to conserve energy
- The purpose and nature of surgical intervention, if appropriate

Because clients with defective or repaired valves are at risk for infective endocarditis, teach them to adhere to the precautions described for endocarditis. Instruct clients to inform all health care providers of the valvular heart disease history; also tell them that they require antibiotic administration before all invasive procedures and tests. Instructions for the client are described in Chart 38-9.

Teach clients taking anticoagulants how to manage their drug therapy successfully, including dietary considerations (if taking warfarin) and the prevention of bleeding. For example, the client should be taught to avoid foods high in vitamin K and to use an electric razor to avoid skin cuts. In addition, the client should report any bleeding or excessive bruising to the health care provider.

CHART 38-9

CLIENT EDUCATION GUIDE
Valvular Heart Disease

- Notify all your health care providers that you have a defective heart valve.
- Remind the health care provider of your valvular problem when you have any dental work (cleaning, filling, or extraction), any examination by instrument (cystoscopy, endoscopy, or sigmoidoscopy), or any other invasive procedure (arteriogram, surgery).
- Request antibiotic prophylaxis before and after these procedures if the health care provider does not offer it.
- Clean all wounds and apply antibiotic ointment to prevent infection.
- Notify your health care provider immediately if you experience fever, petechiae (pinpoint red dots on your skin), or shortness of breath.

Teach clients who have undergone valve surgery how to care for the sternal incision and instruct them to watch for and report any fever, drainage, or redness at the site. Clients can usually return to normal activity after 6 weeks but should avoid heavy physical labor with their upper extremities for 3 to 6 months to allow the sternotomy incision to heal. Clients who have had valvular surgery should also avoid dental procedures for 6 months because of the potential for endocarditis. Some procedures may be done with caution but only if the client takes a course of antibiotic therapy. Those with prosthetic valves need to avoid any procedure using magnetic resonance technology.

Clients with valvular heart disease may have complicated medication schedules as well as long-term antibiotic or anticoagulant therapy. These circumstances potentially can lead to noncompliance. Provide clear, concise instructions about medication schedules, and discuss the risks associated with noncompliance.

The psychological response to valve surgery is similar to that following coronary artery bypass surgery. Clients may experience an altered self-image as a result of the required lifestyle changes or the visible medial sternotomy incision. In addition, clients with prosthetic valves may need to adjust to a soft but audible clicking sound of the prosthetic valve. Encourage clients to verbalize their feelings about the sternotomy incision and the prosthetic heart valve. It is common for clients to display a variety of emotions postoperatively, especially when they get home.

HEALTH CARE RESOURCES

The American Heart Association and the Mended Hearts Club is a community resource that provides information about valvular heart disease. A wallet-sized card can be obtained to identify the client as needing prophylactic antibiotics. An identification bracelet that states the name of the drug the client is taking should also be worn.

INFLAMMATIONS AND INFECTIONS

Infective Endocarditis

PATHOPHYSIOLOGY

Infective endocarditis (previously called *bacterial endocarditis*) refers to a microbial infection (e.g., viruses, bacteria, fungi) involving the endocardium. A healthy, defective, or prosthetic valve can be affected, but infection may also occur in apparently healthy endocardium or in septal defects.

Etiology

Infective endocarditis occurs primarily in clients who abuse IV drugs, have had valve replacements, have experienced systemic infection, or have structural cardiac defects. With a cardiac defect, blood may flow rapidly from a high-pressure area to a low-pressure zone, eroding a section of endocardium. Platelets and fibrin adhere to the denuded endocardium, forming a vegetative lesion. During bacteremia, bacteria become trapped in the low-pressure "sinkhole" and are deposited in the vegetation. Additional platelets and fibrin are deposited, which causes the vegetative lesion to grow; the endocardium and valve are destroyed. Valvular insufficiency may result when the lesion interferes with normal alignment of the valve. If vegetations become so large that blood flow through the valve is obstructed, the valve appears stenotic and then is very likely to *embolize* (i.e., cause emboli to be released).

Possible ports of entry for infecting organisms include the following:

- The oral cavity (especially if dental procedures have been performed)
- Skin rashes, lesions, or abscesses
- Infections (cutaneous, genitourinary, gastrointestinal, systemic)
- Surgery or invasive procedures, including IV line placement

Incidence/Prevalence

The incidence of infective endocarditis is estimated to be 1 per 1000 hospital admissions, with males and females equally affected. Mortality rates for infective endocarditis have remained high–up to 25% despite antibiotic therapy.

COLLABORATIVE MANAGEMENT

Assessment

Because mortality remains high, early detection of infective endocarditis is essential. Unfortunately, many clients (especially older adults) are misdiagnosed. Clinical manifestations usually occur within 2 weeks of a bacteremia (Chart 38-10).

Assessment usually reveals a recurrent fever. Most clients have temperatures from 99° to 103° F (37.2° to 39.4° C). As a result of physiologic changes associated with aging, however, many older adults remain afebrile. The severity of symptoms may depend on the virulence of the infecting organism.

PHYSICAL ASSESSMENT/CLINICAL MANIFESTATIONS

CARDIOVASCULAR MANIFESTATIONS. Assess the client's cardiovascular status. More than 90% of clients with infective endocarditis develop murmurs. Carefully auscultate the precordium, noting and documenting any new murmurs (usually regurgitant in nature) or any changes in the intensity or quality of an old murmur. An S_3 or S_4 heart sound may also be heard.

Heart failure (HF) is the most common complication of infective endocarditis. Assess for right-sided HF (as evidenced by peripheral edema, weight gain, and anorexia) and left-sided HF (as evidenced by fatigue, shortness of breath, and crackles on auscultation of breath sounds). See discussion of HF earlier in this chapter.

CHART 38-10

KEY FEATURES of
Infective Endocarditis

- Fever associated with chills, night sweats, malaise, and fatigue
- Anorexia and weight loss
- Cardiac murmur (newly developed or change in existing)
- Development of heart failure
- Evidence of systemic embolization
- Petechiae
- Splinter hemorrhages
- Osler's nodes
- Janeway's lesions
- Positive blood cultures

EMBOLIC COMPLICATIONS. Arterial embolization is a major complication in up to 50% of clients with infective endocarditis. Fragments of vegetation break loose and travel randomly through the circulation. When the left side of the heart is involved, vegetation fragments are carried to the spleen, kidneys, gastrointestinal (GI) tract, brain, and extremities. When the right side of the heart is involved, emboli enter the pulmonary circulation.

Splenic infarction with sudden abdominal pain and radiation to the left shoulder can also occur. When performing an abdominal assessment, note rebound tenderness on palpation. The classic pain described with renal infarction is flank pain that radiates to the groin and is accompanied by hematuria or pyuria. Mesenteric emboli may result in the client complaining of diffuse abdominal pain, often after eating, and abdominal distention.

Whereas about a third of clients demonstrate neurologic changes, others have signs and symptoms of pulmonary problems. Emboli to the central nervous system cause either transient ischemic attacks (TIAs) or a stroke. Confusion, reduced concentration and aphasia, or dysphagia may occur. Pleuritic chest pain, dyspnea, and cough are symptoms of pulmonary infarction related to embolization.

PERIPHERAL MANIFESTATIONS. **Petechiae** (pinpoint red spots) occur in up to 40% of clients with endocarditis. Examine the mucous membranes, the palate, the conjunctivae, and the skin above the clavicles for small, red, flat lesions. Assess the distal third of the nail bed for **splinter hemorrhages,** which appear as black longitudinal lines or small red streaks.

DIAGNOSTIC ASSESSMENT

A positive blood culture is of prime diagnostic and therapeutic importance. Both aerobic and anaerobic specimens are obtained for culture. Some slow-growing organisms may take 3 weeks and require a specialized medium to isolate. Therefore cultures should be monitored by the laboratory for 3 to 4 weeks. Low hemoglobin and hematocrit levels may also be found.

Echocardiography has improved the ability to diagnose infective endocarditis accurately. Transesophageal echocardiography (TEE) allows visualization of cardiac structures that are difficult to see with transthoracic echocardiography (TTE). TEE provides good resolution and is very sensitive for discovering valvular abnormalities, thereby enabling the clinician to diagnose infective endocarditis more accurately (see Chapter 36).

The most reliable criteria for diagnosing endocarditis include positive blood cultures, a new regurgitant murmur, and evidence of endocardial involvement by echocardiography.

Interventions

Care of the client with endocarditis usually includes antimicrobials, rest balanced with activity, and supportive therapy for HF. If these interventions are successful, surgery is usually not required.

NONSURGICAL MANAGEMENT. The major component of treatment for endocarditis is drug therapy. Other interventions help to prevent the life-threatening complications.

Drug Therapy. Antimicrobials are the mainstay of treatment, with the choice of drug depending on the specific organism involved. Because vegetations surround and protect the offending microorganism, an appropriate medication must be given in a sufficiently high dose to ensure its destruction. Antimicrobials are most often given intravenously, with the course of treatment lasting 4 to 6 weeks. For most bacterial cases, the ideal antibiotic is one of the penicillins or cephalosporins.

Clients may be hospitalized for several days to institute IV therapy and then are discharged for continued IV therapy at home. After hospitalization, most clients who respond to therapy may continue therapy at home when they become afebrile, have negative blood cultures, and have no signs of HF or embolization.

Anticoagulants are of no value in preventing embolization from vegetations. Because they may result in bleeding, they are avoided unless they are required to prevent thrombus formation on a prosthetic valve.

Other Interventions. Complete bedrest need not be enforced unless clients are hemodynamically unstable; however, activities are balanced with adequate rest. Explain proper oral and general body hygiene and consistently use appropriate aseptic technique to protect the client from contact with potentially infective organisms. Nursing assessment for signs of HF (including rapid pulse, fatigue, cough, and dyspnea; new heart murmurs; and early signs of embolization) continues throughout the antimicrobial regimen.

SURGICAL MANAGEMENT. The cardiac surgeon may be consulted if antibiotic therapy is ineffective in sterilizing a valve, if refractory HF develops secondary to a defective valve, if large valvular vegetations are present, or if multiple embolic events occur. Current surgical interventions for infective endocarditis include the following:

- Removing the infected valve (either biologic or prosthetic)
- Repairing or removing congenital shunts
- Repairing injured valves and chordae tendineae
- Draining abscesses in the heart or elsewhere

Preoperative and postoperative care of clients having surgery involving the valves is similar to that described earlier for valve replacement (pp. 766 and 767).

Community-Based Care

Community-based care for clients with infective endocarditis is essential to resolve the problem, prevent relapse, and avoid complications. Clients and families need to be motivated and have the knowledge, physical ability, and resources to administer IV antibiotics at home. The home care nurse may be contacted to complete teaching started in the acute care institution and to monitor client compliance and health status.

The home care nurse and pharmacist arrange for appropriate supplies to be available to the client at home. Supplies include the prepared antibiotic, IV pump with tubing, alcohol wipes, IV access device, normal saline solution, and a heparin or saline lock flush solution drawn up in syringes. A saline lock, peripherally inserted central catheter (PICC line), or central catheter is positioned at a venous site that is easily accessible to the client or a family member.

Teach the client, family members, or a significant other how to administer the antibiotic and care for the infusion site while maintaining aseptic technique. The client or family member demonstrates this technique before the client is discharged from the hospital. Emphasize the importance of maintaining a blood level of the antibiotic by administering the antibiotics as scheduled. After stabilization at home, the health care provider contacts the client every 3 to 7 days to determine whether he or she is able to comply with and benefit from the IV antibiotic therapy.

Encourage proper hygiene, particularly oral hygiene. Clients are advised to use a soft toothbrush, to brush their teeth at least twice per day, and to rinse the mouth with water after brushing. They should not use irrigation devices or floss the teeth because bacteremia may result. Instruct clients to cleanse lacerations well and apply an antibiotic ointment.

Clients must remind health care providers (including their dentists) of their endocarditis and request prophylactic antibiotic coverage for every invasive procedure, including dental care. Such protection is essential because studies have documented low compliance with prophylaxis regimens by health care providers.

Teach self-monitoring for the manifestations of endocarditis, including the complications of HF and embolic phenomena. Instruct clients to monitor and record their temperature daily for up to 6 weeks. Teach clients to report fever, chills, malaise, weight loss, increased fatigue, sudden weight gain, or dyspnea to their primary care provider.

Pericarditis

PATHOPHYSIOLOGY

Acute pericarditis is an inflammation or alteration of the pericardium, the membranous sac that encloses the heart. Acute pericarditis may be fibrous, serous, hemorrhagic, purulent, or neoplastic. Acute pericarditis is most commonly associated with the following:

- Malignant neoplasms
- Idiopathic causes
- Infective organisms (bacteria, viruses, or fungi)
- Postmyocardial infarction (MI) syndrome (Dressler's syndrome)
- Postpericardiotomy syndrome
- Systemic connective tissue disease
- Renal failure

The cause of the pericarditis determines its presentation. Acute viral pericarditis commonly follows a respiratory infection and is more common in men between 20 and 50 years of age. In 5% to 15% of clients who experience an MI, **Dressler's syndrome** occurs from 1 to 12 weeks after the infarction. This syndrome is characterized by pericarditis, fever, and pericardial and pleural effusions. **Postpericardiotomy syndrome** occurs in 10% to 40% of clients after cardiac surgery.

Chronic constrictive pericarditis occurs when chronic pericardial inflammation causes a fibrous thickening of the pericardium. It is caused by tuberculosis, radiation therapy, trauma, renal failure, or metastatic cancer. In chronic constrictive pericarditis, the pericardium becomes rigid, preventing adequate filling of the ventricles and eventually resulting in cardiac failure.

COLLABORATIVE MANAGEMENT

Assessment

Assessment findings include substernal precordial pain that radiates to the left side of the neck, the shoulder, or the back. Pain is classically grating and oppressive and is aggravated by breathing (mainly on inspiration), coughing, and swallowing. The pain is worse when the client is in the supine position and may be relieved by sitting up and leaning forward. Ask all the questions to evaluate chest discomfort because it is important that the pain of pericarditis be differentiated from that of an acute MI (see Chapter 36).

A pericardial friction rub may be heard with the diaphragm of the stethoscope positioned at the left lower sternal border. This scratchy, high-pitched sound is produced when the inflamed, roughened pericardial layers create friction as their surfaces rub together.

Clients with chronic constrictive pericarditis show signs of right-sided HF, elevated systemic venous pressure with jugular distention, hepatic engorgement, and dependent edema. Exertional fatigue and dyspnea are common complications. Thickening of the pericardium is seen on echocardiography or a computed tomography (CT) scan.

Clients with acute pericarditis may have an elevated white blood cell count and usually have a fever. Therefore blood culture and sensitivity may be analyzed in the laboratory. The electrocardiogram (ECG) usually shows ST-T spiking with the onset of inflammation, which returns to baseline with treatment. Atrial fibrillation is also common. Echocardiograms may be used to determine a pericardial effusion.

Interventions

The client with acute pericarditis may be hospitalized for diagnostic evaluation, observation for complications, and symptom relief. The health care provider usually prescribes nonsteroidal anti-inflammatory drugs (NSAIDs) for the relief of pain. Clients who do not obtain pain relief within 48 to 96 hours and who do not have bacterial pericarditis may receive corticosteroid therapy. The nurse assesses for pain relief and assists the client to assume positions of comfort—usually sitting upright and leaning slightly forward. If the pain is not relieved within 24 to 48 hours, the nurse notifies the primary care provider.

The various causes of pericarditis require specific therapies. For example, bacterial pericarditis (acute) usually requires antibiotics and pericardial drainage. The usual clinical course of acute pericarditis is short term (2 to 6 weeks), but episodes may recur. Chronic pericarditis caused by malignant disease may be treated with radiation or chemotherapy, whereas uremic pericarditis is treated by hemodialysis.

The definitive treatment for chronic constrictive pericarditis is surgical excision of the pericardium **(pericardiectomy).**

Monitoring for Complications of Pericarditis. A significant complication of pericarditis is pericardial effusion, which occurs when the space between the parietal and

CHART 38-11

BEST PRACTICE for
Care of the Client with Pericarditis

- Assess the nature of the client's chest discomfort. (Pericardial pain is typically substernal; it is worse on inspiration and decreases when the client leans forward.)
- Auscultate for a pericardial friction rub.
- Assist the client to a position of comfort.
- Provide anti-inflammatory agents as prescribed.
- Explain that anti-inflammatory agents usually decrease the pain within 48 hours.
- Avoid the administration of aspirin and anticoagulants because these may increase the possibility of tamponade.
- Auscultate the blood pressure carefully to detect paradoxical blood pressure (pulsus paradoxus), a sign of tamponade.
  - Palpate the blood pressure and inflate the cuff above the systolic pressure.
  - Deflate the cuff gradually, and note when sounds are first audible on expiration.
  - Identify when sounds are also audible on inspiration.
  - Subtract the inspiratory pressure from the expiratory pressure to determine the amount of pulsus paradoxus (>10 mm Hg is an indication of tamponade).
- Inspect for other indications of tamponade, including jugular venous distention with clear lungs, muffled heart sounds, and decreased cardiac output.
- Notify the physician if tamponade is suspected.

visceral layers of the pericardium fills with fluid. Pericardial effusion puts the client at risk for cardiac tamponade, or excessive fluid within the pericardial cavity. Tamponade, which occurs in 15% of clients with acute pericarditis, restricts diastolic ventricular filling, and cardiac output drops. Findings of cardiac tamponade include the following:

- Jugular venous distention
- Paradoxical pulse (systolic blood pressure 10 mm Hg higher or more on expiration than on inspiration) (Chart 38-11)
- Decreased cardiac output
- Muffled heart sounds
- Circulatory collapse

Emergency Care: Acute Cardiac Tamponade. **Acute cardiac tamponade** may occur when small volumes (20 to 50 mL) of fluid accumulate rapidly in the pericardium. If the fluid accumulates slowly, the pericardium may stretch to accommodate several hundred milliliters of fluid. Report any suspicion of this complication to the physician immediately. *Cardiac tamponade is an emergency!* The physician may initially manage the decreased cardiac output (CO) with increased fluid volume administration while awaiting a chest x-ray or echocardiogram to confirm the diagnosis. Unfortunately, these tests are not always helpful because the fluid volume around the heart may be too small to visualize. Hemodynamic monitoring in a specialized critical care unit usually demonstrates compression of the heart, with all pressures (right atrial, pulmonary artery, and wedge) being similar and elevated (plateau pressures).

The physician may elect to perform a **pericardiocentesis** to relieve the pressure on the heart. Under echocardiographic or fluoroscopic and hemodynamic monitoring, the cardiologist inserts an 8-inch (20.3-cm), 16- or 18-gauge pericardial needle into the pericardial space. The physician and the nurse monitor the needle's position, recognizing that ST-wave and T-wave changes indicate myocardial injury and that the needle must be withdrawn slightly. When the needle is properly positioned, a catheter is inserted and all available pericardial fluid is withdrawn. Monitor the pulmonary artery, wedge, and right atrial pressures during the procedure. The pressures should return to normal as the fluid compressing the heart is removed, and the clinical manifestations of tamponade should resolve. In situations in which the cause of the effusion is unknown, pericardial fluid specimens may be sent to the laboratory for cell count, culture and sensitivity tests, and cytology.

After the pericardiocentesis, closely monitor the client for the recurrence of tamponade. Pericardiocentesis alone often does not resolve acute tamponade. Be prepared to provide adequate fluid volumes to increase CO and to prepare the client for emergency sternotomy if tamponade recurs.

If the client experiences a recurrence of tamponade or recurrent effusions or adhesions from chronic pericarditis, a portion or all of the pericardium may need to be removed to allow adequate ventricular filling and contraction. The surgeon may perform creation of a pericardial window, which involves removing a portion of the pericardium to permit excessive pericardial fluid to drain into the pleural space. In more severe cases, removal of the toughened encasing pericardium (pericardiectomy) may be necessary.

Rheumatic Carditis

PATHOPHYSIOLOGY

Rheumatic carditis, also called *rheumatic endocarditis,* is a sensitivity response that develops after an upper respiratory tract infection with group A beta-hemolytic streptococci, which occurs in about 40% of clients with rheumatic fever and affects more than one million Americans. The precise mechanism by which the infection causes inflammatory lesions in the heart is not established; however, inflammation is evident in all layers of the heart. The inflammation results in impaired contractile function of the myocardium, thickening of the pericardium, and valvular damage.

Rheumatic carditis is characterized by the formation of Aschoff's bodies, small nodules in the myocardium that are replaced by scar tissue. A diffuse cellular infiltrate also develops and appears to be responsible for the HF. The pericardium becomes thickened and covered with exudate, and a serosanguineous pleural effusion may develop. The most serious damage occurs to the endocardium, with inflammation of the valve leaflets developing. Hemorrhagic and fibrous lesions form along the inflamed surfaces of the valves, resulting in stenosis or regurgitation primarily of the mitral and aortic valves.

Rheumatic fever is a complication of about 3% of group A beta-hemolytic throat infections. Although the primary attacks occur most often in childhood, rheumatic fever may occur in adulthood. The incidence of rheumatic carditis had been decreasing consistently until the mid-1980s. At that time, a resurgence of rheumatic fever began in both the United States and Europe.

COLLABORATIVE MANAGEMENT

Rheumatic carditis is one of the major indicators of rheumatic fever. The following are common clinical manifestations:

- Tachycardia
- Cardiomegaly

- Development of a new murmur or a change in an existing murmur
- Pericardial friction rub
- Precordial pain
- Electrocardiogram (ECG) changes (prolonged PR interval)
- Indications of heart failure (HF)
- Evidence of an existing streptococcal infection

Primary prevention is extremely important. Teach all clients to consult their health care providers and receive appropriate antibiotic therapy if they develop the following indications of streptococcal pharyngitis: moderate to high fever, abrupt onset of a sore throat, a reddened throat with exudate, and enlarged and tender lymph nodes. Penicillin is the antibiotic of choice for treatment. Erythromycin (Eryc, Erythromid✱) is the alternative for penicillin-sensitive clients.

The signs of rheumatic carditis must be recognized promptly, and antibiotic therapy must be instituted immediately for secondary prevention. The client is urged to continue the antibiotic administration for the full 10 days to prevent reinfection. Suggest ways to manage the fever, such as maintaining hydration and administering antipyretics. Encourage the client to obtain adequate rest.

Emphasize tertiary prevention in client education, explaining that a recurrence of rheumatic carditis is probable with reinfection by streptococcus. Thus antibiotic therapy is essential for streptococcal infection. Antibiotic prophylaxis is necessary for the rest of his or her life to prevent infective endocarditis (see Infective Endocarditis, p. 768).

CARDIOMYOPATHY

Cardiomyopathy is a subacute or chronic disease of cardiac muscle. It is not common, occurring in only 10 to 20 per 100,000 population and resulting in about 30,000 deaths each year in the United States. The cause is usually unknown.

Cardiomyopathies are classified into three categories on the basis of abnormalities in structure and function: dilated cardiomyopathy, hypertrophic cardiomyopathy, and restrictive cardiomyopathy (Table 38-3).

Dilated Cardiomyopathy

Dilated cardiomyopathy (DCM) is the structural abnormality in 87% of cardiomyopathy cases. DCM involves extensive damage to the myofibrils and interference with myocardial metabolism. There is normal ventricular wall thickness but a dilation of both ventricles and impairment of systolic function. Decreased CO from inadequate pumping of the heart causes the client to experience dyspnea on exertion, decreased exercise capacity, fatigue, and palpitations. With the exception of peripartum cardiomyopathy, DCM is twice as common in men as in women and occurs most often in middle age. Causes may include alcohol abuse and chemotherapy.

Hypertrophic Cardiomyopathy

The cardinal features of **hypertrophic cardiomyopathy (HCM)** are asymmetric ventricular hypertrophy and disarray of the myocardial fibers. Left ventricular hypertrophy leads to a stiff left ventricle that results in diastolic filling abnormalities. Obstruction in the left ventricular outflow tract is seen in 75% to 80% of clients with HCM. In about 50% of clients, HCM is transmitted as a single-gene autosomal dominant trait. The American Heart Association (2002) reports that about 36% of young athletes who die suddenly probably had hypertrophic cardiomyopathy.

Restrictive Cardiomyopathy

Restrictive cardiomyopathy, the rarest of the three cardiomyopathies, results in restriction of filling of the ventricles. It is caused by endocardial or myocardial disease and produces a clinical picture similar to that of constrictive pericarditis.

◆COLLABORATIVE MANAGEMENT

◆Assessment

Findings in cardiomyopathy depend on the structural and functional abnormalities. Left ventricular or biventricular failure is characteristic of *dilated* cardiomyopathy (DCM). Some clients with DCM are asymptomatic for months to years and have left ventricular dilation confirmed on x-ray examination. Other clients experience sudden, pronounced symptoms of left ventricular failure, such as progressive dyspnea on exertion, orthopnea, palpitations, and activity intolerance. Right-sided HF develops late in the disease and is associated with a poor prognosis. Atrial fibrillation occurs in 25% of clients and is associated with embolism.

The clinical picture of *hypertrophic* cardiomyopathy (HCM) results from the hypertrophied septum, which in 80% of cases causes a mechanical obstruction and thereby reduces stroke volume (SV) and CO. Most clients are asymptomatic until late adolescence or early adulthood. The primary symptoms of HCM are exertional dyspnea (90% of clients), angina (75% of clients), and syncope. The chest pain is atypical in that it usually occurs at rest, is prolonged, has no relation to exertion, and is not relieved by the administration of nitrates. A high incidence of ventricular dysrhythmias is associated with HCM. Sudden death occurs and may be the first manifestation of the disease.

The earliest clinical finding in *restrictive* cardiomyopathy is exertional dyspnea. CO cannot increase during periods of exertion because of the fixed ventricular volume. The client also reports weakness, exercise intolerance, palpitations, and syncope.

Echocardiography, radionuclide imaging, and angiocardiography during cardiac catheterization are performed to diagnose and differentiate cardiomyopathies.

◆Interventions

The treatment of choice for the client with cardiomyopathy varies with the type of cardiomyopathy and may include both medical and surgical interventions.

NONSURGICAL MANAGEMENT. The care of clients with dilated or restrictive cardiomyopathy is initially the same as for HF. Drug therapy includes the use of diuretics, vasodilating agents, and cardiac glycosides to increase CO. Because clients are at risk for sudden death, the nurse urges them to report any palpitations, dizziness, or fainting, which might indicate a dysrhythmia. Antidysrhythmic drugs or implantable cardiac defibrillators may be used to control life-threatening dysrhythmias. To block inappropriate sympathetic stimulation and tachycardia, beta blockers (e.g., metoprolol) are used. If cardiomyopathy has developed in response to a toxin, further exposure to that

TABLE 38-3 Pathophysiology, Signs and Symptoms, and Treatment of Cardiomyopathies

	Hypertrophic Cardiomyopathy		
Dilated Cardiomyopathy	**Nonobstructed**	**Obstructed**	**Restrictive Cardiomyopathy**
Pathophysiology			
Fibrosis of myocardium and endocardium Dilated chambers Mural wall thrombi prevalent	Hypertrophy of all walls Hypertrophied septum Relatively small chamber size	Same as for nonobstructed except for obstruction of left ventricular outflow tract associated with the hypertrophied septum and mitral valve incompetence	Mimics constrictive pericarditis Fibrosed walls cannot expand or contract Chambers narrowed; emboli common
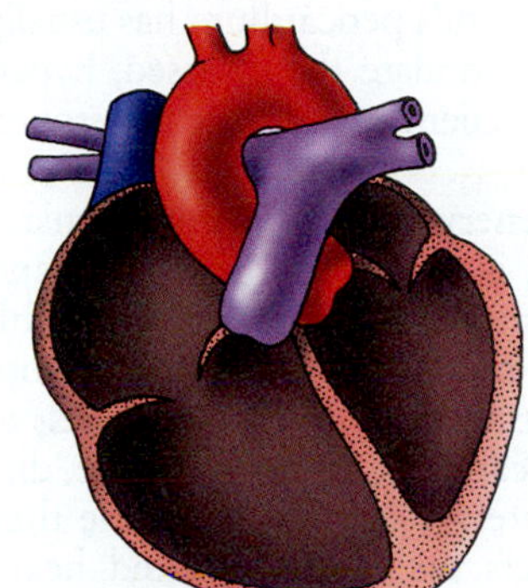		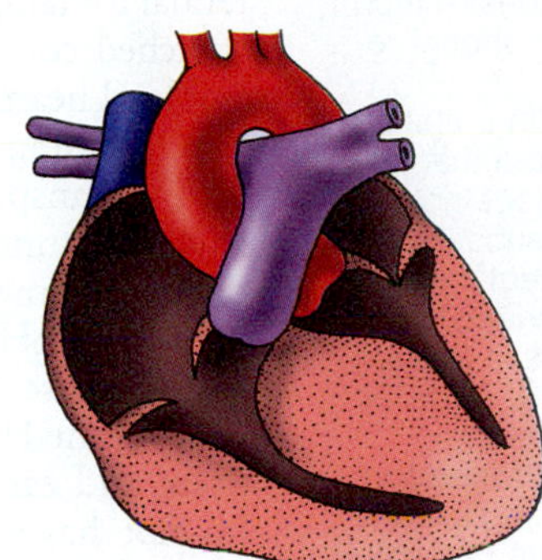	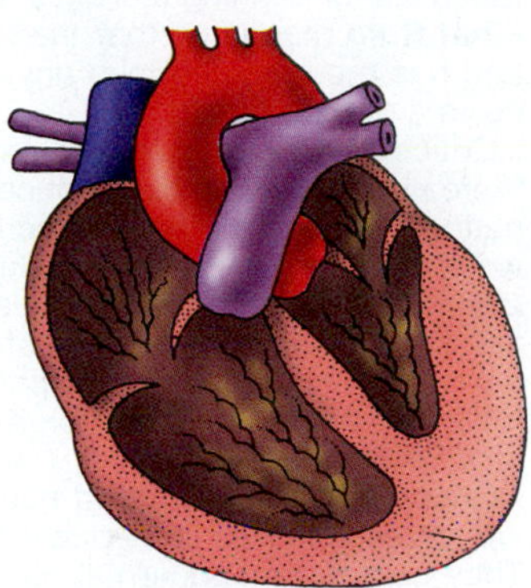
Signs and Symptoms			
Fatigue and weakness Heart failure (left side) Dysrhythmias or heart block Systemic or pulmonary emboli S_3 and S_4 gallops Moderate to severe cardiomegaly	Dyspnea Angina Fatigue, syncope, palpitations Mild cardiomegaly S_4 gallop Ventricular dysrhythmias Sudden death common Heart failure	Same as for nonobstructed except with mitral regurgitation murmur Atrial fibrillation	Dyspnea and fatigue Heart failure (right-sided) Mild to moderate cardiomegaly S_3 and S_4 gallops Heart block Emboli
Treatment			
Symptomatic treatment of heart failure Vasodilators Control of dysrhythmias Surgery: heart transplant	For both: Symptomatic treatment Beta blockers Conversion of atrial fibrillation Surgery: ventriculomyotomy or muscle resection with mitral valve replacement Digitalis, nitrates, and other vasodilators **contraindicated** with the obstructed form		Supportive treatment of symptoms Treatment of hypertension Conversion from dysrhythmias Exercise restrictions Emergency treatment of acute pulmonary edema

Data from Wynne, J., & Braunwald, E. (1992). The cardiomyopathies and myocarditis. In E. Braunwald (Ed.), *Heart disease: A textbook of cardiovascular medicine* (3rd ed.). Philadelphia: W.B. Saunders.

toxin must be avoided. Alcohol ingestion causes cardiac depressant effects and must also be avoided.

Management of obstructive HCM includes administering negative inotropic agents such as beta-adrenergic blocking agents (carvedilol) and calcium antagonists (diltiazem). They decrease the outflow obstruction that accompanies exercise and also decrease HR, resulting in less angina, dyspnea, and syncope. Vasodilators and cardiac glycosides are contraindicated in clients with obstructive HCM because vasodilating and positive inotropic effects may augment the obstruction. Strenuous exercise is also prohibited because it can increase the risk of sudden death.

SURGICAL MANAGEMENT. The type of surgery performed depends on the type of cardiomyopathy.

Excision of Hypertrophied Septum. Surgery may be considered for the small percentage of clients with obstructive HCM who do not respond to medical therapy. The most commonly used surgical treatment **(ventriculomyomectomy)** includes excising a portion of the hypertrophied ventricular septum to create a widened outflow tract. Surgery results in long-term improvement in exercise tolerance in most clients with HCM.

Cardiomyoplasty. Cardiomyoplasty is used when cardiac transplantation is not as option and the client is asymptomatic at rest. The latissimus dorsum muscle is dissected free of its distal insertion and is wrapped around the heart. For the next 2 months, the muscle is stimulated with increasing frequency until it can contract in synchrony with each heartbeat. Six months after surgery, effects of an enhanced cardiac output should be evident. This procedure has produced poor results.

Heart Transplantation. Heart transplantation is the treatment of choice for clients with severe DCM and may be considered for clients with restrictive cardiomyopathy.

LEGAL/ETHICAL ISSUES

TO WHOM SHOULD DONATED HEARTS BE ALLOCATED FOR TRANSPLANTATION?

In 2001, 4096 Americans were waiting for a heart transplant; however, only about 2200 heart transplants are performed each year because of a limited number of donor hearts. In the past, human organ allocation was both by recipient need and by region of the country. The Department of Health and Human Services (DHHS) has created the ***Final Rule,*** which mandates standardized criteria for placing clients on a transplantation list for defining a client's medical status. In addition, the ***Final Rule*** mandates that the person who is the best match and has the greatest need anywhere in the nation should receive a donated heart.

Critics temporarily blocked enactment of the ruling, stating there were serious ethical concerns. First, they noted that donating the heart to the most critically ill person does not always represent good stewardship of resources. In subsequent clarification, DHHS stated, "It is not the Department's intention to require transplantation of clients too ill to benefit; the final rule specifically prohibits policies that might result in such futile transplantations and organ wastage" (*Federal Register,* 42 CFR Part 121).

Critics also argued that a national allocation of transplants would result in less local publicity about transplant recipients. They expressed concern about the already low rate of donations when people are unable to perceive an immediate and local benefit. They feared that only the largest urban transplant centers would survive and that donation rates would drop still further, worsening the scarcity. DHHS responded by recognizing medical factors affecting organ movement, such as the limits of ischemic time. DHHS implemented a monitoring program to ensure that small and medium-sized transplant centers were not adversely affected by the final rule. Closure of such centers can adversely affect client access to transplant services.

The question of how best to allocate donated hearts remains controversial. Should donated hearts be allocated to the sickest person in the nation who is a match? Should the heart be provided to a person who lives in the region, matches the donor, and is most likely to benefit? What are the criteria for benefit? The ethical issue is, How do we decide what is a just or fair way to distribute scarce health care resources? Do we distribute to the person with the greatest need or to the person who is most likely to benefit? Should concerns about how to secure a continuing supply of the scarce resource deserve consideration when deciding how to allocate the resource?

Each year about 2300 clients in the United States receive cardiac transplants, most for DCM (see the Legal/Ethical Issues box above).

Preoperative Care. Criteria for candidate selection include the following:

- Life expectancy less than 1 year
- Age generally less than 65 years
- New York Heart Association (NYHA) class III or IV
- Normal or only slightly increased pulmonary vascular resistance
- Absence of active infection
- Stable psychosocial status
- No evidence of drug or alcohol abuse

Once the candidate is eligible and a heart is available, provide preoperative care as described in Chapter 20.

Operative Procedures. The surgeon transplants a heart from a donor with a comparable body weight and ABO compatibility into a recipient less than 6 hours after procurement. In the most common procedure **(orthotopic transplantation),** the surgeon removes the diseased heart and leaves the posterior walls of the client's atria. The remnant atria serve as the anchor for the donor heart. Anastomoses are made between the recipient and donor atria, aorta, and pulmonary arteries (Figure 38-3). Because the remaining remnant of the recipient's atria contains the sinoatrial node, two unrelated P waves are visible on the ECG.

Postoperative Care. The postoperative care of the heart transplant recipient is similar to that for conventional cardiac surgery; however, the nurse must be especially vigilant to identify occult bleeding into the pericardial sac with the potential for tamponade. The recipient's pericardium has usually stretched considerably to accommodate the diseased, hypertrophied heart, predisposing the client to concealed postoperative bleeding.

The transplanted heart is denervated and is unresponsive to vagal stimulation. The HR is about 100 beats/min and responds slowly to exercise, stress, or position change with increases in HR, contractility, and CO. In the early postoperative phase, the nurse may titrate isoproterenol (Isuprel) to support the HR and maintain cardiac output. Atropine, digitalis, and carotid sinus pressure are not used because they do not have their usual effects on the denervated heart. Denervation of the heart may cause pronounced orthostatic hypotension in the immediate postoperative phase, and the nurse cautions the client to change position slowly. Some clients also require a permanent pacemaker that is rate responsive to the client's activity level. The purpose is to increase CO and improve activity tolerance.

To suppress natural defense mechanisms (especially T- and B-cell function) and prevent transplant rejection, clients require immunosuppressants for the rest of their lives. The foundation of immunosuppressant therapy is large doses of glucocorticoids, such as methylprednisolone (Solu-Medrol) combined with several other drugs. These include monoclonal antibodies (such as OKT 3), tacrolimus (Prograf), and mycophenolate (CellCept). Nurses must be vigilant about handwashing and aseptic technique because clients are immunosuppressed and infection is the major cause of death. Infection usually develops in the immediate post-transplant period or during treatment for acute rejection.

Most clients experience their initial episode of acute rejection in the first 3 months after heart transplantation. Symptoms of rejection are often nonspecific and occur late in the rejection process. They include cardiac dysrhythmias (especially atrial dysrhythmias), hypotension, weakness, fatigue, and dizziness. To detect rejection, the surgeon performs right endomyocardial biopsies at regularly scheduled intervals and whenever symptoms occur.

About 75% of clients survive 3 years after transplantation; most return to NYHA class I or II status (AHA, 1998). Five years after transplantation, many of the surviving clients (20% to 40%) have a form of coronary artery disease (CAD) called **coronary artery vasculopathy (CAV),** which presents as diffuse plaque in the arteries of the donor heart. Because the heart is denervated, clients do not usually experience angina, and regularly scheduled exercise tolerance tests and angiography are required to identify CAV.

To delay the development of CAV, clients are encouraged to follow a prudent lifestyle similar to clients with CAD (see Chapter 41). The physician may prescribe a calcium channel blocker such as diltiazem (Cardizem) to prevent coronary

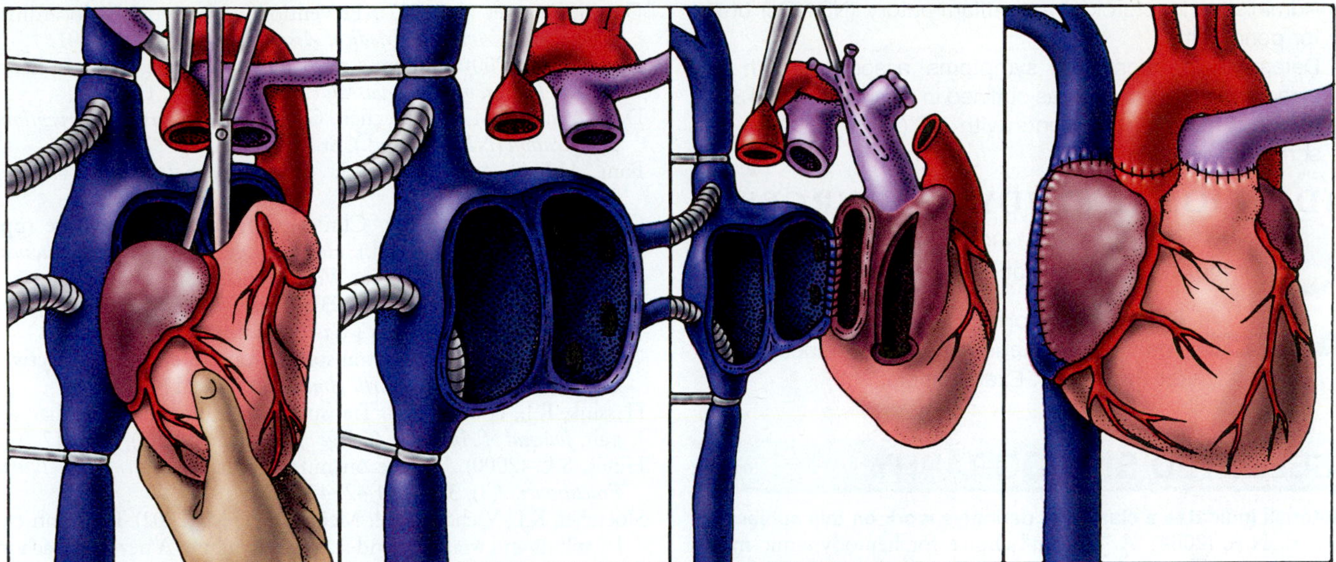

Figure 38-3 ■ Heart transplantation.

spasm and closure. Stress the importance of compliance with dietary modifications and medication regimens. The client is encouraged to participate in a regular exercise program but is cautioned to allow at least 10 minutes of warm up and cool down for the denervated heart to adjust to changes in activity level.

GET READY for the NCLEX Examination!

KEY POINTS

Safe Effective Care Environment

- Monitor the HF client on beta-blockers carefully for hypotension and bradycardia.
- Monitor the pulse of clients taking digitalis preparations before administration, and report a pulse that is not within the desired parameters to the health care provider.
- Monitor for evidence of digitalis toxicity, especially in older clients or in clients with known renal dysfunction (see Chart 38-7).
- Administer long-term antibiotic therapy to clients with valvular disease or cardiac infections.

Health Promotion and Maintenance

- Teach the HF client about a low sodium diet.
- In collaboration with the health care team, teach the HF client to exercise at least 10 minutes 3 to 5 times per week. Have them monitor their pulse and blood pressure. HR should remain within 20 beats/min and BP within 20 mm Hg of baseline.
- Teach clients taking ACE inhibitors to change positions slowly to avoid orthostatic hypotension.
- Teach clients the importance of avoiding respiratory or other infections.
- List foods high in potassium if the client is hypokalemic.
- Teach the client with valvular dysfunction, cardiac infection, or cardiomyopathy the necessity of taking preventive antibiotic therapy before any invasive procedure.

Psychosocial Integrity

- Assess the client for depression resulting from altered self-concept and anxiety.
- Assess the client's coping skills.
- Help the client with strategies for home maintenance to balance rest and activity.
- Help the client develop strategies to manage complex medication regimens.

Physiological Integrity

- Assess the client for symptoms of hypokalemia or hyperkalemia.
- Weigh daily and record.
- Assess for early signs and symptoms of pulmonary edema (e.g., crackles in the lung bases, dyspnea at rest, disorientation, confusion), especially in older adults.
- Assess for symptoms of worsening HF: rapid weight gain (3 pounds in a week), a decrease in exercise tolerance lasting 2 to 3 days, cold symptoms (cough) lasting more than 3 to 5 days, nocturia, development of dyspnea or angina at rest, or unstable angina.
- Monitor the client with valvular dysfunction for atrial fibrillation, which may lead to hemostasis and mural thrombi. Monitor for an irregularly irregular cardiac rhythm and administer warfarin as indicated.
- Assess neurovascular status regularly because emboli may cause strokes.

- Administer nonsteroidal anti-inflammatory (NSAIDs) drugs for pericarditis.
- Determine the signs and symptoms associated with left-sided and right-sided HF as outlined in Charts 38-1 and 38-2.
- Administer drugs for clients with HF (Table 38-2) as prescribed.

ADDITIONAL STUDY RESOURCES

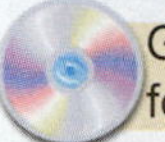

Go to your Student CD-ROM for Review Questions for the NCLEX Examination.

evolve Go to http://evolve.elsevier.com/Iggy/ for Integrated Management of Care Questions for the NCLEX Examination.

SELECTED BIBLIOGRAPHY

Asterisk indicates a classic or definitive work on this subject.

Albert, N.A. (2004). A "current" choice for hemodynamic monitoring. *Nursing 2004, 34*(10), 58-60.

Alderman, L.M. (2000). Congenital heart disease: More than child's play. *Nursing 2000, 30*(5), 41-47.

American Heart Association. (2002). *Heart disease and stroke statistics–2003 update.* Dallas, Texas: American Heart Association.

Ammon, S. (2001). Managing patients with heart failure. *American Journal of Nursing, 101*(12), 34-40.

Artinian, N.T. (2003). The psychosocial aspects of heart failure. *American Journal of Nursing, 103*(12), 32-42.

Augustine, S.M. (2000). Heart transplantation: Long-term management related to immunosuppression, complications, and psychosocial adjustments. *Critical Care Clinics of North America, 12*(1),79-85.

Ayers, D.M.M. (2004). Heart failure. *Nursing 2004, 34*(11), 46-47.

Baker, S., & Graziano, J. (2003). A new device for heart failure. *RN, 66*(3), 32-36.

Bither, C. J., & Apple, S. (2001). Home management of the failing heart. *American Journal of Nursing, 101*(12): 41-47.

Bollinger, K., & Sadar, A.M. (2003). Care and management of the patient with right heart failure secondary to diastolic dysfunction: an advanced practice perspective and case review. *Critical Care Nursing Quarterly, 26*(1), 22-27.

Bond, A.E., et al. (2003). The left ventricular assist device. *American Journal of Nursing, 103*(1), 32-41.

Bosen, D.M. (2003). New strategies for treating patients with heart failure. *Nursing 2003, 33*(12), 44-47.

Buffolo, E., et al. (2003). End-stage cardiomyopathy and secondary mitral insufficiency surgical alternative with prosthesis implant and left-ventricular remodeling. *Journal of Cardiovascular Surgery, 18*(3): 201-205.

Carelock, J., & Clark, A.P. (2003). Heart failure: Pathophysiologic mechanisms. *American Journal of Nursing,* 101(12), 26-35.

Chachques, L.F., et al. (2003). Right ventricular cardiomyopathies: 10 year follow-up. *Annals of Thoracic Surgery, 75*(5), 1464-1468.

Christensen, D.M. (Fall 2004). Managing heart failure: What you need to know. *Med/Surg Insider,* 4-10.

Colbert, K., & Greene, M.H. (2003). Nesiritide (Natrecor): A new treatment for acutely decompensated congestive heart failure. *Critical Care Nursing Quarterly, 26*(1), 40-44.

Coughlin, A.M.C. (2004). Pump away with EECP. *Nursing 2004, 34*(1), 48-49.

Cupples, S.A., & Spruill, L.C. (2000). Evaluation criteria for the pretransplant patient. *Critical Care Clinics of North America, 12*(1), 37-47.

Dahl, J., & Penque, S. (2000). The effects of an advanced practice nurse-directed heart failure program. *Nurse Practitioner, 25*(3), 61-62, 65-66, 68.

*Dajani, A.S., et al. (1997). Prevention of bacterial endocarditis. *Journal of the American Medical Association, 277,* 1794-1801.

Deaton, C. (2000). Outcome measures: self-management in heart failure. *Journal of Cardiovascular Nursing, 14*(4), 116-118.

Dochterman, J.M., & Bulechek, G.M. (2004). *Nursing interventions classification (NIC)* (4th ed.). St. Louis: Mosby.

Fong, H.H.S., & Bauman, J.L. (2002). *Journal of Cardiovascular Nursing,* 16(4), 1-8.

Givertz, M., et al. (2001). Clinical aspects of heart failure (pp. 531-561). In P. Libby (Ed.). *Heart disease: A textbook of cardiovascular medicine.* Philadelphia: W.B. Saunders.

Gorski, L.A., & Johnson, K. (2003). A disease management program for heart failure. *Lippincott's Case Management, 8*(6), 265-273.

Guido, G.W. (2000). Heart transplant from an ethical perspective. *Critical Care Clinics of North America, 12*(1), 111-119.

Hassink, R.J., et al. (2003). Transplantation of cells for cardiac repair. *Journal of American College of Cardiology, 41*(5), 711-717.

Hines, S.E. (2000). Update on mitral prolapse. *Patient Care Nurse Practitioner, 3*(3), 37-37, 41-42, 45-46.

Hoercher, K.J., Vacha, C.J., & McCarthy, P. M. (2002). Left ventricular splints and wraps for end-stage heart failure: A new approach in the new millennium. *Journal of Cardiovascular Nursing, 16*(3), 82-86.

Hussey, C., Hardin, S., & Bla, C. (2002). Outpatient costs of medications for patients with chronic heart failure. *American Journal of Critical Care, 11*(5), 474-478.

Katz, A.M. (2003). Pathophysiology of heart failure: identifying targets for pharmacotherapy. *Medical Clinics of North America, 87*(2), 303-316.

Kearney, K. (2000). Emergency: Digitalis toxicity. *American Journal of Nursing, 100*(6), 51-52.

Khai, P.G., et al. (2000). Infective endocarditis. In T. Nguyen, et al. (Eds.). *Management of complex cardiovascular problems* (pp. 237-250). Armonk, NY: Futura Publishing.

Konick-McMahan, J., Bixby, J., & McKenna, C. (2003). Heart failure in older adults: Providing nursing care to improve outcomes. *Journal of Gerontological Nursing, 29*(12), 35-41.

Krau, S.D. (2000). The evolution of heart transplant. *Critical Care Clinics of North America, 12*(1), 1-9.

Levine, B.S. (2000). Intermittent positive inotrope infusion in the management of end-stage, low-output heart failure. *Journal of Cardiovascular Nursing, 14*(4): 76-93.

Liehr, P., et al. (2003). Addressing current challenges to cardiac rehabilitation care. *AACN Clinical Issues, 14*(1), 13-24.

Lindsey, M. R. (2003). Transmyocardial laser revascularization revisited. *Critical Care Nursing Quarterly, 26*(1), 69-75.

Martin, T. (2003). How heart failure complicates care. *Nursing Management, 34*(5), 27-32.

McCance, K.L., & Huether, S.E. (2002). *Pathophysiology: The biologic basis for disease in adults and children.* (4th ed.). St. Louis: Mosby.

Metra, M., et al. (2003). Marked improvement in left ventricular ejection fraction during long-term beta-blockade in patients with chronic heart failure: clinical correlates and prognostic significance. *American Heart Journal, 145*(2), 292-299.

Milfred-LaForest, S.K. (2000). Pharmacotherapy of systolic heart failure: A review of recent literature and practical applications, *Journal of Cardiovascular Nursing, 14*(4), 57-75.

Morbidity and mortality: 2002 chart book on cardiovascular, lung, and blood diseases. National Institutes of Health, National Heart, Lung, and Blood Institute.

Paul, S. (2000). Impact of a nurse-managed heart failure clinic: A pilot study. *American Journal of Critical Care, 9*(2), 140-146.

Popjes, E.D., & St. John Sutton, M. (2003). Hypertrophic cardiomyopathy. Pathophysiology, diagnosis, and treatment, *Geriatrics, 58*(3), 41-46.

Reeder, D.E., et al. (2000). The impact of angiotensin-converting enzyme inhibitors on managed care: Economic, clinical, and humanistic outcomes. *American Journal of Managed Care, 6*(3 Suppl), S112-131.

*Ritchie, J.L., et al. (1998). *ACC/AHA Guidelines for the management of patients with valvular heart disease–II. General principles: A report of the American College of Cardiology/American Heart Association Task Force on Practice Guidelines (Committee on Management of Patients with Valvular Heart Disease).* American Heart Association. Available at http://www.americanheart.org/reports.

Sanderson, J.E. (2000). Heart failure. In T. Nguyen, et al. (Eds.). *Management of complex cardiovascular problems* (pp. 237-250). Armonk, NY: Futura Publishing.

Saul, L., & Shatzer, M. (2003). B-type natriuretic peptide testing for detection of heart failure. *Critical Care Nursing Quarterly*, *26*(1), 37-39.

Schall, M.B., & Flannery, J. (2004). Undertreatment of women with heart failure: A reversible outcome on hospital readmission. *Lippincott's Case Management: The Journal for Professional Practice, 9*(6), 250-253.

Sherrid M.V., Chaudhry, F.A., & Swistel, D.G. (2003). Obstructive hypertrophic cardiomyopathy: echocardiography, pathophysiology, and the continuing evolution of surgery for obstruction. *Annals of Thoracic Surgery, 75*(2), 620-632.

Smith, A.L., & Brown, C.S. (2003). New advances and novel treatments in heart failure. *Critical Care Nursing Quarterly, 26*(2), 3-15.

Strimike, C.L., & Wojcik, J. (2000). Getting the facts on heart failure treatment. *Nursing 2000, 30*(5), 32hn18-32hn20.

Tarolli, K.A. (2003). Left ventricular systolic dysfunction and nonischemic cardiomyopathy. *Critical Care Nursing Quarterly, 26*(1), 3-15.

Tasota, F.J., & Tate, J. (2000). Assessing digoxin levels. *Nursing 2000, 30*(3), 24.

Tedesco, C., Reigle, J., & Bergin, J. (2000). Sudden cardiac death in heart failure. *Journal of Cardiovascular Nursing, 14*(4), 40-56.

Tokarczyk, T.R. (2003). Cardiac transplantation as a treatment option for the heart failure patient. *Critical Care Nursing Quarterly,* 26(1), 61-68.

Wisniewski, A. (2004). Muscle up your knowledge of myocarditis. *Nursing 2004, 34*(10), 17.

Young, J.B. (2003). Combined cardiac resynchronization and implantable cardioversion defibrillation in advanced chronic heart failure: The MIRACLE ICD trial. *The Journal of the American Medical Association,* 189(20), 1003.

CHAPTER 39

Interventions for Clients with Vascular Problems

DEANNE A. BLACH • DONNA D. IGNATAVICIUS

LEARNING OUTCOMES

After studying this chapter, you should be able to:

1. Explain the pathophysiology of arteriosclerosis and atherosclerosis, including the factors that cause arterial injury.
2. Interpret essential laboratory data related to risk for atherosclerosis.
3. Discuss the role of diet therapy in the management of clients with arteriosclerosis.
4. Describe the differences between essential and secondary hypertension.
5. Develop a collaborative plan of care for a client with essential hypertension.
6. Explain the purpose, action, and nursing implications of drugs used to manage hypertension.
7. Identify cultural considerations that impact care for clients with hypertension.
8. Evaluate the effectiveness of interdisciplinary interventions to improve hypertension.
9. Compare and contrast assessment findings typically present in clients with peripheral arterial and peripheral venous disease.
10. Prioritize postoperative care for clients who have undergone peripheral bypass surgery.
11. Assess clients at risk for venous thromboembolism (VTE) and identify when VTE occurs.
12. Describe nursing interventions used to help prevent venous thromboembolism (VTE).
13. Describe the nurse's role in monitoring clients who are receiving anticoagulants.
14. Develop a continuing care plan for a client who has undergone an abdominal aortic aneurysm repair.
15. Compare and contrast Raynaud's and Buerger's disease.
16. Identify evidence-based practice for care of clients with venous leg ulcers.

Go to your Student CD-ROM for Review Questions for the NCLEX Examination keyed to these Learning Outcomes.

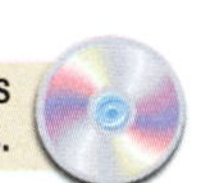

Disease associated with atherosclerosis is the leading cause of death in the United States. More than 1 million people die of heart and blood vessel diseases each year in the United States (American Heart Association, 2003). Atherosclerosis is often a major risk factor for cardiovascular disease, cerebrovascular disease, and peripheral vascular disease (PVD). People with atherosclerosis have an increased risk of developing one or more of these diseases.

Disorders of the vascular system cause many problems and may lead to complete shutdown of all body organs and eventually death. Although vascular disease can affect any portion of the human body, such as the heart, brain, and kidneys, the peripheral vascular system and its associated diseases are described here.

ARTERIOSCLEROSIS AND ATHEROSCLEROSIS

PATHOPHYSIOLOGY

Arteriosclerosis is a thickening, or hardening, of the arterial wall. **Atherosclerosis,** a type of arteriosclerosis, involves the formation of plaque within the arterial wall and is the leading contributor to coronary artery and cerebrovascular disease. The exact pathophysiology of atherosclerosis is not known, but the condition is thought to occur from vascular damage (Figure 39-1). After the vessel becomes inflamed, a fatty streak appears on the intimal surface (inner lining) of the artery. At this stage, the fatty streak may appear flattened

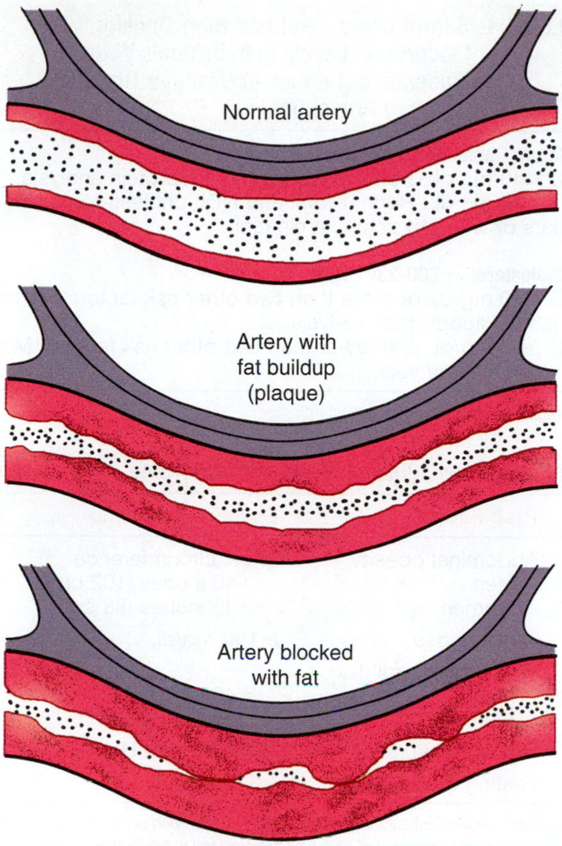

Normal artery

Artery with fat buildup (plaque)

Artery blocked with fat

Figure 39-1 ■ Pathophysiology of atherosclerosis.

or elevated, but it generally does not affect the integrity of the arterial wall.

Next, a stable or unstable plaque develops. *Stable* plaque is a white, glistening, fibrous elevation that covers a lipid (primarily cholesterol) core. By contrast, *unstable* plaque has a liquid lipid core. At this stage, it is elevated enough to partially or completely occlude the blood flow of an artery.

In the final stage, the fibrous lesions become calcified, hemorrhagic, ulcerated, or thrombosed and affect all layers of the vessel. The rate of progression of the process may be influenced by genetic factors, certain chronic diseases (e.g., diabetes mellitus), and lifestyle habits, including smoking, eating habits, and level of exercise. When *stable* plaque ruptures, thrombosis and vasoconstriction obstruct the lumen causing inadequate perfusion to distal tissues. *Unstable* plaque rupture causes more severe damage, such as that seen in acute coronary syndrome (see Chapter 41).

Etiology and Genetic Risk

The exact etiology of atherosclerosis is unknown, but several theories attempt to explain its cause. One theory proposes that an injury to the **intimal** (innermost) **layer** of the artery may initiate the development of atherosclerosis. Another popular theory, known as platelet aggregation, proposes that after the intimal injury has occurred, platelets form a cluster at the arterial wall and produce a peptide that stimulates the proliferation of the smooth muscle cells of the intima. Eventually, this proliferation can narrow the artery enough to compromise the flow of blood or completely occlude arterial blood flow.

Another theory, the *lipid hypothesis,* assumes that after an intimal injury, a group of blood lipids (fats) accumulate. Again, fat accumulation can partially or completely occlude arterial blood flow. The principal lipids involved are cholesterol and triglyceride.

Many theorists believe that a combination of these two events provides the most appropriate explanation of the atherosclerotic process and that the process can occur in any arterial wall of the body. Usually the disease affects the larger arteries, such as the coronary artery beds, the aorta, carotid and vertebral arteries, renal, iliac, and femoral arteries, or any combination of these.

Intimal injury of the major arteries of the body can be attributed to many factors. Hypertension can cause a mechanical injury, whereas elevated levels of low-density lipoprotein cholesterol (LDL-C) and decreased levels of high-density lipoprotein cholesterol (HDL-C) can cause chemical injuries to the intimal wall. (See Chapter 36, which describes cholesterol in more detail.) Chemical injury can also be caused by elevated levels of toxins in the bloodstream, which may occur with renal failure or by carbon monoxide circulating in the bloodstream from cigarette smoking. The intimal wall can be weakened by the natural process of aging or by physiologic disorders, such as diabetes.

Genetic predisposition and diabetes have a fairly direct effect on the development of atherosclerosis. In general, studies have focused on the role of lipoproteins because of their role in the development of atherosclerosis. Some individuals have familial **hyperlipidemia,** an elevation of serum **lipid** (fat) levels. In these people, the liver makes excessive cholesterol and other fats, which accounts for the development of atherosclerosis. In some people with hereditary atherosclerosis, however, the blood cholesterol level is normal. The reason for the development and progression of plaque in these people is not understood.

Clients with severe diabetes mellitus frequently have premature and severe atherosclerosis from microvascular damage. The premature atherosclerosis occurs because diabetes promotes an increase in LDL-C and triglycerides in plasma. In addition, intimal arterial damage may result from the effect of hyperglycemia.

Factors indirectly related to atherosclerosis include obesity, a sedentary lifestyle, smoking, and stress. Clients who are obese or overweight are at greater risk, most often because of associated elevations in cholesterol levels. In general, obesity is defined as a body mass index (BMI) of greater than 30 kg/m^2, and overweight is defined as a BMI of greater than 25 kg/m^2.

CULTURAL CONSIDERATIONS

According to the American Heart Association (2003), African Americans and Hispanics have the highest percentage of people who are overweight and obese. Asian/Pacific Islanders have the smallest percentage. About two thirds of all Americans are overweight or obese.

Smoking causes vessel constriction, which decreases blood flow and tissue perfusion. African American and Native American/American Indian men smoke the most of all ethnic groups. Hispanics and Asian/Pacific Islanders smoke the least.

The causes for differences among groups are unknown. Environmental factors and genetic predisposition may help explain them.

Incidence/Prevalence

It is not known exactly how many people have atherosclerosis, but small plaques are almost always present in the arteries of young adults. The incidence can be better quantified by assessing diseases that result from atherosclerosis. Peripheral vascular disease (PVD) impacts 7 to 12 million people in the United States including many of the over-50 population (Ebersole, Hess, & Luggen, 2004). However, only 50% (5 million) have actual symptoms of the disease. Of the 2.5 million individuals diagnosed with PVD, 2.1 million are medically managed (Society of Interventional Radiology, 2003). Analysis of trends predicts that the number of people affected by atherosclerosis will increase as the population ages.

COLLABORATIVE MANAGEMENT

Assessment

PHYSICAL ASSESSMENT

Because of the high incidence of hypertension in clients with atherosclerosis, assess the blood pressure in both arms. The heart is also thoroughly assessed because associated cardiac disease is often present.

Palpate pulses at all of the major sites on the body and note any differences. Carotid arteries are palpated separately because of the risk of inadequate cerebral perfusion. Also palpate for temperature differences in the lower extremities and check capillary filling. Prolonged capillary filling (greater than 3 seconds in young to middle-aged adults; greater than 5 seconds in older adults) generally indicates poor circulation, although this indicator is not the most reliable. An extremity in a person with significant atherosclerotic disease may be cool or cold, with a diminished or absent pulse.

Many clients with vascular disease have a **bruit** in the larger arteries, which can be heard with a stethoscope or Doppler probe. A bruit is described as a turbulent, swishing sound, which can be soft or loud in pitch. The mere existence of a bruit is considered abnormal, but the role it plays in indicating the severity of vascular disease is not understood. Bruits often occur in the carotid, aortic, femoral, and popliteal arteries and usually indicate some degree of narrowing of the arterial wall. A decrease in intensity and audibility or a complete loss of a pulse may indicate an arterial occlusion.

LABORATORY ASSESSMENT

LIPID PROFILE. Clients with atherosclerosis often have elevated lipids, including cholesterol and triglycerides. Total serum cholesterol levels should be below 200 mg/dL. Elevated cholesterol levels must be validated by HDL and LDL determinations. Elevated low-density lipoprotein cholesterol (LDL-C) ("bad" cholesterol) levels indicate that a person is at an increased risk for atherosclerosis. Low high-density lipoprotein cholesterol ("good" cholesterol) (HDL-C) levels also indicate an increased risk. A desirable LDL-C level is one below 100 mg/dL for all individuals. A desirable HDL-C level is 40 mg/dL or above (Table 39-1).

WOMEN'S HEALTH CONSIDERATIONS

In some people, particularly women, an elevated cholesterol level may be due to an elevated HDL-C level, which is not considered a risk. However, the LDL-C level should also be below 100 to keep the risk of cardiovascular disease low.

TABLE 39-1 Serum Cholesterol and High-Density Lipoprotein Levels in Individuals Without Evidence of Cardiac or Vascular Disease (Primary Prevention)

Total Serum Cholesterol <200 mg/dL
HDL-C <40 mg/dL: Perform full fasting lipoprotein analysis.
HDL-C >40 mg/dL: Repeat total and HDL cholesterol testing in 5 years or with physical examination.

Total Cholesterol = 200-239 mg/dL
HDL-C <40 mg/dL or more than two other risk factors: Perform full fasting lipoprotein analysis.
HDL-C >40 mg/dL and fewer than two other risk factors: Monitor at least every year.

HDL-C, High-density lipoprotein cholesterol.

TABLE 39-2 Recognizing Metabolic Syndrome

Risk Factor	Defining Level
Abdominal obesity	Waist circumference
Men	>40 inches (102 cm)
Women	>35 inches (88 cm)
Triglycerides	≥150 mg/dL
HDL cholesterol	
Men	<40 mg/dL
Women	<50 mg/dL
Blood pressure	≥130/85 mm Hg
Fasting blood sugar	≥110 mg/dL

From National Cholesterol Education Program. (2002). *Third report of the Expert Panel on Detection, Evaluation, and Treatment of High Blood Cholesterol in Adults (Adult Treatment Panel III).* NIH Publication No. 02-5215. Bethesda, MD: National Heart, Lung, and Blood Institute.

Triglyceride levels may also be elevated with atherosclerosis and considered an emerging lipid risk factor by the Adult Treatment Panel (ATP III) Report No. 3 released by the National Heart, Lung, and Blood Institute (2002). A level of 150 mg/dL or above indicates **hypertriglyceridemia.** Elevated triglycerides are considered a marker for other atherogenic lipoproteins and an indicator for the **metabolic syndrome,** which increases the risk for coronary heart disease (Table 39-2).

HOMOCYSTEINE. Homocysteine is an essential sulfur-containing amino acid derived from dietary protein. Studies have shown a positive correlation between increased homocysteine levels and the development of peripheral vascular disease (PVD), coronary artery disease (CAD), stroke, and venous thrombosis. High serum levels of homocysteine can block production of nitric oxide on the vascular endothelium, making the cell walls less elastic and permitting plaque to build up. A serum homocysteine level greater than 15 mmol/L is considered a risk factor. Elevated homocysteine levels may be lowered by a diet enriched with B-complex vitamins, particularly folic acid. Usually, 1 mg or more of supplemental folic acid daily can improve endothelial function and lower homocysteine levels. The American Heart Association (2003) recommends homocysteine screening for high-risk clients who have a family history of premature cardiovascular disease, angina, CAD, or elevated cholesterol.

Interventions

Atherosclerosis progresses for years before clinical manifestations are evident. Adults with or at risk for atherosclerosis can often be identified through cholesterol screening and history.

Because of the high incidence of atherosclerosis in the United States, low-risk individuals 20 years of age and older are advised to have their total serum cholesterol level evaluated at least once every 5 years. More frequent measurements are suggested for individuals with multiple risk factors.

Interventions for individuals with atherosclerosis or who are at high risk for the disease focus on lifestyle changes. Teaching clients about the need for changes and how to make them is crucial. If lipoprotein levels do not improve, the health care provider prescribes medication to lower cholesterol and/or triglycerides.

Diet Therapy. The importance of nutrition should be emphasized for individuals with elevated homocysteine levels. Encourage a diet including enriched or fortified cereals that contain 100% of the daily requirement of folic acid, pyridoxine (vitamin B_6), and cyanocobalamin (vitamin B_{12}). If consumption of vegetables such as fruits, legumes, meats, fish, and fortified cereals and grains do not decrease homocysteine levels, multivitamins containing 0.4 mg of folic acid, 2 mg of pyridoxine, and 6 mcg of cyanocobalamin can be added.

Recent testing and management guidelines from the National Cholesterol Education Program (NCEP) have a major preventive focus for individuals with multiple risk factors (2002). In need of intensified lifestyle changes, these groups of high-risk clients, termed "coronary heart disease equivalents" include the following:

- Those with diabetes but without signs of vascular disease
- Individuals with a Framingham Heart Study 10-year absolute risk score of over 20% for CHD events
- Those identified with multiple metabolic risk factors

The new category groups these people at the same risk level as those who already have vascular disease. Therapeutic lifestyle change recommendations have also been broadened.

The focus of treatment remains on an aggressive approach to lowering LDL-C values and raising HDL-C levels. Having an LDL-C value of less than 100 mg/dL is optimal; values of 100 to 129 mg/dL are near or above optimal. Clients with LDL-C values of 130 to 159 mg/dL (borderline high) are advised to follow a fat-modified diet. In collaboration with the dietitian, instruct your clients with LDL-C values of 160 mg/dL or greater (high or very high) to follow a more structured diet aimed at decreasing saturated fat and cholesterol and, if appropriate, promoting weight loss. The HDL-C level should be greater than 40 mg/dL.

In the United States, 37% of the total caloric intake in the diets of many people is made up of fat. Overconsumption of fat and cholesterol leads to **hypercholesterolemia,** an elevated total blood cholesterol level. Elevated cholesterol levels can often be decreased if fat in the diet is limited to no more than 30% of the caloric intake.

To determine 30% of their caloric intake, clients first need to determine their ideal daily caloric intake. A dietitian can then calculate their fat limit in grams. In addition to tracking fat in grams, people need to assess the fatty acid content of foods.

Step One Diet. The Step One diet of the American Heart Association, often recommended to decrease the serum cholesterol level, calls for a total fat intake of less than 30% of total calories, with less than 10% of total caloric intake coming from saturated fat, up to 10% of total calories coming from polyunsaturated fat, and 10% to 15% coming from monounsaturated fat. The Step One diet limits cholesterol intake to less than 300 mg daily.

In collaboration with the dietitian, educate the client about the fat content of foods in terms of the total amount of fat and saturation. Meats and eggs contain mostly saturated fats. Because canola (grapeseed) oil is rich in monounsaturated fat and safflower and sunflower oil are rich in polyunsaturated oils, they are recommended over highly saturated oils, such as palm or coconut oil. Cholesterol is found only in animal sources, such as meat and eggs, which are also high in saturated fats.

Step Two Diet. The client's serum cholesterol levels are retested 6 and 12 weeks after the initial dietary intervention. If the cholesterol level has not significantly decreased, the client may be referred to a registered dietitian for instruction on a more restricted diet, such as the Step Two diet. The Step Two diet limits saturated fat to less than 7% of total calories and cholesterol to less than 200 mg/day.

In addition to elevated LDL-C values, other variations of hyperlipidemias put clients at risk for atherosclerosis. A low-fat, low-cholesterol, high-fiber diet, however, can play a significant role in improving a lipid profile, regardless of the lipid alteration.

Smoking Cessation. Cigarette smoking lowers levels of high-density lipoprotein (HDL) cholesterol and dramatically increases the rate of progression of atherosclerosis.

Advise all clients who smoke to stop smoking and to avoid secondhand smoke. Describe the relationship of smoking to atherosclerosis, and assess his or her willingness to change the behavior. Health care providers can refer to the Agency for Healthcare Research and Quality's Practice Guidelines on Smoking Cessation (formerly the Agency for Health Care Policy and Research). This reference provides strategies to assist individuals in quitting smoking. A smoking cessation group, such as the American Cancer Society's Fresh Start, may help with this difficult process. Most formal programs encourage people to stop smoking "cold turkey."

Clients may consider using a nicotine patch (Nicoderm, Habitrol, ProStep), which helps relieve nicotine withdrawal symptoms. The patch is about 50% effective in helping clients to stop smoking and is available over the counter. The dose is determined by the client's weight and the extent to which he or she smokes. Clients are urged to stop smoking completely when the nicotine patch is initiated. Inform them that if they continue to smoke while using the patch, their risks for serious adverse effects are increased because the peak levels of nicotine are higher than those experienced from smoking alone. Serious cardiovascular effects, such as angina and dysrhythmias, may result from using the patch while still smoking, although the most common side effect is skin irritation. Many health insurance programs will not cover the costs associated with nicotine patches unless the client is enrolled in a smoking cessation program. In some areas of the country, tobacco settlement money is being used by states to fund cessation programs, provide counseling, patches, and oral medication at no charge to the smoker.

Nicotine gum (Nicorette) also may be used if a client feels the need to smoke. Clients should not chew more than 30 pieces of gum per day. Nicotine lozenges are also available as over-the-counter (OTC) aids. The nasal spray (e.g., Nicotrol) and inhaler forms of nicotine must be prescribed by a health care provider (Bialous & Sarna, 2004).

Some clients need an oral medication, such as bupropion (Wellbutrin, Zyban), to help decrease the urge to smoke. Because these drugs depress the central nervous system, clients taking them are carefully monitored by a health care provider.

Complementary and Alternative Therapies. Some individuals try other methods to help them stop smoking, including acupuncture, acupressure, hypnosis, and biofeedback. Many people have been successful using these methods, as discussed in Chapter 4.

Exercise. Regular exercise is recommended to promote optimal lipid levels and can actually prevent atherosclerosis. Exercise can also lead to regression of atherosclerotic plaque and the building of collateral circulation in people with atherosclerosis. The level of exercise required to provide protection from atherosclerotic disease has not been well established, but it is recommended that individuals get 30 minutes of moderate to vigorous exercise at least three to four times a week. Instruct clients with heart disease and other comorbid conditions, such as hypertension, vascular disease, or diabetes, to undergo an exercise tolerance (treadmill or stress) test before undertaking an exercise program (e.g., aerobics, walking, or running).

Drug Therapy. For clients with elevated total and LDL-C levels that do not respond adequately to dietary intervention, the health care provider prescribes one or more lipid-lowering agents (Chart 39-1). Drug choice is dependent on the lipid levels. Because most of these drugs can produce major side effects, they are generally given only when nonpharmacologic management has been unsuccessful. Bile acid–binding resins, such as cholestyramine (Questran) or colestipol (Colestid), were once given because of their low toxicity, but they are seldom used today.

In the 1980s, many studies reported that a potent and well-tolerated class of drugs called 3-hydroxy-3-methylglutaryl coenzyme A (HMG-CoA) reductase inhibitors (statins) successfully reduced total cholesterol by 20% when used for an extended time period. Medications such as pravastatin (Pravachol), lovastatin (Mevacor), simvastatin (Zocor), rosuvastatin (Crestor), and atorvastatin (Lipitor) lower both LDL-C and triglyceride levels. Statins reduce cholesterol synthesis in the liver and increase clearance of LDL-C from the blood. Therefore they are contraindicated in clients with active liver disease or during pregnancy, because they can cause muscle myopathies and marked decreases in liver function. Statin drugs are discontinued if the client has muscle cramping or elevated liver enzyme levels.

A different type of lipid-lowering agent, ezetimibe (Zetia), has been approved to be used in the place of or in combination with statin-type drugs. This medication inhibits the absorption of cholesterol through the small intestine. Vytorin has recently been approved as a combination drug containing ezetimibe and simvastatin. This medication reduces the absorption of cholesterol while reducing the amount of cholesterol synthesis in the liver.

Nicotinic acid or niacin (Niaspan), a B vitamin, lowers LDL-C and very-low-density lipoprotein (VLDL) cholesterol levels, and increases HDL-C levels. It is used as a single agent or in combination with an acid-binding resin drug or a statin.

CHART 39-1

DRUG THERAPY for Hyperlipidemia/Hypercholesterolemia

Drug	Usual Dosage	Nursing Interventions	Rationales
HMG-CoA reductase inhibitors (statins)			
Lovastatin (Mevacor)	20 mg daily; may increase to 40-80 mg daily	Instruct clients to report muscle tenderness.	Although rare, myopathy has occurred as a side effect, especially when taken with fibric acid.
Simvastatin (Zocor)	5-10 mg daily; may increase to 40 mg daily		
Fluvastatin (Lescol)	20-40 mg daily; not to exceed 80 mg daily	Tell clients to take with evening meal.	Gastrointestinal (GI) disturbances, such as diarrhea, nausea, and vomiting, are common.
Atorvastatin (Lipitor)	10 mg daily; increased to 80 mg daily		
Pravastatin (Pravachol)	10-40 mg daily at bedtime	Monitor liver enzymes.	Minor liver enzyme elevations can occur but are rare.
Rosuvastatin (Crestor)	5-10 mg daily to start; increase to 20 mg daily for very high cholesterol levels; may increase to 40 mg daily	Teach clients to avoid grapefruit juice	Grapefruit juice alters drug metabolism and the drug's effects.
Nicotinic acid (Nicobid, Niaspan, Nia-Bid [niacin])	1.5-3 g daily, with maximum dose of 6 g daily	Encourage clients to take with meals.	Flushing of skin and pruritus are common side effects, which can be minimized when drug is taken with meals.
Fibric acid derivatives (fibrates)			
Gemfibrozil (Lopid)	600 mg twice daily	Instruct clients to take 30 minutes before meals or with meals if nausea or GI discomfort occurs.	Although drug is well tolerated, nausea and GI discomfort may occur and can be prevented if drug is taken with meals.
Fenofibrate (Tricor)	67 mg daily		
Ezetimibe (Zetia)	10 mg daily	Tell clients that they may take drug with or without food. Instruct clients that it is safe to take with HMG-CoA reductase inhibitors, but not with fibric acid derivatives.	GI disturbances are rare and do not depend on food intake.

Med Error Alert! *Write "daily" rather than QD to prevent mistakes.*

Low doses are generally well tolerated, but higher doses can result in an elevation of hepatic enzymes and various other side effects. Gemfibrozil (Lopid) raises HDL-C and lowers triglyceride and VLDL levels, but it is not as effective in lowering LDL-C levels. Fenofibrate (Tricor) inhibits production of LDL-C, which is responsible for triglyceride development.

HYPERTENSION

PATHOPHYSIOLOGY

Hypertension is generally defined as a systolic blood pressure greater than or equal to 135 mm Hg and/or a diastolic blood pressure greater than or equal to 85 mm Hg in individuals who do not have diabetes.

In 2003, the Seventh Report of the Joint National Committee on Prevention, Detection, Evaluation, and Treatment of High Blood Pressure made significant changes in classifying blood pressure in adults. The new classification for **"normal" adult blood pressure** is less than 120 mm Hg systolic *and* less than 80 mm Hg diastolic. Adults with a blood pressure of 120 to 139 mm Hg systolic *or* 80 to 89 mm Hg diastolic, considered "normal" under previous guidelines, are now classified as prehypertensive and are in need of lifestyle changes to prevent cardiovascular complications (Table 39-3). The relationship between hypertension and cardiovascular events is direct and independent of other risk factors. The higher the blood pressure, the greater the chance for coronary, cerebral, renal, and peripheral vascular disease. Control of hypertension, however, has resulted in significant decreases in cardiovascular morbidity and mortality. (See the Meeting Healthy People 2010 Objectives box below.)

TABLE 39-3 Blood Pressure Classification

Classification	Blood Pressure Measurement	Blood Pressure Readings
Normal	Systolic *and* diastolic	<120 mm Hg <80 mm Hg
Prehypertension	Systolic *or* diastolic	120-139 mm Hg 80-89 mm Hg
Stage 1: Hypertension	Systolic *or* diastolic	140-159 mm Hg 90-99 mm Hg
Stage 2: Hypertension	Systolic *or* diastolic	≥160 mm Hg ≥100 mm Hg

From Joint National Committee. (2003). The seventh report of the Joint National Committee on Prevention, Detection, Evaluation, and Treatment of High Blood Pressure. NIH Publication No. 03-5233. Bethesda, MD: National Heart, Lung, and Blood Institute.

Meeting HEALTHY PEOPLE 2010 Objectives

BLOOD PRESSURE

Objective 12.11: Increase the proportion of adults with high blood pressure who are taking action to help control their blood pressure.

- Teach adults with high blood pressure the importance of controlling sodium intake, including reading food labels for sodium content and avoiding high-sodium foods, such as bacon, ham, and processed snacks.
- Refer overweight adults to a support group or weight reduction program.
- Teach about the importance of exercise and increased physical activity to reduce blood pressure.
- For the adult who smokes, teach about the relationship between cardiovascular disease and smoking; refer the individual to a smoking cessation program.
- Participate in community or health care agency health fairs to screen for hypertension and provide community education.
- Teach all adults to have their blood pressure taken at least once every 2 years; for those with hypertension, monitor blood pressure as recommended by the health care provider.

Several other changes were made in the national guidelines for blood pressure management. Thiazide-type diuretics are recommended for initial therapy in most clients with uncomplicated stage 1 hypertension. Stages 2 and 3 hypertension were combined into a single stage 2 category because most hypertensive clients need a combination of two or more drugs for optimal treatment.

The systemic arterial pressure is a product of cardiac output (CO) and total peripheral vascular resistance (PVR) (Figure 39-2). Cardiac output is determined by the stroke volume and heart rate ($CO = SV \times HR$). Control of peripheral vascular resistance, vessel constriction or dilation, is maintained by the autonomic nervous system and circulating hormones, such as norepinephrine and epinephrine. Consequently, any factor producing an increase in peripheral vascular resistance, heart rate, or stroke volume increases the systemic arterial pressure. Conversely, any factor that causes a decrease in peripheral vascular resistance, heart rate, or stroke volume decreases the systemic arterial pressure.

Stabilizing mechanisms exist in the body to exert an overall regulation of systemic arterial pressure and to prevent circulatory collapse. Four control systems play a major role in maintaining blood pressure: the arterial baroreceptor system, regulation of body fluid volume, the renin-angiotensin system, and vascular autoregulation.

Arterial Baroreceptors

The arterial baroreceptors are found primarily in the carotid sinus but also in the aorta and the wall of the left ventricle. The baroreceptors monitor the level of arterial pressure and counteract a rise in arterial pressure through vagally mediated cardiac slowing and vasodilation with decreased sympathetic tone. Therefore reflex control of circulation elevates the systemic arterial pressure when it falls and lowers it when it rises. Why baroceptor control fails in hypertension is unknown. There is evidence for upward resetting of baroreceptor sensitivity so that pressure measures are inadequately sensed even though pressure decreases are not.

Regulation of Body Fluid Volume

Changes in fluid volume also affect the systemic arterial pressure. If there is an excess of sodium and/or water in a person's body, the blood pressure rises through complex physiologic

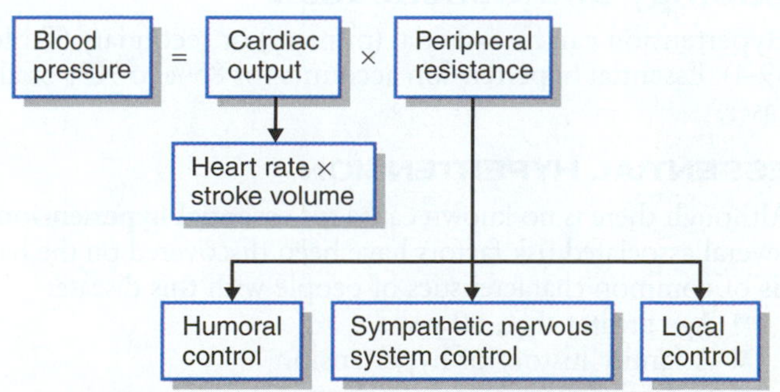

Figure 39-2 ■ The components of blood pressure.

mechanisms that change the venous return to the heart, producing a rise in cardiac output. If the kidneys are functioning adequately, a rise in systemic arterial pressure produces diuresis and a fall in pressure. Pathologic conditions change the pressure threshold at which the kidneys excrete sodium and water, thereby altering the systemic arterial pressure.

Renin-Angiotensin System

Renin, angiotensin, and aldosterone also regulate blood pressure (see discussion in Chapter 14). The kidney produces renin, an enzyme that acts on angiotensinogen (a plasma protein substrate) to split off angiotensin I, which is converted by an enzyme in the lung to form angiotensin II. Angiotensin II has strong vasoconstrictor action on blood vessels and is the controlling mechanism for aldosterone release. Aldosterone then works on the collecting tubules in the kidneys to reabsorb sodium. Sodium retention inhibits fluid loss, thus increasing blood volume and subsequent blood pressure.

Inappropriate secretion of renin may cause increased peripheral vascular resistance in essential (primary) hypertension. In high blood pressure, renin levels should fall because the increased renal arteriolar pressure should inhibit renin secretion. For most people with essential hypertension, however, renin levels are normal.

Vascular Autoregulation

The process of vascular autoregulation, which keeps perfusion of tissues in the body relatively constant, appears to be important in causing hypertension. This mechanism is poorly understood.

Sustained blood pressure elevation in clients with essential (primary) hypertension results in damage to blood vessels in vital organs. Essential hypertension produces medial hyperplasia (thickening) of the arterioles. As the blood vessels thicken and perfusion decreases, body organs are damaged; these changes can result in myocardial infarctions, strokes, peripheral vascular disease (PVD), or renal failure.

Malignant hypertension is a severe type of elevated blood pressure that rapidly progresses. A person with malignant hypertension usually has symptoms such as morning headaches, blurred vision, and dyspnea and/or symptoms of uremia (accumulation in the blood of substances ordinarily eliminated in the urine). Clients are often in their 30s, 40s, or 50s with their systolic blood pressure greater than 200 mm Hg. The diastolic blood pressure is greater than 150 mm Hg or greater than 130 mm Hg when there are pre-existing complications. Unless intervention occurs promptly, a client with malignant hypertension may experience renal failure, left ventricular failure, or stroke.

Etiology and Genetic Risk

Hypertension can be essential (primary) or secondary (Table 39-4). Essential hypertension accounts for 85% to 90% of all cases.

ESSENTIAL HYPERTENSION

Although there is no known cause for **essential hypertension,** several associated risk factors have been discovered on the basis of common characteristics of people with this disease:

- Age greater than 60 years
- A family history of hypertension
- Excessive calorie consumption
- Physical inactivity
- Excessive alcohol intake
- Hyperlipidemia
- African-American ethnicity
- High intake of salt or caffeine; reduced intake of potassium, calcium, or magnesium
- Obesity
- Smoking
- Stress

A family history of hypertension is a major risk factor. In families with hypertension, there may be a defect in renal secretion of sodium or a heightened sympathetic nervous system response to stress.

SECONDARY HYPERTENSION

Specific disease states and medications can increase a person's susceptibility to hypertension; a person with this type of elevation in blood pressure has **secondary hypertension.**

DISEASES. Renal vascular and renal parenchymal diseases are two of the most common causes of secondary hypertension. Hypertension can develop when there is any sudden damage to the kidneys. Renovascular hypertension is associated with narrowing of one or more of the main arteries carrying blood directly to the kidneys. Renal parenchymal diseases are related to infection, inflammation, and changes in kidney structure and function.

Dysfunction of the adrenal medulla or the adrenal cortex can cause secondary hypertension. Adrenal-mediated hypertension is due to primary excesses of aldosterone, cortisol, and catecholamines. In *primary aldosteronism,* excessive aldosterone causes hypertension and hypokalemia (low potassium levels). It usually arises from benign adenomas of the adrenal cortex. *Pheochromocytomas* originate most commonly in the adrenal medulla and result in excessive secretion of catecholamines. In *Cushing's syndrome,* excessive glucocorticoids are excreted from the adrenal cortex. The cause of Cushing's syndrome may be either adrenocortical hyperplasia or adrenocortical adenoma (Chapter 66).

Coarctation of the aorta is a congenital narrowing of the aorta that may cause hypertension. Occurring at any level of

TABLE 39-4 Etiology of Hypertension

Essential (Primary)
- No known cause
- Associated risk factors
  - Family history of hypertension
  - High sodium intake
  - Excessive calorie consumption
  - Physical inactivity
  - Excessive alcohol intake
  - Low potassium intake

Secondary
- Renal vascular and renal parenchymal disease
- Primary aldosteronism
- Pheochromocytoma
- Cushing's disease
- Coarctation of the aorta
- Brain tumors
- Encephalitis
- Psychiatric disturbances
- Pregnancy
- Medications
  - Estrogen (e.g., oral contraceptives)
  - Glucocorticoids
  - Mineralocorticoids
  - Sympathomimetics

the thoracic or abdominal aorta, the narrowing restricts blood flow through the aortic arch, resulting in an elevated blood pressure above the constriction. After surgical repair, the elevation in blood pressure eventually subsides.

Secondary hypertension is also associated with other neurogenic disturbances, such as brain tumors, encephalitis, and psychiatric disturbances.

MEDICATIONS. Medications that can cause secondary hypertension include estrogen, glucocorticoids, mineralocorticoids, sympathomimetics, cyclosporine, and erythropoietin. The use of estrogen-containing oral contraceptives is probably the most common cause of secondary hypertension in women. Discontinuation of medications capable of causing hypertension often reverses this problem.

Incidence/Prevalence

About 50 million Americans, or 1 in every 4 adults, have high blood pressure or are currently being treated for hypertension.

HEALTH PROMOTION/ILLNESS PREVENTION

Teach clients ways to decrease risk factors for hypertension. Risk factor prevention and lifestyle changes are discussed under the nursing diagnosis of Deficient Knowledge on p. 786.

COLLABORATIVE MANAGEMENT

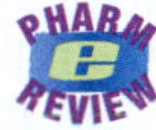

Assessment

HISTORY

During history taking, review the client's risk factors for hypertension. Ascertain the client's age; ethnic origin or race; family history of hypertension; average dietary intake of calories, sodium- and potassium-containing foods, and alcohol; and exercise habits. Also assess any past or present history of renal or cardiovascular disease and current use of medications.

PHYSICAL ASSESSMENT

When a diagnosis of hypertension is made, most clients have no symptoms; however, they may experience headaches, dizziness, or fainting as a result of the elevated blood pressure. Obtain blood pressure readings in both arms. Two or more readings are taken at each visit, with the average of the readings used as the value for the visit (Figure 39-3). To detect postural (orthostatic) changes, also take readings with the client in the supine (lying) or sitting position and at least 2 minutes later with the client standing. **Orthostatic hypotension** is a decrease in blood pressure (20 mm Hg systolic and/or 10 mm Hg diastolic) when the client changes position from lying to sitting.

Funduscopic examination of the eyes to observe vascular changes in the retina is done by a skilled practitioner. The appearance of the retina can be a reliable index of the severity and prognosis of hypertension.

Physical assessment is helpful in diagnosing several conditions that produce secondary hypertension. The presence of abdominal bruits is typical of clients with renovascular disease. Tachycardia, sweating, and pallor may suggest a pheochromocytoma or adrenal medulla tumor. Coarctation of the aorta is often characterized by elevation of blood pressure in the arms, with normal or low blood pressure in the lower extremities. Femoral pulses are also delayed or absent.

PSYCHOSOCIAL ASSESSMENT

Assess for psychosocial stressors that can worsen hypertension and that may affect the client's ability to collaborate in treatment. Job-related, economic, and other life stressors are evaluated, as well as the client's response to these stressors. Some clients may have difficulty coping with the lifestyle changes needed to control hypertension. Be sure to assess the client's past coping strategies.

DIAGNOSTIC ASSESSMENT

Although no laboratory tests are diagnostic of essential hypertension, several laboratory tests can assess possible causes of secondary hypertension. The presence of protein, red blood cells, pus cells, and casts in the urine; elevated levels of blood urea nitrogen (BUN); and elevated serum creatinine levels indicate renal disease. Urinary test results are positive for the presence of catecholamines in clients with a pheochromocytoma (tumor of the adrenal medulla). An elevation in levels of serum corticoids and 17-ketosteroids in the urine is diagnostic of Cushing's disease.

No specific x-ray studies can diagnose hypertension. Routine chest radiography may be of assistance in recognizing cardiomegaly (heart enlargement).

An electrocardiogram (ECG) is of value in determining the degree of cardiac involvement. Left atrial and ventricular hypertrophy is the first ECG sign of cardiac involvement resulting from hypertension. Left ventricular remodeling can be detected on the 12-lead ECG.

Analysis

COMMON NURSING DIAGNOSES AND COLLABORATIVE PROBLEMS

The following are priority nursing diagnoses for clients with hypertension:

1. Deficient Knowledge related to information misinterpretation or unfamiliarity with information resources
2. Risk for Ineffective Therapeutic Regimen Management related to noncompliance with or nonadherence to treatment

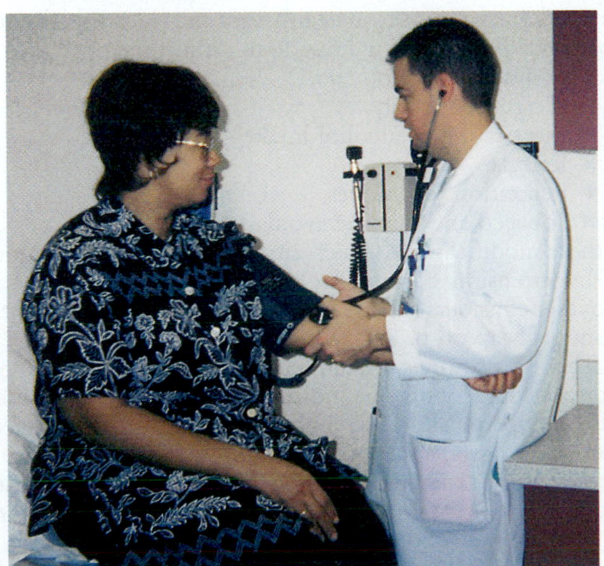

Figure 39-3 ■ Blood pressure screening during routine history and physical examination.

ADDITIONAL NURSING DIAGNOSES AND COLLABORATIVE PROBLEMS

In addition to the common nursing diagnoses, clients with hypertension may have one or more of the following:

- Ineffective Tissue Perfusion (Renal, Cerebral, Cardiopulmonary, and Peripheral) related to decreased blood flow
- Risk for Imbalanced Nutrition: More Than Body Requirements related to learned eating behaviors, ethnic and cultural values, lack of social support for weight loss, and/or imbalance between activity level and caloric intake
- Fatigue related to altered body chemistry (medications) and disease state
- Sexual Dysfunction related to altered body function from drug therapy
- Ineffective Coping related to inadequate level of perception of control
- Excessive Fluid Volume related to compromised regulatory mechanism
- Risk for Noncompliance related to knowledge and skill relevant to the regimen behavior

The following collaborative problems may also occur in some clients with hypertension:

- Potential for Cerebrovascular Hemorrhage
- Potential for Myocardial Infarction
- Potential for Retinal Hemorrhage

Planning and Implementation

DEFICIENT KNOWLEDGE

NOC **PLANNING: EXPECTED OUTCOMES.** The client with hypertension is expected to have an understanding about a specific treatment regimen. Indicators include that the client will be able to extensively describe:

- Specific disease process
- Rationale for treatment regimen
- Self-care responsibilities for ongoing treatment
- Self-monitoring techniques
- Expected effects of treatment
- Benefits of disease management

INTERVENTIONS. For the client with essential hypertension, the nurse or health care provider initially recommends the following lifestyle modifications:

- Sodium restriction
- Weight reduction
- Moderation of alcohol intake
- Exercise
- Relaxation techniques
- Tobacco and caffeine avoidance

If these modifications, which are considered the foundation of hypertension control, are unsuccessful, the health care provider considers the use of antihypertensive drugs (see the Concept Map on p. 787).

There is no surgical treatment for essential hypertension. However, surgery may be indicated for certain causes of secondary hypertension, such as renal vascular disease, coarctation of the aorta, and pheochromocytoma.

Sodium Restriction. In collaboration and consultation with the dietitian, advise all clients with hypertension to decrease their sodium chloride intake from the average of 150 mmol/L (150 mEq/L) to less than 100 mmol/L (100 mEq/L; less than 2.3 g of sodium) per day. To accomplish the goal, clients should avoid adding salt at the table, cooking with salt, or adding seasonings that contain sodium. Teach clients to avoid any food that comes from a factory, except for plain frozen vegetables and fruit.

A dietitian may review a 3-day dietary recall with the client to identify whether sodium intake has been excessive. In collaboration with the dietitian, suggest spices, herbs, fruits, and other non–salt-containing substances, such as powdered garlic and onion, to enhance the flavor of meat, chicken, seafood, and snacks. Instruct clients to read the labels on all food and to avoid those that are high in sodium. Salt substitutes are an alternative to salt. However, some substitutes are high in potassium, and therefore are contraindicated for some clients. Hyperkalemia can also occur in clients who are taking potassium-sparing diuretics, although it is unusual.

Weight Reduction. If a client's body mass index (BMI) is 25 or higher, weight loss is encouraged. Discuss the rationale for reducing or maintaining weight and help plan a weight reduction diet with the client. He or she may be referred to a group or organization for weight reduction. The cost of inactivity was $29 billion in 1987 and nearly $76 billion in 2000. Being active in some form of physical exercise is linked with taking fewer medications, having fewer hospitalizations, and fewer physician visits (CDC, 2003).

Because of the relationship of saturated fat and cholesterol to weight, a weight reduction plan is formulated with the following limits:

- Total fat: less than 30% of daily caloric intake
- Saturated fat: less than 10%
- Cholesterol: less than 300 mg/day

Moderation of Alcohol Intake. In general, instruct clients to limit alcohol intake to no more than 1 ounce of ethanol (2 ounces of liquor, 8 ounces of wine, or 24 ounces of beer) daily. Excessive alcohol consumption may elevate arterial blood pressure and can add "empty" calories.

Exercise. With the physician's approval and in collaboration with the physical therapist, help the client develop a regular exercise program. Exercise is critical for successful weight loss, lowered blood pressure, and increased endurance. The client should start an exercise program slowly and gradually work up to more rigorous activities, such as brisk walking, running, cycling, swimming, or stair climbing, 30 to 45 minutes three to five times a week. Teach the client to stop and notify the physician if severe shortness of breath, fainting, or chest pain occurs.

NIC **Smoking Cessation Assistance.** Although cigarette smoking is not directly related to hypertension, it is a major risk factor for cardiovascular disease. Therefore the client who smokes is strongly urged to stop (Chart 39-2). A smoking cessation program that best fits into his or her lifestyle should be planned. Explain use of nicotine patches and smoking cessation programs and implement follow-up to assess the client's plans for quitting. With the ability to reach many more people than traditional cessation programs, computer cessation programs have been shown to be effective in "precontemplators" who were otherwise not motivated to quit (Etter et al., 2001).

Complementary and Alternative Therapies. In addition to exercise, complementary modalities are often used by clients to reduce stress and thus decrease blood

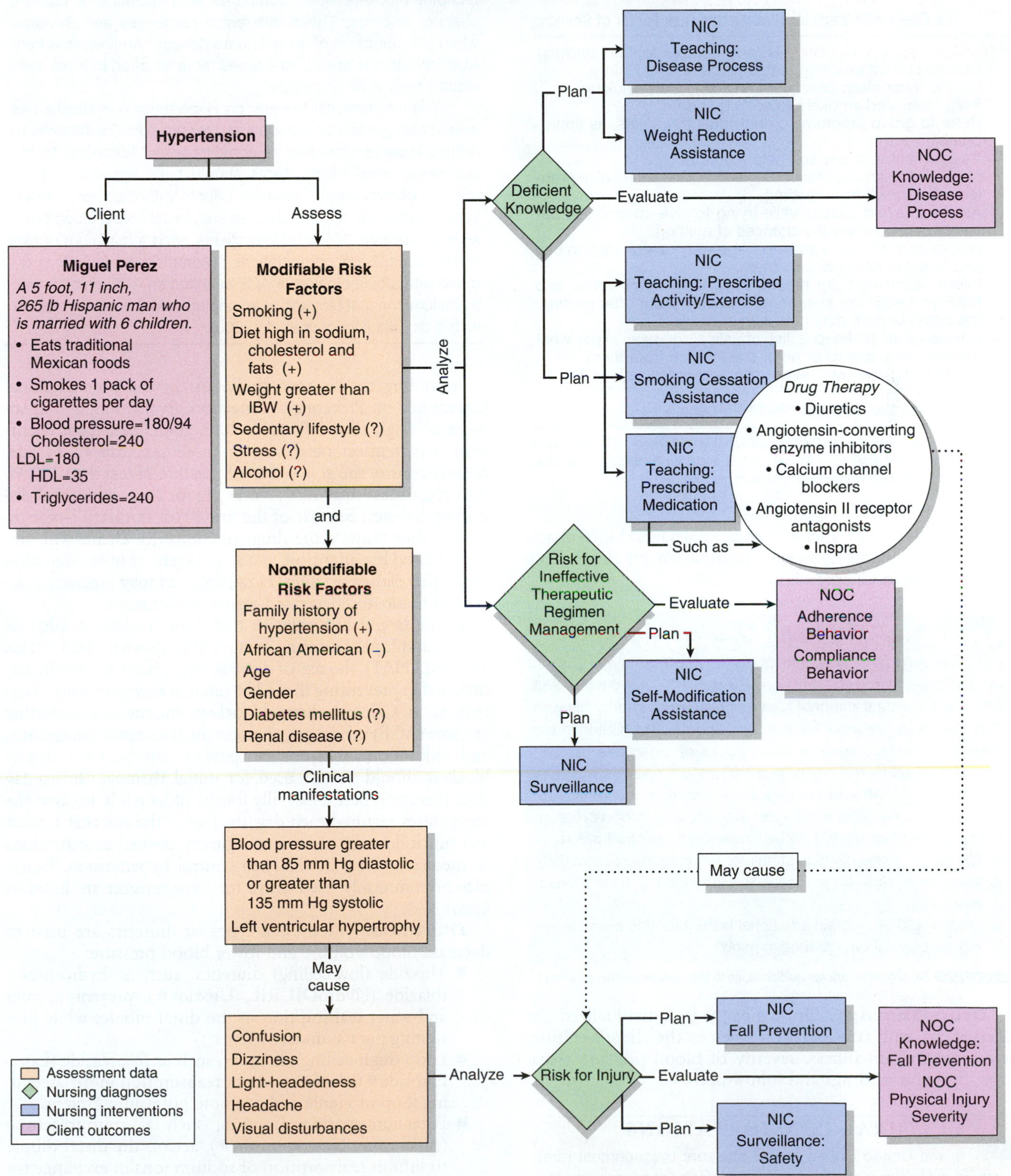

Concept Map by Elaine Bishop Kennedy, EdD, RN

CHART 39-2

NIC INTERVENTION ACTIVITIES for
The Client with Vascular Disease and Risk Factor of Smoking

Smoking Cessation Assistance: *Helping another to stop smoking*
- Record current smoking status and smoking history.
- Give smoker clear, consistent advice to quit smoking.
- Help motivated smokers to set a quit date.
- Refer to group programs or individual therapists, as appropriate.
- Assist client with any self-help methods.
- Help client plan specific coping strategies and resolve problems that result from quitting.
- Advise to avoid dieting while trying to give up smoking because it can undermine chances of quitting.
- Advise to work out a plan to cope with others who smoke and to avoid being around them.
- Inform client that dry mouth, cough, scratchy throat, and feeling on edge are symptoms that may occur after quitting; the patch or gum may help with cravings.
- Advise client to keep a list of "slips" or near slips, what causes them, and what he or she learned from them.
- Contact national and local resource organizations for resource materials.
- Encourage the relapsed client to try again.

NIC intervention activities selected from Dochterman, J.M., & Bulechek, G.M. (Eds.) (2004). *Nursing interventions classification (NIC)* (4th ed.). St. Louis: Mosby.

pressure. Examples include yoga, massage, biofeedback, music therapy, and hypnosis. Information on these therapies is found in Chapter 4.

Critical Thinking Challenge

A middle-aged Hispanic man who speaks minimal English is diagnosed with hypertension. He is 5'10" and weighs 265 pounds. He eats traditional Mexican food prepared by his wife and mother-in-law who live with him and his six children in the inner city. He had smoked three packs of cigarettes per day (ppd) for 22 years and has now cut down to 1 ppd. He is a truck driver, but walking and loading boxes are also part of his job. He arrives at the clinic where you determine his blood pressure is 180/94. He has never had his cholesterol checked before.

1. Explain why this client is at risk for high blood pressure (BP).
2. What other data do you need to complete his initial assessment?
3. How would you obtain additional history for this client, keeping his cultural background in mind?

evolve For suggested answer guidelines, go to http://evolve.elsevier.com/Iggy/.

Drug Therapy. Drug therapy is individualized for each client, with consideration given to the client's culture, age, concomitant illness, severity of blood pressure elevation, and cost of drugs and follow-up.

CULTURAL CONSIDERATIONS

In the United States, blood pressure management rates vary in minorities and are lowest in Mexican Americans and Native Americans/American Indians. Socioeconomic and lifestyle factors may be significant barriers to control blood pressure in some minorities. There is a higher prevalence, incidence, and impact of hypertension among black individuals who also have a decreased treatment response with beta blockers, angiotensin-converting enzyme (ACE) inhibitors, or angiotensin receptor blockers when compared with diuretics or calcium channel blockers. These differential responses are alleviated when the diuretic is of an adequate dosage. Angioedema from ACE inhibitors is seen 2 to 4 times more as often in black individuals than in other groups.

The International Society on Hypertension in Blacks has issued new guidelines personalized for the black community to reduce hypertension and its complications. According to the guidelines, most black clients should have aggressive treatment to control blood pressure. Clients with diabetes, cardiovascular disease, or renal disease should achieve a blood pressure of less than 130/80. Most clients need a minimum of two medications. Drug combinations recommended include a diuretic with a beta blocker or ACE inhibitor, an ACE inhibitor with a calcium channel blocker, or an angiotensin II receptor blocker with a diuretic (Douglas et al., 2003).

According to the Seventh Report of the Joint National Committee on Prevention, Detection, Evaluation, and Treatment of High Blood Pressure 2003 guidelines, most clients with hypertension need two or more medications to adequately control the goal of blood pressure of less than 140/90 mm Hg, or less than 130/80 mm Hg for those with renal disease or diabetes. Because of the lower cost of thiazide-type diuretics, they may be the drugs of choice for clients with uncomplicated hypertension, as a single agent or in combination with other classes of drugs. However, men may experience decreased libido and decreased sexual performance.

In the largest hypertensive trial done to date, Antihypertensive and Lipid Lowering Treatment to Prevent Heart Attack Trial (ALLHAT), the use of diuretics have been practically unmatched in preventing the cardiovascular complications of hypertension. Calcium channel blockers, angiotensin-converting enzyme (ACE) inhibitors, angiotensin II receptor antagonists, and aldosterone receptor antagonists can be tried. Alpha blockers should not be used for initial therapy. Once-a-day drug therapy is best, especially for the older adult, because the more doses required each day, the higher the risk that a client will not follow the treatment regimen. Several classifications of medications are available to control hypertension. Examples of commonly used drugs for hypertension are listed in Chart 39-3.

Diuretics. Three basic types of diuretics are used to decrease blood volume and lower blood pressure:

- Thiazide (low-ceiling) diuretics, such as hydrochlorothiazide (HydroDIURIL, Urozide✱), prevent sodium and water reabsorption in the distal tubules while promoting potassium excretion.
- Loop (high-ceiling) diuretics, such as furosemide (Lasix, Furoside✱), depress sodium reabsorption in the ascending loop of Henle and promote potassium excretion.
- Potassium-sparing diuretics, such as spironolactone (Aldactone, Novospiroton✱), act on the distal tubule to inhibit reabsorption of sodium ions in exchange for potassium, thereby retaining potassium. When used, they are typically in combination with another type of diuretic to conserve potassium.

Diuretics are the drugs of choice for clients who have asthma, chronic airway limitation, and chronic renal disease and for selected clients with heart failure. They are particularly effective

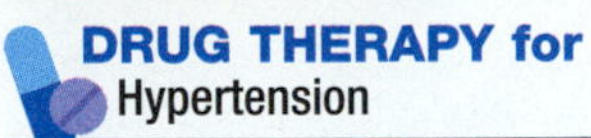

CHART 39-3

DRUG THERAPY for Hypertension

Drug	Usual Dosage	Nursing Interventions	Rationales
Diuretics			
Thiazides (Low-Ceiling)			
Chlorothiazide (Diuril)	125-500 mg daily	Monitor potassium levels and watch for muscle weakness or irregular pulse.	Hypokalemia is a common occurrence.
Hydrochlorothiazide (Esidrix, HydroDIURIL)	12.5-50 mg daily	Encourage intake of foods high in potassium (e.g., bananas and orange juice).	Depleted potassium needs to be replaced.
Loop (High-Ceiling) Diuretics			
[1]Furosemide [2](Lasix, Furoside✱)	20-80 mg PO daily 20-40 mg IV; increase by 20 mg every 2 hr until desired response	Same as for thiazide diuretics. Observe for dehydration, especially in older adults.	Same as for chlorothiazide. Loop diuretics can cause dehydration in older adults.
Bumetanide (Bumex)	0.5-2 mg PO daily or 0.5-1 mg IV; give 2nd or 3rd dose at 2- to 3-hr intervals not to exceed 10 mg daily	Same as for furosemide.	Same as for furosemide.
Potassium-Sparing Diuretics			
Spironolactone (Aldactone)	25-100 mg daily	Monitor potassium levels and watch for muscle weakness or irregular pulse.	Hypokalemia or hyperkalemia may occur.
Triamterene (Dyrenium)	50-100 mg daily		
Calcium Channel Blocking Agents			
[3]Verapamil (Apo-Verap✱, Calan, Calan SR, Isoptin, Isoptin SR)	80 mg q8h or 240 mg SR daily; may titrate upward	Monitor blood pressure (BP) and pulse; change positions slowly. Encourage intake of foods high in fiber.	Hypotension and decreased heart rate may occur. Constipation is a common side effect.
Amlodipine (Norvasc)	5-10 mg daily	Monitor BP and pulse; teach clients to change positions slowly. Use protective clothing or sunscreen when exposed to sun.	Same as verapamil. Photosensitivity is a common side effect.
[4]Diltiazem (Cardizem, Apo-Diltiaz✱, Cardizem CD, Cardizem SR)	30-360 mg daily in divided doses or in extended form	Monitor BP and pulse; teach clients to change positions slowly. Teach clients to avoid grapefruit juice.	Same as verapamil. Increased hypotensive effects may occur as a result of drug-food interaction.
Nicardipine (Cardene, Cardene SR, Cardene IV)	20-40 mg PO three times daily 0.5-2.2 mg/hr IV (for hypertensive crisis)	Do not give with grapefruit juice. Monitor digoxin level if the client is taking this drug.	Grapefruit juice increases drug level and hypotensive effect (applies to most calcium channel blockers). Nicardipine increases the effects of digoxin.
Angiotensin-Converting Enzyme (ACE) Inhibitors			
Captopril (Capoten, Novo-Captopril✱)	25-150 mg two to three times daily	Same as amlodipine. Teach client to report cough.	Same as amlodipine. Coughing is a common side effect of ACE inhibitors; drug is discontinued if this problem occurs.
Enalapril (Vasotec, Vasotec IV)	5-40 mg PO daily; 1.25 mg q6h over 5 min	Same as captopril.	Same as captopril.
Lisinopril (Zestril, Prinivil)	10-40 mg daily; increase to 80 mg daily if needed	Monitor BP and pulse; teach clients to change positions slowly. Monitor for and teach clients to report signs of heart failure (e.g., edema). Teach client to report cough.	Hypotension is a common side effect. This drug can cause heart and renal complications. Cough is a common side effect and requires discontinuation of the drug.

[1]***Med Error Alert!*** *Do not confuse furosemide with torsemide.*

[2]***Med Error Alert!*** *Do not confuse Lasix with Lanoxin.*

[3]***Med Error Alert!*** *Do not crush SR form of drug.*

[4]***Med Error Alert!*** *Do not crush CD or SR forms of drug; do not confuse Cardizem CD and Cardizem SR. Do not confuse with Cardene IV.*

Continued

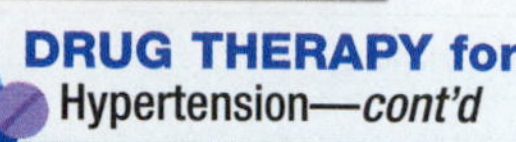

DRUG THERAPY for Hypertension—*cont'd*

Drug	Usual Dosage	Nursing Interventions	Rationales
Angiotensin-Converting Enzyme (ACE) Inhibitors—*cont'd*			
Ramipril (Altace)	2.5-20 mg daily, or twice daily in divided doses	Same as lisinopril.	Same as lisinopril.
Angiotensin II Receptor Antagonists			
Candesartan (Atacand)	8-32 mg daily	Monitor BP and pulse; teach clients to change position slowly.	Hypotension is a common side effect.
		Observe for and teach client to report angioedema (swollen lips, face).	Angioedema is a serious but not common adverse effect of this drug.
Losartan (Cozaar)	25-50 mg daily	Monitor BP and pulse.	Same as above.
		Monitor for and report signs of heart failure, such as edema.	Heart failure can result from taking the drug.
Telmisartan (Micardis)	20-80 mg daily	Same as candesartan.	Same as candesartan.
Aldosterone Receptor Antagonists			
Eplerenone (Inspra)	50 mg daily initially, increased to 100 mg daily if response is not adequate.	Monitor renal function.	Risk of adverse effects increases with deteriorating renal function.
		Monitor triglycerides.	Dose-related adverse effect of hypertriglyceridemia occurred in 15% of study clients.
		Monitor sodium levels.	Hyponatremia may occur when taking this drug.
		Monitor potassium levels every 2 wk for the first few months then every 2 months thereafter.	Potassium imbalances may occur when taking this medication. ▪ Risk of hyperkalemia increases when using ACE inhibitors or angiotensin II receptor antagonists with Inspra. ▪ Do not give with potassium supplements and potassium-sparing diuretics. Client should not take salt substitutes with potassium and other foods rich in potassium.
		Teach client about potential drug and herbal interactions.	Grapefruit juice and St. John's wort, for example, can increase adverse effects.
		Caution client to be careful when getting out of bed, driving, and climbing stairs until the medication's effects are known.	Orthostatic hypotension may occur, especially in older adults.

for black individuals. Caution is indicated in using thiazide diuretics in hypertensive clients with gout or with a history of significant hyponatremia, because these problems can worsen.

Diuretics enhance the antihypertensive effectiveness when using multiple drug therapy combinations and are relatively inexpensive. Adherence to the medication regimen is enhanced because the drug can usually be prescribed on a once-a-day or, at most, twice-a-day schedule. However, the frequent voiding that occurs after a person takes a diuretic may interfere with daily activities. The most frequent side effect associated with diuretics is hypokalemia (low potassium levels). Monitor the serum potassium level and assess for irregular pulse and muscle weakness, which may indicate hypokalemia. Clients receiving potassium-depleting diuretics should eat foods high in potassium, such as bananas and orange juice. However, many individuals need a potassium supplement to maintain adequate serum potassium levels (see Chapter 14). Assess for hypokalemia and hyperkalemia in clients taking potassium-sparing diuretics. Both of these electrolyte disturbances are characterized by weakness and an irregular pulse, and are described in detail in Chapter 15.

Calcium Channel Blocking Agents. Calcium channel blockers, such as verapamil hydrochloride (Calan), amlodipine (Norvasc), and diltiazem (Cardizem), lower blood pressure by interfering with the transmembrane flux of calcium ions. This results in vasodilation and subsequent decrease in blood pressure.

Angiotensin-Converting Enzyme Inhibitors. Angiotensin-converting enzyme (ACE) inhibitors are also used as single or combination agents in the treatment of hyperten-

CHART 39-4

NURSING FOCUS on the OLDER ADULT
Hypertension

- Before initiating drug therapy, obtain blood pressure measurements with the client lying, sitting, and standing to assess for postural changes.
- Monitor the client's standing blood pressure during treatment.
- Instruct the client to avoid caffeine and nicotine for 1 hour before blood pressure measurements to obtain accurate readings.
- Teach the client that dizziness is a symptom of hypotension that should be reported.
- Instruct clients how to avoid orthostatic (postural) hypotension by avoiding sudden changes in position. Clients should arise from bed in three stages: sit in bed for 1 minute; sit on the side of the bed with legs dangling for 1 minute; and stand, holding onto a nonmovable object for 1 minute before walking. Clients should also be cautious about heat exposure (hot tub), alcohol intake, and exercise, which can lead to orthostatic hypotension.

sion. The angiotensin-converting enzyme converts angiotensin I to angiotensin II, one of the most powerful vasoconstrictors in the body, thereby preventing increased blood pressure. ACE inhibitors include captopril (Capoten), enalapril (Vasotec), and lisinopril (Prinivil).

Instruct the client receiving an ACE inhibitor for the first time to get out of bed slowly to avoid the severe hypotensive effect that can occur with initial use. Orthostatic hypotension may occur with subsequent doses, but it is less severe. If dizziness continues or there is a significant decrease in the systolic blood pressure (<20 mm Hg), notify the physician. The older client is at the greatest risk for postural hypotension because of the cardiovascular changes associated with aging. If a cough develops, the drug is discontinued.

CONSIDERATIONS FOR OLDER ADULTS

Seen more often in older adults, orthostatic (postural) hypotension is a decrease in systolic and diastolic blood pressure upon rising (Chart 39-4). When younger individuals stand, the body compensates for the change in gravitational forces when changing positions. Those most susceptible are older adults with systolic hypertension, diabetics, and those taking diuretics, vasodilators, or some psychotropic drugs. Orthostatic hypertension is often accompanied by dizziness, blurring or loss of vision, and syncope or fainting. For this reason, caution is needed to avoid volume depletion and too fast of dosage adjustment with antihypertensive drugs. Wearing elastic venous compression stockings is an effective strategy to reduce the risk of fainting and falls in older adults with postural hypotension.

Angiotensin II Receptor Antagonists. Angiotensin II receptor antagonists, also called angiotensin II receptor blockers (ARBs), make up a group of drugs that selectively block the binding of angiotensin II in the vascular and adrenal tissues by competing directly with angiotensin II but not inhibiting ACE. Examples of drugs in this group are candesartan (Atacand), losartan (Cozaar), and telmisartan (Micardis). Angiotensin II receptor antagonists can be used alone or in combination with other antihypertensive drugs. They are excellent options for clients who complain of cough associated with ACE inhibitors and for those with hyperkalemia. In addition, these drugs do not require initial adjustment of the dose for older adults or for clients with renal impairment.

Aldosterone Receptor Antagonists. In 2002, a new class of antihypertensive drugs was introduced to block the hypertensive effect of the mineralocorticoid hormone, aldosterone. Aldosterone increases sodium reabsorption by the kidney and is a significant contributor to hypertension, cardiac and vascular remodeling, and heart failure. Eplerenone (Inspra) lowers blood pressure by blocking aldosterone binding at the mineralocorticoid receptor sites in the kidney, heart, blood vessels, and brain. The recommended dosage is 50 mg daily, which can be increased to 100 mg daily. Generally well tolerated, eplerenone has dose-related adverse effects of hypertriglyceridemia, hyponatremia, and hyperkalemia. Using concurrent ACE inhibitors increases the risk of hyperkalemia. Monitor potassium levels carefully, initially every 2 weeks for the first few months then monthly thereafter.

When taking eplerenone, itraconazole (Sporanox) and ketoconazole (Nizoral) should not be taken. Drug interactions with these medications are common. Clients taking erythromycin, fluconazole (Diflucan), saquinavir (Fortovase), and verapamil (Isoptin) can take eplerenone but with a reduction in dosage by half to 25 mg daily. Grapefruit juice and the popular herb St. John's wort can also increase the chance of undesirable effects. Like all antihypertensives, clients need to be careful when getting up quickly, driving, or climbing stairs until they are familiar with the effects of the medication.

Other Drugs. *Beta-adrenergic blockers* are categorized as cardioselective (working only on the cardiovascular system) and noncardioselective. Cardioselective beta blockers may be prescribed to lower blood pressure by blocking beta receptors in the heart and peripheral vessels, reducing the cardiac rate and output. By blocking beta-adrenergic receptors in the heart, these drugs decrease heart rate and myocardial contractility. Common side effects of beta blockers include fatigue, weakness, depression, and sexual dysfunction, although the potential for side effects depends on the "selective" blocking effects of the drug.

Clients with diabetes who take beta blockers may not have the usual manifestations of hypoglycemia because the sympathetic nervous system is blocked. Counterregulatory responses to hypoglycemia, such as gluconeogenesis, may also be inhibited by certain beta blockers.

Beta blockers are the drug of choice for hypertensive clients with ischemic heart disease (IHD) because the heart is the most common target of end-organ damage with hypertension. If a beta blocker is not tolerated, a long-acting calcium channel blocker can be used. In clients with unstable angina or myocardial infarction (MI), beta blockers or calcium channel blockers should be used initially in combination with ACE inhibitors, with addition of other drugs if needed to control the blood pressure. Best practice for controlling hypertension in post-MI clients include a combination drug therapy of beta blockers, ACE inhibitors, and aldosterone antagonists plus intense management of lipids and the use of aspirin. Low-dose aspirin should only be considered once the blood pressure is controlled because of the increased risk for hemorrhagic stroke in the presence of uncontrolled hypertension.

Central alpha agonists act on the central nervous system, preventing reuptake of norepinephrine, resulting in lower peripheral vascular resistance and blood pressure. Clonidine (Catapres) is most commonly used in this drug classification, and is usually given as a transdermal patch, providing control of blood pressure for as long as 7 days. Side effects common to clonidine include sedation, postural hypotension, and impotence. This group of drugs is not indicated for first-line management of hypertension.

Alpha-adrenergic agonists, such as prazosin (Minipress), dilate the arterioles and veins. These drugs can lower blood pressure quickly, but their use is limited because of frequent and bothersome side effects.

RISK FOR INEFFECTIVE THERAPEUTIC REGIMEN MANAGEMENT

NOC **PLANNING: EXPECTED OUTCOMES.** The client with hypertension is expected to take personal actions to promote wellness, recovery, and rehabilitation based on professional advice. Indicators include that the client will consistently:

- Discuss prescribed treatment regimen with health care professional
- Perform treatment regimen as prescribed
- Monitor treatment and medication responses
- Keep appointments with health care professional

INTERVENTIONS. Clients who require pharmacologic treatment to control essential hypertension usually need to take medication for the rest of their lives. Frequently, however, some clients stop taking antihypertensive medications because they have no symptoms and experience troublesome side effects.

In the hospital setting, collaboration with the pharmacist is helpful to discuss the goals of therapy with the client, including potential side effects, to help identify potential problems. Assist the client in tailoring the therapeutic regimen to his or her activities of daily living (ADLs).

Clients who do not comply with antihypertensive treatment are at great risk for target organ damage and hypertensive crisis (malignant hypertension) (Chart 39-5). Clients in hypertensive crisis are admitted to critical care units, where they receive intravenous (IV) antihypertensive therapy, such as nitroprusside (Nipride), nicardipine (Cardene IV), fenoldopam (Corlopam), or labetalol (Normodyne). These drugs act quickly as vasodilators to decrease BP. Hospitalization for complications of hypertension can be costly in medical expenses, lost income, and deterioration in the quality of life.

CHART 39-5

BEST PRACTICE for
Emergency Care of Clients with Hypertensive Crisis

EMERGENCY CARE

Assess
- Severe headache
- Extremely high blood pressure
- Dizziness
- Blurred vision
- Disorientation

Intervene
- Place client in a semi-Fowler's position.
- Administer oxygen.
- Administer IV nitroprusside (Nitropress), nicardipine (Cardene IV), or other infusion drug as prescribed (for nitroprusside, cover infusion bag to prevent drug breakdown by light).
- Monitor blood pressure every 5 to 15 minutes until the diastolic pressure is also below 90 and not less than 75; then monitor blood pressure every 30 minutes.
- Observe for neurologic or cardiovascular complications, such as seizures; numbness, weakness, or tingling of extremities; dysrhythmias; or chest pain.

Community-Based Care

HOME CARE MANAGEMENT

Many people do not successfully take medications as prescribed without some intervention designed to enhance adherence. There is no one cause of poor adherence. Clients often stop taking antihypertensive medications with the assumption that the hypertension is under control because they have no symptoms. Some just forget to take their doses. Others may think they are not sick enough. Many clients assume that if their blood pressure returns to normal levels with antihypertensives, they no longer need them. They may also stop taking antihypertensives because of adverse side effects or cost. Evidence-based approaches can be used to improve adherence to taking medications. Reviewing instructions and sending home written instructions appear to have the most impact on improving short-term adherence but less impact on long-term therapy. Self-administration of medications is a behavior that must be learned and most health care professionals have little training in how to assist others in behavior modification. Develop a plan with the client and identify what you will do to encourage adherence, and how other health care providers can also support the goal. Suggest adherence-improving approaches that can be easily incorporated into daily living.

If possible, the client should obtain an ambulatory blood pressure monitoring device (ABPM) for use at home so that the pressure can be checked periodically. Evaluate the client's ability to use this device. If the client cannot monitor the blood pressure, a family member or significant other may be taught how to perform this procedure. If weight reduction is a goal, suggest having a scale in the home for weight monitoring.

HEALTH TEACHING

Instruct the client about sodium restriction, weight maintenance or reduction, alcohol restriction, stress management, and exercise (see Interventions [Arteriosclerosis and Atherosclerosis], p. 780). If necessary, also explain about the need to stop smoking. Provide oral and written information about the indications, dosage, times for administration, side effects, and drug interactions (see Chart 39-3) for antihypertensive medications. Stress that medications must be taken as prescribed and that when all of the medication has been consumed, the prescription must be renewed on a continual basis. Abrupt termination of medications such as beta blockers can result in angina (chest pain), myocardial infarction (MI), or rebound hypertension.

Also urge clients to report unpleasant side effects, such as excessive fatigue, cough, or sexual dysfunction. In many instances, an alternative medication can be prescribed to minimize certain side effects.

Hypertension is a chronic illness. Allow clients to verbalize feelings about the disease and its treatment. Advise them that their involvement in the treatment can lead to control of the disease and can prevent complications.

HEALTH CARE RESOURCES

A home care nurse may be needed for follow-up to monitor the blood pressure. Evaluate the client or family's ability to obtain accurate blood pressure measurements and assess compliance with treatment. The American Heart Association, the Red Cross, or a local pharmacy may be used for free blood pressure checks if clients cannot purchase equipment to monitor their blood pressure.

Evaluation: Outcomes

Evaluate the care of the client with hypertension on the basis of the identified nursing diagnoses and collaborative problems. The expected outcomes are that the client will:

- Understand a specific treatment regimen
- Take personal action to promote wellness, recovery, and rehabilitation based on professional advice

Specific indicators for these outcomes are listed for each nursing diagnosis under the Planning and Implementation section (see earlier).

Critical Thinking Challenge

On a return visit to the clinic, the 48-year-old client's blood pressure is now 166/90. His cholesterol level is 240, LDL-C is 180, and HDL-C is 35. His triglyceride level was 240. His weight is up to 275 pounds.

1. What questions would be important to ask in reviewing his history?
2. What lifestyle behaviors would you further analyze?
3. How can you help this client modify his behaviors?
4. What is the significance of these lipid values and what can be done about them?

evolve For suggested answer guidelines, go to http://evolve.elsevier.com/Iggy/.

PERIPHERAL ARTERIAL DISEASE

Peripheral vascular disease (PVD) includes disorders that alter the natural flow of blood through the arteries and veins of the peripheral circulation. PVD affects the lower extremities much more frequently than the upper extremities. Generally, a client with a diagnosis of PVD implies arterial disease (peripheral arterial disease [PAD]) rather than venous involvement. Some clients have both arterial and venous disease. The cost of PVD is staggering and is expected to rise as "baby boomers" age and obesity in the United States increases (see the Resource Management box above).

PATHOPHYSIOLOGY

PAD is a manifestation of systemic atherosclerosis and is a chronic condition in which partial or total arterial occlusion deprives the lower extremities of oxygen and nutrients. PAD of the lower extremities is sometimes referred to as lower extremity arterial disease (LEAD). Body tissues cannot live without an adequate oxygen and nutrient supply, and tissue eventually dies. Atherosclerosis is the most common cause of chronic altered blood flow. Fatty substances accumulate at the site of vessel wall injury and alter or totally occlude blood flow within the arteries. Tissue damage generally occurs below the arterial obstruction.

Obstructions are classified as inflow or outflow, according to the arteries involved and their relationship to the inguinal ligament (Figure 39-4). *Inflow* obstructions involve the distal end of the aorta and the common, internal, and external iliac arteries. They are located above the inguinal ligament. *Outflow* obstructions involve infrainguinal arterial segments (the femoral, popliteal, and tibial arteries) and are below the superficial femoral artery (SFA). Gradual inflow

RESOURCE MANAGEMENT

PERIPHERAL VASCULAR DISEASE

Cost of Care

- Each year, vascular disorders result in disability or death, and the financial impact on society is overwhelming.
- The cost of cardiovascular disease in 2003 was estimated at $352 billion according to the National Heart, Lung, and Blood Institute and the American Heart Association. This includes direct and indirect health care costs for expenditures such as health care provider fees, hospital care, nursing home services, medications, home care services, durable medical equipment, and loss of productivity to the client, family, and society.
- Case management and the use of critical care pathways by all health care providers decreases the cost of hospital care and helps decrease the length of stay for hospitalized clients.

Implications for Nursing

The medical and nursing management of clients with cardiovascular disease is costly. Research has identified certain risk factors that contribute to the development of cardiac and vascular disease. Be committed to identifying clients at risk and providing teaching and support toward reducing risk factors. Be involved in programs related to smoking cessation, weight reduction, lipid screening, stress reduction, and promoting healthy living behaviors.

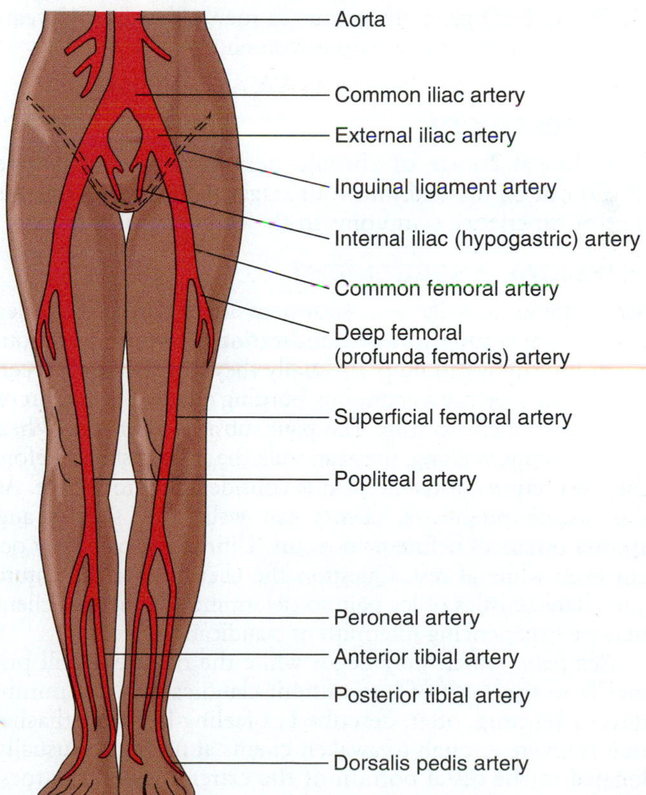

Figure 39-4 ■ Common locations of inflow and outflow lesions.

occlusions may not cause significant tissue damage; gradual outflow occlusions typically do.

Etiology and Genetic Risk

Because atherosclerosis is the most common cause of chronic arterial obstruction, the risk factors for atherosclerosis apply to PAD as well. Risk factors include hypertension, hyperlipidemia, diabetes mellitus, cigarette smoking, obesity, and familial predisposition. Advancing age also increases the risk of disease related to atherosclerosis. Clients with PAD have an increased risk for developing chronic angina, MI, or stroke and are 6 times as likely to die within 10 years compared to those without PAD.

Incidence/Prevalence

About 8 to 10 million people in the United States have PAD. The age-adjusted prevalence rate is 12% increasing to 20% in older adults age 70 years and older (Stewart et al., 2002). The presence of intermittent claudication in peripheral arterial disease is present in 15% to 40% of clients. Diagnosis of PAD is low because measurement of the ankle brachial index (ABI) is not a routine part of a clinic visit and many clients are not diagnosed unless they develop symptomatic leg pain. Black individuals appear to be affected more often than white individuals or Hispanics (Collins et al., 2003). PAD generally occurs in men older than 45 years of age and in postmenopausal women.

COLLABORATIVE MANAGEMENT

Assessment

The clinical course of chronic peripheral arterial disease (PAD) can be divided into four stages (Chart 39-6). Clients do not experience symptoms in the early stages of disease.

PHYSICAL ASSESSMENT

Most clients initially seek treatment for a characteristic leg pain known as **intermittent claudication** (a term derived from a word meaning "to limp"). Usually they can walk only a certain distance before a cramping, burning muscle discomfort or pain forces them to stop. The pain subsides after rest. When clients resume walking, they can walk the same distance before the pain returns; thus the pain is considered reproducible. As the disease progresses, clients can walk only shorter and shorter distances before pain recurs. Ultimately, pain may occur even while at rest. Question the client about the nature and characteristics of leg pain to determine whether the client may be experiencing intermittent claudication.

Rest pain, which may begin while the disease is still primarily in the stage of intermittent claudication, is a numbness or burning, often described as feeling like a toothache, that is severe enough to awaken clients at night. It is usually located in the distal portion of the extremities–in the toes, the foot arches, the forefeet, and the heels, but rarely in the calves or ankles. Clients can sometimes achieve pain relief by keeping the limb in a dependent position. Clients with rest pain often have advanced disease that may result in limb loss.

Clients with **inflow disease** experience discomfort in the lower back, buttocks, or thighs. Lower back or buttock discomfort indicates obstruction at or above the common iliac artery or abdominal aorta. Thigh discomfort indicates obstruction at or above the profunda femoris artery. Clients with *mild* inflow disease experience discomfort after walking about two blocks. This discomfort is not severe but causes the client to stop walking. It is relieved with rest. Clients with *moderate* inflow disease experience pain in these areas after walking about one or two blocks. The discomfort is described as being more like pain, but it subsides with rest most of the time. *Severe* inflow disease causes the client severe pain after walking less than one block. These clients usually have rest pain.

Clients with **outflow disease** describe burning or cramping in the calves, ankles, feet, and toes. Calf discomfort usually indicates arterial obstruction at or below the superficial femoral or popliteal artery. Instep or foot discomfort indicates an obstruction below the popliteal artery. Clients with *mild* outflow disease experience discomfort after walking about five blocks. This discomfort is relieved by rest. Clients with *moderate* outflow disease have pain after walking about two blocks. Intermittent rest pain may be present. Clients with *severe* outflow disease are usually unable to walk more than one-half block and usually experience rest pain. They may hang their feet off the bed at night for comfort. Clients with outflow disease complain more frequently of rest pain than do those with inflow disease.

Specific findings for PAD depend on the severity of the disease. Observe for loss of hair on the lower calf, ankle, and foot; dry, scaly, dusky, pale, or mottled skin; and thickened toenails. With severe arterial disease, the extremity is cold and gray-blue (cyanotic) or darkened. Pallor may occur when the extremity is elevated; dependent **rubor** may occur when the extremity is lowered. Muscle atrophy can accompany prolonged chronic arterial disease.

Palpate all pulses in both legs. The most sensitive and specific indicator of arterial function is the quality of the posterior tibial pulse because the pedal pulse is not palpable in a small percentage of people. The strength of the pulse should be compared bilaterally. Several scales are available for grading pulse strength.

CHART 39-6

KEY FEATURES of Chronic Peripheral Arterial Disease

Stage I: Asymptomatic
- No claudication is present.
- Bruit or aneurysm may be present.
- Pedal pulses are decreased or absent.

Stage II: Claudication
- Muscle pain, cramping, or burning occurs with exercise and is relieved with rest.
- Symptoms are reproducible with exercise.

Stage III: Rest Pain
- Pain while resting commonly awakens the client at night.
- Pain is described as numbness, burning, toothache-type pain.
- Pain usually occurs in the distal portion of the extremity—toes, arch, forefoot, or heel—rarely in the calf or the ankle.
- Pain is relieved by placing the extremity in a dependent position.

Stage IV: Necrosis/Gangrene
- Ulcers and blackened tissue occur on the toes, the forefoot, and the heel.
- Distinctive gangrenous odor is present.

CHART 39-7

KEY FEATURES of
Lower Extremity Ulcers

Feature	Arterial Ulcers	Venous Ulcers	Diabetic Ulcers
History	Client complaints of claudication after walking approximately 1-2 blocks Rest pain usually present Pain at ulcer site Two or three risk factors present	Chronic nonhealing ulcer No claudication or rest pain Moderate ulcer discomfort Client complaints of ankle or leg swelling	Diabetes Peripheral neuropathy No complaints of claudication
Ulcer location and appearance	End of the toes Between the toes Deep Ulcer bed pale, with even edges Little granulation tissue	Ankle area Brown pigmentation Ulcer bed pink Usually superficial, with uneven edges Granulation tissue present	Plantar area of foot Metatarsal heads Pressure points on feet Deep Pale, with even edges Little granulation tissue
Other assessment findings	Cool or cold foot Decreased or absent pulses Atrophy of skin Hair loss Pallor with elevation Dependent rubor Possible gangrene When acute, neurologic deficits noted	Ankle discoloration and edema Full veins when leg slightly dependent No neurologic deficit Pulses present May have scarring from previous ulcers	Pulses usually present Cool or warm foot Painless
Treatment	Treat underlying cause (surgical, revascularization) Prevent trauma and infection Client education, stressing foot care	Long-term wound care (Unna boot, damp-to-dry dressings) Elevate extremity Client education Prevent infection	Rule out major arterial disease Control diabetes Client education regarding foot care Prevent infection

Photographs of arterial ulcer and diabetic ulcer from Callen, J.P., et al. (1993). *Color atlas of dermatology: Slide set.* Philadelphia: W.B. Saunders.

Note early signs of ulcer formation or complete ulcer formation, a complication of PAD. Arterial and venous stasis ulcers differ from diabetic ulcers (Chart 39-7).

Initially, **arterial ulcers** are painful and develop on the toes (often the great toe), between the toes, or on the upper aspect of the foot. With prolonged occlusion, the toes can become gangrenous. Typically, the ulcer is small, round, with a "punched out" appearance and well-defined borders. **Diabetic ulcers** develop on the plantar surface of the foot, over the metatarsal heads, and on the heel anywhere that pressure is exerted. Diabetic ulcers may not be painful because of diabetic neuropathy. **Venous stasis ulcers** cause minimal pain and occur in the ankle area. The foot is warm, and distal pulses are palpable. Note discoloration of the lower extremity at the ulcer site and stasis dermatitis. Skin lesions are discussed in further detail later in this chapter and in Chapter 70.

CULTURAL CONSIDERATIONS

Because only severe cyanosis is evident in the skin of dark-skinned clients, to detect cyanosis assess their skin and nail beds for a dull, lifeless color. The soles of the feet and the toenails are less pigmented and can enable detection of cyanosis or duskiness in the lower extremities.

RADIOGRAPHIC ASSESSMENT

Arteriography of the lower extremities is one x-ray for PAD, but it is not commonly performed today. This procedure involves injecting contrast medium into the arterial system and the risks, which include hemorrhage, thrombosis, embolus, and death, are serious.

OTHER DIAGNOSTIC ASSESSMENTS

The advent of noninvasive evaluation of arterial disease has become a popular method of diagnosis. Noninvasive testing provides information about the arterial system with minimal risk to the client.

SEGMENTAL SYSTOLIC BLOOD PRESSURE MEASUREMENTS. Using a Doppler probe, segmental systolic blood pressure measurements of the lower extremities at the thigh, calf, and ankle are an inexpensive, noninvasive method of assessing PAD. Normally, blood pressure readings in the thigh and calf are higher than those in the upper extremities. With the presence of arterial disease, these pressures are lower than the brachial pressure.

With *inflow* disease, pressures taken at the thigh level indicate the severity of disease. Mild inflow disease may cause a difference of only 10 to 30 mm Hg in pressure on the affected side compared with the brachial pressure. Severe inflow disease can cause a pressure difference of greater than 40 to 50 mm Hg. The ankle pressure is normally equal to or greater than the brachial pressure.

To evaluate *outflow* disease, compare ankle pressure with the brachial pressure, which provides a ratio known as the **ankle-brachial index (ABI).** The value can be derived by dividing the ankle blood pressure by the brachial blood pressure. An ABI of less than 0.9 in either leg is diagnostic of PAD.

EXERCISE TOLERANCE TESTING. Exercise tolerance testing (by stress test or treadmill) may give valuable information about claudication (muscle pain) without rest pain. The technician obtains resting pulse volume recordings and has the client walk on a treadmill until the symptoms are reproduced. At the time of symptom onset or after about 5 minutes, the technician obtains another pulse volume recording. Normally, there may be an increased waveform with minimal, if any, drop in the ankle pressure. In clients with arterial disease, the waveforms are decreased (dampened) and there is a decrease in the ankle pressure of 40 to 60 mm Hg for 20 to 30 seconds in the affected limb. If the return to normal pressure is delayed (longer than 10 minutes), the results suggest abnormal arterial flow in the affected limb.

PLETHYSMOGRAPHY. Plethysmography can also be performed to evaluate arterial flow in the lower extremities. The measurement provides graphs or tracings of arterial flow in the limb. If an occlusion is present, the waveforms are dampened to flattened, depending on the degree of occlusion.

Interventions

First determine whether the altered tissue perfusion is of arterial or venous origin. An accurate assessment often provides this information, but in some people both conditions may exist. In this case, each disease must be considered separately when appropriate interventions are planned.

NONSURGICAL MANAGEMENT. The interventions of exercise, position changes, promotion of vasodilation, drug therapy, and invasive nonsurgical procedures are used to increase arterial flow to the affected limb.

Exercise. Exercise may improve arterial blood flow to the affected limb through buildup of the *collateral* circulation. (Collateral circulation provides blood to the affected area through smaller vessels that develop and compensate for the occluded vessels.) Exercise is individualized for each client, but people with severe rest pain, venous ulcers, or gangrene should not participate. Other clients with peripheral arterial disease (PAD) can benefit from exercise that is initiated gradually and is slowly increased. Instruct the client to walk until the point of claudication, stop and rest, and then walk a little farther. Eventually, clients are able to walk longer distances as collateral circulation develops. Collaborate with the health care provider and physical therapist in determining an appropriate exercise program. Exercise rehabilitation has been used to relieve symptoms but requires a motivated client, and supervised sessions are generally not reimbursed by health care insurance.

Positioning. Positioning of the client to promote circulation has been somewhat controversial. Some clients have swelling in their extremities. Because swelling prevents arterial flow, feet should be elevated. Teach them to refrain from raising their legs above the heart level because extreme elevation *slows* arterial blood flow to the feet.

In severe cases, clients with PAD and swelling may sleep with the affected limb hanging from the bed, or they may sit upright in a chair for comfort. Instruct all clients with PAD to avoid crossing their legs and refrain from wearing restrictive clothing (e.g., garters to hold up hose, particularly common among older women), which interferes with blood flow.

Promoting Vasodilation. Vasodilation can be achieved by providing warmth to the affected extremity and preventing long periods of exposure to cold. Encourage the client to maintain a warm environment at home and to wear socks or insulated shoes at all times. Caution the client to *never* apply direct heat to the limb, such as with the use of heating pads or extremely hot water. Sensitivity is decreased in the affected limb, and the client may get burned without feeling it.

Encourage clients to prevent exposure of the affected limb to the cold because cold temperatures cause vasoconstriction (decreasing of the diameter of the blood vessels) and therefore decrease arterial blood flow. Clients should also drink adequate fluids to prevent increased blood viscosity.

Emotional stress, caffeine, and nicotine also can cause vasoconstriction. Emphasize that complete abstinence from smoking or chewing tobacco is the most effective method of preventing vasoconstriction. The vasoconstrictive effects of each cigarette may last up to 1 hour after the cigarette is smoked.

Drug Therapy. For clients with chronic PAD, prescribed drugs include hemorheologic and antiplatelet agents. Pentoxifylline (Trental) is a hemorheologic agent that increases the flexibility of red blood cells; it decreases blood viscosity by inhibiting platelet aggregation and decreasing fibrinogen, and thus increases blood flow in the extremities. Many clients report limited improvement in their daily lives after taking pentoxifylline. Moreover, clients with extremely limited endurance for walking have reported improvement to the point that they can perform some activities (e.g., walk to the mailbox or dining room) that were previously impossible.

Antiplatelet agents, such as aspirin (acetylsalicylic acid, Ancasal✱) and clopidogrel (Plavix), are commonly used for clients with PAD. Aspirin 325 or 81 mg daily is typically recommended for all clients with chronic PAD. However, in a trial of *c*lopidogrel versus *a*spirin in *p*atients at *r*isk of *i*schemic *e*vents (CAPRIE), clopidogrel demonstrated improvement over aspirin for risk reduction for myocardial infarction (MI), ischemic stroke, and vascular death, but the difference was slight. Therefore clients with peripheral vascular disease (PVD) with no contraindications to platelet therapy should receive either aspirin or clopidogrel.

Controlling hypertension can improve tissue perfusion by maintaining pressures that are adequate to perfuse the periphery but not constrict the vessels. Teach about the effect of blood pressure on the circulation and instruct in methods of control. For example, clients taking beta blockers may experience drug-related claudication or an exacerbation of symptoms. The health care provider closely monitors clients with PAD who are receiving beta blockers.

Percutaneous Transluminal Angioplasty. A nonsurgical but invasive method of improving arterial flow is **percutaneous transluminal angioplasty (PTA)**. One or more arteries are dilated with a balloon catheter advanced through a cannula, which is inserted into or above an occluded or stenosed artery. When the procedure is successful, it opens the vessel lumen and improves arterial blood flow, creating a smooth inner-vessel surface. In addition, **stents** (wirelike devices) may be used along with the PTA to help keep the vessel open. Clients who are candidates for PTA must have occlusions or stenoses that are accessible to the catheter. The physician often uses PTA for those who are poor surgical candidates, who cannot withstand general anesthesia, or for whom amputation may be inevitable. Reocclusion may occur after this procedure, and the procedure may be repeated. Some clients are occlusion free for up to 3 to 5 years, whereas others may experience reocclusion within a year.

During PTA, intravascular stents may be placed to ensure adequate blood flow in a stenosed vessel. Candidates for intravascular stents are individuals with stenosis of the common or external iliac arteries. Intravascular stents are cost-effective and result in shorter hospital stays and earlier recoveries.

Laser-Assisted Angioplasty. Another invasive procedure is **laser-assisted angioplasty.** A laser probe is advanced through a cannula similar to that used for PTA. Laser-assisted angioplasty is usually reserved for clients with smaller occlusions in the distal superficial femoral, proximal popliteal, and common iliac arteries. Heat from the laser vaporizes the arteriosclerotic plaque to open the occluded or stenosed artery. If significant stenosis remains after the artery is opened, a balloon catheter may be inserted to further dilate the artery. Preparation of the client for PTA or laser-assisted angioplasty is similar to that for diagnostic angiography.

The *priority* for postprocedure nursing care is observing for bleeding at the puncture site. Closely observe vital signs and perform frequent checks of the distal pulses in both limbs. Clients are typically restricted to bedrest, with the limb straight for about 6 to 8 hours before ambulation, unless special collagen plugs are used to seal the vessel. Many receive anticoagulant therapy, such as heparin, during the procedure and for a short time after the procedure. Some type of antiplatelet drug is provided for 1 to 3 months after the procedure, however, clients usually take aspirin on a permanent basis.

Atherectomy. The technique of mechanical rotational abrasive **atherectomy** is used to improve blood flow to ischemic limbs in people with PAD. The rotational atherectomy device (Rotablator) is a high-speed rotary, metal burr ranging in size from 1.25 to 4.5 mm in diameter. The distal half of the burr is embedded with fine abrasive bits, which at rotational speeds of 100,000 to 120,000 rotations per minute result in fine-particle destruction of tissue. The Rotablator is designed to preferentially scrape "hard" surfaces (such as plaque) while minimizing damage to the vessel surface.

SURGICAL MANAGEMENT. Clients with severe rest pain or claudication that interferes with the ability to work or threatens loss of a limb become surgical candidates. **Arterial revascularization** is the surgical procedure most commonly used to increase arterial blood flow in an affected limb.

Surgical procedures are classified as inflow or outflow. Inflow procedures involve bypassing arterial occlusions above the superficial femoral arteries (SFAs). Outflow procedures involve surgical bypassing of arterial occlusions at or below the SFAs. For those who have both inflow and outflow problems, the inflow procedure (for larger arteries) is done before the outflow repair.

Inflow procedures include aortoiliac, aortofemoral, and axillofemoral bypasses. Outflow procedures include femoropopliteal and femorotibial bypasses. Inflow procedures are more successful, with less chance of reocclusion or postoperative ischemia. Outflow procedures are less successful in relieving ischemic pain and are associated with a higher incidence of reocclusion.

Graft materials for the bypasses are selected on an individual basis. For outflow procedures, the preferred graft material is an autogenous saphenous vein. However, these clients can experience coronary artery disease and may need this vein for coronary artery bypass. When the saphenous vein is not usable, the cephalic or basilic arm veins may be used.

Grafts made of synthetic materials, such as polytetrafluoroethylene (PTFE), Gore-Tex, and Dacron, have also been used when autogenous veins were not available. Although synthetic grafts have achieved adequate patency in arteries above the knee, they have failed to achieve satisfactory results in infrapopliteal outflow vessels. In addition, autogenous veins are often not long enough for use in these vessels. Composite grafts constructed from multiple vein segments offer even better patency to arteries below the knee.

Preoperative Care. Preparing the client for surgery is similar to procedures described for general or epidural anesthesia (see Chapter 20). Documentation of vital signs and peripheral pulses provides a baseline of information for comparison during the postoperative phase. Depending on the surgical procedure, the client may have an IV line, urinary catheter, central venous catheter, and/or arterial line. To prevent postoperative infection, antibiotic therapy is typically given before the procedure.

Operative Procedures. The anesthesiologist or nurse anesthetist places the client under general, epidural, or spinal anesthesia. Epidural or spinal induction is preferred for older adults to decrease the risk of cardiopulmonary complications in this age group. If arterial bypass is to be accomplished by autogenous grafts, the surgeon excises the appropriate veins through an incision. The occluded artery is then exposed through an incision, and the conduit veins or synthetic graft material is sutured above and below the occlusion to facilitate blood flow around the occlusion.

For *aortoiliac* and *aortofemoral* bypass surgery, the surgeon makes a midline incision into the abdominal cavity to expose the abdominal aorta, with additional incisions into each groin (Figure 39-5). Graft material is tunneled from the aorta to the groin incisions, where it is sutured in place.

In an *axillofemoral* bypass (Figure 39-6), the surgeon makes an incision beneath the clavicle and tunnels graft material sub-

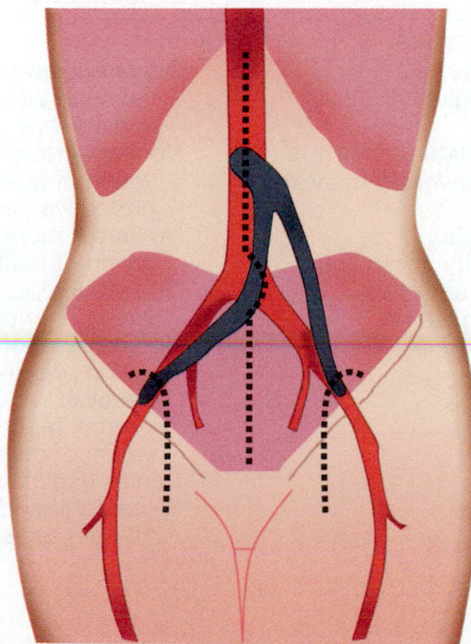

Figure 39-5 ■ In aortoiliac and aortofemoral bypass surgery, a midline incision into the abdominal cavity is required, with an additional incision in each groin.

cutaneously with a catheter from the chest to the iliac crest, into a groin incision, where it is sutured in place. Neither the thoracic nor the abdominal cavity is entered. For that reason, the axillofemoral bypass is used for high-risk clients who cannot tolerate a procedure requiring abdominal surgery.

Postoperative Care. Graft occlusion often occurs within the first 24 hours. Therefore astute nursing care is crucial. The Plan of Care below and on pp. 799-803 highlights the most important aspects of postoperative care.

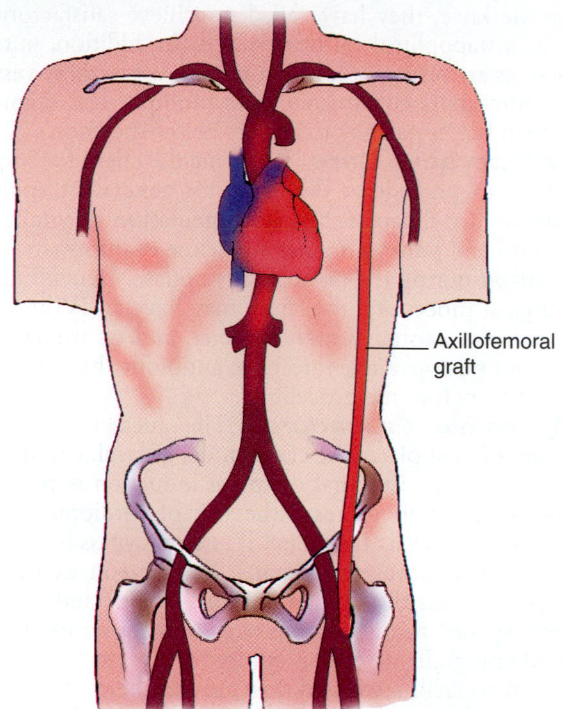

Figure 39-6 ■ An axillofemoral bypass graft.

Assessment for Graft Occlusion. Monitor the patency of the graft by checking the extremity every 15 minutes for the first hour, then hourly, for changes in color, temperature, and pulse intensity. Warmth, redness, and edema of the affected extremity are often expected outcomes of surgery as a result of increased blood flow. Immediately postoperatively, the operating room or postanesthesia care unit (PACU) nurse marks the site where the distal (dorsalis pedis or posterior tibial) pulse is best palpated or heard by Doppler ultrasonography. This information is communicated to the nursing staff on the critical care unit where the client will be sent.

Pain may be one of the first indicators of postoperative graft occlusion. Many people experience a throbbing pain caused by the increased blood flow to the extremity. Because this sensation is different from ischemic pain, be sure to assess the type of pain that the client is experiencing. Pain from occlusion may be masked by patient-controlled analgesia.

Promotion of Graft Patency. To promote graft patency, monitor the client's blood pressure and notify the surgeon if the pressure increases or decreases beyond normal limits. Hypotension may indicate hypovolemia, which can increase the risk of clotting. Range of motion of the affected limb is usually limited, with bending of the hip and knee contraindicated. Consult with the surgeon on a case-by-case basis regarding limitations of movement, including turning. Clients are restricted to bedrest for at least 24 hours postoperatively.

Coughing and deep breathing every 1 to 2 hours and using an incentive spirometer are essential. Clients who have undergone aortoiliac or aortofemoral bypass are allowed nothing by mouth (NPO) for at least 1 day postoperatively. Those who have undergone bypass surgery of the lower extremities not

Text continued on p. 804.

PLAN of CARE — MEDICAL DIAGNOSIS: PERIPHERAL VASCULAR DISEASE

NURSING DIAGNOSIS NO. 1 ■ Chronic Pain

	Expected Outcomes	Nursing Interventions	Rationales
RELATED FACTORS		NIC **Pain Management**	
Chronic physical/psychological disability	No verbal report or observation of alteration in activity level	Perform a comprehensive assessment of pain to include location, characteristics, onset/duration, frequency, quality, intensity or severity of pain, and precipitating factors.	A plan for pain management must be based on the client's unique responses to pain.
DEFINING CHARACTERISTICS	No verbal report or observation of guarding or protective gestures		
Atrophy of involved muscle group	No verbal report or observation of restlessness		
Fear of reinjury	No verbal report or observation of irritability	Determine the needed frequency of assessing client comfort and implement a monitoring plan.	Initial pain management strategies may require frequent evaluation to adjust dosing to maintain adequate comfort.
Altered ability to continue previous activities	No verbal report or observation of self-focusing behavior		
Protective gestures	No verbal report or observation of depression	Reduce or eliminate factors that precipitate or increase the pain experience.	Preventing a pain experience is preferred to trying to control or eliminate pain.
Irritability	Denies experiencing pain greater than 5 on a 0 to 10 pain scale	Select and implement a variety of measures to facilitate pain relief, as appropriate.	Pharmacologic, nonpharmacologic, and interpersonal strategies may provide pain relief depending on the client's unique responses to the therapeutic interventions.
Depression			

PLAN of CARE MEDICAL DIAGNOSIS: PERIPHERAL VASCULAR DISEASE—*cont'd*

NURSING DIAGNOSIS NO. 1 ■ Chronic Pain—*cont'd*

Expected Outcomes	Nursing Interventions	Rationales
	Use pain control measures before pain becomes severe.	Medicating the client in a timely manner prevents pain from reaching acutely unpleasant levels.
	Teach the use of nonpharmacologic techniques before, after and, if possible, during painful activities; before pain occurs or increases; and along with other pain relief measures.	Nonpharmacologic techniques help the client establish a sense of control over his or her pain experience.
	NIC **Analgesic Administration**	
	Administer analgesics around-the-clock.	Administration around-the-clock prevents peaks and troughs of analgesia, especially with severe pain.
	Evaluate the effectiveness of the analgesic at regular frequent intervals after each administration, but especially after the initial dose; also observe for any signs or symptoms of untoward effects.	Frequent evaluation of analgesic effectiveness permits the nurse to adjust the dose and timing interval to the client's need and provides an early warning of adverse responses.
	Document the client's response to the analgesic and any untoward effects.	Documentation provides the health care team with the information needed to evaluate accurately the client's response to the analgesic regimen.
	Implement actions to decrease the untoward effects of analgesics.	Actions taken to prevent the predictable but unwanted effects of narcotic analgesics (e.g., constipation) increase client comfort.
	Collaborate with the physician if drug, dose, route of administration, or interval changes are indicated, making specific recommendations based on equianalgesic principles.	The nurse working with the client is often in the best position to observe his or her response to the analgesic regimen.
	NIC **Progressive Muscle Relaxation**	
	Choose a quiet and comfortable setting, take precautions to prevent interruptions, and seat the client in a reclining chair or otherwise make him or her comfortable.	Ensuring the client's physical comfort and controlling environmental stimuli will aid relaxation efforts.
	Have the client tense, for 5 to 10 sec, each of 8 to 16 major muscle groups.	Tensing the foot muscles for no longer than 5 seconds prevents cramping.
	Terminate the session gradually.	Gradual termination maintains the sense of well-being and relaxation.
	Instruct the client to wear comfortable, nonrestrictive clothing.	The client's personal comfort will facilitate relaxation.

Continued

PLAN of CARE MEDICAL DIAGNOSIS: PERIPHERAL VASCULAR DISEASE—*cont'd*

NURSING DIAGNOSIS NO. 1 ■ Chronic Pain—*cont'd*

	Expected Outcomes	Nursing Interventions	Rationales
		Instruct the client to breathe deeply and to slowly release the breath and tension.	Proper breathing will help the client focus on relaxation rather than on external stimuli.
		Instruct the client to focus on the sensations in the muscles while they are relaxed and while they are tense.	Focusing on the muscle sensations will help build memory that can be called on at later times for relaxation.
		Other Interventions	
		Consider the use of hypnosis, biofeedback, magnetic field therapy, and/or acupuncture to aid in the control of chronic pain.	Cognitive and behavioral strategies may serve as adjuncts to or in place of pharmacologic or surgical interventions for chronic pain. Each therapy has different modes of action, which may or may not benefit the client.
		Refer the client to the Pain Advisory Committee.	The Pain Advisory Committee is a multidisciplinary committee with wide expertise in pain relief interventions.
		Continuing Care Considerations	
		Refer the client to an advanced practice nurse pain specialist, social worker, home care nurse, and/or psychologist, as appropriate.	Health care team members are able to provide continuing support for the client who is facing chronic pain.
		Collaborate with health care team members to secure a referral to a pain management clinic.	Pain management clinics combine many health care disciplines to focus on the management of chronic pain. The client's individual needs and responses to pain are evaluated, and a unique pain management program is initiated and adjusted.

NURSING DIAGNOSIS NO. 2 ■ Ineffective Tissue Perfusion: Peripheral

	Expected Outcomes	Nursing Interventions	Rationales
RELATED FACTORS Hypovolemia Hypervolemia Interruption of flow, arterial Mechanical reduction of venous and/or arterial blood flow Impaired transport of oxygen across the alveolar and/or capillary membrane **DEFINING CHARACTERISTICS** Capillary refill >3 sec Pulses absent or bilaterally unequal Claudication Delayed healing Skin: Pale	Has a pulse that remains strong and equal at all pulse points Has skin with warm undertones No verbal report or observation of delayed healing Denies extremity pain induced by activity No verbal report or observation of irritability	NIC **Circulatory Care: Arterial Insufficiency** D Check peripheral pulses, edema, capillary refill, color, and temperature. D Inspect skin for arterial ulcers or tissue breakdown. Monitor degree of discomfort or pain. D Place the extremity in a dependent position, as appropriate.	 Perform a comprehensive appraisal of peripheral circulation to document arterial sufficiency. Poor oxygenation and nutrition from arterial insufficiency leads to tissure necrosis. Hypoxia from poor oxygenation produces lactic acid, which stimulates pain fibers. A dependent position uses gravity to encourage greater blood flow to the extremity.

D Indicates tasks that can be delegated to unlicensed assistive nursing personnel at the discretion of the nurse.

PLAN of CARE MEDICAL DIAGNOSIS: PERIPHERAL VASCULAR DISEASE—*cont'd*

NURSING DIAGNOSIS NO. 2 ■ Ineffective Tissue Perfusion: Peripheral—*cont'd*

	Expected Outcomes	Nursing Interventions	Rationales
		Administer antiplatelet or anticoagulant medications, as appropriate.	Antiplatelet and anticoagulant medications prevent the formation of blood clots, which further compromise peripheral circulation.
		D Change the client's position at least every 2 hours, as appropriate.	Position changes ensure that pressure does not impede circulation to the tissues.
		Encourage the client to exercise as tolerated.	Exercise causes muscle contraction, which improves blood flow.
		D Place sheepskin under the feet and lower legs, use a footboard/bed cradle at the foot of the bed, and have the client wear well-fitting shoes.	The client's extremity needs protection from injury, which might cause infection.
		D Use additional bed clothes and increase the room temperature, as appropriate.	Additional bed clothes and increased room temperature provide warmth to the extremities.
		Instruct the client regarding smoking, restrictive clothing, exposure to cold temperatures, and crossing of the legs and feet.	The client should avoid actions that interfere with circulation.
		Instruct the client regarding proper foot care.	Proper foot care protects the feet from tissue damage and subsequent infections that heal poorly.
		D Avoid applying direct heat to the extremity.	Poor peripheral circulation causes a diminished ability to determine heat and cold. The client could suffer burns without being aware of it.
		D Maintain adequate hydration.	Adequate hydration decreases blood viscosity, which lowers the risk of thromboembolus.
		Other Interventions	
		Teach the client/family the signs and symptoms of decreased tissue perfusion that need to be reported to the health care provider.	Early intervention may prevent loss of function due to poor tissue perfusion.
		Continuing Care Considerations	
		Monitor the client for adequate tissue perfusion.	Evidence of deteriorating tissue perfusion requires intervention.

NURSING DIAGNOSIS NO. 3 ■ Risk for Injury

	Expected Outcomes	Nursing Interventions	Rationales
RELATED FACTORS		NIC **Surveillance: Safety**	
Tissue hypoxia	Has a pulse that remains strong and equal at all pulse points	Monitor the environment for potential safety hazards.	Removal or modification of the environment will prevent injuries from occurring.
Biochemical, regulatory function (e.g., sensory dysfunction)	No verbal report or observation of delayed healing	Communicate information about the client's risk to other nursing staff.	Caregivers in the environment are better able to prevent injury when high-risk clients are identified and monitored continuously.
Physical (e.g., broken skin, altered mobility)	Denies pain		

Continued

PLAN of CARE — MEDICAL DIAGNOSIS: PERIPHERAL VASCULAR DISEASE—*cont'd*

NURSING DIAGNOSIS NO. 3 ■ Risk for Injury—*cont'd*

	Expected Outcomes	Nursing Interventions	Rationales
		Determine the client's health risk(s), as appropriate.	An appraisal and analysis of the client's risks provide the data for initiating prevention strategies.
		Retrieve and interpret laboratory data; contact the physician, as appropriate.	Laboratory data may provide an early warning of changes in the client's status.
		Compare the client's current status with his or her previous status.	Data comparisons provide ongoing feedback to detect improvements and deterioration in the client's condition.
		Obtain a consultation from the appropriate health care worker to initiate new treatment or to change existing treatments.	Collaboration with health care team members ensures prompt, accurate adjustments to the treatment regimen in an effort to prevent further injury to the client.
		Continuing Care Considerations	
		Educate the client and family about major risk factors and how to avoid/improve them.	The avoidance of injurious agents or activities prevents injury.

NURSING DIAGNOSIS NO. 4 ■ Risk for Peripheral Neurovascular Dysfunction

	Expected Outcomes	Nursing Interventions	Rationales
RELATED FACTORS Trauma or injury Vascular obstruction	Has a pulse that remains strong and equal at all pulse points Has a blood pressure that remains ±10 mm Hg of baseline No verbal report or observation of altered interpretation or response to stimuli No verbal report or observation of guarding or protective gestures Has skin with warm undertones Has a pulse that remains strong and equal at all pulse points No verbal report or observation of delayed healing Denies extremity pain induced by activity No verbal report of altered activity level Denies paresthesias or numbness	NIC **Peripheral Sensation Management**	
		Monitor for paresthesia: numbness, tingling, hyperesthesia, and hypoesthesia.	Changes in sensation are clinical indicators of changes in circulation or nerve functioning.
		D Encourage the client to use the unaffected body part to determine the temperature of food, liquids, bathwater, and so on.	The client's unaffected body part is a better indicator of food or water temperature.
		D Encourage the client to use the unaffected body part to identify the location and texture of objects.	The client's unaffected body part has circulatory and nervous system competence and is better able to discriminate.
		Monitor the fit of bracing devices, prostheses, shoes, and clothing.	Constriction from clothing or abrasion from improperly fitting prostheses can cause skin breakdown.
		D Encourage the use of gloves or other protective clothing over the affected body part.	Protective gear should be worn when the affected body part is in contact with objects that may be potentially hazardous because of their thermal, textural, or other inherent characteristics.
		Avoid or carefully monitor the use of heat or cold, such as heating pads, hot water bottles, and ice packs.	The client/caregiver should monitor heat and cold with a thermometer to prevent thermal injury.
		Monitor for thrombophlebitis and deep vein thrombosis.	Pooling of blood from impaired circulation or impaired mobility facilitates the formation of thrombophlebitis and deep vein thrombosis.

D Indicates tasks that can be delegated to unlicensed assistive nursing personnel at the discretion of the nurse.

PLAN of CARE MEDICAL DIAGNOSIS: PERIPHERAL VASCULAR DISEASE—*cont'd*

NURSING DIAGNOSIS NO. 4 ■ Risk for Peripheral Neurovascular Dysfunction—*cont'd*

Expected Outcomes	Nursing Interventions	Rationales
	Instruct the client to use timed intervals, rather than the presence of discomfort, as a signal to alter position.	Using a time interval for repositioning is a safer standard, because sensation may be diminished.
	Instruct the client or family to examine skin daily for alterations in skin integrity.	Frequent skin inspection may prevent breaks in skin integrity.
	Instruct the client or family to monitor the position of body parts while bathing, sitting, lying, or changing position.	Improper positioning may increase damage to joints or place undue pressure over vulnerable areas of the skin.
	D Use pressure-relieving devices, as appropriate.	Cautious use of pressure-relieving devices may prevent pressure injury.
	Instruct the client to visually monitor the position of body parts.	If proprioception is impaired, the client will need to visually inspect the skin and monitor body position to prevent pressure injury or accidental injuries.
	Other Interventions	
	Assist the client to develop a plan to manage the stress in his or her life.	Emotional stress may cause vasoconstriction.
	Prepare the client for surgical intervention as ordered by the physician.	Procedures such as percutaneous transluminal angioplasty, laser-assisted angioplasty, atherectomy, or arterial revascularization may be needed to restore peripheral tissue perfusion.
	D Instruct the client to avoid crossing the legs.	Crossing the legs will interfere with blood flow.
	Instruct the client to completely abstain from tobacco products.	Nicotine causes vasoconstriction.
	Instruct the client to abstain from caffeine.	Caffeine causes vasoconstriction.
	Continuing Care Considerations	
	Teach the client/family how to assess tissue perfusion to the affected extremity.	Pain, pallor, paresthesias, pulselessness, paralysis, and poikilothermia are indicators of poor tissue perfusion.
	Instruct the client about the therapeutic regimen.	The client needs to follow foot care instructions, cease smoking, and avoid exposure of the affected extremity to heat/cold to prevent further injury to the extremity.
	D Remove safety hazards in the home.	Fall prevention and prevention of injury to the lower extremities is essential if the client has circulatory or nervous system impairments.

CHART 39-8

HOME CARE ASSESSMENT of
Clients with Peripheral Vascular Disease

Assess tissue perfusion to affected extremity(ies), including:
- Distal circulation, sensation, and motion
- Presence of pain, pallor, paresthesias, pulselessness, paralysis, poikilothermia (coolness)
- Ankle-brachial index

Assess adherence to therapeutic regimen, including:
- Following foot care instructions
- Quitting smoking
- Maintaining dietary restrictions
- Participating in exercise regimen
- Avoiding exposure to cold and constrictive clothing

Assess ability to manage wound care and prevent further injury, including:
- Use of compression stockings or compression pumps as directed
- Use of various dressing materials
- Signs and symptoms to report to nurse

Assess coping ability of client and family members.
Assess home environment, including:
- Safety hazards, especially related to falls

CHART 39-9

CLIENT EDUCATION GUIDE
Foot Care for the Client with Peripheral Vascular Disease

- Keep your feet clean by washing them with a mild soap in room-temperature water.
- Keep your feet dry, especially the ankles and between the toes.
- Avoid injury to your feet and ankles. Wear comfortable, well-fitting shoes. Never go without shoes.
- Keep your toenails clean and filed. Have someone cut them if you cannot see them clearly. Cut your toenails straight across.
- To prevent dry, cracked skin, apply a lubricating lotion to your feet.
- Prevent exposure to extreme heat or cold. Never use a heating pad on your feet.
- Avoid constricting garments.
- If a problem develops, see a podiatrist or physician.
- Avoid extended pressure on your feet or ankles, such as occurs when you lean against something.

involving the aorta or abdominal wall (femoropopliteal or femorotibial bypass) may remain NPO status until the first postoperative day when they are allowed clear liquids.

Treatment of Graft Occlusion. If manifestations of graft occlusion occur, notify the surgeon immediately. Perfusion through the graft must be resolved promptly to avoid ischemic injury to the limb. Emergency **thrombectomy** (removal of the clot), which the surgeon may perform at the bedside, is the most common treatment for acute graft occlusion. Thrombectomy is associated with excellent results in prosthetic grafts. Results of thrombectomy in autogenous vein grafts are not as successful and often necessitate graft revision and even replacement.

Local intra-arterial thrombolytic therapy with an agent such as tissue plasminogen activator (t-PA) or an infusion of a platelet inhibitor such as abciximab (ReoPro) may be used for acute graft occlusions in selected clients in settings wherein health care providers are experts on its use. Other antiplatelet drugs, such as the glycoprotein IIb/IIIa inhibitors tirofiban (Aggrastat) or eptifibatide (Integrilin) may be used as alternatives. The physician considers these therapies when the surgical alternative (e.g., thrombectomy with or without graft revision or replacement) carries high morbidity or mortality or when surgery for this type of occlusion has traditionally yielded poor results. When the physician prescribes thrombolytic therapy, closely assess the client for manifestations of bleeding.

Monitoring for Compartment Syndrome. Compartment syndrome occurs when tissue pressure within a confined body space becomes elevated and restricts blood flow. The resultant ischemia can lead to tissue damage and eventually tissue death. Assess the motor and sensory function of the affected extremity. The extremity should also be assessed for worsening pain, fullness, swelling, and tenseness. These symptoms should be reported to the health care provider immediately.

Assessment for Infection. Graft or wound infections can be life threatening and can endanger the client's limb. Use sterile technique when in contact with the incision and observe for symptoms of infection at or around the graft and incision sites. Assess the area for induration, erythema, tenderness, warmth, edema, or drainage. Also monitor for fever and leukocytosis (increased serum white blood cell count). Notify the surgeon if any of these symptoms occur.

Community-Based Care

HOME CARE MANAGEMENT

Peripheral arterial disease (PAD) is a chronic, long-term problem with frequent complications. Clients with PAD may benefit from a case manager who can follow them across the continuum of care. The goal is to maintain the client in the home environment.

Managing the client at home often requires an interdisciplinary team approach. Chart 39-8 outlines the assessment highlights for home care clients with peripheral vascular disease (PVD).

HEALTH TEACHING

Instruct all clients on methods to promote vasodilation. Teach clients to avoid raising their legs above the level of the heart unless venous stasis is also present. Provide written and oral instructions on foot care and methods to prevent injury and ulcer development for all clients (Chart 39-9).

Clients who have had surgery require additional instruction on incision care (see Chapter 22). Encourage all clients to avoid smoking and to limit dietary fat intake to less than 30% of the total daily calories. Remind clients to consume adequate fluids to prevent dehydration.

Clients with chronic arterial obstruction may fear recurrent occlusion or further narrowing of the artery. They often fear that they might lose a limb or become debilitated in other ways. Indeed, chronic PAD may worsen, especially in clients with diabetes mellitus. Reassure them that participation in prescribed exercise, diet, and pharmacologic therapy, along with cessation of smoking, can limit further formation of atherosclerotic plaques.

HEALTH CARE RESOURCES

Clients with arterial compromise may need assistance with activities of daily living (ADLs) if activity is limited by pain. They may need to limit or avoid stair climbing, depending on the severity of disease. Clients who have undergone surgery or need to limit activity usually need temporary help with ADLs.

Clients who must limit activity because of PAD may benefit from the assistance of a home care aide. Those who have undergone surgery may require a home care nurse to assist with incision care. The nurse or case manager arranges for home care resources before the client is discharged.

Critical Thinking Challenge

A 50-year-old African-American man develops diabetes a few years after an injury and is seeking pain relief because of a cramping, burning pain in his calf when he walks any great distance. He describes the pain to be "like a toothache." His blood pressure is 158/90 and his cholesterol is 210.

1. What impact does diabetes have on hypertension?
2. How does diabetes impact the development of peripheral vascular disease?
3. What diagnostic studies would be important for this client?
4. During assessment of this client, what findings would you expect?

evolve For suggested answer guidelines, go to http://evolve.elsevier.com/Iggy/.

ACUTE PERIPHERAL ARTERIAL OCCLUSION

PATHOPHYSIOLOGY

Although chronic peripheral arterial disease (PAD) progresses slowly, the onset of **acute arterial occlusions** may be sudden and dramatic. An embolus is the most common cause of peripheral occlusions, although a local thrombus may be the cause. Occlusion may affect the upper extremities, but it is more common in the lower extremities. Emboli originating from the heart are the most common cause of acute arterial occlusions. Most clients with an embolic occlusion have had an acute myocardial infarction (MI) and/or atrial fibrillation within the preceding weeks.

COLLABORATIVE MANAGEMENT

Clients with an acute arterial occlusion describe severe pain below the level of the occlusion that occurs even at rest. The affected extremity is cool or cold, pulseless, and mottled. Minute areas on the toes may be blackened or gangrenous. Those with acute arterial insufficiency often present with the "six *P*'s" of ischemia:

- *P*ain
- *P*allor
- *P*ulselessness
- *P*aresthesia
- *P*aralysis
- *P*oikilothermia (coolness)

The health care provider must initiate treatment promptly to avoid permanent damage or loss of an extremity. Anticoagulant therapy with unfractionated heparin (UFH; Hepalean✱) is usually the first intervention to prevent further clot formation. A bolus of up to 10,000 units may be prescribed. The client may also undergo angiography.

A surgical thrombectomy or embolectomy with local anesthesia may be performed to remove the occlusion. The physician makes an incision, which is followed by an **arteriotomy** (a surgical opening into an artery). The physician then inserts a Fogarty catheter into the artery and retrieves the embolus. It may be necessary to close the artery with a patch graft.

Postoperatively, monitor the affected extremity for improvement in color, temperature, and pulse, as well as other extremities for manifestations of new thrombi or emboli. Pain should significantly diminish after the surgical procedure, although mild incisional pain remains. Watch closely for complications caused by reperfusing the artery after thrombectomy or embolectomy, which include spasms and swelling of the skeletal muscle. Swelling of the skeletal muscles causing compartment syndrome is characterized by edema, pain on passive movement, poor capillary refill, numbness, and muscle tenseness. Fasciotomy (surgical opening into the tissues) may be necessary to prevent further injury and save the limb.

The use of systemic thrombolytic therapy for acute arterial occlusions has been disappointing because bleeding complications have outweighed the benefits obtained. Local intra-arterial thrombolytic therapy with alteplase (Activase) or t-PA and the use of platelet inhibitors, such as abciximab (ReoPro), have emerged as alternatives to surgical treatment in selected clients in settings where health care providers are familiar with their use and complications. When thrombolytics are given, monitor for manifestations of bleeding, bruising, or hematoma. When a client receives any platelet inhibitor, platelet counts need to be monitored for the first 3, 6, and 12 hours after the start of the infusion. If the platelet count decreases to below 100,000, the abciximab infusion needs to be readjusted or discontinued. If any of these complications occur, notify the physician immediately.

ANEURYSMS OF CENTRAL ARTERIES

PATHOPHYSIOLOGY

An **aneurysm** is a permanent localized dilation of an artery, which enlarges the artery to at least two times its normal diameter. An aneurysm may be described as *fusiform* (a diffuse dilation affecting the entire circumference of the artery) or *saccular* (an outpouching affecting only a distinct portion of the artery). Aneurysms may also be described as true or false. In true aneurysms the arterial wall is weakened by congenital or acquired problems. False aneurysms occur as a result of vessel injury or trauma to all three layers of the arterial wall.

Dissecting hematomas, traditionally called *dissecting aneurysms,* are more accurately described as *aortic dissections* (see the later discussion on p. 809). Aortic dissections differ from aneurysms in that they are formed when blood accumulates in the wall of an artery.

Aneurysms tend to occur at specific anatomic sites (Figure 39-7), most commonly in the abdominal aorta. Aneurysms often occur at a point where the artery is not supported by skeletal muscles or on the lines of curves or flexion in the arterial tree.

An aneurysm forms when the middle layer (media) of the artery is weakened, producing a stretching effect in the inner layer (intima) and outer layers (adventitia) of the artery. As the artery widens, tension in the wall increases and further widening occurs, thus enlarging the aneurysm. Hypertension (high blood pressure) produces more tension and enlargement within the artery. As the aneurysm grows, the risk of arterial rupture increases. When *dissecting* aneurysms occur, the aneurysm enlarges, blood is lost, and blood flow to organs is diminished.

Abdominal aortic aneurysms (AAAs) account for about 75% of all aneurysms. Most of these aneurysms are

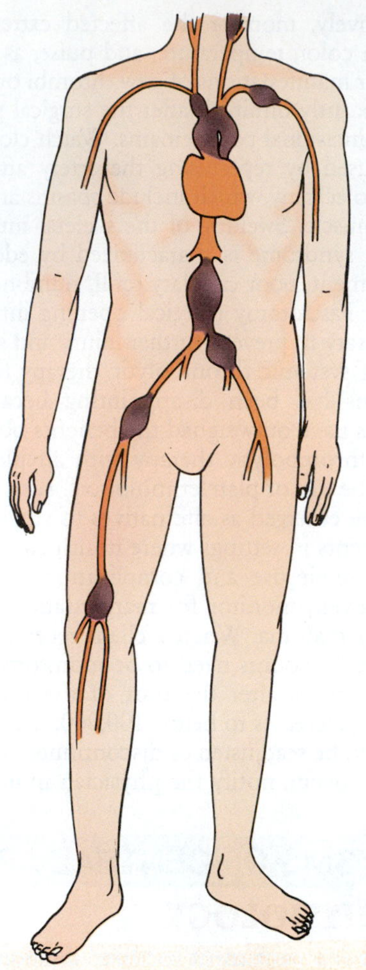

Figure 39-7 ■ Common anatomic sites of arterial aneurysms.

located between the renal arteries and the aortic bifurcation. Of all AAAs greater than 6 cm in diameter, 50% rupture within 1 year; of those aneurysms smaller than 6 cm in diameter, 15% to 20% rupture. Structural changes of the protein matrix in the aortic wall characterize AAAs. Plasma levels of specific biomarkers metalloproteinase-3 and -9 can determine whether AAA repair has been successful. When these markers reappear in the blood following surgery, they may signal a recurrence of the AAA (Sangiorgi et al., 2001).

Thoracic aortic aneurysms account for about 25% of all aneurysms and are frequently misdiagnosed. They are typically discovered when advanced imaging is intended to assess other conditions. Autopsies reveal the diagnosis is missed in about 10% of cases. Thoracic aortic aneurysms commonly develop between the origin of the left subclavian artery and the diaphragm. They are located in the descending, ascending, and transverse sections of the aorta. They can also occur in the aortic arch and are very difficult to manage surgically.

Aneurysms can cause symptoms by exerting pressure on surrounding structures or by rupturing. Rupture of an aneurysm is the most frequent complication and is life threatening because abrupt and massive hemorrhagic shock occurs with the rupture. Thrombi within the wall of an aneurysm can also be the source of emboli in distal arteries below the aneurysm.

Etiology

Atherosclerosis is the most common cause of all aneurysms, with hypertension and cigarette smoking being contributing factors. Syphilis (a sexually transmitted disease), Marfan syndrome (an autoimmune disease), and Ehlers-Danlos syndrome (a rare genetic disorder) are other causes of AAAs.

Incidence/Prevalence

The incidence of AAAs, estimated between 30 and 66 per 1000 persons, is increasing in the Western world. About 15,800 people in the United States die annually of abdominal aneurysms, making it the thirteenth leading cause of death in the United States. (National Heart, Lung, and Blood Institute, 2002). Thoracic aortic aneurysms occur most often in older adults and have a 50% mortality rate even with surgical intervention. AAAs are more common in men than in women (4:1).

◆COLLABORATIVE MANAGEMENT

◆Assessment

Most clients with abdominal or thoracic aneurysms are asymptomatic when their aneurysms are first discovered by routine examination or during radiographic study performed for another reason.

PHYSICAL ASSESSMENT

Because there may be symptoms, assess clients with a known or suspected *abdominal aortic aneurysm (AAA)* for abdominal, flank, or back pain. Pain related to an AAA is usually steady with a gnawing quality, is unaffected by movement, and may last for hours or days.

A pulsation in the upper abdomen slightly to the left of the midline between the xiphoid process and the umbilicus may be present. A detectable aneurysm is at least 5 cm in diameter. Auscultate for a bruit over the mass but avoid palpating the mass because it may be tender and there is a risk of rupture.

Although some clients have symptoms when the aneurysm is intact, many are asymptomatic until the time of rupture. If expansion and impending rupture of an AAA are suspected, assess for sudden and severe pain of sudden onset in the back or lower abdomen, which may radiate to the groin, buttocks, or legs.

Clients with a rupturing AAA are critically ill and in hemorrhagic (hypovolemic) shock. Signs include hypotension, diaphoresis, mental obtundation, oliguria, and dysrhythmias. Retroperitoneal hemorrhage is manifested by hematomas in the flanks. Rupture into the abdominal cavity causes abdominal distention.

When *a thoracic aortic aneurysm* is suspected, assess for back pain and manifestations of compression of the aneurysm on adjacent structures. Signs include shortness of breath, hoarseness, and difficulty swallowing. Thoracic aneurysms are not often detected by physical assessment, but occasionally a mass may be visible above the suprasternal notch. The client with suspected rupture of a thoracic aneurysm is assessed for sudden and excruciating back or chest pain. Rupture of a thoracic aneurysm is also indicated by hemorrhagic shock (see Chapter 40).

DIAGNOSTIC ASSESSMENT

An abdominal x-ray or a lateral x-ray of the spine often shows an AAA. The "eggshell" appearance of the aneurysm is essentially diagnostic.

Computed tomography (CT) scanning is the standard tool for assessing the size and location of an abdominal or thoracic aneurysm. A thoracic aneurysm can be diagnosed by chest x-ray. Aortic arteriography is usually performed for clients who are to undergo surgical repair of a thoracic aneurysm.

Ultrasonography is a noninvasive technique that provides an accurate diagnosis, as well as information about the size and location of an AAA.

Interventions

The size of the aneurysm and the presence of symptoms are the most important parameters in the determination of treatment.

NONSURGICAL MANAGEMENT. The goal of nonsurgical management is to monitor the growth of the aneurysm and maintain the blood pressure at a normal level to decrease the risk of rupture.

Because elevated blood pressure can increase the rate of aneurysmal enlargement, hypertension is an important risk factor for rupture. Clients with hypertension are treated with antihypertensives to decrease the rate of enlargement and the risk for early rupture.

For clients with small or asymptomatic aneurysms, frequent CT scans are necessary to monitor the growth of the aneurysm. Emphasize the importance of following through with scheduled tests to monitor the growth. Also explain the clinical manifestations of aneurysms that need to be promptly reported.

SURGICAL MANAGEMENT. Surgical management of an aneurysm may be an elective or an emergency procedure. For clients with either a *rupturing* abdominal aortic or a thoracic aneurysm, emergency surgery is performed.

Clients with an abdominal aortic aneurysm (AAA) 6 cm in diameter or wider usually undergo elective surgery. Some surgeons favor surgical treatment for clients with aneurysms 4 to 6 cm in diameter if the client is in good health. Clients in good health with aneurysms smaller than 4 cm and clients in poor health with aneurysms 4 to 6 cm in diameter undergo nonsurgical treatment until the aneurysm reaches 6 cm.

Clients with thoracic aortic aneurysms measuring 7 cm or more in diameter and clients with smaller aneurysms that are producing symptoms are advised to have elective surgery. Clients with aneurysms smaller than 7 cm in diameter that are not causing symptoms are treated nonsurgically until symptoms occur or the aneurysm enlarges to 7 cm.

The most common procedure performed for clients with an AAA has traditionally been an AAA resection or repair **(aneurysmectomy).** The mortality rate for elective AAA resection is 2% to 5%. The mortality rate for emergency surgery for expanding AAAs is 5% to 15% and 50% for those that have ruptured.

Newer technology, such as endothelial stent grafts, has improved mortality rates and shortened the hospital stay for selected clients who need aneurysm repair. The stents (wirelike devices) are inserted percutaneously (through the skin), avoiding abdominal incisions and therefore decreasing the risk of a prolonged postoperative recovery. Postoperative care is similar to care required following an arteriogram (angiogram).

Abdominal Aortic Aneurysm Resection. In an AAA resection, the physician excises the aneurysm from the abdominal aorta to prevent or repair the rupture. The goal is to secure stable aortic integrity and tissue perfusion throughout the body.

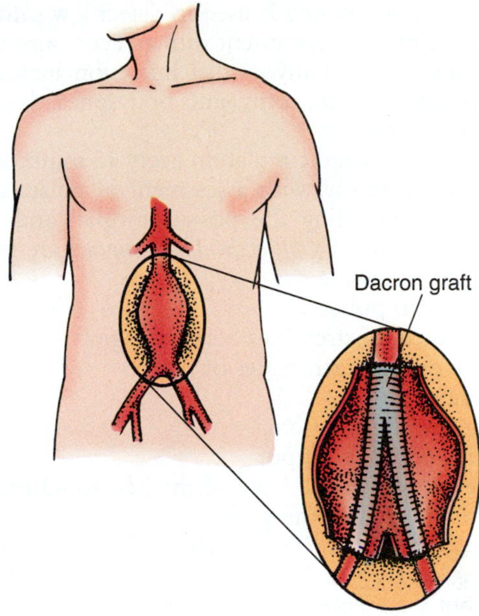

Figure 39-8 ■ Surgical repair of abdominal aortic aneurysm with a woven Dacron graft.

Preoperative Care. Interventions are similar to those for clients undergoing surgery with general anesthesia (see Chapter 20). A bowel preparation and emphasis on coughing and deep breathing are very important. Because significant blood loss may occur during AAA resection, clients planning elective surgery may be advised to bank their blood for autologous (self) transfusions postoperatively.

Assess all peripheral pulses to serve as a baseline for comparison postoperatively. Use a marker to note where the pulse is palpated or heard by Doppler ultrasonography to facilitate locating the pulse postoperatively.

Clients with ruptured aneurysms are brought to the operating suite directly from the emergency department. Preoperative care of clients with ruptured aneurysms involves administration of large volumes of IV fluids to maintain tissue perfusion.

Operative Procedures. The surgeon makes a midline abdominal incision from the xiphoid process to the symphysis pubis, or a wide transverse incision from flank to flank, to expose the aneurysm. Clamps are applied just above and just below the aneurysm, the aneurysm is excised, and a preclotted Dacron graft is sutured in an end-to-end fashion (Figure 39-8).

Postoperative Care. Immediately postoperatively, the client is typically admitted to a critical care unit for 24 hours, depending on his or her age and condition. In addition to providing the routine postoperative care discussed in Chapter 22, assess for and assist in prevention of the postoperative complications that can occur after an AAA repair. Complications include the following:

- Myocardial infarction
- Graft occlusion or rupture causing hemorrhage
- Hypovolemia and/or renal failure
- Respiratory distress
- Paralytic ileus

During the immediate postoperative period, the client's blood pressure is monitored with an arterial catheter. Continuous cardiac monitoring is used to detect any dysrhythmias.

Hemodynamic monitoring is used to detect low cardiac output and other findings consistent with an acute *myocardial infarction.* Other signs of myocardial infarction include chest pain, shortness of breath, complaints of dyspnea, diaphoresis, anxiety, and restlessness.

Assess vital signs and circulation every 15 minutes for the first hour, then hourly, with assessment of pulses distal to the graft site (including the posterior tibial and dorsalis pedis pulses). Signs of *graft occlusion or rupture* are reported, including the following:

- Changes in pulses
- Cool to cold extremities below the graft
- White or blue extremities or flanks
- Severe pain
- Abdominal distention
- Decreased urine output

Limit elevation of the head of the bed to 45 degrees or less to avoid flexion of the graft.

Hypovolemia and renal failure may occur because of blood loss during surgery or before if rupture occurred. Assess urine output via a Foley catheter hourly. If urine output is less than 50 mL/hr, notify the surgeon. Although advances in surgical technique have decreased the risk of renal failure after clamping during surgery, renal failure may occur. Renal failure caused by acute tubular necrosis is more common after emergency surgery. In addition to monitoring urine output, in collaboration with the physician, monitor serum creatinine and blood urea nitrogen (BUN) levels daily.

Assess respiratory rate and depth every hour and auscultate breath sounds every 4 hours to monitor for *respiratory complications.* The client may be maintained on a ventilator, however, early extubation is preferred if the client is stable. Opioids are administered for pain, as prescribed. If the client remains intubated, turning and suctioning are provided as needed. Firm abdominal support of the incision with a pillow or bath blanket during coughing exercises is needed for support. After extubation, assist the client to a bedside chair within 24 hours. Early mobility decreases the risk of atelectasis and deep vein thrombosis.

Paralytic ileus after AAA repair is expected for 2 to 3 days. Clients have a nasogastric tube set to low suction until bowel sounds return. Listen for bowel sounds every 8 hours and report their return to the physician. Prolonged absence of bowel sounds and distention may indicate a prolonged ileus or a bowel infarction.

Thoracic Aortic Aneurysm Repair. Repair of thoracic aneurysms is tailored to each client; the procedure depends on the type and location of the aneurysm. Total cardiopulmonary bypass (CPB) is necessary for excision of aneurysms in the ascending aorta, and partial bypass is often used during excision of aneurysms in the descending aorta.

Preoperative Care. The care of the client undergoing thoracic aneurysm resection is similar to that provided for the client having thoracic surgery.

Operative Procedures. The surgeon uses either a thoracotomy or a median sternotomy approach to enter the thoracic cavity. The surgeon exposes the aneurysm and excises it. After excising the aneurysm, the surgeon usually sews a Dacron graft or prosthesis onto the aorta. Saccular aneurysms, which have an outpouching from a distinct portion of the arterial wall, can sometimes be removed without resection of the aorta. Newer procedures do not remove the aneurysm. Instead, the surgeon cuts into the aneurysm and inserts a graft. The walls of the aneurysm are wrapped around the graft for stability.

Postoperative Care. The care of a client who has undergone thoracic aneurysm repair is similar to that of clients after other chest surgery. Clients who have undergone cardiopulmonary bypass (CPB) receive care similar to that described in Chapter 41. Assess for and assist in the prevention of postoperative complications that can occur after a thoracic aneurysm repair. Complications include:

- Hemorrhage
- Ischemic colitis
- Cerebral and spinal cord ischemia (causing paraplegia)
- Respiratory distress
- Cardiac dysrhythmias

Assess vital signs at least hourly, reporting any signs of *hemorrhage* (e.g., a decrease in blood pressure, an increase in pulse rate, rapid respirations, diaphoresis) to the physician immediately. Assess for bleeding or separation at the graft site by noting significant increases in chest drainage from the chest tubes.

Inadvertent interruption of the blood supply to the spinal cord during thoracic aneurysm repair can result in *paraplegia.* Assess the client hourly for sensation and motion in all extremities and report deficits immediately.

After thoracic aneurysm repair, clients are especially susceptible to *respiratory distress* from atelectasis or pneumonia. This problem occurs as a result of both CPB and incisional discomfort. Both atelectasis and pneumonia may cause shallow breathing and poor cough effort. These clients are often maintained on a ventilator, at least overnight, after surgery. For clients with a median sternotomy, the surgeon firmly splints the incision to prevent separation of the sternum.

Assess all clients recovering from thoracic aneurysm repair for cardiac *dysrhythmias.* The stress of the thoracic surgery, added to the increased incidence of arteriosclerosis in this group, may predispose these clients to a myocardial infarction, cardiac dysrhythmias, or heart failure.

Endovascular Repair of Abdominal Aortic Aneurysms. The repair of AAAs with **endovascular stent grafts** provides an alternative choice for some clients. Clients selected for endovascular repair of AAAs are generally at high risk for major abdominal surgery. Some clients with AAAs may be referred for endovascular repair before the aneurysm reaches the recommended diameter for elective surgery.

There are different designs of endovascular stent grafts for use, depending on the anatomic involvement of the aneurysm. The stent graft is flexible with either Dacron or polytetrafluoroethylene (PTFE) material. It is inserted through a skin incision into the femoral artery by way of a catheter-based system. The catheter is advanced to a level above the aneurysm, away from the renal arteries. The graft is released from the catheter, and the stent graft is deployed into place with a series of hooks. A defined proximal and distal neck is needed for tight seating of the stent to prevent leakage. This procedure is done in collaboration with the vascular surgeon, interventional radiologist, operating room team, and at some centers, vascular medicine physician.

The endovascular repair of AAAs has decreased the

length of hospital stay for clients requiring repair of abdominal aneurysms; however, the client needs to be closely monitored, in the hospital and at home, for the development of complications following the procedure. Expert nursing care is required to allow for early identification of problems and complications that can be resolved in a timely fashion. In addition, expert nursing skills are needed for the coordination and collaboration required for discharge planning and follow-up care for clients at home (see the Clinical Pathway on the Evolve website).

Endovascular stent repair is not without complications. Complications include the need for conversion from an endovascular repair to open surgical repair of the aneurysm, bleeding, aneurysm rupture, peripheral embolization, and misdeployment of the stent graft. All of these complications require surgical intervention.

Community-Based Care

Most clients are discharged to home after aneurysm repair. However, in the absence of family or other support systems, the postoperative client may be discharged to an extended (long-term) care facility for rehabilitation.

If discharged to home, the client must follow the instructions provided by the nurse regarding activity level and incisional care. Because stair climbing may be restricted initially, the client may need a bedside commode if the bathroom is inaccessible.

For clients who have not undergone surgical aneurysm repair, the teaching plan emphasizes the importance of compliance with the schedule of computed tomography (CT) scanning to monitor the size of the aneurysm. Educate the client receiving treatment for hypertension about the importance of continuing to take prescribed medication. Instruct the client and family or significant others about the signs and symptoms that must promptly be reported to the health care provider, which include the following:

- Abdominal fullness or pain, or back pain
- Chest or back pain, shortness of breath, difficulty swallowing, or hoarseness

Teach the client who has undergone repair of the aneurysm about activity restrictions, wound care, and pain management. Clients may not engage in activities that involve lifting heavy objects (usually more than 15 to 20 pounds [6.8 to 9.1 kg]) for 6 to 12 weeks postoperatively. Advise them to use discretion in activities that involve pulling, pushing, or straining. Clients who usually engage in vigorous activities should discuss them with their health care provider. Most individuals are restricted from driving a car for several weeks after discharge.

Clients who have not undergone aneurysm repair may fear rupture and subsequent death. Reinforce the rationales for CT monitoring of the size of the aneurysm and for controlling hypertension and encourages clients to verbalize their fears.

In collaboration with the case manager or social worker, assess the availability of transportation to and from appointments for clients needing CT monitoring. Clients who have undergone surgery may require the services of a home care nurse for assistance with dressing changes. A home care aide may be needed to assist with activities of daily living (ADLs).

ANEURYSMS OF THE PERIPHERAL ARTERIES

PATHOPHYSIOLOGY

Although femoral and popliteal aneurysms are relatively uncommon, they are often associated with an aneurysm in another location of the arterial tree. To detect a popliteal aneurysm, a pulsating mass is seen in the popliteal space. To detect a femoral aneurysm, observe a pulsatile mass over the femoral artery. Both extremities are evaluated because more than one femoral or popliteal aneurysm may be present.

COLLABORATIVE MANAGEMENT

The client may exhibit symptoms of limb ischemia, including diminished or absent pulses, cool to cold skin, and pain. Pain may also be present if an adjacent nerve is compressed. The recommended treatment for either type of aneurysm, regardless of the size, is surgery because of the risk of thromboembolic complications associated with their presence.

To treat a femoral aneurysm, the physician excises the aneurysm and restores circulation using a Dacron graft or an autogenous saphenous vein graft. Most surgeons prefer to bypass rather than resect a popliteal aneurysm.

Postoperatively, monitor for lower limb ischemia. Palpate pulses below the graft to assess graft patency. Often, Doppler ultrasonography is necessary to assess blood flow when pulses are not palpable. Sudden development of pain or discoloration of the extremity is reported immediately to the physician because it may indicate graft occlusion.

AORTIC DISSECTION

PATHOPHYSIOLOGY

Aortic dissection has traditionally been referred to as a dissecting aneurysm. However, because this condition is more accurately described as a dissecting hematoma, the term *aortic dissection* has gained favor.

Aortic dissection is thought to be caused by a sudden tear in the aortic intima, opening the way for blood to enter the aortic wall. Degeneration of the aortic media might be a prerequisite for this condition, with hypertension being an important contributing factor.

Aortic dissection is a relatively common event, occurring in at least 2000 people in the United States annually. It is often associated with connective tissue disorders such as Marfan syndrome (see Chapter 24). It also occurs in older people, peaking in adults in their 50s and 60s, and in women in their third trimester of pregnancy. Because the circulation of any major artery arising from the aorta can be impaired in clients with aortic dissection, this condition is highly lethal and represents an emergency situation.

Proximal dissections occur almost twice as often as distal dissections. Although the ascending aorta and descending thoracic aorta are the most common sites, dissections can also occur in the abdominal aorta and other arteries.

COLLABORATIVE MANAGEMENT

The most common presenting symptom is pain, with painless dissection occurring rarely. The pain is described as "tearing," "ripping," and "stabbing" and tends to move from its point of origin. Depending on the site of dissection, the client may feel pain in the anterior chest, back, neck, throat, jaw, or teeth.

Diaphoresis, nausea, vomiting, faintness, and apprehension are also common. Blood pressure is usually elevated unless complications, such as cardiac tamponade or rupture, have occurred. A decrease or absence of peripheral pulses is common, as is aortic regurgitation, which is characterized by a musical murmur better heard along the right sternal border. Neurologic deficits, such as an altered level of consciousness, paraparesis, and strokes, can also occur.

Chest x-ray, Doppler echocardiogram, computed tomography (CT), and aortic angiography may be used to confirm the diagnosis.

EMERGENCY CARE: AORTIC DISSECTION

The following are goals of emergency treatment:

- Elimination of pain
- Reduction of systolic blood pressure to 100 to 120 mm Hg
- Decrease in the velocity of left ventricular ejection

The physician prescribes IV sodium nitroprusside (Nitropress) or fenoldopam (Corlopam) by continuous drip initially to lower the blood pressure. If this regimen is ineffective, nicardipine hydrochloride (Cardene) may be used.

Subsequent treatment depends on the location of the dissection. Generally, clients receive continued medical treatment for uncomplicated distal dissections and surgical treatment for proximal dissections. For clients receiving long-term medical treatment, the systolic blood pressure must be maintained at or below 130 to 140 mm Hg. Beta blockers (propranolol) and calcium channel antagonists are indicated.

Clients receiving surgical intervention for a proximal dissection always require cardiopulmonary bypass (CPB) (see Chapter 41). The surgeon excises the intimal tear and obliterates entry in the false opening by suturing edges of the dissected aorta. Usually, a prosthetic graft is used.

Critical Thinking Challenge

A middle-aged client arrives at the emergency department complaining of a terrible pain described as a "ripping" sensation in his mid back. He is diaphoretic and very apprehensive. You note his blood pressure is 190/120 and have trouble finding any pedal pulses.

1. What additional assessment data should you collect at this time?
2. What are the priority nursing actions for this client?
3. What collaborative problems are priorities?
4. Should you delegate vital sign monitoring to unlicensed assistive personnel? Why or why not?

evolve For suggested answer guidelines, go to http://evolve.elsevier.com/Iggy/.

BUERGER'S DISEASE

PATHOPHYSIOLOGY

Buerger's disease (thromboangiitis obliterans) is a relatively uncommon occlusive disease limited to the medium and small arteries and veins. The distal upper and lower limbs are the most frequently affected. Typically, Buerger's disease is identified in young adult men who smoke. Larger arteries, such as the femoral and brachial, become involved in the late stages of the disease. The veins are less commonly involved.

The disease often extends into the perivascular tissues, resulting in fibrosis and scarring that binds the artery, vein, and nerve firmly together. For people who have this disease, cessation of cigarette smoking usually arrests the disease process, but persistence in smoking causes occlusion in the more proximal vessels.

The cause of Buerger's disease is unknown, although there is a strong association with tobacco smoking. A familial or genetic predisposition and autoimmune etiologic factors are also possible.

COLLABORATIVE MANAGEMENT

Assessment

The first clinical manifestation of Buerger's disease is usually claudication (pain in the muscles resulting from an inadequate blood supply) of the arch of the foot. Intermittent claudication may occur in the lower extremities. The pain may be ischemic, occurring in the digits while the client is at rest. Often, there is an aching pain that is more severe at night. Paroxysmal shocklike pain can be the result of ischemic neuropathy. Clients often experience increased sensitivity to cold and complain of coldness and numbness. On physical examination, pulses are often diminished in the distal extremities, and the extremities are cool and red or cyanotic in the dependent position.

A diagnosis of Buerger's disease is commonly based on a physical finding of peripheral ischemia, often in association with migratory superficial phlebitis. Ulcerations and gangrene may be seen in the digits. The ulcerations are usually sharply demarcated. The gangrenous lesion can be small or can affect the entire digit.

Arteriograms can be useful in delineating the degree of disease in the arteries. Commonly, arteriography reveals multiple segmental occlusions in the smaller arteries of the forearm, hand, leg, and foot. Plethysmographic studies of the fingers or toes may be diagnostic of the disease in the early stages. These studies can also be useful in following the progression of the disease in more proximal arteries.

Interventions

Nursing interventions are directed at the following:

- Preventing the progression of the disease
- Avoiding vasoconstriction
- Promoting vasodilation
- Relieving pain
- Treating ulceration and gangrene

To prevent the progression of Buerger's disease, complete abstinence from tobacco in all forms is essential. Extreme cold or prolonged exposure to cold should be avoided to prevent vasoconstriction. Instruct the client about medications that are prescribed for vasodilation. The treatment for Buerger's disease is similar to that for peripheral arterial disease (PAD) (see Interventions [Peripheral Arterial Disease], p. 796).

SUBCLAVIAN STEAL

PATHOPHYSIOLOGY

Subclavian steal occurs in the upper extremities from a subclavian artery occlusion or stenosis. The result is altered blood flow and ischemia in the arm. Subclavian steal can occur in people at any age but is more common in those with risk factors for atherosclerosis. Symptoms include tiredness in the arm with exertion, paresthesias, dizziness, and exercise-induced pain in the forearm when the arms are elevated.

COLLABORATIVE MANAGEMENT

Physical examination usually reveals a significant difference in the blood pressures between the arms. A difference greater than 20 mm Hg is considered significant. Another important finding is a subclavian bruit, which can occur on the affected side. The subclavian pulse may be decreased on the occluded side compared with the opposite side. The affected arm may also be discolored or cyanotic; however, this finding generally occurs only in severe cases.

Surgery is the recommended intervention for cyanosis or pain. One of three procedures may be used: endarterectomy of the subclavian artery, carotid-subclavian bypass, or dilation of the subclavian artery with placement of a vascular stent.

Postoperative nursing care of the client includes monitoring of the arterial flow in the affected arm. Check brachial and radial pulses frequently and observe for ischemic changes. Observe the arm for edema, redness, or any other signs.

THORACIC OUTLET SYNDROME

PATHOPHYSIOLOGY

Thoracic outlet syndrome is a compression of the subclavian artery at the thoracic outlet by anatomic structures, such as a rib or muscle. The arterial wall may be damaged, producing thrombosis or embolization to distal arteries of the arms. The three common sites of compression in the thoracic outlet are as follows:

- The interscalene triangle
- Between the coracoid process of the scapula and the pectoralis minor tendon
- Most commonly, the costoclavicular space

COLLABORATIVE MANAGEMENT

Thoracic outlet syndrome is more common in females and in people whose occupations require holding their arms up or leaning over, such as baseball players, golfers, or swimmers. It is also seen in clients who have had trauma such as whiplash or after clavicular fracture. Clients generally complain of neck, shoulder, and arm pain that may be intermittent. They may also have numbness and moderate edema of the extremity. The pain and numbness are worse when the arm is placed in certain positions, such as over the head or out to the side. Clients may have overdeveloped neck and shoulder muscles, and the affected arm may appear cyanotic.

Treatment includes physical therapy, exercises, and avoiding aggravating positions, such as elevating the arms. Surgical treatment involves resection of the anatomic structure that is compressing the artery. Surgery is performed only if a client has severe pain, has lost hand function, or is responding poorly to conservative treatment.

RAYNAUD'S PHENOMENON

PATHOPHYSIOLOGY

Raynaud's phenomenon is caused by vasospasm of the arterioles and arteries of the upper and lower extremities, usually unilaterally. *Raynaud's disease* occurs bilaterally. The two terms are sometimes used interchangeably, but although they are related, there are some differences. Raynaud's phenomenon usually occurs in people older than 30 years of age; Raynaud's disease can occur between the ages of 17 and 50 years of age. Raynaud's phenomenon can occur in either gender, but Raynaud's disease is more common in women.

The pathophysiology is the same for both entities. The etiology is unknown. Clients often have an associated systemic connective tissue disease, such as systemic lupus erythematosus or progressive systemic sclerosis (see Chapter 24).

As a result of vasospasm, the cutaneous vessels are constricted, and blanching of the extremity occurs, followed by cyanosis. When the vasospasm is relieved, the tissue becomes reddened or hyperemic. The client's extremities are numb and cold, and he or she may complain of pain and swelling. Ulcers may also be present. These attacks are intermittent and can be aggravated by cold or stress. In severe cases, the attack lasts longer and gangrene of the digits can occur.

COLLABORATIVE MANAGEMENT

Treatment involves relieving or preventing the vasoconstriction by drug therapy. Commonly prescribed drugs are nifedipine (Procardia), cyclandelate (Cyclospasmol), and phenoxybenzamine (Dibenzyline). These vasodilating agents may help to relieve the symptoms, but they can cause uncomfortable side effects, such as facial flushing, headaches, hypotension, and dizziness.

For severe symptoms that cannot be alleviated by drugs, a lumbar sympathectomy can be performed. The physician cuts the sympathetic nerve fibers that cause vasoconstriction of blood vessels in the lower extremities. This method is effective for foot symptoms. For the upper extremities, a similar procedure–sympathetic ganglionectomy–may provide symptom relief. The long-term effectiveness of these treatments is questionable.

Education of the client is important in prevention of complications. Explain methods to prevent vasoconstriction, such as minimizing exposure to cold, smoking cessation (if client smokes), and decreasing stress. The client is instructed to wear warm clothes, socks, or gloves when exposed to cool or cold temperatures. He or she should keep the home at a comfortably warm temperature and wear gloves to the grocery store. Help the client identify stressors and provide suggestions for reducing them. (See Chapter 24 for further discussion of Raynaud's disease as it relates to connective tissue disease.)

POPLITEAL ENTRAPMENT

Popliteal entrapment causes ischemic symptoms in the affected leg or foot because of anatomic compression of the popliteal artery. Popliteal entrapment occurs in young people, most often in men complaining of intermittent claudication of one or both extremities.

Physical examination may reveal ischemic changes of the affected extremity, with normal function of the unaffected limb. When the client is at rest, the nurse may note diminished distal pulses, although this is a rare finding. Diagnosis of popliteal entrapment is possible only after an accurate history, physical examination, and arteriography.

The recommended treatment is surgical repair of the anatomic compression. Reconstruction of the popliteal artery may be necessary to restore arterial blood flow to the limb. Nursing care involves preventing general postoperative complications and evaluating the patency of the graft or artery postoperatively. Observe for ischemic changes and evaluate distal pulses at frequent intervals postoperatively.

PERIPHERAL VENOUS DISEASE

To function properly, veins must be patent (unobstructed) with competent valves. Vein function also necessitates the assistance of the surrounding muscle beds to help pump blood toward the heart. If one or more veins are not operating efficiently, they become distended and clinical manifestations occur.

Three distinct phenomena alter the blood flow in veins:

- Thrombus formation *(venous thrombosis)* can lead to pulmonary embolism (PE), a life-threatening complication (see Chapter 35). **Venous thromboembolism (VTE)** is the current term that includes both deep vein thrombosis and PE.
- Defective valves lead to *venous insufficiency* and *varicose veins,* which are not life threatening but are problematic.
- Lack of skeletal muscle contractility

Venous Thromboembolism

PATHOPHYSIOLOGY

Venous thromboembolism (VTE) constitutes one of health care's greatest challenges, and includes both thrombus and embolus complications. A **thrombus** (also called a thrombosis) is a blood clot believed to result from an endothelial injury, venous stasis, or hypercoagulability. The thrombosis may not be specifically attributable to one element, or it may involve all three elements. It is often associated with an inflammatory process. When a thrombus develops, inflammation can occur around the clot, thickening the vein wall and consequently leading to embolization (the formation of an **embolus**).

Thrombophlebitis refers to a thrombus that is associated with inflammation; **phlebothrombosis** is a thrombus without inflammation. Thrombophlebitis can occur in superficial veins; however, it most frequently occurs in the deep veins of the lower extremities.

Deep vein thrombophlebitis, commonly referred to as **deep vein thrombosis (DVT),** not only is more common but also is more serious than superficial thrombophlebitis because it presents a greater risk for **pulmonary embolism (PE),** in which a dislodged blood clot travels to the pulmonary artery. DVT develops most often in the legs, but it is becoming more frequently seen due to increased use of central venous devices (Crowther & McCourt, 2004).

Thrombus formation has been associated with stasis of blood flow, endothelial injury, and/or hypercoagulability, known as **Virchow's triad.** The precise cause of these events remains unknown; however, a few predisposing factors have been identified. Thrombosis has commonly occurred in people undergoing certain surgical procedures.

Etiology

The highest incidence of clot formation occurs in clients who have undergone hip surgery, total knee replacement, or open prostate surgery. Other conditions that seem to promote thrombus formation are pregnancy, ulcerative colitis, heart failure, and immobility. Immobility occurs during prolonged bedrest, such as when a client is confined to bed during the perioperative period. Individuals who sit for long periods of time, such as on an airplane, are also at risk for VTE.

Phlebitis (vein inflammation) associated with invasive procedures, such as IV therapy, can predispose clients to thrombosis. Severe infections, systemic lupus erythematosus, polycythemia vera, oral contraceptives, and trauma have also been linked to thrombosis. Cancer, especially adenocarcinoma of the visceral organs, is the most common malignancy associated with DVT. Cancer has been discovered in nearly all people with fatal PEs who did not have other predisposing factors (Horlander et al., 2003).

Incidence/Prevalence

2.5 million individuals in the United States are affected by DVT each year (Day, 2003). It is estimated that 50,000 to 100,000 individuals die each year of pulmonary embolism (Horlander et al., 2003). The largest number of deaths occurred in the 75- to 84-year-old age-group. Black individuals have a high rate of death resulting from PE due to predisposing risk factors and coexisting diseases, such as certain cancers, chronic renal and cardiac failure, and an increased prevalence in smoking.

> **WOMEN'S HEALTH CONSIDERATIONS**
>
> The rate of diagnosis for DVT and PE is higher in women than in men. There have been suggestions that a possible diagnostic disparity exists among men and women for DVT and PE. However, in the United States, Stein and colleagues (2003) found a comparable effort was made to diagnose these venous disorders equally among genders. Duration of hospital stays was comparable with a primary discharge diagnosis of DVT and PE.

HEALTH PROMOTION/ILLNESS PREVENTION

In the community, if a person has a history of VTE, the following precautions should be taken:

- Avoid oral contraceptives.
- Drink adequate fluids to avoid dehydration.
- Exercise legs during long periods of bedrest or sitting.

In the inpatient setting, interventions to prevent VTE include the following:

- Client education
- Leg exercises
- Early ambulation
- Adequate hydration
- Graduated compression stockings (e.g., TEDs)
- Intermittent pneumatic compression, such as sequential compression devices (SCDs)
- Venous plexus foot pump

COLLABORATIVE MANAGEMENT

Assessment

People with DVT may have symptoms or may be asymptomatic. The classic signs and symptoms of DVT are calf or groin tenderness and pain, and sudden onset of unilateral swelling of the leg. Pain in the calf on dorsiflexion of the foot (positive Homan's sign) appears in only 10% of clients with DVT, and false-positive findings are common (Church, 2000). *Therefore checking a Homan's sign is not advised!* Examine the area described as painful, comparing this site with the contralateral limb. Gently palpate the site, observing for induration along the blood vessel, and for warmth and edema. Signs and symptoms, however, may be absent with thrombophlebitis. Because there are often silent clinical findings, have a high index of suspicion for this disorder especially for clients who are likely to develop VTE.

Localized edema in one extremity may suggest thrombophlebitis. Measure and compare right and left calf and thigh circumferences for changes over time as an indicator of DVT or venous insufficiency. However, serial leg measurements may not be the most reliable indicator of DVT.

DVT can also occur in the arm from an indwelling IV catheter or from compression injuries to the arm or subclavian vein by a rib. Although diagnostic tests for DVT are available, physical examination findings are often adequate for diagnosis. If a definitive diagnosis is lacking from physical examination alone, other diagnostic tests may be performed, such as contrast venography, duplex ultrasonography, Doppler flow studies, and impedance plethysmography.

Venography uses contrast medium to visualize clot formation in about 95% of people with DVT. Venography is not performed as frequently but is still considered the "gold standard" by many health care professionals for diagnosing DVT. Besides being painful for the client, complications to a venogram include hypersensitivity to the contrast dye, acute renal failure, extravasation of the medium, especially in those with arterial insufficiency, and precipitation of the thrombosis.

The preferred diagnostic test for DVT if a definitive diagnosis cannot be made by physical examination is **venous duplex ultrasonography**, a noninvasive test. Doppler flow studies may also be useful in the diagnosis of DVT, but they are more sensitive in detecting proximal rather than distal DVT. Normal venous circulation is characterized by audible signals, whereas thrombosed veins produce little or no flow. The accuracy of the duplex ultrasonographic scanning is dependent upon the technical skill of the health care professional performing the test. If the test is negative but a DVT is still suspected, a venogram may be needed to make an accurate diagnosis.

Impedance plethysmography assesses venous outflow and can detect more than 90% of DVTs that are located above the popliteal vein. However, it is not helpful in locating clots in the calf and is less sensitive than Doppler studies (Church, 2000).

Magnetic resonance direct thrombus imaging (MRI), another noninvasive test, is useful in finding a DVT in the proximal deep veins and is better than traditional venography in finding DVT in the inferior vena cava or pelvic veins.

A D-dimer test is a global marker of coagulation activation and measures fibrin degradation products produced from fibrinolysis. The test is widely used for the diagnosis of DVT when the client has few clinical signs and stratifies clients into a high-risk category for reoccurrence. Useful as an adjunct to noninvasive testing, a negative D-dimer test can exclude a DVT without an ultrasound.

Common Nursing Diagnoses and Collaborative Problems

Nursing diagnoses and collaborative problems that may apply to clients with DVT include the following:

1. Risk for Ineffective Tissue Perfusion (Peripheral) related to interruption of venous blood flow
2. Acute Pain related to physical injury agent (thrombus)

The most common collaborative problem is Potential for Embolism.

Interventions

The focus of treatment for thrombophlebitis is to prevent complications, such as pulmonary emboli, prevent further thrombus formation, and prevent an increase in size of the thrombus. Deep vein thrombophlebitis (thrombosis) is the most common type of thrombophlebitis. Clients with deep vein thrombosis (DVT) are often hospitalized for treatment, although this practice is changing as a result of the use of newer drugs.

NONSURGICAL MANAGEMENT. DVT is most often treated medically, using a combination of rest, drug therapy, and preventive measures.

Rest. Supportive therapy for DVT includes bedrest and elevation of the extremity. Some health care providers order intermittent or continuous warm, moist soaks to the affected area. *Do not massage the affected extremity to prevent the thrombus from dislodging and becoming an embolus.* All clients are evaluated for signs and symptoms of pulmonary embolism (PE), which include shortness of breath and chest pain. Emboli may also travel to the brain or heart, but these complications are not as common as PE.

Drug Therapy. Anticoagulants are the drugs of choice for a client with DVT and for clients at risk for DVT. The conventional treatment has been IV unfractionated heparin followed by oral anticoagulation with warfarin (Coumadin). However, unfractionated heparin can be problematic because each client's response to the drug is unpredictable, and hospital admission is usually required for laboratory monitoring and dose adjustments. Today the use of low-molecular weight heparin (LMWH) is changing the management of both DVT and PE.

Unfractionated Heparin Therapy. Many clients with a confirmed diagnosis of an existing blood clot are started on a regimen of IV unfractionated heparin (UFH; Hepalean✱) therapy. UFH is an anticoagulant agent that at low doses interacts with antithrombin III to produce selective inhibition of clotting factors IIa (thrombin) and Xa. At higher doses it inhibits practically all clotting factors. The ultimate result is inhibition of fibrin formation; the drug does nothing to the existing clot. The physician prescribes UFH to prevent the formation of other clots, which often develop in the presence of an existing clot, and to prevent enlargement of the existing clot. Over a long period of time, the existing clot is slowly absorbed by the body.

Before UFH administration, a baseline prothrombin time (PT), activated partial thromboplastin time (aPTT), International Normalized Ratio (INR), complete blood count (CBC) with platelet count, urinalysis, stool for occult blood, and creatinine level are required.

UFH is initially given in a bolus IV dose of about 100 units/kg of body weight, followed by constant infusion. The infusion is regulated by a reliable electronic infusion device that protects against accidental free flow of solution. The physician or clinical pharmacist prescribes concentrations of UFH (in 5% dextrose in water) and the number of units or milliliters per hour needed to maintain a therapeutic aPTT. Measurement of aPTT is obtained daily, or more frequently, and reported to the health care provider as soon as results are available to allow adjustment of heparin dosage. Therapeutic levels of aPTTs are usually 1½ to 2 times normal control levels. Assess clients for signs and symptoms of bleeding, which include hematuria, frank or occult blood in the stool, ecchymosis (bruising), petechiae, an altered level of consciousness, or pain.

UFH can also decrease platelet counts. Mild reductions are common and are resolved with continued heparin therapy. Severe platelet reductions, although rare, result from the development of antiplatelet bodies within 6 to 14 days after the beginning of treatment. Platelets aggregate into "white clots" that can cause thrombosis, usually in the form of an acute arterial occlusion. The provider discontinues heparin administration if severe **heparin-induced thrombocytopenia and thrombosis (HITT)** (>100,000 mm^3), or "white clot syndrome," occurs. LMWH is used more commonly today due to the complications involved with UFH.

Argatroban (Acova) or lepirudin (Refludan) are highly selective direct thrombin inhibitors that may be used as an alternative to heparin or for clients who have had HITT. Like heparin, these drugs increase the client's risk for bleeding. An oral anticoagulant may also be substituted for heparin if necessary.

Ensure that protamine sulfate, the antidote for heparin, is available, if needed, for excessive bleeding. Chart 39-10 highlights information important to nursing care and client education associated with anticoagulant therapy.

To *prevent* DVT, heparin may be given in low doses subcutaneously for high-risk clients, especially after orthopedic surgery. However, other pharmacologic agents are often used for prophylaxis:

- Low-molecular weight heparin (e.g., enoxaparin [Lovenox]) (drug class of choice after orthopedic surgery) (Crowther & McCourt, 2004)
- Selective factor Xa inhibitors (e.g., fondaparinux [Arixtra])
- Warfarin (Coumadin, Warfilone✱)

Prevention of DVT is crucial for clients at risk. Preventive measures are listed earlier under the Health Promotion/Illness Prevention section.

Low-Molecular Weight Heparin. Subcutaneous low-molecular weight heparins (LMWHs), such as enoxaparin (Lovenox), dalteparin (Fragmin), and ardeparin (Normiflo), have a consistent action and are approved for prevention and treatment of DVT. Danaparoid (Orgaran) is also classified as an LMWH but is actually a heparinoid. LMWHs bind less to plasma proteins, blood cells, and vessel walls, resulting in a longer half-life and more predictable response. These drugs inhibit thrombin formation due to reduced factor IIa activity and enhanced inhibition of factor Xa and thrombin.

Some clients may be safely managed at home with daily visits from a home care nurse. Candidates for home LMWH therapy must have stable DVT or PE, low risk for bleeding, adequate renal function, and normal vital signs. They must be willing to learn self-injection or have a family member, friend, or home care nurse administer the subcutaneous injections.

CHART 39-10

BEST PRACTICE for
The Client Receiving Anticoagulant Therapy

- Carefully check the dosage of anticoagulant to be administered, even if the pharmacy prepared the medication.
- Monitor the client for signs and symptoms of bleeding, including hematuria, frank or occult blood in the stool, ecchymosis, petechiae, altered mental status (indicating possible cranial bleeding), or pain (especially abdominal pain, which could indicate abdominal bleeding).
- Monitor vital signs frequently for decreased blood pressure and increased pulse (indicating possible internal bleeding).
- Have antidotes available as needed (e.g., protamine sulfate for heparin and vitamin K for warfarin [Coumadin, Warfilone✱]).
- Monitor activated partial thromboplastin time (aPTT) for clients receiving unfractionated heparin; monitor prothrombin time (PT) or International Normalized Ratio (INR) for clients receiving warfarin or low-molecular weight heparin (LMWH).
- Apply prolonged pressure over venipuncture sites and injection sites.
- When administering *subcutaneous* heparin, apply pressure over the site and do not massage.
- Teach the client going home while taking an anticoagulant to:
  - Use only an electric razor
  - Take precautions to avoid injury; for example, do not use tools such as hammers or saws, where accidents commonly occur
  - Report signs and symptoms of bleeding, such as blood in the urine or stool, nosebleeds, ecchymosis, or altered mental status
  - Take the prescribed dosage of medication at the precise time that it was prescribed to be given
  - Not stop taking the medication abruptly; the physician usually tapers the anticoagulant gradually

Some health care providers place the client on a regimen of IV unfractionated heparin (UFH) for several days, then follow up with an LMWH. In this case, the UFH is discontinued at least 30 minutes before the first LMWH injection. The usual dose of enoxaparin is 1 mg/kg of body weight, not to exceed 90 mg, and is repeated every 12 hours. If the client's creatinine level is greater than 2 mg/dL (indicating renal insufficiency), the health care provider lowers the dose. Dalteparin can be given once daily at 200 units/kg of body weight and does not require dose adjustment for renal insufficiency. The usual dose of ardeparin is 50 units/kg of body weight and is given every 12 hours.

Monitor the INR and stools daily for occult blood. The aPTTs are not checked on an ongoing basis because the doses of LMWH are not adjusted.

Warfarin Therapy. If the client is receiving continuous UFH, warfarin (Coumadin) may be added at least 5 days later. Clients receiving LMWH are placed on a regimen of warfarin after the first dose. Warfarin works in the liver to inhibit synthesis of the four vitamin K–dependent clotting factors and takes 3 to 4 days before it can exert therapeutic anticoagulation. The heparin continues to provide therapeutic anticoagulation until this effect is achieved with warfarin. IV heparin is then discontinued at that time.

Therapeutic levels of warfarin are monitored by measuring prothrombin time (PT) and/or the International Normalized Ratio (INR). Because PTs are often inconsistent and misleading, the INR was developed. Most laboratories report both results. Most clients receiving warfarin should have an INR between 1.5 and 2.0 to prevent recurrent DVT and minimizing the risk of stroke or hemorrhage (Ridker et al., 2003). Warfarin therapy should be started with low doses, at least 5 mg, and gradually titrated up according to the INR. Clients usually receive warfarin for 3 to 6 months after an episode of DVT or longer if no precipitating factors were discovered, with recurrence, or if there are continuing risk factors (Gallus et al., 2000).

Nursing assessment for bleeding is similar to that described for clients receiving heparin. Ensure that vitamin K, the antidote for warfarin, is available in case of excessive bleeding (see Chart 39-10). However, anticoagulation is not possible for 3 weeks after vitamin K administration.

Thrombolytic Therapy. The use of systemic thrombolytic therapy for DVT is effective in dissolving thrombi quickly and completely. The greatest advantage is thought to be the prevention of valvular damage and consequential venous insufficiency, or "postphlebitis syndrome." However, thrombolytic therapy is contraindicated postoperatively, during pregnancy, and after childbirth, trauma, strokes, or spinal injuries. To be most effective, thrombolytic therapy must be initiated within 5 days after the onset of symptoms.

Thrombolytic agents such as recombinant tissue plasminogen activator (t-PA), as well as platelet inhibitors such as abciximab (ReoPro), tirofiban (Aggrastat), and eptifibatide (Integrilin), may be effective in dissolving a clot or preventing new clots during the first 24 hours. Infusion can be given via a catheter so the thrombolytic agent can be injected directly into the thrombus. Compared to giving systemic thrombolytic dosing, this approach decreases the concentration needed and reduces the chance of bleeding. Thrombolytic agents, such as alteplase and reteplase, are used to treat peripheral vascular occlusion. Reteplase is a plasminogen activator that penetrates the clot and causes lysis. It is not compatible with heparin and should not be given in the same IV line. Reteplase has been used successfully in treating coronary thrombosis and use in peripheral vascular occlusion is experimental. The most serious complication from thrombolytic therapy is intracerebral bleeding. Be aware of the importance of thrombolytic therapy, its indications, and its implications for nursing care; closely monitor clients for signs and symptoms of bleeding.

Critical Thinking Challenge

An older adult who had a total hip replacement for osteoarthritis 3 days ago is diagnosed as having DVT of the operative leg calf. She lives alone, but plans to return home while receiving low–molecular weight heparin (LMWH) injections.

1. What health teaching will the client require?
2. What resources will she need at home during her recovery?
3. What laboratory tests will need to be monitored while she is receiving LMWH?

evolve For suggested answer guidelines, go to http://evolve.elsevier.com/Iggy/.

Prevention and Management of Peripheral Edema. The client's legs should be elevated when in bed and when in a chair. To help prevent chronic venous insufficiency, clients with active and resolving DVT are often instructed to wear knee- or thigh-high compression or elastic stockings for an extended period of time.

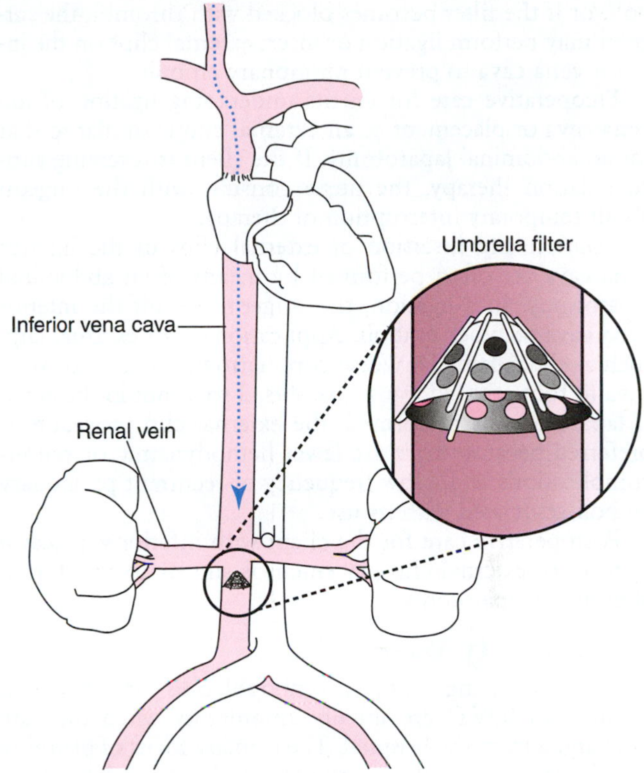

Figure 39-9 ■ An inferior vena caval filter.

SURGICAL MANAGEMENT. A deep vein thrombus is rarely removed surgically unless there is a massive occlusion that does not respond to medical treatment and the thrombus is of recent (1 to 2 days) onset. **Thrombectomy** is the most common surgical procedure for removing the thrombus. Preoperative and postoperative care of clients undergoing thrombectomy are similar to the care for clients undergoing arterial surgery (see earlier discussion under Acute Peripheral Arterial Occlusion, p. 805).

Inferior Vena Caval Interruption. Recurrent deep vein thrombosis (DVT) or pulmonary emboli that do not respond to medical treatment and for clients who cannot tolerate anticoagulation, **inferior vena caval interruption** may be indicated to prevent pulmonary emboli.

Preoperative care is similar to that provided for clients receiving local anesthesia (see Chapter 20). If clients have recently been taking anticoagulants, consult with the physician about interrupting this therapy in the preoperative period to avoid hemorrhage.

The surgeon inserts a filter device, or "umbrella," percutaneously into the inferior vena cava (Figure 39-9). The device is meant to trap emboli in the inferior vena cava before they progress to the lungs. Holes in the device allow blood to pass through, thus not significantly interfering with the return of blood to the heart. Popular inferior vena caval filters include the bird's nest filter and the Greenfield filter.

Postoperatively, inspect the incision on the right side of the chest for bleeding and signs or symptoms of infection. Other postoperative nursing care is similar to that for any client undergoing surgery (see Chapter 22).

Ligation or External Clips. If an inferior vena caval filter is not successful in preventing pulmonary emboli, or if the filter becomes blocked with thrombi, the surgeon may perform ligation or insert external clips on the inferior vena cava to prevent pulmonary emboli.

Preoperative care for clients undergoing ligation of the vena cava or placement of an external clip is similar to that for an abdominal laparotomy. If the client is receiving anticoagulation therapy, the nurse consults with the surgeon about temporary interruption of therapy.

Ligation and insertion of external clips in the inferior vena cava are often performed by means of an abdominal laparotomy. In a ligation, the surgeon ties off the inferior vena cava to block emboli. Application of an external clip, such as the Adams-DeWeese clip, narrows the inferior vena cava to four serrated transverse slits, 3 to 5 mm in diameter. If laparotomy is performed, the external clip procedure is preferred because there are fewer hemodynamic or venous complications and a low frequency of recurrent pulmonary emboli associated with its use.

Postoperative care for the client with inferior vena caval ligation or external clip placement is similar to that for an abdominal laparotomy.

Community-Based Care

Clients recovering from thrombophlebitis or deep vein thrombosis (DVT) are usually ambulatory when they are discharged from the hospital. The primary focus of planning for discharge is to educate the client about the hazards of anticoagulation therapy.

HOME CARE MANAGEMENT

Help the client identify situations and equipment that might cause trauma, such as the use of a straight-edged razor. Help the client and family or significant others to make arrangements to avoid hazardous situations and to procure alternative types of equipment if needed, such as an electric razor.

HEALTH TEACHING

Teach clients recovering from DVT to stop or avoid smoking and to avoid the use of oral contraceptives to decrease the risk of recurrence. Most clients are discharged on a regimen of warfarin (Coumadin, Warfilone✱) or low–molecular weight heparin (LMWH). Instruct clients and their families to avoid potentially traumatic situations, such as participation in contact sports. Provide written and oral information about the signs and symptoms of bleeding (see Chart 39-10). The client must report any of these manifestations to the health care provider immediately.

The anticoagulant effect of warfarin may be reversed by the omission of one or two doses of the drug or by the administration of vitamin K. In case of injury, clients are directed to apply pressure to bleeding wounds and to seek medical assistance immediately. Encourage them to carry an identification card or wear a medical alert bracelet that states that they are taking warfarin.

Also instruct clients to inform their dentist and other health care providers that they are taking warfarin before receiving treatment or prescriptions. Prothrombin times are affected by many prescription and over-the-counter medications, such as antacids, antihistamines, aspirin, mineral oil, oral contraceptives, and large doses of vitamin C. The action of warfarin is also affected by high-fat and vitamin K–rich foods, such as cabbage, cauliflower, broccoli, asparagus, turnips, spinach, kale, fish, and liver. Therefore instruct clients to eat a well-balanced diet with moderate amounts of vitamin K and to avoid taking additional medications without consulting a health care provider. Teach clients to also avoid hydration, alcohol, and sitting for prolonged periods of time. Arrange for clients to have prothrombin time (PT) and International Normalized Ratio (INR) determinations made 1 to 2 weeks after discharge.

Clients receiving subcutaneous LMWH injections at home need instruction on self-injection. Teach the appropriate caregiver and family members or friends, if necessary, to administer the injections

Clients who have experienced DVT may fear recurrence of a thrombus and may also be concerned about treatment with warfarin and the risk for bleeding. Assure them that participation in the prescribed treatment frequently helps in resolving this problem and that ongoing assessment of PTs and INRs should minimize the risks of bleeding.

HEALTH CARE RESOURCES

Clients discharged on a regimen of warfarin need access to a pharmacy to renew prescriptions and, if feasible, obtain a medical alert bracelet. They also need access to a laboratory for frequent monitoring of PTs and INRs.

Venous Insufficiency

PATHOPHYSIOLOGY

Venous insufficiency occurs as a result of prolonged venous hypertension, which stretches the veins and damages the valves. Valvular damage can lead to a backup of blood and further venous hypertension, resulting in edema. Edema occurs as the by-product of red blood cells as they break down and infiltrate the surrounding tissues. Because the client cannot eliminate waste products, they accumulate within the tissues. With time, this stasis (stoppage) results in venous stasis ulcers, swelling, and cellulitis.

Venous efficiency is altered when thrombosis occurs or when valves are not functioning correctly. Defective valves can result from prolonged venous hypertension, which stretches the veins and damages valves. Venous hypertension can occur in people who stand or sit in one position for long periods, such as teachers and office personnel. Pregnancy and obesity can also cause chronically distended veins, which lead to damaged valves. Thrombus formation can contribute to valve destruction. Chronic venous insufficiency often occurs in clients who have had thrombophlebitis.

Venous leg ulcer disease is a major cause of death, pain, and health care costs. The prevalence rate varies from 0.6 to 1.6 per 1000 for adults and increases to 10 to 30 per 1000 in persons older than 85 years of age. Because the ulcers take a great deal of time to heal and often reoccur, between $1.9 and $2.5 billion yearly is spent on venous disease in the United States. Greater than 80% of venous ulcer care is delivered in the community setting by home care nurses (Lorimer et al., 2003).

◆COLLABORATIVE MANAGEMENT

◆Assessment

Venous insufficiency may result in edema of both extremities. There may be **stasis dermatitis** or discoloration along the ankles, extending up to the calf. In people with long-term venous insufficiency, **stasis ulcers** often form. Ulcer formation can result from the edema or from minor injury to the limb. Venous ulcers typically occur over the malleolus, more often medially than laterally. The ulcer usually has irregular borders. In general, these ulcers are chronic and difficult to heal (see Chart 39-7). Many people live with ulcers for years, and recurrence is common. Some may lose one or both limbs if ulcers are not controlled.

Interventions

The focus of treating venous insufficiency is to decrease edema and promote venous return from the affected extremity. Clients are not usually hospitalized for venous insufficiency alone unless it is complicated by an ulcer or another disorder is occurring simultaneously.

NONSURGICAL MANAGEMENT. Treatment of chronic venous insufficiency is primarily nonsurgical, unless it is complicated by a venous stasis ulcer that requires surgical debridement. The goals of managing venous stasis ulcers are to heal the ulcer, prevent infection, and prevent stasis with recurrence of ulcer formation. A wound care specialist, such as a Wound, Ostomy, and Continence nurse, should be contacted to make recommendations for ulcer care. A dietitian can suggest dietary supplements, such as zinc and vitamins A and C, as well as high-protein foods to promote wound healing.

Management of Edema. Clients with chronic venous insufficiency wear elastic or compression stockings, which fit from the middle of the foot to just below the knee or to the thigh. Stockings should be worn during the day and evening. Legs should be elevated for at least 20 minutes four or five times per day. When the client is in bed, the legs should be elevated above the level of the heart (Chart 39-11).

Confer with the physician about the use of intermittent sequential pneumatic compression of the lower extremities or foot plexus pumps for clients with past or present venous stasis ulcers. If an open venous ulcer is present, the device may be applied over a dressing such as an Unna boot. Instruct the client to apply the pump as directed during the period of healing. Because of the high incidence of venous ulcer recurrence, clients with chronic venous insufficiency whose ulcers have healed are encouraged to continue compression therapy for life.

Management of Venous Stasis Ulcers. Venous stasis ulcers are slightly more manageable than ulcers resulting from arterial disease. They are chronic in nature, with some clients manifesting the same ulcer for years. Ulcers often heal, only to recur in the same area several years later.

Two types of occlusive dressings are used for venous stasis ulcers: oxygen permeable dressings and oxygen impermeable dressings. Because the role of atmospheric oxygen in wound healing is controversial, opinions vary with regard to which type of dressing is preferred. An oxygen-permeable polyethylene film and an oxygen-impermeable hydrocolloid dressing (e.g., DuoDerm) are common. Hydrocolloid dressings are left in place for a minimum of 3 to 5 days for best effect. Use strict aseptic technique when changing dressings. If the wound is infected, use contact precautions in addition to standard precautions.

Artificial skin products can be used for difficult-to-heal venous leg ulcers. These first-generation products are very expensive but are laying the foundation in the field with costs anticipated to come down in the future. Except for cultured epithelial autografts, artificial skins are only temporary. Artificial skin serves as a biologic cover to secrete growth factors to promote more growth factor secretion from the client's own skin to speed the wound healing process.

CHART 39-11

CLIENT EDUCATION GUIDE

Venous Insufficiency

Elastic Stockings

- Wear elastic stockings as prescribed, usually during the day and evening.
- Put the stockings on upon awakening and before getting out of bed.
- When applying the stockings, do not "bunch up" and apply like socks. Instead, place your hand inside the stocking and pull out the heel. Then place the foot of the stocking over your foot and slide the rest of the stocking up. Be sure that rough seams on the stocking are on the outside, not next to your skin.
- Do not push stockings down for comfort, because they may function like a tourniquet and further impair venous return.
- Put on a clean pair of stockings each day. Wash them by hand (not in a washing machine) in a gentle detergent and warm water.
- If the stockings seem to be "stretched out," replace them with a new pair.

Do's and Don'ts

- Elevate your legs for at least 20 minutes four or five times a day. When in bed, elevate your legs above the level of your heart.
- Avoid prolonged sitting or standing.
- Do not cross your legs; crossing at the ankles is acceptable for short periods of time.
- Do not wear tight, restrictive pants; avoid girdles and garters.

CONSIDERATIONS FOR OLDER ADULTS

The pedal pulses in older adults may be more difficult to find. Thin, shiny skin, thick ridged nails, and loss of hair on the lower legs are signs of arterial insufficiency associated with normal aging

If the client is ambulatory, an **Unna boot** may be used. An Unna boot dressing is constructed of gauze that has been moistened with zinc oxide. Apply the boot to the affected limb, from the toes to the knee, after the ulcer has been cleaned with normal saline solution. Povidone-iodine (Betadine) and hydrogen peroxide are not used, because they destroy granulation tissue. The Unna boot is then covered with an elastic wrap and hardens like a cast; this promotes venous return and prevents stasis. The Unna boot also forms a sterile environment for the ulcer. The physician or advanced-practice nurse should change the boot about once a week. Instruct the client about what to look for if arterial occlusion occurs from an Unna boot that is too tight.

Drug Therapy. The health care provider may prescribe topical agents, such as Accuzyme, to chemically debride the ulcer, eliminating necrotic tissue and promoting healing. If an infection or cellulitis develops, systemic antibiotics are necessary.

SURGICAL MANAGEMENT. Surgery for chronic venous insufficiency is not usually performed, because historically it has not been successful. Attempts at transplanting vein valves have had limited success. Surgical debridement of venous ulcers is similar to that performed for arterial ulcers (see Chapter 70).

Community-Based Care

The goal for the client with chronic venous insufficiency is to be managed in the home. For clients with frequent acute complications and repeated hospital admissions, case management can help meet appropriate clinical and cost outcomes.

HOME CARE MANAGEMENT

Help clients with chronic venous insufficiency to plan for opportunities and facilities that allow for elevation of the lower extremities in and outside the home. In addition, clients with venous stasis ulcers need to plan for care of the ulcers.

HEALTH TEACHING

Instruct clients with chronic venous stasis to:

- Avoid standing still if possible
- Elevate their legs when sitting
- Avoid crossing their legs
- Avoid wearing tight girdles, tight pants, and narrow-banded knee-high socks

The physician prescribes support hose or antiembolism stockings. Teach clients to apply these stockings before they get out of bed in the morning and to remove them just before going to bed at night (see Chart 39-11). Also advise them that they will probably need to wear these stockings for the rest of their lives.

To improve circulation and aid in weight reduction, prescribe an exercise program on an individual basis with health care provider input. Encourage all clients to maintain an optimal weight and consult with the dietitian to plan a weight reduction diet. Instruct clients with venous stasis ulcers how to care for the ulcers at home.

Clients with venous stasis disease, especially those with venous stasis ulcers, may require long-term emotional support to assist them in meeting long-term needs. They may also need assistance in coping with necessary lifestyle adjustments, such as changes in occupation.

HEALTH CARE RESOURCES

Clients with venous stasis ulcers may need the assistance of a home care nurse to perform dressing changes. Clients with Unna boots need weekly transportation to their health care provider for dressing changes. Arrange for a sequential compression device in the home if the health care provider prescribes one.

VARICOSE VEINS

PATHOPHYSIOLOGY

Varicose veins are distended, protruding veins that appear darkened and tortuous. They can occur in anyone, but they are common in clients older than 30 years of age whose occupations require prolonged standing. Varicose veins are also frequently seen in pregnant women, clients with systemic problems (e.g., heart disease), obese clients, and clients with a family history of varicose veins.

As the vein wall weakens and dilates, venous pressure increases and the valves become incompetent (defective). The incompetent valves enhance the vessel dilation, and the veins become tortuous and distended. The client may complain of pain, especially after standing, and may experience a feeling of fullness in the legs. Nursing assessment reveals distended, protruding veins.

The Trendelenburg test assists with the diagnosis. The client is placed in a supine position with elevated legs. As the client sits up, the veins would normally fill from the distal end; however, if there are varicosities, the veins fill from the proximal end.

◆COLLABORATIVE MANAGEMENT

Conservative measures are the treatment of choice. Measures involve wearing elastic stockings and elevating the extremities as much as possible. Clients who continue to have pain or unsightly veins, despite this treatment, may opt for either sclerotherapy or surgical removal of the vein.

Sclerotherapy is performed on small or a limited number of varicosities. The physician injects a solution, such as sodium tetradecyl, directly into the vein, or he or she may use a laser device. A pressure dressing may be applied over the sclerosed vein to keep vessels free of blood for 24 to 72 hours. The surgeon performs an incision and drainage of trapped blood in the sclerosed vein 14 to 21 days after injection, followed by application of a second pressure dressing for 12 to 18 hours.

Varicose veins are surgically removed when they are larger than 4 mm in diameter or are in clusters. The stab avulsion technique may be used if the saphenous veins are competent. The surgeon exposes varices through 2- to 3-mm stab incisions, grasping the veins with hooks, and dividing and avulsing each vein.

The surgeon may need to strip (remove) affected veins if the saphenous vein is incompetent. The surgeon threads a long wire through an incision above an affected vein, pulling it down through the vein and out through an incision below the vein. After this procedure, the legs are bandaged with firm elastic (Ace) bandages.

Postoperatively, assess the groin and entire leg for bleeding through the elastic bandage. Instruct the client to keep the legs elevated and to perform range-of-motion exercises of the legs at least hourly. Clients are ambulatory and are often discharged from the hospital by the first postoperative day. At this time, instruct clients to continue to wear elastic stockings, walk, limit sitting, avoid standing in one place, and elevate their legs when sitting.

Application of RF (radio frequency) energy is a new technique done as an alternative to surgery. The vein is heated from the inside by the RF energy and shrinks. Collateral veins nearby take over.

Laser treatment is another alternative to surgery. Performed by interventional radiologists, the EndoVenous Laser Treatment uses a laser fiber to heat and close the main vessel that is contributing to the varicosity.

PHLEBITIS

Phlebitis is an inflammation of the superficial veins caused by an irritant, such as IV therapy (see Chapter 17). The client has a reddened, warm area radiating up an extremity, commonly an arm. Pain, soreness, and swelling of the extremity may also occur.

Management generally takes place at home and involves application of warm, moist soaks, which dilate the vein and promote circulation. Sometimes a heating unit is used to keep the soaks warm. Rarely, ice packs are used. Apply the soaks, making sure that the temperature is not hot enough to burn the client, and assess for complications, such as tissue necrosis, infection, or pulmonary embolus. After a few days of conservative therapy, the inflammation usually subsides. Elastic stockings may be prescribed.

VASCULAR TRAUMA

PATHOPHYSIOLOGY

Many types of trauma can result in vascular injury. Injuries to the blood vessels in the upper and lower extremities account for about 70% of all vascular injuries to the human body. Vascular injuries to the blood vessels include punctures, lacerations, and transections. Acute blunt or penetrating trauma may result in a false aneurysm or hematoma. Arteriovenous fistulas may be seen after penetrating injuries. The more common causes of penetrating injuries to the blood vessels are gunshot and knife wounds.

Blunt trauma, which is less common, can result from high-speed automobile accidents as a result of the shearing force of rapid deceleration. Vascular trauma can also occur during arterial puncture for arteriographic or hemodynamic studies in which a dissection, hematoma, or occlusive lesion occurs.

COLLABORATIVE MANAGEMENT

The history and physical examination aid in establishing the diagnosis in the client with vascular injury. Question the client or family about the mechanism of injury, the site of injury, the amount of blood loss, and symptoms present after the injury.

Assess for circulatory, sensory, or motor impairment but be aware that, despite significant trauma, impairment may not be apparent, especially if deep vessels have been injured. Arteriography provides essential information about the vascular injury. Emergency or urgent surgical intervention is needed for ischemia to maximize successful revascularization.

Management of vascular injuries is often initiated in a hospital emergency department. Careful triage of all clients is crucial. The most important principles in the management of vascular trauma are establishment of a patent airway, control of bleeding, and restoration of blood flow.

The method of repair varies with the type of vascular injury. Techniques include vein bypass grafting, lateral suture repair, thrombectomy (excision of blood clot), resection with end-to-end anastomosis, and vein patch grafting.

GET READY for the NCLEX Examination!

KEY POINTS

Safe Effective Care Environment

- In collaboration with the health care team, assess the home environment of the client with peripheral vascular disease for potential safety hazards, place high-risk clients on a fall prevention program.
- To reduce the risk of injury, caution clients about orthostatic hypertension when taking antihypertensive medications, especially diuretics.
- For clients with leg ulcers, initiate a consult with a Wound, Ostomy, and Continence Nurse or other wound specialist.
- Use contact precautions for infected, draining wounds.
- Use strict aseptic technique for changing dressings over open ulcers.
- Teach the client to report excessive drainage from the wound, development of redness, warmth, pain, or induration, and a temperature greater than 100° F.
- Insertion sites for IV lines, central line catheters, arterial lines, and Foley catheters should be cared for meticulously and observed for signs of infection.

Health Promotion and Maintenance

- In collaboration with the dietitian, assist the client to incorporate healthy eating behaviors to lower cholesterol and saturated fats, and increase fresh fruits, vegetables, and fiber in the diet. For overweight clients, assist in a weight reduction plan. Assist the diabetic client with maintaining normal blood glucose levels to enhance wound healing. For clients on warfarin, instruct on diet interaction, vitamin K moderation, and avoiding alcohol.
- Teach clients taking statin-type drugs to report adverse effects to their health care provider as described in Chart 39-1.
- For clients with wounds, collaborate with the dietitian to promote adequate intake of protein, vitamins C and A, and zinc to enhance wound healing.
- Teach clients ways to prevent deep vein thrombosis and subsequent embolism; in the hospital setting, provide measures, such as wearing compression stockings, to prevent or manage DVT.
- Encourage your client to stop smoking, take a daily walk, care for his or her feet and skin carefully, eat healthy, and drink plenty of fluids (also see Chart 39-2).
- For smoking or tobacco-chewing clients, initiate a consult to begin a tobacco cessation program.
- Assess the client for modifiable and nonmodifiable risk factors for cardiovascular disease and be ready to teach health promotion behaviors to the client and family. Pay particular attention to the client with a family history of cardiovascular disease.
- For clients with vascular disorders, teach them the importance of each medication, review the mechanism of action, potential side effects, and the duration for taking the medications. Instruct the client to report to the health care provider before stopping any medications.
- To prevent reoccurrence of leg ulcers, teach the client about avoiding trauma to the extremities, proper foot and skin care, proper clothing and footwear, applying prescribed compression stockings, and appropriate activity and extremity positioning.

Psychosocial Integrity

- Encourage the client to verbalize fears about facing sudden death and clarify misconceptions. Applying diversional activities if indicated for a prolonged hospital stay.
- Encourage biofeedback, relaxation therapy and assist clients with coping strategies to reduce stress.
- Monitor the client's response to stress to determine whether the behavior is a typical reaction or an unusual reaction to a

stressful situation. Report any unusual behavior immediately for appropriate intervention.

- Identify and address clients' concerns that could hinder learning.

Physiological Integrity

- Closely observe the client receiving anticoagulants or thrombolytics for signs of bleeding and monitor appropriate laboratory values.
- Assess respiratory, cardiovascular, gastrointestinal, renal, circulatory and neurovascular status closely on all postprocedure or postsurgical clients.
- Administer antihypertensives or vasopressors as prescribed to maintain sufficient pressure for adequate renal perfusion, graft patency, and cardiovascular status, including heart rate and blood pressure (see Chart 39-3).
- Monitor for indications of aneurysm rupture: diaphoresis, nausea, vomiting, pallor, hypotension, tachycardia, severe pain, and decreased level of consciousness, or a pulsating abdominal mass.
- Document assessment findings completely.
- Assess and manage pain effectively.

ADDITIONAL STUDY RESOURCES

Go to your Student CD-ROM for Review Questions for the NCLEX Examination.

evolve Go to http://evolve.elsevier.com/Iggy/ for Integrated Management of Care Questions for the NCLEX Examination.

SELECTED BIBLIOGRAPHY

ALLHAT Officers and Coordinators for the ALLHAT Collaborative Research Group. (2002a). Major outcomes in high-risk hypertensive patients randomized to Angiotensin-converting enzyme inhibitor or calcium channel blocker vs diuretic. The Antihypertensive and Lipid-Lowering Treatment to Prevent Heart Attack Trial (ALLHAT). *Journal of the American Medical Association, 288*(23), 2981-2997.

ALLHAT Officers and Coordinators for the ALLHAT Collaborative Research Group. (2002b). Major outcomes in moderately hypercholesterolemic, hypertensive patients randomized to pravastatin vs usual care. The Antihypertensive and Lipid-Lowering Treatment to Prevent Heart Attack Trial (ALLHAT-LLT). *Journal of the American Medical Association, 288*(23), 2998-3007.

American College of Chest Physicians. (2001). Sixth ACCP consensus conference on antithrombotic therapy. *Chest, 119*(1, suppl.)1S-370S.

American Heart Association. (2003). *Heart Disease and Stroke Statistics-2003 Update.* Dallas: American Heart Association.

Aquila, A. (2001). Deep venous thrombosis. *Journal of Cardiovascular Nursing, 15*(4), 25-44.

Ayello, E.A. (2000). On the lookout for peripheral vascular disease. *Nursing2000, 30*(6), 64hh1-64hh4.

Baumann, L.C., Chang, M.W., & Hoebeke, R. (2002). Clinical outcomes for low-income adults with hypertension and diabetes. *Nursing Research, 51*(3), 191-197.

Bialous, S.A., and Sarna, L. (2004). Sparing a few minutes for tobacco cessation. *American Journal of Nursing, 104*(12), 54-59.

Bussard, M.E. (2002). Reteplase: nursing implications for catheter-directed thrombolytic therapy for peripheral vascular occlusions. *Critical Care Nurse, 22*(3), 57-63.

Bussey, H. (2002). Traditional anticoagulant therapy: Why abandon half a century of success? *American Journal of Health-System Pharmacy, 59*(20), S3-S6.

Byrne, B. (2001). Deep vein thrombosis prophylaxis: the effectiveness and implications of using below-knee or thigh-length graduated compression stockings. *Heart and Lung,* 30(4), 277-284.

Church, V. (2000). Staying on guard for DVT and PE. *Nursing2000, 30*(2), 34-44.

Coffey, M., Crowder, G.K., & Check, D.J. (2003). Reducing coronary artery disease by decreasing homocysteine levels. *Critical Care Nurse, 23*(1), 25-30.

Collins, T.C., et al. (2003). The prevalence of peripheral arterial disease in a racially diverse population. *Archives of Internal Medicine, 163*(12), 1469-1474.

Crowther, M., & McCourt, K. (2004). Get the edge on deep vein thrombosis. *Nursing Management, 35*(1), 22-29.

Day, M.W. (2003). Recognizing and managing deep vein thrombosis. *Nursing2003, 33*(5), 36-42.

Douglas, J.G., et al. (2003). Consensus Statement of the Hypertension in African Americans Working Group of the International Society on Hypertension in Blacks. Management of high blood pressure in African Americans. *Archives of Internal Medicine, 163*(5) 525-541.

Ebersole, P., Hess, P., & Luggen, A.S. (2004). *Toward healthy aging* (6th ed.). St. Louis: Mosby.

Eichinger, S., et al. (2003). D-Dimer levels and risk of recurrent venous thromboembolism. *Journal of the American Medical Association, 290*(8), 1071-1074.

Etter, J.K., & Perneger, T.V. (2001). Effectiveness of a computer-tailored smoking cessation program. *Archives of Internal Medicine, 161*(21), 2696-2601.

Forette, F., et al. (2002). The prevention of dementia with antihypertensive treatment. New Evidence from the Systolic Hypertension in Europe (Syst-Eur) Study. *Archives of Internal Medicine, 162*(18), 2046-2052.

Gallus, A.S., et al. (2000). Consensus guidelines for warfarin therapy. An article published on the Internet by *The Medical Journal of Australia.* Available at http://www.mja.com.au.

Gerstein, H.C., et al. (2001). Albuminuria and risk of cardiovascular events, death, and heart failure in diabetic and nondiabetic individuals. *Journal of the American Medical Association,* 286(4), 421-426.

Heart Protection Study Collaborative Group (2003). MRC/BHF Heart Protection Study of cholesterol-lowering with simvastatin in 5963 people with diabetes: A randomized placebo-controlled trial. *Lancet 361*, 2005-2016.

Hess, C.T. (2003). Managing your patient's arterial ulcer. *Nursing2003, 33*(5), 17.

Horlander, K.T., Mannino, D.M., & Leeper, K.V. (2003). Pulmonary embolism mortality in the United States, 1979-1998. *Archives of Internal Medicine, 163*(14), 1711-1717.

Jarvis, C. (2004). *Physical examination and health assessment* (4th ed.). St. Louis: Mosby.

Joint National Committee. (2003). *The seventh report of the Joint National Committee on Prevention, Detection, Evaluation, and Treatment of High Blood Pressure.* NIH Publication No. 03-5233. Bethesda, MD: National Heart, Lung, and Blood Institute..

Kaatz, S. (2000). The venous side: Current directions in anticoagulant therapy. *J Am Osteopath Assoc,* 100(11), s17-s21.

Klompas, M. (2002). Does this patient have an acute thoracic aortic dissection? *Journal of the American Medical Association, 287*(17), 2262-2272.

Kuncl, N., & Nelson, K.M. (2000). Getting the skinny on lipid-lowering drugs. *Nursing2000, 30*(7), 52-53.

Lorimer, K.R., et al. (2003). Venous leg ulcer care: How evidence-based is nursing practice? *Journal of Wound, Ostomy, and Continence Nursing 30*(3), 132-142.

Luggen, A.S., & Meiner, S.E. (2001). *NGNA core curriculum for gerontological nursing* (2nd ed.). St. Louis: Mosby.

Maas, M.L., et al. (2001). *Nursing care of older adults: Diagnoses, outcomes, and interventions.* St. Louis: Mosby.

Malacaria, B., & Feloney, C.D.H. (2003). Going with the flow of anticoagulant therapy. *Nursing2003, 33*(3), 36-42.

McCance, K.L., & Huether, S.E. (2002). Pathophysiology: The biologic basis for disease in adults and children. St. Louis: Mosby.

National Cholesterol Education Program. (2002). *Third report of the Expert Panel on Detection, Evaluation, and Treatment of High Blood Cholesterol in Adults (Adult Treatment Panel III).* NIH Publication No. 02-5215. Bethesda, MD: National Heart, Lung, and Blood Institute.

National Heart, Lung, and Blood Institute. (2002). *Morbidity and mortality 2002 chartbook on cardiovascular, lung and blood diseases.* Washington, DC: National Institutes of Health, Public Health Service, U.S. Department of Health and Human Services.

National High Blood Pressure Education Program. (2002). Primary prevention of hypertension: Clinical and public health advisory. NIH Publication No. 02-5076. Bethesda, MD: National Heart, Lung, and Blood Institute.

Ridker, P.M., et al. (2003). Long term therapy, low-intensity warfarin therapy for the prevention of recurrent venous thromboembolism. *The New England Journal of Medicine, 348*(15), 1425-1434.

Sangiorgi, G., et al. (2001). Plasma levels of metalloproteinases-3 and -9 as markers of successful abdominal aortic aneurysm exclusion after endovascular graft treatment. *Circulation, 104*(suppl. 1), 288I-296I.

Sever, P.S., et al. (2003). Prevention of coronary and stroke events with atorvastatin in hypertensive patients who have average or lower than average cholesterol concentrations, in the Anglo-Scandinavian cardiac outcomes trial-lipid lowering arm (ASCOT-LLA): A multicentre randomized controlled trial. *The Lancet, 361,* 1149-1158.

Society of Interventional Radiology. (2003). Peripheral vascular disease statistics. Retrieved September 4, 2003, from http://www.sirweb.org.

Stein, P.D., et al. (2003). Venous thromboembolic disease. *Archives of Internal Medicine 163*(14), 1689-1694.

Stewart, K.J., et al. (2002). Exercise training for claudication. *The New England Journal of Medicine, 347*(24), 1941-1951.

White, W.B. (2003). Selective aldosterone blockage in hypertension: Clinical benefits across patient populations. Available at Medscape at http://www.medscape.com.

Woods, A. (2004). Loosening the grip of hypertension. *Nursing 2004, 34*(12), 36-43.

CHAPTER

40 Interventions for Clients with Shock

M. LINDA WORKMAN

LEARNING OUTCOMES

After studying this chapter, you should be able to:

1. Describe the clinical manifestations associated with the compensatory mechanisms for shock.
2. Identify clients at risk for hypovolemic shock.
3. Use laboratory data and clinical manifestations to determine the effectiveness of therapy for shock.
4. Explain the basis for intravenous therapy for shock.
5. Describe the mechanisms of action, side effects, and nursing implications for pharmacologic management of shock.
6. Prioritize nursing care for the client experiencing the nonprogressive stage of hypovolemic shock.
7. Compare the pathophysiology and clinical manifestations of the hyperdynamic and hypodynamic phases of septic shock.
8. Identify clients at risk for septic shock.
9. Identify nursing practices to reduce infection risk in an immunocompromised client.
10. Explain the rationale for the drug therapy for septic shock.
11. Prioritize nursing care for the client experiencing the hyperdynamic stage of septic shock.
12. Prioritize nursing care for the client experiencing the hypodynamic stage of septic shock.
13. Develop a community-based teaching plan for the client at risk for septic shock.

Go to your Student CD-ROM for Review Questions for the NCLEX Examination keyed to these Learning Outcomes.

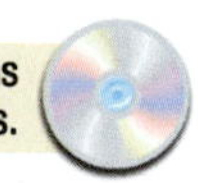

Shock, the whole-body response to poor tissue oxygenation, is a condition rather than a disease. Any problem that impairs oxygen delivery to tissues and organs can start the syndrome of shock and lead to a life-threatening emergency. Clients in acute care settings are at higher risk, but shock can occur in any setting. When compensation or interventions are not effective and shock progresses, hypoxia can lead to multiple organ dysfunction syndrome (MODS) and death.

PATHOPHYSIOLOGY

Organs, tissues, and cells need a continuous supply of oxygen to function properly. The lungs first bring oxygen into the body. The cardiovascular system (heart, blood, and blood vessels) delivers oxygen to all tissues and removes cellular wastes. When any part of the cardiovascular system does not function properly for any reason, shock can result.

Shock begins with abnormal cellular metabolism, which occurs when too little oxygen is delivered to the tissues (McCance & Huether, 2002). In the past shock was classified as hypovolemic, cardiogenic, vasogenic, or septic, which indicated the origin of the problem causing the shock. Shock is now classified by the specific functional impairment caused: hypovolemic shock, cardiogenic shock, distributive shock, and obstructive shock (Effron & Chernow, 1992). Table 40-1 compares both classification systems and common problems leading to each shock category. The functional classification is used by researchers and guides clinicians and therefore is used in this chapter.

Many manifestations of shock are similar regardless of what starts the process or which tissues are affected first. These common manifestations are due to physiologic compensatory mechanisms. Manifestations unique to any one type of shock result from specific tissue dysfunction. The common features of shock are listed in Chart 40-1.

Review of Tissue Perfusion

Tissue oxygenation depends on how much oxygen from arterial blood perfuses the tissue. Organ perfusion is related to mean arterial pressure (MAP). Because the cardiovascular

TABLE 40-1 Comparison of New and Old Shock Classification Systems

Classification by Functional Impairment			
Hypovolemic Total body fluid decreased (in all fluid compartments) ▪ Hemorrhage ▪ Dehydration	***Cardiogenic*** Direct pump failure Fluid volume not affected ▪ Myocardial infarction ▪ Valvular problems Stenosis Incompetence ▪ Myopathies ▪ Dysrhythmias ▪ Cardiac arrest	***Distributive*** Fluid shifted from central vascular space Total body fluid volume normal or increased ▪ Neural-induced loss of vascular tone ▪ Chemical-induced loss of vascular tone Sepsis Anaphylaxis Capillary leak	***Obstructive*** Cardiac function decreased by non-cardiac factors Total body fluid volume not affected Central volume decreased ▪ Pulmonary hypertension ▪ Tension pneumothorax ▪ Pericarditis ▪ Thoracic tumor ▪ Tamponade
Classification by Site of Origin			
Hypovolemic Central vascular volume decreased Total body fluid may or may not be decreased ▪ Hemorrhage ▪ Dehydration ▪ Fluid shifts Trauma Burns Anaphylaxis	***Cardiogenic*** Direct pump failure Indirect pump failure Decreased cardiac output Total body fluid not decreased ▪ Valvular problems Stenosis Incompetence ▪ Myocardial infarction ▪ Myopathies ▪ Dysrhythmias ▪ Cardiac arrest ▪ Tamponade ▪ Pericarditis ▪ Pulmonary hypertension ▪ Pulmonary emboli	***Vasogenic*** Loss of vascular tone Total body fluid not decreased ▪ Neurogenic Head trauma Vasovagal response ▪ Vessel dilation Anaphylaxis Inflammation	***Septic*** Loss of vascular tone Eventual reduced cardiac output Seen as a more intense type of vasogenic shock ▪ Infection

CHART 40-1

KEY FEATURES of Shock

Cardiovascular Manifestations
- Decreased cardiac output
- Increased pulse rate
- Thready pulse
- Decreased blood pressure
- Narrowed pulse pressure
- Postural hypotension
- Low central venous pressure
- Flat neck and hand veins in dependent positions
- Slow capillary refill in nail beds
- Diminished peripheral pulses

Respiratory Manifestations
- Increased respiratory rate
- Shallow depth of respirations
- Decreased $Paco_2$
- Decreased arterial Pao_2
- Cyanosis, especially around lips and nail beds

Neuromuscular Manifestations
- Early
  - Anxiety
  - Restlessness
  - Increased thirst
- Late
  - Decreased central nervous system activity (lethargy to coma)
  - Generalized muscle weakness
  - Diminished or absent deep tendon reflexes
  - Sluggish pupillary response to light

Renal Manifestations
- Decreased urine output
- Increased specific gravity
- Sugar and acetone present in urine

Integumentary Manifestations
- Cool to cold
- Pale to mottled to cyanotic
- Moist, clammy
- Mouth dry; pastelike coating present

Gastrointestinal Manifestations
- Decreased motility
- Diminished or absent bowel sounds
- Nausea and vomiting
- Constipation

$Paco_2$, Partial pressure of arterial carbon dioxide; *Pao_2,* partial pressure of arterial oxygen.

system is a closed but continuous circuit, the factors that influence MAP include the following:
- Total blood volume
- Cardiac output
- Size of the vascular bed

Total blood volume and cardiac output are directly related to MAP so that increases in either total blood volume or cardiac output raise MAP. Decreases in either total blood volume or cardiac output lower MAP.

The size of the vascular bed is inversely (negatively) related to MAP. This means that increases in the size of the vascular bed lower MAP and decreases raise MAP (Figure 40-1). Blood vessels, especially small arteries and veins connected to capillaries, can increase in diameter by relaxing the smooth muscle in vessel walls (dilating) or decrease in diameter by contracting the muscle **(vasoconstriction).** When blood vessels dilate and total blood volume remains the same, blood pressure decreases and blood flow is slower. When blood vessels constrict

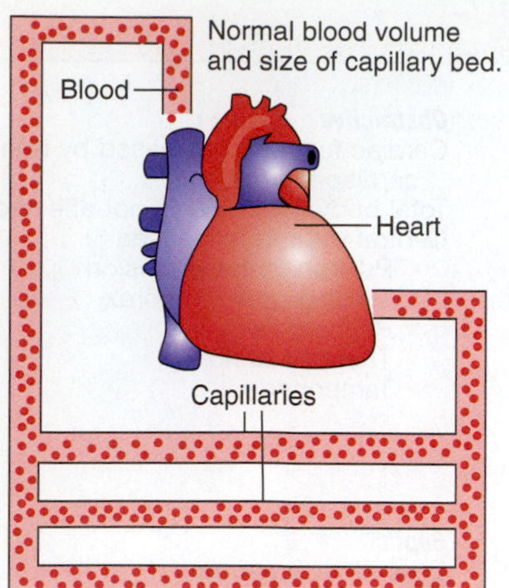

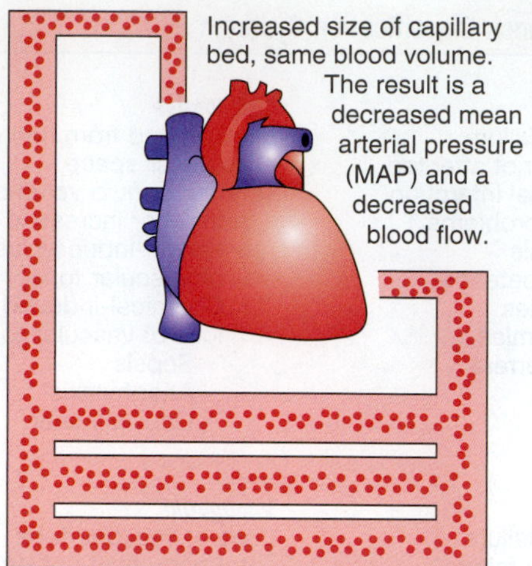

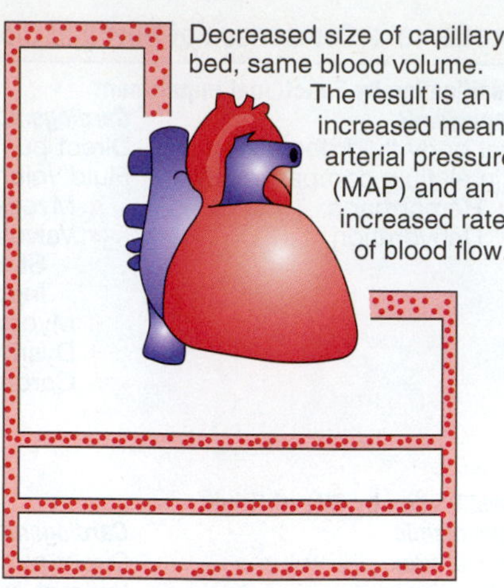

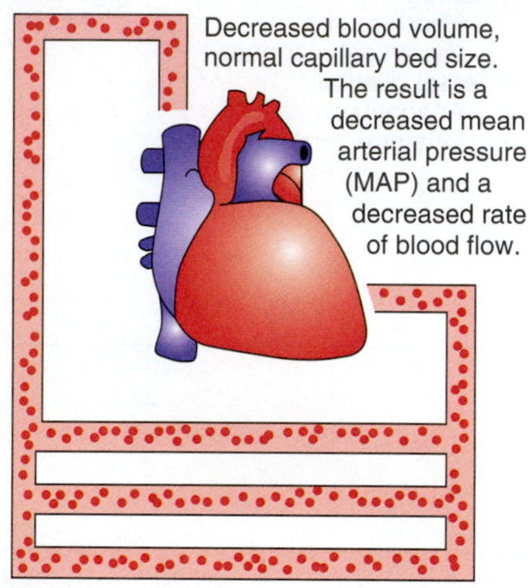

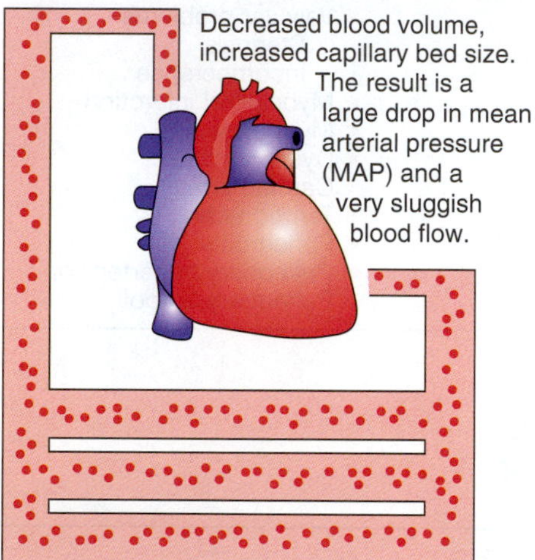

Figure 40-1 ■ Interaction of blood volume and the size of the capillary bed affecting mean arterial pressure.

and total blood volume remains the same, blood pressure increases and blood flow is faster.

Blood vessels contain nerves from the sympathetic division of the autonomic nervous system. Some nerves continuously stimulate vascular smooth muscle so that the blood vessels are normally partially constricted. This state of partial blood vessel constriction is called **sympathetic tone.** Increases in sympathetic stimulation constrict blood vessel smooth muscle even more, raising MAP. Decreases in sympathetic tone relax blood vessel smooth muscle, dilating them and lowering MAP.

Blood flow to organs varies and adjusts to changes in tissue oxygen needs. The body can selectively increase blood flow to some areas while reducing blood flow to others. Some organs, such as the skin and skeletal muscles, can tolerate low levels of oxygen for hours without dying or being damaged. Other organs (e.g., heart, brain, liver) tolerate **hypoxic** conditions (low levels of tissue oxygenation) poorly, and even just a few minutes without adequate oxygen results in serious or permanent damage.

The Processes of Shock

The problems common to all types of shock, regardless of cause, are the effects of **anaerobic cellular metabolism** (metabolism without oxygen). These effects are caused by inadequate tissue oxygenation and lead to impaired tissue function. The body begins to compensate to maintain or restore tissue perfusion and oxygenation even while the causes of shock are still present.

When the conditions that cause shock remain uncorrected, shock progresses through the following stages:

1. Initial stage
2. Nonprogressive stage
3. Progressive stage
4. Refractory stage

These stages of shock are classified on the basis of the following:

- How well compensatory mechanisms are working
- The severity of the clinical manifestations
- Whether tissue damage is reversible

The main trigger leading to shock is a sustained decrease in mean arterial pressure (MAP) that results from decreased cardiac output, decreased circulating blood volume, or expansion of the vascular bed. A decrease in MAP of 5 to 10 mm Hg below the client's baseline value is detected by pressure-sensitive nerve receptors **(baroreceptors)** in the aortic arch and carotid sinus (Berne, et al., 2004). These data are transmitted to brain centers, which stimulate compensatory mechanisms. These mechanisms ensure continued blood flow and oxygen delivery to vital organs while limiting blood

TABLE 40-2 Physiologic Events During Shock

Initial Stage
Decrease in baseline mean arterial pressure (MAP) of 5-10 mm Hg
Increased sympathetic stimulation
- Mild vasoconstriction
- Increase in heart rate

Nonprogressive Stage
Decrease in MAP of 10-15 mm Hg from the client's baseline value
Continued sympathetic stimulation
- Moderate vasoconstriction
- Increased heart rate
- Decreased pulse pressure

Chemical compensation
- Renin, aldosterone, and antidiuretic hormone secretion
  - Increased vasoconstriction
  - Decreased urine output
  - Stimulation of the thirst reflex

Some anaerobic metabolism in nonvital organs
- Mild acidosis
- Mild hyperkalemia

Progressive Stage
Decrease in MAP of >20 mm Hg from the client's baseline value
Anoxia of nonvital organs
Hypoxia of vital organs
Overall metabolism is anaerobic
- Moderate acidosis
- Moderate hyperkalemia
- Tissue ischemia

Refractory Stage
Severe tissue hypoxia with ischemia and necrosis
Release of myocardial depressant factor from the pancreas
Buildup of toxic metabolites
Multiple organ dysfunction syndrome (MODS)
Death

flow to less vital areas. Moving oxygenated blood into selected areas while bypassing others **(shunting)** causes the manifestations of shock.

If the events that caused the initial decrease in MAP are halted at this point, the compensatory mechanisms can return the body to a normal perfused and oxygenated state, even without outside intervention. If the initiating events continue and MAP decreases further, some tissues function under anaerobic conditions. This condition creates an increase in lactic acid levels and other harmful metabolites (e.g., protein-destroying enzymes and oxygen radicals). These substances cause electrolyte and acid-base imbalances with tissue-damaging effects and depressed heart muscle activity. Such effects are temporary and reversible if the cause of shock is corrected within 1 to 2 hours after onset. When such conditions continue for longer periods without help, the resulting acid-base imbalance, electrolyte imbalances, and increased metabolites cause so much cell damage in vital organs that multiple organ dysfunction syndrome (MODS) occurs and full recovery from shock is no longer possible. Table 40-2 lists the progression of shock.

INITIAL STAGE OF SHOCK (EARLY SHOCK)

The **initial** (early) stage of shock is present when the client's baseline MAP is decreased by less than 10 mm Hg. During this stage, compensatory mechanisms are so effective at returning MAP to normal levels that oxygenated blood flow to all vital organs is maintained. The cellular change in this stage is increased anaerobic metabolism with production of lactic acid, although overall cellular metabolism is still aerobic. Compensation (vascular constriction and increased heart rate) is effective, and both cardiac output and MAP are maintained within the normal range. Because vital organ function is not disrupted, the manifestations of shock are difficult to detect. *An increase in heart and respiratory rate from the client's baseline level or a slight increase in diastolic blood pressure may be the only objective manifestations of this early stage of shock.*

NONPROGRESSIVE STAGE (COMPENSATORY STAGE)

The **nonprogressive** (compensatory) stage of shock occurs when MAP decreases 10 to 15 mm Hg from baseline. Kidney and hormonal mechanisms are activated because cardiovascular compensation alone is not enough to maintain MAP and supply needed oxygen to the vital organs.

The kidneys and baroreceptors sense an ongoing decrease in MAP and trigger the release of renin, antidiuretic hormone (ADH), aldosterone, epinephrine, and norepinephrine. Kidney compensation occurs through the actions of renin, aldosterone, and ADH (see Chapter 14). Renin, secreted by the kidney, starts the reactions to decrease urine output, increase sodium reabsorption, and cause widespread blood vessel constriction (see Chapter 14, Figure 14-8). ADH is secreted by the posterior pituitary gland. ADH increases water reabsorption in the kidney and causes blood vessel constriction in the skin and other less vital tissue areas. Together these actions compensate for shock by keeping volume in the central blood vessels.

Tissue hypoxia occurs in nonvital organs and in the kidney, but it is not great enough to cause permanent damage. Because some metabolism is anaerobic, acid-base and electrolyte changes occur in response to the buildup of metabolites. Changes include **acidosis** (low blood pH) and **hyperkalemia** (increased blood potassium level) (see Chapters 16 and 19).

If the client is stable and compensatory mechanisms are supported by interventions, he or she can remain in this stage for hours without having permanent damage. Stopping the conditions that started the shock and providing supportive interventions can prevent the shock from progressing. The cellular effects of this stage are reversible with intervention.

PROGRESSIVE STAGE OF SHOCK (INTERMEDIATE STAGE)

The **progressive** stage of shock occurs when there is a sustained decrease in MAP of more than 20 mm Hg from baseline. In this stage compensatory mechanisms are functioning but no longer deliver sufficient oxygen, even to vital organs. Compensatory mechanisms use large amounts of oxygen in some tissues, which worsens the problem of general poor oxygenation. Vital organs develop hypoxia, and less vital organs become **anoxic** (no oxygen) and **ischemic** (cell dysfunction or death from lack of oxygen). As a result of poor oxygenation and a buildup of toxic metabolites, some tissues have severe cell damage and die.

The progressive stage of shock is a life-threatening emergency. Vital organs can tolerate this situation for only a short time before being damaged permanently. Immediate interventions are needed to reverse the effects of this stage of shock. Tolerance varies from person to person and depends on pre-existing health. The client's life usually can be saved if the conditions causing shock are corrected within 1 hour of the onset of the progressive stage.

REFRACTORY STAGE OF SHOCK (IRREVERSIBLE STAGE)

Formerly called the **irreversible stage,** the **refractory stage** of shock occurs when too much cell death and tissue damage results from too little oxygen reaching the tissues. Vital organs have overwhelming damage. This stage is termed *refractory* because the body is unable to respond effectively to interventions, and shock continues. The remaining cells metabolize anaerobically. *Therapy is not effective in saving the client's life, even if the cause of shock is corrected and MAP temporarily returns to normal.* So much tissue damage has occurred with widespread release of toxic metabolites and destructive enzymes that cell damage in vital organs continues.

MULTIPLE ORGAN DYSFUNCTION SYNDROME

The sequence of cell damage caused by the massive release of toxic metabolites and enzymes is termed **multiple organ dysfunction syndrome (MODS).** Once the damage has started, the sequence becomes a vicious cycle as more dead cells break open and release harmful metabolites. The metabolites trigger small clots *(microthrombi)* to form. The clots block tissue oxygenation and damage more cells, thus continuing the devastating cycle. MODS occurs first in the liver, heart, brain, and kidney. In septic shock, the lungs also are affected. The most profound change is damage to the heart muscle. One cause of this damage is the release of myocardial depressant factor (MDF) from the ischemic pancreas.

Etiology

Because shock is a manifestation of a pathologic condition rather than a disease state, its causes vary. Specific problems leading to different types of shock are listed in Table 40-3. *More than one type of shock can be present at the same time.* For example, trauma caused by a car accident may trigger hemorrhage (leading to hypovolemic shock) and a myocardial infarction (leading to cardiogenic shock).

TABLE 40-3 Causes of Shock

Hypovolemic Shock	Distributive Shock
Overall Cause	***Overall Cause***
Body fluid depletion	Decreased vascular volume or tone
Hemorrhage	***Specific Cause or Risk Factors***
▪ Trauma	Neural-induced
▪ Gastrointestinal ulcer	▪ Pain
▪ Surgery	▪ Anesthesia
▪ Inadequate clotting	▪ Stress
Hemophilia	▪ Spinal cord injury
Liver disease	▪ Head trauma
Malnutrition	Chemical-induced
Bone marrow suppression	▪ Anaphylaxis
Cancer	▪ Sepsis
Anticoagulation therapy	▪ Capillary leak
Dehydration	Burns
▪ Vomiting	Extensive trauma
▪ Diarrhea	Hepatic dysfunction
▪ Heavy diaphoresis	Hypoproteinemia
▪ Diuretic therapy	
▪ Nasogastric suction	**Obstructive Shock**
▪ Diabetes insipidus	***Overall Cause***
▪ Hyperglycemia	Indirect pump failure
Cardiogenic Shock	***Specific Cause or Risk Factors***
Overall Cause	Cardiac tamponade
Direct pump failure	Arterial stenosis
Specific Cause or Risk Factors	Pulmonary embolus
Myocardial infarction	Pulmonary hypertension
Cardiac arrest	Constrictive pericarditis
Ventricular dysrhythmias	Thoracic tumors
▪ Fibrillation	Tension pneumothorax
▪ Tachycardia	
Cardiac amyloidosis	
Cardiomyopathies	
▪ Viral	
▪ Toxic	
Myocardial degeneration	

HYPOVOLEMIC SHOCK

Hypovolemic shock occurs when too little circulating blood volume causes a MAP decrease so that the body's total need for oxygen is not met. Common problems leading to hypovolemic shock are hemorrhage (external or internal) and dehydration.

Hypovolemic shock caused by external hemorrhage is common after trauma and surgery. Hypovolemic shock caused by internal hemorrhage occurs with blunt trauma, gastrointestinal (GI) ulcers, and poor control of surgical bleeding. External and internal hemorrhage can be caused by any problem that reduces the levels of clotting factors (see Table 40-3). Hypovolemia as a result of dehydration can be caused by any problem that decreases fluid intake or increases fluid loss (see Table 40-3).

CARDIOGENIC SHOCK

Cardiogenic shock occurs when the actual heart muscle is unhealthy and pumping is directly impaired. Table 40-3 lists the common causes of direct pump failure. These conditions decrease cardiac output and afterload, thus reducing MAP. Chapter 41 discusses cardiogenic shock resulting from myocardial infarction.

DISTRIBUTIVE SHOCK

Distributive shock is caused by a loss of sympathetic tone, blood vessel dilation, pooling of blood in venous and capillary beds, and increased blood vessel permeability (capillary leak). All these factors can decrease mean arterial pressure (MAP) and may be started by nerve changes (neural-induced) or the presence of chemicals (chemical-induced).

NEURAL-INDUCED DISTRIBUTIVE SHOCK. Neural-induced loss of MAP occurs when sympathetic nerve impulses controlling blood vessel smooth muscle are decreased and the smooth muscles of blood vessels relax, causing vasodilation. This blood vessel dilation can be a normal local response to injury, but shock results when the vasodilation is widespread or systemic. Common problems that can cause a systemic loss of sympathetic tone are listed in Table 40-3.

CHEMICAL-INDUCED DISTRIBUTIVE SHOCK. Chemical-induced distributive shock has three common origins: anaphylaxis, sepsis, and capillary leak syndrome. Chemical-induced distributive shock occurs when certain chemicals or foreign substances within the blood and blood vessels start widespread changes in blood vessel walls. The chemicals are usually **exogenous** (originate outside the body), but this type of shock also can be induced by substances normally found in the body **(endogenous).**

ANAPHYLAXIS. Anaphylaxis is one result of type I allergic reactions (see Chapter 26). It begins within seconds to minutes after exposure to a specific allergen. It is termed *delayed,* however, because this type of reaction rarely occurs the first time a person encounters the allergen. It occurs on repeated exposure to the same allergen (McCance & Huether, 2002). Table 26-2 lists common allergens that can cause anaphylaxis.

Anaphylaxis is due to an antigen-antibody reaction that occurs in blood vessels throughout the body in response to contact with a substance to which the person has a severe allergy. This widespread reaction involves the interaction of the allergen, immunoglobulin E (IgE), basophils, and mast cells. It occurs within the walls of blood vessels, heart muscle cells, and bronchial tubes (see Chapters 23 and 26).

Anaphylaxis damages cells and causes the release of large amounts of histamine and other inflammatory chemicals. These natural chemicals move rapidly in the blood, causing massive blood vessel dilation and increased capillary leak. These responses result in severe hypovolemia and vascular collapse. Decreased cardiac contraction and dysrhythmias occur during anaphylaxis. These symptoms may be the result of heart-muscle changes induced by the antigen-antibody reaction, or they may result from the profound hypovolemia and resulting tissue hypoxia. Antigen-antibody reactions in the bronchial tissues cause severe edema and obstruction, which reduce gas exchange. The pulmonary problems, together with reduced circulation, cause extreme whole-body hypoxia. *Without intervention, this condition results in death.*

SEPSIS. Sepsis leading to distributive shock occurs when organisms are present in the blood. This form of shock is most commonly called **septic shock.** Sepsis often occurs with disseminated intravascular coagulation (DIC). Septic shock (sepsis-induced distributive shock) occurs most often with bacterial infection and has also been reported among clients with viral and yeast sepsis. Common organisms causing sepsis include gram-negative bacteria (*Pseudomonas aeruginosa, Escherichia coli,* and *Klebsiella pneumoniae*) and gram-positive bacteria (*Staphylococcus* and *Streptococcus*). Table 40-4 lists some of the health problems that increase the risk for septic shock.

Septic shock occurs when large amounts of toxins and endotoxins produced by bacteria are released into the blood, causing a whole-body inflammatory reaction. These substances react with blood vessels and cell membranes. Through the activity of white blood cells, the reactions start inflammatory and immune events known as the **systemic inflammatory response syndrome (SIRS).** These toxin-host actions activate complement, cause small clots to form within the capillaries of vital organs, increase capillary leakiness, injure cells (especially endothelial cells of blood vessels), and increase cell metabolism. Damage to endothelial cells reduces anticlotting actions and triggers the formation of small clots. Metabolism becomes anaerobic because of decreased MAP, clot formation in capillaries, and poor cell uptake of oxygen.

CAPILLARY LEAK SYNDROME. Capillary leak syndrome leading to distributive shock occurs when fluid shifts from the blood to the interstitial space. Such shifts are caused by increased size of capillary pores, loss of plasma osmolarity, and increased hydrostatic pressure in the blood. Problems causing fluid shifts include severe burns, liver disorders, ascites, peritonitis, paralytic ileus, severe malnutrition, large wounds, hyperglycemia, kidney disease, hypoproteinemia, and trauma.

TABLE 40-4 Conditions Predisposing to Sepsis-Induced Distributive Shock (Septic Shock)

- Malnutrition
- Immunosuppression
- Large, open wounds
- Mucous membrane fissures in prolonged contact with bloody or drainage-soaked packing
- Gastrointestinal ischemia
- Loss of gastrointestinal integrity
- Exposure to invasive procedures
- Malignancy
- Over 85 years of age
- Infection with resistant microorganisms
- Receiving cancer chemotherapy

OBSTRUCTIVE SHOCK

Obstructive shock is caused by problems that impair the ability of the normal heart muscle to pump effectively. The heart itself is normal, but conditions outside the heart prevent either adequate filling of the heart or adequate contraction of the healthy heart muscle. Common causes of obstructive shock are listed in Table 40-3.

Incidence/Prevalence

The exact incidence of shock is not known because it is a response rather than a disease. Shock is a common complication among hospitalized clients. Hypovolemic shock is most common among clients in emergency departments and after surgery or invasive procedures. Cardiogenic shock is the most common complication of myocardial infarction (MI) in clients who have damage to 40% or more of the heart muscle. Distributive shock from sepsis, which has a 40% to 85% mortality rate, is increasing among clients who are immunocompromised or have infections.

This chapter presents the collaborative management of clients with hypovolemic shock caused by hemorrhage and distributive shock caused by sepsis. Chapter 26 discusses anaphylaxis, and Chapter 41 discusses care of the client with cardiogenic shock as a result of MI.

HEALTH PROMOTION/ILLNESS PREVENTION

Hypovolemic Shock

Although hypovolemic shock often occurs as a complication of surgical intervention or trauma, primary prevention is possible. Chart 40-2 lists interventions to prevent shock. Teach all people to prevent dehydration by having an adequate fluid intake during exercise or when in hot, dry environments. Urge people to prevent trauma and hemorrhage by using proper safety equipment, seat belts, and being aware of hazards in the home or workplace.

Secondary prevention of hypovolemic shock is a major nursing responsibility. Keep in mind that just being a client

CHART 40-2

NIC **INTERVENTION ACTIVITIES for Shock Prevention**

Shock Prevention: *Detecting and treating a client at risk for impending shock*

- Monitor circulatory status: BP, skin color, skin temperature, heart sounds, heart rate and rhythm, presence and quality of peripheral pulses, and capillary refill.
- Monitor for signs of inadequate tissue oxygenation.
- Monitor for apprehension, increased anxiety, and changes in mental status.
- Monitor temperature and respiratory status.
- Monitor intake and output.
- Monitor laboratory values, especially hemoglobin and hematocrit levels, clotting profile, ABG and electrolyte levels, cultures, and chemistry profile.
- Note bruising, petechiae, and condition of mucous membranes.
- Note color, amount, and frequency of stools, vomitus, and nasogastric drainage.
- Test urine for blood, glucose, and protein, as appropriate.
- Monitor abdominal pain and girth.
- Monitor for early compensatory responses to fluid loss: increased heart rate, decreased BP, orthostatic hypotension, decreased urinary output, narrowed pulse pressure, decreased capillary refill, apprehension, pale and cool skin, and diaphoresis.
- Monitor for early signs of septic shock: warm, flushed, dry skin; increasing cardiac output and temperature; and declining SVR and PAP.
- Monitor for possible sources of fluid loss: chest tube, wound, and nasogastric drainage; diarrhea; vomiting; and increasing abdominal and extremity girth.
- Place client in supine position with legs elevated to increase preload, as appropriate.
- Administer IV and/or oral fluids, as appropriate.
- Initiate early administration of antimicrobial agents and closely monitor their effectiveness, as appropriate.

NIC intervention activities selected from Dochterman, J.M., & Bulechek, G.M. (Eds.). (2004). *Nursing interventions classification (NIC)* (4th ed). St. Louis: Mosby.

PAP, Pulmonary artery pressure; *SVR,* systemic vascular resistance.

in the acute care setting is a risk factor. Identify clients at risk for dehydration and assess for early manifestations. This is especially important for those who have reduced cognition or reduced mobility or who are on nothing-by-mouth (NPO) status.

Assess all clients who have invasive procedures or trauma for obvious or occult bleeding. Compare pulse quality and rate to baseline. Compare urine output to fluid intake. Check vital signs for clients who have persistent thirst. Assess for shock in any client who develops a change in mental status, an increase in pain, or an increase in anxiety.

Septic Shock

Identify clients at risk for sepsis. Use aseptic technique during invasive procedures and when working with nonintact skin and mucous membranes in immunocompromised clients. Remove indwelling urinary catheters and intravenous (IV) access lines as soon as they are no longer needed. Contact with potted plants and cut flowers has been considered a source of potential infection and sepsis for susceptible clients. Restriction of these items in hospital units to prevent infection is controversial (see the Evidence-Based Practice for Nursing box above).

EVIDENCE-BASED PRACTICE for Nursing

Flowers and plants as sources of infection

LaCharity, L., & McClure, E. (2003). Are plants vectors for transmission of infection in acute care? *Critical Care Nursing Clinics of North America, 15*(1), 119-124.

This research is an analysis of the evidence regarding potted plants and cut flowers as infection sources in acute care settings, especially for clients at higher risk for infection. The authors reviewed current and historical nursing and medical literature. The review revealed that many health care professionals, hospitals, professional organizations, and the Centers for Disease Control and Prevention continue to recommend restriction of cut flowers and potted plants in rooms of clients at risk for infection and sepsis. These recommendations, however, were not based on clinical evidence. Few prospective clinical studies in which organisms were cultured from plants, soil, cut flowers, or vase water and compared with the organisms present in client wounds, drainage, or blood have been completed. Some recently published studies examined plant, soil, flower, and water environments under controlled conditions.

Soil of potted plants was found to contain bacteria and fungus. Standing vase water contained the largest variety and greatest quantities of microorganisms. Adding hydrogen peroxide to vase water reduced the number of organisms and did not adversely affect cut flowers. Using sterile or distilled water in vases did not reduce the growth of organisms.

Level of Evidence: 1—Quantitative systematic review.

Critique. Clinical studies are needed to compare organisms found in clients with infections who also have plants or flowers in the room to the organisms in the plant and flower environments. Studies are also needed that examine the presence of specific organisms on the hands of persons handling potted plants and flowers in the acute care setting and whether standard handwashing is effective in removing these organisms.

Implications for Nursing. Although no clear evidence links the actual transmission of infectious organisms from plants and flowers to clients, it seems reasonable for nurses to restrict these items from the rooms of clients who are immunocompromised or who have open wounds. Other precautionary recommendations include teaching the client to refrain from caring for plants or flowers, having personnel handling plants or flowers not have direct contact with clients, changing vase water at least every 3 days, and adding hydrogen peroxide to vase water. The use of good handwashing after handling flowers remains a major anti-infection strategy for nursing personnel and clients.

Early detection of septic shock is a major nursing responsibility. Because septic shock can be a complication of many conditions found in acute care settings, always consider the possibility of septic shock. Assess vital signs often (at least twice per shift) for changes from baseline levels. Review laboratory data for changes in total white blood cell count and in the differential. The hallmark of sepsis is a decreasing segmented neutrophil level with a rising band neutrophil level. This change is called a **left shift** (see Chapter 23).

COLLABORATIVE MANAGEMENT: HYPOVOLEMIC SHOCK

The Concept Map on p. 829 addresses assessment and nursing care issues related to clients with hypovolemic shock.

Assessment

HISTORY

Collect data on risk factors and causative factors related to hypovolemic shock. If the client is alert and stable, question him or her directly. If the client is not alert or if his or her

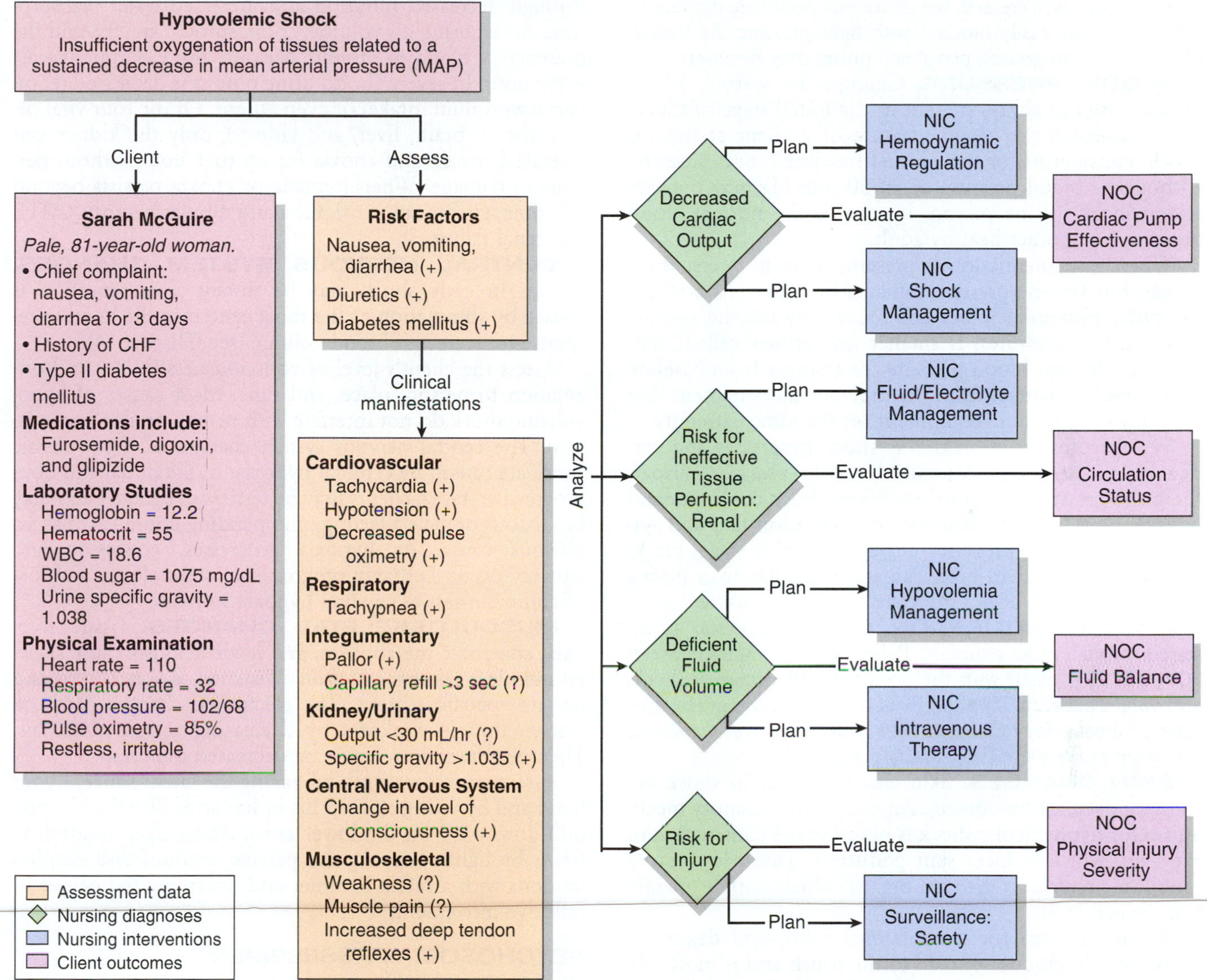

Concept Map by Elaine Bishop Kennedy, EdD, RN

condition is not stable, collect information from family members. *Age* is important because hypovolemic shock from trauma is more common in young adults, whereas sepsis is more common among older adults. Ask clients specific questions about recent illness, trauma, procedures, or chronic health problems that may lead to shock. Such problems include GI ulcers, general surgery, hemophilia, liver disorders, prolonged vomiting, and prolonged diarrhea. Ask about the use of drugs such as aspirin, diuretics, and antacids that may cause changes leading to hypovolemic shock or may indicate the presence of a problem that can contribute to shock.

Ask about fluid intake and output during the previous 24 hours. *Information about urine output is especially important because urine output is reduced during the first stages of shock, even when fluid intake is normal.*

Assess the client for obvious signs of factors that can lead to shock. Areas to examine for signs of hemorrhage include the gums, wounds, and sites of dressings, drains, and vascular accesses. Also check *under* the client for blood. Observe for any swelling or skin discoloration that may indicate an internal hemorrhage.

PHYSICAL ASSESSMENT/CLINICAL MANIFESTATIONS

Most manifestations of hypovolemic shock are caused by the changes resulting from compensatory efforts. **Compensation** or **compensatory mechanisms** are physiologic responses that try to keep an adequate blood flow to vital organs. Signs of shock are first evident as changes in cardiovascular function. As shock progresses, changes in the kidney, respiratory, integumentary, musculoskeletal, and central nervous systems become evident.

CARDIOVASCULAR CHANGES. Shock decreases mean arterial pressure (MAP), and the resulting early compensation is cardiovascular. Thus the earliest clinical signs of hypovolemic shock are cardiovascular.

PULSE. Assess the central and peripheral pulses for rate and quality. In the initial stage of hypovolemic shock, the pulse rate increases to keep cardiac output and MAP at normal levels, even though the actual **stroke volume** (amount of blood pumped out from the heart) per beat is decreased. Because stroke volume is decreased, the peripheral pulses are difficult to palpate and are easily blocked with light pressure. As hypovolemic shock progresses, peripheral pulses may be absent.

BLOOD PRESSURE. Changes in systolic blood pressure are not always present in the initial stage of shock. When assessing the blood pressure of a client at risk for shock, consider his or her normal baseline blood pressure. Although a blood pressure of 90/50 mm Hg may indicate severe shock in one person, it may be the normal blood pressure for another healthy adult.

When vasoconstriction is present, diastolic pressure increases but systolic pressure remains the same. As a result, the **pulse pressure,** or the difference between the systolic and diastolic pressures, is smaller (sometimes called "narrower"). Monitor blood pressure for changes from baseline levels and for changes from the previous measurement. For accuracy use the same equipment on the same extremity.

Systolic pressure decreases as shock progresses and cardiac output decreases. A reduced systolic pressure narrows the pulse pressure even further. When shock continues and interventions are not adequate, compensation fails and systolic and diastolic pressures decrease. At this stage, blood pressure is difficult to hear. Palpation or a Doppler device may be needed to detect the systolic blood pressure.

OXYGEN SATURATION. Oxygen saturation is assessed through pulse oximetry. Pulse oximetry values between 90% and 95% occur with the nonprogressive stage of shock, and values between 75% and 80% occur with the progressive stage of shock. *Any value below 70% is considered a life-threatening emergency and may signal the refractory stage of shock.*

SKIN CHANGES. Skin changes occur in shock because of decreased perfusion. An early compensatory mechanism for hypovolemic shock is blood vessel constriction in the skin, which reduces skin perfusion. This allows more blood to circulate to the vital organs, which cannot tolerate low oxygen levels.

Assess the skin for temperature, color, and degree of moisture. It feels cool or cold to the touch and is moist. As shock progresses, color changes are first evident in the mucous membranes and in the skin around the mouth. Pallor or cyanosis is best assessed in the oral mucous membranes in dark-skinned clients. Color changes in clients with lighter skin are noted first in the extremities and then in the central trunk area. The skin feels clammy or moist to the touch, not because sweating increases but because the normal fluid lost through the skin does not evaporate quickly on cold skin.

Evaluate capillary refill time by pressing on the client's fingernail until it blanches and then observing how fast the nail bed resumes color when pressure is released. Normally the nail bed capillaries resume color as soon as pressure is released. With shock, capillary refill is slow or is sometimes absent. Capillary refill may not be a reliable indicator for peripheral blood flow in older clients or those with anemia, diabetes mellitus, or peripheral vascular disease.

RESPIRATORY CHANGES. Assess the rate, depth, and ease of respiration and also auscultate the lungs for abnormal breath sounds. Respiratory rate increases during hypovolemic shock. This increase is a compensatory mechanism to provide oxygen to the critical tissues. When shock progresses to the stage at which lactic acidosis is present, the respiratory depth also increases.

RENAL/URINARY CHANGES. The renal system compensates for decreased MAP by saving body water through decreased filtration and increased water reabsorption. Assess urine for volume, color, specific gravity, and the presence of blood or protein. Measure urine output at least every hour. In severe shock, urine output is decreased (compared with fluid intake) or even absent. Of the four vital organs (heart, brain, liver, and kidney), only the kidney can tolerate hypoxia and anoxia for up to 1 hour without permanent damage. When hypoxia or anoxia persists beyond this time, clients are at risk for acute tubular necrosis (ATN) and renal failure.

CENTRAL NERVOUS SYSTEM CHANGES. Clients in early shock may be thirsty. This sensation is caused by stimulation of the thirst centers in the brain in response to decreased blood volume (see Chapter 14).

Assess the client's level of consciousness (LOC) and orientation to person, place, and time. Most causes of hypovolemic shock do not interfere with nerve impulse transmission. The central nervous system changes of hypovolemic shock are caused by cerebral hypoxia. In the initial and nonprogressive stages, clients may be restless or agitated and may be anxious or have a feeling of impending doom that has no obvious cause. As hypoxia progresses, confusion and lethargy occur. Lethargy progresses to somnolence and loss of consciousness as cerebral hypoxia worsens.

MUSCULOSKELETAL CHANGES. Tissue hypoxia, anaerobic metabolism, and lactic acidosis cause skeletal muscle weakness and pain. Weakness is generalized and has no specific pattern. The electrolyte changes of shock worsen muscle weakness by decreasing action potentials. Then deep tendon reflexes are decreased or absent.

Assess muscle strength by having the client squeeze your hand and by trying to keep his or her arms flexed while you pull downward on the lower arms. Assess deep tendon reflexes by lightly tapping the patellar tendons and Achilles tendons with a reflex hammer and observing the degree of reflexive movement.

PSYCHOSOCIAL ASSESSMENT

Changes in mental status and behavior may be early signs of shock. Observe the client closely and document behavior. Assess current mental status by evaluating LOC and noting whether the client is asleep or awake. If the client is asleep, attempt to awaken him or her and document how easily he or she is aroused. If the client is awake, determine whether he or she is oriented to person, time, and place. Avoid asking questions that can be answered with a "yes" or a "no" response. Consider the following points during assessment:

- Is it necessary to repeat questions to obtain a response?
- Does the response answer the question asked?
- Does the client have difficulty making word choices?
- Is the client irritated or upset by the questions?
- Can the client concentrate on a question long enough to answer appropriately, or is the attention span limited?

If possible, talk with family members to determine whether the client's behavior and mental status are typical or represent a change.

LABORATORY ASSESSMENT

Although no single laboratory finding confirms or rules out shock, changes in laboratory data may support the diagno-

CHART 40-3

LABORATORY PROFILE
Hypovolemic Shock

Test	Normal Range for Adults	Significance of Abnormal Findings
pH (arterial)	7.35-7.45	Decreased: insufficient tissue oxygenation causing anaerobic metabolism and acidosis
Pao_2	80-100 mm Hg	Decreased: anaerobic metabolism
$Paco_2$	35-45 mm Hg	Increased: anaerobic metabolism
Lactic acid (arterial)	0.3-0.8 mmol/L	Increased: anaerobic metabolism with buildup of metabolites
Hematocrit	*Females:* 37%-47% *Males:* 42%-52%	Increased: fluid shift, dehydration Decreased: hemorrhage
Hemoglobin	*Females:* 12-16 g/dL *Males:* 14-18 g/dL	Increased: fluid shift, dehydration Decreased: hemorrhage
Potassium	3.5-5.0 mEq/L or mmol/L	Increased: dehydration, acidosis

Data from Pagana, K., & Pagana, T. (2002). *Mosby's manual of diagnostic and laboratory tests* (2nd ed.). St. Louis: Mosby.
Pao_2, Partial pressure of arterial oxygen; *$Paco_2$*, partial pressure of arterial carbon dioxide.

sis of hypovolemic shock. (Chart 40-3 lists common laboratory findings occurring with hypovolemic shock.) As shock progresses, arterial blood gas values become abnormal. The pH decreases, the partial pressure of arterial oxygen (Pao_2) decreases, and the partial pressure of arterial carbon dioxide ($Paco_2$) increases. Changes in other laboratory values may occur with specific causes of hypovolemic shock.

Hematocrit and hemoglobin levels decrease if shock is caused by hemorrhage. When shock is caused by dehydration or a fluid shift, hematocrit and hemoglobin levels are elevated.

Common Nursing Diagnoses and Collaborative Problems

Nursing diagnoses that may apply to clients with hypovolemic shock include the following:

- Anxiety related to potential for death
- Deficient Fluid Volume related to active fluid volume loss
- Decreased Cardiac Output related to hypovolemia
- Ineffective Tissue Perfusion (General) related to hypovolemia
- Disturbed Thought Processes related to decreased cerebral perfusion

Critical Thinking Challenge

Your client is a 33-year-old woman who is returned to your outpatient unit after having a surgical tubal ligation by colposcopy. After moving her from the stretcher to her bed, you take her vital signs. Her pulse is 110 and thready, blood pressure is 90/72, respiratory rate is 28, and pulse oximetry is 89%. When you shake her shoulder, she opens her eyes but does not answer any questions.

1. What should you do first?
2. What other assessment data should you obtain?
3. Given the type of surgery, where would you expect bleeding to occur and what manifestations would you expect to find?
4. She still has an IV in her left hand infusing dextrose 5% in 0.45% saline. The postsurgical orders indicate that it should be removed when she is stable. Should you remove it now? Why or why not?

evolve For suggested answer guidelines, go to http://evolve.elsevier.com/Iggy/.

CHART 40-4

BEST PRACTICE for
The Client in Hypovolemic Shock

- Ensure a patent airway.
- Start an IV catheter or maintain an established catheter.
- Administer oxygen.
- Elevate the client's feet, keeping his or her head flat or elevated to a 30-degree angle.
- Examine the client for overt bleeding.
- If overt bleeding is present, apply direct pressure to the site.
- Administer medications as prescribed.
- Increase the rate of IV fluid delivery.
- Do not leave the client.

CHART 40-5

NIC **INTERVENTION ACTIVITIES for**
The Client with Hypovolemic Shock

Shock Management: Volume: *Promotion of adequate tissue perfusion for a client with severely compromised intravascular volume*

- Monitor for signs and symptoms of persistent bleeding (e.g., check all secretions for frank or occult blood).
- Monitor the client closely for hemorrhage.
- Prevent blood volume loss (e.g., apply pressure to site of bleeding).
- Administer IV fluids, as appropriate.
- Note hemoglobin/hematocrit level before and after blood loss, as indicated.
- Administer blood products (e.g., platelets or fresh frozen plasma), as appropriate.
- Monitor coagulation studies, including prothrombin time (PT), partial thromboplastin time (PTT), fibrinogen, fibrin degradation/split products, and platelet counts, as appropriate.

NIC intervention activities selected from Dochterman, J.M., & Bulechek, G.M. (Eds.). (2004). *Nursing interventions classification (NIC)* (4th ed.). St. Louis: Mosby. No part of this work is to be altered without prior written permission from the Publisher.

Interventions

Interventions for clients in hypovolemic shock focus on reversing the shock, restoring fluid volume, and preventing complications through supportive and drug therapies. Surgery may be needed to correct the problem leading to hypovolemic shock. Chart 40-4 lists best practices for clients in hypovolemic shock. Chart 40-5 lists NIC interventions for clients with hypovolemic shock.

NONSURGICAL MANAGEMENT. The goals of shock management are to maintain tissue oxygenation, increase vascular volume to normal range, and support compensatory mechanisms. Oxygen therapy, fluid replacement therapy, and drug therapies are useful for this problem.

Oxygen Therapy. Oxygen therapy is useful whenever shock is present. Oxygen can be delivered by mask, hood, nasal cannula, nasopharyngeal tube, endotracheal tube, and tracheostomy tube. Oxygen is given in L/min (when using a cannula) or concentration by percentage (when using a mask).

Intravenous Therapy. Colloids and crystalloids are the two types of fluids used for volume replacement during hypovolemia. Colloid solutions contain large molecules (usually proteins or starches) (see Chapter 14). Crystalloid solutions contain nonprotein substances (e.g., minerals, salts, sugars).

Colloid Fluids. Protein-containing colloid fluids help restore osmotic pressure and fluid volume. Blood and blood products are often used for this purpose when shock is caused by blood loss. These fluids include whole blood, packed red blood cells, plasma, plasma fractions, and synthetic plasma expanders.

Whole blood and packed red blood cells increase hematocrit and hemoglobin levels along with fluid volume. Whole blood is used to replace large volumes of blood loss because it increases volume and improves the oxygen-carrying capacity of the blood. Packed red cells are given for moderate blood loss because they restore the red blood cell deficit and improve oxygen-carrying capacity without adding excessive fluid volume. Chapter 43 discusses nursing care issues when giving blood or blood products.

Human plasma, an acellular blood product containing some clotting factors, is given to restore osmotic pressure when hematocrit and hemoglobin levels are within normal ranges. Plasma protein fractions (e.g., Plasmanate) and synthetic plasma expanders (e.g., hetastarch [hydroxyethyl starch, Hespan]) increase plasma volume and are used as early treatment for hypovolemic shock before a cause has been established.

Crystalloid Fluids. Crystalloid fluids are given to help maintain an adequate fluid and electrolyte balance. Two common solutions are Ringer's lactate and normal saline. Ringer's lactate contains sodium, chloride, calcium, potassium, and lactate dissolved in water. This isotonic solution expands volume, and the lactate buffers any acidosis. Normal saline (0.9% sodium chloride in water) is a fluid replacement used to increase plasma volume when there has been no loss of red blood cells.

Drug Therapy. Drugs may be needed if the volume deficit is severe and the client does not respond sufficiently to the replacement of fluid volume and blood products. The actions of drugs for shock increase venous return, improve cardiac contractility, or improve cardiac perfusion by dilating the coronary vessels. Chart 40-6 lists the drugs used to treat hypovolemic shock.

Vasoconstricting Drugs. Many drugs stimulate venous return by constricting blood vessels and decreasing venous pooling of blood. These actions increase cardiac output and mean arterial pressure (MAP), which helps to improve tissue perfusion and oxygenation. Such agents include dopamine (Intropin, Revimine✱) and norepinephrine (Levophed). These drugs can produce serious side effects, and their dosages must be carefully calculated on the basis of the client's size and response to treatment (see Chart 40-6).

Drugs Enhancing Myocardial Contractility. Some drugs directly stimulate adrenergic receptor sites on the heart muscle (beta$_1$ receptors) and improve heart muscle cell contraction. Other drugs enhance cardiac contraction by slowing heart rate and allowing the left ventricle a longer filling time. When filling time is increased, more blood enters the left ventricle and stretches the muscle fibers. Thus greater recoil occurs, and more blood leaves the left ventricle during contraction. Some of these drugs also stimulate the ventricles. Drugs with these actions include dobutamine (Dobutrex) and milrinone (Primacor).

Drugs Enhancing Myocardial Perfusion. It is important to ensure that the heart is well perfused, especially when giving drugs to improve cardiac contraction, so that aerobic metabolism is maintained in the heart cells and maximum contractility can occur. Drugs that dilate coronary blood vessels while minimally dilating systemic vessels are used for this purpose. A common drug with this action is sodium nitroprusside (Nitropress, Nipride✱). *Care is taken because these drugs can cause systemic vasodilation and increase shock if the client is volume depleted.*

Monitoring. A major nursing action in caring for clients in hypovolemic shock is monitoring vital signs and level of consciousness (LOC). Monitor the following vital signs:

- Pulse
- Blood pressure
- Pulse pressure
- Central venous pressure (CVP)
- Respiratory rate
- Skin and mucosal color
- Oxygen saturation

Assess parameters at least every 15 minutes until the shock is controlled and the client's condition improves. Hemodynamic monitoring in critical care settings includes intra-arterial monitoring, mixed venous oxygen saturation (SvO_2), pulmonary artery monitoring, and pulmonary capillary wedge pressures. Table 40-5 compares the changes in hemodynamic patterns seen with different types of shock.

Insertion of a CVP catheter allows pressure to be monitored in the client's right atrium or superior vena cava while providing venous access. Changes in CVP reflect hypovolemic shock. As circulating volume decreases, the amount of blood returning to the right atrium also decreases, causing the CVP to decrease from baseline levels.

Intra-arterial catheters allow continuous monitoring of blood pressure and are an access for arterial blood sampling. Intra-arterial catheters are inserted into an artery (radial, brachial, femoral, or dorsalis pedis). The catheter is attached to pressure tubing and a transducer. The transducer converts pressure in the artery into an electrical signal that is seen as a visible waveform on an oscilloscope and as digital numeric value.

SURGICAL MANAGEMENT. The nonsurgical interventions described above are used to stabilize the client's hemodynamic status. After a cause has been established, surgical intervention may be needed to correct the cause of shock. Such procedures include vascular repair or revision, surgical hemostasis of major wounds, closure of bleeding ulcers, and chemical scarring (chemosclerosis) of varicosities.

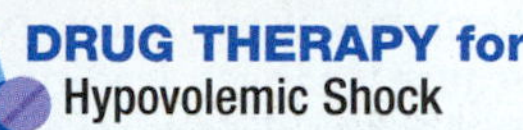

CHART 40-6

DRUG THERAPY for Hypovolemic Shock

Drug	Usual Dosage	Nursing Interventions	Rationales
Vasoconstrictors			
Dopamine hydrochloride (Intropin, Revimine✱)	5-30 mcg/kg/min IV (for hypotension)	Assess the client for chest pain.	Dopamine increases myocardial oxygen consumption.
	2-5 mcg/kg/min IV (for renal perfusion)	Monitor urine output hourly.	Higher doses decrease renal perfusion and urine output.
		Assess blood pressure every 15 min.	Hypertension is a symptom of overdose.
		Assess the client for headache.	Headache is an early symptom of drug excess.
Epinephrine (Adrenalin)	0.5-1 mg IV initially, followed by 0.5 mg q5min	Monitor the client for dysrhythmias.	Epinephrine may cause ventricular tachydysrhythmias.
	May also be given by intracardiac injection	Assess the client for chest pain.	Vasoconstriction may impair cardiac oxygenation.
Norepinephrine (Levophed)	0.5-1 mcg/kg/min continuous IV infusion to maintain blood pressure at 90-100 mm Hg	Assess for extravasation.	Norepinephrine can cause severe tissue damage and necrosis.
		Observe the client's extremities for color and perfusion.	Norepinephrine can cause such vasoconstriction that peripheral ischemia may result.
Phenylephrine (Neo-Synephrine)	80-200 mcg/min IV	Assess for chest pain.	Vasoconstriction may impair cardiac oxygenation.
Agents Enhancing Contractility			
Milrinone (Primacor)	50 mcg/kg bolus over 10 min; 0.3-0.75 mcg/kg/min continuous IV infusion	Assess blood pressure every 15 min.	Hypertension is a symptom of overdose.
Atropine sulfate	0.5-1 mg IV q5min, up to a total of 2 mg	Take pulse every 5 min.	Atropine sulfate may cause a rebound tachycardia.
		Monitor urine output every 30 min.	Atropine sulfate may cause urinary retention.
		Administer cautiously to clients with glaucoma.	Atropine sulfate may precipitate an episode of acute angle-closure glaucoma.
Dobutamine hydrochloride (Dobutrex)	2.5-20 mcg/kg/min continuous IV infusion	Assess the client for chest pain.	Dobutamine increases myocardial oxygen consumption.
		Assess blood pressure every 15 minutes.	Hypertension is a symptom of overdose.
Agents Enhancing Myocardial Perfusion			
Sodium nitroprusside (Nitropress, Nipride✱)	0.5-10 mcg/kg/min continuous IV infusion	Assess blood pressure every 15 min.	Hypotension may result from the systemic dilation of veins and arteries.

Med Error Alert! *Dopamine, norepinephrine, milrinone, dobutamine, and nitroprusside are all administered in doses of micrograms, not milligrams.*

Critical Thinking Challenge

Your client who had the tubal ligation by colposcopy has no external bleeding, but her abdomen is enlarging and you observe skin discoloration on her lower back.

1. Is oxygen an appropriate therapy for her? Why or why not?
2. Should you apply pressure to the abdominal-pelvic region? Why or why not?
3. What type(s) of IV solutions should you be prepared to give? Provide a rationale for your choice. (You may need to refer to the blood therapy section of Chapter 43.)

evolve For suggested answer guidelines, go to http://evolve.elsevier.com/Iggy/.

COLLABORATIVE MANAGEMENT: SEPSIS-INDUCED DISTRIBUTIVE SHOCK (SEPTIC SHOCK)

PHARM e REVIEW

Assessment

Distributive shock caused by sepsis does not resemble other types of shock in that it has two distinctive phases (Figure 40-2). The first phase can be long, often lasting from hours to a day or longer. Manifestations during this phase are subtle. The chance for recovery is good when the client is recognized as being in the first phase of septic shock and appropriate interventions are started. The second phase of septic shock has a sudden onset and a rapid downhill course. If septic shock progresses to the second phase, chances for recovery are poor. Identifying clients in the first phase of septic shock can make the greatest difference in survival.

HISTORY

Collect data about risk factors and causative factors related to septic shock. Age is important because sepsis develops more easily among older, debilitated clients who are immunosuppressed. Chart 40-7 lists factors that increase the older adult's risk for shock. Ask about recent illness, trauma, invasive procedures, or chronic conditions that may lead to sepsis. Check which drugs the client has used in the past week. Some drugs may directly cause changes leading to shock. Also, a drug regimen may indicate a disease or problem that can contribute to septic shock. Such drugs include aspirin and aspirin-containing drugs, antibiotics, and cancer therapy drugs.

TABLE 40-5 Hemodynamic Pattern Changes Associated with Different Types of Shock

Type of Shock	Cardiac Output (CO)	Central Venous Pressure (CVP)	Pulmonary Artery Pressure (PAP)	Pulmonary Capillary Wedge Pressure (PCWP)
Hypovolemic	↓	↓	↓	↓
Cardiac	↓	↑	↑	↑
Obstructive	↓	↑	↑	↑
Distributive				
Anaphylactic	↓	↓	↓	↓
Sepsis (early)	↑	Ø	Ø or ↑	Ø or ↑
Sepsis (late)	↓	↓	↓	↓

Data from Jones, K. (1996). Shock. In J. Clochesy, et al. (Eds.). *Critical care nursing* (2nd ed., pp. 1371-1381). Philadelphia: W.B. Saunders.
↑, Increased; ↓, decreased; Ø, normal or unchanged.

PHYSICAL ASSESSMENT/CLINICAL MANIFESTATIONS

Manifestations of the first phase are unique to septic shock and are often opposite from those seen with all other types of shock. Chart 40-8 lists the manifestations of the first (hyperdynamic) phase of septic shock. These changes are caused by the body's response to endotoxins and affect most body systems.

CARDIOVASCULAR CHANGES. Endotoxins in the blood interact with white blood cells and blood vessel walls to trigger an inflammatory reaction. Some endotoxins also stimulate the heart muscle directly. As a result, cardiac output *increases* during the first phase of septic shock. This phase is hyperdynamic and also may be called the **high-output** or **warm-shock phase.** Increased cardiac output is reflected by tachycardia, increased stroke volume, a normal-to-elevated systolic blood pressure, and a normal CVP. Increased cardiac output and vasodilation make the skin color appear normal with pink mucous membranes and may feel warm to the touch. This situation is temporary and eventually the cardiac output is greatly reduced.

As septic shock progresses, disseminated intravascular coagulation (DIC) may occur. The endotoxins and inflamma-

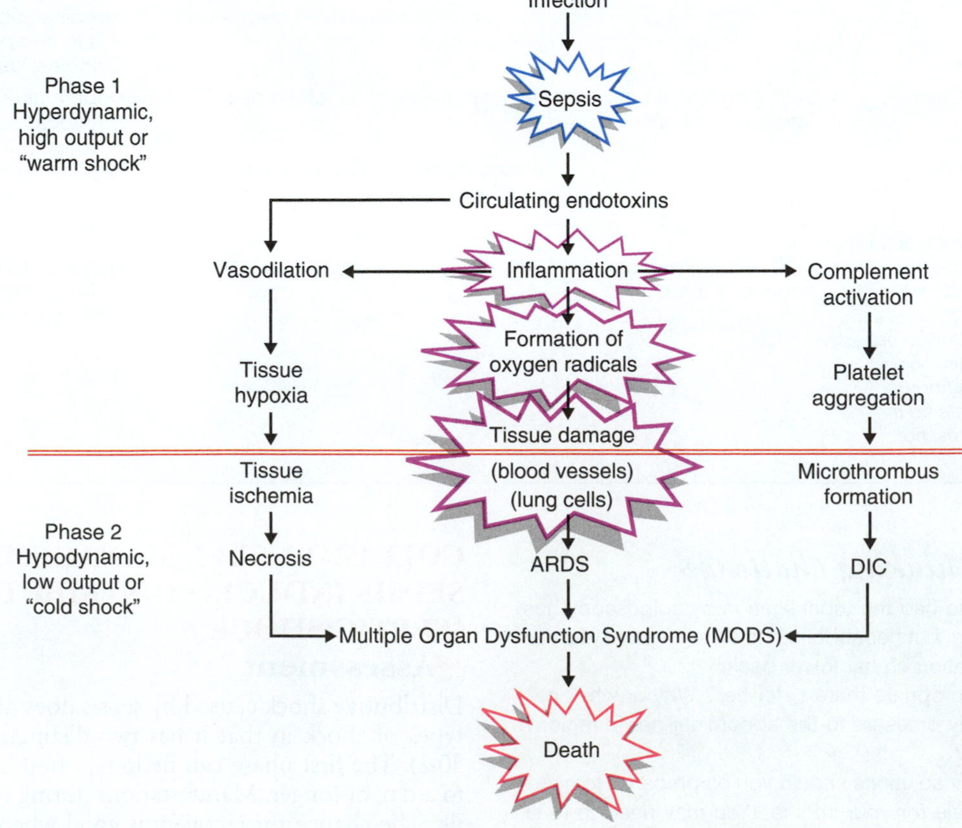

Figure 40-2 ■ The sequence of sepsis-induced distributive shock, septic shock. *ARDS,* Acute respiratory distress syndrome; *DIC,* disseminated intravascular coagulation.

tory reactions trigger complement activation (see Chapter 23). These actions damage endothelial cells of blood vessels, which then allows thousands of small clots to form in the tiny capillaries of the liver, kidney, brain, spleen, and heart. These small clots reduce oxygenation in those organs, causing hypoxia and ischemia and making overall metabolism anaerobic. This huge number of small clots uses clotting factors and fibrinogen faster than they can be produced by the liver. This problem makes clients much more susceptible to hemorrhage. Reduction of clotting factors and fibrinogen mark the beginning of the second phase of septic shock.

Because many small clots have formed, the clotting factors have been used and the blood vessels are dilated. Clients are hypovolemic in this phase of septic shock. Cardiac output, blood pressure, and pulse pressure decrease dramatically. This phase is called the **hypodynamic, low-output,** or **cold-shock phase** of septic shock. The manifestations of this phase are the same as those of the later stages of hypovolemic shock.

RESPIRATORY CHANGES. In the hyperdynamic phase of septic shock, respiratory rate and depth are increased, leading to respiratory alkalosis. When septic shock progresses to the hypodynamic phase, the life-threatening lung complication of acute respiratory distress syndrome (ARDS) may occur. ARDS in septic shock is caused by the continued systemic inflammatory response syndrome (SIRS)

CHART 40-7

NURSING FOCUS on the OLDER ADULT

Risk Factors for Shock

Hypovolemic Shock
- Diuretic therapy
- Diminished thirst reflex
- Immobility
- Use of aspirin-containing products
- Use of integrative therapies such as gingko biloba
- Anticoagulant therapy

Cardiogenic Shock
- Diabetes mellitus
- Presence of cardiomyopathies

Distributive Shock
- Diminished immune response
- Reduced skin integrity
- Presence of cancer
- Peripheral neuropathy
- Strokes
- Institutionalization (hospital or extended care facility)
- Malnutrition
- Anemia

Obstructive Shock
- Pulmonary hypertension
- Presence of cancer

CHART 40-8

KEY FEATURES of

Hyperdynamic Phase of Sepsis-Induced Distributive Shock (Septic Shock)

Assessment	Findings
General	
Assess the mental status and level of consciousness.	Irritability, restlessness, lethargy, disorientation, and inappropriate euphoria
Check the oral temperature.	Normal, subnormal, or elevated temperature
Cardiovascular System	
Check the pulse and blood pressure. Document the pulse pressure with each blood pressure reading.	Tachycardia: normal mean arterial blood pressure; widening pulse pressure
Check peripheral pulses.	"Bounding" peripheral pulses
Auscultate heart sounds at four valvular sites, and record the onset of murmur or gallop.	No murmur or gallop
Respiratory System	
Observe the rate, rhythm, and effort of breathing. Observe the symmetry of chest expansion.	Tachypnea, hyperventilation
Percuss and auscultate the lungs. Note the onset of adventitious sounds.	Crackles and decreased breath sounds
Check blood gas levels.	Respiratory alkalosis
Integumentary System	
Inspect and palpate the skin. Note color, vascularity, moisture, temperature, texture, thickness, mobility, and turgor. Assess the oral mucosa.	Warm, flushed skin and peripheral edema Pink oral mucous membranes
Immune System	
Check complete white blood count with differential and IL-6 levels.	Abnormal total white blood cell count "Left shift" (decreasing segmented neutrophils; rising band neutrophils) Rising IL-6 levels
Hematologic System	
Check platelets and clotting factors.	Decreasing fibrinogen levels Decreasing platelet levels Decreasing activated protein C Rising plasma D-dimer levels

IL-6, Interleukin-6.

increasing the formation of oxygen free radicals, which damage the lung cells. Oxygen free radicals also can form as a result of oxygen therapy and in response to release of oxidizing enzymes from damaged cells. *The presence of ARDS in a client with septic shock has a high mortality rate.*

SKIN CHANGES. It may be difficult to recognize the hyperdynamic phase of septic shock, often because the skin is warm and no cyanosis is evident. The normal appearance of the skin and mucous membranes leads health care professionals to believe circulation is unimpaired. When septic shock progresses so that circulation is compromised in the hypodynamic phase, the skin is cool and clammy, and pallor or cyanosis is present. In clients with DIC, petechiae and ecchymoses can occur anywhere. Blood may ooze from the gums, other mucous membranes, and venipuncture sites as well as around IV catheters.

PSYCHOSOCIAL ASSESSMENT

The indicator that clients may be in the beginning of septic shock is often a change in affect or behavior. Compare the client's current behavior, verbal responses, and general affect with those assessed earlier in the day or the day before. Clients may seem just slightly different in their reactions to greetings, comments, or jokes. They may be less patient than usual or act restless or fidgety. They may make statements such as, "I feel as if something is wrong, but I don't know what." If this behavior is a change from prior assessments, consider the possibility of sepsis and shock.

LABORATORY ASSESSMENT

The presence of bacteria in the blood supports the diagnosis of sepsis. Obtain specimens of urine, blood, sputum, and any drainage for culture to identify the causative organisms. Other abnormal laboratory findings that occur with septic shock include changes in the white blood cell count; the differential leukocyte count may show a left shift (see Chapter 23). Changes in hematocrit and hemoglobin levels usually are not present until late in septic shock. At that point, the hematocrit and hemoglobin levels, fibrinogen levels, and platelet count are low.

Another indicator of sepsis and septic shock is a reduction in the blood levels of **activated protein C.** This protein is an enzyme that helps prevent inappropriate clot formation. It is activated when it binds to healthy endothelial cells of blood vessels. In septic shock, the endothelial cells injured by endotoxins cannot activate protein C and thousands of small clots form in the capillaries of vascular organs. Decreasing levels of activated protein C indicate the beginning of septic shock even before other manifestations are evident (Kleinpell, 2003a).

Other biologic indicators of sepsis and septic shock are changes in plasma D-dimer levels and specific cytokine (interleukin-6 [IL-6] and interleukin-10 [IL-10]) levels. Plasma D-dimer levels rise during sepsis as the fibrin in clots is broken down. IL-6 is a proinflammatory cytokine and IL-10 is an anti-inflammatory cytokine. In sepsis, IL-6 levels rise and IL-10 levels either remain normal or decrease.

Analysis

A common collaborative problem for clients with septic shock is Potential for Multiple Organ Dysfunction Syndrome (MODS).

Planning and Implementation

POTENTIAL FOR MULTIPLE ORGAN DYSFUNCTION SYNDROME

NOC **PLANNING: EXPECTED OUTCOMES.** The client in septic shock is expected to have normal aerobic cellular metabolism. Indicators include the following:

- Arterial blood gases (pH, PaO_2, and $PaCO_2$) within the normal range
- Maintenance of a urine output of at least 20 mL/hr
- Maintenance of mean arterial blood pressure within 10 mm Hg of baseline
- Absence of multiple organ dysfunction syndrome (MODS)
- States measures to reduce the risk for sepsis

INTERVENTIONS. Interventions for septic shock focus on correcting the conditions causing shock and on preventing complications. Chart 40-9 lists the best practices for clients with septic shock.

Interventions for fluid volume deficit are the same as for hypovolemic shock.

Oxygen Therapy. Oxygen therapy is useful whenever poor tissue perfusion and poor oxygenation are present. Oxygen is delivered in the same ways as for hypovolemic shock.

Drug Therapy. The same drugs used to enhance cardiac output and restore vascular volume in hypovolemic shock are used for septic shock. A major focus of drug therapy is antibiotics to combat sepsis. In addition, drugs to counteract disseminated intravascular coagulation (DIC) may be needed. Septic shock and DIC have two distinctly different phases, and the drugs for each phase of septic shock are different. Drug therapy in the first phase is aimed at preventing coagulation by administering heparin. Drug therapy in the second, late phase of septic shock is aimed at increasing the blood's ability to clot. This therapy consists of clotting factors, plasma, platelets, or other blood products.

Antibiotics. Although septic shock can be caused by any organism, the most common agents are gram-negative

CHART 40-9

BEST PRACTICE for
The Client in Sepsis-Induced Distributive Shock (Septic Shock)

- Ensure a patent airway.
- Start or maintain an established IV catheter.
- Administer oxygen.
- Administer antibiotics.
- Obtain specimens of blood, urine, wound drainage, and sputum for culture.
- Increase the rate of IV fluid delivery.
- Use aseptic technique for any invasive procedure.
- Handle the client gently.
- Examine the client for overt bleeding, especially of gums, injection sites, and IV sites.
- Elevate the client's feet, keeping his or her head flat or elevated to a 30-degree angle.
- Take the client's vital signs every 5 minutes until they are stable.
- Administer medications as prescribed:
  - Heparin during phase 1
  - Clotting factors, platelets, and plasma during phase 2
- Do not leave the client.

bacteria. When blood cultures have identified specific bacteria, IV antibiotics with known activity against the bacteria are given. Multiple drugs with wide activity are prescribed when the causative organism is not known. Drugs and drug categories commonly used for septic shock include vancomycin, aminoglycosides, systemic penicillin or cephalosporins, macrolides, and quinolones.

Anticoagulants. When clients are in the early phase of septic shock and are beginning to form many small clots, heparin may be given to limit unneeded clotting and to prevent the consumption of clotting factors.

Clotting Factors and Blood Products. When septic shock progresses to the late phase and small clots have formed to such an extent that the client no longer has enough clotting factors to prevent hemorrhage, clotting factors are infused. These factors (cryoprecipitate) are obtained from pooled human serum. Infusing fresh frozen plasma (FFP) also helps to replace clotting factors. Platelets or other blood products also may be needed.

Activated Protein C. Synthetic activated protein C has been shown to stop the inflammatory responses and small clot formation of septic shock (Kleinpell, 2003a). This drug, drotrecogin alpha (Xigris), is given as a continuous infusion over 4 days.

Antibodies. Antibodies against the body's mediators for inflammation are being tested for their effectiveness in septic shock. Antibodies have been developed against the some proinflammatory cytokines, particularly interleukin-1 (IL-1), interleukin-6 (IL-6), and tumor necrosis factor (TNF). This experimental therapy shows promise in reducing the extensive mortality associated with septic shock.

CHART 40-10

HOME CARE ASSESSMENT of
Clients at Risk for Sepsis

Assess the client for any clinical manifestations of infection, including the following:
- Temperature, pulse, respiration, and blood pressure
- Color of skin and mucous membranes
- The mouth and perianal area for fissures or lesions
- Any nonintact skin area for the presence of exudates, redness, increased warmth, swelling
- Any pain, tenderness, or other discomfort anywhere
- Cough or any other symptoms of a cold or the flu
- Urine; or ask client whether urine is dark or cloudy, has an odor, or causes pain or burning during urination

Assess client's and caregiver's adherence to and understanding of infection prevention techniques.

Assess home environment, including the following:
- General cleanliness
- Kitchen and bathroom facilities, including refrigeration
- Availability and type of soap for handwashing
- Presence of pets, especially cats, rodents, or reptiles

CHART 40-11

CLIENT EDUCATION GUIDE
Infection Precautions

- Avoid crowds and other large gatherings of people, who might be ill.
- Do not share eating utensils or personal toilet articles (e.g., toothbrushes, toothpaste, washcloths, or deodorant sticks) with others.
- If possible, bathe daily.
- Wash the armpits, groin, genitals, and rectal area at least twice a day with an antimicrobial soap.
- Clean your toothbrush daily by either running it through the dishwasher or rinsing it in liquid laundry bleach.
- Wash your hands thoroughly with an antimicrobial soap before you eat or drink, after touching a pet, after shaking hands with anyone, as soon as you come home from any outing, and after using the toilet.
- Wash dishes between use with hot, sudsy water, or use a dishwasher.
- Do not drink water that has been standing for longer than 15 minutes.
- Do not reuse cups and glasses without washing them.
- Do not change pet litter boxes.
- Take your temperature at least once a day.
- Refrigerate and prepare food appropriately. Do not eat raw or undercooked meat, fish, poultry, or eggs.
- Report any of the following signs or symptoms of infection to your physician immediately:
  - Temperature greater than 100° F (38° C)
  - Persistent cough (with or without sputum)
  - Pus or foul-smelling drainage from any open skin area or normal body opening
  - Presence of a boil or abscess
  - Urine that is cloudy or foul-smelling or causes burning on urination
- Do not dig in the garden or work with houseplants.
- Use antibacterial cleansers to clean kitchen and bathroom surfaces at least twice each week. If you clean these areas yourself, wear rubber or vinyl work gloves while cleaning.
- Use a condom when having sex.
- Take all medications as prescribed.

Community-Based Care

Shock is a complication of another condition and is resolved before clients are discharged from the acute care setting. Because more clients are receiving treatment on an outpatient basis and are being discharged earlier from acute care settings, more clients at home are at increased risk for infection and septic shock.

HOME CARE MANAGEMENT

Evaluate the home environment for safety regarding infection hazards. Note the general cleanliness, especially in the kitchen and bathrooms. Chart 40-10 lists focused client and environmental assessment data to obtain during a home visit.

HEALTH TEACHING

Protecting vulnerable clients from infection and sepsis at home is an important nursing function. Instruct about the importance of self-care strategies, such as good hygiene, handwashing, balanced diet, rest, and exercise, skin care, and mouth care. If clients or family members do not know how to take a temperature or read a thermometer, teach them and obtain a return demonstration. Instruct clients to notify the health care provider immediately if fever or other signs of infection appear. Specific recommendations for infection precautions for clients at risk for sepsis are listed in Chart 40-11.

Evaluation: Outcomes

Evaluate the care of the client with sepsis-induced distributive shock. The expected outcome is that the client will maintain normal aerobic cellular metabolism.

Specific indicators for these outcomes are listed for the collaborative problem under the Planning and Implementation section (see earlier).

GET READY for the NCLEX Examination!

KEY POINTS

Safe Effective Care Environment

- Use strict aseptic techniques when performing invasive procedures, dressing changes, or handling nonintact skin.
- Use good handwashing techniques before providing any care to a client who is either immunocompromised or immunodeficient.

Health Promotion and Maintenance

- Encourage all adult clients to know their immunization history for tetanus.
- Identify clients at high risk for infection as a result of age, disease, work environment, or leisure activities.
- Teach the client and family about the clinical manifestations of infection and when to seek medical advice.
- Teach clients at risk for bleeding the precautions to take to avoid injury (see Chart 28-10).

Psychosocial Integrity

- Assess all clients at risk for shock for a change in affect, reduced cognition, altered level of consciousness, and increased anxiety.
- Stay with the client in shock.
- Explain all diagnostic procedures, restrictions, and follow-up care to the client scheduled for tests.
- Reassure clients who are in shock that the appropriate interventions are being instituted.

Physiological Integrity

- Assess the immunocompromised client every shift for infection.
- Assess the skin integrity of the client with reduced immune function at least every shift.
- Immediately assess vital signs of clients who have a change in level of consciousness, increased thirst, or anxiety.
- Assess for changes in pulse rate and quality rather than blood pressure as an indicator of shock.
- Give oxygen to any client in shock.
- Assess hourly urine output for adequacy of treatment for hypovolemic shock.

ADDITIONAL STUDY RESOURCES

Go to your Student CD-ROM for Review Questions for the NCLEX Examination.

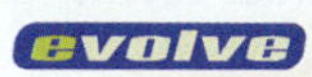
Go to http://evolve.elsevier.com/Iggy/ for Integrated Management of Care Questions for the NCLEX Examination.

SELECTED BIBLIOGRAPHY

Asterisk indicates a classic or definitive work on this subject.

Abbas, A., & Lichtman, A. (2003). *Cellular and molecular immunology* (5th ed.). Philadelphia: W.B. Saunders.

Ackley, B., & Ladwig, G. (2002). *Nursing diagnosis handbook: A guide to planning care* (5th ed.). St. Louis: Mosby.

Ahrens, T., & Vollman, K. (2003). Severe sepsis management: Are we doing enough? *Critical Care Nurse (Supplement October), 23*(5), 2-15.

Atassi, K., & Harris, M. (2001). Action stat: Disseminated intravascular coagulation. *Nursing 2001, 31*(3), 64.

Beery, T. (2003). Sex differences in infection and sepsis. *Critical Care Nursing Clinics of North America, 15*(1), 55-62.

Berne, R., et al. (2004). *Physiology* (5th ed.). St. Louis: Mosby.

Berry, B., & Pinard, A. (2002). Assessing tissue oxygenation. *Critical Care Nurse, 22*(3), 22-39.

Chavez, J., & Brewer, C. (2002). Stopping the shock slide. *RN, 65*(9), 30-35.

Cheek, D. et al. (2005). Sepsis: Taking a deeper look. *Nursing 2005, 35*(1), 38-42.

Dettenmeier, P., et al. (2003). Role of activated protein C in the pathophysiology of severe sepsis. *American Journal of Critical Care, 12*(6), 518-524.

Diehl-Oplinger, L. (2004). Choosing the right fluid to counter hypovolemic shock. *Nursing 2004, 34*(3), 52-54.

Dochterman, J., & Bulechek, G. (Eds.). (2004). *Nursing interventions classification (NIC)* (4th ed.). St. Louis: Mosby.

Dressler, D. (2004). DIC: Coping with a coagulation crisis. *Nursing 2004, 34*(5), 58-62.

Ebersole, P., Hess, P., & Luggen, A. (2004). *Toward healthy aging: Human needs and nursing response* (6th ed.). St. Louis: Mosby.

*Effron, M., & Chernow, B. (1992). Shock. In E. Rubenstein & D. Federman (Eds.), *Scientific American: Medicine* (pp. I card III Shock 1-12). New York: Scientific American.

Facts and Comparisons. (2004). *Drug facts and comparisons* (58th ed.). St. Louis: Author.

Felblinger, D. (2003). Malnutrition, infection, and sepsis in acute and chronic illness. *Critical Care Nursing Clinics of North America, 15*(1), 71-78.

Hadaway, L. (2003). Infusing without infecting. *Nursing 2003, 33*(10), 58-63.

Holcomb, S. (2002). Helping your patient conquer cardiogenic shock. *Nursing 2002, 32*(9), 32cc1-32cc6.

Kleinpell, R. (2003a). Advances in treating patients with severe sepsis: Role of drotrecogin alfa (activated). *Critical Care Nurse, 23*(3), 16-29.

Kleinpell, R. (2003b). The role of the critical care nurse in the assessment and management of the patient with severe sepsis. *Critical Care Nursing Clinics of North America, 15*(1), 27-34.

LaCharity, L., & McClure, E. (2003). Are plants vectors for transmission of infection in acute care? *Critical Care Nursing Clinics of North America, 15*(1), 119-124.

McCance, K., & Huether, S. (2002). *Pathophysiology: The biologic basis for disease in adults and children* (4th ed.). St. Louis: Mosby.

Mehta, M. (2003). Assessing cardiovascular status. *Nursing 2003, 33*(1), 56-58.

Moorhead, S., Johnson, M., & Maas, M. (Eds.). (2004). *Nursing outcomes classification (NOC)* (3rd ed.). St. Louis: Mosby.

Mower-Wade, D., & Kang, T. (2004). Sepsis: When defense turns deadly. *Nursing 2004, 34*(7), 32cc1-32cc4.

Mower-Wade, D., Bartley, M., & Chiari-Allwein, J. (2001). How to respond to shock. *Dimensions in Critical Care Nursing, 20*(2), 22-27.

O'Neill, D. (2001). The right plasma volume expander. *Nursing Times, 97*(27), 38-39.

Pagana, K., & Pagana, T. (2002). *Mosby's manual of diagnostic and laboratory tests* (2nd ed.). St. Louis: Mosby.

Paminter, S. (2001). Hands on detection of systemic circulatory deterioration. *Nursing Times, 97*(27), 40-42.

Ross, V. (2003). Uncertainty about the clinical detection of sepsis. *Journal of Infusion Nursing, 26*(1), 23-28.

Rudnicke, C. (2003). Transfusion alternatives. *Journal of Infusion Nursing, 26*(1), 29-33.

Sarvis, C. (2004). The role of bacterial toxins in wounds. *Nursing 2004, 34*(7), 68.

Sommers, M. (2003). The cellular basis of septic shock. *Critical Care Nursing Clinics of North America, 15*(1), 13-25.

*Stengle, J., & Dries, D. (1994). Sepsis in the elderly. *Critical Care Nursing Clinics of North America, 6*(2), 421-427.

Workman, M.L. (2003). The cellular basis of bacterial infection. *Critical Care Nursing Clinics of North America, 15*(1), 1-11.

CHAPTER 41

Interventions for Critically Ill Clients with Acute Coronary Syndromes

WADE HAGAN • DONNA D. IGNATAVICIUS

LEARNING OUTCOMES

After studying this chapter, you should be able to:

1. Describe the relationship between coronary artery disease (CAD) and acute coronary syndromes (ACS).
2. Explain the pathophysiology of ACS.
3. Compare and contrast stable angina, unstable angina, and myocardial infarction (MI).
4. Identify modifiable and nonmodifiable risk factors for ACS.
5. Interpret physical and diagnostic assessment findings in clients who have ACS.
6. Describe the psychosocial aspects of ACS.
7. Prioritize nursing care for clients who have ACS.
8. Identify the life-threatening complications of ACS.
9. Explain the advantages of thrombolysis for a client experiencing an MI.
10. Compare and contrast the drug classifications used to treat ACS.
11. Describe the appropriate nursing interventions for monitoring clients receiving drug therapy for ACS.
12. Develop a plan of care for the client who has undergone a percutaneous transluminal coronary angioplasty.
13. Manage care for the client who has undergone coronary artery bypass graft (CABG) surgery.
14. Discuss the differences between CABG surgery, minimally invasive direct coronary artery bypass, off-pump CABG, and transmyocardial laser revascularization.
15. Develop a discharge plan for the client with ACS.

Go to your Student CD-ROM for Review Questions for the NCLEX Examination keyed to these Learning Outcomes.

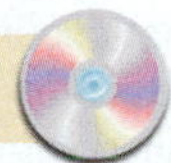

CORONARY ARTERY DISEASE

Coronary artery disease (CAD), also called coronary heart disease (CHD), is the single largest killer of American men and women in all cultural groups (American Heart Association [AHA], 2003). According to the AHA, CHD caused more than 1 of every 5 deaths in the United States in 2000. From 1990 to 2000, the death rate from CAD declined 25%. Multiple factors can be identified as contributing to the decline in CAD. These factors include more effective medical treatment and an increased awareness and emphasis on reducing the major modifiable cardiovascular risk factors (e.g., high blood pressure [BP], smoking, high cholesterol, obesity, diabetes).

PATHOPHYSIOLOGY

Coronary artery disease (CAD) is a broad term that includes stable angina pectoris and acute coronary syndromes. CAD affects the arteries that provide blood, oxygen, and nutrients to the myocardium. When blood flow through the coronary arteries is partially or completely blocked, ischemia and infarction of the myocardium may result. **Ischemia** occurs when insufficient oxygen is supplied to meet the requirements of the myocardium. **Infarction** (necrosis, or cell death) occurs when severe ischemia is prolonged and irreversible damage to tissue results.

CULTURAL CONSIDERATIONS

Several groups have a higher genetic risk for CAD than others. Black and Hispanic women have higher CAD risk factors than white women of comparable socioeconomic status. Of Native Americans/American Indians/Alaskan Natives 18 years of age and older, 63.7% of men and 81.4% of women have one or more CAD risk factors (hypertension [HTN], smoking, high cholesterol, excess weight, or diabetes mellitus). The leading cause of death for both men and women in the most prevalent ethnic groups is cardiac disease even though there are genetic predispositions to develop risk factors (AHA, 2003).

Stable Angina Pectoris

Angina pectoris means "strangling of the chest." Angina is a temporary imbalance between the coronary arteries' ability to supply oxygen and the cardiac muscle's demand for oxygen. Ischemia that occurs with angina is limited in duration, and it does not cause permanent damage of myocardial tissue.

Angina may be of two predominant types: stable angina and unstable angina. **Stable angina** is chest discomfort that occurs with moderate to prolonged exertion in a pattern that is familiar to the client. The frequency, duration, and intensity of symptoms remain stable over the preceding several months. Stable angina results in only slight limitation of activity and is usually associated with a stable atherosclerotic plaque. It is usually relieved by nitroglycerin or rest and often is managed medically with agents such as calcium channel blockers and beta-blocking medications. Rarely does stable angina require aggressive treatment. **Unstable angina** is discussed below under Acute Coronary Syndromes.

WOMEN'S HEALTH CONSIDERATIONS

More women than men have angina; many women experience **atypical angina.** Atypical angina can manifest itself as indigestion, pain between the shoulders, an aching jaw, or a choking sensation that occurs with exertion. Angina in women has often been diagnosed as panic disorder, stress, menopause-related problems, gastrointestinal disease, or hypochondriasis (*Harvard Heart Letter,* 2003).

Acute Coronary Syndromes

In **acute coronary syndromes,** it is believed that the atherosclerotic plaque in the coronary artery ruptures, resulting in platelet aggregation ("clumping"), thrombus (clot) formation, and vasoconstriction (Figure 41-1). The amount of disruption of the atherosclerotic plaque determines the degree of obstruction of the coronary artery and the specific disease process (unstable angina or myocardial infarction [MI]). Between 10% and 30% of clients with unstable angina progress to having an MI in 1 year, and 29% die of MI in 5 years (AHA, 2003).

UNSTABLE ANGINA PECTORIS

Unstable angina (as it is usually called), or USA, is chest pain or discomfort that occurs at rest or with exertion and causes marked limitation of activity. An increase in the

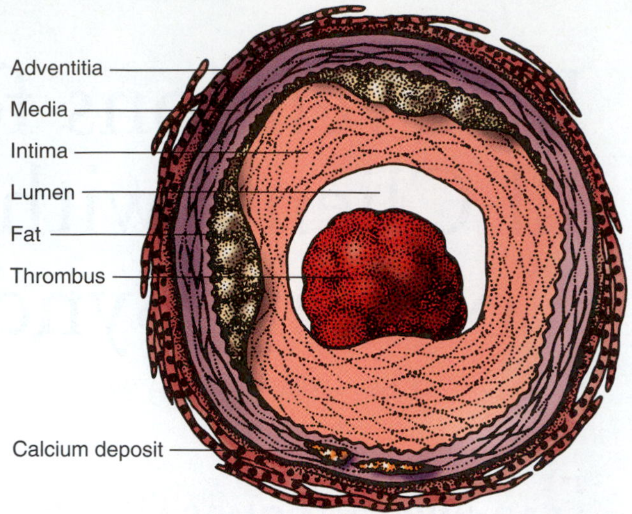

Figure 41-1 ■ A cross section of an atherosclerotic coronary artery.

number of attacks and an increase in the intensity of the pain characterize USA. The pain may last longer than 15 minutes, or it may be poorly relieved by rest or nitroglycerin. USA describes a broad spectrum of disorders, including *new-onset angina, variant (Prinzmetal's) angina, preinfarction angina,* and *crescendo angina.* The term used to describe the disorders that include unstable angina, subendocardial MI, and MI is **acute coronary syndromes.**

MYOCARDIAL INFARCTION

The most serious acute coronary syndrome is MI, often referred to as a "heart attack." Undiagnosed or untreated angina can lead to this very serious health problem.

Myocardial infarction (MI) occurs when myocardial tissue is abruptly and severely deprived of oxygen. When blood flow is acutely reduced by 80% to 90%, ischemia develops. Ischemia can lead to injury and necrosis **(infarction)** of myocardial tissue if blood flow is not restored. Most MIs are the result of atherosclerosis of a coronary artery, rupture of the plaque, subsequent thrombosis, and occlusion of blood flow. Other factors may be implicated, however, such as coronary artery spasm, platelet aggregation, and emboli from mural thrombi (thrombi lining the walls of the cardiac chambers).

Often MIs begin with infarction **(necrosis)** of the subendocardial layer of cardiac muscle. This layer has the longest myofibrils in the heart, the greatest oxygen demand, and the poorest oxygen supply. Around the initial area of infarction (zone of necrosis) in the subendocardium are two other zones: (1) the zone of injury, tissue that is injured but not necrotic, and (2) the zone of ischemia, tissue that is oxygen deprived. This pattern is illustrated in Figure 41-2.

PROCESS OF INFARCTION. Infarction is a dynamic process that does not occur instantly; rather, it evolves over a period of several hours. **Hypoxia** (decreased oxygen) from ischemia may lead to local vasodilation of blood vessels and acidosis. Potassium, calcium, and magnesium imbalances, as well as acidosis at the cellular level, may lead to suppression of normal conduction and contractile functions. Automaticity and ectopy are enhanced. Catecholamines (epinephrine and norepinephrine) released in

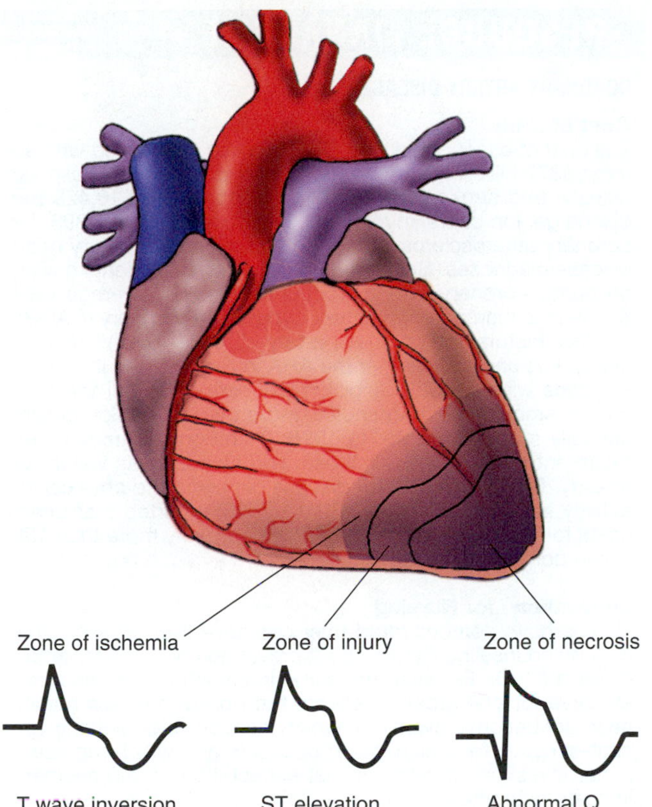

Figure 41-2 ■ Electrocardiographic changes and patterns associated with myocardial infarction.

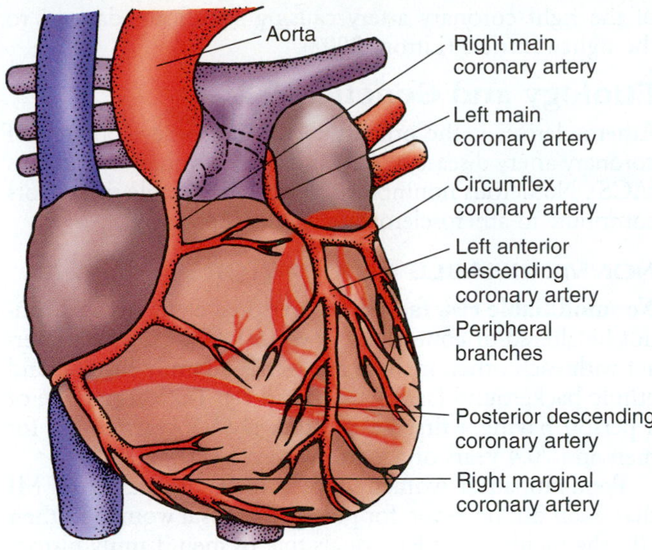

Figure 41-3 ■ Coronary arterial system.

TABLE 41-1 Major Coronary Vessels and the Structures They Perfuse

Left Anterior Descending Coronary Artery
- Most of the left ventricular muscle mass and septum

Left Circumflex Coronary Artery
- Posterior wall of the left ventricle
- SA node in 39% of clients
- AV node in 12% of clients
- Left ventricular muscle in 10% of clients

Right Coronary Artery
- Right ventricle
- Inferior portion of the left ventricle
- SA node in 59% of clients
- AV node in 88% of clients

SA, Sinoatrial; *AV*, atrioventricular.

response to hypoxia and pain may increase the heart's rate and contractility and afterload. These factors increase oxygen requirements in tissue that is already oxygen deprived. The area of infarction may extend into the zones of injury and ischemia. The actual extent of the zone of infarction depends on three factors: collateral circulation, anaerobic metabolism, and workload demands on the myocardium.

The infarction may involve only the subendocardium (called a **subendocardial MI**), or it may spread to the epicardium or to all three layers of cardiac muscle. When all three layers are involved, the MI is termed **transmural.** Subendocardial MIs have less effect on wall motion and cardiac output than do transmural infarctions.

PHYSIOLOGIC RESPONSE TO INFARCTION. Obvious physical changes do not occur in the heart until 6 hours after the infarction, when the infarcted region appears blue and swollen. After 48 hours, the infarct turns gray with yellow streaks as neutrophils invade the tissue and begin to remove the necrotic cells. By 8 to 10 days after infarction, granulation tissue forms at the edges of the necrotic tissue. Over a 2- to 3-month period, the necrotic area eventually develops into a shrunken, thin, firm scar. Scar tissue permanently changes the size and shape of the entire left ventricle **(ventricular remodeling).** Remodeling may decrease left ventricular function, cause heart failure, and increase morbidity and mortality.

CLASSIFICATION OF MYOCARDIAL INFARCTION BY LOCATION. The client's response to an MI also depends on which coronary artery or arteries were obstructed and which part of the left ventricle wall was damaged: anterior, lateral, septal, inferior, or posterior. Figure 41-3 details the major coronary arteries, and Table 41-1 describes the structures they perfuse.

Obstruction of the left anterior descending (LAD) artery causes anterior or septal MIs because the LAD artery perfuses the anterior wall and most of the septum of the left ventricle. Anterior wall MIs (AWMIs) account for 25% of all MIs and have the highest mortality rate. Clients with anterior MIs are most likely to experience left ventricular heart failure and ventricular dysrhythmias because a large segment of the left ventricle wall may have been damaged.

The circumflex artery supplies the lateral wall of the left ventricle and possibly portions of the posterior wall or the sinoatrial (SA) and atrioventricular (AV) nodes. Clients with obstruction of the circumflex artery may experience a posterior wall MI (PWMIs) or a lateral wall MI (LWMIs) and sinus dysrhythmias.

In most people, the right coronary artery perfuses the SA and AV nodes as well as the right ventricle and inferior or diaphragmatic portion of the left ventricle. Clients with obstruction of the right coronary artery often have **inferior wall MIs.** Inferior wall MIs (IWMIs) account for about 17% of all MIs and have a mortality rate of about 10%. Up to 50% of all inferior wall MIs are associated with an occlusion of the right coronary artery causing significant damage to the right ventricle (Litton, 2002).

Etiology and Genetic Risk

Atherosclerosis is the primary factor in the development of coronary artery disease (CAD) and acute coronary syndromes (ACS). Numerous nonmodifiable and modifiable risk factors contribute to atherosclerosis (also see Chapter 39).

NONMODIFIABLE RISK FACTORS

Nonmodifiable risk factors are personal elements that cannot be altered or controlled. These risk factors, which interact with each other, include age, gender, family history, and ethnic background (as discussed earlier). The average age of a person having a first heart attack is 65.8 years of age for men and 70.4 years of age for women (AHA, 2003).

Premenopausal women have a lower incidence of MI than men do; however, for postmenopausal women in their 70s, the incidence of MI equals that of men. Family history is also a risk factor; people whose parents had CAD are more susceptible.

Incidence/Prevalence

In 2000, the total mortality of those experiencing MI in the United States was 239,000. About every 29 seconds, an American suffers a coronary event, and about every minute someone will die of one. About half of the people who experience an MI in a given year will die of it.

Many people die from coronary heart disease without being hospitalized. Most of these are sudden deaths caused by cardiac arrest, usually resulting from ventricular fibrillation.

Ninety-five percent of sudden cardiac arrest victims die before reaching the hospital. To help combat this problem, automatic external defibrillators (AEDs) are found in many public places, such as in shopping centers and on airplanes. Employees are taught how to use these devices if a sudden cardiac arrest occurs.

WOMEN'S HEALTH CONSIDERATIONS

Twenty-five percent of men and 40% of women die within 1 year after having an initial recognized MI. Because women have heart attacks at older ages than men do, they are more likely to die from them within a few weeks.

Studies have shown that women do not realize that heart disease is the number one killer among women (AHA, 2003). More disturbing are the recent findings that combined hormone replacement therapy (HRT) does not protect cardiac health in postmenopausal women; however, HRT has other protective effects, such as osteoporosis prevention. HRT is discussed in detail in Chapter 78.

Causes of MI may be different in women, perhaps explaining the atypical presentations. Bursting plaques may not be as important for women as men because women distribute atherosclerosis more evenly through the arteries. Some women have narrow arteries that indicate, in general, a lower dose of blood thinning medications and the use of smaller catheters and stents. Women also tend to develop less collateral circulation than men. For more information, contact www.womenheart.org (Gorman et al., 2003).

Many clients who survive MIs are not able to return to work. CAD is the leading cause of premature, permanent disability in the United States Labor Force, accounting for 19% of disability allowances by the Social Security. The direct cost of cardiovascular disease and stroke in the United States in 2003 was estimated at $371.8 billion dollars (AHA, 2003) (see the Resource Management box above).

RESOURCE MANAGEMENT

CORONARY ARTERY DISEASE

Cost of Care

The cost of cancer care was $202.2 billion, compared with almost $372 billion spent to care for clients with cardiovascular disease and stroke (AHA, 2003). Medicare paid $10,428 per discharge for acute myocardial infarction (MI), $11,399 for coronary atherosclerosis, and $3617 for other coronary heart disease diagnoses. Becker (2003) reported that clients having off-pump coronary artery procedures had an average cost $1839 less than coronary artery bypass graft surgery (CABG).

Risk factors for coronary artery disease (CAD) are also costly. It is unclear whether the AHA included these individual statistics with the $371.8 billion estimate. In 2000, the total cost of smoking cost Americans more than 157 billion dollars annually in medical care. In 1996, 31 billion dollars was the treatment cost of CAD for those who have excess weight or obesity. The annual cost for disease connected to physical inactivity is 76 billion dollars. Gentz (2000) reported that direct costs for testing clients with CAD are currently more than 150 billion dollars each year.

Implications for Nursing

Nurses have demonstrated they can save lives at a minimal cost by counseling clients about prevention of coronary artery disease (CAD). Because the same intervention may be cost-effective for one group of clients but not for another, nurses need to become aware of which cardiac interventions are cost-effective for which group of clients and which represent major investments with minimal expectation of improvement in client outcomes.

HEALTH PROMOTION/ILLNESS PREVENTION

MODIFIABLE RISK FACTORS

Modifiable risk factors include elevated serum cholesterol levels, cigarette smoking, hypertension, impaired glucose tolerance, obesity, physical inactivity, and stress. Individuals who have one or more of these risk factors should modify or eliminate them to decrease their chances of myocardial infarction (MI). For clients at risk for coronary artery disease (CAD), especially MI, assess which factors they have and teach ways that the factor(s) can be modified. A complete discussion of health teaching for decreasing risk factors may be found in Chapter 39 under the discussion of Arteriosclerosis/Atherosclerosis.

CULTURAL CONSIDERATIONS

Modifiable risk factors vary for people of different racial and ethnic backgrounds. A comparison of risk factors by racial/ethnic group is found in Table 41-2. Some of the differences may be explained by lack of access to health care for some groups or genetic factors. Native Americans/American Indians, for example, have the highest percentage of smokers among women and men; however, many of these individuals have poor access to care or language barriers in a predominantly English-speaking, white health care system. Dietary preferences may also explain some of the differences. For instance, according to the AHA (2003), high cholesterol is more common in black and Hispanic populations. Diets higher in fat and cholesterol are often less expensive and may be a factor in explaining differences. Genetics may also contribute to the differences among ethnic groups. Obesity is also greater in these groups.

ELEVATED SERUM CHOLESTEROL LEVELS. The risk of CAD rises as serum cholesterol levels increase. It is estimated that around 97 million people have total cholesterol levels of greater than 200 mg/dL (Allen, 2000). In addition to measuring the total serum cholesterol, low-density lipoprotein (LDL) and high-density lipoprotein (HDL) levels are just as important in assessing risk for CAD and potential MI. LDL cholesterol has been termed "bad" and HDL cholesterol has been termed "good." Elevated levels of LDL combined with low levels of HDL increase the risk of MI. Total serum cholesterol levels put the individual at a higher risk of developing an MI. According to the AHA (2003), a 10% reduction in serum cholesterol may result in an estimated 30% reduction in the incidence of CAD and MI. The goal for LDL levels in clients who have existing CAD or diabetes mellitus is less than 100 mg/dL. HDL cholesterol levels should be above 40 mg/dL. Approaches to decrease cholesterol are focused on diet and medications that lower cholesterol levels.

CIGARETTE SMOKING. An estimated 25.7% of men and 21% of women smoke putting them at increased risk of MI (AHA, 2003). About five million American men and women are chewing tobacco, with the highest rates in the South and rural areas. **Passive smoking** from "second-hand smoke" substantially reduces blood flow velocity in the coronary arteries of healthy young adults, causing about 37,000 deaths annually (AHA, 2003).

Cigarette smoking accounts for 30% of the mortality rate from CAD. Smoking enhances the process of atherosclerosis through mechanisms that are still poorly understood. Nicotine initiates the release of catecholamines, resulting in an increased heart rate and peripheral vasoconstriction. This action causes increases in BP, cardiac afterload, and oxygen consumption. Cigarette smoking has also been found to cause endothelial dysfunction and increased vessel wall thickness. This process increases the risk for clot formation and vessel occlusion. Another factor of cigarette smoking is carbon monoxide, which has been found to decrease the oxygen content in arterial blood. The resulting hypertension may exacerbate the atherosclerotic process by increasing vessel wall permeability. The good news is that when cigarette smoking is stopped, the risk for CAD decreases. A person who stops smoking may decrease the risk of CAD by as much as 80% in 1 year. Reducing the tar and nicotine content of the cigarettes smoked does not reduce the risk of CAD (AHA, 2003).

PHYSICAL INACTIVITY. Physical inactivity may be the most important risk factor for the general population. Less active, less-fit persons have a 30% to 50% greater risk of developing high BP, which predisposes to CAD. Physical inactivity is more prevalent among women than men, among blacks and Hispanics than whites, among older than younger adults, and among the less affluent than the more affluent (AHA, 2003). Regular physical activity helps maintain body weight and muscle mass while optimizing BP and lipid values.

For women, studies have shown that moderate-intensity physical activity, such as walking, is associated with a substantial reduction in risk. Another study of men suggested, however, that intense exercising may contribute to plaque rupture and increase the number of cardiac episodes (Cadroy et al., 2003). Participating in physical exercise can reduce hypertension and increase secretions of endorphins, leading to less smoking and eating, improved metabolism, and a stronger feeling of well-being. Other benefits include decreased blood clotting and higher plasma HDL levels. Physical activity does not increase collateral circulation or reduce the size of existing plaques. Benefits include increased heart volume, increased cardiac capillary vascularity, and decreased heart rate.

The individual's response to stress may be associated with heart disease. Some evidence indicates that job stress may be associated with left ventricular hypertrophy.

TABLE 41-2 Comparison of the Incidence of Smoking, Leisure Activity, Cholesterol Level, and Body Mass Index (BMI) Among Selected Racial/Ethnic Groups

	Men (%)	Women (%)
Smoking		
Hispanics	24.1	12.3
Asian/Pacific Islanders	24.3	7.1
Native Americans/American Indians	40.9	40.8
Blacks	26.1	20.8
Whites	25.8	21.6
No Leisure Activity		
Hispanics	48.9	57.4
Blacks	55.2	44.1
Asian/Pacific Islanders	30.9	45.5
Native Americans/American Indians	16.8	19.6
Whites	32.5	36.2
Cholesterol >200 mg/dL or higher*		
Hispanics	53	48
Blacks	45	45
Asian/Pacific Islanders	not reported	not reported
Native Americans/American Indians	35.7	35.6
Whites	52	49
BMI >30		
Hispanics	28.9	39.7
Blacks	28.1	49.7
Native Americans/American Indians	35.5	41.2
Asian/Pacific Islanders	36.7	27.1
Whites	27.3	30.1

Modified from the American Heart Association (2003).

*NOTE: A 10% decrease in total cholesterol levels may result in a 30% reduction in the incidence of coronary heart disease.

OTHER FACTORS

One in five Americans has hypertension (HTN). *Hypertension* increases the workload of the heart, which increases the risk of myocardial infarction (MI). The cause of 90% to 95% of HTN is not known; however, it is easily detected and usually controllable. About 50% of clients having a first MI have a BP greater than 160/95 mm Hg.

CULTURAL CONSIDERATIONS

The prevalence of hypertension (HTN) among blacks and whites in the Southeastern United States is greater than among those in other regions of the country. Blacks have the highest prevalence in the United States and are among the highest in the world. They develop HTN earlier in life, and the average blood pressures (BP) are much higher than other groups (AHA, 2003). The causes for differences are not known but may be related to genetics or diet.

WOMEN'S HEALTH CONSIDERATIONS

For women, *impaired glucose tolerance* (e.g., diabetes) seriously increases the risk of CAD. *Obesity* is associated with increased serum cholesterol, elevated BP, and abnormal glucose tolerance. It may also have an independent effect on the risk of CAD. The distribution of adipose tissue seems to be important; women with fat deposited around the waist rather than the hips often have unfavorable lipid profiles and higher rates of CAD.

Elevated levels of serum *homocysteine,* an amino acid, are believed by some researchers to be associated with an increased risk of CAD. Clients with multiple risk factors have several times the risk of CAD as those without these characteristics. Although many factors place a person at risk for heart disease, there are well-documented, effective ways of promoting cardiovascular health. Some of these interventions, including health teaching, are described in Chart 41-1. Additional information is found in Chapter 39 under Arteriosclerosis/Atherosclerosis.

COLLABORATIVE MANAGEMENT

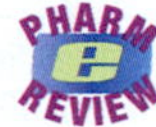

Assessment

HISTORY

If chest discomfort or other symptom is present at the time of the interview, collection of historical data is delayed until interventions for pain, vital sign instability, and dysrhythmias are initiated and the discomfort resolves. If possible, ask about how clients have managed the current episode of chest discomfort and which medications they are taking. When the client is *pain free,* information about family history and modifiable risk factors, including eating habits, lifestyle, and physical activity levels, is obtained.

PHYSICAL ASSESSMENT/CLINICAL MANIFESTATIONS

PAIN ASSESSMENT. Ask the client to describe his or her immediate concerns. The presence of chest, epigastric, jaw, back, or arm discomfort is noted. The client is asked to rate the discomfort on a scale of 0 to 10, with 10 being the highest level of discomfort. Clients often describe the discomfort as tightness, a burning sensation, pressure, or indigestion. Clients are asked what they have already done to try to relieve the pain. Pain management is described in detail in Chapter 7.

Rapid assessment of client with chest pain is crucial. It is important to differentiate among the types of chest pain and to identify the source. Question the client to determine the characteristics of the discomfort. Appropriate questions to ask concerning the discomfort include onset, location, radiation, intensity, duration, precipitating, and relieving factors.

CHART 41-1

CLIENT EDUCATION GUIDE
Prevention of Coronary Artery Disease

Smoking
- If you smoke, quit.
- If you don't smoke, don't start.

Diet
- Consume sufficient calories for your body:
  - 50% to 55% from carbohydrates
  - 30% to 35% from complex carbohydrates
  - 10% from simple sugars
  - Less than 30% from fat
  - 15% from monounsaturated fat
  - 10% from polyunsaturated fat
  - The remainder (5% to 10%) from saturated fat
  - 12% to 20% from protein
- Limit your cholesterol intake to less than 300 mg/day.
- Limit your sodium intake as specified by your health care provider.

Cholesterol
- Have your cholesterol and low-density lipoprotein (LDL) levels checked regularly.
- If your cholesterol and LDL levels are elevated, follow your health care provider's advice.

Physical Activity
- If you are middle-aged or older or have a history of medical problems, check with your health care provider before starting an exercise program.
- Appropriate exercise should be enjoyable, burn 400 calories per session, and sustain a heart rate of 120 to 150 beats/min, depending on your age.
- Exercise moderately at least three times each week, preferably five.
- Exercise periods should be at least 20 to 30 minutes long with 10-minute warm-up and 5-minute cool-down periods.
- If you are unable to exercise moderately three to five times each week, walk daily for 30 minutes at a comfortable pace.
- If you are unable to walk 30 minutes daily, walk any distance you can (e.g., park farther away from a site than necessary; use the stairs, not the elevator, to go one floor up or two floors down).

Diabetes
- Manage your diabetes with your health care provider.

Blood Pressure
- Have your blood pressure checked regularly.
- If your blood pressure is elevated, follow your health care provider's advice.
- Continue to monitor your blood pressure at regular intervals.

Obesity
- Avoid severely restrictive or fad diets.
- Consider a restriction in intake of saturated fats, simple sugars, and cholesterol-rich foods.
- Increase your physical activity.

Chart 41-2 compares and contrasts anginal and infarction pain. Because anginal pain is ischemic pain, it usually improves when the imbalance between oxygen supply and demand is resolved. For example, rest reduces tissue demands, and nitroglycerin improves oxygen supply. Discomfort from an MI does not usually resolve with such simple measures. Also noted is the presence of any associated symptoms, including nausea, vomiting, diaphoresis, dizziness, weakness, palpitations, and shortness of breath.

CHART 41-2

KEY FEATURES of
Angina and Myocardial Infarction

Angina	Myocardial Infarction
Substernal chest discomfort: ▪ Radiating to the left arm ▪ Precipitated by exertion or stress ▪ Relieved by nitroglycerin or rest ▪ Lasting <15 min Few associated symptoms	Substernal chest pressure: ▪ Radiating to the left arm, back, or jaw ▪ Occurring without cause, usually in the morning ▪ Relieved only by opioids ▪ Lasting 30 min or more Frequent associated symptoms: ▪ Nausea ▪ Diaphoresis ▪ Dyspnea ▪ Feelings of fear and anxiety ▪ Dysrhythmias ▪ Fatigue ▪ Epigastric distress ▪ Feeling "short of breath"

CULTURAL CONSIDERATIONS

Black individuals experience longer delays in seeking treatment for MI and higher mortality rates than white individuals. One factor thought to contribute to this delay is a greater incidence of dyspnea as an acute symptom of MI among both black males and black females rather than the more classic chest discomfort.

CONSIDERATIONS FOR OLDER ADULTS

The presence of the associated symptoms without chest discomfort is also significant. In 15% to 25% of all clients with MI, primarily older adults and clients with diabetes, chest pain or discomfort may be mild or absent, and clients may complain primarily of the associated symptoms. Some older clients may think they are experiencing indigestion and therefore not recognize that they are having an MI. Twenty-five percent of older adults experiencing an MI complain only of shortness of breath. The major manifestation of MI in people older than 80 years of age may be disorientation or confusion due to poor cardiac output.

CARDIOVASCULAR ASSESSMENT. Immediate assessment of BP, determination of heart rate, interpretation of cardiac rhythm, and presence of dysrhythmias is crucial. Sinus tachycardia with premature ventricular contractions (PVCs) frequently occurs in the first few hours after an MI.

Next assess distal peripheral pulses and skin temperature. The skin should be warm, with all pulses palpable. In the client with unstable angina or MI, poor cardiac output may be manifested by cool, diaphoretic skin, and diminished or absent pulses.

Auscultate for an S_3 gallop, which often indicates heart failure, a serious and common complication of MI. Also assess the respiratory rate and breath sounds for signs of heart failure. An increased respiratory rate is common because of anxiety and pain, but crackles or wheezes may indicate heart failure. Auscultation of an S_4 heart sound is a common finding in the client who has had a previous MI or hypertension.

The client with MI may experience a temperature elevation for several days after infarction. Temperatures as high as 102° F (40.9° C) may occur in response to myocardial necrosis.

PSYCHOSOCIAL ASSESSMENT

Denial is a common early reaction to chest discomfort associated with angina or MI. On average, the client with an acute MI waits more than 2 hours before seeking medical attention. Often the client rationalizes that symptoms are due to indigestion or overexertion. In some situations, denial is a normal part of adapting to a stressful event; however, denial that interferes with identification of a symptom, such as chest discomfort, can be harmful. Explain the significance of reporting any discomfort, emphasizing that the health care provider will immediately attempt to relieve the discomfort.

Fear, anxiety, and anger are other common reactions of clients and families. Nursing assessment focuses on assisting the client and family members in identifying these feelings. Allow the client and family time to explain their understanding of the event and clarify any misconceptions.

Critical Thinking Challenge

A 55-year-old female client visits an urgent care center with a complaint of burning epigastric pain. She states that she believes it is a bad case of persistent heartburn. Assessment findings show slight shortness of breath, diaphoresis, and nausea and vomiting. Vital signs are BP 122/78, P 82, R 20, T 98.2. She is 5 feet 2 inches tall and weighs 168 pounds. Her tentative diagnosis is to "r/o MI."

1. What additional data and assessments should you collect at this time?
2. What risk factors may have contributed to this health problem?
3. How do this client's initial symptoms differ from those of a male client who has an MI?

evolve For suggested answer guidelines, go to http://evolve.elsevier.com/Iggy/.

LABORATORY ASSESSMENT

At present no single ideal test to diagnose MI exists. Health care providers use a series of different blood tests to diagnose a MI. The most common diagnostic tests include troponin T and I, creatinine kinase-MB (CK-MB), and myoglobin. These tests are described in Chapter 36.

RADIOGRAPHIC ASSESSMENT

Unless there is associated cardiac dysfunction (e.g., valvular disease) or heart failure, a chest x-ray is not diagnostic for angina or MI.

OTHER DIAGNOSTIC ASSESSMENTS

ELECTROCARDIOGRAPHY. Twelve-lead electrocardiograms (ECGs) allow the health care provider to examine the heart from varying perspectives and to note both the occurrence and the location of ischemia (angina) or necrosis (infarction).

An ischemic myocardium does not repolarize normally. Thus 12-lead ECGs obtained during an anginal episode reveal ST depression, T-wave inversion, or both. **Variant angina,** caused by coronary vasospasm (vessel spasm), usually causes elevation of the ST segment during anginal attacks.

These ST- and T-wave changes usually subside when the ischemia is resolved and the pain is relieved; however, the T wave may remain flat or inverted for a period of time. If the client is not experiencing angina at the moment of the test, the ECG for the client with angina is usually normal unless the client has evidence of an old MI.

When infarction occurs, three ECG changes are usually observed: ST-segment elevation, T-wave inversion, and an abnormal Q wave (wider than 0.04 seconds or more than one third the height of the QRS complex). Women who have a myocardial infarction (MI), however, may not have an ST-segment elevation (Cheek & Cesan, 2003). Figure 41-2 shows the usual ECG changes seen in MI.

The **Q wave** develops because necrotic cells do not conduct electrical stimuli. Hours to days after the MI, the ST-segment and T-wave changes will return to normal, but the Q wave usually remains permanently. By identifying the lead in which the ECG changes are occurring, the health care provider can identify the location and extent of the infarction.

STRESS TEST. After the acute stages of an anginal episode or MI, the health care provider often orders an **exercise tolerance test (stress test)** to assess for ECG changes consistent with ischemia, evaluate medical therapy, and identify those who might benefit from referral for invasive therapy (see Chapter 36). Pharmacologic stress testing using agents, such as adenosine (Adenocard) or dobutamine (Dobutrex), may also be used. Women are better diagnosed using an echocardiography stress test rather than the thallium stress test (Cheek & Cesan, 2003).

MYOCARDIAL PERFUSION IMAGING (MPI). *Thallium* scans use radioisotope imaging to assess for ischemia or necrotic muscle tissue related to angina or myocardial infarction (MI). Areas of decreased or absent perfusion, referred to as *cold spots,* identify ischemia or infarction. Thallium may also be used with the exercise tolerance test. Dipyridamole thallium scanning (DTS) may also be used.

MAGNETIC RESONANCE IMAGING (MRI). Contrast-enhanced cardiovascular magnetic resonance (CMR) may also be used as a noninvasive approach to detect MI (Rademaker, 2003).

CARDIAC CATHETERIZATION. This procedure may be performed to determine the extent and exact location of obstructions of the coronary arteries. Cardiac catheterization allows the cardiologist and cardiac surgeon to identify clients who might benefit from percutaneous transluminal angioplasty (PCTA) or coronary artery bypass grafting (CABG). Each of the diagnostic tests in this section is described in detail in Chapter 36.

Analysis

The client with coronary artery disease (CAD) may have either angina or MI. If MI is suspected or cannot be completely ruled out, the client is admitted to a telemetry unit for continuous monitoring or to a critical care unit if hemodynamically unstable.

COMMON NURSING DIAGNOSES AND COLLABORATIVE PROBLEMS

The following are priority nursing diagnoses for clients with CAD:

1. Acute Pain related to biologic injury agents (imbalance between myocardial oxygen supply and demand)
2. Ineffective Tissue Perfusion (Cardiopulmonary) related to interruption of arterial blood flow
3. Activity Intolerance related to fatigue (caused by imbalance between oxygen supply and demand)
4. Ineffective Coping related to effects of acute illness and major changes in lifestyle

For the client experiencing an MI, the following are the most important collaborative problems:

1. Potential for Dysrhythmias
2. Potential for Heart Failure
3. Potential for Recurrent Symptoms and Extension of Injury

ADDITIONAL NURSING DIAGNOSES AND COLLABORATIVE PROBLEMS

In addition to the common nursing diagnoses and collaborative problems, clients with CAD may have one or more of the following:

- Ineffective Sexuality Patterns related to pain and effects of illness
- Impaired Physical Mobility related to pain or fear of movement
- Potential for Acute Renal Failure

Planning and Implementation

ACUTE PAIN

PLANNING: EXPECTED OUTCOMES. The client with CAD is expected to state that pain, if present, is relieved. Older women may not experience the characteristic chest pain and may have silent myocardial ischemia or silent MI (Chart 41-3).

INTERVENTIONS. The objective of management is to eliminate discomfort by providing pain relief modalities, decreasing myocardial oxygen demand, and increasing myocardial oxygen supply.

NIC **PAIN MANAGEMENT.** Evaluate chest or other complaints of pain, obtain vital signs, ensure the patency of IV accesses, and notify the health care provider of the client's condition. Chart 41-4 summarizes the appropriate interventions for the client with symptoms of CAD.

Drug Therapy. Pain relief helps to increase the oxygen supply and decrease myocardial oxygen demand. The Amer-

CHART 41-3

NURSING FOCUS on the OLDER ADULT

Silent Myocardial Ischemia/Silent Myocardial Infarction

Silent myocardial ischemia and silent myocardial infarction (MI), once believed relatively rare, are now recognized to affect 21% to 68% of older adults with coronary artery disease (CAD) (Aronow, 2003). Reasons for the frequent absence of chest pain in older adults with CAD may be due to cognitive impairment and inability to verbalize sensations of pain, has more collateral circulation, and a reduced sensitivity to pain. Older clients with acute MI also delay longer in seeking assistance.

Silent myocardial ischemia increases the incidence of new coronary events in older clients with CAD and should be treated aggressively. The prevalence of clinical unrecognized MI diagnosed by routine ECGs in older persons varies from 21% to 68%. Older persons with clinically unrecognized MI have a similar or higher incidence of new coronary events and mortality compared with those with unrecognized MI. They should be aggressively treated with antiplatelet drugs, beta blockers, angiotensin converting enzymes, and statins if necessary.

ican Heart Association (AHA) recommends several strategies, including morphine sulfate and oxygen. In addition, aspirin 325 mg may be administered orally (chewed) immediately to prevent future occlusions. At home or in the hospital, the client may use nitroglycerin to relieve anginal pain.

Nitroglycerin. **Nitroglycerin (NTG),** a nitrate often referred to as "nitro," increases collateral blood flow, redistributes blood flow toward the subendocardium, and causes dilation of the coronary arteries. Instruct the client to hold the tablet under the tongue and drink 5 mL of water, if necessary, to allow the tablet to dissolve. NTG spray is also available and is more quickly absorbed. Pain relief should begin within 1 or 2 minutes and should be clearly evident in 3 to 5 minutes. After 5 minutes, recheck the client's pain intensity and vital signs. If the blood pressure (BP) is less than 100 mm Hg systolic or 25 mm Hg lower than the previous reading, lower the head of the bed and notify the health care provider. If the client is experiencing some but not complete relief and vital signs remain stable, another NTG tablet or spray may be used. In 5-minute increments, a total of three doses may be administered in an attempt to relieve anginal pain.

Angina usually responds to NTG. The client typically states that the pain is relieved or markedly diminished. When simple measures, such as taking three sublingual nitroglycerin tablets one after the other, do not relieve chest discomfort, the client may be experiencing an MI. Immediately inform the health care provider and prepare the client for transfer to a specialized unit where close monitoring and appropriate management can be provided. If the client is at home or in the community, the client or family should call 911 for transfer to the closest emergency department.

In a specialized unit the health care provider may prescribe IV NTG for management of the chest pain. Begin the drug infusion slowly, checking the BP and pain level every 3 to 5 minutes. The nitroglycerin dose is increased until the pain is relieved, the BP falls excessively, or the maximum prescribed dose is reached. The BP is monitored continuously (Chart 41-5).

When the pain has subsided and the client is stabilized, the health care provider may change the medication to an oral or topical nitrate. During administration of long-term oral and topical nitrates, a 12-hour nitrate-free period should be maintained to prevent tolerance. The client may complain initially of headache. The health care provider may prescribe acetaminophen (Tylenol, Exdol✱) to be taken before the nitrate to ease some of this discomfort.

Morphine Sulfate. The health care provider usually prescribes morphine sulfate (MS) to relieve chest discomfort that is unresponsive to nitroglycerin. Morphine relieves MI pain, decreases myocardial oxygen demand, relaxes smooth muscle, and reduces circulating catecholamines. It is usually administered in 2- to 10-mg doses intravenously every 5 to 15 minutes until the maximum prescribed dose is reached or until the client experiences relief or signs of toxicity. Adverse effects of morphine include respiratory depression, hypotension, bradycardia, and severe vomiting. Treatment for morphine toxicity consists of administering naloxone (Narcan) 0.2 to 0.8 mg intravenously, vasopressors, administration of IV fluids, and oxygen therapy. Monitor the client's vital signs and cardiac rhythm every few minutes.

These strategies are often enough to relieve the pain. If these methods are not adequate, additional interventions, identified later under Ineffective Tissue Perfusion (Cardiopulmonary), may be attempted.

Other Interventions. Several interventions may assist in relieving chest pain. Supplemental oxygen may increase the amount of oxygen available to myocardial tissue. Therefore oxygen is often prescribed and administered at a flow of 2 to 4 L/min by nasal cannula titrated to maintain an arterial oxygen saturation (SaO_2) equal to or greater than 95%. If the BP is stable, assist the client in assuming any position of comfort. Placing the client in semi-Fowler's position often enhances comfort and tissue oxygenation. A quiet, calm environment and explanations of interventions often reduce anxiety and assist in relief of chest pain. If needed, instruct the client to take several deep breaths to increase oxygenation.

CHART 41-4

BEST PRACTICE for
Emergency Care of the Client with Chest Discomfort

EMERGENCY CARE

- Obtain the client's description of the chest discomfort.
- Obtain the client's vital signs (blood pressure, pulse, respiration).
- Assess the client's vascular access.
- Consult standing orders or notify the physician for specific intervention.
- Obtain a 12-lead electrocardiogram if indicated.
- Provide pain relief medication and aspirin as prescribed.
- Administer oxygen therapy as prescribed.
- Remain calm; stay with the client if possible.
- Assess the client's vital signs and intensity of pain 5 minutes after administration of medication.
- Remedicate with prescribed medications (if vital signs remain stable), and check the client every 5 minutes.
- Notify the physician if vital signs deteriorate or pain is not relieved after three doses of nitroglycerin.

Critical Thinking Challenge

Five hours ago, a 48-year-old African-American man becomes nauseated and short of breath while mowing his yard. His wife brings him to the emergency department with excruciating pain between his shoulders. He states that the pain is a 10 on a scale of 0 to 10 and radiates down his left arm.

1. What are four essential components you should include in your initial assessment of this client?
2. What diagnostic testing will most likely be done?
3. What are the priorities of care for this client over the next 4 hours?

evolve For suggested answer guidelines, go to http://evolve.elsevier.com/Iggy/.

INEFFECTIVE TISSUE PERFUSION (CARDIOPULMONARY)

NOC **PLANNING: EXPECTED OUTCOMES.** The client with coronary artery disease (CAD) is expected to have adequate blood flow through the coronary vasculature to maintain heart function. Indicators include the following uncompromised measurements in the client:

- Ejection fraction
- Pulmonary wedge pressure
- Cardiac enzymes
- Apical heart rate
- Systolic and diastolic blood pressure
- Additionally, the client will have no:
  Angina
  Profuse diaphoresis

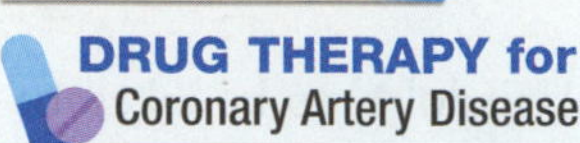

CHART 41-5

DRUG THERAPY for Coronary Artery Disease

Drug	Usual Dosage	Nursing Interventions	Rationales
Nitrates			
Nitroglycerin (Nitrostat, NitroQuick)	0.3-0.4 mg sublingually q5min; up to 3 tablets over 15 min	Instruct the client to lie down with the head of the bed at a level of comfort when taking the sublingual form.	Hypotension can be dramatic, immediate, and intensified by the upright position.
Nitrolingual translingual spray	0.4 mg/metered spray	Monitor BP. Pay attention to orthostatic changes.	A decrease in BP occurs with vasodilation.
		Instruct the client to allow the sublingual tablet to dissolve and to avoid swallowing the tablet.	The sublingual dose is absorbed through the sublingual mucous membranes.
		Check the expiration date on sublingual tablets and sprays. Tablets should be replaced every 3-5 mo.	The efficacy of the tablets decreases with time.
		Determine whether pain is relieved.	Additional medication may be required to relieve pain.
		Monitor for headache.	Vasodilation is generalized.
Isosorbide dinitrate (Isordil, Iso-Bid)	2.5 mg sublingually q4-6h; 5-40 mg PO four times daily 40 to 80 mg sustained-release tablet q8-12h	Instruct the client taking sublingual forms to lie down before administration.	The hypotensive effect can be dramatic and immediate with sublingual administration.
		Monitor BP and assess for dizziness.	A decrease in BP occurs with vasodilation.
Isosorbide mononitrate (Imdur)	60-mg extended-release tablet daily	Schedule sustained-release form with an 8- to 12-hr dose-free interval.	Tolerance may develop.
Nitroglycerin patch (Minitran, Nitro-Dur, Nitrek)	Transdermally started at 5 mg/24 hr (10-cm^2 system)	Remove the patch from the client before defibrillation.	The client may develop a burn.
		Rotate application sites.	Rotation prevents skin irritation.
		Apply the patch to a clean, dry, hairless area.	The drug is better absorbed when the skin is clean, dry, and hairless.
		Remove patch after 12-14 hr each day.	Removal prevents drug tolerance.
Beta Blockers			
Propranolol (Inderal, Inderal LA, Novo-Pranol)	80-320 mg twice daily to four times daily 1-3 mg IV at rate not to exceed 1 mg/min	Assess heart rate before administration.	Beta-blocking effects cause a decrease in heart rate.
		Monitor BP.	The hypotensive effect is due to a decrease in cardiac output, suppressed renin activity, and beta-blocking effects.
		Observe for signs of heart failure.	Heart failure may occur as a result of a decrease in cardiac output.
		Assess for shortness of breath and wheezing.	Beta$_2$-blocking effects in the lungs can cause bronchoconstriction.
Metoprolol (Lopressor, Toprol XL, Betaloc✱), a cardioselective beta-adrenergic blocker	*Angina*: 100 mg daily *MI*: 100 mg twice daily; 5 mg IV over 2 min may be repeated twice for a total of 15 mg	Assess heart rate before administration; do not administer if heart rate $<$50 beats/min.	Beta blockers may cause further decreases in heart rate.
		Monitor BP and hold for systolic $<$90 mm Hg.	Decreased BP pressure is an anticipated effect.
		Assess client for cough, shortness of breath, edema, and weight gain.	These are indications of heart failure.
Calcium Channel Blockers			
Nifedipine (Adalat, Adalat CC, Adalat XL, Procardia, Procardia XL, Nu-Nifed✱)	10-30 mg PO three times daily 30-60 mg daily for XL and CC	Monitor BP and assess for dizziness.	Vasodilation can cause dramatic hypotension, which occurs within minutes.
		Assess for headache and edema of the lower extremities.	These are common side effects.
		Tell client that empty shell of med may be in stool (for XL drugs).	Shell encases active part of medication and is not absorbed by the body.
Verapamil (Calan, Isoptin)	40-80 mg PO four times daily or 120- to 240-mg sustained-release tablet once daily 5-10 mg IV over 2 min	Monitor heart rate.	This agent slows SA and AV node conduction.
		Monitor blood pressure and assess for dizziness.	Vasodilation decreases BP.
		Assess for constipation.	This is a common side effect.

SA, Sinoatrial; *AV*, atrioventricular.

CHART 41-5

DRUG THERAPY for Coronary Artery Disease—*cont'd*

Drug	Usual Dosage	Nursing Interventions	Rationales
Calcium Channel Blockers—*cont'd*			
Diltiazem (Cardizem, Cardizem CD, Cardizem SR, Dilacor-XR, Tiazac, Apo-Diltiaz✱)	30-60 mg PO four times daily or 120- to 480-mg sustained-release tablet once daily; increase dose slowly	Monitor BP and assess for dizziness.	Vasodilation decreases blood pressure.
		Monitor heart rate.	This drug slows SA and AV node conduction, but the decrease is not as great as that which occurs with verapamil.
		Teach client to avoid grapefruit juice.	Drug's hypotensive effects increase.
Amlodipine (Norvasc)	5-10 mg daily	Monitor BP and pulse.	Like all drugs in this class, SA node conduction is slower and vessels dilate.
		Teach client to observe for signs and symptoms of heart failure, such as sudden weight gain, dyspnea, edema.	Drug can cause heart failure.
[1]Bepridil (Vascor)	200-400 mg daily	Instruct client to avoid grapefruit juice.	This juice increases the hypotensive effects.
		Monitor liver function tests (LFTs).	Drug can increase LFTs.
		Do not break, chew, or crush tablet.	Drug is long-acting and releases slowly.
		Monitor BP and pulse.	Same as diltiazem.
Felodipine (Plendil, Renedil✱)	5-10 mg daily	Same as most calcium channel blockers.	Same as most calcium channel blockers
Isradipine (DynaCirc, DynaCirc CR)	2.5 mg twice daily, increase up to 10 mg twice daily	Do not break, chew, or crush CR form.	Same as bepridil.
		Notify health care provider if signs and symptoms of heart failure.	Same as bepridil.
		Monitor blood pressure and pulse.	Same as diltiazem.
[2]Nicardipine (Cardene, Cardene SR, Cardene IV)	20-40 mg PO three times daily 0.5-2.2 mg/hr IV	Same as isradipine.	Same as isradipine.
Antiplatelet Agents			
Aspirin (Empirin, Apo-ASA✱, Ecotrin)	81-650 PO daily	Suggest that the client take the daily dose with food.	Gastric irritation may occur.
		Question the client about ringing in the ears.	Tinnitus may occur with aspirin toxicity.
		Emphasize to the client that aspirin is an important cardiac medication and should be continued unless the client is told to stop.	Studies document significantly better survival rates for clients with coronary artery disease receiving aspirin.
Ticlopidine (Ticlid)	250 mg twice daily	Teach client to take drug with food.	Drug can cause diarrhea and other GI disturbances.
		Inform client to report any usual bleeding or bruising.	Drug prevents platelet aggregation, thus slowing down clot formation.
[3]Clopidogrel (Plavix)	*Recent MI:* 75 mg daily *Acute coronary syndrome:* 300 mg, then 75-150 mg daily	Same as ticlopidine.	Same as ticlopidine.

[1]***Med Error Alert!*** *Do not confuse bepridil and prepidil.*

[2]***Med Error Alert!*** *Do not confuse Cardene and Cardizem.*

[3]***Med Error Alert!*** *Do not confuse Plavix with Paxil.*

INTERVENTIONS. Because myocardial infarction (MI) is a dynamic process, restoration of perfusion to the injured area often limits the amount of extension and improves left ventricular function. Complete, sustained reperfusion of coronary arteries in the first few hours after an MI has decreased mortality in clients with MI.

Thrombolytic Therapy. Fibrinolytics are used to dissolve thrombi in the coronary arteries and restore myocardial blood flow. Examples of these agents, which target the fibrin component of the coronary thrombosis, include tissue plasminogen activator (t-PA, alteplase [Activase]), anisoylated plasminogen-streptokinase activator complex (APSAC), and reteplase (Retavase). The health care provider may prescribe the administration of fibrinolytics intravenously or by the intracoronary route during cardiac catheterization. Thrombolytic agents are most effective when administered within the first 6 hours of a coronary event. Thrombolytics are underused nationwide in men and women, young and old.

Thrombolytic therapy should be given in a unit where the client can be continuously monitored. It is indicated for clients who have chest pain of greater than 30 minutes' duration that is unrelieved by nitroglycerin, with indications of transmural ischemia and injury as shown by the ECG. Contraindications include recent abdominal surgery or stroke because bleeding may occur when fresh clots are lysed (broken down). Table 41-3 lists the current contraindications to thrombolytic therapy.

Clients who weigh less than 65 kg may need to have their dose of thrombolytic weight adjusted to lessen the likelihood of bleeding. During administration, the nurse immediately reports any indications of bleeding to the health care provider. After administration, observe for signs of bleeding by doing the following:

- Documenting the client's neurologic status
- Observing all IV sites for bleeding and patency
- Monitoring clotting studies
- Observing for signs of internal bleeding (watching hemoglobin and hematocrit)
- Testing stools, urine, and emesis for occult blood

TABLE 41-3 Contraindications to Thrombolytic Therapy

Absolute
Active internal bleeding
Known allergy to streptokinase products
Recent head trauma
Known bleeding disorders
Suspected aortic dissection
Increased blood pressure 200/120 mm Hg
Pregnancy or recent delivery
Cerebrovascular processes: recent stoke (within 2 mo). Recent spinal or cerebral surgery, cranial neoplasm
Prolonged cardiopulmonary resuscitation

Relative
Endocarditis or pericarditis
Hemostatic defects
Severe uncontrolled hypertension
Trauma within last 10 days
Surgery within the last 10 days
Current use of oral anticoagulants
Active peptic ulcer disease

Data from Lapchak, P.A., et al. (2002). The nonpeptide glycoprotein IIb/IIIa platelet receptor antagonist SM-20302 reduces tissue plasminogen activator-induced intracerebral hemorrhage after thromboembolic stroke. *Stroke, 35*(1), 147-152.

Some concerns in thrombolytic administration are associated with the specific agent. For example, *streptokinase*, a first-generation thrombolytic agent, is not fibrin specific; thus it may create systemic bleeding problems. Therefore, it is not used as commonly as other agents.

Second- and third-generation fibrinolytics include tissue plasminogen activator (t-PA, alteplase [Activase]), reteplase (Retavase), tenecteplase (TNKase), and t-PA. These drugs are fibrin specific, have a short half-life (3 to 5 minutes), and lack antigenicity. Because some studies have associated t-PA with a more frequent occurrence of cerebrovascular bleeding, carefully document neurologic findings. Reteplase can be given in two boluses ½ hour apart, needs not be weight adjusted, and results in greater rates of reperfusion than t-PA.

Tenecteplase (TNKase) is a newer fibrinolytic to be approved for use in clients with MIs. This drug has some advantages over other fibrinolytics. First, it can be easily administered as a single bolus over 5 seconds. Tenecteplase also targets clots more specifically than other fibrinolytics, resulting in slightly less overall bleeding. Bleeding is still possible, however, and nursing considerations are similar to the other fibrinolytics. Dosage is based on the client's weight. Use the utmost caution in administering these agents to avoid administration errors and prevent complications. Research continues to investigate and develop new, improved thrombolytic agents.

Glycoprotein IIb/IIIa Inhibitors. Glycoprotein (GP) IIb/IIIa inhibitors target the platelet component of the thrombus. Abciximab (ReoPro), eptifibatide (Integrilin), and tirofiban (Aggrastat) are administered intravenously to prevent fibrinogen from attaching to activated platelets at the site of a thrombus. These medications have been used in acute coronary syndromes (especially unstable angina and non–Q-wave MI). They are also administered before and during percutaneous transluminal coronary angioplasty (PTCA) to ensure patency of the newly opened artery and in conjunction with fibrinolytic agents following MI. If the GP IIb/IIIa inhibitors are used with a fibrinolytic agent, then the dose of the thrombolytic should be reduced by 25% to 50% to decrease the likelihood of bleeding. During the administration of GP IIb/IIIa inhibitors, assess the client closely for indications of bleeding or hypersensitivity reactions. If either occurs, the health care provider is notified immediately regarding administration of the appropriate medications (e.g., antihistamines or corticosteroids) for a hypersensitivity response.

For some clients experiencing an MI, primary PTCA may be used to reopen the thrombosed coronary artery. PTCA has been associated with excellent return of blood flow through the coronary artery when it can be performed within 70 minutes of the onset of chest discomfort by an interventional cardiologist. Most community hospitals are now capable of performing emergent PTCA. When primary PTCA is not available, clients with MI should receive immediate thrombolytic agents if they are an appropriate candidate and then transferred to a facility that can perform PTCA. This procedure is described in detail later in this chapter.

Identification of Coronary Artery Reperfusion. Monitor the client for indications that the clot has been lysed and the artery reperfused. These indications include the following:

- Abrupt cessation of pain or discomfort
- Sudden onset of ventricular dysrhythmias

- Resolution of ST-segment depression
- A peak at 12 hours of markers of myocardial damage

After clot lysis with thrombolytics, large amounts of thrombin are released into the system, increasing the risk of vessel reocclusion. To maintain the patency of the coronary artery after thrombolytic therapy, the health care provider usually prescribes aspirin and IV heparin. Monitor the activated partial thromboplastin time (aPTT)–the usual appropriate range is $1\frac{1}{2}$ to $2\frac{1}{2}$ times the control sample)–and maintain the heparin infusion for 3 to 5 days as prescribed. Low-molecular-weight heparin (enoxaparin [Lovenox]) may be substituted for IV heparin.

Oral Drug Therapy. Clients who have had an MI, whether or not they are receiving thrombolytics, should begin aspirin therapy unless contraindicated. They may receive a chewable aspirin immediately and then an enteric-coated aspirin (Ancasal✱, Ecotrin) 80 to 325 mg daily or every other day to prevent platelet aggregation at the site of the obstruction.

Beta-adrenergic blocking agents (e.g., metoprolol [Lopressor, Toprol XL, Betaloc✱]) decrease the size of the infarct, ventricular dysrhythmias, and mortality rates in clients with MI. The physician usually prescribes a cardioselective beta-blocking agent within the first 24 hours after a myocardial infarction (MI). Beta blockers slow the heart rate and decrease the force of cardiac contraction (see Chart 41-5). Thus these agents prolong the period of diastole and increase myocardial perfusion while reducing the force of myocardial contraction. With beta blockade, the heart is capable of performing 25% to 30% more work without ischemia. During beta-blocking therapy, do the following:

- Monitor the heart rate (bradycardia is common)
- Check the BP
- Check the level of consciousness
- Monitor for any chest discomfort

Assess the lungs for crackles (indicative of heart failure) and wheezes (indicative of bronchospasm). Hypoglycemia, depression, nightmares, and forgetfulness are also problems with beta blockade, especially in older clients. Many of these side effects decrease with time, however.

Health care providers frequently prescribe angiotensin-converting enzyme (ACE) inhibitors within 48 hours of an MI to prevent ventricular remodeling and the development of heart failure. ACE inhibitors have been demonstrated to increase survival after an MI. Monitor the client for decreased urine output, hypotension, cough, and changes in serum potassium, creatinine, and blood urea nitrogen. (See Chapters 38 and 39 for a more detailed discussion of ACE inhibitors.)

For clients with angina, the health care provider may prescribe calcium channel blockers to enhance vasodilation and myocardial perfusion. Calcium channel blockers are indicated for clients with variant angina or for those who are hypertensive and continue to have angina despite therapy with beta blockers. They are not indicated after an MI. Monitor the client for hypotension and peripheral edema, and review the frequency of anginal episodes.

The recent Clopidogrel in Unstable Angina to Prevent Recurrent Ischemic Events (CURE) study showed that the combination of clopidogrel (Plavix) and aspirin was more effective in reducing death, MI, and stroke compared with aspirin alone. The risk of bleeding from using two antiplatelet agents together was not significantly increased (Palatnik, 2001).

Enhanced External Counterpulsation. Enhanced external counterpulsation (EECP) is a noninvasive procedure that may be used to manage the symptoms of chronic, stable angina. It works by increasing blood flow to the ischemic areas of the myocardium. The EECP device consists of a series of compressive cuffs that are placed around the client's calves and thighs (Figure 41-4). Teach clients that this procedure may be repeated as needed.

ACTIVITY INTOLERANCE

PLANNING: EXPECTED OUTCOMES. The client with coronary artery disease (CAD) is expected to walk at least 200 feet four times a day without chest discomfort or shortness of breath.

INTERVENTIONS. Activity intolerance is reduced by a planned program of cardiac rehabilitation implemented primarily by the nurse and physical therapist and continued after discharge.

NIC **Cardiac Care: Rehabilitative.** **Cardiac rehabilitation** is the process of actively assisting the client with cardiac disease in achieving and maintaining a vital and productive life while remaining within the limits of the heart's ability to respond to increases in activity and stress. It can be divided into three phases. *Phase 1* begins with the acute illness and ends with discharge from the hospital. *Phase 2* begins after discharge and continues through convalescence at home. *Phase 3* refers to long-term conditioning.

In the acute phase (phase 1), promote rest and ensure some limited mobility. Assistance may be needed for some activities of daily living (ADLs), such as assistance in ambulating to the bathroom. Clients progress at their own rate to increasing levels of activity, depending on their clinical status, age, and physical capabilities.

The next step in phase 1 is independent ambulation of the client in the room and to the bathroom. Encourage progressive ambulation in the hallway, usually 50, 100, and then 200 feet three times a day. In addition, the client may begin showering for 5 or 10 minutes with warm water; a stool should be available to facilitate rest and maintain balance.

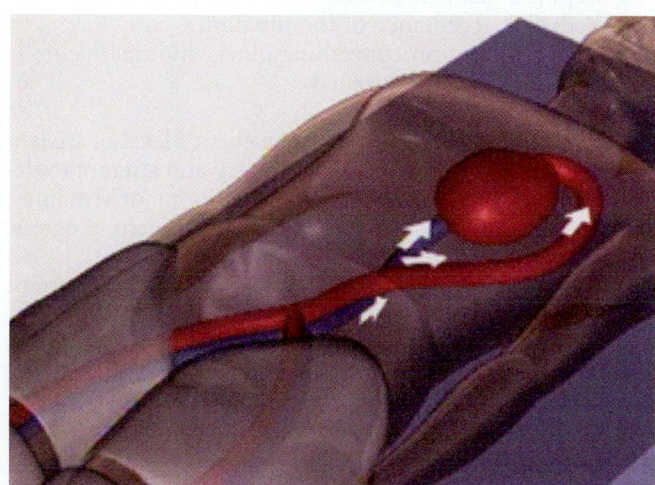

Figure 41-4 ■ Enhanced external counterpulsation device. This noninvasive procedure supplies blood and oxygen to the heart, reduces workload, and eases anginal symptoms.

CHART 41-6

NURSING FOCUS on the OLDER ADULT
Coronary Artery Disease

- Recognize that chest pain may not be evident in the older client; associated symptoms, such as unexplained dyspnea, confusion, or GI symptoms.
- Although older adults have a greater reduction in mortality from myocardial infarction (MI) with the use of thrombolytics, they also have the most severe side effects. Monitor older clients receiving thrombolytics extremely carefully.
- Dysrhythmia may be a normal age-related change rather than a complication of MI. Determine whether the dysrhythmia is causing significant symptoms, then notify the physician.
- If beta blockers are used, assess the client carefully for the development of side effects. Exacerbation of the depression already present in older adults is a significant problem with beta blockade.
- Plan slow, steady increases in activity. Older adults with minimal previous exercise show particular benefit from a gradual increase in activity.
- Older adults should plan longer warm-up and cool-down periods when participating in an exercise program. Their pulse rates may not return to baseline until 30 minutes or longer after exercise.

Assess the client's heart rate, blood pressure (BP), respiratory rate, and level of fatigue with each higher level of activity. Decreases greater than 20 mm Hg in the systolic BP, changes of 20 beats/min in the pulse rate, and complaints of dyspnea or chest pain indicate intolerance of activity. When such signs and symptoms develop, notify the health care provider and do not advance the client to the next level. Older adults with CAD often have needs and concerns different from those of younger adults, as described in Chart 41-6.

INEFFECTIVE COPING

NOC **PLANNING: EXPECTED OUTCOMES.** The client with CAD is expected to take personal actions to manage stressors related to CAD. Indicators include that the client will consistently be able to do the following:

- Identify effective coping patterns
- Verbalize a sense of control
- Report a decrease in stress
- Verbalize acceptance of the situation
- Seek information concerning illness and treatment
- Modify lifestyle as needed
- Adapt to life changes

INTERVENTIONS. Assess the client's level of anxiety while allowing expressions of any anxiety and attempt to define its origin. Simple, repeated explanations of therapies, expectations, and surroundings, as well as client progress, may help relieve anxiety.

NIC **Coping Enhancement.** Identify the client's current coping mechanisms; the most common are denial, anger, and depression. Denial allows the client to minimize a threat and use problem-focused coping mechanisms. The client may avoid discussing what has happened and yet comply with treatment regimens. This type of denial decreases anxiety and should not be discouraged; however, denial that results in a client's "acting out" and refusing to follow treatment regimens can be harmful. Because this behavior is usually due to extreme anxiety or fear, threats only worsen the behavior. Remain calm and avoid confronting the client.

CHART 41-7

NIC **INTERVENTION ACTIVITIES for**
Clients with Coronary Artery Disease

Pain Management: *Alleviation of pain or a reduction in pain to a level of comfort that is acceptable to the client*

- Perform a comprehensive assessment of pain to include location, characteristics, onset/duration, frequency, quality, intensity or severity of pain, and precipitating factors.
- Verify level of discomfort with client, note changes in the medical record, inform other health professionals working with the client.
- Ensure that client receives attentive analgesic care.
- Determine the needed frequency of making an assessment of client comfort and implement monitoring plan.
- Evaluate the effectiveness of the pain control measures used while performing thorough ongoing assessment of the pain experience.

Cardiac Care: Rehabilitative: *Promotion of maximum functional activity level for a client who has experienced an episode of impaired cardiac function that resulted from an imbalance between myocardial oxygen supply and demand*

- Monitor the client's activity tolerance.
- Maintain ambulation schedule, as tolerated.
- Instruct the client and family on the exercise regimen, including warm-up, endurance, and cool-down, as appropriate.
- Instruct the client and family on any lifting/pushing weight limitations, if appropriate.
- Encourage realistic expectations for the client and family.

Coping Enhancement: *Assisting a client to adapt to perceived stressors, changes, or threats that interfere with meeting life demands and roles*

- Appraise the client's understanding of the disease process.
- Use a calm, reassuring approach.
- Provide an atmosphere of acceptance.
- Assist the client in developing an objective appraisal of the event.
- Help client to identify the information he or she is most interested in obtaining.
- Provide factual information concerning diagnosis, treatment, and prognosis.
- Foster constructive outlets for anger and hostility.
- Explore with the client previous methods of dealing with life problems.
- Support the use of appropriate defense mechanisms.

NIC intervention activities selected from Dochterman, J.M., & Bulechek, G.M. (2004). *Nursing interventions classification (NIC)* (4th ed.). St. Louis: Mosby.

Clearly indicate when a behavior is not acceptable and is potentially harmful as a result of noncompliance.

Anger may represent an attempt to regain control of life. Encourage the client to verbalize the source of frustration and provide opportunities for decision making and control.

Depression may be a client's response to grief and loss of function. Listen as the client verbalizes feelings of loss, being careful not to offer false or general reassurances. Depression is acknowledged, but the client is expected to perform ADLs and other activities within restrictions. Identify all improvements in the client's condition and share them. Chart 41-7 summarizes the major NIC intervention activities for clients with CAD.

POTENTIAL FOR DYSRHYTHMIAS

PLANNING: EXPECTED OUTCOMES. The client with CAD is expected to resume a normal sinus rhythm or normal rhythm and to be hemodynamically stable.

INTERVENTIONS. Dysrhythmias are the leading cause of death in most clients with myocardial infarction (MI) who die before they can be hospitalized. Even in the early period of hospitalization, 70% to 90% of clients with MI experience some abnormality of cardiac rhythm. Whenever a dysrhythmia develops in a client with CAD:

- Identify the dysrhythmia
- Assess hemodynamic status
- Evaluate for discomfort

Dysrhythmias are treated when they are causing hemodynamic compromise, are increasing myocardial oxygen requirements, or predispose to lethal ventricular dysrhythmias.

Typical dysrhythmias for the client with an *inferior* MI are bradycardias and second-degree AV blocks resulting from ischemia of the AV node. These rhythms tend to be transient. Monitor the cardiac rhythm and rate and the hemodynamic status. If the client becomes hemodynamically unstable, a temporary pacemaker may be necessary.

The client with an *anterior* MI is likely to exhibit ventricular irritability (premature ventricular contractions [PVCs]). Third-degree or bundle branch block is a serious complication in the client with an anterior MI because it indicates that a large portion of the left ventricle is involved. The health care provider may insert a pacemaker. Observe the client closely to detect the development of heart failure. Appropriate interventions for dysrhythmias are described in Chapter 37.

POTENTIAL FOR HEART FAILURE

PLANNING: EXPECTED OUTCOMES. The client with coronary artery disease (CAD) is expected to regain hemodynamic stability as evidenced by the following:

- BP and pulse rate within the client's acceptable range and adequate for metabolic demands
- Adequate urine output
- Mental alertness
- Clear lungs on auscultation
- Palpable peripheral pulses

INTERVENTIONS. Decreased cardiac output related to heart failure is a relatively common complication after an MI resulting from left ventricular dysfunction, rupture of the intraventricular septum, papillary muscle rupture with valvular dysfunction, or right ventricular infarction The most severe form of heart failure, *cardiogenic shock*, discussed on p. 854, accounts for most in-hospital deaths after an MI. The type of management used to increase cardiac output depends on the location of the MI and the type of heart failure that resulted from the infarction.

MANAGING LEFT VENTRICULAR FAILURE. When a client with MI experiences damage to the left ventricle, rupture of the intraventricular septum, or tear of a papillary muscle, a reduction occurs in the amount of blood that the heart can eject. When volume and pressure are markedly increased in the pulmonary vasculature, pulmonary complications develop.

Nursing Assessment and Monitoring. The development of left ventricular failure and pulmonary edema is assessed by auscultating for crackles and identifying their location in the lung fields. Wheezing, tachypnea, and frothy sputum may also occur with pulmonary edema. Auscultate the heart, paying particular attention to the presence of an S_3 heart sound.

Monitor for the following signs of poor organ perfusion that may result from decreased cardiac output:

- A change in orientation or mental status
- Urine output less than 1 mL/kg/hr or less than 30 mL/hr
- Cool, clammy extremities with decreased or absent pulses
- Unusual fatigue
- Recurrent chest pain

In specialized units, hemodynamic monitoring may be instituted to assess the client's preload, afterload, and cardiac output; however, hemodynamic monitoring in the hospital requires the insertion of a pulmonary artery catheter (see Chapter 36). Obtain and record hemodynamic measurements, which include the following:

- Right atrial pressure
- Pulmonary artery systolic and diastolic pressures
- Pulmonary artery wedge pressure (PAWP) (a measure of preload)
- Pulmonary vascular resistance
- Systemic vascular resistance (a measure of afterload)
- Cardiac output
- Central venous pressure (CVP)
- Cardiac index

Single values of these measurements are less significant than the trend of values combined with the client's clinical manifestations. These measurements help health care providers to identify heart failure and guide the administration of fluids and vasoactive drugs.

Classification of Postmyocardial Infarction Heart Failure. Killip categorized heart failure after an MI into four classes based on prognosis (Table 41-4).

Class I. Clients with class I heart failure often respond well to reduction in preload with IV nitrates and diuretics. Monitor the urine output hourly, check vital signs hourly, continue to assess for signs of heart failure, and review the serum potassium level.

Class II and Class III. Clients with class II and class III heart failure may require diuresis and more aggressive medical intervention, such as afterload reduction and contractility or enhancement of contractility. IV nitroprusside or nitroglycerin may be used to decrease both preload and afterload. These drugs are administered as continuous infusions in specialized units where the PAWP and BP can be closely monitored. The BP can drop in response to excessive vasodilation (see Chart 41-5).

Clients in class II and III are usually started on low dose beta blockers (usually Lopressor or Coreg). Dosing is titrated depending on goal achievement and drug tolerance. Other medications, including angiotensin-converting enzyme (ACE) inhibitors and angiotensin receptor blockers (ARBs), are commonly prescribed to promote ventricular remodeling. These medications are described in Chapter 38.

TABLE 41-4 Killip Classification of Heart Failure

Class	Description
I	Absent crackles and S_3
II	Crackles in the lower half of the lung fields and possible S_3
III	Crackles more than halfway up the lung fields and frequent pulmonary edema
IV	Cardiogenic shock

Positive inotropes, dobutamine (Dobutrex), and milrinone (Primacor), increase the force of cardiac contraction. They are administered by continuous IV infusion. The effects of these drugs on the vasculature and heart rate vary and may be dose dependent. An understanding of the anticipated effect of the drug and the desired dosage range is imperative. The infusions are titrated to optimize cardiac output. Use caution when administering these drugs because of the potential risk of increasing myocardial oxygen consumption and further decreasing cardiac output. The client is frequently monitored, paying particular attention to the development of chest pain (Chart 41-8).

Class IV: Cardiogenic Shock. Class IV heart failure is cardiogenic shock. In **cardiogenic shock,** necrosis of more than 40% of the left ventricle has occurred. Most clients have a stuttering pattern of chest pain, resulting in piecemeal extension of the MI. Manifestations of cardiogenic shock include the following:

- Tachycardia
- Hypotension
- BP less than 90 mm Hg or 30 mm Hg less than the client's baseline
- Urine output less than 30 mL/hr
- Cold, clammy skin with poor peripheral pulses
- Agitation, restlessness, or confusion
- Pulmonary congestion
- Tachypnea
- Continuing chest discomfort

Early detection is essential because established cardiogenic shock has a mortality rate of 65% to 100%.

Medical Management. Medical interventions aim to relieve pain and decrease myocardial oxygen requirements through preload and afterload reduction (see Charts 41-5 and 41-7). The health care provider prescribes IV morphine, which is used to decrease pulmonary congestion and relieve pain. Oxygen is administered; intubation and ventilation may be necessary.

Use the information gained from hemodynamic monitoring to titrate drug therapy. Preload reduction may be cautiously attempted with diuretics or nitroglycerin, as described for clients with Killip class III heart failure. (See Chapter 36 for a complete discussion of preload and afterload.) Monitor systolic pressure constantly, because vasodilation may result in a further decline in BP. Vasopressors and positive inotropes may be used to maintain organ perfusion, but such drugs increase myocardial oxygen consumption and can worsen ischemia. Use utmost caution in medication administration.

Use of an Intra-Aortic Balloon Pump. When clients do not respond to drug therapy with improved tissue perfusion, decreased workload of the heart, and increased cardiac contractility, an **intra-aortic balloon pump (IABP)** may be inserted. Insertion of an intra-aortic counterpulsation device, such as the IABP, is an invasive intervention that is used to improve myocardial perfusion during an acute MI, reduce preload and afterload, and facilitate left ventricular ejection.

The health care provider can insert an IABP percutaneously or through a surgical cutdown. Inflation of the IABP during diastole augments the diastolic pressure and improves coronary perfusion by increasing blood flow to the arteries. Deflation of the balloon just before systole reduces afterload at the time of systolic contraction. This action facilitates emptying of the left ventricle and improves cardiac output. The balloon catheter is attached to a pump console, which is triggered by an electrocardiogram (ECG) tracing and arterial waveform.

Immediate Reperfusion. Immediate reperfusion is an invasive intervention that shows some promise for clients with cardiogenic shock. The client is taken to the cardiac catheterization laboratory, and an emergency left-sided heart catheterization is performed. If the client has a treatable lesion or lesions, the surgeon performs an immediate percutaneous transluminal coronary angioplasty (PTCA or stent placement) in the catheterization laboratory, or the client is transferred to the operating suite for a coronary artery bypass graft (CABG).

MANAGING RIGHT VENTRICULAR FAILURE. Conditions other than left ventricular failure may result in decreased cardiac output after an MI. In about 30% of clients with inferior MIs, right ventricular infarction and failure develop. In this instance, the right ventricle fails independently of the left. Decreased cardiac output with a paradoxical pulse, clear lungs, and jugular venous distention results when the client is in semi-Fowler's position.

A right ventricular MI may be documented by echocardiography and by an ECG using right-sided precordial leads. The goal of medical management is to improve right ventricular stroke volume by increasing right ventricular fiber stretch or preload. To enhance right ventricular preload, the nurse administers sufficient fluids (as much as 200 mL/hr) to increase right atrial pressure to 20 mm Hg, as ordered. Monitor the pulmonary artery wedge pressure (PAWP) (attempting to maintain it below 15 to 20 mm Hg), and auscultate the lungs to ensure that left-sided failure is not developing. The client's cardiac output is monitored to ensure that fluid administration is having the desired effect.

POTENTIAL FOR RECURRENT SYMPTOMS AND EXTENSION OF INJURY

PLANNING: EXPECTED OUTCOMES. The client with coronary artery disease (CAD) is expected to experience minimal angina while engaging in activities of daily living (ADLs) and an exercise program.

INTERVENTIONS. Recurrent discomfort despite medical therapy is one of the major indications for surgical management of CAD. Clients who continue to have chest discomfort despite medical therapy or ischemia during a stress test may require invasive correction by PTCA or CABG to resolve angina or prevent myocardial infarction (MI). Before invasive treatment, a left-sided cardiac catheterization with coronary angiogram (see Chapter 36) is performed to document that the lesions are correctable and that left ventricular pump function is adequate.

Percutaneous Transluminal Coronary Angioplasty. **Percutaneous transluminal coronary angioplasty (PTCA)** is an invasive but nonsurgical technique. It is performed to reduce the frequency and severity of discomfort for clients with angina and to bridge clients to coronary bypass graft surgery.

Indications. Clients who are most likely to benefit from PTCA have single- or double-vessel disease with discrete, proximal, noncalcified lesions. This procedure often will not open complex lesions. When identifying which lesions are

CHART 41-8

DRUG THERAPY for
Commonly Used Intravenous Vasodilators and Inotropes

Drug	Usual Dosage	Nursing Interventions	Rationales
Nitrates			
Nitroprusside sodium (Nipride, Nitropress)	IV only by infusion device. Begin with 0.4-0.5 mcg/kg/min. May increase gradually to 10 mcg/kg/min.	Monitor BP q2-5 min when initiating therapy. If BP drops excessively, elevate the legs, decrease the dose, and increase fluids per unit policy.	This agent is a potent, rapidly reversible vasodilator acting on both peripheral venous and arterial musculature. BP may drop in 2 min.
		Monitor PAWP, SVR, BP, heart rate, urine output frequently.	
		Titrate medication to obtain the desired effect.	
		Protect from light.	This agent is light sensitive.
		Maintain dose at less than 3 mcg/min if possible.	Doses >3 mcg/min are associated with thiocyanate or cyanide toxicity.
		In clients requiring doses >3 mcg/min for >24-36 hr, monitor for metabolic acidosis, confusion, or hyperreflexia. Examine blood thiocyanate level.	These are indications of the toxic effects of cyanide.
Nitroglycerin (Tridil)	IV only by infusion device started at 5 mcg/min and gradually increased in increments of 5 q3-5min. If no response after 20 mcg/min, increase by 10-20 mcg until desired response.	Monitor BP q1-3 min when initiating therapy. If BP drops excessively, elevate the legs and decrease the dose according to unit policies.	This agent dilates coronary arteries. It is a more potent systemic venodilator than an arterial vasodilator. BP may drop in 1 min.
		Monitor RAP, PAWP, SVR, BP, heart rate, and urine output frequently.	
		Titrate medication to obtain the desired effect.	
		Intermittent administration of IV nitroglycerin should be considered.	Tolerance may develop rapidly to nitroglycerin administered by continuous IV.
		Monitor the client for headache.	Headache is a frequent side effect of initial nitroglycerin therapy.
Milrinone (Primacor)	IV bolus 50 mcg/kg given over 10 min; start infusion of 0.375-0.75 mcg/kg/min; reduce dose in renal impairment.	Assess BP and pulse q5min. If BP drops 30 mm Hg, stop infusion and call health care provider.	Hypotension is a common adverse effect.
		Monitor I&O and weight.	The drug causes diuresis.
Fenoldopam (Corlopam)	0.01-1.6 mcg/kg/min IV.	Assess BP and pulse q5min, then q1h × 2, then q4h, or according to agency policy.	Same as milrinone.
		Monitor I&O and assess for signs of dehydration.	
		Observe IV site for extravasation.	
Sympathomimetics			
Dopamine (Intropin)	IV only by infusion device. Starting dose 2-5 mcg/kg/min. Titrate up to 50 mcg/kg/min.	Determine the reason for use and the expected result.	This agent is a dose-dependent activator of alpha, beta, and dopaminergic receptors.
		Observe the client's heart rate, ECG, BP, PAWP, SVR, cardiac output, and urine output q5min to q1h.	2-5 mcg/kg/min stimulates dopaminergic receptors, which promotes renal and mesenteric blood flow.
		Titrate the dose carefully to maintain the dose range and obtain the desired effect.	5 mcg/kg/min stimulates beta receptors. This increases heart rate and contractility >10-15 mcg/kg/min, alpha effects predominate. This causes peripheral constriction.
		Infuse through a central catheter.	Extravasation can cause tissue necrosis and sloughing.
		Monitor the client for ectopy and angina.	These are adverse effects.
Dobutamine (Dobutrex)	IV only by infusion device, 2-10 mcg/kg/min. May increase to 40 mcg/kg/min.	Observe the client continuously during administration.	This agent is a very strong $beta_1$-receptor activator and a moderately strong $beta_2$-activator.
		Titrate the drug on the basis of heart rate, ECG findings, BP, PAWP, cardiac output, SVR, and urine output.	
		Monitor for atrial and ventricular ectopy.	Dysrhythmias are an adverse effect.

ECG, electrocardiogram; *I&O*, input and output; *PAWP*, pulmonary artery wedge pressure; *RAP*, right atrial pressure; *SVR*, systemic vascular resistance.

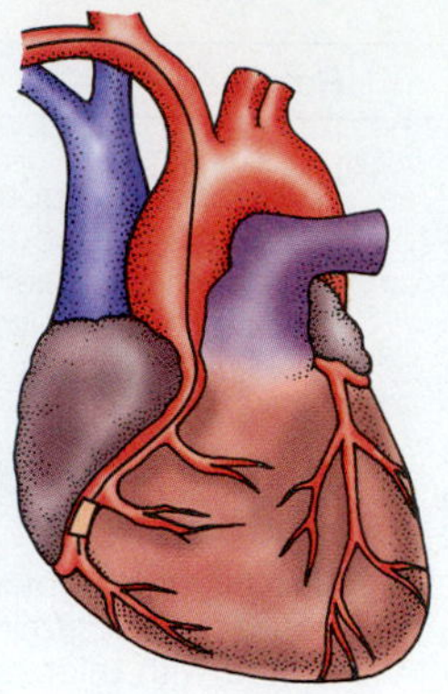

1. The balloon-tipped catheter is positioned in the artery.

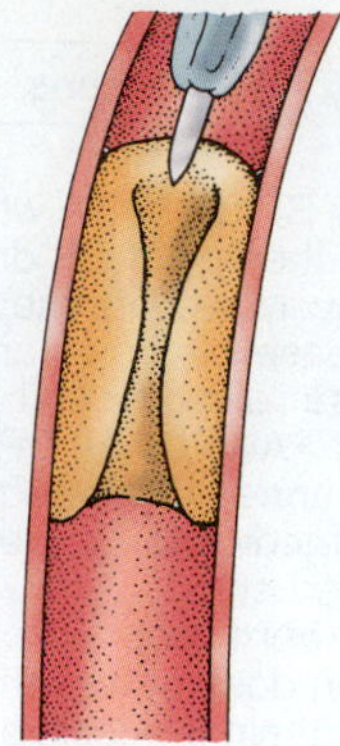

2. The uninflated balloon is centered in the obstruction.

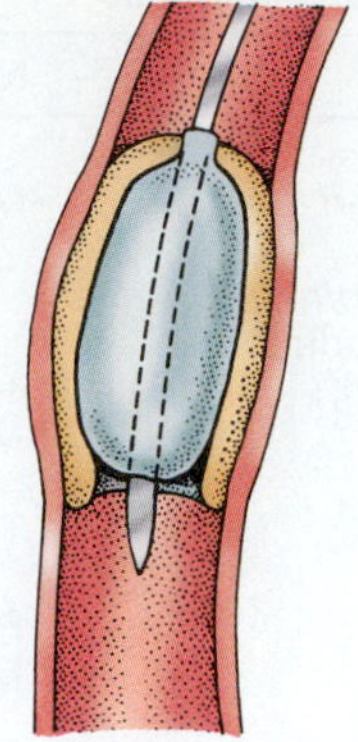

3. The balloon is inflated, which flattens plaque against the artery wall.

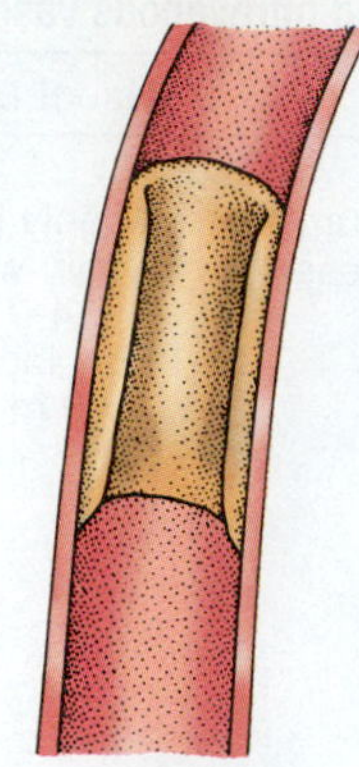

4. The balloon is removed, and the artery is left unoccluded.

Figure 41-5 ■ Percutaneous transluminal coronary angioplasty.

treatable with PTCA, the cardiologist considers the lesion's complexity and location as well as the amount of myocardium at risk. Treating lesions located in the left main artery would place a large amount of myocardial tissue at risk should the vessel close acutely; therefore these lesions are rarely treated with PTCA.

Percutaneous transluminal coronary angioplasty may also be used for the client with an evolving acute MI, either alone or in conjunction with thrombolytic therapy or glycoprotein (GP) IIb/IIIa inhibitor, to reperfuse the damaged myocardium. About 50% of clients needing revascularization are initially treated with PTCA.

Procedure. The physician performs PTCA under fluoroscopic guidance in the cardiac catheterization laboratory. A balloon-tipped catheter is introduced through a guidewire to the occlusion in the coronary artery. The physician activates a compressor that inflates the balloon at 4 to 14 atmospheres of pressure. This process compresses the plaque against the vessel wall, thus dilating the wall, and reduces or eliminates the occluding lesion (Figure 41-5). Balloon inflation may be repeated until angiography indicates a decrease in the stenosis (narrowing) to less than 50% of the vessel's diameter.

Following the procedure, IV heparin is administered in a continuous infusion to prevent thrombus formation. IV or intracoronary nitroglycerin or diltiazem (Cardizem) is given to prevent coronary vasospasm. PTCA initially reopens the vessel in more than 90% of appropriately selected clients. Within the first 24 hours, however, a small percentage of clients experience restenosis. At 6 months, restenosis or neointimal proliferation has an incidence of 20% to 50% (Grech, 2003c). GPIIb/IIIa inhibitors are also administered to prevent restenosis and maintaining the patency of the artery, reduce nonfatal MIs, and prevent deaths following PTCA.

Other techniques being used to ensure continued patency of the vessel are laser angioplasty, arthrectomy, and stents. Lasers may be used alone to remove atherosclerotic material from coronary arteries, or they may be used in conjunction with balloon angioplasty to create a smooth lumen about the size of the balloon. Arthrectomy devices can either excise and retrieve plaque or emulsify it. One of the advantages of arthrectomy is that it creates a less bulky vessel with better elastic recoil. **Stents** are used to maintain the patent lumen obtained by angioplasty or arthrectomy. By providing a supportive scaffold, stents prevent acute closure of the vessel from arterial dissection or vasospasm. Figure 41-6 depicts a stent positioned in a coronary artery.

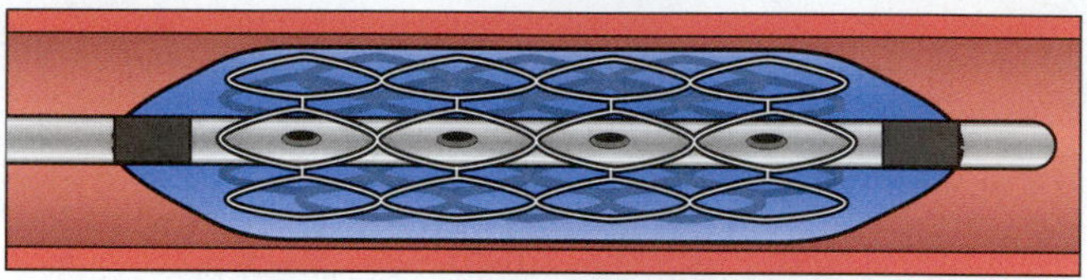

Figure 41-6 ■ A coronary stent open after balloon inflation.

Stents are an expandable mesh alloy tube placed at the site of the vessel lesion. The incidence of restenosis following placement of a stent is about 20% to 30%. Stents coated with drugs inhibit new cell and tissue growth and prevent neointimal hyperplasia are showing positive results. Sirolimus, paclitaxel, everolimus, and tacrolimus are some of the agents being used to reduce restenosis. Other therapies include brachytherapy (radiation) to prevent intimal artery hyperplasia (overgrowth) at the site of the stent. Rheolytic thrombectomy (e.g., AngioJet or Vortex) uses low-pressure, high-speed saline jets to disintegrate a thrombus. Endicor X-sizer lances and aspirates a clot simultaneously. Copper chelation, with the reagent tetrathiomolybdate (TTM), slows or stops cell proliferation, which can lead to restenosis.

Gene therapy has demonstrated that injecting vascular endothelial growth factor (VEGF) during angioplasty increased perfusion to the wall of the heart. Also, VEGF helps to initiate new blood vessel growth and development, which results in increased blood supply to cardiac muscle.

Postprocedure Care. Monitor for potential problems, which include acute closure of the vessel, bleeding from the insertion site, reaction to the dye used in angiography, hypotension, hypokalemia, and dysrhythmias.

The health care provider usually prescribes a long-term nitrate, calcium channel blocker, and aspirin therapy for clients after PTCA. A beta blocker and an angiotensin-converting enzyme (ACE) inhibitor may be added for clients who have had primary angioplasty following an MI. Many clients continue to have infusions of GPIIb/IIIa inhibitors during the initial hours after PTCA. Some clients may experience hypokalemia after the procedure and require careful monitoring and supplementation of potassium. Those who have intracoronary stents inserted may require clopidogrel (Plavix) for 6 to 9 months to prevent platelet aggregation. The nursing interventions for clients receiving these medications are described in Chart 41-5. Provide careful explanations of drug therapy and any recommended lifestyle changes.

Critical Thinking Challenge

Immediately following a PTCA and stent placement, the 48-year-old client admitted to your care arrives from the cardiology laboratory. The client denies any chest discomfort or shortness of breath. Heparin 1000 units/hr and normal saline 100 mL/hr are infusing. Laboratory results indicate an activated partial thromboplastin time (aPTT) value of 52 seconds.

1. What are three nursing priority assessments or interventions for a client following a PTCA or placement of a stent?
2. Which clients are most likely to benefit from a PTCA or stent?
3. What is the role of GPIIb/IIIa inhibitor administration following PTCA?

evolve For suggested answer guidelines, go to http://evolve.elsevier.com/Iggy/.

Coronary Artery Bypass Graft Surgery. Between 500,000 and 800,000 **coronary artery bypass graft** (CABG) surgeries were performed in the United States in 2001. It is the most common type of cardiac surgery and the most common procedure for older adults. Almost half of all CABGs are performed on clients older than 65 years of age. The occluded coronary arteries are bypassed with the client's own venous or arterial blood vessels or synthetic grafts. The internal mammary artery (IMA) is the current graft of choice because it has a 90% patency rate at 12 years after the procedure.

Coronary artery bypass graft is indicated when clients do not respond to medical management of CAD or when disease progression is evident. The decision for surgery is based on the client's symptoms and the results of cardiac catheterization. Candidates for surgery are clients who have the following:

- Angina with greater than 50% occlusion of the left main coronary artery
- Unstable angina with severe two-vessel or moderate three-vessel disease
- Ischemia with heart failure
- Acute MI
- Signs of ischemia or impending MI after angiography or PTCA
- Valvular disease
- Cardiogenic shock
- Coronary vessels unsuitable for PTCA

The vessels to be bypassed should have proximal lesions occluding more than 70% of the vessel's diameter but with good distal runoff. Bypass of less occluded vessels may result in poor perfusion through the graft and early obstruction. CABG is most effective when good ventricular function remains and the ejection fraction is more than 40% to 50%. Clients with lower ejection fractions are subject to develop more complications.

For most clients, the risk is low and the benefits of bypass surgery are clear. Surgical treatment of CAD does not appear to affect the life span. Early mortality rates are 1% to 2%. Left ventricular function is the most important long-term indicator of survival. CABG does improve the quality of life for most clients; 80% to 90% of clients are pain free at 1 year after CABG, and 70% remain pain free at 5 years after the procedure. The percentage of clients experiencing some pain increases sharply after 5 years.

LEGAL/ETHICAL ISSUES

IS INFORMED CONSENT POSSIBLE IN EMERGENT SITUATIONS?

Twenty-five years ago, physicians consistently provided care with a paternalistic "father knows best" approach. They decided what care was best for their clients and provided it with little input from them. For the past 15 years, however, there has been a movement toward client autonomy—the belief that clients should have the final say in their medical care. To ensure that they understand their options, many ethicists, lawyers, and health care providers have supported the concept of informed consent.

Informed consent has three important components: clients must be competent, must understand treatment options, and must make their choice freely without coercion by family or health care providers. The information provided to the client should include the following:

- Nature and purpose of the proposed treatment
- Expected outcome and likelihood of success
- Risks involved
- Alternatives to treatment
- Effect of not undergoing treatment

Unfortunately, health care is frequently provided in an emotionally charged atmosphere with clients in pain, hypoxic, or incapacitated. In addition, care to clients experiencing a myocardial infarction (MI) must be provided almost immediately, and there is little opportunity for them to weigh and evaluate options.

Some ethicists would argue that asking a client experiencing pain and anxiety to make a decision about care represents a distortion of informed consent. They might argue that clients presented themselves for emergent care and were therefore implying consent to standard treatment for that emergency. Benjamin and Curtis (1992) contended that it is appropriate for health care providers to act paternalistically and make health care decisions for clients in the following limited situations:

- If the client is incompetent or incapacitated and unable to make a rational decision
- If there is likely to be significant harm to the client if a decision is not made
- If clients are likely to approve of the decision when and if their capacity to make rational decisions is restored

Clients would meet Benjamin and Curtis's criteria for a paternalistic decision. In addition, *Heart Disease Weekly* (2003) presented research that would support clients at least remembering the details of informed consent. Six weeks after hospital discharge, 42% of clients who had angioplasty could not identify any risks and 41% could not identify any benefits. For coronary artery bypass graft (CABG) procedures, 45% could not identify any risks and 22% could not identify any benefits. However, in both groups, there was a high percentage (94%) of satisfaction with their decisions.

Implications for Nursing

In collaboration with the health care provider, it is the nurse's responsibility to be sure that the client desires and comprehends the medical and nursing care that is being provided. That usually entails ensuring that the client is fully informed and voluntarily consenting to the treatment. However, in some emergent situations or incapacitated clients, fully informed consent may not be reasonable or possible. In such situations, Benjamin and Curtis's criteria for making a paternalistic decision might be applied.

TABLE 41-5 Medication Administration Before Coronary Artery Bypass Graft Surgery

Medications Often Discontinued
- Digitalis 12 hr before surgery
- Diuretics 2 to 3 days before surgery
- Aspirin and anticoagulants 1 wk before surgery

Medications Often Administered
- Potassium chloride to maintain potassium between 3.5 and 4.0 mEq/L
- Scheduled beta blockers
- Scheduled calcium channel blockers
- Scheduled antidysrhythmics
- Scheduled antihypertensives
- Prophylactic antibiotic 20 to 30 min before surgery

Preoperative Care. CABG surgery may be planned as an elective procedure or performed on an emergency basis. (See the Legal/Ethical Issues box on p. 857 for a discussion of the dilemma of requiring a patient to provide informed consent under stressful conditions.) Clients undergoing elective surgery are often admitted on the morning of the surgery. Preoperative preparations and teaching are completed during prehospitalization interviews (see the Clinical Pathway on the Evolve website). Clients must understand that some medications will need to be adjusted because of the surgery. Ensure that appropriate medications have been discontinued preoperatively and that the necessary ones have been administered (Table 41-5).

Prehospital Preparation. Familiarize the client and family with the cardiac surgical critical care environment and prepare the client for postoperative care. If the procedure is elective, demonstrate and have the client return a demonstration of how to splint the chest incision, cough, deep breathe, and perform arm and leg exercises (see Chapter 20). Stress the following:

- The client should identify any pain to the nursing staff.
- Most of the pain will be in the site where the vein was harvested.
- Pain medication will be available.
- Coughing and deep breathing are important in preventing pulmonary complications.

Explain that the client should expect to have a sternal incision, possibly a leg incision, one or two chest tubes, a Foley catheter, pacemaker wires, and hemodynamic monitoring. An endotracheal tube will be connected to a ventilator for several hours postoperatively. The client and family must understand that the client will not be able to talk while the endotracheal tube is in place. The client should breathe with the ventilator and not fight it. When describing the postoperative course, emphasize that close monitoring and the use of sophisticated equipment are standard treatment.

Preoperative anxiety is common. An appropriate nursing assessment should identify the level of anxiety and the coping methods clients have used successfully in the past. Some clients may find it helpful to define their fears. Common sources of fear include fear of the unknown, fear of bodily harm, and fear of death.

In elective procedures, clients may benefit from detailed information about the surgery. Some may feel overwhelmed by so much material. Some need to discuss their feelings in detail or describe the experiences of people they know who have undergone CABG. Assess clients' anxiety level and helps them to cope.

Operative Procedures. Coronary artery bypass surgery is performed with the client under general anesthesia and for cardiopulmonary bypass or off-pump surgery. The anesthesiologist or nurse anesthetist administers anesthesia and intubates the client. The cardiac surgical team begins the procedure with a median sternotomy incision and visualization of the heart and great vessels. Another surgical team may begin harvesting the saphenous vein if it is to be used for the graft.

Cardiopulmonary bypass (CPB) is accomplished by cannulation of the inferior and superior venae cavae. The purpose of CPB is to provide oxygenation, circulation, and hypothermia during induced cardiac arrest. Blood is diverted from the heart to the bypass machine, where it is heparinized, oxygenated, and returned to the circulation through a cannula placed in the ascending aortic arch or femoral artery (Figure 41-7). During bypass, the client's core temperature is cooled to 90° F (32° C). Cooling decreases the rate of metabolism and demand for oxygen. The heart is perfused with a cardioplegic solution containing potassium, which decreases myocardial oxygen consumption and causes the heart to stop during diastole. This process ensures a motionless operative field and prevents myocardial ischemia.

Once the heart is arrested, the grafting procedure can begin. The surgeon uses the internal mammary artery (IMA), a saphenous vein, or both or a radial artery to bypass lesions in the coronary arteries (Figure 41-8). The distal end of the IMA is dissected and attached below the lesion on the coronary artery. If the surgeon uses a venous graft or the radial artery, it is anastomosed (sutured) proximally to the aorta and distally to the coronary artery just beyond the occlusion, thus improving myocardial perfusion. After flow rates through the grafts are measured, the heart is rewarmed slowly. The cardioplegic solution is flushed from the heart. The heart regains its rate and rhythm, or it may be defibrillated to return it to a normal rhythm. When the procedure is completed, the client is rewarmed by CPB and weaned from the bypass machine while the grafts are observed for patency and leakage. The surgeon may place atrial and ventricular pacemaker wires and mediastinal and pleural chest tubes. Finally, the surgeon closes the sternum with wire sutures.

Postoperative Care. After surgery the client is transported to a post–open heart surgery unit. There the client undergoes mechanical ventilation for 3 to 6 hours. The client requires highly skilled nursing care from a nurse qualified to provide post–cardiac surgery care, including routine postoperative care described in Chapter 22. The mediastinal tubes are connected to water-seal drainage systems and ground the epicardial pacer wires by connecting them to the pacemaker generator. Monitor pulmonary artery and arterial pressures as well as the heart rate and rhythm, which are displayed on a monitor (see the Clinical Pathway on the Evolve website).

Closely assess the client for dysrhythmias, such as ventricular ectopic rhythms, bradydysrhythmias, atrial fibrillation, or heart block. Treat symptomatic dysrhythmias according to unit protocol or the health care provider's order. Hypoxemia and hypokalemia are frequent causes of ventricular dysrhythmias. If the client has symptomatic bradydysrhythmias or heart block, turn on the pacemaker and adjust the pacemaker settings as ordered (see Chapter 37). Also,

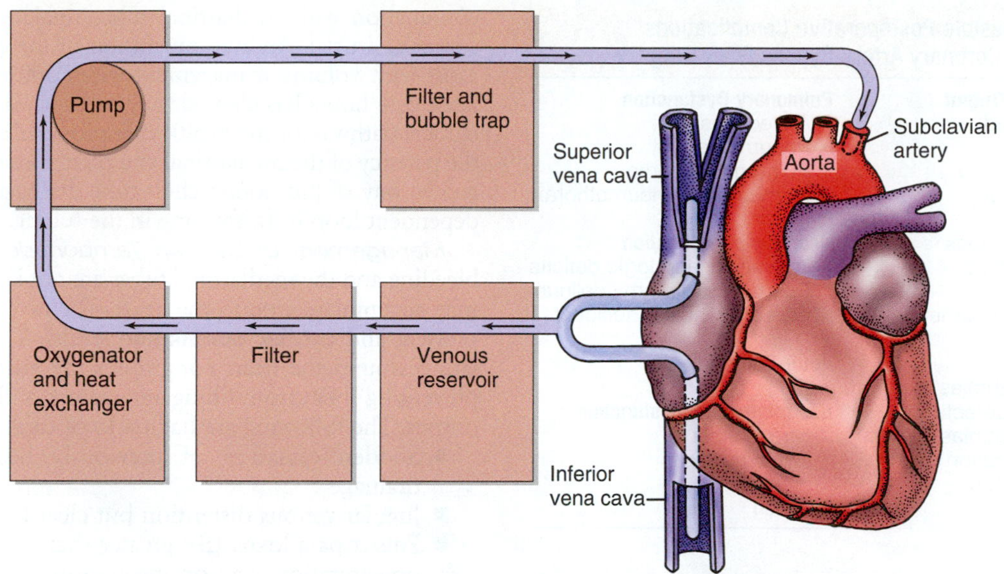

Figure 41-7 ■ Heart-lung bypass circuitry used during cardiopulmonary bypass.

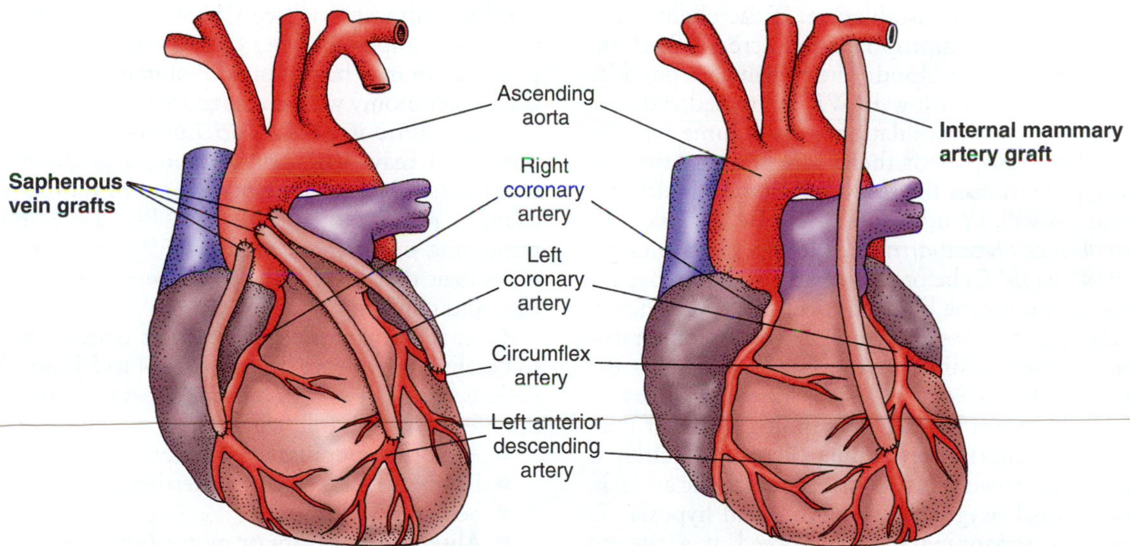

Figure 41-8 ■ Two methods of coronary artery bypass grafting. The procedure used depends on the nature of the coronary artery disease, the condition of the vessels available for grating, and the client's health status.

monitor for other complications of CABG, including fluid and electrolyte imbalance, hypotension, hypothermia, hypertension, bleeding, cardiac tamponade, and altered cerebral perfusion. Table 41-6 lists some of the possible postoperative complications of CABG.

Management of Fluid and Electrolyte Imbalance. Assessing fluid and electrolyte balance is a high priority in the early postoperative period. Edema is common; however, decisions concerning fluid administration are made on the basis of the blood pressure (BP), pulmonary artery wedge pressure (PAWP), right atrial pressure, cardiac output, cardiac index, systemic vascular resistance, blood loss, and urine output. An experienced nurse interprets the assessment findings and adjusts fluid administration on the basis of standing unit policies or specific orders from the physician.

Serum electrolytes (especially calcium, magnesium, and phosphorus) may be reduced postoperatively and are monitored carefully by both the physician and the nurse. Because the serum potassium level can fluctuate dramatically, electrolyte levels are checked frequently. Potassium and magnesium depletion is common and may result from hemodilution or diuretic therapy.

If the serum potassium level is depleted, the health care provider may order IV potassium replacement. The dose of potassium administered exceeds the usual recommended level of no more than 20 mEq of potassium per hour. For a potassium bolus, as much as 40 to 80 mEq may be mixed in 100 mL of IV solution and given at a rate as high as 40 mEq/hr. The drug must be given through a central catheter, and the rate of administration must be controlled by an infusion pump. The client must be placed on a cardiac monitor for intense, focused observation.

Management of Hypotension. Hypotension (systolic BP less than 90 mm Hg) is a significant problem because it

TABLE 41-6 Possible Postoperative Complications of Coronary Artery Bypass Graft Surgery

Decreased Cardiac Output
- Reduced preload
  - Hypovolemia
  - Hemorrhage
- Increased preload
  - Heart failure
  - Cardiogenic shock
- Increased afterload
  - Hypothermia
  - Increased sympathetic activity
- Dysrhythmias
  - Bradydysrhythmias
  - Conduction defects
  - Tachydysrhythmias
- Myocardial infarction

Pulmonary Dysfunction
- Atelectasis
- Pneumonia
- Pulmonary edema
- Hemothorax/pneumothorax

Neurologic Dysfunction
- Transient neurologic deficits
- Postpericardiotomy delirium
- Cerebrovascular accident

Acute Renal Failure

Gastrointestinal Dysfunction
- Stress ulcer
- Paralytic ileus

Infection

may result in the collapse of a vein graft. Review the assessment parameters to identify what might be causing the hypotension. Decreased preload (decreased PAWP) can result from hypovolemia or vasodilation. If the client is hypovolemic, it might be appropriate to increase fluid administration or administer blood. The health care provider may treat the client with a low PAWP, decreased systemic vascular resistance, and vasodilation with volume replacement followed by vasopressor therapy to increase the BP; however, if hypotension is the result of left ventricular failure (increased PAWP), IV inotropes might be necessary.

Management of Hypothermia. Although the client is rewarmed to 98.6° F (35° C) before being removed from bypass, it is not uncommon for the body temperature to drift downward after the client leaves the surgical suite. Monitor the body temperature and institute rewarming procedures if the temperature drops below 96.8° F (36° C). Rewarming may be accomplished with warm blankets, rewarming lights, or thermal blankets. The danger of rewarming clients too quickly is that they may begin shivering, resulting in metabolic acidosis, increased myocardial oxygen consumption, and hypoxia. To prevent shivering, rewarming should proceed at a rate no faster than 1.8° F (1° C)/hr. Discontinue rewarming when the body temperature approaches 98.6° F (35° C) and the client's extremities feel warm.

Management of Hypertension. Hypothermia is a significant risk for the client following CABG surgery because it promotes vasoconstriction and hypertension. Other factors contributing to hypertension in the CABG client include CPB, medications, and the client's own sympathetic nervous system activity.

Postoperatively, many CABG clients experience hypertension (if hypertension is defined as a systolic BP greater than 140 to 150 mm Hg). Hypertension is dangerous because increased pressure promotes leakage from suture lines and may cause bleeding.

Management of Bleeding. Postoperative bleeding occurs to a limited extent in all clients. Mediastinal and pleural chest tube drainage is measured at least hourly, and drainage exceeding 150 mL/hr is reported to the surgeon. Clients with IMA grafts may have more chest drainage than those with saphenous vein grafts. To access the IMA, the pleural space has to be entered and will necessitate a pleural chest tube in conjunction with mediastinal tubes, making pulmonary assessment crucial. An autotransfusion of the chest drainage to assist with volume management when 500 mL has accumulated or 4 hours has elapsed may be done, depending on the clinical pathway or the health care provider's order. Maintain the patency of the mediastinal and pleural chest tubes. One effective way of promoting chest tube drainage is to prevent a dependent loop from forming in the tubing.

Management of Cardiac Tamponade. If the client is bleeding and the mediastinal tubes are not kept patent, blood may accumulate around the heart. The myocardium is compressed, and **cardiac tamponade** results. The fluid accumulating around the heart compresses the atria and ventricles, preventing them from filling adequately, and reduces cardiac output. The following are hallmarks of cardiac tamponade:

- Sudden cessation of previously heavy mediastinal drainage
- Jugular venous distention but clear lung sounds
- Pulsus paradoxus (BP greater than 10 mm Hg higher on expiration than on inspiration)
- An equalizing of PAWP and right atrial pressure
- Cardiovascular collapse

Tamponade can be confirmed by echocardiogram or chest x-ray. Pericardiocentesis (see Chapter 38) may not be appropriate for tamponade after CABG because the blood in the pericardium may have clotted. Volume expansion and emergency sternotomy with drainage are the treatments of choice.

Management of Altered Levels of Consciousness. The client may demonstrate changes in the level of consciousness, which may be permanent or transient. Transient changes related to anesthesia, CPB, air emboli, or hypothermia occur in as many as 75% of clients. Transient neurologic deficits may include slowness to arouse, memory loss, and confusion.

Clients with transient neurologic deficits usually return to baseline neurologic status within 4 to 8 hours. Permanent deficits associated with an intraoperative stroke may be manifested by the following:

- Abnormal pupillary response
- Failure to awaken from anesthesia
- Seizures
- Absence of sensory or motor function

Check the client's neurologic status every 30 to 60 minutes until the client has awakened from anesthesia; then check every 2 to 4 hours or per agency policy.

Pain Management. Differentiate between sternotomy pain, which is expected after CABG, and anginal pain, which might indicate graft failure. Typical sternotomy pain is localized, does not radiate, and often becomes worse when the client coughs or breathes deeply. The client may describe the pain as sharp, aching, or burning. Pain may stimulate the sympathetic nervous system, which increases the heart rate and vascular resistance while decreasing cardiac output. Administer the prescribed medication, in adequate doses, frequently enough to limit pain. During the process of weaning the client from mechanical ventilation, however, it may be necessary to use short-acting analgesics and to limit pain medication because of the respiratory depressant effects of analgesia.

Transfer from the Special Care Unit. Ventilation is usually provided for 3 to 6 hours postoperatively, until the client is breathing adequately and is hemodynamically stable. During the first day, the client usually has pacer wires, hemodynamic monitoring lines, and mediastinal tubes removed and is transferred to an intermediate care unit. All CABG clients, especially those with IMA grafts, are at high risk for atelectasis, the number one complication. Encourage clients to splint, cough, turn, and deep breathe to raise secretions. Guide them in a gradual resumption of activity. Two hours after extubation, clients should be dangled as tolerated and turned side to side. Within 4 to 8 hours after extubation, clients should be out of bed in a chair. By the first day after surgery, clients should be out of bed in a chair and ambulating 25 to 100 feet three times a day as tolerated. Continue to monitor for decreased cardiac output, pain, dysrhythmias, and infection.

Monitor the neurovascular status of the donor arm of clients who have had the radial artery used as a conduit in CABG. Assess the hand color, temperature (pulse both ulnar and radial stump), and capillary refill every hour initially. In addition, check the fingertips, hand, and arm for sensation and mobility at least every 4 hours. Intravenous nitroglycerin is often given for the first 24 hours postoperatively to promote vasodilation in the donor arm and therefore maintain circulation.

Many clients experience supraventricular dysrhythmias (especially atrial fibrillation) during the postoperative period, most commonly on the second or third postoperative day. Examine the monitor pattern for atrial fibrillation. When auscultating the heart, listen for an irregular rhythm. (See Chapter 37 for interventions for atrial fibrillation.)

Sternal wound infections develop between 5 days and several weeks postoperatively in about 3% of clients and are responsible for increased costs and longer length of stays. Be alert for the presence of **mediastinitis** (infection of the mediastinum) by the presence of the following:

- Fever continuing beyond the first 4 days after CABG
- Instability (bogginess or stepping) of the sternum
- Redness, induration, swelling, or drainage from suture sites
- An increased white blood cell count

The health care provider may perform a needle biopsy to confirm a sternal infection. Surgical debridement, antibiotic wound irrigation, and IV antibiotics are usually indicated. Four to 6 weeks of IV antibiotics are required if sternal osteomyelitis has developed. The mortality rate among clients with sternal surgical wound infections has been reported to range from 14% to 42% (Kohli et al., 2003). Prophylactic use of mupirocin (Bactroban) intranasally may be prescribed to decrease the incidence of sternal wound infection.

Postpericardiotomy syndrome is a source of chest discomfort in 10% to 40% of post–cardiac surgery clients. The syndrome is characterized by pericardial and pleural pain, pericarditis, a friction rub, an elevated temperature and white blood cell count, and dysrhythmias. Postpericardiotomy syndrome may occur days to weeks after surgery and seems to be associated with blood remaining in the pericardial sac. Observe for the development of pericardial or pleural pain. For most clients, the syndrome is mild and self-limiting; however, the client may require treatment similar to that for pericarditis. Be prepared to detect acute cardiac (pericardial) tamponade (see Chapter 38).

CONSIDERATIONS FOR OLDER ADULTS

Older adults may have different needs and experience slightly different problems after CABG. Special nursing concerns related to the older CABG client are detailed in Chart 41-9.

CHART 41-9

NURSING FOCUS on the OLDER ADULT

Coronary Artery Bypass Graft Surgery

- Be aware that perioperative mortality rates are higher for the older client (4% to 9%) than for the client younger than 60 years of age (1% to 2%).
- Monitor neurologic and mental status carefully because older adults are more likely to have transient neurologic deficits after coronary artery bypass graft (CABG) surgery than younger adults are.
- Observe for side effects of cardiac drugs because older clients are more likely to develop toxic effects from positive inotropes (dobutamine) and potent antihypertensives (nitroglycerin or nitroprusside).
- Monitor the client closely for dysrhythmias because older adults are more likely to have dysrhythmias, such as atrial fibrillation or supraventricular tachycardia, after CABG surgery.
- Be aware that recuperation after CABG surgery is slower for older clients and that their average length of hospital stay is longer.
- Teach the client and family that during the first 2 to 5 weeks after discharge, fatigue, chest discomfort, and lack of appetite may be particularly bothersome for older clients.
- Let someone know where you are when you are walking.

Minimally Invasive Direct Coronary Artery Bypass. The **minimally invasive direct coronary artery bypass (MIDCAB)** may be indicated for clients with a lesion of the left anterior descending (LAD) artery. In one of the most common MIDCAB procedures, after a 2-inch left thoracotomy incision is made and the fourth rib is removed, the left internal mammary artery (IMA) is dissected and attached to the still-beating heart below the level of the lesion in the LAD. Cardiopulmonary bypass (CPB) is not required. Postoperatively assess for chest pain and electrocardiogram (ECG) changes (Q waves and ST-segment and T-wave changes in leads V_2 to V_6) because occlusion of the IMA graft occurs acutely in 10% of clients. If there is any question of acute graph closure, immediately notify the health care provider. Clients tend to have more incisional pain after MIDCAB than after traditional CABG surgery, but the pain can usually be managed with oxycodone or codeine. Because they have a thoracotomy incision and a chest tube or smaller-lumen vacuum chest device, clients are encouraged to cough, deep breathe, and use an incentive spirometer for a week postoperatively. Most clients spend less than 6 hours in a critical care unit and are discharged in 2 or 3 days.

Transmyocardial Laser Revascularization. Transmyocardial laser revascularization is a new procedure for clients with unstable angina and inoperable CAD with areas of reversible myocardial ischemia. After a single-lung intubation, a left anterior thoracotomy is performed and the heart is visualized. A laser is used to create 20 to 24 long, narrow channels through the left ventricular muscle to the left ventricle. These channels will eventually allow oxygenated blood to flow during diastole from the left ventricle to nourish the muscle. After the surgery, the client is transported to a critical care unit, where hemodynamic monitoring is instituted for assessment of anginal episodes and bleeding disturbances. Although many clients report decreases in anginal episodes following the procedure, researchers have been unable to document why clients experience such an improvement.

Off-Pump Coronary Artery Bypass. Off-pump coronary artery bypass (OPCAB) is a procedure in which open heart surgery is performed without the use of a heart-lung bypass machine. Advantages include shorter hospital stays and decreased mortality, risk of infection, and cost. OPCAB does have some risk, for example, increased skill and steeper learning curve for surgeons to master the technique and inaccessible surgery sites.

Robotics. Robotic heart surgery is a new step toward less invasive open heart surgery. Surgeons operate endoscopically through 8- to 10-mm long incisions in the chest wall. Use of robotics provides surgeons with capabilities that simplify the surgical process, eliminates tremors that can exist with human hands, increases the ability to reach inaccessible sites, and improves depth perception and visual acuity.

Other advantages of robotic procedures include shorter hospital stays (average stay is 3 days), less pain due to smaller incisions, no need for heart-lung bypass machine, less anxiety for the client, and greater client acceptance. Also, the use of robotics will enable surgeons to perform telesurgery, performing heart procedures over long distances.

Disadvantages include computer failure, the skill and ability of the surgeon, and the length of surgery time (the time is about 50 minutes longer than the conventional surgery).

Community-Based Care

HOME CARE MANAGEMENT

Case management is most appropriate for clients who meet high-cost, high-volume, and high-risk criteria. Clients with coronary artery disease (CAD) clearly meet all these criteria. Clinical pathways and case management programs for clients who have CAD are in effect in most U.S. hospitals. By focusing on cardiovascular risk reduction and improving the continuity of care, health care professionals have reduced the length and cost of hospital stays. Posthospital case management should reduce hospital readmission rates and improve client health.

Clients who have experienced a myocardial infarction (MI), angina, or coronary artery bypass graft (CABG) surgery are usually discharged to home or to a subacute care setting with pharmacologic therapy and specific activity prescriptions. Depending on the procedure, hospital stays may be 4 to 7 days for clients with MI or those undergoing CABG and only 2 days for those undergoing percutaneous transluminal coronary angioplasty (PTCA); therefore clients are still recovering when they are discharged.

WOMEN'S HEALTH CONSIDERATIONS

A large number of middle-aged and older women who have had coronary artery bypass graft (CABG) surgery are living alone, and this number is expected to increase as baby boomers age. Few studies have been done to examine their special needs. Robinson (2002) conducted a qualitative descriptive study of 12 postoperative women in rural southwestern Louisiana living at home alone. All these women were white except one African American. Most reported educational levels ranging between the third and eighth grades. The researcher found four primary themes that described their at-home experience:

- Relief and gratitude that they had survived the surgery
- A need to continue living a full life
- A sense of vulnerability (feeling that they might have more heart problems)
- Regained independence, increasing self-worth and personal freedom

Robinson also noted that the knowledge of their surgery and heart disease was inadequate.

A home care nurse may be required for assessment and teaching following discharge and an aide for assistance with activities of daily living (ADLs) if clients are older or weaker (Chart 41-10). In addition, women, who tend to be older and living alone when coronary events occur, may have a greater need for home assistance after CABG surgery. Clients who were residents in long-term care may be returned there after hospitalization for unstable angina, MI, or CABG surgery.

Cardiac rehabilitation is available in many communities for clients after an MI or CABG surgery, but only 10% to 30% of clients participate in structured rehabilitation programs (Yates, Braklow-Whitton, & Agrawal, 2003). The most frequently cited reasons for nonparticipation are lack of insurance coverage, a physician's directive that it is unnecessary, and the client's decision that it is not necessary. Clients who participate in structured rehabilitation programs report greater improvement in exercise tolerance and improved ability to control stress. However, no difference in their return to work has been seen.

HEALTH TEACHING

The need for health teaching depends in part on the treatment plan or type of procedure that the client had. Cronin et al.

CHART 41-10

HOME CARE ASSESSMENT of
The Client Who Has Had a Myocardial Infarction

Assess cardiovascular function, including the following:
- Current vital signs (compare with previous to identify changes)
- Recurrence of discomfort (characteristics, frequency, onset)
- Indications of heart failure (weight gain, crackles, cough, or dyspnea)
- Adequacy of tissue perfusion (mentation, skin temperature, peripheral pulses, urine output)
- Indications of serious dysrhythmia (very irregular pulse, palpitations with fainting or near fainting)

Assess coping skills, including the following:
- Is client displaying denial, anger, or fear?
- Is the caregiver providing adequate support?
- Are the client and caregiver having disagreements about treatment?

Assess functional ability, including the following:
- Activity tolerance (examine the client's activity diary: review distance, duration, frequency, and symptoms occurring during exercise)
- Activities of daily living (is any assistance needed?)
- Household chores (who performs them?)
- Does client plan to return to work? When?

Assess nutritional status, including the following:
- Food intake (review client's intake of fats and cholesterol)

Assess client's understanding of illness and treatment, including the following:
- How to treat chest discomfort
- Signs and symptoms to report to health care provider
- Dosage, effects, and side effects of medications
- How to advance and when to limit activity
- Modification of risk factors for coronary artery disease

(2000) found that short hospital stays following a percutaneous transluminal coronary angioplasty (PTCA) did not allow enough time to educate adequately clients having the procedure (see the Evidence-Based Practice for Nursing box below). Because hospital stays are short and clients are quite ill during hospitalization, most in-hospital education programs concentrate on the skills essential for self-care after discharge.

As part of home visits or a cardiac rehabilitation program, identify the additional educational needs of the client and family as well as their readiness to learn. Develop a teaching plan, which usually includes education about the normal anatomy and physiology of the heart, the pathophysiology of angina and MI, risk factor modification, activity and exercise protocols, cardiac medications, and when to seek medical assistance. Clients are taught that myocardial healing after an MI begins early and is usually complete in 6 to 8 weeks. Those who have undergone CABG are told that the sternotomy should heal in about 6 to 8 weeks, but upper body exercise needs to be limited for several months.

Clients who have undergone CABG require instruction on incisional care for the sternum and the graft site. They should inspect the incisions daily for any redness, swelling, or drainage. The leg of a saphenous vein donor site is often edematous. Instruct clients to avoid crossing legs, to wear elastic stockings until the edema subsides, and to elevate the surgical limb when sitting in a chair. Clients who have had a radial artery graft are instructed to open and close the hand vigorously 10 times every 2 hours.

RISK FACTOR MODIFICATION. Modification of risk factors is a necessary part of a clients' management and involves changing their health maintenance patterns. Such modifications may include smoking cessation, altered dietary habits, regular exercise, BP control, and blood glucose control.

SMOKING CESSATION. For clients who smoke, explain the detrimental effects on the cardiovascular system of smoking tobacco, especially cigarettes. Many clients spontaneously quit smoking soon after an MI. Nurse counseling has been demonstrated to be a cost-effective way to assist clients to stop smoking. See Chapter 39 for more discussion. Other methods of smoking cessation include acupuncture, acupressure, and hypnosis.

DIET CONTROL. The mainstays of cholesterol control are diet therapy and administration of anti-hyperlipidemic agents. Research is being conducted to determine genetic implications for familial hypercholesterolemia. See Chapter 39 for a discussion of ways to lower cholesterol.

Also instruct clients not to add salt in food preparation or when beginning the meal. A reduction of 80 mg/day of sodium can reduce the systolic blood pressure (SBP) by 5 mm Hg and 3 mm Hg for the diastolic blood pressure (DBP). Maintain adequate dietary potassium, calcium, and magnesium intake. Increasing potassium to 80 mEq/day may reduce the SBP by 8 mm Hg (Zanabria & Welch, 2003). Booklets and cookbooks that can assist the client in learning to cook with reduced fats, oils, and salt are available from the American Heart Association (AHA).

Complementary and Alternative Therapies. The use of antioxidants (such as vitamin E) is an area of controversy. Some researchers report that the use of such agents counteracts the adverse effects of oxygen free radicals (derived from high cholesterol levels) on blood vessels and protects arteries. Other reports point out that excessive vitamin E increases the risk for liver damage and that the long-term effects of antioxidants are not known.

PHYSICAL ACTIVITY. Collaborate with the physical therapist to establish an activity and exercise schedule as part of client rehabilitation. Instruct the client to remain near home during the first week after discharge and to continue a walking program. Clients may engage in light housework or any activity done while sitting and that does not precipitate angina. During the second week, they are encouraged to increase social activities and possibly to return to work part-time. By the third week, they may begin to lift objects as

EVIDENCE-BASED PRACTICE for Nursing

What are the client's education needs in discharge teaching following PTCA?

Cronin, S.N., Freeman, L.H., Ryan, G., & Drake, D.M. (2000). Recovery after percutaneous transluminal coronary angioplasty: Assessment after discharge. *Critical Care Nurse, 20*(2), 70-76.

The concern that prompted this study was motivated by short hospital stays associated with percutaneous transluminal coronary angioplasty (PCTA), leaving insufficient time to assess the client's knowledge level, the need for teaching, and evaluating assimilation of the information. After discharge, clients may not respond appropriately to recurrences of chest pain. Clients may perceive that their hearts have been repaired and subsequent chest pain may be ignored as a result of client denial. The perception that their problem has been fixed may influence their reactions of modifying risk factors or making lifestyle changes. The purpose of the study was to examine these factors: prevalence and response to chest pain, the need for information, determination of concerns, and evaluation of lifestyle modifications.

The study was a descriptive, cross-sectional design that included the responses of 105 clients. Thirty-five subjects each were selected from clients who previously experienced PTCA at 1, 3, and 6 months. Clients had to be a minimum of 21 years of age, speak and understand English, able to participate in and respond to an interview format, have a home telephone, and first-time recipients of PTCA. A specific tool was used to obtain information about recurrent chest pain.

Level of Evidence: 5—This study used a cross-sectional design with an adequate sample size.

Critique. Demographics of the sample did not equally represent gender and race. Discrepancy in gender was greatest in groups 1 and 3. Group 1 was 1-month postprocedure, and group 3 was 6 months postprocedure. The most significant problem with the study was that the group's composition was 97.1% white and only 2.9% were African American. Ethnicity could play an important part in processing and acting on information. There could be a bigger impact on lifestyle changes in the African American group. Another limitation could be that the learning styles of the recipients were not assessed. Knowledge of specific learning styles could influence how instruction is delivered to the participants and impact retention.

Implications for Nursing

- Be aware that clients do experience chest pain following PTCA.
- Essential discharge teaching should include information regarding chest pain recurrence and specific instructions on necessary interventions.
- The number one learning need identified by clients was how to deal with feelings of depression and anxiety.
- Clients need information about taking over-the-counter medications.
- Be sure to include information on necessary modifications in diet, exercise, prescribed medications, and stress management.

CHART 41-11

CLIENT EDUCATION GUIDE
Activity for the Client with Coronary Artery Disease

- Begin by walking the same distance at home as in the hospital (usually 400 feet) three times each day.
- Carry nitroglycerin with you.
- Check your pulse before, during, and after the exercise.
- Stop the activity for a pulse increase of more than 20 beats/min, shortness of breath, angina, or dizziness.
- Exercise outdoors when the weather is good.
- Gradually increase the walking until the distance is ¼ mile twice daily (usually the end of the second week).
- After an exercise tolerance test and with your physician's approval, walk at least three times each week, increasing the distance by ½ mile every other week, until the total distance is 2 miles.
- Avoid straining (lifting, pushups, pull-ups, and straining at bowel movements).

CHART 41-12

CLIENT EDUCATION GUIDE
Management of Chest Pain at Home

- Keep fresh nitroglycerin available for immediate use.
- At the first indication of chest discomfort, cease activity and sit or lie down.
- Place one nitroglycerin tablet or spray under your tongue, allowing the tablet to dissolve.
- Wait 5 minutes for relief.
- If no relief results, repeat the nitroglycerin and wait 5 more minutes.
- If there is no relief, repeat and wait 5 more minutes.
- If there is still no relief, call for transportation to a health care facility.
- Carry a medical identification card or wear a bracelet or necklace that identifies a history of heart problems.

heavy as 15 pounds (such as 2 gallons of milk) but should avoid lifting or pulling heavier objects for the first 6 to 8 weeks. Chart 41-11 lists suggested instructions for exercise.

Clients may begin a simple walking program by walking 400 feet twice a day at the rate of 1 mile/hr the first week after discharge and increasing the distance and rate as tolerated, usually weekly, until they can walk 2 miles at 3 to 4 miles/hr. Instruct clients to take their pulse reading before, halfway through, and after exercise. The client should stop exercising if the target pulse rate is exceeded or if dyspnea or angina develops.

After a limited exercise tolerance test, the physical therapist or nurse encourages the client to join a formal exercise program, ideally one that assists the client in monitoring cardiovascular progress. The program should include 5- to 7-minute warm-up and cool-down periods, as well as 30 minutes of aerobic exercise. The client should engage in aerobic exercise a minimum of three (and preferably five) times a week.

The benefits of lowering BP following exercise were reported by Zanabria and Welch (2003). After 30 to 45 minutes, SBP was lowered by 10 to 20 mm Hg. This effect usually lasts for 9 hours. BP changes can be seen as soon as 3 weeks to 3 months after beginning an exercise program.

Complementary and Alternative Therapies. Additional therapies can aid in reducing the client's anxiety about progressive activity both in the immediate postoperative period and during the rehabilitation phase. The overall use of complementary and alternative medicine is about 75% in clients undergoing heart surgery procedures (*Heart Disease Weekly,* 2000). However, many clients do not share with their health care providers that they use complementary therapies. Techniques such as progressive muscle relaxation, guided imagery, music therapy, pet therapy, and therapeutic touch have been shown to decrease anxiety, reduce depression, and increase compliance with activity/exercise regimens after heart surgery. A recent study examined the use of therapeutic touch as a relaxation intervention to lessen perceived stress, heart rate variability, and BP following surgery (Sneed et al., 2001).

SEXUAL ACTIVITY. Sexual activity is often a subject of great concern to clients and their partners. Inform the client and partner that engaging in their usual sexual activity is unlikely to cause any damage to the heart. Clients can resume sexual intercourse on the advice of the health care provider, usually after an exercise tolerance assessment. In general, clients who can walk one block or climb two flights of stairs without symptoms can usually safely resume sexual activity.

Suggest that initially clients schedule intercourse after a period of rest. They might try having intercourse in the morning when they are well rested or wait 1½ hours after exercise or a heavy meal. The position selected should be comfortable for both the client and his or her partner so that no undue stress is placed on the heart or suture line.

BLOOD PRESSURE CONTROL. Make arrangements for the client to have blood pressure (BP) measurements taken at regular intervals, and collaborate with the health care provider to establish parameters for reporting the BP. Lifestyle modifications such as weight reduction, physical activity, and reduced-sodium diets may assist in the management of hypertension. If the client is taking medication, assess compliance with the medication regimen.

BLOOD GLUCOSE CONTROL. Clients with diabetes mellitus are assessed for their participation in efforts to control hyperglycemia. Review the prescribed dosage of insulin or oral hypoglycemic agents with the client and family. The client should demonstrate accurate testing of blood for glucose levels.

CARDIAC MEDICATIONS. Assist the client in understanding the type of cardiac medications prescribed, the benefit of each drug, potential side effects, and the correct dosage and time of day to take each drug. Medication regimens vary considerably; however, many clients with angina are discharged while taking aspirin, a beta blocker, a calcium channel blocker, an anti-hyperlipidemic agent, and a nitrate. Clients who have experienced an MI may require aspirin, a beta blocker, an anti-hyperlipidemic agent, and an angiotensin-converting enzyme (ACE) inhibitor. The regimen can be complex. Determine whether the client can comply with the instructions.

Use of sublingual or spray nitroglycerin (NTG) deserves special attention. Instruct the client to carry NTG at all times. Keep the tablets in a glass, light-resistant container. NTG should be replaced every 3 to 5 months, before it loses its potency or stops producing a tingling sensation when placed under the tongue. Chart 41-12 gives instructions for clients for management of chest discomfort at home.

SEEKING MEDICAL ASSISTANCE. Clients are encouraged to notify their health care provider if they experience the following:

- Heart rate remaining less than 50 after arising
- Wheezing or difficulty breathing

- Weight gain of 3 pounds in 1 week or 1 to 2 pounds overnight
- Show persistent increase in NTG use
- Dizziness, faintness, or shortness of breath with activity

Clients are encouraged to call for transportation to the hospital if they experience the following:

- Chest discomfort that does not improve after 20 minutes or three NTG tablets
- Extremely severe chest or epigastric discomfort with weakness, nausea, or fainting
- Other symptoms that are particular to the client, such as fatigue and nausea

HEALTH CARE RESOURCES

The AHA is an excellent source for booklets, films, videocassettes, cookbooks, and professional service referrals for the client with CAD. Many local affiliates have their own cardiac rehabilitation programs.

Within the community, cardiac rehabilitation programs may be affiliated with local hospitals, community centers, or other facilities, such as clinics. Many shopping malls open before shopping hours to allow a measured walking program indoors; this is particularly popular with older clients because it provides a good support group and allows for an appropriate place to exercise in inclement weather.

Mended Hearts is a nationwide program with local chapters that provides education and support to CABG clients and their families. Smoking-cessation programs and clinics as well as weight-reduction programs are found within the community. Many hospitals also sponsor health fairs, BP screening, and risk factor modification programs.

Evaluation: Outcomes

Evaluate the client with CAD on the basis of the identified nursing diagnoses and collaborative problems. The expected outcomes are that the client will:

- State that discomfort or other symptoms are alleviated
- Have adequate blood flow through the coronary vasculature to ensure heart function
- Walk 200 feet four times a day without discomfort, shortness of breath, or other symptoms of CAD
- Take personal actions to manage stressors related to CAD

Specific indicators for these outcomes are listed for each nursing diagnosis and collaborative problem under the Planning and Implementation section (see earlier).

GET READY for the NCLEX Examination!

KEY POINTS

Safe Effective Care Environment

- Manage and use aseptic techniques when caring for all sternal and leg wound incisions, and any invasive lines.
- Refer clients who have had heart surgery for consultation with interdisciplinary health care team members (e.g., physical therapist, case manager, and home care providers).
- Evaluate the client's support options for meeting self-care needs.
- Interview the client and assess the client's home for environmental hazards and accessibility.
- Assist clients in securing personal medical identification alert devices that provide information regarding their heart conditions.

Health Promotion and Maintenance

- In collaboration with the dietitian, identify a healthy pattern of eating that helps reduce the incidence of CAD.
- In collaboration with the multidisciplinary health team, assess the client for activity tolerance and help design an appropriate exercise regimen.
- Teach the client about the signs and symptoms of cardiovascular disease and when to seek medical assistance.
- Assess the client for lifestyle risk factors of coronary artery disease (CAD), such as obesity, smoking, positive family history, cholesterol management, and the diagnosis and treatment of hypertension.
- Teach clients ways to decrease their risk for CAD.
- Teach clients about drug therapy, including therapeutic and adverse effects.
- Refer clients to appropriate community programs and support groups.

Psychosocial Integrity

- Allow clients to verbalize and express feelings of fear, anxiety, anger, denial, and grief regarding their CAD.
- Address the needs of the family and significant others and provide teaching and information regarding the disease process; clarify any misconceptions.
- Explain to the client the significance of reporting any pain or discomfort, and help identify barriers in seeking medical assistance.
- Identify and explain various diagnostic tests and procedures for clients experiencing cardiac compromise. Examples include electrocardiography, stress and exercise testing, nuclear scans, and cardiac catheterization.

Physiological Integrity

- Identify and interpret diagnostic values for cardiac enzymes and other indicators of CAD.
- Monitor clients receiving thrombolytics and anticoagulants, such as heparin, for bleeding.
- For clients undergoing invasive cardiac procedures, assess for signs and symptoms of active bleeding.
- Interpret and assess the client with CAD for dysrhythmias.
- Evaluate the client for pain characteristics (e.g., type, location, duration, cause, intensity, and measures taken to relieve symptoms).
- Identify and assess for complications for post–cardiac surgical clients, especially stroke, heart failure, bleeding, and pulmonary dysfunction.

ADDITIONAL STUDY RESOURCES

Go to your Student CD-ROM for Review Questions for the NCLEX Examination.

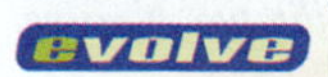

Go to http://evolve.elsevier.com/Iggy/ for Integrated Management of Care Questions for the NCLEX Examination.

SELECTED BIBLIOGRAPHY

Asterisk indicates a classic or definitive work on this subject.

Allen, J.K. (2000). Cholesterol management: An opportunity for nurse case managers. *Journal of Cardiovascular Nursing, 14*(2), 50-58.

Angioplasty: Copper chelation holds promise for clogged arteries. (2003). *Heart Disease Weekly, June 28,* 3-4.

Angioplasty: Gene therapy during procedure improves blood flow. (2003). *Heart Disease Weekly, June 15,* 10-11.

Aronow, W.S. (2003). Silent MI: Prevalence and prognosis in older patients diagnosed by routine electrocardiogram. *Geriatrics, 59*(1), 24-40.

Becker, C. (2003). Bypassing the pump. *Modern Healthcare, 35*(10), 36-40.

Bialous, S.A., & Sarna, L. (2004). Sparing a few minutes for tobacco cessation. *American Journal of Nursing, 104*(12), 54-60.

Boersma, E., et al. (2003). Acute myocardial infarction. *Lancet, 361*(9630), 847-859.

Cadroy, Y., et al. (2003). Strenuous activity may pose a risk of plaque injury. *Journal of Applied Physiology, 93*(3), 829-835.

Cardiac medication: Study newer anticoagulation is as effective as gold standard. (2003). *Heart Disease Weekly, March 23,* 22-23.

Cheek, D., & Cesan, A. (2003). What's different about heart disease in women? *Nursing 2003, 33*(8), 36-42.

Chen-Scarabelli, C. (2002). Beating-heart coronary artery bypass surgery: Indications, advantages, and limitations. *Critical Care Nurse, 22*(5), 44-58.

Clinical trials: Enrollment completed for gamma in-stent restenosis study. (2002). *Heart Disease Weekly, March 3,* 7-8.

Coronary artery bypass surgery versus percutaneous coronary intervention with stent implantation in patients with multivessel coronary artery disease. (2002). *Lancet, 360*(9360), 965-971.

Coronary artery occlusion: Heart attack victims to benefit from drug-coated stents. (2003). *Heart Disease Weekly, June 8,* 25-26.

Coronary bypass: Procedure without general anesthesia studied. (2000). *Heart Disease Weekly, October 15,* 11-12.

Cronin, S.N., et al. (2000). Recovery after percutaneous transluminal coronary angioplasty: Assessment after discharge. *Critical Care Nurse, 20*(2), 70-84.

Crumlish, C.M., et al. (2000). When time is muscle. *American Journal of Nursing, 100*(1), 26-36.

Daly, J., et al. (2000). Health status, perceptions of coping, and social support immediately after discharge of survivors of acute myocardial infarction. *American Journal of Critical Care, 9*(1), 62-69.

Davis, S.L. (2002). How the heart failure picture has changed. *Nursing, 32*(11), 36-44.

Ditlea, S. (2000). Robosurgeons. *Technology Review, 103*(6), 74-82.

Estabrooks, P.A., Glasgow, R.E., & Dzewaltowski, D.A. (2003). Physical activity promotion. *JAMA, 289*(22), 2913-2917.

Furry, B., & House-Fancher, M.A. (2000). Reviewing the drug lineup against AMI. *Nursing 2000, 30*(7), 32hn1-32hn3.

Futterman, L.G., & Lemberg, L. (2000). Update on management of acute myocardial infarction: Facilitated percutaneous coronary intervention. *American Journal of Critical Care, 9*(1), 70-76.

Gentz, C.A. (2000). Perceived learning needs of the patient undergoing coronary angioplasty: An integrative review of the literature. *Heart and Lung, 29*(3), 161-172.

Gorman, C., et al. (2003). The no. 1 killer of women. *Time Canada, 161*(17), 42-49.

Gradman, J. H., & Schell, M. (2002). *Managing cardiac emergencies.* Eau Claire, WI: PESI HealthCare.

Graham, H. (2003). A conceptual map for studying long-term exercise adherence in a cardiac population. *Rehabilitation Nursing, 28*(3), 80-86.

Grech, E. (2003a). ABC of interventional cardiology: Pathophysiology and investigation of coronary artery disease. *British Medical Journal, 326*(7399), 1027-1030.

Grech, E. (2003b). Percutaneous coronary intervention. I: History and development. *British Medical Journal, 326*(7398), 1080-1083.

Grech, E. (2003c). Percutaneous coronary intervention. II: The procedure. *British Medical Journal, 326*(7359), 1135-1141.

Grech, E., & Ramsdale, D. (2003). ABC of interventional cardiology: Acute coronary syndrome, unstable angina and non-ST segment elevation myocardial infarction. *British Medical Journal, 326*(7359), 1259-1261.

Hamilton, A. (2001). Forceps! Scalpel! Robot! *Time, 157*(22), 64-66.

Heart disease and stroke statistics–2003 update. (2003). Dallas: American Heart Association.

Heart disease mortality: Gene for cellular receptors could be key for lower heart risk. (2003). *Genomics & Genetics Weekly, May 2,* 19-20.

Henke, K., & Eigsti, J. (2003). After cardiopulmonary bypass: Watching for complications. *Nursing, 35*(3), cc1-cc4.

Here's a pet therapy for stressed caregivers. (2001). *Work & Family Life, 2.*

High cholesterol: Gene therapy lowers cholesterol in a model of familial hypercholesterolemia. (2003). *Heart Disease Weekly, June 22,* 36-35.

Hooker, S., Holbrook, L. F., & Stewart, P. (2002). Pet therapy research: A historical review. *Holistic Nursing Practice, 17*(1), 17-23.

Hussey, L. C., Hynan, L., & Leeper, B. (2001). Risk factors for sternal wound infection in men versus women. *American Journal of Critical Care, 10*(2), 112-116.

Hyett, J.M. (2004). Caring for a patient after CABG surgery, *Nursing 2004, 34*(7), 48-49.

Intracoronary radiation: Intima may become so thin that stent struts are exposed, may lead to thrombosis. (2003). *Heart Disease Weekly, June 1,* 53-54.

Kohli, M., et al. (2003). A risk index for sternal surgical wound infection after cardiovascular surgery. *Infection Control and Hospital Epidemiology, 24*(1), 17-22.

Lapchak, P.A., et al. (2002). The nonpeptide glycoprotein IIb/IIIa platelet receptor antagonist SM-20302 reduces tissue plasminogen activator-induced intracerebral hemorrhage after thromboembolic stroke. *Stroke, 35*(1), 147-152.

Litton, K. (2002). Left vs. right ventricular MI: Which is it? *RN, 65*(5), 36ac5-36ac10.

Liu, E.H. (2000). Use of alternate medicine by patients undergoing cardiac surgery. *Journal Thoracic Cardiovascular Surgery, 120*(2), 355-361.

Low-cost intranasal antibiotic reduces sternal wound infections in open-heart surgery patients. (2001). *Formulary, 36*(7), 483-484.

Madias, J. E. (2000). Killip and Forrester classifications: Should they be abandoned, kept, reevaluated, or modified? *Chest, 117*(5), 1223-1226.

Manson, J.E., et al. (2001). Heart disease in older women. *Patient Care for the Nurse Practitioner, 4*(5), 28-40.

McAvoy, J.A. (2000). Cardiac pain: Discover the unexpected. *Nursing 2000, 30*(3), 36-40.

McCance, K., & Huether, S. (2002). *Pathophysiology: The biologic basis for disease in adults* (4th ed.). St. Louis: Mosby.

Meadows, M. (2002). Robots lend a helpful hand to surgeons. *FDA Consumer,36*(3), 10-16.

Nguyen, T., et al. (2000). Catheter based interventions in acute myocardial infarction. In T. Nguyen et al. (Eds.), *Management of complex cardiovascular problems* (pp. 35-56). Armonk, NY: Futura Publishing.

O'Toole, L., Grech, E., & Grech, E. (2003). ABC of interventional cardiology. Chronic stable angina: Treatment options. *British Medical Journal, 326*(7400), 1185-1189.

Pagana, K.D., & Pagana, T.J.(2002). *Mosby's manual of diagnostic and laboratory tests* (2nd ed.). St. Louis: Mosby.

Palatnik, A.M. (2001). Acute coronary syndrome: New advances and nursing strategies. *Nursing 2001, 31*(5), 32cc1-32cc6.

Peterson, D.A. (2000). Managing hypotension after cardiac surgery: An algorithm for treatment. *Critical Care Nurse, 20*(2), 36-49.

Quality assurance: Half of heart patients unable to recall details of informed consent. (2003). *Heart Disease Weekly, April 20,* 74-75.

Rademaker, F.E. (2003). Magnetic resonance imaging in cardiology. *Lancet, 361*(9355), 359-361.

Richards, S.B., Funk, M., & Milner, K.A. (2000). Differences between blacks and whites with coronary artery disease in initial symptoms and delay in seeking care. *American Journal of Critical Care, 9*(4), 235-244.

Riemsma, R.P., et al. (2003). Systematic review of the effectiveness of stage based interventions to promote smoking cessation. *British Medical Journal, 326*(74), 1175-1178.

Robinson, A.W. (2002). Older women's experiences if living alone after heart surgery. *Applied Nursing Research, 15*(3), 118-125.

Robotic heart surgery (2002). *Science News, 162*(23), 365.

Ryan, D. (2000). Is it an MI? A lab primer for myocardial infarction. *RN, 63*(1), 26-31.

Sadovsky, R. (2003a). Clopidogrel vs. aspirin in preventing acute MI. *American Family Physician, 67*(5), 1085.

Sadovsky, R. (2003b). Preventing plaque rupture: New clinical strategies. *American Family Physician, 67*(6), 1362-1365.

Sakallaris, et al. (2000). Same-day transfer of patients to the cardiac telemetry unit after surgery: The rapid after bypass back into telemetry (Rabbit) program. *Critical Care Nurse, 20*(2), 50-68.

Skidmore-Roth, L. (2002). *Mosby's nursing drug reference.* St. Louis: Mosby.

Sneed, N.V., et al. (2001). Influence of a relaxation intervention on perceived stress and power spectral analysis of heart rate variability. *Progress in Cardiovascular Nursing, 16*(2), 57-62.

Solomon, A.J., & Gersh, B.J. (2000). Unstable coronary artery disease. In T. Nguyen et al. (Eds.), *Management of complex cardiovascular problems* (pp. 1-14). Armonk, NY: Futura Publishing.

Verosky, D. (2003). Using pharmacologic stress testing to evaluate cardiac perfusion. *Nursing 2003, 33*(8), 68.

Watson, R.D., Chin, B.S.P., & Lip, G.Y.H. (2002). ABC of antithrombotic therapy. *British Medical Journal, 325*(7356), 1348-1352.

*Wenger, N.K., et al. (1995). *Cardiac rehabilitation as secondary prevention. Clinical practice guideline. Quick reference guide for clinicians, No. 17.* AHCPR Pub. No. 96-0673. Rockville, MD: Agency for Health Care Policy and Research and National Heart, Lung, and Blood Institute, Public Health Service, U.S. Department of Health and Human Services.

Wilson, J. (2000). Beating-heart surgery. *Popular Mechanics, 177*(4), 50-52.

Women and heart disease. (2003). *Harvard Heart Letter, 13*(9), 7.

Woods, A. (2004). Loosening the grip of hypertension. *Nursing 2004, 34*(12), 36-43.

Yates, B.C., Braklow-Whitton, J.L., & Agrawal, S. (2003). Outcomes of cardiac rehabilitation participants and nonparticipants in a rural area. *Rehabilitation Nursing, 28*(2), 57-64.

Yoshihiro, M. (2002). Coronary artery disease: Repeat stenting not always durable. *Heart Disease Weekly, June 16,* 12-13.

Zanabria, E., & Welch, G. (2003). Hypertension and exercise. *American Fitness, 21*(2), 56-60.

Zepf, B. (2003a). Walking vs. vigorous exercise for heart health in women. *American Family Physician, 67*(3), 599.

Zepf, B. (2003b). Choosing anticoagulation or aspirin after heart attack. *American Family Physician, 67*(6), 1399.

UNIT **NINE**

PROBLEMS of TISSUE PERFUSION

Management of Clients with Problems of the Hematologic System

CHAPTER

42

Assessment of the Hematologic System

M. LINDA WORKMAN

LEARNING OUTCOMES

After studying this chapter, you should be able to:

1. Describe the hematologic changes associated with aging.
2. Explain the process of erythrocyte maturation.
3. Describe the role of platelets in hemostasis.
4. Compare the structure and function of platelet plugs and fibrin clots.
5. Interpret blood cell counts and clotting tests to assess the client's hematologic status.
6. Compare the actions and uses of anticoagulants, fibrinolytics, and inhibitors of platelet activity.
7. Develop a community-based teaching plan for the client on anticoagulant therapy at home.
8. Prioritize nursing care for the client after bone marrow aspiration.

Go to your Student CD-ROM for Review Questions for the NCLEX Examination keyed to these Learning Outcomes.

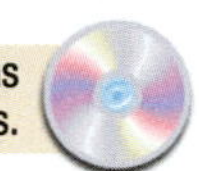

The hematologic system is the blood, blood cells, lymph, and organs involved with blood formation or blood storage. All systems depend on circulation; thus any problem of the hematologic system affects total body health and well-being. This chapter, together with Chapter 23, reviews the normal physiology of the hematologic system and assessment of hematologic status.

ANATOMY AND PHYSIOLOGY REVIEW

Bone Marrow

Bone marrow is the blood-forming **(hematopoietic)** organ. It produces most of the cells of the blood, including red blood cells **(RBCs, erythrocytes),** white blood cells (WBCs), and platelets. Bone marrow also is involved in the immune responses (see Chapter 23).

Each day the bone marrow in a healthy adult releases about 2.5 billion RBCs, 2.5 billion platelets, and one billion white blood cells **(leukocytes)** per kilogram of body weight.

In the fetus, blood components are formed in the liver and spleen and, by the last trimester, the bone marrow. At birth, blood-producing marrow is present in every bone. The flat bones (sternum, skull, pelvic and shoulder girdles) contain active blood-producing marrow throughout life. As a person ages, the amount of blood-producing marrow decreases in the long bones and in small, irregularly shaped bones. By the age of 18 years, blood production is limited to the ends of the long bones. During adulthood, fatty tissue replaces inactive bone marrow. In older adults the amount of fatty marrow increases and only a small portion of the remaining marrow continues with active blood production.

The bone marrow first produces stem cells. Stem cells are immature, undifferentiated cells that are capable of maturing into any one of several types of blood cells: RBCs, WBCs, or platelets, depending on the body's needs (Figure 42-1).

The next stage in blood cell development is the committed stem cell (also called the precursor cell or the unipotent stem cell). A committed stem cell enters one maturational pathway and can at that point differentiate into only one cell type. Committed stem cells actively divide but require the presence of a specific growth factor for maturation. For example, **erythropoietin** is a growth factor made in the kidneys that is specific for the RBC. Many different growth factors influence WBC and platelet maturation (see Chapters 23, 28, and 43).

Blood Components

Blood is composed of plasma and cells. Plasma is part of the body's extracellular fluid. It is similar to the interstitial fluid found between tissue cells, but plasma contains several times more protein than interstitial fluid contains. The three major types of plasma proteins are albumin, globulins, and fibrinogen.

Albumin increases the osmotic pressure of the blood, which prevents the plasma from leaking into the tissues (see

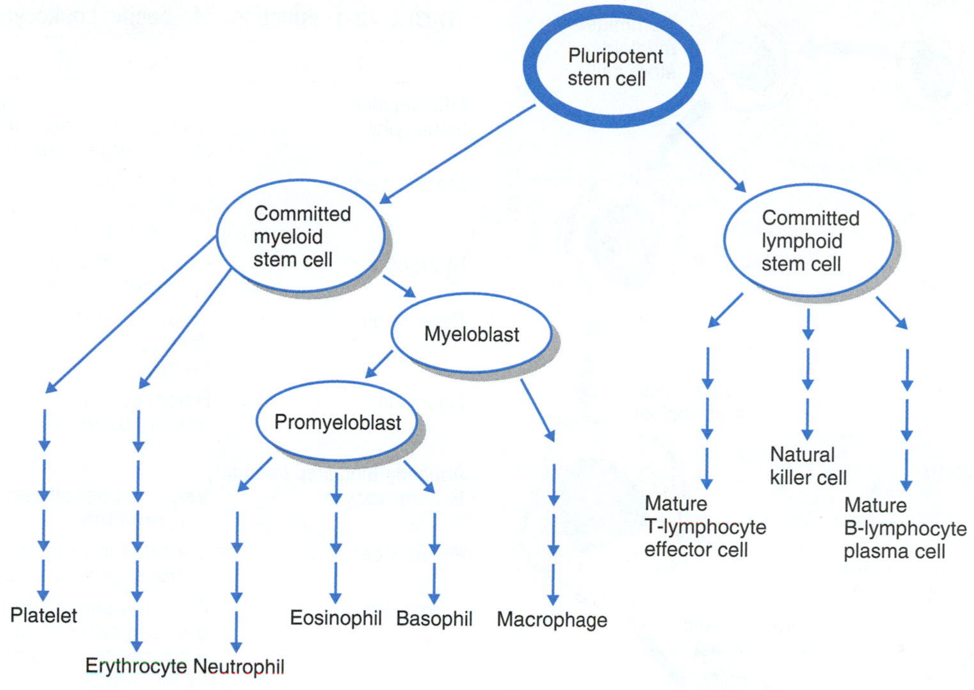

Figure 42-1 ■ Bone marrow cell differentiation and maturational pathways.

Chapter 14). Globulins have many functions, such as transporting other substances and protecting the body against infection. Globulins are also the main component of antibodies. **Fibrinogen** is a protein molecule that can be activated to form fibrin. Fibrin molecules assemble together to form structures important in the blood clotting process.

The blood cells include RBCs, WBCs, and platelets. These cells differ in structure, site of maturation, and function.

RED BLOOD CELLS (ERYTHROCYTES)

Red blood cells, or **erythrocytes,** are the largest proportion of blood cells. Mature RBCs have no nucleus and have a biconcave disk shape. Together with a flexible membrane, this feature allows RBCs to change their shape without breaking as they pass through narrow, winding capillaries. The number of RBCs a person has varies according to gender, age, and general health, but the normal range is from 4,200,000 to 6,100,000/mm^3.

As shown in Figures 42-1 and 42-2, RBCs start out as stem cells, enter the myeloid pathway, and progress in stages to the mature RBC (i.e., the erythrocyte). Healthy, mature RBCs have a life span of about 120 days after being released into the blood. As RBCs age, their membranes become more fragile. These old cells are trapped and destroyed in the tissues, spleen, and liver. Some parts of destroyed RBCs (e.g., iron), are recycled and used to make new RBCs.

The RBCs produce hemoglobin (Hgb). Each normal mature RBC contains thousands of hemoglobin molecules (Berne et al., 2004). The heme part of each hemoglobin molecule needs a molecule of iron. Only when the heme molecule is complete with iron can it transport up to four molecules of oxygen. *Therefore iron is a critical component of hemoglobin.* The globin portion of hemoglobin carries carbon dioxide. RBCs also are buffers and help maintain acid-base balance.

The most important feature of hemoglobin is its ability to combine loosely with oxygen. With only a small drop in oxygen level in the tissues, a greater increase in the transfer of oxygen from hemoglobin to tissues occurs. This transfer is also known as **oxygen dissociation.** Some problems change the speed and amount of oxygen released to the tissues.

The total number of RBCs a person has is carefully controlled through **erythropoiesis** (selective maturation of stem cells into mature erythrocytes). This process ensures that enough RBCs are present for good oxygenation without having too many cells that could "thicken" the blood and slow its flow. The trigger for control of erythropoiesis is tissue oxygenation. The kidney produces the RBC growth factor erythropoietin at the same rate as RBC destruction occurs to maintain a constant normal level of circulating RBCs. When tissue oxygenation is less than normal **(hypoxia),** the kidney increases the production of erythropoietin. This growth factor stimulates the bone marrow to increase RBC production. When tissue oxygenation is normal or high, the kidney reduces erythropoietin levels, slowing the production of RBCs. Synthetic erythropoietin (Procrit, Epogen, EPO) has the same effect on bone marrow as the naturally occurring erythropoietin.

Many substances are needed to form hemoglobin and RBCs, including iron, vitamin B_{12}, folic acid, copper, pyridoxine, cobalt, and nickel. A lack of any of these substances can lead to anemia. Anemia is the result of any problem that reduces the function or the number of erythrocytes to the point that tissue oxygen demands are not completely met (see Chapter 43).

WHITE BLOOD CELLS (LEUKOCYTES)

White blood cells (WBCs), or leukocytes, perform actions critical to inflammation or immunity (Table 42-1). The many types of WBCs all have specialized functions. Most

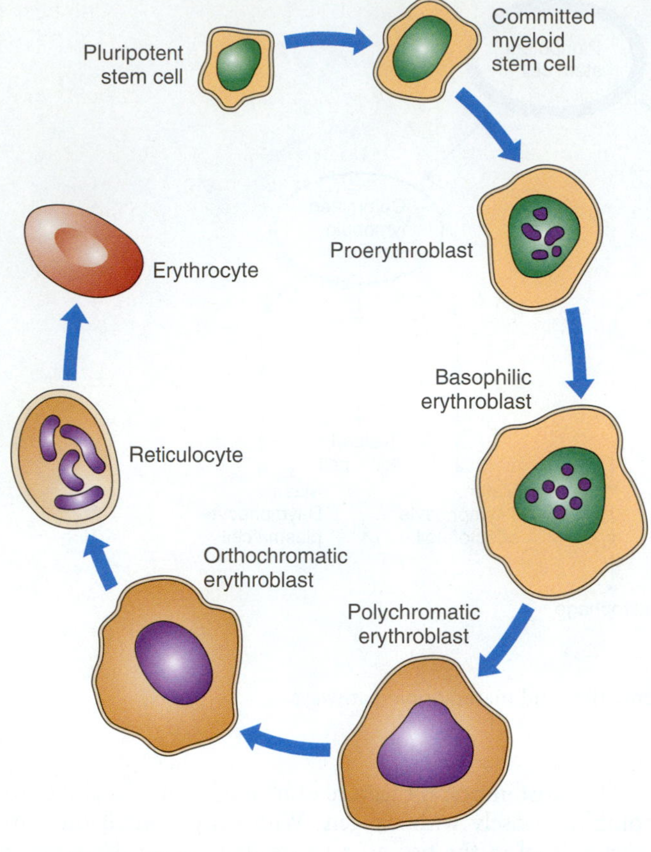

Figure 42-2 ■ Erythrocyte maturational pathway.

WBCs are formed in the bone marrow and are part of the hematopoietic system. WBC function is presented in Chapter 23 because these cells provide immunity and protect against invasion and infection.

PLATELETS

Platelets are the third type of blood cells. They are the smallest of the blood cells, formed as fragments of a giant precursor cell in the bone marrow, the **megakaryocyte.** Figure 42-1 shows the overall blood cell developmental pathway, and Figure 42-3 shows specific platelet development.

Platelets stick to injured blood vessel walls and form platelet plugs that can stop the flow of blood from the injured site. They also produce substances important to coagulation. Platelets help keep blood vessels intact by beginning the repair of damage to small blood vessels. They perform most of their functions by **aggregation** (clumping).

Bone marrow production of platelets also is precisely controlled by growth factors (thrombopoietin). After platelets leave the bone marrow, they are stored in the spleen and then released slowly to meet the body's needs. Normally 80% of platelets circulate and 20% are stored in the spleen. Each platelet has a life span of 1 to 2 weeks.

Accessory Organs of Hematopoiesis

The spleen and liver are important accessory organs of the hematopoietic system. They help to regulate the maturation of blood cells to help maintain hematologic homeostasis.

TABLE 42-1 Functions of Specific Leukocytes

Leukocyte	Function
Inflammation	
Neutrophil	Nonspecific ingestion and phagocytosis of microorganisms and foreign protein
Macrophage	Nonspecific recognition of foreign proteins and microorganisms; ingestion and phagocytosis
Monocyte	Destruction of bacteria and cellular debris; matures into macrophage
Eosinophil	Weak phagocytic action, releases vasoactive amines during allergic reactions
Basophil	Releases histamine and heparin in areas of tissue damage
Antibody-Mediated Immunity	
B-lymphocyte	Becomes sensitized to foreign cells and proteins
Plasma cell	Secretes immunoglobulins in response to the presence of a specific antigen
Memory cell	Remains sensitized to a specific antigen and can secrete increased amounts of immunoglobulins specific to the antigen
Cell-Mediated Immunity	
T-lymphocyte helper/ inducer T-cell	Enhances immune activity through the secretion of various factors, cytokines, and lymphokines
Cytotoxic-cytolytic T-cell	Selectively attacks and destroys non-self cells, including virally infected cells, grafts, and transplanted organs
Natural killer cell	Nonselectively attacks non-self cells, especially body cells that have undergone mutation and become malignant; also attacks grafts and transplanted organs

SPLEEN

The spleen is located under the diaphragm to the left of the stomach. It contains three types of tissue: white pulp, red pulp, and marginal pulp. These tissues all help to balance blood cell production with blood cell destruction and assist with immunity. White pulp is filled with white blood cells (WBCs), especially lymphocytes and macrophages. As whole blood filters through the white pulp, unwanted cells (such as bacteria and old RBCs) are removed. Red pulp contains vascular enlargements **(sinuses)** that store RBCs and platelets. Marginal pulp contains the ends of many arteries and other blood vessels.

The spleen destroys old or imperfect RBCs, breaks down the hemoglobin released from these destroyed cells, stores platelets, and filters antigens. A client who has had a splenectomy has reduced immune functions. Thus, after a splenectomy, clients are not as efficient at ridding the body of disease-causing organisms and are at greater risk for infection and sepsis.

LIVER

The liver is the main production site for prothrombin and most of the blood clotting factors. In addition, proper liver function and bile production are critical to the formation of vitamin K in the intestinal tract. (Vitamin K is essential for

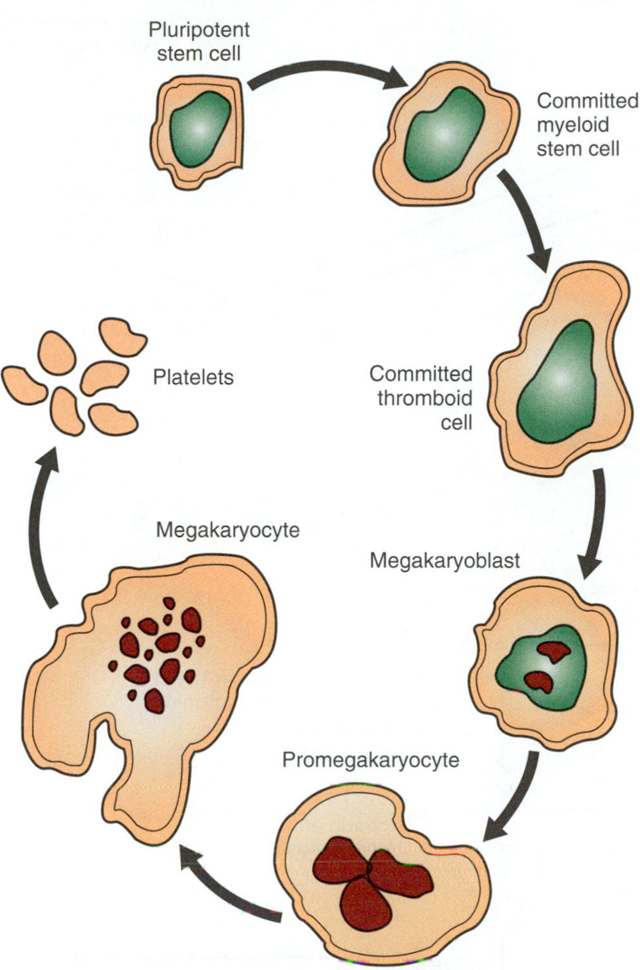

Figure 42-3 ■ Platelet maturational pathway.

producing blood clotting factors VII, IX, and X and prothrombin.) Large quantities of whole blood and blood cells can be stored in the liver. The liver also converts bilirubin (one end product of hemoglobin breakdown) to bile and stores extra iron within the protein ferritin. Small amounts of erythropoietin are produced in the liver.

Hemostasis/Blood Clotting

In hemostasis, localized blood clotting occurs in damaged blood vessels while blood continues to circulate to all other areas. Hemostasis is a complex process that balances the production of clotting and dissolving factors. It begins with the formation of a platelet plug and continues with a series of events that eventually cause the formation of a fibrin clot. Intrinsic and extrinsic factors are involved in blood clotting. Three sequential processes result in blood clotting: platelet aggregation with formation of a platelet plug, the blood clotting cascade, and the formation of a complete fibrin clot.

PLATELET AGGREGATION

Forming a platelet plug by causing platelets to clump together is essential for blood clotting. Platelets normally circulate as individual cell-like structures. They are not attracted to each other and do not clump together until activated. Usually activation causes platelet membranes to become sticky, allowing clumping to occur. When platelets become activated and clump, they form large, semisolid plugs within the lumens and walls of blood vessels and disrupt local blood flow. *These platelet plugs are not clots and cannot provide complete hemostasis.*

Some substances that cause platelets to clump include adenosine diphosphate (ADP), calcium, thromboxane A_2, and collagen. Platelets themselves can be stimulated to secrete some of these substances, whereas other substances that activate platelets are exogenous. Platelet plugs start the cascade reaction that leads to fibrin clot formation and blood coagulation.

THE BLOOD CLOTTING CASCADE

The blood clotting cascade is triggered by the formation of a platelet plug. Platelet plugs can occur from both intrinsic and extrinsic factors. The beginning of the blood clotting cascade is rapidly amplified or enhanced; that is, the final result is much larger than the triggering event. Cascades work like a landslide. A few small pebbles rolling down a steep hillside can dislodge large rocks and pieces of soil, causing a final enormous movement of earth. Just like landslides, cascade reactions are hard to stop once set into motion.

Intrinsic Factors

Intrinsic factors are problems or substances directly in the blood itself that first make platelets clump and then activate the blood clotting cascade (Figure 42-4). These factors or conditions include antigen-antibody reactions, circulating debris, prolonged venous stasis, and bacterial toxins. Continuing the cascade to the point of fibrin clot formation depends on the presence of sufficient amounts of all the various clotting factors and cofactors (Table 42-2).

Extrinsic Factors

Platelet plugs also can form as a result of changes in the blood vessels rather than in the blood. When platelet plugs form in response to blood vessel changes, the response is said to be caused by **extrinsic factors** (outside the blood). The most common extrinsic event is trauma that damages blood vessels and exposes the platelets to collagen. Collagen then activates platelets and causes clumping. The platelet plug is formed within seconds of the trauma. The blood clotting cascade is started sooner by the extrinsic pathway because some of the steps of the intrinsic pathway are bypassed.

Whether the platelet plugs were formed because of abnormal blood (intrinsic factors) or by exposure of substances from damaged blood vessels (extrinsic factors), the end result of the cascade is the same: *formation of a fibrin clot and coagulation.*

Many steps of the cascade that occur between the formation of a platelet plug and the formation of a fibrin clot are dependent on the presence of specific clotting factors as well as calcium and more platelets.

Clotting factors (see Table 42-2) are inactive enzymes that become activated in a sequence. The last part of the sequence is the activation fibrinogen into fibrin. At each step, the activated enzyme from the previous step activates the next enzyme. The last two steps in the cascade are the activation of thrombin from prothrombin and the conversion (by thrombin) of fibrinogen into fibrin. Only fibrin molecules can begin the formation of a true clot.

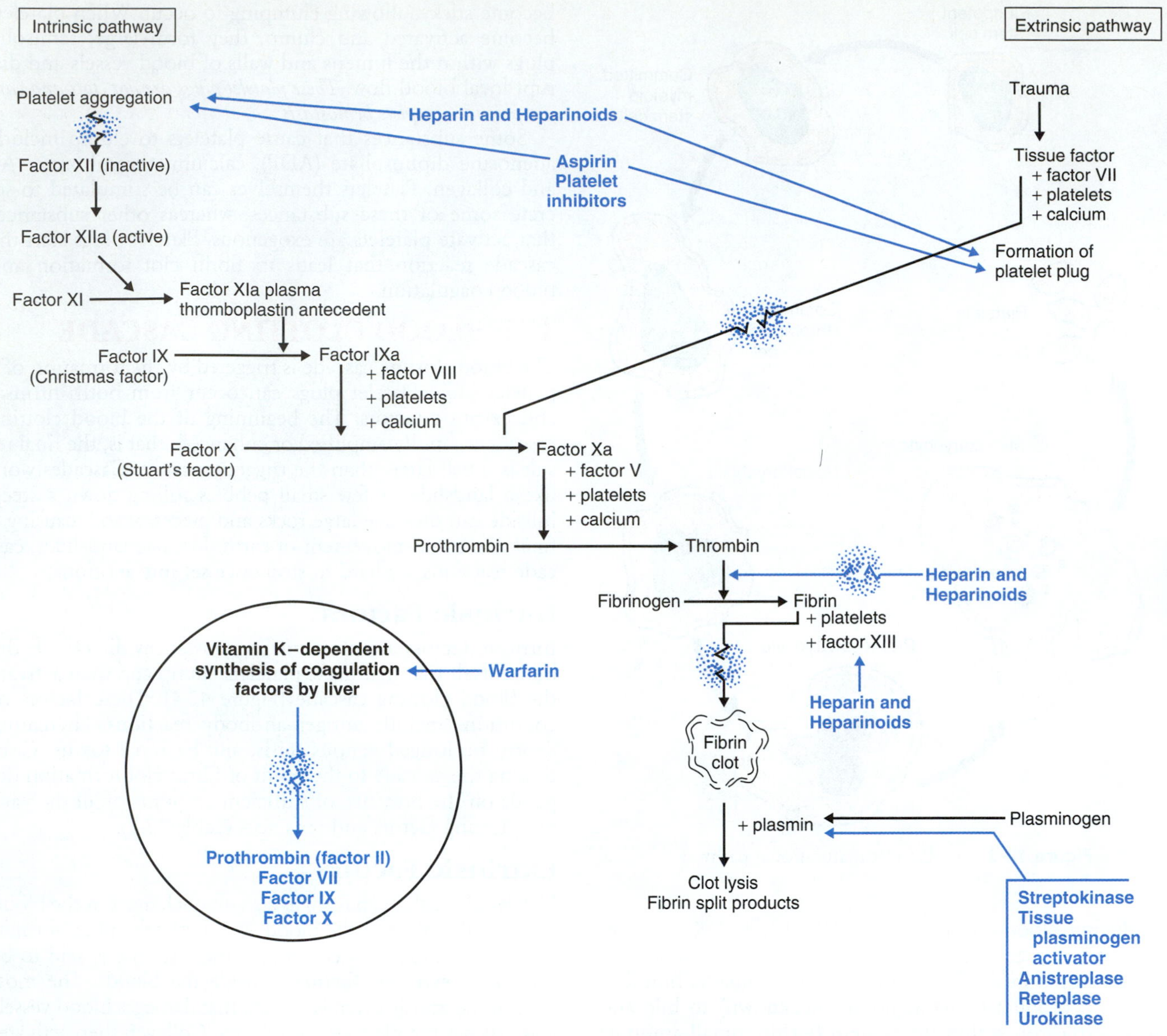

Figure 42-4 ■ Summary of blood clotting cascade.

FIBRIN CLOT FORMATION

Fibrinogen is a large, inactive protein made in the liver. The enzyme thrombin removes the end portions of fibrinogen, converting it to active fibrin. Individual fibrin molecules link together to form fibrin threads. The fibrin threads make a netlike meshwork that forms the base of a blood clot (Figure 42-5).

After the fibrin mesh is formed, clotting factor XIII tightens up the mesh, making it more dense and stable. More platelets stick to the threads of the mesh and attract other blood cells and proteins to form an actual blood clot. As this clot retracts, the **serum** (plasma without the clotting factors) is extruded, and clot formation is complete.

FIBRINOLYSIS

Because blood clotting occurs through a rapid cascade process, in theory it keeps forming fibrin clots whenever the cascade is set into motion until all blood throughout the entire body has coagulated. Such widespread clotting would lead to death. Therefore, whenever the blood clotting cascade is started, counterclotting or **anticoagulant** forces are also started. These forces limit clot formation to damaged areas only so that normal blood flow is maintained everywhere else. When blood clotting and anticlotting actions are normal and balanced, clotting occurs only where it is needed and normal blood flow elsewhere is maintained.

The fibrinolytic system dissolves the fibrin clot with special enzymes (Figure 42-6). The key to fibrinolysis is activating plasminogen to plasmin. Plasmin, an active enzyme, then digests fibrin, fibrinogen, and prothrombin, thus breaking down the fibrin clot.

Hematologic Changes Associated with Aging

Aging changes the cellular and plasma components of blood. Chart 42-1 lists assessment tips for older adults. Sev-

TABLE 42-2 The Clotting Factors

Factor	Action
I: Fibrinogen	Factor I is converted to fibrin by the enzyme thrombin. Individual fibrin molecules form fibrin threads, which are the scaffold for clot formation and wound healing.
II: Prothrombin	Factor II is the inactive precursor of thrombin. Prothrombin is activated to thrombin by coagulation factor X (Stuart-Prower factor). After it is activated, thrombin converts fibrinogen (coagulation factor I) into fibrin and activates factors V and VIII. Synthesis is vitamin K–dependent.
III: Tissue thromboplastin	Factor III interacts with factor VII to initiate the extrinsic clotting cascade.
IV: Calcium	Calcium (Ca^{2+}), a divalent cation, is a cofactor for most of the enzyme-activated processes required in blood coagulation. Calcium also enhances platelet aggregation and makes red blood cells clump together.
V: Proaccelerin	Factor V is a cofactor for activated factor X, which is essential for converting prothrombin to thrombin.
VI: Discovered to be an artifact	No factor VI is involved in blood coagulation.
VII: Proconvertin	Factor VII activates factors IX and X, which are essential in converting prothrombin to thrombin. Synthesis is vitamin K–dependent.
VIII: Antihemophilic factor	Factor VIII together with activated factor IX enzymatically activates factor X. In addition, factor VIII combines with another protein (von Willebrand's factor) to help platelets adhere to capillary walls in areas of tissue injury. A lack of factor VIII is the basis for classic hemophilia (hemophilia A).
IX: Plasma thromboplastin component (Christmas factor)	Factor IX, when activated, activates factor X to convert prothrombin to thrombin. This factor is essential in the common pathway between the intrinsic and extrinsic clotting cascades. A lack of factor IX is the basis for hemophilia B. Synthesis is vitamin K–dependent.
X: Stuart-Prower factor	Factor X, when activated, converts prothrombin into thrombin. Synthesis is vitamin K–dependent.
XI: Plasma thromboplastin antecedent	Factor XI, when activated, assists in the activation of factor IX. However, a similar factor must exist in tissues. People who are deficient in factor XI have mild bleeding problems after surgery but do not bleed excessively as a result of trauma.
XII: Hageman factor	Factor XII is critically important in the intrinsic pathway for the activation of factor XI.
XIII: Fibrin-stabilizing factor	Factor XIII assists in forming cross-links among the fibrin threads to form a strong fibrin clot.

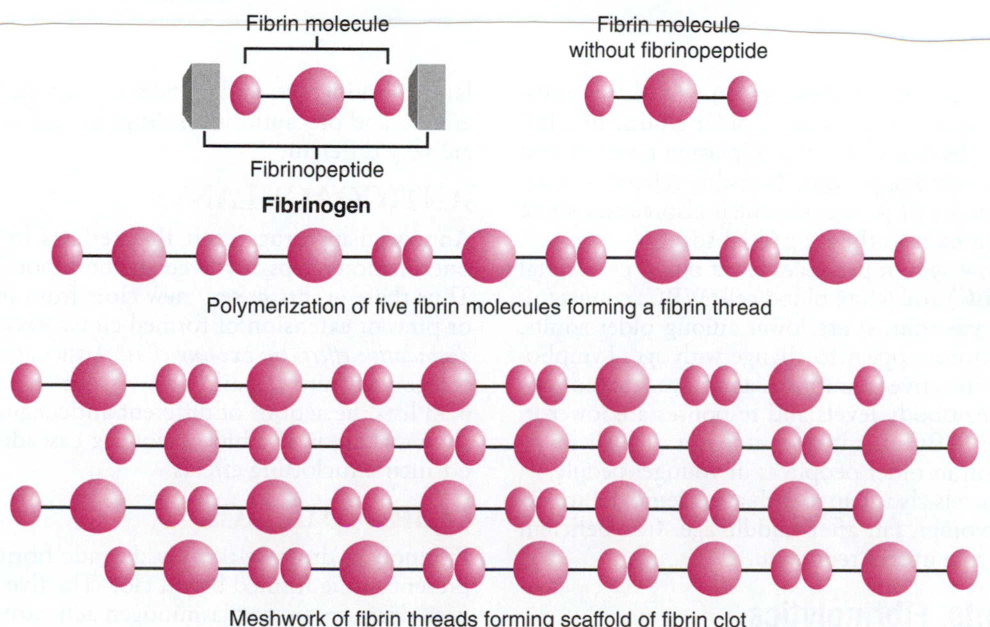

Figure 42-5 ■ Activation and polymerization of fibrin to form fibrin clot.

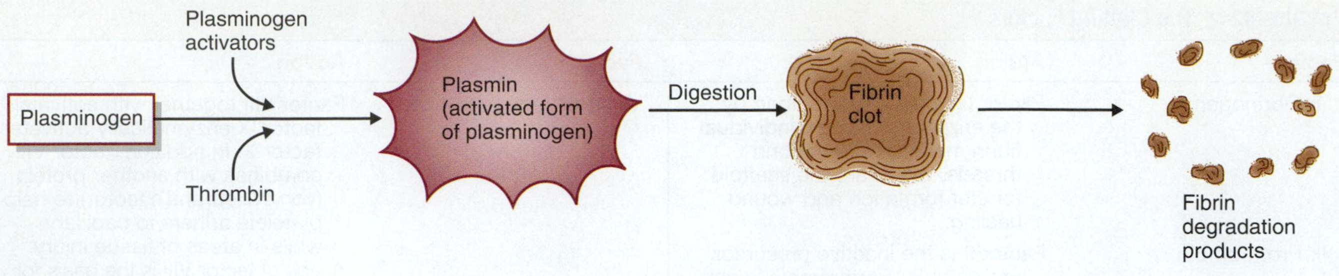

Figure 42-6 ■ The process of fibrinolysis.

CHART 42-1

NURSING FOCUS on the OLDER ADULT

Hematologic Assessment

Findings in Hematologic Disorders	Normal Changes in the Older Adult	Significance/Alternatives
Nail Beds (for Capillary Refill)		
Pallor or cyanosis may indicate a hematologic disorder.	Thickened or discolored nails make visualization of skin color beneath the nails impossible.	Use another body area, such as the lip, to assess central capillary refill.
Hair Distribution		
Thin or absent hair on the trunk or extremities may indicate poor circulation to a particular area.	Progressive loss of body hair is a normal facet of aging.	A relatively even pattern of hair loss that has occurred over an extended period is not significant.
Skin Moisture		
Skin dryness may indicate any of a number of hematologic disorders.	Skin dryness is a normal result of aging.	Skin moisture is not usually a reliable indicator of an underlying pathologic condition in the older adult.
Skin Color		
Skin color changes, especially pallor and jaundice, are associated with some hematologic disorders.	Pigment loss and skin yellowing are common changes associated with aging.	Pallor in an older adult may not be a reliable indicator of anemia; laboratory testing is required. Yellow-tinged skin in an older adult may not be a reliable indicator of increased serum bilirubin levels; laboratory testing is required.

eral factors cause a decreased blood volume in older adults. Total body water is decreased among older adults. In addition, they tend to have lower levels of plasma proteins and decreased plasma osmotic pressure (possibly related to a decreased dietary intake of proteins), which also causes some loss of blood volume into the interstitial space.

As bone marrow ages, it produces fewer blood cells. Total red blood cell (RBC) and white blood cell (WBC) counts (especially lymphocyte counts) are lower among older adults. Platelet counts do not appear to change with age. Lymphocytes become less reactive to antigens and have a loss of immune function. Antibody levels and responses are lower in older adults. The WBC count does not rise as high in response to infection in older people as in younger people.

Hemoglobin levels also change with age. Hemoglobin levels in men and women fall after middle age. Iron-deficient diets may play a role in this reduction.

Anticoagulants, Fibrinolytics, and Platelet Inhibitors

Drug therapy is used to reduce clotting ability or to destroy existing clots when circulation is at risk. The broad categories of drugs that perform these functions are anticoagulants, fibrinolytics, and platelet inhibitors. The actions, side effects, and precautions for drugs in each of these categories are very different.

ANTICOAGULANTS

Anticoagulant drugs exert their effects by interfering with one or more steps involved in the blood clotting cascade. Thus these agents *prevent* new clots from forming and limit or prevent extension of formed clots. *Anticoagulants have no degradative effects on existing clots.* Anticoagulants are further categorized into heparin and vitamin K antagonists. Table 42-3 lists the actions of different anticoagulants. Figure 42-4 shows where in the blood clotting cascade these agents exert their anticlotting effects.

FIBRINOLYTICS

Fibrinolytic drugs selectively degrade fibrin threads already present in the formed blood clot. The five most commonly used drugs are tissue plasminogen activator (t-PA), streptokinase (SK), reteplase, anistreplase, and urokinase. The mechanism to start fibrin degradation is activation of the inactive tissue protein **plasminogen** to its active form, **plasmin**. Plasmin directly attacks and degrades the fibrin molecule, having fewer effects on the fibrinogen molecule. Thus the ac-

TABLE 42-3 Anticoagulants, Fibrinolytics, and Platelet Inhibitors

Agent	Mechanism of Action	Side Effects/Precautions	Nursing Implications
Anticoagulants			
Heparin (Calciparin, Hepalean✱)	Potentiates the inhibiting actions of antithrombin III Interferes with thrombin formation Prevents conversion of fibrinogen to fibrin	Prevents clot formation	Check client for bleeding
		Has no effect on existing clots	Used for prevention of clot formation or extension
		Must be given parenterally	Teach client proper technique for home administration
		Antidote is protamine sulfate	Keep protamine sulfate on the unit when a client is receiving heparin
		Half-life is 1 to 6 hr	Client is most at risk for excessive bleeding in the first few hours after administration
		Derived from animal sources	Check client for possible allergic reactions
		Can induce thrombocytopenia	Monitor platelet count, monitor for blood in urine, stool, emesis; check skin for increasing bruises or petechiae
Low-Molecular-Weight Heparins			
Enoxaparin (Lovenox)	Same as heparin	Same as heparin, less allergenic, does not alter laboratory value	Does not require monitoring of drug levels or aPTT Same as for heparin
Dalteparin (Fragmin, Tedelparin)	Similar to heparin Also inhibits clotting factor Xa	Same as for enoxaparin	Same as for enoxaparin
Vitamin K Antagonists			
Warfarin (Coumadin, Warfilone✱)	Disrupts liver synthesis of vitamin K–dependent clotting factors (factors II, VII, IX, X)	Requires 48-96 hr to peak effect	May be started while the client is still receiving heparin
		Requires 1 wk to clear after drug is discontinued	Instruct client that bleeding precautions are still needed for at least a week after stopping the drug
		Anticoagulation is additive to that of platelet inhibitors	Warn clients not to take aspirin or other platelet inhibitors unless prescribed by the health care provider who also prescribed the warfarin
		Blood levels fluctuate with diet and other factors	Instruct clients to keep all appointments for drug level checks and not to self adjust drug dosages
Fibrinolytics			
Reteplase (Retavase)	Activates plasminogen into plasmin, which breaks degrades fibrin, disintegrating clots	Peak activity is immediate, lasting about an hour	Avoid venipunctures during and for one hour after administration
		May induce intracranial hemorrhage in older clients	Do not place clients in a position in which the head is dependent to the body; assess neurologic status every 30 minutes for the first 3 hours after administration
		Affects all existing clots <24 hr old	Assess any incisions, venipuncture sites, previous areas of trauma for bleeding
Anistreplase (Eminase)	Binds with plasminogen to form a complex that digests fibrin	Activity persists for 2-4 hr after administration	Avoid venipunctures during and for 4 hours after drug administration
		Others same as for reteplase	Same as for reteplase
Alteplase (Activase)	Same as for reteplase	Same as for reteplase	Same as for reteplase
Streptokinase (Streptase)	Same as for anistreplase	Made from exogenous substances and is allergenic	Check client for mild and severe allergic reactions during and after treatment (rash, hypotension, difficulty breathing, wheezing); keep emergency equipment and medications in client's room
		Not clot specific, also disrupts clotting cascade-greater risk for hemorrhage	Use bleeding precautions when handling the client; assess for excessive bleeding at least every 15 minutes during and for 2 hours after drug administration
		May not be effective in clients who have had multiple *Streptococcal* infections	Assess for drug effectiveness during administration

Data from Facts and Comparisons. (2004). *Drug facts and comparisons* (58th ed.). St. Louis: Author.

Continued

TABLE 42-3 Anticoagulants, Fibrinolytics, and Platelet Inhibitors—*cont'd*

Agent	Mechanism of Action	Side Effects/Precautions	Nursing Implications
Fibrinolytics—*cont'd*			
Urokinase (Abbokinase)	Same as for reteplase	Fibrinogen levels remain low for 12-24 hr	Use bleeding precautions for at least 24 hours after drug administration; assess for bleeding at least every 2 hours for the first 24 hours.
		Produced by cultured human cells, thus has the potential to transmit infectious disease	Assess client for manifestations of infection at least every shift during hospitalization; teach client to have regular monitoring for blood-borne diseases for at least 1 year after therapy.
Platelet Inhibitors			
Aspirin	Disrupts production of thromboxane A-2, preventing platelets aggregation	Can trigger asthma when taken frequently or in high doses	Instruct clients to stop aspirin if wheezing occurs
		Platelet aggregation is affected for up to 10 days after a single dose	Instruct clients to discontinue aspirin at least a week before scheduled dental work, surgery and other invasive procedures
		Irritates gastric lining and promotes gastrointestinal ulceration	Teach clients to take drug with food and to observe stools for evidence of bleeding (bright red blood, black tarry-looking stools)
Abciximab (ReoPro)	Is an antibody that binds to the receptors on the platelet surface that normally bind the sticky glycoproteins, preventing platelet adhesion	Contains human and mouse proteins that may induce an allergic reaction	Teach client to observe for any skin rashes, swelling, or difficulty breathing that may indicate an allergy to the drug
Clopidogrel (Plavix)	Prevents ADP from binding to platelet receptors, inhibiting platelet activation	Platelet function remains low for up to 5 days after the drug is discontinued	Instruct clients to avoid dental work and invasive procedures while taking this drug or to inform health care professionals that he or she is taking the drug
		Irritates gastric lining and promotes gastrointestinal ulceration	Teach clients to take drug with food and to observe stools for evidence of bleeding (bright red blood, black tarry-looking stools)
		Prolongs bleeding	Same as for aspirin
Dipyridamole (Persantine)	Increases levels of adenosine which then inhibits ADP formation and platelet activation	Produces peripheral vasodilation	Teach clients that their blood pressure could be lower than normal during position changes and that they should move slowly when changing from a sitting or lying position to a standing position
		Prolongs bleeding	Same as for aspirin

Data from Facts and Comparisons. (2004). *Drug facts and comparisons* (58th ed.). St. Louis: Author.

tion of fibrinolytic drugs is the selective breakdown of formed fibrin clots with less effect on clot formation.

The use of fibrinolytic drugs results in the best clot breakdown with less disruption of blood clotting. These drugs are the first-line therapy for problems caused by small, localized formed clots such as myocardial infarction (MI), limited arterial thrombosis, and thrombotic strokes. For some problems, such as MI, these drugs are only given within the first 6 hours after the onset of symptoms. This time limitation is not related to drug activity because fibrinolytic agents can break down clots older than 6 hours. Rather, the tissue that has been anoxic for more than 6 hours as a result of an acute event is not likely to benefit from this therapy, making the risks to the client greater than the advantages.

Fibrinolytic therapy has a limited role when clotting is extensive, such as in deep vein thrombophlebitis. With these problems, clots are very large compared with the size of the clots found in the coronary arteries. The amount of drug and the duration of therapy needed for breakdown of such large clots are cost prohibitive and risky. Many of these clots are not easily accessed for direct infusion of the fibrinolytic drug. In addition, these clots are large and the drug response creates many small clots that can enter circulation **(emboli).** These emboli could potentially occlude other blood vessels. The chance of emboli formation is much greater when degrading large venous clots than it is for degrading smaller arterial clots. In such cases, mechanical thrombolytic devices may be able to debulk the clot. These devices remove debris or break it into fragments small enough to pass through capillary beds without causing vessel occlusion.

One exception for using fibrinolytics in large clots is the newly approved use of urokinase for adults who have massive pulmonary emboli with obstruction of blood flow either to an entire lobe or to multiple segments (see Chapter 35 for further discussion of pulmonary emboli therapy).

PLATELET INHIBITORS

Platelet inhibitors are drugs that either prevent platelets from becoming active or prevent activated platelets from clumping together. The most widely used drug for this effect is aspirin, which inhibits the production of substances that can trigger platelet activation, such as thromboxane. Other drugs change the platelet membrane, reducing its "stickiness," or prevent activators from binding to platelet receptor sites. Table 42-3 lists the actions and nursing implications for specific platelet inhibitors.

ASSESSMENT TECHNIQUES

History

DEMOGRAPHIC DATA

Chart 42-2 lists questions based on Gordon's Functional Health Patterns to ask during assessment of hematologic function. Age and gender are important variables to obtain when assessing the client's hematologic status. Bone marrow and immune activity diminish with age.

WOMEN'S HEALTH CONSIDERATIONS

At all ages, women have lower blood cell counts than do men. This difference is greater during menstrual years. This gender difference may be related to a blood dilution caused by fluid retention from female hormones or to differences in bone marrow activity.

FAMILY HISTORY AND GENETIC RISK

Obtaining an accurate family history is important because many bleeding disorders are inherited. Ask whether anyone in the family has had hemophilia, frequent nosebleeds, postpartum hemorrhages, excessive bleeding after tooth extractions, or heavy bruising after relatively mild trauma. Obtain family information about sickle cell disease or sickle cell trait. Although sickle cell disease is seen most often among African Americans, anyone can have the trait.

PERSONAL HISTORY

Personal factors to be included in the hematologic assessment are liver function, the presence of known immunologic or hematologic disorders, and current drug use. Because the liver makes clotting factors, ask about manifestations that may indicate liver problems, such as jaundice, anemia, and gallstones.

Ask the client about use of blood "thinners" such as warfarin (Coumadin, Warfilone✱), aspirin, and other nonsteroidal anti-inflammatory drugs (NSAIDs). A person who takes aspirin daily may have bleeding problems, and many over-the-counter drugs contain aspirin or other drugs that disrupt platelet clumping. Check all drugs that the client is using or has used in the past 3 weeks. Ask about the use of antibiotics because prolonged antibiotic therapy can lead to clotting problems or bone marrow depression. Table 42-4 lists drugs known to change hematologic function. Previous radiation therapy may result in some permanent impairment of hematologic function if marrow-forming bones were in the radiation path.

It is also important to collect information about occupation, hobbies, and the location of housing. This information may indicate an exposure to agents or chemicals that affect bone marrow growth and hematologic function.

CHART 42-2

Hematologic Assessment
USING GORDON'S FUNCTIONAL HEALTH PATTERNS

Activity-Exercise Pattern

- How does your energy level seem to you compared with last year at this time?
- Do you feel rested after a typical night's sleep?
- Have you experienced any dizziness or light-headedness?
- Does your heart ever seem to pound?
- How much exercise do you get? How often? What type?
- Do you feel you have enough energy to do what you want or need to do?

Nutrition-Metabolic Pattern

- Have you noticed any change in your skin lately?
- How easily do you bruise?
- Do your gums ever bleed? Under what conditions?
- How much meat do you eat in a week?
- How often do you eat salads or other green leafy vegetables?
- Are you taking any vitamin or mineral supplements?
- Do your feet and hands usually feel warm or cold?
- Has your weight changed by 5 pounds or more this year?
- How often do you take aspirin or any other nonsteroidal anti-inflammatory drug?
- What medications do you take daily?

Modified from Gordon, M. (2002). *Manual of nursing diagnosis* (10th ed.). St. Louis: Mosby.

DIET HISTORY

Dietary pattern can alter cell quality and affect blood clotting. Ask clients to record everything eaten during the previous week. Use this information to determine the causes of anemias and of protein, mineral, or vitamin deficiencies. Diets high in fat and carbohydrates and low in protein, iron, and vitamins can cause many types of anemia and decrease the functions of all blood cells.

Ask the clients about alcohol consumption. Chronic alcoholism can cause nutritional deficiencies and liver impairment, both of which reduce blood clotting.

Certain dietary habits can enhance blood clotting. Diets high in vitamin K may increase the rate of blood clotting. Assess the amount of raw, leafy green vegetables that the client eats and whether he or she routinely takes supplemental vitamins. Also assess the amount of calcium in the diet or in supplements.

SOCIOECONOMIC STATUS

Assess the client's ability to understand and follow instructions related to diet, procedures and tests, and therapeutic regimens. Ask about personal resources, such as finances and social support. A person with a poor income may have a diet low in iron and protein.

CURRENT HEALTH PROBLEMS

Determine whether the client has had swelling of lymph nodes or excessive bruising or bleeding and whether the bleeding was spontaneous or induced by trauma. Ask about the amount and duration of bleeding after routine dental work.

TABLE 42-4 Drugs Impairing the Hematologic System

Generic Name	Common Trade Names
Drugs Causing Bone Marrow Suppression	
Altretamine	Hexalen, Hexastat🍁
Amphotericin B	Fungizone
Azathioprine	Imuran
Chemotherapeutic agents*	
Chloramphenicol	Chloromycetin, Novochlorocap🍁
Chromic phosphate	Phosphocol
Colchicine	(Generic only)
Didanosine	Videx
Eflornithine	Ornidyl
Foscarnet sodium	Foscavir
Ganciclovir	Cytovene
Interferon alfa	Actimmune, Alferon, Intron-A, Roferon-A, Wellferon
Pentamidine	Pentam 300, NebuPent, Pentacarinat🍁
Sodium iodide	Iodopen
Zalcitabine	HIVID
Zidovudine	AZT, Retrovir, Novo-AZT🍁
Drugs Causing Hemolysis	
Acetohydroxamic acid	Lithostat
Chlorpropamide	Diabinese, Glucamide, Novo-Propamide🍁
Doxapram	Dopram
Glyburide	DiaBeta, Micronase, Euglucon🍁
Mefenamic acid	Ponstel, Ponstan🍁
Menadiol diphosphate	Synkayvite
Methyldopa	Aldomet, Dopamet🍁
Nitrofurantoin	Macrodantin, Novo-Furantoin🍁
Amoxicillin	Amoxil, Augmentin, Apo-Amoxi🍁
Drugs Causing Hemolysis—*cont'd*	
Penicillin G benzathine	Bicillin, Crystapen
Penicillin V	Pen-Vee K, Pen Vee, Nu-Pen-VK🍁
Primaquine	(Generic only)
Procainamide hydrochloride	Procan-SR, Promine, Pronestyl
Quinidine polygalacturonate	Cardioquin, Quinalan, Novoquinidin🍁
Quinine	Legatrin, Quindan
Sulfonamides	Sulfamethoxazole (Gantanol), sulfisoxazole (Gantrisin, Novo-Soxazole🍁)
Tolbutamide	Oramide, Orinase, Apo-Tolbutamide🍁, Mobenol🍁
Vitamin K	AquaMEPHYTON, Konakion
Drugs Disrupting Platelet Action	
Aspirin	Anacin, Ascriptin, Bufferin, Ecotrin, Entrophen🍁, Riphen🍁, Triaphen🍁
Carbenicillin	Geopen, Pyopen🍁
Carindacillin	Geocillin
Dipyridamole	Persantine, Apo-Dipyridamole🍁, Novo-Dipiradol🍁
Moxalactam	Moxam
Pentoxifylline	Trental
Sulfinpyrazone	Anturane, Antazone🍁, Novopyrazone🍁
Ticarcillin	Ticar
Ticlopidine	Ticlid
Valproic acid	Dalpro, Depakene, Epival🍁

Data from United States Pharmacopeia Dispensing Information (USP DI): Vol. I. *Drug information for the health care professional* (20th ed.). Englewood, CO: Micromedex.
* General categories of chemotherapeutic agents include alkylating agents, antimitotics, antitumor antibiotics, and antimetabolites.

Determine whether a woman has **menorrhagia** (excessive menstrual flow). Ask her to estimate the number of pads or tampons used during the most recent menstrual cycle and whether this amount represents a change from her usual pattern of menstrual flow. Determine whether clots are present in menstrual blood. If the client has had menstrual clots, ask her to estimate clot size using coins or fruit for comparison ("clots are dime-sized" or "clots are the size of lemons").

Assess whether the client has dyspnea on exertion, palpitations, frequent infections, fevers, recent weight loss, headaches, or paresthesias. Any or all of these symptoms may occur with hematologic disease.

The single most common symptom of anemia is fatigue. Ask clients about feeling tired, needing more rest, or losing endurance during normal activities. Ask them to compare their activities during the past month with those of the same month a year ago. Determine whether they have other symptoms of anemia, such as vertigo, tinnitus, and a sore tongue.

Physical Assessment

Assess the whole body; hematologic dysfunction affects all systems. Certain problems are specific for hematologic assessment in older adults (see Chart 42-1).

SKIN ASSESSMENT

Inspect the color of the skin for pallor or jaundice and of the mucous membranes and nail beds for pallor or cyanosis. Pallor of the gums, conjunctivae, and palmar creases indicates decreased hemoglobin levels. Assess the gums for active bleeding in response to light pressure or brushing the teeth with a soft-bristled brush and any lesions or draining areas. Inspect for petechiae and large bruises **(ecchymoses). Petechiae** are pinpoint hemorrhagic lesions in the skin. Bruises may be confluent or clustered. For hospitalized clients, determine whether there is bleeding from sites such as nasogastric tubes, endotracheal tubes, central lines, peripheral intravenous (IV) sites, or Foley catheters. Check the skin turgor and ask about itching because dry skin or itching can indicate hematologic disease.

CULTURAL CONSIDERATIONS

Pallor and cyanosis are more easily detected in people with darker skin by examining the oral mucous membranes and the conjunctiva of the eye. Jaundice can be seen more easily on the roof of the mouth. Petechiae may be visible only on the palms of the hands or the soles of the feet. Bruises can be seen as darker areas of skin and palpated as slight swellings or irregular skin surfaces. Ask the client about pain when skin surfaces are touched lightly or palpated. (Chapter 69 provides tips for assessing darker skin.)

HEAD AND NECK ASSESSMENT

Check for pallor or ulceration of the oral mucosa. The tongue may be completely smooth in pernicious anemia and iron deficiency anemia or smooth and red in nutritional deficiencies. These manifestations may occur with fissures at the corners of the mouth. Assess for jaundice of the sclera.

Inspect and palpate all lymph node areas. Document any lymph node enlargement, including whether palpation of the enlarged node causes pain. It is important to determine whether the enlarged node moves or remains fixed with palpation.

RESPIRATORY ASSESSMENT

Assess the rate and depth of respiration while the client is at rest as well as during and after mild physical activity (e.g., walking 20 steps in 10 seconds). Note whether the client can complete a 10-word sentence without stopping for a breath. Assess whether the client is fatigued easily, has shortness of breath at rest or on exertion, or needs extra pillows to sleep comfortably at night. Many anemias cause these symptoms.

CARDIOVASCULAR ASSESSMENT

Observe for heaves, distended neck veins, edema, or signs of phlebitis. Auscultate for murmurs, gallops, irregular rhythms, and abnormal blood pressure (BP). Systolic BP tends to be lower than normal in clients with anemia. If hypercellularity is present, BP is higher than normal. Severe anemias can cause enlargement of the right ventricle and heart disease.

RENAL AND URINARY ASSESSMENT

The kidneys have many blood vessels, and bleeding problems may manifest as overt or occult **hematuria** (blood in the urine). Inspect a voided sample of urine for color. Hematuria may appear as grossly bloody red or dark brownish gold urine. Test the urine for proteins with a urine test dipstick because hematologic problems may increase the protein content of the urine. Also test the urine sample for occult blood (Hemoccult test).

MUSCULOSKELETAL ASSESSMENT

Rib or sternal tenderness is an important sign of hematologic malignancy. Examine the superficial surfaces of all bones, including the ribs and sternum, by applying intermittent firm pressure with the fingertips. Assess the range of joint motion and document any swelling or joint pain.

ABDOMINAL ASSESSMENT

The normal adult spleen is usually not palpable. An enlarged spleen, however, occurs with many hematologic problems. An enlarged spleen may be detected by percussion, although palpation is more reliable. The spleen lies just beneath the abdominal wall, under the ribs on the left side. When it is enlarged, the spleen can be identified by its movement during respiration. During palpation have the client lie in a relaxed, supine position while you stand on the client's right and palpate the left upper quadrant. *Palpate gently and cautiously because an enlarged spleen may be tender and easily ruptured.*

Palpating the edge of the liver in the right upper quadrant of the abdomen can detect hepatic enlargement, which is often associated with hematologic problems. The normal liver may be palpable as much as 4 to 5 cm below the right costal margin but is usually not palpable in the epigastrium.

A common cause of anemia among older adults is a chronically bleeding gastrointestinal lesion. If the lesion or open area is located in the stomach or the small intestine, obvious blood may not be visible in the stool, or such a small amount is passed each day that the client is not aware of it. Therefore obtain a stool specimen for occult blood testing.

CENTRAL NERVOUS SYSTEM ASSESSMENT

Examination of cranial nerves and neurologic function is important in hematologic assessment because some problems cause specific nervous system manifestations. Vitamin B_{12} deficiency impairs cerebral, olfactory, spinal cord, and peripheral nerve function, and severe chronic deficiency may cause permanent neurologic degeneration. Many neurologic problems can develop in clients who have hematologic malignancies as a consequence of bleeding, infection, or tumor spread. When the client with a known or suspected bleeding disorder has any head trauma, expand the assessment to include frequent neurologic checks and mental status examinations (see Chapter 44).

Other clinical manifestations that occur with impaired hematologic function include fever, chills, and night sweats.

Psychosocial Assessment

The client with hematologic problems may have a chronic illness (e.g., hemophilia or cancer) or an acute episode of a chronic disease (e.g., pernicious anemia). In either case, each person brings his or her own coping style to the illness. Develop a rapport with the client and learn what coping mechanisms he or she has used successfully during past illness or crises.

Ask the client and family members about social support networks, community resources, and financial health. A problem in any of these areas can interfere with the client's adherence to therapy and, ultimately, recovery.

Critical Thinking Challenge

The client is a 22-year-old woman who is in the emergency room for an ankle injury that occurred while she was playing volleyball at a family picnic. Her complete blood count indicates a total white blood count of 8000, erythrocyte count of 200,000, hematocrit of 22%, and hemoglobin level of 8.5 g. She says she is very tired and has palpitations on exertion. Her vital signs are P 94, R 26, BP 102/70. Her oxygen saturation measured by pulse oximetry is 98% on room air.

1. Are these counts considered normal or abnormal? If any are abnormal, are they high or low?
2. Do her vital signs indicate any type of hematologic problem? Explain why or why not.
3. What specific questions regarding family history, recent health history, diet history, and personal history should you ask?

evolve For suggested answer guidelines, go to http://evolve.elsevier.com/Iggy/.

Diagnostic Assessment

LABORATORY TESTS

In hematologic disease, the most definitive signs are often the laboratory test results. Chart 42-3 lists laboratory data associated with hematologic function.

CHART 42-3

LABORATORY PROFILE
Hematologic Assessment

Test	Reference	Range	International Reference Units	Significance of Abnormal Findings
Red blood cell (RBC) count	18-64 yr	*Females:* 4.2-5.4 million/μL	4.2-5.4 × 10^{12} cells/L	*Decreased levels* indicate possible anemia or hemorrhage.
		Males: 4.7-6.1 million/μL	4.7-6.1 × 10^{12} cells/L	*Increased levels* indicate possible chronic hypoxia or polycythemia vera.
	>64 yr	*Females:* 3.8-5.2 million/μL	3.8-5.2 × 10^{12} cells/L	
		Males: 3.8-5.8 million/μL	3.8-5.8 × 10^{12} cells/L	
Hemoglobin (Hgb)	18-64 yr	*Females:* 12-16 g/dL	112-160 g/L	Same as for RBC.
		Males: 14-18 g/dL	140-180 g/L	
	>64 yr	*Females:* 11.7-16.1 g/dL	117-161 g/L	
		Males: 12.6-17.4 g/dL	126-174 g/L	
Hematocrit (Hct)	18-64 yr	*Females:* 37-47%	0.37-0.47 fraction	Same as for RBC.
		Males: 42-52%	0.42-0.52 fraction	
	>64 yr	*Females:* 35%-47%	0.35-0.47 fraction	
		Males: 37%-51%	0.37-0.51 fraction	
Mean cell hemoglobin (MCV)		80-95 mm³	Same as reference range	*Increased levels* indicate macrocytic cells, possible anemia. *Decreased levels* indicate microcytic cells, possible iron deficiency anemia.
Mean cell hemoglobin (MCH)		27-31 pg/cell	Same as reference range	Same as for MCV.
Mean cell hemoglobin concentration (MCHC)		32-36 g/dL cells	320-370 g/L	*Increased levels* may indicate spherocytosis or anemia. *Decreased levels* may indicate iron deficiency anemia or a hemoglobinopathy.
White blood cell (WBC) count		5000-10,000/μL	5.0-10.0 × 10^9 cells/L	*Increased levels* are associated with infection, inflammation, autoimmune disorders, and leukemia. *Decreased levels* may indicate prolonged infection or bone marrow suppression.
Reticulocyte count		0.5%-0.2% of RBCs	0.005-0.020 fraction	*Increased* levels may indicate chronic blood loss. *Decreased levels* indicate possible inadequate RBC production.
Total iron binding capacity (TIBC)		250-460 mcg/dL	45-82 μmol/L	*Increased levels* indicate iron deficiency. *Decreased levels* may indicate anemia, hemorrhage, hemolysis.
Iron (Fe)		*Females:* 60-160 mcg/dL *Males:* 80-180 mcg/dL	11-29 μmol/L 14-32 μmol/L	*Increased levels* indicate iron excess, hemochromocytosis, liver disorders, megaloblastic anemia. *Decreased levels* indicate possible iron deficiency anemia, hemorrhage.
Serum ferritin		*Females:* 10-150 ng/mL *Males:* 12-300 ng/mL	Same as reference range	Same as for iron.
Platelet count		150,000-400,000 mm³	150-400 × 10^9/L	*Increased levels* may indicate polycythemia vera or malignancy. *Decreased levels* may indicate bone marrow suppression, autoimmune disease, hypersplenism.
Hemoglobin electrophoresis		Hgb A_1: 95%-98% Hgb A_2: 2%-3% Hgb F: 0.8%-2% Hgb S: 0% Hgb C: 0%	>0.95 fraction 0.020-0.030 fraction <0.02 fraction 0.0 fraction 0.0 fraction	*Variations* indicate hemoglobinopathies.

Values for people over 64 years from Tietz, N. (1995). *Clinical guide to laboratory tests* (3rd ed.). Philadelphia: W.B. Saunders.
pg, picogram; *INR*, International Normalized Ratio.

CHART 42-3

LABORATORY PROFILE

Hematologic Assessment—*cont'd*

Test	Reference Range	International Reference Units	Significance of Abnormal Findings
Direct Coombs' and indirect Coombs' test	Negative	Negative	*Positive findings* indicate antibodies to RBCs.
Prothrombin time (PT)	11-12.5 sec	Patient PT/normal PT (INR)	*Increased time* indicates possible deficiency of clotting factors V and VII. *Decreased time* may indicate vitamin K excess.
Bleeding time	1-9 min	Same as reference range	*Increased time* may indicate inadequate platelet function or number, clotting factor deficiencies.
Fibrin degradation products	<10 mcg/mL	<10 mg/L	*Increased levels* may indicate disseminated intravascular coagulation of fibrinolysis.

Tests of Cell Number and Function

COMPLETE BLOOD COUNT

A complete blood count (CBC) includes a number of studies: red blood cell (RBC) count, white blood cell (WBC) count, hematocrit, and hemoglobin level. The RBC count measures circulating RBCs in 1 mm^3 of blood. The WBC count measures all leukocytes present in 1 mm^3 of blood. To determine the percentages of different types of leukocytes circulating in the blood, a WBC count with differential leukocyte count is performed (Chapter 23). The hematocrit (Hct) is calculated as the percentage of red blood cells in the total blood volume. The hemoglobin level is the total amount of hemoglobin in blood.

The CBC can measure other variables of the RBCs, including mean corpuscular volume (MCV), mean corpuscular hemoglobin (MCH), and mean corpuscular hemoglobin concentration (MCHC). MCV measures the average volume or size of a single RBC and is useful for classifying anemias. When the MCV is elevated, the cell is abnormally large **(macrocytic)**, as seen in megaloblastic anemias. When the MCV is decreased, the cell is abnormally small **(microcytic)**, as seen in iron deficiency anemia. The MCH is the average amount of hemoglobin by weight in a single RBC. The MCHC measures the average amount of hemoglobin by percentage in a single RBC. When the MCHC is decreased, the cell has a hemoglobin deficiency and is hypochromic, as in iron deficiency anemia.

RETICULOCYTE COUNT

Another hematologic test helpful in determining bone marrow function is the reticulocyte count. A reticulocyte is an immature RBC that still has its nucleus. An elevated reticulocyte count indicates increased RBC production by the bone marrow. Normally about 2% of circulating RBCs are reticulocytes. An elevated reticulocyte count is desirable in an anemic client or after hemorrhage because this indicates that the bone marrow is responding appropriately to a decrease in the total RBC mass. An elevated reticulocyte count without a precipitating cause usually indicates health problems, such as polycythemia vera.

HEMOGLOBIN ELECTROPHORESIS

Hemoglobin electrophoresis detects abnormal forms of hemoglobin, such as hemoglobin S in sickle cell disease. Hemoglobin A is the major type of hemoglobin in the normal RBC from an adult. Decreased hemoglobin A levels with increasing levels of other types of hemoglobin indicate some hematologic problems, such as sickle cell disease.

LEUKOCYTE ALKALINE PHOSPHATASE

Leukocyte alkaline phosphatase (LAP) is an enzyme produced by normal mature neutrophils. Elevated LAP levels occur during episodes of infection or stress. An elevated neutrophil count without an elevation in LAP level occurs with chronic myelogenous leukemia

COOMBS' TEST

The two Coombs' tests (direct and indirect) are used for blood typing. The direct test detects the presence of antibodies (also called antiglobulins) against RBCs that may be attached to a person's RBCs. Although healthy people can make these antibodies, in certain diseases (e.g., systemic lupus erythematosus, mononucleosis, lymphomas) these antibodies are directed against the client's own RBCs. The presence of these antibodies usually causes a hemolytic anemia.

The indirect Coombs' test detects the presence of circulating antiglobulins. The test is used to determine whether the client has serum antibodies to the type of RBCs that he or she is about to receive by blood transfusion.

SERUM FERRITIN, TRANSFERRIN, AND TOTAL IRON-BINDING CAPACITY

Serum ferritin, transferrin, and the total iron-binding capacity (TIBC) tests measure iron levels. Abnormal levels of iron and TIBC occur with hematologic problems, including iron deficiency anemia.

The serum ferritin test measures the amount of iron present as free iron in the plasma. The amount of serum ferritin is related to the amount of intracellular iron and represents 1% of the total body iron stores. Therefore the serum ferritin level provides a means to assess total iron stores. People with serum ferritin levels within 10 g of the normal range for their gender have adequate iron stores; people with levels 10 g or more lower than the normal range have inadequate iron stores and have difficulty recovering from any hemorrhagic event.

Transferrin is a protein that transports iron from the intestines to cell storage sites. Transferrin is not easily measured, but by measuring the amount of iron that can be bound to serum transferrin indirectly one can determine whether an adequate amount of transferrin is present. This test is the total iron binding capacity (TIBC) test. In healthy people only about 30% of the transferrin is bound to iron in the blood. TIBC is measured by taking a sample of blood and adding measured amounts of iron to it. TIBC is calculated when the blood no longer binds the iron but allows it to precipitate. TIBC increases when a person is deficient in serum iron and stored iron levels. Such a value indicates that an adequate amount of transferrin is present but less than 30% of it is bound to serum iron.

Tests Measuring Bleeding and Coagulation

CAPILLARY FRAGILITY TEST

The capillary fragility test, or Rumpel-Leede test, measures vascular hemostatic function. The intracapillary pressure in the arm is increased by occluding venous outflow or by applying controlled negative pressure to a skin area. A blood pressure cuff is usually inflated to a pressure halfway between the systolic and diastolic pressures. This pressure is maintained for 5 minutes and the petechiae that appear distal to the cuff are counted. Normally 5 to 10 petechiae appear. When the number of petechiae that form increases, the cause of excessive bleeding or bruising is capillary fragility rather than poor platelet action.

BLEEDING TIME TEST

The bleeding time test evaluates vascular and platelet activity during hemostasis. A special spring-loaded lancet that makes a uniform wound depth is applied to the forearm while a blood pressure cuff remains inflated at 40 mm Hg. Blood is blotted from the site at 30-second intervals, and the time required for the bleeding to stop is recorded. Normal bleeding time ranges from 1 to 9 minutes.

PROTHROMBIN TIME

The prothrombin time (PT) measures how long blood takes to clot. This test reflects how much of the clotting factors II, V, VII, and X is present and how well they are functioning. When enough of these clotting factors are present and functioning, the PT shows blood clotting between 11 and 13 seconds or within 85% to 100% of the time needed for a control sample of blood to clot. PT is prolonged when one or more clotting factors is deficient, such as when liver disease is present. Sodium warfarin (Coumadin, Warfilone✱) therapy is also monitored using PT levels. Usually warfarin therapy is considered appropriate when the PT is prolonged by one and a half to two times the client's normal PT value.

Facilities are using the PT test less often to assess blood clotting because control blood is taken from different people and may not be the same even in one laboratory from one day to the next. To reduce PT errors as a result of control blood variation or in some of the chemicals used in the test, the **International Normalized Ratio (INR)** is used to assess clotting time.

INTERNATIONAL NORMALIZED RATIO

The INR measures the same process as the PT in a slightly different way: by establishing a normal mean or standard for PT. The INR is calculated by dividing the client's PT by the established standard PT. A normal INR ranges between 0.7 and 1.8. When using the INR to monitor warfarin therapy, the goal is usually to maintain the client's INR is between 2.0 and 3.0 regardless of the actual PT in seconds. It is important to remember, however, that the desired INR range for any client is individualized for specific client factors.

PARTIAL THROMBOPLASTIN TIME

The partial thromboplastin time (PTT) assesses the intrinsic clotting cascade and evaluates the action of factors II, V, VIII, IX, XI, and XII. PTT is prolonged whenever any of these factors is deficient, such as in hemophilia or disseminated intravascular coagulation (DIC). Because factors II, IX, and X are vitamin K–dependent and are produced in the liver, liver disease can decrease their levels and prolong the PTT. Heparin (Calciparin, Hepalean✱) therapy is monitored by PTT. Desired therapeutic ranges for anticoagulation are 1.5 to 2.0 times normal values.

Controversy exists as to whether this test is accurate when the blood sample is taken through a vascular access device (e.g., arterial line or a normal saline lock) instead of through a separate new venipuncture. With an appropriate discard, samples obtained through vascular access devices accurately reflect the client's aPTT.

PLATELET AGGLUTINATION/AGGREGATION

Platelet aggregation, or the ability to clump, is tested by mixing the client's plasma with a substance called ristocetin. The degree of clumping is noted. Aggregation can be impaired in von Willebrand's disease and during the use of drugs such as aspirin, anti-inflammatory agents, psychotropic agents, and platelet inhibitors.

RADIOGRAPHIC EXAMINATIONS

Assessment of the client with a suspected hematologic abnormality can include radioisotopic imaging. Isotopes are used to evaluate the bone marrow for sites of active blood cell formation and sites of iron storage. Radioactive colloids are used to determine organ size and liver and spleen function.

The client is given a radioactive isotope intravenously about 3 hours before the procedure. The client is then taken to the nuclear medicine department for the scan, where he or she must lie still for about an hour. No special client preparation or follow-up care is needed for these tests.

Standard x-rays may be used to diagnose some hematologic disorders. For example, multiple myeloma causes characteristic bone destruction, with a "Swiss cheese" appearance on x-ray.

BONE MARROW ASPIRATION AND BIOPSY

Bone marrow aspiration or biopsy is often performed to evaluate the client's hematologic status when other tests show persistent abnormal findings. Results can provide important information about bone marrow function, including the production of red blood cells (RBCs), white blood cells (WBCs), and platelets. Bone marrow aspiration and bone marrow biopsy are similar invasive procedures. In a bone marrow aspiration, cells and fluids are suctioned from the bone marrow. In a bone marrow biopsy, solid tissue and cells are obtained by coring out an area of bone marrow with a large-bore needle.

A physician's order and a signed informed consent are obtained from the client before a bone marrow aspiration or biopsy is performed. Bone marrow aspiration may be performed by a physician, a sanctioned clinical nurse specialist, a nurse practitioner, or a physician assistant, depending on the agency's policy and regional law. The procedure may be performed at the client's bedside, in an examination room, or in a laboratory.

After learning what specific tests will be performed on the marrow, check the facility's procedure manual and the hematology laboratory to determine how to handle the specimen. Some tests require that heparin or other solutions be added to the specimen.

CLIENT PREPARATION. Most clients have anxiety or fear before a bone marrow aspiration. Clients who have had a bone marrow aspiration in the past may have less anxiety or more anxiety, depending on their previous experience. You can help reduce anxiety and allay fears by providing accurate information and emotional support. Some clients like to have their hand held during the procedure; others may want you to hug or hold their entire upper body.

Explain the procedure to the client and tell him or her that you will stay during the entire procedure. Occasionally a friend or family member is permitted to be present to hold the client's hand and provide additional emotional support. If a local anesthetic is used, tell the client that the injection will feel like a stinging or burning sensation. Tell him or her to expect a heavy sensation of pressure and pushing while the needle is being inserted. Some clients also can hear a crunching sound or feel a scraping sensation as the needle punctures the bone. Explain that a brief sensation of painful pulling will be experienced as the marrow is being aspirated by mild suction in the syringe. If a biopsy is performed, the client may feel more pressure and discomfort as the needle is rotated into the bone.

The client is assisted onto an examining table, and the site (most commonly the iliac crest) is exposed. If this site is not available or if more marrow is needed, the sternum can be used. If the iliac crest is the site, the client is usually placed in the prone position or, occasionally, in the side-lying position. Depending on the tests to be performed on the specimen, a laboratory technician may also be present to ensure appropriate handling of the specimen.

PROCEDURE. The procedure usually lasts from 5 to 15 minutes. Clients may have pain. The type and the amount of anesthesia or sedation depend on the physician's preference, the client's preference and previous experience with bone marrow aspiration and biopsy, and the setting.

A local anesthetic agent is injected into the skin around the site. The client may also receive a mild tranquilizer or a rapid-acting sedative, such as midazolam (Versed) or lorazepam (Ativan, Apo-Lorazepam♣, Novo-Lorazem♣). Some clients do well with guided imagery or autohypnosis.

Aspiration or biopsy procedures are invasive, and sterile precautions are observed. The skin over the site is cleaned with a disinfectant solution. For an aspiration, the needle is inserted with a twisting motion and the marrow is aspirated by pulling back on the plunger of the syringe. When sufficient marrow has been aspirated to ensure accurate analysis, the needle is rapidly withdrawn while the tissues are supported at the site. For a biopsy, a small skin incision is made and the biopsy needle is inserted through the skin opening. Pressure and several twisting motions are needed to ensure coring and loosening of an adequate amount of marrow tissue. Apply external pressure to the site until hemostasis is ensured. A pressure dressing or sandbags may be applied to reduce bleeding at the site.

FOLLOW-UP CARE. Cover the site with a dressing after bleeding is controlled, and closely observe it for 24 hours for signs of bleeding and infection. A mild analgesic (aspirin free) may be given for discomfort, and ice packs can be placed over the site to limit bruising. Instruct the client to inspect the site every 2 hours for the first 24 hours and to note the presence of active bleeding or bruising. Advise him or her to avoid contact sports or any activity that might result in trauma to the site for 48 hours.

Information obtained from bone marrow aspiration or biopsy reflects the degree and quality of bone marrow activity present. The counts made on a marrow specimen can indicate whether stem cells, blast cells, committed cells, and more mature cell forms are present in the expected quantities and proportions. In addition, bone marrow aspiration or biopsy can confirm the spread of cancer cells from other tumor sites.

Critical Thinking Challenge

The client is a 70-year-old man who is scheduled to have a bone marrow aspiration in 1 week to determine the cause of abnormal white blood cell and red blood cell counts. He has been healthy otherwise, and his only drugs are a daily multiple vitamin and one aspirin per day (81 mg). He is very concerned about the pain of the procedure and the possible results. In addition, he wants to travel by air to attend his grandson's graduation in 10 days.

1. What is your care priority for this client?
2. What will you tell him regarding pain or pain management?
3. What should you tell him about air travel within 4 days after having the procedure?

evolve For suggested answer guidelines, go to http://evolve.elsevier.com/Iggy/.

GET READY for the NCLEX Examination!

KEY POINTS

Safe Effective Care Environment

- Use good handwashing techniques before providing any care to a client who is either immunocompromised or immunodeficient.
- Use bleeding precautions (see Chart 43-11) for any client with a bleeding problem or who is receiving anticoagulants, thrombolytics, or platelet inhibitors.

Health Promotion and Maintenance

- Teach people to avoid unnecessary contact with environmental chemicals or toxins. If contact cannot be avoided, teach people to use safety precautions.
- Instruct clients about the importance of eating a diet with adequate amounts of foods that are good sources of iron, folic acid, and vitamin B_{12}.
- Teach clients who are taking anticoagulants or platelet inhibitors on a daily basis to use a soft-bristled toothbrush and to avoid flossing.
- Encourage clients who are confined to bed for any reason or who are recovering from surgery to turn and perform leg exercises at least every 2 hours.
- Instruct clients to stop taking aspirin, aspirin-containing products, or most nonsteroidal anti-inflammatory drugs (NSAIDs) 10 days to 2 weeks before having surgery or dental work.

Psychosocial Integrity

- Explain all procedures, restrictions, medications, and follow-up care to the client and family.
- Ask clients about their activity level and whether they are satisfied with the energy they have for activities.

Physiological Integrity

- Teach the side effects of the drugs to clients who are taking anticoagulants or platelet inhibitors at home.
- Teach clients who are taking anticoagulants or platelet inhibitors to assess themselves daily for increased bleeding. They should check their gums and toothbrush for fresh bleeding, look at voided urine or evacuated stool for color changes indicating bleeding, and examine their skin for the presence of bruises or petechiae.
- Stress the importance of keeping all appointments for blood testing for clients who are receiving anticoagulation therapy.
- Instruct clients taking warfarin to keep a food diary to determine whether eating habits are influencing blood clotting (especially keeping track of the amount of leafy, green raw vegetables).
- Apply an ice pack to the needle site after a bone marrow aspiration or biopsy.
- Check the needle site at least every 2 hours after a bone marrow aspiration or biopsy. If the client is going home, teach the client and family how to assess the site for bleeding and when to seek assistance.
- Instruct clients to avoid activities that may traumatize the site after a bone marrow aspiration or biopsy.

ADDITIONAL STUDY RESOURCES

Go to your Student CD-ROM for Review Questions for the NCLEX Examination.

evolve Go to http://evolve.elsevier.com/Iggy/ for Integrated Management of Care Questions for the NCLEX Examination.

SELECTED BIBLIOGRAPHY

Beitz, J. (2004). Anticoagulant-induced skin necrosis. *American Journal of Nursing, 104*(4), 31-32.

Berne, R., et al. (2004). *Physiology* (5th ed.). St. Louis: Mosby.

Buchsel, P., Murphy, B., & Newton, S. (2002). Epoetin alfa: Current and future indications and nursing implications. *Clinical Journal of Oncology Nursing, 6*(5), 261-267.

Cagen, D., Franco, M., & Vasquez, D. (2002). The ABCs of low blood cell count. *Clinical Journal of Oncology Nursing, 6*(1), 34-36.

Cleveland, K. (2003). Argatroban: A new treatment option for heparin-induced thrombocytopenia. *Critical Care Nurse, 23*(6), 61-66.

Ebersole, P., Hess, P., & Luggen, A. (2004). *Toward healthy aging: Human needs and nursing response* (6th ed.). St. Louis: Mosby.

Facts and Comparisons. (2004). Drug facts and comparisons (58th ed.). St. Louis: Author.

Gibbar-Clements, T., et al. (2000). The challenge of warfarin therapy. *American Journal of Nursing, 100*(3), 38-40.

Gordon, M. (2002). *Manual of nursing diagnosis* (10th ed.). St. Louis: Mosby.

Hirsh, J., Dalen, J., & Guyatt, G. (2001). Oral anticoagulants: Mechanisms of action, clinical effectiveness, and optimal therapeutic range. *Chest, 119*(Suppl 1), 8S-21S.

Horner, B., & Myers, S. (2004). Don't miss HIT (heparin-induced thrombocytopenia). *Burns, 30*(1), 88-90.

Jarvis, C. (2004). *Physical examination and health assessment* (4th ed.). Philadelphia: W. B. Saunders.

McCance, K., & Huether, S. (2002). *Pathophysiology: The biologic basis for disease in adults and children* (4th ed.). St. Louis: Mosby.

Mullaney, S., Letizia, M., & Jennrich, J. (2001). Enoxaparin (Lovenox): An effective and convenient anticoagulant. *MEDSURG Nursing, 10*(6), 326-329.

Nussbaum, R., McInnes, R., & Willard, H. (2001). *Thompson & Thompson: Genetics in medicine* (6th ed.). Philadelphia: W.B. Saunders.

Ogedegbe, H. (2002). Your lab focus: An overview of hemostasis. *Laboratory Medicine, 948-953*, 955-956.

O'Malley, P. (2003). Clotting and bleeding: Anticoagulation update for the clinical nurse specialist. *Clinical Nurse Specialist, 17*(2), 83-85.

Pagana, K., & Pagana, T. (2002). *Mosby's manual of diagnostic and laboratory tests* (2nd ed.). St. Louis: Mosby.

Rempher, K., & Little, J. (2004). Assessment of red blood cell and coagulation laboratory data. *AACN Clinical Issues, 15*(4), 622-637.

Stevens, S. (2000). Heparin-induced thrombocytopenia. *Journal of Vascular Nursing, 18*(2), 54-58.

Trewhitt, K. (2001). Bone marrow aspiration and biopsy: Collection and interpretation. *Oncology Nursing Forum, 28*(9), 1409-1416.

Weitz, J., & Hirsh, J. (2001). New anticoagulant drugs. *Chest, 119*(Suppl 1), 95S-107S.

Wheatley, M., Cox, J., & Nemis-White, J. (2003). Optimizing anticoagulation therapy. *Canadian Nurse, 99*(6), 16-19.

Woodrow, P. (2003). Assessing blood results in older people: Haematology and liver function tests. *Nursing Older People, 15*(3), 29-31.

CHAPTER 43

Interventions for Clients with Hematologic Problems

CONSTANCE VISOVSKY

LEARNING OUTCOMES

After studying this chapter, you should be able to:

1. Identify three clinical manifestations common to clients who have any type of anemia.
2. Explain the pattern of inheritance for sickle cell disease.
3. Prioritize nursing care for the client who has sickle cell disease.
4. Plan a diet for a client who has iron deficiency anemia or vitamin B_{12} deficiency anemia.
5. Explain the mechanism of action and potential side effects of epoetin alpha therapy.
6. Compare the pathologic mechanisms of hemolytic anemia versus aplastic anemia.
7. Compare leukemia and lymphoma for etiology, pathophysiology, and clinical manifestations.
8. List four risk factors for the development of leukemia.
9. Analyze laboratory data and clinical manifestations to determine the presence of infection in a client who has neutropenia.
10. Compare the purposes and scheduling of induction therapy, consolidation therapy, and maintenance therapy for leukemia.
11. Prioritize nursing interventions for the client with neutropenia.
12. Prioritize nursing interventions for the client with thrombocytopenia.
13. Develop a community-based teaching plan for a client with thrombocytopenia.
14. Prioritize nursing responsibilities during transfusion therapy.
15. Identify clients at risk for complications of transfusion therapy.

Go to your Student CD-ROM for Review Questions for the NCLEX Examination keyed to these Learning Outcomes.

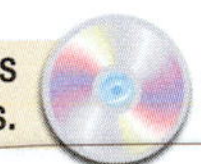

Hematologic disorders or diseases are the result of impaired production or function, or the abnormal destruction of any type of blood cell. The type and severity of the disorder determine the impact it has on the health of individuals. This chapter discusses mild hematologic disorders and those that are potentially life threatening, such as sickle cell disease and leukemia.

Red Blood Cell Disorders

Red blood cells (RBCs), also known as **erythrocytes**, are the major cell in the blood. Tissue oxygenation depends on keeping the circulating number of RBCs within the normal range for the person's age and gender. Tissue oxygenation also depends on the ability of RBCs to perform their normal functions. RBC disorders include problems in production, function, and destruction. Problems may result in a deficient number or poor function of RBCs **(anemia)** or an excess of RBCs **(polycythemia).**

ANEMIA

Anemia is a reduction in either the number of RBCs, the amount of hemoglobin, or the **hematocrit** (percentage of packed RBCs per deciliter of blood). Anemia is a clinical sign, not a specific disease, because it is a manifestation of several abnormal conditions. Anemia can result from dietary problems, genetic disorders, bone marrow disease, or excessive bleeding. Gastrointestinal bleeding is the most common reason for anemia in adults.

There are many types and causes of anemia. Some anemias are caused by a deficiency in one or more of the components needed to make fully functional RBCs. Such anemias can be caused by deficiencies of iron, vitamin B_{12}, folic acid, or intrinsic factor. Other causes include a decreased rate of RBC

TABLE 43-1 Common Causes of Anemia

Type of Anemia	Common Causes
Sickle cell disease	Autosomal recessive inheritance of two defective gene alleles for hemoglobin synthesis
Glucose-6-phosphate dehydrogenase (G6PD) deficiency anemia	X-linked recessive deficiency of the enzyme G6PD
Autoimmune hemolytic anemia	Abnormal immune function in which a person's immune reactive cells fail to recognize his or her own red blood cells as self cells
Iron deficiency anemia	Inadequate iron intake caused by ▪ Iron-deficient diet ▪ Chronic alcoholism ▪ Malabsorption syndromes ▪ Partial gastrectomy Rapid metabolic (anabolic) activity caused by ▪ Pregnancy ▪ Adolescence ▪ Infection
Vitamin B_{12} deficiency anemia	Dietary deficiency Failure to absorb vitamin B_{12} from intestinal tract as a result of ▪ Partial gastrectomy ▪ Pernicious anemia
Folic acid deficiency anemia	Dietary deficiency Malabsorption syndromes Drugs ▪ Oral contraceptives ▪ Anticonvulsants ▪ Methotrexate
Aplastic anemia	Exposure to myelotoxic agents ▪ Radiation ▪ Benzene ▪ Chloramphenicol ▪ Alkylating agents ▪ Antimetabolites ▪ Sulfonamides ▪ Insecticides Viral infection (unproven) ▪ Epstein-Barr virus ▪ Hepatitis B ▪ Cytomegalovirus

production and increased RBC destruction. Table 43-1 lists common causes of many anemias. Despite the many causes of anemia, the effects of anemia on the client (Chart 43-1) and the nursing care needed are similar for all types of anemia.

ANEMIAS RESULTING FROM INCREASED DESTRUCTION OF RED BLOOD CELLS

Sickle Cell Disease

PATHOPHYSIOLOGY

Sickle cell disease is a genetic disorder that results in chronic anemia, pain, disability, organ damage, increased risk for infection, and early death. There is a difference between sickle cell disease state and sickle cell trait. In addition, there is great variation among clients in how severe the disease is and when complications start.

CHART 43-1

KEY FEATURES of Anemia

Integumentary Manifestations
- Pallor, especially of the ears, the nail beds, the palmar creases, the conjunctiva, and around the mouth
- Cool to the touch
- Intolerance of cold temperatures
- Nails become brittle and may lose the normal convex shape; over time, nails become concave and fingers assume clublike appearance

Cardiovascular Manifestations
- Tachycardia at basal activity levels, increasing with activity and during and immediately after meals
- Murmurs and gallops heard on auscultation when anemia is severe
- Orthostatic hypotension

Respiratory Manifestations
- Dyspnea on exertion
- Decreased oxygen saturation levels

Neurologic Manifestations
- Increased somnolence and fatigue
- Headache

The main problem in this disorder is the formation of abnormal hemoglobin chains. In adults, the normal hemoglobin molecule has two alpha chains and two beta chains of amino acids. This normal adult hemoglobin is called **hemoglobin A (HbA).** Normal adult hemoglobin usually contains 98% to 99% HbA, with a small percentage of a fetal form of hemoglobin (HbF).

In sickle cell disease, at least 40% of the total hemoglobin contains an abnormality of the beta chains, known as hemoglobin S (HbS). HbS is sensitive to changes in the oxygen content of the RBC. When RBCs having large amounts of HbS are exposed to decreased oxygen states, the abnormal beta chains contract and pile together within the cell, distorting the shape of the RBC. These cells assume a sickle shape, become rigid, clump together, and form masses of sickled RBCs that block blood flow (Figure 43-1). Thus blood vessel obstruction leads to further tissue **hypoxia** (reduced oxygen supply) and more sickling, with more blood vessel obstructions and ischemia in the affected tissues. Repeated episodes of ischemia lead to progressive organ damage from infarction (Larsen, Neverett, & Larsen, 2001). Conditions that cause sickling include hypoxia, dehydration, infections, venous stasis, low environmental or body temperatures, acidosis, strenuous exercise, and anesthesia.

Usually, sickled cells go back to normal shape when the low oxygen condition is removed and proper oxygenation occurs. Although the cells then appear normal, at least some of the hemoglobin remains twisted, decreasing cell flexibility. The cell membranes become damaged over time, and cells are permanently sickled. The membranes of cells with HbS are more fragile and more easily broken. The average life span of an RBC containing 40% or more of HbS is about 12 to 15 days, much less than the 120-day life span of normal RBCs. This reduced RBC life span causes **hemolytic** (blood cell–destroying) anemia in clients with sickle cell disease.

The client with sickle cell disease has periodic episodes of extensive cellular sickling, called **crises.** The crises have a

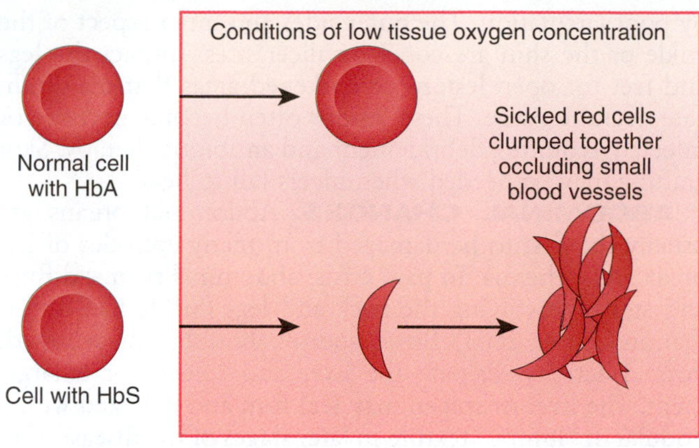

Figure 43-1 ■ Red blood cell actions under conditions of low tissue oxygenation. *HbA,* Hemoglobin A; *HbS,* hemoglobin S.

CHART 43-2

KEY FEATURES of Sickle Cell Disease

Hematologic Manifestations
- Fragile red blood cells that sickle and clump under conditions of low tissue oxygenation, venous stasis, lower environmental or body temperature
  - Anemia
- Tissue hypoxia and ischemia
  - Pain
  - Hardened, enlarged spleen

Respiratory Manifestations
- Pulmonary infarcts
  - Chest pain
  - Pneumonia

Genitourinary Manifestations
- Renal ischemia
  - Decreased urine concentration
- Priapism

Cardiovascular Manifestations
- Cardiac ischemia
  - Myocardial infarctions
  - Chest pain
  - Heart failure
- Strokes

Musculoskeletal Manifestations
- Necrosis of femur head
- Pain in extremities with moderate physical exercise
- Delayed growth—small stature

Integumentary Manifestations
- Leg ulcers
- Pale, cyanotic skin

sudden onset and can occur as often as weekly or as seldom as once a year. Many clients are in good health much of the time, with crises occurring only in response to conditions that cause local or systemic **hypoxemia** (deficient oxygen in the blood).

Repeated occlusions of larger blood vessels have long-term poor effects on tissues and organs (Chart 43-2). Most effects occur as a result of blood vessel occlusion leading to tissue hypoxia, anoxia, ischemia, and cell death. Tissues and organs begin to have small infarcted areas. Eventually, enough healthy cells are destroyed that organ failure results. Organs most often affected in this way are the spleen, liver, heart, kidney, brain, bones, and retina.

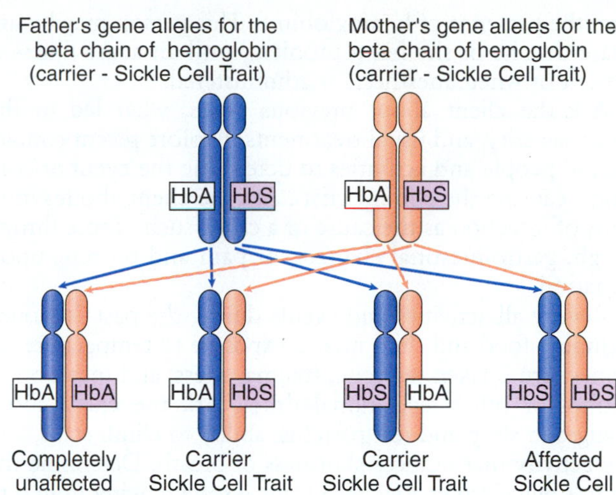

Figure 43-2 ■ Inheritance pattern for sickle cell disease.

Etiology and Genetic Risk

Sickle cell disease is a genetic disorder with an autosomal recessive pattern of inheritance (see Chapter 11). The formation of the beta chains of the hemoglobin molecule is dependent on a pair of gene alleles. A mutation in these alleles leads to the formation of hemoglobin S (HbS) instead of HbA. In sickle cell disease, the client has inherited one hemoglobin S gene allele from each parent, resulting in 80% to 100% of the total hemoglobin containing HbS. Clients with sickle cell disease have severe manifestations of the disease, even under mild precipitating conditions. If a client with sickle cell disease has children, each child will inherit one of the two abnormal gene alleles and at least have sickle cell trait.

In sickle cell trait, one normal gene allele and one abnormal gene allele are inherited, so that only half of the hemoglobin chains produced will be abnormal. The client is a carrier of the HbS gene allele (Figure 43-2). The client can pass the trait on to his or her children, but the client has only mild manifestations of the disease under severe precipitating conditions because less than 40% of the hemoglobin is abnormal.

Incidence/Prevalence

Sickle cell trait and different forms of sickle cell disease occur in people of all races and ethnicities but less often among white individuals. In the United States, about 70,000 people have sickle cell disease, most commonly in African Americans (Sickle Cell Information Center, 2003). Sickle cell disease occurs in 1 in 400 African Americans, and 8% to 10% of all African Americans are carriers of one sickle cell gene allele and have sickle cell trait (Platt et al., 2002).

◆COLLABORATIVE MANAGEMENT

◆Assessment

HISTORY

An adult with sickle cell disease usually has a long-standing diagnosis of the disorder. Adults with sickle cell trait usually have no symptoms or abnormal laboratory findings other than the presence of hemoglobin S. This person may be unaware that he or she has a problem until an acute illness is present or when anesthesia is administered.

Ask the client about previous crises, what led to the crises, severity, and usual treatments. Explore recent contact with ill people and activities to determine the event or condition causing the current crisis. Ask the client about symptoms of infection as the cause of a crisis, such as sore throat, cough, gastrointestinal changes, or pain and burning upon urination.

Review all activities and events during the past 24 hours, including food and fluid intake, exposure to temperature extremes, drugs taken, exercise, trauma, stress, and ingestion of alcohol or other recreational drugs. Ask the client about changes in sleep and rest patterns, ability to climb stairs, and any activity that induces shortness of breath. Determine the client's perceived energy level using a scale ranging from 0 to 10 (0 = not tired with plenty of energy; 10 = total exhaustion) to evaluate the degree of fatigue. This activity review provides important information about fatigue, activity tolerance, and participation in activities of daily living (ADLs).

PHYSICAL ASSESSMENT/CLINICAL MANIFESTATIONS

Pain is the most common symptom of sickle cell crisis. Jaundice may also be present as a result of RBC destruction and release of bilirubin. Other manifestations vary with the site of tissue damage.

CARDIOVASCULAR CHANGES. Clients with sickle cell disease are at risk for high output heart failure because of the anemia. Assess the client for shortness of breath, dyspnea upon exertion, and weakness. Other problems may include murmurs and the presence of an S_3 heart sound. Assess the client's cardiac and vascular status by comparing peripheral pulses, temperature, and capillary refill in all extremities. Extremities distal to blood vessel occlusion are cool to the touch with slow capillary refill and may have reduced or absent pulses. The heart rate may be rapid and the blood pressure low to average, with a decreased pulse pressure, because breakage of RBCs leads to anemia.

SKIN CHANGES. The skin may be pale or cyanotic because of decreased perfusion and anemia. Examine the lips, tongue, nail beds, conjunctivae, palms, and soles of the feet at least once per shift for subtle color changes. With cyanosis, the lips and tongue are gray, and the palms, soles, conjunctivae, and nail beds have a bluish tinge.

Another skin manifestation of sickle cell disease is jaundice. Bilirubin, present inside RBCs, is released when fragile cells are damaged, leading to jaundice. Assess for jaundice in clients with darker skin by inspecting the roof of the mouth for yellow discoloration. Yellow-tinged sclera may be misleading because of normal deposits of fat that appears yellowish in contrast to the dark skin around the eye. Examine the sclera closest to the cornea to assess jaundice more accurately. The palms and soles of dark-skinned clients may appear yellow if callused and should not be mistaken for jaundice. Jaundice often causes intense itching.

Despite the anemia, clients with sickle cell disease usually are not iron deficient. In fact, with increased RBC production and destruction, iron released from the cells may increase the pigmentation of the skin.

As many as 75% of adult clients with sickle cell disease have open sores or ulcers on the lower legs that are caused by poor circulation. The outer sides and inner aspect of the ankle or the shin are common ulcer sites. Inspect the legs and feet for open lesions or darkened areas that may indicate necrotic tissue. These lesions often become necrotic or infected, requiring debridement and antibiotic therapy. Skin grafting may be needed when ulcers fail to heal.

ABDOMINAL CHANGES. Abdominal organs are usually the first to be damaged from many episodes of hypoxia and ischemia. In pain crisis, abdominal pain is diffuse and steady, involving the back and legs (Sickle Cell Information Center, 2003). Bowel sounds should be present with normal activity. Palpate the liver and spleen for enlargement. The liver or spleen may feel firm and enlarged with a nodular or "lumpy" texture in later stages of the disease. Observe whether the client has guarding or rebound tenderness to palpation. A rapidly enlarging liver or spleen that occurs with increasing jaundice may indicate blood trapping in those organs.

MUSCULOSKELETAL CHANGES. Arms and legs are common sites of blood vessel occlusion in clients with sickle cell disease. Joints also may be damaged from many hypoxic episodes and have necrotic degeneration. Inspect the arms and legs for symmetry and record any areas of swelling or color difference. Ask clients to move all joints and record the range of motion and any pain with movement.

CENTRAL NERVOUS SYSTEM CHANGES. Changes in central nervous system (CNS) function may occur in sickle cell disease. During crises, clients may have a low-grade fever. If the CNS has infarcts or repeated episodes of hypoxia, clients may have seizures or manifestations of a stroke. Assess hand grasps on both sides. Also assess the client's gait and coordination.

PSYCHOSOCIAL ASSESSMENT

Psychosocial assessment is important because behavioral changes are early manifestations of cerebral hypoxia. Observe the client and document behavior. Ask family members whether the current behavior and mental status are usual for the client.

Sickle cell disease is a chronic, painful, life-limiting disorder that can be passed on to one's children. Assess the client's psychosocial needs in terms of new factors, established support systems, previous and current coping patterns, and disease progression. Ask the client about how he or she views the disease and what changes in lifestyle have been made as limitations increased.

LABORATORY ASSESSMENT

The diagnosis of sickle cell disease is based on the large percentage of hemoglobin S (HbS) seen on electrophoresis. A person who has sickle cell trait usually has less than 40% HbS, and the client with sickle cell disease may have 80% to 100% HbS. *This percentage does not change during crises.* Another indicator of sickle cell disease is the number of RBCs with permanent sickling. This value is less than 1% among people who do not have sickle cell disease, is 5% to 50% among people with sickle cell trait, and may exceed 90% among clients with sickle cell disease.

Other laboratory tests can indicate the problems or complications of the disease, especially during crises. The hematocrit of clients with sickle cell disease is low (between 20% and 30%). This value decreases even more during crises or when the bone marrow fails to produce cells during stress (aplastic crisis). The reticulocyte count is high, indicating anemia of long duration. Often the mean corpuscular hemoglobin concentration (MCHC) and total bilirubin levels are high in clients with sickle cell disease.

The total white blood cell (WBC) count is usually elevated in clients with sickle cell disease. This elevation is related to chronic inflammation caused by tissue hypoxia and ischemia.

RADIOGRAPHIC ASSESSMENT

Bone changes occur as a result of chronically stimulated marrow and hypoxic bone tissue. The skull may show changes on x-ray as a result of chronic bone surface cell destruction and new growth, giving the skull a "crew cut" appearance on x-ray. X-rays of joints may show necrosis and destruction.

OTHER DIAGNOSTIC ASSESSMENTS

Electrocardiographic (ECG) changes document cardiac infarcts and tissue damage. Specific ECG changes are related to the area of the heart that has been damaged. Ultrasonography, computed tomography (CT), positron emission tomography (PET), and magnetic resonance imaging (MRI) may show soft-tissue and organ changes from poor oxygenation and chronic inflammation.

Common Nursing Diagnoses and Collaborative Problems

Nursing diagnoses and collaborative problems that may apply to clients with sickle cell disease include the following:

- Acute Pain related to poor tissue oxygenation
- Chronic Pain related to joint destruction
- Potential for Sepsis
- Potential for Multiple Organ Dysfunction and Death

Interventions

PAIN. The most common problem of sickle cell disease is pain. The pain with sickle cell crisis is the result of ischemic tissue injury caused by obstructed blood flow. At times, clients have mild pain episodes that can be managed at home. However, pain is often severe enough to require hospitalization and large doses of opioid analgesics. Acute pain episodes have a sudden onset, usually involving the chest, back, abdomen, and extremities (Platt et al., 2002). Complications of sickle cell disease, such as bone necrosis, can cause severe, chronic pain, requiring large doses of opioid analgesics.

Ask the client if the pain is typical of past pain episodes. If not, other pain causes or disease complications must be explored. Use of a pain rating scale can help proper pain management. Ask the client to rate pain on a scale ranging from 0 to 10 and evaluate the effectiveness of interventions based on the ratings.

Concerns about substance abuse can lead to inadequate pain treatment in these clients. Opioid addiction is rare, occurring in only 2% to 5% of clients with sickle cell disease (Platt et al., 2002). Treatment of pain is based on past pain history, previous drug use, disease complications, and current pain assessment. Health care providers must be aware of their own attitudes when caring for this population. If substance abuse is suspected, the treatment of addiction is incorporated into the client's overall treatment plan. Treatment of substance abuse and sickle cell disease pose many challenges, because the client usually cannot be expected to be totally opioid-free. Addicted clients with acute pain crisis may need opioids for short periods. The use of individual contracts as plans for pain control can also be helpful.

Drug Therapy. Clients in acute sickle cell crisis often need at least 48 hours of intravenous (IV) analgesics. (Chart 43-3 lists best practices for nursing care of the client in sickle cell crisis.) Morphine and hydromorphone (Dilaudid) are given IV on a routine schedule, or by infusion pump using patient-controlled analgesia (PCA) (see Chapter 7). Once relief is obtained, the IV dose can be tapered and the drug given orally. Avoid "as needed" (PRN) schedules because they do not provide adequate relief. Avoid intramuscular (IM) injections because absorption is impaired by poor circulation and sclerosed skin. Moderate pain may be treated with oral doses of opioids or nonsteroidal anti-inflammatory drugs (NSAIDs). (See Chapter 7 for more information on pain management.)

Hydroxyurea (Droxia) has been successfully used to reduce the number of sickling and pain episodes. Hydroxyurea works by stimulating fetal hemoglobin (HbF) production. HbF is present during fetal development, but production of hemoglobin F is turned off before birth. Increasing the level of HbF reduces sickling of red blood cells in persons with sickle cell disease. However, this drug is associated with an increased incidence of leukemia (Weiner & Brugnara, 2003). Long-term complications should be discussed with the client before this therapy is started. Hydroxyurea also suppresses bone marrow function, and regular follow-up to monitor complete blood counts (CBCs) for drug toxicity is important. *Hydroxyurea also causes birth defects, thus female clients of childbearing age should use at least two methods of birth control while taking this drug.*

Oral Hydration. Oral or IV hydration helps reduce the duration of pain episodes. Urge the client to drink water or juices. Hydration with hypotonic fluids, such as dextrose 5% with water (D_5W) or with dextrose 5% in 0.45% sodium chloride, is infused at 250 mL/hr for 4 hours. The IV rate is then reduced to 125 mL/hr if more hydration is needed.

Complementary and Alternative Therapies. Complementary therapies and other measures, such as keeping the room warm, using distraction and relaxation tech-

CHART 43-3

BEST PRACTICE for
Care of the Client in Sickle Cell Crisis

- Administer oxygen.
- Administer pain medication as prescribed.
- Hydrate the client with normal saline intravenously and with beverages of choice (without caffeine) orally.
- Remove any constrictive clothing.
- Encourage the client to keep extremities extended to promote venous return.
- Do not raise the knee gatch of the bed.
- Elevate the head of the bed no more than 30 degrees.
- Keep room temperature at or above 72° F (22.2° C).
- Avoid taking blood pressure with external cuff.
- Check circulation in extremities every hour:
  - Pulse oximetry of fingers and toes
  - Capillary refill
  - Peripheral pulses
  - Toe temperature

niques, positioning with support for painful areas, aromatherapy, therapeutic touch, and warm soaks or compresses all help reduce pain perception. *Do not assume that these methods alone will provide adequate pain relief. Analgesics are needed to treat sickle cell pain.*

POTENTIAL FOR SEPSIS. The client with sickle cell disease is at greater risk for infection by such organisms as *Streptococcus pneumoniae* and *Haemophilus influenzae,* because of decreased spleen function. Interventions aim at preventing infection, controlling infection, and initiating early treatment for specific infections. The client who develops a fever should have diagnostic testing for sepsis including CBC with differential, blood cultures, reticulocyte count, urine culture, and a chest x-ray. Usually, these clients are started on prophylactic antibiotics.

Prevention/Early Detection. A major objective is to protect the client in sickle cell crisis from infection. Frequent, thorough handwashing is of the utmost importance. Any person with an upper respiratory tract infection who must enter the client's room wears a mask. Use strict aseptic technique for all invasive procedures.

Continually assess the client for infection and monitor the daily complete blood count (CBC) with differential WBC count. Inspect the mouth during every shift for lesions indicating fungal or viral infection. Auscultate the lungs every 8 hours for crackles, wheezes, or reduced breath sounds. Each time the client voids, inspect the urine for odor and cloudiness, and ask about urgency, burning, or pain during urination. Take vital signs at least every 4 hours to assess for fever.

Drug Therapy. Drug therapy is a major defense against the infections that develop in the client with sickle cell disease. Prophylactic therapy with twice-daily oral penicillin reduces the number of pneumonia and other streptococcal infections. Encourage yearly influenza vaccination. Drug therapy for an actual infection can control infection and prevent sepsis. Agents used depend on the sensitivity of the specific organism causing the infection as well as on the extent of the infection.

POTENTIAL FOR MULTIPLE ORGAN DYSFUNCTION. Continued blood vessel occlusion by clumping of sickled cells increases the risk for multiple organ dysfunction. Management of sickle cell disease focuses on prevention of blood vessel occlusion and promotion of oxygenation.

The client in sickle cell crisis is admitted to the acute care hospital. Assess for adequacy of circulation to all body areas. Remove restrictive clothing and instruct the client to avoid flexing the knees and hips.

Hydration. Dehydration increases cell sickling and must be avoided. Assist the client in maintaining adequate hydration. The client in acute crisis needs an oral or IV intake of at least 200 mL/hr.

Oxygen Therapy. Oxygen is given during crises because deoxygenation is the main cause of sickling. Ensure that oxygen therapy is delivered with nebulization to prevent dehydration. Monitor oxygen saturation using pulse oximetry. Clients with low oxygen saturation should have an arterial blood gas (ABG) drawn and a chest x-ray obtained.

Transfusion Therapy. RBC transfusions can be helpful to increase HbA levels and dilute HbS levels. During transfusion, monitor the client for complications of the procedure (discussed under Transfusion Reactions, p. 916).

Transfusions are prescribed cautiously to prevent iron overload with repeated transfusions. Iron overload damages the heart, liver, and endocrine organs (Sickle Cell Information Center, 2003). Monitor the client's serum ferritin, serum iron (Fe), and total iron binding capacity (TIBC). Deferoxamine mesylate (Desferal, Desferrioxamine) may be prescribed to treat transfusion-induced iron overload.

In some treatment centers, bone marrow transplantation is performed to correct abnormal hemoglobin permanently. Because bone marrow transplantation is expensive and may result in chronic and life-threatening complications, its risks and benefits need to be considered for each client.

Critical Thinking Challenge

A 20-year-old African-American woman with sickle cell disease comes to the outpatient clinic with complaints of joint and back pain, cough, runny nose, and a temperature of 100° F (38° C). She states her pain level is 7/10.

1. What questions related to pain would you ask this client?
2. What drugs and by which route would you expect this client to receive?
3. What diagnostic tests would you expect to be ordered for this client?
4. What nursing assessments would be most important for you to make at this time?

evolve For suggested answer guidelines, go to http://evolve.elsevier.com/Iggy/.

Community-Based Care

Sickle cell disease is progressive with periods of disease exacerbation. Rarely is there a true remission, although the number of crisis episodes may be reduced. Care focuses on prevention of complications. The client with sickle cell disease may receive care in a variety of settings, including acute care, subacute care, extended or assistive care, and home care.

Teach the client to avoid specific activities that lead to hypoxia and hypoxemia. (See the Resource Management box on p. 893.) Emphasize the recognition of the early manifestations of crisis so that treatment can be started early to prevent undue pain, complications, and permanent tissue damage. The client is often given opioid analgesics for self-management of sickle cell crises at home. Teach the client and family about the correct use of these drugs. In addition, counsel clients about the hereditary aspects of sickle cell disease, and provide information about prenatal diagnosis, birth control methods, and pregnancy options.

WOMEN'S HEALTH CONSIDERATIONS

Pregnancy in women with sickle cell disease may be life threatening. Clients who have damage to vital organs are advised against becoming pregnant. Usually, barrier methods of contraception (cervical cap, diaphragm, or condoms with or without spermicides) are recommended for women with sickle cell disease. The use of oral contraceptives (OCs) among these women is controversial, however. OCs may increase clot formation, especially among smokers, predisposing them to crises. However, the use of oral contraceptives also can reduce menstrual blood loss and decrease the degree of anemia. The risks versus benefits of OCs must be examined for each client.

RESOURCE MANAGEMENT

SICKLE CELL DISEASE

Cost of Care

- Each year in the United States, an average of 75,000 hospitalizations are due to sickle cell disease, costing about $475 million.
- The National Institutes of Health report that about $47 million per year is spent on sickle cell research.
- In pharmacies, the average price of 100 capsules of hydroxyurea is between $121 and $164.
- Most clients take two to three capsules daily, which would cost about $100 per month.

Implications for Nursing

The costs related to the treatment of sickle cell disease are the direct result of the need for frequent health-related interventions and hospitalizations related to a lifelong chronic disease. Preventive educational interventions aimed at ways to prevent pain crisis may assist in reducing the costs related to hospitalizations.

Data from Sickle Cell Information Center. (2004). Emory University, Atlanta, GA. Available at http://www.scinfo.org.

Glucose-6-Phosphate Dehydrogenase Deficiency Anemia

PATHOPHYSIOLOGY

Many forms of **hemolytic** (blood cell–destroying) anemia are present from birth as a result of defects or deficiencies of one or more enzymes within the red blood cell (RBC). More than 200 such disorders have been identified. Most of these enzymes are needed to complete some critical step in RBC energy production. The most common type of congenital hemolytic anemia is the deficiency of the enzyme glucose-6-phosphate dehydrogenase (G6PD). This disease is inherited as an X-linked recessive disorder and affects about 10% of all African Americans (McCance & Huether, 2002).

G6PD stimulates reactions in glucose metabolism. RBCs contain no **mitochondria** (sites of production of adenosine triphosphate [ATP]), so active glycolysis is needed for energy metabolism. Newly produced RBCs from clients with G6PD deficiency have sufficient levels of G6PD; however, as the cells age, the level decreases rapidly. Cells with reduced amounts of G6PD break more easily during exposure to some drugs (e.g., phenacetin, sulfonamides, aspirin, quinine derivatives, and thiazide diuretics) and toxins.

The client is usually asymptomatic until exposed to these agents or when a severe infection develops. After exposure to any of these agents, clients have acute breakage of RBCs lasting from 7 to 12 days. During this acute phase, anemia and jaundice develop. The hemolytic reaction is limited because only older RBCs, containing less G6PD, are destroyed.

COLLABORATIVE MANAGEMENT

It is critical that the drug or toxin responsible for the hemolytic reaction be identified and totally removed. People should be screened for this deficiency before donating blood, because cells deficient in G6PD can be hazardous for the recipient.

Hydration is essential during an episode of hemolysis to prevent precipitation of debris and hemoglobin in the kidney tubules, which can lead to acute tubular necrosis. Osmotic diuretics, such as mannitol (Osmitrol), may help prevent this complication. Transfusion therapy is needed when anemia is present and kidney function is normal. Table 43-6 lists indications for transfusion with various types of blood components (see discussion under Transfusion Therapy, p. 913).

Immunohemolytic Anemia

PATHOPHYSIOLOGY

Increased RBC destruction through hemolysis occurs in response to many situations, including trauma, malarial infection, and autoimmune reactions. All increase the rate of RBC destruction by causing membrane **lysis** (breakage). The most common types of hemolytic anemias in North America are the immunohemolytic anemias, also referred to as autoimmune hemolytic anemias (McCance & Huether, 2002).

In immunohemolytic anemia, immune system products attack a person's own RBCs for unknown reasons. Some hemolytic anemias occur with other autoimmune disorders (e.g., systemic lupus erythematosus). Regardless of the cause, RBCs are viewed as non-self by the immune system and are destroyed.

There are two types of immunohemolytic anemia: warm antibody anemia and cold antibody anemia. **Warm antibody anemia** occurs with immunoglobulin G (IgG) antibody excess. These antibodies are most active at 98° F (37° C) and may be triggered by drugs, chemicals, or other autoimmune problems. **Cold antibody anemia** occurs with complement protein fixation on immunoglobulin M (IgM) and occurs most at 86° F (30° C). This problem often occurs with a Raynaud-like response in which the arteries in the hands and feet constrict profoundly in response to cold temperatures or stress.

COLLABORATIVE MANAGEMENT

Treatment depends on symptom severity. Steroid therapy to cause immunosuppression is the first line of treatment and is temporarily effective in most clients. Splenectomy and more intense immunosuppressive therapy with cyclophosphamide (Cytoxan, Procytox✱) and azathioprine (Imuran) may be used if steroid therapy fails. Plasma exchange therapy to remove attacking antibodies is effective for clients who do not respond to immunosuppressive therapy.

ANEMIAS RESULTING FROM DECREASED PRODUCTION OF RED BLOOD CELLS

Anemias caused by decreased red blood cell (RBC) production can occur in response to many problems. Some anemias are caused by failure or inability of the bone marrow to properly produce RBCs. Other anemias are caused by failure of the body to make or absorb a substance needed for RBC production.

CONSIDERATIONS FOR OLDER ADULTS

Older clients often have restricted diets and may be unable to eat meat because of tooth loss or economic reasons, and thus are at risk for iron deficiency anemia (McCance & Huether, 2002). Ask about a family history of anemia. B_{12} deficiency anemia often occurs in clients 50 to 80 years of age and may be genetically transmitted.

Iron Deficiency Anemia

PATHOPHYSIOLOGY

Adults usually have between 2 and 6 g of iron, depending on the size of the person and the amount of hemoglobin in the cells. About two thirds of this iron is contained in hemoglobin; the other one third is stored in the bone marrow, spleen, liver, and muscle (see Chapter 42). With iron deficiency, the iron stores are depleted first, followed by the hemoglobin stores. As a result, RBCs are small **(microcytic),** and the client has mild manifestations of anemia, including weakness and pallor. In iron deficiency anemia, serum ferritin values are less than 12 g/L.

Iron deficiency anemia is a common type of anemia and can result from blood loss, poor intestinal absorption, and an inadequate diet. The basic problem is a decreased iron supply for the developing RBC. Iron deficiency anemia can occur at any age but is more frequent in women, older adults, and people with poor diets.

COLLABORATIVE MANAGEMENT

Any adult with iron deficiency should be evaluated for abnormal bleeding, especially from the gastrointestinal tract. The treatment of iron deficiency anemia is to increase the oral intake of iron from common food sources (Table 43-2). An adequate diet supplies about 10 to 15 mg of iron per day. However, only 5% to 10% of dietary iron is absorbed. This amount is enough to meet the needs of men and women after childbearing age but is not sufficient to supply the greater needs of menstruating women. Fortunately, if iron intake is inadequate, or if bleeding or pregnancy occurs, the intestinal tract increases iron absorption to about 20% to 30% of the total daily intake (McCance & Huether, 2002).

If iron losses are mild, oral iron supplements, such as ferrous sulfate, are started. This treatment should cause the hemoglobin level to rise about 2 g/dL in 4 weeks. Treatment continues until the hemoglobin level returns to normal. When iron deficiency anemia is severe, iron solutions can be given IM. These solutions must be given using the Z-track best practice method outlined in Chart 43-4.

TABLE 43-2 Common Food Sources of Iron, Vitamin B_{12}, and Folic Acid

Iron	Vitamin B_{12}
▪ Liver (especially pork and lamb)	▪ Liver
▪ Red meat	▪ Organ meats
▪ Organ meats	▪ Dried beans
▪ Kidney beans	▪ Nuts
▪ Whole-wheat breads and cereals	▪ Green leafy vegetables
▪ Leafy green vegetables	▪ Citrus fruit
▪ Carrots	▪ Brewer's yeast
▪ Egg yolks	**Folic Acid**
▪ Raisins	▪ Liver
	▪ Organ meats
	▪ Eggs
	▪ Cabbage
	▪ Broccoli
	▪ Brussels sprouts

Data from Pennington, J. (1998). *Bowe's and Church's food values of portions commonly used* (17th ed.). Philadelphia: J. B. Lippincott.

CHART 43-4

BEST PRACTICE for
Administering Intramuscular Medications by the Z-Track Method

- Draw the medication up into the syringe using aseptic technique.
- Add 0.25 mL of air to the syringe.
- Discard the needle used to draw up the medication.
- Place a new needle (22-gauge, 2 to 3 inches long) on the syringe.
- Make certain that the injection site is in bright light.
- *Select the dorsal gluteal site only.*
- Identify appropriate landmarks for administration into the upper, outer quadrant.
- Once the site is selected, pull the skin and subcutaneous tissues sideways away from the muscle.
- Clean the site while holding the skin and subcutaneous tissues off to the side.
- Insert the needle deeply into the muscle tissue.
- Aspirate to determine needle placement.
- Iron dextran is black; look very closely to determine whether or not blood is being aspirated into the syringe.
- If blood is aspirated, withdraw the needle and begin the procedure again from the first step.
- If no blood is aspirated, inject the medication slowly, followed by injection of the air bubble.
- Quickly withdraw the needle.
- Release the skin and subcutaneous tissue.
- *Do not massage the injection site.*

Vitamin B_{12} Deficiency Anemia

PATHOPHYSIOLOGY

Proper production of RBCs depends on adequate **deoxyribonucleic acid (DNA)** synthesis in the precursor cells so that cell division and growth into functional RBCs can occur. All cell division requires adequate amounts of folic acid to make DNA. One function of vitamin B_{12} is to activate the enzymes that move folic acid into the cell, where DNA synthesis occurs. Vitamin B_{12} deficiency causes anemia by inhibiting folic acid transport and reducing DNA synthesis in precursor cells. These precursor cells then undergo improper DNA synthesis and increase in size. Only a few are released from the bone marrow. This type of anemia is called **megaloblastic (macrocytic)** because of the large size of these abnormal cells.

Vitamin B_{12} deficiency results result from poor intake of foods containing vitamin B_{12}. This can occur with vegetarian diets or diets lacking dairy products. Conditions such as small bowel resection, diverticula, tapeworm, or overgrowth of intestinal bacteria can lead to poor absorption of vitamin B_{12}. Anemia caused by failure to absorb vitamin B_{12} **(pernicious anemia)** is caused by a deficiency of **intrinsic factor** (a substance normally secreted by the gastric mucosa), which is needed for intestinal absorption of vitamin B_{12}.

Vitamin B_{12} deficiency anemia may be mild or severe, usually develops slowly, and produces few symptoms. Clients usually have pallor and jaundice, as well as **glossitis** (a smooth, beefy-red tongue), fatigue, and weight loss. Because vitamin B_{12} is needed for normal nerve function, clients with pernicious anemia may also have **paresthesias** (abnormal sensations) in the feet and hands and poor balance (Chart 43-5).

COLLABORATIVE MANAGEMENT

When anemia is caused by a dietary deficiency, the client must increase the intake of foods rich in vitamin B_{12} (animal proteins, eggs, dairy products). Vitamin supplements may

CHART 43-5

KEY FEATURES of
Vitamin B_{12} Deficiency Anemia

- Severe pallor
- Slight jaundice
- Smooth, beefy red tongue
- Fatigue
- Weight loss
- Paresthesias of the hands and feet
- Difficulty with gait

be prescribed when anemia is severe. Vitamin B_{12} and folic acid levels are monitored. Clients who may have pernicious anemia, are tested using the Shilling test of vitamin B_{12} absorption. Clients who have pernicious anemia are given vitamin B_{12} injections weekly at first, then monthly for maintenance.

Folic Acid Deficiency Anemia

PATHOPHYSIOLOGY

Folic acid deficiency can also cause megaloblastic anemia. Manifestations are similar to those of vitamin B_{12} deficiency but nervous system functions remain normal, because folic acid does not affect nerve function. The absence of neurologic problems helps distinguish folic acid deficiency from vitamin B_{12} deficiency. The disease develops slowly, and symptoms may be attributed to other problems or diseases.

The three common causes of folic acid deficiency are poor nutrition, malabsorption, and drugs. Poor nutrition, especially a diet lacking green leafy vegetables, liver, yeast, citrus fruits, dried beans, and nuts, is the most common cause. Malabsorption syndromes, such as Crohn's disease, are the second most common cause. Chronic alcohol abuse with malnutrition is another cause. Anticonvulsants and oral contraceptives slow or prevent the absorption and conversion of folic acid to its active form, leading to folic acid deficiency and anemia.

COLLABORATIVE MANAGEMENT

Prevention of folic acid deficiency anemia is aimed at identifying high-risk clients, such as older, debilitated clients with alcoholism; clients susceptible to malnutrition; and those with increased folic acid requirements. A diet high in folic acid and vitamin B_{12} prevents a deficiency (see Table 43-2). By assessing dietary habits for all clients, you can determine which clients are at risk for diet-induced anemias. This type of anemia is treated with scheduled folic acid replacement therapy.

Aplastic Anemia

PATHOPHYSIOLOGY

Aplastic anemia is a deficiency of circulating red blood cells (RBCs) because of failure of the bone marrow to produce these cells. It is caused by an injury to the hematopoietic precursor cell, the **pluripotent stem cell.** Although aplastic anemia sometimes occurs alone, it usually occurs with **leukopenia** (a reduction in white blood cells) and **thrombocytopenia** (a reduction in platelets). These three problems occur together because the damaged bone marrow loses the ability to produce any of these cells. **Pancytopenia** (a deficiency of all three cell types) is common in aplastic anemia. The onset of aplastic anemia may be slow or rapid.

Aplastic anemia may be caused by long-term exposure to toxic agents, ionizing radiation, or infection (see Table 42-4). In about 50% of cases, the cause of aplastic anemia is unknown. Aplastic anemia may follow viral infection (McCance & Huether, 2002), but the exact mechanism of bone marrow damage is unknown.

COLLABORATIVE MANAGEMENT

Assess for symptoms of bone marrow failure such as weakness, pallor, and petechiae or ecchymosis. A complete blood count (CBC) shows severe macrocytic anemia, leukopenia and thrombocytopenia. A bone marrow biopsy may show replacement of cells by fat.

Blood transfusions are the mainstay of treatment for clients with aplastic anemia. Transfusion is used only when the anemia causes disability or when bleeding is life threatening because of thrombocytopenia. Unnecessary transfusion, however, increases the chances of developing immune reactions to platelets and shortens the life span of the transfused cell. Transfusions are discontinued as soon as the bone marrow begins to produce RBCs.

Immunosuppressive therapy helps clients who have the types of aplastic anemia with a disease course similar to that of autoimmune problems. Agents that suppress lymphocyte activity, such as antilymphocyte globulin (ALG), antithymocyte globulin (ATG), and cyclosporine (Sandimmune), have brought about partial or complete remissions. In more severe cases, stronger immunosuppressive agents, such as prednisone and cyclophosphamide (Cytoxan, Procytox✱), have been effective.

Splenectomy (removal of the spleen) may be performed for clients with an enlarged spleen that is either destroying normal RBCs or suppressing their development. Bone marrow transplantation replaces defective stem cells and can cure the disorder. Cost, availability, and complications limit this treatment of aplastic anemia.

POLYCYTHEMIA

In polycythemia, the number of red blood cells (RBCs) in the blood is greater than normal. The blood of a client with polycythemia is **hyperviscous** (thicker than normal blood). The problem may be temporary (occurring as a result of other conditions) or chronic. One type of polycythemia, polycythemia vera (PV), is fatal if left untreated.

Polycythemia Vera

PATHOPHYSIOLOGY

Polycythemia vera (PV) is a disease with a sustained increase in blood hemoglobin levels to 18 g/dL, an RBC count of 6 million/mm^3, or a hematocrit of 55% or greater. PV is a cancer of the RBCs with three major hallmarks: massive production of RBCs, excessive leukocyte production, and excessive production of platelets. Extreme **hypercellularity** (cell excess) of the peripheral blood occurs in people with PV (Chart 43-6).

At the time of diagnosis, the client's facial skin and mucous membranes have a dark, flushed **(plethoric)** appearance. These

CHART 43-6

KEY FEATURES of
Polycythemia Vera

- Persistently elevated hematocrit value (>55%)
- Hypertension
- Dark, flushed appearance of the hands and face
- Distention of superficial veins
- Weight loss
- Fatigue
- Intense itching
- Enlarged hemorrhoids
- Swollen, painful joints
- Enlarged, firm spleen
- Infarctions of the heart
    - Chest pain
    - Heart failure
- Strokes
- Bleeding tendency

CHART 43-7

CLIENT EDUCATION GUIDE
Polycythemia Vera

- Drink at least 3 L of liquids each day.
- Avoid tight or constrictive clothing, especially garters or girdles.
- Wear gloves when outdoors in temperatures lower than 50° F (10° C).
- Keep all health care–related appointments.
- Contact your physician at the first sign of infection.
- Take anticoagulants as prescribed.
- Wear support hose or stockings while you are awake and up.
- Elevate your feet whenever you are seated.
- Exercise slowly and only on the advice of your physician.
- Stop activity at the first sign of chest pain.
- Use an electric shaver.
- Use a soft-bristled toothbrush to brush your teeth.
- Do not floss between your teeth.

areas appear purplish or cyanotic because the blood in these tissues is poorly oxygenated. Many clients have intense itching caused by dilated blood vessels and varied tissue oxygenation. Blood viscosity is increased, causing an increase in peripheral resistance. Superficial veins are visibly distended. The thick blood moves more slowly through all tissues and places increased demands on the heart, resulting in hypertension. In some highly vascular areas, blood flow may become so slow that stasis occurs. Vascular stasis causes **thrombosis** (clot formation) within the smaller vessels, occluding blood vessels. The blood vessel occlusion leads to tissue hypoxia, anoxia and, later, to infarction and necrosis. Tissues most at risk for this problem are the heart, spleen, and kidneys, although infarction and damage can occur in any organ or tissue.

Because the actual number of cells in the blood is greatly increased and the cells are not completely normal, cell life spans are shorter. The shorter life spans and increased cell production cause a rapid turnover of circulating blood cells. This rapid turnover increases the amount of cell debris (released when cells die) in the blood, adding to the general "sludging" of the blood. This debris includes uric acid and potassium, which cause the symptoms of gout and **hyperkalemia** (elevated serum potassium level).

Other manifestations of PV are related to abnormal RBCs. Even though the number of RBCs is greatly increased, their oxygen-carrying capacity is impaired, and clients have severe hypoxia. Clients with PV also have bleeding problems because of platelet impairment (McCance & Huether, 2002).

COLLABORATIVE MANAGEMENT

Polycythemia vera (PV) is a malignant disease that progresses in severity over time. If left untreated, few people with PV live longer than 2 years after diagnosis. Monitor the CBC to assess response to treatment. Conservative treatment of repeated phlebotomies (two to five times per week) can prolong life for 10 to 20 years. (**Phlebotomy** is the blood drawing with removal of the client's RBCs to decrease the number of RBCs and reduce blood viscosity.) Increasing hydration and promoting venous return help prevent clot formation. Therapy aims to prevent clot formation and includes the use of anticoagulants. Chart 43-7 lists health tips for clients with PV.

As the disease progresses, more intensive therapies are needed to suppress bone marrow activity. Therapy includes oral chemotherapy agents and radiation therapy with injections of radioactive phosphorus. Bone marrow transplantation is promising, but the results are too limited to determine its application to PV. A significant number of clients with PV go on to develop acute leukemia.

MYELODYSPLASTIC SYNDROME

PATHOPHYSIOLOGY

Myelodysplastic syndromes (MDS) are a group of disorders caused by the formation of abnormal cells in the bone marrow. These abnormal cells are usually destroyed shortly after they are released into the blood. As a result, clients with MDS have decreases in the type of blood cell lines affected. MDS occurs in about 5 per 100,000 people, with older adults being affected more frequently (National Comprehensive Cancer Network, 2004). Although not officially a type of cancer, MDS has cancer-like features and is considered to be a precursor to cancer. Like cancer, MDS arises from a single population of abnormal cells. About 30% of all clients with MDS do eventually have acute leukemia. There are many subtypes of MDS and problems can range from unresponsive anemia to cytopenia with increased numbers of blast cells.

Diagnosis is made by examination of the chromosomes and the genes within the chromosomes (cytogenetic testing) of the bone marrow cells. Peripheral blood smears are used to assess marrow cell maturation and the degree of abnormal cells present.

COLLABORATIVE MANAGEMENT

Supportive care of the client with MDS includes blood transfusions for anemia and platelet transfusions for severe thrombocytopenia. Erythropoietin may be given in addition to transfusions. Clients with neutropenia may receive granulocyte colony stimulating factor (G-CSF) or granulocyte-monocyte colony-stimulating factor (GM-CSF). Treatment can include low-dose chemotherapy. For clients with more advanced disease and a high risk for leukemia, bone marrow transplantation is considered.

TABLE 43-3 Differentiating Characteristics of the Four Types of Leukemia

Age at Onset (yr)	Gender Predilection	Racial Predilection	Cell of Origin	Specific Markers	Comments
Acute Lymphocytic (ALL)					
<15	Males	White	B-cell	CALLA+ Hyperdiploidy TDT+	Prognosis poorer for adults than for children Prognosis better than in AML Curable in children
Acute Myelogenous (AML)					
15-39	Equal incidence	None	Myelocyte Promyelocyte Myelomonocyte	TDT− t(9;22) t(15;17)	Prognosis generally poor Heterogeneous tumor cell populations Best prognosis with bone marrow transplant
Chronic Myelogenous (CML)					
>50	Males	None	Myeloid cell	Ph[1] chromosome	Prognosis generally poor; worse if no Ph[1] chromosome No blockage of maturation of nonmalignant leukocytes Blastic crisis indicative of more acute disease
Chronic Lymphocytic (CLL)					
>50	Males	White	B-cell	Trisomy 12	Prognosis poor Long (4-10 yr) course with rare conversion to acute form Only leukemia with a possible genetic predisposition

White Blood Cell Disorders

As discussed in Chapter 23, white blood cells (WBCs), or **leukocytes,** provide protection from infection and cancer development. These protective functions depend on maintaining normal numbers and ratios of the different mature, circulating WBCs. When any one type of WBC is present in either abnormally high or abnormally low amounts, immune function is altered to some degree, as are the functions of oxygen transport and blood clotting, placing clients at risk for many complications. This section covers the changes and nursing care for clients with disorders involving overgrowth of specific types of WBCs. (See Chapter 25 for the problems and care needs for clients with immunodeficiency.)

LEUKEMIA

PATHOPHYSIOLOGY

Leukemia is a type of cancer with uncontrolled production of immature WBCs (usually blast cells) in the bone marrow. As a result, the bone marrow becomes overcrowded with immature, nonfunctional cells and production of normal blood cells is greatly decreased. **Leukemia** may be **acute,** with a sudden onset and short duration, or **chronic,** with a slow onset and symptoms that persist for a period of years.

Leukemias are classified by cell type. Abnormal leukemic cells coming from the lymphoid pathways (see Figure 23-3) are **lymphocytic** or **lymphoblastic.** Leukemias in which the abnormal cells come from the myeloid pathways are **myelocytic** or **myelogenous.** Several subtypes exist for each of these diseases, which are classified according to the degree of maturity of the abnormal cell and the specific cell type involved (Table 43-3).

With leukemia, cancer occurs in the stem cells or early precursor leukocyte cells, causing excessive growth of a specific type of leukocyte. These cells are abnormal and their excessive production in the bone marrow stops normal bone marrow production of red blood cells, platelets, and mature leukocytes. Anemia, thrombocytopenia, and leukopenia result. The number of immature, abnormal WBCs in the blood is greatly elevated. Leukemic cells can also be found in the spleen, liver, lymph nodes and central nervous system. Without treatment, the client dies of infection or hemorrhage. For clients with acute leukemia, these changes occur rapidly and, without intervention, progress to death. Chronic leukemia may be present for years before changes appear.

Etiology and Genetic Risk

The exact cause of leukemia is unknown, although many genetic and environmental factors are involved in its development. The basic mechanism involves damage to genes controlling cell growth. This damage then changes cells from a normal to a **malignant** (cancer) state. Analysis of the bone marrow of a client with acute leukemia shows abnormal chromosomes about 50% of the time (McCance & Huether, 2002). Possible risk factors for the development of leukemia include ionizing radiation, exposure to chemicals and drugs, bone marrow **hypoplasia** (reduced production blood cells), genetic factors, immunologic factors, environmental factors, and the interaction of these factors.

Ionizing radiation exposures such as radiation therapy for cancer treatment or environmental irradiation (e.g., the atomic bomb at Hiroshima or the nuclear accident at Chernobyl) increase the risk for leukemia development, particularly acute myelogenous leukemia (AML) (Stone, 2002).

Certain chemicals and drugs have been linked to the development of leukemia because of their ability to damage DNA. Previous treatment for cancer that included melphalan, cyclophosphamide, doxorubicin, and etoposide poses risks for leukemia development about 5 to 8 years after treatment (Stone, 2002). Table 42-4 lists chemicals and drugs that increase the risk for leukemia.

Bone marrow hypoplasia can increase leukemia risk by reducing or changing bone marrow cell production. Disorders that have marrow hypoplasia and may lead to leukemia development include Fanconi's anemia, paroxysmal nocturnal hemoglobinuria, and myelodysplastic syndromes.

Genetic factors influence leukemia development. There is an increased incidence of the disease among clients with hereditary conditions such as Down syndrome, Bloom syndrome, Klinefelter syndrome, and Fanconi's anemia. Identical siblings of clients with leukemia have a higher incidence of leukemia than does the general population.

Immunologic factors, especially immune deficiencies, may promote the development of leukemia. Leukemia among immunodeficient people may be a result of immune surveillance failure, or the same mechanisms that cause the immune deficiency may also trigger cancer in the WBC population.

Interaction of many host and environmental factors may result in leukemia. Because each person tolerates the interaction of these factors differently, it is difficult to determine the origin of any specific leukemia.

Incidence/Prevalence

Leukemia accounts for 2% of all new cases of cancer and for 4% of all deaths from cancer (American Cancer Society, 2005). The incidence depends on many factors, including the type of WBC affected, age, gender, race, and geographic locale.

In the United States, about 28,800 new cases of leukemia occur each year (American Cancer Society, 2005), with most cases occurring among adults older than 60 years of age (Stone, 2002). Leukemia is classified into any one of four types based on the cell type affected and the rate of progression of the leukemia:

- *Acute myelogenous leukemia (AML)* is the most common form of adult leukemia. *Acute promyelocytic leukemia (APL)* is a subtype of AML that makes up about 10% of adult-onset AML.
- *Acute lymphocytic leukemia (ALL)* constitutes about 10% of adult leukemias but is most common in children.
- *Chronic myelogenous leukemia (CML)* constitutes about 20% of adult leukemias, occurring more often in people older than 50 years of age.
- *Chronic lymphocytic leukemia (CLL)* is the rarest type of leukemia and occurs most often in people older than 50 years of age.

Features of and risk factors for leukemia are listed in Table 43-3.

◆COLLABORATIVE MANAGEMENT

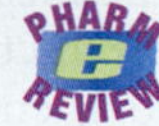

◆Assessment

HISTORY

Ask the client about exposure to risk factors and related genetic factors. Age is important because the risk for adult leukemia increases with age. Occupation and hobbies may also reveal exposure to agents that increase the risk for leukemia. Previous illnesses and the medical history may reveal exposure to ionizing radiation or drugs that increase risk.

Changes in immune function increase the risk for infection in the client with leukemia. Ask about the frequency and severity of infections, such as colds, influenza, pneumonia, bronchitis, or unexplained fevers, during the preceding 6 months.

Platelet function is reduced with leukemia. Ask the client about any excessive bleeding episodes, such as the following:

- A tendency to bruise easily
- Nosebleeds
- Increased menstrual flow
- Bleeding from the gums
- Rectal bleeding
- Hematuria (blood in the urine)
- Prolonged bleeding after minor abrasions or cuts

If the client has experienced such an episode, ask whether this type and extent of bleeding is his or her usual response to injury or represents a change.

The client with leukemia often has weakness and fatigue from anemia and increased metabolism of the leukemic cells. Ask whether the client has had any of the following:

- Headaches
- Behavior changes
- Increased somnolence
- Decreased alertness
- Decreased attention span
- Lethargy, muscle weakness
- Loss of appetite
- Weight loss
- Increased fatigue

Listing activities in the previous 24 hours may reveal information about activity intolerance, changes in behavior, and unexplained fatigue. Determine how long the client has had any of these debilitating symptoms.

PHYSICAL ASSESSMENT/CLINICAL MANIFESTATIONS

Leukemia affects all blood cells, and blood influences the health and function of all organs and systems, thus many body areas and systems cells may be affected (Chart 43-8). The following manifestations occur with the acute leukemias (McCance & Huether, 2002). Some of these findings may also be present in the client with chronic leukemia in the blast phase.

CARDIOVASCULAR CHANGES. Cardiovascular changes are usually related to anemia. The heart rate is increased and blood pressure is decreased. **Murmurs** (abnormal blood flow sounds through the heart) and **bruits** (abnormal blood flow sounds heard over arteries) may be present. Capillary filling time is increased.

RESPIRATORY CHANGES. Respiratory changes are related to anemia and infections. The respiratory rate increases as anemia becomes more severe. If respiratory infections are present, the client may have manifestations of pneumonia, including cough and shortness of breath. Abnormal breath sounds are present on auscultation.

SKIN CHANGES. The skin may be pale and cool to the touch as a result of anemia. Pallor is most evident on the face, around the mouth, and in the nail beds. The conjunctiva of the eye also is pale, as are the creases on the palm of the hand (most evident when the skin over the palm of the

CHART 43-8

KEY FEATURES of
Acute Leukemia

Integumentary Manifestations
- Ecchymoses
- Petechiae
- Open infected lesions
- Pallor of the conjunctiva, nail beds, palmar creases, and around the mouth

Gastrointestinal Manifestations
- Bleeding gums
- Anorexia
- Weight loss
- Enlarged liver and spleen

Renal Manifestations
- Hematuria

Cardiovascular Manifestations
- Tachycardia at basal activity levels
- Orthostatic hypotension
- Palpitations

Respiratory Manifestations
- Dyspnea on exertion

Neurologic Manifestations
- Fatigue
- Headache
- Fever

Musculoskeletal Manifestations
- Bone pain
- Joint swelling and pain

hand is stretched). **Petechiae** (raised red spots) may be present on any area of skin surface, especially the legs and feet. The petechiae may be unrelated to any obvious trauma. Inspect for skin infections or injured areas that have failed to heal. Inspect the mouth for gum bleeding and any sore or lesion of the oral cavity indicating infection.

INTESTINAL CHANGES. Intestinal manifestations may be related to an increased bleeding tendency and to fatigue. Weight loss, nausea, and anorexia are common. Examine the rectal area for fissures and test the stool for occult blood. Many clients with leukemia have reduced bowel sounds and constipation. Enlargement of the liver and spleen and abdominal tenderness also may be present from leukemic infiltration of abdominal viscera.

CENTRAL NERVOUS SYSTEM CHANGES. Cranial nerve disturbances, headache, and papilledema may occur as a result of leukemic invasion of the central nervous system (CNS). In advanced cases, seizures and coma may occur. Clients often have fever, although this is more related to infection than to changes in the CNS.

MISCELLANEOUS CHANGES. Other problems include bone and joint tenderness as the marrow is damaged and the bone resorbs. Leukemic cells invade lymph nodes, causing enlargement or masses.

PSYCHOSOCIAL ASSESSMENT

The client with newly diagnosed leukemia is very anxious and fearful of the disease outcome. Current therapies have greatly improved the prognoses of leukemia. Spend time with the client and family to assess what the diagnosis means to them and what they expect in the future. Without knowing the client's expectations and feelings, you cannot educate and provide individualized support.

A diagnosis of leukemia has serious consequences for a person's lifestyle. Hospitalization for initial treatment often lasts weeks and may result in boredom, loneliness, isolation, and financial stress. Assess coping patterns, including activities that the client finds enjoyable and methods that help the client relax. After initial therapy, the client may be able to resume work, depending on his or her occupation. Often the client must make adjustments for changes in functional status. Repeated hospitalizations for complications are common.

LABORATORY ASSESSMENT

The client with acute leukemia usually has decreased hemoglobin and hematocrit levels, a low platelet count, and an abnormal white blood cell (WBC) count. The WBC count may be low, normal, or elevated but usually is quite high, with counts of 20,000 to 100,000. The client with a high WBC count at diagnosis has a poorer prognosis.

The definitive test for leukemia is an examination of cells obtained from bone marrow aspiration and biopsy. The bone marrow is full of leukemic **blast phase cells** (immature cells that are dividing). The proteins **(antigens)** on the surfaces of the leukemic cells help diagnose the type of leukemia. These proteins are "markers" of certain types of leukemia or may indicate prognosis. Such markers include the T11 protein, terminal deoxynucleotidyl transferase (TDT), the common acute lymphoblastic leukemia antigen (CALLA), and the CD33 antigen.

Blood-clotting times and factors are usually abnormal with acute leukemia. Reduced levels of fibrinogen and other clotting factors are common. Whole blood–clotting time (Lee-White clotting test) is increased, as is the activated partial thromboplastin time (aPTT).

Chromosome analysis (cytogenetic studies) of the leukemic cells may identify marker chromosomes to help diagnose the type of leukemia, predict the prognosis, and determine therapy effectiveness. An example is the Philadelphia chromosome, which is important in the diagnosis and treatment of chronic myelogenous leukemia (CML).

RADIOGRAPHIC ASSESSMENT

Specific manifestations determine the need for specific tests. For example, in a client with dyspnea, a chest x-ray is needed to determine whether leukemic infiltrates are present in the lung. Skeletal x-rays may help determine whether bone **resorption** (loss of bone minerals and density) is present.

Critical Thinking Challenge

The client is a 44-year-old man who has been recently diagnosed with acute myelogenous leukemia (AML). His past medical history includes Hodgkin's disease at 22 years of age, for which he was treated with chemotherapy and radiation. He also has hypertension, gout, and hypercholesterolemia. He is admitted to your unit to begin induction chemotherapy.

1. What risk factors would predispose this client to development of AML?
2. What are some of the physical findings you would expect to see when examining him?
3. What abnormalities would you expect when reviewing his laboratory tests and bone marrow biopsy?

evolve For suggested answer guidelines, go to http://evolve.elsevier.com/Iggy/.

Analysis

COMMON NURSING DIAGNOSIS AND COLLABORATIVE PROBLEMS

The following are priority nursing diagnoses for adult clients with acute myelogenous leukemia (AML), the most common type of adult leukemia:

1. Risk for Infection related to decreased immune response
2. Risk for Injury related to thrombocytopenia
3. Fatigue related to decreased tissue oxygenation and increased energy demands

The primary collaborative problem is Potential for Antineoplastic Therapy Adverse Effects.

ADDITIONAL NURSING DIAGNOSES AND COLLABORATIVE PROBLEMS

In addition to the common nursing diagnoses and collaborative problems, clients with AML may have one or more of the following:

- Impaired Skin Integrity related to prolonged immobility
- Impaired Oral Mucous Membrane related to effects of chemotherapy and pancytopenia
- Self-Care Deficit (Total) related to progressive debilitation and weakness
- Imbalanced Nutrition: Less Than Body Requirements related to anorexia, nausea, and vomiting
- Anxiety related to fear of death
- Powerlessness related to an inability to control disease progression
- Interrupted Family Processes related to acute, life-threatening illness of a family member
- Ineffective Role Performance related to perceived inability to fulfill parental and other family roles and prolonged hospitalization
- Deficient Diversional Activity related to prolonged hospitalization.

Planning and Implementation

RISK FOR INFECTION

NOC **PLANNING: EXPECTED OUTCOMES.** The client with leukemia is expected to remain free from infection. Indicators include the following:

- Absence of fever and foul-smelling or purulent drainage
- Absence of cough, chest pain, and dyspnea
- Absence of urinary frequency, urgency, or pain and burning

INTERVENTIONS. Infection is a major cause of death in the client with leukemia, and sepsis is a common complication. Infection occurs through both **autocontamination** (normal flora overgrows and penetrates the internal environment) and **cross-contamination** (organisms from another person or the environment are transmitted to the client). The three most common sites of infection are the skin, respiratory tract, and intestinal tract.

Gram-negative bacteria are the most common cause of infection, although other infections do occur. Interventions aim to halt infection and control specific infections early. Chart 43-9 lists areas to assess for the client at risk for infection.

Drug Therapy for Acute Leukemia. Drug therapy for clients with AML is divided into three distinctive phases: induction, consolidation, and maintenance.

CHART 43-9

FOCUSED ASSESSMENT of
Hospitalized or Home Care Clients with Potential or Actual Risk for Infection

General Condition
- Age, fatigue, malaise
- History of allergies
- History of chemotherapy, radiation therapy, or other immunosuppressive therapies, such as steroid use
- Chronic diseases
- History of febrile neutropenia and associated symptoms
- Nutritional status
- Functional status—problems with immobility
- Tobacco use—cigarettes, pipe, cigars, oral
- Recreational drug use
- Alcohol use
- Prescribed and over-the-counter medication use
- Baseline and ongoing vital signs—blood pressure, heart rate, respiratory rate, and temperature

Skin and Mucous Membranes
- Thorough inspection of all skin surfaces with special attention to axilla, perineum (particularly the anorectal area), and under breasts; inspection of skin for color, vascularity, bleeding, lesions, edema, moist areas, excoriation, irritation, erythema; general condition of hair and nails, pressure areas, swelling, pain, tenderness, biopsy or surgical sites, wounds, enlarged lymph nodes, catheters, or other devices
- Inspection of oral cavity, including lips, tongue, mucous membranes, gingiva, teeth, and throat—color, moisture, bleeding, ulcerations, lesions, exudate, mucositis, stomatitis, plaque, swelling, pain, tenderness, taste changes, amount and character of saliva, ability to swallow, changes in voice, dental caries, client's oral hygiene routine
- History of current skin disorders or problems with mucous membranes

Head, Eyes, Ears, Nose
- Pain, tenderness, exudate, crusting, enlarged lymph nodes

Cardiopulmonary
- Respiratory rate and pattern, breath sounds (presence/absence, adventitious sounds), quantity and characteristics of sputum, shortness of breath, use of accessory muscles, dysphagia, diminished gag reflex, tachycardia, blood pressure

Gastrointestinal
- Pain, diarrhea, bowel sounds, character and frequency of bowel movements, constipation, rectal bleeding, hemorrhoids, change in bowel habits, sexual practices, erythema, ulceration

Genitourinary
- Dysuria, frequency, urgency, hematuria, pruritus, pain, vaginal or penile discharge, vaginal bleeding, burning, lesions, ulcerations, characteristics of urine

Central Nervous System
- Cognition, level of consciousness, personality, behavior

Musculoskeletal
- Tenderness, pain, loss of function

Modified from Dean, G.E., Haeuber, D., & Rivera, L.M. (1996). Infection. In R. McCorkle, et al. (Eds.), *Cancer nursing: A comprehensive textbook* (2nd ed., p. 975). Philadelphia: W. B. Saunders.

Induction Therapy. Induction therapy is intensive and consists of combination chemotherapy started at the time of diagnosis. The goal of this therapy is to achieve a rapid, complete remission of all manifestations of disease. Agencies and physicians differ in drugs used and the treatment schedule. A commonly prescribed course of aggressive chemotherapy includes continuous IV cytosine arabinoside for 7 days together with a brief infusion of daunorubicin for the first 3 days. Fifty percent to 90% of clients receiving this therapy achieve a complete remission (Scigliano et al., 2001).

A major side effect of this therapy is severe bone marrow suppression. As a result, the client is at even more risk for infection than before the treatment started. Prolonged hospitalizations are common while the client is immunosuppressed. Recovery of bone marrow function requires at least 2 to 3 weeks, during which time the client must be protected from life-threatening infections. Other side effects include nausea, vomiting, diarrhea, **alopecia** (hair loss), **stomatitis** (mouth sores), kidney toxicity, liver toxicity, and cardiac toxicity. (See Chapter 28 for information on effects of anticancer agents.) Older clients have a greater infection-related death rate during this phase than do younger clients (Stone, 2002).

For clients with APL type of AML, induction therapy typically consists of all-trans retinoic acid (ATRA) plus combination chemotherapy. If a remission of APL is not achieved with induction, the client may be treated with arsenic trioxide (Trisenox), or referred for bone marrow transplantation.

Consolidation Therapy. Consolidation therapy often consists of another course of either the same drugs used for induction at a different dosage or a different combination of chemotherapeutic agents. This treatment occurs early in remission, and its intent is to cure. Consolidation therapy may be either a single course of chemotherapy or repeated courses of chemotherapy for 1 to 2 years.

Maintenance Therapy. Maintenance therapy may be prescribed for months to years after successful induction and consolidation therapies. It is indicated for clients with acute lymphocytic leukemia (ALL) and acute promyelocytic leukemia (APL). The purpose is to maintain the remission achieved through induction and consolidation. Maintenance agents for ALL are milder and are often given orally for 2 to 5 years. Not all types of leukemia respond to maintenance therapy.

Maintenance therapy for clients with APL may consist of additional chemotherapy with mercaptopurine plus methotrexate and/or ATRA (National Comprehensive Cancer Network, 2004). Older clients who have a relapse of previously treated AML may be treated with gemtuzumab ozogamicin (Mylotarg), a monoclonal antibody-based chemotherapy agent.

New Drug Therapies. Currently, clinical trials are underway exploring the use of such therapies as targeted therapy, radioimmunotherapy, and tumor vaccines in the treatment of leukemia. See Chapter 28 for further information on cancer therapies. Imatinib mesylate (Gleevec) is targeted therapy for chronic myelogenous leukemia (CML) that is Philadelphia chromosome positive. This drug prevents the activation of an enzyme (tyrosine kinase) needed for growth of CML cells.

Drug Therapy for Infection. Drug therapy is the main defense against infections that develop in clients undergoing therapy for AML. Agents used depend on the sensitivity of the organism causing the infection, as well as infection severity. Drugs for infection are classified as antibacterial, antiviral, or antifungal. Figure 43-3 outlines the drug therapy for management of the febrile neutropenic client.

Antibiotic and Antibacterial Agents. Antibiotic and antibacterial drugs used for prevention or treatment of infection in clients with AML usually include an aminoglycoside antibiotic (amikacin, gentamicin, and tobramycin) and a penicillin, or a third-generation cephalosporin (ceftazidime). Additional, powerful antibiotics used may include vancomycin in cases of methicillin-resistant *Staphylococcus aureus* or when indwelling venous catheter infection is suspected (Peterson, 2003; Moran & Camp-Sorrell, 2002).

Antifungal Agents. Systemic antifungal agents are used when a fungal infection has been diagnosed or is strongly suggested, or when a neutropenic client remains febrile 4 to 7 days after starting antibiotic therapy. Common antifungal drugs include amphotericin B, ketoconazole (Nizoral), voriconazole (Vfend), and nystatin (Mycostatin, Nadostine✱, Nilstat). In neutropenic clients, antifungal creams (e.g., miconazole nitrate) are given intravaginally to prevent yeast infections.

Antiviral Agents. Antiviral agents are used in clients with leukemia to prevent and treat viral infections. Acyclovir is given at the start of chemotherapy, especially for clients who are cytomegalovirus (CMV) positive. If a viral infection is suspected or diagnosed, drug treatments may include ganciclovir, foscarnet, or steroids. The antivirals, although helpful in combating severe infections, have serious adverse effects, especially **ototoxicity** (disruption of hearing and/or balance) and **nephrotoxicity** (disruption of kidney function). Carefully monitor the client treated with such drugs for signs of hearing impairment and renal insufficiency.

NIC **Infection Protection.** A major objective in caring for the client with leukemia is protection from infection. Chart 43-10 lists NIC interventions for the client with leukemia. All personnel must use extreme care during all nursing procedures. Frequent, thorough handwashing is of the utmost importance. Anyone with an upper respiratory tract infection who must enter the client's room must wear a mask. Observe strict procedures when performing dressing changes or accessing a central venous catheter. Maintain strict aseptic technique in the care of these catheters at all times.

If possible, ensure that the client is in a private room to reduce cross-contamination. Other environmental precautions are used, such as allowing no standing collections of water in vases, denture cups, or humidifiers in the client's room, because they are excellent breeding grounds for organisms.

Some treatment centers prescribe a "minimal bacteria diet" during the neutropenic period. Any uncooked foods, such as raw fruits and vegetables, and pepper are removed from the diet because they contain large numbers of organisms. Whether clients benefit from this diet is controversial.

The immunosuppressed client may be placed in a room with a high-efficiency particulate air (HEPA) filtration or laminar airflow system. These systems decrease the number of airborne pathogens. Again, whether these systems benefit clients is not known.

Continually assess the client for the presence of infection. This task is difficult because manifestations may not be obvious in the client with leukopenia. The development of fever and the formation of pus (both common indicators of infection) depend on the presence of white blood cells (WBCs). The client with leukopenia may have a severe infection without pus and with a relatively low fever.

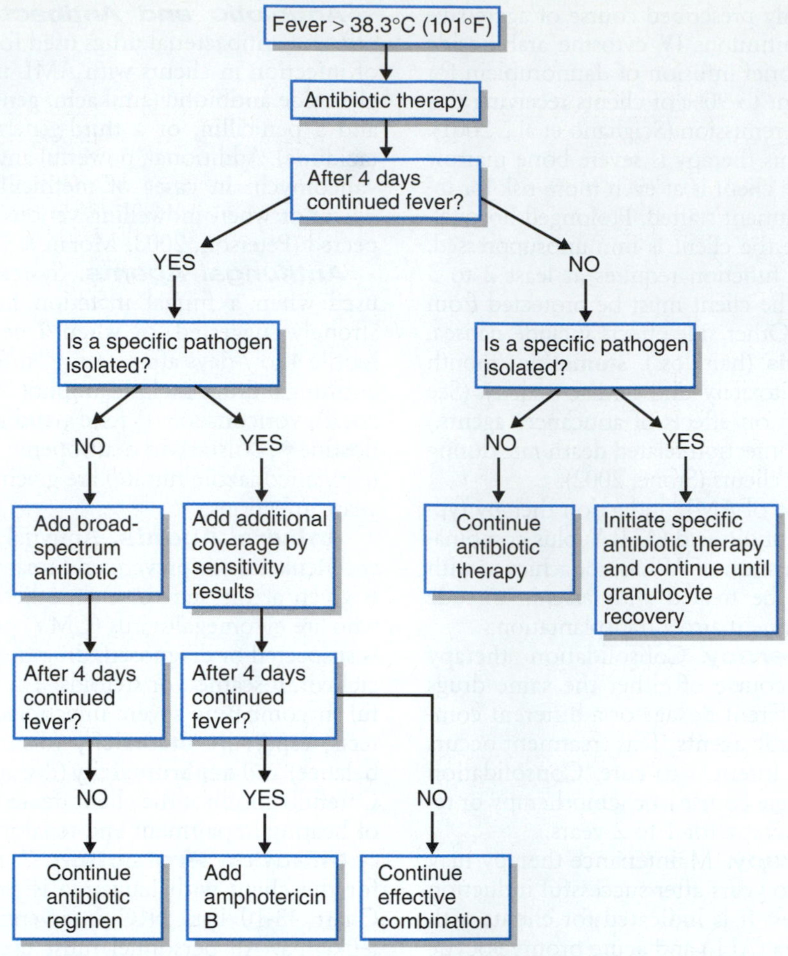

Figure 43-3 ■ Example of antibiotic management for fever in the neutropenic client.

Monitor the client's daily CBC with differential WBC count. Inspect the oral mucosa during every shift for lesions. Auscultate the lungs every 8 hours for crackles, wheezes, or reduced breath sounds. Each time the client voids, assess the urine for odor and cloudiness. Ask the client about any urgency, burning, or pain present on urination.

Take vital signs at least every 4 hours to assess for fever. A temperature elevation of even 0.5° F (or 0.5° C) above baseline is significant for a client with leukopenia and indicates infection until it has been proved otherwise.

Many hospital units that specialize in the care of clients with neutropenia have specific protocols for antibiotic therapy if infection is suspected. Usually, the health care provider is notified immediately, and specific specimens are obtained for culture. Obtain blood for bacterial and fungal cultures from peripheral sites and from the central venous catheter. Obtain urine specimens, sputum specimens, and specimens from open lesions for culture. Chest x-rays are taken. After the specimens are obtained, the client begins IV antibiotics.

Skin Care. Skin care is important for preventing infection in the client with leukemia. The skin may be the only intact defense. Teach the client about thorough hygiene care and encourage daily bathing. If the client is immobile, turn him or her every hour and apply skin lubricants.

Respiratory Care. Perform pulmonary hygiene every 2 to 4 hours. Auscultate the lungs for crackles, wheezes, or reduced breath sounds. Urge the client to cough and deep breathe or to perform sustained maximal inhalations every hour while awake.

Critical Thinking Challenge

The previously described client has completed induction therapy for 7 days. A few days later, he has a temperature of 38.4° C. He complains of having sores in his mouth and a burning sensation in his throat when he swallows.

1. What assessments should you make at this time?
2. What infection protection measures should be instituted for this client?
3. What is the most likely source of the client's infection?

evolve For suggested answer guidelines, go to http://evolve.elsevier.com/Iggy/.

Bone Marrow Transplantation. Bone marrow transplantation (BMT) is a standard treatment for leukemia. BMT is the treatment of choice for the client with leukemia who has a closely matched donor and who is in temporary remission after induction therapy. This therapy is also used for lymphoma, aplastic anemia, sickle cell disease, and many solid tumors.

The bone marrow is the actual site of production of leukemic cells. It can be difficult to ensure that all leukemic cells have been eradicated during induction therapy; therefore, before BMT, additional chemotherapy treatments and total body irradiation are given to purge (condition) the marrow

CHART 43-10

NIC **INTERVENTION ACTIVITIES for**
The Client with Leukemia or the Client Undergoing Bone Marrow/Stem Cell Transplantation

Infection Protection: *Prevention and early detection of infection in a client at risk*
- Monitor absolute granulocyte count, WBC count, and differential results.
- Screen all visitors for communicable disease.
- Maintain asepsis for client at risk.
- Inspect skin and mucous membranes for redness, extreme warmth, or drainage.
- Obtain cultures, as needed.
- Promote sufficient nutritional intake.
- Encourage fluid intake, as appropriate.
- Encourage deep breathing and coughing, as appropriate.
- Instruct client to take antibiotics as prescribed.
- Teach the client and family about signs and symptoms of infection and when to report them to health care provider.
- Remove fresh flowers and plants from client areas, as appropriate.
- Provide private room, as needed.

Bleeding Precautions: *Reduction of stimuli that may induce bleeding or hemorrhage in at-risk clients*
- Monitor the client closely for hemorrhage.
- Note hemoglobin/hematocrit levels before and after blood loss, as indicated.
- Monitor for signs and symptoms of persistent bleeding (e.g., check all secretions for frank or occult blood).
- Monitor coagulation studies, including prothrombin time (PT), partial thromboplastin time (PTT), fibrinogen, fibrin degradation/split products, and platelet counts, as appropriate.
- Administer blood products (e.g., platelets and fresh frozen plasma), as appropriate.
- Protect the client from trauma, which may cause bleeding.
- Avoid injections (IV, IM, or SC), as appropriate.
- Use soft toothbrush or toothettes for oral care.
- Use electric razor, instead of straight-edge, for shaving.
- Instruct client to avoid aspirin or other anticoagulants.
- Instruct client to increase intake of foods rich in vitamin K.
- Avoid constipation (e.g., encourage fluid intake and stool softeners), as appropriate.
- Instruct the client and/or family on signs of bleeding and appropriate actions (e.g., notify the nurse), should bleeding occur.

Energy Management: *Regulating energy use to treat or prevent fatigue and optimize function*
- Determine client's/significant other's perception of causes of fatigue.
- Encourage verbalization of feelings about limitations.
- Monitor nutritional intake to ensure adequate energy resources.
- Monitor/record client's sleep pattern and number of sleep hours.
- Limit number of visitors and interruptions by visitors, as appropriate.
- Provide calming diversionary activities to promote relaxation.
- Encourage an afternoon nap, if appropriate.
- Avoid care activities during scheduled rest periods.
- Plan activities for periods when the client has the most energy.
- Monitor client's oxygen response (e.g., pulse rate, cardiac rhythm, and respiratory rate) to self-care or nursing activities.
- Instruct client/significant other to recognize signs and symptoms of fatigue that require reduction in activity.

NIC intervention activities selected from Dochterman, J.M., & Bulechek, G.M. (2004). *Nursing interventions classification (NIC)* (4th ed.). St. Louis: Mosby. No part of this work is to be altered without prior written permission from the Publisher.
WBC, White blood cell.

of leukemic cells. These treatments are lethal to the bone marrow, and without replacement of bone marrow through transplantation, the client would die of infection or hemorrhage.

After conditioning, new, healthy marrow is given to the client. The new marrow then begins the process of hematopoiesis, which results in normal, properly functioning cells and, ideally, a permanent cure.

BMT units are commonplace, even in community hospital settings. With long-term survival after transplantation increasing, nurses can expect to be caring for these people, if not during the actual transplantation or recovery period, then during the post-transplantation period, in a variety of health care settings.

Sources of Stem Cells. BMT started with the use of **allogeneic bone marrow transplantation** (transplantation of bone marrow from a sibling) and has advanced to the use of human leukocyte antigen (HLA)-matched stem cells from the umbilical cords of unrelated donors. Transplants are classified by the source of stem cells. In **autologous transplants,** clients receive their own stem cells (which were collected before high-dose therapy). **Syngeneic transplants** are those with the stems cells taken from the client's own identical sibling. In **allogeneic transplants,** a closely HLA-matched sibling or an unrelated but matched donor provides the stem cells. Stem cells for transplantation may be obtained by bone marrow harvest, peripheral stem cell pheresis, or umbilical cord blood stem cell banking. Table 43-4 lists the types of transplants.

TABLE 43-4 Classification of Transplants

Type of Transplant	Sources of Stem Cells
Autologous	
Self-donation	Bone marrow harvest Peripheral stem cell pheresis Umbilical cord blood
Syngeneic	
Client's HLA identical twin	Bone marrow harvest Peripheral stem cell pheresis
Allogeneic	
HLA-matched relative, usually a sibling Unrelated HLA-matched donor Mismatched or partially HLA-matched family member or unrelated donor (donor registries)	Bone marrow harvest Peripheral stem cell pheresis Umbilical cord blood

HLA, Human leukocyte antigen.

Transplantation has five phases: stem cell obtainment, conditioning regimen, transplantation, engraftment, and post-transplantation recovery.

Obtaining the Stem Cells. Bone marrow is taken either from the client directly (autologous marrow) or from an HLA-matched person (allogeneic marrow). For allogeneic marrow, a donor is selected from family members tested for HLA type. The best results occur when the donor is an HLA-identical sibling, but BMT can also be successful between those with closely matched HLA types. The chance of matching with any given sibling is 25%.

Donor registries keep records of people willing to donate marrow to provide marrow for clients who do not have a family member HLA match. The chance of matching with an unrelated donor is one in 5000.

CULTURAL CONSIDERATIONS

About 70% of people on the bone marrow donor lists are white. It is estimated that the chance of finding an HLA-matched unrelated donor is 30% to 40% for white individuals, but for African Americans the chance is less than 20% because there are fewer African Americans among registered donors. Unlike blood types, which are present in all racial groups, tissue types can be very different among racial and ethnic groups. Nationally, efforts are made to publicize the need for donors from all cultural backgrounds.

After a suitable donor is identified by tissue typing, the donor is taken to the operating room, where sufficient marrow for transplant is removed through multiple aspirations from the iliac crests. About 500 to 1000 mL of marrow is aspirated; this amount is about 5% to 10% of the donor's marrow supply and regrows within a few weeks. The marrow is then filtered and, if autologous, is treated to rid the marrow of any remaining cancer cells. Allogeneic marrow is transfused into the recipient immediately; autologous marrow is frozen for later use.

Monitor the donor for manifestations of fluid loss, assess for complications of anesthesia, and manage postoperative pain. During surgery, donors may lose a large amount of fluid in addition to the volume of marrow donated. Donors are hydrated with saline infusions before and immediately after surgery. Occasionally the donor may need an RBC transfusion. Assess the harvest sites to ensure that the dressings are dry and intact and that the donor is not bleeding excessively.

Marrow donation is usually a same-day surgical procedure. Teach the donor to inspect the harvest sites for bleeding and to take analgesics for pain. Pain at the harvest sites (hip) is common and is managed with oral non–aspirin-containing analgesics. Some donors may require opioid analgesics for pain control.

There are three phases to obtaining **peripheral blood stem cells (PBSCs):** mobilization, collection, and reinfusion. During the mobilization phase, chemotherapy or hematopoietic growth factors are given to the client. These agents increase the numbers of stem cells and WBCs in the peripheral blood. The stem cells are then collected by **pheresis** (withdrawing whole blood, filtering out the cells, and returning the plasma to the client). One to five pheresis procedures, each lasting 2 to 4 hours, are usually needed to obtain enough stem cells for transplantation. The stem cells are then frozen and stored for reinfusion after the conditioning regimen.

Monitor the client closely during pheresis. Complications include catheter clotting and hypocalcemia (caused by anticoagulants). Hypocalcemia may cause chills, numbness, abdominal or muscle cramping, or chest pain. Oral calcium supplements may be used to manage these symptoms. Monitor vital signs at least every hour during pheresis. The client may become hypotensive from fluid volume changes during the procedure.

Stem cells may also be obtained from umbilical cord blood of newborns. This blood has a high concentration of stem cells. Umbilical stem cells are obtained via a simple phlebotomy procedure. After birth, before the placenta detaches, a syringe is used to withdraw 43 to 150 mL of blood from the umbilical vein from the placenta. The syringes are placed in a kit, which is returned to the Cord Blood Registry for processing and storage. The stem cells may be used later for an unrelated recipient or stored in case the infant develops a serious illness later in life and needs them. The cost of banking and processing umbilical cord stem cells is about $1500, with an additional charge of $100 per year for storage. Umbilical stem cells can last for years when stored properly in liquid nitrogen.

Conditioning Regimen. Figure 43-4 outlines the timing and steps involved in BMT. The day the client receives the bone marrow is day T-0. The pretransplantation conditioning days are counted in reverse order from T-0, just like a rocket countdown. Post-transplantation days are counted in order from the day of transplantation.

The client must first undergo a conditioning regimen, which varies with the diagnosis and type of transplant to be received. The conditioning regimen serves two purposes: (1) to "wipe out" the client's own bone marrow, thus preparing the client for optimal graft take and (2) to give higher than normal doses of chemotherapy and/or radiotherapy to rid the person of cancer cells (myeloablation). Usually a period of 5 to 10 days is required. The regimen usually includes high-dose chemotherapy and sometimes includes total-body irradiation (TBI). Each conditioning regimen is individually tailored, with the client's specific disease, overall health, and previous treat-

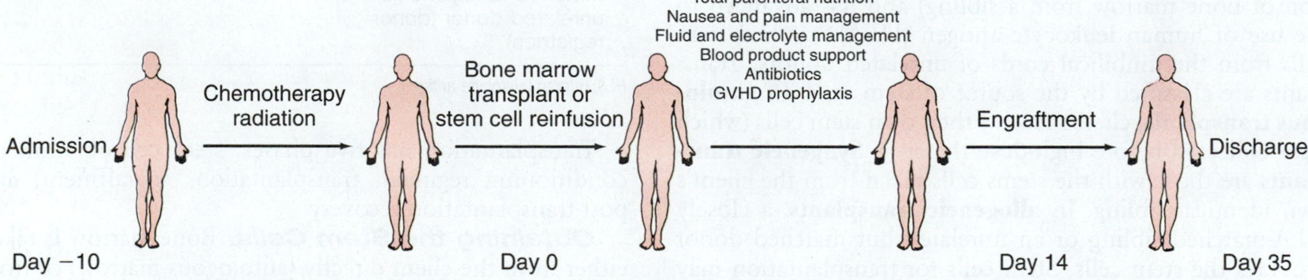

Figure 43-4 ■ Timing and steps of allogeneic bone marrow transplantation. *GVHD,* Graft-versus-host disease.

ment taken into account. A typical conditioning regimen for an adult with acute myelogenous leukemia (AML) receiving an allogenic BMT for treatment is as follows:

- *Days T-7 through T-5:* High-dose chemotherapy to obliterate the client's own bone marrow cells and to kill off any remaining leukemic cells. Specific agents include busulfan, carmustine, cyclophosphamide, cytosine arabinoside, etoposide, and melphalan. The dosages are much higher than those used for normal chemotherapy.
- *Days T-4 through T-2:* Delivery of TBI. The total radiation dose for TBI is 1200 rads given as 200 rads twice daily over 3 days.

Because of the morbidity and mortality associated with this conditioning regimen, a nonmyeloablative approach is being studied. There are many variations in nonmyeloablative conditioning regimens. This approach uses lower chemotherapy doses and low-dose TBI to reduce side effects (Kim, 2002).

During conditioning, bone marrow and normal tissues respond immediately to the chemotherapy and radiation. The client has all of the expected side effects associated with both therapies. When chemotherapy is given in high doses, these side effects are more intense than those seen with standard doses. Side effects include nausea and vomiting, mucositis, capillary leak syndrome, diarrhea, and bone marrow suppression.

Late effects from the conditioning regimen are also common, occurring as late as 3 to 10 years after transplantation. These problems include veno-occlusive disease (VOD), skin toxicities, cataracts, lung fibrosis, second cancers, cardiomyopathy, endocrine complications, and neurologic complications.

Transplantation. Day T-0, the day of transplantation, is separated from the conditioning by at least 2 days to ensure that the chemotherapy drugs have been cleared and will not kill off the transplanted stem cells. The client has few circulating WBCs, indicating successful conditioning.

The transplantation itself is very simple. Frozen marrow, PBSCs, or umbilical cord blood cells are thawed and then infused through the client's central catheter like an ordinary blood transfusion *(but not using blood administration tubing).* Usually the marrow is infused over a 30-minute period, although it can be given by IV push directly into the central catheter. In nonablative transplants, the new marrow plus stem cells from the umbilical cord are also infused.

Side effects of all types of stem cell transfusions are similar. The client may have fever and hypertension as a reaction to the preservative used in stem cell storage. To prevent these reactions, acetaminophen (Tylenol), hydrocortisone, and diphenhydramine (Benadryl) are given before the infusion. Antihypertensives or diuretics may be needed to treat fluid volume changes. The client may have red urine as a result of red blood cell hemolysis in the infused stem cells.

Engraftment. The transfused PBSCs and marrow cells circulate briefly in the peripheral blood. The stems cells find their way to the marrow-forming sites of the client's bones and establish residency there. How the donated marrow cells "home in" on the bone marrow sites is not yet understood.

Engraftment, successful "take" of the transplanted cells in the client's bone marrow, is key to the whole transplantation process. For the donated marrow or stem cells to "rescue" the client after large doses of chemotherapy or radiotherapy have wiped out his or her own bone marrow, the transfused stem cells must survive and grow in the client's bone marrow sites. Engraftment takes 8 to 12 days for peripheral blood stem cell transplantation and 12 to 28 days for bone marrow stem cell transplantation. To aid engraftment, growth factors, such as granulocyte colony-stimulating factor or granulocyte-macrophage colony-stimulating factor, may be given. When engraftment occurs, the client's WBC, RBC, and platelet counts begin to rise.

Prevention of Complications. The period after transplantation is difficult. Infection and bleeding are severe problems because the client remains without any natural immunity until the transfused stem cells grow and engraftment occurs. The nursing care for this client is the same as for the client during induction therapy for AML. Helping the client to maintain hope through this long recovery period is difficult. Complications are often severe and life threatening. Help the client to have a positive attitude and be involved in his or her own recovery.

In addition to the problems related to the period of **pancytopenia** (too few circulating blood cells), other complications of BMT include failure to engraft, development of graft-versus-host disease (GVHD), and VOD.

Failure to Engraft. Sometimes the donated marrow or stem cells fail to engraft. This possibility is discussed in advance with the client and the donor. Failure to engraft occurs more often with transplants using allogeneic stem cells than those using autologous stem cells. The causes include insufficient numbers of cells transplanted, attack or rejection of donor cells by the remaining immune system cells of the recipient, infection of transplanted cells, and unknown biologic factors. If the transplanted cells fail to engraft, the client will die unless another transplantation is successful.

Graft-Versus-Host Disease. Graft-versus-host disease (GVHD) occurs mostly in allogeneic transplants. The immunocompetent cells of the donated marrow recognize the client's (recipient) cells, tissues, and organs as foreign and start an immunologic attack against them. The graft is actually trying to attack the host tissues and cells.

Although all host tissues can be attacked and harmed, the tissues usually damaged are the skin, intestinal tract, and liver. About 25% to 50% of all allogeneic BMT recipients have some degree of GVHD, and more than 15% of the clients who develop GVHD die of its complications. The presence of some GVHD indicates successful engraftment.

Management of GVHD involves limiting the activity of donor T-cells by using immunosuppressive drugs such as cyclosporine, methotrexate, corticosteroids, and antithymocyte globulin (Kim, 2002). Care is taken to avoid suppressing the new immune system to the extent that either the client is at risk for infection or the transplanted cells stop engrafting.

Veno-occlusive Disease. Veno-occlusive disease (VOD) is the occlusion of liver blood vessels by clotting and inflammation (phlebitis). This problem occurs in up to 20% of clients who undergo BMT. Problems usually begin within the first 30 days after transplantation. Clients who received high doses of chemotherapy, especially alkylating agents, are at risk for life-threatening liver complications. Manifestations include jaundice, pain in the right upper quadrant, ascites, weight gain, and liver enlargement.

There is no known way of opening the liver vessels, thus treatment is supportive. Early detection improves the chance for survival. Fluid management is also crucial. Assess the client daily for weight gain, fluid retention, increases in abdominal girth, and hepatomegaly.

RISK FOR INJURY

Normal bone marrow production of platelets is severely limited with acute myelogenic leukemia (AML), leading to thrombocytopenia. The client is at great risk for excessive bleeding in response to minimal trauma. Thrombocytopenia can also be caused by induction therapy for AML or high-dose chemotherapy for transplantation.

NOC **PLANNING: EXPECTED OUTCOMES.** The client with leukemia is expected to remain free from bleeding. Indicators include the following:

- Maintenance of hematocrit and hemoglobin within normal limits
- Absence of frank bleeding, petechiae, or ecchymosis

INTERVENTIONS. The client's platelet count is decreased as a side effect of chemotherapy. During the period of greatest bone marrow suppression (the **nadir**), the platelet count may be very low (<10,000/mm^3). The client is at extreme risk for bleeding once the platelet count falls below 50,000/mm^3, and spontaneous bleeding often occurs when the platelet count is lower than 20,000/mm^3.

NIC **Bleeding Precautions.** The goals are to protect the client from injury with bleeding and to closely monitor any bleeding that does occur (see Chart 43-10). Assess the client at least twice per shift for evidence of bleeding: oozing, enlarging bruises, petechiae, or purpura. Inspect all stool, urine, drainage, and vomitus for blood and test for occult blood. Measure any blood loss as accurately as possible and measure the client's abdominal girth daily. Increases in abdominal girth can indicate internal hemorrhage. Institute bleeding precautions (Chart 43-11).

CHART 43-11

BEST PRACTICE for
The Client with Thrombocytopenia

- Handle the client gently.
- Use a lift sheet when moving and positioning in bed.
- Avoid IM injections and venipunctures.
- When injections or venipunctures are necessary, use the smallest-gauge needle for the task.
- Apply firm pressure to the needle stick site for 10 minutes or until the site no longer oozes blood.
- Apply ice to areas of trauma.
- Test all urine and stool for the presence of occult blood.
- Observe IV sites every 2 hours for bleeding.
- Avoid trauma to rectal tissues:
  - Do not take temperatures rectally.
  - Do not give enemas.
  - Administer well-lubricated suppositories with caution.
  - Advise client not to have anal intercourse.
- Measure abdominal girth daily.
- Advise the client to use an electric shaver.
- Teach the client to avoid mouth trauma:
  - Use soft-bristled toothbrush or tooth sponges.
  - Do not floss between teeth.
  - Avoid dental work, especially extractions.
  - Avoid hard foods.
  - Make sure that dentures fit and do not rub.
- Encourage the client not to blow the nose or insert objects into the nose.
- Advise the client to avoid contact sports.
- Teach client to wear shoes with firm soles whenever ambulating.

Monitoring. Monitor laboratory values daily. Review CBC results daily to determine the risk for bleeding, as well as actual blood loss. The client with a platelet count below 20,000/mm^3 may need a platelet transfusion. Oprelvekin (Neumega), a platelet (thrombopoietic) growth factor, may be prescribed to induce platelet growth after the completion of chemotherapy. For the client with severe blood loss, packed RBCs may be prescribed (see later discussion under Red Blood Cell Transfusions, p. 914).

FATIGUE

Normal production of red blood cells is limited in leukemia, causing anemia, which results in fatigue. Additionally, leukemic cells have high rates of metabolism, increasing fatigue in the anemic client with leukemia. Anemia may also occur as a side effect of chemotherapy treatment.

NOC **PLANNING: EXPECTED OUTCOMES.** The client with leukemia is expected to have no increase in fatigue. Indicators include that the client consistently demonstrates the following behaviors:

- Participation in self-care
- Recognition of symptoms of fatigue and alteration of activity before fatigue becomes excessive

NIC **INTERVENTIONS.** Interventions aim to reduce fatigue through energy management (see Chart 43-10) and improving red blood cell (RBC) counts.

Diet Therapy. The client must eat enough calories to meet at least basal energy requirements, but increasing dietary intake can be difficult when the client is fatigued. Provide small, frequent meals high in protein and carbohydrates. Food items that are liquid or semisolid require less effort to eat.

Blood Replacement Therapy. Blood transfusions are sometimes indicated for the client with fatigue. Transfusions increase the blood's oxygen-carrying capacity and replace missing RBCs. For the client with leukemia who has fatigue related to anemia, packed RBCs are the blood component choice. (See Table 43-6 under Transfusion Therapy, p. 913, for a discussion of nursing care during transfusions.)

Drug Therapy. Clients may receive colony-stimulating factors to reduce the severity and duration of anemia and/or neutropenia following intensive chemotherapy. For anemia, subcutaneous injections of epoetin alfa (Epogen or Procrit) 50 to 100 units/kg may be given three times per week, or darbepoetin alfa (Aranesp) 2 to 2.5 mcg/kg may be given subcutaneously weekly. This growth factor boosts the production of RBCs. This agent causes a stinging sensation when injected. Assess for side effects such as hypertension, headaches, fever, **myalgia** (muscle aches), and rashes. (See Chapter 28 for information on hematopoietic growth factors.)

Energy Conservation. Examine the client's schedule of prescribed and routine activities. Assess those activities that do not have a direct positive effect on the client's condition in terms of their usefulness. If the benefit of an activity is less than its worsening of fatigue, consult with other members of the health care team about eliminating or postponing it. Candidates for cancellation or postponement include physical therapy and any invasive diagnostic tests not needed for assessment or treatment of current problems.

Community-Based Care

The client with leukemia is discharged after induction chemotherapy and recovery of blood cell production. Follow-up care continues on an outpatient basis. Although many transplant centers discharge clients following engraftment, some centers give high-dose chemotherapy and stem cell infusion on an outpatient basis. This plan involves daily clinic visits and frequent follow-up by nurses in the home care setting.

HOME CARE MANAGEMENT

Planning for home care for the client with leukemia begins as soon as remission is achieved. The client will need help at home until the condition improves. Assess the available support mechanisms. Many clients need a visiting nurse to assist with dressing changes for central venous catheters, hyperalimentation infusions, platelet infusions, and to answer questions. Home transfusion therapy for blood components may be needed.

The home care team is critical for the client receiving stem cell transplantation in the home setting. Potential candidates are evaluated in advance. Criteria include a knowledgeable caregiver, a clean home environment, location near the hospital, telephone access, and emotional stability on the part of the client and caregiver.

Home care nurses give chemotherapy and monitor the client for complications. Nurses visit the client once or twice per day and spend between 4 and 8 hours per day in the home. The client receives the stem cell transplant infusion in the outpatient clinic. Nursing care is similar to that provided in the hospital. If complications such as sepsis or veno-occlusive disease (VOD) occur, the client is admitted to the inpatient facility.

HEALTH TEACHING

Instruct the client and family about the importance of continuing therapy and medical follow-up. Many clients go home with a central venous catheter in place and need instructions about its care. Chart 43-12 lists guidelines for central venous catheter care at home. These guidelines may be altered depending on the home setting, assistance available, and agency policy.

Protecting the client from infection at home is just as important as it was during hospitalization. (See Chart 43-9 for focused assessment for the client at risk for infection.) Urge the client to use proper hygiene and to avoid crowds or others with infections. Neither the client nor any household member should receive live virus immunization (poliomyelitis, measles, or rubella) for 2 years after transplantation. Instruct the client to continue mouth care regimens at home. Emphasize that the client should immediately notify the physician if he or she has a fever or any other sign of infection. Chart 43-13 lists guidelines for clients for infection prevention.

Many clients return home still at risk for bleeding because platelet recovery is slower than recovery of white blood cells (WBCs). Platelet levels may be low for 6 months after transplantation. Reinforce safety and bleeding precautions, and emphasize that the client must follow these precautions until the platelet count is above 50,000/mm^3. Instruct the client and family to assess for petechiae, avoid trauma and sharp objects, apply pressure to wounds for 10 minutes, and report blood in the stool or urine, or headache that does not respond to acetaminophen. Chart 43-14 lists guidelines for clients at risk for bleeding.

PSYCHOSOCIAL PREPARATION

A diagnosis of leukemia threatens self-esteem and the family role. The client faces the possibility of death, and treatment causes major changes in self-image. The client and family also experience changes in the client's body image,

CHART 43-12

CLIENT EDUCATION GUIDE
Home Care of the Central Venous Catheter

- To maintain patency, flush the catheter briskly with heparinized saline (10 units/mL) once a day and after completing infusions.
- Change the Luer-Lok cap on each catheter lumen weekly.
- Change the dressing every other day:
  - Use clean technique with thorough handwashing.
  - Clean the exit site with alcohol and povidone-iodine (Betadine).
  - Apply antibacterial ointment to the site.
  - Cover the site with dry sterile gauze dressing, taped securely, or with transparent adherent dressing.
- To prevent tension, always tape the catheter to yourself.
- Look for and report any signs of infection (redness, swelling, or drainage at the exit site).
- In case of a break or puncture in the catheter lumen, immediately clamp the catheter between yourself and the opening. *Notify your physician immediately.*

CHART 43-13

CLIENT EDUCATION GUIDE
Prevention of Infection

- Avoid crowds and other large gatherings of people who might be ill.
- Do not share personal toilet articles, such as toothbrushes, toothpaste, washcloths, or deodorant sticks, with others.
- If possible, bathe daily.
- Wash the armpits, groin, genitals, and anal area at least twice a day with an antimicrobial soap.
- Clean your toothbrush daily by either running it through the dishwasher or rinsing it in liquid laundry bleach and water.
- Wash your hands thoroughly with an antimicrobial soap before you eat or drink, after touching a pet, after shaking hands with anyone, as soon as you come home from any outing, and after using the toilet.
- Eat a low-bacteria diet, and avoid salads, raw fruits and vegetables, undercooked meat, pepper, and paprika.
- Wash dishes between uses with hot, sudsy water, or use a dishwasher.
- Do not drink water that has been standing for longer than 15 minutes.
- Do not reuse cups and glasses without washing.
- Avoid changing pet litter boxes. If unavoidable, use gloves or wash hands immediately.
- Avoid keeping turtles and reptiles as pets.
- Do not feed pets raw or undercooked meat.
- Take your temperature at least twice a day.
- Report any of the following manifestations of infection to your physician immediately:
  - Temperature greater than 100° F (38° C)
  - Persistent cough (with or without sputum)
  - Pus or foul-smelling drainage from any open skin area or normal body opening
  - Presence of a boil or abscess
  - Urine that is cloudy or foul smelling, or burning on urination
- Take all medications as prescribed.
- Do not dig in the garden or work with houseplants.
- Avoid travel to areas of the world with poor sanitation or less-than-adequate health care facilities.

CHART 43-14

CLIENT EDUCATION GUIDE
The Client at Risk for Bleeding

- Use an electric shaver.
- Use a soft-bristled toothbrush, and do not floss.
- Do not have dental work done without consulting your doctor.
- Do not take aspirin or any aspirin-containing products. Read the label to be sure that the product does not contain aspirin or salicylates.
- Do not participate in contact sports or any activity likely to result in your being bumped, scratched, or scraped.
- If you are bumped, apply ice to the site for at least 1 hour.
- Notify your doctor if you:
  - Experience an injury and persistent bleeding results
  - Have excessive menstrual bleeding
  - See blood in your urine or bowel movement
  - Have a headache that does not respond to acetaminophen.
- Avoid anal intercourse.
- Take a stool softener to prevent straining during a bowel movement.
- Do not use enemas or rectal suppositories.
- Avoid bending over at the waist.
- Do not wear clothing or shoes that are tight or that rub.
- Avoid blowing your nose or placing objects in your nose. If you must blow your nose, do so gently without blocking either nasal passage.

level of independence, and lifestyle. Some feel threatened by their environment, seeing everything as potentially infectious. Clients who are cared for in protective isolation may feel lonely and isolated. Help the client and family define priorities, understand the illness and its treatment, and find hope. Make referrals to support groups sponsored by organizations such as the American Cancer Society ("I Can Cope" and "Make Today Count"), which may benefit both the client and the family. (See the Evidence-Based Practice for Nursing box at right.)

HEALTH CARE RESOURCES

The client with limited social support may need help at home until strength and energy return. A home care aide may suffice for some clients, whereas for others a visiting nurse may be needed to reinforce teaching. The client may also need equipment for activities of daily living (ADLs) and ambulation. Assess financial resources. Cancer treatment is expensive, and you must work closely with the social services department to ensure that insurance is adequate. If the client is uninsured, explore other sources, such as drug company-sponsored compassionate aid programs. The Leukemia Society of America offers limited financial help for clients with leukemia, sponsors support groups, and provides information for clients and families.

Prolonged outpatient contact and follow-up is necessary and clients need transportation to the outpatient facility. Many local units of the American Cancer Society offer free transportation to clients with cancer, including leukemia.

Critical Thinking Challenge

The client has received a bone marrow transplant for treatment of leukemia.

1. For what complications from this procedure should you assess?
2. What discharge instructions should be given to this client?

evolve For suggested answer guidelines, go to http://evolve.elsevier.com/Iggy/.

EVIDENCE-BASED PRACTICE for Nursing

What is the best measure of quality of life for clients undergoing bone marrow or peripheral blood stem cell transplantation?

Danaher Hacker, E. (2003). Quantitative measurement of quality of life in adult patients undergoing bone marrow transplant or peripheral blood stem cell transplant: A decade in review. *Oncology Nursing Forum, 30*(4), 613-629.

The evaluation of quality of life (QOL) becomes important as cancer treatments impact all aspects of a person's life. The purpose of this review was to evaluate the quantitative means of measuring QOL in clients undergoing bone marrow transplantation (BMT) or peripheral blood stem cell transplantation (PBSCT) over the past 10 years. Thirty-two research studies were included in the review. In terms of sample size, 22 studies (69%) had more than 100 participants, whereas 10 studies (31%) had fewer than 100 participants. Eighty-eight percent of the studies evaluated QOL in clients who had undergone BMT, but only 9% (n = 3) focused on QOL following PBSCT. In 66% of the studies, QOL was measured only once, from 1 to 5 years after transplantation. Two studies measured QOL in long-term transplant survivors, and 34% measured QOL before transplantation, 100 days after transplantation, and 1 year after transplantation. Most studies used measurement tools that captured the multidimensional nature of QOL. The severe toxicities associated with transplant underscore the need to assess the client's QOL as well as overall survival and disease-free survival when looking at client outcomes. Controversy remains regarding whether to use one or more instruments to measure QOL, and no gold standard measure for QOL, either in research or practice, yet exists.

Level of Evidence: 1—Quantitative systematic review.

Critique. Few studies had actually defined QOL, and a lack of consensus remains as to what QOL represents. Study sample sizes were relatively small, limiting the generalizability of the study findings. The majority of the studies used a cross-sectional design, measuring QOL only once rather than over time. A review of a decade of research fails to resolve the controversy regarding the use of single or multiple instruments to measure QOL.

Implications for Nursing. The assessment of QOL as a client outcome of transplantation is receiving increased attention. Therefore the inclusion of a QOL measure that captures the multidimensional nature of QOL, but is not too burdensome for the client should be a consideration in clinical practice and research. The determination of research findings that are clinically relevant regarding QOL in transplant recipients will provide the basis for evidence-based nursing practice and ultimately improve care for transplant recipients.

Evaluation: Outcomes

Evaluate the care of the client with leukemia on the basis of the identified nursing diagnoses and collaborative problems. The expected outcomes include that the client will:

- Remain free of infection and sepsis
- Not experience episodes of bleeding
- Be able to balance activity and rest
- Use energy conservation techniques
- Adapt lifestyle to energy level

Specific indicators for these outcomes are listed for each nursing diagnosis and collaborative problem under the Planning and Implementation section (see earlier).

MALIGNANT LYMPHOMA

Malignant lymphomas are the abnormal overgrowth of one type of leukocyte, the lymphocyte. They differ from the leukemias in the degree of maturation of the affected cells and the location of cancer cell production. Lymphomas are cancers of committed lymphocytes rather than stem cell precursors (as in leukemia). This growth occurs in lymphoid tissues scattered throughout the body, especially the lymph nodes and spleen, rather than in the bone marrow. Lymphomas are solid tumors rather than cellular suspensions within the blood and bone marrow. There are two major categories of lymphoma among adults: Hodgkin's lymphoma (HL) and non-Hodgkin's lymphoma (NHL).

Hodgkin's Lymphoma

PATHOPHYSIOLOGY

Hodgkin's lymphoma (HL) is a cancer that can affect any age-group. It occurs most often in people in their mid to late 20s and in people older than 50 years of age (McCance & Huether, 2002). HL equally affects younger men and women, but the disease is more prevalent in men in the older group.

Possible causes of HL include viral infections and exposure to chemical agents. This cancer usually starts in a single lymph node or a single chain of nodes. The tissue in the node becomes cancerous. These nodes contain a specific cancer cell type, the **Reed-Sternberg cell,** a marker for Hodgkin's lymphoma. The disease first spreads in a predictable manner to nearby lymph tissues and eventually invades nonlymphoid tissues.

COLLABORATIVE MANAGEMENT

Assessment

The most common first assessment finding is a large but painless lymph node or nodes, usually in the neck. The client also often has fever, malaise, and night sweats (Table 43-5). Specific manifestations depend on the site and extent of disease.

Diagnosis and grade are established when biopsy of a node or mass reveals Reed-Sternberg cells (McCance & Huether, 2002). The client then undergoes staging procedures to determine the extent of disease. Staging is detailed and accurate because the treatment regimen is determined by the extent of disease. Staging procedures for HL include biopsies of distant lymph nodes, computed tomography (CT) of the chest and abdomen, laparotomy, a complete blood count (CBC), liver function studies, and bilateral bone marrow biopsies.

TABLE 43-5 Manifestations and Staging Criteria for Hodgkin's Lymphoma

Stage Ia
Disease is confined to a single lymph node region or only one extranodal site.

Stage Ib
Disease is confined to a single lymph node region or only one extranodal site. The client also experiences some or all of the following systemic symptoms: persistent fever, night sweats, and significant weight loss (>10%).

Stage IIa
Disease is confined to either two or more lymph node regions on the same side of the diaphragm or contiguous extranodal sites on the same side of the diaphragm.

Stage IIb
Disease is confined to either two or more lymph node regions on the same side of the diaphragm or contiguous extranodal sites on the same side of the diaphragm. Client also experiences some or all of the following systemic symptoms: persistent fever, night sweats, and significant weight loss (>10%).

Stage IIIa
Disease extends to lymph node regions on both sides of the diaphragm.

Stage IIIb
Disease extends to lymph node regions on both sides of the diaphragm. The client also experiences some or all of the following systemic symptoms: persistent fever, night sweats, and significant weight loss (>10%).

Stage IIIc
Disease extends to lymph node regions on both sides of the diaphragm. The client also experiences some or all of the following systemic symptoms: persistent fever, night sweats, and significant weight loss (>10%). The spleen is also involved in disease.

Stage IV
Disease has widely disseminated foci of involvement, including one or more extranodal tissues and organs.

Interventions

Hodgkin's lymphoma (HL) is one of the most curable types of cancer. Generally, for stage I and stage II disease, the treatment of choice is external radiation of involved lymph node regions. With more extensive disease, radiation is used along with combination chemotherapy to achieve a cure. (See Chapter 28 on general care of clients receiving radiation and chemotherapy.)

Nursing management of the client undergoing treatment for HL focuses on the side effects of therapy, especially the following:

- Drug-induced pancytopenia, which increases the risk for infection, bleeding, and anemia
- Severe nausea and vomiting
- Skin problems at the site of radiation
- Impaired hepatic function either by metastasis to the liver or by multiagent chemotherapy
- Permanent sterility for male clients receiving radiation to the abdominopelvic region in the pattern of an inverted Y in combination with specific chemotherapeutic agents (The client is informed of this side effect and given the option to store sperm in a sperm bank before treatment.)
- Secondary cancer development as a result of HL treatment (Long-term follow-up includes screening for recurrence, as well as the possible development of a secondary cancer.)

Non-Hodgkin's Lymphoma

PATHOPHYSIOLOGY

Non-Hodgkin's lymphoma (NHL) includes all lymphoid cancers that do not have the Reed-Sternberg cell. There are more than 12 subtypes of NHL, including low-grade, intermediate, and high-grade lymphomas. NHLs arise from altered B or T lymphocytes. The low-grade lymphomas usually arise from B-cell lymphocytes and progress slowly. Although clients with low-grade lymphomas have longer survival rates, the diseases are less responsive to treatment and cures are rare (Strauss, 2003).

High-grade lymphomas are aggressive tumors of mixed cell types with rapid growth. High-grade lymphomas are more responsive to chemotherapy, and the chances for a long-term cure are greater. A low-grade lymphoma can convert to a higher-grade lymphoma. When this occurs, the prognosis is poor.

NHL is the sixth most common cause of cancer-related death in the United States (American Cancer Society, 2005). The disease is more common in men, white individuals, and people older than 50 years of age. The long-term prognosis is better for women and clients younger than 65 years of age. Most NHLs start in lymph nodes, but they can originate in any tissue or organ. NHL may be related to inherited problems that result in gene damage. Gene damage may result in loss of tumor suppressor gene function, allowing cancer development to occur. Viral infection, autoimmune disease, and exposure to radiation or to toxic chemicals have all been implicated in the development of NHL.

◆COLLABORATIVE MANAGEMENT

Enlarged lymph nodes may be the only manifestation of lymphoma because these nodes can arise from lymphoid cells in any tissue and can spread to any organ. Painless swelling of the cervical, axillary, inguinal, and femoral nodes are most often seen. Diagnosis is made from the histologic features of cells obtained by biopsy of a node or mass. Classification of the lymphoma subtype is based on a complex grading of surface markers, chromosomes, cell size, and presence of viral antigens. Staging is similar to that for Hodgkin's lymphoma (HL) (see Table 43-5).

Treatment consists of radiation therapy and multiagent chemotherapy, or single-agent therapy with fludarabine. In relapsed disease, newer agents including monoclonal antibodies (e.g., rituximab and alemtuzumab) and radiolabeled antibodies (^{131}I tositumomab and ^{90}Y ibritumomab) are being used. Nursing care needs are similar to those for clients with HL, with additional organ-specific problems taken into account if the disease is widely spread.

Multiple Myeloma

PATHOPHYSIOLOGY

Multiple myeloma is a white blood cell (WBC) cancer that involves a more mature lymphocyte than either leukemia or lymphoma. There is overgrowth of B-lymphocyte plasma cells in the bone marrow. These cells normally make antibodies. When they become cancerous, these plasma cells overproduce both complete and incomplete antibodies or gamma globulins. Thus the disorder is called a "gammopathy." Similar to the leukemias, when the myeloma cells are overproduced, fewer functional red blood cells (RBCs), WBCs, and platelets are produced.

In addition to the excess antibodies, multiple myeloma cells also produce excess cytokines (see Chapter 23) that increase the cancer cell growth rates and destroy bone. The excess antibodies are released into the blood, increasing the serum protein levels and clogging blood vessels in the kidney and other organs. Without treatment, the disease causes progressive bone destruction, bleeding problems, kidney failure, immunosuppression, and death.

Multiple myeloma is an uncommon cancer, accounting for 1% of all cancers (Rice & Sheridan, 2001). This disorder occurs mostly in people older than 50 years of age and is about twice as common among African Americans as white individuals. It occurs equally in men and women. The cause of multiple myeloma is unknown, although radiation and chemical exposure may be risk factors.

◆COLLABORATIVE MANAGEMENT

The client with multiple myeloma usually first notices fatigue, easy bruising, and bone pain. Other manifestations, such as bone fractures, hypertension, increased infection, hypercalcemia, and fluid imbalance, occur as the disease progresses. Diagnosis is made by bone marrow biopsy, x-ray findings of bone thinning with areas of bone loss that resemble "Swiss cheese," electrophoresis of plasma proteins, and the presence of "Bence-Jones" protein in the urine.

Standard treatment for multiple myeloma is chemotherapy. Agents most commonly used are melphalan, prednisone, vincristine, cyclophosphamide, doxorubicin, and carmustine. Recently, thalidomide is showing promise in controlling the disease. Autologous bone marrow transplantation is being used with clients who have a good response to the chemotherapy. For client's whose disease progresses despite treatment, a recently approved proteasome inhibitor, bortezomib (Velcade), may be used. Bortezomib acts by blocking processes needed for the cancer cells' growth and survival. Side effects include fatigue, nausea, diarrhea, neuropathy, thrombocytopenia, and neutropenia.

Coagulation Disorders

Coagulation disorders are bleeding disorders with increased bleeding resulting from defects in one or more components regulating the blood clotting system. Bleeding disorders may be spontaneous or traumatic, localized or generalized, lifelong or acquired. They can arise from a defect in the clotting processes at the vascular, platelet, or clotting factor level. Figure 43-5 outlines the blood-clotting cascade and sites where specific defects and drugs disrupt the clotting processes.

PLATELET DISORDERS

Platelets have a vital role in blood clotting. Blood clotting always starts with platelets sticking together and forming a platelet plug. Any condition that either reduces the number of platelets or interferes with their ability to adhere (to one another, blood vessel walls, collagen, or fibrin threads) can result in increased bleeding. Platelet disorders can be inherited, acquired, or temporarily induced by drugs that limit platelet production or inhibit aggregation.

A decrease in the number of platelets below the level needed for normal coagulation is called **thrombocytopenia.** Thrombocytopenia may occur as a result of other conditions or treatments that suppress general bone marrow activity. It also can occur through processes that limit platelet formation or increase the rate of platelet destruction. The two thrombocytopenic conditions affecting adults are autoim-

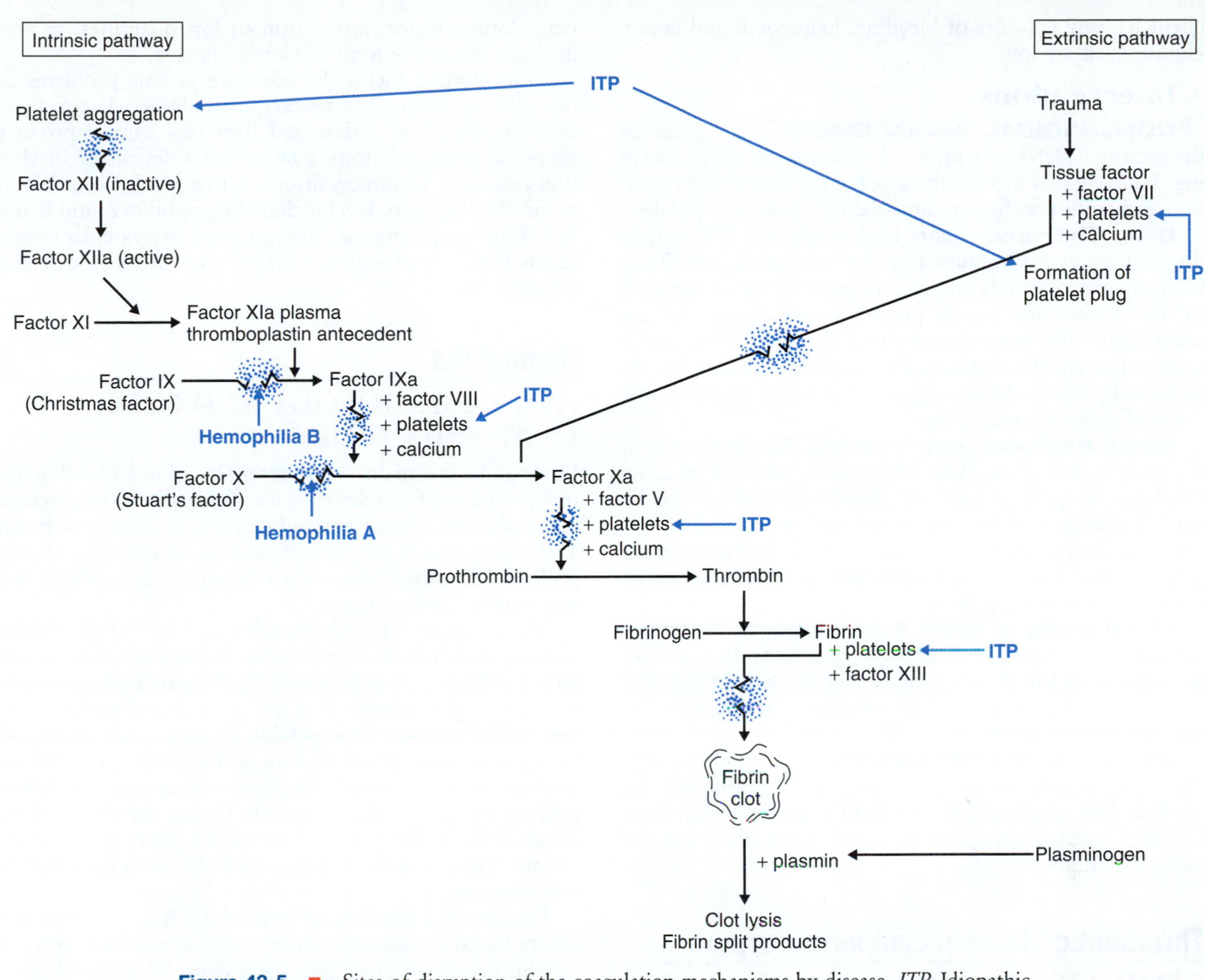

Figure 43-5 ■ Sites of disruption of the coagulation mechanisms by disease. *ITP,* Idiopathic thrombocytopenic purpura.

mune thrombocytopenic purpura and thrombotic thrombocytopenic purpura.

Autoimmune Thrombocytopenic Purpura

PATHOPHYSIOLOGY

Autoimmune thrombocytopenic purpura is also called idiopathic thrombocytopenic purpura (ITP). The total number of circulating platelets is greatly reduced in ITP, even though platelet production in the bone marrow is normal.

Clients with this disorder make an antibody directed against the surface of their own platelets (an antiplatelet-antibody). This antibody coats the surface of the platelets, making them more likely to be destroyed by macrophages (see Chapter 23). The spleen contains a large number of macrophages and the blood vessels of the spleen are long and twisted. Both of these conditions allow antibody-coated platelets to be destroyed in the spleen (Blackwell, 2003). When the rate of platelet destruction exceeds that of production, the number of circulating platelets decreases and blood clotting slows.

Although the cause of this disorder is autoimmune, the trigger for the production of autoantibodies is unknown. ITP is most common among women between the ages of 20 and 40 and among people who have other autoimmune disorders, such as systemic lupus erythematosus (McCance & Huether, 2002).

COLLABORATIVE MANAGEMENT

Assessment

Clinical manifestations of ITP are at first limited to the skin and mucous membranes: large **ecchymoses** (bruises) or a petechial rash on the arms, legs, upper chest, and neck. Mucosal bleeding occurs easily. If the client has had significant blood loss, anemia may also be present.

A rare complication is an intracranial bleed–induced stroke. Assess for neurologic function and mental status (see Chapter 44). Ask family members whether the client's behavior and responses to questions are typical or represent a change.

ITP is diagnosed by a decreased platelet count and large numbers of megakaryocytes in the bone marrow. Antiplatelet antibodies may be detected in the blood. If the client has any episodes of bleeding, hematocrit and hemoglobin levels are low.

Interventions

NONSURGICAL MANAGEMENT. As a result of the decreased platelet count, the client is at great risk for bleeding. Interventions include therapy for the underlying condition and protection from trauma-induced bleeding episodes.

Drug Therapy. Agents used to control ITP include drugs that suppress immune function to some degree. Drugs such as corticosteroids and azathioprine (Imuran) are used to inhibit immune system production of antiplatelet autoantibodies. IV immunoglobulin and IV anti-Rho can be used to prevent the destruction of antibody-coated platelets (Blackwell, 2003). More aggressive therapy involves low doses of chemotherapy drugs.

Blood Replacement Therapy. For the client with a platelet count of less than 20,000/mm^3 who has an acute life-threatening bleeding episode, platelet transfusions may be needed. Platelet transfusions are not performed routinely because the donated platelets are just as rapidly destroyed by the spleen as the client's own platelets (see later discussion under Platelet Transfusions, p. 915).

Maintaining a Safe Environment. The major goals are to protect the client from conditions that can lead to bleeding and to closely monitor the amount of bleeding that is occurring. (For nursing care actions, see Risk for Injury [Leukemia], p. 906.)

SURGICAL MANAGEMENT. For the client who does not respond to drug therapy, splenectomy may be needed. After splenectomy, the client is at increased risk for infection because the spleen performs many protective immune functions.

Thrombotic Thrombocytopenic Purpura

PATHOPHYSIOLOGY

Thrombotic thrombocytopenic purpura (TTP) is a rare disorder in which platelets clump together abnormally in the capillaries and too few platelets remain in circulation. The client has inappropriate clotting, yet the blood fails to clot properly when trauma occurs. The underlying cause of TTP appears to be an autoimmune reaction in blood vessel cells (endothelial cells) that makes platelets clump together in very small blood vessels. As a result, tissues become ischemic. Manifestations include renal failure, myocardial infarction, and stroke. If left untreated, this condition is often fatal within 3 months.

COLLABORATIVE MANAGEMENT

Treatment for the client with TTP focuses on preventing platelet clumping and stopping the underlying autoimmune process. Treatment consists of plasma pheresis and the infusion of fresh frozen plasma. This treatment provides platelet aggregation inhibitors. Drugs that inhibit platelet clumping, such as aspirin, alprostadil (Prostin), and plicamycin, also may be helpful. Immunosuppressive therapy reduces the intensity of this disorder.

CLOTTING FACTOR DISORDERS

Coagulation or bleeding disorders can result from a clotting factor defect. Defects include the inability to produce a specific clotting factor, production of low quantities, or producing a less active form of clotting factors.

Most clotting factor disorders are genetic problems of one clotting factor. The few acquired clotting factor disorders are related to a damaged liver that cannot produce proper amounts of clotting factors or a deficiency of clotting cofactors. Common disorders that result from defects at the clotting factor level include hemophilias A and B and von Willebrand's disease. Disseminated intravascular coagulation (DIC) is closely associated with septic shock (see Chapter 40).

Hemophilia

PATHOPHYSIOLOGY AND GENETICS OF THE DISORDER

Hemophilia is actually two different hereditary bleeding disorders resulting from deficiencies of specific clotting factors. Hemophilia A (classic hemophilia) is a deficiency of factor VIII and accounts for 80% of cases of hemophilia. Hemophilia B (Christmas disease) is a deficiency of factor IX and accounts for 20% of cases.

The incidence of both disorders is 1 in 10,000. Hemophilia is an X-linked recessive trait. Women who are carriers have a 50% chance of transmitting the gene for hemophilia to their daughters (who then are carriers) and to their sons (who will have overt hemophilia). Hemophilia A mostly affects males, none of whose sons will have the gene for hemophilia and all of whose daughters will be **carriers** (able to pass on the gene without actually having the disorder). In about 30% of clients with hemophilia, there is no family history, and it is presumed that their disease is the result of a new mutation.

The bleeding disorder of hemophilia A is so severe that before blood transfusions were available, children with hemophilia rarely survived past age 3 years. With blood transfusion and factor VIII therapy, survival time has increased so greatly that hemophilia now is often seen among adult clients.

The clinical pictures of hemophilia A and B are identical. The client has abnormal bleeding in response to any trauma because of a deficiency of the specific clotting factor. Clients with hemophilia do not bleed more frequently or even more rapidly than those without the disease, but they do bleed for a longer period. Hemophiliacs form platelet plugs at the bleeding site, but the clotting factor deficiency impairs the clotting response and stable fibrin clots do not form. This allows excessive bleeding, which may be mild, moderate, or severe, depending on the degree of factor deficiency.

COLLABORATIVE MANAGEMENT

Assessment

Assessment of the client with hemophilia shows the following:

- Excessive hemorrhage from minor cuts, bruises, or abrasions (as a result of abnormal platelet function)
- Joint and muscle hemorrhages that lead to disabling long-term problems
- A tendency to bruise easily
- Prolonged and potentially fatal postoperative hemorrhage

The laboratory test results for a client with hemophilia show a prolonged partial thromboplastin time (PTT), a normal bleeding time, and a normal prothrombin time (PT). The most common problem that occurs with hemophilia is degenerating joint function as a result of chronic bleeding into the joints, especially at the hip and knee.

Interventions

The bleeding problems of hemophilia A are managed by either regularly scheduled IV infusions of factor VIII cryoprecipitate (Bioclate, Helixate, ReFacto) or intermittent infusions as needed (see Cryoprecipitate Transfusions, p. 915). The cost of cryoprecipitate is prohibitive for many people with hemophilia. In addition, because the precipitated clotting factors are made from pooled human serum, a risk for viral contamination remains, even with the use of heat-inactivated serum. Infectious complications of hemophilia therapy include hepatitis B, hepatitis C, cytomegalovirus, and human immunodeficiency virus (HIV). Although newer serum processing techniques have reduced these risks, they have not yet been eliminated.

Transfusion Therapy

Any blood component may be removed from a donor and transfused to a recipient. Components may be transfused individually or collectively, with varying degrees of benefit to the recipient. Table 43-6 lists indications for transfusion therapy.

PRETRANSFUSION RESPONSIBILITIES

Nursing actions during transfusions aim at prevention or early recognition of adverse transfusion reactions. Preparation of the client for transfusion therapy is imperative, and institutional blood product administration procedures must be carefully followed. Before administering any blood product, review the agency's policies and procedures. Chart 43-15 lists best practices for transfusion therapy.

Legally, a physician's prescription is needed to administer blood or its components. The prescription specifies the type of component, the volume, and any special conditions the physician judges to be important. Verify the prescription for accuracy and completeness. In many hospitals a separate consent form must be obtained before a transfusion is performed.

A blood specimen is obtained for crossmatching (testing of the donor's blood and the recipient's blood for compatibility). The procedure and responsibility for obtaining this specimen are specified by hospital policy. The laboratory requires at least 45 minutes to complete the crossmatch testing. In most hospitals a new crossmatching specimen is required at least every 48 hours.

Blood components are viscous, requiring that a large needle (at least 20-gauge) be used, whenever possible, for venous access. Both Y-tubing and straight tubing sets are used for blood component infusion. A blood filter (about 170 μm) to remove sediment from the stored blood products is included with blood administration sets and must be used to transfuse most blood products. In massive transfusion, a microaggregate filter (20 to 43 μm) may be used.

Use normal saline as the solution to administer with blood products. Ringer's lactate and dextrose in water are not used for infusion with blood products because they cause clotting or hemolysis of blood cells. *Never add drugs to blood products.*

Before the transfusion is started, it is essential to determine that the blood component delivered is correct and that identification of the client is correct. Check the physician's prescription simultaneously with another registered nurse to determine the client's identity and whether the hospital identification band name and number are identical to those on the blood component tag. *Checking the client's room number is not an acceptable form of identification* (Joint Commission on Accreditation of Healthcare Organizations, 2004). Examine the blood bag label, the attached tag, and the requisition slip to ensure that the ABO and Rh types are compatible. Check the expiration date and inspect the product for discoloration, gas bubbles, or cloudiness, all indicators of bacterial growth or hemolysis.

TRANSFUSION RESPONSIBILITIES

Before starting the transfusion, explain the procedure to the client. Take the vital signs, including temperature, immediately before starting the transfusion. Begin the infusion slowly. Remain with the client for the first 15 to 30 minutes. Any severe reaction usually occurs with infusion of the first 50 mL of blood. Ask the client to report unusual

TABLE 43-6 Indications for Treatment with Blood Components

Component	Volume	Infusion Time	Indications
Packed red blood cells (PRBCs)	200-250 mL	2-4 hr	Anemia; hemoglobin <6 g/dL, 6-10 g/dL, depending on symptoms
Washed red blood cells (WBC-poor PRBCs)	200 mL	2-4 hr	History of allergic transfusion reactions Bone marrow transplant clients
Platelets			
Pooled	About 300 mL	15-30 min	Thrombocytopenia, platelet count <20,000 Clients who are actively bleeding with a platelet count <80,000
Single donor	200 mL	30 min	History of febrile or allergic reactions
Fresh frozen plasma	200 mL	15-30 min	Deficiency in plasma coagulation factors Prothrombin or partial thromboplastin time 1.5 times normal
Cryoprecipitate	10-20 mL/unit	15-30 min	Hemophilia VIII or von Willebrand's disease Fibrinogen levels <100 mg/dL
White blood cells (WBCs)	400 mL	1 hr	Sepsis, neutropenic infection not responding to antibiotic therapy

CHART 43-15

BEST PRACTICE for
Transfusion Therapy

Nursing Actions	Rationales
Before Infusion	
1. Assess laboratory values.	Many institutions have specific guidelines for blood product transfusions (i.e., platelet count <20,000 or hemoglobin <6 g/dL).
2. Verify the medical prescription.	Legally, a physician's prescription is required for transfusions. The order should state the type of product, dose, and transfusion time.
3. Assess the client's vital signs, urine output, skin color, and history of transfusion reactions.	Determine whether the client can tolerate infusion. Baseline information may be needed to help identify transfusion reactions.
4. Obtain venous access. Use a central catheter or 19-gauge needle if possible.	The larger-bore needle allows cells to flow more easily without occluding the lumen of the catheter.
5. Obtain blood products from a blood bank. Transfuse immediately.	Once a blood product has been released from the blood bank, the product should be transfused as soon as possible (e.g., red blood cell transfusions should be completed within 4 hours of removal from refrigeration).
6. With another registered nurse, verify the client by name and number, check blood compatibility, and note expiration time.	Human error is the most common cause of ABO incompatibility reactions.
During Infusion	
7. Administer the blood product using the appropriate filtered tubing.	Filters are needed to remove aggregates and possible contaminants.
8. If the blood product needs to be diluted, use only normal saline solution.	Hemolysis occurs if any other IV solution is used.
9. Remain with the client during the first 15 to 30 minutes of the infusion.	Hemolytic reactions occur most often within the first 50 mL of the infusion.
10. Infuse the blood product at the prescribed rate.	Fluid overload is a potential complication of rapid infusion.
11. Monitor vital signs.	Vital sign changes often indicate transfusion reactions.
After Infusion	
12. When the transfusion is completed, discontinue infusion and dispose of the bag and tubing properly.	Bloodborne pathogens may be spread inadvertently through improper disposal.
13. Document.	The client record should indicate the type of product infused, product number, volume infused, time of infusion, and any adverse reactions.

sensations such as chills, shortness of breath, hives, or itching. Assess vital signs 15 minutes after starting the transfusion to detect signs of a reaction. If there are none, the infusion rate can be increased to transfuse 1 unit in about 2 hours (depending on the client's cardiac status). Take vital signs every hour throughout the transfusion or as specified by agency policy.

Blood components without large amounts of red blood cells (RBCs) can be infused more quickly. The identification checks are the same as for RBC transfusions. It may be necessary to infuse blood products at a slower rate for older clients. Best practices related to the nursing care needs of older clients during transfusion therapy are listed in Chart 43-16.

TYPES OF TRANSFUSIONS

Red Blood Cell Transfusions

RBCs are given to replace cells lost as a result of trauma or surgery. Clients with problems that destroy RBCs or impair RBC maturation also may benefit from RBC transfusions. Packed RBCs, supplied in 250-mL bags, are a concentrated source of RBCs and are the most common component given to RBC-deficient clients. Packed RBCs are given to clients with a hemoglobin level less than 6 g/dL (or a hemoglobin value of 6 to 10 g/dL if manifestations are present).

Blood transfusions are actually transplantations of tissue from one person to another. The donor and recipient blood must thus be carefully checked for compatibility to prevent lethal reactions (Table 43-7). Compatibility is determined by two different types of antigen systems (cell surface proteins): the ABO system antigens and the Rh antigen, which is present on the membrane surface of RBCs.

RBC antigens are inherited. For the ABO antigen system, a person inherits one of the following:

- A antigen (type A blood)
- B antigen (type B blood)
- Both A and B antigens (type AB blood)
- No A or B antigens (type O blood)

Within the first few years of life, circulating antibodies develop against the blood type antigens that were not inherited. For example, a person with type A blood forms antigens against type B blood. A person with type O blood has not inherited either A or B antigens and will form antibodies against RBCs that have either A or B antigens. If RBCs that contain an antigen are infused into a recipient who does not share the antigen, the donated tissue is recognized by the immune system of the recipient as non-self, and the recipient has a reaction to the transfused products.

CHART 43-16

BEST PRACTICE for

The Older Adult Receiving a Transfusion

- Assess the client's circulatory, renal, and fluid status before initiating the transfusion.
- Use no larger than a 19-gauge needle.
- Try to use blood that is less than 1 week old. (Older blood cell membranes are more fragile, break easily, and release potassium into the circulation.)
- Take vital signs (especially pulse, blood pressure, and respiratory rate) every 15 minutes throughout the transfusion. Changes in these parameters can indicate fluid overload and may also be the only indicators of adverse transfusion reactions.

Overload
- Rapid bounding pulse
- Hypertension
- Swollen superficial veins

Transfusion Reaction
- Rapid thready pulse
- Hypotension
- Increased pallor, cyanosis
- Administer blood slowly, taking 2 to 4 hours for each unit of whole blood, packed red blood cells, or plasma.
- Avoid concurrent fluid administration into any other IV site.
- If possible, allow 2 full hours after the administration of 1 unit of blood before administering the next unit.

The Rh antigen system is slightly different. An Rh-negative person is born without the Rh-antigen on his or her RBCs and does not form antibodies unless he or she is specifically sensitized to it. Sensitization can occur with RBC transfusions from an Rh-positive person or from exposure during pregnancy and birth. Once an Rh-negative person has been sensitized and antibody development has occurred, any exposure to Rh-positive blood can cause a transfusion reaction. Antibody development can be prevented by giving Rh-immune globulin as soon as exposure to the Rh antigen is suspected. *People who have Rh-positive blood can receive an RBC transfusion from an Rh-negative donor, but Rh-negative people should not receive Rh-positive blood.*

Platelet Transfusions

Platelets are given to clients with platelet counts below 20,000 mm³ and to clients with thrombocytopenia who are actively bleeding or are scheduled for an invasive procedure. Platelet transfusions are usually pooled from as many as 10 donors and do not have to be of the same blood type as the client. For clients who are going to receive a bone marrow transplant (BMT) or who need multiple platelet transfusions, single-donor platelets may be prescribed. Single-donor platelets are taken from just one donor and decrease the amount of antigen exposure to the recipient, helping to prevent the formation of platelet antibodies. The chances of allergic reactions to future platelet transfusions are thus reduced.

Platelet infusion bags usually contain 300 mL for pooled platelets and 200 mL for single-donor platelets. Platelets are fragile and must be infused immediately after being brought to the client's room, usually over a 15- to 30-minute period. A special transfusion set with a smaller filter and shorter tubing is used. *Standard transfusion sets are not used with platelets because the filter traps the platelets, and the longer tubing increases platelet adherence to the lumen.* Additional platelet filters help remove white blood cells (WBCs) from the platelet concentrate. These filters are connected directly to the platelet transfusion set and are used for clients who have a history of febrile reactions or who need multiple platelet transfusions.

TABLE 43-7 Compatibility Chart for Red Blood Cell Transfusions

	Recipient			
Donor	A	B	AB	O
A	X		X	
B		X	X	
AB			X	
O	X	X	X	X

Take the vital signs before the infusion, 15 minutes after the infusion is initiated, and at its completion. The client may be premedicated with meperidine (Demerol) or hydrocortisone to reduce the chances of a reaction. He or she can become febrile and have **rigors** (severe chills) during transfusion, but these symptoms are not considered a true transfusion reaction. IV infusion of amphotericin B (Amphotec, Fungizone), an antifungal agent given to many clients with leukemia, is discontinued during platelet transfusion and not resumed for at least 1 hour after transfusion. This drug can cause severe allergic reactions that are difficult to distinguish from transfusion reactions.

Plasma Transfusions

Plasma infusions may be given fresh to replace blood volume. More commonly, plasma is frozen immediately after donation, forming **fresh frozen plasma (FFP)**. Freezing preserves the clotting factors, and the plasma can then be used for clients with clotting disorders. Infuse FFP immediately after thawing while the clotting factors are still active. Clients who are actively bleeding with a prothrombin time (PT) or partial thromboplastin time (PTT) greater than 1.5 times normal are candidates for an FFP infusion.

ABO compatibility is required for transfusion of plasma products. The infusion bag contains about 200 mL. Infuse FFP as rapidly as the client can tolerate, generally over a 30- to 60-minute period, through a regular Y-set or straight-filtered tubing.

Cryoprecipitate Transfusions

Cryoprecipitate is a product derived from plasma. Clotting factors VIII and XIII, von Willebrand's factor, and fibrinogen are precipitated from pooled plasma to produce cryoprecipitate. Clients with a fibrinogen level of less than 100 mg/dL are candidates for a cryoprecipitate infusion. Give this highly concentrated blood product to clients with clotting factor disorders at a volume of 10 to 15 mL/unit. Although cryoprecipitate can be infused, it is usually given by IV push within 3 minutes. Dosages are individualized, and it is best if the cryoprecipitate is ABO compatible.

Granulocyte (White Cell) Transfusions

At some centers, neutropenic clients with infections receive white blood cell (WBC) replacement transfusions. This practice is controversial because the potential benefit to the client must be weighed against the potential severe reactions that often occur with WBC transfusions. The surfaces of WBCs contain many antigens that can cause severe reactions when infused into a client whose immune system recognizes these antigens as non-self. In addition, transfused WBCs have a short life span and provide minimal protection (see Chapter 23).

WBCs are suspended in 430 mL of plasma and should be infused over a 45- to 60-minute period. Agency policies often require more stringent monitoring of clients receiving WBCs. A physician may need to be present in the hospital unit, and vital signs may need to be taken every 15 minutes throughout the transfusion. Amphotericin B infusion and WBC transfusions should be separated by 4 to 6 hours.

CULTURAL CONSIDERATIONS

Although transfusion with blood products is common in acute care settings, you must remain sensitive to those clients who view receiving blood or blood products of others as repugnant, even sinful. More than 800,000 Jehovah's Witnesses live in the United States. A belief of Jehovah's Witnesses is that receiving autotransfusion or donated blood is the same as "consuming" blood, an act specifically prohibited in the Old Testament. Often Jehovah's Witnesses will accept the use of dialysis and heart-lung equipment, as well as intraoperative blood salvage if the blood outside the body remains intact with circulatory system. Whenever possible, transfusion therapy with human blood products is avoided for this group. If in an emergency situation, clients are transfused with blood products against their will, show respect for the client's distress and religious beliefs (Glendenning, 2002).

Newer therapies for clients with anemia or hypovolemia may reduce the need for transfusion of human blood products. One therapy is the use of hemoglobin substitutes, also known as "artificial blood," which increases the oxygen-carrying power of the client's own blood. In addition, pretreating or treating these clients with epoetin alfa (Procrit) or darbepoetin alfa (Aranesp) can reduce the recovery time from blood loss without transfusion.

TRANSFUSION REACTIONS

Clients can develop any of the following transfusion reactions: hemolytic, allergic, febrile, or bacterial reactions; circulatory overload; or transfusion-associated graft-versus-host disease (GVHD). Remain vigilant during transfusions to prevent complications through early detection and initiation of appropriate treatment.

Hemolytic Transfusion Reactions

Hemolytic transfusion reactions are caused by blood type or Rh incompatibility. When blood containing antigens different from the client's own antigens is infused, antigen-antibody complexes are formed in the client's blood. These complexes destroy the transfused cells and start inflammatory responses in the client's blood vessel walls and organs. The reaction may be mild, with fever and chills, or life threatening, with disseminated intravascular coagulation (DIC) and circulatory collapse. Other manifestations include the following:

- Apprehension
- Headache
- Chest pain
- Low back pain
- Tachycardia
- Tachypnea
- Hypotension
- Hemoglobinuria
- A sense of impending doom

The onset of a hemolytic reaction may be immediate or may not occur until subsequent units have been transfused (McConnell, 2000; Atterbury, 2001).

Allergic Transfusion Reactions

Allergic transfusion reactions are most often seen in clients with a history of allergy. They may have urticaria, itching, bronchospasm, or anaphylaxis. Onset of this type of reaction usually occurs during or up to 24 hours after the transfusion. Clients with a history of allergy can be given leukocyte-reduced or washed red blood cells (RBCs) in which the white blood cells (WBCs) and plasma have been removed. This procedure reduces the possibility of an allergic reaction.

Febrile Transfusion Reactions

Febrile transfusion reactions occur most often in the client with anti-WBC antibodies, a situation that can develop after multiple transfusions. The recipient develops the following:

- Chills
- Tachycardia
- Fever
- Hypotension
- Tachypnea

Giving leukocyte-reduced blood or single-donor HLA-matched platelets reduces the risk for this type of reaction. WBC filters may be used to trap WBCs and prevent their infusion into the client (Baldwin, 2002).

Bacterial Transfusion Reactions

Bacterial transfusion reactions occur as a result of infusion of contaminated blood products. Usually a gram-negative organism is the source because these bacteria grow rapidly in blood stored under refrigeration. Symptoms include the following:

- Tachycardia
- Hypotension
- Fever
- Chills
- Shock

The onset of a bacterial transfusion reaction is rapid. (See Chapter 40 for care of the client experiencing septic shock.)

Circulatory Overload

Circulatory overload can occur when a blood product is infused too quickly. This complication is most common with whole-blood transfusions or when the client requires multiple transfusions. Older adults are most at risk for this condition (see Chart 43-16). Symptoms include the following:

- Hypertension
- Bounding pulse
- Distended jugular veins
- Dyspnea

- Restlessness
- Confusion

You can both manage and prevent this complication by monitoring intake and output, infusing blood products more slowly, and giving diuretics. (See Chapter 15 for management of clients with fluid overload.)

Transfusion-Associated Graft-Versus-Host Disease

Transfusion-associated graft-versus-host disease (TA-GVHD) is a rare but life-threatening problem that can occur in both immunosuppressed and immunocompetent clients. Its cause in immunosuppressed clients is similar to that of GVHD that occurs with allogeneic bone marrow transplantation (BMT), discussed on p. 902, in which donor T-cell lymphocytes attack host tissues.

Manifestations usually occur within 1 to 2 weeks and include thrombocytopenia, anorexia, nausea, vomiting, chronic hepatitis, weight loss, and recurrent infection.

TA-GVHD has a 90% mortality rate but can be prevented by using irradiated blood products. Irradiation destroys T-cells and their cytokine products.

AUTOLOGOUS BLOOD TRANSFUSIONS

Autologous blood transfusions involve collection and infusion of the client's own blood. This type of transfusion eliminates compatibility problems and reduces the risk for transmitting bloodborne diseases. The four types of autologous blood transfusions are preoperative autologous blood donation, acute normovolemic hemodilution, intraoperative autologous transfusion, and postoperative blood salvage.

Preoperative autologous blood donation, the most common type of autologous blood transfusion, involves collection of whole blood from the client, division into components, and then storage for later use (e.g., after a scheduled surgical procedure). As long as hematocrit and hemoglobin levels are within a safe range, the client can donate blood on a weekly basis until the prescribed amount of blood is obtained. Fresh packed RBCs may be stored for 43 days. For clients with rare blood types, blood may be frozen for up to 10 years. Platelets and plasma may be collected by pheresis. Some cardiac problems and bacteremia are contraindications for autologous blood donation.

Acute normovolemic hemodilution involves withdrawal of a client's RBCs and volume replacement just before a surgical procedure. The goal is to decrease RBC loss during surgery. The blood is stored at room temperature for up to 6 hours and reinfused after surgery. This type of autologous transfusion is contraindicated for anemic clients or those with poor renal function.

Intraoperative autologous transfusion and postoperative blood salvage are the recovery and reinfusion of a client's own blood, collected either from an operative field or from a bleeding wound. Special devices collect, filter, and drain the blood into a transfusion bag. This autologous blood is often used for trauma or surgical clients with severe blood loss. The salvaged blood must be reinfused within 6 hours.

Transfuse autologous blood products using the guidelines previously described. Although the client receiving autologous blood is not at risk for most types of transfusion reactions, you must still assess for circulatory overload or bacterial transfusion reactions that occur as a result of contamination.

GET READY for the NCLEX Examination!

KEY POINTS

Safe Effective Care Environment

- Use aseptic technique during all central line dressing changes or any invasive procedure.
- Use standard precautions for all clients regardless of age, gender, race or ethnicity, sexual orientation, education level, and profession.
- Ask all clients about advance directives and document their status.
- Use good handwashing techniques before providing any care to a client who is either immunocompromised or immunodeficient.
- Use bleeding precautions for any client with thrombocytopenia pancytopenia (see Chart 43-10).
- Verify prescriptions for transfusion of blood products with another registered nurse.
- Use at least two forms of identification for the client who is to receive a blood product transfusion (name and identification number). *Do not use a room number to identify the client.*

Health Promotion and Maintenance

- Teach people to avoid unnecessary contact with environmental chemicals or toxins. If contact cannot be avoided, teach people to use safety precautions.
- Identify clients at high risk for infection because of disease or therapy.
- Teach the client and family about the manifestations of infection and when to seek medical advice.
- Instruct clients who have anemia as a result of dietary deficiency which foods are good sources of iron, folic acid, and vitamin B_{12}.
- Teach precautions to take to avoid injury (Chart 43-14) to clients at risk for bleeding.

Psychosocial Integrity

- Allow the client the opportunity to express fear or anxiety regarding the diagnosis of leukemia or lymphoma or the treatment regimen, including bone marrow transplantation.
- Explain all procedures, restrictions, medications, and follow-up care to the client and family.
- Offer alternative therapies for relaxation, pain reduction, and distraction, such as massage, music therapy, and guided imagery.
- Refer clients and family members to local cancer resources and support groups.
- Reassure clients having pain that using opioid analgesics for needed pain relief is not drug abuse.

Physiological Integrity

- Teach the client about any medications to be continued after discharge from the hospital.
- Instruct the client and family in the manifestations of complications and when to seek assistance.
- Pace nonurgent health care activities to reduce the risk for fatigue among clients with anemia or pancytopenia.

- Assess the client in the induction phase of chemotherapy and those after BMT every shift for manifestations of infection.
- Assess the skin integrity of the perianal region of a client with leukemia after every bowel movement.
- Administer analgesics on a schedule rather than PRN.
- Use normal saline as the solution infusing with blood products.
- Transfuse blood products more slowly to older clients or those who have a cardiac problem.
- Remain with the client during the first 15 minutes of infusion of any blood product.
- Do not administer any drugs with infusing blood products.

ADDITIONAL STUDY RESOURCES

Go to your Student CD-ROM for Review Questions for the NCLEX Examination.

evolve Go to http://evolve.elsevier.com/Iggy/ for Integrated Management of Care Questions for the NCLEX Examination.

SELECTED BIBLIOGRAPHY

Asterisk indicates a classic or definitive work on this subject.

American Cancer Society. (2005). *Cancer facts and figures 2005.* Report No. 01-300M-No. 5008.05. Atlanta: Author.

Anastasia, P. (2001). Nursing considerations for managing topotecan- related hematologic side effects. *Clinical Journal of Oncology Nursing, 5*(1), 9-13.

Applebaum, F. (2003). Update on treatment for acute myeloid leukemia. *Oncology (Special Edition),* 6, 45-49.

Atterbury, C. (2001). Blood transfusions. *Nursing Times, 97*(27), 45-46.

Baldwin, P. (2002). Febrile nonhemolytic transfusion reactions. *Clinical Journal of Oncology Nursing,* 6(3), 171-172.

Bedell, C. (2003). Pegfilgrastim for chemotherapy-induced neutropenia. *Clinical Journal of Oncology Nursing, 7*(1),55-64.

Bennett, C., & Schumock, G. (2003). Cost analyses of adjunct colony stimulating factors for older patients with acute myeloid leukemia: Can they improve clinical decision making? *Drugs & Aging,* 20(7), 479-483.

*Bilodeau, B.B., & Fessele, K.L. (1998). Non-Hodgkin's lymphoma. *Seminars in Oncology Nursing, 14*(4), 273-283.

Birner, A. (2003). Safe administration of oral chemotherapy. *Clinical Journal of Oncology Nursing, 7*(2), 158-162.

Blackwell, J. (2003). Diagnosis and treatment of idiopathic thrombocytopenia purpura. *Journal of the American Academy of Nurse Practitioners, 15*(6), 244-245.

Blash, J. (2002). Systemic candida infections in patients with leukemia: An overview of drug therapy. *Clinical Journal of Oncology Nursing,* 6(6), 323-331.

Brown, C., & Yoder, L. (2002). Stomatitis: An overview. *American Journal of Nursing, 102*(4), 20-23.

Buchsel, P., Murphy, B., & Newton, S. (2002). Epoetin Alfa: Current and future indications and nursing implications. *Clinical Journal of Oncology Nursing,* 6(5), 261-267.

Cagen, D., Franco, M., & Vasquez, D. (2002). The ABCs of low blood cell count. *Clinical Journal of Oncology Nursing,* 6(1), 34-36.

*Callaghan, M. (1998). Hodgkin's disease. *Seminars in Oncology Nursing 14*(4), 262-272.

*Chielens, D. (1999). Chronic myelogenous leukemia. In C. Miaskowski & P. Buchsel (Eds.), *Oncology nursing: Assessment and clinical care* (pp. 1239-1250). St. Louis: Mosby.

Clark, P., & Gomez, E. (2001). Details on demand: Consumers, cancer information, and the Internet. *Clinical Journal of Oncology Nursing, 5*(1), 19-26.

Cleveland, K. (2003). Argatroban: A new treatment option for heparin-induced thrombocytopenia. *Critical Care Nurse, 23*(6), 61-66.

Cook, L. (2000). A simple case of anemia: Pathophysiology of a common symptom. *Journal of Intravenous Nursing, 23*(5), 271-281.

Cope, D. (2002). Patients' and physicians' experiences with sperm banking and infertility issues related to cancer treatment. *Clinical Journal of Oncology Nursing,* 6(5), 293-295, 309.

D'Arcy, Y. (2004). Managing sickle-cell crisis. *Nursing2004, 34*(1), 24-25.

Davey, M. (2002). Imatinib mesylate. *Clinical Journal of Oncology Nursing,* 6(2), 118-120

Day, S., & Wynn, L. (2000). Sickle cell pain & hydroxyurea. *American Journal of Nursing, 100*(11), 34-39.

Decker, G. (2000). Pharmacologic and biologic therapies in cancer care. *Clinical Journal of Oncology Nursing,* 4(5), 242-244.

Dillman, R. (2001). Monoclonal antibody therapy for lymphoma. *Cancer Practice,* 9(2), 71-80.

Dochterman, J.M., & Bulechek, G.M. (2004). *Nursing interventions classification (NIC)* (4th ed.). St. Louis: Mosby.

Ebersole, P., Hess, P., & Luggen, A. (2004). *Toward healthy aging: Human needs and nursing response* (6th ed.). St. Louis: Mosby.

Facts and Comparisons. (2004). *Drug facts and comparisons* (58th ed.). St. Louis: Author.

Folloder, J. (2005). Effects of darbepoetin alfa administration every two weeks on hemoglobin and quality of life of patients receiving chemotherapy. *Oncology Nursing Forum, 32*(1), 81-89.

Franck, L., et al. (2002). Assessment of sickle cell pain in children and young adults using the Adolescent Pediatric Pain Tool. *Journal of Pain and Symptom Management, 23*(2), 114-120.

Garcia-Manero, G., & Kantarjian, H. (2003). Treatment innovations in chronic myelogenous leukemia. *Oncology (Special Edition), 6,* 25-30.

Giving Z-track injections. (2002). *Nursing2002, 32*(9), 81.

Glendenning, J. (2002). Refusal of blood because of religious beliefs: A patient's right to die. *Journal of Emergency Nursing, 28*(3), 196-198.

Golden, C. (2003). Polycythemia: A review. *Clinical Journal of Oncology Nursing, 7*(5), 553-556.

Goldman, D. (2000). Chronic lymphocytic leukemia and its impact on the immune system. *Clinical Journal of Oncology Nursing,* 4(5), 233-236.

Hacker, E.D. (2003). Quantitative measurement of quality of life in adult patients undergoing bone marrow transplant or peripheral blood stem cell transplant: A decade in review. *Oncology Nursing Forum, 30*(4). 613-629.

Hadaway, L. (2002). What you can do to decrease catheter-related infections. *Nursing2002, 32*(9), 46-48.

Hadaway, L. (2004). Preventing extravasation from a central line. *Nursing2004, 34*(6), 22-23.

Hendrix, C., deLeon, C., & Dillman, R. (2002). Radioimmunotherapy for non-Hodgkin's lymphoma with yttrium 90 ibritumomab tiuxetan. *Clinical Journal of Oncology Nursing,* 6(3), 144-148.

Hood, L. (2003). Chemotherapy in the elderly: Supportive therapy for chemotherapy-induced myelotoxicity. *Clinical Journal of Oncology Nursing, 7*(2), 185-190.

Horrell, C., & Rothman, J. (2000). Establishing the etiology of thrombocytopenia. *The Nurse Practitioner, 25*(6), 68-77.

Iovino, C. (2003). Acute myeloid leukemia: A classification and treatment update. *Clinical Journal of Oncology Nursing, 7*(5), 535-540.

Joint Commission on Accreditation of Healthcare Organizations (2004). National Patient Safety Goals. Patient Identification. Available at http://www.jcaho.com.

Kantarjian, H., et al. (2002). Hematologic and cytogenetic responses to imatinib mesylate in chronic myelogenous leukemia. *The New England Journal of Medicine, 346*(9), 645-652.

Kemp, J. (2002). Interdisciplinary modular teaching for patients undergoing progenitor cell transplantation. *Clinical Journal of Oncology Nursing,* 6(3), 157-160.

Kim, H. (2002). Mini-allogeneic stem cell transplantation. *Cancer Practice, 10*(3), 170-172.

Kirschman, A. (2004). Finding alternatives to blood transfusions. *Nursing2004, 34*(6), 58-62.

Kosits, C. (2000). Rituximab: A new monoclonal antibody therapy for non-Hodgkin's lymphoma. *Oncology Nursing Forum*, 27(1), 51-59.

Larsen, L., Neverett, S., & Larsen, R. (2001). Clinical nurse specialist as facilitator of interdisciplinary collaborative program for adult sickle cell population. *Clinical Nurse Specialist, 15*(1), 15-22.

Lynn, A., et al. (2003). Treatment of chronic lymphocytic leukemia with alemtuzumab: A review for nurses. *Oncology Nursing Forum, 30*(4), 689-696.

Maloy, B. (2000). Hematopoiesis, stem cells, and transplantation. *Journal of Intravenous Nursing, 23*(5), 298-303.

Mayorga, J., Richardson-Hardin, C., & Dicke, K. (2002). Arsenic trioxide as effective therapy for relapsed acute promyelocytic leukemia. *Clinical Journal of Oncology Nursing, 6*(6), 341-346.

McCance, K., & Huether, S. (2002). *Pathophysiology: The biologic basis for disease in adults and children* (4th ed.). St. Louis: Mosby.

McConnell, E. (2000). Infusion perfusion: IV pumps for every need. *Nursing Management, 31*(10), 49-50.

McGuire, D. (2002). Mucosal tissue injury in cancer therapy. *Cancer Practice, 10*(4), 179-191.

McSweeney, P., et al. (2001). Hematopoietic cell transplantation in older patients with hematologic malignancies: Replacing high-dose cytotoxic therapy with graft-versus-tumor effects. *Blood*, 97, 3390-3400.

Moorhead, S., Johnson, M., & Maas, M. (Eds.). (2004). *Nursing outcomes classification (NOC)* (3rd ed.). St. Louis: Mosby.

Moran, A., & Camp-Sorrell, D. (2002). Maintenance of venous access devices in patients with neutropenia. *Clinical Journal of Oncology Nursing, 6*(3), 126-130.

Mower-Wade, D., Bartley, M., & Chiari-Allwein, J. (2001). How to respond to shock. *Dimensions of Critical Care Nursing, 20*(2), 22-27.

National Comprehensive Cancer Network. (2004). Clinical practice guidelines in oncology nursing. Available at http://www.nccn.org.

Nussbaum, R., McInnes, R., & Willard, H. (2001). *Thompson & Thompson: Genetics in medicine* (6th ed.). Philadelphia: W. B. Saunders.

O'Malley, P. (2003). Clotting and bleeding. *Clinical Nurse Specialist, 17*(2), 83-85.

Ott, M. (2002). Complementary and alternative therapies in cancer symptom management. *Cancer Practice, 10*(3), 162-166.

Parker, D., Deel, P., & Arner, S. (2004). Iron out the details of therapeutic phlebotomy. *Nursing2004, 34*(2), 46-47.

Parmar, K., & King, R. (2001). Imatinib mesylate: A new pill for chronic myelogenous leukemia. *Cancer Practice, 9*(5), 263-265.

Pearl, R., & Pohlman, A. (2002). Understanding and managing anemia in critically ill patients. *Critical Care Nurse, Supp* (December), 1-14.

Penwarden, L., & Montgomery, P. (2002). Developing a protocol for obtaining blood cultures from central venous catheters and peripheral sites. *Clinical Journal of Oncology Nursing, 6*(5), 268-270.

Peterson, K. (2003). Central line sepsis. *Clinical Journal of Oncology Nursing, 7*(2), 218-221.

Plaisance, L., & Ellis, J. (2002). Opioid-induced constipation. *American Journal of Nursing, 102*(3), 72-73.

Platt, A., et al. (2002). Treating sickle cell pain: An update from the Georgia Comprehensive Sickle Cell Center. *Journal of Emergency Nursing, 28*(4), 297-303.

Pohlman, A., Carven, J., & Lindsay, K. (2001). Conserving blood in the intensive care unit. *Critical Care Nurse, Supp* (December), 1-6.

Rice, D., & Sheridan, C. (2001). Nursing care of patients with multiple myeloma: A paradigm for the needs of a special population. *Clinical Journal of Oncology Nursing, 5*(3), 89-93.

Rudnicke, C. (2003). Transfusion alternatives. *Journal of Infusion Nursing, 26*(1), 29-33.

Scigliano, E., et al. (2001). The leukemias. In Rubin & Williams (Eds.). *Clinical oncology: A multidisciplinary approach for physicians & students.* Philadelphia: W. B. Saunders.

Seeley, K., & DeMeyer, E. (2002). Nursing care of patients receiving Campath. *Clinical Journal of Oncology Nursing, 6*(3), 138-143.

Shannon-Dorcy, K. (2002). Nursing implications of Mylotarg: A novel antibody-targeted chemotherapy for CD 33+ acute myeloid leukemia in first relapse. *Oncology Nursing Forum, 29*(4), 52-57.

Sickle Cell Information Center. (2003). Emory University. Atlanta, GA. Available at http://www.scinfo.org.

Simmons, P. (2003). A primer for nurses who administer blood products. *MEDSURG Nursing, 12*(3), 184-192.

Sorokin, P. (2002). New agents and future directions in biotherapy. *Clinical Journal of Oncology Nursing, 6*(1), 19-26.

Stevens, S. (2000). Heparin-induced thrombocytopenia. *Journal of Vascular Nursing, 18*(2), 54-68.

Stone, R. (2002). The difficult problem of acute myeloid leukemia in the older adult. *CA: A Cancer Journal for Clinicians, 52*(6), 363-372.

Strauss, D. (2003). Therapeutic strategies for indolent B-cell non-Hodgkin's lymphoma: Toward a cure. *Oncology Special Edition*, 6, 33-37.

Tariman, J. (2003). Thalidomide: Current therapeutic uses and management of its toxicities. *Clinical Journal of Oncology Nursing, 7*(2), 143-147.

Tasota, F., & Tate, J. (2001). Interpreting the highs and lows of platelet counts. *Nursing2001, 31*(2), 25.

Tennant, L. (2001). Chronic myelogenous leukemia: An overview. *Clinical Journal of Oncology Nursing, 5*(5), 218-220.

Triesh, I. (2000). Targeting leukemia cells with gemtuzumab ozogamicin. *Cancer Practice*, 8(5), 254-256.

Tuinstra, N. (2003). Outpatient administration of radiolabeled monoclonal antibodies. *Clinical Journal of Oncology Nursing, 7*(1), 106-111.

Vernon, S., & Pfeifer, G. (2003). Blood management strategies for critical care patients. *Critical Care Nurse, 23*(6), 34-41.

Viele, C. (2002). Gentuzumab ozogamicin. *Clinical Journal of Oncology Nursing, 6*(5), 298-299, 304.

Wagner, H., et al. (2002). Administration guidelines for radioimmunotherapy of non-Hodgkin's lymphoma with ^{90}Y-labeled anti CD20 monoclonal antibody. *The Journal of Nuclear Medicine, 43*(2), 267-272.

Waldman, A. (2003). Understanding non-Hodgkin's lymphomas. *Clinical Journal of Oncology Nursing, 7*(1), 93-96.

Weiner, D., & Brugnara, C. (2003). Hydroxyurea and sickle cell disease: A chance for every patient. *Journal of the American Medical Association, 289*(13), 1692-1694.

White, C. (2002). Painful lesions in a pancytopenic patient. *Clinical Journal of Oncology Nursing, 6*(1), 47-49, 51.

Witt, J. (2002). Living with fatigue. *American Journal of Nursing, 102*(4), 28-31.

Witzig, T, et al. (2002). Randomized controlled trial of Yttrium-90-labeled ibritumomab immunotherapy for patients with relapsed or refractory low-grade, follicular, or transformed B-cell non-Hodgkin's lymphoma. *Journal of Clinical Oncology, 20*(10), 2453-2463.

Wolff, S., et al. (2000). Fluconazole vs low-dose amphotericin for the prevention of fungal infections in patients undergoing bone marrow transplantation: A study of the North American Marrow Transplant Group. *Bone Marrow Transplantation, 25*, 853-859.

Wu, H. (2002). Tretinoin for the treatment of acute promyelocytic leukemia. *Cancer Practice, 10*(2), 109-111.

Young, J. (2000). Transfusion reaction. *Nursing2000, 30*(12), 33.

Zitella, L. (2000). Tyrosine kinase inhibitors: A cure for chronic myeloid leukemia? *Clinical Journal of Oncology Nursing, 4*(5), 227-231.

Index

b indicates boxed material, *c* indicates charts, *f* indicates illustrations, and *t* indicates tables.

H

J

K

M

Q

S

T

U

Communication Quick Reference for Spanish-Speaking Clients–cont'd

OBTAINING BLOOD FROM A FINGER STICK

I need to take a few drops of blood from your finger.	Necesito sacarle unas gotas de sangre de uno de sus dedos.	*Neh-seh-SEE-toh sah-KAHR-leh OO-nahs GOH-tahs deh SAHN-greh deh OO-noh deh soos DEH-dohs.*

OBTAINING A URINE SAMPLE

We also need a urine sample.	También necesitamos una muestra de la orina.	*Tahm-BYEHN neh-seh-see-TAH-mohs OO-nah MWEHS-trah deh lah oh-REE-nah.*
It has to be from the middle of the stream.	Tiene que ser de la mitad del chorro.	*TYEH-neh keh sehr deh lah mee-TAHD dehl CHOH-rroh.*
Put the urine in this cup.	Ponga la orina en este vaso.	*POHN-gah lah oh-REE-nah ehn EHS-teh VAH-soh.*

OBTAINING A STOOL SPECIMEN

I need a sample of your stool.	Necesito una muestra de su excremento.	*Neh-seh-SEE-toh OO-nah MWEHS-trah deh soo ehks-kreh-MEN-toh.*
Please put a small amount in this cup.	Por favor ponga un poco en este vaso.	*Pohr fa-VOHR POHN-gah oon POH-koh ehn EHS-teh VAH-soh.*

OBTAINING A SPUTUM SPECIMEN

I need a sample of your sputum.	Necesito una muestra de su esputo.	*Neh-seh-SEE-toh OO-nah MWEHS-trah deh soo ehs-POO-toh.*
Please spit in this cup.	Por favor, escupa en este vaso.	*Pohr fah-VOHR, ehs-KOO-pah ehn EHS-teh VAH-soh.*

ORDERS

You need . . .	Necesita . . .	*Neh-seh-see-TAH . . .*
a bandage.	un vendaje.	*oon behn-DAH-heh.*
a blood transfusion.	una transfusión de sangre.	*OO-nah trahns-foo-SEE-ohn deh SAHN-greh.*
a cast.	una armadura de yeso.	*OO-nah ahr-mah-DOO-rah deh YEH-soh.*
gauze.	la gasa.	*lah GAH-sah.*
intensive care.	el cuidado intensivo.	*ehl kwee-DAH-doh een-tehn-SEE-boh.*
intravenous fluids.	los líquidos intravenosos.	*lohs LEE-kee-dohs een-trah-beh-NOH-sohs.*
an operation.	una operación.	*OO-nah oh-peh-rah-see-OHN.*
physical therapy.	la terapia física.	*lah teh-RAH-pee-ah FEE-see-kah.*
a shot.	una inyección.	*OO-nah een-yehk-see-OHN.*
x-rays.	los rayos equis.	*lohs RAH-yohs EH-kees.*
We're going to . . .	Vamos a . . .	*VAH-mohs ah . . .*
change the bandage.	cambiarle el vendaje.	*kahm-bee-AHR-leh ehl behn-DAH-heh.*
give you a bath.	darle un baño.	*DAHR-leh oon BAH-nyoh.*
take out the I.V.	sacarle el tubo intravenoso.	*sah-KAHR-leh ehl TOO-boh een-trah-beh-NOH-soh.*

DESCRIPTION OF TUBES

The tube in your . . .	El tubo en su . . .	*Ehl TOO-boh ehn soo . . .*
arm is for I.V. fluids.	brazo está para los líquidos intravenosos.	*BRAH-soh ehs-TAH PAH-rah LEE-kee-dohs een-trah-beh-NOH-sohs.*
bladder is for urinating.	vejiga es para orinar.	*beh-HEE-gah ehs PAH-rah oh-ree-NAHR.*
stomach is for the food.	estómago es para la comida.	*ehs-TOH-mah-goh ehs PAH-rah lah koh-MEE-dah.*
throat is for breathing.	garganta es para respirar.	*gahr-GAHN-tah ehs PAH-rah rehs-pee-RAHR.*

Communication Quick Reference for Spanish-Speaking Clients

THE BODY • EL CUERPO (ehl KWEHR-poh)

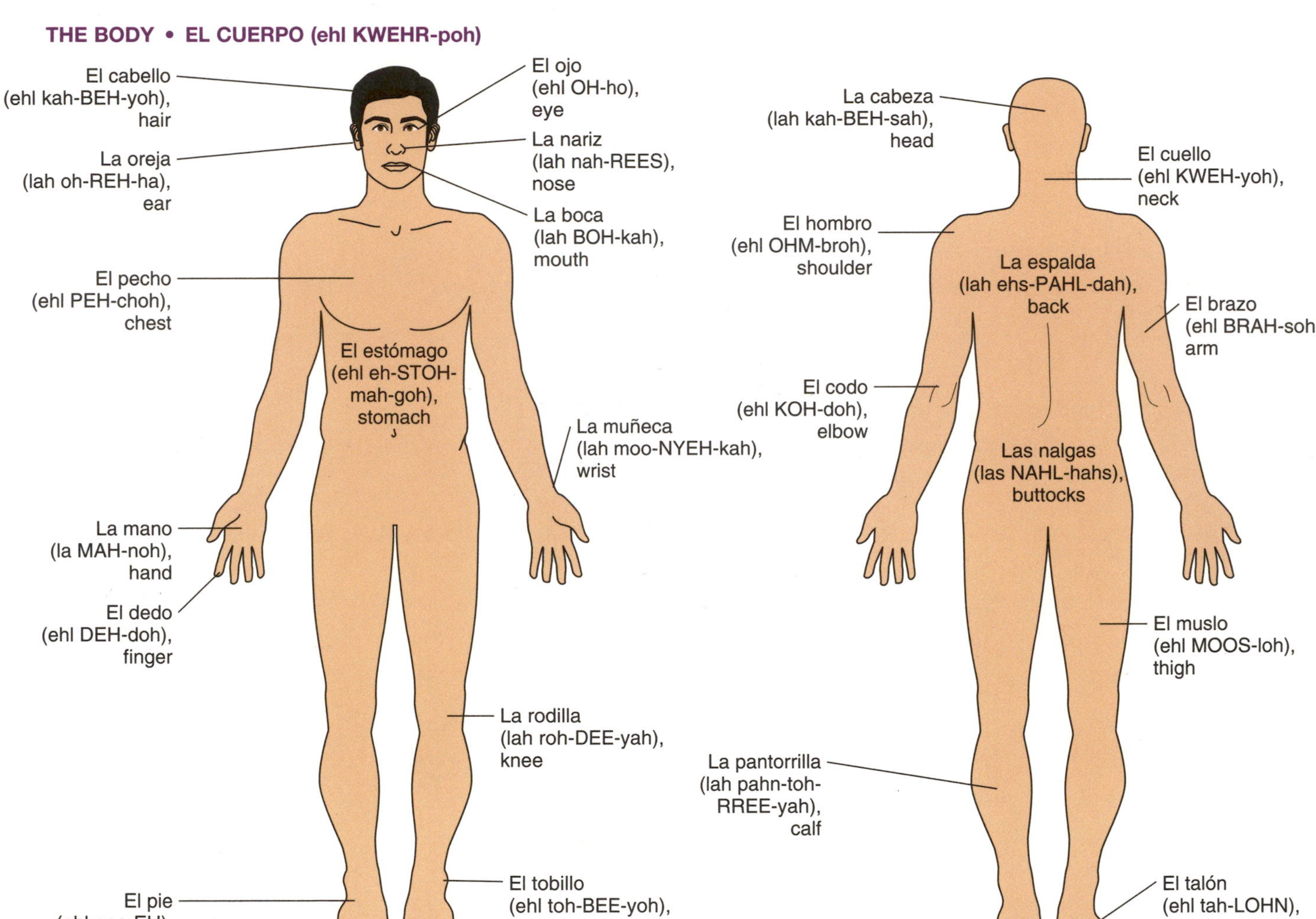

COMMON INSTRUCTIONS TO BE USED WITH THE BODY PARTS

Move the, Mueva *(mooh-EH-bah)*
Touch the, Toque *(TOH-keh)*
Point to the, Señale *(seh-NYAH-leh)*

MORE PARTS OF THE BODY

Armpit, la axila *(lah ahk-SEE-lah)*
Breasts, los senos *(lohs SEH-nohs)*
Collarbone, la clavícula *(lah klah-BEE-koo-lah)*
Diaphragm, el diafragma *(ehl dee-ah-FRAH-mah)*
Forearm, el antebrazo *(ehl ahn-teh-BRAH-soh)*
Groin, la ingle *(lah EEN-gleh)*
Hip, la cadera *(lah kah-DEH-rah)*
Kneecap, la rótula *(lah ROH-too-lah)*
Nail, la uña *(lah OON-yah)*
Pelvis, la pelvis *(lah PEHL-beece)*
Rectum, el recto *(ehl REHK-toh)*
Rib, la costilla *(lah koh-STEE-yah)*
Spine, el espinazo *(ehl ehs-pee-NAH-soh)*
Throat, la garganta *(lah gahr-GAHN-tah)*
Tongue, le lengua *(lah LEHN-gwah)*

ORGANS

Appendix, el apéndice *(ehl ah-PEHN-dee-seh)*
Bladder, la vejiga *(lah beh-HEE-gah)*
Brain, el cerebro *(ehl seh-REH-broh)*
Colon, el colon *(ehl KOH-lohn)*
Esophagus, el esófago *(ehl eh-SOH-fah-goh)*
Gallbladder, la vesícula biliar *(lah beh-SEE-koo-lah bee-lee-AHR)*
Genitals, los genitales *(lohs heh-nee-TAH-lehs)*
Heart, el corazón *(ehl koh-rah-SOHN)*
Kidney, el riñón *(ehl ree-NYOHN)*
Large intestine, el intestino grueso *(ehl een-tehs-TEE-noh groo-EH-so)*
Liver, el hígado *(ehl EE-gah-doh)*
Lungs, los pulmones *(lohs pool-MOH-nehs)*
Pancreas, el páncreas *(ehl PAHN-kreh-ahs)*
Small intestine, el intestino delgado *(ehl een-tehs-TEE-noh dehl-GAH-doh)*
Spleen, el bazo *(ehl BAH-soh)*
Thyroid gland, la tiroides *(lah tee-ROH-ee-dehs)*
Tonsils, las amígdalas *(lahs ah-MEEG-dah-lahs)*
Uterus, el útero *(ehl OO-teh-roh)*